Chronic Obstructive
Pulmonary Disease

Chronic Obstructive Pulmonary Disease

Professor Robert A. Stockley

Professor of Medicine
Department of Medicine
Queen Elizabeth Hospital
Birmingham
B15 2TH
UK

Professor Stephen I. Rennard

Pulmonary & Critical Care Medicine Section
University of Nebraska Medical Center
985125 Nebraska Medical Center
800 South 42nd Street
Omaha
NE 68198-5300

Professor Klaus Rabe

Dept of Pulmonology
Leiden Universtiy Medical Centre
Albinusdreef 2, C3-P
Postbox 9600
2300 RC
Leiden
Netherlands

Professor Bartolome Celli

Division of Pulmonary and Critical Care
St Elizabeth's Medical Centre
736 Cambridge Street
Tufts University
Boston
MA 02135-2907

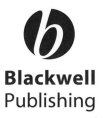

Blackwell
Publishing

© 2007 by Blackwell Publishing Ltd

Blackwell Publishing, Inc., 350 Main Street, Malden, Massachusetts 02148-5020, USA
Blackwell Publishing Ltd, 9600 Garsington Road, Oxford OX4 2DQ, UK
Blackwell Publishing Asia Pty Ltd, 550 Swanston Street, Carlton, Victoria 3053, Australia

The right of the Author to be identified as the Author of this Work has been asserted in
accordance with the Copyright, Designs and Patents Act 1988.

First published 2007

Library of Congress Cataloging-in-Publication Data

Chronic obstructive pulmonary disease / [edited by] Robert Stockley . . . [*et al.*].
        p. ; cm.
     Includes bibliographical references and index.
     ISBN-13: 978-1-4051-2289-4
     ISBN-10: 1-4051-2289-7
     1. Lungs-Diseases, Obstructive.   I. Stockley, Robert A.
     [DNLM: 1. Pulmonary Disease, Chronic Obstructive.   WF 600 C55165 2006]
     RC776.O3C47423 2006
     616.2′4–dc22   2005012341

ISBN-13: 978-1-4051-2289-4
ISBN-10: 1-4051-2289-7

A catalogue record for this title is available from the British Library

Set in 9/12pt Meridien by Graphicraft Limited, Hong Kong

Printed and bound in Singapore by Fabulous Printers Pte Ltd

Commissioning Editor: Maria Khan
Development Editor: Rebecca Huxley
Production Controller: Debbie Wyer

For further information on Blackwell Publishing, visit our website:
http://www.blackwellpublishing.com

The publisher's policy is to use permanent paper from mills that operate a sustainable
forestry policy, and which has been manufactured from pulp processed using acid-free and
elementary chlorine-free practices. Furthermore, the publisher ensures that the text paper
and cover board used have met acceptable environmental accreditation standards.

Contents

Section 4: Pathogenesis

Section 5: Clinical Considerations and Complications

Section 6: Current and Future Treatment

Section 7: Pharmacotherapy: Developing Therapies

Colour plate section falls between pp. 354 and 355

Contributors

Loutfi S. Aboussouan
Associate Professor of Medicine
Division of Pulmonary and Critical
    Care Medicine
Wayne State University School of Medicine
Harper University Hospital, 3-Hudson
Detroit, Michigan
USA

Lewis Adams
School of Physiotherapy and Exercise Science
Griffith University – Gold Coast Campus
Southport, Queensland
Australia

Antonio Anzueto
Associate Professor Medicine
University of Texas San Antonio
Division of Pulmonary Diseases and
    Critical Care Medicine
Audie L. Murphy Memorial Veterans Hospital
South Texas Veterans Healthcare System
San Antonio, Texas
USA

Lorenzo Appendini
Fondazione Salvatore Maugeri IRCCS
Veruno
Italy

David H. Au
Health Services Research and Development
VA Puget Sound Health Care System
Division of Pulmonary and Critical
    Care Medicine
University of Washington
Seattle, Washington
USA

Simonetta Baraldo
Padua University School of Medicine
Department of Cardio-Thoracic and
    Vascular Sciences
Section of Respiratory Diseases
University of Padua
Padua
Italy

Joan Albert Barberà
Associate Professor of Medicine
Pneumology Service
Hospital Clinic
Institut d'Investigacions Biomèdiques August
    Pi i Sunyer (IDIBAPS)
University of Barcelona
Barcelona
Spain

Peter J. Barnes
Department of Thoracic Medicine
National Heart and Lung Institute
Imperial College
London
UK

Barbara Bartalesi
Department of Physiopathology
Experimental Medicine and Public Health
University of Siena
Siena
Italy

Dirk Bredenbröker
ALTANA Pharma AG
Konstanz
Germany

Daniela S. Bundschuh
ALTANA Pharma AG
Konstanz
Germany

Peter M. A. Calverley
Professor of Medicine (Pulmonary and
    Rehabilitation)
Department of Medicine
Clinical Sciences Centre
University Hospital Aintree
Liverpool
UK

Rick Carter
Chair and Professor
Health, Exercise and Sport Sciences
Texas Tech University
Lubbock, Texas
USA

Bartolome R. Celli
Professor of Medicine
Tufts University
Chief, Pulmonary Critical Care Medicine
Caritas St Elizabeth's Medical Center
Boston, Massachusetts
USA

Hugues Chanteux
Pulmonary and Microbiology Department
University of Louvain
Louvain
Belgium

Cheng Chen
Developmental Biology Program
Saban Research Institute of Children's
    Hospital
University of Southern California, Los Angeles
Keck School of Medicine
Los Angeles, California
USA and
Developmental Biology Division
China Medical University
Shenyang
China

Andrew Churg
Professor of Pathology
University of British Columbia
Vancouver, British Columbia
Canada

Christelle Coraux
INSERM UMR-S, 514
IFR 53
Reims
France

Gerard J. Criner
Professor of Medicine
Temple Lung Center
Division of Pulmonary and Critical Care
    Medicine
Temple University School of Medicine
Philadelphia, Pennsylvania
USA

Sven-Erik Dahlén
Experimental Asthma and Allergy Research
The National Institute of Environmental
    Medicine
The Centre for Allergy Research
Karolinska Institutet
Stockholm
Sweden

Philip Davies
Department of Immunology
Merck Research Laboratories
Rahway, New Jersey
USA

Marc Decramer
Respiratory Rehabilitation and Respiratory
    Division
University Hospitals
Katholieke Universiteit Leuven
Leuven
Belgium

John K. DiBaise
Associate Professor of Medicine
Division of Gastroenterology and Hepatology
Mayo Clinic
Scottsdale, Arizona
USA

Kenneth Donaldson
Professor of Respiratory Toxicology
ELEGI Colt Laboratory
Wilkie Building
University of Edinburgh Medical School
Teviot Place
Edinburgh
UK

Claudio F. Donner
Medical Director
Mondo Medico
Multidisciplinary and Rehabilitation
    Outpatient Clinic
Via Monsignor Cavigioli 10
Borgomanero (NO)
Italy

Sarah E. Dunsmore
Department of Medicine (Pulmonary Division)
Brigham and Women's Hospital
Boston, Massachusetts
USA

Andrés Echazarreta
Servicio de Neumonología
Hospital San Martín
La Plata
Argentina

Souheil El-Chemaly
Clinical Fellow
Pulmonary Critical Care Medicine Branch
NHLBI, National Institutes of Health
10 Center Drive
Bethesda, Maryland
USA

Jack A. Elias
Section of Pulmonary & Critical Care Medicine
Dept of Internal Medicine
Yale University School of Medicine
New Haven, Connecticut
USA

Mark W. Elliott
St James's University Hospital
Beckett Street
Leeds
UK

Alan M. Fein
Professor of Medicine
NYU School of Medicine
Chief of Pulmonary, Sleep & Critical Care
    Medicine
ProHealth Care Associates
2800 Marcus Avenue
Suite 202
Lake Success
New York
USA

Daryl Freeman
General Practice Airways Group Research
    Fellow in Primary Care Respiratory Medicine
GP and GP Specialist in Respiratory Medicine
North Norfolk
UK

Joe G. N. Garcia
Division of Pulmonary and Critical Care
    Medicine
Center for Translational Respiratory Medicine
Johns Hopkins University School of Medicine
Baltimore, Maryland
USA

Ghislaine Gayan-Ramirez
Respiratory Rehabilitation and Respiratory
    Division
University Hospitals
Katholieke Universiteit Leuven
Leuven
Belgium

Colin Gelder
Department of Infection and Immunity
University of Wales College of Medicine
Heath Park
Cardiff
UK

Federico P. Gómez
Pneumology Service
Hospital Clinic
Institut d'Investigacions Biomèdiques August
    Pi i Sunyer (IDIBAPS)
University of Barcelona
Barcelona
Spain

Diana C. Grootendorst
Department of Pulmonology and Clinical
    Epidemiology
Leiden University Medical Center
Leiden
The Netherlands

Hélène Levrey Hadden
Pulmonary, Allergy and Critical Care Medicine
University of Minnesota Medical School
Minneapolis, Minnesota
USA

Armin Hatzelmann
ALTANA Pharma AG
Konstanz
Germany

Ann L. Heffner
Division of Pulmonary and Critical Care
Medical University of South Carolina
Charleston, South Carolina
USA

John E. Heffner
Professor of Medicine
Division of Pulmonary and Critical Care
Medical University of South Carolina
Charleston, South Carolina
USA

Lisa M. Hepp
Pulmonary and Critical Care Medicine
University of Nebraska Medical Center
    985885 Nebraska Medical Center
Omaha, Nebraska

Craig P. Hersh
Channing Laboratory
Department of Medicine
Brigham and Women's Hospital
Boston, Massachusetts
USA

Marshall I. Hertz
Pulmonary, Allergy and Critical Care Medicine
University of Minnesota Medical School
Minneapolis, Minnesota
USA

Sam Hibbitts
Department of Medical Microbiology
University of Wales College of Medicine
Heath Park
Cardiff
UK

Robert J. Homer
Associate Professor of Pathology
Yale University School of Medicine
New Haven, Connecticut
Director of Anatomic Pathology
VA Connecticut HealthCare System
West Haven, Connecticut
USA

Suzanne S. Hurd
Scientific Director
Global Initiative for Chronic Obstructive Lung
    Disease (GOLD)
Gaithersburg, Maryland
USA

Bruce D. Johnson
Division of Cardiovascular Disease
Mayo Clinic
Rochester, Minnesota
USA

Malcolm Johnson
GlaxoSmithKline Research and Development
Greenford
Middlesex
UK

Kellie R. Jones
Assistant Professor
Pulmonary and Critical Care Division
Department of Internal Medicine
Oklahoma University of Oklahoma Health
    Sciences Center
Oklahoma
USA

Paul W. Jones
Professor of Respiratory Medicine
St George's Hospital Medical School
London
UK

Jill P. Karpel
Professor of Medicine
Albert Einstein College of Medicine
Medical Director
Beth Thalheim Asthma Center
Department of Medicine
North Shore-Long Island Jewish Medical
    Center
North Shore University Hospital
New York
USA

Marcus P. Kennedy
Division of Pulmonary and Critical Care
    Medicine
University of North Carolina
Chapel Hill, North Carolina
USA

Michael R. Knowles
Division of Pulmonary and Critical Care
    Medicine
University of North Carolina
Chapel Hill, North Carolina
USA

Marian Kollarik
John Hopkins Asthma & Allergy Center
John Hopkins School of Medicine
Baltimore, Maryland
USA

Antonia Koutsoukou
Critical Care Department and Pulmonary
    Services
Evangelismos General Hospital
University of Athens Medical School
Athens
Greece

Geoffrey J. Laurent
Centre for Cardiopulmonary Biochemistry
    and Respiratory Medicine
Royal Free and University College Medical
    School
The Rayne Institute
London
UK

Claude Lenfant
Former Director
National Heart, Lung, and Blood Institute
National Institutes of Health, DHHS
Bethesda, Maryland
USA

Monica Lucattelli
Department of Physiopathology
Experimental Medicine and Public Health
University of Siena
Siena
Italy

Giuseppe Lungarella
Department of Physiopathology
Experimental Medicine and Public Health
University of Siena
Siena
Italy

Malcolm MacCoss
Department of Medicinal Chemistry
Merck Research Laboratories
Rahway, New Jersey
USA

William MacNee
Professor of Respiratory and Environmental
    Medicine
ELEGI, Colt Research Laboratories
MRC Centre for Inflammation Research
University of Edinburgh Medical School
Edinburgh
UK

Donald A. Mahler
Professor of Medicine
Dartmouth Medical School
Lebanon, New Hampshire
USA

Fernando J. Martinez
Professor of Medicine
Division of Pulmonary and Critical Care
    Medicine
University of Michigan School of Medicine
Taubman Center 3916
Ann Arbor, Michigan
USA

Piero A. Martorana
Department of Physiopathology
Experimental Medicine and Public Health
University of Siena
Siena
Italy

Frank McCaughan
Clinical Research Fellow
Department of Thoracic Medicine
University College London NHS Trust
London
UK

Jordan P. Metcalf
Associate Professor
Pulmonary and Critical Care Division
Department of Internal Medicine
Oklahoma University of Oklahoma Health
  Sciences Center
Oklahoma
USA

Joseph Milic-Emili
Meakins-Christie Laboratories
McGill University
Montreal
Quebec
Canada

Norman R. Morris
School of Physiotherapy and Exercise Science
Griffith University – Gold Coast Campus
Southport, Queensland
Australia

Bernd Muller
Laboratory of Respiratory Cell Biology
University of Giessen and Marburg
Philipps University of Marburg Dept of
  Internal Medicine
Division of Respiratory Medicine
Marburg
Germany

Richard Mumford
Department of Immunology
Merck Research Laboratories
Rahway, New Jersey
USA

Stephen P. Newman
Scientific Consultant
Nottingham
UK

Michael S. Niederman
Chairman, Department of Medicine
Winthrop-University Hospital
Mineola, NY and
Professor of Medicine
Vice-Chairman, Department of Medicine
SUNY at Stony Brook, New York
USA

Dennis E. Niewoehner
Chief Pulmonary Section
Minneapolis Veterans Affairs Medical Center
  and Professor of Medicine
University of Minnesota
Minneapolis, Minnesota
USA

Stephanie A. Nonas
Division of Pulmonary and Critical Care
  Medicine
Center for Translational Respiratory Medicine
Johns Hopkins University School of Medicine
Baltimore, Maryland
USA

Irina Petrache
Division of Pulmonary and Critical Care
  Medicine
Center for Translational Respiratory Medicine
Johns Hopkins University School of Medicine
Baltimore, Maryland
USA

Charles Pilette
Pulmonary and Microbiology Department
University of Louvain
Louvain
Belguim

Guido Polese
Pulmonary Division
Ospedali Riuniti di Bergamo
Bergamo
Italy

David Price
General Practice Airways Group Professor of
  Primary Care Respiratory Medicine
Department of General Practice and Primary
  Care
University of Aberdeen
Foresterhill Health Centre
Aberdeen
UK

Edith Puchelle
INSERM UMR-S, 514
IFR 53
Reims
France

Klaus F. Rabe
Department of Pulmonology
Leiden University Medical Center
Leiden
The Netherlands

Maria Rappai
Instructor of Medicine
Division of Pulmonary, Critical Care
  and Sleep Medicine
Department of Medicine
University of Mississippi Medical Center
Jackson, Mississippi
USA

Stephen I. Rennard
Professor of Medicine
Pulmonary and Critical Care Medicine Section
University of Nebraska Medical Center
Omaha, Nebraska
USA

Robert Rodriguez-Roisin
Professor of Medicine
Pneumology Service
Hospital Clinic
Institut d'Investigacions Biomèdiques August
  Pi i Sunyer (IDIBAPS)
University of Barcelona
Barcelona
Spain

Duncan F. Rogers
Thoracic Medicine
National Heart and Lung Institute
Imperial College London
London
UK

Andrea Rossi
Pulmonary Division
Ospedali Riuniti di Bergamo
Bergamo
Italy

Bruce K. Rubin
Professor and Associate Chair for Research
Department of Pediatrics
Professor of Physiology and Pharmacology
Wake Forest University School of Medicine
Winston-Salem, North Carolina
USA

Marina Saetta
Padua University School of Medicine
Department of Cardio-Thoracic and Vascular
  Sciences
Section of Respiratory Diseases
University of Padua
Padua
Italy

Matthias Salathe
Associate Professor of Medicine
Division of Pulmonary and Critical Care
  Medicine
University of Miami
Miami, Florida
USA

Christian Schudt
ALTANA Pharma AG
Konstanz
Germany

Carola Seifart
University of Giessen and Marburg
Philipps University of Marburg
Dept of Internal Medicine
Division of Respiratory Medicine
Marburg
Germany

Olof Selroos
Associate Professor of Pulmonary Medicine
Helsinki University
Helsinki
Finland

Sanjay Sethi
Associate Professor of Medicine
Division of Pulmonary, Critical Care and
    Sleep Medicine
University of Buffalo
State University of New York and
VA Western New York Healthcare System
Buffalo, New York
USA

Martin Sevenoaks
Department of Medicine
Queen Elizabeth Hospital
Edgbaston
Birmingham
UK

J. Graham Sharp
Professor
Genetics Cell Biology & Anatomy
University of Nebraska Medical Center 986395
    Nebraska Medical Center
Omaha, Nebraska

Richard deShazo
Professor of Medicine and Pediatrics
Division of Allergy and Clinical Immunology
Department of Medicine and Pediatrics
University of Mississippi Medical Center
Jackson, Mississippi
USA

Wei Shi
Developmental Biology Program
Saban Research Institute of Children's
    Hospital
University of Southern California, Los Angeles
Keck School of Medicine
Los Angeles, California
USA

Yves Sibille
Pulmonary and Microbiology Department
University of Louvain
Louvain
Belguim

Edwin K. Silverman
Channing Laboratory and Division of
    Pulmonary and Critical Care Medicine
Department of Medicine
Brigham and Women's Hospital
Boston, Massachusetts
USA

Joan B. Soriano
Head, Programme of Epidemiology and
    Clinical Research
Fundació Caubet-CIMERA Illes Balears
International Centre for Advanced Respiratory
    Medicine
Recinte Hospital Joan March, Carretera Soller
    Km 12
07110 Bunyola, Mallorca, Illes Balears
Spain

Stephen G. Spiro
Department of Thoracic Medicine
University College London NHS Trust
London
UK

Robin Stevenson
Department of Respiratory Medicine
Glasgow Royal Infirmary
Glasgow
UK

Robert A. Stockley
Professor of Medicine
Department of Medicine
Queen Elizabeth Hospital
Edgbaston
Birmingham
UK

James K. Stoller
Professor of Medicine, Cleveland Clinic Lerner
    School of Medicine
Vice Chairman, Division of Medicine
Head, Section of Respiratory Therapy
Department of Pulmonary and Critical Care
    Medicine, A-190
Associate Chief of Staff
Cleveland Clinic Foundation
Cleveland, Ohio
USA

Anita L. Sullivan
Department of Respiratory Medicine
Queen Elizabeth Hospital
Edgbaston
Birmingham
UK

Sean D. Sullivan
Pharmaceutical Outcomes Research and Policy
    Program
Department of Pharmacy
University of Washington
Seattle, Washington
USA

Victor F. Tapson
Professor of Medicine
Division of Pulmonary and Critical Care
Duke University Medical Center
Durham, North Carolina
USA

Hermann Tenor
ALTANA Pharma AG
Konstanz
Germany

Brian Tiep
Respiratory Disease Management Institute
Irwindale, California
Western University of Health Sciences
Pomona, California
Pulmonary Rehabilitation
City of Hope National Cancer Center
Duarte, California
USA

Philip Tønnesen
Chair, Department of Pulmonary Medicine
Gentofte University Hospital
Copenhagen
Denmark

Jean-Marie Tournier
INSERM UMR-S, 514
IFR 53
Reims
France

Stephen R. Tudhope
Bayer Plc
Stoke Court
Stoke Poges
Buckinghamshire
UK

Bradley J. Undem
John Hopkins Asthma & Allergy Center
John Hopkins School of Medicine
Baltimore, Maryland
USA

Jørgen Vestbo
Professor of Respiratory Medicine
North West Lung Centre
South Manchester University Hospital
Southmoor Road
Manchester
UK and
Department of Heart and Lung Diseases
Hvidovre University Hospital
Kettegaard Alle 30
Hvidovre
Denmark

Norbert F. Voelkel
Professor of Medicine
The Hart Family Professor of Emphysema
   Research
Director, COPD Center
Pulmonary Hypertension Center
University of Colorado Health Sciences Center
Denver, Colorado

Adam Wanner
Professor of Medicine
Division of Pulmonary and Critical Care
   Medicine
University of Miami
Miami, Florida
USA

David Warburton
Developmental Biology Program
Saban Research Institute of Children's
   Hospital
University of Southern California, Los Angeles
Keck School of Medicine
Los Angeles, California
USA

Andrew J. Wardlaw
Professor of Respiratory Medicine and
Director of Institute for Lung Health
Institute for Lung Health
Department of Infection, Immunity
   and Inflammation
Leicester University Medical School
Leicester
UK

Idelle M. Weisman
PfizerGlobal Pharmaceuticals
Pfizer Inc.
New York
USA

Robert Wilson
Consultant Physician
Royal Brompton Hospital
Sydney Street
London
UK

Theodore J. Witek, Jr
Boehringer Ingelheim, Lda – Portugal
Av. António Augusto de Aguiar nº 104-1º
1069-029 Lisboa
Portugal

Ian S. Woolhouse
Consultant Physician and Honorary Senior
   Clinical Lecturer
Department of Respiratory Medicine
University Hospital Birmingham
Birmingham
UK

Emile F. M. Wouters
Professor of Medicine
Department of Respiratory Medicine
University Hospital Maastricht
Maastricht
The Netherlands

Jean-Marie Zahm
INSERM UMR-S, 514
IFR 53
Reims
France

Maria Elena Zanin
Padua University School of Medicine
Department of Cardio-Thoracic and
   Vascular Sciences
Section of Respiratory Diseases
University of Padua
Padua
Italy

Renzo Zuin
Padua University School of Medicine
Department of Cardio-Thoracic and Vascular
   Sciences
Section of Respiratory Diseases
University of Padua
Padua
Italy

Richard ZuWallack
Professor of Clinical Medicine
University of Connecticut School of Medicine
Associate Chief, Pulmonary and Critical Care
Hartford, Connecticut
USA

Preface

In recent years COPD has become widely recognised as a major healthcare problem. This has led to an increase in interest of the clinical manifestations, management and pathophysiology of the condition. The increase in interest has been mirrored by dramatic increase in publications and research into COPD. Following on from this there has also been an increase in books dedicated to COPD.

Several years ago Steve Rennard and I noted that although there were several textbooks on COPD there were many facets of the condition that required alternative literature searches and turning to more books, particularly those of basic physiology. With this in mind we perceived that there was a need for a comprehensive textbook that covered normal and abnormal physiology, the latter being particularly related to COPD patients and that a spectrum from basic to clinical science was missing. Therefore we embarked upon a project to produce as comprehensive a book as possible.

However, it became clear that such a book would be extensive and would require the involvement of more editors. For this reason we were very pleased that we persuaded both Bart Celli and Klaus Rabe to join us in this task. The complexities resulted in a long gestation period, however the persistence of all of the editors and publishers eventually led to the development of this text. We recognize that any book of this sort should be regarded as a 'work in progress', since the field of COPD research is advancing steadily, but we greatly appreciate the work of the authors of the chapters to keep the book as up to date as possible.

We hope this text will provide background and update necessary for physicians/scientists/healthcare workers with an interest in COPD.

Robert Stockley
Stephen Rennard
November 2006

SECTION 1
Physiology

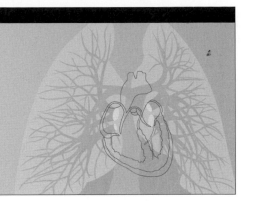

CHAPTER 1

Structure–function relationships: the pathophysiology of airflow obstruction

Dennis E. Niewoehner

A decrease in maximal expiratory flow rates is the cardinal physiological abnormality associated with chronic obstructive pulmonary disease (COPD). Expiratory flow obstruction is deemed to be so important that the presence and severity of COPD is commonly defined in terms of the forced expiratory pressure in 1 second (FEV_1) and of the ratio of the FEV_1 to the forced vital capacity (FVC) [1]. The morphological features thought responsible for expiratory airflow obstruction also play a prominent part in the causation of other physiological derangements in COPD, such as hyperinflation and uneven ventilation. These various functional abnormalities largely reflect the passive mechanical properties of the lung, namely the elastic behaviour of lung parenchyma and airways, and the flow-restrictive characteristics of the bronchial tree. The pathological lesions found in the lungs of COPD patients have been described in some detail, and they can be broadly classified into those that principally affect lung elastic recoil (emphysema) and others that primarily affect the flow-restrictive properties of the bronchi and bronchioles (airways disease). Ideally, an expert pathologist would be able to estimate accurately the degree of airflow obstruction from a comprehensive quantitative assessment of the diseased lung. This can be accomplished in rather broad terms, but the state-of-the-art falls well short of the ideal. The physiologist's assessment of disease severity in the individual case may be markedly discrepant from that of the pathologist. These failures reflect our incomplete understanding of basic pathophysiology in COPD, as well as the formidable methodological problems in studying an organ so structurally and functionally complex as the lung. This chapter describes some of the interrelationships of pathology with physiology in COPD.

Pathology

Emphysema

Patients with symptomatic COPD nearly always have some emphysematous involvement of their lungs, although the extent may vary widely among patients who have the same degree of spirometric impairment. Patients are sometimes labelled with a clinical diagnosis of 'emphysema', but this usage is discouraged because emphysema has a stricter, pathological definition. An expert committee has defined emphysema as 'a condition characterized by abnormal enlargement of the airspaces distal to the terminal bronchiole, accompanied by destruction of their walls, and without obvious fibrosis' [1]. Enlargement of the parenchymal airspaces within the gas exchange region of the lung (alveolus, alveolar duct and respiratory bronchiole) is the seminal feature of emphysema (Fig. 1.1). Airspace enlargement may be caused by actual departitioning and fenestration of the alveolar walls or by a simpler structural rearrangement of the normal acinus. Airspace enlargement is a normal feature of the ageing lung ('senile emphysema'), and it may also be observed in diseases such as interstitial fibrosis. Focal areas of fibrosis may be found in many lungs that are judged to have predominantly emphysema, particularly of the centriacinar subtype. Consequently, it may be difficult to ascertain the presence of mild grades of emphysema in the lungs of older patients, and in some instances there may be confusion as to whether airspace enlargement should be attributed to emphysema or to a separate disease process.

Pathologists recognize two principal subtypes of emphysema. Centriacinar, or centrilobular, emphysema is characterized grossly by discrete, enlarged airspaces, usually measuring 1–10 mm in diameter, which tend to be most prominent in the upper lobes. Microscopically, these

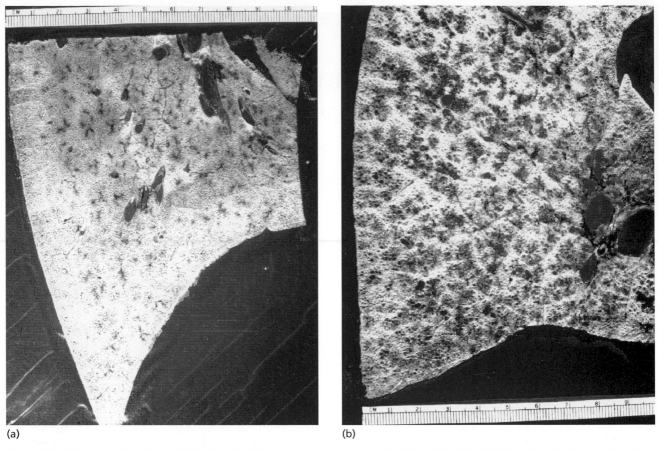

(a)

(b)

Figure 1.1 Macroscopic sections of inflation-fixed lungs comparing a normal subject (a) with a COPD patient having moderately severe emphysema (b). The emphysema has both centriacinar and panacinar features.

lesions may be seen in the proximal parts of the respiratory bronchiole, which is the partially alveolated airway immediately distal to the terminal bronchiole. Alveolar structures in the more distal acinus are usually well preserved, although very large centriacinar emphysema lesions may obliterate much of the acinus. Focal areas of inflammation, fibrosis and carbonaceous pigment are commonly present in adjacent alveolar and bronchiolar walls.

As the name implies, panacinar, or panlobular, emphysema, more uniformly involves the entire acinus. Macroscopically, mild panacinar emphysema appears as a subtle diffuse enlargement of airspaces, which resembles the aged lung. With progression of the disease, single lesions coalesce to form airspaces measuring millimeters to centimeters in diameter; large bullae may form in severe cases. Microscopically, alveolar ducts are diffusely enlarged, and adjacent alveoli become effaced to the extent that individual units cannot be identified. Panacinar emphysema involves all regions of the lung, and some patients, particularly those with severe α_1-antitrypsin deficiency, may exhibit a basal predominance.

When lung sections are appropriately stained, a dense labyrinth of elastic fibres becomes visible within alveolar walls and around peripheral airways (Fig. 1.2). This intricate elastic fibre network helps maintain normal parenchymal structure and contributes importantly to the lung's distinctive elastic recoil properties. The prevailing theory is that emphysema develops from an elastase–antielastase imbalance causing damage to the elastic fibres within the lung parenchyma. Despite their presumed importance in the pathogenesis of emphysema, surprisingly little is known about the state of elastic fibres and other extracellular matrix components in severe human emphysema. Existing studies are mostly descriptive and such basic information as the elastin content of the emphysematous lung is not available.

Emphysema is an anatomical entity, so that estimates of prevalence and severity can be directly made only from specimens obtained by surgical resection or at autopsy. Because reliable estimates of emphysema severity require that specimens be fixed in a uniformly inflated state, whole lungs or lobes are generally more satisfactory than smaller lung samples. The most widely used and accepted method for estimating emphysema severity utilizes a standard panel

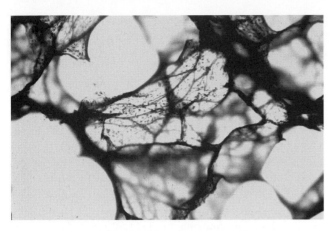

Figure 1.2 Thick histological section of normal human lung stained for elastic fibres. Elastic fibres appear as a lacy network of thin dark lines when an alveolar wall is viewed *en face*. Thicker elastic fibres surround the ostia connecting alveolar ducts with individual aveoli. Elastic fibres are major contributors to lung elastic recoil.

that depicts whole lung sections with increasing degrees of emphysema [2]. The lung section in question is subjectively scored by direct comparison against the panel. Determination of a mean linear intercept (average distance between alveolar walls) is the preferred method for evaluating emphysema severity from histological sections. This method has the advantage of being truly quantitative, but it is time and resource intensive and, because of sampling issues, it is limited in its capability for distinguishing mild emphysema from normal lung [3]. Milder forms of emphysema may be focal in their distribution, and can usually be best appreciated from visualization of whole-lung slices. Estimates of emphysema severity by the picture panel and the mean linear intercept methods are generally in good agreement, but for most purposes the picture panel method is considered the gold standard.

There is now good evidence that reliable estimates of emphysema severity may be made indirectly from computed tomography (CT). Studies to date have consistently shown a good correlation between regions of reduced lung tissue density found on CT scan and the presence of anatomical emphysema [4]. CT scans are highly specific, but they lack sensitivity in detecting very mild grades of emphysema. This is an evolving technology, with issues relating to sensitivity, specificity and standardization currently being addressed.

Airways disease

Much confusion attends the terminology associated with airways disease in COPD. The term 'chronic bronchitis' has been widely used but with a variety of meanings. Strictly speaking, 'chronic bronchitis' refers to an inflammatory condition involving the bronchi, which are the more central, larger and cartilage-containing airways. (The more peripheral airways without cartilage are termed bronchioles.) However, pathologists sometimes refer to bronchial mucous gland enlargement as 'chronic bronchitis'. To complete this rather illogical pattern, the term has also used to define a 'clinical disorder characterized by excessive mucus secretion in the bronchial tree, manifested by chronic or recurrent productive cough on most days for a minimum of 3 months per year for not less than 2 successive years' [5]. Experts arrived at this definition when excess mucus secretion was thought to have a central role in the development of airflow obstruction in COPD. This is no longer thought to be the case, but the definition persists to the bewilderment of several generations of medical students and residents. To avoid this confusion, all pathological changes within the bronchial tree that have been implicated in the pathophysiology of COPD will be called simply 'airways disease'. For reasons that will later become evident, it is appropriate to distinguish pathological changes that primarily involve the central bronchi from those found in the peripheral bronchioles.

Central airways disease

Mucus lines the airway lumens of the bronchial tree and serves an important role in host defence against the environment. Mucous glands, containing both mucous and serous cells, are found between the epithelial basement membrane and the cartilage plates of the central bronchial tree. Mucus is actively secreted into the bronchial lumen via specialized ducts. Modest enlargement of the bronchial mucous glands is found in the lungs of many patients with COPD but not all. Bronchial mucous gland enlargement correlates with cough and excess sputum production [6]. The Reid Index was the first described method for quantifying the degree of mucous gland enlargement [7]. In this technique, the width of the mucous gland is compared with the width of the bronchial wall between the basal lamina and the perichondrium. This method has been largely supplanted by better methods which quantify area proportions. The volume of bronchial mucous gland may increase by 50–100% in selected cases of severe COPD (Fig. 1.3).

In addition to the mucous glands, mucus-secreting goblet cells are found in airway epithelium at all levels of the conducting airways. The population of epithelial goblet cells may expand in the larger airways of COPD patients, but existing studies are mostly descriptive. Epithelial metaplasia and loss of cilia have also been described. It is not clear whether the proportions of smooth muscle and cartilage are abnormal in lungs of COPD patients. COPD is commonly associated with a low-grade inflammatory response within the epithelium and submucosa of the more central

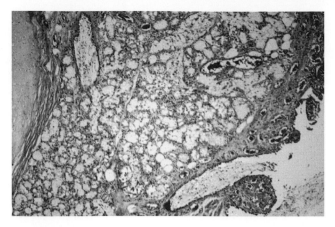

Figure 1.3 Histological section of a cartilaginous bronchus from a COPD patient with chronic cough and sputum production shows marked mucous gland enlargement. Mucous glands normally occupy but a small part of the area between cartilage and epithelium. A low-grade inflammatory reaction commonly accompanies mucous gland enlargement.

bronchi. Neutrophils, macrophages and CD8[+] T lymphocytes are the predominant inflammatory cells [8].

Peripheral airways disease

The pathological changes seen in the peripheral airways of COPD patients are multiple and relatively non-specific (Fig. 1.4). The earliest abnormalities seen in lungs from young smokers are focal collections of brown-pigmented macrophages in the proximal respiratory bronchioles [9]. In older patients with established COPD, the walls of membranous bronchioles frequently contain a low-grade inflammatory response that includes scattered neutrophils, macrophages and lymphocytes [10]. Additional abnormalities include fibrosis, goblet cell and squamous cell metaplasia of the lining epithelium, smooth muscle enlargement and scattered aggregations of mucus within the lumen. Most of this pathology can probably be directly attributed to the toxic effects of cigarette smoke, but peripheral airways in the lungs of elderly lifelong non-smokers may exhibit some of the same abnormalities [11].

Measurements in lungs obtained at surgery and at autopsy indicate that the internal calibre of fully distended peripheral bronchioles is smaller in COPD patients compared with normal subjects [11,12]. In addition, the walls of bronchioles from COPD patients are abnormally thickened, with the increased width being caused by epithelial, smooth muscle and connective tissue elements [13]. Abnormally thickened airway walls may take on added functional significance at smaller lung volumes, because the peripheral airways shorten and narrow as the lung deflates. Figure 1.5 illustrates this point. In the example shown, the abnormal airway has a wall that is twice the

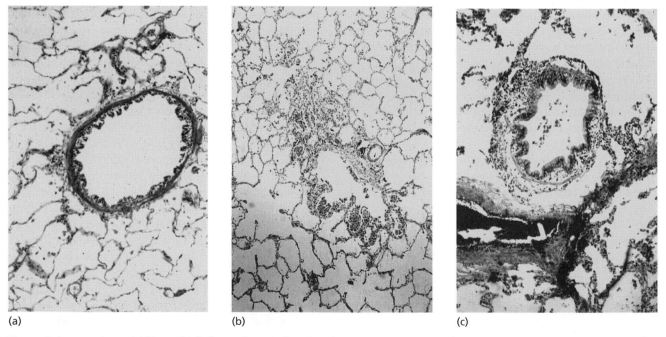

(a)   (b)   (c)

Figure 1.4 Normal terminal bronchiole from a human lung is a thin-walled structure with an internal diameter of approximately 0.5 mm (a). Section through the junction of a membranous and respiratory bronchiole from the lung of a young adult shows the typical inflammatory lesion caused by cigarette smoking (b). Clusters of brown-pigmented macrophages are visible in the respiratory bronchiole and a few mixed inflammatory cells are present within the walls of the membranous bronchiole. In patients with established COPD, membranous bronchioles may exhibit thickened walls and narrowed distorted lumens (c).

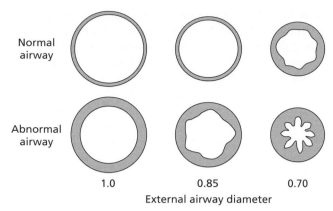

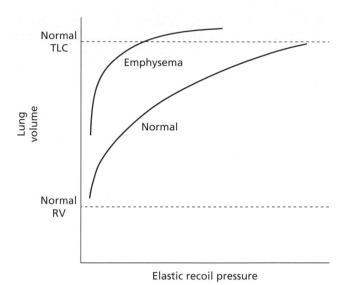

Figure 1.5 External airway diameter decreases as lung volume becomes smaller. Because the volume of the airway wall remains constant, the wall becomes thicker at smaller lung volumes, with a disproportionate reduction in the calibre of the lumen. At very small lung volumes, longitudinal folds may develop along the inner wall of the airway. Abnormally thick airway walls, as occurs in COPD, may exaggerate this effect.

Figure 1.6 Lung volume as a function of lung elastic recoil pressure in a normal subject and in a COPD patient with extensive emphysema. At any particular lung volume, lung elastic recoil pressure is reduced with emphysema. In addition, the pressure–volume curve in the emphysema patient exhibits greater concavity towards the pressure axis. RV, residual volume; TLC, total lung capacity.

normal thickness. For the same change in external diameter, the lumen of the abnormal airway wall narrows to a far greater extent because the constant volume of excess tissue tends to bulge inward. This effect is greatly magnified at very small lung volumes, where the development of longitudinal folds along the inner surface may predispose to complete airway closure.

The accurate assessment of diverse pathological features that are widely distributed among tens of thousands of individual airways presents a formidable problem. Standardized scoring systems and direct quantitative approaches that measure the dimensions and volume components of the airways have largely supplanted earlier descriptive studies [11,12,14]. However carefully they are performed, assessments of airways in fixed tissues may poorly reflect their functional behaviour during the respiratory cycle. There have been efforts to image airways with CT and ultrasound during life [15,16]. These methods are interesting and promising, but they have yet to be fully validated. The major issue is whether they are capable of adequately resolving the dimensions of the smaller airways.

Physiological abnormalities

Lung elastic recoil

Lung elastic recoil refers to the lung's intrinsic tendency to deflate after it has been inflated. This relationship is commonly expressed by plotting lung volume as a function of transpulmonary pressure under the condition of no airflow

(Fig. 1.6). Transpulmonary pressure is defined as the pressure differential between the inside and the outside of the pleura. Pressure in the pleural space may be roughly estimated from a balloon catheter placed in the mid-oesophagus. In normal young adults, transpulmonary pressure at total lung capacity (TLC) is typically in excess of 35 cm H_2O and at functional residual capacity (FRC) is approximately 5 cm H_2O. Lung elastic recoil is sometimes defined in terms of compliance, defined as the change in lung volume relative to the change in pressure. The pressure–volume relationship is curvilinear through its entirety, and as a result, compliance has a unique value at each lung volume. There has been some success in fitting empirical mathematical models to the pressure–volume curve so that the entire relationship can be described by estimation of one or two parameters [17,18]. For most purposes lung elastic recoil can be adequately described in terms of the transpulmonary pressure at some specified lung volumes, TLC and FRC being most commonly used.

Loss of lung elastic recoil is one of the distinguishing features of ageing. This occurs in a manner so predictable that age can be estimated with fair accuracy from the pressure–volume characteristics of a postmortem lung [17]. Age-related losses in lung elasticity probably explain much of the decrease in spirometric function that occurs with advancing age.

Lung elastic recoil may be divided into two components: one resulting from tissue elasticity and a second attributable to the air–liquid interface at the alveolar surface. Tissue elasticity arises from the rich network of elastic fibres within lung parenchyma, from other components of the extracellular matrix, and from the geometrical arrangements of these elements. Isolated elastic fibres behave much like rubber bands, snapping back to their original position upon being stretched to twice their resting length. Alveolar structures are sufficiently small that surface tension at the air–liquid interface creates significant pressure within the alveolar spaces, even in the presence of the surface tension-lowering substance, surfactant. This relationship is defined by the law of Laplace, which states that the pressure within a wetted sphere is proportional to the tension within the lining liquid film and inversely proportional to the radius of curvature. Comparing pressure–volume curves from air- and fluid-filled lungs delineates the contribution of tissue elements and of surface tension. Both make substantial contributions in the human lung. Hence, damage to matrix elements and loss of alveolar surface area would both be expected to reduce lung elastic recoil.

Because damage to elastic fibres and loss of alveolar surface area are the characteristic pathological features of emphysema, a decrease in lung elastic recoil would be anticipated. This prediction has been fully confirmed and Figure 1.5 illustrates the typical abnormality. Compared with normal, the severely emphysematous lung exhibits a substantial loss in elastic recoil pressure at all lung volumes. In addition, the pressure–volume curve in severe emphysema exhibits a shape change, being somewhat more convex with respect to the pressure axis. These altered lung elastic properties might be viewed as the primary functional defect associated with human emphysema.

Airflow resistance

The human bronchial tree is a complex structure. Starting with the trachea, conducting airways branch in an irregularly dichotomous pattern. Different pathways from trachea to terminal membranous bronchiole may encompass as few as 10 generations or as many as 25. Further branching occurs within the partly alveolated respiratory bronchioles distal to the terminal bronchiole. The internal diameter of the adult trachea is approximately 2 cm. Airway calibre decreases with each succeeding generation to a miniscule 0.5 mm at the level of the terminal bronchiole. Because there are approximately 50 000 terminal bronchioles in each human lung, total cross-sectional area at this level of the bronchial tree exceeds that of the trachea by about two orders of magnitude. Hence, the velocity of airflow during the breathing cycle is substantially larger in the central airways compared with the peripheral airways.

A pressure differential is necessary to generate airflow through a cylinder. The ratio of the longitudinal pressure difference to the flow rate defines airflow resistance. The magnitude of airflow resistance varies with the flow profile (laminar versus non-laminar), the physical properties of the gas and the dimensions of the cylinder. The many airways comprising the bronchial tree can be viewed as resistive elements existing in series and in parallel.

As is true for lung parenchyma, airways exhibit intrinsic elastic behaviour which allows them to widen or narrow in response to traction and pressure differentials. Because of the cartilaginous rings within their walls, proximal bronchi are relatively rigid structures. However, the membranous posterior portion is easily deformed, and it will bow inward to occlude the airway lumen when subjected to large compressive pressures. Peripheral bronchioles have little inherent rigidity. The relatively thin, cartilage-free walls of these airways are embedded within lung parenchyma, and they depend upon the tethering effect from alveolar wall attachments to maintain patent lumens. The outward tension exerted by alveolar walls is a function of lung volume; the bigger the volume, the larger the lung elastic recoil, and the greater the tension within each alveolar attachment. If the lung were to exhibit perfect isotropy, a 50% reduction in lung volume would be associated with a 21% reduction in airway calibre.

Assessment of airflow resistance requires simultaneous measurements of airflow at the mouth and of pressure differential between the mouth and the alveolus. Alveolar pressures can be estimated either with an oesophageal balloon or by a plethysmographic method. Figure 1.7 compares

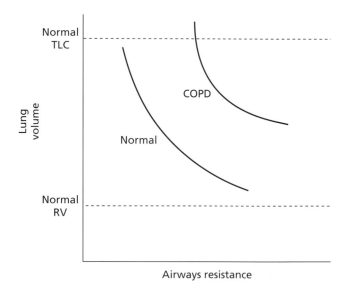

Figure 1.7 Lung volume as a function of airways resistance in a normal subject and in a COPD patient. In both patients airways resistance increases as lung volume becomes smaller. At any given lung volume, airways resistance is considerably larger in the COPD patient. RV, residual volume; TLC, total lung capacity.

typical airflow resistance as a function of lung volume in a normal subject with that in a COPD patient with emphysematous lungs. There is a strong volume dependence of airflow resistance in both subjects, this reflecting the decrease in lung elastic recoil and consequent reduction in airway calibre at smaller lung volumes. Airflow resistance is substantially higher at comparable lung volumes in the patient with COPD, and this might be attributed to two distinct mechanisms. At the same lung volumes, lung elastic recoil would be less in the emphysematous lungs, with the expectation that airways would be narrower and airflow resistance would be higher. It is possible to negate this effect by comparing airflow resistance in different lungs at the same lung elastic recoil pressures. Under these conditions, airflow resistance is still substantially higher in COPD compared with normal. This strongly suggests structural and functional abnormalities inherent to the conducting airways cause increased airflow resistance in COPD.

The dominant site of airflow resistance within the pulmonary airways is not intuitively obvious. The bronchial tree is a complex structure and pathological changes have been described at all levels in lungs from patients with COPD. The peripheral bronchioles are much smaller than the proximal bronchi, but there are a great many of them. Total cross-sectional area at the level of the terminal bronchiole is larger than the trachea by orders of magnitude. However, this tells us little about the relative flow-resistive properties at the two levels, because area changes as the square of airway radius while resistance changes as the fourth power or higher.

Studies with a retrograde catheter in excised animal and human lungs provide an invaluable clue to the site and nature of increased airflow resistance in COPD [19,20]. The catheter was placed at a site in the bronchial tree where airflow resistance in airways less than 2 mm diameter could be partitioned from resistance in airways with a diameter of greater than 2 mm. The first studies were performed in normal dogs and they yielded results that at the time were considered rather surprising [19]. The peripheral component accounted for only approximately 10% of total airflow resistance, a value much smaller than had been suggested by earlier studies.

Retrograde catheter studies of central and peripheral airflow resistance were subsequently made in postmortem lungs from subjects with and without COPD [20]. As was the case in dog lungs, the peripheral component of total airflow resistance in normal human lungs appeared quite low, representing only 10–20% of the total. In lungs from COPD patients, the central component of airflow resistance was only slightly increased from that in normal lungs. However, the peripheral component was increased by factor of between 10 and 20. These observations added enormously to our understanding of the pathophysiology of COPD, because they indicated that it was disease in the distal airways and not the large bronchi that was principally responsible for increased airflow resistance in COPD.

The partitioning of airflow resistance in normal and diseased human lungs also led to a novel idea about the natural history of COPD, which in turn spawned a large and mostly futile research effort. The retrograde catheter studies indicated peripheral airflow resistance was negligible in normal lungs, but predominant in severe COPD. Therefore, early stages of the disease might be associated with pathological changes in the peripheral airways that had minimal effect on standard tests of lung function, such as the FEV_1. It was further reasoned that these early changes might better be detected with more sensitive, non-standard tests. Considerable effort was expended in developing and evaluating newer, so-called 'tests of small airways disease', including the frequency dependence of dynamic lung compliance, the single breath nitrogen washout test, and spirometry with exotic gas mixtures. These tests have long been abandoned, because a variety of epidemiological and pathological–physiological correlative studies indicated that these newer, specialized tests offered little advantage over the FEV_1 in detecting the earliest stages of COPD [21–24].

These newer tests failed in part because they were based on a faulty rationale. Studies by other investigators indicated that the original retrograde catheter studies were subject to methodological errors that led to a systematic underestimate of peripheral airflow resistance in both normal and COPD lungs [25,26]. Repeat measurements in human lungs indicated that the peripheral component represents approximately 90% of total airflow resistance in the normal lung [27]. Additionally, studies in normal postmortem lungs demonstrated a remarkably good correlation between total airflow resistance and the diameter of the peripheral airways, but not with the diameter of the proximal airways [28].

These findings have important implications regarding our understanding of COPD. They lend strong support to the concept that the peripheral airways, and not the central airways, are principally responsible for the increased airflow resistance in COPD. If the peripheral airways determine levels of ventilatory function in the normal lung, it logically follows that relatively minor pathological changes in those same airways take on added functional significance in disease states.

Maximal expiratory airflow limitation

Spirometry is recommended as the single best test for the diagnosis of COPD. During this procedure maximal expiratory airflow is measured as a function of time, and the result is graphically displayed as either a volume–time or flow–volume plot. The two plots contain identical

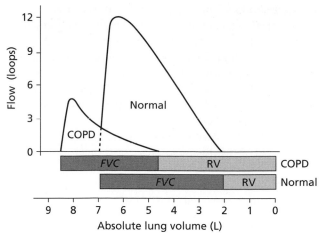

Figure 1.8 Expiratory flow–volume loops as a function of absolute lung volume in a normal subject and in a patient with COPD. This figure illustrates the cardinal functional abnormalities associated with COPD, expiratory airflow limitation and hyperinflation. *FVC*, forced vital capacity; RV, residual volume.

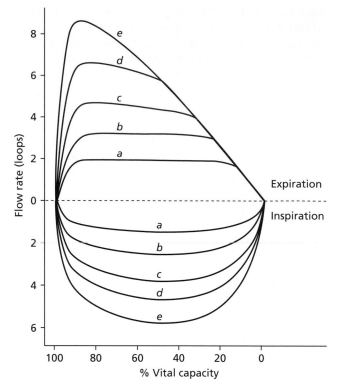

Figure 1.9 A normal subject performed a series of full inspiratory and expiratory manoeuvres with graded effort (*a–e*). On the expiratory limbs, flow rates are independent of effort at smaller lung volumes. This phenomenon, described as 'flow limitation' or 'effort-independence', is not seen with inspiratory manoeuvres.

information. The most common parameters extracted from the spirogram are the FEV_1 and the *FVC*. The expiratory flow rate between 200 and 1200 mL of the *FVC*, the mid-expiratory forced expiratory flow rate between 25% and 75% of the *FVC*, and other less frequently used spirometric parameters contain little additional diagnostic information and have fallen out of favour. A decrease in the FEV_1, best expressed as the percentage of predicted, and a decrease in the ratio of the FEV_1 to the *FVC* (FEV_1/*FVC*) are the hallmark spirometric abnormalities of COPD.

Figure 1.8 shows representative flow–volume curves from a normal subject and from a patient with COPD. At any given fraction of *VC*, maximal expiratory flow rates are smaller in the COPD patient. In this example, flow rates are shown as a function of absolute lung volume to illustrate another of the cardinal physiological abnormalities in COPD. The COPD patient exhibits hyperinflation in that both the TLC and residual volume (RV) are shifted to larger lung volumes.

Forced expiratory flow–volume curves exhibit a phenomenon that is termed airflow limitation. The principle can be demonstrated by having a normal subject perform a series of full inspiratory and expiratory breathing manoeuvres between RV and TLC, each with a different strength of effort. Figure 1.9 depicts these graded efforts (*a* increasing through *e*) as a family of flow–volume loops. Greater effort during the inspiratory phase yields larger flow rates, and these increases are roughly proportional at all lung volumes. On the expiratory cycle, greater effort also generates larger flow rates, but only at the higher lung volumes. At intermediate and low lung volumes, airflow

increases with added effort, but only up to a certain point. At that point the tracing superimposes those from other individual efforts. Over the lower two-thirds of the vital capacity a ceiling becomes evident, beyond which airflow does not increase further however great the expiratory effort. Expiratory flow rates at these lung volumes are sometimes described as being 'flow limited' or 'effort independent'.

The principle of flow limitation can be demonstrated in somewhat better detail from what are called isovolume pressure–flow diagrams (Fig. 1.10). Inspiratory and expiratory flow are plotted as a function of alveolar pressure at specified lung volumes. The pressure differential between the mouth and the alveolar space, or driving pressure, generates airflow though the bronchial tree. Alveolar pressure is negative with respect to the mouth during inspiration and positive with expiration. During inspiration, airflow remains linear with driving pressure at each of the indicated lung volumes, meaning that airflow resistance remains nearly constant. Hence, inspiratory flow is largely limited by the magnitude of the applied pressure, which is largely a function of respiratory muscle strength. Differences in

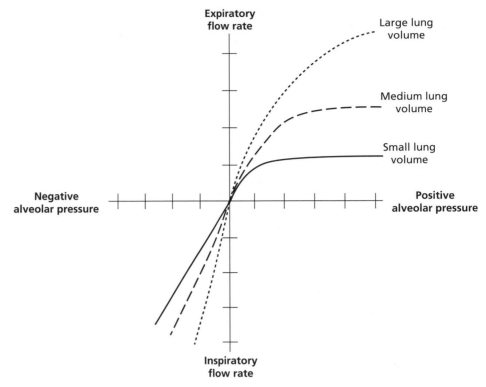

Figure 1.10 Relationship of inspiratory and expiratory airflow rates to alveolar pressure at various lung volumes. With inspiration, flow increases proportionally to alveolar pressure. With expiration, flow increases with alveolar pressure only to a certain point, beyond which flow remains constant despite greater alveolar pressures. This effect, flow limitation, is most pronounced at smaller lung volumes.

the slopes of the pressure–flow relationships at the three different lung volumes indicate that airflow resistance becomes greater as lung volumes become smaller.

The patterns obtained during expiration are qualitatively different in that relationships between the pressure differential and airflow are curvilinear rather than linear. This is most obvious at smaller lung volumes where a fairly sharp inflection occurs at a relatively low driving pressure. Beyond this inflection, the relationship assumes a plateau shape, meaning that airflow is independent of changes in driving pressure. In other words, greater expiratory effort creates greater airflow resistance with no increase in airflow. Limitations to expiratory airflow are set by the mechanical properties of lung parenchyma and bronchial tree.

The relevance of expiratory airflow limitation to clinical disability can be appreciated by comparing flow–volume loops from a COPD patient with that of a normal subject. Figure 1.11 shows inspiratory and expiratory flow–volume loops during tidal breathing at rest and with maximal effort in the two subjects. Note that the normal subject has enormous reserve and from the resting state is able to increase minute ventilation by a large factor in response to increased metabolic demands. Consequently, ventilation is not a limiting factor, even with very vigorous exercise. In contrast, maximal inspiratory and expiratory flow rates are much smaller in the patient with COPD, expiration typically being more severely affected than inspiration. Most importantly, a large portion of the expiratory flow–volume loop

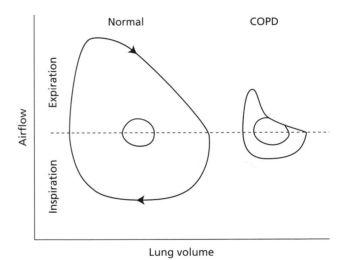

Figure 1.11 Inspiratory and expiratory flow–volume loops in a normal subject and in a patient with severe COPD. The outer loops represent maximal efforts and the loops represent tidal breathing. In the patient with COPD, expiration is flow limited even during a tidal breath.

obtained during tidal expiration superimposes that from a forced expiration. Severe COPD patients exhibit flow limitation even while meeting the minimal ventilatory requirements of the resting state. These patients have only limited capability for increasing minute ventilation in response to exercise. Their only effective strategy for increasing minute ventilation is to shift tidal breathing to larger lung volumes where higher expiratory flow rates can be achieved. Clinical studies have shown that hyperinflation is a common response to increased workload in COPD patients [29]. Unfortunately, this compensatory mechanism comes with a price, because the lung and the thoracic cage both become stiffer at larger volumes. This increases the elastic workload of the respiratory muscles and is an important component in generating the sensation of breathlessness.

Mechanism of expiratory airflow limitation

Models of varying complexity have been used to analyse the physical behaviour of the lung in an effort to explain flow limitation during forced expiratory manoeuvres. A relatively simple model is described that provides some insight into this mechanism. The interested reader is referred elsewhere for more detailed and rigorous approaches to the subject [30–32].

The model shown in Figure 1.12 includes an expandable balloon to represent lung parenchyma. The balloon is contained within a box that depicts the thoracic cage. The space between the box and the balloon may be viewed as the pleural space. An airway with semi-rigid walls connects the balloon to the exterior. Up or down movement of the piston, representing the function of respiratory muscles, activates the model by altering intrapleural pressure (Ppl). The centrally directed arrows on the interior of the balloon symbolize lung elastic recoil.

Figure 1.12(a) shows the model at a fixed volume with no airflow. Under these static conditions, there is no gradient along the length of the airway and alveolar pressure (Palv) is equal to the reference pressure at the airway opening (Pao). The intrapleural pressure required to keep the lung statically inflated (arbitrarily chosen to be -10 cm H_2O in this example) is equal in magnitude but opposite in sign to the lung elastic recoil pressure (Pel). Hence, Palv is the algebraic sum of Ppl and Pel.

Downward motion of the piston creates a more negative Ppl. Palv now becomes negative with respect to Pao and air flows into the lung. On expiration, muscles relax and the lung typically contracts passively because of its inherent elastic recoil. As Ppl becomes less negative (-10 cm H_2O increasing to -5 cm H_2O), Palv becomes positive with respect to Pao and the lung exhales air (Fig. 1.12b). During the normal tidal breathing cycle, Ppl fluctuates by only a few centimetres H_2O and it remains negative even during expiration. As a result, pressure at each point within the conducting airway remains positive with respect to Ppl during the entire inspiratory and expiratory cycle. Consequently, an outwardly directed transmural pressure gradient expands the airway along its entire length, an effect that is greater during inspiration.

However, a forced expiratory effort creates a strongly positive Ppl that reverses the usual transmural pressure gradient along a segment of the airway. Figure 1.12(c) illustrates these pressure relationships during a submaximal forced expiration. Respiratory muscles generate sufficient force to increase Ppl to $+10$ cm H_2O. From the algebraic sum of Ppl and Pel, Palv now becomes $+20$ cm H_2O. The alveolar driving pressure dissipates along the length of airway lumen and at some point becomes equal to Ppl so that the transmural pressure gradient is zero. This is sometimes described as the 'equal-pressure point' (EPP). The EPP has no fixed anatomical site. Direct measurements suggest that the EPP is located in the central cartilaginous airways during the early stages of the maximal expiratory manoeuvre, but then migrates peripherally at lower lung volumes. Downstream from the EPP, intraluminal pressures become negative with respect to Ppl, creating a compressive force on the airway. Because the airway is not a rigid tube, compressive pressures narrow the lumen to some degree, thereby increasing airflow resistance. The length of compressed airway is referred to as the 'flow-limiting segment'.

Figure 1.12(d) illustrates the same relationships but with a more forceful expiratory effort. In this example, Ppl increases to $+20$ cm H_2O and the alveolar driving pressure, Palv, now enlarges to $+30$ cm H_2O. Because of the higher Ppl, compressive transmural pressures downstream from the EPP are now twice as large as in Figure 1.12(c). This further narrows the airway lumen with a corresponding increase in airflow resistance. In other words, greater expiratory effort increases the pressure head between alveolus and airway opening, but it also increases flow resistance because of greater compression of the airway downstream from the EPP. The result is little net change in expiratory airflow. This type of feedback mechanism for limiting flow is sometimes referred to as a Starling resistor, of which there are examples in other organ systems. It bears emphasizing that these relationships are exceedingly complex when analysed from first principles and no physical law requires that changes in Palv and airflow resistance need be strictly proportional. However, empirical observations indicate that these changes are roughly proportional in most human subjects.

The illustrated model permits some insight into other factors that might influence the flow-limiting airway segment. It is intuitively evident that a less rigid airway would narrow to a greater extent in response to the same transmural compressive pressure differential. Other conditions being equal, excessively compliant central airways would fix maximal expiratory airflow at a lower level. It is unclear from existing studies whether bronchial compliance is abnormal in well-defined patients with COPD.

Airflow resistance in more distal portions of the conducting airways may accentuate compressive effects on the

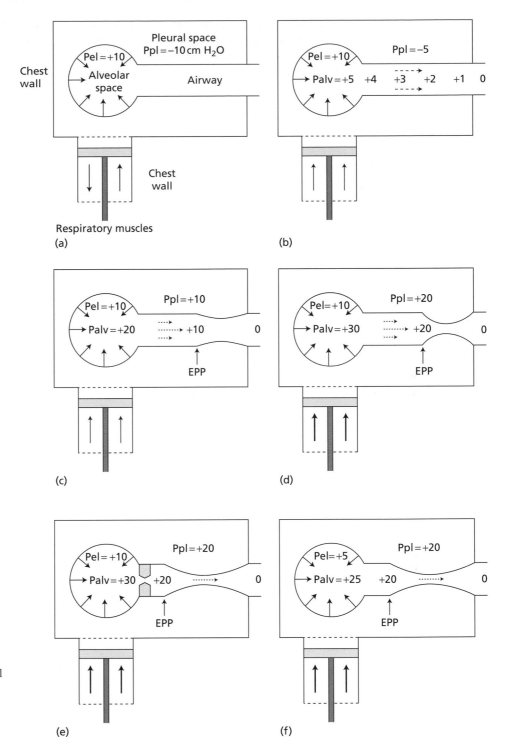

Figure 1.12 Model of expiratory flow limitation. See text for detailed explanation. (a) Description of static model. (b) Expiration during tidal breath. (c) Submaximal forced expiration. (d) Submaximal forced expiration but with greater effort than in (c). (e) Forced expiration with increase in peripheral airways resistance. (f) Forced expiration with decreased lung elastic recoil pressure. EPP, equal-pressure point; Palv, alveolar pressure; Pel, elastic recoil pressure; Ppl, intrapleural pressure.

more proximal flow-limiting airway segment. This is illustrated in Figure 1.12(e), which depicts partial obstruction in the most distal part of the airway. Peripheral airway narrowing may occur as a consequence of pathological features such as inflammation and excess mucus. As as result of the increase in peripheral airflow resistance, a greater portion of the driving pressure between alveolus and airway dissipates over the obstructed segment of airway. Hence, the EPP migrates distally and a longer segment of the more proximal airway is subjected to compressive pressures. Total airway resistance would increase and maximal expiratory airflow would be expected to decrease.

Loss of lung elastic recoil also has an impact on maximal expiratory airflow limitation. One mechanism relates to the effects of lung elastic recoil on the diameter of the intra-parenchymal airways, which are not shown in the model. A decrease in lung elastic recoil at any specified lung volume will reduce airway calibre and increase peripheral airflow resistance. The effect on maximal expiratory airflow will be similar to that shown in Figure 1.12(e).

Another effect of elastic recoil on maximal airflow limitation is less intuitive. Note that an arbitrary value of 10 cm H_2O is assigned to Pel in Figure 1.12(a–e). Note also that when flow limitation becomes evident, as in Figure 1.12(d and e), the difference between Palv and the intra-airway pressure at the EPP has the same magnitude as Pel (10 cm H_2O). Viewed in this manner, lung elastic recoil effectively keeps airways open by opposing the high compressive pressures that develop in the pleural space during forced expiration. Figure 1.12(f) illustrates the effect of decreased lung elastic recoil on flow limitation. In this example, a Pel of 5 cm H_2O has been assigned to an 'emphysematous balloon'. With the same force exerted by respiratory muscles on the pleural space (Ppl = 20 cm H_2O), Palv now increases to only 25 cm H_2O instead of 30 cm H_2O. There is a corresponding decrease in the intra-airway pressure that opposes airway compression. Consequently, the EPP migrates distally, the compressed segment of airway becomes longer, with a corresponding decrease in maximal expiratory airflow.

Lung hyperinflation

A second characteristic and very important physiological abnormality in COPD is hyperinflation. This is variably defined as abnormally large TLC, FRC or RV. Lung volumes can be measured either by the washin or the washout of tracer gases, such as helium, or by plethysmography. Because tracer-gas methods require long equilibration times in the presence of severe COPD, plethysmography is the more accurate method. In clinical practice the diagnosis of COPD can usually be made from clinical and spirometric findings alone, but lung volume measurements may be useful in selected patients.

Figure 1.8 illustrates both the expiratory airflow abnormalities and the hyperinflation that are typical of COPD. As the FEV_1 and the FVC decrease, RV and TLC increase. Indices of hyperinflation, particularly the RV and RV/TLC, track closely with spirometric measures of expiratory airflow obstruction across a broad range of COPD severity [33]. This suggests that the functional and structural features that relate to expiratory airflow obstruction, namely loss of lung elastic recoil and increased peripheral airway resistance, are also responsible for an abnormally large RV.

RV is sometimes termed the 'volume of trapped air', a description that is probably apt. As described previously, lung volume, lung elastic recoil and peripheral airway resistance are intimately interrelated. As lung volume becomes smaller, elastic recoil decreases and the attendant loss of radial tension causes narrowing of the peripheral airways. At some point, resistance effectively becomes infinite and flow ceases. Several lines of indirect evidence suggest that peripheral airways in humans may actually close at lung volumes near RV, a phenomenon that has been directly observed in experimental animal lungs [34]. Calculations suggest that surface tension at the air–liquid interface on the epithelial surface of peripheral airways may be substantial as the lung volume nears RV, so that an intact surfactant system may be essential if the terminal bronchioles are to remain patent [35].

Structural correlates of expiratory airflow limitation

Expiratory airflow limitation is functionally related both to a loss of lung elastic recoil and to an increase in airflow resistance through the bronchial tree. Emphysema is presumed to be the morphological equivalent of abnormal lung elastic recoil, while a variety of pathological changes, particularly those in the peripheral airways, are thought to be responsible for increased airflow resistance through the bronchial tree. Consequently, there is the expectation that a detailed quantitative assessment of emphysema and airways disease in a lung from a COPD patient should allow a reasonably accurate prediction of spirometric function. Over the past several decades, numerous efforts to show such pathological and physiological correlations have yielded rather disappointing results.

Investigators have utilized several approaches when undertaking correlative structure–function studies, and each of these has certain advantages and limitations. Most commonly, investigators have compared lung tissue obtained at necropsy with function tests performed prior to death. Patients with severe disease tend to be heavily over-represented in this type of study and the interval between the last pulmonary function test and death is variable. Tissue may also be acquired from patients undergoing lung resection surgery, which is usually performed for localized carcinomas. This approach has the major advantage of allowing detailed pulmonary function testing shortly prior to the scheduled surgery. It has the disadvantage of providing only a limited amount of tissue in most patients, with attendant problems in achieving uniform inflation and fixation. Also, potential surgical candidates must have sufficiently good lung function if they are to tolerate resection, which excludes most patients with severe COPD. Lung-volume-reduction surgery provides new opportunities for obtaining resected lung tissue from patients with severe disease, but the samples are relatively small and they may be poorly representative of the remaining lung. Correlation studies have also been carried out in postmortem lungs. Tests of mechanical function performed in carefully selected postmortem lungs are reproducible, and forced expiratory flow rates obtained from such studies correspond quite closely with those obtained in living, age-matched adults [36]. The major disadvantage is in not knowing how severely postmortem changes might affect the results. Finally, CT imaging permits an accurate, indirect assessment of emphysema severity that can be compared against tests of function.

Efforts to show a correlation between emphysema severity and the FEV_1 have yielded inconsistent results [11,37–39]. Most published reports demonstrated either a relatively weak inverse relationship or one that was not statistically significant. Trivial degrees of emphysema may be associated with severe airflow obstruction in selected patients, while others may have normal or near-normal spirometry in the face of fairly advanced emphysema. In the largest series yet published, the Vancouver group of investigators found no statistically significant relationship between emphysema severity and the FEV_1 in 407 patients with mild-to-moderate COPD who were tested shortly before surgery for lung resection [38].

Efforts to show correlations between airflow obstruction and the severity of pathological changes in the conducting airways have fared no better. Numerous efforts to show correlations between expiratory airflow obstruction in COPD with mucous gland enlargement and other pathological features in the cartilaginous airways have been for the most part unsuccessful [40]. These results are perhaps not surprising in light of the retrograde catheter studies, which suggested that the principal pathological changes accounting for increased airflow resistance in COPD were to be found in the peripheral airways [20,27]. Those studies raised an expectation that careful assessments of peripheral airways disease, including features such as inflammation, fibrosis and smooth muscle enlargement, might show closer correlations with spirometric abnormalities. Early, small studies appeared to show such associations [10,41]. However, in the previously cited studies of 407 patients by the Vancouver group, no statistically significant relationship was found between the FEV_1 and total pathology score, or any of its components, for either the membranous or the respiratory bronchiole [38].

Thus, the largest and best available correlative studies indicate that the relationship of FEV_1 with either airway pathology or emphysema is at best tenuous. It bears emphasizing that most existing studies sampled only one part of the continuum between normal lung and severe COPD, and this provides a somewhat restricted view of the larger picture. For example, the Vancouver study included very few non-smokers and no patients with severe disease [38]. Many other studies have been restricted to patients with severe disease [37,39]. When a broader assessment is made in age-matched groups who may be presumed to have increasing levels of ventilatory dysfunction (never smokers, smokers without known COPD, and smokers with severe COPD), emphysema severity and multiple elements of airways disease were found to progress in parallel [11]. In addition, a wealth of circumstantial evidence from human studies and more direct evidence from experimental animal studies indicate that emphysema and some elements of airways disease are important morphological determinants of expiratory airflow obstruction. These considerations not withstanding, the ability to estimate the magnitude of ventilatory impairment in COPD from the most detailed pathological assessments is surprisingly poor. One can only speculate as to the reasons.

Ventilation distribution and gas exchange

COPD is characterized by progressive blood gas abnormalities. Mild hypoxaemia may be present in the early stages of COPD, and it usually progresses as the disease worsens. Hypercapnia may accompany more severe disease. Untreated hypoxaemia and hypercapnia can cause pulmonary hypertension and cor pulmonale, which contribute to the morbidity and mortality associated with this disease. The structural derangements and specific mechanisms responsible for gas exchange abnormalities in COPD are exceedingly complex and imperfectly understood.

Gas exchange within the lung is most efficient when the ratio of ventilation/perfusion ($\dot{V}/\dot{Q}$) remains close to unity within all lung regions. It is obvious that no gas exchange can occur if a ventilated zone receives no blood supply. A relative excess of ventilation is described as 'alveolar dead space', 'wasted ventilation' or a 'high $\dot{V}/\dot{Q}$ abnormality'. Such regions behave functionally as though some portion of the lung region received normal blood flow while the remainder received none. An increase in the dead space/tidal volume ratio (V_D/V_T) reflects lung zones with an abnormally high $\dot{V}/\dot{Q}$. V_D/V_T is usually 0.3–0.4 in normal subjects, but it may increase to as much as 0.7–0.8 in patients with severe COPD. In those patients the major portion of each inspired breath represents 'wasted ventilation'.

Alveolar regions that are underventilated in relation to their blood supply are described as low $\dot{V}/\dot{Q}$ zones. The proportion of cardiac output that passes through a completely unventilated lung region is termed the shunt fraction, and the admixture of shunted blood with other pulmonary venous blood is manifest as arterial hypoxaemia. A $\dot{V}/\dot{Q}$ region of less than 1 but greater than zero behaves as though some part of the region received normal ventilation and the remainder received none. Lung regions with low

$\dot{V}/\dot{Q}$ abnormalities are thought to be the principal cause of hypoxaemia in COPD.

Pathological states affecting either ventilation or perfusion homogeneity might in theory cause regional $\dot{V}/\dot{Q}$ to deviate from unity. Radioactive scanning and other techniques show that COPD is characterized by abnormal patterns involving both ventilation and perfusion. It is generally believed that pathological changes occur initially on the ventilation side and that abnormal perfusion patterns may partly result from compensatory flow regulation. Disease in the peripheral airways and alveolar spaces creates regions of both hyperventilation and hypoventilation. Hypoventilation causes localized hypoxia, which in turn stimulates a vasocontrictor response in the neighbouring arteries. The attendant reduction in blood flow re-establishes a regional $\dot{V}/\dot{Q}$ that is close to unity. Long periods of hypoxia may induce tissue remodelling in small pulmonary arteries, such as intimal fibrosis and smooth muscle hypertrophy, which lead to irreversible pulmonary hypertension. Because abnormalities in the pulmonary vascular bed may be regarded as secondary events, attention is directed to mechanisms by which abnormal ventilation patterns arise in COPD.

Ventilation is the process by which ambient air is transported to the alveolar spaces and resident air is removed to the environment. It is defined as the fractional turnover of inspired gas volume to resident gas volume for any given portion of the lung. Under normal resting conditions, each breath replaces approximately 10–15% of the resident gas volume. Gas is transported from the airway opening to the alveolar–capillary interface by convection and by diffusion. Transport within the proximal airways occurs by convection predominantly, whereas diffusion is more important within the alveolated gas-exchanging regions of the lung. Diffusion is not thought to be an important rate-limiting step for gas transport in the distal airways under normal conditions, but it may become so when diseases such as emphysema cause extensive anatomical rearrangements.

The compliance of a lung region and the change in transpleural pressure to which it is subjected determine ventilation. For a given change in transpleural pressure, a relatively more compliant lung region expands to a greater degree and receives more ventilation than does a less compliant region. An example is to be found in the normal human lung. As shown in Figure 1.6, the lung becomes progressively stiffer as it expands. As a result of gravity effects, a pleural pressure gradient develops from apex to base with apical pressures being more negative. Because the lung apex is subjected to a larger transpleural pressure, it is overinflated relative to the lung base. Consequently, the apex is less compliant and it receives a relatively smaller volume of each inspired breath than does the lung base. Non-homogeneous lung elastic behaviour brought about

by any pathological condition could cause uneven ventilation by a similar mechanism.

Emphysema is a prototype of diseases that cause abnormal lung elasticity. Emphysema tends to be non-uniform in its distribution, both within a single region and between regions. Large emphysema lesions may reside immediately adjacent to apparently normal lung parenchyma. Because of differences in the shape of their respective pressure–volume characteristics, an emphysematous region might be either hyperventilated or hypoventilated relative to normal adjacent lung. This occurs because the pressure–volume curve of the emphysematous lung exhibits greater concavity towards the pressure axis (see Fig. 1.6). Consequently, it is overly compliant at low lung volumes but abnormally stiff at high lung volumes. If a discrete emphysema lesion were located at the lung apex so that it were subjected to a relatively large transpleural pressures, it would overexpand and be less compliant than surrounding normal lung. Therefore, this region would receive less ventilation with each tidal breath. By a parallel argument, the same emphysematous region might be abnormally compliant and overventilated if located at the lung base.

Existing evidence suggests that most emphysematous regions may be relatively underventilated, as shown in Figure 1.13 [42]. Other variables remaining constant, this should give rise to a low $\dot{V}/\dot{Q}$ zone. However, emphysematous regions also tend to be underperfused because a portion of the capillary bed has been lost. Thus, focal emphysematous regions could represent a broad range of $\dot{V}/\dot{Q}$ zones, both high and low, depending upon several critical variables.

Figure 1.13 illustrates another mechanism by which emphysema might cause uneven ventilation. In this example, the destructive change of early centriacinar emphysema is associated with a substantial enlargement of the respiratory bronchiole. Distal portions of the acinus remain largely intact. Enlargement of the proximal airway effectively increases the volume of 'dead space' ventilation to the more distal portions of that transport pathway. At end expiration, all gas-transport pathways contain resident gas. With the next inspiration, the 'dead-space' must be cleared before inspired air reaches the gas-exchanging region. With a larger 'dead space', a given volume of inspired air penetrates less deeply into the acinus. As a result, it is expected that the proximal emphysema lesion might be relatively overventilated while the more distal acinar regions might be underventilated.

Airways disease probably also contributes to $\dot{V}/\dot{Q}$ disturbances in the lungs of COPD patients, though little is known of specific mechanisms. Theoretical considerations suggest that at resting ventilation rates, severe airway narrowing or even complete closure would be necessary to substantially decrease ventilation to lung parenchyma

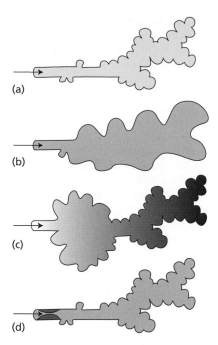

Figure 1.13 Postulated mechanisms for uneven ventilation in COPD. Dark shading indicates resident gas. Light shading represents inspired air. (a) Inspired breath is uniformly distributed in a normal lung unit. (b) Panacinar emphysema lesion is less compliant than normal lung and is less well ventilated, even though inspired air is uniformly distributed. (c) Centriacinar emphysema lesion increases 'dead space' so that distal portion of the unit is underventilated. (d) Obstruction of terminal bronchiole causes underventilation of distal alveolated structures.

subtended by a particular airway. Large plugs of mucus may sometimes occlude a proximal bronchus in patients with COPD, but the peripheral airways are probably more important as a cause of ventilation heterogeneity. Although never directly visualized, inflammatory exudate or excess mucus might well cause intermittent or complete obstruction of terminal bronchioles, resulting in an underventilated region (see Fig. 1.13). If the bronchiole were to remain occluded for an extended period, atelectasis might not occur because of ventilation via collateral channels.

Gas exchange is dependent on numerous other factors, including pulmonary blood flow distribution, neural control of breathing, chest wall mechanics, systemic haemodynamics, metabolic demands and respiratory muscle function. The final common expressions of disordered gas exchange in COPD, arterial hypoxaemia and hypercapnia represent a summation of multiple complex mechanisms.

Clinical and pathological subtypes of COPD

Older studies suggested that some patients with COPD could be fitted into so-called emphysematous and bronchitic

subtypes, based upon certain distinguishing clinical, pathological and physiological criteria [43]. At one time this idea enjoyed widespread currency and the subject is still presented as established fact in some standard textbooks. As implied by their names, either predominant anatomical emphysema or predominant bronchitis (airways disease) was thought to provide the morphological basis for distinguishing clinical and physiological features. The patient with the emphysematous subtype of COPD was sometimes described as 'type A' or 'pink puffer', while the terms 'type B' or 'blue bloater' depicted the bronchitic subtype.

The typical emphysematous patient was described as a cachectic elderly individual who related a long history of progressive and unrelenting breathlessness. Sputum production and recurrent chest infections were notable by their absence. The chest roentgenogram revealed a small cardiac silhouette along with the roentgenographical signs of advanced emphysema and lung hyperinflation. Arterial blood gases showed only mild hypoxaemia and hypercapnia and cor pulmonale was not a prominent clinical feature. A decrease in lung elastic recoil and a severely impaired diffusing capacity for carbon monoxide reflected the severe underlying emphysema.

The typical patient with predominant bronchitis was described as overweight, if not obese, with plethoric facies and obvious cyanosis. Chronic cough and sputum production were considered an essential feature of the bronchitic subtype. The other prominent aspects of the bronchitis patient were severe hypoxaemia, an accompanying hypercapnia, and consequent to the deranged blood gases, cor pulmonale and polycythaemia. Cor pulmonale was manifest clinically as peripheral oedema, cardiac enlargement and electrocardiographical signs of right ventricular enlargement. Reflecting the lack of severe emphysema, lung elastic recoil and diffusing capacity for carbon monoxide were normal or near normal.

The clinical features that distinguish COPD subtypes may be recognizable in selected patients, but most patients with COPD cannot be so simply categorized. It has been proposed that COPD represents a spectrum, with the emphysematous patients at one end and the bronchitic patients at the other. Because of extensive overlap between the two groups, clinical investigations have compared only those patients at the extreme ends of the spectrum. Subgroup distinctions have usually been made on clinical and physiological grounds, which have not been uniform.

Efforts to correlate lung pathology with the clinical subtype of COPD have generally been contradictory and inconclusive. Claims to the existence of the emphysematous and bronchitis subtypes of COPD rest largely on a single small study in which clinical data were compared with autopsy findings [43]. These findings could not be confirmed in subsequent similar studies by others [44,45]. Cor pulmonale is generally considered an essential feature of the bronchitic patient but not the emphysematous patient. Consistent with this concept, small necropsy studies have shown little relationship between right ventricular weight and emphysema severity [46–48]. Similarly, the extent of emphysema as defined by CT imaging bears little relationship to the severity of blood gas or pulmonary haemodynamic abnormalities [49]. However, neither is there a strong relationship between mucous gland enlargement, long considered the essential lesion of the bronchitic subtype, and right ventricular weight [48,50,51]. Correlations of peripheral airways disease with right ventricular weight has been found by some investigators but not others [48,50].

Patients with COPD vary in their propensity for developing hypoxaemia, hypercapnia and pulmonary hypertension, so that the terms 'pink puffer' and 'blue bloater' may have some validity as clinical descriptive terms. However, very little is known as to why these differences exist. There is clearly no scientific justification for describing such patients as having either the emphysematous or bronchitic subtype of COPD.

References

1 National Heart, Lung and Blood Institute, Division of Lung Diseases. Workshop report: The definition of emphysema. *Am Rev Respir Dis* 1985;**132**:182–5.

2 Thurlbeck WM, Dunnill MS, Hartung W *et al.* A comparison of three methods for measuring emphysema. *Hum Pathol* 1970;**1**:215–26.

3 Thurlbeck WM. Internal surface area and other measurements in emphysema. *Thorax* 1967;**22**:483–96.

4 Müller NL, Coxson H. Chronic obstructive pulmonary disease. IV. Imaging the lungs in patients with chronic obstructive pulmonary disease. *Thorax* 2002;**57**:982–5.

5 Ciba Guest Symposium Report. Terminology, definitions and classification of chronic pulmonary emphysema and related conditions. *Thorax* 1959;**14**:286–99.

6 Jamal K, Cooney JK, Fleetham JA, Thurlbeck WM. Chronic bronchitis: correlation of morphologic findings to sputum production and flow rates. *Am Rev Respir Dis* 1984;**129**: 719–22.

7 Reid L. Measurement of the bronchial mucous gland layer: a diagnostic yardstick in chronic bronchitis. *Thorax* 1960;**15**: 132–41.

8 Saetta M, Di Stefano A, Maestrelli P *et al.* Activated T-lymphocytes and macrophages in bronchial mucosa of subjects with chronic bronchitis. *Am Rev Respir Dis* 1993;**147**:301–6.

9 Niewoehner DE, Kleinerman J, Rice DB. Pathologic changes in the peripheral airways of young cigarette smokers. *N Engl J Med* 1974;**291**:755–8.

10 Cosio M, Ghezzo H, Hogg JC *et al.* The relations between structural changes in small airways and pulmonary-function tests. *N Engl J Med* 1978;**298**:1277–81.

11 Hale KA, Ewing SL, Gosnell BA *et al.* Lung disease in long-term cigarette smokers with and without chronic air-flow obstruction. *Am Rev Respir Dis* 1984;**130**:716–21.

12 Matsuba K, Wright JL, Wiggs BR *et al.* The changes in airways structure associated with reduced forced expiratory volume in one second. *Eur Respir J* 1989;**2**:934–9.

13 Bosken CH, Wiggs BR, Paré PD *et al.* Small airway dimensions in smokers with obstruction to airflow. *Am Rev Respir Dis* 1990;**142**:563–70.

14 Wright JL, Cosio M, Wiggs B *et al.* A morphologic grading scheme for membranous and respiratory bronchioles. *Arch Pathol Lab Med* 1985;**109**:163–5.

15 Nakano Y, Muro S, Sakai H *et al.* Computed tomographic measurements of airways dimensions and emphysema in smokers: correlation with lung function. *Am J Respir Crit Care Med* 2000;**162**:1102–8.

16 Sharma V, Shaaban AM, Berges G *et al.* The radiological spectrum of small-airway diseases. *Semin Ultrasound CT MR* 2002;**23**:339–51.

17 Niewoehner DE, Kleinerman J, Liotta L. Elastic behavior of postmortem human lungs: effects of aging and mild emphysema. *J Appl Physiol* 1975;**39**:943–9.

18 Colebatch HJH, Greaves IA, Ng CKY. Exponential analysis of elastic recoil and aging in healthy males and females. *J Appl Physiol* 1979;**47**:683–91.

19 Macklem PT, Mead J. Resistance of central and peripheral airways measured by retrograde catheter. *J Appl Physiol* 1967;**22**:395–401.

20 Hogg JC, Macklem PT, Thurlbeck WM. Site and nature of airway obstruction in chronic obstructive lung disease. *N Engl J Med* 1968;**278**:1355–60.

21 Knudson RJ, Lebowitz MD. Comparison of flow–volume and closing volume variables in a random population. *Am Rev Respir Dis* 1977;**116**:1039–45.

22 Oxhoj H, Bake B, Wilhelmensen L. Ability of spirometry, flow–volume curves, and the nitrogen closing volume test to detect smokers: a population study. *Scand J Respir Dis* 1977; **58**:80–96.

23 Cosio M, Ghezzo H, Hogg JC *et al.* The relation between structural changes in small airways and pulmonary function tests. *N Engl J Med* 1978;**298**:1277–81.

24 van de Woestijne KP. Are the small airways really quiet? *Eur J Respir Dis* 1982;**63**(Suppl 121):19–25.

25 Hoppin FG Jr, Green M, Morgan MS. Relationship of central and peripheral resistance to lung volume in dogs. *J Appl Physiol: Respirat Environ Exercise Physiol* 1978;**44**:728–37.

26 Kappos AD, Rodarte JR, Lai-Fook JS. Frequency dependence and partitioning of respiratory impedance in dogs. *J Appl Physiol: Respirat Environ Exercise Physiol* 1981;**51**:621–9.

27 van Brabrandt H, Cauberghs M, Verbeken E, *et al.* Partitioning of pulmonary impedance in excised human and canine lungs. *J Appl Physiol* 1983;**55**:1733–42.

28 Niewoehner DE, Kleinerman J. Morphologic basis of pulmonary resistance in the human lung and effects of aging. *J Appl Physiol* 1974;**36**:412–8.

29 O'Donnell DE, Revill SM, Webb KA. Dynamic hyperinflation and exercise intolerance in chronic obstructive pulmonary disease. *Am J Respir Crit Care Med* 2001;**164**:770–7.

30 Mead J, Turner JM, Macklem PT, Little JD. Significance of the relationship between lung recoil and maximum expiratory flow. *J Appl Physiol* 1967;**22**:95–108.

31 Dawson SV, Elliot EA. Wave-speed limitation on expiratory flow: a unifying concept. *J Appl Physiol* 1977;**43**:498–515.

32 Elad D, Kamm RD, Shapiro AH. Mathematical simulation of forced expiration. *J Appl Physiol* 1988;**65**:14–25.

33 Dykstra BJ, Scanlon PD, Kester MM *et al.* Lung volumes in 4774 patients with obstructive lung disease. *Chest* 1999;**115**:68–74.

34 Hughes JMB, Rosenzweig DY, Kivitz PB. Site of airway closure in excised dog lungs: histologic demonstration. *J Appl Physiol* 1970;**29**:340–4.

35 Hill MJ, Wilson TA, Lambert RK. Effects of surface tension and intraluminal fluid on mechanics of small airways. *J Appl Physiol* 1997;**82**:233–9.

36 Niewoehner DE, Kleinerman J, Knoke J. Peripheral airways as a determinant of ventilatory function in the human lung. *J Clin Invest* 1977;**60**:139–51.

37 Nagai A, West WW, Thurlbeck WM. The National Institute of Health Intermittent Positive-Pressure Breathing Trial: pathology studies. II. Correlation between morphologic findings, clinical findings and evidence of expiratory airflow obstruction. *Am Rev Respir Dis* 1985;**132**:946–53.

38 Hogg JC, Wright JL, Wiggs BR *et al.* Lung structure and function in cigarette smokers. *Thorax* 1994;**49**:473–8.

39 Gelb AF, Hogg JC, Muller NL *et al.* Contribution of emphysema and small airways in COPD. *Chest* 1996;**109**:353–9.

40 Thurlbeck WM. Chronic airflow obstruction. In: Petty TL, ed. *Chronic Obstructive Lung Disease*, 2nd edn. New York: Marcel Dekker, 1985: 129–204.

41 Berend N, Wright JL, Thurlbeck WM *et al.* Small airways disease: reproducibility of measurements and correlation with lung function. *Chest* 1981;**79**:263–8.

42 Hogg JC, Nepszy SJ, Macklem PT *et al.* Elastic properties of the centrilobular emphysematous space. *J Clin Invest* 1969; **48**:1306–12.

43 Burrows B, Fletcher C, Heard BE *et al.* The emphysematous and bronchial types of chronic airways obstruction: a clinicopathological study of patients in London and Chicago. *Lancet* 1966;**1**:830–5.

44 Cullen JH, Kaemmerlen JT, Assaad D *et al.* A prospective clinical–pathologic study of the lungs and heart in chronic obstructive lung disease. *Am Rev Respir Dis* 1970;**102**:190–204.

45 Mitchell RS, Stanford RE, Johnson JM *et al.* The morphologic features of the bronchi, bronchioles, and alveoli in chronic airway obstruction: a clinicopathologic study. *Am Rev Respir Dis* 1976;**114**:137–45.

46 Cromie JB. Correlation of anatomic pulmonary emphysema and right ventricular hypertrophy. *Am Rev Respir Dis* 1961; **84**:657–62.

47 Hasleton PS. Right ventricular hypertrophy in emphysema. *J Pathol* 1973;**110**:27–36.

48 Mitchell RS, Stanford RE, Silvers GW *et al.* The right ventricle in chronic airway obstruction: a clinicopathologic study. *Am Rev Respir Dis* 1976;**114**:147–54.

49 Biernacki W, Gould GA, Whyte KF *et al.* Pulmonary haemodynamics, gas exchange, and the severity of emphysema as assessed by quantitative CT scan in chronic bronchitis and emphysema. *Am Rev Respir Dis* 1989;**139**:1509–15.

50 Bignon J, Andre-Bougaran J, Brouet G. Parenchymal, bronchiolar, and bronchial measurements in centrilobular emphysema: relation to weight of right ventricle. *Thorax* 1970;**25**:556–67.

51 Thurlbeck WM, Henderson JA, Fraser RG *et al.* Chronic obstructive lung disease: a comparison between clinical, roentgenologic, functional, and morphologic criteria in chronic bronchitis, emphysema, asthma, and bronchiectasis. *Medicine* 1970;**49**:81–145.

CHAPTER 2
The physiology of breathlessness

Donald A. Mahler

Under normal conditions respiration is an unconscious activity regulated by automatic control centres in the brainstem as well as by voluntary output from the cerebral cortex. A variety of abnormalities that affect the respiratory controller, tracheobronchial tree, the alveolar–capillary membrane, and/or the muscles of respiration can contribute to a conscious awareness of breathing experienced as unpleasant or uncomfortable. A respiratory 'sensation' is considered to be the neural activation resulting from the stimulation of a receptor, whereas the 'perception' is the individual's reaction to the sensation [1]. The individual typically describes the experience as 'I am short of breath' or 'I can't get enough air', whereas physicians and investigators commonly identify the patient's complaint by the word dyspnoea.

Various definitions of breathlessness, or dyspnoea (used synonymously in this chapter), have been proposed. These include: 'difficult or laboured breathing' [2], 'an awareness of respiratory distress' [3], 'the sensation of feeling breathless or experiencing air hunger' [4], and 'an uncomfortable sensation of breathing' [5]. However, in 1999 a committee of experts supported by the American Thoracic Society proposed the following definition of dyspnoea [1]: 'A subjective experience of breathing discomfort that consists of qualitatively distinct sensations that vary in intensity'. This experience results from interactions between multiple physiological, psychological, social and environmental factors that may produce behavioural responses.

This chapter is divided into five sections. First, the neurophysiological model for our current understanding of dyspnoea is described. Secondly, I consider the possible mechanisms contributing to this perception in patients with COPD. Thirdly, the various descriptors of breathing discomfort are discussed as they represent a unique language. The different descriptors of breathlessness selected by patients with specific respiratory diseases support our understanding of the mechanisms contributing to dyspnoea. Fourthly,

I review briefly the ability of patients with COPD to perceive breathlessness in response to the addition of respiratory loads or after the acute administration of an inhaled bronchodilator. Finally, I describe how different treatment strategies might provide relief of dyspnoea in patients with COPD.

Neurophysiological model for dyspnoea

Figure 2.1 summarizes the putative pathways of the neurophysiological model for understanding dyspnoea [1,6–8]. The location and presumed stimuli of the receptors that cause dyspnoea are summarized in Table 2.1.

Receptors

There is strong evidence that dyspnoea is directly affected by inputs from chemoreceptors. Peripheral chemoreceptors are located in the carotid bodies and are stimulated predominantly by hypoxia to increase respiration. Furthermore, hypercapnia, as modulated by an increase in H^+ ions, can stimulate central chemoreceptors located in the medulla. However, chemoreceptors are not considered

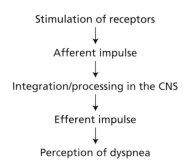

Figure 2.1 A summary of the putative pathways of the neurophysiological model for understanding dyspnoea.

Table 2.1 Location and presumed or major stimuli of receptors that cause dyspnoea. (From American Thoracic Society [1] and Comroe [6] with permission.)

Location	Presumed or major stimulus
Chemoreceptor	
Central medulla	Hypercapnia/acidosis
Carotid body	Hypoxaemia
Mechanoreceptor	
Upper airway and face	Mouthpiece; lack of airflow
Lung	Lung inflation; inhalation of irritants; interstitial congestion; dynamic airway compression
Chest wall	
Joints	Alteration and/or distension
Tendons	Alteration and/or distension
Muscles	Alteration and/or distension

essential for the development of breathlessness. Many patients with COPD, as well as those with other respiratory diseases, experience dyspnoea despite adequate oxygen tensions and eucapnia.

Pulmonary mechanoreceptors respond to mechanical stimuli that are distributed throughout the respiratory system (airway and lung parenchyma). These receptors respond to both chemical (e.g. irritants such as dust or smoke) and mechanical stimuli that can cause broncho-constriction. Pulmonary stretch receptors in the airways respond to lung inflation. C-fibres (unmyelinated nerve endings) located in the alveolar wall and blood vessels are stimulated by interstitial congestion. The corresponding afferent pathways of these mechanoreceptors project to the brain via the vagal nerve. There is evidence that vagal information not only influences the level and pattern of breathing, but may also contribute to the sensation of dyspnoea.

Mechanoreceptors are also located in the joints, tendons and muscles of the chest wall and can play a part in respiratory sensations. Studies involving voluntary constrained breathing, constrained thoracic expansion, as well as chest wall vibration, support the concept that chest wall receptors can cause or contribute to breathlessness.

Central nervous system

The sensory inputs from the various receptors must reach the cerebral cortex in order to be experienced as 'difficult breathing'. Respiratory neurons located in the brainstem project corollary discharges to the sensory cortex; this process contributes to the sense of breathing effort [9]. In addition, there is evidence that conscious awareness of the outgoing respiratory motor command to the ventilatory muscles is important. In fact, current evidence suggests that the pressure generated by the inspiratory muscles, as a ratio of maximal inspiratory pressure capacity, is related to the intensity of the central respiratory motor command [10,11].

Over 40 years ago Campbell and Howell [12,13] proposed 'length–tension inappropriateness' of the respiratory muscles as an explanation for dyspnoea. This theory has subsequently been expanded to include not only information arising from the ventilatory muscles, but also afferent information originating from receptors throughout the respiratory system (see Table 2.1). Our current understanding is that the perception of dyspnoea results from a dissociation or 'mismatch' between the outgoing motor command from the central nervous system and the incoming afferent information from receptors in the airways, lungs and chest wall. The afferent feedback from sensory receptors may allow the brain to assess the effectiveness of the motor commands issued to the ventilatory muscles (i.e. the appropriateness of the response in terms of flow and volume). For any change in respiratory pressures, airflow or movement of the lungs and/or chest wall that is not considered appropriate for the outgoing motor command, the individual may experience breathlessness or an increase in its intensity. This theory has been referred to as both 'efferent–afferent dissociation' [14] and 'neuroventilatory dissociation' [15]. Thus, under certain conditions, the brain 'expects' a certain pattern of breathing or level of ventilation and a corresponding afferent feedback. Any deviation may thus cause or intensify dyspnoea.

Possible mechanisms contributing to dyspnoea in COPD

Several mechanisms may contribute to the experience of breathlessness in those with COPD [16–19] (Table 2.2). Typically, patients with COPD develop dyspnoea when they perform physical activities. The activity may be as minimal as a person taking a few steps on a level surface.

Increased ventilatory demand

Any physical exertion will increase minute ventilation to a significantly greater extent in patients with COPD compared with healthy subjects of comparable age. Although an increased physiological dead space is the major reason for the increased ventilation, hypoxaemia or an early onset of lactic acidosis may also contribute to the increased ventilatory demand. In addition, weakness of the limb muscles requires an increased ventilatory response to exertion; this weakness could result from various causes including deconditioning, systemic effects of COPD or poor nutrition.

Table 2.2 Possible mechanisms contributing to dyspnoea in patients with COPD.

Increased ventilatory demand
    Increased physiological dead space
    Hypoxaemia
    Early onset of lactic acidosis
    Limb muscle weakness resulting from deconditioning,
        systemic effects of COPD and/or poor nutrition
Dynamic airway compression
Dynamic hyperinflation
    Inspiratory threshold loading
    Shortening of the vertical muscle fibres of the diaphragm
        (functional weakness)
Increased airway hyperreactivity
Respiratory muscle weakness

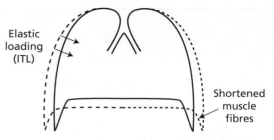

VT occurs on the stiffer portion of *P/V* relationship
↓Effectiveness of SCM and scalene muscles

Figure 2.2 The major consequences of dynamic hyperinflation include an inspiratory threshold load (ITL) resulting from enhanced elastic recoil as well as shortening of the vertical muscle fibres of the diaphragm. P, pressure; SCM, sternocleido-mastoid; V, volume; VT, tidal volume.

Dynamic airway compression

In patients with expiratory airflow obstruction any increase in expiratory effort above the critical transpulmonary pressure can result in dynamic airway compression of airways downstream from the flow limitation. This airway distortion and collapse may stimulate mechanoreceptors in the airway and lead to breathlessness. Evidence to support this proposed mechanism comes from laboratory studies, which applied negative expiratory pressure (NEP) via a mouthpiece in patients with COPD [20]. However, the relative contribution of dynamic airway compression to breathlessness experienced by patients with COPD during daily activities is not clear.

Hyperinflation

Some patients with very severe COPD may be hyperinflated at rest. This finding may be evident by a 'barrel chest' on physical examination as well as a depressed or 'flat' diaphragm on the lateral chest radiograph. Hyperinflation develops as a consequence of the patient's inability to exhale completely because of expiratory flow limitation. One proposed method to examine expiratory flow limitation is the application of NEP [21]. Eltayara *et al.* [22] found that flow limitation as determined by NEP was a better predictor of dyspnoea than standard spirometric measures.

Moreover, various studies have demonstrated that many patients with COPD develop *dynamic hyperinflation* during exertion because of expiratory flow limitation [23,24]. When normal healthy individuals exercise they generally decrease end-expiratory lung volume (EELV); in contrast, EELV frequently increases in patients with COPD during exertion because lung emptying is incomplete because of the expiratory airflow limitation. Although the magnitude of the increase is variable, investigators have reported a

change in the range of 300–600 mL for EELV during exercise in those with COPD [18]. This increase in EELV may be determined non-invasively by having the individual patient perform serial inspiratory capacity (IC) manoeuvres during exercise.

The major consequences of dynamic hyperinflation include an inspiratory threshold load because of increased elastic recoil as well as shortening of the vertical muscle fibres of the diaphragm (Fig. 2.2). The shortened muscle fibres compromise the ability of the diaphragm to generate pressure (i.e. functional weakness). The net effect of dynamic hyperinflation is a constrained tidal volume response despite vigorous inspiratory effort [18].

Airway reactivity

Many patients with COPD report that various 'triggers' cause breathlessness including exposure to cold air, inhalation of dusts and other airborne irritants, respiratory tract infections, in addition to physical exertion. In Lung Health Study I, appproximately 70% of the 5887 smokers, aged 35–60 years, with spirometric evidence of early COPD exhibited a 20% decrease in forced expiratory volume in 1 second (FEV_1) at a dose of 25 mg/mL methacholine [25]. This finding suggests a high percentage of patients with at least early COPD have some degree of airway hyperreactivity.

Respiratory muscle weakness

The muscles of respiration may become weak in patients with COPD [26,27]. The causes are likely multifactorial including deconditioning, poor nutrition and possible systemic manifestations of COPD. There is evidence that inflammation, oxidative stress, etc., which occur in patients with advanced COPD, can affect both skeletal and respiratory muscle function. Certainly, weak respiratory muscles could contribute to a 'mismatch' between the outgoing central motor command and the ventilatory response that would cause breathlessness.

In many patients with COPD a combination of the above factors may act concurrently to contribute to breathing difficulty.

Qualities of dyspnoea

Different pathophysiological processes appear to cause distinct qualitative sensations that reflect the experience of breathing discomfort in healthy individuals as well as in patients with respiratory disease [5,28–31]. For patients with COPD the following descriptors of breathlessness were selected in response to specific questionnaires:
• In the UK, 'distress' associated with breathing was identified [29].
• In the USA, three descriptors: 'My breathing requires effort' (51%); 'I feel out of breath' (49%), and 'I cannot get enough air in' (38%) were indicated [5].
• In Canada, 'increased inspiratory difficulty' and 'unsatisfied inspiratory effort' were chosen [30].

The descriptors selected by patients living in different countries with distinct cultures illustrate a common theme – those with COPD sense breathlessness as part of inspiratory muscle contraction. Further support for this concept is that patients with COPD report that breathing difficulty occurs 'when breathing in' far more frequently than 'when breathing out' [5,30].

These collective findings support the concept that inspiratory 'work/effort' associated with breathing contributes to the breathlessness experienced by patients with COPD. Although expiratory airflow obstruction is the major pathological abnormality in COPD, the consequent resting and/or dynamic hyperinflation result in an 'elastic load' as well as shortening of the vertical muscle fibres of the diaphragm, which clearly contribute to the experience of dyspnoea in COPD.

Perception of breathlessness

One method to examine respiratory perception is to ask subjects to estimate the magnitude of breathlessness while breathing through a system of resistive breathing loads. Mahler et al. [32] reported that patients with COPD showed similar exponents of the psychophysical power function for loads (range, 10–85 cm $H_2O/L/s$) compared with healthy subjects of comparable age. Thus, patients with COPD perceived breathlessness in response to the added loads in a manner similar to control subjects. However, both groups exhibited a large range of magnitude estimation responses.

In another study, Noseda et al. [33] asked patients with COPD to indicate any changes in shortness of breath at rest after inhaling normal saline and then after inhaling the bronchodilator terbutaline. These investigators found that 50% (eight of 16 subjects) reported marked relief in breathlessness and were called 'high perceivers'. In contrast, the other 50% showed little or no perceptual change after inhaled normal saline and terbutaline; they were considered 'low perceivers'.

Van Schayck et al. [34] suggested that poor perception of dyspnoea in patients with obstructive airways disease contributed, in part, to the failure of these patients to report this symptom to their primary care physicians. Such patient behaviour could lead to underdiagnosis of airways disease in the general population.

Possible mechanisms for relief of dyspnoea with specific interventions

At the present time the relief of dyspnoea is directed at the treatment of the underlying pathophysiology of the disease. As the mechanisms causing breathlessness are multifactorial and interdependent, the primary cause(s) of dyspnoea (see Table 2.2) may be different for individual patients with COPD. Furthermore, responses to a specific therapy may vary considerably between patients. The presumed mechanisms whereby different treatments relieve dyspnoea in patients with COPD are listed in Table 2.3.

The information in Table 2.3 is based on current knowledge and understanding of how different treatments work in patients with COPD. Moreover, different mechanisms can clearly be interrelated. For example, improvement in ventilatory capacity may concomitantly reduce hyperinflation and thereby allow the vertical muscle fibres of the diaphragm to lengthen. The enhanced position of the diaphragm promotes an increase in functional strength.

Various clinical trials have demonstrated that bronchodilators can relieve breathlessness by one or more mechanism: increase ventilatory capacity; reduce dynamic airway compression; reduce resting and dynamic hyperinflation; and increase the length of the vertical muscles of the diaphragm [18,23,35,36]. Inhaled corticosteroids provide modest increases in lung function and also decrease airway reactivity [37–39]. Whether the reduction in hyperreactivity with inhaled corticosteroids attenuates dynamic airway compression is unclear.

For decades it has been recognized that oxygen therapy acts on the peripheral chemoreceptor and thereby reduces minute ventilation. However, two recent studies have shown that hyperoxia reduced hyperinflation, as measured by inspiratory capacity manoeuvres, both at rest [40] and during exercise [41]. More importantly, there were

Table 2.3 Putative mechanisms whereby specific treatments provide relief of dyspnoea.

	Ventilatory		↓ Airway compression	↓ Hyperinflation	↓ Airway hyperreactivity	↑ Respiratory muscle function
	↑ Capacity	↓ Requirement				
BD	X		X	X		X*
ICS	X		X†		X	
Exercise training		X				X
IMT						X
Oxygen		X		X		
CPAP/BiPAP			X			X‡
LVRS	X			X		X*

BD, bronchodilators; BiPAP, bilevel positive airway pressure; CPAP, continuous positive airway pressure; ICS, inhaled corticosteroids; IMT, inspiratory muscle training; LVRS, lung volume reduction surgery.
* Increased length of the vertical muscle fibres of the diaphragm by reducing hyperinflation.
† Inhaled corticosteroids have been shown to decrease airway reactivity; whether this affects dynamic airway compression is unclear.
‡ Unloads the respiratory muscles.

concomitant improvements in the severity of dyspnoea with oxygen therapy in both studies, which may, in part, be related to the benefits on hyperinflation.

In addition, it is possible that some of these strategies may alter the processing and perception of breathlessness in the central nervous system. More detailed information about these specific treatments is available in the relevant chapters of this book.

References

1 American Thoracic Society. Dyspnea: mechanisms, assessment, and management. *Am J Respir Crit Care Med* 1999;**159**: 321–40.

2 Schwartzstein RM. Language of dyspnea. In: Mahler DA, O'Donnell DE, eds. *Dyspnea: Mechanisms, Measurement, and Management*, 2nd edn. New York: Taylor & Francis, 2005: 115–45.

3 Wasserman K, Casaburi R. Dyspnoea: physiological and pathophysiological mechanisms. *Annu Rev Med* 1988;**39**: 503–15.

4 Simon PM, Schwartzstein RM, Weiss JW *et al.* Distinguishable sensations of breathlessness in normal volunteers. *Am Rev Respir Dis* 1989;**140**:1021–7.

5 Mahler DA, Harver A, Lentine T *et al.* Descriptors of breathlessness in cardiorespiratory diseases. *Am J Respir Crit Care Med* 1996;**154**:1357–63.

6 Comroe JH. Some theories of the mechanism of dyspnea. In: Howell JB, Campbell EJM, eds. *Breathlessness*. Boston: Blackwell Scientific Publications, 1966: 1–7.

7 Tobin MJ. Dyspnea: pathophysiologic basis, clinical presentation, and management. *Arch Intern Med* 1990;**150**:1604–13.

8 Manning HL, Schwartzstein RM. Pathophysiology of dyspnoea. *N Engl J Med* 1995;**333**:1547–53.

9 Killian KJ, Gandevia SC, Summer E, Campbell EJM. Effect of increased lung volume on perception of breathlessness, effort and tension. *J Appl Physiol* 1984;**57**:686–91.

10 El-Manshawi A, Killian KJ, Summers E, Jones NL. Breathlessness during exercise with and without resistive loading. *J Appl Physiol* 1986;**61**:896–905.

11 O'Donnell DE, Webb KA. Exertional breathlessness in patients with chronic airflow limitation. *Am Rev Respir Dis* 1993;**148**:1351–7.

12 Campbell EJM, Howell JBL. The sensation of breathlessness. *Br Med Bull* 1963;**19**:36–40.

13 Howell JBL, Campbell EJM (eds). *Breathlessness*. Philadelphia: FA Davis, 1966.

14 Banzett RB, Lansing RW, Brown R. 'Air hunger' from increased P_{CO_2} persists after complete neuromuscular block in humans. *Respir Physiol* 1990;**81**:1–17.

15 O'Donnell DE. Exertional breathlessness in chronic respiratory disease. In: Mahler DA, ed. *Dyspnea*. New York: Marcel Dekker, 1998: 97–147.

16 Killian KJ, LeBlanc P, Martin DH *et al.* Exercise capacity and ventilatory, circulatory, and symptom limitation in patients with chronic airflow limitation. *Am Rev Respir Dis* 1992;**146**: 935–40.

17 Mahler DA. Dyspnoea in chronic obstructive pulmonary disease. *Monaldi Arch Chest Dis* 1998;**53**:669–71.

18 O'Donnell DE. Assessment and management of dyspnea in chronic obstructive pulmonary disease. In: Similowski T, Whitelaw WA, Derenne JP, eds. *Clinical Management of Chronic Obstructive Pulmonary Disease*. New York: Marcel Dekker, 2002: 113–70.

19 Killian KJ, Jones NJ. Respiratory muscles and dyspnoea. *Clin Chest Med* 1988;**9**:237–48.

20 O'Donnell DE, Sanii R, Anthonisen NR, Younes M. Effect of dynamic airway compression on breathing pattern and respiratory sensation in severe chronic obstructive pulmonary disease. *Am Rev Respir Dis* 1987;**135**:912–8.

21 Koulouris NG, Valta P, Lavoie A *et al.* A simple method to detect expiratory flow limitation during spontaneous breathing. *Eur Respir J* 1995;**8**:306–13.

22 Eltayara L, Becklake MR, Volta CA, Milic-Emili J. Relationship between chronic dyspnea and expiratory flow limitation in patients with chronic obstructive pulmonary disease. *Am J Respir Crit Care Med* 1996;**154**:1726–34.

23 Belman MJ, Botnick WC, Shin JW. Inhaled bronchodilators reduce dynamic hyperinflation during exercise in patients with chronic obstructive pulmonary disease. *Am J Respir Crit Care Med* 1996;**153**:967–75.

24 O'Donnell DE, Lam M, Webb KA. Measurement of symptoms, lung hyperinflation and endurance during exercise in chronic obstructive pulmonary disease. *Am J Respir Crit Care Med* 1998;**158**:1557–65.

25 Anthonisen NR, Connett JE, Kiley JP *et al.* for the Lung Health Study Research Group. Effects of smoking intervention and the use of an inhaled anticholinergic bronchodilator on the rate of decline of *FEV*$_1$. *JAMA* 1994;**272**:1497–505.

26 Martinez FJ, Montes de Oca M, Whyte RI *et al.* Lung-volume reduction improves dyspnoea, dynamic hyperinflation and respiratory muscle function. *Am J Respir Crit Care Med* 1997;**155**:1984–90.

27 Rochester DF. The diaphragm in COPD: better than expected, but not good enough. *N Engl J Med* 1991;**325**:961–2.

28 Simon PM, Schwartzstein RM, Weiss JW *et al.* Distinguishable types of dyspnoea in patients with shortness of breath. *Am Rev Respir Dis* 1990;**142**:1009–14.

29 Elliott MW, Adams L, Cockcroft A *et al.* The language of breathlessness: use of verbal descriptors by patients with cardiorespiratory disease. *Am Rev Respir Crit Care Med* 1991;**144**:826–32.

30 O'Donnell DE, Bertley JC, Chau LKL, Webb KA. Qualitative aspects of exertional breathlessness in chronic airflow limitation: pathophysiological mechanisms. *Am J Respir Crit Care Med* 1997;**155**:109–15.

31 Harver A, Mahler DA, Schwartzstein RM, Baird JC. Descriptors of breathlessness in healthy individuals: distinct and separable constructs. *Chest* 2000;**118**:679–90.

32 Mahler DA, Rosiello RA, Harver A *et al.* Comparison of clinical dyspnea ratings and psychophysical measurements of respiratory sensation in obstructive airway disease. *Am Rev Respir Dis* 1987;**135**:1229–33.

33 Noseda A, Schmerber J, Prigogine T, Yernault JC. Perceived effect on shortness of breath of an acute inhalation of saline or terbutaline: variability and sensitivity of a visual analogue scale in patients with asthma or COPD. *Eur Respir J* 1992;**5**:1043–53.

34 van Schayck CP, van der Heijden FMMA, van den Boom G, Tirimanna PRS, van Herwaarden CLA. Underdiagnosis of asthma: is the doctor or the patient to blame? The DIMCA project. *Thorax* 2000;**55**:562–5.

35 Ramirez-Venegas A, Ward J, Lentine T, Mahler DA. Salmeterol reduces dyspnea and improves lung function in patients with COPD. *Chest* 1997;**112**:336–40.

36 Casaburi R, Mahler DA, Jones P *et al.* A long-term evaluation of once-daily inhaled tiotropium in chronic obstructive pulmonary disease. *Eur Respir J* 2002;**19**:217–24.

37 Burge PS, Calverly PMA, Jones PW *et al.* Randomized, double blind, placebo controlled study of fluticasone propionate in patients with moderate to severe chronic obstructive pulmonary disease: the ISOLDE trial. *BMJ* 2000;**320**:1297–303.

38 The Lung Health Study Research Group. Effect of inhaled triamcinolone on the decline in pulmonary function in chronic obstructive pulmonary disease. *N Engl J Med* 2000;**343**:1902–9.

39 Mahler DA, Wire P, Horstman D *et al.* Effectiveness of fluticasone propionate and salmeterol combination delivered by the Diskus Device in the treatment of chronic obstructive pulmonary disease. *Am J Respir Crit Care Med* 2002;**166**:1084–91.

40 Valentina A, Mirkovic T, Nesme P, Guerin C, Milic-Emili J. Acute effects of hyperoxia on dyspnoea in hypoxaemia patients with chronic airway obstruction at rest. *Chest* 2003;**123**:1038–46.

41 Somfay A, Porszasz J, Lee SM, Casaburi R. Dose–response effect of oxygen on hyperinflation and exercise endurance in non-hypoxaemic COPD patients. *Eur Respir J* 2001;**18**:77–84.

CHAPTER 3
The physiology of muscle

Ghislaine Gayan-Ramirez and Marc Decramer

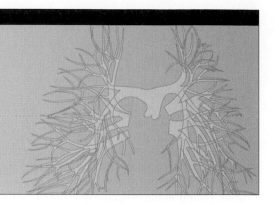

Chronic obstructive pulmonary disease (COPD) is a multi-organ system disease in which dyspnoea, decreased exercise capacity and impairment of quality of life are common. Importantly, the decrease in exercise performance is associated with mortality in these patients. In response to COPD, the respiratory muscles that are working against increased mechanical loads adapt to cope with this chronic load. In addition to respiratory muscle dysfunction, there is accumulating evidence that peripheral muscle dysfunction is also present in COPD patients. Adaptation of peripheral muscles in response to COPD, however, differs from the adaptation of respiratory muscles.

The aim of this chapter is to summarize the knowledge of the physiological adaptations of different respiratory and peripheral muscles in response to COPD.

Muscle dysfunction in COPD patients

Muscle activity and recruitment

Respiratory muscles
In COPD patients, both the respiratory muscle strength and the load to the respiratory muscles are altered. Indeed, the inspiratory muscles have to cope with a higher resistive load (higher airway resistance) and a higher elastic load (resulting from a decrease in the dynamic compliance). In addition, in patients with more severe COPD, the action of the inspiratory muscles is confronted by the charge due to the intrinsic positive end-expiratory pressure (PEEPi) and to the posterior movement of the rib cage at end-expiratory volume when the latter is above the relaxation volume of the rib cage. As a consequence, an imbalance between the respiratory muscle capacity and the load they have to deal with develops. Therefore, in order to maintain adequate ventilation, the central command to the respiratory mus-

cles is increased in COPD patients. Electromyographical studies [1,2] and data on discharge frequency [3] revealed that the motor command to the diaphragm is increased at rest in patients with severe COPD but the contribution of the diaphragm to tidal volume in these patients decreased [4]. Also, the discharge frequency of the parasternal intercostals is elevated in patients with severe COPD compared with controls [5]. Similarly, the discharge frequency of the scalenes and also the number of recruited motor units are enhanced in COPD patients [5]. By contrast, the sternocleidomastoids are not recruited during quiet breathing [6], but only during exercise [7]. Activation of the abdominal muscles is frequent in COPD patients. This activation mainly concerns the transversus abdominis whose recruitment is proportional to the level of airway obstruction [8]. This activation leads to an increase in abdominal pressure at the end of expiration in patients with severe COPD [4], contributing thereby to the PEEPi described in these patients [9].

Peripheral muscles
Very few data are available concerning the activity and recruitment of peripheral muscles in COPD. Actually, modification of the electrical activity of the quadriceps was demonstrated in patients with COPD compared with healthy subjects [10]. M-wave duration was increased from exercise onset but its amplitude was decreased [10]. This indicates that the muscle excitability propagation was impaired in these patients [10]. However, in another study, M-wave amplitude was shown to be unchanged post-exercise [11]. On the other hand, abnormalities in the surface electromyography of the quadriceps appeared very soon after exercise onset in COPD patients compared with healthy individuals [10]. Interestingly, 3 weeks of endurance training normalized the electrical activity abnormalities in the muscles of these patients [12].

Muscle mass

Respiratory muscles

Concerning the mass of the diaphragm, the literature is still controversial. While in one study the mass and the thickness of the diaphragm were reported to be increased in patients with COPD [13], a reduction in the volume and the thickness of the diaphragm was observed in another study [14]. According to Arora and Rochester [15], the diaphragm dimensions of COPD patients are likely to be similar to those of patients without chronic pulmonary diseases.

There are no data available concerning the mass of the respiratory muscles other than the diaphragm in COPD patients.

Peripheral muscles

The prevalence of peripheral muscle wasting in COPD patients is estimated to be 30% and this increases with disease severity. Even if body weight is well preserved, muscle mass may be low [16]. Only indirect evaluations of peripheral muscle mass are available for COPD patients. Fat-free mass is usually used as a marker for muscle mass. Using bioelectrical impedance analysis, fat-free mass has been reported to be decreased in COPD patients [17]. Interestingly, a strong correlation between mean fibre cross-sectional area of the vastus lateralis and fat-free mass was found in COPD patients [18]. Magnetic resonance imaging revealed a lower cross-sectional area of the calf muscles (−13%) in patients with COPD compared with control subjects [19]. More recently, using computed tomography, a decrease in the thigh muscle cross-sectional area (approximately 30%) has been reported in COPD patients compared with healthy age-matched controls [20]. It is important to mention that muscle mass loss in COPD patients is associated with muscle weakness [20,21] and poor exercise tolerance [22]. It is also a predictor of mortality independently of lung function [23].

Muscle fibre type and size

Based on their physiological and metabolic properties, the different fibre types of skeletal muscles are classified as type I (slow oxidative fibre), type IIa (fast oxidative and glycolytic fibre), and type IIx and IIb (fast glycolytic) fibres. The fibre profile of a muscle is a determinant of its metabolic capacity and can be assessed classically with ATPase staining or by separating the different myosin heavy-chain isoforms by electrophoresis or western blotting. Immunohistochemistry determines the presence of hybrid fibres, namely fibres co-expressing different myosin heavy-chain isoforms.

Respiratory muscles

In the diaphragm of COPD patients, the proportion of the slow myosin heavy-chain isoform (MHC-I) is increased at the expense of the fast MHC-IIa and MHC-IIb [24–27] (Fig. 3.1). A positive correlation between the proportion of the diaphragm MHC-I and total lung capacity (TLC) and functional residual capacity (FRC) has been found, while an inverse relationship is present with the forced expiratory volume in 1 second (FEV_1) [25]. More recently, Levine *et al.* [28] showed that the relationship between the proportion of pure type I fibres in the costal diaphragm of COPD patients and FEV_1 was exponential. Thus, when FEV_1 fell

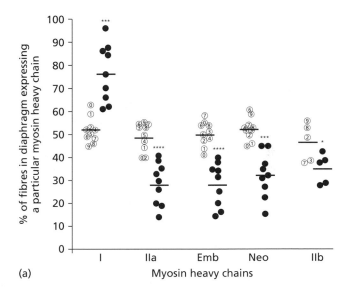

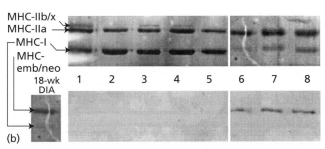

Figure 3.1 (a) Proportion of diaphragm fibre containing slow (I), type IIa, embryonic (Emb), neonatal (neo) and type IIb myosin heavy chain isoforms in control subjects (open circles) and in COPD patients (closed circles). Circles represent individual values. Number in circles indicates specific individuals. * P < 0.05; *** P < 0.001; **** P < 0.0001 vs controls. (b) Representative SDS-PAGE and immunoblotting of diaphragm myosin heavy-chain (MHC) isoforms from controls (lanes 1, 3, 4), COPD (lanes 2 and 5), 18-week-old fetus (lane 6) and 28-week-old fetus (lanes 7 and 8). The immunoblotting is specific for the embryonic MHC isoform. (From Nguyen *et al.* [26] with permission.)

below 60% of the predicted value, an increase in type I fibres developed in the costal diaphragm of COPD patients [28]. Like the diaphragm of healthy subjects, the diaphragm of COPD patients contains neonatal and embryonic MHC [26]. As for the MHCs, the proportion of the slow myosin light-chain (MLC) isoforms is increased in the diaphragm of COPD patients along with a decrease in the fast MLC isoforms [24]. The diaphragmatic fibre diameters are reduced in COPD patients compared with patients with normal lung function, this decreased diameter being correlated with vital capacity (VC) and FEV_1 [29]. An atrophy of type II fibres correlated with the amount of weight loss has also been reported in patients with COPD [30].

For the external and internal intercostal muscles, in contrast to the diaphragm, the proportion of type II fibres and fast MHC isoforms increased in COPD patients, the percentage of type II fibres being inversely related to the level of airway obstruction [31]. Moreover, an atrophy of type II fibres is also present in these muscles [30,32] and was shown to be correlated with weight loss [30].

Only a few data are available for the sternocleidomastoid muscle adaptation in COPD and these data are controversial. In one study, a decrease in the fibre size was described in these muscles [33], while in another no changes in dimension were reported [34]. There are no data available concerning the fibre profile of the other respiratory muscles in COPD patients.

Peripheral muscles

The changes in muscle fibre phenotype depend on disease severity. In patients with moderate COPD, the fibre proportion of the quadriceps does not change [30,35] while significant type II atrophy is observed, this atrophy consistently correlated with weight loss [30]. In advanced COPD, a decrease in type I fibre proportion together with a reciprocal increase in type II fibre proportion were reported in the vastus lateralis [35–41] (Fig. 3.2), while both fibre types atrophied [18,36]. No correlation was found between this shift in fibre proportion and exercise capacity [35,37]. An increased proportion of MHC-IIb as well as of fast MLCs was also observed in the vastus lateralis of COPD patients [35]. Positive correlations were found between VC and FEV_1 and the proportion of slow MHC [35]. A selective type IIx atrophy with a shift from type I to IIx fibre type was recently reported in the vastus lateralis biopsies obtained from weight-stable COPD patients [42]. In addition, the low oxidative capacity of the vastus lateralis was closely related to the proportion of type I fibres [41]. The adaptation of the vastus lateralis in response to COPD is thus clearly different from the adaptation occurring in the diaphragm.

For the biceps, while fibre proportions remained unchanged, the diameter of all fibre types and more particularly of the type II fibres was reduced in severe COPD

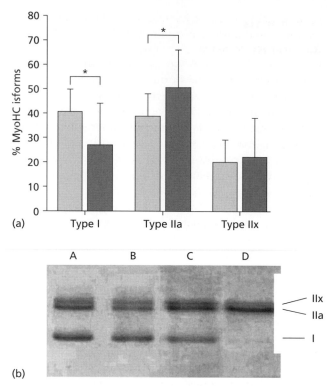

Figure 3.2 (a) Proportion of the myosin heavy-chain (MyoHC) isoforms of the vastus lateralis in normal subjects (light bars) and in COPD patients (dark bars). Values are means and SD. * $P < 0.05$ vs controls. (b) Representative SDS-PAGE of MyoHC isoforms (slow: I, type IIa and type IIx) separation from vastus lateralis of normal subjects (lanes A and B) and COPD patient (lanes C and D). (From Maltais *et al.* [37] with permission.)

compared with control subjects. Decreased diameters were correlated with the amount of weight loss and reduction in FEV_1 (percentage of predicted value; % pred) [43]. Also, a type II atrophy correlated with weight loss was reported in the latissimus dorsi of COPD patients [30].

Recent data revealed that neither the size nor the proportion of the fibres of the deltoid muscle was affected in COPD patients compared with controls [44]. However, there was a trend to increased type I fibres with increased air trapping (as represented by residual volume (RV)/TLC ratio) but this did not reach statistical significance [44].

Muscle capillarity

Respiratory muscles

In COPD patients, the number of capillaries in the diaphragm increases proportionally with disease severity. A relationship is thus present between the number of capillaries in the diaphragm and FEV_1 (% pred) [45]. This probably represents a structural adaptation of the diaphragm in response to the increased chronic load.

The number of capillaries per fibre is higher in the external intercostal muscles of patients with severe COPD and was inversely related to FEV_1 [46].

Peripheral muscles

A reduction of 53% in the number of capillaries per unit cross-sectional area was observed with electron microscopy in the vastus lateralis of patients with COPD compared with age-matched controls [47]. Similar data were reported by others using histological techniques [38]. Moreover, the capillary/mitochondria ratio was decreased in the vastus lateralis of these COPD patients as the number of mitochondria per unit surface was unchanged [47]. Data are controversial concerning the capillary/fibre ratio in the vastus lateralis of COPD patients, as this ratio was reported to be lower in one study [38] but unchanged in another [36]. The number of capillary contacts for both type I and II fibres were significantly lower in patients with COPD but, when normalized for fibre cross-sectional area, the number of capillary contacts for each fibre type was similar in COPD patients and control subjects [36]. Reduced oxygen delivery within muscle in COPD patients may be related to the lower number of capillary contacts, together with a lower myoglobulin level as found in the vastus lateralis of these patients [47].

To the best of our knowledge, there are no data available concerning the number of capillary contacts in the lower limb muscles other than the vastus lateralis and in the upper limb muscles.

Metabolic enzymes

The metabolic properties of a muscle depend on its fibre composition. To evaluate the oxidative or glycolytic potential of a muscle, the content in mitochondria and the concentration of several enzymes are measured. These include the enzymes specific for the oxidative capacity (e.g. citrate synthase, succinate dehydrogenase, 3-hydroxylacyl coenzyme A dehydrogenase) and the enzymes representative of the glycolytic capacity (e.g. lactate dehydrogenase, phosphofructokinase, hexokinase).

Respiratory muscles

It seems that the oxidative capacity of the diaphragm in COPD is better preserved than the glycolytic capacity. Compared with subjects with normal lung function, the activities of hexokinase and lactate dehydrogenase were decreased in the diaphragm of patients with moderate COPD [48]. A twofold increase in succinate dehydrogenase activity in all diaphragm fibre types along with an increase in the succinate dehydrogenase to myosin/ATPase ratio was reported in severe COPD patients compared with patients with mild pulmonary impairment [27]. In severe COPD, the phosphofructokinase activity in the diaphragm is decreased but the citrate synthase activity is unaffected [49]. The activity of the phosphofructokinase was inversely related to static lung volume and to diaphragm type II proportion [49].

The oxidative capacity as well as the hexokinase activity of the internal and external intercostal muscles are increased in COPD patients [50]. In fact, according to Pasto *et al.* [51], the oxidative capacity of the external intercostals is preserved in COPD patients and glycolytic activity increased proportionally to disease severity.

Peripheral muscles

In agreement with the changes in fibre profile, the oxidative capacity of the quadriceps is reduced in patients with COPD compared with controls [52–54]. Citrate synthase and, to a lesser extent, 3-hydroxyacyl coenzyme A dehydrogenase were lower in patients with COPD. In addition, citrate synthase activity was significantly correlated with peak $\dot{V}o_2$, and this independently of lung function [53]. No significant differences were seen in glycolytic enzyme activities in COPD patients except for phosphofructokinase, which increased significantly in one study [52] but remained unchanged in another [53]. Surprisingly, elevated activity of the cytochrome-c oxidase (a key enzyme of the electron transport chain) has been found in the quadriceps of COPD patients compared with healthy controls [55], but it is believed that the activities of all mitochondrial enzymes would respond in a similar way to a given situation.

Few data are available on metabolic enzymes in the upper limb muscles of COPD patients. It seems that the citrate synthase activity of the deltoid is preserved or increased in patients with severe COPD compared with subjects with normal lung function [44]. Interestingly, the activity of lactate dehydrogenase (a glycolytic enzyme) was significantly higher in the deltoid of these patients [44]. An inverse relationship was also found between citrate synthase or lactate dehydrogenase activity and FEV_1 (% pred) as well as with air trapping (represented by RV/TLC) [44].

Structural alterations

Respiratory muscles

Sarcomere length in the diaphragm of patients with COPD is shorter than that of subjects with normal lung function [56]. An inverse relationship was also found between diaphragm sarcomere length and TLC and RV [56]. Although sarcomere disruption was observed in normal diaphragm, the number of disrupted sarcomeres was significantly higher in the diaphragm of COPD patients [57]. An increase in the number of mitochondria was found in the diaphragm of COPD patients, the concentration of mitochondria was inversely related to the severity of airways obstruction, while a direct relationship was found with air trapping [56]. Recently, the degree of airflow obstruction was shown to be inversely related to abnormal diaphragm [58]. Finally, the diaphragm of COPD patients showed more irregular-shaped fibres as well as more smaller fibres compared with non-COPD patients undergoing thoracotomy [59]. Increased content of β-spectrin was also present in the diaphragm of these COPD patients, indicating alterations in the spectrin–cytoskeletal complex [59].

For the other respiratory muscles, the shortening occurring in the muscle fibres when the volume moves from FRC to TLC is minimal for the parasternal intercostals, the scalenes and the sternocleidomastoids [34,60]. Therefore, the fibre length of these muscles is better preserved than in the diaphragm of patients with COPD. The fibre size of the external intercostal muscles correlated with P_{Imax} values [61].

Peripheral muscles

Myopathological examination of the vastus lateralis revealed only the presence of a slight increase in fibrosis and fat cell replacement in COPD patients compared with age-matched controls [42]. In addition, in COPD patients with low body mass index (BMI), apoptosis in the quadriceps has been demonstrated, BMI being inversely related to apoptosis [62].

There were no structural alterations in the deltoid of patients with COPD compared with control individuals [63]. The frequency histograms of the deltoid fibre diameters, however, demonstrated a multimodal distribution with higher standard deviation values, wider range of diameters and a greater proportion of both atrophic and hypertrophic fibres [63].

Muscle strength

Respiratory muscles

At FRC, the maximal inspiratory static pressure as well as oesophagal pressure are reduced in patients with COPD compared with healthy subjects [64]. Along the same lines, the transdiaphragmatic pressure developed during electrical [64] or magnetic [65] stimulation of the phrenic nerves is lower in these patients, while the function of the expiratory muscles seems to be well preserved although the maximal expiratory static pressure is normal [66]. In contrast to healthy subjects, body position has an effect on maximal inspiratory pressure in COPD patients in whom this pressure is higher in the sitting position than the lying position, especially in advanced disease [67]. Furthermore, it was recently shown in diaphragm single fibres that maximal specific force generation of both the MHC-slow and the MHC-IIa isoforms was reduced as was the myofibrillar calcium sensitivity [68].

The decrease in diaphragm force is related to the fact that the length of the diaphragmatic fibres is shorter in COPD [69], such that the diaphragm is contracting on the ascending branch of its length–tension relationship. Animal models have shown that diaphragm adapted to chronic hyperinflation by losing sarcomeres in series such that the diaphragm force–length relationship is preserved and is shifted to shorter length [70]. Whether this phenomenon is present in the diaphragm of patients with COPD has never been demonstrated but, interestingly, at a given lung volume, these patients are able to generate maximal inspiratory pressures that are higher than those developed by healthy subjects [64].

There are no data available concerning the force of other respiratory muscles in COPD patients.

Peripheral muscles

The decreased muscle strength in patients with COPD is now well documented [20,71,72]. Quadriceps force is reduced by 30% in patients with moderate to severe COPD [20,72] and also the strength of the shoulder girdle muscles (pectoralis major: −40%; latissimus dorsi: −48%) [20] (Fig. 3.3) and of the handgrip and elbow flexion muscles [73] has been reported to be reduced. In addition to reduced strength, the cross-sectional area of the thigh, measured by computed tomography scanning, is considerably reduced in COPD patients [20] (Fig. 3.4). The reduction in strength was, however, proportional to the reduction in thigh area [20], suggesting that the loss in muscle force was entirely a result of muscle atrophy. Furthermore, quadriceps strength and muscle cross-sectional area were positively correlated with FEV_1 [20]. Quadriceps force also correlated with exercise capacity and 6-min walking distance [20,72]. Interestingly, because the contractile properties of the

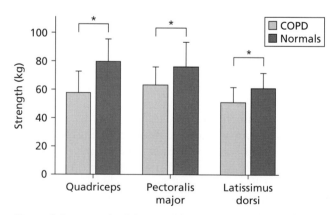

Figure 3.3 Strength of the quadriceps, the pectoralis major and the latissimus dorsi muscles obtained in normal subjects (light bars) and in COPD patients (dark bars). Values are mean and SD. * $P < 0.005$ vs controls. (From Bernard *et al.* [20] with permission.)

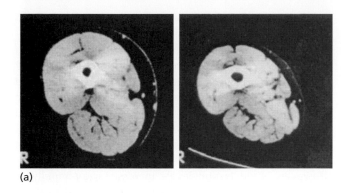

(a)

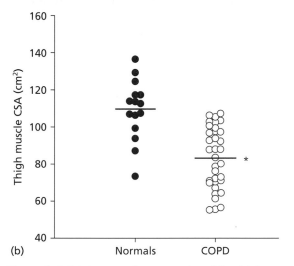

(b)

Figure 3.4 (a) Computed tomography of the thigh cross-sectional area of the vastus lateralis in a representative normal subject (*left*) and a representative patient with COPD (*right*). (b) Individual values of the thigh cross-sectional area (CSA) of the vastus lateralis obtained in normal individuals (closed circles) and in COPD patients (open circles). The horizontal lines represent the mean of each group. * P < 0.0001 vs controls. (From Bernard *et al.* [20] with permission.)

vastus lateralis are preserved in patients with COPD, the reduction in quadriceps strength in these patients is unlikely to be explained by an alteration of the contractile apparatus [40]. Finally, force impairment was more severe for the lower limb muscles than for the upper limb muscles, probably because of a greater reduction in activity of the lower limbs in these patients [20,72].

Muscle endurance

Respiratory muscles

Because the diaphragm of COPD patients is working against increased mechanical loads, it has been suggested that such a loading would result in chronic endurance training of the diaphragm. Thus, information on muscle endurance capacity can be derived from muscle metabolic measurements.

The diaphragm adapts to chronically increased workload induced by obstruction and hyperinflation by shifting from fast to slow fibre type, by increasing oxidative enzymes consistent with an increase in mitochondrial density. The degree of adaptation is correlated with disease severity. Also, increased efficiency of mitochondrial ATP production is present in these patients [74]. Interestingly, the increase in oxidative capacity of the diaphragm (when represented by $\dot{V}_{max}$: maximal respiratory rate of the mitochondrial respiration) in COPD patients [74] was approaching values obtained for the vastus lateralis muscle after 6 weeks of endurance training [75].

Endurance data for the respiratory muscles other than the diaphragm are not yet available.

Peripheral muscles

The data available on peripheral muscle endurance in COPD patients are contradictory. Thus, while 35% [76] and 65% [77] reductions in the endurance of the vastus lateralis in COPD patients were reported by some researchers, no changes were observed in another study [78]. Discrepancies between these studies may be attributed to the fact that endurance measurement is strongly dependent on motivational factors so variability may be high. On the other hand, these discrepant data may simply reflect heterogeneity in skeletal muscle function between COPD patients. Further, it was shown that the quadriceps endurance in patients with COPD was impaired to a greater extent than the quadriceps muscle strength of these patients [79]. More recently, a decrease in quadriceps endurance was reported in COPD patients and was associated with an increase in oxidative stress in the vastus lateralis of these patients. Endurance time was correlated with lipid peroxidation and oxidized protein [80].

Data on upper limb muscles are also not clear. Endurance of the elbow flexor muscle seems to be preserved [81] while that of the adductor pollicis muscle is slightly reduced [78].

Fatigability

Respiratory muscles

An imbalance between load and capacity is present in the respiratory muscles of COPD patients. Fatigue has been induced separately in the diaphragm and the rib cage muscles in volunteers breathing against resistance [82,83]. Further, it has been hypothetized that COPD patients develop respiratory muscle fatigue during exacerbations, leading to ventilatory failure and hypercapnia. However, it was not possible to prove the presence of respiratory muscle fatigue. Actually, it is believed that rapid shallow breathing as chosen by COPD patients would represent a way to avoid respiratory muscle fatigue but at the expense of hypercapnia [84].

Peripheral muscles

A significant reduction in quadriceps twitch force (more than 15%) was found after high-intensity cycle exercise in 58% of COPD patients [11]. This was subsequently confirmed in another study where it was also shown that potentiated quadriceps twitch force was decreased in 81% of these patients after exercise [85], suggesting that potentiated twitch was a more sensitive index of contractile fatigue. Quadriceps fatigue following exercise affected patients with more severe disease (FEV_1 < 40% pred) (seven out of nine) as much as those with milder disease (10 out of 12), although exercise in severe COPD was performed at lower intensities [85]. Of interest, while quadriceps low-frequency fatigue after cycling is frequent in COPD patients, such fatigue is not observed after exhaustive walking, suggesting that symptom limitation in COPD is exercise-specific [86].

In stable COPD patients, mechanical efficiency of the upper limb muscles has been shown to be preserved during submaximal exercise [87]. Differences in muscle fibre composition as well as differences in training status between upper and lower limbs probably contributed to the observation that arm exercise tolerance is less impaired than leg exercise tolerance in COPD patients.

Muscle bioenergetics

Respiratory muscles

An increase in maximal oxidative capacity was reported in the costal diaphragm of COPD patients compared with control subjects [74]. In addition, inverse relationships were found between diaphragm maximal oxidative capacity and FEV_1 (% pred) and RV/TLC [74]. These data suggest that the improvement in oxidation and phosphorylation implies an increased efficiency of ATP production by the mitochondria. A twofold increase in succinate dehydrogenase activity, an indicator of mitochondrial oxidative capacity, of each fibre type was observed in the diaphragm biopsies of patients with severe COPD compared with age-matched controls [27]. In addition, mitochondrial oxidative capacity relative to ATP demand was higher in each of the fibre types in the diaphragm of COPD patients [27]. These data show that patients with severe COPD have an increased capacity to generate ATP through aerobic oxidative pathways [27]. ATP and creatine phosphate content is decreased in the internal and external intercostal muscles of COPD patients, these decreases being related to the level of airway obstruction [32].

Peripheral muscles

^{31}P magnetic resonance spectroscopy is a non-invasive method used to measure muscle metabolism. The ratio of intracellular phosphocreatine/inorganic phosphate is generally measured with this technique as it is related to that of ATP/ADP. This measure seems to be representative of the mitochondrial phosphorylation potential. In patients with COPD, reduced phosphocreatine and ATP contents and a decrease in intracellular pH have been found in skeletal muscles under resting conditions while lactate and inorganic phosphate concentrations are increased [39,88–90]. In addition, during exercise, a greater decline in muscle intracellular pH and phosphocreatine/inorganic phosphate ratio is observed in these patients [19,91–93]. However, blood lactate levels increased very rapidly at low levels of exercise in patients with COPD [19,94,95]. These data show evidence of impaired oxidative phosphorylation and abnormal metabolic regulation in COPD patients.

Potential causes of muscle dysfunction in COPD patients

Alterations in muscle environment

COPD

Muscle metabolism is altered in COPD patients but the mechanisms underlying the muscle abnormalities are still unknown. However, several factors related to COPD such as hypoxia, hypercapnia, inflammation, undernutrition and oxidative stress may contribute to these alterations.

Hypoxia
Chronic hypoxia is well known to exert adverse effects on skeletal muscles. Its role in muscle deconditioning in COPD patients is probably essential as hypoxia reduces exercise performance. Reduction in maximal force and endurance has been reported in the diaphragm, the adductor pollicis and vastus lateralis of hypoxaemic COPD patients [78,96]. A positive correlation was even reported between arterial partial pressure of oxygen and percentage of type I fibres in the vastus lateralis of COPD patients [39]. Even if it remains difficult to be certain about the degree of tissue hypoxia in COPD patients, the fact that capillary/fibre ratio is reduced further impaired oxygen delivery to muscle tissue in these patients.

Hypercapnia
Acute or chronic hypercapnia frequently occurs in COPD patients with acute or chronic respiratory insufficiency. Marked reduction in ATP and phosphocreatine concentrations and intracellular acidosis were observed in the quadriceps of COPD patients with acute respiratory failure [88,89]. A decrease in maximal inspiratory muscle strength was described in COPD patients with chronic hypercapnia compared with normocapnic COPD patients [97].

Inflammation

Pro-inflammatory cytokines such as tumor necrosis factor α (TNF-α) and interleukin 6 (IL-6) can induce muscle wasting in animals [98,99]. An increase in serum levels of TNF-α and its soluble receptors has been reported in malnourished COPD patients [100–102] but also in COPD patients with normal BMI [103]. However, this increase in circulating cytokines seems not to be linked to a decrease in dietary energy intake [104]. Also, increases in IL-6 serum levels [103,105,106], or its soluble receptors [103], were observed in COPD patients where the IL-6/dehydroepiandrosterone (DEHA) ratio, a marker of the catabolic/anabolic balance, was significantly correlated with the mid-thigh muscle cross-sectional area [106]. A relationship was found between the reduced creatinine–height index (used as an index of skeletal muscle mass) and the increased circulating levels of IL-6, TNF-α and their soluble receptors [103], supporting a contributory role for systemic inflammation in muscle wasting in COPD patients. Recently, enhanced serum levels of IL-8 were reported in patients with stable COPD and in those hospitalized for acute exacerbation [107]. In these patients, the force of the quadriceps was inversely related to log IL-8, suggesting a contributory role for systemic inflammation in skeletal muscle weakness [107]. In addition, increased levels of TNF-α in the quadriceps muscle of stable COPD patients were recently reported [108]. The molecular mechanisms by which inflammation may lead to muscle atrophy are still unknown. However, there are several ways by which TNF-α may affect muscle cells. For example, TNF-α is known to activate the nuclear transcription factor NF-κB and to induce the expression of a variety of genes including the inducible form of nitric oxidase synthase (iNOS). This is particularly interesting as activation of NF-κB and upregulation of iNOS expression have been demonstrated in the quadriceps muscles of COPD patients with low BMI [109]. Increased oxidative stress was also shown in the quadriceps muscle of stable COPD patients in whom iNOS and nitrotyrosine protein levels were increased compared with healthy sedentary subjects [108].

Nutritional imbalance

The incidence of undernutrition in COPD patients varies between 25 and 50%, depending on disease severity. Nutritional depletion is associated with a poorer outcome in COPD patients [110,111]. Because increases in daily and resting energy expenditure are frequent in COPD patients, they may contribute to body weight and muscle mass loss especially in severe COPD patients in whom the caloric intake decreased [112,113]. Depletion of high-energy phosphate compound (ATP and phosphocreatine) and cations (magnesium and potassium) in the respiratory muscles is particularly severe in undernourished patients

with respiratory failure resulting from acute or chronic lung disease [114]. The effect of nutritional status on respiratory muscle function in COPD patients is, however, still controversial. Indeed, it remains difficult to determine the additive role of undernutrition in the observed respiratory muscle weakness, especially because nutritional support failed to increase lean body mass in these patients [115], suggesting that other factors are probably involved in muscle wasting and dysfunction in COPD patients. Even when assessing diaphragm contractility with magnetic phrenic nerve stimulation, a test that is independent of patient effort, Hamnegård *et al.* [116] did not find any differences in diaphragm strength of severe COPD patients, either undernourished or normally nourished.

Oxidative stress

The term oxidative stress refers to alterations caused by the reactive oxygen species. Under physiological conditions, the generation of reactive oxygen species is removed by the cellular antioxidant systems which include antioxidant vitamins, protein and non-protein thiols, and antioxidant enzymes. Excessive production of reactive oxygen species may lead to an imbalance between oxidant–antioxidant such that extensive cell and tissue damage may occur.

Actually, there are only a few studies reporting the level of oxidative stress in the diaphragm of COPD patients. Thus, compared with control subjects, severe COPD patients showed an increase in protein oxidation in their diaphragm [117]. This increased expression was, moreover, inversely related to disease severity. Immunohistochemistry revealed an increased level of 4-hydroxy-2-nonenal, a marker of lipid peroxidation in the diaphragm of COPD patients [59].

Total glutathione has been shown to be reduced in leg muscles of COPD patients compared with control subjects [118]. An increase in lipid peroxidation and Mn-superoxide dismutase (an enzyme involved in dismutation of superoxide anions) have been found in the quadriceps of COPD patients when compared with controls [119]. Protein oxidation and catalase were similar in the two groups as were the expressions of neuronal NOS and endothelial NOS isoforms. Interestingly, 3-nitrotyrosine levels were also significantly elevated in the quadriceps of the patients with COPD and these levels were positively correlated with the degree of airflow obstruction [119].

Comorbid conditions

Electrolyte disturbances

Although electrolyte disturbances may affect muscle function, few studies have examined these effects in COPD patients. In case electrolyte disturbances are severe, cell destruction, myopathy and rhabdomyolysis may occur especially with hypokalaemia and hypophosphataemia.

Hypokalaemia is frequently caused by diuretic therapy.

Potassium deficiency alters membrane electrical properties of the muscle cells towards hyperpolarization [120]. In addition, hypokalaemia is associated with glycogen depletion which in turn affects muscle contraction under anaerobic conditions [120]. This latter observation is particularly important for COPD patients in whom the oxidative capacity is already reduced.

Hypophosphataemia in COPD patients may be frequent and is caused by malnourishment or by renal reabsorption failure brought about by some medication (theophylline, diuretic, corticosteroids, β-agonist) [121]. Hypophosphataemia is associated with a reduction in diaphragmatic function [122,123] and serum levels of phosphate are related to transdiaphragmatic pressure [122]. Further administration of phosphate to COPD patients with hypophosphatemia improves diaphragmatic function [122,123].

Deconditioning

COPD patients are subjected to various degrees of deconditioning, ranging from reduced activity to prolonged bed rest. Deconditioning is the adaptive response of muscle to disuse. Signs of deconditioning are present in the peripheral muscles of COPD patients. These include reduced oxidative enzyme capacity, atrophy of type I fibres and reduction in type I fibre proportion. It is important to mention that physical activity in daily life is an important predictor of risk of readmission to hospital and mortality in patients with COPD [124,125]. Patients' estimation of time spent in physical activities in daily life is, in fact, not accurate when compared with objective assessment [126]. Compared with matched healthy subjects, stable COPD patients are effectively less active, walking less and lying down more than controls [127]. Inactivity is worsened during hospitalization resulting from acute exacerbation and, although recovery occurs, the levels of inactivity in these patients is still significantly reduced 1 month after discharge compared with stable COPD patients [128].

Cardiac failure

There are no data available on the effects of cor pulmonale on muscle function in COPD patients. In patients with congestive heart failure, inspiratory muscle weakness is present and is more pronounced than that observed in peripheral muscles [129–132]. In the diaphragm, the proportion of type I fibres decreased and there is also a disproportionate atrophy of type I and II fibres while the activity and the protein levels of the sarcoplasmatic endoplasmatic reticulum calcium ATPase (SERCA) pump diminished [24,133,134]. A downward displacement of the diaphragm occurs at the end of expiration in patients with chronic heart failure which was strongly correlated with the changes of left ventricular morphology [135].

For peripheral muscles, strength was found to be decreased or unchanged [136–138]. Structural changes and fibre shift towards type II [139] as well as type IIb and/or type IIa atrophy were reported [140,141]. This was associated with a reduction in oxidative enzyme capacity but glycolytic enzyme function was preserved [140,141].

Ageing

It is well known that muscle force and muscle mass decrease with age because of a reduction in fibre cross-sectional area, mainly of the type II fibres [142]. Although COPD affects elderly individuals, peripheral muscle dysfunction in these patients is unlikely to be accounted for by the ageing process alone, because the muscle abnormalities seen in these patients are clearly more pronounced than those in age-matched individuals.

Anabolic hormones

Growth hormone, insulin-like growth factor I (IGF-I) and androgenic steroids are stimulators of muscle growth and development. In healthy elderly individuals, the circulating levels of IGF-I are decreased [143,144]. In COPD patients, the serum levels of IGF-I tended to be lower than aged-matched individuals [107,145,146]. A positive correlation was also found between circulating IGF-I and quadriceps peak force in COPD patients [107].

Testosterone has been shown to exert its anabolic properties by increasing the fractional synthesis rates of actin and MHC and by stimulating protein synthesis, resulting in muscle hypertrophy [147,148]. In men testosterone levels decline with age and in women testosterone levels start to decrease with the menopause. In addition, sex hormone binding globulin, to which testosterone is bound, increases with age and postmenopausally in females such that free testosterone is substantially reduced in these individuals [149,150]. In acutely ill, hospitalized COPD patients, levels of testosterone are low and are correlated with the severity of arterial hypoxaemia and hypercapnia [151]. In men with COPD, levels of testosterone are considerably lower than those of aged-matched subjects [152].

References

1 Druz WS, Sharp JT. Electrical and mechanical activity of the diaphragm accompanying body position in severe chronic obstructive pulmonary disease. *Am Rev Respir Dis* 1982;**125**: 275–80.

2 Gorini M, Spinelli A, Ginanni R *et al.* Neural respiratory drive and neuromuscular coupling in patients with chronic obstructive pulmonary disease (COPD). *Chest* 1990;**98**: 1179–86.

3 De Troyer A, Leeper JB, McKenzie DK, Gandevia SC. Neural drive to the diaphragm in patients with severe chronic obstructive pulmonary disease. *Am J Respir Crit Care Med* 1997;**155**:1335–40.

4 Martinez FJ, Couser JI, Celli BR. Factors influencing venti-latory muscle recruitment in patients with chronic airflow obstruction. *Am Rev Respir Dis* 1990;**142**:276–82.

5 Gandevia SC, Leeper JB, McKenzie DK, De Troyer A. Discharge frequencies of parasternal intercostal and scalene motor units during breathing in normal and COPD subjects. *Am J Respir Crit Care Med* 1996;**153**:622–8.

6 De Troyer A, Peche R, Yernault JC, Estenne M. Neck muscle activity in patients with severe chronic obstructive pulmonary disease. *Am J Respir Crit Care Med* 1994;**150**:41–7.

7 Wilson SH, Cooke NT, Moxham J, Spiro SG. Sternomastoid muscle function and fatigue in normal subjects and in patients with chronic obstructive pulmonary disease. *Am Rev Respir Dis* 1984;**129**:460–4.

8 Ninane V, Rypens F, Yernault JC, De Troyer A. Abdominal muscle use during breathing in patients with chronic airflow obstruction. *Am Rev Respir Dis* 1992;**146**:16–21.

9 Ninane V, Yernault JC, De Troyer A. Intrinsic PEEP in patients with chronic obstructive pulmonary disease: role of expiratory muscles. *Am Rev Respir Dis* 1993;**148**:1037–42.

10 Gosselin N, Matecki S, Poulain M *et al.* Electrophysiologic changes during exercise testing in patients with chronic obstructive pulmonary disease. *Muscle Nerve* 2003;**27**:170–9.

11 Jeffery MM, Kufel TJ, Pineda L. Quadriceps fatigue after cycle exercise in patients with chronic obstructive pulmonary disease. *Am J Respir Crit Care Med* 2000;**161**(2 Part 1):447–53.

12 Gosselin N, Lambert K, Poulain M *et al.* Endurance training improves skeletal muscle electrical activity in active COPD patients. *Muscle Nerve* 2003;**28**:744–53.

13 Scott KWM, Hoy J. The cross-sectional area of diaphragmatic muscle fibre in emphysema, measured by an automated image analysis system. *J Pathol* 1976;**120**:121–8.

14 Steele RH, Heard BE. Size of the diaphragm in chronic bronchitis. *Thorax* 1973;**28**:55–60.

15 Arora NS, Rochester DF. COPD and human diaphragm muscle dimensions. *Chest* 1987;**91**:719–24.

16 Schols AMWJ, Soeters PB, Dingemans AM *et al.* Prevalence and characteristics of nutritional depletion in patients with stable COPD eligible for pulmonary rehabilitation. *Am Rev Respir Dis* 1993;**147**:1151–6.

17 Schols AMWJ, Wouters EFM, Soeters PB, Westerterp KR. Body composition by bioelectrical impedance analysis compared to deuterium dilution and skinfold anthropometry in patients with chronic obstructive pulmonary disease. *Am J Clin Nutr* 1991;**53**:421–4.

18 Gosker HR, Engelen MP, van Mameren H *et al.* Muscle fibre type IIX atrophy is involved in the loss of fat-free mass in chronic obstructive pulmonary disease. *Am J Clin Nutr* 2002;**76**:113–9.

19 Wuyam B, Payen JF, Levy P *et al.* Metabolism and aerobic capacity of skeletal muscle in chronic respiratory failure related to chronic obstructive pulmonary disease. *Eur Respir J* 1992;**5**:157–62.

20 Bernard S, Leblanc P, Whittom F *et al.* Peripheral muscle weakness in patients with chronic obstructive pulmonary disease. *Am J Respir Crit Care Med* 1998;**158**:629–34.

21 Engelen MP, Schols AM, Baken WC, Wesseling GJ, Wouters EF. Nutritional depletion in relation to respiratory and peripheral skeletal muscle function in out-patients with COPD. *Eur Respir J* 1994;**7**:1793–7.

22 Schols AM, Mostert R, Soeters PB, Wouters EF. Body composition and exercise performance in patients with chronic obstructive pulmonary disease. *Thorax* 1991;**46**:695–9.

23 Wilson DO, Rogers RM, Wright EC, Anthonisen NR. Body weight in chronic obstructive pulmonary disease. The National Institutes of Health Intermittent Positive-Pressure Breathing Trial. *Am Rev Respir Dis* 1989;**139**:1435–8.

24 Levine S, Kaiser L, Leferovich J, Tikunov B. Cellular adaptations in the diaphragm in chronic obstructive pulmonary disease. *N Engl J Med* 1997;**337**:1799–806.

25 Mercadier JJ, Schwartz K, Schiaffino S *et al.* Myosin heavy chain gene expression changes in the diaphragm of patients with chronic lung hyperinflation. *Am J Physiol* 1998;**274**:L527–34.

26 Nguyen T, Shrager J, Kaiser L *et al.* Developmental myosin heavy chains in the adult human diaphragm: coexpression patterns and effect of COPD. *J Appl Physiol* 2000;**88**:1446–56.

27 Levine S, Gregory C, Nguyen T *et al.* Bioenergetic adaptation of individual human diaphragmatic fibres to severe COPD. *J Appl Physiol* 2002;**92**:1205–13.

28 Levine S, Nguyen T, Kaiser LR *et al.* Human diaphragm remodeling associated with chronic obstructive pulmonary disease: clinical implications. *Am J Respir Crit Care Med* 2003;**168**:706–13.

29 Tikunov BA, Kaiser L, Nguyen T, Levine S. Myosin light chain and regulatory protein composition of lateral costal diaphragm in normal subjects and in patients with chronic obstructive pulmonary disease. *Am J Respir Crit Care Med* 1997;**155**:A510.

30 Hughes RL, Katz H, Sahgal V *et al.* Fibre size and energy metabolites in five separate muscles from patients with chronic obstructive lung disease. *Respiration* 1983;**44**:321–8.

31 Gea J, Orozco-Levi M, Aguar C *et al.* Adaptive changes concerning the type of fibres and isoforms of myosin in the external intercostal muscle of COPD patients. *Eur Respir J* 1996;**9**:160S.

32 Campbell JA, Hughes RL, Sahgal V, Frederiksen J, Schields TW. Alterations in intercostal muscle morphology and biochemistry in patients with obstructive lung disease. *Am Rev Respir Dis* 1980;**122**:679–86.

33 Arora NS, Rochester DF. Effect of chronic pulmonary disease on sternocleid mastoid muscle. *Am Rev Respir Dis* 1982;**125**:252.

34 Peche R, Estenne M, Genevois PA *et al.* Sternomastoid muscle size and strength in patients with severe chronic obstructive pulmonary disease. *Am J Respir Crit Care Med* 1996;**153**:422–5.

35 Satta A, Migliori GB, Spanevello A *et al.* Fibre types in skeletal muscles of chronic obstructive pulmonary disease patients related to respiratory function and exercise tolerance. *Eur Respir J* 1997;**10**:2853–60.

36 Whittom F, Jobin J, Simard P-M *et al.* Histochemical and morphological characteristics of the vastus lateralis muscle in COPD patients. *Med Sci Sports Exerc* 1998;**30**:1467–74.

37 Maltais F, Sullivan MJ, Leblanc P *et al.* Altered expression of myosin heavy chain in the vastus lateralis muscle in patients with COPD. *Eur Respir J* 1999;**13**:850–4.

38 Jobin J, Maltais F, Doyon JF *et al.* Chronic obstructive pulmonary disease: capillarity and fibre-type characteristics of skeletal muscle. *J Cardiolpulm Rehabil* 1998;**18**:432–7.

39 Jakobsson P, Jorfeldt L, Brundin A. Skeletal muscle metabolites and fibre types in patients with advanced chronic obstructive pulmonary disease (COPD), with and without chronic respiratory failure. *Eur Respir J* 1990;**3**:192–6.

40 Debigare R, Cote CH, Hould FS, Leblanc P, Maltais F. *In vitro* and *in vivo* contractile properties of the vastus lateralis muscle in males with COPD. *Eur Respir J* 2003;**21**:273–8.

41 Gosker HR, van Mameren H, van Dijk PJ *et al.* Skeletal muscle fibre-type shifting and metabolic profile in patients with chronic obstructive pulmonary disease. *Eur Respir J* 2002;**19**:617–25.

42 Gosker HR, Kubat B, Schaart G *et al.* Myopathological features in skeletal muscle of patients with chronic obstructive pulmonary disease. *Eur Respir J* 2003;**22**:280–5.

43 Sato Y, Asoh T, Honda Y *et al.* Morphologic and histochemical evaluation of muscle in patients with chronic obstructive pulmonary disease related to respiratory function and exercise tolerance. *Eur Neurol* 1997;**37**:116–21.

44 Gea JG, Pasto M, Carmona MA *et al.* Metabolic characteristics of the deltoid muscle in patients with chronic obstructive pulmonary disease. *Eur Respir J* 2001;**17**:939–45.

45 Orozco-Levi M, Gea J, Aguar C *et al.* Changes in the capillary content in the diaphragm of COPD patients: a sort of muscle remodelling? *Am J Respir Crit Care Med* 1996;**153**:A298.

46 Jimenez-Fuentes MA, Gea J, Aguar C *et al.* Densidad capilar y función respiratoria en el músculo intercostal externo. *Arch Bronchoneumol* 1999;**35**:471–6.

47 Simard C, Maltais F, Leblanc P, Simard P-M, Jobin J. Mitochondrial and capillarity changes in vastus lateralis muscle of COPD patients: electron microscopy study. *Med Sci Sports Exerc* 1996;**28**:S95.

48 Sanchez J, Bastien C, Medrano G, Riquet M, Derenne JP. Metabolic enzymatic activities in the diaphragm of normal men and patients with moderate chronic obstructive pulmonary disease. *Bull Eur Physiopathol Respir* 1984;**20**:535–40.

49 Gea J, Felez M, Carmona MA *et al.* Oxidative capacity is preserved but glycolytic activity is reduced in the diaphragm of severe COPD. *Am J Respir Crit Care Med* 1999;**159**:A579.

50 Sanchez J, Brunet A, Medrano G, Debesse B, Derenne JP. Metabolic enzymatic activities in the intercostal and serratus muscles and in the latissimus dorsi of middle-aged normal men and patients with moderate obstructive pulmonary disease. *Eur Respir J* 1988;**1**:376–83.

51 Pasto M, Gea J, Blanco M *et al.* Metabolic activity of the external intercostal muscle of patients with COPD. *Arch Bronconeumol* 2001;**37**:108–14.

52 Jakobsson P, Jorfeldt L, Henriksson J. Metabolic enzyme activity in the quadriceps femoris muscle in patients with severe chronic obstructive pulmonary disease. *Am J Respir Crit Care Med* 1995;**151**:374–7.

53 Maltais F, Simard AA, Simard C *et al.* Oxidative capacity of the skeletal muscle and lactic acid kinetics during exercise in normal subjects and in patients with COPD. *Am J Respir Crit Care Med* 1996;**153**:288–93.

54 Maltais F, Leblanc P, Whittom F *et al.* Oxidative enzyme activities of the vastus lateralis muscle and the functional status in patients with COPD. *Thorax* 2000;**55**:848–53.

55 Sauleda J, Garcia-Palmer F, Wiesner RJ *et al.* Cytochrome oxidase activity and mitochondrial gene expression in skeletal muscle of patients with chronic obstructive pulmonary disease. *Am J Respir Crit Care Med* 1998;**157**(5 Part 1):1413–7.

56 Orozco-Levi M, Gea J, Lloretay JL *et al.* Subcellular adaptation of the human diaphragm in chronic obstructive pulmonary disease. *Eur Respir J* 1999;**13**:371–8.

57 Orozco-Levi M, Gea J, Aguar C *et al.* Sarcomere disruption in the diaphragm of COPD patients: a sign of muscle injury? *Am J Respir Crit Care Med* 2001;**155**:A510.

58 Macgowan NA, Evans KG, Road JD, Reid WD. Diaphragm injury in individuals with airflow obstruction. *Am J Respir Crit Care Med* 2001;**163**:1654–9.

59 Wijnhoven JH, Jansen AJM, van Kuppevelt TH, Rodenburg RJT, Dekhuijzen PNR. Metabol capacity of the diaphragm in patients with COPD. *Respir Med* 2005 (in press).

60 De Troyer A, Legrand A, Genevois PA, Wilson TA. Mechanical advantage of the human parasternal intercostal and triangularis sterni muscles. *J Physiol (Lond)* 1998;**513**:915–25.

61 Sauleda J, Gea J, Orozco-Levi M *et al.* Structure and function relationships of the respiratory muscles. *Eur Respir J* 1998;**11**:906–11.

62 Agusti AG, Sauleda J, Miralles C *et al.* Skeletal muscle apoptosis and weight loss in chronic obstructive pulmonary disease. *Am J Respir Crit Care Med* 2002;**166**:485–9.

63 Hernandez N, Orozco-Levi M, Belalcazar V *et al.* Dual morphometrical changes of the deltoid muscle in patients with COPD. *Respir Physiol Neurobiol* 2003;**134**:219–29.

64 Similowski T, Yan S, Gauthier AP, Macklem PT, Bellemare F. Contractile properties of the human diaphragm during chronic hyperinflation. *N Engl J Med* 1991;**325**:917–23.

65 Polkey MI, Kyroussis D, Hamnegard C-H *et al.* Diaphragm strength in chronic obstructive pulmonary disease. *Am J Respir Crit Care Med* 1996;**154**:1310–7.

66 Morrison NJ, Richardson J, Dunn L, Pardy RL. Respiratory muscle performance in normal elderly subjects and patients with COPD. *Chest* 1989;**95**:90–4.

67 O'Neill S, McCarthy DS. Postural relief of dyspnoea in severe chronic airflow limitation: relationship to respiratory muscle strength. *Thorax* 1983;**38**:595–600.

68 Ottenheijm CAC, Heunks LM, Sieck GC *et al.* Diaphragm dysfunction in chronic obstructive pulmonary disease. *Am J Respir Crit Care Med* 2005;**172**:200–5.

69 Cassart M, Pettiaux N, Genevois PA, Paiva M, Estenne M. Effect of chronic hyperinflation on diaphragm length and surface area. *Am J Respir Crit Care Med* 1997;**156**:504–8.

70 Farkas GA, Roussos C. Diaphragm in emphysematous hamsters: sarcomere adaptability. *J Appl Physiol* 1983;**54**:1635–40.

71 Hamilton AL, Killian KJ, Summers E, Jones NL. Muscle strength, symptom intensity, and exercise capacity in patients with cardiorespiratory disorders. *Am J Respir Crit Care Med* 1995;**152**(6 Part 1):2021–31.

72 Gosselink R, Troosters T, Decramer M. Peripheral muscle weakness contributes to exercise limitation in COPD. *Am J Respir Crit Care Med* 1996;**153**:976–80.

73 Gosselink R, Troosters T, Decramer M. Distribution of muscle weakness in patients with stable chronic obstructive pulmonary disease. *J Cardiolpulm Rehabil* 2000;**20**:353–60.

74 Ribera F, N'Guessan B, Zoll J *et al*. Mitochondrial electron transport chain function is enhanced in inspiratory muscles of patients with chronic obstructive pulmonary disease. *Am J Respir Crit Care Med* 2003;**167**:873–9.

75 Walsh B, Tonkonogi M, Sahlin K. Effect of endurance training on oxidative and antioxidative function in human permeabilized muscle fibres. *Pflugers Arch* 2001;**442**:420–5.

76 Serres I, Gautier V, Varray AL, Préfaut CG. Impaired skeletal muscle endurance related to physical inactivity and altered lung function in COPD patients. *Chest* 1998;**113**:900–5.

77 Couillard A, Koechlin C, Cristol JP, Varray A, Prefaut C. Evidence of local exercise-induced systemic oxidative stress in chronic obstructive pulmonary disease patients. *Eur Respir J* 2002;**20**:1123–9.

78 Zattara-Hartmann MC, Badier M, Guillot C, Tomei C, Jammes Y. Maximal force and endurance to fatigue of respiratory and skeletal muscles in chronic hypoxemic patients: the effects of oxygen breathing. *Muscle Nerve* 1995;**18**:495–502.

79 Van't Hul A, Harlaar J, Gosselink R *et al*. Quadriceps muscle endurance in patients with chronic obstructive pulmonary disease. *Muscle Nerve* 2004;**29**:267–74.

80 Couillard A, Maltais F, Saey D *et al*. Exercise-induced quadriceps oxidative stress and peripheral muscle dysfunction in patients with chronic obstructive pulmonary disease. *Am J Respir Crit Care Med* 2003;**167**:1664–9.

81 Newell SZ, McKenzie DK, Gandevia SC. Inspiratory and skeletal muscle strength and endurance and diaphragmatic activation in patients with chronic airflow limitation. *Thorax* 1989;**44**:903–12.

82 Fitting JW, Bradley TD, Easton PA *et al*. Dissociation between diaphragmatic and rib cage muscle fatigue. *J Appl Physiol* 1988;**64**:959–65.

83 Zocchi L, Fitting JW, Majani U *et al*. Effect of pressure and timing of contraction on human rib cage muscle fatigue. *Am Rev Respir Dis* 1993;**147**:857–64.

84 Begin P, Grassino A. Chronic alveolar hypoventilation helps to maintain the inspiratory muscle effort of COPD patients within sustainable limits. *Chest* 2000;**117**(5 Suppl 1):271–3S.

85 Mador MJ, Kufel TJ, Pineda LA *et al*. Effect of pulmonary rehabilitation on quadriceps fatiguability during exercise. *Am J Respir Crit Care Med* 2001;**163**:930–5.

86 Man WD, Soliman MG, Gearing J *et al*. Symptoms and quadriceps fatigability after walking and cycling in chronic obstructive pulmonary disease. *Am J Respir Crit Care Med* 2003;**168**:562–7.

87 Franssen FM, Wouters EF, Baarends EM, Akkermans MA, Schols AM. Arm mechanical efficiency and arm exercise capacity are relatively preserved in chronic obstructive pulmonary disease. *Med Sci Sports Exerc* 2002;**34**:1570–6.

88 Fiaccadori E, Del Canale S, Vitali P *et al*. Skeletal muscle energetics, acid–base equilibrium and lactate metabolism in patients with severe hypercapnia and hypoxemia. *Chest* 1987;**92**:883–7.

89 Gertz I, Hedenstierna G, Hellers G, Wahren J. Muscle metabolism in patients with chronic obstructive lung disease and acute respiratory failure. *Clin Sci Mol Med* 1977;**52**:396–403.

90 Pouw EM, Schols AM, van der Vusse GJ, Wouters EF. Elevated inosine monophosphate levels in resting muscle of patients with stable chronic obstructive pulmonary disease. *Am J Respir Crit Care Med* 1998;**157**:453–7.

91 Kutsuzawa T, Shioya S, Kurita D *et al*. ^{31}P-NMR study of skeletal muscle metabolism in patients with chronic respiratory impairment. *Am Rev Respir Dis* 1992;**146**:1019–24.

92 Payen JF, Wuyam B, Levy P *et al*. Muscular metabolism during oxygen supplementation in patients with chronic hypoxemia. *Am Rev Respir Dis* 1993;**147**:592–8.

93 Tada H, Kato H, Misawa T *et al*. ^{31}P-nuclear magnetic resonance evidence of abnormal skeletal muscle metabolism in patients with chronic lung disease and congestive heart failure. *Eur Respir J* 1992;**5**:163–9.

94 Casaburi R, Patessio A, Ioli F *et al*. Reductions in exercise lactic acidosis and ventilation as a result of exercise training in patients with obstructive lung disease. *Am Rev Respir Dis* 1991;**143**:9–18.

95 Maltais F, Jobin J, Sullivan MJ *et al*. Metabolic and hemodynamic responses of lower limb during exercise in patients with COPD. *J Appl Physiol* 1998;**84**:1573–80.

96 Incalzi RA, Fuso L, Ricci T *et al*. Acute oxygen supplementation does not relieve the impairment of respiratory muscle strength hypoxemic COPD. *Chest* 1998;**113**:334–9.

97 Scano G, Spinelli A, Duranti R *et al*. Carbon dioxide responsiveness in COPD patients with and without chronic hypercapnia. *Eur Respir J* 1995;**8**:78–85.

98 Buck M, Chojkier M. Muscle wasting and dedifferentiation induced by oxidative stress in a murine model of cachexia is prevented by inhibitors of nitric oxide synthesis and antioxidants. *EMBO J* 1996;**15**:1753–65.

99 Janssen SP, Gayan-Ramirez G, Van den Bergh A *et al*. Interleukin-6 causes myocardial failure and skeletal muscle atrophy in rats. *Circulation* 2005;**111**:996–1005.

100 Di Francia M, Barbier D, Mege JL, Orehek J. Tumor necrosis factor alpha levels and weight loss in chronic obstructive pulmonary disease. *Am J Respir Crit Care Med* 1994;**150**:1453–5.

101 Schols AMWJ, Buurman WA, Staal-van den Brekel AJ, Dentener MA, Wouters EFM. Evidence for a relation between metabolic derangements and increased levels of inflammatory mediators in a subgroup of patients with chronic obstructive pulmonary disease. *Thorax* 1996;**51**:819–24.

102 Creutzberg EC, Schols AM, Weling-Scheepers CA, Buurman WA, Wouters EF. Characterization of non-response to high

caloric oral nutritional therapy in depleted patients with chronic obstructive pulmonary disease. *Am J Respir Crit Care Med* 2000;**161**(3 Part 1):745–52.

103 Eid AA, Ionescu AA, Nixon LS *et al*. Inflammatory response and body composition in chronic obstructive pulmonary disease. *Am J Respir Crit Care Med* 2001;**164**(8 Part 1):1414–8.

104 Godoy I, Campana AO, Geraldo RR, Padovani CR, Paiva SA. Cytokines and dietary energy restriction in stable chronic obstructive pulmonary disease patients. *Eur Respir J* 2003;**22**:920–5.

105 Malo O, Sauleda J, Busquets X *et al*. Systemic inflammation during exacerbations of chronic obstructive pulmonary disease. *Arch Bronconeumol* 2002;**38**:172–6.

106 Debigare R, Marquis K, Cote CH *et al*. Catabolic–anabolic balance and muscle wasting in patients with COPD. *Chest* 2003;**124**:83–9.

107 Spruit MA, Gosselink R, Troosters T *et al*. Muscle force during an acute exacerbation in hospitalized patients with COPD and its relationship with CXCL8 and IGF-I. *Thorax* 2003;**58**:752–6.

108 Torres SH, MontesdeOca M, De Sanctis JB *et al*. Oxidative stress, nitric oxide and nytrotyrosine production in the skeletal muscle of COPD patients. *Am J Respir Crit Care Med* 2004;**169**:A902.

109 Agusti A, Morla M, Sauleda J, Saus C, Busquets X. NF-κB activation and iNOS upregulation in skeletal muscle of patients with COPD and low body weight. *Thorax* 2004;**59**: 483–7.

110 Gray-Donald K, Gibbons L, Shapiro SH, Macklem PT, Martin JG. Nutritional status and mortality in chronic obstructive pulmonary disease. *Am J Respir Crit Care Med* 1996;**153**:961–6.

111 Shoup R, Dalsky G, Warner S *et al*. Body composition and health-related quality of life in patients with obstructive airways disease. *Eur Respir J* 1997;**10**:1576–80.

112 Baarends EM, Schols AM, Pannemans DL, Westerterp KR, Wouters EF. Total free living energy expenditure in patients with severe chronic obstructive pulmonary disease. *Am J Respir Crit Care Med* 1997;**155**:549–54.

113 Schols AM, Soeters PB, Mostert R, Saris WH, Wouters EF. Energy balance in chronic obstructive pulmonary disease. *Am Rev Respir Dis* 1991;**143**:1248–52.

114 Fiaccadori E, Zambrelli P, Tortorell G. Physiopathology of respiratory muscles in malnutrition. *Minerva Anestesiol* 1995;**61**:93–9.

115 Ferreira IM, Brooks D, Lacasse Y, Goldstein RS. Nutritional support for individuals with COPD: a meta-analysis. *Chest* 2000;**117**:672–8.

116 Hamnegård CH, Bake B, Moxham J, Polkey MI. Does undernutrition contribute to diaphragm weakness in patients with severe COPD? *Clin Nutr* 2002;**21**:239–43.

117 Barreiro E, Sanchez D, Minguella J *et al*. Protein oxidation in the diaphragm of patients with COPD. *Eur Respir J* 2003;**22**:358S.

118 Engelen MP, Schols AM, Does JD, Deutz NE, Wouters EF. Altered glutamate metabolism is associated with reduced muscle glutathione levels in patients with emphysema. *Am J Respir Crit Care Med* 2000;**161**:98–103.

119 Barreiro E, Gea J, Corominas JM, Hussain SN. Nitric oxide synthases and protein oxidation in the quadriceps femoris of patients with chronic obstructive pulmonary disease. *Am J Respir Cell Mol Biol* 2003;**29**:771–8.

120 Knochel JP. Neuromuscular manifestations of electrolyte disorders. *Am J Med* 1982;**72**:521–35.

121 Fiaccadori E, Coffrini E, Ronda N *et al*. Hypophosphatemia in course of chronic obstructive pulmonary disease: prevalence, mechanisms, and relationships with skeletal muscle phosphorus content. *Chest* 1990;**97**:857–68.

122 Aubier M, Murciano D, Lecocguic Y *et al*. Effect of hypophosphatemia on diaphragmatic contractility in patients with acute respiratory failure. *N Engl J Med* 1985;**313**:420–4.

123 Marchesani F, Valerio G, Dardes N, Viglianti B, Sanguinetti CM. Effect of intravenous fructose 1,6-diphophate administration in malnourished chronic obstructive pulmonary disease patients with chronic respiratory failure. *Respiration* 2000;**67**:177–82.

124 Garcia-Aymerich J, Farrero E *et al*. Risk factors of readmission to hospital for a COPD exacerbation: a prospective study. *Thorax* 2003;**58**:100–5.

125 Kessler R, Faller M, Fourgaut G, Mennecier B, Weitzenblum E. Predictive factors of hospitalization for acute exacerbation in a series of 64 patients with chronic obstructive pulmonary disease. *Am J Respir Crit Care Med* 1999;**159**:158–64.

126 Pitta F, Troosters T, Spruit MA, Decramer M, Gosselink R. Activity monitoring for assessment of physical activities in daily life in patients with chronic obstructive pulmonary disease. *Arch Phys Med Rehabil* 2005;**86**:1979–85.

127 Pitta F, Troosters T, Spruit MA *et al*. Characteristics of physical activities in daily life in chronic obstructive pulmonary disease. *Am J Respir Crit Care Med* 2005;**171**:972–7.

128 Pitta F, Troosters T, Probst VS *et al*. Physical activity and hospitalization for exacerbation of COPD. *Chest* 2006;**129**: 536–44.

129 Mancini DM, Henson D, Lamanca J, Levine S. Respiratory muscle function and dyspnea in patients with chronic congestive heart failure. *Circulation* 1992;**86**:909–18.

130 McParland C, Resch EF, Krishnan B *et al*. Inspiratory muscle weakness in chronic heart failure: role of nutrition and electrolyte status and systemic myopathy. *Am J Respir Crit Care Med* 1995;**151**:1101–7.

131 Hammond MD, Bauer KA, Sharp JT, Rocha RD. Respiratory muscle strength in congestive heart failure. *Chest* 1990;**98**: 1091–4.

132 Lindsay DC, Lovegrove CA, Dun MJ *et al*. Histological abnormalities of muscle from limb, thorax and diaphragm in chronic heart failure. *Eur Heart J* 1996;**17**:1239–50.

133 Peters DG, Mitchell HL, McCune SA *et al*. Skeletal muscle sarcoplasmic reticulum Ca^{2+}-ATPase gene expression in congestive heart failure. *Circ Res* 1997;**81**:703–10.

134 Simonini A, Long CS, Dudley GA *et al*. Heart failure in rats causes changes in skeletal muscle morphology and gene expression that are not explained by reduced activity. *Circ Res* 1996;**79**:128–36.

135 Caruana L, Petrie MC, McMurray JJ, MacFarlane NG. Altered diaphragm position and function in patients with chronic heart failure. *Eur J Heart Fail* 2001;**3**:183–7.

136 Buller NP, Jones D, Poole-Wilson PA. Direct measurement of skeletal muscle fatigue in patients with chronic heart failure. *Br Heart J* 1991;**65**:20–4.

137 Minotti JR, Pillay P, Chang L, Wells L, Massie BM. Neurophysiological assessment of skeletal muscle fatigue in patients with congestive heart failure. *Circulation* 1992;**86**: 903–8.

138 Minotti JR, Christoph I, Oka R *et al.* Impaired skeletal muscle function in patients with congestive heart failure: relationship to systemic exercise performance. *J Clin Invest* 1991;**88**:2077–82.

139 Drexler H, Riede U, Munzel T *et al.* Alterations of skeletal muscle in chronic heart failure. *Circulation* 1992;**85**:1751–9.

140 Sullivan MJ, Green HJ, Cobb FR. Skeletal muscle biochemistry and histology in ambulatory patients with long-term heart failure. *Circulation* 1990;**81**:518–27.

141 Mancini DM, Coyle E, Coggan A *et al.* Contribution of intrinsic skeletal muscle changes to ^{13}P NMR skeletal muscle metabobic abnormalities in patients with congestive heart failure. *Circulation* 1989;**80**:1338–46.

142 Brooks SV, Faulkner JA. Effect of aging on the structure and function of skeletal muscle. In: Roussos C, ed. *The Thorax.* New York: Marcel Dekker, 1995: 295–312.

143 Abbasi AA, Drinka PJ, Mattson DE, Rudman D. Low circulating levels of insulin-like growth factors and testosterone in chronically institutionalized elderly men. *J Am Geriatr Soc* 1993;**41**:975–82.

144 Rudman D, Mattson DE. Serum insulin-like growth factor I

145 Scalvini S, Volterrani M, Vitacca M *et al.* Plasma hormone levels and haemodynamics in patients with chronic obstructive lung disease. *Monaldi Arch Chest Dis* 1996;**51**:380–6.

146 Hjalmarsen A, Aasebo U, Birkeland K, Sager G, Jorde R. Impaired glucose tolerance in patients with chronic hypoxic pulmonary disease. *Diabetes Metab* 1996;**22**:37–42.

147 Brodsky IG, Balagopal P, Nair KS. Effects of testosterone replacement on muscle mass and muscle protein synthesis in hypogonadal men: a clinical research center study. *J Clin Endocrinol Metab* 1996;**81**:3469–75.

148 Ferrando AA, Tipton KD, Doyle D *et al.* Testosterone injection stimulates net protein synthesis but not tissue amino acid transport. *Am J Physiol* 1998;**275**(5 Part 1):E864–71.

149 Gambera A, Scagliola P, Falsetti L, Sartori E, Bianchi U. Androgens, insulin-like growth factor-I (IGF-I), and carrier proteins (SHBG, IGFBP-3) in postmenopause. *Menopause* 2004;**11**:159–66.

150 Muller M, den Thijssen JH, Grobbee DE, van der Schouw YT. Endogenous sex hormones in men aged 40–80 years. *Eur J Endocrinol* 2003;**149**:583–9.

151 Semple PD, Beastall GH, Watson WS, Hume R. Serum testosterone depression associated with hypoxia in respiratory failure. *Clin Sci (Lond)* 1980;**58**:105–6.

152 Casaburi R, Goren S, Bhasin S. Substantial prevalence of low anabolic hormone levels in COPD undergoing rehabilitation. *Am J Respir Crit Care Med* 1996;**153**;A128.

in healthy older men in relation to physical activity. *J Am Geriatr Soc* 1994;**42**:71–6.

CHAPTER 4

Exercise limitations and cardiopulmonary exercise testing in COPD

Norman R. Morris, Lewis Adams, Bruce D. Johnson and Idelle M. Weisman

Chronic obstructive pulmonary disease (COPD) is a progressive disorder that leads to a gradual deterioration of lung mechanics and gas exchange. Early manifestations include mild exertional dyspnoea and reduced activity levels [1,2]. As the disease progresses, with further lung tissue destruction and remodelling, there are additional losses in lung elastic recoil, altered ventilation and perfusion relationships, an increased work and cost of breathing, and dyspnoea that becomes more prominent with activity [3,4]. There may be further functional limitations imposed by progressive pulmonary hypertension and by production of cytokines and inflammatory mediators that may impair skeletal muscle function (beyond the results of inactivity) with the disease appearing a more systemic illness than previously appreciated [5–7]. The focus of this chapter is to discuss practical aspects of clinical exercise testing, to review components of exercise limitation in patients with COPD and address current therapeutic strategies in this population.

Clinical exercise testing modalities

There are several modalities of exercise testing used in clinical practice. Some provide basic information, require minimal technical expertise and are simple to perform; while others provide a more complete assessment of all the components involved in exercise and require more complex technology. The following are the most popular exercise tests used in the clinical setting in order of increasing complexity: (i) 6-minute walk test; (ii) shuttle walk test; (iii) cardiac stress test, when cardiac ischaemia needs to be ruled out; and (iv) the cardiopulmonary exercise test (CPET), which may on occasion include arterial blood gas assessment. The CPET typically includes electrocardiographic assessment along with measurements of expired gas exchange. The reader is referred to other sources for a discussion of these different exercise testing modalities [8,9] as this review primarily focuses on the information gained from the more comprehensive but commonly used non-invasive CPET.

Indications

CPET involves the measurement of oxygen uptake ($\dot{V}O_2$), carbon dioxide output ($\dot{V}CO_2$), minute ventilation ($\dot{V}_E$), and other variables in addition to the monitoring of a 12-lead electrocardiogram (ECG), blood pressure, and pulse oximetry (SaO_2) during a maximal symptom-limited incremental exercise test on the cycle ergometer or on the treadmill [10]. When appropriate, the additional measurement of arterial blood gases provides important information on pulmonary gas exchange and many automated systems now allow measurement of the tidal flow–volume loop placed according to a measured inspiratory capacity (IC) within the maximal flow–volume envelope (MFVL) to help better assess the degree of mechanical constraint to breathing [11].

CPET is clinically useful in the evaluation of patients with COPD and permits:

1 Objective determination ($\dot{V}O_{2max}$) of functional capacity or impairment;

2 Evaluation of the mechanisms of exercise limitation, such as the contribution of different organ systems involved in exercise (e.g. heart, lungs, blood and/or skeletal muscles);

3 Differentiation between heart and lung disease;

4 Monitoring of disease progression and response to treatment;

5 Determination of the appropriate intensity needed to perform prolonged exercise (for constant load testing); and

6 Exercise prescription for cardiopulmonary rehabilitation. Maximal exercise testing can be safely performed in the vast majority of patients with respiratory disease with careful monitoring of the ECG and arterial oxygen saturation (Sao_2).

CPET is important in relating symptoms to exercise limitation, especially when exertional symptoms are disproportionate to resting pulmonary function tests (PFTs) and when hypoxaemia may contribute to exercise limitation and O_2 requirements need to be directly quantified. Furthermore, CPET permits the evaluation of therapeutic interventions on exercise capacity, relief of dyspnoea and improvement in exercise tolerance. The efficacy of CPET in monitoring a variety of treatment modalities (bronchodilators, exercise training, lung volume reduction surgery (LVRS), continuous positive airway pressure (CPAP) and proportional assist ventilation (PAV)) directed at improving breathing strategy and/or reducing dynamic hyperinflation, thus resulting in improved breathlessness and exercise capacity, has been demonstrated [12–17]. CPET complements other clinical and diagnostic modalities and by directly quantifying work capacity improves the diagnostic accuracy of impairment–disability evaluation.

Methodology (CPET)

Commercially available automated systems process four primary signals: air flow, O_2, CO_2 and heart rate, which form the basis for the determination of all the measured and derived cardiopulmonary variables [18]. The current systems are technically advanced and provide online analysis of expired respiratory gas exchange using either breath-by-breath or modern mixing chamber techniques [19,20]. Both are acceptable for clinical exercise testing [18]. The more popular breath-by-breath technique is associated with a high degree of breath-to-breath variability 'noise' which can be minimized by 30–60-s interval averaging of the data [21]. Cardiopulmonary measurements obtained during maximal CPET in both control subjects and patients are reproducible provided that calibration and quality assurance procedures are followed [18,22].

Exercise testing can be performed using either a cycle ergometer or a treadmill. Traditionally, exercise testing in respiratory patients has used cycle ergometry. However, depending on the reasons for which CPET was requested, a treadmill might be an acceptable alternative. For clinical CPET purposes, electronically braked cycle ergometry, which maintains a given work level independent of cycling frequency, may be preferable to treadmill testing. Advantages of using cycle ergometry include: direct quantitation of work rate, less noise (artefact) on ECG, ease in collection of blood samples during exercise, expense and safety [18]. However, one important limitation using the cycle is that the $\dot{V}o_{2max}$ achieved is usually 5–11% less than

on a treadmill, which is likely because of more local fatigue and less muscle mass involved in exercise as well as the electrically propelled treadmill possibly pushing patients beyond usual comfort or motivation levels.

Protocols

There are several symptom-limited protocols that can be used with either the cycle ergometer or the treadmill (Fig. 4.1) [18,23]. These include incremental protocols in which the work intensity is increased in a square wave fashion, from 5 W every 1–3 min for debilitated patients to 25 W every 1–3 min for mild disease or healthy subjects, and the ramp protocol in which the power is increased continuously. Both should be programmed to achieve maximal aerobic capacity in 8–12 min [24]. The comparability of these protocols for metabolic and cardiopulmonary measurements is well established [20,25,26]. Subsequently, these results can be used to establish constant work ('steady-state') protocols (see below). CPET results are quite reproducible although, like most physiological tests, there appears to be a learning curve and most subjects will tend to perform slightly better or be willing to work slightly harder on subsequent studies [21,23].

Increasingly, constant work exercise at a standardized submaximal work load (based on an initial incremental exercise test) is being utilized to evaluate the impact of therapeutic interventions including exercise training, oxygen therapy, bronchodilators and LVRS. Recent work

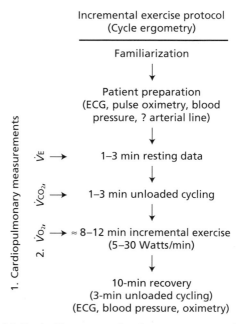

Figure 4.1 Typical incremental cycle ergometer exercise protocol used for clinical testing. ECG, electrocardiogram.

has suggested that Borg dyspnoea ratings, measurements of IC (as a reflection of dynamic hyperinflation) and endurance times during submaximal exercise are reproducible and sensitive in patients with severe COPD [27–29]. Furthermore, constant work endurance times were more sensitive than 6-minute walk test in determining therapeutic effectiveness of pharmacological intervention [29]. More recent work would suggest, however, that endurance shuttle walk tests are sufficiently sensitive to detect changes after bronchodilatation, which may reflect in part differences in quadriceps femoris muscle fatigue occurring more frequently with cycling than walking [9].

An exercise intensity of 65–80% of the maximum work rate achieved during the incremental exercise test has been used for the constant work rate test, which results in $\dot{V}_{O_{2peak}} > 90\%$ of the value obtained in the maximal exercise evaluation [14,30]. To evaluate therapeutic effectiveness of various interventions, it should be kept in mind that intensity of exercise can influence the study outcome. For example, low level activity (e.g. < 50% of peak work) in patients with moderate–severe COPD may result in patients being limited primarily by the endurance capabilities of their peripheral muscles, while exercise > 70% of peak work should result in a sufficient ventilatory stimulus so that most patients would come close to reaching the mechanical limits imposed by their airways. Thus, to examine an intervention aimed at improving maximal expiratory airflows, a higher intensity of exercise should likely be chosen [28].

Patient safety

Extensive literature documents that symptom-limited exercise testing is safe with the risk of medical complications during exercise testing related to the underlying disease, with morbidity for patients in the range of 2–5 per 100 000 clinical exercise tests [31–35]. Advantages to performing CPET over less structured exercise tests include not only the extensive amount of physiological information gained, but also safety. Typically, trained personnel, physicians, exercise physiologists and nurses, carry out exercise testing under controlled and stable conditions for temperature and humidity, with emergency equipment and a bed available, while carefully monitoring the electrocardiogram, blood pressure, symptoms and O_2 saturation [23,36,37]. These trained individuals should be knowledgeable about the conduct and risks of testing, contraindications to testing and the criteria for terminating exercise tests.

Measurements

Computerized metabolic systems allow for an impressive number of variables to be measured or derived during exercise (Table 4.1). The number of variables actually used will vary and be a function of the reasons for exercise testing. The most commonly measured variables are listed below. Figure 4.2 shows an example of the normal cardiopulmonary responses to exercise in a healthy adult.

Oxygen consumption ($\dot{V}_{O_2}$)

$\dot{V}_{O_2}$ rises linearly with increases in work rate to a maximal value. The measurement of $\dot{V}_{O_{2max}}$ or $\dot{V}_{O_{2peak}}$ remains the best available index for the assessment of aerobic capacity [24]. $\dot{V}_{O_{2peak}}$ can be estimated from work rate; however, previous studies have suggested such estimates may not always be reliable [38]. $\dot{V}_{O_{2peak}}$ may be expressed in absolute values (L/min), per kilogram body weight (mL/kg/min) and as percentage of predicted. The optimal normalization for body mass remains somewhat controversial.

Table 4.1 Cardiopulmonary variables measured during exercise testing. (Modified from Zeballos and Weisman [21].)

Variables	Non-invasive	Invasive
Work	Work rate	
Metabolic	$\dot{V}_{O_2}$, $\dot{V}_{CO_2}$, R, AT (a.k.a. LT)	Lactate
Cardiovascular	HR, HRR, ECG, BP, O_2 pulse	
Respiratory	$\dot{V}_E$, V_T, fb, VR, $P_{ET}O_2$, $P_{ET}CO_2$	
Pulmonary gas exchange	Sp_{O_2}, $\dot{V}_E/\dot{V}_{CO_2}$, $\dot{V}_E/\dot{V}_{O_2}$	Sa_{O_2}, Pa_{O_2}, $P(A-a)_{O_2}$, V_D/V_T
Acid–base		pH, Pa_{CO_2}, HCO_3^-
Symptoms	Dyspnoea, leg fatigue, chest pain	

Abnormality of a variable does not necessarily define exercise limitation in that category.
AT, anaerobic threshold; BP, blood pressure; ECG, electrocardiogram; fb, breathing frequency; HCO_3^-, bicarbonate; HR, heart rate; HRR, heart rate reserve; O_2, oxygen; $P(A-a)_{O_2}$, alveolar-arterial oxygen difference; Pa_{CO_2}, arterial partial pressure of carbon dioxide; Pa_{O_2}, arterial partial pressure for oxygen; $P_{ET}CO_2$, end tidal partial pressure for carbon dioxide; $P_{ET}O_2$, end tidal partial pressure for oxygen; R, respiratory exchange ratio; Sa_{O_2}, arterial oxygen saturation; Sp_{O_2}, oxygen saturation; $\dot{V}_{CO_2}$, carbon dioxide production; V_D/V_T, dead space to tidal volume ratio; $\dot{V}_E$, minute ventilation; $\dot{V}_E/\dot{V}_{CO_2}$, ventilatory equivalents for carbon dioxide; $\dot{V}_E/\dot{V}_{O_2}$, ventilatory equivalents for oxygen; $\dot{V}_{O_2}$, oxygen uptake; VR, ventilatory reserve; V_T, tidal volume.

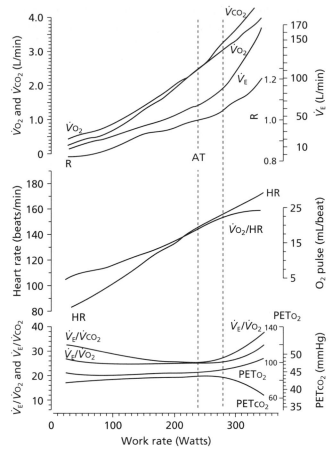

Figure 4.2 Results of a maximal, minute-by-minute, incremental, cardiopulmonary exercise test of a young, healthy, physically active person. The upper panel shows response of O_2 uptake ($\dot{V}O_2$), CO_2 output ($\dot{V}CO_2$), minute ventilation ($\dot{V}_E$) and respiratory exchange ratio (R) to the progressive increase in work rate. The middle panel shows the responses of heart rate (HR) and O_2 pulse ($\dot{V}O_2$/HR) and the lower panel the responses of the ventilatory equivalent for O_2 ($\dot{V}_E/\dot{V}O_2$), ventilatory equivalent for CO_2 ($\dot{V}_E/\dot{V}CO_2$), end-tidal pressure for O_2 (PETO_2) and end-tidal pressure for CO_2 (PETCO_2). Also shown is the transition zone corresponding to the anaerobic threshold (AT).

In addition to the typical expression in mL/kg/min (e.g. American Heart Association, American College of Sports Medicine), others have expressed $\dot{V}O_2$ relative to body mass index (kg/m^2) or for fat-free mass (mL/kg/min) [39]. $\dot{V}O_{2max}$ values have been regarded as most reliable when $\dot{V}O_2$ does not increase (plateau) despite further increase in work rate [25,40]. Such a plateau, however, especially in COPD patients, is not often observed, and the maximum $\dot{V}O_2$ achieved has been called $\dot{V}O_{2peak}$ [41]. This implies that if a subject could be pushed harder, there may be a small further increase in the peak value. For practical purposes, however, $\dot{V}O_{2peak}$ is likely quite close to $\dot{V}O_{2max}$ and thus they are often used interchangeably.

A reduced $\dot{V}O_{2peak}$ (defined by the Fick equation, $\dot{V}O_2 = HR \times SV \times$ a-$\dot{V}O_2$ diff) reflects problems with O_2 delivery (heart, lung, systemic and pulmonary circulation; and blood) and/or peripheral abnormalities (reduced O_2 utilization and/or muscle dysfunction) [42–44]. A reduced $\dot{V}O_{2peak}$ may also reflect poor effort. $\dot{V}O_{2peak}$ is modulated by physical activity and, as such, has been the gold standard for the evaluation of fitness. A number of normative studies have derived predicted equations based on age and gender [20,45]. A normal $\dot{V}O_{2peak}$ reflects a normal aerobic power and exercise capacity and suggests that no significant functional abnormality exist. In some subjects, however, even though the $\dot{V}O_{2peak}$ may be near normal, exercise testing may reveal other abnormalities (e.g. abnormal breathing patterns) that may be of diagnostic value [28,46,47]. A reduced $\dot{V}O_{2peak}$ is usually the starting point in the evaluation of a cardiopulmonary exercise test [48].

Although $\dot{V}O_{2peak}$ is most commonly reported, it may also be of interest to assess the slope of rise in $\dot{V}O_2$ relative to work. In health, this slope is approximately a rise in $\dot{V}O_2$ of 10 mL for every watt increase in work. Clinically, an abnormal slope of this relationship is most often caused by O_2 transport dysfunction (heart failure and pulmonary hypertension); less commonly O_2 utilization dysfunction may also be associated with a reduced slope of this relationship [49,50]. Obese individuals may show an increase in $\dot{V}O_2$ for a given external work rate, but the slope of the relationship is usually normal [24].

Carbon dioxide production ($\dot{V}CO_2$)

Paralleling the changes in $\dot{V}O_2$ with exercise are the changes in the volume of CO_2 expired. At low levels of exercise, the volume of CO_2 expired tends to be slightly less than the uptake of O_2; however, this becomes equimolar in moderate exercise and exceeds O_2 uptake with moderate to heavy exercise. The relationship of $\dot{V}CO_2$ to $\dot{V}O_2$ is known as the respiratory exchange ratio (R). Under steady-state conditions, this ratio may reflect the fuels being consumed at the muscle (similar to the respiratory quotient, RQ). However, with non-steady-state or heavy exercise this more accurately reflects transient changes in CO_2 stores and exceeds 1.0 when lactate buffering occurs and when pH falls causing a significant hyperventilation [51,52]. Anxiety-related hyperventilation will also cause a high R. As noted, $\dot{V}CO_2$ is typically assessed in combination with $\dot{V}O_2$ or with minute ventilation ($\dot{V}_E$).

Heart rate (HR)

The best index for the evaluation of cardiac function during exercise would be the measurement of cardiac output. However, this is not routinely performed in the clinical exercise laboratory. It is well established that increases in cardiac output are initially accomplished by increases in stroke volume and heart rate (HR), and then at higher work rates almost exclusively by increases in HR [24]. Achievement of age-predicted values for heart rate typically reflects maximal or near maximal effort and presumably signals attainment of $\dot{V}_{O_{2max}}$ and, in turn, maximal cardiac output [53]. For interpretative purposes, it is extremely important to remember that there is considerable variability (10–20 b/min) within an age group when estimates of maximal HR are used. The difference between the age-predicted maximal HR and the maximum HR achieved during exercise is referred to as the HR reserve (HRR) [20]. Normally, at maximal exercise, there is little or no HRR. In patients with COPD, the achievement of peak heart rate during exercise may vary considerably depending on the disease severity and medications. Marked mechanical constraints to breathing may result in a submaximal HR attained during exercise.

Oxygen pulse (O₂ pulse)

The O₂ pulse is the $\dot{V}_{O_2}$ divided by HR. This is equivalent to the product of stroke volume multiplied times the arterial–mixed venous oxygen difference (a-$\dot{V}_{O_2}$ diff, extraction). Some studies have suggested that the O₂ pulse may be a good non-invasive estimate of stroke volume because the degree of extraction tends to reach similar levels in multiple populations [48]. The classic response is an initial linear rise with workload followed by a gradual plateauing as exercise intensity increases.

Ventilation ($\dot{V}_E$)

Minute ventilation (expressed in L/min) is typically determined from respiratory rate and tidal volume. Ventilation includes both alveolar and dead space ventilation and is most often expressed relative to ventilatory capacity (see Ventilatory reserve below) or metabolic demand (see Ventilatory efficiency below).

Ventilatory reserve (VR)

This concept is used to determine the degree of mechanical limitation or constraint to breathing during exercise. It is typically expressed as the maximal ventilation achieved during exercise relative to the maximal voluntary ventilation ($\dot{V}_E$/MVV) or some estimate of the MVV (e.g. forced expiratory in 1 s (FEV_1) multiplied times 35–40) used as an index of ventilatory capacity [45]. VR is dependent on many factors responsible for altering ventilatory capacity and ventilatory demand. Those influencing ventilatory demand include metabolic demand (fitness), body weight, mode of testing, dead space ventilation as well as neuroregulatory and behavioural considerations. Ventilatory capacity, in turn, is influenced by multiple factors including ventilatory muscle function, genetic endowment, ageing and disease [54–57]. The ventilatory capacity may also vary during exercise depending on bronchodilatation or bronchoconstriction and the regulation of the operational lung volume (where one breathes relative to the constraints imposed by the boundaries of the maximal flow–volume envelope (see below)) [11].

A high $\dot{V}_E$/MVV is one of the criteria often used to indicate encroachment on the ventilatory reserve and increasing ventilatory constraint to breathing. A reduced or absent ventilatory reserve especially when accompanied by other respiratory abnormalities (and an inability to achieve maximal HR) increases the likelihood that respiratory limitation may be a significant contributing factor to exercise limitation.

Limitations to the use of classical VR

Although widely used and practical, MVV may not always be a reliable indicator of the maximal available ventilation nor provide adequate insight into abnormalities in breathing strategy [11]. The MVV is typically a 15-s test, and patients will typically produce pulmonary pressures in excess of those produced even during maximal exercise [58]. In addition, patients have a tendency to perform the MVV at higher lung volumes than those achieved during exercise, taking advantage of the higher available maximal expiratory flows at the higher lung volumes. However, this can increase the work and cost of breathing because of the increased elastic load as one approaches total lung capacity (TLC).

A more comprehensive assessment of the degree of ventilatory constraint can be gained by comparison of the exercise tidal flow–volume loop to the maximal volitional flow–volume envelopes [11]. This display of the exercise breathing pattern provides visual insight into the degree of ventilatory constraint and the strategies used to achieve a given level of ventilation relative to that which is available. Quantification of the degree of constraint from the tidal flow and volume responses to exercise relative to the MFVL has been suggested (Fig. 4.3). In addition to a more in depth assessment of ventilatory constraint during exercise, a more precise assessment of ventilatory capacity (VECAP) can be obtained. This assessment of ventilatory capacity takes into account the tidal volume, the operational lung volume (end-expiratory lung volume, EELV) and the constraints imposed by the maximal expiratory flow–volume curve. To account for changes in ventilatory capacity during exercise (i.e. brochodilation or constriction), comparisons can be made to an MFVL obtained during or immediately post exercise [11]. Exercise tidal flow–volume loop analysis has been applied in several clinical settings [55–57,59–61].

Anaerobic threshold (AT)

With progressive increases in work intensity, there is a work intensity or $\dot{V}_{O_2}$ where lactate would begin to accumulate. This was termed the lactate threshold and subsequently it was determined that non-invasive gas exchange measurements could fairly closely approximate these changes in lactate accumulation. Although the exact

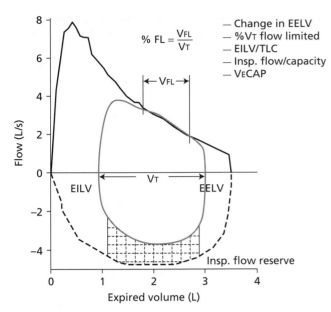

Figure 4.3 Defining expiratory flow limitation. Tidal exercise flow–volume loops are aligned within maximal expiratory flow–volume envelope according to a measured end-expiratory lung volume (EELV). The percentage of the tidal breath (VFL) that expiratory air flows meet or exceed the maximal expiratory flows are used as an estimate as to the degree of expiratory flow limitation. EILV, end-inspiratory lung volume [11].

mechanism for the rise remains somewhat controversial and may vary depending on disease population, the lactate rise in health most likely reflects accumulative recruitment of glycolytic fibres [54,62,63]. The lactic acid is subsequently buffered by bicarbonate and the by-product becomes CO_2 production in excess of typical metabolic CO_2 production. This results in a rise in the $\dot{V}CO_2$ and a parallel increase in minute ventilation to maintain iso-pH.

Current knowledge suggests that the AT may be affected by factors that impact both O_2 delivery and O_2 utilization processes, pattern of muscle fibre recruitment, and possibly others [64]. The AT usually occurs at 50–70% $\dot{V}O_{2max}$ in sedentary individuals and higher in fit individuals [45]. There is a wide range of normal predicted values (35–70%) making its usefulness in clinical decision making somewhat limited [23,34].

Although there are several ways to determine the AT non-invasively, none appears consistently superior. Currently, the modified V-slope method ($\dot{V}CO_2$ vs $\dot{V}O_2$ plot) is most popular [65]. The AT, using the ventilatory equivalents method, is defined as the lowest (nadir) for $\dot{V}_E/\dot{V}O_2$ and end tidal partial pressure for oxygen (PETO$_2$) before beginning to consistently increase, while $\dot{V}_E/\dot{V}CO_2$ and PETCO$_2$ remain unchanged, and R is approximately 1.0. An approach that combines the modified V-slope and the ventilatory

equivalents method is recommended [21]. Blood samples for standard bicarbonate or lactates help avoid false-positive non-invasive AT determinations that have been reported in COPD [66]. The AT determination is helpful as an indicator of level of fitness and to monitor the effect of physical training [67]. The AT is reduced in a wide spectrum of clinical entities (e.g. heart disease, lung disease, deconditioning, post lung and heart transplantation, muscle abnormalities (metabolic myopathy)) and therefore may be of limited discriminatory value in interpretative schemes [68].

Ventilatory efficiency ($\dot{V}_E/\dot{V}CO_2$ and $\dot{V}_E/\dot{V}O_2$)

Ventilatory efficiency is determined by how much ventilation is achieved for a given level of metabolic demand (i.e. $\dot{V}_E/\dot{V}CO_2$ and/or $\dot{V}_E/\dot{V}O_2$). Because $\dot{V}_E$ is more closely linked to $\dot{V}CO_2$, the relationship of $\dot{V}_E$ to $\dot{V}CO_2$ has typically been reported [51]. In healthy subjects, it typically requires approximately 25 L of ventilation for every 1 L of carbon dioxide produced. $\dot{V}_E/\dot{V}CO_2$ and $\dot{V}_E/\dot{V}O_2$ are typically similar until near where the AT occurs and then $\dot{V}_E/\dot{V}CO_2$ tends to stay constant while $\dot{V}_E/\dot{V}O_2$ starts to rise [69]. The degree of ventilation produced is best described in the alveolar air equation where $\dot{V}_E = K \times \dot{V}CO_2/(PaCO_2 \times (1 - V_D/V_T))$ [54]. Thus, the relationship of $\dot{V}_E/\dot{V}CO_2$ is critically influenced by dead space ventilation, and arterial CO_2 levels. A high dead space ventilation increases the $\dot{V}_E : \dot{V}CO_2$ ratio as does hyperventilation (reduced PaCO$_2$ values). An inadequate hyperventilation during exercise (high or rising PaCO$_2$) may result in a low $\dot{V}_E : \dot{V}CO_2$ particularly if the V_D/V_T is normal. Various $\dot{V}_E : \dot{V}CO_2$ values have been reported, including, the lowest point in an incremental test, at or near the AT, the slope of $\dot{V}_E$ relative to $\dot{V}CO_2$ and peak. For most purposes, the $\dot{V}_E/\dot{V}CO_2$ nadir occurs near the AT where it is usually reported since during heavy exercise, it is more susceptible to variation in the degree of hyperventilation, altered breathing pattern, anxiety and the degree of acidosis [69]. Under some circumstances, the peak values may be important as when a relatively sudden increase in $\dot{V}_E/\dot{V}CO_2$ with heavier exercise occurs in patients with pulmonary hypertension, likely related to the high pulmonary pressures and the shunting of blood through a patent foramen ovale [70]. Examining the PETCO$_2$, or preferably PaCO$_2$ (if available), is useful in distinguishing between a hyperventilation-induced increase in $\dot{V}_E/\dot{V}CO_2$ versus that related to a high dead space.

Blood gases

In the clinical laboratory when more specific gas exchange information is needed, direct arterial blood gas (ABG) sampling during exercise should be considered. This may be useful in a patient with significant oxygen desaturation (< 85%) during a non-invasive cardiopulmonary exercise test or in patients with a markedly elevated $\dot{V}_E/\dot{V}CO_2$. It may also be of importance in patients where it is difficult to obtain clean non-invasive gas exchange data because of problems with the mouthpiece or non-invasive estimates of oxygen saturation.

Measurements of Pa_{O_2}, Pa_{CO_2}, combined with ventilatory measurements also allows the assessment of the alveolar (PA_{O_2})–arterial (Pa_{O_2}) oxygen pressure difference (AaD_{O_2}) and physiological dead space to tidal volume ratio (V_D/V_T) [71]. V_D/V_T determined non-invasively using PET_{CO_2} can often yield unreliable results [72]. Abnormal widening of the AaD_{O_2} with exercise, usually reflects ventilation–perfusion (V/Q) mismatching, but may also be a result of diffusion abnormalities, anatomical shunt and/or reduced O_2 saturation in mixed venous blood (thereby worsening the V/Q mismatching shunt effect) [73]. Failure of V_D/V_T to decrease normally with exercise is indicative of V/Q abnormalities caused by increases in physiological dead space (wasted ventilation).

Pulse oximetry (Sp_{O_2})

Sp_{O_2} is only an estimation of the arterial O_2 saturation with actual $Sa_{O_2} \pm 4\%$ of the pulse oximetry readings [74]. Each laboratory should validate its pulse oximeter(s) with arterial oxygen saturation. This is important because some pulse oximeters underestimate and others overestimate true arterial oxygen saturation, especially at $Sa_{O_2} < 88\%$ [75]. Caution should be exercised in the use of pulse oximetry in darker skinned subjects, because the inaccuracies reported in Caucasians appear to be exaggerated [76]. Pulse oximeters cannot be used in patients with high levels of carboxyhaemoglobin, resulting from smoking or CO exposure, as COHb is not measured. Pulse oximeters measure functional Sa_{O_2} and not fractional saturation as do CO-Oximeters. Care should be exercised in interpreting changes obtained by pulse oximetry alone. Significant desaturation, defined as change in $Sp_{O_2} > 5\%$, should be confirmed with arterial blood gases [77].

Clinical signs and symptoms

In a symptom-limited test it is important to describe and characterize signs and symptoms limiting the test (e.g. chest pain, breathlessness, leg fatigue, wheezing, diaphoresis, arrhythmia) [43]. Ratings of perceived exertion symptoms (breathlessness, fatigue, chest pain) using the Borg Scale (0–10) or other rating scores including visual analogue scales should be noted with the physiological measurements [78–81] (see section on Dyspnoea under Exercise limitations in COPD below).

Exercise limitations in COPD

As COPD progresses, there is a gradual loss of lung elastic recoil, a destruction of lung parenchyma and inhomogeneities in the compliance characteristics of the lung. This leads to airway narrowing or collapse (airflow limitation) at higher and higher lung volumes, progressive air trapping, a maldistribution of ventilation, areas of hypoxic pulmonary vasoconstriction, pulmonary hypertension and ventilation–perfusion mismatching resulting in a high dead space ventilation and areas of effective shunt, leading to progressive hypoxaemia. In mild to moderate disease, blood gas homeostasis may be preserved, while the dominant effect is the altered lung mechanics. Given the large reserves of the pulmonary system, at rest many of these changes may not render the patient particularly symptomatic; however, with activity and the increased ventilatory demands required to maintain arterial P_{O_2} and eliminate metabolic CO_2, patients become symptomatic. Table 4.2 summarizes factors involved in limiting exercise tolerance in patients with COPD.

Table 4.2 Factors contributing to exercise limitations in patients with COPD.

Lung mechanics
Tissue destruction (alveolar)
Loss of parenchymal elastic recoil
- Expiratory flow limitation
- Hyperinflation
- Increased inspiratory elastic load
- High work and cost of breathing

Gas exchange
Tissue destruction (alveolar–capillary)
Loss of elastic recoil
Ventilation–perfusion abnormalities
- High dead space ventilation
- Widened alveolar–arterial difference
- Hypoxaemia

Cardiovascular
Hyperinflation
Reduced intrathoracic space
Reduced venous return
- Reduced cardiac output

Hypoxaemia
Pulmonary hypertension
- Reduced cardiac output

Peripheral muscles
Deconditioning
Inflammation
Competition for blood flow

Dyspnoea
Respiratory drive
Central perception
Inspiratory muscles
Chemoreceptors

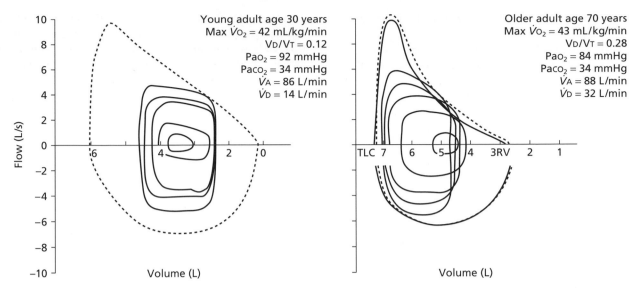

Figure 4.4 Flow–volume response to exercise in the average fit healthy young adult during incremental exercise plotted within the maximal expiratory flow–volume (MFVL). In this population, end-expiratory lung volume (EELV) progressively decreases with exercise and expiratory flow limitation is only present near EELV over a small portion of the tidal volume. Considerable room exists to increase ventilation even at peak exercise.

Lung mechanics

In health, with large pulmonary reserves, the ventilatory demands of exercise (required to maintain blood gas homoeostasis) are met with a fairly efficient breathing pattern and strategy, which minimizes the work and cost of breathing [54]. The ventilatory response to exercise in young and older healthy subjects is shown in Figure 4.4. Classically tidal volume increases and EELV falls as expiratory muscles are recruited, optimizing inspiratory muscle length. As exercise intensity increases, tidal volume continues to increase up to approximately 50% of the vital capacity (VC), which is followed by predominantly a breathing frequency response. EELV may drop further (0.5–1 L) and there is some encroachment on the inspiratory reserve volume (IRV); however, the alinear portions of the pressure–volume relationship of the lungs and chest wall are avoided and, even at maximal exercise, expiratory flow rates typically only approach the maximal available flow rate near EELV. Inspiratory pleural pressures continue to become more negative and approach –20 to –30 cm H_2O and only approach a small percentage of the available capacity for producing inspiratory pressure [60]. Even with maximal exercise, the cost of breathing is estimated to only approach 5–7% of the whole body $\dot{V}_{O_2}$ in the average fit young adult [59,82].

With healthy ageing, there is some loss in pulmonary reserves so that the typical 70-year-old male will have an approximately 25–30% decline in VC and a similar decline in maximal expiratory flow rates ($FEF_{25–75}$), primarily because a loss of lung elastic recoil [83]. Despite this loss

in ventilatory reserve, the healthy older adult is able to increase ventilation with exercise with minimal increments in ventilatory cost relative to the younger adult. Only with very heavy exercise and with sustained high levels of physical training (increased metabolic demands), might the older adult reach significant mechanical limitations to breathing, typically associated with a mild to moderate degree of dynamic hyperinflation and expiratory flows that approach or reach the maximal available flows over a portion of the tidal breath (typically over the later half of the tidal breath, near EELV) [55].

The aged adult would therefore develop a breathing pattern and strategy that would be similar to a younger person with mild COPD (e.g. 15–30% reduction in FEV_1). Typically, older subjects will approach expiratory flow limitation at a $\dot{V}_E$ of approximately 50–70 L/min and will need to increase EELV slightly to produce ventilations beyond 70 L/min. With more moderate lung disease, 40–50% reductions in FEV_1, patients will approach expiratory flow limitation over a portion of the tidal breath even at rest. Thus, with exercise, to be able to increase ventilation, they will need to dynamically hyperinflate almost immediately to take advantage of the shape of the maximal expiratory flow–volume envelope and the available flows at the higher lung volumes [84,85]. However, as EELV starts to rise, it becomes more difficult to maintain tidal volume because of a shrinking IRV. As end inspiratory lung volume approaches TLC, the elastic load begins to rise as patients move away from the linear portion of the pressure–volume characteristics of the lung and chest wall. In addition, expiratory muscles need to be heavily recruited to produce large

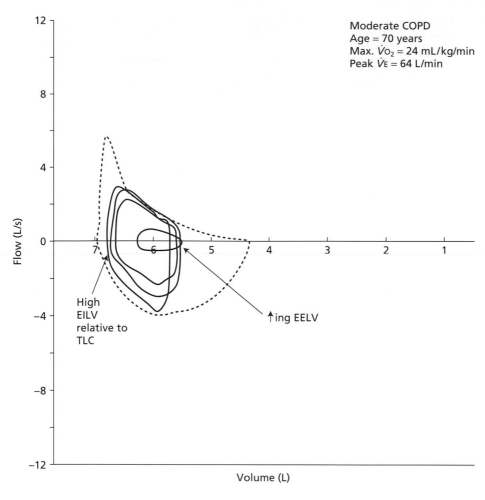

Moderate COPD
Age = 70 years
Max. $\dot{V}_{O_2}$ = 24 mL/kg/min
Peak $\dot{V}_E$ = 64 L/min

Figure 4.5 Patient with history of moderate COPD (forced expiratory flow at 50% of VC = 35% of predicted for age). End-expiratory lung volume (EELV) increases from the onset of exercise and expiratory flow limitation is present over > 80% of the V_T by peak exercise. Inspiratory flows approach those available over the higher lung volumes. Little room exists to increase ventilation. EILV, end-inspiratory lung volume; TLC, total lung capacity.

expiratory flows early in expiration and thus the work and cost of breathing begins to rise substantially. Previous studies have suggested that this cost of breathing may approach approach 15% of the whole body $\dot{V}_{O_2}$ in older, relatively fit adults and as much as 30–50% of the whole body $\dot{V}_{O_2}$ in patients with severe COPD at ventilations of 30–40 L/min [85]. In terms of cardiac output and blood flow distribution, this would be a large percentage of blood flow unavailable to the muscles of locomotion, as previous work in animals and humans have suggested that the respiratory muscles will preferentially recruit blood flow at the expense of the locomotor muscles [86,87]. This reflex reduction in blood flow to locomotor muscles, along with the deconditioning process, may contribute to the symptoms of leg fatigue rather than dyspnoea as a primary limiting factor during exercise. Figure 4.5 is an example of the flow–volume responses to exercise in a relatively active older patient with moderate COPD.

Gas exchange

In healthy humans, the partial pressure of oxygen in the arterial blood (Pa_{O_2}) generally remains close to resting values, even during heavy exercise [88]. Arterial CO_2 (Pa_{CO_2}) also is maintained relatively close to resting values through precise ventilatory control mechanisms. Only with heavy exercise is there a compensatory increase in ventilation that is out of proportion to the CO_2 produced resulting in a fall in Pa_{CO_2} [54]. The alveolar (PA_{O_2}) to arterial oxygen difference (AaD_{O_2}) tends to remain constant or in some cases fall slightly with very light exercise and then increases primarily as a result of a rise in PA_{O_2} [89]. In some healthy, typically endurance trained subjects with heavier exercise, Pa_{O_2} may fall despite a rising PA_{O_2} [60]. The widening of the AaD_{O_2} in these healthy subjects has been considered to be related to a lack of time for end-capillary diffusion (resulting from a high cardiac output), interregional ventilation perfusion inhomogeneities and a 1–2% shunt due to the thebesian and bronchial circulations, which becomes more prominent as the mixed venous P_{O_2} falls [89]. The ventilatory dead space to tidal volume ratio (V_D/V_T) in healthy younger adults is approximately 0.20–0.30 and falls with exercise as the tidal volume increases. With healthy ageing, there tends to be a decline in resting Pa_{O_2} values likely resulting from more inhomogeneities in ventilation–perfusion relationships [83]. There is also a rise in V_D/V_T.

However, during exercise older healthy adults tend to do a relatively good job at maintaining Pao_2 values, although the $AaDo_2$ tends to widen at a lower intensity of exercise than in young adults [90].

COPD is associated with relatively variable blood gas responses, with some patients having a well-preserved response to exercise and others with marked declines in Pao_2 [91,92]. In general, however, there is a much greater widening of the $AaDo_2$ at much lower work intensities than in age- and gender-matched controls. CO_2 elimination is also variable, from a relatively normal fall in $Paco_2$ with heavy exercise to a rise in $Paco_2$, likely because subjects cannot increase alveolar ventilation enough to achieve adequate CO_2 removal. V_D/V_T can be quite high in patients with COPD so that they need to attain a much higher total ventilation than in healthy subjects to achieve a similar level of alveolar ventilation. Arterial hypoxaemia during exercise is primarily a result of ventilation–perfusion mismatching, with a contribution in some subjects from a diffusion limitation as well as increased shunt [89]. The hypoxaemia not only contributes to the sensation of dyspnoea, but may also result in worsening pulmonary hypertension that in turn may influence cardiac function and contribute to a reduced exercise tolerance. Previous studies have suggested that treadmill walking may be associated with more exercise-induced hypoxaemia than cycling [93].

Dyspnoea

Clinically, dyspnoea is a term for shortness of breath that is commonly found in COPD patients. The American Thoracic Society defines dyspnoea as 'a term used to characterize a subjective experience of breathing discomfort that is comprised of qualitatively distinct sensations that vary in intensity' [94]. The experience derives from interactions among multiple physiological, psychological, social and environmental factors, and may induce secondary physiological and behavioural responses. Dyspnoea is extremely distressing for the patient and is typically described as 'having to fight for every breath' or 'a sense of impending doom'.

Many patients with COPD fall into a spiral of increasing levels of dyspnoea and decreasing levels of physical activity (Fig. 4.6). As the spiral progresses, dyspnoea arises at increasingly lower levels of exertion, and patients decrease the level of physical activity in an effort to avoid the sensation of dyspnoea. This decrease in the level of activity leads to further deconditioning. Eventually, this spiral will lead to dyspnoea impacting on activities of daily living (ADL) including basic functions such as washing and dressing. As a result, patients have a significant loss of quality of life. Interventions for COPD patients focus on dyspnoea as a key outcome measure often over and above any improvement in functional capacity [95,96].

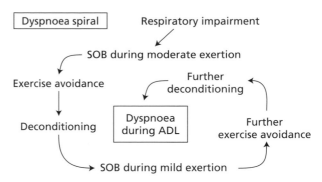

Figure 4.6 The cycle of decline associated with COPD. ADL, activity of daily living; SOB, Shortness of breath.

Pathophysiology

The recent evolution of functional brain mapping techniques of positron emission tomography (PET) and functional magnetic resonance imaging (fMRI) have provided new insights into dyspnoea perception. Using different technologies, these brain mapping techniques have suggested that the sensation of dyspnoea is associated with a pattern of activation of phylogenically ancient limbic and paralimbic cortical structures (e.g. anterior insular cortex, anterior cingulate gyrus and amygdala) [97–101].

As far as the respiratory system is concerned it seems that dyspnoea perception depends more on the degree to which the brainstem respiratory complex is stimulated than on the movement of the ventilatory apparatus. Thus, increases in ventilation associated with exercise, hypoxia, hypercapnia and metabolic acidosis are associated with dyspnoea while volitional ventilation is not [102]. Most interestingly, this is the case even in patients with severe COPD [103,104]. In addition, dyspnoea accompanies central respiratory stimulation in the absence of a ventilatory response in subjects with high spinal cord transection [105] or following experimental respiratory muscle paralysis [106,107]. For patients with COPD, one may hypothesize that exertional dyspnoea could be a manifestation of the increased central respiratory activity necessary to achieve adequate ventilation in the face of respiratory mechanical impairment. This hypothesis fits with the finding that progressive hyperinflation in COPD patients leads to increasing dyspnoea as greater respiratory muscle activity is required to ventilate at high lung volumes where compliance is low [108]. Support for this idea is provided in the study by Lahrmann *et al.* [109] who showed that a decrease in dyspnoea following LVRS was accompanied by a decrease in lung hyperinflation and a reduced neural activity in the diaphragm. It also could explain the observation that exertional dyspnoea in COPD patients is lessened when non-invasive ventilatory support is provided [110].

An individual's personality, emotional state and cognitive function seem likely to impact on their experience of dyspnoea [111]. Dyspnoea has been reported in both hyperventilation syndrome and in those individuals prone to panic attacks [112,113]. There is evidence that patients with airflow limitation perceive dyspnoea less intensively when they become familiar with the situation that is giving rise to their dyspnoea [112].

Assessment scales that rate dyspnoea

A number of instruments are available that allow reasonably reproducible rating of the intensity of dyspnoea during exercise or in response to specific questions. Two of the most common scales used to rate dyspnoea are the visual analogue scale (VAS) and the Borg scale. VAS is a horizontal or a vertical line, usually 10 cm long, anchored at either end with words such as 'no dyspnoea' and 'maximal dyspnoea'. In response to a question (e.g. 'How short of breath are you?'), the subject marks a point along the line so that the length reflects the intensity of the sensation [114,115]. This scale was first used for rating the sensation associated with increased airway resistance and was only later adopted for the quantification of breathlessness [80,116].

The Borg scale is a 12-point category scale with extremes of 'nothing at all' and 'maximal' [79]. Unlike the VAS, the Borg scale includes verbal descriptors (e.g. 'slight', 'severe') to assist in rating the symptom. Like the VAS, the Borg scale has good reproducibility but the proximity of the terms 'slight' and 'severe' in the Borg scale may reduce its sensitivity and discourage subjects from using the whole scale as they do the VAS [114,115,117]. Although researchers have utilized the Borg and the VAS scales, clinicians often rely on a simple verbal numerical rating scale ranging from zero to 10 [118].

Importantly, there appears to be good correlation among the various rating scales, even when used in mechanically ventilated patients [119]. Moreover, it has been shown that patients can reliably use such dyspnoea ratings to reach a predetermined level of exercise and oxygen consumption [120]. Notably, there has been some development of new scales to assess dyspnoea such as the word-labelled visual analogue scale (LVAS) [121].

Exercise performance as an assessment of dyspnoea

In patients with COPD, exercise testing is used to quantify the degree of functional impairment. It has been presumed that there is an association between functional capacity and the severity of dyspnoea, with those individuals with the poorest exercise capacity having the highest ratings of dyspnoea. However, such a presumption may be somewhat simplistic and the performance in such a test is likely to reflect a complex interaction of physiological limitations, associated symptoms and cognitive factors, especially motivation. Simple questionnaires designed to assess dyspnoea severity have required patients to assess their own exercise tolerance compared with their peers (e.g. Medical Research Council American Thoracic Society (ATS) scale) [122]. Although such scales are simple and widely used, they are insensitive, require individuals to make comparisons with others, and cannot measure changes with therapeutic interventions. The traditional test is the Baseline Dyspnoea Index, a rate-administered test, developed to rate patients with regard not only to the 'magnitude of the task' that elicits dyspnoea (e.g. hills compared with level ground) but also to the impact of dyspnoea on activities of daily living and the effort expended before dyspnoea occurs [123]. Similar and easier to use self-administered questionnaires have been developed, but these have not been widely used [124].

Peripheral muscle dysfunction

For patients with COPD, limited exercise capacity is a major cause of morbidity. While many early studies in patients with COPD focused on the central limitations to exercise capacity such as ventilation and gas exchange, the large degree of variation in exercise capacity for given level of airflow limitation and the reduced exercise tolerance following lung transplantation suggests that peripheral factors such as skeletal muscle dysfunction may also have a role (Fig. 4.7) [125]. In particular, there appears to be either impaired oxygen utilization associated with a greater reliance on glycolytic activity and/or an abnormal redistribution of blood flow to the exercising muscle in these patients [126,127].

Changes in skeletal muscle structure and function with COPD

Muscle mass and cross-sectional area
Compared with healthy age-matched controls, patients with

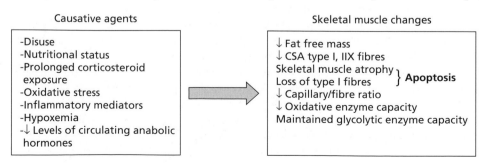

Figure 4.7 Factors contributing to skeletal muscle abnormalities in patients with COPD. CSA, cross-sectional area.

COPD have a reduced skeletal muscle fat-free mass (FFM) and cross-sectional area of type I and IIa fibres [128–131]. Using dual-energy X-ray absorptiometry (DEXA), Gosker *et al.* [132] reported a lower FFM in 15 patients with COPD (49.5 ± 8.2 kg) compared with 15 age-matched controls (58.7 ± 10.8 kg; $P = 0.03$). Moreover, COPD patients had a lower mean fibre cross-sectional area (CSA) than healthy subjects (COPD patients 3839 μm^2; healthy controls 4428 μm^2; $P = 0.037$).

The reduction in FFM has been cited as a strong predictor of decreased exercise capacity ($\dot{V}o_{2peak}$) and muscle strength of individuals with COPD [133]. In a group of 25 subjects with severe COPD ($FEV_1 = 32 \pm 11\%$ predicted), $\dot{V}o_{2peak}$ was significantly correlated with FFM ($r = 0.56$; $P < 0.005$) [129,132]. However, this study reported that the relationship was weaker in the COPD group than for healthy age- and gender-matched controls ($r = 0.84$; $P < 0.001$ for controls), suggesting that other factors apart from the loss of FFM are involved in the decreased exercise capacity in COPD patients.

Skeletal muscle morphology
Morphological changes in skeletal muscle have traditionally been determined using needle biopsy techniques. Recent studies of needle biopsy samples taken from the vastus lateralis muscle in COPD patients have shown significant muscle fibre atrophy [131,132,134], changes in fibre composition with a selective loss of type I fibres [132,134–137], reduced capillary to fibre ratio [131,138] and a reduction in oxidative enzyme capacity [139–141] compared with healthy controls.

In one of the original investigations of skeletal muscle dysfunction in patients with COPD, Jakobsson *et al.* [135] found atrophy and loss of type I fibres in 18 patients with COPD, eight of whom had severe COPD with chronic respiratory failure. These results were supported in a later study by Whittom *et al.* [131] who reported a selective loss of type I fibres in patients with COPD compared with controls and a decrease in the cross-sectional area of type I, IIa and IIab fibres. However this finding has not been a universal, with others reporting selective decrease in the cross sectional area of Type IIa and IIX fibres in COPD patients [132]. In addition, Whittom *et al.* [131] reported that the percentage of type IIb fibres (fast twitch glycolytic) was higher in COPD patients compared with controls and that cross-sectional area of the IIb fibres was retained. The results of these studies suggest that there is selective loss of the oxidative fibres of the vastus lateralis in patients with COPD (type I and IIa fibres) with a concomitant loss of cross-sectional area. At the same time, there appears to be an increase in the size and percentage of IIb fibres with COPD.

The change in the skeletal muscle fibre type with COPD appears consistent with the changes in activities of enzymes associated with ATP production. Several studies have reported a decrease in the activity of mitochondrial enzymes such as citrate synthase (CS) and β-hydroxyacyl CoA-dehydrogenanse (HAD) [127,137,139,141] in COPD patients. While there has been some evidence to suggest that the decrease in the activity of oxidative enzymes is associated with an increase in the activity of enzymes associated with glycolysis such as phosphofuctokinase (PFK) and lactate dehydrogenase (LDH), this finding has not been universal [137,139]. For example, Maltais *et al.* [127] reported that there was a decrease in the activity of CS and HAD in COPD patients compared with healthy controls. However, there was no reported change in the activity glycolytic enzymes such as PFK, LDH and hexokinase.

Interestingly, the functional and morphological changes in skeletal muscle with COPD appear to be confined to the lower limb. The study by Gea *et al.* [142] examined the metabolic characteristics of the deltoid muscle in the upper limb of 10 patients with COPD and nine healthy age-matched controls. While finding that exercise capacity (measured using cycle ergometry) was significantly reduced in COPD patients, these authors found that handgrip strength was essentially preserved in COPD patients when compared with healthy subjects. In addition, this study reported the activities of CS and PFK were the same in COPD and control subjects and that the activity of LDH was elevated in COPD patients compared with controls. These authors concluded that the upper limbs of patients with COPD had an essentially unchanged metabolic profile whereas (based on the findings in other studies) the lower limb had an altered metabolic profile with lower levels of oxidative enzymes.

In addition to impaired oxygen utilization of oxygen, COPD patients have altered delivery of oxygen at the level of the skeletal muscle. Jobin *et al.* [138] reported a decrease in the number of capillaries to fibre ratio in COPD subjects compared with controls (0.83 ± 0.05 COPD, 1.56 ± 0.10 controls; $P < 0.001$). Another study reported a trend for lower capillary to fibre ratio ($P = 0.15$) and a reduction in the number of capillaries in contact with skeletal muscle fibres in patients with COPD compared with healthy individuals [131]. The reduction in the number of capillaries in contact was greatest in the more oxidative fibres (type I, IIa) in the COPD patients. However, this study correctly noted that when the number of capillaries in contact was corrected for the differences in cross-sectional area the differences between the healthy and COPD patients was removed.

It is not clear what impact COPD has on the maximal vasodilatory capacity of the lower limb in COPD patients. The maximal vasodilatory capacity is an indicator of the ability to vasodilatate the local vascular bed following during reactive hyperaemia. In healthy older individuals, vasodilatory capacity tends to decrease with age and is correlated with exercise capacity [143]. Moreover, vasodilatory capacity has been shown to increase with endurance training in young and older individuals [144]. While it may be hypothesized that the decline in physical activity with COPD may in turn result in a decrease in the vasodilatory capacity, Sabapathy *et al.* [145] have recently reported no significant difference in the peak calf blood flow responses between age- and gender-matched controls and COPD patients. This may suggest that there is a time lag for the reduction in peak calf blood flow responses and while not present in patients with moderate COPD, individuals with severe COPD may well have reduced vasodilatory capacity in association with significant reductions physical activity levels.

Recent studies have suggested that COPD patients develop a greater degree of fatigue in skeletal muscle during endurance exercise when compared with healthy controls [146,147]. Endurance cycle ergometry induces quadriceps twitch muscle fatigue and a locus of symptom limitation (legs) that is different from the predominance of dyspnoea and absence of quadriceps twitch leg fatigue reported in COPD with walking which may partially explain the difference [7,9]. There appears to be some debate on the actual mechanism for greater development of fatigue in skeletal muscle in COPD. Allaire *et al.* [148] suggested that the limitation in skeletal muscle endurance in COPD patients was related to lower levels of oxidative enzymes (CS) and independent of the cross-sectional area of the skeletal muscle. Most recently, Saey *et al.* [149] have suggested that the greater contractile fatigue found in some COPD patients following constant work cycling exercise is because of the greater reliance on glycolytic (non-aerobic) metabolism during exercise.

Proposed mechanisms of skeletal muscle dysfunction in COPD

While it is now accepted that COPD is associated with an inherent skeletal muscle dysfunction, the underlying mechanism for this dysfunction has yet to be elucidated. It has been suggested that skeletal muscle dysfunction associated with COPD may be the result of several factors including deconditioning, malnutrition, skeletal muscle myopathy and low levels of circulating anabolic hormones [150–152].

Generally speaking, the changes in skeletal muscle morphology with deconditioning are similar to those seen with COPD. Following a period of bedrest, microgravity or detraining, there is a reported decrease in the number and CSA of type I fibres and a decrease in the activity of mitochondrial enzymes CS, HAD and succinate dehydrogenanse (SDH) [153–155]. However, unlike COPD patients, deconditioning in healthy individuals is not typically associated with an increase in the activity of glycolytic enzymes PFK and LDH. Indeed, some studies examining the changes in enzyme activity following a period of leg immobilization reported a decrease in both CS and LDH [154,156].

Poor nutritional status is common in COPD patients, with one pulmonary rehabilitation programme reporting that 35% of patients entering the programme were nutritionally depleted [157]. This reduction in nutritional status in COPD patients has been associated with a decreased skeletal muscle strength and endurance [158].

Prolonged exposure to high-dose corticosteriods can result in significant myopathy in COPD patients [159]. While the role of prolonged hypoxia, hypercapnia and oxidative stress are less clear, there is emerging evidence that some if not all of these factors may combine to result in significant myopathic changes in skeletal muscle for patients with COPD [150].

It should be noted that not all studies have reported significant myopathic changes in COPD patients. Recently, Heijdra *et al.* [160] reported that a group ($n = 32$) of COPD subjects (FEV_1 38 ± 11% predicted) had a similar FFM index (FFMI) as age-matched controls ($n = 36$). Moreover, these authors reported similar phase II steady-state oxygen uptake kinetics ($\tau = 72 \pm 32$ s COPD patients; $\tau = 78 \pm 37$ s controls). These authors questioned the existence of underlying skeletal muscle myopathy in COPD patients given that normal and healthy groups had similar oxygen uptake kinetics.

The role of oxidative stress as a causative factor for the myopthatic changes in skeletal muscle in patients with COPD has received recent attention. Couillard *et al.* [161,162] examined whether oxidative stress was involved in the myopathy typically associated with COPD. These authors found that local muscle activity induced oxidative stress in COPD patients and that this in turn was associated with decreased muscle endurance. Local exercise-induced oxidative stress failed to raise antioxidant activity in COPD patients, in contrast to controls where an elevation of antioxidants was observed. These observations are consistent with increased oxidative stress in the mypopathic changes in skeletal muscle in COPD.

There is evidence to suggest that the level of circulating anabolic hormones, such as insulin-like growth factor (IGF)-I and testosterone, are low in patients with COPD [163,164]. Recently, Debigare *et al.* [134] reported that there was a significant disturbance in catabolic–anabolic metabolism in COPD, with a distinct shift toward catabolism, which may contribute to skeletal muscle wasting in patients with COPD.

Cardiovascular abnormalities

Although the progressive loss of lung function remains the primary limitation in COPD, there is also evidence that significant cardiovascular limitations exist in this population, particularly in more severe patients [165]. A study by Montes de Oca *et al.* [166] found oxygen pulse measured

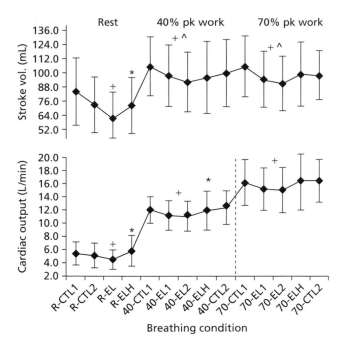

Figure 4.8 Influence of an expiratory load on stroke volume (SV) and cardiac output (CO) in healthy subjects. SV and CO are shown for each breathing condition (CTL, control; EL, expiratory loading; ELH, expiratory loading + voluntary hyperinflation) at three workloads. Vertical dotted lines indicate change in workload. Significance $P < 0.05$. (+) Average of two CTL conditions compared to EL (rest) or average EL conditions (exercise). (*) EL condition (rest) or average of EL conditions (exercise) compared with ELH condition. (#) ELH condition compared with average of two CTL conditions. (^) EL1 compared with EL2 (exercise) [169].

during exercise to be the best predictor of peak $\dot{V}_{O_2}$ in patients with an average FEV_1 of 0.79 L. Oelberg *et al.* [167] found a blunted cardiac output during exercise in patients with COPD relative to normal subjects. During activity, patients with COPD experience increased expiratory loads as well as progressive hyperinflation as ventilatory demands increase. In the resting state, expiratory loads created by positive pressure breathing reduce cardiac output likely via an effect of increasing pleural pressure and right atrial pressure and subsequently reducing venous return [168]. We recently studied healthy subjects to determine the influence of a small expiratory load (10 cm H_2O) on cardiac function during exercise (Fig. 4.8) [169]. We found a small but consistent drop in cardiac output (15–20%) resulting from a fall in stroke volume without complete compensation in heart rate. In COPD patients during exercise, studies have suggested some subjects may produce expiratory pressures > 20–30 cm H_2O [170]. Thus, it would be expected that these loads may further inhibit increases in stroke volume and possibly cardiac output during exercise.

There is also the potential separate influence of a chronic hyperinflation combined with a dynamic hyperinflation during exercise on cardiac output [170]. Because the heart and lungs share a common surface area, a progressive hyperinflation with chronic disease or dynamically with exercise may increase competition for intrathoracic space and inhibit cardiac filling via a change in cardiac compliance. We previously observed a significant fall in cardiac output with chest wall restriction (40% decline in VC) in healthy subjects [171]. This level of heart and lung competition for intrathoracic space may be similar to that observed in patients with severe COPD and hyperinflation.

Other changes associated with COPD also occur that may further reduce cardiac output responses to exercise in COPD patients. This includes a progressive pulmonary hypertension and right heart failure, polycythaemia and ineffective negative intrathoracic pressure generation by the diaphragm muscles [172,173].

CPET in evaluation of therapeutic interventions

Lung volume reduction surgery

The potential utility of CPET is highlighted by its emergence as an important tool in the evaluation of patients being considered for LVRS. The range of application of CPET in this patient group includes the determination of cardiopulmonary functional status and assessment of potential operative risk prior to surgery; the determination of exercise training prescription before and after LVRS; quantification and monitoring of the clinical response to surgery; and also definition of the underlying pathophysiologic mechanisms responsible for improvements in exercise performance resulting from LVRS [16,174–177].

In several studies, exercise capacity has been shown to improve after LVRS. This has been attributed to reduced hyperinflation, improved inspiratory muscle pressure generation (reduced drive to breathe), reduced oxygen cost of breathing and/or improved blood gas homoeostasis, all leading to reductions in the perception of dyspnoea [15,178]. The NETT was a large National Institutes of Health (NIH) funded trial of a total of 1218 patients with severe emphysema who underwent pulmonary rehabilitation and were randomly assigned to undergo LVRS or to receive continued medical treatment [16]. Overall in this trial, LVRS increased the chance of improved exercise capacity but did not bestow a survival advantage over medical therapy. It did yield a survival advantage for patients with both predominantly upper lobe emphysema and low baseline exercise capacity. Patients previously reported to be at high risk and those with non-upper-lobe emphysema and high baseline exercise capacity were considered poor candidates for LVRS because of increased mortality and insignificant functional gain. A 10-W change in cycle ergometry work rate was determined as a minimally clinically significant difference in this study in determining the impact of pulmonary rehabilitation on exercise tolerance.

Exercise training

Exercise training is a recommended, integral component of comprehensive pulmonary rehabilitation in patients with COPD and other chronic lung diseases [31,152,179,180]. CPET provides valuable information prior to exercise training to determine exercise capacity, anaerobic threshold, safety (ischaemia, arrhythmias, O_2 desaturation) and training intensity [181,182], and can be repeated following training to document improvement objectively and to refine training levels.

Exercise training to relieve dyspnoea

The goal of exercise training in lung disease patients is to carry improvement in performance and dyspnoea that is achieved with one form of exercise (e.g. treadmill walking) into activities of daily living. However, only since 1989 have controlled trials of rehabilitation regularly included measures of dyspnoea [183,184]. Exercise training appears to be a critical part of pulmonary rehabilitation programmes for reduction in dyspnoea [184,185].

Importantly, exercise training may decrease dyspnoea even when it does not improve exercise performance or mechanical efficiency [186]. Although most studies have utilized treadmills or cycles, weight training is also effective. Home-based exercise training has also been shown to improve dyspnoea and exercise performance [187].

Most commonly, exercise training for COPD patients is incorporated into a pulmonary rehabilitation programme that includes an education as well as an exercise component. A programme of dyspnoea management (including relaxation, breathing retraining, pacing, self-talk and panic control) without an exercise component was compared with general health education; neither improved dyspnoea nor 6-minute walking distance [188]. One study showed that treadmill training with or without nurse coaching was equally effective in reducing dyspnoea during exercise testing and with activities of daily living [189].

Several studies have recently explored intermittent exercise training as an alternative to continuous exercise training for COPD patients [190,191]. Healthy older individuals performing intermittent or continuous exercise training at the same absolute intensity with the same total work completed resulted in similar training adaptations [192]. Intermittent exercise performed at the same intensity as continuous exercise has been associated with lower ratings of perceived exertion and degree of dynamic hyperinflation in COPD patients [193]. It remains to be seen if intermittent exercise is a better mode of endurance exercise training in COPD patients. Two recent studies compared training adaptations with high-intensity intermittent (90 and 100% of W_{max}, respectively) with low-intensity continuous (60 and 50% of W_{peak}, respectively [190,191]). Both studies reported that both intermittent and continuous exercise training resulted in similar reductions in ratings of breathlessness during submaximal exercise.

Exercise training and skeletal muscle

Given that deconditioning of the skeletal muscle as a result of disuse is believed to be a major contributing factor to skeletal muscle dysfunction, it is no surprise that endurance exercise training is a significant component of any pulmonary rehabilitation programme. However, endurance training as a method of reversing skeletal muscle deconditioning has not always been an accepted part of pulmonary rehabilitation and has only recently become accepted practice (ATS guidelines) [31]. Indeed, in an early study of only seven COPD patients, Belman and Kendregan [194] reported that there were no significant changes in lower limb skeletal muscle enzymes following 6 weeks of endurance training (leg cycling). This led these authors to conclude that COPD patients were unable to exercise at an intensity high enough to induce a classic training response.

However, more recent studies have clearly demonstrated that endurance exercise training improves both the maximal and the submaximal exercise response in COPD patients [67,195,196]. In addition, endurance exercise training has been shown to alter both the morphological and histochemical properties of skeletal muscle [131,197]. In an important study, Maltais et al. [197] reported that 11 patients with severe COPD ($36 \pm 11\%$ FEV_1 % predicted) had a significant increase in the activity of CS and HAD following 12 weeks of cycle training (30 min, three times per week). The activity of other glycolytic enzymes PFK, LDH and HK did not change with endurance training.

In a similar study, Whittom et al. [131] examined the changes in fibre type proportions, the CSA of muscle fibres and the capillary to fibre ratio following 12 weeks of endurance training in 12 patients with COPD ($37 \pm 11\%$ FEV_1 % predicted). This study reported an 11% increase in $\dot{V}O_{2peak}$ and a significant increase in the CSA of the type I and IIa fibres. However, the proportion of type I, IIa, IIb, IIab fibres remained unchanged and there was no significant change in the number of capillaries per fibre.

Given the well-documented reductions in lower limb muscle strength with COPD, there have been few studies examining the effect of strength training in patients with COPD. In an early study, Simpson et al. [186] reported that 8 weeks of lower limb strength training in a group of 14

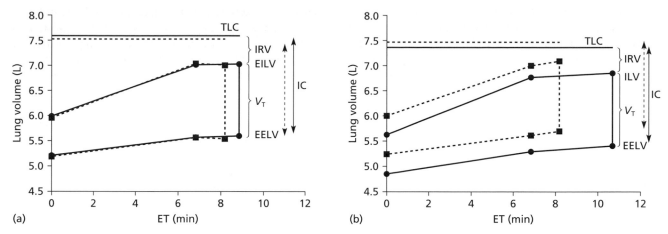

Figure 4.9 Operating lung volumes at rest and during exercise at baseline (■---) and after 42 days (●—) of treatment with placebo (a; $n = 91$) and tiotropium (b; $n = 96$). EELV, end-expiratory lung volume; EILV, end-inspiratory lung volume; IC, inspiratory capacity; IRV, inspiratory reserve volume; TLC, total lung capacity; V_T, tidal volume [14].

COPD patients resulted in a 16–44% increase in the maximal voluntary contraction (MVC). The resistance training consisted of three sets of 10 repetitions of three lower limb exercises. Subjects commenced training at 50% of one-repetition maximum (1-RM) and progressed to 85% of 1-RM in the final weeks. There were no significant changes in the MVC of 18 COPD patients who acted as a control.

Bernard *et al.* [198] compared the impact of 12 weeks of aerobic training with 12 weeks of strength and aerobic training in two groups of patients with moderate to severe COPD. Each training group completed 30 min of cycling exercise at 80% of the peak power achieved during the pretraining peak exercise test. The strength and aerobic training group completed an additional four strengthening exercises (two upper and two lower limb). While each group had a similar and significant increase in $\dot{V}O_{2peak}$ and 6-minute walking distance, the aerobic plus strengthening exercise group had a greater increase in quadriceps strength and cross-sectional area compared with the aerobic training alone group. These authors noted that strength training was well tolerated and elicited less dyspnoea than aerobic training in the subjects who participated in the study. Importantly, strength training provided some diversity to the training programme and tended to maintain motivation and interest in the participants.

A recent interesting study by Casuburi *et al.* [199] examined the effect of strength training in 47 men with COPD with and without testosterone supplementation. Subjects all had low testosterone levels prior to commencing the study. Subjects completed either 10 weeks of strength training or control (no strength training) with or without testosterone supplementation. The authors reported that the testosterone injections were well tolerated by all subjects. Testosterone injections alone resulted in a 2.3-kg increase in lean body mass (as measured using DEXA) and a

17% increase in the lower limb 1-RM (leg press). On the other hand, testosterone plus strength training resulted in a significantly greater increase in lean body mass (3.3 kg) and lower limb 1-RM (26.8%).

Bronchodilators

A number of studies have used CPET as a measure if effectiveness of pharmacological treatment [12–14,28,84, 200–203]. Both short- and long-acting β-agonists as well as short- and long-acting anticholinergic agents have been shown to improve exercise tolerance. This appears to be particularly true for the long-acting anticholinergic agents while the evidence for improved exercise capacity regarding the use of long-acting β₂-mimetics is not as clear [12]. In a randomized, double-blind, placebo-controlled, parallel group study, the long-acting anticholinergic agent tiotropium was shown to reduce chronic hyperinflation, allow for greater tidal volumes during exercise, reduce dyspnoea and improve endurance time (Fig. 4.9) [14,28]. At a standardized time point (isotime), IC was also greater consistent with reduced dynamic hyperinflation, despite an increase in $\dot{V}_E$. A second study has confirmed these data for improvements in chronic and exercise-induced dynamic hyperinflation, dyspnoea, endurance time and IC measured at isotime as well as demonstrating a sustained effect over 8 h [203]. Improvements in lung mechanics and the ventilatory responses to exercise were also observed in a study by O'Donnell *et al.* [13] using salmeterol and are also consistent with earlier work using shorter acting agents [84].

Interestingly, tiotropium combined with classic pulmonary rehabilitation has been shown to improve and, furthermore, enabled sustained (3 months after cessation of a 25-week pulmonary rehabilitation programme) improvement in exercise capacity (treadmill endurance time) beyond that achieved by rehabilitation by itself with usual treatment [204]. Presumably, more consistent management of airway patency attributed to longer acting anticholinergic agents appears to facilitate training by allowing higher intensity training associated with greater physiological benefit and then sustaining its effect at least in the short term after cessation of formal pulmonary rehabilitation in this challenging patient population. Future exercise training studies should evaluate the pharmacological agents providing maximal bronchodilatation combined with treatments described below in order to optimize therapeutic strategies.

Oxygen and low-density gas therapy

Oxygen therapy reduces pulmonary vascular resistance (in patients with hypoxaemia and pulmonary hypertension), reduces minute ventilation and likely reduces the peripheral chemoreceptor stimulation resulting from hypoxia [17,167,205–207]. All of these appear to lead to a substantial improvement in exercise capacity. There is also evidence that supplemental oxygen during exercise may be beneficial in non-hypoxaemic COPD patients [208,209]. This may also be because of a reduction in ventilation and dyspnoea, a blunting of respiratory drive as well as a mild bronchodilatation. By reducing $\dot{V}_E$ demand, the degree of expiratory flow limitation and lung hyperinflation is reduced [206].

Helium gas (79%) combined with oxygen (21%, heliox), results in a gas density that is approximately one-third that of air. Flow increases, particularly at the higher lung volumes, as a result of decreased turbulence with the large airways. This leads to a general reduction in the resistive work of breathing and increases the size of the maximal flow volume envelope in most patients with COPD. Palange *et al.* [30] found that, in a group of moderate to severe COPD patients exercising at 80% of their maximum power output, heliox resulted in a twofold increase in exercise endurance capacity. This was because of an increase in $\dot{V}_E$ and tidal volume during exercise and to a significant reduction in lung hyperinflation and dyspnoea at isotime. Other studies have combined increased inspired oxygen gases with low-density gases in an attempt to optimize benefits from both gases with beneficial results. Such a strategy used during rehabilitation may help achieve a greater skeletal muscle stimulus for training [17].

Pressure support ventilation

The application of inspiratory pressure support during exercise increases endurance, reduces dyspnoea, unloads the respiratory muscles and prolongs the development of exercise-induced lactataemia [210,211]. Proportional assist ventilation (PAV), a mode of ventilation that matches ventilator output to patient effort, is more tolerable for patients with COPD and is as effective at prolonging exercise as conventional inspiratory pressure support [212]. Hawkins *et al.* [213] used PAV as an aid to exercise training in patients with severe COPD and found that mean training intensity was 15% higher in the group that used ventilatory assistance vs subjects training without assistance. In addition, the group with PAV had a 33% increase in exercise capacity vs the non-PAV group which had a 15% increase post training. Although the number of subjects in this study was limited and it is difficult to perform a blinded study with this type of intervention, the findings of this study and previous work on exercise capacity with pressure support breathing suggest this may (along with oxygen, pharmacological treatment and low-density gases) provide a method to help minimize the cycle of decline in patients with COPD.

Conclusions

CPET has an integral role in assessing the health status of patients with COPD. Exercise tolerance may decline rapidly, and CPET provides important prognostic information as well as practical information regarding primary sources of limitation, degree of mechanical constraint, hypoxaemia and guidelines for exercise training. It also plays an important part in evaluating response to therapy using endurance cycle and treadmill protocols; however, future clinical trials may also use endurance shuttle walk tests as an assessment tool as they are sufficiently sensitive in discerninig response to bronchodilatator therapy in patients with COPD. Although patients with COPD are limited by marked reductions in maximal expiratory airflows, a progressive hyperinflation, ineffective inspiratory muscles and a rising elastic load (work and cost of breathing), the illness becomes a systemic syndrome resulting in deterioration of skeletal muscle function and cardiac limitations to exercise. Pharmacological management aimed at maximally maintaining airway patency and reducing hyperinflation, exercise training as a part of a comprehensive pulmonary rehabilitation programme, oxygen therapy and, finally, surgical therapies help to improve exercise capacity in this population and limit the rapid decline in functional capacity.

References

1 Wolkove N, Dajczman E, Colacone A *et al.* The relationship between pulmonary function and dyspnea in obstructive lung disease. *Chest* 1989;**96**:1247–51.

2 Hodgev VA, Kostianev SS, Torosian AA *et al.* Long-term changes in dyspnea lung function and exercise capacity in COPD patients. *Folia Med (Plovdiv)* 2004;**46**:12–7.

3 Pitcher WD, Cunningham HS. Oxygen cost of increasing tidal volume and diaphragm flattening in obstructive pulmonary disease. *J Appl Physiol* 1993;**74**:2750–6.

4 Gibson GJ. Pulmonary hyperinflation a clinical overview. *Eur Respir J* 1996;**9**:2640–9.

5 Agusti AG. Systemic effects of chronic obstructive pulmonary disease. *Novartis Found Symp* 2001;**234**:242–9; discussion 250–4.

6 Bernard S, LeBlanc P, Whittom F *et al.* Peripheral muscle weakness in patients with chronic obstructive pulmonary disease. *Am J Respir Crit Care Med* 1998;**158**:629–34.

7 Man WD, Soliman MG, Nikoletou D *et al.* Non-volitional assessment of skeletal muscle strength in patients with chronic obstructive pulmonary disease. *Thorax* 2003;**58**: 665–9.

8 Zeballos R, Weisman I. Modalities of clinical exercise testing. In: Weisman IM, Zeballos RJ, eds. *Clinical Exercise Testing.* Basel: Karger, 2002.

9 Pepin V, Saey D, Whittom F, LeBlanc P, Maltais F. Walking versus cycling: sensitivity to bronchodilation in chronic obstructive pulmonary disease. *Am J Respir Crit Care Med* 2005;**172**:1517–22.

10 Jones NL. *Clinical Exercise Testing*, 3rd edn. Philadelphia: Saunders, 1988: 325.

11 Johnson BD, Weisman IM, Zeballos RJ, Beck KC. Emerging concepts in the evaluation of ventilatory limitation during exercise: the exercise tidal flow–volume loop. *Chest* 1999; **116**:488–503.

12 Liesker JJ, Wijkstra PJ, Ten Hacken NH *et al.* A systematic review of the effects of bronchodilators on exercise capacity in patients with COPD. *Chest* 2002;**121**:597–608.

13 O'Donnell DE, Voduc N, Fitzpatrick M, Webb KA. Effect of salmeterol on the ventilatory response to exercise in chronic obstructive pulmonary disease. *Eur Respir J* 2004;**24**:86–94.

14 O'Donnell DE, Fluge T, Gerken F *et al.* Effects of tiotropium on lung hyperinflation dyspnoea and exercise tolerance in COPD. *Eur Respir J* 2004;**23**:832–40.

15 Tschernko EM, Gruber EM, Jaksch P *et al.* Ventilatory mechanics and gas exchange during exercise before and after lung volume reduction surgery. *Am J Respir Crit Care Med* 1998;**158**:1424–31.

16 Fishman A, Martinez F, Naunheim K *et al.* A randomized trial comparing lung-volume-reduction surgery with medical therapy for severe emphysema. *N Engl J Med* 2003;**348**: 2059–73.

17 Palange P, Crimi E, Pellegrino R, Brusaco V. Supplemental oxygen and heliox: 'new' tools for exercise training in chronic obstructive pulmonary disease. *Curr Opin Pulm Med* 2005;**11**:145–8.

18 Beck KC, Weisman IM. Methods for cardiopulmonary exercise testing. In: Weisman IM, Zeballos RJ, eds. *Clinical Exercise Testing.* Basel: Karger 2002: 43–59.

19 Beaver WL, Wasserman K, Whipp BJ. On-line computer analysis and breath-by-breath graphical display of exercise function tests. *J Appl Physiol* 1973;**34**:128–34.

20 Jones NL. *Clinical Exercise Testing*, 4th edn. Philadelphia: Saunders, 1997: xi; 259.

21 Zeballos RJ, Weisman IM. Behind the scenes of cardiopulmonary exercise testing. *Clin Chest Med* 1994;**15**:193–213.

22 Marciniuk DD, Watts RE, Gallagher CG. Reproducibility of incremental maximal cycle ergometer testing in patients with restrictive lung disease. *Thorax* 1993;**48**:894–8.

23 American Thoracic Society, American College of Chest Physicians. ATS/ACCP statement on cardiopulmonary exercise testing. *Am J Respir Crit Care Med* 2003;**167**:211–77.

24 Åstrand P-O, Rodahl K. *Textbook of Work Physiology: Physiological Bases of Exercise*, 3rd edn. McGraw-Hill series in health education physical education and recreation. New York: McGraw Hill, 1986: xii; 756.

25 Åstrand P-O, Rodahl K. *Textbook of Work Physiology: Physiological Bases of Exercise*, 2nd edn. New York: McGraw Hill, 1977: xviii; 681.

26 Jones NL, Makrides L, Hitchcock C, Chypchar T, McCartney N. Normal standards for an incremental progressive cycle ergometer test. *Am Rev Respir Dis* 1985;**131**:700–8.

27 O'Donnell DE, Lam M, Webb KA. Spirometric correlates of improvement in exercise performance after anticholinergic therapy in chronic obstructive pulmonary disease. *Am J Respir Crit Care Med* 1999;**160**:542–9.

28 O'Donnell DE, Magnussen H, Aguilaniu B *et al.* Spiriva (Tiotropium) improves exercise tolerance in COPD. *Am J Resp Crit Care Med* 2002;**165**:A227.

29 Oga T, Nishimura K, Tsukino M *et al.* The effects of oxitropium bromide on exercise performance in patients with stable chronic obstructive pulmonary disease: a comparison of three different exercise tests. *Am J Respir Crit Care Med* 2000;**161**:1897–901.

30 Palange P, Valli G, Onorati P *et al.* Effect of heliox on lung dynamic hyperinflation dyspnea and exercise endurance capacity in COPD patients. *J Appl Physiol* 2004;**97**:1637–42.

31 American Thoracic Society. Pulmonary rehabilitation – 1999. *Am J Respir Crit Care Med* 1999;**159**:1666–82.

32 ACC/AHA panel prepares guidelines for exercise testing. *Am Fam Physician* 1998;**57**:563–5.

33 European Respiratory Society. Clinical exercise testing. In: Roca J, Whipp BJ, eds. *European Respiratory Monograph* 1997: 164.

34 ERS Task Force on Standardization of Clinical Exercise Testing. Clinical exercise testing with reference to lung diseases: indications standardization and interpretation strategies. *Eur Respir J* 1997;**10**:2662–89.

35 Meyer T, Broocks A. Therapeutic impact of exercise on psychiatric diseases: guidelines for exercise testing and prescription. *Sports Med* 2000;**30**:269–79.

36 American College of Sports Medicine. *ACSM's Guidelines for Exercise Testing and Prescription*, 6th edn. Baltimore, MD: Williams & Wilkins, 2000: xvi; 368.

37 American College of Sports Medicine. *ACSM's Guidelines for Exercise Testing and Prescription*, 4th edn. Philadelphia: Lea & Febiger, 1991: xv; 314.

38 ACC/AHA guidelines for exercise testing: executive summary. A report of the American College of Cardiology/American Heart Association Task Force on Practice Guidelines (Committee on Exercise Testing) *Circulation* 1997;**96**:345–54.

39 Cotes JE. *Lung Function: Assessment and Application in Medicine*, 5th edn. Oxford: Blackwell Scientific Publications, 1993: 54–8.

40 Shepard RJ. Tests of maximum oxygen intake: a critical review. *Sports Med* 1984;**1**:99–124.

41 Cumming GR, Borysyk LM. Criteria for maximum oxygen uptake in men over 40 in a population survey. *Med Sci Sports* 1972;**4**:18–22.

42 Dempsey JA, Babcock MA. An integrative view of limitations to muscular performance. *Adv Exp Med Biol* 1995;**384**: 393–9.

43 Hamilton AL, Killian KJ, Summers E, Jones NL. Muscle strength symptom intensity and exercise capacity in patients with cardiorespiratory disorders. *Am J Respir Crit Care Med* 1995;**152**:2021–31.

44 Jones NL, Killian KJ. Exercise limitation in health and disease. *N Engl J Med* 2000;**343**:632–41.

45 Wasserman K *et al. Principles of Exercise Testing and Interpretation: Including Pathophysiology and Clinical Applications*, 3rd edn. Philadelphia: Lippincott Williams & Wilkins, 1999: 556.

46 Weisman IM, Zeballos RJ. Cardiopulmonary exercise testing. *Pulm Crit Care Update* 1995;**11**:1–9.

47 O'Donnell DE, Sanii R, Anthonisen NR, Younes M. Effect of dynamic airway compression on breathing pattern and respiratory sensation in severe chronic obstructive pulmonary disease. *Am Rev Respir Dis* 1987;**135**:912–8.

48 Wasserman K. *Principles of Exercise Testing and Interpretation*, 2nd edn. Philadelphia: Lea & Febiger, 1994: 479.

49 Flaherty KR, Wald J, Weisman IM *et al.* Unexplained exertional limitation: characterization in a large cohort discovered to have mitchondrial myopathy. *Am J Respir Crit Care Med* 2001;**164**:425–32.

50 Moser C, Tirakitsoontorn P, Nussbaum E, Newcomb R, Cooper DM. Muscle size and cardiorespiratory response to exercise in cystic fibrosis. *Am J Respir Crit Care Med* 2000; **162**:1823–7.

51 Wasserman K, Hansen JE, Sue DY, Whipp BJ, Casaburi R. *Principles of Exercise Testing and Interpretation*. Philadelphia: Lea & Febiger, 1987: 274.

52 Wasserman K. Coupling of external to cellular respiration during exercise: the wisdom of the body revisited. *Am J Physiol* 1994;**266**:E519–39.

53 American College of Sports Medicine, *ACSM's Guidelines for Exercise Testing and Prescription*, 5th edn. Baltimore: Williams & Wilkins, 1995: 373.

54 Johnson BD, Beck KC. Respiratory system responses to dynamic exercise. In: Weiler JM, ed. *Allergic and Respiratory Disease in Sports Medicine*. New York: Marcel Dekker, 1997: 1–34.

55 Johnson BD, Reddan WG, Seow KC, Dempsey JA. Mechanical constraints on exercise hyperpnea in a fit aging population. *Am Rev Respir Dis* 1991;**143**:968–77.

56 Johnson BD, Scanlon PD, Beck KC. Regulation of ventilatory capacity during exercise in asthmatics. *J Appl Physiol* 1995;**79**:892–901.

57 Babb TG. Mechanical ventilatory constraints in aging lung disease and obesity: perspectives and brief review. *Med Sci Sports Exerc* 1999;**31**:S12–22.

58 Klas JV, Dempsey JA. Voluntary versus reflex regulation of maximal exercise flow: volume loops. *Am Rev Respir Dis* 1989;**139**:150–6.

59 Aaron EA, Johnson BD, Seow CK, Dempsey JA. Oxygen cost of exercise hyperpnea: measurement. *J Appl Physiol* 1992;**72**:1810–7.

60 Johnson BD, Saupe KW, Dempsey JA. Mechanical constraints on exercise hyperpnea in endurance athletes. *J Appl Physiol* 1992;**73**:874–86.

61 Babb TG, Viggiano R, Hurley B, Staats B, Rodarte JR. Effect of mild-to-moderate airflow limitation on exercise capacity. *J Appl Physiol* 1991;**70**:223–30.

62 Brooks GA. Anaerobic threshold: review of the concept and directions for future research. *Med Sci Sports Exerc* 1985;**17**: 22–34.

63 Brooks GA. Current concepts in lactate exchange. *Med Sci Sports Exerc* 1991;**23**:895–906.

64 Myers J, Ashley E. Dangerous curves: a perspective on exercise lactate and the anaerobic threshold. *Chest* 1997;**111**:787–95.

65 Sue DY, Wasserman K, Moricca RB, Casaburi R. Metabolic acidosis during exercise in patients with chronic obstructive pulmonary disease: use of the V-slope method for anaerobic threshold determination. *Chest* 1988;**94**:931–8.

66 Wagner PD. Determinants of maximal oxygen transport and utilization. *Annu Rev Physiol* 1996;**58**:21–50.

67 Casaburi R, Patessio A, Ioli F *et al.* Reductions in exercise lactic acidosis and ventilation as a result of exercise training in patients with obstructive lung disease. *Am Rev Respir Dis* 1991;**143**:9–18.

68 Weisman IM, Zeballos RJ. Integrative approach to the interpretation of cardiopulmonary exercise testing in clinical exercise testing progress. In: Weisman IM, Zeballos RJ, eds. *Respiratory Research*, vol 32. Basel: Karger, 2002: 300–22.

69 Sun XG, Hansen JE, Garatachea N, Storer TW, Wasserman K. Ventilatory efficiency during exercise in healthy subjects. *Am J Respir Crit Care Med* 2002;**166**:1443–8.

70 Sun XG, Hansen JE, Oudiz RJ, Wasserman K. Gas exchange detection of exercise-induced right-to-left shunt in patients with primary pulmonary hypertension. *Circulation* 2002; **105**:54–60.

71 Anthonisen NR, Fleetham JA. Ventilation: total alveolar and dead space. In: Fishman AP, ed. *Handbook of Physiology: The Respiratory System: Gas Exchange*. Bethesda MD: American Physiological Society, 1987: 113–7.

72 Lewis DA, Sietsema KE, Casaburi R, Sue DY. Inaccuracy of noninvasive estimates of VD/VT in clinical exercise testing. *Chest* 1994;**106**:1476–80.

73 Wagner PD. Ventilation–perfusion matching during exercise. *Chest* 1992;**101**:192S–8S.

74 Ries AL, Farrow JT, Clausen JL. Accuracy of two ear oximeters at rest and during exercise in pulmonary patients. *Am Rev Respir Dis* 1985;**132**:685–9.

75 Severinghaus JW, Naifeh KH, Koh SO. Errors in 14 pulse oximeters during profound hypoxia. *J Clin Monit* 1989;**5**: 72–81.

76 Zeballos RJ, Weisman IM. Reliability of noninvasive oximetry in black subjects during exercise and hypoxia. *Am Rev Respir Dis* 1991;**144**:1240–4.

77 American Association for Respiratory Care. AARC Clinical Practice Guideline. Exercise testing for evaluation of hypoxemia and/or desaturation. *Respir Care* 1992;**37**:907–12.

78 Borg G. Subjective effort and physical activities. *Scand J Rehab Med* 1978;**6**:108–13.

79 Borg GA. Psychophysical bases of perceived exertion. *Med Sci Sports Exerc* 1982;**14**:377–81.

80 Aitken RC. Measurement of feelings using visual analogue scales. *Proc R Soc Med* 1969;**62**:989–93.

81 Mahler DA, Guyatt GH, Jones PW. Clinical measurement of dyspnea in dyspnea lung biology. In: Mahler DA, ed. *Health and Disease*, vol III. New York: Marcel Dekker, 1998: 149–98.

82 Aaron EA, Seow KC, Johnson BD, Dempsey JA. Oxygen cost of exercise hyperpnea: implications for performance. *J Appl Physiol* 1992;**72**:1818–25.

83 Johnson BD, Dempsey JA. Demand vs capacity in the aging pulmonary system. *Exerc Sport Sci Rev* 1991;**19**:171–210.

84 Belman MJ, Botnick WC, Shin JW. Inhaled bronchodilators reduce dynamic hyperinflation during exercise in patients with chronic obstructive pulmonary disease. *Am J Respir Crit Care Med* 1996;**153**:967–75.

85 O'Donnell DE, Lam M, Webb KA. Measurement of symptoms lung hyperinflation and endurance during exercise in chronic obstructive pulmonary disease. *Am J Respir Crit Care Med* 1998;**158**:1557–65.

86 Musch TI. Elevated diaphragmatic blood flow during submaximal exercise in rats with chronic heart failure. *Am J Physiol* 1993;**265**:H1721–6.

87 Harms CA, Wetter TJ, St Croix CM, Pegelow DF, Dempsey JA. Effects of respiratory muscle work on exercise performance. *J Appl Physiol* 2000;**89**:131–8.

88 Dempsey JA, Johnson BD. Demand vs capacity in the healthy pulmonary system. *Schweiz Z Sportmed* 1992;**40**: 55–64.

89 Dempsey JA. JB Wolffe Memorial Lecture: Is the lung built for exercise? *Med Sci Sports Exerc* 1986;**18**:143–55.

90 Johnson BD, Badr MS, Dempsey JA. Impact of the aging pulmonary system on the response to exercise. *Clin Chest Med* 1994;**15**:229–46.

91 Barbera JA, Roca J, Ramirez J *et al.* Gas exchange during exercise in mild chronic obstructive pulmonary disease: correlation with lung structure. *Am Rev Respir Dis* 1991; **144**:520–5.

92 Yamamoto T, Kimura H, Okada O *et al.* Arterial and mixed venous oxygen desaturation during incremental exercise in patients with chronic pulmonary disease. *Intern Med* 1998; **37**:280–5.

93 Christensen CC, Ryg MS, Edvardsen A, Skjonsberg OH. Effect of exercise mode on oxygen uptake and blood gases in COPD patients. *Respir Med* 2004;**98**:656–60.

94 American Thoracic Society. Dyspnea mechanisms assessment and management: a consensus statement. *Am J Respir Crit Care Med* 1999;**159**:321–40.

95 ZuWallack RL, Mahler DA, Reilly D *et al.* Salmeterol plus theophylline combination therapy in the treatment of COPD. *Chest* 2001;**119**:1661–70.

96 Gelb AF, McKenna RJ Jr, Brenner M, Epstein JD, Zamel N. Lung function 5 yr after lung volume reduction surgery for emphysema. *Am J Respir Crit Care Med* 2001;**163**:1562–6.

97 Corfield DR, Fink GR, Ramsey SC *et al.* Evidence for limbic system activation during CO_2-stimulated breathing in man. *J Physiol* 1995;**488**:77–84.

98 Liotti M, Brannan S, Egan G *et al.* Brain responses associated with consciousness of breathlessness (air hunger). *Proc Natl Acad Sci U S A* 2001;**98**:2035–40.

99 Peiffer C *et al.* Neural substrates for the perception of acutely induced dyspnea. *Am J Respir Crit Care Med* 2001;**163**:951–7.

100 Brannan S, Liotti M, Egan G *et al.* Neuroimaging of cerebral activations and deactivations associated with hypercapnia and hunger for air. *Proc Natl Acad Sci U S A* 2001;**98**:2029–34.

101 Parsons LM, Egan G, Liotti M *et al.* Neuroimaging evidence implicating cerebellum in the experience of hypercapnia and hunger for air. *Proc Natl Acad Sci U S A* 2001;**98**:2041–6.

102 Lane R, Adams L. Metabolic acidosis and breathlessness during exercise and hypercapnia in man. *J Physiol (Lond)* 1993;**461**:47–61.

103 Freedman S, Lane R, Guz A. Breathlessness and respiratory mechanics during reflex or voluntary hyperventilation in patients with chronic airflow limitation. *Clin Sci* 1987;**73**: 311–8.

104 Lane R, Adams L, Guz A. Is low-level respiratory resistive loading during exercise perceived as breathlessness? *Clin Sci* 1987;**73**:627–34.

105 Banzett RB, Lansing RW, Reid MB, Adams L, Brown R. 'Air hunger' arising from increased P_{CO_2} in mechanically ventilated quadriplegics. *Respir Physiol* 1989;**76**:53–68.

106 Banzett RB, Lansing RW, Brown R *et al.* 'Air hunger' from increased P_{CO_2} persists after complete neuromuscular block in humans. *Respir Physiol* 1990;**81**:1–17.

107 Gandevia SC, Killian K, McKenzie DK *et al.* Respiratory sensations cardiovascular control kinaesthesia and transcranial stimulation during paralysis in humans. *J Physiol (Lond)* 1993;**470**:85–107.

108 O'Donnell DE, Webb KA. Exertional breathlessness in patients with chronic airflow limitation: the role of lung hyperinflation. *Am Rev Respir Dis* 1993;**148**:1351–7.

109 Lahrmann H, Wild M, Wanke T *et al.* Neural drive to the diaphragm after lung volume reduction surgery. *Chest* 1999 **116**:1593–600.

110 van't Hul A, Kwakkel G, Gosselink R. The acute effects of noninvasive ventilatory support during exercise on exercise endurance and dyspnea in patients with chronic obstructive pulmonary disease: a systematic review. *J Cardiopulm Rehabil* 2002;**22**:290–7.

111 Chetta A, Gerra G, Foresi A *et al.* Personality profiles and breathlessness perception in outpatients with different gradings of asthma. *Am J Respir Crit Care Med* 1998;**157**:116–22.

112 Belman MJ, Brooks LR, Ross DJ, Mohsenifar Z. Variability of breathlessness measurement in patients with chronic obstructive pulmonary disease. *Chest* 1991;**99**:566–71.

113 Smoller JW, Pollack MH, Otto MW, Rosenbaum JF, Kradin RL. Panic anxiety dyspnea and respiratory disease: theoretical and clinical considerations. *Am J Respir Crit Care Med* 1996;**154**:6–17.

the nature of the mechanical impediment to breathing which leads to ventilatory failure in COPD patients is now better understood, and FEV_1 is no longer considered a useful marker of respiratory loading.

Theory and methods of control of breathing

Mouth occlusion pressure

Responses to various stimuli are expressed quantitatively by the 'sensitivity' or input–output relationship of the system that controls breathing. The input can be simplified by carrying out experiments in which a single stimulus, such as P_{CO_2} or P_{O_2}, is the only important variable, but it has been more difficult to find a good measure of the output of the system. In general, however, the most commonly used output variable is pulmonary ventilation. It has long been recognized that in the presence of mechanical loading of breathing (e.g. increased elastance and flow resistance of the respiratory system), the ventilatory output reflects both how much the patient 'wants' to breathe, an issue directly involving respiratory control, and how much his or her mechanical abnormality 'allows' him or her to breathe in response to a given level of respiratory stimulation, an issue that involves control of breathing only indirectly. To circumvent this problem, responses to respiratory stimuli have been assessed in terms of oxygen consumption of the respiratory muscles, mechanical work rate of the respiratory muscles, pleural pressure swings and diaphragmatic electromyography (EMG). All of these output variables involve measurements that are technically complex and, with the exception of the O_2 cost of breathing, cause discomfort to patients, for these measurements involve the use of oesophageal balloons or electrodes. The mouth pressure generated by the inspiratory muscles against an airway occluded at end-expiration has been proposed as a useful alternative [8]. The subject is allowed to breathe through a mouthpiece with a valve arranged so that he or she breathes in through one tube and out through another. Taking care that the subject cannot see them and is unable to anticipate the manoeuvre, the operator closes off the inspiratory tube while the subject is breathing out. Unaware of this manoeuvre, the subject begins his or her next inspiration in the usual way, but now generates negative pressure in the mouthpiece instead of taking in air. After a short interval he or she realizes that the tube is blocked and makes some abnormal movement, but the pressure generated in the first 0.1 second ($P_{0.1}$) is an expression of the force generated by his or her inspiratory muscles in a more or less isometric contraction, under the same respiratory neural stimulus as the preceding unobstructed

breaths. Reduced to its essentials, the apparatus required to measure the mouth occlusion pressure consists only of a mouthpiece, valve, pressure transducer and recorder, and it can easily be brought to a patient on the ward. Unlike inspiratory work or diaphragm EMG it requires no oesophageal balloons or electrodes, and a minimum of electronic apparatus and skill. In fact, it offers no more trouble than the conventional spirometric methods.

A full account and critique of the mouth occlusion pressure technique is provided elsewhere [8,9]. Briefly, $P_{0.1}$ depends on both: (a) the neural drive to the inspiratory muscles (a summation of the chemical, reflex, higher nervous, brainstem and spinal inputs which are eventually integrated at the level of the inspiratory motor neurons in the spinal cord); and (b) the effectiveness of the inspiratory muscles as pressure generators. The latter depends on the lung volume and geometry of the respiratory system [10]. In general, with increasing lung volume, the diaphragmatic and extradiaphragmatic inspiratory muscle fibres become shorter, and hence develop less force for a given neural drive (force–length relationship). Furthermore, with increasing lung volume, the radius of curvature (r) of the diaphragm increases (flatter diaphragm) and hence, because of the Laplace relationship ($P = 2T/r$), for a given tension T (which is related to force) less pressure is developed. Thus, $P_{0.1}$ is an index of *neuromuscular inspiratory drive* representing the pressure available to produce the changes in lung volume or ventilation.

Analysis of the respiratory cycle

The breathing movements can be regarded as a mechanical event in the respiratory control mechanism, which is both an expression of 'output' and a source of 'input' to the respiratory controller. The spirogram, simple as it looks, is the result of an extremely complex process which, to some extent, can be decoded by appropriate analysis. Further, it is the manifestation of control of breathing that is most accessible to clinical observation.

The respiratory cycle consists of an ascending limb, inspiration, and a descending limb, expiration. It can be characterized schematically by the volume displaced (V_T), duration of inspiration (T_I) and duration of expiration (T_E), as well as by the mean inspiratory flow (V_T/T_I). There is ample evidence that T_I, T_E and V_T/T_I can be independently controlled by various mechanisms such as reflexes and chemoreceptor stimulation [11–16]. The interaction of these mechanisms results in a given breathing cycle. Although the nature of the interaction is not fully understood, as a first useful approximation one can regard the breathing cycle as the result of a 'driving mechanism' (inspiratory neurons firing) turned on and off by cyclic 'timing mechanisms' [14–16].

Ventilation equations

The classic equation defines ventilation ($\dot{V}_E$) as the product of tidal volume and respiratory frequency (f):

$$\dot{V}_E = V_T \times f \tag{5.1}$$

However, considering the breathing cycle as being the result of a 'driving' and a 'timing' mechanism, another equation to partition ventilation has been proposed [17]:

$$\dot{V}_E = (V_T/T_I) \times (T_I/T_{TOT}) \tag{5.2}$$

where T_I/T_{TOT} is the ratio of inspiratory to total breathing cycle duration and is commonly referred to as the inspiratory duty cycle.

The advantage of analysing ventilation by equation 5.2 is that it partitions ventilation into two components: one related to neuromuscular inspiratory drive (V_T/T_I) and the other (T_I/T_{TOT}) reflecting the timing mechanism. A change in pulmonary ventilation can result from a change in V_T/T_I or in T_I/T_{TOT}, or both.

Alveolar ventilation equation

Clinical evaluation of control of breathing has often been based on measurement of the ventilatory response to CO_2 [18], hypoxia [19] and muscular exercise. While these responses provide useful information, assessment of control of breathing during air breathing at rest is the fundamental first step. In fact, having defined ventilatory failure in terms of an increased Pa_{CO_2} *during resting breathing*, it seems imperative to explain how this is brought about. Clearly, this requires the study of control of breathing under the conditions prevailing at the time when the blood sample was taken to obtain the Pa_{CO_2}.

The Pa_{CO_2} is given by the ratio of metabolic CO_2 production ($\dot{V}_{CO_2}$) to alveolar ventilation, and can be expressed in the following form:

$$Pa_{CO_2} = k \times \dot{V}_{CO_2}/\dot{V}_E (1 - V_D/V_T) \tag{5.3}$$

where k is constant, $\dot{V}_E$ is minute ventilation, V_T is tidal volume and V_D is physiological dead space. The latter can be computed from measurements of the other variables in equation 5.3.

Inspection of equation 5.3 reveals that the breathing pattern plays an important part in determining Pa_{CO_2}; for a given $\dot{V}_E$ and V_D, the alveolar ventilation will decrease the smaller the V_T (and hence the higher the respiratory frequency).

Mechanical impediment to breathing

The problem in maintaining a normal Pa_{CO_2} in COPD is due to impaired respiratory mechanics. Implicit in the definition of this disease, there is initially increased inspiratory and expiratory flow-resistance, but the latter reverts in time to tidal expiratory flow limitation with concurrent dynamic pulmonary hyperinflation. It is this that causes the main impediment to breathing in COPD. In this disease the abnormalities in respiratory statics are not by themselves severe, although with severe hyperinflation the compliance may be reduced because tidal breathing occurs in the flat upper portion of the static volume–pressure curve of the respiratory system. Although the inspiratory flow-resistance may be markedly increased, the resistive inspiratory work during resting breathing is relatively low because at rest the inspiratory flow is low. In COPD the main impediment to breathing is neither elastic nor resistive but is represented by an inspiratory threshold load (i.e. intrinsic positive end-expiratory pressure, PEEPi), which is brought about by dynamic hyperinflation.

Dynamic hyperinflation (DH). In normal individuals at rest, the end-expiratory lung volume (functional residual capacity, FRC) corresponds to the relaxation volume (Vr) of the respiratory system (i.e. the lung volume at which the elastic recoil pressure of the respiratory system is zero) [20]. Pulmonary hyperinflation, which is defined as an increase in FRC above the predicted normal range, may be caused by increased Vr as a result of loss of lung recoil (e.g. emphysema) and/or dynamic pulmonary hyperinflation, which is said to be present when the FRC exceeds Vr. Dynamic hyperinflation exists whenever the duration of expiration is insufficient to allow the lungs to deflate to Vr prior to the next inspiration. This may occur when expiratory flow is impeded (e.g. increased airway resistance) and/or expiratory time shortened (e.g. increased breathing frequency). Expiratory flow may also be reduced by other mechanisms, such as persistent contraction of the inspiratory muscles during expiration and expiratory narrowing of the glottic aperture. In COPD patients hyperinflation is very common, and is mainly caused by tidal expiratory flow limitation [21–23].

Expiratory flow limitation (EFL). The term expiratory flow limitation should be used only to describe a condition in which expiratory flow cannot be augmented at a given lung volume by further increasing pleural and therefore alveolar pressure. This phenomenon is exhibited by both normal subjects and patients with respiratory disorders during correctly performed maximal forced expiratory manoeuvres in which, from peak expiratory flow, expiratory flow rates cannot be increased by increasing the expiratory effort and, thus, are maximal [24,25].

While normal subjects and athletes do not exhibit EFL even during maximal exercise [26], in COPD patients tidal EFL is commonly present even at rest [21,22].

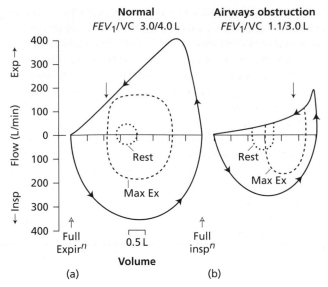

Figure 5.2 Flow–volume curves of a normal subject (a) and a patient with severe COPD (b). Tidal flow–volume loops at rest (dotted lines) and maximum exercise (Max ex, dashed lines) are compared with maximum flow–volume loops (outer solid lines). Forced expiratory volume in 1 s (FEV_1) (vertical arrows) is below the resting end-expiratory volume in the normal subject but well above in the COPD patient. Expir[n], expiration; insp[n], inspiration; VC, vital capacity. (From Leaver and Pride [27] with permission.)

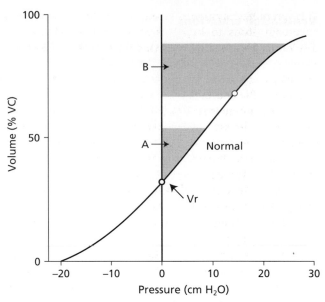

Figure 5.3 Static volume–pressure diagram of relaxed respiratory system showing the increase in work caused by dynamic hyperinflation. VC, vital capacity; Vr, relaxation volume of respiratory system. A: elastic work of breath started from relaxation volume (normal); B: work of similar breath to A but started from higher volume than Vr. In case B, the intrinsic positive end-expiratory pressure is 15 cm H_2O. See text for further information.

Two main mechanisms promote the occurrence of tidal EFL: reduction of expiratory flow reserve and increase in ventilatory (flow) requirements. The expiratory flow reserve in the tidal volume range is given by the difference between the maximal flows available and the actual tidal flows developed during expiration. In normal individuals at rest the expiratory flow reserve is very high (Fig. 5.2a), while in patients with severe COPD there may not be any flow reserve left even at rest (Fig. 5.2b). In the latter condition, ventilation can only be increased by augmenting the operating lung volume with a concurrent increase in expiratory flow reserve, or by decreasing the duration of inspiration with a concurrent increase in time available for expiration.

Because the FRC is lower in the supine position than sitting [20], with a concomitant reduction in expiratory flow reserve, tidal EFL is an earlier manifestation in the supine position [21,22]. With ageing, there is a preferential decrease of maximal expiratory flow at low lung volume [28], which makes elderly individuals more susceptible to developing tidal EFL, particularly in the supine position.

The increased ventilatory requirements of COPD patients [7] augment the expiratory flow requirements because of greater tidal volume and faster respiratory frequency, promoting tidal EFL. In COPD patients who do not exhibit EFL at rest but have little expiratory flow reserve, EFL will occur at relatively low levels of exercise, while patients with larger flow reserve may achieve greater exercise levels without developing EFL [23].

Effects of dynamic hyperinflation on inspiratory work. Figure 5.3 illustrates the pressure required to overcome the static recoil of the respiratory system for the same tidal volume (20% of vital capacity, VC) inhaled from Vr (34% VC) and from an increased end-expiratory lung volume corresponding to 67% VC. As shown by the hatched areas in Figure 5.3, the static work increases approximately fivefold when the breath is inhaled from 67% VC (case B) relative to the breath taken from the Vr (case A). Clearly, dynamic hyperinflation implies an increase in static work of breathing (WOB). Furthermore, as lung volume increases, there is a decreased effectiveness of the inspiratory muscles as pressure generators because their fibres become shorter (force–length relationship) and their geometrical arrangement changes [10]. Thus, in COPD patients there is a vicious cycle: the inspiratory flow-resistive WOB is invariably increased because of airway obstruction but, more importantly, as a result of hyperinflation, there is increase in WOB resulting from PEEPi (see below) and impairment of the mechanical performance of the inspiratory muscles.

This promotes dyspnoea and exercise limitation, and eventually leads to hypercapnic ventilatory failure and inspiratory muscle fatigue [10,21,29].

Intrinsic positive end-expiratory pressure (PEEPi). Under normal conditions, the end-expiratory elastic recoil pressure of the respiratory system is zero (see Fig. 5.3, case A). In this case, the alveolar pressure becomes sub-atmospheric and gas flows into the lungs as soon as the inspiratory muscles contract. When breathing takes place at lung volumes greater than Vr, the end-expiratory elastic recoil pressure of the respiratory system is positive (15 cm H_2O in case B of Fig. 5.3). The elastic recoil pressure present at end-expiration has been termed auto- or intrinsic positive end-expiratory pressure (PEEPi) [30,31]. When PEEPi is present, onset of inspiratory muscle activity and inspiratory flow are not synchronous; inspiratory flow starts only when the pressure developed by the inspiratory muscles exceeds PEEPi and hence the alveolar pressure becomes sub-atmospheric. In this respect, PEEPi acts as an inspiratory threshold load, which increases the inspiratory effort. This places a major burden on the inspiratory muscles. In fact, the work performed by PEEPi in case B of Figure 5.3 is given by the product of PEEPi and V_T, which represents most of the hatched area. The remainder of this area is elastic work.

Because the static volume–pressure relationship of the respiratory system is approximately linear (see Fig. 5.3), PEEPi is approximated by the product of the static elastance of respiratory system (Est, rs, the reciprocal of the slope in Fig. 5.3) and the magnitude of dynamic hyperinflation (i.e. the increase of FRC above Vr):

$$PEEPi = Est, rs \ (FRC - Vr) \qquad (5.4)$$

This implies that dynamic hyperinflation (FRC – Vr) and PEEPi are closely related indices. However, in actively breathing subjects it is very difficult to determine PEEPi [32], whereas the degree of dynamic hyperinflation can be readily assessed from measurements of the inspiratory capacity (see below).

Methods for assessing EFL. Comparison between maximal and tidal flow–volume loops has been widely used to detect EFL, which is assumed to be present when the tidal expiratory flow impinges on or exceeds the maximal expiratory flow–volume curve (see Fig. 5.2b) [22,24]. However, this method is not valid because of the different volume and time history between resting breathing and the FVC manoeuvre [21,22,33]. In fact, because the inflation volume and speed of inspiration during resting breathing are necessarily different from those obtained during the FVC manoeuvre, it is axiomatic that detection of flow-limitation based on comparison of tidal with maximal flow–volume curves is not valid.

Recently, the negative expiratory pressure (NEP) method has been introduced to detect EFL [22,34]. A small negative pressure is applied during tidal expiration, thus widening the pressure gradient between the alveoli and the airway opening. In the absence of EFL, with NEP there is an increase in expiratory flow compared with the preceding control breath. In contrast, in the presence of EFL the expiratory flow does not increase throughout the entire or part of the tidal expiration over that of the preceding control expiration. With the NEP method the volume and time history is not a problem because these are necessarily the same during the control and NEP test breaths.

Methods for assessing pulmonary hyperinflation. Pulmonary hyperinflation is commonly assessed through the measurement of the FRC with body plethysmography. In patients with severe airway obstruction, however, this method may overestimate the actual FRC because during the panting manoeuvre the transmission of alveolar pressure to the mouth is delayed by increased airway resistance [35]. On the other hand, measurements with the nitrogen washout or helium dilution methods may underestimate the FRC because of gas trapping in the lung. However, in patients with tidal EFL at rest the increase of FRC is accompanied by a reduction in resting inspiratory capacity (IC). In contrast to FRC, measurement of IC is simple, cheap and reliable, providing a useful tool for the indirect assessment of pulmonary hyperinflation [36]. Indeed, in COPD patients a reduction of IC implies dynamic hyperinflation.

Assessment of control of breathing in COPD

Stable patients at rest

Chronic obstructive lung disease is characterized by: (a) impaired pulmonary gas exchange; (b) changes in the mechanical properties of the ventilatory apparatus which increase the load on the respiratory muscles; and (c) decreased effectiveness of the inspiratory muscles as pressure generators as a result of thoracic overinflation. Despite these disadvantages, some patients are able to maintain adequate ventilation while others develop hypercapnia. Originally, it was suggested that patients who do not develop CO_2 retention are 'fighters', because they increase sufficiently the inspiratory drive to compensate for their impaired respiratory function, while the 'non-fighters' have defective inspiratory drive, and hence exhibit CO_2 retention [6]. If this hypothesis is correct, patients with CO_2 retention should have high $P_{0.1}$ values, while patients with CO_2 retention should exhibit $P_{0.1}$ values lower than the non-CO_2 retainers. However, Šorli *et al.* [7] showed that there

Table 5.1 Mean values (± SD) of pulmonary gas exchange data in 15 stable COPD patients breathing air at rest. (From Šorli *et al.* [7] with permission.)

	Pa_{CO_2} (mmHg)	$\dot{V}_E$ (L/min)	V_T (L)	V_D (L)	$\dot{V}_{CO_2}$ (L/min)	$P_{0.1}$ (cm H_2O)
Group A ($n = 8$)	38 ± 4	10.6 ± 1.8	0.71 ± 0.09	0.37 ± 0.07	0.26 ± 0.03	3.3 ± 0.10
Group B ($n = 7$)	50 ± 9	9.4 ± 1.0	0.56 ± 00.07	0.32 ± 0.05	0.28 ± 0.05	4.3 ± 0.13
Group A vs group B	$P < 0.005$	NS	$P < 0.01$	NS	NS	NS

$P_{0.1}$, mouth occlusion pressure at 0.1 s; $\dot{V}_{CO_2}$, carbon dioxide output; V_D, physiologic dead space; $\dot{V}_E$, pulmonary ventilation; V_T, tidal volume.

was no difference in $P_{0.1}$ between hypercapnic and non-hypercapnic patients (Table 5.1), both exhibiting higher $P_{0.1}$ values than normal individuals ($P < 0.001$). Why then do some patients retain CO_2? This can be answered by analysis according to equation 5.3. As shown in Table 5.1, there is no difference in $\dot{V}_E$, V_D and $\dot{V}_{CO_2}$ between patients without and with CO_2 retention, although the values are higher than normal. Tidal volume, on the contrary, is significantly lower in the hypercapnic patients (group B). Thus, by use of equation 5.3, it is possible to conclude that CO_2 retention in COPD patients is closely associated with decreased V_T. A decreased V_T, however, can be caused by decreased inspiratory flow or shortened inspiratory duration, or both. As shown in Figure 5.4, the mean inspiratory flow (V_T/T_I) does not differ between patients with and without CO_2 retention; in both it is higher than normal.

That V_T is significantly smaller in hypercapnic compared with non-hypercapnic patients has been confirmed by several cross-sectional studies [37–41]. Furthermore, in a longitudinal investigation it has been shown that the increase in Pa_{CO_2} is associated with a decrease in V_T, with no significant change in respiratory frequency [42]. However, some evidence suggests that in patients with severe hypercapnia ($Pa_{CO_2} > 55$ mmHg) a reduction of $\dot{V}_E$ may contribute to hypercapnia [40].

As shown in Figure 5.4, the reduction of V_T in the hypercapnic patients (group B) is caused entirely by reduced T_I, while V_T/T_I is actually higher than normal. This was initially attributed to vagally mediated reflexes originating from the irritant and J-receptors within the lung [7]. While such mediation is not excluded, it is likely that it mainly reflects uncoupling of neuromuscular and spirometric timing resulting from the presence of DH and PEEPi [43]. As a result of PEEPi, there is a delay between the onset of inspiratory muscle activity, as reflected by negative swing in pleural pressure, and the onset of inspiratory flow, the time-lag depending on the time taken by the pressure developed by the inspiratory muscles to balance PEEPi [32,43]. Thus, spirometric T_I underestimates the neuromuscular T_I, and the opposite occurs in terms of T_E. In contrast, in the absence of DH and PEEPi, the onset of neuromuscular and spirometric inspiration are essentially synchronous, and the pressure developed by the inspiratory muscles is expended solely to overcome the elastance and resistance offered by the respiratory system. Thus, in patients with PEEPi, a large part of the inspiratory muscle effort may be wasted in overcoming PEEPi and, as a result, V_T is reduced. In fact, Haluszka *et al.* [44] found a significant correlation between Pa_{CO_2} and PEEPi in stable COPD patients. In line with Šorli *et al.* [7], they also observed that V_T was significantly lower in the hypercapnic patients, and interpreted their results as follows. Increasing severity of COPD results in increased flow resistance leading eventually to tidal EFL, which in turn causes DH and PEEPi. Pulmonary hyperinflation results not only in increased work of breathing because of PEEPi but also in decreased

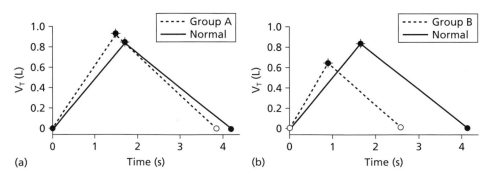

(a)   (b)

Figure 5.4 Average spirograms at rest in non-hypercapnic (a) and hypercapnic (b) COPD patients compared with normal subjects. Bars placed at peak inspiration indicate 1 SD. Mean inspiratory flow (V_T/T_I) is represented by slope of ascending limb of schematic spirogram. V_T, tidal volume. (From Šorli *et al.* [7] with permission.)

effectiveness of the inspiratory muscles as a pressure generators [10]. When DH and PEEPi reach a critical level, an adequate V_T can no longer be maintained because of impending inspiratory muscle fatigue [45]. Thus, patients reduce tidal volume and alveolar ventilation, with a concomitant increase in $Paco_2$. If hypercapnic COPD patients are asked to voluntarily restore V_T to normal values, they invariably develop diaphragmatic fatigue, suggesting that shallow breathing may be an adaptive strategy used to avoid inspiratory muscle fatigue. Regional differences in PEEPi enhance maldistribution of pulmonary ventilation and impaired gas exchange, contributing to increased $Paco_2$ and decreased Pao_2 [46]. In short, DH and PEEPi have a pivotal role in causing hypercapnic ventilatory failure in COPD.

In actively breathing subjects in whom assessment of PEEPi is not feasible [32], the decrease in IC is commonly used as a surrogate marker of DH and PEEPi. Because in COPD the respiratory elastance is essentially normal (~10 cm H_2O/L), according to equation 5.4 a decrease in IC of 1 L implies a PEEPi of approximately 10 cm H_2O.

Diaz *et al.* [47] found a significant correlation of $Paco_2$ to IC in stable COPD patients at rest, and suggested that the difference between 'blue bloaters' and 'pink puffers' was mainly caused by the presence or absence of DH and PEEPi. This is supported by the highly significant linear correlation of $Paco_2$ to PEEPi [44] and IC (% pred) [47] found in COPD patients. In 'blue bloaters', the small V_T (see Fig. 5.4) reflects the 'tip of the iceberg', with most of the inspiratory effort being expended against PEEPi. In contrast, in 'pink puffers', PEEPi is absent and hence there is no 'iceberg' penalty. Nevertheless, the 'pink puffers' also exhibit an increased $P_{0.1}$ which is not chemoreceptor-mediated because the $Paco_2$ is normal or below normal (see Table 5.1) and the hypoxic drive is modest [7].

The premorbid response to CO_2 has been advocated as a determinant of hypercapnia in COPD. This is an attractive hypothesis, based on the wide variation of ventilatory response to CO_2 observed among normal individuals [48]. Thus, individuals with low ventilatory response to CO_2 when developing lung disease with mechanical impairment should retain CO_2, whereas those with high ventilatory responses would avoid CO_2 retention by increasing ventilation. However, this theory does not explain why the $Paco_2$ is either normal or below normal in the 'pink puffers'.

Relationship between $Paco_2$ and FEV_1. Inspection of Figure 5.1 shows that FEV_1 is *not* a good marker of hypercapnia. This is further confirmed by the fact that high $Paco_2$ values can often be found in stable patients with FEV_1 higher than 1.5 L (Fig. 5.5) [40]. Furthermore, in a longitudinal study of COPD patients it was found that the variations in $Paco_2$ were independent of the evolution of FEV_1 and VC [42].

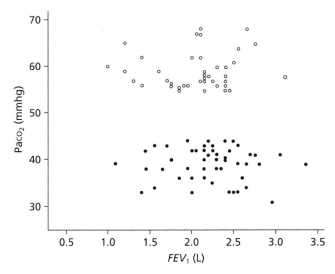

Figure 5.5 Relationship between arterial Pco_2 ($Paco_2$) and FEV_1 in stable hypercapnic (○) and non-hypercapnic (●) COPD patients. (From Parot *et al.* [39] with permission.)

This is not surprising because in COPD patients the FEV_1 describes events that occur at volumes well above FRC (see Fig. 5.2b) and hence is of little or no consequence in terms of regulation of $Paco_2$ at rest.

Assessment of severity of COPD. The severity of COPD is commonly based on the value of FEV_1, expressed as percentage predicted. To the extent that 'severity' implies curtailment of exercise capacity and increased dyspnoea, the choice of FEV_1 is not appropriate in view of the very poor correlation of this parameter to both exercise capacity [49,50] and chronic dyspnoea [21]. Assessment of severity of COPD according to IC (% pred) or presence or absence of EFL at rest appears to be more appropriate [47,49,50].

Stratification of COPD patients into two severity categories – those with and those without EFL sitting at rest – appears to be clinically very useful because the EFL patients not only have severe curtailment of exercise capacity and marked chronic dyspnoea, but also exhibit increased $Paco_2$ and decreased Pao_2 both at rest and during exercise [47,49]. Thus, this category of patients exhibits the altered blood gases that categorize the 'blue bloaters'. It should also be noted that this stratification also reflects patients with and without a reduction of resting IC [47].

Orthopnoea. In stable COPD patients with tidal EFL in sitting and/or supine position at rest, there is a high prevalence of orthopnoea, which mainly results from increased inspiratory effort resulting from PEEPi in the supine position [51]. However, increased airway resistance in recumbency also contributes to orthopnoea.

Stable patients during exercise

A detailed description of exercise physiology is provided in Chapter 4 of this book. This brief account is designed to provide a coherent link between the control of breathing at rest and during exercise in COPD patients. During exercise in normal subjects, V_T increases at the expense of both the inspiratory and expiratory reserve volumes (see Fig. 5.2a), and hence the work of breathing is shared among the inspiratory and expiratory muscles. In contrast, in COPD patients in whom EFL is present at rest, the increase in V_T during exercise occurs entirely at the expense of the inspiratory reserve volume with a concurrent increase in FRC (see Fig. 5.2b). In this case all the work of breathing is sustained solely by the inspiratory muscles, whose burden is markedly increased through increased PEEPi and respiratory elastance, as patients now breathe along a flatter portion of the static volume–pressure curve (see Fig. 5.3). Furthermore, the increase in lung volume during exercise is associated with a further expansion of the thoracic cage to a point where the inspiratory muscles may operate very inefficiently [10]. More important, however, is the fact that in such patients the maximal tidal volume during exercise (V_{Tmax}) is limited by the reduced IC. This implies that exercise capacity and V_{Tmax} should be lower in COPD patients with than those without tidal EFL at rest. This was confirmed by Diaz *et al.* [47] who studied the breathing pattern and gas exchange at peak exercise in stable COPD patients with ($n = 29$) and without ($n = 23$) tidal EFL at rest. They did not measure $P_{0.1}$ because this variable is not reliable during exercise [9]. The maximal oxygen uptake ($\dot{V}O_{2max}$) was significantly lower in the EFL patients, and in all of them was below the normal limits. In contrast, 35% of the non-EFL patients had $\dot{V}O_{2max}$ within the normal limits. The lower $\dot{V}O_{2max}$ in the EFL patients was associated with lower ventilation, mainly as a result of lower V_T. In fact, there was a significant correlation of $\dot{V}O_{2max}$ to V_{Tmax} ($r = 0.7$, $P < 0.0001$). Because T_I was the same, the lower V_{Tmax} in the patients with tidal EFL at rest was caused entirely by lower V_T/T_I (Fig. 5.6). This is contrary to results obtained at rest (see Fig. 5.4), and suggests that in the EFL patients the exercise-induced increase in inspiratory load resulting from PEEPi becomes so large that an adequate V_T/T_I can no longer be achieved [47].

In the above study, the EFL patients exhibited higher Pa_{CO_2} and lower Pa_{O_2} at rest than the non-EFL patients. At peak exercise, the former subjects exhibited a further significant increase in Pa_{CO_2} and decrease in Pa_{O_2}, while in the non-EFL patients these variables did not change. Because V_D and $\dot{V}CO_2/\dot{V}_E$ were similar in the two groups of patients, it follows from equation (5.3) that the increase in Pa_{CO_2} during exercise was caused by lower V_{Tmax}.

The results of Diaz *et al.* [47] are similar to those obtained

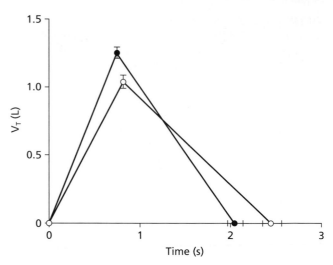

Figure 5.6 Average spirograms during maximal exercise in COPD patients without (●) and with (○) tidal expiratory flow limitation at rest. V_T, tidal volume. (From Diaz *et al.* [47] with permission.)

on a smaller number of patients by Koulouris *et al.* [23], who also showed that most COPD patients who were not EFL at rest become EFL during exercise. One of the most important findings by Diaz *et al.* [47,49] was a close correlation of resting IC to V_{Tmax} ($r = 0.77$, $P < 0.0001$) and $\dot{V}O_{2max}$ ($r = 0.75$, $P < 0.001$). The latter implies that when cardiopulmonary exercise testing (CPET) is not available or is contraindicated, the exercise capacity may be predicted to a useful approximation by simple measurement of IC.

Inspiratory capacity and exercise tolerance

Because in COPD patients reduced exercise capacity shows a weak link to FEV_1 and forced vital capacity (FVC) [47,49,50], it has been suggested that factors other than lung function impairment (e.g. deconditioning and peripheral muscle dysfunction) are the predominant contributors to reduced exercise tolerance [52–54]. Recent studies based on assessment of IC and FEV_1/FVC ratio, however, indicate that lung function impairment is the major contributor to reduced exercise tolerance in COPD [47,49,55]. In fact, because the IC and FEV_1/FVC ratio together account for 72% of the variance in $\dot{V}O_{2max}$ [49], only 28% of the variance can be ascribed to other factors such as deconditioning and peripheral muscle dysfunction, or decreased cardiac output as a result of PEEPi [47]. These considerations pertain to average values; in individual patients the contribution of these factors may be different.

Figure 5.7 illustrates the relationship between $\dot{V}O_{2max}$ during incremental, symptom-limited exercise on a cycle ergometer and IC in ambulatory COPD patients [47]. The patients were stratified according to the presence or

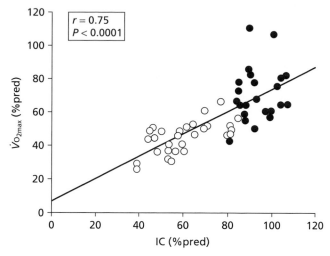

Figure 5.7 Relationship of maximal oxygen uptake during exercise ($\dot{V}o_{2\text{max}}$) to resting inspiratory capacity (IC) in 52 COPD patients with (○) and without (●) tidal expiratory flow limitation at rest. (From Diaz *et al.* [49] with permission.)

absence of EFL during resting breathing in a sitting position. In the absence of EFL the IC was within normal limits and, with two exceptions, the $\dot{V}o_{2\text{max}}$ was either normal or the reduction was mild to moderate ($\dot{V}o_{2\text{max}}$ between 77 and 56% pred) [56]. In contrast, in all EFL patients IC was below the normal limits and the reduction in $\dot{V}o_{2\text{max}}$ was severe to very severe. Figure 5.7 also shows that in EFL subjects the $\dot{V}o_{2\text{max}}$ decreases approximately linearly with increasing severity of dynamic hyperinflation, as reflected by decreased IC. There were no patients with IC below 40% pred because such patients require domiciliary oxygen therapy, as a result of markedly reduced Pao_2 at rest or exercise. Supplemental oxygen elicits an increase in IC, with concurrent improvement of dyspnoea, through a reduction of ventilation and bronchodilation caused by removal of hypoxia [57,58]. An increase of IC can also be obtained with bronchodilators [cf. 2,59]. Eventually, however, dynamic hyperinflation may become so severe that patients require mechanical ventilation [32; see Chapter 48 of this book].

Finally, it should be stressed that in other forms of chronic airways obstruction, such as bronchiectasis [60] and asthma [61], the control of breathing differs from COPD, the main difference being in that tidal EFL is less common.

Dyspnoea

Together with decreased exercise tolerance, dyspnoea is the predominant complaint of patients with COPD. Because it correlates poorly with FEV_1 and FVC, it has been suggested that dyspnoea and lung function should be considered as separate factors, which independently characterize the severity of COPD [62]. In reality, however, the poor correlation is caused by the fact that FEV_1 and FVC are poor predictors of dynamic hyperinflation, which is the major cause of dyspnoea [21]. There is a good correlation between chronic dyspnoea measured with the modified Medical Research Council (MRC) scale to various indices of dynamic hyperinflation [21], including IC [59].

A close correlation (r = 0.86) has recently been found between maximal exercise power and MRC dyspnoea score in stable patients with COPD [63] and bronchiectasis [60]. This suggests that the MRC dyspnoea scale is designed to assess exercise capacity rather than severity of dyspnoea per se. Further studies are required to confirm these observations, which implies that when CPET is not available or contraindicated, the maximum exercise capacity may be predicted to a good approximation by using the MRC dyspnoea questionnaire.

Mechanisms contributing to shallow breathing

The mechanisms leading to alterations in respiratory timing and consequently to shallow breathing in stable COPD patients have not yet been clearly defined. The fact that most hypercapnic COPD patients can achieve normocapnia by voluntarily increasing their ventilation [6] and that stable COPD patients, by voluntarily deep breathing, can bring the inspiratory muscles near fatigue in a few minutes [64], has led to the speculation that hypercapnic COPD patients choose 'wisely' to hypoventilate to avoid inspiratory muscle fatigue.

Because under conditions of increased load and/or reduced efficiency, the strain on the diaphragm that is required to maintain an adequate alveolar ventilation has been shown to lead to myofibril membrane damage and sarcomere disruption [65,66], it is likely that a protective mechanism might exist in order to protect the respiratory muscles from such damage. The functional elements of this protective mechanism (i.e. the way in which peripheral and mechanical stimuli are transmitted and modify the breathing pattern) have not been fully elucidated.

Small myelinated and non-myelinated phrenic afferent fibres (types III and IV, respectively) have been found to influence the central inspiratory neural activity in anesthetized cats, in which it was shown that selective stimulation of these fibres results in changes in the respiratory rhythm (altering the T_I/T_{TOT}) and, hence, in the central inspiratory activity [67]. Under states of severe respiratory stress (muscle tension, local ischaemia, accumulation of toxic metabolites) afferents from the respiratory muscles may have a predominant role in the genesis of shallow breathing [67,68].

A direct link between stimulation of group III and IV afferents and the central processing of endogenous opioids has been postulated [69], given that in anesthetized dogs respiratory depression persisted even after withdrawal of afferent fibre stimulation, whereas the magnitude of the respiratory depression was significantly reduced by naloxone. Other investigators have confirmed these results in cats and demonstrated that the phenomenon involved a supraspinal mechanism [70], which could be prevented by pretreatment with naloxone [71]. This strongly suggests involvement of endogenous opioid pathways. The fact that in COPD patients with absent respiratory response to flow-resistive loading the response could be acutely restored by administration of naloxone [72], suggests that in these patients the chronic increase in airway resistance may generate endogenous opioids to lessen the stress of prolonged dyspnoea.

The source of endogenous opiods during strenuous inspiratory resistive breathing remains elusive, and both central sites such as the hypothalamic–pituitary–adrenal (HPA) axis, and peripheral sites such as the spinal cord and peripheral nerves have been implicated [73].

Recently, it has been shown that in normal humans strenuous resistive breathing leads to a significant rise in the levels of proinflammatory cytokines (interleukins IL-1b, IL-6), adenocorticotrophic hormone (ACTH) and β-endorphin [74]. The strong correlation between the rise in the β-endorphin and ACTH and the preceding increase in circulating IL-6 allowed the authors to conclude that pro-inflammatory cytokines are responsible for the activation of the HPA axis, leading eventually to an increase in plasma β-endorphin and ACTH. It is tempting to suggest that the mechanism accounting for the increase of β-endorphin and ACTH could be the stimulation of small afferent nerve fibres by the cytokines that are produced during resistive breathing, given that global depletion of small afferent fibres inhibits the plasma ACTH response to intravenous IL-1b [75].

Although the stimuli for the production of the cytokines are not known, reactive oxygen species produced during fatiguing resistive breathing [76,77] could be responsible. Even though the time profile (brief) and intensity (much greater) of the increased loading of breathing in the above mentioned models are different from those in patients with chronic CO_2 retention, given that strenuous breathing causes diaphragm muscle fibre injury one could speculate that strenuous resistive breathing through reactive oxygen species induces plasma cytokine production, which in turn modulates the respiratory controllers either directly through the blood or more likely the small afferents, or via the HPA axis. The ensuing production of β-endorphins, by altering the breathing pattern, results in reduced load and alleviation of fatigue, thus protecting the ventilatory pump

from exhaustion [78]. In the last analysis, however, PEEPi and its 'tip of the iceberg' effect are probably the main reasons for the reduced V_T and dyspnoea exhibited by COPD patients with CO_2 retention at rest and during exercise.

Acknowledgement

The authors thank Ms Karyn Mitchell for typing the manuscript.

References

1 Cherniack NS. Control of breathing in chronic obstructive pulmonary disease. In: Altose MD, Kowakami Y, eds. *Control of Breathing in Health and Disease*. New York: Marcel Dekker, 1999: 423–37.

2 O'Donnell D. Assessment and management of dyspnoea in chronic obstructive pulmonary disease. In: Similowski T, Whitelow WA, Derenne J-Ph, eds. *Clinical Management of Chronic Obstructive Pulmonary Disease*. New York: Marcel Dekker, 2002: 114–70.

3 Hertle FH, Georg R, Lange HJ. Arterial blood partial pressure as related to age and anthropometric data. *Respiration* 1971; **28**:1–30.

4 Sorbini CA, Grassi V, Solinas E, Muiesan G. Arterial oxygen tension in relation to age in healthy subjects. *Respiration* 1968;**25**:3–13.

5 Lane DJ, Howell JBL, Giblin B. Relationship between airways obstruction and carbon dioxide tension in patients with obstructive pulmonary disease. *BMJ* 1965;**38**:707–9.

6 Robin ED, O'Neill RP. The fighter versus the non-fighter. *Arch Environ Health* 1963;**7**:125–9.

7 Šorli J, Grassino A, Lorange G *et al.* Control of breathing in patients with chronic obstructive lung disease. *Clin Sci* 1978; **54**:295–304.

8 Whitelaw WA, Derenne JP, Milic-Emili J. Occlusion pressure as a measure of respiratory center output in conscious man. *Respir Physiol* 1975;**23**:181–99.

9 Whitelaw WA, Derenne JP. Airway occlusion pressure. *J Appl Physiol* 1993;**74**:1475–83.

10 Rochester DF. Effects of COPD on the respiratory muscles. In: Cherniack NS, ed. *Chronic Obstructive Pulmonary Disease*. Philadelphia: WB Saunders, 1991: 134–57.

11 Bradley GW, von Euler C, Martilla I *et al.* A model of the central and reflex inhibition of inspiration in the cat. *Biol Cybern* 1975;**19**:105–16.

12 Cohen MI, Feldman JL. Models of respiratory phase-switching. *Fed Proc* 1977;**36**:2367–74.

13 von Euler C. On the neural organization of the motor control of the diaphragm. *Am Rev Respir Dis* 1979;**19**:45–50.

14 Remmers JE. Analysis of ventilatory response. *Chest* 1976;**70** (Suppl):134–7.

15 Wyman RJ. Neural generation of the breathing rhythm. *Annu Rev Physiol* 1975;**39**:417–48.

16 Clark F, von Euler C. On the regulation of depth and rate of breathing. *J Physiol* 1972;**222**:267–95.

17 Milic-Emili J, Grunstein MM. Drive and timing components of ventilation. *Chest* 1976;**70**(Suppl):131–3.

18 Read DJC. A clinical method for assessing the ventilatory response to carbon dioxide. *Aust Ann Med* 1967;**16**:20–32.

19 Rebuck AW, Campbell EJM. A clinical method for assessing the ventilatory response to hypoxia. *Am Rev Respir Dis* 1974;**109**:345–50.

20 Agostoni E, Mead J. Statics of the respiratory system. In: Macklem PT, Mead J, eds. *Handbook of Physiology*. Section 3, vol. I. *The Respiratory System: Mechanics of Breathing*. Bethesda MD: American Physiological Society, 1964: 387–409.

21 Eltayara L, Becklake MR, Volta CA, Milic-Emili J. Relationship between chronic dyspnoea and expiratory flow-limitation in patients with chronic obstructive pulmonary disease. *Am J Respir Crit Care Med* 1996;**154**:1726–34.

22 Koulouris NG, Valta P, Lavoie A *et al*. A simple method to detect expiratory flow limitation during spontaneous breathing. *Eur Respir J* 1995;**8**:306–13.

23 Koulouris NG, Dimopoulou I, Valta P *et al*. Detection of expiratory flow limitation during exercise in COPD patients. *J Appl Physiol* 1997;**82**:723–31.

24 Hyatt RE. The interrelationship of pressure, flow and volume during various respiratory maneuvers in normal and emphysematous patients. *Am Rev Respir Dis* 1961;**83**:676–83.

25 Volta CA, Ploysongsang Y, Eltayara L *et al*. A simple method to monitor performance of forced vital capacity. *J Appl Physiol* 1996;**80**:693–8.

26 Mota S, Casan P, Drobnic E *et al*. Expiratory flow limitation during exercise in competition cyclists. *J Appl Physiol* 1999;**86**:611–6.

27 Leaver DG, Pride NB. Flow–volume curves and expiratory pressures during exercise in patients with chronic airways obstruction. *Scand J Respir Dis Suppl* 1971;**77**:23–7.

28 Knudson RJ. Physiology of the aging lung. In: Crystal RG, West JB *et al*., eds. *The Lung: Scientific Foundations*. New York: Raven Press, 1991: 1749.

29 Pride NB, Milic-Emili J. Lung mechanics. In: Calverley PMA, Pride NB, eds. *Chronic Obstructive Pulmonary Disease*. London: Chapman & Hall, 1995: 135–60.

30 Pepe PE, Marini JJ. Occult positive end-expiratory pressure in mechanically ventilated patients with airflow obstruction. *Am Rev Respir Dis* 1982;**126**:166–70.

31 Rossi A, Gottfried SB, Zocchi L *et al*. Measurement of static compliance of the total respiratory system in patients with acute respiratory failure during mechanical ventilation: the effect of intrinsic PEEP. *Am Rev Respir Dis* 1985;**131**:672–7.

32 Rossi A, Polese G, Milic-Emili J. Monitoring respiratory mechanics in ventilator-dependent patients. In: Tobin MJ, ed. *Principles and Practice of Intensive Care Monitoring*. New York: McGraw-Hill, 1998: 553–616.

33 D'Angelo E, Prandi E, Marazzini L, Milic-Emili J. Dependence of maximal flow–volume curves on time course of preceding inspiration in patients with chronic obstructive lung disease. *Am J Respir Crit Care Med* 1994;**150**:1581–6.

34 Valta P, Corbeil C, Lavoie A *et al*. Detection of expiratory flow limitation during mechanical ventilation. *Am J Respir Crit Care Med* 1994;**150**:1311–7.

35 Shore SA, Huk O, Marmixs S, Martin JG. Effect of panting frequency on plethysurographic determination of thoracic gas volume in chronic obstructive pulmonary disease. *Am Rev Respir Dis* 1983;**128**:54–9.

36 Yan S, Kaminski D, Sliwinski P. Reliability of inspiratory capacity for estimating end-expiratory lung volume changes during exercise in patients with chronic obstructive pulmonary disease. *Am J Respir Crit Care Med* 1997;**156**:55–9.

37 Loveridge B, West P, Kryger MH, Anthonisen NR. Alteration in breathing pattern with progression of chronic obstructive pulmonary disease. *Am Rev Respir Dis* 1986;**134**:930–4.

38 Burrows B, Saksena FB, Diener CF. Carbon dioxide retention and ventilatory mechanics in chronic obstructive lung disease. *Ann Intern Med* 1966;**65**:685–700.

39 Parot S, Miara B, Milic-Emili J, Gautier H. Hypoxemia, hypercapia and breathing pattern in patients with chronic obstructive pulmonary disease. *Am Rev Respir Dis* 1982;**126**:882–6.

40 Parot S, Saunier C, Gautier H *et al*. Breathing pattern and hypercapnia in patients with obstructive pulmonary disease. *Am Rev Respir Dis* 1980;**121**:985–91.

41 Bradley CA, Fleetham JA, Anthonisen NR. Ventilatory control in patients with hypoxemia due to obstructive lung disease. *Am Rev Respir Dis* 1979;**120**:21–30.

42 Parot S, Saunier C, Schrijen F, Gautier H, Milic-Emili J. Concomitant changes in function tests, breathing pattern and $Paco_2$ in patients with chronic obstructive pulmonary disease. *Bull Eur Physiopathol Respir* 1982;**18**:145–51.

43 Murciano D, Aubier M, Bussi S *et al*. Comparison of esophageal, tacheal, and mouth occlusion pressure in patients with chronic obstructive pulmonary disease during acute respiratory failure. *Am Rev Respir Dis* 1982;**128**:837–41.

44 Haluszka J, Chartrand DA, Grassino AE, Milic-Emili J. Intrinsic PEEP and arterial Pco_2 in stable patients with chronic obstructive pulmonary disease. *Am Rev Respir Dis* 1990;**141**:1194–7.

45 Bellemare F, Grassino A. Effect of pressure and timing of contraction on human diaphragm fatigue. *J Appl Physiol* 1982;**53**:1190–5.

46 Rossi A, Santos C, Roca J *et al*. Effects of PEEP on V/Q mismatching in ventilated patients with chronic airflow obstruction. *Am J Respir Crit Care Med* 1994;**149**:1077–84.

47 Diaz O, Villafranca C, Ghezzo H *et al*. Breathing pattern and gas exchange at peak exercise in COPD patients with and without tidal flow limitation at rest. *Eur Respir J* 2001;**17**:1120–7.

48 Read DJ. A clinical method for assessing the ventilatory response to carbon dioxide. *Australas Ann Med* 1967;**16**:20–32.

49 Diaz O, Villafranca C, Ghezzo H *et al*. Exercise tolerance in COPD patients with and without tidal expiratory flow limitation at rest. *Eur Respir J* 2000;**16**:269–75.

50 Murariu C, Ghezzo H, Milic-Emili J, Gauthier H. Exercise limitation in obstructive lung disease. *Am Rev Respir Dis* 1987;**135**:1069–74.

51 Eltayara L, Ghezzo H, Milic-Emili J. Orthopnoea and tidal expiratory flow limitation in patients with stable COPD. *Chest* 2001;**119**:99–104.

52 Hamilton N, Killian KJ, Summers E, Jones NL. Muscle strength, symptom intensity, and exercise capacity in patients with cardio-respiratory disorders. *Am J Respir Crit Care Med* 1995;**152**:2021–31.

53 Gosselink R, Troosters T, Decramer M. Peripheral muscle weakness contributes to exercise limitation in COPD. *Am J Respir Crit Care Med* 1996;**153**:976–80.

54 Maltais F, Simard AA, Simard C *et al.* Oxidative capacity of the skeletal muscle and lactic acid kinetics during exercise in normal subjects and in patients with COPD. *Am J Respir Crit Care Med* 1996;**153**:288–93.

55 O'Donnell D, Revill S, Webb K. Dynamic hyperinflation and exercise intolerance in chronic obstructive pulmonary disease. *Am J Respir Crit Care Med* 2001;**164**:770–7.

56 American Thoracic Society. Standards for the diagnosis and care of patients with chronic obstructive pulmonary disease (COPD) and asthma. *Am Rev Respir Dis* 1987;**135**:1069–174.

57 Alvisi V, Mirkovic T, Nesme P *et al.* Acute effects of hyperoxia on dyspnoea in hypoxemic patients with chronic airway obstruction at rest. *Chest* 2003;**123**:1038–46.

58 Coe CL, Pride NB. Effects of correcting arterial hypoxaemia on respiratory resistance in patients with chronic obstructive pulmonary disease. *Clin Sci (Lond)* 1993;**136**:325–9.

59 Tantucci C, Duguet A, Similowski T *et al.* Effect of salbutamol on dynamic hyperinflation in chronic obstructive pulmonary disease in patients. *Eur Respir J* 2001;**12**:799–804.

60 Koulouris NG, Retsou S, Kosmas E *et al.* Tidal expiratory flow limitation, dyspnoea, and exercise capacity in patients with biloteral bronchiectasis. *Em Respir J* 2003;**21**:743–8.

61 Kosmas EN, Milic-Emili J, Polychronaki A *et al.* Exercise-induced flow limitation, dynamic hyperinflation and exercise capacity in patients with asthma. *Eur Respir J* 2004;**24**:378–84.

62 Mahler DA, Harver A. A factor analysis of dyspnoea ratings, respiratory muscle strength, and lung function in patients with chronic obstructive pulmonary disease. *Am Rev Respir Dis* 1992;**145**:467–70.

63 Kontogiorgi M, Kosmas EN, Gaga M *et al.* Exercise capacity, tidal expiratory flow limitation and chronic dyspnoea in patients with stable COPD. *Am J Respir Crit Care Med* 2003;**167**:A293.

64 Bellemare F, Grassino A. Force reserve of the diaphragm in patients with chronic obstructive pulmonary disease. *J Appl Physiol* 1983;**55**:8–15.

65 Zhu E, Petrof BJ, Gea J, Comtois N, Grassino AE. Diaphragm muscle fiber injury after inspiratory resistive breathing. *Am J Resp Crit Care Med* 1997;**155**:1110–6.

66 Jiang T-X, Reid WD, Road JD. Delayed diaphragm injury and diaphragm force production. *Am J Resp Crit Care Med* 1998;**157**:736–42.

67 Jammes Y, Buchler B, Delpierre S *et al.* Phrenic afferents and their role in inspiratory control. *J Appl Physiol* 1986;**60**:854–60.

68 Hussain SNA, Magder S, Chatillon A, Roussos C. Chemical activation of thin fiber phrenic afferents: respiratory responses. *J Appl Physiol* 1990;**69**:1002–11.

69 Kumazawa T, Tadaki E, Kim K. A possible participation of endogenous opiates in respiratory reflexes induced by thin fiber muscular afferents. *Brain Res* 1980;**199**:244–8.

70 Waldrop TG, Eldridge FL, Milhorn DE. Prolonged poststimulus inhibition of breathing following stimulation of afferents from muscle. *Respir Physiol* 1982;**50**:239–54.

71 Waldrop TG, Eldridge FL, Milhorn DE. Inhibition of breathing after stimulation of muscle is mediated by endogenous opiates and GABA. *Respir Physiol* 1983;**54**:211–22.

72 Santiago TV, Remolina C, Scoles Veldeman NH. Endorphins and the control of breathing: ability of naloxone to restore flow-resistive load compensation in chronic obstructive pulmonary disease. *N Engl J Med* 1981;**304**:1190–5.

73 Petrozzino JJ, Scardella AT, Edelman NH, Santiago TV. Respiratory muscle acidosis stimulates endogenous opioids during inspiratory loading. *Am Rev Respir Dis* 1993;**144**: 607–15.

74 Vassilakopoulos T, Zakynthinos S, Roussos C. Strenuous resistive breathing induces pro-inflammatory cytokines and stimulates the HPA axis in humans. *Am J Physiol* 1999;**277**: 1013–9.

75 Watanabe TA, Morimoto A, Tan N *et al.* ACTH response induced in capsaicin-desensitized rats by interleukin-1 or prostaglandin E. *J Physiol (Lond)* 1994;**457**:139–45.

76 Anzuetto A, Andrate FH, Maxwell LC *et al.* Resistive breathing activates the glutathione redox cycle and impairs performance of the rat diaphragm. *J Appl Physiol* 1992;**72**:529–34.

77 Anzuetto A, Supinski GS, Levine SM, Jekinson SG. Methods of disease: are oxygen derived free radicals involved in diaphragmatic dysfunction? *Am J Respir Crit Care Med* 1994;**149**:1048–52.

78 Roussos C, Koutsoukou A. Respiratory failure. *Eur Respir J* 2003;**22**:1–12S.

CHAPTER 6
Physiology and pathobiology of the lung circulation

Norbert F. Voelkel

How normal lung circulation works

Design

The lung circulation is designed as a low-pressure low-resistance system, whereas the bronchial circulation is systemic and under high pressure. The blood flow through the lung had been thought to be controlled by gravitational forces and therefore, according to West [1], apical–basal zonal patterns. However, more recent studies by Glenny et al. [2] indicate that lung blood flow is fractal and largely determined by the design of the vascular tree [2]. Thus, the branching pattern (branching angle and variation of branch lumen diameter of segments of the same generation) appears to determine how the blood flows through the lung circulation. 'At the end of the day, the lung is designed as an efficient gas exchanger, and it needs to stay dry' (John T. Reeves, personal communication).

Wagner et al. [3] have studied recruitment of unperfused lung vessels, which is likely maximal with maximal exercise. This opening and perfusion of a large number of 'reserve capillaries' likely explains why the lung circulation can accommodate fold increases in cardiac output without a substantial increase in pulmonary artery pressure [4].

Ventilation–perfusion matching

As the primary function of the lung organ is that of an efficient gas exchanger, mechanisms are needed – and exist – to match ventilation–air flow with blood flow. Hypoxic vasoconstriction – originally termed alveolar – capillary 'reflex' by von Euler and Liljestrand [5] – is perhaps the most recognized and best-studied aspect of ventilation–perfusion (V/Q) matching. The principle is, simply stated: what is not ventilated must not be perfused. Studies designed and performed several decades ago showed con-vincingly that vasodilator drugs decrease the Pa_{O_2} significantly by allowing perfusion of non-ventilated areas of the lung [6]. Regional hypoxia results in regional pulmonary vasoconstriction, limiting blood flow to under- or unventilated areas. Hypoxic vasoconstriction is nearly instantaneous after the occurrence of alveolar hypoxia [7], hence the original term 'reflex'.

Hypoxic vasoconstriction may be the most important mechanism of V/Q matching, but there may be other mechanisms. These are likely endogenous vasoconstriction and vasodilator agents, which modulate pulmonary vascular tone hypoxia independently. For example, Walker et al. [8] showed that a cyclo-oxygenase inhibitor (meclofenamate) increased pulmonary artery pressure in trained awake dogs, indicating that a cyclo-oxygenase product was involved in the normal control of the lung circulation.

Interestingly, Naeiji et al. [9] treated COPD patients with supplemental oxygen to 'remove' hypoxic vasoconstriction and then documented a fall in the pulmonary artery pressure after prostaglandin E$_2$ infusion – indicating that these patients had an element of hypoxia-independent vasoconstriction – which presumably contributed to V/Q matching.

Lung circulation in COPD/emphysema

Most of the traditional lung function studies assess variables of airway disease, flow–volume, airway resistance–reactivity or trapped air–hyperinflation. The high-resolution chest computed tomography (CT) scan can assess thickened airway walls and the degree of lung tissue, and also vessel loss in emphysematous areas. Pulmonary angiography, still occasionally performed to rule out pulmonary embolism, can show the pruning of the subpleural vessels, the diffusion capacity and, when corrected for alveolar volume, can provide information regarding the loss of alveolar capillaries.

Conclusions

There can be no doubt that COPD is also a pulmonary vascular disease [33] and skeletal muscle vessels may also be impaired [34]. Immune mechanisms likely involved in the pathogenesis of COPD/emphysema need to be vigorously explored to better understand the so-called pulmonary vascular remodelling of the precapillary arterioles and the disappearance of lung capillaries. The factors that control the development of pulmonary hypertension in COPD remain complex.

References

1 West JB. Regional differences in the lung. *Chest* 1978;**74**: 426–37.

2 Glenny RW, Robertson HT, Hlastala MP. Vasomotor tone does not affect perfusion heterogeneity and gas exchange in normal primate lungs during normoxia. *J Appl Physiol* 2000;**89**:2263–7.

3 Wagner WW Jr, Latham LP, Gillespie MN, Guenther JP, Capen RL. Direct measurement of pulmonary capillary transit times. *Science* 1982;**218**:379–81.

4 Grunig E, Koehler R, Miltenberger-Miltenyi G *et al.* Primary pulmonary hypertension in children may have a different genetic background than in adults. *Pediatr Res* 2004;**56**: 571–8.

5 von Euler U, Liljestrand G. Observations on the pulmonary arterial blood pressure in the cat. *Acta Physiol Scand* 1946; **12**:301–20.

6 Motley HL, Cournand A, Werko L, Himmelstein A, Dresdale D. The influence of short periods of induced acute anoxia upon pulmonary artery pressures in man. *Am J Physiol* 1947; **150**:315–20.

7 Jensen KS, Micco AJ, Czartolomna J, Latham L, Voelkel NF. Rapid onset of hypoxic vasoconstriction in isolated lungs. *J Appl Physiol* 1992;**72**:2018–23.

8 Walker BR, Voelkel NF, Reeves JT. Pulmonary pressor response after prostaglandin synthesis inhibition in conscious dogs. *J Appl Physiol* 1982;**52**:705–9.

9 Naeiji R, Melot C, Mols P, Hallemans R. Reduction in pulmonary hypertension by prostaglandin E$_1$ in decompensated chronic obstructive pulmonary disease. *Am Rev Respir Dis* 1982;**125**:1–5.

10 Liebow AA. Pulmonary emphysema with special reference to vascular changes. *Am Rev Respir Dis* 1959;**80**:67–93.

11 Wright JL, Petty T, Thurlbeck WM. Analysis of the structure of the muscular pulmonary arteries in patients with pulmonary hypertension and COPD: National Institutes of Health nocturnal oxygen therapy trial. *Lung* 1992;**170**: 109–24.

12 Barbera JA, Riverola A, Roca J *et al.* Pulmonary vascular abnormalities and ventilation–perfusion relationships in mild chronic obstructive pulmonary disease. *Am J Respir Crit Care Med* 1994;**149**:423–9.

13 Peinado VI, Barbera JA, Abate P *et al.* Inflammatory reaction in pulmonary muscular arteries of patients with mild chronic obstructive pulmonary disease. *Am J Respir Crit Care Med* 1999;**159**:1605–11.

14 Santos S, Peinado VI, Ramirez J *et al.* Characterization of pulmonary vascular remodelling in smokers and patients with mild COPD. *Eur Respir J* 2002;**19**:632–8.

15 Kasahara Y, Tuder RM, Cool CD *et al.* Endothelial cell death and decreased expression of vascular endothelial growth factor and vascular endothelial growth factor receptor 2 in emphysema. *Am J Respir Crit Care Med* 2001;**163**:737–44.

16 Lee JD, Taraseviciene-Stewart L, Keith R, Geraci MW, Voelkel NF. Is prostacyclin (PGI2) part of the adult lung structure program? *Am J Respir Crit Care Med* 2005;**169**:A842.

17 Hoshikawa Y, Nana-Sinkam P, Moore MD *et al.* Hypoxia induces different genes in the lungs of rats compared with mice. *Physiol Genomics* 2003;**12**:209–19.

18 Tuder RM, Flook BE, Voelkel NF. Increased gene expression for VEGF and the VEGF receptors KDR/Flk and Flt in lungs exposed to acute or to chronic hypoxia: modulation of gene expression by nitric oxide. *J Clin Invest* 1995;**95**: 1798–807.

19 Voelkel NF, Tuder RM. Hypoxia-induced pulmonary vascular remodeling: a model for what human disease? *J Clin Invest* 2000;**106**:733–8.

20 Peinado VI, Barbera JA, Ramirez J *et al.* Endothelial dysfunction in pulmonary arteries of patients with mild COPD. *Am J Physiol* 1998;**274**:L908–13.

21 Dinh-Xuan AT, Higenbottam TW, Clelland CA *et al.* Impairment of endothelium-dependent pulmonary-artery relaxation in chronic obstructive lung disease. *N Engl J Med* 1991;**324**:1539–47.

22 Burrows B, Kettel LJ, Niden AH *et al.* Patterns of cardiovascular dysfunction in chronic obstructive lung disease. *N Engl J Med* 1972;**286**:912–8.

23 Weitzenblum E, Schrijen F, Mohan-Kumar T, Colas des Francs V, Lockhart A. Variability of the pulmonary vascular response to acute hypoxia in chronic bronchitis. *Chest* 1988; **94**:772–8.

24 Kessler R, Faller M, Weitzenblum E *et al.* 'Natural history' of pulmonary hypertension in a series of 131 patients with chronic obstructive lung disease. *Am J Respir Crit Care Med* 2001;**164**:219–24.

25 Weitzenblum E, Chaouat A, Kessler R, Beau-Faller M. Pulmonary hypertension and cor pulmonale in chronic obstructive pulmonary disease. In: Voelkel NF, MacNee W, eds. *Chronic Obstructive Lung Disease*. London: Decker, 2002: 306–18.

26 Voelkel NF, Cool CD. Pulmonary vascular involvement in chronic obstructive pulmonary disease. *Eur Respir J Suppl* 2003;**46**:28–32.

27 Voelkel NF. Cor pulmonale with a normal chest radiograph. In: Schwarz MI, ed. *Pulmonary Grand Rounds*. Ontario: Decker, 1990: 3–11.

28 Catterall JR, Calverley PM, MacNee W *et al.* Mechanism of transient nocturnal hypoxemia in hypoxic chronic bronchitis and emphysema. *J Appl Physiol* 1985;**59**:1698–703.

29 Douglas NJ, Calverley PM, Leggett RJ *et al.* Transient

hypoxaemia during sleep in chronic bronchitis and emphysema. *Lancet* 1979;**1**:1–4.

30 Zielinski J. Effects of intermittent hypoxia on pulmonary haemodynamics: animal models versus studies in humans. *Eur Respir J* 2005;**25**:173–80.

31 O'Donnell DE, Lam M, Webb KA. Measurement of symptoms, lung hyperinflation, and endurance during exercise in chronic obstructive pulmonary disease. *Am J Respir Crit Care Med* 1998;**158**:1557–65.

32 Tashkin DP. Is a long-acting inhaled bronchodilator the first agent to use in stable chronic obstructive pulmonary disease? *Curr Opin Pulm Med* 2005;**11**:121–8.

33 Voelkel NF, Taraseviciene-Stewart L, Tuder R. Emphysema: a vascular disease? *Drug Discovery Today: Disease Mechanisms* 2004;**1**:145–9.

34 Tang K, Breen EC, Gerber HP, Ferrara NM, Wagner PD. Capillary regression in vascular endothelial growth factor-deficient skeletal muscle. *Physiol Genomics* 2004;**18**:63–9.

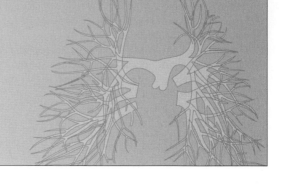

CHAPTER 7
Sleep in patients with COPD

Mark W. Elliott

During sleep there are profound physiological changes. This is particularly true of breathing, and in a number of conditions this has important implications. The sleep apnoea hypopnoea syndrome (SAHS) is increasingly recognized and in this condition the symptoms and other adverse health consequences (e.g. hypertension) are a result of what happens when the individual is asleep. In other conditions, changes happening during sleep exacerbate daytime function; in patients with heart failure and Cheyne–Stokes breathing, the abnormality of respiration during sleep contributes to daytime symptoms of tiredness and fatigue and is associated with a worse prognosis [1]. In patients with chest wall deformity and neuromuscular disease, nocturnal hypoventilation is important in the pathogenesis of daytime symptoms, respiratory failure and cor pulmonale [2]. Repeated episodes of hypoxaemia and hypercapnia during sleep lead, in time, to the development of daytime respiratory failure, pulmonary hypertension, right heart failure and death [3].

Breathing alters according to the state of consciousness. In healthy subjects, ventilation falls with the onset of sleep and is reduced during all phases of sleep compared with waking levels [4]. Alterations in the pattern of breathing occur, including periodic breathing, apnoea and hypopnoea, particularly with the onset of sleep and during stages I and II. Upper airway resistance may increase [5]. The changes are generally more marked during rapid eye movement (REM) sleep than non-rapid eye movement (NREM) sleep.

NREM sleep is associated with a decrease in respiratory frequency and a small increase in tidal volume. A reduction in central drive during sleep has been postulated to explain these differences. However, ventilation has been shown to fall despite an increase in occlusion pressure [6]. In awake supine humans, movements of the ribcage and abdomen account for 40 and 60% of the tidal volume, respectively. In NREM sleep, ribcage movement accounts for 65% of the tidal volume, suggesting increased intercostal activity [7].

In cats, expiratory intercostal muscle activity increases throughout NREM sleep and although its significance is not known, this increase indicates that at least some of the NREM changes are not simply a reduction of central drive compared with that during waking. By contrast to NREM sleep, during REM sleep respiratory frequency is often greater and tidal volume lower than during wakefulness and atonia of the intercostal muscles reduces or eliminates costal breathing. Ventilatory responses to chemical stimuli and other respiratory reflexes are also impaired during phasic REM sleep [8,9]. During NREM sleep the decrease in alveolar ventilation is relatively small, but this may be much more marked during REM sleep, particularly during bursts of eye movement [10], when alveolar ventilation may fall by as much as 40% of waking levels (Fig. 7.1). In healthy subjects, an increment in CO_2 tension of up to 6 mmHg above waking levels is normal [11], but this degree of hypoventilation is insufficient to cause any appreciable degree of oxygen desaturation. However, in patients with little respiratory reserve, more marked hypercapnia can occur together with significant oxygen desaturation.

Sleep in patients with COPD

Polysomnographic studies have shown that oxygen desaturation may occur in patients with COPD, and that this is particularly marked during REM sleep [12,13] (Fig. 7.2). Carbon dioxide tensions may rise; in one recent study, 47% of COPD patients had an increment in transcutaneous P_{CO_2} greater than 1.33 kPa (10 mmHg) above waking levels (see Fig. 7.2). This was correlated with diurnal Pa_{CO_2}, body mass index and percentage of time spent in REM sleep [14]. Alveolar hypoventilation is the dominant mechanism, with ventilation falling in one study by 18%, compared with wakefulness, during NREM sleep and 35% during REM sleep [15]. The effects of sleep on breathing in normal

Figure 7.1 This shows a 30-s epoch from an overnight polysomnogram of a patient with severe COPD. There is a period of apnoea associated with reduced chest and abdominal wall motion leading to marked oxygen desaturation. Note the phasic movements in the electro-oculograms (EOR and EOL). (C4, EEG; EMG, submental electromyogram; So_2, oxygen saturation; AFL, oronasal airflow; CMV and AMV, chest and abdominal wall motion, respectively.)

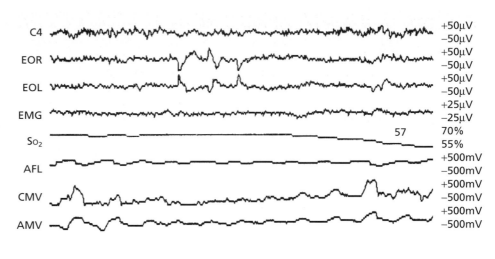

Figure 7.2 Overnight monitoring of oxygen saturation (Sao_2) and transcutaneous carbon dioxide tension ($Ptcco_2$). Note the reduction in Sao_2 at sleep onset and the episodes of marked worsening over a period of 15–20 min. These correspond to episodes of REM sleep. $Ptcco_2$ also rises with sleep onset and is much more marked during the episodes of REM sleep. Over the course of the night it can be seen that the $Ptcco_2$ gradually rises.

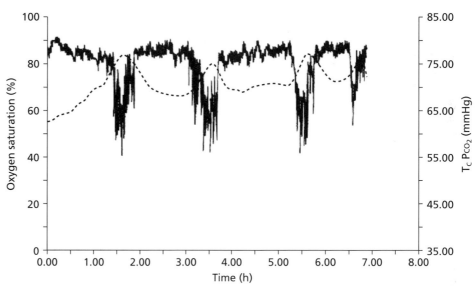

subjects discussed above, are much more marked in COPD. Patients with COPD have a higher physiological dead space than normal subjects and therefore the rapid shallow breathing that occurs in REM sleep will produce an even greater decrease in alveolar ventilation [16]. In addition, hyperinflated patients with COPD, like scoliotic patients, are more dependent upon intercostal and accessory muscle activity than normal subjects and during REM sleep, the diaphragm alone is unable to maintain ventilation [17]. In addition, contraction of the low flat diaphragm against a flaccid lower chest wall will result in costal indrawing, and a possible further reduction in ventilation. Lower respiratory system resistance rises during sleep, independent of sleep stage, because of an increase in cholinergic tone [18] and this may compromise effective ventilation still further. A reduction in functional residual capacity (FRC), because of reduced muscle tone, occurs in normal subjects and

probably in patients with COPD. The effect of this will be to increase airway closure, elevate closing capacity above FRC with consequent changes in ventilation/perfusion ($\dot{V}/\dot{Q}$) relationships, but this remains to be proved [19]. Many investigators [13,20,21] have stated that $\dot{V}/\dot{Q}$ imbalance is a major cause of REM-related hypoxaemia in patients with COPD. However, the argument that because Pao_2 falls more than $Paco_2$ rises, changes in $\dot{V}/\dot{Q}$ must be important, cannot be sustained because this is exactly what happens during transient hypoventilation because the body has the capacity to store relatively large amounts of CO_2 [22]. Nevertheless, it is likely that changes in $\dot{V}/\dot{Q}$ do play some part. Increased upper airway resistance [23], or frank obstruction, or the change in the ventilatory response to increased upper airway resistance [24] may impact upon gas exchange during sleep and affect diurnal arterial blood gas tensions.

In a study comparing patients with airflow obstruction of similar severity, the presence of upper airway dysfunction together with increased alcohol consumption was more likely to be associated with daytime hypercapnia [25]. In another study of patients with severe SAHS and COPD, those with hypercapnia while awake were heavier, had smaller upper airway dimensions on CT scanning and a greater alcohol intake than those who were normocapnic. There was no difference in the severity of SAHS on the basis of the apnoea hypopnoea index (AHI) [26]. However, the 35% reduction in ventilation during REM sleep described above [15] occurred despite 4 cm H_2O continuous positive airway pressure (CPAP), suggesting that upper airway obstruction is not a major factor, although 4 cm H_2O CPAP may not have been sufficient to completely abolish this.

Changes in oxygen consumption, carbon dioxide production [27] and in cardiac output may also contribute to worsening of arterial blood gas tensions during sleep. Abnormal ventilatory control during wakefulness has also been implicated in the sleep hypoxaemia of COPD. Various workers have shown correlations between reduced ventilatory and occlusion pressure responses to hypoxia and hypercapnia and sleep-related oxygen desaturation [28–31]. However, it is also possible that changes in daytime ventilatory control occur as a consequence of the changes at night. Nocturnal hypoventilation causes Pa_{CO_2} to rise with renal retention of bicarbonate ions to compensate for the resulting respiratory acidosis. The effect of an elevated bicarbonate is to buffer the pH changes associated with an acute rise in Pa_{CO_2} and reduce the ventilatory response to CO_2 [32]. Secondly, sleep disruption reduces the daytime ventilatory response to both hypercapnia and hypoxia [33].

Patients with COPD may also complain of night-time cough. There is no correlation between apnoea or hypoxaemia and cough, which seldom occurs during sleep and only rarely awakens patients [34].

Effects of sleep-disordered breathing in COPD

It is clear that significant abnormalities of arterial blood gas tensions occur during sleep in patients with COPD and that, regardless of the exact mechanism, alveolar hypoventilation is a major contributor. However, the affect of these derangements during sleep upon survival and daytime function is not well known. Impaired sleep quality is well recognized in COPD compared with age-matched controls [35], and experience from SAHS suggests that sleep disruption is associated with impaired neuropsychiatric functioning and reduced quality of life [36]. However, there is no evidence as yet that poor sleep in patients with COPD causes excessive daytime sleepiness [37].

Nocturnal hypoxaemia has been postulated to be important in the genesis of pulmonary hypertension during the day in COPD [38]. REM-related falls in oxygen saturation may be associated with rises in pulmonary artery pressure (PAP) of up to 20 mmHg [39]. However, the effect of transient rises in PAP during sleep is not clear. Higher mean PAP and red cell mass were found in 36 patients with COPD and mild to moderate oxygen desaturation (desaturation to at least 85% and at least 5 min spent with Sa_{O_2} less than 90%) than in 30 patients who did not desaturate. However, there were also significant differences in their awake oxygenation [40]. The effect of the interaction between hypoxia and hypercapnia upon the human pulmonary circulation is not well known. However, in isolated animal preparations hypercapnia, in the presence of hypoxia, leads to a variety of different responses in the pulmonary circulation: vasoconstriction (dogs), vasodilatation (rats) or a biphasic response (cats) [41]. In humans, acidosis is a potent vasoconstrictor and therefore transient rises in CO_2 during sleep may exacerbate the vasoconstrictor response to hypoxia.

COPD and sleep apnoea hypopnoea syndrome (SAHS)

These are common conditions and available data suggest that they coexist in approximately 10% of patients [42]. Patients with COPD and impaired respiratory drive and those who have the normal risk factors for SAHS, particularly obesity, are more likely to have both conditions. The added load on the respiratory muscle pump of an increase in upper airway resistance during sleep produces acute CO_2 retention [43]. Acute derangement of gas exchange, which occurs in a patient with SAHS but normal lungs, would usually correct rapidly with termination of the apnoea and the hyperventilation that follows. However, in a patient with airflow limitation this may not be the case and, as a consequence, CO_2 retention occurs which may persist into wakefulness. Patients with both COPD and SAHS typically develop more severe hypoxia during sleep and as a result they are more prone to complications such as fluid retention and polycythaemia with less severely impaired lung function than would normally be the case [42]. Patients with SAHS and COPD and hypercapnia were found to be heavier than those who were normocapnic [44]. COPD patients without SAHS but who were hypercapnic had a smaller upper airway size, more snoring and a higher long-term alcohol consumption than those who were normocapnic [45]. These studies taken together suggest that upper airway changes during sleep are one factor contributing to diurnal respiratory failure in patients with COPD.

Table 7.1 Sleep studies in patients with COPD.

Suspected sleep apnoea syndrome
 Excessive daytime sleepiness on a background of heavy
 snoring
Oedema or polycythaemia that are unexpected for the
 degree of airflow obstruction
Respiratory variable only study usually sufficient
Monitoring of transcutaneous carbon dioxide tensions
 maybe useful, particularly if patient is receiving
 supplemental oxygen

Who needs a sleep study? (Table 7.1)

Sleep studies are not routinely indicated in patients with COPD. The awake blood gas tensions provide a good indicator of likely sleep-related disturbances of gas exchange [46]. Overnight monitoring should be performed if there is the clinical suspicion of coexistent sleep apnoea syndrome or there is fluid retention or polycythaemia that are unexpected for the severity of airflow obstruction. In most cases, a limited respiratory variable only study will suffice and full polysomnography is seldom, if ever, necessary.

Treatment of sleep-disordered breathing and nocturnal hypoxia

Oxygen therapy during sleep

Long-term oxygen therapy (LTOT) has been shown to prolong life in patients with sustained daytime hypoxia [47,48]. The question of whether patients with mild to moderate daytime hypoxaemia (arterial oxygen tension [Pao_2] in the range 7.4–9.2 kPa [56–69 mmHg]) and sleep-related oxygen desaturation should be given oxygen was addressed in a study of nocturnal oxygen therapy (NOT) alone [49]. Seventy-six patients with COPD and no polysomnographical evidence of SAHS were randomized to NOT ($n = 41$) adjusted to achieve an arterial oxygen saturation of > 90% throughout the night, or to no supplemental oxygen ($n = 35$). The mean daytime Pao_2 was 8.4 ± 0.4 kPa at baseline. There were no differences between the groups in need for LTOT, evolution of pulmonary artery pressure or survival although the study was not adequately powered to exclude an effect of NOT. Twenty-two patients (12 in the NOT group and 10 in the control group, $P = 0.98$) required LTOT during an average follow-up of 3 years. Sixteen patients died, nine in the NOT group and seven in the control group ($P = 0.84$). After 2 years, pulmonary haemodynamics were reassessed in a subgroup of patients. In the control group ($n = 22$), mean resting pulmonary artery pressure increased from 19.8 ± 5.6 to 20.5 ± 6.5 mmHg, which was not different from the change in mean pulmonary artery pressure in the NOT group ($n = 24$) from 18.3 ± 4.7 to 19.5 ± 5.3 mmHg ($P = 0.79$). These results suggest that the prescription of NOT to improve survival is not justified in patients with COPD.

The effect of oxygen on sleep quality is contentious, with some investigators showing an improvement [50] and others no benefit [51]. In neither of these studies was CO_2 tension measured and although severe hypoxia ($SaO_2 < 70\%$) may not cause arousal in humans [52], acute hypercapnia, with a rise in $Paco_2$ of 6–15 mmHg, has been shown to be a reliable and powerful arousal stimulus [53]. The arousal response to hypercapnia varies between REM and NREM sleep, with arousal occurring at a much lower level of $Paco_2$ during REM than NREM sleep [54]. A rise in $Paco_2$ appears therefore to be more important in disrupting sleep than hypoxaemia.

Drugs

Drugs have been used in patients with COPD, targeted upon improving gas exchange and sleep quality. The rationale behind the use of protriptyline is specifically its effect upon sleep architecture. Ten to 20 mg of protriptyline taken at bed time has been shown to reduce the proportion of the night spent in REM sleep, when the most severe derangements of blood gas tensions occur, from 22 to 12% in eight patients with restrictive chest wall disorders [55]. The total amount of sleep time spent with a Sao_2 less than 80% decreased and there was a reduction in the maximum CO_2 tension reached during the night. The magnitude of the reduction in oxygen desaturation was correlated with the decrease in REM. The Pao_2 during the day increased by approximately 1 kPa but the changes in $Paco_2$ and base excess failed to reach statistical significance. Similar results have been reported in COPD [56,57]. Series *et al.* [56] studied 14 patients with stable COPD in an open study. Patients took 20 mg protriptyline each night and were studied before starting treatment and after 2 and 10 weeks. There was a reduction in the percentage of sleep spent in REM from 11.1 to 4.2% but there were no other changes in sleep time or architecture. While taking protriptyline, the lowest sleep Sao_2 increased from mean 64.5% to mean 77.4% and the amount of time with Sao_2 below a given level of saturation was significantly decreased for all values greater than 65%. Arterial blood gas tensions by day showed an increase in Pao_2 from 57 to 66 mmHg and a nonsignificant fall in $Paco_2$ from 52 to 48 mmHg. There were no changes in arterial pH or bicarbonate ion concentration. Clinical state and treatment were unchanged for 4 weeks before the start of the study and, although no control group was studied, the benefits seen probably reflect the action of protriptyline.

Carroll *et al.* [57] recruited 18 patients with severe stable COPD to a randomized double-blind cross-over study of 10 mg protriptyline and placebo. Each limb of the study lasted 6 weeks, with assessments made before starting and after 6 and 12 weeks' treatment. Each polysomnographic study was preceded by an acclimatization night and the percentage of total sleep time (TST) spent in REM sleep was 16% on entry, 15% during the placebo phase and 8.8% while taking protriptyline ($P < 0.001$). The percentage of TST spent with Sao_2 less than 90%, 80% and 70% were all improved but only the change in %TST with $Sao_2 < 90\%$ reached statistical significance. The maximum increase in transcutaneous carbon dioxide tension ($Ptcco_2$) was similar during both phases of the trial; however, as REM time was reduced during the protriptyline limb, the total time with $Ptcco_2$ greater than awake baseline was reduced. $Paco_2$ during spontaneous breathing fell from 6.4 kPa (5.2–8.5 kPa) to 5.8 kPa (5–8.1 kPa), $P < 0.01$ and Pao_2 increased from 6.9 kPa (4.8–10.1 kPa) to 7.8 kPa (5.1–10 kPa), $P = NS$. There were statistically significant increases in 6 minute walking distance and maximal inspiratory mouth pressures.

The beneficial effects of protriptyline upon daytime arterial blood gas tensions and function were attributed to the reduction in arterial oxygen desaturation. However, abolition of nocturnal oxygen desaturation by supplemental oxygen does not improve daytime arterial blood gas tensions. Simonds *et al.* [55] found a significant reduction in maximum $Ptcco_2$ in a group of patients with extrapulmonary restrictive disorders and Carroll *et al.* [57], in patients with COPD, noted a reduction in the time spent with $Ptcco_2$ above baseline levels, both suggesting that nocturnal hypoventilation was reduced. This may have contributed to the improved daytime arterial blood gas tensions by allowing renal excretion of bicarbonate, thereby restoring central ventilatory drive. However, the ventilatory response to carbon dioxide was not measured and a direct effect of protriptyline upon ventilatory response cannot be excluded. The anticholinergic side-effects of protriptyline were a major problem in all the studies. In the study by Carroll *et al.* [57], five of 12 male patients expressed reluctance to take protriptyline on a long-term basis, primarily because of urinary difficulties. With the advent of newer antidepressants, protriptyline has largely been withdrawn from the market and although a potent REM-suppressing and beneficial effect on sleep-disordered breathing has been demonstrated with the selective serotonin uptake inhibitor fluoxetine in obese patients [58] its use in patients with COPD has not been evaluated.

There are few studies of the effects of either oral or inhaled long-acting bronchodilators during sleep in patients with COPD. The studies are small and the results variable.

In a cross-over study of 20 patients with COPD, evening administration of theophylline resulted in less time with $Sao_2 < 90\%$ than QDS salbutamol and there was subjectively less nocturnal wheeze but no changes in sleep quality [59]. In another study, higher concentrations of theophylline resulted in a greater improvement in spirometric variables at 7 a.m. but no difference in oxygen saturation or sleep quality [60]. Mulloy and McNicholas [61] found that theophylline increased oxygen saturation and decreased transcutaneous CO_2 overnight but at the expense of impaired sleep quality in 10 stable patients. They also found beneficial effects upon exercise and a reduction in hyperinflation. Worse sleep quality was seen in another study without beneficial effects on gas exchange [62]. In patients with asthma, salmeterol but not theophylline has been shown to improve the patient's perception of sleep [63–65] but the differences are small. To date there have been no similar studies in patients with COPD. Tiotropium, a once-a-day long-acting anticholinergic agent, improves nocturnal FEV_1 compared with placebo [66] and increases nadir oxygen saturation without compromising sleep quality.

Respiratory stimulants such as medroxyprogesterone acetate, acetazolamide and almitrine have been shown to improve arterial blood gas tensions during wakefulness and sleep in some studies [67–69] but the results are not consistent [68,70] and side-effects have precluded widespread use.

Assisted ventilation during sleep

A number of studies have shown that non-invasive positive pressure ventilation (NPPV) is feasible at home during sleep in patients with COPD [71–77] and that abnormal physiology can be corrected using NPPV. However, there have been few controlled trials and most of these had small numbers of patients followed over a short period of time [78–81]. They have generally been characterized by no significant advantage from NPPV [78–80], poor tolerance [78] and worse sleep efficiency [80]. However, Meecham Jones *et al.* [79] showed improvements in daytime arterial blood gas tensions, sleep quality and quality of life during the pressure support (PSV) limb of a cross-over study comparing PSV and oxygen with oxygen alone. This was the only study in which the overnight control of nocturnal hypoventilation was confirmed and the improvement in daytime $Paco_2$ correlated with a reduction in overnight transcutaneous CO_2. Sleep quality was shown to improve in another uncontrolled study in which an overnight reduction in transcutaneous CO_2 tension was confirmed [72]. The reason for improved sleep quality is not clear. It is likely to be multifactorial and may include better oxygenation, the reduction in CO_2, but also offloading of the respiratory muscles. In patients with SAHS, it is the increased effort of breathing against an occluded airway that is a major stimulus causing arousal [82], and the reduction in respiratory muscle effort [83,84], which can be achieved with non-invasive ventilation, may be important in improving sleep quality.

In a 1-year controlled trial, Casanova *et al.* [85] randomized 52 patients with severe stable COPD to either NPPV plus 'standard care' or to standard care alone. The adequacy of ventilation was determined by close observation of the patient, during the day and night, but was not confirmed objectively. The level of support was modest, with a mean inspiratory positive airway pressure (IPAP) of 12 ± 2 cm H_2O. One-year survival was similar in both groups (78%) as was the number of acute exacerbations. The number of hospital admissions was less at 3 months in the NPPV group (5 vs 15%, $P < 0.05$), but this difference was not seen at 6 months (18 vs 19%, respectively). There was either no or little difference between the groups in dyspnoea scales, gas exchange, haematocrit, pulmonary function, cardiac function and neuropsychological performance. However, the number of patients was too small to avoid a type II error and the period of follow-up too short to evaluate the effect upon outcome fully.

Clini *et al.* [86] reported a prospective randomized controlled trial of NPPV during sleep in chronic stable COPD patients, with a significant number of patients followed for a reasonable period of time. One hundred and twenty-two patients with stable chronic hypercapnia who had been on LTOT for at least 6 months were considered and 90 randomized to continuing LTOT or LTOT and NPPV. Compliance with LTOT was excellent and amongst NPPV patients the mean night-time use of 9 h compares very favourably with reported use in other studies. There were small improvements in the NPPV group in resting $Paco_2$ and dyspnoea and health-related quality of life, but no improvement in survival or hospital stay, although there was a trend towards a lesser time in hospital in the NPPV group compared with an increase in the LTOT group when compared with the period before the study. ICU stay was reduced in both groups, but more in the NPPV than in the LTOT group. The effect of NPPV upon sleep quality and quantity was not evaluated. In common with most other studies, there was inadequate confirmation that effective ventilation had been delivered. NPPV was deemed to be adequate when the $Paco_2$ was reduced by 5% during wakefulness; this reduction in CO_2 during NPPV when awake is very modest. The changes in diurnal $Paco_2$, which was the primary endpoint that informed the power calculation, were small and it remains to be seen whether more aggressive ventilation would have resulted in a bigger change in this and other endpoints. The average IPAP was 14 ± 3 and expiratory positive airway pressure (EPAP) 2 ± 1 cm H_2O,

suggesting that there was room to increase the pressures, at least to levels closer to those seen in the study of Meecham Jones *et al.* [79]. The fact that the effectiveness of ventilation during sleep was not confirmed is an important limitation of the study and it is possible that there was in fact no change in $Paco_2$ overnight, given that the pressures used were comparable with those used in the study of Lin [80] in which no effect of NPPV was seen upon nocturnal hypoventilation. If this is correct, the question arises as to why patients reported less dyspnoea and an improved quality of life. First, this could have been a placebo effect, as was seen in the study of Gay *et al.* [81]. A significant placebo effect has been seen with sham CPAP [87] and the placebo effect of a 'breathing machine' should not be underestimated. Secondly, exacerbations have been shown to have a detrimental effect upon quality of life [88] in patients with COPD. NPPV offloads the respiratory muscles [89] and reduces the sensation of dyspnoea [90,91] associated with an acute exacerbation at ventilator settings similar to those used in this study. It is possible that NPPV therefore reduced the impact of exacerbations upon the patient; this may also have contributed to the trend towards reduced hospitalization. Compliance was considered to be acceptable if NPPV use was greater than 5 h/day on average; in fact the mean daily use in those who achieved this minimum usage was much higher at 9 ± 2 h/day. This suggests that at least some patients were using the ventilator during wakefulness, which lends some support to this hypothesis. Thirdly, no data are given about input from health-care workers, which may impact upon quality of life and dyspnoea [92]. It is possible that patients receiving NPPV, which requires considerable staff input at least initially, had greater contact with medical and paramedical staff than those on LTOT alone.

Most studies suggest that it is the patients with more severe hypercapnia who are likely to benefit and there is no place for nocturnal NPPV, at present, in those without sustained daytime hypercapnia. On the basis of current knowledge, a trial of NPPV can only be justified in patients with COPD who have symptoms of nocturnal hypoventilation (morning headaches, daytime sleepiness, etc.) despite maximal bronchodilator therapy or who cannot tolerate LTOT, even with careful administration using Venturi masks or a low flow meter. It should also be considered in patients with repeated episodes of hospitalization with hypercapnic ventilatory failure requiring acute NPPV [93]. Adequate control of nocturnal hypoventilation should be confirmed as this has been a feature of the studies in which benefit has been seen [72,79].

However, NPPV does not have to be delivered during sleep to improve both daytime and sleep parameters. In a carefully designed study of patients with extrapulmonary lung restriction, NPPV was delivered either during sleep or during the day for a 1-month period [94]. In the latter group, patients were prevented from sleeping by having to respond to intermittent prompts by pressing a button when a light came on. There were no differences between the two groups, with each showing improved diurnal blood gas tensions, increased respiratory muscle strength and a slight reduction in the occlusion pressure 100 ms after the onset of inspiratory flow (pressure generated in the first 0.1 s, $P_{0.1}$), a measure of central drive. Overnight Sao_2 and transcutaneous CO_2 tensions were also improved in both groups at the end of the study during spontaneous breathing overnight. Sleep quality was also shown to improve in a small subgroup who underwent full polysomnography. Diaz et al. [95] also showed significant increases in daytime Pao_2 (mean increase 1.14 kPa) and $Paco_2$ (mean decrease -1.12 kPa) when patients with COPD were ventilated for 2 h/day 5 days/week for 3 weeks. Although the effect upon sleep was not evaluated, they found that the improvement in $Paco_2$ correlated with changes in dynamic hyperinflation, intrinsic positive end-expiratory pressure (PEEP), inspiratory lung impedance, tidal volume and functional residual capacity. There was no demonstrable effect upon tests of respiratory muscle function. They concluded that the primary effect of NPPV was upon respiratory system load. Daytime ventilation may be an option in patients who cannot tolerate NPPV during sleep, but again this warrants much more detailed evaluation before this strategy becomes widespread.

The use of CPAP overnight in patients with COPD has also been evaluated and while no effect upon gas exchange or sleep quality has been demonstrated, an improvement in inspiratory muscle strength and endurance as well as walking distance has been demonstrated [96], presumably a consequence of reducing the work of breathing [97]. In patients with a combination of SAHS and COPD, CPAP improves blood gas tensions and FEV_1 [98,99] and reduces the need for hospitalization [98]. The benefit seemed to be greatest in patients with hypercapnia [99].

Conclusions

Significant changes in respiratory function take place during sleep in normal subjects. These do not usually impact upon daytime function. However, in the patient with COPD the effect may be sufficient to worsen ventilation to the point at which diurnal ventilatory failure occurs. In patients with combined SAHS and COPD, more severe derangements of daytime blood gas tensions are seen than would be expected for the degree of airflow limitation. Whether other effects such as minor degrees of sleep disruption are clinically important remains to be seen. With the increasing recognition of patients with SAHS, abnormalities occurring solely during sleep are increasingly recognized and their implications and hence management requires further study.

References

1 Kohnlein T, Welte T, Tan LB, Elliott MW. Central sleep apnoea syndrome in patients with chronic heart disease: a critical review of the current literature. *Thorax* 2002;**57**:547–54.

2 Mezon BL, West P, Israels J, Kryger M. Sleep breathing abnormalities in kyphoscoliosis. *Am Rev Respir Dis* 1980;**122**: 617–21.

3 Guilleminault C, Kurlan G, Winkle R, Miles LE. Severe kyphoscoliosis, breathing and sleep: the Quasimodo syndrome during sleep. *Chest* 1981;**79**:626–30.

4 Douglas NJ, White DP, Pickett CK, Weil J, Zwillich CW. Respiration during sleep in normal man. *Thorax* 1982;**37**: 840–4.

5 Sullivan CE, Issa FG, Berthon-Jones M, Saunders NA. Pathophysiology of sleep apnea. In: Saunders NA, Sullivan CE, eds. *Sleep and Breathing*. New York: Marcel Dekker, 1984: 299–364.

6 White DP. Occlusion pressure and ventilation during sleep in normal humans. *J Appl Physiol* 1986;**61**:1279–87.

7 Tabachnick E, Muller N, Levison H, Bryan AC. The behaviour of the respiratory muscles during sleep. *Physiologist* 1980; **23**:1.

8 Douglas NJ, White DP, Weil JV *et al.* Hypoxic ventilatory response decreases during sleep in normal men. *Am Rev Respir Dis* 1982;**125**:286–9.

9 Douglas N, White DP, Weil JV, Pickett CK, Clifford WZ. Hypercapnic ventilatory response in sleeping adults. *Am Rev Resp Dis* 1982;**126**:758–62.

10 Gould GA, Gugger M, Molloy J *et al.* Breathing pattern and eye movement density during REM sleep in humans. *Am Rev Respir Dis* 1988;**138**:874–7.

11 Stradling JR, Chadwick GA, Frew AJ. Changes in ventilation and its components in normal subjects during sleep. *Thorax* 1985;**40**:364–70.

12 Douglas NJ, Calverley PMA, Leggett RJE *et al.* Transient hypoxaemia during sleep in chronic bronchitis and emphysema. *Lancet* 1979;**1**:1–4.

13 Fletcher EC, Gray BA, Levin DC. Non-apneic mechanisms of arterial oxygen desaturation during rapid-eye-movement sleep. *J Appl Physiol* 1983;**54**:632–9.

14 O'Donoghue FJ, Catcheside PG, Ellis EE *et al.* Sleep hypoventilation in hypercapnic chronic obstructive pulmonary disease: prevalence and associated factors. *Eur Respir J* 2003;**21**: 977–84.

15 Becker HF, Piper AJ, Flynn WE *et al.* Breathing during sleep in patients with nocturnal desaturation. *Am J Respir Crit Care Med* 1999;**159**:112–8.

16 Catterall JR, Calverley PM, Macnee W *et al.* Mechanism of transient nocturnal hypoxemia in hypoxic chronic bronchitis and emphysema. *J Appl Physiol* 1985;**59**:1698–703.

17 White JE, Drinnan MJ, Smithson AJ, Griffiths CJ, Gibson GJ. Respiratory muscle activity during rapid eye movement (REM) sleep in patients with chronic obstructive pulmonary disease. *Thorax* 1995;**50**:376–82.

18 Ballard RD, Clover CW, Suh BY. Influence of sleep on respiratory function in emphysema. *Am J Respir Crit Care Med* 1995;**151**:945–51.

19 Douglas NJ, Flenley DC. Breathing during sleep in patients with obstructive lung disease. *Am Rev Respir Dis* 1990;**141**: 1055–70.

20 Koo KW, Sax DS, Snider GL. Arterial blood gas tensions and pH during sleep in chronic obstructive pulmonary disease. *Am J Med* 1975;**58**:663–70.

21 Leitch AG, Clancy LJ, Leggett RJE *et al*. Arterial blood gas-tensions, hydrogen ion and electroencephalogram during sleep in patients with chronic ventilatory failure. *Thorax* 1976; **31**:730–5.

22 Millman RP, Knight H, Kline LR *et al*. Changes in compartmental ventilation associated with eye movements during REM sleep. *J Appl Physiol* 1988;**65**:1196–202.

23 Hudgel DW, Martin RJ, Johnson B, Hill P. Mechanics of the respiratory system and breathing pattern during sleep in normal humans. *J Appl Physiol* 1984;**56**:133–7.

24 Wiegand L, Zwillich CW, White DP. Sleep and the ventilatory response to resistive loading in normal men. *J Appl Physiol* 1988;**64**:1186–95.

25 Chan CS, Bye PT, Woolcock AJ, Sullivan CE. Eucapnia and hypercapnia in patients with chronic airflow limitation: the role of the upper airway. *Am Rev Respir Dis* 1990;**141**:861–5.

26 Chan CS, Grunstein RR, Bye PT, Woolcock AJ, Sullivan CE. Obstructive sleep apnea with severe chronic airflow limitation: comparison of hypercapnic and eucapnic patients. *Am Rev Respir Dis* 1989;**140**:1274–8.

27 White DP, Weil JV, Zwillich CW. Metabolic rate and breathing during sleep. *J Appl Physiol* 1985;**59**:384–91.

28 Flenley DC, Millar JS. Ventilatory response to oxygen and carbon dioxide in chronic respiratory failure. *Clin Sci* 1967;**33**: 319–34.

29 Littner NR, McGinty DJ, Arand DL. Determinants of oxygen desaturation in the couse of ventilation during sleep in chronic obstructive pulmonary disease. *Am Rev Respir Dis* 1980;**122**:849–57.

30 Tatsumi K, Kimura H, Kunitomo F *et al*. Sleep arterial oxygen desaturation and chemical control of breathing during wakefulness in COPD. *Chest* 1986;**90**:68–73.

31 Fleetham JA, Mezon B, West P *et al*. Chemical control of ventilation and sleep arterial oxygen desaturation in patients with COPD. *Am Rev Respir Dis* 1980;**122**:583–9.

32 Elliott MW, Mulvey DA, Moxham J, Green M, Branthwaite MA. Domiciliary nocturnal nasal intermittent positive pressure ventilation in COPD: mechanisms underlying changes in arterial blood gas tensions. *Eur Respir J* 1991;**4**:1044–52.

33 White DP, Douglas NJ, Pickett CK, Zwillich CW, Weil JV. Sleep deprivation and control of ventilation. *Am Rev Respir Dis* 1983;**128**:984–6.

34 Power JT, Stewart IC, Connaughton JJ *et al*. Nocturnal cough in patients with chronic bronchitis and emphysema. *Am Rev Respir Dis* 1984;**130**:999–1001.

35 Arand DL, McGinty DJ, Littner MR. Respiratory patterns associated with hemoglobin desaturation during sleep in chronic obstructive pulmonary disease. *Chest* 1981;**80**:183–90.

36 Singh B. Sleep apnea: a psychiatric perspective. In: Saunders NA, Sullivan CE, eds. *Sleep and Breathing*. New York: Marcel Dekker, 1984: 403–22.

37 Orr WC, Shamma-Othman Z, Levin D, Othman J, Rundell OH. Persistent hypoxemia and excessive daytime sleepiness in chronic obstructive pulmonary disease (COPD). *Chest* 1990;**97**:583–5.

38 Boysen PG, Block AJ, Wynne JW, Hunt LA, Flick MR. Nocturnal pulmonary hypertension in patients with chronic obstructive pulmonary disease. *Chest* 1979;**76**:536–42.

39 Coccagna G, Lugaresi E. Arterial blood gases and pulmonary and systemic arterial pressure during sleep in chronic obstructive pulmonary disease. *Sleep* 1978;**1**:117–24.

40 Fletcher EC, Costarangos C, Miller T. The rate of fall of arterial oxyhemoglobin saturation in obstructive sleep apnea. *Chest* 1989;**96**:717–22.

41 Emery CJ, Sloan PJ, Mohammed FH, Barer GR. The action of hypercapnia during hypoxia on pulmonary vessels. *Bull Eur Physiopathol Respir* 1977;**13**:763–76.

42 Chaouat A, Weitzenblum E, Krieger J *et al*. Association of chronic obstructive pulmonary disease and sleep apnea syndrome. *Am J Respir Crit Care Med* 1995;**151**:82–6.

43 Henke KG, Dempsey JA, Kowitz JM, Skatrud JB. Effects of sleep-induced increases in upper airway resistance on ventilation. *J Appl Physiol* 1990;**69**:617–24.

44 Chan CS, Grunstein RR, Bye PT, Woolcock AJ, Sullivan CE. Obstructive sleep apnea with severe chronic airflow limitation: comparison of hypercapnic and eucapnic patients. *Am Rev Respir Dis* 1989;**140**:1274–8.

45 Chan CS, Bye PT, Woolcock AJ, Sullivan CE. Eucapnia and hypercapnia in patients with chronic airflow limitation: the role of the upper airway. *Am Rev Respir Dis* 1990;**141**(4 Pt 1): 861–5.

46 Piper AJ, Parker S, Torzillo PJ, Sullivan CE, Bye PT. Nocturnal nasal IPPV stabilizes patients with cystic fibrosis and hypercapnic respiratory failure. *Chest* 1992;**102**:846–50.

47 Nocturnal Oxygen Therapy Trial Group. Continuous or nocturnal oxygen therapy in hypoxaemic chronic obstructive lung disease. *Ann Intern Med* 1980;**93**:391–8.

48 Medical Research Council Working Party Report. Long-term domiciliary oxygen therapy in chronic hypoxic cor pulmonale complicating chronic bronchitis and emphysema. *Lancet* 1981;**i**:681–5.

49 Chaouat A, Weitzenblum E, Kessler R *et al*. A randomized trial of nocturnal oxygen therapy in chronic obstructive pulmonary disease patients. *Eur Respir J* 1999;**14**:1002–8.

50 Calverley PMA, Brezinova V, Douglas NJ, Catterall JR, Flenley DC. The effect of oxygenation on sleep quality in chronic bronchitis and emphysema. *Am Rev Respir Dis* 1982;**126**:206–10.

51 Fleetham JA, West P, Mezon B *et al*. Sleep, arousals, and oxygen desaturation in COPD. *Am Rev Respir Dis* 1982;**126**: 429–33.

52 Berthon-Jones M, Sullivan CE. Ventilatory and arousal

responses to hypoxia in sleeping humans. *Am Rev Respir Dis* 1982;**125**:632–9.

53 Hedemark L, Kronenberg R. Ventilatory responses to hypoxia and CO_2 during natural and flurazepam induced sleep in normal adults. *Am Rev Respir Dis* 1981;**123**:190 [Abstract].

54 Berthon-Jones M, Sullivan CE. Ventilation and arousal responses to hypercapnia in normal sleeping humans. *J Appl Physiol* 1984;**57**:59–67.

55 Simonds AK, Parker RA, Sawicka EH, Branthwaite MA. Protriptyline for nocturnal hypoventilation in restrictive chest wall disease. *Thorax* 1986;**41**:586–90.

56 Series F, Cormier Y, La Forge J. Changes in day and night time oxygenation with protriptyline in patients with chronic obstructive lung disease. *Thorax* 1989;**44**:275–9.

57 Carroll N, Parker RA, Branthwaite MA. The use of protriptyline for respiratory failure in patients with chronic airflow limitation. *Eur Respir J* 1990;**3**:746–51.

58 Kopelman PG, Elliott MW, Simonds A *et al*. Short-term use of fluoxetine in asymptomatic obese subjects with sleep-related hypoventilation. *Int J Obes Relat Metab Disord* 1992;**16**:825–30.

59 Man GC, Champman KR, Ali SH, Darke AC. Sleep quality and nocturnal respiratory function with once-daily theophylline (Uniphyl) and inhaled salbutamol in patients with COPD. *Chest* 1996;**110**:648–53.

60 Martin RJ, Pak J. Overnight theophylline concentrations and effects on sleep and lung function in chronic obstructive pulmonary disease. *Am Rev Respir Dis* 1992;**145**:540–4.

61 Mulloy E, McNicholas WT. Theophylline improves gas exchange during rest, exercise, and sleep in severe chronic obstructive pulmonary disease. *Am Rev Respir Dis* 1993;**148**(4 Pt 1):1030–6.

62 Sacco C, Braghiroli A, Grossi E, Donner CF. The effects of doxofylline versus theophylline on sleep architecture in COPD patients. *Monald Arch Chest Dis* 1995;**50**:98–103.

63 Selby C, Engleman HM, Fitzpatrick MF *et al*. Inhaled salmeterol or oral theophylline in nocturnal asthma? *Am J Respir Crit Care Med* 1997;**155**:104–8.

64 Wiegand L, Mende CN, Zaidel G *et al*. Salmeterol vs theophylline: sleep and efficacy outcomes in patients with nocturnal asthma. *Chest* 1999;**115**:1525–32.

65 Fitzpatrick MF, Mackay T, Driver H, Douglas NJ. Salmeterol in nocturnal asthma: a double blind, placebo controlled trial of a long acting inhaled beta-2 agonist. *BMJ* 1990;**301**:1365–8.

66 Calverley PM, Lee A, Towse L *et al*. Effect of tiotropium bromide on circadian variation in airflow limitation in chronic obstructive pulmonary disease. *Thorax* 2003;**58**:855–60.

67 Skatrud JB, Dempsey JA, Iber C, Berssenbrugge A. Correction of CO_2 retention during sleep in patients with chronic obstructive pulmonary diseases. *Am Rev Respir Dis* 1981;**124**:260–8.

68 Skatrud JB, Dempsey JA. Relative effectiveness of acetazolamide versus medroxyprogesterone acetate in correction of carbon dioxide retention. *Am Rev Respir Dis* 1983;**127**:405–12.

69 Connaughton JJ, Douglas NJ, Morgan AD *et al*. Almitrine improves oxygenation when both awake and asleep in patients with hypoxia and carbon dioxide retention caused by chronic bronchitis and emphysema. *Am Rev Respir Dis* 1985;**132**:206–10.

70 Dolly FR, Block AJ. Medroxyprogesterone acetate and COPD: effect on breathing and oxygenation in sleeping and awake patients. *Chest* 1983;**84**:394–8.

71 Carroll N, Branthwaite MA. Control of nocturnal hypoventilation by nasal intermittent positive pressure ventilation. *Thorax* 1988;**43**:349–53.

72 Elliott MW, Simonds AK, Carroll MP, Wedzicha JA, Branthwaite MA. Domiciliary nocturnal nasal intermittent positive pressure ventilation in hypercapnic respiratory failure due to chronic obstructive lung disease: effects on sleep and quality of life. *Thorax* 1992;**47**:342–8.

73 Marino W. Intermittent volume cycled mechanical ventilation via nasal mask in patients with respiratory failure due to COPD. *Chest* 1991;**99**:681–4.

74 Leger P, Bedicam JM, Cornette A *et al*. Nasal intermittent positive pressure ventilation: long-term follow-up in patients with severe chronic respiratory insufficiency. *Chest* 1994;**105**:100–5.

75 Simonds AK, Elliott MW. Outcome of domiciliary nasal intermittent positive pressure ventilation in restrictive and obstructive disorders. *Thorax* 1995;**50**:604–9.

76 Sivasothy P, Smith IE, Shneerson JM. Mask intermittent positive pressure ventilation in chronic hypercapnic respiratory failure due to chronic obstructive pulmonary disease. *Eur Respir J* 1998;**11**:34–40.

77 Jones SE, Packham S, Hebden M, Smith AP. Domiciliary nocturnal intermittent positive pressure ventilation in patients with respiratory failure due to severe COPD: long-term follow-up and effect on survival. *Thorax* 1998;**53**:495–8.

78 Strumpf DA, Millman RP, Carlisle CC *et al*. Nocturnal positive-pressure ventilation via nasal mask in patients with severe chronic obstructive pulmonary disease. *Am Rev Respir Dis* 1991;**144**:1234–9.

79 Meecham Jones DJ, Paul EA, Jones PW, Wedzicha JA. Nasal pressure support ventilation plus oxygen compared with oxygen therapy alone in hypercapnic COPD. *Am J Respir Crit Care Med* 1995;**152**:538–44.

80 Lin CC. Comparison between nocturnal nasal positive pressure ventilation combined with oxygen therapy and oxygen monotherapy in patients with severe COPD. *Am J Respir Crit Care Med* 1996;**154**:353–8.

81 Gay PC, Hubmayr RD, Stroetz RW. Efficacy of nocturnal nasal ventilation in stable, severe chronic obstructive pulmonary disease during a 3-month controlled trial. *Mayo Clin Proc* 1996;**71**:533–42.

82 Black JE, Guilleminault C, Colrain IM, Carrillo O. Upper airway resistance syndrome: central electroencephalographic power and changes in breathing effort. *Am J Respir Crit Care Med* 2000;**162**(2 Pt 1):406–11.

83 Elliott MW, Mulvey DA, Moxham J, Green M, Branthwaite MA. Inspiratory muscle effort during nasal intermittent positive pressure ventilation in patients with chronic obstructive airways disease. *Anaesthesia* 1993;**48**:8–13.

84 Carrey Z, Gottfried SB, Levy RD. Ventilatory muscle support in respiratory failure with nasal positive pressure ventilation. *Chest* 1990;**97**:150–8.

85 Casanova C, Celli BR, Tost L *et al*. Long-term controlled trial of nocturnal nasal positive pressure ventilation in patients with severe COPD. *Chest* 2000;**118**:1582–90.

86 Clini E, Sturani C, Rossi A *et al*. The Italian multicentre study on non-invasive ventilation in chronic obstructive pulmonary disease patients. *Eur Respir J* 2002;**20**:529–38.

87 Jenkinson C, Davies RJ, Mullins R, Stradling JR. Comparison of therapeutic and subtherapeutic nasal continuous positive airway pressure for obstructive sleep apnoea: a randomised prospective parallel trial. *Lancet* 1999;**353**:2100–5.

88 Seemungal TA, Donaldson GC, Paul EA *et al*. Effect of exacerbation on quality of life in patients with chronic obstructive pulmonary disease. *Am J Respir Crit Care Med* 1998;**157**(5 Pt 1): 1418–22.

89 Appendini L, Patessio A, Zanaboni S *et al*. Physiologic effects of positive end-expiratory pressure and mask pressure support during exacerbations of chronic obstructive pulmonary disease. *Am J Respir Crit Care Med* 1994;**149**:1069–76.

90 Bott J, Carroll MP, Conway JH *et al*. Randomised controlled trial of nasal ventilation in acute ventilatory failure due to chronic obstructive airways disease. *Lancet* 1993;**341**:1555–7.

91 Plant PK, Owen JL, Elliott MW. Early use of non-invasive ventilation for acute exacerbations of chronic obstructive pulmonary disease on general respiratory wards: a multicentre randomised controlled trial. *Lancet* 2000;**355**:1931–5.

92 Cockcroft A, Bagnall P, Heslop A *et al*. Controlled trial of respiratory health worker visiting patients with chronic respiratory disability. *BMJ* 1987;**294**:225–8.

93 Clinical indications for non-invasive positive pressure ventilation in chronic respiratory failure due to restrictive lung disease, COPD, and nocturnal hypoventilation: a consensus conference report. *Chest* 1999;**116**:521–34.

94 Schonhofer B, Geibel M, Sonnerborn M, Kohler D. Daytime mechanical ventilation in chronic respiratory insufficiency. *Eur Respir J* 1997;**10**:2840–6.

95 Diaz O, Begin P, Torrealba B, Jover E, Lisboa C. Effects of non-invasive ventilation on lung hyperinflation in stable hypercapnic COPD. *Eur Respir J* 2002;**20**:1490–8.

96 Mezzanotte WS, Tangel DJ, Fox AM, Ballard RD, White DP. Nocturnal nasal continuous positive airway pressure in patients with chronic obstructive pulmonary disease: influence on waking respiratory muscle function. *Chest* 1994;**106**: 1100–8.

97 Petrof BJ, Kimoff RJ, Levy RD, Cosio MG, Gottfried SB. Nasal continuous positive airway pressure facilitates respiratory muscle function during sleep in severe chronic obstructive pulmonary disease. *Am Rev Respir Dis* 1991;**143**:928–35.

98 Mansfield D, Naughton MT. Effects of continuous positive airway pressure on lung function in patients with chronic obstructive pulmonary disease and sleep disordered breathing. *Respirology* 1999;**4**:365–70.

99 de Miguel J, Cabello J, Sanchez-Alarcos JM *et al*. Long-term effects of treatment with nasal continuous positive airway pressure on lung function in patients with overlap syndrome. *Sleep Breath* 2002;**6**:3–10.

CHAPTER 8
The physiology of cough

Marian Kollarik and Bradley J. Undem

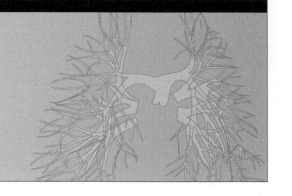

The problem of cough is often underestimated when considering life-threatening diseases such as COPD. Yet chronic and non-relenting cough can substantially diminish the quality of life of those suffering from this disease [1]. In patients with COPD, cough is often a natural consequence of the mucus hypersecretion and airway obstruction that typify their disease. In some patients with inflammatory airways disease, however, the neurophysiology of the cough reflex may be pathologically altered, leading to an exaggerated sensitivity of the reflex pathways. An inappropriately sensitized cough reflex may lead to persistent 'urge to cough' sensations which result in cough in excess of functional requirements. In this review we discuss the basic physiological concepts of the cough reflex. Emphasis is placed on the nature of the afferent (sensory) neural pathways involved in the initiation of the cough response, and the potential mechanisms by which these pathways can become altered in inflammatory airways diseases such as COPD.

The cough reflex

The basic function of cough is to remove excessive or irritant material from the airways. This is achieved by the interaction of the airflow with the mucus lining the airway wall. The physical characteristics of the airflow and mucus are critical determinants of cough efficacy. A key factor underlying the clearing effect of cough is the extraordinary high linear velocity of the airflow that acts to remove irritants and mucus from the airways. The linear velocity of the airflow equals the airflow rate divided by the airway cross-sectional area (linear velocity = airflow rate/cross-sectional area). The effectors of the cough reflex (i.e. respiratory and laryngeal muscles) are activated in a highly coordinated and stereotypic pattern to generate high intrapleural pressure, which is responsible for both high airflow rate and the reduction in airway cross-sectional area.

Cough can be described in three separate phases: 'inspiratory', 'compressive' and 'expulsive' [2]. The inspiratory phase denotes the rapid inspiration of a variable tidal volume, usually larger than the eupnoeic tidal volume. This phase depends on the proper action of inspiratory muscles. Larger end-inspiratory volume inhaled during the inspiratory phase improves contractility of the expiratory muscles by improving their length–tension relationships (the length–tension relationship is optimal at higher lung volumes). Thus, larger end-inspiratory volume helps to generate the intrapleural pressure required during the subsequent phases. Cough can also occur in the absence of the inspiratory phase. This type of cough is often referred to as an 'expiration reflex'. An initial expiration reflex is often followed by bouts of more traditional coughing [2].

During the compressive phase of the cough, expiratory muscles are activated and the glottis closes (for ~0.2 s). The glottis closure allows for a great rise of intrapleural pressure (reported up to 300 mmHg ~ 40 kPa) (Fig. 8.1). The onset of the expulsive phase is marked by the opening of the glottis. When the glottis opens, the high pressure gradient between atmospheric pressure and the pressure in the airways results in a rapid expiratory airflow. The pressure gradient between intrapleural pressure and the pressure in the airways causes substantial dynamic compression of the airways as the pressure in the airways drops. The high values of the intrapleural pressure are important to achieve substantial dynamic compression of the airways. The dynamic compression is initiated early in the expulsive phase in the trachea and extends to the more peripheral airways as air is expelled. The cross-sectional area of the trachea can be reduced as much as fivefold, which leads to the fivefold increase in the linear velocity of the airflow (reported up to 25 m/s) [3]. Because the kinetic energy of a gas increases with the square of the linear velocity of the airflow, the fivefold increase in the linear velocity results in a 25-fold increase in the kinetic energy of expelled

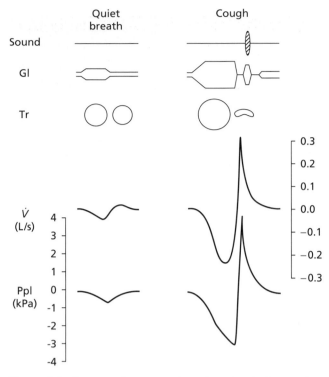

Figure 8.1 The acoustic, geometric and mechanical events in quiet breath and cough. Changes in cough sound, glottal (Gl) and tracheal (Tr) cross-sectional areas, airflow ($\dot{V}$; scale on the right) and intrathoracic pressure (Ppl; scale on the left). Note dramatic reduction in the tracheal cross-sectional area in cough as a result of dynamic compression. The traces were obtained from an anaesthetized cat. (Modified from Korpas and Tomori [2].)

gas which is available to interact with the mucus on the airway wall.

The expulsive phase of cough may be interrupted by the repeated glottis closures into the series of short expiratory efforts, each having compressive and expulsive components. It has been speculated that this interruptive pattern of coughing enhances clearance of the smaller airways [4]. Although all three phases are typically described, cough can be effective without complete glottis closure. Effective coughing was also reported in intubated patients and in patients with tracheostomies, who cannot achieve extreme values of intrathoracic pressure because of the functional absence of the glottis [5].

Cough is effective in clearing the mucus from the central airways but not the more peripheral airways. Theoretical estimates suggest that coughing is only effective to the 7th or 12th generation of the airways [6]. Thus, mucus from the more peripheral airways must be removed by mucociliary transport in order to be 'coughed up'.

Although the high linear velocity of the airflow is an essential prerequisite for effective coughing, the quantity and quality of mucus are also critical factors of the cough efficacy. At high linear velocities of the airflow, mucus is torn from the airway wall and the droplets are aerosolized into the airway lumen (described as a misty flow). This phenomenon is greatly affected by the physical properties of mucus. Increased thickness of the mucus layer promotes the formation of misty flow while increased cohesiveness and adhesiveness of the mucus have the opposite effect [7]. The effect of cough on airway clearance is typically measured by the clearance of inhaled radioactive particles. This technique showed that cough improves airway clearance in COPD patients with increased mucus production [8–10]. In contrast, most studies agree that cough has little effect on airway clearance in subjects, including COPD patients, without mucus hypersecretion (unproductive cough) [8,11]. A modest benefit from cough without clinically detectable mucus secretion has occasionally been reported [12].

Other physical factors may also contribute to effective coughing. Airways are not rigid tubes and probably vibrate during the expulsive phase of the cough reflex. Cough often occurs as a succession of interrupted expirations instead of a single forced expiration. Airway wall vibration and rapid pressure swings acting on the airway wall during coughing may help to loosen the mucus from the airway wall [4]. Many stimuli that evoke cough also induce bronchoconstriction. It has been speculated that the airway smooth muscle contraction may prevent the collapse of the small diameter airways and thus facilitate the clearing of the more distal airways [13].

Neurophysiology of cough

The cough reflex is a *polysynaptic* reflex consisting of the primary afferent pathways, integration in the central nervous system, and the efferent motor pathways. Much of the current knowledge of the cough reflex neurophysiology is derived from animal models. Studies on humans are limited to morphological (bronchial biopsies in patients with cough), functional and pharmacological studies (mostly the inhalation aerosol challenges) from which only indirect inferences can made about the cough reflex neural circuits. Additional information indicating involvement of certain neural pathways in the cough reflex in humans comes from studies in heart–lung transplant patients. The neurophysiology of cough has been more directly studied using various animal models including dogs, cats, rabbits and guinea pigs. In general terms, stimuli that provoke cough in humans also cause cough in these animals, and drugs that inhibit cough in humans also show efficacy in the various animal models.

Primary afferent (sensory) nerves

Primary afferent neurons have their cell bodies situated in sensory ganglia outside the central nervous system (CNS). The axon leaves the cell body and after a short distance bifurcates with one end innervating the peripheral target (e.g. airways, lungs) and the other end projecting centrally where it forms a synapse with secondary sensory neurons in the CNS. Information in the form of action potentials is transmitted from the periphery to the CNS along the axon. There is overwhelming experimental evidence that the afferent pathways involved in the initiation of cough are contained in the vagi nerves [14]. In humans, the relevant structures supplied by the vagi nerves include the lower part of the oropharynx, the larynx, the lower respiratory tract and the lung parenchyma. The cell bodies of the vagal afferent neurons are located in the superior (jugular) and inferior (nodose) vagal ganglia. These ganglia can be visualized as swellings along cervical portions of the vagi nerves.

Sensory nerves are subclassified based on the velocity at which they conduct action potentials along their axons. Myelinated fibres conduct action potentials at relatively high velocities (4–60 m/s). These fibres are referred to as 'A-fibres'. The other subset of vagal afferent nerve fibres are non-myelinated and conduct action potentials at a slow rate (< 2 m/s). The slow conducting fibres are referred to as sensory 'C-fibres'. It has been estimated that approximately 80% of the vagal afferent nerves innervating the respiratory system are C-fibres [15]. Most A-fibres in the respiratory system are low-threshold mechanosensors. In contrast, C-fibres are relatively insensitive to mechanical perturbation (i.e. high-threshold mechanosensors), but are readily stimulated by noxious stimuli and inflammatory mediators [16–18]. The C-fibres are therefore often referred to as 'nociceptive' or nociceptive-like C-fibres, inasmuch as they respond to noxious stimuli.

Regardless of the fibre type, in order to evoke activation, the stimuli interact with receptors or ion channels on the peripheral terminals of the afferent fibre causing a membrane depolarization. This membrane depolarization (generator potential) spreads along the nerve fibre to an active zone where, if of sufficient magnitude, it leads to production of action potentials that travel in an all or none fashion to the central terminals of the nerve.

Vagal afferent A-fibres

With few exceptions, myelinated A-fibres innervating the respiratory system are sensitive to mechanical distortion of their receptive fields [19,20]. Many of the A-fibres in the intrapulmonary airways are sufficiently sensitive to mechanical distension of the surrounding tissue that they are activated by the cyclic changes in stretch occurring during eupnoeic breathing. These fibres are therefore characterized as 'pulmonary stretch receptors' and are found within the lungs of all mammals studied to date.

The pulmonary A-fibre stretch receptors are subclassified based on their ability to adapt to a prolonged suprathreshold stretch stimulus (Fig. 8.2) [21]. Some stretch receptors respond to the sustained lung inflation with a burst of action potential discharge which adapts rapidly (within seconds). These fibres are referred to as rapidly adapting stretch receptors (RARs). At the other end of the spectrum are stretch receptors that respond continuously through a prolonged suprathreshold lung inflation. These are referred to as slowly adapting stretch receptors (SARs). There are also subsets of A-fibres that are difficult to categorize as stretch receptors (either RAR or SAR). A significant proportion of the pulmonary stretch receptors are activated by bronchospasm resulting from the airway smooth-muscle contraction [14]. The activity of some RARs is inversely related to lung compliance [22]. In addition, some RARs can be activated by changes in the pulmonary extravascular space produced by mild elevations of left atrial pressure [23]. Lung deflation and certain inhaled irritants including cigarette smoke and ammonia also activate RARs [19,20, 24,25].

Activation of SARs is thought to lead to the Hering–Breuer reflex and to inhibition of parasympathetic outflow [20]. By contrast, RAR activation can evoke tachypnoeic responses and increases in parasympathetic outflow [19].

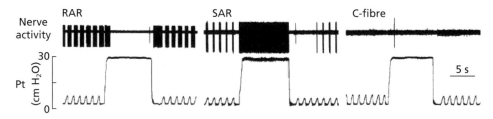

Figure 8.2 Representative traces of tracheal pressure (Pt) and single unit recording of action potential discharge of a rapidly adapting stretch receptor (RAR), slowly adapting stretch receptor (SAR), and C-fibre in the anaesthetized rat. Note that the C-fibre does not respond to the lung distension during tidal breathing, or even when the lungs are overinflated (this fibre responded vigorously to capsaicin, not shown). The RAR and SAR both responded to the lung distension caused by tidal breathing; the difference in adaptation is obvious when the lung is overinflated for 10 s. (Modified from Ho *et al.* [90].)

Both types of stretch receptors may contribute to the cough reflex.

Vagal afferent A-fibres with characteristics similar to the pulmonary stretch receptors are less often encountered in the extrapulmonary airways [26,27]. In the dog and guinea pig, a subset of A-fibres situated in the extrapulmonary airways is exquisitely sensitive to a focal mechanical stimulus, but responds poorly to stretch or to changes in airway luminal pressure (see Plate 8.1; colour plate section falls between pp. 354 and 355) [26–28]. These extrapulmonary A-fibre mechanosensors do not fit into the classically defined categories of stretch receptors. Particularly relevant to the present discussion is the observation that activation of these extrapulmonary A-fibre mechanosensors effectively evokes coughing (see below) [27]. These low threshold A-fibre mechanosensors are relatively unimodal in their activation profile, with few other stimuli effective in evoking action potential discharge from their nerve endings [18,29]. Hypertonic saline solutions are poor activators of the extrapulmonary A-fibre mechanosensors in the guinea pig trachea; however, hypotonic solutions are effective stimuli (perhaps through mechanical means). At least a proportion of the extrapulmonary A-fibre mechanosensors can be directly activated by a modest reduction in pH (and this activation evokes cough in experimental animals) [27,30, 31]. The molecular mechanism of acid-evoked activation of these A-fibres has not been elucidated, but mechanistic studies suggest that this activation may be mediated by certain acid-sensing ion channels (ASICs) [30]. The mechanisms by which the mechanical stimulus is translated into a generator potential in the nerve terminals is not yet understood. A large and growing number of mechanically sensitive ion channels have been identified [32], but the role of these channels in vagal bronchopulmonary afferent mechanotransduction is yet to be explored.

Vagal afferent C-fibres

The majority of afferent nerves innervating the respiratory system are unmyelinated slow conducting C-fibres [15,16]. C-fibres innervate the airways from the nose to the terminal bronchi. In addition, C-fibres are thought to innervate structures associated with the alveolus (juxta-capilliary receptors, or J-receptors) [33]. The C-fibres innervating the conducting airways are referred to as bronchial C-fibres, whereas those deeper in the lung tissue are referred to as pulmonary C-fibres [16]. In either case, the C-fibres are poorly responsive to mechanical perturbation (i.e. they are high-threshold mechanosensors) and are quiet during normal respiration. Unlike A-fibres with their structurally more defined nerve terminals, C-fibres, at least in the conducting airways, form a lattice-like plexus within and just beneath the epithelium [34]. An example of the difference between the morphology of nociceptive-like C-fibres and

mechanosensitive A-fibres in the guinea pig trachea can be seen in Plate 8.1 (colour plate section falls between pp. 354 and 355).

Virtually all vagal bronchopulmonary C-fibres can be activated by capsaicin. In addition, C-fibres are responsive to many chemicals and autacoids associated with inflammation, with bradykinin, adenosine triphosphate (ATP), serotonin (5-HT) and acids being the most commonly studied [16,35]. Activation of C-fibres can lead to reflex responses that include increases in parasympathetic outflow (and consequent bronchoconstriction and mucus secretion), apnoea, bradycardia and, as discussed below, cough [36].

Afferent fibres that trigger cough

Based on the rather simplified categorization scheme of respiratory afferent nerves (A-fibre subtypes, C-fibres), it would seem a trivial task to label one or the other afferent nerve type as the 'cough receptor'. Despite several decades of laboratory investigation, however, the fibre type(s) involved in initiation of the cough reflex has remained difficult to pin down. The reason for the difficulty comes from a confluence of variables that confuse the issue. The variables that confound the identification of the subtype of afferent nerves initiating the cough reflex include the nature of the tussigenic stimulus, the location from which the cough is initiated, the state of consciousness, the role of competing or facilitating reflexes, and the degree of integration by the CNS of the information arising from each fibre subtype.

Subconscious cough

Experimentally, the most straightforward cough reflex to study with respect to afferent nerve pathways is that evoked in an anaesthetized animal by punctate mechanical stimulation. Mechanically probing of the larynx, trachea, carina or large bronchi leads to a cough reflex in most mammals studied (humans, monkeys, dogs, cats, rabbits, guinea pigs). There would appear to be no exception to the conclusion that the afferent fibre type responsible for cough under these conditions is a mechanically sensitive (by definition) vagal A-fibre. Cooling the vagus nerve to a temperature that blocks conduction of all A-fibres but leaves unimpeded the conduction of C-fibres, abolishes this type of cough reflex [31,37].

Vagal A-fibre mechanosensors comprise stretch receptors (pulmonary RAR and SAR), as well as extrapulmonary A-fibre mechanosensors. Several studies indicate that SARs do not directly trigger cough reflex [14]. Moreover, in a species such as the guinea pig, there are few A-fibres with the characteristics consistent with SARs in the regions of the airways that lead to cough upon mechanical stimulation (larynx, trachea, carina, main bronchi) [18]. Studies in dogs and cats have led to the conclusion that the cough evoked by mechanical perturbation of the trachea is secondary to RARs [14,37]. In the guinea pig, the extrapulmonary cough-evoking A-fibres that are exquisitely sensitive to a punctate mechanical stimulus can also be activated by tussigenic concentrations of hypotonic and acidic solutions [18,30]. The focal mechanical stimulus-induced action potential discharge in these fibres adapts rapidly (see Plate 8.1; colour plate section falls between pp. 354 and 355) and thus one might be tempted to classify these A-fibres as a subtype of RARs. In so doing, however, one quickly gets into a nomenclature thicket. In the guinea pig and dog, there are relatively few fibres in the larynx, trachea, carina or mainstem bronchus that have characteristics of RARs (i.e. exquisite sensitivity to tissue distention) [26,38]. Moreover, although the cough-evoking fibres in the guinea pig are myelinated A-fibres, they conduct action potentials relatively slowly, only at approximately 3–6 m/s compared with 15–20 m/s for guinea pig pulmonary stretch receptors (RARs and SARs) [27]. There are also intrinsic differences in the pharmacological properties between the cough-evoking extrapulmonary A-fibre mechanosensors and the intrapulmonary stretch receptors [27]. Rather than confusing the issue with subtypes of RARs, these fibres are perhaps better left diffusely characterized as extrapulmonary A-fibre mechanosensors. In the guinea pig, these cough-provoking fibres are not found within the epithelium, but rather are situated just beneath the basement membrane [39]. Extrapulmonary A-fibre mechanosensors appear to be limited to the larynx, trachea and large bronchi, and not appreciably found in the peripheral airways or lung parenchyma [27].

In contrast to the extrapulmonary A-fibre mechanosensors, activation of extrapulmonary or intrapulmonary C-fibres is relatively ineffective in evoking cough reflexes in anaesthetized animals. Bradykinin and capsaicin are potent C-fibre activators and evoke bursts of action potentials in tracheobronchial C-fibres, but rather than cough, this is followed by apnoeic reflexes and increases in parasympathetic tone [27]. In fact, the propensity of C-fibres in the extrapulmonary airways to evoke apnoeic reflexes may inhibit the cough reflex in the anaesthetized animals. In humans under light anaesthesia, applying water to the airway mucosa leads to cough, respiratory irregularity and apnoea [40]. As the anaesthesia is deepened, the cough reflex is blocked but the apnoeic response persists [40].

Based on data from experimental animals as well as clinical studies in humans, one can conclude that cough evoked by mechanical perturbation of the extrapulmonary airways of anaesthetized animals is brought about by a single class of mechanically sensitive vagal A-fibres. A study in conscious volunteers, where a nebulized solution of tartaric acid pulsed onto the larynx triggered a cough (expiration) reflex within 20 ms of application also directly indicates A-fibre involvement [41]. Inasmuch as the cough evoked by activation of this fibre type can be obtained in deeply anaesthetized animals as well as in anaesthetized humans and comatose patients, this is unlikely to be a reflex that can be voluntarily controlled [42]. This type of immediate cough reflex likely underlies the vigorous cough response to aspiration and possibly to mechanical effects of mucus abutting the epithelium of large airways.

Conscious cough

A 'productive' cough is evoked upon aspiration or increased mucus secretions abutting mechanosensors. This cough is termed productive because it serves the purpose of removing the provocative substance from the airways. However, some airway pathologies are associated with so-called non-productive cough. In this case, afferent nerves are signalling urge to cough sensations, despite nothing in the airways to 'cough up'. Non-productive cough is a common experience. An irritating, itchy sensation in the throat builds up until relief by a cough is demanded. The temporary relief caused by the cough is only to be followed by the return of the building itch sensations and another cough, and so on. This type of cough often follows upper respiratory tract viral infections or other airway inflammatory conditions. In some patients these irritating sensations can occur chronically for extended periods of time. The resultant chronic coughing can have deleterious effects both physically and emotionally. The afferent neurophysiology of this type of cough is poorly understood, but it is intuitively obvious that this reflex is qualitatively different from the violent cough observed within milliseconds of aspiration. The evidence to date implicates activation of C-fibres as contributors to this type of cough.

Inhalation of C-fibre stimulants such as capsaicin and bradykinin evokes cough in most awake mammals including humans [43,44]. In human studies, intravenous injection of the nicotinic receptor agonist, lobeline (a C-fibre stimulant) leads to strong 'need to cough' sensations which are absent in lung transplant subjects [45]. With the assumption that lobeline, bradykinin and capsaicin are selective for activating C-fibres, these data indicate that bronchopulmonary vagal C-fibre activation can lead to urge to cough sensations in humans.

The location of C-fibres responsible for non-productive cough is difficult to address experimentally. Monitoring the respiratory deposition of particles released from different nebulizers revealed that prostaglandin E_2 (a C-fibre stimulant) was relatively ineffective in evoking cough when the particles were deposited primarily in the more peripheral airways [46]. By contrast, cough was effectively evoked with larger particles that were deposited mainly in the more central airways. Lung transplant patients failed to cough with inhaled capsaicin, yet their upper trachea and larynx were innervated and cough could be evoked from these regions by direct stimulation with water [47,48]. These types of studies hint that the relevant C-fibres are those found primarily innervating the conducting airways (i.e. bronchial C-fibres).

CNS integration of primary afferent input and central sensitization

We have discussed the potential roles of A-fibres and C-fibres in initiating the cough reflex. It must be kept in mind, however, that the afferent fibres comprise a sensory nervous *system*. The bronchopulmonary afferent fibres are never acting alone, and their activity must be interpreted within the context of an integrated nervous system. The question as to the specific type of afferent nerve that alone can lead to cough may be less relevant than questions pertaining to the nature of the integrated input to the CNS that lead to cough.

The central terminals of primary vagal airway afferent nerves synapse with secondary neurons situated in the brainstem within the nucleus tractus solitarius (NTS) [49]. The RARs as well as low threshold extrapulmonary A-fibre mechanosensors use the excitatory amino acid glutamate as their central neurotransmitter. Pharmacologically blocking the glutamate receptors in the brainstem blocks cough and profoundly disrupts normal respiration [49,50]. Bronchopulmonary C-fibres use certain sensory neuropeptides such as neurokinins and calcitonin gene-related peptide (CGRP) as central transmitters. The synaptic input of one vagal fibre type may enhance or inhibit the input from another type. In the field of pain research, for example, much attention has been given to the ability of nociceptive C-fibre input to enhance (sensitize) the input form fast-conducting mechanosensitive A-fibres [51]. One mechanism involved in the C-fibre-induced increase in synaptic transmission occurs as a result of neurokinins released from the central terminals of C-fibres. Neurokinins stimulate receptors on secondary neurons in the CNS leading to long-lasting increases in their neuronal excitability and a consequent increase in synaptic efficacy. This sensitizing process of converging inputs may involve many other distinct mechanisms, but regardless of mechanism, has been termed 'central sensitization'. It is likely that central sensitizing processes contribute to the excessive coughing in COPD patients.

Central sensitization has helped provide mechanistic insights into states of both hyperalgesia (states of a decreased threshold for pain), as well as allodynia. Allodynia is a pain syndrome where a normally painless stimulus (e.g. brushing your hair) becomes inappropriately painful. These conditions may provide useful analogies when it comes to understanding the hypertussiveness seen in many COPD patients. In some cases a subject may be simply more sensitive to a cough stimulus (i.e. a leftward shift in an inhaled capsaicin–cough response curve, Fig. 8.3), but in others an 'urge to cough' sensation may occur to a stimulus that is ordinarily not a cough stimulus, resulting in non-productive cough (by analogy 'an allotussive state'). Airway inflammation leads to accumulation of mediators that are known to be capable of activating bronchopulmonary C-fibres. One might speculate by analogy from the somatosensory research that this activation could lead to central sensitization of the constant synaptic input from pulmonary stretch receptors (e.g. certain RARs) resulting in a poorly defined irritating itch sensation.

By considering the processes of central sensitization, one is less inclined to conclude that cough associated with

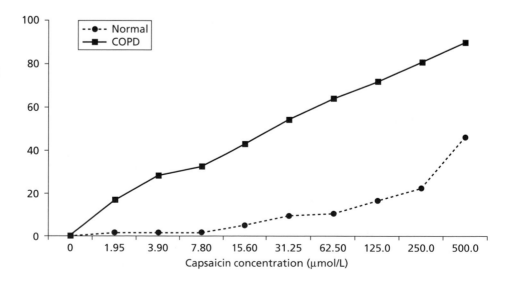

Figure 8.3 Cumulative concentration–response curve for capsaicin inhalation-induced cough in subjects with COPD compared with healthy volunteers. The cumulative percentage of subjects who coughed is expressed as a function of capsaicin concentration. These data support the hypothesis that subjects with COPD have a heightened cough reflex sensitivity to the C-fibre stimulant capsaicin. (Modified from Doherty *et al.* [68].)

airway inflammation is specifically a C-fibre or A-fibre phenomenon, but rather an integrated process. Experimental studies support the hypothesis that different types of bronchopulmonary afferent nerves functionally converge in the NTS [52,52]. For example, the C-fibres from the larynx, which alone have little effect on airway parasympathetic tone, substantially enhance the parasympathetic drive that is increased secondary to pulmonary RAR activation [52]. In the studies of cough in anaesthetized animals, stimulation of bronchopulmonary C-fibres fails to evoke cough; however, their activation quite impressively decreases the amount of the extrapulmonary A-fibre input to the NTS required to evoke the cough reflex [54]. This occurs whether the C-fibre activation occurs in the trachea or within the lungs. Indeed, activation of C-fibres within the oesophagus can sensitize the extrapulmonary A-fibre mechanosensor initiated cough reflex via central sensitizing mechanisms (B.J. Canning, personal observation). Likewise, indirect studies support the hypothesis that SARs alone do not evoke cough, but may enhance the cough reflex [55]. The extensive integration of afferent inputs at the level of the CNS may contribute to the difficulty in precisely localizing the cough stimulus within the lungs. Kinasewitz *et al.* [56] used a fibreoptic bronchoscope to deliver a unilateral mechanical tussive stimulus. All subjects coughed, but most were unable to determine which side of the lungs the tussigenic stimulus was applied.

In addition to the secondary neurons in the NTS, the cough reflex involves many complex neural pathways within the CNS. These include premotor inspiratory and expiratory neurons in the medulla, and a group of neural pathways referred to as the cough-pattern generator system. An overview of the central neural pathways involved in this 'cough centre' can be found elsewhere [50,57]. Functionally, the cough pattern generator is made up of a network of the multifunctional respiratory-related neurons in the medulla oblongata. Cortical inhibitory inputs into the cough centre are also important as evidenced by the powerful effect of placebo in controlling certain types of cough [58]. These inputs have yet to be critically defined.

Motor pathways

Although many different types of stimuli, and afferent nerve types, may initiate cough reflexes, the final efferent pathway seems to be, for the most part, common to all cough. The efferent pathways of the cough reflexes are well defined and reviewed in more detail elsewhere [13]. These pathways include the motor neurons to the respiratory muscles originating in cervical spinal cord for the phrenic nerve and thoracic segment for other respiratory muscles and the motor neurons to larynx originating in the nucleus ambiguus.

Cough in the COPD patient

Triggers of the cough reflex in COPD

The two major types of stimuli that initiate cough reflexes are mechanical perturbations and stimuli that activate nociceptive-like C-fibres. It is likely that both mechanisms are involved in initiating the excessive coughing in COPD.

Low-threshold mechanosensor activation

Mechanical probing of mucosal surface of the larynx, trachea and large bronchi evokes cough. The nerve fibres involved are myelinated low-threshold mechanosensitive A-fibres. It is likely that mucus traversing along the large airways serves as a mechanical stimulus needed to activate this mechanosensor-evoked cough. The mechanosensors are also likely activated by aspiration of foreign substances in the airways. In addition, tracheal mechanosensors can be stimulated by rapid decreases in pH, but whether the changes in local concentrations of endogenous protons are sufficient to activate afferent nerves in the inflamed airway is unknown. Finally, pulmonary RARs are activated by cigarette smoke, an observation particularly relevant to COPD [24].

C-fibre activators

Unlike the low-threshold mechanosensors that have a rather limited activation profile, C-fibres in the lungs can be activated by many types of stimuli. For this reason they are referred to as 'polymodal' nerve fibres. The stimuli may even include mechanical distortion, which is normally ineffective in activating C-fibres, because the excitability of C-fibres at sites of inflammation can be enhanced enough to respond to physiologically relevant mechanical stretch.

Capsaicin, the active ingredient in hot peppers, is a chemical used to define nociceptive C-fibres. Nearly all bronchopulmonary C-fibres in experimental animals respond vigorously to capsaicin application. Capsaicin evokes a generator potential by binding to the vanilloid receptor TRPV1 (formerly VR1). The vanilloid receptor TRPV1 is not only gated by vanilloids such as capsaicin but, importantly, can also be activated by endogenous stimuli within the lungs. These stimuli include lipoxygenase products of arachidonic acid, anandamide and hydrogen ions (pH threshold ~5.0) [59]. Moreover, there is some indication that G-protein coupled receptors such as the bradykinin B_2 receptor may lead to TRPV1 activation via various second messenger systems [60,61].

Serotonin (5-HT) can activate C-fibres in the airways via interaction with 5-HT$_3$ receptors [62,63]. Extracellular ATP is an effective activator of many C-fibres, and this occurs through interaction with purinergic receptors of the

P2X subtype [64,65]. Both 5-HT$_3$ and P2X receptors, like TRPV1, are non-selective cation channels that depolarize the nerve terminals by allowing the influx of sodium and calcium across the nerve membrane.

Bronchopulmonary C-fibres are also stimulated by mediators that act on 7 transmembrane G-protein linked receptors. Examples here include certain prostanoids, bradykinin acting through the B$_2$ receptor, and adenosine acting through adenosine A receptors [16,35]. The mechanisms by which activation of the G-protein linked receptor is transduced into a depolarizing generator potential has not yet been elucidated.

Mechanisms of enhanced cough in COPD

Increases in afferent activators

In most patients with COPD, the amount of coughing falls well outside the normal range. This may simply be because of more primary afferent stimulators in the COPD lung than in the healthy lung. In the first instance, the increased mucus secretion may lead to mechanically evoked cough. The physical characteristics of the mucus, combined with weakened respiratory muscles, may decrease the effectiveness of cough, leading to increased bouts of coughing.

Changes in pulmonary vascular pressure as well as the altered mechanics of breathing in the COPD patient may contribute to excessive coughing. In experimental animals both SAR and RAR type pulmonary stretch receptors may contribute to central sensitization and increased coughing, especially in the presence of inflammation and C-fibre activation. The activity of RARs may be enhanced as a consequence of increases in pulmonary vascular pressure [23]. By breathing at higher lung volumes and higher rates, both RAR and SAR activity may be enhanced in COPD patients. In clinical studies, bronchodilators have been shown to reduce cough reflexes [66]. Thus, the decreased airway calibre in COPD may indirectly contribute to excessive coughing. One can envision certain positive feedback loops operating in COPD. For example, the increase in afferent activity coming from the lungs of the COPD patient may increase reflex parasympathetic tone, and consequently increase airway smooth-muscle contractions and mucus secretion that in turn could increase need to cough sensations.

Many airway mechanosensors are imbedded in the airway wall. The stress–strain properties of the tissue will influence the efficacy of mechanical transduction in the nerve terminal. It is possible that the remodelling of the airways seen in COPD may affect the efficacy of mechanical activation of some types of bronchopulmonary afferent nerve fibres. This could indirectly increase or decrease the cough sensation arising from the lungs of the COPD patient. It should be kept in mind that these issues are extremely difficult to address experimentally, and thus remain mere speculation.

The C-fibres lining the airways of COPD patients are likely to contribute to the excessive coughing, especially during acute exacerbations of the disease. Various inflammatory mediators may be constantly evoking action potential discharge in bronchopulmonary C-fibres leading to increases in need to cough sensations. In addition, a decrease in the pH at the site of inflammation may also contribute to bronchopulmonary C-fibre activation [30,67].

Plasticity and enhanced afferent excitability

There is sound reason to suppose that part of the excessive coughing in COPD patients can be explained by the increased amount of primary afferent nerve activators that are present within the inflamed respiratory system. In addition to this, however, the afferent nerves may be *hypersensitive* to a given amount of stimuli. That is, the amount of afferent activation required to trigger cough (cough threshold) may be decreased. This can occur through changes in excitability and plasticity of the afferent nerves. This concept finds experimental support in clinical studies of cough evoked by inhalation of defined concentrations of tussigenic stimuli. Cough reflex sensitivity to both capsaicin and citric acid is increased in patients with COPD (see Fig. 8.3) [68,69]. This increase cannot be explained by the sensitizing effect of cigarette smoke in smokers with COPD because cough hypersensitivity has not been found in smokers with normal lung function [70].

Electrical excitability

An increase in electrical excitability of the afferent nerve membrane will increase the amplitude of the depolarizing receptor potential, or increase the ability of the depolarization to lead to regenerative action potentials (i.e. lower action potential threshold). In addition, changes in electrical excitability can alter the frequency of action potential discharge by modulating the relative refractory period of the nerve fibre. The manifold mechanisms underlying changes in electrical excitability involve changes in the function of various ion channels situated within the afferent nerve membrane [71].

Many inflammatory mediators can act on receptors through various second messengers to modulate ion channel function. Classic second messenger pathways such as cyclic AMP-dependent kinases, phospholipase C and activation of various isoforms of protein kinase C can all lead to phosphorylation of ion channels and consequent alterations in their function [51]. This often leads to an overall increase in excitability of the afferent nerve. This has been repeatedly observed in experimental animals where, for example, certain inflammatory mediators increase the excitability of high-threshold C-fibres to the extent that they may become activated by the mechanical forces that occur during eupnoeic breathing [35]. The increase in electrical excitability of an afferent nerve is often non-selective in that it results in enhanced activation regardless of whether the stimulus is mechanical or chemical. There are more examples published on the increases by inflammatory mediators of electrical excitability seen among C-fibre afferents than A-fibre afferent nerves; nevertheless, the mechanical threshold of extrapulmonary A-fibre mechanosensors in the guinea pig trachea (those that directly lead to cough) can be substantially reduced in the presence of allergic inflammation [72]. Many inflammatory mediators acting in concert may participate in increasing afferent nerve excitability [73]. Clinical pharmacological studies have suggested that inhibition of thromboxanes or cysteinyl leukotriene receptors can inhibit increased cough sensitivity in some subjects [74]. However, because multiple inflammatory mediators are increased in the airways of patients with chronic cough, it is unlikely that inhibition of a single mediator would normalize cough sensitivity in all COPD patients [75].

Afferent nerve plasticity

The changes in electrical excitability caused by inflammatory mediators and various second messenger systems are often short-lived, lasting only as long as the presence of the causative agent. In chronic disease, there may be more persistent 'plastic' changes that occur in the nervous system [76]. There is much attention given to the role of airway wall remodelling in the pathophysiology of airways inflammatory disease. In the same way, the nervous system within the airways may be qualitatively 'remodelled'. In this case, chemical and mechanical interactions within the bronchopulmonary nerve endings are transduced into changes in gene expression within the cell nucleus situated in the distant vagal ganglia. This can lead to changes in the afferent nerve sprouting and density, as well as to changes in the expression of neurotransmitters, receptors, ion channels and other molecules.

There have been no published studies that have rigorously addressed the hypothesis that increased afferent nerve density is related to increased cough specifically in COPD. However, studies have been carried out that have quantified nerve density in subjects with chronic cough. In one study bronchial biopsies were obtained from subjects with idiopathic persistent non-productive cough and from healthy volunteers [77]. The subjects with persistent coughing were more sensitive to inhaled capsaicin than control subjects. The overall density of nerves in the bronchial epithelium was similar between the two groups. However, there were more neuropeptide (CGRP) containing nerves in the coughing subjects compared with controls. In another study bronchial biopsies were obtained from healthy volunteers, typical asthmatic patients, and subjects with cough variant asthma [78]. Nerve densities were not assessed, but again significantly more neuropeptide (substance P) containing nerves were noted in the epithelium of the cough variant asthma subjects than in either of the two other groups. These types of studies focus on the epithelial nerve plexus, and thus likely pertain only to the C-fibre population of nerves. A change in nerve density of the low-threshold A-fibres would be also relevant, if found in the cough region of the respiratory tract. These fibres are likely found beneath the mucosa.

The studies that evaluated nerves in the epithelium of subjects with persistent cough noted changes in the amount of neuropeptides within airway nerves, without a change in nerve density per se. Inflammation in the upper or lower airways of animal models has been noted to increase the expression of neuropeptide synthesizing genes (e.g. preprotachykinin A) in vagal sensory neurons [79–82]. The increased amount of neuropeptides in the central terminals of bronchopulmonary afferent nerves can lead to central sensitization by increasing synaptic efficacy in the brainstem and consequently increasing cough reflexes [49]. The question arises as to how inflammation in the lungs can lead to changes in gene expression in the nerve cell bodies situated in the distant sensory ganglia? The neurotrophins, exemplified by nerve growth factor (NGF), are a family of molecules adept at regulating neural gene expression by interactions with specific neurotrophin receptors located at the distant nerve terminals [83]. In this light it is worth noting that several neurotrophins including NGF are increased in the lungs during inflammatory airways disease [84,85].

A chronic change in the quantity and quality of afferent input into the CNS may also lead to plastic changes within the brainstem. This has been noted in the somatosensory system where inflammation can lead to long-lasting changes in spinal cord neurophysiology [86]. Consistent with this idea, persistent airway inflammation evoked by ozone inhalation in infant primates caused neuroplastic changes in the synaptic physiology within the nucleus of the solitary tract [87].

Treatment of cough in COPD

Therapeutic strategies aimed at inhibiting excessive coughing in COPD are generally based on the premise that cough is the natural consequence of the underlying inflammation and airway obstruction. Treatment of cough is thus appropriately integrated within the treatment of the inflammation and obstruction. While it is true that the coughing will decrease with overall improvement of the disease, in some cases it may be informative to consider the pathophysiology of cough per se as part of the pathophysiological process in the COPD. If the neurophysiology of the cough reflex is deranged by the chronic inflammatory condition such that the cough is persistent and non-productive, it would be useful to have selective antitussive therapies available that target the hypersensitive component of the cough reflex. Regrettably, such therapies are not yet available [88].

The antitussive drugs currently available for use in the clinic have not changed appreciably over the past couple of decades [88]. Codeine is perhaps the most effective antitussive agent available, although its utility is limited by the bothersome and sometimes serious unintended consequences of central opiate action. Codeine inhibits cough mainly through interaction with µ-opioid receptors in the CNS [89]. Both δ- and κ-opioid receptor agonists are also effective in inhibiting cough in experimental animals [89]. Dextromethorphan is the most commonly used antitussive drug in use today, and is thought to work either through activation of subsets of central glutamate receptors, or opiate-like σ-receptors [89]. Dextromethorphan has fewer side-effects than codeine, but is also less efficacious in inhibiting cough than codeine and related opioids. In addition to these antitussive compounds, mucolytic agents have been used with variable success in the treatment of chronic cough.

The availability of novel effective antitussive treatments is limited, but not for lack of interest by the pharmaceutical industry. Within the pharmaceutical 'pipeline' are many interesting compounds aimed at strategically decreasing the afferent nerve excitability and cough hypersensitivity that accompany various airway inflammatory diseases. As promising as some of these compounds appear in pre-clinical studies, the propensity for novel therapies to be shipwrecked on the shoals of evidence-based medicine makes a discussion of their potential use in cough therapy premature and unproductive. Suffice it to say, it is hoped that this section on cough therapy in COPD will be first in the present textbook to be outdated.

Conclusions

In summary, cough is a complex reflex that is initiated by activation of primary vagal afferent nerves within the respiratory tract. Both low-threshold mechanosensitive A-fibres and nociceptive-like C-fibres can contribute to the initiation of cough reflexes. A consideration of the convergence of these types of afferent inputs within the CNS may help explain the cough in excess of functional demand that is commonly associated with COPD and other airways inflammatory diseases.

When the coughing becomes non-relenting and non-productive, it can have a deleterious effect on quality of life, and potentially the health of the individual. Coughing in patients with COPD occurs because at any given time they are more apt to have excessive mechanical and chemical tussigenic stimuli within their respiratory systems. In addition, the indirect evidence indicates that many subjects with COPD suffer from an increased sensitivity to a given amount of a tussive stimulus. Although difficult to prove experimentally, evidence from various animal models indicate that an increase in cough sensitivity likely stems from increases in electrical excitability of the sensory nerve terminals, plastic changes in the cough reflex afferent pathways, and sensitizing events occurring at synapses within the CNS. These effects are likely a consequence of certain aspects of the inflammatory processes occurring in the lungs, but relatively little is yet known about the specific mechanisms involved.

References

1 Irwin RS, French CT, Fletcher KE. Quality of life in coughers. *Pulm Pharmacol Ther* 2002;**15**:283–6.

2 Korpas M, Tomori Z. *Cough and Other Respiratory Reflexes*. Basel: S. Karger, 1979.

3 Irwin RS, Boulet LP, Cloutier MM *et al*. Managing cough as a defense mechanism and as a symptom. A consensus panel report of the American College of Chest Physicians. *Chest* 1998;**114**(2 Suppl Managing):133–81S.

4 Sant'Ambrogio G. Coughing: an airway defensive reflex. In: Andrews P, Widdicombe JG, eds. *Pathophysiology of the Gut and Airways*. London: Portland Press and Chapel Hill, 1993: 124.

5 Gal TJ. Effects of endotracheal intubation on normal cough performance. *Anesthesiology* 1980;**52**:324–9.

6 Scherer PW. Mucus transport by cough. *Chest* 1981;**80** (6 Suppl):830–3.

7 Albers GM, Tomkiewicz RP, May MK, Ramirez OE, Rubin BK. Ring distraction technique for measuring surface tension of sputum: relationship to sputum clearability. *J Appl Physiol* 1996;**81**:2690–5.

8 Camner P, Mossberg B, Philipson K, Strandberg K. Elimination of test particles from the human tracheobronchial tract by voluntary coughing. *Scand J Respir Dis* 1979;**60**:56–62.

9 Oldenburg FA Jr, Dolovich MB, Montgomery JM, Newhouse MT. Effects of postural drainage, exercise, and cough on mucus clearance in chronic bronchitis. *Am Rev Respir Dis* 1979;**120**:739–45.

10 Agnew JE, Little F, Pavia D, Clarke SW. Mucus clearance from the airways in chronic bronchitis: smokers and ex-smokers. *Bull Eur Physiopathol Respir* 1982;**18**:473–84.

11 Pavia D, Agnew JE, Clarke SW. Cough and mucociliary clearance. *Bull Eur Physiopathol Respir* 1987;**23**(Suppl 10):41–5S.

12 Hasani A, Pavia D, Agnew JE, Clarke SW. Regional mucus transport following unproductive cough and forced expiration technique in patients with airways obstruction. *Chest* 1994;**105**:1420–5.

13 Fontana GA. Motor mechanisms and the mechanics of cough. In: Boushey HA, Chung F, Widdicombe JG, eds. *Cough: Causes, Mechanisms and Therapy*. Oxford: Blackwell Publishing, 2003: 193–205.

14 Widdicombe JG. Afferent receptors in the airways and cough. *Respir Physiol* 1998;**114**:5–15.

15 Agostoni E, Chinnock JE, De Burgh Daly M, Murray JG. Functional and histological studies of the vagus nerve and its branches to the heart, lungs and abdominal viscera in the cat. *J Physiol* 1957;**135**:182–205.

16 Coleridge JC, Coleridge HM. Afferent vagal C-fibre innervation of the lungs and airways and its functional significance. *Rev Physiol Biochem Pharmacol* 1984;**99**:1–110.

17 Widdicombe J. Airway receptors. *Respir Physiol* 2001;**125**: 3–15.

18 Undem BJ, Carr MJ, Kollarik M. Physiology and plasticity of putative cough fibres in the guinea pig. *Pulm Pharmacol Ther* 2002;**15**:193–8.

19 Sant'Ambrogio G, Widdicombe J. Reflexes from airway rapidly adapting receptors. *Respir Physiol* 2001;**125**:33–45.

20 Schelegle ES, Green JF. An overview of the anatomy and physiology of slowly adapting pulmonary stretch receptors. *Respir Physiol* 2001;**125**:17–31.

21 Knowlton GC, Larabee MG. A unitary analysis of pulmonary volume receptors. *Am J Physiol* 1946;**147**:100–14.

22 Pisarri TE, Jonzon A, Coleridge JC, Coleridge HM. Rapidly adapting receptors monitor lung compliance in spontaneously breathing dogs. *J Appl Physiol* 1990;**68**:1997–2005.

23 Kappagoda CT, Ravi K. Plasmapheresis affects responses of slowly and rapidly adapting airway receptors to pulmonary venous congestion in dogs. *J Physiol* 1989;**416**:79–91.

24 Ravi K, Singh M, Julka DB. Properties of rapidly adapting receptors of the airways in monkeys (*Macaca mulatta*). *Respir Physiol* 1995;**99**:51–62.

25 Ravi K, Kappagoda CT. Airway rapidly adapting receptors: sensors of pulmonary extravascular fluid volume. *Indian J Physiol Pharmacol* 2002;**46**:264–78.

26 Lee BP, Sant'Ambrogio G, Sant'Ambrogio FB. Afferent innervation and receptors of the canine extrathoracic trachea. *Respir Physiol* 1992;**90**:55–65.

27 Canning BJ, Mazzone SB, Meeker SN *et al.* Identification of the tracheal and laryngeal afferent neurons mediating cough in anaesthetized guinea-pigs. *J Physiol* 2004;**557**:543–58.

28 McAlexander MA, Myers AC, Undem BJ. Adaptation of guinea-pig vagal airway afferent neurones to mechanical stimulation. *J Physiol* 1999;**521**:239–47.

29 Sampson SR, Vidruk EH. Properties of 'irritant' receptors in canine lung. *Respir Physiol* 1975;**25**:9–22.

30 Kollarik M, Undem BJ. Mechanisms of acid-induced activation of airway afferent nerve fibres in guinea-pig. *J Physiol* 2002;**543**:591–600.

31 Tatar M, Sant'Ambrogio G, Sant'Ambrogio FB. Laryngeal and tracheobronchial cough in anesthetized dogs. *J Appl Physiol* 1994;**76**:2672–9.

32 Gillespie PG, Walker RG. Molecular basis of mechanosensory transduction. *Nature* 2001;**413**:194–202.

33 Paintal AS. Some recent advances in studies on J-receptors. *Adv Exp Med Biol* 1995;**381**:15–25.

34 Baluk P, Nadel JA, McDonald DM. Substance P-immunoreactive sensory axons in the rat respiratory tract: a quantitative study of their distribution and role in neurogenic inflammation. *J Comp Neurol* 1992;**319**:586–98.

35 Lee LY, Pisarri TE. Afferent properties and reflex functions of bronchopulmonary C-fibers. *Respir Physiol* 2001;**125**:47–65.

36 Coleridge HM, Coleridge JC. Pulmonary reflexes: neural mechanisms of pulmonary defense. *Annu Rev Physiol* 1994; **56**:69–91.

37 Widdicombe JG. Receptors in the trachea and bronchi of the cat. *J Physiol* 1954;**123**:71–104.

38 Riccio MM, Kummer W, Biglari B, Myers AC, Undem BJ. Interganglionic segregation of distinct vagal afferent fibre phenotypes in guinea-pig airways. *J Physiol* 1996;**496**: 521–30.

39 Hunter DD, Undem BJ. Identification and substance P content of vagal afferent neurons innervating the epithelium of the guinea pig trachea. *Am J Respir Crit Care Med* 1999;**159**: 1943–8.

40 Nishino T, Hiraga K, Mizuguchi T, Honda Y. Respiratory reflex responses to stimulation of tracheal mucosa in enflurane-anesthetized humans. *J Appl Physiol* 1988;**65**:1069–74.

41 Addington WR, Stephens RE, Widdicombe JG *et al.* Electrophysiologic latency to the external obliques of the laryngeal cough expiration reflex in humans. *Am J Phys Med Rehabil* 2003;**82**:370–3.

42 Moulton C, Pennycook AG. Relation between Glasgow coma score and cough reflex. *Lancet* 1994;**343**:1261–2.

43 Choudry NB, Fuller RW, Pride NB. Sensitivity of the human cough reflex: effect of inflammatory mediators prostaglandin E$_2$, bradykinin, and histamine. *Am Rev Respir Dis* 1989;**140**: 137–41.

44 Forsberg K, Karlsson JA. Cough induced by stimulation of capsaicin-sensitive sensory neurons in conscious guinea-pigs. *Acta Physiol Scand* 1986;**128**:319–20.

45 Butler JE, Anand A, Crawford MR *et al.* Changes in respiratory sensations induced by lobeline after human bilateral lung transplantation. *J Physiol* 2001;**534**:583–93.

46 Higenbottam T. Chronic cough and the cough reflex in common lung diseases. *Pulm Pharmacol Ther* 2002;**15**:241–7.

47 Higenbottam T, Jackson M, Woolman P, Lowry R, Wallwork J. The cough response to ultrasonically nebulized distilled water in heart–lung transplantation patients. *Am Rev Respir Dis* 1989;**140**:58–61.

48 Hathaway TJ, Higenbottam TW, Morrison JF, Clelland CA, Wallwork J. Effects of inhaled capsaicin in heart–lung transplant patients and asthmatic subjects. *Am Rev Respir Dis* 1993;**148**:1233–7.

49 Mazzone SB, Canning BJ. Central nervous system control of the airways: pharmacological implications. *Curr Opin Pharmacol* 2002;**2**:220–8.

50 Pantaleo T, Bongianni F, Mutolo D. Central nervous mechanisms of cough. *Pulm Pharmacol Ther* 2002;**15**:227–33.

51 Woolf CJ, Salter MW. Neuronal plasticity: increasing the gain in pain. *Science* 2000;**288**:1765–9.

52 Mazzone SB, Canning BJ. Synergistic interactions between airway afferent nerve subtypes mediating reflex bronchospasm in guinea pigs. *Am J Physiol Regul Integr Comp Physiol* 2002;**283**:R86–98.

53 Canning BJ. Interactions between vagal afferent nerve subtypes mediating cough. *Pulm Pharmacol Ther* 2002;**15**:187–92.

54 Mazzone SB, Mori N, Canning BJ. Synergistic interaction between airway afferent nerve subtypes regulating the cough reflex in guinea-pigs. *J Physiol* 2005;**569**:559–73.

55 Hanacek J, Davies A, Widdicombe JG. Influence of lung stretch receptors on the cough reflex in rabbits. *Respiration* 1984;**45**:161–8.

56 Kinasewitz GT, Long RJ, George RB. Inability of awake patients to correctly locate a cough stimulus. *South Med J* 1985;**78**:970–1.

57 Bolser DC, Davenport PW. Functional organization of the central cough generation mechanism. *Pulm Pharmacol Ther* 2002;**15**:221–5.

58 Eccles R. The powerful placebo in cough studies? *Pulm Pharmacol Ther* 2002;**15**:303–8.

59 Caterina MJ, Julius D. The vanilloid receptor: a molecular gateway to the pain pathway. *Annu Rev Neurosci* 2001;**24**:487–517.

60 Shin J, Cho H, Hwang SW et al. Bradykinin-12-lipoxygenase-VR1 signaling pathway for inflammatory hyperalgesia. *Proc Natl Acad Sci U S A* 2002;**99**:10150–5.

61 Carr MJ, Kollarik M, Meeker SN, Undem BJ. A role for TRPV1 in bradykinin-induced excitation of vagal airway afferent nerve terminals. *J Pharmacol Exp Ther* 2003;**304**:1275–9.

62 Coleridge HM, Coleridge JC. Impulse activity in afferent vagal C-fibres with endings in the intrapulmonary airways of dogs. *Respir Physiol* 1977;**29**:125–42.

63 Undem BJ, Carr MJ. Pharmacology of airway afferent nerve activity. *Respir Res* 2001;**2**:234–44.

64 Pelleg A, Hurt CM. Mechanism of action of ATP on canine pulmonary vagal C-fibre nerve terminals. *J Physiol* 1996;**490**:265–75.

65 Dunn PM, Zhong Y, Burnstock G. P2X receptors in peripheral neurons. *Prog Neurobiol* 2001;**65**:107–34.

66 Lowry R, Wood A, Johnson T, Higenbottam T. Antitussive properties of inhaled bronchodilators on induced cough. *Chest* 1988;**93**:1186–9.

67 Fox AJ, Urban L, Barnes PJ, Dray A. Effects of capsazepine against capsaicin- and proton-evoked excitation of single airway C-fibres and vagus nerve from the guinea-pig. *Neuroscience* 1995;**67**:741–52.

68 Doherty MJ, Mister R, Pearson MG, Calverley PM. Capsaicin responsiveness and cough in asthma and chronic obstructive pulmonary disease. *Thorax* 2000;**55**:643–9.

69 Wong CH, Morice AH. Cough threshold in patients with chronic obstructive pulmonary disease. *Thorax* 1999;**54**:62–4.

70 Dicpinigaitis PV. Cough reflex sensitivity in cigarette smokers. *Chest* 2003;**123**:685–8.

71 Kollarik M, Undem BJ. Plasticity of vagal afferent fibres mediating cough. In: Boushey HA, Chung F, Widdicombe JG, eds. *Cough: Causes, Mechanisms and Therapy.* Oxford: Blackwell Publishing, 2003: 181–92.

72 Riccio MM, Myers AC, Undem BJ. Immunomodulation of afferent neurons in guinea-pig isolated airway. *J Physiol* 1996;**491**:499–509.

73 Carr MJ, Ellis JL. The study of airway primary afferent neuron excitability. *Curr Opin Pharmacol* 2002;**2**:216–9.

74 Ishiura Y, Fujimura M, Yamamori C et al. Thromboxane antagonism and cough in chronic bronchitis. *Ann Med* 2003;**35**:135–9.

75 Birring SS, Parker D, Brightling CE et al. Induced sputum inflammatory mediator concentrations in chronic cough. *Am J Respir Crit Care Med* 2004;**169**:15–9.

76 Li Y, Owyang C. Musings on the wanderer: what's new in our understanding of vago-vagal reflexes? V. Remodeling of vagus and enteric neural circuitry after vagal injury. *Am J Physiol Gastrointest Liver Physiol* 2003;**285**:G461–9.

77 O'Connell F, Springall DR, Moradoghli-Haftvani A et al. Abnormal intraepithelial airway nerves in persistent unexplained cough? *Am J Respir Crit Care Med* 1995;**152**:2068–75.

78 Lee SY, Kim MK, Shin C et al. Substance P-immunoreactive nerves in endobronchial biopsies in cough-variant asthma and classic asthma. *Respiration* 2003;**70**:49–53.

79 Hunter DD, Castranova V, Stanley C, Dey RD. Effects of silica exposure on substance P immunoreactivity and prepro-tachykinin mRNA expression in trigeminal sensory neurons in Fischer 344 rats. *J Toxicol Environ Health A* 1998;**53**:593–605.

80 Fischer A, McGregor GP, Saria A, Philippin B, Kummer W. Induction of tachykinin gene and peptide expression in guinea pig no dose primary afferent neurons by allergic airway inflammation. *J Clin Invest* 1996;**98**:2284–91.

81 Carr MJ, Hunter DD, Jacoby DB, Undem BJ. Expression of tachykinins in non-nociceptive vagal afferent neurons during respiratory viral infection in guinea pigs. *Am J Respir Crit Care Med* 2002;**165**:1071–5.

82 Myers AC, Kajekar R, Undem BJ. Allergic inflammation-induced neuropeptide production in rapidly adapting afferent nerves in guinea pig airways. *Am J Physiol Lung Cell Mol Physiol* 2002;**282**:L775–81.

83 Chao MV. Neurotrophins and their receptors: a convergence point for many signalling pathways. *Nat Rev Neurosci* 2003;**4**:299–309.

84 Joos GF, De Swert KO, Schelfhout V, Pauwels RA. The role of neural inflammation in asthma and chronic obstructive pulmonary disease. *Ann NY Acad Sci* 2003;**992**:218–30.

85 Virchow JC, Julius P, Lommatzsch M et al. Neurotrophins are increased in bronchoalveolar lavage fluid after segmental allergen provocation. *Am J Respir Crit Care Med* 1998;**158**:2002–5.

86 Willis WD. Role of neurotransmitters in sensitization of pain responses. *Ann NY Acad Sci* 2001;**933**:142–56.

87 Chen CY, Bonham AC, Plopper CG, Joad JP. Neuroplasticity in nucleus tractus solitarius neurons after episodic ozone exposure in infant primates. *J Appl Physiol* 2003;**94**:819–27.

88 McLeod RM, Tulshian DB, Hey JA. Novel pharmacological targets and progression of new antitussive drugs. *Expert Opin Ther Patents* 2003;**13**:1501–12.

89 Kotzer CJ, Hay DW, Dondio G et al. The antitussive activity of delta-opioid receptor stimulation in guinea pigs. *J Pharmacol Exp Ther* 2000;**292**:803–9.

90 Ho CY, Gu Q, Lin YS, Lee LY. Sensitivity of vagal afferent endings to chemical irritants in the rat lung. *Respir Physiol* 2001;**127**:113–24.

91 Lamb JP, Sparrow MP. Three-dimensional mapping of sensory innervation with substance P in porcine bronchial mucosa: comparison with human airways. *Am J Respir Crit Care Med* 2002;**166**:1269–81.

CHAPTER 9

The physiology of gas exchange

Robert Rodriguez-Roisin, Andrés Echazarreta, Federico P. Gómez and Joan Albert Barberà

The major goal of the respiratory system is to exchange physiological (respiratory) blood gases, namely oxygen (O_2) and carbon dioxide (CO_2), to cope with the metabolic needs of the body. To exchange these two respiratory gases adequately, alveolar ventilation and pulmonary blood flow must be properly balanced and matched within the lung, such that alveolar ventilation to pulmonary blood flow ($\dot{V}a/\dot{Q}$) mismatching emerges as the most influential mechanism determining abnormal arterial blood gases in chronic obstructive pulmonary disease (COPD), both in stable and acute (exacerbation) conditions. In contrast, the role of the other two intrapulmonary determinants of physiological respiratory gases (alveolar to end-capillary diffusion impairment to oxygen and increased intrapulmonary shunt) (i.e. zero $\dot{V}a/\dot{Q}$ ratios), are almost negligible. Indeed, there is no diffusion limitation to oxygen in COPD and intrapulmonary shunt is only present marginally during exacerbations, even in the most life-threatening critical conditions. By contrast, the influence of the major extrapulmonary factors modulating respiratory gases, namely the inspired fraction of oxygen, overall ventilation, cardiac output and oxygen consumption (uptake), are the major determinants during exacerbations [1]. The inspired fraction of oxygen in particular has a major influence on the value of Pao$_2$, cardiac output and oxygen consumption interact mutually via the arterial–mixed venous oxygen content difference (i.e. Fick principle), and overall ventilation governs CO_2 by means of the alveolar gas equation for carbon dioxide.

The two most characteristic pathological features of COPD, obstructive airway changes and pulmonary emphysema, in addition to varying degrees of pulmonary vascular structural abnormalities, in particular vascular wall remodelling, contribute to the development of $\dot{V}a/\dot{Q}$ mismatching even in the earliest stages of the disease. Alveolar hypoventilation also contributes to the development of hypercapnia in these patients [2,3].

This chapter reviews the physiological frontiers of pulmonary gas exchange abnormalities in COPD, mainly through the research carried out over the last 25 years with the multiple inert gas exchange technique (MIGET). This approach, originally designed by Wagner *et al.* [4,5], extended and complemented the relatively simple tools conventionally devoted in respiratory medicine to the assessment of the $\dot{V}a/\dot{Q}$ relationship, becoming central to understanding the complexity of the interplay between and within the intrapulmonary and extrapulmonary determinants of pulmonary gas exchange in acute and chronic pulmonary diseases. Moreover, the extent of $\dot{V}a/\dot{Q}$ inequalities detected by MIGET is better than that derived from topographical measurements with radioactive particles using scans and computed tomograms, or positron emission tomography (PET). This is especially true when used in patients with COPD [6], as imaging techniques underestimate the intraregional $\dot{V}a/\dot{Q}$ abnormalities and have limited spatial resolution.

Gas exchange approach

The advantages and limitations of MIGET have been extensively addressed over recent years and will not be discussed here [4,7,8]. Complete technical details of MIGET have been reported at length elsewhere [1–4,8,9] and will only be briefly explained here. The arterial, mixed venous and mixed expired concentrations of six infused inert gases, determined by gas chromatography, are used to calculate the ratio of arterial to mixed venous pressures (retention) and the ratio of mixed expired or alveolar to mixed venous pressure (excretion). Retention and excretion are then used to compute multicompartmental $\dot{V}a/\dot{Q}$ distributions. The six gases used include a wide variety of solubilities, from the more insoluble gas (sulphur hexafluoride) to the most soluble (acetone) through those

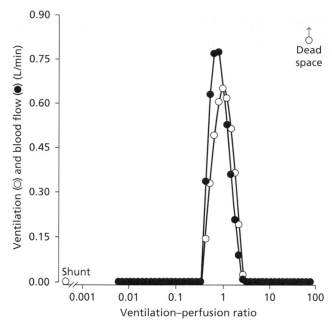

Figure 9.1 Representative ventilation–perfusion distributions, using the multiple inert gas methodology, in a healthy individual (see text for further explanation).

of intermediate solubility (ethane, cyclopropane, enfluorane or halothane and ether). The use of these inert gases overcomes the common limitations derived from a nonlinear dissociation curve on gas exchange observed for respiratory gases. Moreover, the large range of solubilities facilitates a better assessment of $\dot{V}a/\dot{Q}$ relationships as it is known that the gas exchange in the presence of $\dot{V}a/\dot{Q}$ abnormalities, is a function of its solubility [8–10]. Figure 9.1 illustrates a classic distribution of $\dot{V}a/\dot{Q}$ ratios in a young healthy non-smoker at rest, in a semi-recumbent position, breathing room air. The sum (distributions) of alveolar ventilation and of pulmonary perfusion (ordinate) is plotted against a broad range of 50 $\dot{V}a/\dot{Q}$ (from 0 to infinity) on a logarithmic scale (abscissa). Each data point indicates a specific amount of alveolar ventilation or pulmonary blood flow while the lines have been drawn to facilitate visual interpretation. Total blood flow or total alveolar ventilation corresponds to the sum of all data points for their respective distributions.

The use of logarithmic rather than linear axis of $\dot{V}a/\dot{Q}$ ratios is based on conventional practice in the field of pulmonary gas exchange. A logarithmic normal distribution of ventilation and blood flow is one of the simplest distributions and allows the spread to be defined by a simple variable that is the standard deviation (SD) on a logarithmic scale. Both distributions are unimodal with three major common findings: symmetry, location around an 'ideal' mean $\dot{V}a/\dot{Q}$ ratio of 1.0, and a narrow dispersion (between 0.1 and 10.0). Therefore, in young healthy individuals

there is no blood flow spread left to a zone of low $\dot{V}a/\dot{Q}$ ratios (poorly ventilated lung units) nor ventilation distributed to the right to a zone of high $\dot{V}a/\dot{Q}$ ratios (incompletely perfused, but still finite, lung units). Intrapulmonary shunt (detected by MIGET) is identified as areas with zero $\dot{V}a/\dot{Q}$ (in practice < 0.005) ratio (0% of cardiac output). The normal value of inert physiological dead space with infinite (in practice > 100) $\dot{V}a/\dot{Q}$ ratio (approximately 30% of alveolar ventilation) is also less than that computed with the traditional Bohr equation, because the inert gas approach represents only the dead space-like effects of those alveoli whose $\dot{V}a/\dot{Q}$ ratios are > 100. The second moment (or dispersion) of each distribution (log SD) is the common way to assess the degree of $\dot{V}a/\dot{Q}$ disturbances and corresponds precisely to the square root of the pulmonary blood flow (log SD$\dot{Q}$ and that of alveolar ventilation (log SD$\dot{V}$) distributions, reflecting the variance (standard deviation) of $\dot{V}a/\dot{Q}$ ratios about the mean. In an ideal, perfectly homogeneous lung, both log SD$\dot{Q}$ and log SD$\dot{V}$ should be zero; in practice, in a normal healthy individual they are in the range 0.30–0.60 in young individuals and 0.70–0.75 in older people [10]. West [11] demonstrated that log SD$\dot{Q}$ or log SD$\dot{V}$ values of 1.0 and 1.5 entail moderate and severe degrees of $\dot{V}a/\dot{Q}$ mismatch, respectively. The degree of $\dot{V}a/\dot{Q}$ inequality can also be expressed as the total percentage of ventilation–perfusion in distinct regions of the $\dot{V}a/\dot{Q}$ range, such that the percentage of blood flow distributed in areas of $\dot{V}a/\dot{Q}$ ratios < 0.1 and > 0.005 and, consequently, excluding intrapulmonary shunt, is conventionally named 'low $\dot{V}a/\dot{Q}$ mode' while the amount of ventilation diverted to the region of $\dot{V}a/\dot{Q}$ ratios located between 10.0 and 100 (and, therefore, excluding dead space) is viewed as a 'high $\dot{V}a/\dot{Q}$ mode' [1,8]. Arterial–alveolar difference averaged for the whole range of inert gases also can be calculated and employed to give indirect estimates of the level of $\dot{V}a/\dot{Q}$ abnormalities, such as an overall index of $\dot{V}a/\dot{Q}$ heterogeneity (DISP R-E*), which includes all inert gas retention and excretion differences except the excretion of acetone [12].

In summary, using MIGET, $\dot{V}a/\dot{Q}$ imbalance has been shown to explain the measured Pao_2 and $Paco_2$ comprehensively through the influence of the intrapulmonary factors of pulmonary gas exchange while unravelling the hierarchy with the vital extrapulmonary determinants in respiratory medicine [12].

Stable conditions

Types and severities of $\dot{V}a/\dot{Q}$ imbalance found in patients with COPD differ between patients and change with time in accordance with the natural history of the disease and the clinical state of the individual patient.

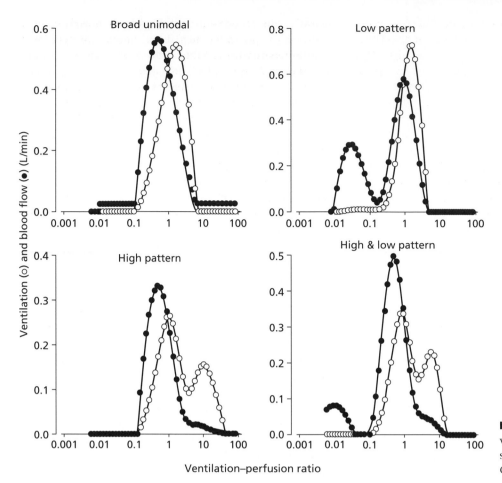

Figure 9.2 Typical profiles of ventilation–perfusion inequality shown in patients with stable COPD.

Severe stages

In the late 1970s, stable patients with advanced COPD (forced expiratory pressure in 1 s, $FEV_1 < 60\%$ predicted: GOLD stage II) with mild to severe hypoxaemia and hypercapnia representing the two classic clinical phenotypes (types A and B) were studied [13]. In these patients, distributions of $\dot{V}a/\dot{Q}$ ratios were extremely abnormal, and exhibited three different $\dot{V}a/\dot{Q}$ patterns (Fig. 9.2). The first $\dot{V}a/\dot{Q}$ profile showed the presence of lung units with very high $\dot{V}a/\dot{Q}$ ratios or a 'high $\dot{V}a/\dot{Q}$ mode' (type H), a pattern in which most of the ventilation was diverted to the zone of higher $\dot{V}a/\dot{Q}$ ratios. The second pattern was characterized by a large proportion of blood flow perfusing alveolar units with low $\dot{V}a/\dot{Q}$ ratio, named 'low $\dot{V}a/\dot{Q}$ mode' (type L). The third pattern was a mixed 'high/low $\dot{V}a/\dot{Q}$ mode' (type H-L), including additional modes above and below the main $\dot{V}a/\dot{Q}$ distribution. In general, the distributions of blood flow or ventilation, or both, showed moderate to severe increases. These findings suggested that type A COPD patients were more likely to have high $\dot{V}a/\dot{Q}$ areas and were unlikely to have low $\dot{V}a/\dot{Q}$ areas, unless they also had clinical evidence of type B COPD. The belief was that the type H of the $\dot{V}a/\dot{Q}$ profile was caused by constant ventilation of zones with reduced blood flow, possibly corresponding to emphysematous areas with alveolar wall destruction and pulmonary capillary network loss. In contrast, COPD patients of the type B subset usually had distinct either low or high $\dot{V}a/\dot{Q}$ areas, or both, even though there was more variability within this patient population. Accordingly, the investigators suggested that type L likely reflected airways occluded by inspissated mucus secretions and luminal plugging, smooth muscle hypertrophy, wall oedema, bronchospasm, distortion, or some mixture of these abnormalities. The lack of increased intrapulmonary shunt was ascribed to the vigorous efficiency of both collateral ventilation and hypoxic pulmonary vasoconstriction such that airways obstruction was never complete, and the coexistence of mild to moderate increased dead space were two conspicuous complementary $\dot{V}a/\dot{Q}$ features.

Several studies [14–29] including more than 100 patients with stable severe or very severe airflow obstruction (mean FEV_1 approximately 36% predicted: GOLD stages III–IV), many of them hypoxaemic, with or without chronic hypercapnia, have reported abnormal $\dot{V}a/\dot{Q}$ patterns similar to those documented in the study above [13]. However, the association shown with the clinical COPD types could not be established as clearly. Similarly, the levels of blood flow or ventilation diverted to regions with low or high $\dot{V}a/\dot{Q}$ ratios, respectively, were modest (range $\leq 10\%$ of cardiac output) in almost all the reports.

Of note is the potential modulation of an increased CO_2 output on $Paco_2$ and its relationship with nutritional status, a clinical phenotype in COPD with poor prognosis [30]. Under physiological conditions, the amount of CO_2 produced per unit of time is a function of the metabolic rate and the substrate used for fuel. In healthy individuals, the absorption and metabolism of carbohydrate induces an increase in CO_2 production (up to 70–100% of the oxygen uptake) because the entire body fuel utilization is transformed from predominantly fat to essentially carbohydrate in addition to the thermogenic effects of food. Malnutrition, currently considered to be one of the most characteristic features of systemic involvement in COPD patients, has been associated with poor prognosis and contributes to complications and increased mortality [30]. Other non-pulmonary (systemic) complications, including increased resting and total energy expenditure, systemic inflammatory response, cardiovascular involvement, cachexia and anorexia, have been proposed to explain malnutrition in COPD. Body weight and body composition are important in assessment of COPD patients, because loss of fat-free mass is not limited to underweight COPD patients, but also occurs in some 'normal weight' COPD patients [31]. Nutritional support has been recommended to improve clinical state and/or exercise capacity in stable COPD. However, it often fails, especially in those patients with a considerable systemic involvement. The potential pulmonary functional implications of nutritional regimens with high percentage of fat in hospitalized COPD patients are uncertain. Total caloric intake is probably a more important determinant of the magnitude of added CO_2 production than the single proportion of carbohydrate [32].

Mild to moderate stages

Over 24 patients with mild COPD (mean FEV_1 approximately 75% predicted) have been studied (see below) [17]. In general, the distribution of ventilation and blood flow were mildly abnormal (log $SDQ < 1.0$ each), although intrapulmonary shunt was absent and dead space was within the normal range. Blood flow distributions were mostly unimodal in two-thirds of patients and discretely bimodal in the remaining one-third. By contrast, the ventilation distribution patterns were never bimodal, with no regions of high $\dot{V}a/\dot{Q}$ ratios.

There is only one preliminary study in patients with small airways disease [33]. A few patients (GOLD stage 0) with functional criteria compatible with small airways

disease ($FEV_1 > 80\%$ predicted with abnormal maximal expiratory flow rates and single breath nitrogen test) were compared with healthy individuals with normal lung function and also with COPD patients with $FEV_1 < 80\%$ predicted. Patients with small airways disease had normal Pao_2 and showed a mild but significant increase in the alveolar–arterial Po_2 difference with little $\dot{V}a/\dot{Q}$ mismatch, as expressed by small increases in the dispersions of both blood flow and ventilation, compared with controls. Yet, there were no differences in these functional outcomes between these patients with mild airways dysfunction and those with early COPD and established airflow obstruction. The contention was that functional abnormalities in peripheral small airways can induce maldistribution of ventilation and $\dot{V}a/\dot{Q}$ mismatching in the face of a normal Pao_2.

A retrospective analysis of almost 90 patients in a stable condition studied at our centre, including all clinical phenotypes of COPD, showed four different patterns of $\dot{V}a/\dot{Q}$ distribution [34]: a broad unimodal distributions of both blood flow and ventilation (45% of the patients); a bimodal blood flow distribution, with both normal and low $\dot{V}a/\dot{Q}$ areas (type L) (23% of patients); a bimodal distribution of ventilation, with normal and high $\dot{V}a/\dot{Q}$ areas (type H) (18% of patients); and both bimodal blood flow and ventilation distribution patterns (type H-L) (14% of patients). This wide variety of patterns of $\dot{V}a/\dot{Q}$ distributions is interpreted as a reflection of the heterogeneity of the underlying pulmonary pathological derangement and the efficiency of compensatory mechanisms, essentially collateral ventilation and hypoxic vasoconstriction. Although the correlations between the abnormalities in the two most representative descriptors of $\dot{V}a/\dot{Q}$ inequality in stable COPD (log SDQ and log SDV) and the degree of abnormal FEV_1 are present, the levels of significance are usually modest [2].

Exacerbations

Exacerbations of COPD provoke further $\dot{V}a/\dot{Q}$ imbalance, which can improve significantly after 4–6 weeks of an effective and appropriate treatment [35], indicating that an important component of the $\dot{V}a/\dot{Q}$ mismatching under these critical conditions is a result of partially reversible airway narrowing, such as mucus impaction, bronchial wall oedema, bronchoconstriction, lung hyperinflation and air trapping. Different studies have shown more severe, but qualitatively similar, patterns of $\dot{V}a/\dot{Q}$ imbalance in COPD patients needing mechanical ventilation than in those breathing spontaneously (Fig. 9.3) [35–38]. By contrast, the presence of an increased intrapulmonary shunt (4–10% of cardiac output), more evident in the more life-threatening conditions, indicates that some airways are completely occluded by inspissated secretions. It is

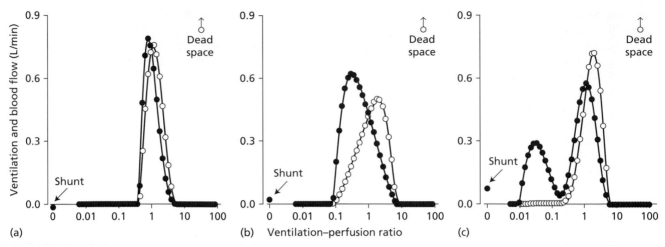

Figure 9.3 Most common patterns of ventilation/perfusion mismatching observed in patients with COPD during exacerbations.

plausible, however, that the efficiency of collateral ventilation and that of hypoxic vasoconstriction along with the influence of breathing hyperoxic mixtures on critical inspired $\dot{V}a/\dot{Q}$ ratios interact together, contributing to this disrupted gas exchange state.

It has been shown that, in COPD patients during exacerbations while breathing spontaneously, the main determinants of hypoxaemia are the levels of $\dot{V}a/\dot{Q}$ mismatching (approximately 50%), increased oxygen consumption (approximately 25%), likely related to an increased work of breathing, an overuse of short-acting β-agonists, and an amplifying deleterious effect of a decreased mixed venous Po_2 on $\dot{V}a/\dot{Q}$ imbalance (approximately 25%), not sufficiently offset by the simultaneous increased cardiac output. Interestingly, the role of overall ventilation was negligible. During COPD exacerbations, the extrapulmonary factors in addition to $\dot{V}a/\dot{Q}$ imbalance are modulating the endpoint of pulmonary gas exchange state [35], unlike in stable COPD patients. Similarly, in COPD patients requiring mechanical ventilatory support, either invasively [36,37] or non-invasively [38], the principal determinants of gas exchange in conjunction with $\dot{V}a/\dot{Q}$ inequality (cardiac output, overall ventilation and oxygen uptake) also have a vital role.

Non-invasive ventilation

This is particularly evident while using non-invasive ventilation in which the detrimental effects of a rapid and shallow breathing on $Paco_2$ and acid–base status are replaced by a more physiological pattern, such that both CO_2 and pH decrease while Pao_2 increases (Fig. 9.4a) [35]. Interestingly, the simultaneous decrease in cardiac output, induced by the increased intrathoracic pressure, is not sufficient to limit the significant improvement of Pao_2. It is also of note that,

during the application of non-invasive ventilation, $\dot{V}a/\dot{Q}$ imbalance remains essentially unchanged. This highlights the key influence of extrapulmonary factors, essentially represented by the efficiency of the ventilatory pattern, while the role of cardiac output is here less relevant (Fig. 9.4b).

Recently, the combined use of long-term oxygen therapy and nocturnal non-invasive mechanical ventilation in advanced COPD patients with hypercapnic respiratory failure for a period of 6 months improved both hypoxaemia and hypercapnia [39]. Moreover, the descriptors of $\dot{V}a/\dot{Q}$ mismatch improved remarkably towards normal. The relevance of this preliminary data is unique in that it is highly likely that $\dot{V}a/\dot{Q}$ abnormalities ameliorated because of an efficacious structural–functional remodelling in the airways and the pulmonary vessels under some special controlled circumstances of both nocturnal long-term oxygen therapy and non-invasive ventilation. However, this noticeable $\dot{V}a/\dot{Q}$ improvement in this trial in a few patients with stable advanced hypercapnic COPD remains intriguing, raising several hypotheses.

Invasive ventilation

During conventional ventilation, the abnormal $\dot{V}a/\dot{Q}$ patterns do not differ from those shown while breathing spontaneously and therefore do not share any special features, even in the face of the current diversity of ventilatory modalities [40]. This clinical scenario needs to be differentiated, however, from that of non-invasive ventilation, more specifically during weaning where $\dot{V}a/\dot{Q}$ patterns are not normal [37]. When mechanical support is discontinued, the abrupt increase in venous return because of the reduction in intrathoracic pressure provokes a significant increase in cardiac output without changes in total ventilation, although both the reduction in tidal volume and the

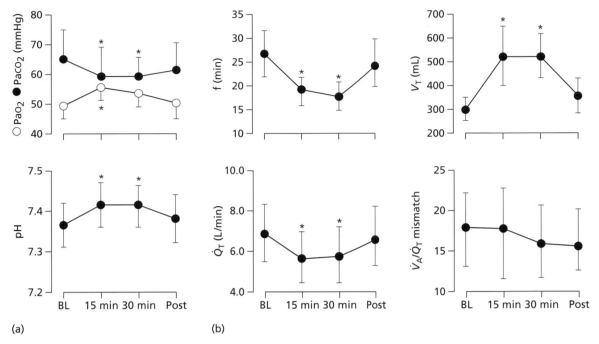

(a)   (b)

Figure 9.4 (a) Changes in Pa_{O_2}, Pa_{CO_2} and pH before, during a 30-min period, and then 30 min after the application of non-invasive ventilation in patients with COPD exacerbations. (b) Changes in the ventilatory pattern (top) and in cardiac output and an overall index of ventilation/perfusion heterogeneity (bottom) following the same time-course and identical non-invasive ventilatory support.

increase in respiratory frequency become less efficient. As a result, both the dispersion of alveolar ventilation and the overall $\dot{V}a/\dot{Q}$ heterogeneity increase, resulting in more $\dot{V}a/\dot{Q}$ inequalities (Fig. 9.5).

An intriguing finding was that there was only a small increase in intrapulmonary shunt from mechanical ventilation to spontaneous breathing, despite the substantial increases in cardiac output and mixed venous P_{O_2}. This was at variance with the poorly understood, strong linear relationship between increase in pulmonary blood flow and shunt fraction commonly observed in patients with acute lung injury [41]. The use of inert gas and radionuclide data showed that the critical alteration in ventilation during ventilator weaning resulted in the development of very low $\dot{V}a/\dot{Q}$ ratios in the basal lung regions [42]. Another striking observation during weaning was that respiratory blood gases were unchanged despite increases in mixed venous P_{O_2} and oxygen delivery. In other words, the potentially beneficial effect of the increased cardiac output on Pa_{O_2}, through its positive impact on mixed venous P_{O_2}, was offset by the detrimental influence of the change in ventilatory pattern on Pa_{O_2}. Despite these problems, weaning in these patients was successful. When patients were removed from the ventilator in this study, oxygen consumption did not change. Other investigators [43] have also stressed the role of cardiac output variations and other haemodynamic changes together with an increase in oxygen uptake as cause of

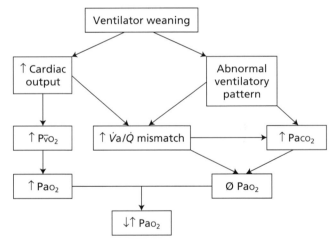

Figure 9.5 Interplay between increased cardiac output and deteriorated ventilatory pattern (extrapulmonary factors) and further ventilation–perfusion imbalance (intrapulmonary factor) during weaning in a COPD patient after 7 days of conventional invasive ventilation. The endpoint Pa_{O_2} remains unchanged. ($P\bar{v}_{O_2}$, mixed venous P_{O_2}.)

unsuccessful weaning. In patients with severe COPD with coexisting myocardial infarction and left ventricular dysfunction, oxygen consumption usually increases during weaning, which would tend to induce a decrease in Pa_{O_2}.

We have also investigated the effects of positive end-expiratory pressure (PEEP) and those of intrinsic (auto) PEEP (PEEPi) on $\dot{V}a/\dot{Q}$ mismatching in mechanically ventilated COPD patients, with the contention that a low PEEP can improve rather than impair lung mechanics as PEEP can replace PEEPi [37]. It was shown that PEEP levels approximately 50% of the initial PEEPi improved the gas exchange state without affecting lung mechanics or haemodynamics adversely. Furthermore, the application of 'controlled hypoventilation' along with low PEEPi levels considerably reduced intrathoracic pressure, while increasing cardiac output and systemic oxygen delivery, a practice that could be recommended during exacerbations.

Taken together, these findings indicate that arterial hypoxaemia and hypercapnia during exacerbations are the integrative endpoint of $\dot{V}a/\dot{Q}$ abnormalities in conjunction with the active interplay of extrapulmonary indices of gas exchange, namely overall ventilation, cardiac output and oxygen uptake.

Bronchodilators

Both short-acting and long-acting β_2-agonists are mainstays in the therapeutic strategy of COPD [44]. Yet, it is conventionally known that they may induce a decrease in arterial oxygenation, generally rapidly offset by short-term oxygen therapy. Moreover, these mild to moderate deleterious oxygenation defects, of the order of 5 mmHg in most of the studies, are well tolerated.

Intravenous terbutaline in patients with advanced COPD and mild chronic respiratory failure increased cardiac output [26], mixed venous Po_2 and oxygen delivery, while Pao_2, systemic blood pressure and pulmonary vascular resistance decreased in the face of an improved FEV_1. In parallel, there was further $\dot{V}a/\dot{Q}$ worsening (the perfusion to regions of low $\dot{V}a/\dot{Q}$ units increased) and this was not counterbalanced by hyperventilation and/or the potential of an active reduction in pulmonary vascular tone (Fig. 9.6). In contrast, in most severe COPD, with more airflow obstruction, hypoxaemia, hypercapnia and more pronounced pulmonary hypertension, cardiac output increased without pulmonary vascular changes. Furthermore, ventilation increased modestly but without improving airflow limitation; however, Pao_2 and the underlying $\dot{V}a/\dot{Q}$ mismatching remained stable. Gas exchange state during agent administration was not disturbed in these patients, conceivably because hypoxic pulmonary vasoconstriction was less active or even absent because of more intense structural pulmonary vascular remodelling. This would be in keeping with the concept that the progressive increase of pulmonary vascular resistance seen in advanced COPD is not only caused by irreversible structural vascular

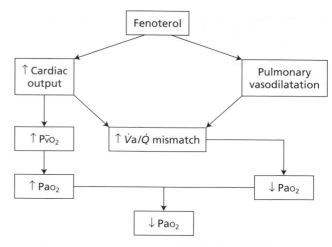

Figure 9.6 Interaction between increased cardiac output and further pulmonary vasodilation (extrapulmonary factor) and ventilation–perfusion deterioration (intrapulmonary factor) during the infusion of terbutaline in stable advanced COPD with reactive pulmonary vasculature. The endpoint Pao_2 ultimately decreased. ($P\bar{v}o_2$, mixed venous Po_2.)

lesions, but also by a reversible component [45]. In more severe advanced COPD, the pulmonary vascular tone seems to be more altered, more rigid and fixed, and therefore less liable to be dilated by selective β-agonists.

The short-term effect on gas exchange of nebulized fenoterol, a non-selective short-acting bronchodilator [29], in stable COPD patients demonstrated only a slight reduction in Pao_2 caused by further $\dot{V}a/\dot{Q}$ deterioration. After ipratropium, gas exchange was unaltered, hence indicating that the pulmonary vascular tone was disturbed following inhaled fenoterol resulting in further $\dot{V}a/\dot{Q}$ imbalance. The impact of intravenous aminophylline on $\dot{V}a/\dot{Q}$ mismatching has been also assessed in COPD patients recovering from a severe exacerbation [15]. Aminophylline improved spirometry but did not adversely affect arterial blood gases or the underlying $\dot{V}a/\dot{Q}$ disturbances. Although therapeutic doses of aminophylline can increase $\dot{V}a/\dot{Q}$ mismatching in some patients, the overall effect is in general modest and of little clinical significance in patients with advanced COPD. No inert gas studies are available using long-acting β-agonist and anticholinergic bronchodilators. A preliminary analysis of an ongoing study in COPD during the first days of hospitalization for exacerbations in our centre highlights no deterioration of $\dot{V}a/\dot{Q}$ imbalance in the face of a simultaneous moderate increased cardiac output (approximately 15%), with marginal changes in the other extrapulmonary factors governing gas exchange. In contrast, when these patients become stable, $\dot{V}a/\dot{Q}$ mismatching further deteriorated and Pao_2 significantly decreased, suggesting active release of hypoxic pulmonary vasoconstriction.

Structure and gas exchange

COPD encompasses an abnormal inflammatory response of the lungs that involves alveolar spaces (emphysema), small and large airways (bronchiolitis) and pulmonary vessels (remodelling) [44]. This widespread structural derangement will ultimately result in alveolar ventilation to pulmonary blood flow imbalance, particularly in severe and very severe stages of the disease. A recent study in a cohort of more than 600 COPD patients, 37% with severe to very severe disease, showed that 61% died from respiratory failure [46].

Alveoli

The influence of pulmonary emphysema and small airway disarrangement on $\dot{V}a/\dot{Q}$ mismatching has been investigated extensively in patients with mild to moderate COPD [17]. It has been shown that emphysema was positively correlated with the alveolar–arterial oxygen partial pressure difference (AaPo$_2$) but negatively for Pao$_2$. Moreover, the levels of emphysema severity showed a positive correlation with the dispersion of blood flow (log SDQ) and that of alveolar ventilation (log SDV). In essence, the more severe the degree of emphysema, the more abnormal the $\dot{V}a/\dot{Q}$ mismatch. The degree of abnormality in the log SDQ suggests the preferential development of regions with lower than normal $\dot{V}a/\dot{Q}$ ratios. These findings indicate therefore that poorly ventilated lung units associated with emphysema could be one of the structural determinants of abnormal Pao$_2$ in these patients. Thus, arterial hypoxaemia may be related to the loss of alveolar attachments of bronchiolar walls shown in emphysema, resulting in both distortion and narrowing of the lumen of bronchioles. This leads to impairment of alveolar ventilation in many regions of the lung and, consequently, to the presence of low $\dot{V}a/\dot{Q}$ ratios (Fig. 9.7; see also Plate 9.1; colour plate section falls between pp. 354 and 355) [47]. Similarly, it has been observed that areas of centrilobular emphysema have a greater residual volume (air trapping) and lower compliance, resulting in a reduction of ventilation/volume ratio. Accordingly, this could be an additional mechanism of reduction of effective ventilation in peripheral alveolar units. There is also a close correlation between the degree of emphysema and the abnormalities in the dispersion of alveolar ventilation (log SDV). This may be caused, at least in part, by wasted ventilation related to the dysfunction and/or loss of pulmonary capillary network of emphysematous spaces. This in turn induces the development of regions with lung units with high $\dot{V}a/\dot{Q}$ ratios, hence increasing the dispersion of ventilation. In this regard, the bimodal $\dot{V}a/\dot{Q}$ pattern of the ventilation distribution alluded to above, with a major amount of ventilation to high $\dot{V}a/\dot{Q}$ ratios (type H) observed in patients with advanced type A COPD, would be an extension of this finding, likely reflecting large areas of destroyed parenchyma.

Airways

Bronchiolar lesions were found to be related to $\dot{V}a/\dot{Q}$ imbalance as shown by the correlation between the airway inflammation score and the dispersion of ventilation (log SD$\dot{V}$). This finding reflects a heterogeneous distribution of inspired air to alveolar spaces caused by airway obstruction secondary to bronchiolar damage, thereby inducing the increase in the dispersion of ventilation (see Fig. 9.7; see also Plate 9.1; colour plate section falls between pp. 354 and 355). In contrast, there was no correlation between these chronic alterations in peripheral small airways and arterial blood gases, an observation akin to the deficient relationship between these structural changes and the dispersion of blood flow (log SDQ). Notwithstanding, the lack of correlation between small airways abnormalities and both the dispersion of blood flow and the percentage of perfusion to regions with low $\dot{V}a/\dot{Q}$ ratios cannot be extrapolated to the typical $\dot{V}a/\dot{Q}$ findings in patients with highly developed COPD, principally during exacerbations [35–38]. In severe to very severe stages of COPD, a bimodal blood flow $\dot{V}a/\dot{Q}$ profile may be more common and can be attributed to an acute superimposition of abrupt, potentially reversible airway changes (such as bronchial wall oedema or inspissated mucus plugging) on the chronic airways abnormalities.

In summary, these data suggest that there is a wide variety of $\dot{V}a/\dot{Q}$ abnormalities in patients with COPD. At one end of the spectrum are those patients with mild to moderate COPD and mild arterial blood gas abnormalities, with modest $\dot{V}a/\dot{Q}$ inequality, mainly characterized by broadly unimodal $\dot{V}a/\dot{Q}$ patterns of the dispersions of blood flow and alveolar ventilation. At the other end of the spectrum are those patients with severe advanced COPD and abnormal arterial blood gases who show dramatic $\dot{V}a/\dot{Q}$ imbalance, with bimodal $\dot{V}a/\dot{Q}$ patterns of either pulmonary blood flow or alveolar ventilation distributions, or both, depending on clinical conditions and reflecting different levels of COPD progression. Ultimately, historical type B COPD patients with regions of high $\dot{V}a/\dot{Q}$ ratios share emphysema as well as chronic bronchitis areas, whereas type A COPD patients with regions with low $\dot{V}a/\dot{Q}$ ratios are seldom detected. The latter patients usually have increased dead space and sporadically modest levels of increased intrapulmonary shunt, in particular during exacerbations. In between these two extremes there are many patients with different degrees of $\dot{V}a/\dot{Q}$ imbalance, depending on progression, clinical status and therapy.

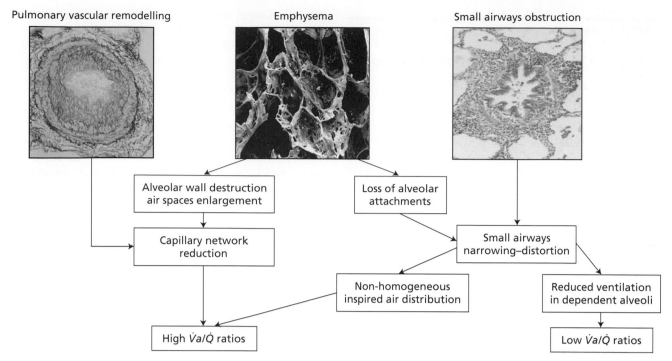

Figure 9.7 Schematic diagram of the correlations between key pathological features of COPD (small airways obstruction, pulmonary emphysema and vascular remodelling) and pulmonary gas exchange state (ventilation–perfusion imbalance) in stable advanced COPD. See also Plate 9.1; colour plate section falls between pp. 354 and 355.

Vessels

The relationship between the pulmonary vascular abnormalities and the $\dot{V}a/\dot{Q}$ relationships in COPD patients has been investigated [48]. It has been shown that the lower the degree of response to 100% oxygen (a relatively simple tool to assess the state of pulmonary vascular reactivity), the greater the thickness of the intimal layer of the pulmonary muscular arteries. Furthermore, the width of the intima was correlated with some gas exchange abnormalities, namely Pao_2 and the amount of $\dot{V}a/\dot{Q}$ mismatch, as expressed by both the dispersion of alveolar ventilation and an overall descriptor of $\dot{V}a/\dot{Q}$ imbalance. It was also correlated with the underlying degree of bronchiolar inflammation, a finding that can be considered central to the development of further abnormal $\dot{V}a/\dot{Q}$ progression (see Fig. 9.7; see also Plate 9.1; colour plate section falls between pp. 354 and 355). Moreover, in patients with mild COPD, the intimal enlargement in pulmonary arteries coexists with a superior $\dot{V}a/\dot{Q}$ impairment and this arterial wall thickness in small vessels may minimize the response of pulmonary vascular reactivity to the breathing of different oxygen concentrations.

Using a multivariate analysis, it has been shown that two of the best independent predictors of hospitalization for exacerbations in patients with moderate to severe COPD were pulmonary artery pressure value > 18 mmHg and $Paco_2$ > 44 mmHg [49]. Thus, pulmonary vascular pressures could represent an outcome of the deleterious effects of alveolar hypoxia on the pulmonary vessels, indicating the individual's vulnerability to arterial hypoxaemia. It is well established that both anatomical and functional pulmonary vascular derangements that result in pulmonary hypertension are characteristic features of the natural progression of COPD. Plausible mechanisms of the development of pulmonary hypertension in COPD include remodelling of pulmonary vessels, hypoxic pulmonary vasoconstriction, polycythaemia and emphysematous damage of the capillary network. Pulmonary vascular remodelling appears to be one of the central causative factors of pulmonary hypertension in COPD, as suggested by its failure to resolve after arterial hypoxaemia correction during acute or continuous oxygen administration.

Patients with severe emphysema with air trapping had a mean pulmonary artery pressure > 20 mmHg and a normal cardiac index [50]. Nevertheless, the pulmonary artery pressure correlated negatively with Pao_2 and with the severity of emphysema, and a subsequent multiple stepwise regression analysis demonstrated that Pao_2 was not an independent predictor of elevated pulmonary artery pressure. This finding led to the conclusion that in patients with severe emphysema, the commonly increased pulmonary artery pressure is not related to hypoxaemia or impaired systemic oxygen transport.

Altogether these data point to the central role of pulmonary vascular remodelling as part of the repair response to acute and/or chronic injury. This remodelling appears to be one of the key pathobiological determinants of pulmonary hypertension development in COPD, being manifested throughout the spectrum of disease severity. Moreover, structural changes of pulmonary vasculature in COPD preferentially affect the pulmonary muscular arteries as well as the pre-capillary vessels. In patients with end-stage COPD, the media is commonly normal or atrophic while the intimal coat is thickened by deposition of longitudinal muscle, fibrosis and elastosis in pulmonary muscular arteries resulting in cor pulmonale [51]. At the pre-capillary level, the formation of a medial coat of circular smooth muscle is surrounded by a new internal elastic lamina, and occasionally the lumen is subdivided into parallel tubes.

In a seminal study on the pulmonary vascular state in cystic fibrosis patients undergoing lung transplantation [52], it was observed that endothelial pulmonary vascular dysfunction correlated linearly to pre-transplantation Pa_{O_2}. This suggested that chronic hypoxaemia may have a detrimental influence on endothelial cell metabolism and possibly the synthesis of endogenous nitric oxide (NO) production, probably having a crucial role in the pulmonary vascular remodelling process in COPD. Although chronic hypoxaemia may explain the impairment of endothelial dysfunction in advanced COPD, the mechanisms operating in mild COPD without coexisting hypoxaemia remain unknown. It has been shown that endothelial dysfunction of pulmonary arteries is already active in early mild COPD [45]. These patients exhibit a significantly reduced vascular dilation in response to increasing concentrations of acetylcholine (ACh) and adenosine diphosphate (ADP) early in the natural history of COPD. The maximal pulmonary vascular dilation correlated significantly with the FEV_1/FVC ratio, indicating that endothelial dysfunction may be enhanced by COPD progression. These data are similar to the findings observed in end-stage cystic fibrosis [52], except for the fact that mild COPD patients do not have associated arterial hypoxaemia. Interestingly, both patients with COPD and smokers with normal lung function demonstrated the same severity of intimal thickening in pulmonary arteries. These findings suggest that structural vascular changes might be initiated well before the impairment of pulmonary vascular reactivity or lung function, and that cigarette smoking may coexist with structural abnormalities of the pulmonary vasculature related to the remodelling process, even in the absence of reduced airflow. The presence of gas exchange abnormalities in some patients with mild to moderate COPD out of proportion to the severity of airflow

obstruction may be explained by the finding that the severity of intimal thickening in the pulmonary arteries in these patients correlates with the severity of the inflammatory infiltrate in small airways, suggesting a common inflammatory process [48].

It was also shown in both mild COPD patients and smokers with normal lung function that the number of inflammatory cells in the adventitia of pulmonary muscular arteries is increased [53]. This inflammatory infiltrate is mainly composed of activated T lymphocytes, driven by a higher proportion of the $CD8^+$ subset, resulting in a reduced $CD4^+/CD8^+$ ratio, similar to that shown in large and peripheral airways and in the alveolar septa [54,55]. The severity of the inflammatory pulmonary vascular wall reaction correlated with the FEV_1/FVC ratio, the severity of endothelium dysfunction and also with the extent of the intimal thickness of the pulmonary vessels.

It has been suggested that the reduction in NO synthesis or release by the pulmonary endothelium may contribute to the structural and functional abnormalities of the pulmonary vasculature shown in the early stages of COPD. Patients with mild COPD, compared with non-smokers, expressed less endothelial NO synthase (eNOS) in their pulmonary arteries and this finding was correlated with endothelial dysfunction and enlargement of the intimal coat of pulmonary arteries [56]. It is of note that in smokers with normal lung function the expression of eNOS adopted an intermediate position between non-smokers and COPD patients, suggesting that inhibition of eNOS by the components of cigarette smoking in the pulmonary vasculature may precede the development of an established COPD phenotype. In contrast, no differences were observed in endothelin-1 (ET-1). Similar data on eNOS have been recently confirmed in lung tissue specimens excised by lung volume reduction surgery (LVRS) [57].

In addition, the smooth muscle cell proliferation and extracellular matrix deposition shown in the intimal layer of pulmonary muscular arteries in moderate COPD [58] may be linked to an enhanced expression of vascular endothelial growth factor (VEGF) associated with arterial wall enlargement in early mild COPD [59]. In severe emphysema the immunohistochemical expression of VEGF in pulmonary arteries and its protein content in lung tissue tend to be down-regulated despite intense vascular remodelling [57]. This is consistent with the reduction of VEGF expression in the lungs from emphysematous patients [60]. At an early COPD stage, VEGF might be a key signalling molecule linking changes in endothelial function with vascular remodelling. In COPD patients with advanced disease including emphysema, the vascular expression of VEGF is reduced, consistent with the anatomical changes that take place in the underlying lung parenchyma.

These findings suggest that cigarette smoke can be explicitly implicated very early in the pathogenesis of pulmonary vascular abnormalities in COPD. It can be hypothesized therefore that a chronic CD8+ T-cell inflammatory process, CD8+ accompanied by the release of a cascade of inflammatory mediators (including interleukin 8 [IL-8], leukotriene B_4 and tumour necrosis factor α [TNF-α]) is influentially involved in the development of the structural and functional disturbances of the pulmonary vasculature in mild COPD. Recently, a negative correlation has been demonstrated between the levels of Pao_2 and TNF-α *in vivo* [61]. This suggests that TNF-α contributes to weight loss and the systemic effects. Likewise, a direct effect of cigarette smoke might induce the thickening of the intimal coat through cell proliferation, resulting in pulmonary vascular remodelling which ultimately leads to pulmonary hypertension. As disease progresses, the coexistence of chronic severe hypoxaemia in more advanced COPD may further amplify and/or enhance this pulmonary vascular effect.

Future prospects

The study of human lung tissue is a critical research area in COPD [62]. One of the most appropriate sources of tissue for study is surgically explanted specimens from patients undergoing lung transplantation, although it only reflects accelerated end-stage COPD. Mild pulmonary hypertension is a common complication in COPD. However, characterization of the inflammatory pulmonary vascular process by advanced cellular, molecular and histopathological tools has received relatively little attention to date. Pulmonary hypertension is associated with shorter survival rates and is a predictive factor of worse clinical condition in COPD. The actual incidence of pulmonary hypertension in COPD is insufficiently known but varies from 20 to 91% in advanced emphysematous phenotypes [63]. Unfortunately, the therapeutic options available to patients with COPD are limited, and no pharmacological therapy is available as yet to slow down the progressive decline in FEV_1. Domiciliary long-term oxygen therapy appears to be the only medical therapy to improve survival in advanced COPD with chronic respiratory failure.

Given the relative ineffectiveness of current therapeutic modalities, substantial progress in COPD treatment will require novel therapies. Recent advances in the understanding of the pathophysiological processes underlying COPD, as discussed in this chapter, may help to identify potential therapeutic approaches in the future. One example [64] could be based on the finding that treatment of rats with a VEGF blocker causes emphysema associate with endothelial cell apoptosis and with enhanced oxidative stress but is not accompanied by inflammation. Oxidative stress decreases VEGF, and the expression of both VEGF and its receptor are decreased in emphysema [60]. A reduction in VEGF might be implicated in the apoptotic changes that take place in the alveolar septa of emphysematous lungs. As a result, pharmacological inhibition of apoptosis might prevent loss of alveoli. Similarly, it is conceivable that agents that modulate the vasoconstrictor–dilator balance could be beneficial in COPD patients with pulmonary vascular involvement. Pulmonary gas exchange pathobiology in COPD encompasses a multidimensional process involving large and small airways, alveolar walls and pulmonary arteries, resulting in a wide spectrum of $\dot{V}a/\dot{Q}$ imbalance in accordance with the underlying degree of airflow obstruction. Ultimately, the structural and functional correlations may help to foster new and specific therapeutic targets.

Acknowledgements

The authors thank Laura Morte for her administrative support.

The authors were supported by Red Respira-ISCIII-RTIC-03/11, Fondo de Investigación Sanitaria (FIS-050208) and Generalitat de Catalunya (2005S6R00822). The author R. Rodríguez-Roisin also holds a career scientist award from the Generalitat de Catalunya (2001–07).

References

1 Glenny R, Wagner PD, Roca J, Rodriguez-Roisin R. Gas exchange in health: rest, exercise, and aging. In: Roca J, Rodriguez-Roisin R, Wagner PD, eds. *Pulmonary and Peripheral Gas Exchange in Health and Disease*. New York: Marcel Dekker, 2000: 121–48.

2 Barbera JA. Chronic obstructive pulmonary disease. In: Roca J, Rodriguez-Roisin R, Wagner PD, eds. *Pulmonary and Peripheral Gas Exchange in Health and Disease*. New York: Marcel Dekker, 2000: 229–61.

3 Begin P, Grassino A. Inspiratory muscle dysfunction and chronic hypercapnia in chronic obstructive pulmonary disease. *Am Rev Respir Dis* 1991;**143**:905–12.

4 Wagner PD, Saltzman HA, West JB. Measurement of continuous distributions of ventilation/perfusion ratios: theory. *J Appl Physiol* 1974;**36**:588–99.

5 Wagner PD, Naumann PF, Laravuso RB. Simultaneous measurement of eight foreign gases in blood by gas chromatography. *J Appl Physiol* 1974;**36**:600–5.

6 Brudin LH, Rhodes CG, Valind SO *et al.* Regional structure–function correlations in chronic obstructive lung disease measured with positron emission tomography. *Thorax* 1992;**47**:914–21.

7 Evans JW, Wagner PD. Limits on Va/Q distributions from analysis of experimental inert gas elimination. *J Appl Physiol* 1977;**42**:889–98.

8 Roca J, Wagner PD. Contribution of multiple inert gas elim-

ination technique to pulmonary medicine. I. Principles and information content of the multiple inert gas elimination technique. *Thorax* 1994;**49**:815–24.

9 Wagner PD, Laravuso RB, Uhl RR, West JB. Continuous distributions of ventilation/perfusion ratios in normal subjects breathing air and 100% O$_2$. *J Clin Invest* 1974;**54**:54–68.

10 Ketty SS. The theory and applications of the exchange of inert gas at the lungs and tissues. *Pharmacol Rev* 1951;**3**:1–41.

11 West JB. Ventilation/perfusion inequality and overall gas exchange in computer models of the lung. *Respir Physiol* 1969;**7**:88–110.

12 Hiastala MP, Robertson HT. Inert gas elimination characteristics of the normal and abnormal lung. *J Appl Physiol* 1978;**44**:258–66.

13 Wagner PD, Dantzker DR, Dueck R, Clausen JL, West JB. Ventilation/perfusion inequality in chronic obstructive pulmonary disease. *J Clin Invest* 1977;**59**:203–16.

14 Agusti AG, Barberà JA, Roca J *et al.* Hypoxic pulmonary vasoconstriction and gas exchange during exercise in chronic obstructive pulmonary disease. *Chest* 1990;**97**:268–75.

15 Barberà JA, Reyes A, Roca J *et al.* Effect of intravenously administered aminophylline on ventilation/perfusion inequality during recovery from exacerbations of chronic obstructive pulmonary disease. *Am Rev Respir Dis* 1992;**145**:1328–33.

16 Barberà JA, Roger N, Roca J *et al.* Worsening of pulmonary gas exchange with nitric oxide inhalation in chronic obstructive pulmonary disease. *Lancet* 1996;**347**:436–40.

17 Barberà JA, Ramirez J, Roca J *et al.* Lung structure and gas exchange in mild chronic obstructive pulmonary disease. *Am Rev Respir Dis* 1990;**141**:895–901.

18 Bratel T, Hedenstierna G, Nyquist O, Ripe E. The use of a vasodilator, felodipine, as an adjuvant to long-term oxygen treatment in COLD patients. *Eur Respir J* 1990;**3**:46–54.

19 Castaing Y, Manier G, Guenard H. Effect of 26% oxygen breathing on ventilation and perfusion distribution in patients with COLD. *Bull Eur Physiopathol Respir* 1985;**21**:17–23.

20 Castaing Y, Manier G, Guenard H. Improvement in ventilation/perfusion relationships by almitrine in patients with chronic obstructive pulmonary disease during mechanical ventilation. *Am Rev Respir Dis* 1986;**134**:910–6.

21 Dantzker DR, D'Alonzo GE. The effect of exercise on pulmonary gas exchange in patients with severe chronic obstructive pulmonary disease. *Am Rev Respir Dis* 1986;**134**:1135–9.

22 Gunnarsson L, Tokics L, Lundquist H *et al.* Chronic obstructive pulmonary disease and anaesthesia: formation of atelectasis and gas exchange impairment. *Eur Respir J* 1991;**4**:1106–16.

23 Marthan R, Castaing Y, Manier G, Guenard H. Gas exchange alterations in patients with chronic obstructive lung disease. *Chest* 1985;**87**:470–5.

24 Melot C, Naeije R, Rothschild T *et al.* Improvement in ventilation/perfusion matching by almitrine in COPD. *Chest* 1983;**83**:528–33.

25 Melot C, Hallemans R, Naeije R, Mols P, Lejeune P. Deleterious effect of nifedipine on pulmonary gas exchange in chronic obstructive pulmonary disease. *Am Rev Respir Dis* 1984;**130**:612–6.

26 Ringsted CV, Eliasen K, Andersen JB, Heslet L, Qvist J. Ventilation/perfusion distributions and central hemodynamics in chronic obstructive pulmonary disease: effects of terbutaline administration. *Chest* 1989;**96**:976–83.

27 Roca J, Montserrat JM, Rodriguez-Roisin R *et al.* Gas exchange response to naloxone in chronic obstructive pulmonary disease with hypercapnic respiratory failure. *Bull Eur Physiopathol Respir* 1987;**23**:249–54.

28 Roger N, Barbera JA, Roca J *et al.* Nitric oxide inhalation during exercise in chronic obstructive pulmonary disease. *Am J Respir Crit Care Med* 1997;**156**:800–6.

29 Viegas CA, Ferrer A, Montserrat JM *et al.* Ventilation/perfusion response after fenoterol in hypoxemic patients with stable COPD. *Chest* 1996;**110**:71–7.

30 Schols AM, Slangen J, Volovics L, Wouters EF. Weight loss is a reversible factor in the prognosis of chronic obstructive pulmonary disease. *Am J Respir Crit Care Med* 1998;**157**:1791–7.

31 Wouters EF. Nutrition and metabolism in COPD. *Chest* 2000;**117**:274S–80S.

32 Talpers SS, Romberger DJ, Bunce SB, Pingleton SK. Nutritionally associated increased carbon dioxide production: excess total calories vs high proportion of carbohydrate calories. *Chest* 1992;**102**:551–5.

33 Barbera JA, Roca J, Rodriguez-Roisin R *et al.* Gas exchange in patients with small airways dysfunction. *Eur Respir J* 1988;**1**:27S [Abstract].

34 Barbera JA, Rodriguez-Roisin R. Ventilation/perfusion mismatch. In: Voelkel NF, MacNee W, eds. *Chronic Obstructive Pulmonary Disease*. Hamilton: BC Decker, 2002: 292–305.

35 Barbera JA, Roca J, Ferrer A *et al.* Mechanisms of worsening gas exchange during acute exacerbations of chronic obstructive pulmonary disease. *Eur Respir J* 1997;**10**:1285–91.

36 Diaz O, Iglesia R, Ferrer M *et al.* Effects of non-invasive ventilation on pulmonary gas exchange and hemodynamics during acute hypercapnic exacerbations of chronic obstructive pulmonary disease. *Am J Respir Crit Care Med* 1997;**156**:1840–5.

37 Rossi A, Santos C, Roca J *et al.* Effects of PEEP on $\dot{V}a/\dot{Q}$ mismatching in ventilated patients with chronic airflow obstruction. *Am J Respir Crit Care Med* 1994;**149**:1077–84.

38 Torres A, Reyes A, Roca J, Wagner PD, Rodriguez-Roisin R. Ventilation/perfusion mismatching in chronic obstructive pulmonary disease during ventilator weaning. *Am Rev Respir Dis* 1989;**140**:1246–50.

39 Robinson TD, Collins ER, Sullivan CE, Young IH. Long-term nocturnal non-invasive ventilation (NIV) improves hypercapnia in patients with COPD by reducing alveolar dead space. *Am J Respir Crit Care Med* 1994;**163**:A501 [Abstract].

40 Ferrer M, Iglesia R, Roca J *et al.* Pulmonary gas exchange response to weaning with pressure-support ventilation in exacerbated chronic obstructive pulmonary disease patients. *Intensive Care Med* 2002;**28**:1595–9.

41 Wagner PD, Rodriguez-Roisin R. Clinical advances in pulmonary gas exchange. *Am Rev Respir Dis* 1991;**143**:883–8.

42 Beydon L, Cinotti L, Rekik N *et al.* Changes in the distribution of ventilation and perfusion associated with separation from mechanical ventilation in patients with obstructive pulmonary disease. *Anesthesiology* 1991;**75**:730–8.

43 Lemaire F, Teboul JL, Cinotti L *et al*. Acute left ventricular dysfunction during unsuccessful weaning from mechanical ventilation. *Anesthesiology* 1988;**69**:171–9.

44 National Institutes of Health. Global initiative for chronic obstructive lung disease. Global strategy for the diagnosis, management, and prevention of chronic obstructive pulmonary disease. National Heart, Lung and Blood Institute. Updated July 2004. www.goldcopd.com. 2004.

45 Peinado VI, Barbera JA, Ramirez J *et al*. Endothelial dysfunction in pulmonary arteries of patients with mild COPD. *Am J Physiol* 1998;**274**:L908–13.

46 Celli BR, Cote CG, Marin JM *et al*. The body-mass index, airflow obstruction, dyspnea, and exercise capacity index in chronic obstructive pulmonary disease. *N Engl J Med* 2004; **350**:1005–12.

47 Saetta M, Ghezzo H, Kim WD *et al*. Loss of alveolar attachments in smokers: a morphometric correlate of lung function impairment. *Am Rev Respir Dis* 1985;**132**:894–900.

48 Barbera JA, Riverola A, Roca J *et al*. Pulmonary vascular abnormalities and ventilation/perfusion relationships in mild chronic obstructive pulmonary disease. *Am J Respir Crit Care Med* 1994;**149**:423–9.

49 Kessler R, Faller M, Fourgaut G, Mennecier B, Weitzenblum E. Predictive factors of hospitalization for acute exacerbation in a series of 64 patients with chronic obstructive pulmonary disease. *Am J Respir Crit Care Med* 1999;**159**:158–64.

50 Scharf SM, Iqbal M, Keller C *et al*. Hemodynamic characterization of patients with severe emphysema. *Am J Respir Crit Care Med* 2002;**166**:314–22.

51 Wilkinson M, Langhorne CA, Heath D, Barer GR, Howard P. A pathophysiological study of 10 cases of hypoxic cor pulmonale. *Q J Med* 1988;**66**:65–85.

52 Dinh-Xuan AT, Higenbottam TW, Clelland CA *et al*. Impairment of endothelium-dependent pulmonary-artery relaxation in chronic obstructive lung disease. *N Engl J Med* 1991;**324**:1539–47.

53 Peinado VI, Barbera JA, Abate P *et al*. Inflammatory reaction in pulmonary muscular arteries of patients with mild chronic obstructive pulmonary disease. *Am J Respir Crit Care Med* 1999;**159**:1605–11.

54 O'Shaughnessy TC, Ansari TW, Barnes NC, Jeffery PK. Inflammation in bronchial biopsies of subjects with chronic bronchitis: inverse relationship of CD8$^+$ T lymphocytes with *FEV*$_1$. *Am J Respir Crit Care Med* 1997;**155**:852–7.

55 Saetta M, Turato G, Facchini FM *et al*. Inflammatory cells in the bronchial glands of smokers with chronic bronchitis. *Am J Respir Crit Care Med* 1997;**156**:1633–9.

56 Barbera JA, Peinado VI, Santos S *et al*. Reduced expression of endothelial nitric oxide synthase in pulmonary arteries of smokers. *Am J Respir Crit Care Med* 2001;**164**:709–13.

57 Santos S, Peinado VI, Ramirez J *et al*. Characterization of pulmonary vascular remodelling in smokers and patients with mild COPD. *Eur Respir J* 2002;**19**:632–8.

58 Santos S, Peinado VI, Ramirez J *et al*. Enhanced expression of vascular endothelial growth factor in pulmonary arteries of smokers and patients with moderate chronic obstructive pulmonary disease. *Am J Respir Crit Care Med* 2003;**167**:1250–6.

59 Melgosa T, Peinado VI, Santos S *et al*. Expression of endothelial nitric oxide synthase (eNOS) and endothelin-1 (ET-1) in pulmonary arteries of patients with severe COPD. *Eur Respir J* 2002;**22**:20S [Abstract].

60 Kasahara Y, Tuder RM, Cool CD *et al*. Endothelial cell death and decreased expression of vascular endothelial growth factor and vascular endothelial growth factor receptor 2 in emphysema. *Am J Respir Crit Care Med* 2001;**163**:737–44.

61 Takabatake N, Nakamura H, Abe S *et al*. The relationship between chronic hypoxemia and activation of the tumor necrosis factor-α system in patients with chronic obstructive pulmonary disease. *Am J Respir Crit Care Med* 2000;**161**: 1179–84.

62 Croxton TL, Weinmann GG, Senior RM, Hoidal JR. Future research directions in chronic obstructive pulmonary disease. *Am J Respir Crit Care Med* 2002;**165**:838–44.

63 Barbera JA, Peinado VI, Santos S. Pulmonary hypertension in chronic obstructive pulmonary disease. *Eur Respir J* 2003;**21**:892–905.

64 Croxton TL, Weinmann GG, Senior RM *et al*. Clinical research in chronic obstructive pulmonary disease: needs and opportunities. *Am J Respir Crit Care Med* 2003;**167**: 1142–9.

SECTION 2
COPD and allied conditions

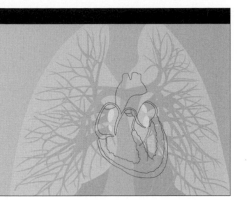

COPD and allied conditions

CHAPTER 10
The natural history of COPD

Jørgen Vestbo

Our knowledge about the natural history of COPD comes mainly from large epidemiological studies over the last four decades describing aspects of the natural history of chronic respiratory symptoms and of obstructive lung function impairment. This has mainly been a result of the development of standardized questionnaires and the application of spirometry in large-scale studies. Although no single study has followed its participants with lung function measurements from birth to old age, it is possible to put the information from studies covering different parts of life together and present a relatively clear picture of the natural history of forced expiratory volume in 1 s (FEV_1), and other lung function measures [1].

The natural history of COPD should include two distinctly different time periods:

1 Growth of lung function, from pre-birth to the values reached at age 20–25 years

2 Decline in lung function in adult life.

This is illustrated in Figure 10.1 and implies that reduced lung function may be caused by inadequate growth of the lungs during childhood (or even *in utero*) and adolescence, premature start of decline in FEV_1 in early adulthood, accelerated decline after the age of 30 years throughout middle and old age, or even a combination of all these factors [2].

Previously, growth of lung function was generally ignored when considering COPD. However, it has become apparent that the maximally attained FEV_1 prior to the normal decline from adulthood is important [3]. Even a normal decline in FEV_1 may result in reduced lung function in old age if the starting point at age 25 years is very low. As with other chronic diseases, such as ischaemic heart disease, genetic and non-genetic prenatal factors as well as perinatal factors may be of importance. Our knowledge of genetic determinants of a low maximally attained lung function is poor and in COPD genetic determinants mainly point to genetic products that may affect the individual's susceptibility to smoking and presumably other environmental

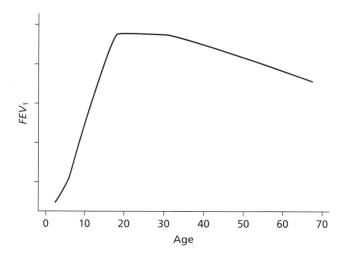

Figure 10.1 Growth of forced expiratory volume in 1 s (FEV_1), the plateau phase and the decline with age in a normal individual.

factors. Both family and twin studies have confirmed a significant genetic contribution to the variance in pulmonary function [4–7] but, other than α_1-antitrypsin, few strong specific genetic factors are known.

In some studies low birth weight has been shown to predict low lung function in adult life, consistent with the theory connecting pre- and perinatal events with many chronic diseases proposed by Barker *et al.* [8,9]. However, it can be difficult to separate the effects of perinatal events from those of other strong risk factors, especially socio-economic status [10,11], maternal smoking status [12,13] and subsequent smoking habits [14]. In the study by Barker *et al.* [8], the effect of birth weight was not limited to lung function in adult life, but was also related to subsequent death from COPD. Le Souëf [15] has pointed out that a disease such as COPD, which is generally considered a disease secondary to adult smoking, in fact has its roots in childhood. Smoking during pregnancy affects both growth

117

in general and lung growth *in utero* and leads to decreased lung function at birth [12,13,16]. An altered growth of lung function, resulting from genetics, perinatal factors or exposures during childhood and adolescence, such as recurrent infections [17,18] or smoking [14], will result in a suboptimal level of lung function in early adulthood. Evidence of mild airway obstruction and slowed growth of lung function was found in smoking American adolescents [14] and this is in accordance with a previous study showing a slowing of growth of FEV_1 in smoking adolescents with respiratory symptoms [19]. Depending on subsequent lifestyle, this may increase the risk of developing COPD. Likewise, a recent study showed effects of air pollution on lung function, including FEV_1, in school children in California [20]. An effect on growth of lung function resulting from exposures such as smoking and air pollution is likely to be larger in subjects from lower socioeconomic strata. This could potentially explain why the effects of socioeconomic status on lung function are obvious even in early adult life [10].

The growth phase of FEV_1 continues until approximately the age of 20–25 years, when the maximum values are reached. Thereafter follows a phase of quite stable lung function, the so-called 'plateau phase', which may last until approximately 35 years of age. Subsequently, as part of the ageing process, the FEV_1 starts to decline in an accelerating fashion. This is the most well-described part of the lung function curve and the decline in FEV_1 is often reported in millilitres per year rather than as percentage change of FEV_1 by year. The mean values of FEV_1 decline in healthy men and women approximately 30 mL/year and 25 mL/year, respectively [1]. This means that an average reduction in FEV_1 for a healthy non-smoking man is approximately 1.2 L from the 40th to the 80th year of life. An interesting observation from longitudinal studies is the phenomenon of tracking, which means that a measurement of FEV_1 before the age of 10 years is a strong predictor of the level of FEV_1 in early adulthood and probably even in old age, a finding similar to the course of body height throughout life.

The lung function impairment that usually characterizes COPD is generally believed to be the result of changes over decades. The most important and also best investigated deviation from the normal course of changes in lung function is the accelerated decline of FEV_1 in the middle-aged or elderly smoker. Adult smokers experience on average an FEV_1 decline of 40–50 mL/year, an excess of the normal annual decline of 15–20 mL/year. Yet, the FEV_1 of some smokers may decline by 80–100 mL/year. Thus, although the rate of decline in FEV_1 shows considerable interindividual variation in the literature, the notion of rapid decliners seems justified. The smokers who are most susceptible to the deleterious effects of tobacco may lose 3–4 L of FEV_1 during four decades, a process with devastating clinical consequences. Most studies link COPD to cigarette smoking, mainly because cigarettes are smoked much more often than cigars, cheroots or pipes. From studies including all types of smokers it seems that the type of tobacco smoked has a minor role, if any [21]. The crucial factor seems to be the amount smoked and the extent of inhalation [22]. Filter cigarettes do not differ significantly from non-filter cigarettes, presumably because the substances causing lung function impairment originate from the volatile part of cigarettes which is not reduced by filters.

The role of environmental tobacco smoking (ETS) has been more difficult to comprehend. In a recent review on the effect of passive smoking on children [23], it was concluded that maternal smoking is associated with small but statistically significant deficits in FEV_1 and other spirometric indices and that the association was almost certainly causal. In adults, the role of ETS is less clear. The effect of ETS on lung function and COPD seems to depend strongly on the setting in which it is studied and in particular in which country ETS is studied. Even if studies from China, which show the largest effects, are excluded, a possible effect of ETS seems to be present [24].

Smoking cessation has in several surveys been shown to reduce both the prevalence of respiratory symptoms and the decline in FEV_1 [22,25–28]. The first change in lung function seen after smoking cessation is a small increase, usually in the region of 30–50 mL for FEV_1. This is presumably because of the disappearance of the acute inflammatory oedema in the smoker's airways. The favourable change in subsequent decline in lung function is seen in younger subjects and in those without apparent COPD, whereas the beneficial changes are less apparent in older subjects with overt COPD [22,26]. In young and middle-aged subjects, it is a matter of debate whether the decline in FEV_1 after smoking cessation normalizes completely. At present it seems that in general quitters continue to have an FEV_1 decline that is slightly larger than that seen in those who have never smoked [23,26,27]. Whether this is because a small number of the quitters have continuous respiratory symptoms indicating an ongoing inflammation in the airways remains to be seen.

Besides smoking other exposures may accelerate FEV_1 decline. The association between occupational exposures and excess decline in lung function has previously been the topic of heated debate, but presumably weaknesses in early study designs have led to an underestimation of the role of occupational exposures in COPD [29]. An important milestone in demonstrating the role of occupational exposures was the study of Paris area workers, in which working men with exposure to gases, dust or heat had an accelerated decline in FEV_1 [30]. In this study, the effect of different exposures on FEV_1 decline was examined and on average the exposed men had 5–15 mL/year excess decline in FEV_1

resulting from the exposure. These and other findings from both occupational cohorts and general population samples have led to a general acceptance of a causal relationship between occupational exposure to dust and development of COPD [31–36].

Chronic mucus hypersecretion and recurrent lower respiratory tract infections have also been proposed as events accelerating FEV_1 decline. This point is discussed in more detail in the last part of this chapter.

Asthma is generally regarded as distinctly different from COPD. Longitudinal population studies have, however, shown that asthmatics may have a more rapid decline in FEV_1 than non-asthmatics [37–39]. This is likely to be seen in only a proportion of asthmatics but indeed demonstrates a group with presumed increased susceptibility to exposures leading to loss of lung function. Asthma patients also have an increased mortality risk, primarily because of an increased COPD mortality [40]. It has been argued that features usually associated with asthma – such as airway hyperresponsiveness – determines susceptibility to extrinsic exposures leading to COPD and thus are central in the natural history of COPD. This is usually referred to as the 'Dutch hypothesis' and is dealt with separately later.

Once airway obstruction has developed the further course of disease is characterized by accelerated decline of lung function and the development of dyspnoea. In addition, patients with chronic mucus hypersecretion are particularly prone to recurrent lower airways infections, resulting in acute exacerbations with a frequency up to several exacerbations each year. At this stage it is now generally accepted that many patients show signs of systemic disease, reflected in measurable systemic inflammation, loss of body mass and changes in other organs such as skeletal muscle [41–43]. Along with the progressive decline of FEV_1, and especially recurrent exacerbations, patients experience the gradual loss of health status or health-related quality of life [44,45]. Late in the course of the disease disability is present as a result of the severely reduced lung function. The progressive loss of FEV_1 may be accompanied by a decrease in the volume adjusted diffusion capacity (diffusion constant) brought about by emphysema.

With more decreased lung function, hypoxaemia develops and, secondary to this, elevation of the pulmonary arterial pressure. In severe COPD, the mean pulmonary artery pressure increases approximately 0.5–3 mmHg/year. As a consequence of the high pressure in the pulmonary vascular bed, right ventricular hypertrophy, 'cor pulmonale', develops. Because severe COPD is the disease of current and former elderly smokers, comorbidities caused by other smoking-related diseases such as ischaemic heart disease, general atherosclerosis and cancer are important features of COPD [46]. Although many COPD patients may die from cardiovascular diseases, the risk of dying from respiratory failure or respiratory infections is high, especially in patients with chronic hypoxaemia [47,48].

Reduced FEV_1 is a strong predictor of morbidity and mortality in established COPD. Survival is more closely related to postbronchodilator FEV_1 than to the prebronchodilator value [49], whereas it is unclear whether bronchodilator reversibility as such is a significant predictor of prognosis [50]. COPD patients with peripheral oedema resulting from cor pulmonale have a 5-year survival of 30–40% [51]. Other predictors of mortality in established COPD include smoking, low body weight for height, dyspnoea, chronic mucus hypersecretion, signs of ischaemic heart disease and male gender. Low body weight, expressed as low body mass index (BMI), is an indicator of malnutrition and probably systemic disease in patients with COPD. Low BMI (< 20 kg/m^2) interacts with the level of FEV_1 with regard to mortality, being a much stronger predictor of death in severe COPD than in mild or moderate disease [52]. Recently, an index combining lung function, dyspnoea, body mass and exercise tolerance has been shown to be a better prognostic indicator than staging of COPD based on lung function alone [53].

The British and Dutch hypotheses in COPD

So far, attempts to understand the natural history of COPD have been influenced by the prevalent description of anatomy and physiology as well as the clinical description of the disease. In addition, the heterogeneity of COPD, covering a spectrum from a disease of the airways resembling asthma to a disease of the pulmonary parenchyma, has made it difficult to provide a single hypothesis describing the development and progression of the disease.

Initially, COPD was not defined but described as 'obstructive bronchitis' in contrast to 'simple bronchitis'. This was the basis for the 'British hypothesis', which claimed that chronic mucus hypersecretion (CMH), by setting the stage for recurrent airway infection, was causative in the development of airway obstruction. In the 1960s, Fletcher *et al.* performed a 7-year longitudinal study of a working population consisting of 30–60-year-old men, mostly heavy smokers and all of whom lived in London in a period of heavy air pollution. The seminal work by Fletcher *et al.* [54] rejected the 'British hypothesis' by showing that in middle-aged men CMH and progressive airway obstruction were two separate entities, although often occurring concomitantly because of a common risk factor – smoking. Whereas the progressive airway obstruction was the most important disease process resulting in progressive disability in COPD patients, the presence of mucus hypersecretion clearly predisposed to recurrent bronchopulmonary infections causing increased morbidity and absence from work.

However, it is likely that these findings have been over-interpreted. Fletcher et al. [55] clearly state that 'In the preclinical stages of these disorders, which we have studied, we find no causal relationship between them, for neither mucus hypersecretion nor clinical chest illnesses cause accelerated loss of FEV'. Whereas it seems likely that the progressive loss of lung function is not initiated by recurrent lower respiratory tract infections, the study by Fletcher et al. cannot describe the role of infection in later stages of COPD. Also, the fact that the London study, and other studies with similar findings, was conducted in selected occupational cohorts may have skewed the picture.

Within the last 15 years several studies have shown CMH and lower respiratory tract infections (LRTIs) to be less innocent. Mortality studies have all shown an association between CMH and overall mortality [56,57] as well as COPD mortality [58,59]. In the latter study, the excess risk of mortality associated with CMH was caused by an increased risk of death associated with infection [60]. Regarding an association between CMH and development of COPD, fewer studies have confirmed an association between CMH and FEV_1. Sherman et al. [61] reported an excess FEV_1 decline in men with CMH in the US Six Cities Study but the association was weak. In the Copenhagen City Heart Study, Vestbo et al. [62] showed that CMH was associated with an excess FEV_1 decline: 22.8 mL/year in men; 12.6 mL/year in women. CMH was also associated with an increased risk of subsequent hospitalization resulting from COPD. This raised the possibility that CMH accelerates progression of disease. However, the association may only be present in established COPD as the same group has shown that CMH in subjects with normal lung function does not seem to predispose to airflow obstruction [63]. The effect of CMH on COPD morbidity is also present in the elderly [64]. The mechanism in established COPD is still not entirely clear but it is most likely the increased risk of exacerbations or LRTIs associated with CMH that may lead to an excess decline in FEV_1 in this random population sample. Support for this comes from 5-year data from the US Lung Health Study. Kanner et al. [65] showed that LRTIs, which in this study were associated with CMH, were linked with lung function decline in patients with mild COPD: every 1 LRTI/year in smokers was associated with a decrease in FEV_1 of approximately 7 mL. This decrease may seem small but in a patient with 2–3 exacerbations per year the excess decline would be approximately 20 mL/year. These findings were further supported by a smaller 4-year UK study of patients with moderate to severe COPD [66]. In this study, patients with frequent exacerbations (median 4.2/year) showed a more rapid decline in FEV_1 (difference 8 mL/year) than infrequent exacerbators (median 1.9/year).

In terms of the percentage decline, FEV_1 fell by 4.2%/year in frequent exacerbators compared with 3.6%/year in infrequent exacerbators.

Thus, the pendulum seems to have swung regarding our view on CMH, exacerbations and progression of COPD [67]. CMH and LRTIs may not have a role in initiating changes leading to fixed airflow obstruction. In established COPD, however, CMH increases the risk of exacerbations and the most recent data seem to show that this impacts on the natural history of COPD.

With the initial rejection of the 'British hypothesis' a new approach to the understanding of factors related to the development of chronic bronchitis and emphysema was possible. In 1961 a group of Dutch investigators put forward the hypothesis that various forms of airways obstruction such as asthma, chronic bronchitis and even emphysema should be considered as different expressions of the same underlying abnormality and introduced the term 'chronic non-specific lung disease'. They suggested that host factors, airway hyperresponsiveness and allergy define suscepti-bility to the development of airways obstruction by inter-acting with environmental factors such as smoking and air pollution. This was subsequently named the 'Dutch hypothesis' [68–70]. Although the idea of combining asthma with bronchitis and emphysema into a single dis-ease category has not gained wide acceptance outside the Netherlands, several prospective studies have until now shown that airway hyperresponsiveness is a significant predictor of FEV_1 decline, development of respiratory symptoms and even mortality from COPD [71–77]. One of the problems of interpreting the role of airway hyperre-sponsiveness as a host susceptibility factor for the develop-ment of COPD is the fact that airway hyperresponsiveness may develop secondary to development of airways obstruc-tion resulting from changes in airway geometry. Yet it seems that airway hyperresponsiveness is a significant pre-dictor of both the preclinical and clinical course of COPD and asthma, even after some adjustment for the impact of airway geometry. With regard to allergy, which in epidemio-logical studies is usually measured as skin prick test posi-tivity or elevated levels of IgE, it has been shown that these allergy markers may interact with smoking in predicting FEV_1 decline and survival. Based on the analyses of survival and the course of lung function of the participants in the longitudinal Tucson respiratory study, Burrows et al. [78] suggested that the 'Dutch hypothesis' is valid for the sub-group of COPD patients with obstructive lung function impairment mainly caused by airways disease: patients who clinically share some common characteristics with asthma and that the term asthmatic bronchitis is a relevant description of this group. On the other hand, the 'Dutch hypothesis' is probably less relevant to COPD patients with a more 'malignant type of disease', where emphysema is the main cause of airways obstruction. An important consequence of the 'Dutch hypothesis' is that asthma could be regarded as a risk factor for COPD. As long-standing asthma does not result in emphysema in the absence of smoking, it may well be that the risk factors of the emphysematous type of COPD are different and in general much more research is needed regarding the natural history of different subtypes of COPD [79]. However, this may prove to be difficult to disentangle as most patients cannot be clearly subtyped into bronchitic or emphysematous, most patients in fact have features of both, *and* small airways disease. Postma and Boezen [70] have suggested that mapping of genes in asthma and COPD may eventually show if the 'Dutch hypothesis' is a suitable explanation for the pathogenesis of COPD.

In conclusion, we have quite detailed knowledge on the natural history of COPD although the majority of studies to date have used FEV_1 as a proxy for COPD. The future challenge will be to disentangle the different phenotypes of COPD and gain more knowledge on the factors differentiating these phenotypes.

References

1 Anto JM, Vermeire P, Vestbo J, Sunyer J. Epidemiology of chronic obstructive pulmonary disease. *Eur Respir J* 2001;**17**: 982–94.

2 Rijcken B, Britton J. Epidemiology of chronic obstructive pulmonary disease. *Eur Respir Mon* 1998;**7**:74–83.

3 Kerstjens HAM, Rijcken B, Schouten JP, Postma DS. Decline of FEV_1 by age and smoking status: facts, figures, and fallacies. *Thorax* 1997;**52**:820–7.

4 Larson RK, Barman ML, Kueppers F, Fudenberg HH. Genetic and environmental determinants of chronic obstructive pulmonary disease. *Ann Intern Med* 1970;**72**:627–32.

5 Kueppers F, Miller RD, Gordon H, Hepper NG, Offord K. Familial prevalence of chronic obstructive pulmonary disease in a matched pair study. *Am J Med* 1977;**63**:336–42.

6 Cohen BH, Ball WC Jr, Brashears S *et al.* Risk factors in chronic obstructive pulmonary disease (COPD). *Am J Epidemiol* 1977;**105**:223–32.

7 Silverman EK, Chapman HA, Drazen JM *et al.* Genetic epidemiology of severe, early-onset chronic obstructive pulmonary disease: risk to relatives for airflow obstruction and chronic bronchitis. *Am J Respir Crit Care Med* 1998;**157**: 1770–8.

8 Barker DJ, Godfrey KM, Fall C *et al.* Relation of birth weight and childhood respiratory infection to adult lung function and death from chronic obstructive airways disease. *BMJ* 1991;**303**:671–5.

9 Stein CE, Kumaran K, Fall CH *et al.* Relation of fetal growth to adult lung function in south India. *Thorax* 1997;**52**:895–9.

10 Prescott E, Lange P, Vestbo J and the Copenhagen City Heart Study Group. Socio-economic status, lung function, and admission to hospital for COPD: results from the Copenhagen City Heart Study. *Eur Respir J* 1999;**13**:1109–14.

11 Prescott E, Vestbo J. Socioeconomic status and chronic obstructive pulmonary disease. *Thorax* 1999;**54**:737–41.

12 Hanrahan JP, Tager IB, Segal MR *et al.* The effect of maternal smoking during pregnancy on early infant lung function. *Am Rev Respir Dis* 1992;**145**:1129–35.

13 Carlsen HCL, Jaakkola JJK, Nafstad P, Carlsen K-H. *In utero* exposure to cigarette smoking influences lung function at birth. *Eur Respir J* 1997;**10**:1774–9.

14 Gold DR, Wang X, Wypij D *et al.* Effects of cigarette smoking on the pulmonary function in adolescent boys and girls. *N Engl J Med* 1996;**335**:931–7.

15 Le Souëf PN. Tobacco related lung diseases begin in childhood. *Thorax* 2000;**55**:1063–7.

16 Tager IB, Ngo L, Hanrahan JP. Maternal smoking during pregnancy: effects on lung function during the first 18 months of life. *Am J Respir Crit Care Med* 1995;**152**:977–83.

17 Gold DR, Tager IB, Weiss ST, Tosteson TD, Speizer FE. Acute lower respiratory illness in childhood as a predictor of lung function and chronic respiratory symptoms. *Am Rev Respir Dis* 1989;**140**:877–84.

18 Shaheen SO, Barker DJ, Shiell AW *et al.* The relationship between pneumonia in early childhood and impaired lung function in late adult life. *Am J Respir Crit Care Med* 1994; **149**:616–9.

19 Sherrill DL, Lebowitz MD, Knudson RJ, Burrows B. Smoking and symptom effects on the curves of lung function growth and decline. *Am Rev Respir Dis* 1991;**144**:17–22.

20 Gauderman WJ, Avol E, Gilliland F *et al.* The effect of air pollution on lung development from 10 to 18 years of age. *N Engl J Med* 2004;**351**:1057–67.

21 Lange P. Development and prognosis of chronic obstructive pulmonary disease with special reference to the role of tobacco smoking. *Dan Med Bull* 1992;**39**:30–48.

22 Lange P, Groth S, Nyboe J *et al.* Effects of smoking and changes in smoking habits on the decline of FEV_1. *Eur Respir J* 1989;**2**:811–6.

23 Cook DG, Strachan DP. Summary of parental smoking on the effects of parental smoking on the respiratory health of children and implications for research. *Thorax* 1999;**54**:357–66.

24 Jaakkola MS. Environmental tobacco smoke and respiratory diseases. *Eur Respir Mon* 2000;**15**:322–83.

25 Royal College of Physicians of London. *Health or Smoking?* Follow-up report of the Royal College of Physicians. London: Pitman, 1983.

26 Camilli AE, Burrows B, Knudson RJ, Lyle SK, Lebowitz MD. Longitudinal changes in forced expiratory volume in one second in adults. *Am Rev Respir Dis* 1987;**135**:794–9.

27 Anthonisen NR, Connett JE, Kiley JP *et al.* Effects of smoking intervention and the use of an inhaled anticholinergic bronchodilator on the rate of decline of FEV_1: the Lung Health Study. *JAMA* 1994;**272**:1497–505.

28 Anthonisen NR, Connett JE, Murray RP, for the Lung Health Study Research Group. Smoking and lung function of Lung Health Study participants after 11 years. *Am J Respir Crit Care Med* 2002;**166**:675–9.

29 Hendrick DJ. Occupation and chronic obstructive pulmonary disease. *Thorax* 1996;**51**:947–55.

30 Kauffmann F, Drouet D, Lellouch J, Brille D. Occupational exposure and 12-year spirometric changes among Paris area workers. *Br J Ind Med* 1982;**39**:221–32.

31 Becklake MR. Occupational exposures: evidence for a causal association with chronic obstructive pulmonary disease. *Am Rev Respir Dis* 1989;**140**:S85–91.

32 Heederik D. Epidemiology of occupational respiratory diseases and risk factors. *Eur Respir Mon* 2000;**15**:429–47.

33 Krzyzanowski M, Jedrychowski W, Wysocki M. Factors associated with the change in ventilatory function and the development of chronic obstructive pulmonary disease in a 13-year follow-up of the Cracow study. *Am Rev Respir Dis* 1986;**134**:1011–9.

34 Korn RJ, Dockery DW, Speizer FE, Ware JH, Ferris BG Jr. Occupational exposures and chronic respiratory symptoms: a population-based study. *Am Rev Respir Dis* 1987;**136**:298–304.

35 Heederik D, Pouwels H, Kromhout H, Kromhout D. Chronic non-specific lung disease and occupational exposures estimated by means of a job exposure matrix: the Zutphen Study. *Int J Epidemiol* 1989;**18**:382–9.

36 Humerfelt S, Gulsvik A, Skjærven R *et al.* Decline in FEV_1 and airflow limitation related to occupational exposures in men of an urban community. *Eur Respir J* 1993;**6**:1095–103.

37 Peat JK, Woolcock AJ, Cullen K. Rate of decline of lung function in subjects with asthma. *Eur J Respir Dis* 1987;**70**:171–9.

38 Lange P, Parner J, Vestbo J, Jensen G, Schnohr P. A 15-year follow-up of ventilatory function in adults with asthma. *N Engl J Med* 1998;**339**:1194–200.

39 Silva GE, Sherrill DL, Guerra S, Barbee RA. Asthma as a risk factor for COPD in a longitudinal study. *Chest* 2004;**126**:59–65.

40 Lange P, Ulrik CS, Vestbo J, for the Copenhagen City Heart Study Group. Mortality in adults with self-reported bronchial asthma: a study of the general population. *Lancet* 1996;**347**:1285–9.

41 Wouters EFM. A wasting disease. In: Voelkel NF, MacNee W, eds. *Chronic Obstructive Lung Disease.* Hamilton, London: BC Dekker, 2002.

42 Agusti AG, Noguera A, Sauleda J *et al.* Systemic effects of chronic obstructive pulmonary disease. *Eur Respir J* 2003;**21**:347–60.

43 Agusti AG, Sauleda J, Miralles C *et al.* Skeletal muscle apoptosis and weight loss in chronic obstructive pulmonary disease. *Am J Respir Crit Care Med* 2002;**166**:485–9.

44 Burge PS, Calverley PM, Jones PW *et al.* Randomised, double blind, placebo controlled study of fluticasone propionate in patients with moderate to severe chronic obstructive pulmonary disease: the ISOLDE trial. *BMJ* 2000;**320**:1297–303.

45 Spencer S, Calverley PM, Burge PS, Jones PW, on behalf of the ISOLDE Study Group. Health status deterioration in patients with chronic obstructive pulmonary disease. *Am J Respir Crit Care Med* 2001;**163**:122–8.

46 Mapel DW, Hurley JS, Frost FJ *et al.* Health care utilization in chronic obstructive pulmonary disease: a case–control study in a health maintenance organization. *Arch Intern Med* 2000;**160**:2653–8.

47 Zielinski J, MacNee W, Wedzicha W *et al.* Causes of death in patients with COPD and chronic respiratory failure. *Monaldi Arch Chest Dis* 1997;**52**:43–7.

48 Incalzi RA, Fuso L, De Rosa M *et al.* Comorbidity contributors to predict mortality of patients with chronic obstructive pulmonary disease. *Eur Respir J* 1997;**10**:2794–800.

49 Anthonisen NR, Wright EC, Hodking JE. Prognosis in chronic obstructive pulmonary disease. *Am Rev Respir Dis* 1986;**133**:14–20.

50 Hansen EF, Phanareth K, Laursen LC, Kok-Jensen A, Dirksen A. Reversible and irreversible airflow obstruction as predictor of overall mortality in asthma and chronic obstructive pulmonary disease. *Am J Respir Crit Care Med* 1999;**159**:1267–71.

51 Weitzenblum E, Hirth C, Ducolone A *et al.* Prognostic value of pulmonary artery pressure in chronic obstructive pulmonary disease. *Thorax* 1981;**36**:752–8.

52 Landbo C, Prescott E, Lange P, Vestbo J, Almdal TP. Prognostic value of nutritional status in chronic obstructive pulmonary disease. *Am J Respir Crit Care Med* 1999;**160**:1856–61.

53 Celli BR, Cote CG, Marin JM *et al.* The body-mass index, airflow obstruction, dyspnea, and exercise capacity index in chronic obstructive pulmonary disease. *N Engl J Med* 2004;**350**:1005–12.

54 Fletcher CM, Peto R, Tinker CM, Speizer FE. *The Natural History of Chronic Bronchitis and Emphysema.* Oxford: Oxford University Press, 1976.

55 Fletcher CM, Peto R. The natural history of chronic airflow obstruction. *BMJ* 1977;**i**:1645–8.

56 Annesi I, Kauffmann F. Is respiratory mucus hypersecretion really an innocent disorder? *Am Rev Respir Dis* 1986;**134**:688–93.

57 Vollmer WM, McCamant LE, Johnson LR, Buist AS. Respiratory symptoms, lung function, and mortality in a screening center cohort. *Am J Epidemiol* 1989;**129**:1157–69.

58 Speizer FE, Fay ME, Dockery DW, Ferris BG Jr. Chronic obstructive pulmonary disease mortality in six US cities. *Am Rev Respir Dis* 1989;**140**(Suppl):S49–55.

59 Lange P, Nyboe J, Appleyard M, Jensen G, Schnohr P. The relation of ventilatory impairment and of chronic mucus hypersecretion to mortality from obstructive lung disease and from all causes. *Thorax* 1990;**45**:579–85.

60 Prescott E, Lange P, Vestbo J. Chronic mucus hypersecretion in COPD and death from pulmonary infection. *Eur Respir J* 1995;**8**:1333–8.

61 Sherman CB, Xu X, Speizer FE *et al.* Longitudinal lung function decline in subjects with respiratory symptoms. *Am Rev Respir Dis* 1992;**46**:855–9.

62 Vestbo J, Prescott E, Lange P, and the Copenhagen City Heart Study Group. Association of chronic mucus hypersecretion with FEV_1 decline and COPD morbidity. *Am J Respir Crit Care Med* 1996;**153**:1530–5.

63 Vestbo J, Lange P. Can GOLD Stage 0 provide information of prognostic value in chronic obstructive pulmonary disease? *Am J Respir Crit Care Med* 2002;**166**:329–32.

64 Lange P, Parner J, Prescott E, Vestbo J. Chronic bronchitis in an elderly population. *Age Ageing* 2003;**32**:636–42.

65 Kanner RE, Anthonisen NR, Connett JE, for the Lung Health Study Research Group. Lower respiratory illnesses promote FEV_1 decline in current smokers but not ex-smokers with mild chronic obstructive pulmonary disease. *Am J Respir Crit Care Med* 2001;**164**:358–64.

66 Donaldson GC, Seemungal TAR, Bhomik A, Wedzicha JA. Relationship between exacerbation frequency and lung function decline in chronic obstructive pulmonary disease. *Thorax* 2002;**57**:847–52.

67 Anthonisen NR. The British hypothesis revisited. *Eur Respir J* 2004;**23**:657–8.

68 Orie NGM, Sluiter HJ, de Vries K, Tammeling GJ, Witkop J. The host factor in bronchitis. In: Orie NGM, Sluiter HJ, eds. *Bronchitis: an International Symposium.* Assen, Netherlands: Royal van Gorcum, 1961.

69 Vestbo J, Prescott E. An update on the Dutch hypothesis and chronic respiratory disease. *Thorax* 1998;**53**(Suppl 2):S15–9.

70 Postma DS, Boezen HM. Rationale for the Dutch hypothesis: allergy and airway hyperresponsiveness as genetic factors and their interaction with environment in the development of asthma and COPD. *Chest* 2004;**126**:96–104S.

71 Hospers JJ, Postma DS, Rijcken B, Weiss ST, Schouten JP. Histamine airway hyperresponsiveness and mortality from chronic obstructive pulmonary disease: a cohort study. *Lancet* 2000;**356**:1313–7.

72 Vestbo J, Hansen EF. Airway hyperresponsiveness and COPD mortality. *Thorax* 2001;**56**(Suppl 2):11–4.

73 Rijcken B, Scouten JP, Xu X, Rosner B, Weiss ST. Bronchial hyperresponsiveness to histamine is associated with accelerated decline of FEV_1. *Am J Respir Crit Care Med* 1995;**151**: 1377–82.

74 Villar MT, Dow L, Coggon D, Lampe FC, Holgate ST. The influence of increased bronchial responsiveness, atopy, and serum IgE on decline in FEV_1: a longitudinal study in the elderly. *Am J Respir Crit Care Med* 1995;**151**:656–62.

75 Parker DR, O'Connor GT, Sparrow D, Segal MR, Weiss ST. The relationship of non-specific airway responsiveness and atopy to the rate of decline of lung function: the normative aging study. *Am Rev Respir Dis* 1990;**141**:589–94.

76 O'Connor GT, Sparrow D, Weiss ST. A prospective study of methacholine airway responsiveness as a predictor of pulmonary function decline: the Normative Aging Study. *Am J Respir Crit Care Med* 1995;**152**:87–92.

77 Tashkin DP, Altose MD, Connett JE *et al.* for the Lung Health Study Research Group. Methacholine reactivity predicts chages in lung function over time in smokers with early chronic obstructive pulmonary disease. *Am J Respir Crit Care Med* 1996;**153**:1802–11.

78 Burrows B, Bloom JW, Traver GA, Cline MG. The course and prognosis of different forms of chronic airways obstruction in a sample of the general population. *N Engl J Med* 1987; **317**:1309–14.

79 Kondoh Y, Taniguchi H, Yokoyama S *et al.* Emphysematous change in chronic asthma in relation to cigarette smoking: assessment by computed tomography. *Chest* 1990;**97**:845–9.

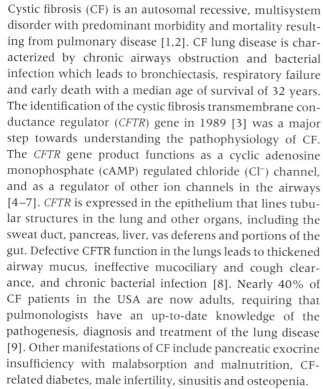

CHAPTER 11
Cystic fibrosis

Marcus P. Kennedy and Michael R. Knowles

Cystic fibrosis (CF) is an autosomal recessive, multisystem disorder with predominant morbidity and mortality resulting from pulmonary disease [1,2]. CF lung disease is characterized by chronic airways obstruction and bacterial infection which leads to bronchiectasis, respiratory failure and early death with a median age of survival of 32 years. The identification of the cystic fibrosis transmembrane conductance regulator (*CFTR*) gene in 1989 [3] was a major step towards understanding the pathophysiology of CF. The *CFTR* gene product functions as a cyclic adenosine monophosphate (cAMP) regulated chloride (Cl⁻) channel, and as a regulator of other ion channels in the airways [4–7]. *CFTR* is expressed in the epithelium that lines tubular structures in the lung and other organs, including the sweat duct, pancreas, liver, vas deferens and portions of the gut. Defective CFTR function in the lungs leads to thickened airway mucus, ineffective mucociliary and cough clearance, and chronic bacterial infection [8]. Nearly 40% of CF patients in the USA are now adults, requiring that pulmonologists have an up-to-date knowledge of the pathogenesis, diagnosis and treatment of the lung disease [9]. Other manifestations of CF include pancreatic exocrine insufficiency with malabsorption and malnutrition, CF-related diabetes, male infertility, sinusitis and osteopenia.

In the USA, there are approximately 120 specialized CF clinical centres sponsored by the Cystic Fibrosis Foundation (CFF). These centres offer high-quality clinical care and also coordinate clinical research on various aspects of the disease. A number of comprehensive consensus statements have been published as a combined effort between the CFF and physicians at CF centres, which outline recommended diagnostic and treatment protocols for various aspects of the disease, of which some are cited here [10–17]. The CFF foundation website (http://www.cff.org/) also contains information on all aspects of the disease with links to related websites.

Epidemiology and genetics

CF is a recessive genetic disorder, reflecting mutations in the *CFTR* gene. CF occurs in 1 in 3000 live births in Caucasian populations, but is much less common in African and Asian Americans. Approximately 5% of Caucasians are carriers, and it has been suggested that the preponderance of heterozygotes (carriers) reflects protection from chloride-secreting diarrhoeal infection in the distant past [18,19].

The *CFTR* gene is located on the long arm of human chromosome 7. It consists of 250 kB of genomic DNA containing 27 exons. CFTR is a 1480 amino acid membrane protein with 12 membrane-spanning regions. Heterozygote carriers of a *CFTR* mutation are asymptomatic, without evidence of disease. This suggests that 50% of the normal level of functional CFTR is enough to prevent the CF phenotype. More than 1000 distinct mutations have been described in the CF gene. The most common mutation is the ΔF508 mutation, which reflects deletion of three bases and leads to a loss of a single phenylalanine. This results in misfolding and cellular degradation of the protein, and absence of functional CFTR on the apical membrane of airway epithelia. The ΔF508 mutation accounts for 70% of the CF alleles, and 50% of CF patients are homozygous for the ΔF508 mutation [1]. Depending on the molecular abnormality in CFTR, there is a spectrum of consequences from 'severe' loss of function mutations to 'mild' mutations with partial and/or residual function.

This heterogeneity of molecular defects leads to a spectrum of clinical disease. At one end of the spectrum, 'severe' mutations resulting in absence of functional CFTR correlate strongly with pancreatic exocrine insufficiency, but less strongly with severity of lung disease. 'Mild' mutations with residual function of CFTR are associated with pancreatic

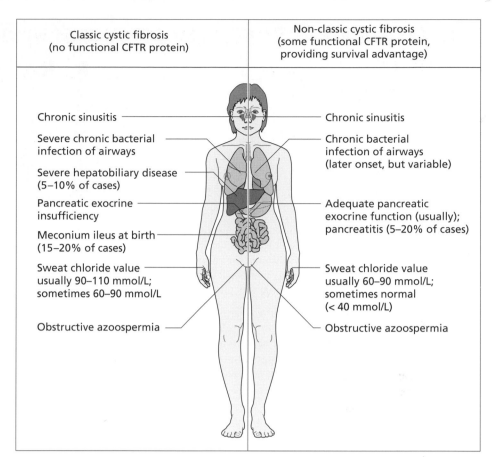

Classic cystic fibrosis (no functional CFTR protein)	Non-classic cystic fibrosis (some functional CFTR protein, providing survival advantage)
Chronic sinusitis	Chronic sinusitis
Severe chronic bacterial infection of airways	Chronic bacterial infection of airways (later onset, but variable)
Severe hepatobiliary disease (5–10% of cases)	
Pancreatic exocrine insufficiency	Adequate pancreatic exocrine function (usually); pancreatitis (5–20% of cases)
Meconium ileus at birth (15–20% of cases)	
Sweat chloride value usually 90–110 mmol/L; sometimes 60–90 mmol/L	Sweat chloride value usually 60–90 mmol/L; sometimes normal (< 40 mmol/L)
Obstructive azoospermia	Obstructive azoospermia

Figure 11.1 Classic (left-side) and non-classic (right-side) cystic fibrosis. Non-classic cystic fibrosis patients usually have better overall survival with later onset and more slowly progressive lung disease, and better nutritional status.

exocrine sufficiency and milder pulmonary disease. From these observations, 'classic' CF is associated with two loss-of-function mutations, and 'non-classic' CF patients have at least one copy of a mutant gene that confers partial function of CFTR. Figure 11.1 compares the classic and non-classic phenotypes [20]. There are also 'mono-organ' forms of disease associated with mild mutations in *CFTR*, including congenital bilateral absence of the vas deferens [21], and idiopathic chronic pancreatitis [22,23]. Screening for 25 of the more common mutations is recommended for all pregnant women or women planning pregnancy by the National Institutes of Health [24].

The variability in clinical phenotype extends beyond the type of mutation in *CFTR* and reflects environmental and non-*CFTR* genetic influences (modifier genes). An initial report investigated the influence of variants in 10 genes other than *CFTR* on the severity of pulmonary disease in a large population of CF patients and identified that genetic variation in transforming growth factor β1 (*TGF β1*) modified disease severity in cystic fibrosis [25,26]. Investigation of other genes is in progress.

Pulmonary disease

Pulmonary disease is the chief cause of morbidity and mortality in CF. In this section, an overview of the key aspects of pulmonary disease is described, including a discussion of normal airway epithelial ion transport, defective ion transport in CF, cellular and organ-level pathophysiology, clinical features, microbiology and complications.

Normal airway epithelial ion transport

Airway surface liquid (ASL) plays a key part in mucociliary clearance, which is an important airway host defence mechanism. In normal airway epithelia, the ASL is comprised of a periciliary layer (PCL) and a mucus layer, and tight regulation of the volume and composition of ASL is required for optimal function [5,6,8,27]. The low-viscosity PCL layer allows effective ciliary movement and mucociliary clearance. As the volume of surface liquid is moved by mucociliary clearance from the large surface area of

Normal

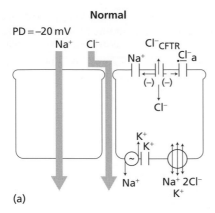

Cystic fibrosis

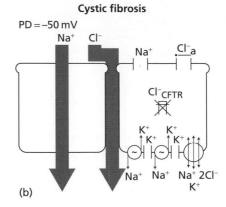

Figure 11.2 Airway epithelial ion transport: cell models display the location of key ion transport proteins. (a) In normal airway epithelia, Na^+ enters the cell through apical amiloride-sensitive Na^+ channels (ENaC) and is extruded across the basolateral membrane by Na^+-ATPase; Cl^- follows through the paracellular pathway to maintain electrical neutrality. The 'alternative' calcium activated channel (Cl_a^-) is closed under basal circumstances. (b) In cystic fibrosis, the apical membrane Na^+ conductance is large, because of the loss of the tonic inhibitory effect of *CFTR*, leading to increased net Na^+ (and Cl^-) absorption. PD, transepithelial potential difference.

the distal airways to the much smaller surface area of the proximal airways, isotonic volume absorption occurs via active ion transport. The lung is often depicted as an inverted funnel, reflecting the relative surface area of the distal versus proximal airways.

Sodium (Na^+) absorption is the dominant ion transport pathway in the airway surface epithelium of adult humans [28]. Figure 11.2(a) depicts basal ion transport across the proximal airway epithelium in a normal lung. Active Na^+ absorption, dependent on apical membrane Na^+ channels (EnaC) and the Na^+-K^+-ATPase pump, mediates ASL volume absorption under basal conditions. This Na^+ absorption is inhibited by luminal amiloride, acting on amiloride-sensitive epithelial channels (EnaC). Chloride (Cl^-) ion follows through the paracellular pathway to maintain electrical neutrality. Under some circumstances, normal airway epithelia can slow Na^+ absorption and induce Cl^- secretion via apical Cl^- channels, with Cl^- entry from the basolateral Na^+-K^+-$2Cl^-$ transporter. Water permeability of airway epithelium appears to be high relative to other barrier epithelia, and water follows the movement of salt by osmosis; thus, there is net volume absorption under basal conditions [29–31].

Defective ion transport in cystic fibrosis

Ion transport in CF is abnormal. A loss of funtional *CFTR* affects both the Na^+ and Cl^- ion transport pathways. CF airway epithelia have an accelerated basal rate of Na^+ (and volume) absorption that reflects the absence of the tonic inhibitory effect of CFTR on epithelial Na^+ channel (EnaC) activity [4,8]. Figure 11.2(b) highlights the abnormal basal ion transport in cystic fibrosis airways, with unabated

Na^+ (and volume) absorption via an increase in the apical membrane Na^+ conductance, and increased basolateral Na^+-K^--ATPase pump activity. This acceleration of Na^+ (and volume absorption) results in depletion of the ASL. In the face of ASL volume depletion, CF airway epithelia are also missing the capacity to add liquid back to airway surfaces, because of the absence of CFTR functioning as a 'secretory' Cl^- channel. Nasal epithelial potential difference (PD) is one tool to assess normal and defective CFTR function. In normal epithelia, perfusion of the luminal surface with a Cl^--free (containing amiloride) solution results in a hyperpolarization of transepithelial PD (resulting from a Cl^- diffusion potential). This hyperpolarization ('secretion of Cl^-') is further augmented via addition of a β-agonist (isoprotenerol) to increase cellular cAMP and thereby increase *CFTR* activity. In CF epithelia, the basal PD is raised (accelerated Na^+ transport) and there is no hyperpolarization in response to luminal Cl^--free solution and isoprotenerol [32]. Thus, the predominant defect from loss of *CFTR* function is hyperabsorption of salt (and liquid) from the luminal surface of airways, coupled to an inability to secrete Cl^- and liquid.

Pathophysiology at microcellular level

Figure 11.3 highlights the consequences of loss of *CFTR* function in the airways. Excessive volume absorption, loss of PCL and continuous build-up of mucus allows gel-forming mucins (MUC5AC and MUC5B) in the mucus layer to adhere to luminal surface glycoproteins, including tethered epithelial surface mucins (MUC1 and MUC4). Despite the fact that mucus plugs are a major component of CF-related lung disease, there have been no defined

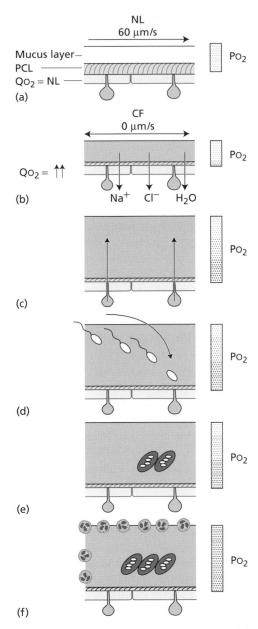

primary genetic abnormalities in mucus [33,34]. There may be some secondary changes in glycosylation, sulfation or other post-translational modifications of mucins secondary to abnormal *CFTR* function [35]. 'Abnormal mucus' is primarily a function of excessive concentration of macromolecules in the mucus layer, reflecting defective ion (and liquid) transport [8]. Taken together, these effects lead to loss of both mucociliary and cough clearance. Furthermore, this viscous mucus is a nidus for early bacterial infection.

Initial pathogenic organisms include *Staphylococcus aureus* and *Haemophilus influenza*, with eventual chronic infection with Gram-negative organisms, including *Pseudomonas aeruginosa* and *Burkholderia cepacia*. Figure 11.3 highlights mechanistic steps in the progression of *P. aeruginosa* infection. Raised oxygen consumption in stagnant mucus on the respiratory cell surface is an ideal niche for *P. aeruginosa*, which can use nitrogen-based compounds as an alternative energy source [36,37]. Macrocolonies develop, and have increased alginate production in this hypoxic environment [36], with resistance to secondary defences, including a slowing of the influx of neutrophils [38]. Formation of macrocolonies down-regulates many bacterial cell functions in an energy-conserving fashion, including loss of 'O' side-chains [39], flagellum and pili [40] and down-regulation of the production of toxins [41]. As described in Figure 11.3, a host inflammatory response occurs in an attempt to counteract infection with a massive recruitment of neutrophils, release of oxidase products and proteases, and upon cellular decomposition, DNA. Airway macrophages are also involved with release of tumour necrosis factor (TNF), interleukin 1 (IL-1) and IL-8, which contribute to the overall chemotactic and neutrophil-activating activity in the CF lung [42]. The presence of an increasing macrocolony density and infiltration of neutrophils adds to the hypoxia of the airway surface mucus layer.

Pathophysiology at macro-organ level

Compromise of CFTR function leads to a number of complications depending on the organ system involved. Loss of CFTR function has its most severe consequences in the lungs. CF neonates have normal lungs at birth, but radiological evidence of abnormalities in the distal conducting

Figure 11.3 Schematic model of the pathogenesis of chronic *Pseudomonas aeruginosa* infection in cystic fibrosis (CF) patients. (a) Normal airway epithelia, a thin mucus layer (clear) resides atop the periciliary layer (PCL) (tinted stripes). Efficient mucociliary clearance, denoted by the vector is facilitated by the presence of low viscosity PCL. A normal rate of epithelia O_2 consumption (Qo_2; left) produces no O_2 gradients within this thin ASL (denoted by light spotted bar). (b–f) CF airway epithelia. (b) Excessive CF volume depletion (denoted by vertical arrows) removes the PCL, mucus becomes adherent to epithelial surfaces and mucus transport slows or stops (bidirectional vector). Raised O_2 consumption occurs. (c) Persistent mucus secretion (denoted as mucus secretory gland/goblet cell units; dark grey) with time increases the height of the luminal mucus masses/plugs. Raised epithelial Qo_2 generates steep hypoxic gradients (dark spotted in bar) in

thickened mucus masses. (d) *P. aeruginosa* bacteria penetrate into hypoxic zones within the mucus masses. (e) *P. aeruginosa* adapts to hypoxic niches within mucus masses with increased alginate formation and the creation of macrocolonies. (f) Macrocolonies resist secondary defences, including neutrophils, setting the stage for chronic infection. The presence of increased macrocolony density and, to a lesser extent, neutrophils render the mucopurulent mass hypoxic (dark spotted bar).

airways occurs early in life [43,44]. Obstruction of the conducting airways occurs, secondary to a gradual build-up of thickened mucus, and secondary bacterial infection. The inflammatory response, secondary to neutrophil infiltration, leads to protease and elastase release with tissue breakdown. Remodelling is associated with fibrosis and ectasia of the airways (bronchiectasis).

Pulmonary function testing is compatible with disease in the conducting airways [45]. There is obstruction to airflow and air trapping. Reduction in the maximal mid-expiratory flow (MMEF) occurs first, then in the forced expiratory volume (*FEV*), and finally in the forced vital capacity (*FVC*), with increased residual volume and forced residual capacity. The alveolar space is relatively preserved, as is the diffusing capacity (DLCO). As disease progresses, pulmonary function worsens, with a variable pattern of loss of lung function, which can be linear or stepwise, slow or rapid. Acute reductions in FEV_1 and FVC often herald pulmonary exacerbations, which require intensified treatment.

Chronic infection with an associated chronic inflammatory response leads to gradual loss of lung function, bronchiectasis and, eventually, end-stage disease with respiratory failure.

Clinical manifestations

Chronic suppurative airway disease is present in more than 98% of adults who have CF, and over 90% of deaths are related to progressive pulmonary insufficiency. Respiratory symptoms start with a recurrent cough and sputum production, which is sometimes associated with wheezing. The cough eventually occurs on a daily basis, becoming productive of mucopurulent secretions. Damage to the conducting airways via the inflammatory response occurs, and hyperinflation and the clinical findings of a barrel-shaped chest are similar to COPD patients. Airway reactivity is a common finding, with one study highlighting wheezing in 50% of young children with CF [46]. The chest X-ray may appear normal initially, or may show subtle changes of hyperinflation. Eventually, hyperinflation with interstitial markings develops. With progression of disease, peribronchial cuffing, 'tram tracks' and rounded shadows of saccular bronchiectasis occur, eventually leading to changes consistent with bronchiectasis, cyst formation and fibrosis. Abnormalities tend to be more prominent in the upper lobes. Chest computed tomography (CT) allows greater detail and assessment of bronchiectasis and recent studies demonstrate that bronchiectasis commonly begins before the age of 5 years [43].

Ultimately, there is progressive decline in lung function with frequent exacerbations, which are heralded by clinical features including increased sputum production, loss of appetite and worsening in pulmonary function. Signific-

antly, fever is relatively uncommon. Progression leads to loss of function of the conducting airways with bronchiectasis, and eventually hypoxia (initially, with or without hypercarbia) and respiratory failure.

Microbiology

Bacteriology

Mortality in CF is predominantly a function of chronic airway infection and tissue damage from the host inflammatory response. *S. aureus* and *P. aeruginosa* are the primary aetiological agents of pulmonary infection in adults with CF. Before effective antistaphylococcal therapy became available, *S. aureus*-related pulmonary infection was the leading cause of death. With effective therapy, morbidity is reduced. However, the emergence of methacillin-resistant *S. aureus* (MRSA) has led to 10–20% of adults being infected with this agent, and necessitating the use of intravenous therapy with exacerbations. The effect of MRSA infection in one case–control study was more frequent antibiotic treatment, although there was not worsening in lung function [47].

Chronic bacterial infection of the airways with *P. aeruginosa* occurs in more than 80% of adults and adolescents with CF [35]. Although the burden of *P. aeruginosa* is high (10^8 per millilitre of airway secretions), sepsis associated with *Pseudomonas* infection is rare in CF. The development of chronic *Pseudomonas* infection has been described in the pathophysiology section and is illustrated in Figure 11.3. The potential risk for emergence of drug-resistant organisms is high in patients with *P. aeruginosa* infection, because eradication of the organism from adults is impossible. The adaptation of bacteria to a heterogeneous and changing environment promotes the selection of hypermutatable strains, as evident in isolates from CF versus non-CF patients. These strains contribute to the emergence of antibiotic-resistant organisms [48].

Other bacteria, such as *H. influenza*, *Moraxella catarrhalis*, *Stenotrophomonas maltophilia*, *Alcaligenes xylosidans* and Enterobacteriaceae are being recovered with increased frequency as life expectancy increases. Multidrug-resistance patterns to these organisms are developing. *B. cepacia* is found in approximately 10% of CF adults. It can be divided into nine different genomovars by molecular analysis, with *B. multivorans* and *B. cenocepacia* comprising 90% of the isolates in CF [49]. Infection is associated with an accelerated decline in lung function and shortened survival in a subset of patients. *B. cenocepacia* is associated with poor outcomes post lung transplant and is considered a contraindication to transplant in some centres [50,51]. *B. cepacia* also causes the 'cepacia syndrome', with rapid deterioration in lung function, bacteraemia and death within 6 months occurring in adolescent and young adult CF patients [52].

Mycobacteriology

In a recent multicentre trial, non-tuberculous mycobacteria (NTM) have been found in sputum of 13% of 1000 CF patients older than 10 years, with 72% being *Mycobacterium avium* complex (MAC) and 18% having *Mycobacterium abscessus* [53]. Diagnosis of NTM is challenging, because infection can mimic worsening of CF seen in chronic *Pseudomonas* infection. Improvement in culture techniques [54,55], repeating cultures and CT scanning [56] has helped this diagnostic challenge. The clinical course of CF is often minimally affected by MAC [53], and treatment has become more feasible. For *M. abscessus*, the clinical course is usually worse, and eradication is difficult to achieve and requires prolonged intravenous therapy.

Treatment of NTM in CF can also be difficult because of altered drug absorption and metabolism [57]. Follow-up of CT findings and acid-fast bacilli (AFB) cultures are recommended for a single NTM isolate from sputum in the absence of a decline in clinical course or if CT findings are not suggestive of infection [53,58].

Aspergillus

Approximately 50% of CF adults will periodically culture *Aspergillus fumigatus*, but only a small subgroup develops allergic bronchopulmonary aspergillosis (ABPA). ABPA should be suspected in any patient with pulmonary infiltration or deterioration not responding to conventional therapy. Testing of immunoglobulin E (IgE) and IgG specific for *Aspergillus* is useful; routine screening for ABPA in CF with total IgE level has been recommended with specific *Aspergillus* serology obtained only if the total IgE level exceeds 500 IU/mL [10,59,60]. Systemic steroid therapy is often sufficient to treat APBA, but side-effects occur; some advocate itraconazole treatment in addition, which may reduce the average daily oral steroid dose and occurrence of acute exacerbations [10,59]. Invasive aspergillosis is very uncommon in CF patients, although it may occur in the immunocompromised post-transplant population [13]. Some advocate antiaspergillus treatment prior to lung transplant in patients with evidence of *Aspergillus* colonization [61,62].

Complications

The major pulmonary complications [14,63] include respiratory failure, pneumothorax and haemoptysis (Table 11.1).

Respiratory failure

This complication leads to death in more than 90% of CF patients. The slowly progressive airways disease and bronchiectasis lead to both hypoxic and hypercapnic respiratory failure. Airway obstruction from mucosal oedema, thickened airway secretions and bronchoconstriction leads

Table 11.1 Clinical disease in cystic fibrosis.

Complication	Life time prevalence (%)
Pulmonary	
Respiratory failure	100
Pneumothorax	1.4
Massive haemoptysis	1.8
Extrapulmonary	
Male infertility	99
Sinusitis	>90
Pancreatic exocrine insufficiency	85
Osteopenia	>70
Cystic fibrosis-related diabetes	30
Nasal polyposis	25
Distal intestinal obstructive syndrome (DIOS)	20
Cholelithiasis	12
Clinical cirrhosis	5
Cystic fibrosis arthropathy	5

to ventilation/perfusion mismatch and hypoxaemic respiratory failure, with secondary pulmonary hypertension. Adequate supplemental oxygen is usually sufficient to prevent fluid retention, and limit adverse effects of pulmonary hypertension. Hypercapnia occurs late in the disease. Alveolar hypoventilation occurs secondary to air trapping, increased dead space and reduced vital capacity, as well as muscle weakness and fatigue. Acute respiratory failure can occur during exacerbations of bronchiectatic infection and some patients with respiratory failure resulting from reversible causes benefit from mechanical ventilation, but aggressive management (including intensive airway clearance) is necessary to wean as rapidly as possible [64]. Individuals with progressive respiratory failure, despite appropriate ongoing treatment, do not usually respond to mechanical ventilation [63]. Non-invasive ventilation devices have been used with some success, avoiding intubation in some patients, although close monitoring by trained staff is required [65,66]. For patients with end-stage disease, daily/nocturnal non-invasive ventilation (BIPAP) is frequently useful to bridge to transplantion [65].

Haemoptysis

Massive haemoptysis, defined as bleeding of more than 240 mL blood in a 24-hour period, occurs in 1.8% of CF adults per year [17] and previously had a high mortality rate before bronchial artery embolization (BAE) was available [67,68]. Haemoptysis can be successfully managed in most CF patients with BAE [68], but a recent review in a specialized CF centre revealed a mortality of 9% during

23 ICU admissions for massive haemoptysis [64]. Recurrent episodes of moderate haemoptysis (three or more bouts of 100 mL/day blood within a week) are also considered a major bleeding event and require admission and consideration for urgent therapy and haemorrhage control [63,68]. The source of this bleeding is usually enlarged tortuous bronchial arteries secondary to chronic inflammation. Initial treatment measures include a brief period of bed rest and cough suppression, along with intravenous antibiotics. BAE has proven to be effective for most episodes of major haemoptysis, and surgical intervention is rarely indicated [68].

Pneumothorax

The incidence of spontaneous pneumothorax in adults is 1.4% per year [17]. A high incidence of subpleural air cysts has been found. Caution is taken with CF patients with pneumothorax and most are admitted for observation. Although the rate of recurrence approaches 50%, most authors recommend a conservative initial approach to treatment: observation, aspiration or chest tube drainage depending on size [69]. Pleurodesis is recommended only for persistent air leak or recurrence [63]. Pleurodesis is not an absolute contraindication to lung transplantation, although surgical pleurodesis is preferred to chemical methods [69].

Diagnosis

Diagnosis is based on a combination of pertinent clinical findings, plus biochemical evidence (CFTR dysfunction; abnormal sweat test) or genetic testing. Abnormal CFTR function can be documented by elevated sweat chloride concentrations or abnormal nasal potential difference (NPD). Where sweat chloride tests are normal or borderline, and two mutations are not identified, abnormal nasal potential difference measurements can be used as evidence of CFTR dysfunction [12,32].

Sweat chloride

This is the gold standard test in experienced hands. Sweat is collected by iontophoresis and the chloride concentration is determined. A value of greater than 60 meq/L is consistent with CF and distinguishes CF from normal controls in adults. A lower cut-off point (< 40 meq/L) is necessary for diagnosis in children. Accuracy is greatly increased when experienced technicians in specialized CF centres perform the test under stringent conditions [70,71]. A false-negative rate occurs in only 1% of subjects in experienced laboratories. Patients are frequently referred to CF centres with a misdiagnosis of CF based upon an elevation in sweat

chloride level that reflects faulty technique. A number of other conditions are associated with a false-positive sweat chloride test, including hypothyroidism and adrenal insufficiency [12].

Nasal potential difference

The nasal transepithelial potential difference can also identify abnormal CFTR function. This test needs to be performed in specialized centres, as standardization of measurements is critical. Nasal potential difference measurements (including responses to amiloride, chloride-free solution and isoproterenol) may demonstrate abnormal *CFTR* function even when sweat Cl⁻ values are normal [72,73].

Genetic/molecular diagnosis

Genetic testing for common mutations is effective at documenting CF mutations on both alleles in the vast majority of CF patients [1,2]. Most laboratories in the USA screen for 20–30 of the most common mutations, which identifies the causative mutations in 90% of CF patients [1,74]. Ethnic differences in mutations should be considered in every patient. In patients with clinical features of CF with but only one *CFTR* mutation defined by screening, intensive genetic testing is likely to identify a second *CFTR* mutation or polymorphism [75].

Treatment of lung disease

The goals of therapy are to slow the progression of pulmonary disease by removing viscous, infected mucus, treating infection and improving nutritional status [17,76]. Other aspects of care include treatment of sinus disease, diagnosis and treatment of diabetes mellitus and addressing psychosocial issues.

A multidisciplinary approach coordinated by a specialized centre is recognized as the most effective method. There are over 100 specialized centres throughout the USA that are standardized and monitored by the CFF. This team approach involves physicians, nurses, dietitians, social workers and physical and respiratory therapists with overlapping responsibilities. It has been demonstrated that patients attending specialized centres have better outcomes [77].

Airway clearance

Although large randomized control trials are unavailable, physiotherapy is considered a cornerstone of therapy in CF [78]. A meta-analysis from 1995 compared modalities available at that time and concluded that no method of physiotherapy was beneficial over other methods, but all were better than no physiotherapy [79].

A variety of traditional techniques are used, including postural drainage, percussion, vibration techniques, breathing exercises and directed cough. Newer techniques include the forced expiration technique and autogenic drainage. Recently, devices have become available to help mucus clearance, including positive expiratory pressure (PEP) masks, flutter devices and external percussive vests. Physical exercise has a central role in the management of patients with CF [80,81].

Inhaled hypertonic saline

One approach that targets the basic pathophysiology (Figs 11.2 and 11.3) is aerosolized hypertonic saline, which hydrates the mucosal surface and improves mucus clearance [82]. A recent long-term placebo controlled trial of 7% hypertonic saline in CF identified that it is an inexpensive, safe, and effective additional therapy with reduction in exacerbations and decline in lung function over 48 week period [83].

Nutrition

Chronic malnutrition with significant weight retardation and linear growth failure has been recognized as a general problem among CF patients [15,84]. Malnutrition results from increased caloric expenditure associated with chronic respiratory disease, decreased caloric intake and malabsorption of ingested nutrients because of pancreatic exocrine insufficiency.

Abnormal liver function and vitamin deficiencies secondary to pancreatic insufficiency are contributing components. To maintain their ideal body weight, patients are encouraged to eat a diet that provides 120–150% of the recommended energy intake of normal age- and sex-matched controls [85]. Nocturnal enteral feeding is considered if weight falls below 85% of the ideal body weight [15]. Gastrostomy feeding is much preferred to long-term parenteral feeding, and has been demonstrated to result in sustained weight gain and a slowing in decline of respiratory function [86]. Prevention of malnutrition from the time of diagnosis is associated with better lung function and improved survival [87]. No single strategy of treatment works for all patients and it is essential that an experienced dietitian gives individually tailored nutritional advice to each patient [88].

Antibiotic therapy

The frequent and targeted use of antibiotics improves survival in CF [1,89]. Antibiotic management in CF targets signs of pulmonary exacerbations, which include increased production of sputum, cough, dyspnoea and sometimes a low-grade fever. Antibiotic guidance is based on sputum cultures and sensitivities and clinical response [76,90]. Mild exacerbations are often treated with an oral agent with or without an inhaled agent for 14–21 days. Intravenous antibiotics are used if the patient fails oral therapy, culture reveals an organism resistant to available oral therapies or the exacerbation is severe. Double antibiotic coverage is used against Gram-negative organisms because of a synergistic effect and to reduce the development of drug resistance, which occurs more frequently with monotherapy. A usual combination against *P. aeruginosa* is an aminoglycoside, plus a cephalosporin or broad-spectrum penicillin derivative. In more advanced disease, courses of up to 3 weeks may be required. An important development in parenteral antibiotic therapy is improved delivery systems and availability of home health services, transferring the administration of intravenous antibiotics from an inpatient to an outpatient setting and reducing inpatient stay and cost.

An important aspect of antibiotic therapy in CF patients is pharmacokinetics, because there is increased plasma clearance of almost all hydrophilic antibiotics (aminoglycosides, penicillins and cephalosporins) in CF patients [91,92]. This rapid elimination dictates the use of larger (and sometimes more frequent) doses of antimicrobials. Renal clearance of aminoglycosides is accelerated for unclear reasons, and CF patients require at least 6 mg/kg/day in divided doses. Patients are at risk of renal and ototoxicity from aminoglycosides, and monitoring of serum aminoglycoside levels is required.

Infection with *B. cepacia* is difficult to treat because of intrinsic resistance to aminoglycosides and polymixins. Initial isolates can be sensitive to antipseudomonal β-lactams and co-trimoxazole, but resistance develops rapidly, with eventual resistance to all available antimicrobials.

Aerosolized antibiotics are being now used both as treatment and prophylaxis. Tobramycin prophylaxis has been shown to reduce hospital admissions by 25% after 10 weeks of therapy [93]. Colistin is another available nebulized antibiotic; resistance is uncommon, and it is rarely used as an intravenous agent because of side-effects [94–96].

Macrolide therapy

Chronic macrolide therapy appears to improve lung function [97–99] and reduce exacerbations in both adults and children with chronic *P. aeruginosa*. The standard dose for adults is 500 mg azithromycin three times per week. It is unclear whether the improvement is related to an anti-inflammatory or antimicrobial effect, or both. Cultures for AFB need to be checked prior to commencement of macrolide

Table 11.2 Predictors of worse outcome in cystic fibrosis after lung transplantation [101].

Adverse prognostic factors	
Female gender	Older age
Diabetes mellitus	Pancreatic insufficiency
Low weight-for-age score	*Burkholderia cepacia* infection
Frequency of pulmonary exacerbations	Low FEV_1

FEV_1, forced expiratory volume in 1 s.

therapy, to prevent development of infection with non-tuberculous mycobacteria that is macrolide resistant.

Aerosolized DNAase

The endonuclease DNAase I cleaves denatured DNA in mucus and improves the clearance of airway secretions. Chronic use of DNAase improves FEV_1 and reduces the frequency of exacerbations [100]. DNAase is not useful in patients with severe lung disease [101].

Bronchodilator therapy

A subgroup of CF patients has bronchoconstriction secondary to airway hyperreactivity, and these patients often respond to inhaled bronchodilator therapy [1,2]. Large trials testing the long-term effects of inhaled bronchodilator on the progression of disease are not available for either short- or long-acting β-agonists. Clinical practice is to continue usage required for symptomatic relief.

Anti-inflammatory therapy

Controlling the magnitude of the inflammatory response in the airways is likely to be useful in CF. Early studies showed that prednisone slowed the loss of lung function in CF children, but side-effects (including diabetes, growth failure and cataract development) were unacceptable [102,103]. Studies of inhaled corticosteroid have been underpowered, therefore it is not clear whether they benefit CF lung disease or not. Like bronchodilators, they are used for symptomatic benefit. Ibuprofen (high dose) is beneficial in slowing the decline of lung function of children less than 13 years of age, but there is no evidence of benefit in adults [104].

Vaccinations

Annual influenza vaccinations are recommended, but pneumococcal vaccine is not routinely indicated because of the relative absence of *Streptococcus pneumoniae* as an infectious organism in CF adults.

Lung transplantation

Approximately one-third of all double lung transplants in adults are performed for CF [13]. Overall, the 5-year survival post-transplant is approximately 50% but there are several predictors of mortality in lung transplantation (Table 11.2). An $FEV_1 < 30\%$ is used as a threshold for referral for transplantation [13,105].

Extrapulmonary manifestations

Impaired *CFTR* function leads to abnormal secretory function and associated clinical disease in other organ systems. Table 11.1 highlights common clinical features of CF.

Pancreatic disease

The pancreas in CF patients is destroyed by autodigestion *in utero*, reflecting a defect in Cl⁻ (liquid) secretion to flush digestive enzymes from the pancreatic ducts into the intestinal lumen. The lack of pancreatic enzyme secretion into the gastrointestinal tract leads to malabsorption of protein and fat with steatorrhoea. This leads to failure to thrive in children, deficiencies in fat-soluble vitamins (A, D, E and K) and malabsorption and malnutrition. Management of pancreatic exocrine deficiency involves enteral replacement of enzymes (lipase, protease and amylase). The dosage depends on patients' weight and dietary fat intake [15,84].

Damage to the endocrine function of the pancreas also occurs and CF-related diabetes occurs in up to 35% of adults at age 25 [16,106]. CF-related diabetes is usually treated with insulin replacement. Glucose intolerance often worsens with exacerbations in pulmonary disease and with steroid therapy. Long-term survival is worse for patients with CF-related diabetes mellitus [16].

Interestingly, 'non-classic' CF patients with mild mutations usually have residual pancreatic exocrine function and can suffer from pancreatitis, whereas 'classic' (e.g. homozygous ΔF508) patients have complete loss of pancreatic function and never have pancreatitis [20,22].

Gastrointestinal disease

Meconium ileus (MI) is the neonatal presentation of CF in approximately 15–20% of patients. An equivalent called 'distal intestinal obstructive syndrome' (DIOS) occurs in approximately 20% of adults [107]. DIOS involves impaction of inspissated intestinal contents in the terminal ileum, caecum and proximal colon. It can present as colicky abdominal pain, intestinal obstruction, abdominal distension or bilious vomiting, with various clinical signs that can mimic appendicitis, colonic strictures and volvulus. If appropriate medical management is initiated (including nasogastric tube, treating electrolyte imbalance, fluid replacement and enemas), surgical intervention is rarely required [108].

Hepatobiliary disease includes cholelithiasis and cirrhosis, which reflects obstruction of biliary flow secondary to abnormal *CFTR*. Management includes optimization of nutrition status, replacement of fat-soluble vitamins and cholecystectomy if necessary. Liver transplantation may be needed in end-stage disease, which occurs in 2–5% of patients [11].

Gastroesophageal reflux disease occurs more frequently in CF patients [109], which can be also a cause of chronic cough.

Sinus disease

Panopacification of the paranasal sinuses occur in > 90% of patients at 8 months of age, with nasal polyposis in 10–30% of patients [110]. Despite this, the frequency of symptoms is lower than expected in adults (24%) [111]. Surgery is reserved for severe disease and symptomatic nasal polyposis.

Reproductive system

Reduced fertility occurs in females (approximately 20% are infertile), which is often a consequence of secondary amenorrhoea from chronic systemic illness, although cervical mucus abnormalities are also involved [112]. An FEV_1 of greater than 50% predicts better maternal and fetal outcome in pregnancy [113]. Males are usually infertile as a result of complete absence of the vas deferens, although men with a splice mutation have been reported to father children [73,114].

Osteoporosis

There is a high risk of osteopenia-associated bone fractures in CF adults, which reflects multifactorial causes related to delayed puberty, malabsorption, reduced vitamin D, glucocorticoid treatment and chronic lung infection [115,116].

Musculoskeletal system

Clubbing of both fingers and toes is common in patients with CF. Some develop hypertrophic osteoarthropathy. CF-associated arthropathy occurs in 2–9% of patients [117].

Cystic fibrosis in comparison with COPD

End-stage lung disease occurs in CF and COPD, but the time course and most clinical features are different (Table 11.3).

CF is a genetic disease of the conducting airways with morbidity usually commencing early in life. Smoke-induced COPD progresses over decades, and the alveolar destruction of emphysema contrasts with the airways disease and bronchiectasis of CF. Chronic bronchitis (CB) leads to an obstructive lung disease with some similarities to CF. Specifically, both CF and CB have 'abnormal mucus' in the airways with recurrent cough, sputum production and exacerbations of bacterial infection of the airways. For CF, the abnormal mucus reflects defective ion transport rather than primary (genetic) abnormalities in mucus [8,33,34], but the aetiology of abnormal mucus in CB is not well understood. It may reflect complex genetic and/or environmental interactions that lead to changes in the species or glycoforms of mucins produced in response to the irritant stimuli. Recent studies in an animal (mouse) model of accelerated Na^+ transport [118] resemble aspects of CB, raising the possibility that the inflammatory stimulus of cytokines associated with CB may secondarily modify ion transport in an adverse fashion and contribute to the pathophysiology of CB.

Despite the differences in clinical phenotype between CF and COPD, there are likely some common genetic and pathophysiological links between the airways disease in these two disorders. As summarized in Chapter 37 by Hersh and Silverman, there are many candidate genes that have been associated with several pathways in COPD, including proteases–antiproteases, oxidant–antioxidants, inflammatory cytokines, and the β_2-adrenergic receptor. Many of these genes have been implicated as genetic modifiers of the lung disease in CF [119–121], but the only proven genetic risk factor for COPD (severe α_1-antitrypsin deficiency) [122,123] has been shown to have no association with worse lung disease in CF [124–127]. Nonetheless, we predict that ongoing studies in large populations of COPD and CF patients are likely to identify some common genetic variants (e.g. gluthathione S-transferases, matrix metalloproteinases and inflammatory cytokines), which have an adverse role in the airways disease of both disorders. In fact, recent studies have suggested that genetic variants in *TGFβ1* may influence phenotypic severity in both CF and COPD [25,26,128].

Prospects for the future

CF life expectancy has improved considerably over recent decades, with a current medial survival age of 32 years. Lung transplantation programmes are achieving 5-year survival of 50%. The effect of early-targeted therapy to prevent and treat infection and inflammation is being assessed and will likely bear fruit over the next decade. Developments in antimicrobial and anti-inflammatory therapy are occurring at a rapid pace. Therapies targeting

Table 11.3 Comparison of cystic fibrosis and chronic obstructive pulmonary disease. **Similarities are in bold type**.

	Cystic fibrosis	COPD
Age of onset	Childhood	Adulthood
Genetics	Autosomal recessive	Complex environmental and genetic interaction
Pathophysiology	**Obstructive airway disease** secondary to *CFTR* malfunction, with viscous sputum and chronic infection leading bronchiectasis No alveolar disease	**Obstructive airways disease** secondary to increased mucus production, tissue damage and inflammation secondary to cigarette smoke Alveolar disease (emphysema)
Pulmonary symptoms	**Cough** **Sputum production** (large volume, purulent; bronchiectasis)	**Cough** **Sputum production** (smaller volume, usually mucopurulent)
Pulmonary signs	**Dyspnoea** **Hyperinflation** **Wheeze** Inspiratory crackles	**Dyspnoea** **Hyperinflation** **Wheeze**
Pulmonary function tests	**Obstructive defect** **High residual volume** Normal diffusion capacity	**Obstructive defect** **High residual volume** Reduced diffusion capacity
Microbiology	*Staphylococcus aureus* *Pseudomonas aeruginosa* *Burkholderia cepacia* NTM ABPA	*Streptococcus pneumonia* *Haemophilus influenza* *Moraxella catarrhalis*
Diagnosis	Sweat test Genetic testing Nasal potential difference	Clinical features Radiography Pulmonary function tests
Radiology	Cystic bronchiectasis Upper lobe predominance	Bronchial thickening Increased lung markings, Translucency in advanced emphysema
Treatment of pulmonary disease	Airway clearance **Antibiotics** (inhaled and intravenous) **Bronchodilator therapy** DNAase Macrolides	**Antibiotics** (oral) **Bronchodilator therapy** Anti-inflammatory therapy Volume reduction surgery

ABPA, allergic bronchopulmonary aspergillosis; NTM, non-tuberculous mycobacteria.

altered ion transport and abnormal mucus clearance are being investigated.

Successful transfer of the *CFTR* gene to *CFTR*-deficient cultured cells with production of effective chloride channels has been performed [129], but progress in gene transfer *in vivo* has been less successful [130]. Improvement in duration of expression, vector delivery and production and reduction in inflammatory responses are needed to progress this ultimate cure of CF.

References

1 Welsh MJ, Ramsey BW, Accurso FJ, Cutting GR. Cystic fibrosis. In: Scriver CR, Beaudet AL, Sly WS, Valle D, eds. *The Metabolic and Molecular Bases of Inherited Disease*. New York: McGraw-Hill, 2001: 5121–88.
2 Boucher RC, Knowles MR, Yankaskas JR. Cystic fibrosis. In: Murray JF, Nadel JA, eds. *Textbook of Respiratory Medicine*. New York: WB Saunders, 2000: 1291–323.

3 Kerem B, Rommens JM, Buchanan JA *et al*. Identification of the cystic fibrosis gene: genetic analysis. *Science* 1989;**245**: 1073–80.

4 Stutts MJ, Canessa CM, Olsen JC *et al*. *CFTR* as a cAMP-dependent regulator of sodium channels. *Science* 1995;**269**: 847–50.

5 Boucher RC. Human airway ion transport. Part 1. *Am J Respir Crit Care Med* 1994;**150**:271–81.

6 Boucher RC. Human airway ion transport. Part 2. *Am J Respir Crit Care Med* 1994;**150**:581–93.

7 Bear CE, Li C, Kartner N *et al*. Purification and functional reconstitution of the cystic fibrosis transmembrane conductance regulator (CFTR). *Cell* 1992;**68**:809–18.

8 Knowles MR, Boucher RC. Mucus clearance as a primary innate defense mechanism for mammalian airways ('Perspective'). *J Clin Invest* 2002;**109**:571–7.

9 Yankaskas JR, Knowles MR, eds. *Cystic Fibrosis in Adults*. Philadelphia: Lippincott-Raven, 1999.

10 Stevens DA, Moss RB, Kurup VP *et al*. Allergic bronchopulmonary aspergillosis in cystic fibrosis: state of the art. Cystic Fibrosis Foundation Consensus Conference. *Clin Infect Dis* 2003;**37**(Suppl 3):S225–64.

11 Sokol RJ, Durie PR. Recommendations for management of liver and biliary tract disease in cystic fibrosis. Cystic Fibrosis Foundation Hepatobiliary Disease Consensus Group. *J Pediatr Gastroenterol Nutr* 1999;**28**:S1–13.

12 Rosenstein BJ, Cutting GR. The diagnosis of cystic fibrosis: a consensus statement. Cystic Fibrosis Foundation Consensus Panel. *J Pediatr* 1998;**132**:589–95.

13 Yankaskas JR, Mallory GB Jr. Lung transplantation in cystic fibrosis. Consensus Conference Statement. *Chest* 1998;**113**: 217–26.

14 Schidlow DV, Taussig LM, Knowles MR. Cystic Fibrosis Foundation Consensus Conference Report on pulmonary complications of cystic fibrosis. *Pediatr Pulmonol* 1993;**15**: 187–98.

15 Ramsey BW, Farrell PM, Pencharz P. Nutritional assessment and management in cystic fibrosis: a consensus report. The Consensus Committee. *Am J Clin Nutr* 1992;**55**: 108–16.

16 Moran A, Hardin D, Rodman D *et al*. Diagnosis, screening and management of cystic fibrosis related diabetes mellitus: a Consensus Conference Report. *Diabetes Res Clin Pract* 1999; **45**:61–73.

17 Yankaskas JR, Marshall BC, Sufian B, Simon RH, Rodman D. Cystic fibrosis adult care: Consensus Conference Report. *Chest* 2004;**125**(1 Suppl):S1–39.

18 Pier GB, Grout M, Zaidi T *et al*. *Salmonella typhi* uses CFTR to enter intestinal epithelial cells. *Nature* 1998;**393**:79–82.

19 Quinton PM. What is good about cystic fibrosis? *Curr Biol* 1994;**4**:742–3.

20 Knowles MR, Durie PR. What is cystic fibrosis? *N Engl J Med* 2002;**347**:439–42.

21 Mak V, Zielenski J, Tsui LC *et al*. Cystic fibrosis gene mutations and infertile men with primary testicular failure. *Hum Reprod* 2000;**15**:436–9.

22 Noone PG, Zhou Z, Silverman LM *et al*. Cystic fibrosis gene mutations and pancreatitis risk: relation to epithelial ion transport and trypsin inhibitor gene mutations. *Gastroenterology* 2001;**121**:1310–9.

23 Noone PG, Knowles MR. 'CFTR-opathies': disease phenotypes associated with cystic fibrosis transmembrane regulator gene mutations. *Respir Res* 2001;**2**:328–32.

24 NIH Consensus Statement. *Genetic Testing for Cystic Fibrosis*. 1997;**15**:200.

25 Drumm ML, Konstan MW, Schluchter MD *et al*. Gene Modifier Study Group. Genetic modifiers of lung disease in cystic fibrosis. *N Engl J Med* 2005;**353**(14):1443–53.

26 Haston CK, Hudson TJ. Finding genetic modifiers of cystic fibrosis. *N Engl J Med* 2005;**353**(14):1509–11.

27 Knowles MR, Noone PG, Bennett WD, Boucher RC. Mucociliary and cough clearance: role of ion transport and the P_2Y_2 receptor-mediated system. In: Baum GL, Priel Z, Roth Y, Liron N, Ostfeld E, eds. *Cilia, Mucus, and Mucociliary Interactions*. New York: Marcel Dekker, 1998: 307–15.

28 Stutts MJ, Boucher RC. Cystic fibrosis gene and functions of *CFTR*: implications of dysfunctional ion transport for pulmonary pathogenesis. In: Yankaskas JR, Knowles MR, eds. *Cystic Fibrosis in Adults*. Philadelphia: Lippincott-Raven, 1999: 3–25.

29 Matsui H, Randell SH, Peretti SW, Davis CW, Boucher RC. Coordinated clearance of periciliary liquid and mucus from airway surfaces. *J Clin Invest* 1998;**102**:1125–31.

30 Matsui H, Davis CW, Tarran R, Boucher RC. Osmotic water permeabilities of cultured, well-differentiated normal and cystic fibrosis airway epithelia. *J Clin Invest* 2000;**105**: 1419–27.

31 Tarran R, Grubb BR, Parsons D *et al*. The CF salt controversy: *in vivo* observations and therapeutic approaches. *Mol Cell* 2001;**8**:149–58.

32 Knowles MR, Paradiso AM, Boucher RC. *In vivo* nasal potential difference: techniques and protocols for assessing efficacy of gene transfer in cystic fibrosis. *Hum Gene Ther* 1995;**6**:447–57.

33 Leigh MW. Airway secretions. In: Yankaskas JR, Knowles MR, eds. *Cystic Fibrosis in Adults*. Philadelphia: Lippincott-Raven, 1999: 69–92.

34 Voynow JA, Selby DM, Rose MC. Mucin gene expression (MUC1, MUC2, and MUC5/5AC) in nasal epithelial cells of cystic fibrosis, allergic rhinitis, and normal individuals. *Lung* 1998;**176**:345–54.

35 Scanlin TF. Terminal glycosylation in cystic fibrosis. *Biochim Biophys Acta* 1999;**1455**:241–53.

36 Worlitzsch D, Tarran R, Ulrich M *et al*. Effects of reduced mucus oxygen concentration in airway *Pseudomonas* infections of cystic fibrosis patients. *J Clin Invest* 2002;**109**:317–25.

37 Yoon SS, Hennigan RF, Hilliard GM *et al*. *Pseudomonas aeruginosa* anaerobic respiration in biofilms: relationships to cystic fibrosis pathogenesis. *Dev Cell* 2002;**3**:593–603.

38 Matsui H, Verghese MW, Boucher RC. Low motility in thick mucus prevents neutrophils from catching bacteria. *Pediatr Pulmonol Suppl* 2002;**24**:265.

39 Hancock RE, Mutharia LM, Chan L *et al*. *Pseudomonas aeruginosa* isolates from patients with cystic fibrosis: a class of serum-sensitive, non-typable strains deficient in lipopolysaccharide O side chains. *Infect Immun* 1983;**42**:170–7.

40 Mahenthiralingam E, Campbell ME, Speert DP. Non-motility and phagocytic resistance of *Pseudomonas aeruginosa* isolates from chronically colonized patients with cystic fibrosis. *Infect Immun* 1994;**62**:596–605.

41 Raivio TL, Ujack EE, Rabin HR, Storey DG. Association between transcript levels of the *Pseudomonas aeruginosa* Rega, Regb, and Toxa genes in sputa of cystic-fibrosis patients. *Infect Immun* 1994;**62**:3506–14.

42 Chmiel JF, Berger M, Konstan MW. The role of inflammation in the pathophysiology of CF lung disease. *Clin Rev Allergy Immunol* 2002;**23**:5–27.

43 Helbich TH, Heinz-Peer G, Eichler I *et al.* Cystic fibrosis: CT assessment of lung involvement in children and adults. *Radiology* 1999;**213**:537–44.

44 Zuelzer WW, Newton WA Jr. The pathogenesis of fibrocystic disease of the pancreas: a study of 36 cases with special reference to the pulmonary lesions. *Pediatrics* 1949;**4**:53–69.

45 Davis PB, Drumm M, Konstan MW. Cystic fibrosis: state of the art. *Am J Respir Crit Care Med* 1996;**154**:1229–56.

46 Hiatt P, Eigen H, Yu P, Tepper RS. Bronchodilator responsiveness in infants and young children with cystic fibrosis. *Am Rev Respir Dis* 1988;**137**:119–22.

47 Miall LS, McGinley NT, Brownlee KG, Conway SP. Methicillin-resistant *Staphylococcus aureus* (MRSA) infection in cystic fibrosis. *Arch Dis Child* 2001;**84**:160–2.

48 Oliver A, Canton R, Campo P, Baquero F, Blazquez J. High frequency of hypermutable *Pseudomonas aeruginosa* in cystic fibrosis lung infection. *Science* 2000;**288**:1251–4.

49 LiPuma JJ, Spilker T, Gill LH *et al.* Disproportionate distribution of *Burkholderia cepacia* complex species and transmissibility markers in cystic fibrosis. *Am J Respir Crit Care Med* 2001;**164**:92–6.

50 Aris RM, Routh JC, LiPuma JJ, Heath DG, Gilligan PH. Lung transplantation for cystic fibrosis patients with *Burkholderia cepacia* complex: survival linked to genomovar type. *Am J Respir Crit Care Med* 2001;**164**:2102–6.

51 Chaparro C, Maurer J, Gutierrez C *et al.* Infection with *Burkholderia cepacia* in cystic fibrosis: outcome following lung transplantation. *Am J Respir Crit Care Med* 2001;**163**:43–8.

52 Lewin LO, Byard PJ, Davis PB. Effect of *Pseudomonas cepacia* colonization on survival and pulmonary function of cystic fibrosis patients. *J Clin Epidemiol* 1990;**43**:125–31.

53 Olivier KN, Weber DJ, Wallace RJ Jr *et al.* Non-tuberculous mycobacteria in cystic fibrosis. I. Multicenter prevalence study of a potential pathogen in a susceptible population. *Am J Respir Crit Care Med* 2003;**167**:835–40.

54 Kennedy MP, O'Connor TM, Ryan C *et al.* Non-tuberculous mycobacteria: incidence in Southwest Ireland from 1987 to 2000. *Respir Med* 2003;**97**:257–63.

55 Woods GL. The mycobacteriology laboratory and new diagnostic techniques. *Infect Dis Clin North Am* 2002;**16**:127–44.

56 Ellis SM, Hansell DM. Imaging of non-tuberculous (atypical) mycobacterial pulmonary infection. *Clin Radiol* 2002;**57**:661–9.

57 Olivier KN, Yankaskas JR, Knowles MR. Non-tuberculous mycobacterial pulmonary disease in cystic fibrosis. *Semin Respir Infect* 1996;**11**:272–84.

58 Olivier KN, Weber DJ, Lee JH *et al.* Non-tuberculous mycobacteria. II. Nested cohort study of impact on cystic fibrosis lung disease. *Am J Respir Crit Care Med* 2003;**167**:835–40.

59 Nepomuceno IB, Esrig S, Moss RB. Allergic bronchopulmonary aspergillosis in cystic fibrosis: role of atopy and response to itraconazole. *Chest* 1999;**115**:364–70.

60 Steinbach WJ, Stevens DA, Denning DW, Moss RB. Advances against aspergillosis. *Clin Infect Dis* 2000;**37**:(Suppl 3):S155–6.

61 Kramer MR, Marshall SE, Starnes VA *et al.* Infectious complications in heart–lung transplantation: analysis of 200 episodes. *Arch Intern Med* 1993;**153**:2010–6.

62 Paradis IL, Williams P. Infection after lung transplantation. *Semin Respir Infect* 1993;**8**:207–15.

63 Yankaskas JR, Egan TM, Mauro MA. Major complications. In: Yankaskas JR, Knowles MR, eds. *Cystic Fibrosis in Adults*. Philadelphia: Lippincott-Raven, 1999: 175–93.

64 Sood N, Paradowski LJ, Yankaskas JR. Outcomes of intensive care unit care in adults with cystic fibrosis. *Am J Respir Crit Care Med* 2001;**163**:335–8.

65 Piper AJ, Parker S, Torzillo PJ, Sullivan CE, Bye PTP. Nocturnal nasal IPPV stabilizes patients with cystic fibrosis and hypercapnic respiratory failure. *Chest* 1992;**102**:846–50.

66 Hodson ME, Madden BP, Steven MH, Tsang VT, Yacoub MH. Non-invasive mechanical ventilation for cystic fibrosis patients: a potential bridge to transplantation. *Eur Respir J* 1991;**4**:524–7.

67 Wholey MH, Chamorro HA, Rao G, Ford WB, Miller WH. Bronchial artery embolization for massive hemoptysis. *JAMA* 1976;**236**:2501–4.

68 Brinson GM, Noone PG, Mauro MA *et al.* Bronchial artery embolization for the treatment of hemoptysis in patients with cystic fibrosis. *Am J Respir Crit Care Med* 1998;**157**:1951–8.

69 Flume PA. Pneumothorax in cystic fibrosis. *Chest* 2003;**123**:217–21.

70 LeGrys VA. Sweat testing for the diagnosis of cystic fibrosis: practical considerations. *J Pediatr* 1996;**129**:892–7.

71 Legrys VA. Assessment of sweat-testing practices for the diagnosis of cystic fibrosis. *Arch Pathol Lab Med* 2001;**125**:1420–4.

72 Knowles MR, Buntin WH, Bromberg PA, Gatzy JT, Boucher RC. *In vivo* measurements of tracheal and bronchial transepithelial electric potential difference (PD) in human subjects. *Am Rev Respir Dis* 1982;**125**:242.

73 Highsmith WE, Burch LH, Zhou Z *et al.* A novel mutation in the cystic fibrosis gene in patients with pulmonary disease but normal sweat chloride concentrations. *N Engl J Med* 1994;**331**:974–80.

74 Grody WW, Cutting GR, Klinger KW *et al.* Laboratory standards and guidelines for population-based cystic fibrosis carrier screening. *Genet Med* 2001;**3**:149–54.

75 Groman JD, Meyer ME, Wilmott RW, Zeitlin PL, Cutting GR. Variant cystic fibrosis phenotypes in the absence of *CFTR* mutations. *N Engl J Med* 2002;**347**:401–7.

76 Ramsey BW. Management of pulmonary disease in patients with cystic fibrosis. *N Engl J Med* 1996;**335**:179–88.

77 Mahadeva R, Webb K, Westerbeek RC *et al.* Clinical outcome

in relation to care in centres specialising in cystic fibrosis: cross-sectional study. *BMJ* 1998;**316**:1771–5.

78 Reisman JJ, Rivington-Law B, Corey M *et al*. Role of conventional physiotherapy in cystic fibrosis. *J Pediatr* 1988;**113**: 632–6.

79 Thomas J, Cook DJ, Brooks D. Chest physical therapy management of patients with cystic fibrosis: a meta-analysis. *Am J Respir Crit Care Med* 1995;**151**(3 Pt 1):846–50.

80 Williams MT. Chest physiotherapy and cystic fibrosis: why is the most effective form of treatment still unclear? *Chest* 1994;**106**:1872–82.

81 Alison JA, Donnelly PM, Lennon M *et al*. The effect of a comprehensive, intensive inpatient treatment program on lung-function and exercise capacity in patients with cystic-fibrosis. *Phys Ther* 1994;**74**:583–93.

82 Donaldson SH, Bennett WD, Zeman KL *et al*. Mucus clearance and lung function in cystic fibrosis with hypertonic saline. *N Engl J Med*;**354**(3):241–50.

83 Elkins MR, Robinson M, Rose BR *et al*. National Hypertonic Saline in Cystic Fibrosis (NHSCF) Study Group. A controlled trial of long-term inhaled hypertonic saline in patients with cystic fibrosis. *N Engl J Med* 2006;**354**(3):229–40.

84 Kalnins D, Stewart C, Tullis E, Pencharz PB. Nutrition. In: Yankaskas JR, Knowles MR, eds. *Cystic Fibrosis in Adults*. Philadelphia: Lippincott-Raven, 1999: 289–307.

85 Littlewood JM, Macdonald A. Rationale of modern dietary recommendations in cystic-fibrosis. *J R Soc Med* 1987;**80**: 16–24.

86 Williams SG, Ashworth F, McAlweenie A *et al*. Percutaneous endoscopic gastrostomy feeding in patients with cystic fibrosis. *Gut* 1999;**44**:87–90.

87 Merelle ME, Schouten JP, Dankert-Roelse JE. Long-term prognosis of patients with cystic fibrosis in relation to early detection by neonatal screening. *Am J Respir Crit Care Med* 1999;**159**:A897.

88 Erdman SH. Nutritional imperatives in cystic fibrosis therapy. *Pediatr Ann* 1999;**28**:129–36.

89 Michel BC. Antibacterial therapy in cystic fibrosis: a review of the literature published between 1980 and 1987. *Chest* 1988;**94**: S129–40.

90 Noone PG, Knowles MR. Standard therapy of cystic fibrosis lung disease. In: Yankaskas JR, Knowles MR, eds. *Cystic Fibrosis in Adults*. Philadelphia: Lippincott-Raven, 1999: 145–73.

91 Kavanaugh RE, Unadkat JD, Smith AL. Drug disposition in cystic fibrosis. In: Davis PB, ed. *Cystic Fibrosis*. New York: Marcel Dekker, 1993: 91–136.

92 Smith A, Cohen M, Ramsey B. Pharmacotherapy. In: Yankaskas JR, Knowles MR, eds. *Cystic Fibrosis in Adults*. Philadelphia: Lippincott-Raven, 1999: 345–64.

93 Ramsey BW, Pepe MS, Quan JM *et al*. Intermittent administration of inhaled tobramycin in patients with cystic fibrosis. The Cystic Fibrosis Inhaled Tobramycin Study Group. *N Engl J Med* 1999;**340**:23–30.

94 Ryan G. Update: nebulized anti-pseudomonal antibiotics for cystic fibrosis. In: Mukhopadhay S, Singh M, eds. *Cochrane Data Base Syst Rev* 3, cd001021, 2003.

95 Jensen T, Pedersen SS, Garne S *et al*. Colistin inhalation therapy in cystic fibrosis patients with chronic *Pseudomonas*

96 Littlewood JM, Koch C, Lambert PA *et al*. A 10 year review of colomycin. *Respir Med* 2000;**94**:632–40.

97 Equi A, Balfour-Lynn IM, Bush A, Rosenthal M. Long-term azithromycin in children with cystic fibrosis: a randomised, placebo-controlled crossover trial. *Lancet* 2002;**360**:978–84.

98 Wolter J, Seeney S, Bell S *et al*. Effect of long-term treatment with azithromycin on disease parameters in cystic fibrosis: a randomised trial. *Thorax* 2002;**57**:212–6.

99 Saiman L, Marshall BC, Mayer-Hamblett N *et al*. Azithromycin in patients with cystic fibrosis chronically infected with *Pseudomonas aeruginosa*: a randomized controlled trial. *JAMA* 2003;**290**:1749–56.

100 Fuchs HJ, Borowitz DS, Christiansen DH *et al*. Effect of aerosolized recombinant human DNase on exacerbations of respiratory symptoms and on pulmonary function in patients with cystic fibrosis. The Pulmozyme Study Group. *N Engl J Med* 1994;**331**:637–42.

101 Hodson ME. Clinical studies of rhDNase in moderately and severely affected patients with cystic-fibrosis: an overview. *Respiration* 1995;**62**:29–32.

102 Auerbach HS, Williams M, Kirkpatrick JA, Colten HR. Alternate-day prednisone reduces morbidity and improves pulmonary function in cystic fibrosis. *Lancet* 1985;**ii**: 686–8.

103 Eigen H, Rosenstein BJ, FitzSimmons S, Schidlow DV. A multicenter study of alternate-day prednisone therapy in patients with cystic fibrosis. Cystic Fibrosis Foundation Prednisone Trial Group. *J Pediatr* 1995;**126**:515–23.

104 Konstan MW, Byard PJ, Hoppel CL, Davis PB. Effect of high-dose ibuprofen in patients with cystic fibrosis. *N Engl J Med* 1995;**332**:848–54.

105 Liou TG, Adler FR, FitzSimmons SC *et al*. Predictive 5-year survivorship model of cystic fibrosis. *Am J Epidemiol* 2001;**153**:345–52.

106 Lanng S. Glucose intolerance in cystic fibrosis patients. *Paediatr Respir Rev* 2001;**2**:253–9.

107 di Sant'Agnese PA, Davis PB. Cystic fibrosis in adults: 75 cases and a review of 232 cases in the literature. *Am J Med* 1979;**66**:121–32.

108 Cleghorn GJ, Stringer DA, Forstner GG, Durie PR. Treatment of distal intestinal obstruction syndrome in cystic fibrosis with a balanced intestinal lavage solution. *Lancet* 1986;**1**:8–11.

109 Eggermont E. Gastrointestinal manifestations in cystic fibrosis. *Eur J Gastroenterol Hepatol* 1996;**8**:731–8.

110 Ramsey B, Richardson MA. Impact of sinusitis in cystic-fibrosis. *J Allergy Clin Immunol* 1992;**90**:547–52.

111 Stern RC, Jones K. Nasal and sinus disease. In: Yankaskas JR, Knowles MR, eds. *Cystic Fibrosis in Adults*. Philadelphia: Lippincott-Raven, 1999: 221–31.

112 Gervais R, Dumur V, Letombe B *et al*. Hypofertility with thick cervical mucus: another mild form of cystic fibrosis? *JAMA* 1996;**276**:1638.

113 Goss CH, Rubenfeld GD, Otto K, Aitken ML. The effect of pregnancy on survival in women with cystic fibrosis. *Chest* 2003;**124**:1460–8.

aeruginosa lung infection. *J Antimicrob Chemother* 1987;**19**: 831–8.

114 Dreyfus DH, Bethel R, Gelfand EW. Cystic fibrosis 3849+ 10 kb C > T mutation associated with severe pulmonary disease and male fertility. *Am J Respir Crit Care Med* 1996;**153**: 858–60.

115 Aris RM, Stephens AR, Ontjes DA *et al.* Adverse alterations in bone metabolism are associated with lung infection in adults with cystic fibrosis. *Am J Respir Crit Care Med* 2000; **162**:1674–8.

116 Aris RM, Lester GE, Dingman S, Ontjes DA. Altered calcium homeostasis in adults with cystic fibrosis. *Osteoporos Int* 1999;**10**:102–8.

117 Merkel PA. Rheumatic disease and cystic fibrosis. *Arthritis Rheum* 1999;**42**:1563–71.

118 Mall M. Overexpression of ENaC in mouse airways: a novel animal model for chronic bronchitis and cystic fibrosis lung disease. *Pediatr Pulmonol Suppl* 2003;**25**:121.

119 Arkwright PD, Pravica V, Geraghty PJ *et al.* End-organ dysfunction in cystic fibrosis: association with angiotensin I converting enzyme and cytokine gene polymorphisms. *Am J Respir Crit Care Med* 2003;**167**:384–9.

120 Hull J, Thomson AH. Contribution of genetic factors other than *CFTR* to disease severity in cystic fibrosis. *Thorax* 1998;**53**:1018–21.

121 Buscher R, Eilmes KJ, Graseman H *et al.* Beta-2 adrenoceptor gene polymorphisms in cystic fibrosis lung disease. *Pharmacogenetics* 2002;**12**:347–53.

122 Silverman EK, Pierce JA, Province MA, Rao DC, Campbell EJ. Variability of pulmonary-function in α_1-antitrypsin deficiency: clinical correlates. *Ann Intern Med* 1989;**111**: 982–91.

123 Laurell CB, Eriksson S. The electrophoretic α_1-globulin pattern of serum in α_1-antitrypsin deficiency. *Scand J Clin Lab Invest* 1963;**15**:132–40.

124 Doring G, Krogh-Johansen H, Weidinger S, Hoiby N. Allotypes of α_1-antitrypsin in patients with cystic fibrosis, homozygous and heterozygous for ΔF508. *Pediatr Pulmonol* 1994;**18**:3–7.

125 Frangolias DD, Ruan J, Wilcox PJ *et al.* α_1-Antitrypsin deficiency alleles in cystic fibrosis lung disease. *Am J Respir Cell Mol Biol* 2003;**29**:390–6.

126 Mahadeva R, Stewart S, Bilton D, Lomas DA. α_1-Antitrypsin deficiency alleles and severe cystic fibrosis lung disease. *Thorax* 1998;**53**:1022–4.

127 Mahadeva R, Westerbeek RC, Perry DJ *et al.* α_1-Antitrypsin deficiency alleles and the Taq-I G $\rightarrow$ A allele in cystic fibrosis lung disease. *Eur Respir J* 1998;**11**:873–9.

128 Celedon JC, Lange C, Raby BA *et al.* The transforming growth factor-betal (*TGFβ1*) gene is associated with chronic obstructive pulmonary disease (COPD). *Hum Mol Genet* 2004; **13**(15):1649–56.

129 Drumm ML, Pope HA, Cliff WH *et al.* Correction of the cystic fibrosis defect *in vitro* by retrovirus-mediated gene transfer. *Cell* 1990;**62**:1227–33.

130 Johnson LG, Knowles MR. New therapeutic strategies for cystic fibrosis lung disease. In: Yankaskas JR, Knowles MR, eds. *Cystic Fibrosis in Adults*. Philadelphia: Lippincott-Raven, 1999: 233–58.

CHAPTER 12

Bronchiectasis and COPD

Robert Wilson

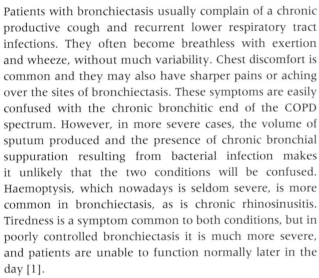

Patients with bronchiectasis usually complain of a chronic productive cough and recurrent lower respiratory tract infections. They often become breathless with exertion and wheeze, without much variability. Chest discomfort is common and they may also have sharper pains or aching over the sites of bronchiectasis. These symptoms are easily confused with the chronic bronchitic end of the COPD spectrum. However, in more severe cases, the volume of sputum produced and the presence of chronic bronchial suppuration resulting from bacterial infection makes it unlikely that the two conditions will be confused. Haemoptysis, which nowadays is seldom severe, is more common in bronchiectasis, as is chronic rhinosinusitis. Tiredness is a symptom common to both conditions, but in poorly controlled bronchiectasis it is much more severe, and patients are unable to function normally later in the day [1].

Most patients diagnosed with bronchiectasis are non-smokers. This may be influenced by current medical practice, in that an opinion is more likely to be sought and investigations performed in non-smoking patients who have a productive cough. Patients often have symptoms from an early age, which are very different from COPD, and make it less likely that patients will begin smoking. A history of wheezy bronchitis in childhood may be present, and in some patients bronchiectasis (and the consequent symptoms) occurs following a childhood pneumonia. Similarly, hereditary causes of bronchiectasis such as cystic fibrosis and primary ciliary dyskinesia have symptoms from birth or soon after.

Other features of the two conditions are similar. Symptoms of anxiety or depression may be present as in any chronic illness. We have found that in bronchiectasis depression correlates with severity of disease, but the level of anxiety may be much higher than is appropriate [2]. Exercise tolerance, the frequency of exacerbations, requirement for hospital admission, the presence or absence of

Pseudomonas aeruginosa infection, and raised systemic markers of inflammation in the stable state are the best predictors of quality of life in bronchiectasis [3–5], which is not dissimilar to studies of this type in COPD [6].

The prevalence of severe cystic bronchiectasis has decreased since the introduction of vaccination against childhood infections, improved socioeconomic conditions and the availability of antibiotics, but in parts of the world where social conditions are poor and health care less available, bronchiectasis remains a much more common cause of morbidity and mortality. The availability of high-resolution computed tomography (CT) has increased the recognition of milder forms of disease. This cylindrical or tubular form has been termed 'modern' bronchiectasis [7]. The disease is usually bilateral and may be widespread, although the lower lobes are usually worst affected. Progression of disease may be bimodal, with most patients stable or declining slowly, whereas a smaller number progress more rapidly for reasons that are not clear at present.

The findings on examination are similar to COPD. Coarse inspiratory crackles are sometimes heard over the site of bronchiectasis but quite often, particularly in milder cases, there are no signs in the lung to suggest the diagnosis. Wheezes and squeaks may be heard as a result of obstructed airways, and patients may have signs of hyperinflation. Clubbing is quite unusual, because it only occurs in severe cases with cystic bronchiectasis, which are less prevalent than in the past.

Pathology

Bronchiectasis results from loss of structural proteins such as elastin from the bronchial wall, and the muscle and cartilage layers also show signs of damage. These changes lead to abnormal chronic dilation of the affected bronchi. Copious secretions may be produced by increased numbers of goblet cells and hypertrophic submucosal glands, and these are poorly cleared and hence partially obstruct the airway lumen. Mucociliary clearance is delayed for several reasons: there is pooling of excess secretions in abnormal dilated airways; ciliated cells are lost when the epithelium is damaged and they are replaced by goblet cells; purulent mucus is less elastic and more viscous, making it difficult to clear by both ciliary beat and coughing. Side branches of the tortuous airways are frequently obliterated, and there may be complete fibrosis of small airways. There may be peribronchial pneumonic changes with evidence of parenchymal damage.

Lymphocytes predominate in the bronchial wall, which contains lymphoid follicles and nodes, whereas neutrophils are abundant in the lumen. As well as B lymphocytes, plasma cells and CD4+ T lymphocytes in the follicles, there is a well-developed cell-mediated immune response, with increased numbers of activated T lymphocytes, mainly of the suppressor/cytotoxic CD8+ phenotype, antigen-processing cells and mature macrophages [8].

Pathogenesis

We remain ignorant of the cause of bronchiectasis in up to half of cases. The more important causes that have been identified are listed in Table 12.1. Broadly speaking, the host defences are usually impaired in some way, and this may either be a systemic problem or one that is local in the lung, and it may be hereditary or acquired. Whatever the cause, inhaled bacteria that are normally cleared are able to persist and multiply in the airway lumen. Neutrophils are then attracted to this site by products of bacteria themselves, and also by mediators released from host cells (e.g. interleukin 8 [IL-8], C5a and LTB$_4$). Serum levels of the adhesion molecules E-selectin, ICAM-1 and VCAM-1 are elevated, suggesting that endothelial activation occurs, probably within the lung [9]. Many patients with bronchiectasis have chronic bacterial infection of the airway, and the failure of the inflammation to eradicate the infection is partly caused by the impaired defences, but also by the number of bacteria present and their pathogenic determinants [10].

Chronic neutrophilic inflammation has the potential to cause tissue damage via spillage of proteolytic enzymes such as elastase and reactive oxygen species, which overwhelm the lung's ability to neutralize them. Immune complexes, which are formed between bacterial antigens and antibodies (produced locally and by protein transudation), trigger other inflammatory cascades. Infection and inflammation may spread to involve adjacent areas of normal bystander lung. The lung's defences are further weakened by damage to both the surface epithelium and deeper structures of the bronchial wall, leading to the accumulation

Table 12.1 Causes of bronchiectasis.

Congenital
e.g. defective bronchial wall (Mounier–Kuhn syndrome and others), pulmonary sequestration

Postinfective
e.g. tuberculosis, whooping cough, non-tuberculous mycobacteria especially *Mycobacterium avium complex* and adenoviruses

Mechanical obstruction/bronchial stenosis
e.g. within lumen (tumour) or external compression (lymph node)

Deficient immune response
e.g. common variable immunodeficiency, HIV, acute or chronic lymphocytic leukaemia

Inflammatory pneumonitis
e.g. aspiration of gastric contents, inhalation of toxic gases

Excessive immune response
e.g. allergic bronchopulmonary aspergillosis, lung transplant rejection, chronic graft-versus-host disease

Abnormal mucociliary clearance
e.g. primary ciliary dyskinesia, cystic fibrosis, Young's syndrome

Fibrosis traction
e.g. cryptogenic fibrosing alveolitis, sarcoidosis, radiation pneumonitis

Associated with inflammatory bowel disease
Especially ulcerative colitis, also Crohn's disease and coeliac disease

Associated with connective tissue disorders
Especially rheumatoid arthritis, also Sjögren's syndrome and SLE

Others
e.g. diffuse panbronchiolitis, yellow nail syndrome, associated with α_1-antiproteinase deficiency

HIV, human immunodeficiency virus; SLE, systemic lupus erythematosus.

of mucus-containing bacteria in the lumen. These changes in turn promote continued infection and this perpetuates chronic inflammation. Epithelial cells, lymphocytes and macrophages release mediators that orchestrate this sequence of events (Fig. 12.1), which has been called a 'vicious circle' [7]. Bacterial numbers are higher during an exacerbation, either because a new strain is not constrained by the immune defences, or the defences are further impaired (e.g. because of a viral infection), and this leads to an increase in the amount of inflammation.

In COPD, tobacco smoke is the predominant cause of

A vicious circle of infection and inflammation

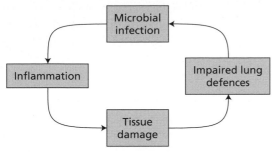

Figure 12.1 A 'vicious circle' of bacteria-stimulated host-mediated lung damage, which may occur with chronic bacterial infection of the airways or with frequent bacterial infective exacerbations.

lung damage and impaired airway defences against inhaled matter including bacteria. Bacteria are isolated in half or more of exacerbations [11], and isolation of a new bacterial strain makes the chances of an exacerbation twice as likely as when this is not the case [12]. Evidence is accumulating that exacerbations contribute to disease progression when they are frequent, and that lower airway bacterial colonization (LABC) in the stable state, which is present more often in patients with frequent exacerbations, stimulates chronic inflammation [13–16]. An animal model of chronic exposure of the lung to bacterial lipolysaccharide has shown changes characteristic, in some ways, of those seen in both COPD and bronchiectasis in terms of inflammatory cells, cytokine expression and pathological changes in both airways and alveoli [17]. Therefore, bacterial infections and LABC in stable state COPD patients have been linked to airway inflammation in a way similar to bronchiectasis, and one study has shown a more rapid decline in forced expiratory volume in 1 s (FEV_1) in patients with LABC [18]. Bacterial numbers isolated when LABC is present correlate with markers of inflammation, including the important neutrophil chemoattractant IL-8 [15,18,19].

A 'vicious circle' similar to that proposed in bronchiectasis might therefore operate in some patients with COPD [20], particularly those patients with frequent exacerbations and LABC. If this were the case one would expect high-resolution CT scans to reveal evidence of bronchiectasis, although the predominant pattern might still be of COPD. In these circumstances, sputum bacteriology might reflect this shift in disease pattern. Several recent studies have shown that Gram-negative species (e.g. *P. aeruginosa*), more commonly associated with bronchiectasis and cystic fibrosis, are isolated in COPD patients [21–23]. The risk factors for isolation of *P. aeruginosa* include severe airflow obstruction and frequent prior courses of antibiotics. *P. aeruginosa* isolation in bronchiectasis is similarly associated with more severe disease and airflow obstruction [24].

Investigations

Suspicion of the presence of bronchiectasis should lead to investigation of possible causes, and an assessment of the extent of disease and functional impairment, before a management plan is constructed. This advice is unchanged if significant bronchiectasis is found in a COPD patient, because cigarette smoking does not cause this type of airway disease. The protocol of investigations performed in our unit is given in Table 12.2. Using a similar protocol, Pasteur *et al.* [25] found a cause that influenced management in approximately one-third of cases.

A chest radiograph is an insensitive test for bronchiectasis. In one study, less than 50% of patients who subsequently had positive bronchography were detected [26]. Therefore, to investigate the prevalence of bronchiectasis in COPD would require high-resolution thin section (1–2 mm) CT scans, and this would not be justifiable as a screening method because of radiation exposure. However, CT is now regarded as the 'gold' standard for establishing the diagnosis and extent of disease, and bronchography is

Table 12.2 Investigation of bronchiectasis.

All patients
Chest radiograph (PA and lateral)
Sinus radiographs
High-resolution thin-section computed tomography scan
Respiratory function tests
Blood investigations*
Sputum microscopy including eosinophils
Sputum culture and sensitivities
Sputum smear and culture for acid-fast bacilli
Skin tests (atopy, *Aspergillus*)
Sweat test (nasal potential difference, genotyping)
Nasal mucociliary clearance and nasal nitric oxide and proceed to cilia studies if these tests are abnormal

Selected patients
Fibreoptic bronchoscopy
Barium swallow (video fluoroscopy)
Respiratory muscle function
Semen analysis for ciliary function
Tests for associated conditions
Blood tests for rarer immune deficiencies

* To include: differential white cell count; erythrocyte sedimentation rate and C-reactive protein; total immunoglobulin (Ig) levels of IgG, IgM, IgA, and IgE; specific antibodies to bacterial polysaccharide and protein antigens, e.g. pneumococcal and tetanus antibodies, repeat after vaccination if low; Aspergillus radioallergosorbent RAST test and precipitins; autoantibodies including rheumatoid factor; α_1-antiproteinase.

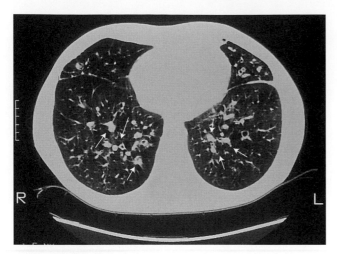

Figure 12.2 High-resolution computed tomography of lung of patient with COPD, rheumatoid arthritis and *Pseudomonas aeruginosa* infection showing bronchiectasis (arrow).

almost never undertaken. CT scans are performed with a fast scan time (1 s or less) to reduce artefacts from respiratory motion and cardiac pulsation. The whole of the lung should be examined with 10-mm intersection spacing. The characteristic features are lack of bronchial tapering as the airways progress to the outside of the lung. The easiest method of ascertaining whether a bronchus is dilated is to compare it with the adjacent pulmonary artery. Dilated bronchi that are perpendicular to the scanning plane have a circular appearance, and then the smaller pulmonary artery gives a 'signet ring' appearance. Mucus-filled bronchi appear as branching tubules or nodules, and there may be a 'tree-in-bud' appearance indicating exudative bronchiolitis. End-expiratory scans identify increased transradiency in areas where air-trapping has occurred because of obstruction of small airways. Because the gas trapping is usually patchy, this gives a pattern of mosaic perfusion.

An example of bronchiectasis in a COPD patient with a long smoking history is shown in Figure 12.2. However, this patient also had rheumatoid arthritis (see Table 12.1), which may have influenced his lung disease. Although certain features on CT may suggest a cause of bronchiectasis (e.g. cystic fibrosis, upper lobe disease), allergic bronchopulmonary aspergillosis (proximal disease), non-tuberculous mycobacteria (diffuse mild disease with peripheral nodules that might be cavitating) or diffuse panbronchiolitis (widespread small nodules), they do not usually allow a confident diagnosis [27]. Several new volumetric techniques have improved accuracy in the assessment of bronchiectasis, but all have required increased doses of radiation which is unlikely to be justifiable [28].

Lung function tests provide a measure of functional impairment and an assessment of change with time. Airflow obstruction, which is largely fixed, and gas trapping

are very common as in COPD. However, unlike COPD, where there is often a component of emphysema, gas transfer values that have been adjusted for alveolar volume are usually well perseveed unless the disease is severe. We also include a measure of exercise capacity in our assessment, because this has a strong correlation with quality of life scores [3].

Variable immune (antibody) deficiency is a relatively common cause of bronchiectasis. Immunoglobulin G (IgG) subclass deficiency by itself is not a cause of susceptibility to infection. Specific antibody levels should be measured, and if these are low the ability to respond appropriately to vaccination with polysaccharide (pneumococcal and *Haemophilus influenzae* type b) and protein (tetanus) antigens should be tested. All cases of immune deficiency may be secondary to malignancy, particularly of the lymphoreticular system, so a high index of suspicion must be maintained [1].

Sputum should be examined by microscopy as well as culture for respiratory pathogens including fungi and mycobacteria, because eosinophils can cause mild purulence, and their presence would indicate asthma or allergic bronchopulmonary aspergillosis. *H. influenzae*, *H. parainfluenzae* and *P. aeruginosa* are the species identified most frequently, but *Streptococcus pneumoniae* and *Moraxella catarrhalis* are also common isolates, so the microbiology of COPD and bronchiectasis is similar. In a CT study, the extent and severity of bronchiectasis, the severity of bronchial wall thickening and the extent of decreased attenuation were strikingly greater in the patients who cultured *P. aeruginosa* [24], but it is not clear whether isolation of this bacterium is simply a marker of disease severity, as it seems to be in COPD [21–23]. *Staphylococcus aureus* is less commonly isolated in both diseases, and we found regular isolation of this pathogen in bronchiectasis to predict allergic bronchopulmonary aspergillosis or atypical cystic fibrosis [29].

Prevalence of bronchiectasis in COPD

The prevalence of bronchiectasis in the community is unknown and will remain so until a cheap and safe screening tool is developed. Magnetic resonance scans would be ideal, but have not to date proved useful, although new approaches might hold some promise [30]. Possibly, low-dose CT could screen for the 'signet ring' appearance of bronchiectatic airways, in the same way as nodules are screened for in a smoking population. Empirically one would expect the pick-up rate of bronchiectasis to be increased by targeting patients with daily sputum production of significant volumes. Munro *et al.* [31] investigated 27 patients with such a history, 11 of whom were ex-smokers and 10 had an $FEV_1 \leq 80\%$. Bronchiectasis was identified in 15. Chronic mucus hypersecretion in COPD has been associated with more frequent exacerbations, excess decline in FEV_1 and mortality resulting from an infectious cause [32–34], and it is likely that such patients have a high prevalence of bronchiectasis.

However, in the largest CT study of the prevalence of bronchiectasis in COPD performed so far, this expected association with sputum production was not found in milder cases of cylindrical bronchiectasis. O'Brien *et al.* [35] studied 110 patients aged 40–80 years old who had been diagnosed as having COPD by their primary care physician. Patients were in a stable condition at the time of the study, and had a high-resolution CT scan and full lung function tests. The finding of a wide variation in the severity of airflow obstruction was to be expected, as was the finding of emphysema in 51% of CT scans. Bronchiectasis was found in 29%, a much higher proportion than expected. In 23 patients this was tubular bronchiectasis, but in five it was cystic and in four varicose (i.e. more severe forms of disease). Six of the patients with tubular bronchiectasis had no history of sputum production. This result suggests that in the future when designing studies on the role of bacterial infection in COPD consideration will have to be given to performing CT scans on all patients to ensure that comparisons are made of like with like.

The East London Group have published many studies of their hospital clinic-based COPD population. An overt history of bronchiectasis is one of the exclusion factors for participation in their studies. Despite this, they have recently reported the results of high-resolution CT scans in 54 subjects from this population of older patients (mean age 69 years) with severe COPD (mean FEV_1 0.96 L, 38.1% predicted). Bronchiectasis was present in 72.2%, usually mild tubular disease in the lower lobes. Interestingly, these patients with bronchiectasis had more severe exacerbations, with greater rise in symptom scores and slower rates of recovery of peak flow [36]. Our own anecdotal experience at the Royal Brompton Hospital, London, is similar to this, bronchiectasis by CT scan criteria is common in COPD patients selected because of recurrent bacterial chest infections confirmed by sputum culture and particularly isolation of *P. aeruginosa*.

More studies are required before the prevalence of bronchiectasis in COPD is determined, particularly studies of unselected patients from primary care. The results of the studies performed so far suggest that bronchiectasis by CT scan criteria will be quite commonly found. This is not surprising given evidence of the role of neutrophilic inflammation during exacerbations and in the stable state. A more difficult question is the clinical relevance of this finding. The study of the East London Group showing that these patients have more severe exacerbations, suggest that the presence of bronchiectasis may influence management.

Two recent studies have shown a prolonged infection-free interval following treatment of an infective exacerbation with quinolone antibiotics which also achieved superior bacteriological eradication compared with comparator antibiotics [37,38]. Therefore, antibiotic treatment could influence exacerbation frequency, and in this way slow decline in FEV_1 [16,39]. The presence of bronchiectasis might identify patients in whom bacterial infection has an important role in provoking heightened airway inflammation and frequent exacerbations [19,40]. It is our practice to carry out a high-resolution CT scan in patients with documented frequent (more than four per year) bacterial infective exacerbations of COPD if this does not respond to appropriate antibiotic management and optimization of other aspects of treatment, particularly if *P. aeruginosa* is isolated. Other causes of increased susceptibility to infection should be screened for in such patients.

We have studied serial change in lung function and CT scans in bronchiectasis over time [41], and overall most patients show little change. FEV_1 correlated best with mosaic attenuation (small airways disease) in the CT scans, and this feature rarely regressed. When change did occur in FEV_1, it correlated with changes in mucus plugging (small and large airways) seen on CT. Finally, when patients' disease progressed, an increased bronchiectasis score went hand in hand with increased mucus plugging and bronchial wall thickening, which is thought to reflect airway inflammation. Therefore, knowledge that a COPD patient has bronchiectasis should focus attention on efforts to improve mucus clearance and reduce airway inflammation by controlling bacterial infection.

Non-antibiotic management of bronchiectasis and its applications to COPD

Poor clearance of mucus from bronchiectatic airways is probably the fundamental reason that patients become colonized. Therefore, physiotherapy exercises to clear secretions are a critical aspect of management. Patients are advised to perform postural drainage at least once daily, and increase the frequency to twice or three times daily if they suffer an exacerbation. Patients know from experience their most productive time of day to perform the exercises. They should be taught by a trained physiotherapist to adopt the correct position to drain an affected area identified by CT scan, and clear mucus by controlled breathing techniques (e.g. active cycle of breathing and huffing), sometimes assisted by chest clapping from the patient themselves or a partner. Approximately 10 min in any one productive position is required so, understandably, compliance with physiotherapy is poor because of the nature of the process and the time involved. Evidence of benefit from physiotherapy is largely anecdotal, but the importance of mucus clearance is emphasized by patients with primary ciliary dyskinesia who have widespread bronchiectasis, and by a group of patients in whom cough suppression had an adverse effect on their clinical condition [42]. Medical staff should regularly remind patients of the importance of physiotherapy. Controlled breathing techniques to clear mucus may be performed more conveniently in a sitting position, and physical exercise is also an effective way of encouraging mucus clearance. These latter methods should be encouraged in COPD patients with daily mucus production.

Any asthmatic component of bronchiectasis should be treated in the usual way. Systemic corticosteroids have unacceptable side-effects when used long term to try to reduce airway inflammation, although they are used for short periods during severe exacerbations. Inhaled corticosteroids are commonly prescribed to bronchiectasis patients in an attempt to reduce airway inflammation and relieve airflow obstruction [43], but unlike COPD there is no evidence that they reduce exacerbation frequency, nor that they influence disease progression. If they are used, an objective assessment of symptoms and lung function tests should be made several months after their introduction to justify continuation. Treatment of allergic bronchopulmonary aspergillosis with high-dose inhaled corticosteroids may prevent exacerbations and airway wall damage, but in some patients systemic corticosteroids are required. The antifungal antibiotic itraconazole may be used as a steroid-sparing agent [44]. Acid reflux and rhinosinusitis should be treated if present and influenza (annual) and pneumococcal vaccinations should be encouraged. Nebulized saline may be given in an attempt to promote cough clearance by liquefying secretions in some patients, although mucolytic agents have no proven benefit. This includes nebulized recombinant DNase which improves lung function and may decrease exacerbation frequency in cystic fibrosis, but not in other forms of bronchiectasis [45].

The only curative treatment of bronchiectasis is surgical resection. 'Modern' cylindrical bronchiectasis is usually bilateral and surgery is rarely considered for this reason and because it is a less problematic type to the patient. Palliative resection may be considered if a localized area of severe bronchiectasis defies medical management and acts as a sump for infection, even if less severe disease is present elsewhere. Nasal intermittent positive pressure ventilation is often surprisingly well tolerated despite sinusitis and excess bronchial secretions, and is used in patients with respiratory failure and bronchiectasis [46]. Lung transplantation is used to treat end-stage respiratory failure resulting from bronchiectasis. This is usually bilateral or heart–lung transplantation, otherwise infection in the remaining lung may spread to the new organ.

Antibiotic management of bronchiectasis and its application to COPD

When bronchiectasis is mild to moderate, antibiotic treatment reduces the bacterial numbers in the airway to low levels and can even achieve sterility, leading to resolution of the bronchial inflammation and symptoms. The next exacerbation occurs either with a new bacterial infection, or if residual bacterial numbers increase for some reason (e.g. a reduction in the host defences with a concomitant viral infection, or a change in the bacterial strain allowing it to escape the host defences). When bronchiectasis is more severe, the airways are usually chronically colonized and the symptoms of an exacerbation may recur soon after stopping the antibiotic. In these different circumstances, antibiotics may be needed only during an infective exacerbation when there is a change in sputum production, breathlessness or malaise, or at the other end of the spectrum continuously if relapse is rapid following treatment.

LABC in bronchiectasis and COPD probably represents a balance in which the impaired host defences are able to limit the number of bacteria, such that they do not stimulate an overt inflammatory response sufficient to generate symptoms of an exacerbation [47–49]. LABC is a dynamic process, multiple strains may be present and changes may occur in both their genotype and phenotype over time; strains may be carried for variable periods of time before being lost and replaced by others [50]. Acquisition of a new strain, which is not constrained by the immune system, may lead to an exacerbation associated with an increase in bacterial numbers [12]. The total bacterial load in the bronchial tree is a very important parameter in determining the level of inflammation [19], but other factors such as the species involved may be influential, and even different strains in the same species vary in their ability to elicit an inflammatory response [51]. Some patients with COPD behave in a similar fashion to those with bronchiectasis, having LABC and repeated chest infections. Their antibiotic management can therefore be planned in a similar way. These patients are probably best recognized clinically by frequent (more than four in 12 months) exacerbations associated with purulent sputum production.

The choice of antibiotic is influenced by the high frequency of β-lactamase production by strains of *H. influenzae* and *M. catarrhalis* in patients who have taken frequent antibiotic courses in the past, and the presence or absence of *P. aeruginosa* that is resistant to oral antibiotics other than ciprofloxacin [52]. Co-amoxiclav and ciprofloxacin are our first-line choices. Dosage is usually at the higher end of the options available, to ensure good concentrations are achieved in bronchial secretions, and the length of the course should be determined by resolution of symptoms (particularly sputum purulence) rather than fixed at a certain number of days. Although initial antibiotic choice may be empirical, sputum culture should always be performed in cases of treatment failure.

If patients are severely unwell at presentation or infected by resistant strains, intravenous antibiotics are necessary. These should be commenced in hospital where supportive treatment such as physiotherapy can also be given, but increasingly patients are being taught to administer their own injections, so that when their condition is improving their hospital stay can be shortened by finishing the course at home. Ceftriaxone (non-*P.aeruginosa* patients) and ceftazidime plus an aminoglycoside (*P. aeruginosa* patients) are our first-line antibiotics with piperacillin–tazobactam and meropenem second-line.

Patients with frequent exacerbations who relapse quickly following antibiotic treatment may be considered for long-term prophylactic antibiotics, in some cases restricted to the winter months when infective exacerbations are more frequent. This approach should only be taken after careful consideration, and only after other aspects of management have been optimized. There are several concerns about antibiotic prophylaxis: development of resistance in the strains already present; promotion of infection by more antibiotic-resistant species (e.g. *P. aeruginosa*); and antibiotic-induced side-effects (e.g. *Clostridium difficile* infection). Three different approaches to antibiotic prophylaxis have been used: oral antibiotics, which can either be with a single antibiotic, or a rotation of several antibiotics from different classes [53]; inhaled antibiotics given as an isotonic solution via a nebulizer [54]; and regular pulsed courses of intravenous antibiotics [55]. The first two approaches have been shown to reduce exacerbation frequency, although doubts have been expressed about the third [56]. Other benefits have also been shown in various aspects of patient well-being. In broad terms, we use oral prophylaxis in patients not infected with *P. aeruginosa,* nebulized antibiotics for patients with chronic *P. aeruginosa* infection, and pulsed intravenous antibiotics for patients with most severe disease in whom other forms of prophylaxis have failed.

Continuous treatment with macrolide antibiotics has been used effectively to treat diffuse panbronchiolitis, even when there is chronic infection with *P. aeruginosa*. This conditions was first described in Japan [57], where it seems to be much more common. There are unique radiological and histological features, but clinically many features are similar to idiopathic bronchiectasis. The benefit of macrolides seem certain to be more than simple antibacterial effect, although azithromycin is active against *P. aeruginosa* with prolonged courses. Macrolides also affect *P. aeruginosa* virulence determinants including biofilm made of growth. However, it is more likely that the anti-inflammatory properties of the macrolide class are responsible [58]. A recent study has shown promising results in cystic fibrosis, and further studies in bronchiectasis and COPD are planned [59,60].

References

1 Wilson R. Bronchiectasis. In: Gibson GJ, Geddes DM, Costabel U, Sterk PJ, Corrin B, eds. *Respiratory Medicine*, vol. 2, 3rd edn. Saunders/Elsevier Science, 2003:1445–64.

2 O'Leary CJ, Wilson CB, Hansell DM *et al.* Relationship between psychological well-being and lung health status in patients with bronchiectasis. *Respir Med* 2002;**96**:686–92.

3 Wilson CB, Jones PW, O'Leary CJ *et al.* Health status assessment in bronchiectasis using the St George's Respiratory Questionnaire. *Am J Respir Crit Care Med* 1997;**156**;536–41.

4 Wilson CB, Jones PW, O'Leary CJ *et al.* Effect of sputum bacteriology on the quality of life of patients with bronchiectasis. *Eur Respir J* 1998;**12**:820–4.

5 Wilson CB, Jones PW, O'Leary CJ *et al.* Systemic markers of inflammation in stable bronchiectasis. *Eur Respir J* 1998;**12**: 820–4.

6 Seemungal TAR, Donaldson GC, Bhowmik A *et al.* Time course and recovery of exacerbations in patients with chronic obstructive pulmonary disease. *Am J Respir Crit Care Med* 2000;**161**:1608–13.

7 Cole PJ. Bronchiectasis. In: Brewis RAL, Corrin B, Geddes AM, Gibson GJ, eds. *Respiratory Medicine*, 2nd edn. London: WB Saunders, 1995: 1286–317.

8 Lapa e Silva JR, Jones JAH, Cole PJ, Poulter PW. The immunological component of the cellular inflammatory infiltrate in bronchiectasis. *Thorax* 1989;**44**:668–73.

9 Zheng L, Tipoe G, Lam WK *et al.* Upregulation of circulating adhesion molecules in bronchiectasis. *Eur Respir J* 2000;**16**: 691–6.

10 Wilson R, Dowling R, Jackson AD. The biology of bacterial colonization and invasion of the respiratory mucosa. *Eur Respir J* 1996;**9**:523–30.

11 Monso E, Ruiz J, Rosell A *et al.* Bacterial infection in chronic obstructive pulmonary disease: a study of stable and exacerbated patients using the protected specimen brush. *Am J Respir Crit Care Med* 1995;**152**:1316–20.

12 Sethi S, Evans N, Brydon JB, Murphy TF. New strains of bacteria and exacerbations of chronic obstructive pulmonary disease. *N Engl J Med* 2002;**347**:465–71.

13 Wilson R. Bacterial infection and chronic obstructive pulmonary disease. *Eur Respir J* 1999;**13**:233–5.

14 Soler N, Eurig S, Torres A *et al.* Airway inflammation and bronchial microbial patterns in patients with stable chronic obstructive pulmonary disease. *Eur Respir J* 1999;**14**:1015–22.

15 Patel IS, Seemungal TAR, Wilks M *et al.* Relationship between bacterial colonisation and the frequency, character and severity of COPD exacerbations. *Thorax* 2002;**57**:759–64.

16 Donaldson GC, Seemungal TAR, Bhomik A, Wedzicha JA. The relationship between exacerbation frequency and lung

function decline in chronic obstructive pulmonary disease. *Thorax* 2002;**57**:847–52.

17 Vernooy J, Dentener MA, Vam Smylen RJ, Buurman WA, Wouters EM. Long term intratracheal lipopolysaccharide exposure in mice results in chronic lung inflammation and persistent pathology. *Am J Respir Cell Mol Biol* 2002;**26**: 152–9.

18 Wilkinson TMA, Patel IS, Wilks M, Donaldson GC, Wedzicha JA. Airway bacterial load and FEV_1 decline in patients with chronic obstructive pulmonary disease. *Am J Respir Crit Care Med* 2003;**167**:1090–5.

19 Hill AT, Campbell EJ, Hill SL *et al.* Association between airway bacterial load and markers of inflammatory in patients with stable chronic bronchiectasis. *Am J Med* 2000;**109**:288–95.

20 Wilson R. The pathogenesis and management of bronchial infections: the vicious circle of respiratory decline. *Rev Contemp Pharacother* 1992;**3**:103–12.

21 Eller J, Ede A, Schaberg T *et al.* Infective exacerbations of chronic bronchitis: relationship between bacteriological aetiology and lung function. *Chest* 1998;**113**:1542–8.

22 Miravitlles M, Espinosa C, Fernandez-Laso E *et al.* Relationship between bacterial flora in sputum and functional impairment in patients with acute exacerbations of COPD. *Chest* 1999;**115**:40–6.

23 Soler N, Torres A, Eurig S *et al.* Bronchial microbial pattersn in severe exacerbations of chronic obstructive pulmonary disease (COPD) requiring mechanical ventilation. *Am J Respir Crit Care Med* 1998;**157**:1498–1505.

24 Wells CT, Miszkiel KA, Wells AU *et al.* Effects of airway infection by *Pseudomonas aeruginosa*: a computed tomography study. *Thorax* 1997;**52**:260–4.

25 Pasteur MC, Helliwell S, Houghton SJ *et al.* An investigation into causative factors in patients with bronchiectasis. *Am J Respir Crit Care Med* 2000;**162**:1277–84.

26 Curry DC, Cooke JC, Morgan AD *et al.* Interpretation of bronchograms and chest radiographs in patients with chronic sputum production. *Thorax* 1987;**42**:278.

27 Reiff DB, Wells AU, Carr DH *et al.* CT findings in bronchiectasis: limited value in distinguishing between idiopathic and specific types. *Am J Roentgenol* 1995;**165**:261–7.

28 Engeler CE, Tashijian JH, Engeler CM *et al.* Volumetric highresolution CT in the diagnosis of interstitial lung disease and bronchiectasis: diagnostic accuracy and radiation dose. *Am J Roentgenol* 1994;**163**:31–5.

29 Mawdsley S, Nash K *et al. Staphylococcus aureus* in patients with bronchiectasis: identification of disease associations. *Eur Respir J* 1998;**12**:1340–4.

30 Biederer J, Both M, Graessner J *et al.* Lung morphology: fast MR imaging assessment with volumetric interpolated breathhold technique – initial experience with patients. *Radiology* 2003;**226**:242–9.

31 Munro NC, Cooke JC, Currie DC, Strickland B, Cole PJ. Comparison of thin-section computed tomography with bronchography for identifying bronchiectatic segments in patients with chronic sputum production. *Thorax* 1990;**45**: 135–9.

32 Seemungal TAR, Donaldson GC, Paul EA *et al.* Effect of exacerbation on quality of life in patients with chronic obstructive pulmonary disease. *Am J Respir Crit Care Med* 1998;**157**: 1418–22.

33 Vesto J, Prescott E, Longe P. Association between chronic mucus hypersecretion with FEV_1 decline and chronic obstructive pulmonary disease morbidity. *Am J Respir Crit Care Med* 1996;**153**:1530–5.

34 Prescott E, Lange P, Vestbo J. Chronic mucus hypersecretion in COPD and death from pulmonary infection. *Eur Respir J* 1995;**8**:1333–8.

35 O'Brien C, Guest PJ, Hill SH *et al.* Physiological and radiological characterisation of patient diagnosed with chronic obstructive pulmonary disease in primary care. *Thorax* 2000; **55**:635–42.

36 Patel IS, Vlahos I, Wilkinson TMA *et al.* Bronchiectasis, exacerbation indices and inflammation in COPD. *Am J Respir Crit Care Med* 2004;**170**:400–7.

37 Wilson R, Schentag JJ, Ball P, Mandell L. A comparison of gemifloxacin and clarithromycin in acute exacerbations of chronic bronchitis and long term outcomes. *Clin Ther* 2002; **24**:639–52.

38 Wilson R, Allegra L, Huchon G *et al.* Short and long term outcomes of moxifloxacin in acute exacerbations of chronic bronchitis. *Chest* 2004;**125**:953–64.

39 Kanner RE, Anthonisen NR, Connett JE. Lower respiratory illnesses promote FEV_1 decline in current smokers but not ex-smokers with mild chronic obstructive pulmonary disease. *Am J Respir Crit Care Med* 2001;**164**:358–64.

40 Bhowmik A, Seemungal TAR, Sapsford RJ, Wedzicha JA. Relation of sputum inflammatory markers to symptoms and lung function changes in COPD exacerbations. *Thorax* 2000; **55**:114–20.

41 Sheehan RE, Wells AU, Copley SJ *et al.* A comparison of serial computed tomography and functional change in bronchiectasis. *Eur Respir J* 2002;**20**:581–7.

42 Wells A, Rahman A, Woodhead M *et al.* Voluntary cough suppression associated with chronic pulmonary suppuration: a new syndrome. *Eur Respir J* 1992;**5**(Suppl 15):141S.

43 Tsang KWT, Ho PL, Lam WK *et al.* Inhaled fluticasone reduces sputum inflammatory indices in severe bronchiectasis. *Am J Respir Crit Care Med* 1998;**158**:723–7.

44 Stevens DA, Schwartz HJ, Lee JY *et al.* A randomised trial of itraconazole in allergic bronchopulmonary aspergillosis. *N Engl J Med* 2000;**342**:756–62.

45 O'Donnell AE, Barker AF, Howke JS, Fick RB. Treatment of idiopathic bronchiectasis with recombinant human DNase. *Chest* 1998;**113**:1329–34.

46 Grascouin A, Desrues B, Lena H *et al.* Long term nasal intermittent positive pressure ventilation (NIPPV) in sixteen consecutive patients with bronchiectasis: a retrospective study. *Eur Respir J* 1996;**9**:1246–50.

47 Monso E, Rosell AI, Boret G *et al.* Risk factors of lower airway bacterial colonisation in chronic bronchitis. *Eur Respir J* 1999;**13**:338–42.

48 Zalacain R, Sobradillo V, Anilibia J *et al.* Predisposing factors to bacterial colonisation in chronic obstructive pulmonary disease. *Eur Respir J* 1999;**13**:348–8.

49 Soler N, Ewig S, Torres A *et al.* Airway inflammation and

bronchial microbial patters in patients with stable chronic obstructive pulmonary disease. *Eur Respir J* 1999;**14**:1015–22.

50 Murphy TF, Sethi S, Klingman KL *et al*. Simultaneous respiratory tract colonization by multiple strains of non-typable *Haemophilus influenzae* in chronic obstructive pulmonary disease: implications for antibiotic therapy. *J Infect Dis* 1999;**180**:404–9.

51 Bresser P, van Alphen L, Habets FJM. Persisting *Haemophilus influenzae* strains induce lower levels of interleukin-6 and interleukin-8 in H292 lung epithelial cells than non-persisting strains. *Eur Respir J* 1997;**10**:2319–26.

52 Angrill J, Agusti C, de Celis R *et al*. Bacterial colonisation in patients with bronchiectasis: microbiological pattern and risk factors. *Thorax* 2002;**57**:15–9.

53 Rayner CFJ, Tillotson G, Cole PJ, Wilson R. Efficacy and safety of long term ciprofloxacin in the management of severe bronchiectasis. *J Antimicrob Chemother* 1994;**34**:149–56.

54 Mukopadhyay S, Singh M, Cater J *et al*. Nebulised antipseudomonal antibiotic therapy in cystic fibrosis: a meta-analysis of benefits and risks. *Thorax* 1996;**51**:364–8.

55 Szaff M, Hoiby N, Flensborg EW. Frequent antibiotic therapy improves surval of cystic fibrosis patients with chronic *Pseudomonas aeruginosa* infection. *Acta Paediatr Scand* 1983;**72**:651–7.

56 Elborn JS, Prescott RJ, Stack BHR *et al*. Elective versus symptomatic antibiotic treatment in cystic fibrosis patients with chronic *Pseudomonas* infection of the lungs. *Thorax* 2000;**55**:355–8.

57 Labro MT, Abdelghaffar H. Immunomodulation by macrolide antibiotics. *J Chemother* 2001;**13**:3–8.

58 Howe RA, Spencer RC. Macrolides for the treatment of *Pseudomonas aeruginosa* infections? *J Antimicrob Chemother* 1997;**40**:153–5.

59 Wolter J. Effect of long term treatment with azithromycin on disease parameters in cystic fibrosis: a randomised trial. *Thorax* 2002;**57**:212–6.

60 Davies G, Wilson R. Prophylactic antibiotic treatment of bronchiectasis with azithromycin. *Thorax* 2004;**59**:540–1.

CHAPTER 13

Obliterative bronchiolitis

Hélène Levrey Hadden and Marshall I. Hertz

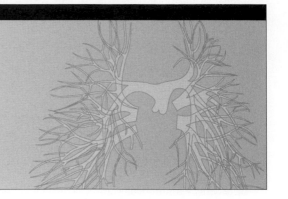

The term 'obliterative bronchiolitis' refers to a specific histopathological pattern resulting from fibroproliferation in the walls and lumen of bronchioles; and to the clinical syndrome which results from these abnormalities. In general, obliterative bronchiolitis results from airway epithelial injury, leading to a lymphocytic and/or neutrophilic inflammatory reaction, with subsequent fibroproliferation around and within affected airways. Obliterative bronchiolitis is a distinct entity from bronchiolitis obliterans organizing pneumonia ('BOOP') and several other clinico-pathological entities characterized by inflammation of small airways. The clinical, histological, radiographical and therapeutic aspects of obliterative bronchiolitis are reviewed in this chapter.

Aetiology and clinical associations

Obliterative bronchiolitis can result from direct airway injury from external agents, including viral infections and toxic inhalations, and from autoimmune and alloimmune reactions taking place within airway structures.

Postinfectious obliterative bronchiolitis

Airway infections frequently result in airway epithelial inflammation and injury. However, given the very high frequency of these infections in normal populations, evolution into obliterative bronchiolitis is uncommon. In children, obliterative bronchiolitis can follow acute bronchiolitis caused by adenovirus, but it is a very unusual complication, occurring in less than 1% of cases. Adenovirus serotypes 3, 7 and 21 have been particularly associated with the development of obliterative bronchiolitis [1–3]. Influenza virus, parainfluenza virus, measles, pertussis and *Mycoplasma pneumoniae* alone or in combination with an adenovirus have also been reported as preludes to the disease [2,4–6].

Although respiratory syncytial virus (RSV) is the most common cause of acute bronchiolitis in infancy, and may be followed by recurrent wheezing and airflow obstruction, little information is available to directly link RSV to the later development of obliterative bronchiolitis [5,7].

Adults with postinfectious obliterative bronchiolitis have usually been reported as isolated cases with a diversity of agents, including adenovirus, parainfluenza virus, cytomegalovirus and *Mycoplasma pneumoniae* [8]. Occasionally, adult patients present with a clinical syndrome suggesting lower respiratory infection, followed by progressive dyspnoea and irreversible progressive airflow obstruction; airway infections are frequently implicated as causative of this syndrome based on clinical suspicion, despite negative cultures and serological studies.

Toxin inhalation

Inhalation of chemical fumes may lead to bronchiolar epithelial injury and inflammation, followed by airway fibroproliferation. The prototype of this mechanism of injury is the syndrome of silo filler's lung, in which inhalation of silo gas containing high concentrations of nitrogen dioxide leads to respiratory illness [9,10]. Depending on the severity of the exposure, the clinical syndrome may range from mild to severe, and from slowly progressive to fulminant. In severe cases, lung injury usually overshadows the bronchiolar abnormalities, and may lead to respiratory failure and death. After milder exposures, cough and dyspnoea are often accompanied by nausea, vomiting, headache and other non-specific symptoms. After recovery from the acute illness, progressive dyspnoea and decreased pulmonary function tests signal bronchiolar inflammation and obliteration. Corticosteroids are generally recommended for patients with significant exposures to inhaled nitrogen dioxide; they should be started as soon after exposure as possible and the duration of therapy is usually at least 8 weeks.

Anhydrous ammonia and sulphur dioxide are much more water-soluble than nitrogen dioxide; therefore, they usually dissolve in secretions on the mucus membranes of the upper airways and bronchial tree and may cause intense irritation. Eye irritation, laryngitis, cough, wheezing and airflow obstruction often follow exposure, and obliterative bronchiolitis may ensue [11,12].

An outbreak of obliterative bronchiolitis has been reported in patients who had all worked at a microwave popcorn production plant. This was believed to have been caused by the inhalation of diacetyl, a volatile artificial butter flavouring agent [13].

Toxin ingestion

Obliterative bronchiolitis resulting from ingested toxins is rare. Several cases have been reported from Taiwan and China which were associated with consumption of the plant *Sauropus androgynous* [14]. Although the syndrome is hypothesized to result from the papaverine contained in the plant, papaverine has not been shown to lead to obliterative bronchiolitis in experimental animals. This injury has proven to be quite resistant to therapy, and several affected patients have undergone lung transplantation [15].

Connective tissue disease

Obliterative bronchiolitis is one of many pulmonary problems that occur in patients with connective tissue disease [16,17]. This problem complicates rheumatoid arthritis in a small proportion of patients [18] and systemic lupus erythematosus even more infrequently. Although bronchial inflammation may occur in Sjögren syndrome, progressive systemic sclerosis and other connective tissue syndromes, obliterative bronchiolitis is rarely observed. Treatment with penicillamine may contribute to the development of obliterative bronchiolitis, although the literature is not clear as to whether the penicillamine or the underlying connective disease is the causative factor [19]. Evidence against penicillamine as a causative agent is the failure to observe obliterative bronchiolitis in patients treated with penicillamine for Wilson disease.

Alloimmune reactions

Lung transplant recipients now constitute the largest population of patients with obliterative bronchiolitis, with a cumulative incidence of approximately 50% during the first 5–8 years after transplantation [20]. The exact pathogenesis of this problem is not clear, although an alloimmune-mediated mechanism is almost certainly involved [21,22]. The occurrence of acute lung rejection, especially when episodes are recurrent or severe, is a major statistical risk factor for the subsequent development of obliterative bronchiolitis [23]. Infections, including cytomegalovirus, and the community respiratory viruses respiratory syncytial virus, parainfluenza virus and influenza may also contribute in some patients [24]. Gastroesophageal reflux has recently been identified as a risk factor for obliterative bronchiolitis after lung transplantation; it has been suggested, but not yet conclusively proven, that antireflux surgery may reduce the incidence of this problem in selected patients [25,26].

Obliterative bronchiolitis may also complicate allogeneic and autologous bone marrow transplantation [27]. Although this occurs much less frequently than in lung transplant patients, the incidence of this problem may be higher than previously appreciated [28]. The disease is usually seen in the setting of chronic graft-versus-host disease, but it is less common than other clinical manifestations of graft-versus-host disease, including skin and gastrointestinal manifestations.

Histopathology

Histopathological findings of obliterative bronchiolitis mirror the clinical manifestations, with anatomical obstruction of bronchioles resulting from fibroproliferation in the airway walls and lumen [29] (Fig. 13.1). The lesions primarily affect terminal bronchioles. A spectrum of histopathological abnormalities is seen, ranging from inflammation and fibrosis of the bronchial wall, sometimes referred to as 'constrictive bronchiolitis', to fibroproliferation within of the lumen, referred to as 'proliferative bronchiolitis'. Although these histopathological patterns may coexist, one or the other tends to predominate within the lungs of an affected individual. In many cases, the process is spatially inhomogeneous, with diseased and apparently normal bronchioles appearing in the same anatomical area. The airway epithelium is often disrupted and abnormalities ranging from none, to squamous metaplasia, to complete absence of epithelium are seen. Eventually, affected bronchioles are replaced by a small nubbin of a scar, which may be quite inapparent on lung biopsy. In postinfectious obliterative bronchiolitis, fibroblasts, leucocytes and fibrin partially or fully obstruct the airway lumen, and signs of active inflammation may still be present several years after the initial illness [30]. In many cases, abnormalities of the large airways coexist with bronchiolitis, resulting in bronchiectasis and a chronic bronchitis-like clinical picture. Inflammation of the alveolar ducts and alveoli is not a primary manifestation of obliterative bronchiolitis, but may occur if bronchopneumonia results from obstruction of more proximal airways.

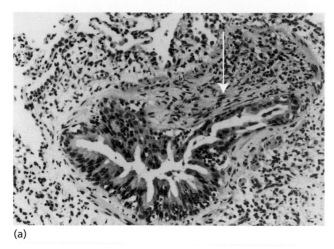

(a)

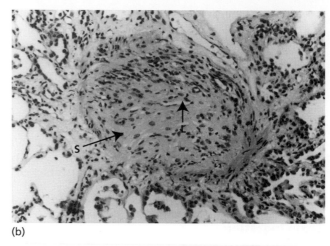

(b)

Figure 13.1 Histology of bronchiolitis obliterans. (a) 'Constrictive' obliterative bronchiolitis. Peribronchiolar lymphocytic inflammation is accompanied by an increase in the number of mesenchymal cells and their connective tissue products in the lamina propria (arrow), compromising the airway lumen in an eccentric, constrictive fashion. An inflammatory infiltrate comprised of small round cells can be appreciated in the bronchial epithelium, and in the advancing fibrous tissue. (b) 'Proliferative' obliterative bronchiolitis, in which granulation tissue comprised of mesenchymal cells and capillary loops virtually fill the lumen (L, airway lumen; S, airway smooth muscle).

Clinical presentation

Progressive dyspnoea on exertion is the hallmark symptom of obliterative bronchiolitis. Cough, which may be productive at first, is often the presenting complaint. Wheezing may be present and the condition is often initially diagnosed as asthma. In cases associated with known causes, such as infections and toxic gas inhalation, the clinical symptoms generally appear within weeks of the initial insult. In general, systemic complaints and fever are absent unless secondary infections supervene.

The clinical course and progression of the disease are variable. In children with postinfectious obliterative bronchiolitis and patients with toxic gas inhalations, the clinical and radiographical features of the disease may wax and wane for several weeks or months, sometimes with recurrent episodes of atelectasis, pneumonia and wheezing. Some patients recover completely [30,31], while others display permanent obstructive airways disease that is only partially reversible [4]. In some cases patients die of progressive respiratory failure [30]. This variability in the clinical course presumably reflects a variable balance between reversible inflammation and irreversible fibroproliferation in the lower airways.

In patients with obliterative bronchiolitis resulting from alloimmune or autoimmune reactions, the course of the disease tends to be more relentlessly downhill. Periods of relative quiescence may be punctuated by bouts resembling acute exacerbations of COPD, often resulting in further irreversible loss of lung function. Although stabilization of

pulmonary function may occur, significant recovery of lost lung function is unusual.

Differential diagnosis

It is important to differentiate bronchiolitis obliterans from many other entities with similar names, physiological findings and histopathology. Other forms of COPD, including chronic bronchitis, emphysema and chronic asthma, generally evolve over a much longer time than does obliterative bronchiolitis. Obliterative bronchiolitis is not associated with cigarette smoking, and demonstrates minimal, if any, response to bronchodilator medications. Often, a history of infection or exposure to another known causative agent is present in patients with obliterative bronchiolitis.

Respiratory bronchiolitis with interstitial lung disease (RBILD) primarily affects alveolar ducts and respiratory bronchioles [32]. An increased number of alveolar macrophages is a characteristic biopsy finding. This syndrome is most often associated with cigarette smoking, and usually improves or resolves with smoking cessation. Pulmonary function tests reflect a restrictive ventilatory abnormality. High-resolution computed tomography (HRCT) scans can be very helpful in differentiating these entities, because RBILD may be characterized by extensive ground glass opacities, which are not typical of obliterative bronchiolitis.

Bronchiolitis obliterans organizing pneumonia (BOOP) is a distinct entity characterized by polyps of loose connective tissue in alveolar ducts, in association with alveolar inflammation [33]. Although BOOP and obliterative bronchiolitis share associations with many causative agents and conditions, they are distinct clinically, radiographically, histologically and in their response to treatment. It is not clear whether these differences result from the location and severity of the initial insult, or differential healing responses between individuals. The histological lesions of BOOP may be seen in association with almost any insult known to cause obliterative bronchiolitis. However, an underlying aetiology is often not apparent, and the illness is called 'idiopathic BOOP' or 'cryptogenic organizing pneumonia'. Idiopathic BOOP is often accompanied by signs of systemic illness, including fever, malaise and weight loss. The chest radiographical findings are quite variable, but a normal radiograph is unusual. In BOOP, pulmonary function testing generally demonstrates a restrictive ventilatory abnormality with decreased diffusing capacity. In some patients with only segmental involvement, pulmonary function is normal [4].

Diffuse panbronchiolitis is a relatively common condition in Japan, China and Korea, but rare in other parts of the world [34,35]. It is most often associated with chronic sinusitis and productive cough, features that are not characteristic of obliterative bronchiolitis. Pulmonary function tests usually show airflow obstruction and a reduction in diffusing capacity. Radiographically, the disease is characterized by small nodular opacities and peripheral linear densities. Because this syndrome is quite unusual outside of Asia, it rarely confuses the diagnosis of obliterative bronchiolitis in Western countries.

Swyer-James, or MacLeod, syndrome is a variant of postinfectious bronchiolitis. It usually develops as a sequela of pulmonary infection in infancy or early childhood and leads to alveolar destruction and obliterative bronchiolitis. This may prevent the normal development of the affected lung, resulting in decreased lung volumes and blood flow, which is characterized radiographically by a unilateral hyperlucent lung with normal or reduced lung volume during inspiration and air trapping during expiration.

Diagnostic testing

Physical examination

On physical examination, affected patients may appear normal, or may display varying degrees of dyspnoea and decreased oxygen saturation, depending on the severity of their disease. Percussion of the chest may demonstrate hyperresonance, but not usually to the degree observed in patients with emphysema. Auscultation usually shows decreased inspiratory breath sounds, and end-inspiratory squeaks and crackles may be heard. Expiratory wheezes may be present, but are often absent, even in advanced disease. Clubbing is generally absent.

Pulmonary function

Pulmonary function tests typically show airflow obstruction with decreased forced expiratory volume in 1 s (FEV_1), FEV_1 : FVC (forced vital capacity) ratio and mid-expiratory flow rates. There is characteristically minimal response to inhaled bronchodilators. Lung volumes are usually normal or increased, although in some cases total lung capacity (TLC) is reduced. The diffusing capacity for carbon monoxide is normal or mildly reduced. Some patients with obliterative bronchiolitis demonstrate a restrictive pattern of pulmonary function abnormalities with reduced FEV_1, FVC and TLC; presumably the anatomical lesions in these individuals are primarily of the proliferative type, with complete obstruction of bronchiolar lumena.

Chest radiograhy

The plain chest radiograph is the most common noninvasive diagnostic test in obliterative bronchiolitis. Typically, pulmonary parenchymal opacities are absent, unless pneumonia complicates the picture. Hyperinflation may be apparent, and bronchial markings may be accentuated.

In children with postinfectious bronchiolitis, five radiographical patterns have been recognized [4]:
1 bilateral hyperlucent lungs;
2 unilateral hyperlucency and expansion of all or part of a lung;
3 unilateral hyperlucency of a small to normal-sized lung with air trapping on expiration (Swyer-James or MacLeod syndrome);
4 persistent complete collapse of the affected lobe; and
5 a mixed pattern of persistent collapse, hyperlucency and peribronchial thickening.

High-resolution computed tomography

The advent of HRCT has markedly improved the accuracy of non-diagnostic testing. Patients with obliterative bronchiolitis may show mosaic perfusion, with variable opacity in different lung zones reflecting hypoperfusion of some anatomical regions. Comparing inspiratory and expiratory HRCT scans can be very useful when inhomogeneous emptying of alveolar structures is seen, reflecting patchy air trapping. Finally, HRCT images may show peripheral branching structures that are thought to represent collapsed or fluid-filled small airways distal to obstructed bronchioles [36,37].

The use of ultrafast HRCT scans is feasible in children too young or too sick to hold their breath and allows early detection and accurate characterization of the lung process [38,39]. HRCT findings include varying degrees of bronchial wall thickening and bronchial dilatation, pulmonary vascular attenuation and areas of collapse, hyperlucency and air trapping on expiration.

Treatment

Obliterative bronchiolitis is generally poorly responsive to treatment with bronchodilators, corticosteroids and other medical therapeutics. Clearly, when a treatable infection is identified, it should be treated; however, even when the aetiology of obliterative bronchiolitis is known, specific therapy is difficult because the lesion evolves long after the initial insult. For example, there may be a hiatus of several weeks between toxic fume inhalation or respiratory viral infection and the development of progressive airflow limitation.

Bronchodilator therapies are relatively ineffective because the lesions are the result of fibroproliferation with anatomical obstruction, rather than of bronchoconstriction resulting from smooth muscle contraction. Corticosteroids are often administered, with variable results; undoubtedly they are more helpful in the early stages of the disease when anti-inflammatory therapy might be expected to be of benefit. As the disease progresses, corticosteroids are less effective. Corticosteroids are administered routinely in patients with silo filler's lung and other non-infectious inhalational airway injuries. They are also used frequently in obliterative bronchiolitis associated with connective tissue syndromes.

Erythromycin and other macrolide antibiotics have anti-neutrophil properties, and are used routinely in patients with diffuse panbronchiolitis. They have also been reported to benefit some patients with lung transplant-associated obliterative bronchiolitis [40].

Immune modulatory therapies are the mainstay of treatment for obliterative bronchiolitis resulting from alloimmune reactions. Immunosuppressive medications employed include ciclosporin, tacrolimus, mycophenolate mofetil, methotrexate and cyclophosphamide. There is evidence in the lung transplant literature that each of these agents is effective in stopping the progression of the disease in some patients, although reversal of established airflow obstruction is unusual [21]. Photochemotherapy (photopheresis) has also been shown to be beneficial in slowing disease progression in some patients [41,42].

Because the end lesion of obliterative bronchiolitis results from fibroproliferation, one would expect that antiproliferative therapies might be useful. Thalidomide has been used in some cases of chronic graft-versus-host disease after bone marrow transplantation, but its efficacy in treating obliterative bronchiolitis in that setting has not been established [43–45]. Rapamycin, a relatively new medication with immunosuppressive and antiproliferative properties, is also promising on theoretical grounds [46]. However, its clinical efficacy for obliterative bronchiolitis is also unknown at this point.

The treatment of postinfectious obliterative bronchiolitis in children is mostly supportive, consisting of oxygen therapy, bronchodilators, antibiotics for secondary infections and regular chest physiotherapy, especially if bronchiectasis is present. Despite the persisting inflammatory lesions still present at a late stage, the use of corticosteroids remains controversial, and no clinical trials in children are available. Treatment with non-steroidal anti-inflammatory therapies has been reported, as has intravenous gammaglobulin infusion.

Lung transplantation is a therapeutic option for obliterative bronchiolitis patients with severe airflow obstruction not responsive to medical therapy. The Registry of the International Society for Heart and Lung Transplantation indicates that 263 single or bilateral lung transplants were performed between January 1995 and June 2004 for patients with obliterative bronchiolitis; this represents approximately 2% of all lung transplants during that time interval [20]. Of these, approximately half were retransplant procedures for patients with obliterative bronchiolitis after lung transplantation. Recurrent obliterative bronchiolitis after repeat lung transplantation does not appear to occur with increased frequency relative to that seen in patients undergoing repeat lung transplantation for other indications [47].

References

1 Chuang YY, Chiu CH, Wong KS *et al*. Severe adenovirus infection in children. *J Microbiol Immunol Infect* 2003;**36**:37–40.

2 Kim CK, Kim SW, Kim JS *et al*. Bronchiolitis obliterans in the 1990s in Korea and the United States. *Chest* 2001;**120**:1101–6.

3 Sly PD, Soto-Quiros ME, Landau LI, Hudson I, Newton-John H. Factors predisposing to abnormal pulmonary function after adenovirus type 7 peumonia. *Arch Dis Child* 1984;**59**:935–9.

4 Chang AB, Masel JP, Masters B. Post-infectious bronchiolitis obliterans: clinical, radiological and pulmonary function sequelae. *Pediatr Radiol* 1998;**28**:23–9.

5 Mauad T, Dolhnikoff M. Histology of childhood bronchiolitis obliterans. *Pediatr Pulmonol* 2002;**33**:466–74.

6 Isles AF, Masel J, O'Duffy J. Obliterative bronchiolitis due to *Mycoplasma pneumoniae* infection in a child. *Pediatr Radiol* 1987;**17**:109–11.

7 Milner AD, Murray M. Acute bronchiolitis in infancy: treatment and prognosis. *Thorax* 1989;**44**:1–5.

8 Penn CC, Liu C. Bronchiolitis following infection in adults and children. *Clin Chest Med* 1993;**14**:645–54.

9 Douglas WW, Hepper NG, Colby TV. Silo-filler's disease. *Mayo Clin Proc* 1989;**64**:291–304.

10 Milne JE. Nitrogen dioxide inhalation and bronchiolitis obliterans: a review of the literature and report of a case. *J Occup Med* 1969;**11**:538–47.

11 Hahn IH, Muhammad A. Does nebulized corticosteroid ther-

apy have an effect on ammonia-induced pulmonary injury? *J Toxicol Clin Toxicol* 2000;**38**:79.

12 Ward K, Murray B, Costello GP. Acute and long-term pulmonary sequelae of acute ammonia inhalation. *Ir Med J* 1983;**76**:279–81.

13 Kreiss K, Gomaa A, Kullman G *et al.* Clinical bronchiolitis obliterans in workers at a microwave-popcorn plant. *N Engl J Med* 2002;**347**:330–8.

14 Lai R-S, Chiang AA, Wu M-T *et al.* Outbreak of bronchiolitis obliterans associated with consumption of *Sauropus androgynus* in Taiwan. *Lancet* 1996;**348**:83–5.

15 Luh SP, Lee YC, Chang YL *et al.* Lung transplantation for patients with end-stage *Sauropus androgynus*-induced bronchiolitis obliterans (SABO) syndrome. *Clin Transplant* 1999; **13**:496–503.

16 Hakala M, Paakko P, Sutinen S *et al.* Association of bronchiolitis with connective tissue disorders. *Ann Rheum Dis* 1986; **45**:656–62.

17 Wells AU, du Bois RM. Bronchiolitis in association with connective tissue disorders. *Clin Chest Med* 1993;**14**:655–66.

18 Geddes DM, Corrin B, Brewerton DA, Davies RJ, Turner-Warwick M. Progressive airway obliteration in adults and its association with rheumatoid disease. *Q J Med* 1977;**46**:427–44.

19 Epler GR, Snider GL, Gaensler EA *et al.* Bronchiolitis and bronchitis in connective tissue disease: a possible relationship to the use of penicillamine. *JAMA* 1979;**242**:528–32.

20 Trulock EP, Edwards LB, Taylor DO *et al.* Registry of the International Society for Heart and Lung Transplantation: twenty-second official adult lung and heart-lung transplant report—2005. *J Heart Lung Transplant* 2005;**24**(8):956–67.

21 Estenne M, Hertz MI. Bronchiolitis obliterans after human lung transplantation. *Am J Respir Crit Care Med* 2002;**166**:440–4.

22 Neuringer IP, Chalermskulrat W, Aris R. Obliterative bronchiolitis or chronic lung allograft rejection: a basic science review. *J Heart Lung Transplant* 2005;**24**(1):3–19.

23 Bando K, Paradis IL, Similo S *et al.* Obliterative bronchiolitis after lung and heart–lung transplantation: an analysis of risk factors and management. *J Thorac Cardiovasc Surg* 1995; **110**:4–13.

24 Billings JL, Hertz MI, Savik K, Wendt CH. Respiratory viruses and chronic rejection in lung transplant recipients. *J Heart Lung Transplant* 2002;**21**:559–66.

25 Lau CL, Palmer SM, Howell DN *et al.* Laparoscopic antireflux surgery in the lung transplant population. *Surg Endosc* 2002;**16**:1674–8.

26 Cantu E, 3rd, Appel JZ, 3rd, Hartwig MG *et al.* Early fundoplication prevents chronic allograft dysfunction in patients with gastroesophageal reflux disease. *Ann Thorac Surg* 2004; **78**(4):1142–51.

27 Philit F, Wiesendanger T, Archimbaud E *et al.* Post-transplant obstructive lung disease ('bronchiolitis obliterans'): a clinical comparative study of bone marrow and lung transplant patients. *Eur Respir J* 1995;**8**:551–8.

28 Chien JW, Martin PJ, Gooley TA *et al.* Airflow obstruction after myeloablative allogeneic hematopoietic stem cell transplantation. *Am J Respir Crit Care Med* 2003;**168**:208–14.

29 Colby TV. Bronchiolitis: pathologic considerations. *Am J Clin Pathol* 1998;**109**:101–9.

30 Zhang L, Irion K, Kozakewich H *et al.* Clinical course of postinfectious bronchiolitis obliterans. *Pediatr Pulmonol* 2000;**29**:341–50.

31 Hodges IGC, Milner AD, Groggins RC, Stokes GM. Causes and management of bronchiolitis with chronic obstructive features. *Arch Dis Child* 1982;**57**:495–9.

32 King TE Jr. Respiratory bronchiolitis-associated interstitial lung disease. *Clin Chest Med* 1993;**14**:693–8.

33 Epler GR. Bronchiolitis obliterans organizing pneumonia [Review]. *Semin Respir Infect* 1995;**10**:65–77.

34 Sugiyama Y. Diffuse panbronchiolitis. *Clin Chest Med* 1993; **14**:765–72.

35 Fitzgerald JE, King TE Jr, Lynch DA, Tuder RM, Schwarz MI. Diffuse panbronchiolitis in the United States. *Am J Respir Crit Care Med* 1996;**154**(2 Pt 1):497–503.

36 Bankier AA, Van Muylem A, Knoop C, Estenne M, Gevenois PA. Bronchiolitis obliterans syndrome in heart–lung transplant recipients: diagnosis with expiratory CT. *Radiology* 2001;**218**:533–9.

37 Jensen SP, Lynch DA, Brown KK, Wenzel SE, Newell JD. High-resolution CT features of severe asthma and bronchiolitis obliterans. *Clin Radiol* 2002;**57**:1078–85.

38 Zhang L, Irion K, da Silva Porto N, Abreu e Silva F. High-resolution computed tomography in pediatric patients with postinfectious bronchiolitis obliterans. *J Thorac Imaging* 1999;**14**:85–9.

39 Lynch DA, Brasch RC, Hardy KA, Webb WR. Pediatric pulmonary disease: assessment with high-resolution ultrafast CT. *Radiology* 1990;**176**:243–8.

40 Gerhardt SG, McDyer JF, Girgis RE *et al.* Maintenance azithromycin therapy for bronchiolitis obliterans syndrome: results of a pilot study. *Am J Respir Crit Care Med* 2003;**168**: 121–5.

41 Salerno CT, Park SJ, Kreykes NS *et al.* Adjuvant treatment of refractory lung transplant rejection with extracorporeal photopheresis. *J Thorac Cardiovasc Surg* 1999;**117**:1063–9.

42 Khuu HM, Desmond R, Huang ST, Marques MB. Characteristics of photopheresis treatments for the management of rejection in heart and lung transplant recipients. *J Clin Apheresis* 2002;**17**:27–32.

43 Heaton DC. Failure of thalidomide to control bronchiolitis obliterans post bone marrow transplant. *Bone Marrow Transplant* 1989;**4**:598.

44 Rovelli A, Arrigo C, Nesi F *et al.* The role of thalidomide in the treatment of refractory chronic graft-versus-host disease following bone marrow transplantation in children. *Bone Marrow Transplant* 1998;**21**:577–81.

45 Mehta P, Kedar A, Graham-Pole J, Skoda-Smith S, Wingard JR. Thalidomide in children undergoing bone marrow transplantation: series at a single institution and review of the literature. *Pediatrics* 1999;**103**:E44.

46 Saunders RN, Metcalfe MS, Nicholson ML. Rapamycin in transplantation: a review of the evidence. *Kidney Int* 2001; **59**:3–16.

47 Novick RJ, Stitt LW, Al-Kattan K *et al.* Pulmonary retransplantation: predictors of graft function and survival in 230 patients. Pulmonary Retransplant Registry. *Ann Thorac Surg* 1998;**65**:227–34.

CHAPTER 14

Asthma

Diana C. Grootendorst and Klaus F. Rabe

A major differential diagnosis in patients with COPD is asthma (Fig. 14.1) [1]. Although these diseases are clearly different, in some patients with chronic asthma a clear distinction from COPD is not possible [2], even when history, physical examination, physiology testing and imaging are used. A minority of patients with asthma develop irreversible airflow obstruction and other features of COPD over time [3]. Asthma is assumed to coexist with COPD in these patients and management is highly similar in severe forms of the disease(s) [1]. This chapter presents an overview of the current knowledge on aetiology, pathology, pathogenesis, pathophysiology and treatment of asthma, and discusses the possible (dis)similar pathways underlying asthma and COPD.

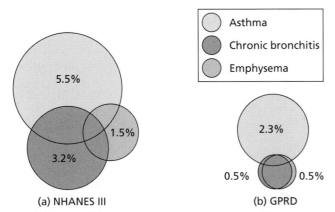

Figure 14.1 Proportional Venn diagram of obstructive lung disease (asthma, chronic bronchitis and emphysema) (a) in the USA (National Health and Nutrition Examination Survey [NHANES] III surveys from 1988 to 1994) and (b) in the UK (UK General Practices Research Database [GPRD] in 1998) for all ages. (From Soriano *et al.* [164] with permission.)

Definition

Asthma is a chronic inflammatory disease of the airways, characterized by variable airflow obstruction and bronchial hyperresponsiveness to a variety of stimuli. Symptoms of asthma include episodes of wheeze, breathlessness, chest tightness and cough, particularly at night and/or in the early morning [4]. Usually, the airflow limitation observed in asthma is (at least partly) reversible either spontaneously or following treatment [4].

Diagnosis

The clinical diagnosis of asthma is usually prompted by symptoms such as episodic breathlessness, wheezing, chest tightness and cough. These are often more pronounced at night and in the early hours of the morning [4]. Although the diagnosis of asthma can be made on the basis of symptoms alone, the accuracy is improved when objectified by lung function measurements, including the assessment of airflow limitation together with the reversibility and variability of airflow limitation.

Measurement of the forced expiratory volume in 1 second (FEV_1) and forced vital capacity (FVC) by flow–volume curves is used for the assessment of airflow limitation [5]. FEV_1 and FVC values below 80% of the reference value are usually considered as abnormal [5]. In addition, when FEV_1 normalized for FVC ($FEV_1 : FVC$) is below 75%, this is indicative or airflow limitation or airways obstruction.

Variability in airflow limitation is most frequently tested by measuring the response of FEV_1 to an inhaled bronchodilator such as the β_2-agonist salbutamol [5]. An improvement in FEV_1 and/or FVC following the administration of a bronchodilator by more than 12% predicted and 200 mL or in peak expiratory flow rate by more than

60 L/min is considered an unambiguous bronchodilator response [5], fitting in with the diagnosis of asthma. Even in the absence of a bronchodilator response, the airflow limitation can be reversible after a short course of prednisolone [4]. In addition to reversibility testing, daily recording of the peak expiratory flow rate can be used to assess (daily) variability in lung function. Daily variability in peak expiratory flow rate > 20% is usually considered as a sign of unstable asthma, requiring a change in treatment [4].

Variable airways obstruction can be mimicked in the lung function laboratory by challenge tests with bronchoconstrictive stimuli such as histamine or methacholine [6]. In subjects with airways hyperresponsiveness, an exaggerated response to the bronchoconstrictor can be observed. The response to a bronchoconstrictor is usually expressed as the provocative dose or concentration of bronchoconstrictor causing a fall in FEV_1 of > 20% from baseline (PD_{20} or PC_{20}). In normal subjects, the PC_{20} is > 8 mg/mL ($PD_{20} > 7.8$ µmol) of histamine or methacholine.

Having a bronchodilator response or airways hyperresponsiveness is considered to be indicative for asthma. However, absence of these features does not exclude the possibility of asthma. Furthermore, each of these features can also be present in patients with COPD [7]. Other patient characteristics, such as the presence of atopy or a positive smoking status or history, are helpful to increase or decrease the diagnostic probability for asthma instead of COPD.

Epidemiology

Bronchial asthma is one of the most common chronic diseases in high-income countries, affecting over 100 million people [4]. Reported prevalence rates for asthma show a wide variation. In adults, the prevalence of symptoms of wheeze varies from 4.1 to 32.0%, whereas the prevalence of diagnosis of current asthma varies between 2.0 and 11.9% [8]. The international patterns in asthma prevalence show that prevalences are highest among English-speaking countries (UK, New Zealand, Australia, USA and Canada) and Western Europe, and much lower in Eastern and Southern Europe [9]. During the last decades, not only the prevalence and but also the severity of asthma has increased [10,11]. Recent studies, however, show trends for a plateau in the prevalence of asthma [12].

Aetiology

Several risk factors for the development of asthma have been described. The strongest predisposing factor associated with the development of asthma, and in particular childhood-onset asthma, is atopy [4]. Approximately 50% of asthma cases are attributable to atopic sensitization [13].

Atopic sensitization

Up to 90% of children with asthma are sensitized to common airborne allergens such as domestic mites, furred animals, fungi and pollens [14]. In particular, sensitization to house dust mite [15], *Alternaria* [16] and cockroach [17] has been shown to be associated with an increased risk for asthma in children. The relation between *level* of exposure and *development* of asthma is far from clear and seems rather controversial. In one study, the risk for the development of asthma in house dust mite sensitized children doubled with every doubling of indoor house dust mite level [18], although this dose–response relation was not confirmed in another large study [19]. Furthermore, being allergic to cat dander is a risk factor for the development of asthma, but having a cat in the house may be protective for the development of asthma [20]. Several studies have also suggested a relation between *level* of exposure to allergens and *severity* of asthma. First, patients with severe asthma are exposed to higher levels of domestic allergens to which they are sensitized, compared with patients with mild asthma [21,22]. In addition, sensitization to the moulds *Alternaria alternata* and *Cladosporium herbarum* occurs more frequently in patients with severe asthma, while this is not the case for sensitization to grass and tree pollens [23]. Secondly, seasonal variation in, for instance, house dust mites is associated with changes in peak expiratory flow rates [24] and airways hyperresponsiveness [25]. Taken together, these studies show that allergic sensitization is not only an important precursor of developing asthma, but also is associated with severity of the disease.

Genetic predisposition

In addition to atopic sensitization, asthma, which develops during childhood, has a clear genetic component [4]. Children from allergic and/or asthmatic parents have an increased risk for asthma [26,27]. Several gene loci have been linked to atopy and asthma, including chromosome 5q31 (IgE), chromosome 5q31–33 (multiple genes modulating atopic responses: IL-4, IL-13, IL-5, CD14 and GM-CSF), major histocompatibility complex region on chromosome 6, several genes on chromosome 7 (atopy, asthma and eosinophilia), chromosome 11q13 (atopy, high affinity receptor for IgE), chromosome 13q (atopy), chromosome 14, chromosome 16 [28] and the ADAM33 gene on chromosome 20p13 [29]. Genetic background and environment may interact in the development of asthma: high levels of cat allergen in the house are associated with a reduced risk of wheezing in childhood in children from mothers with no history of asthma, whereas this is related to an increased risk for wheezing in children from mothers with a history of asthma [30].

Socioeconomic status

Another important determinant of childhood asthma may be socioeconomic status. Recently, it has been shown that the increase in incidence of asthma is driven by factors associated with improved social circumstances (higher income and education of parents, less unemployment, welfare and overcrowding), whereas severity of asthma is related to factors associated with poverty [31].

Late-onset asthma

In asthma that starts later in life, the role of atopy is less clear. The prevalence of being non-atopic is higher in adult-onset asthma than in childhood-onset asthma, and prevalences of atopy ranging from 25–30% [32] to more than 60% [33] have been described in adult-onset asthmatics. Non-atopic adult-onset asthma is known to have a more severe clinical presentation and to be less responsive to standard therapy [34]. This type of asthma may also be associated with the rapid development of persistent airflow limitation [35], indicating a worse prognosis when compared with childhood asthma. As such, late-onset asthma may be more difficult to distinguish from COPD. Factors implicated in causing adult-onset asthma include aspirin sensitivity [36], rhinitis and chronic sinusitis [37], occupational exposure to chemicals [38], exposure to fungi on the skin and nails [39], and persistent infection with respiratory pathogens [40].

Pathology

The pathology underlying the clinical presentation of both asthma and COPD is chronic inflammation of the airways [41,42]. However, even in patients with comparable fixed airflow obstruction, patients with a history of asthma have distinct pathological characteristics compared with those with COPD (see Plate 14.1; colour plate section falls between pp. 354 and 355) [2].

In general, the inflammatory infiltrate in the airway wall mucosa of patients with asthma (mainly) consists of eosinophils, mast cells and lymphocytes [43]. These features can even be found in subjects with newly diagnosed asthma [44]. Interestingly, lymphocytic and mast cell inflammation seems to be associated specifically with childhood-onset asthma, and not with late-onset asthma [45].

In patients with severe asthma, increased neutrophil numbers have been found in the lamina propria [46].

Moreover, an increase in neutrophils in the submucosa has also been implicated in sudden-onset, fatal attacks of asthma [47]. Other pathological changes of the airways that have been described in association with asthma include loss of epithelial integrity [48], smooth muscle hypertrophy and hyperplasia [49], changes in the vasculature including neovascularization, dilation and leakage [50], and thickening of the reticular layer beneath the basement membrane [48]. In patients with late-onset asthma without eosinophilia in the airways, however, subepithelial basement membrane thickening is not present, suggesting a different pathological process in these patients [45].

In addition to inflammation in airway tissue, changes in cellular infiltrate in the airway lumen are present in patients with asthma. As in bronchial biopsies, an increase in eosinophils and mast cells characterizes the inflammatory infiltrate in both bronchoalveolar lavage fluid [51,52] and induced sputum [53], with an additional increase in sputum neutrophil numbers in patients with severe asthma [54]. Furthermore, an increase in a variety of cytokines, chemokines and markers of microvascular leakage can be found in the sputum of patients with asthma, including eosinophil cationic protein (ECP), fibrinogen, albumin and interleukin 8 (IL-8) [55,56].

Pathogenesis

How do each of these factors interact and contribute to clinical asthma? It is clear that the presence of both host and environmental factors are needed for the transition from sensitization alone to allergic asthma. According to current concepts, these include dysregulation of immunological control mechanisms within the airway mucosa, and a series of environmental factors [57,58].

Initial priming of T helper (Th) cells against environmental allergens occurs *in utero*, presumably by means of transplacental transport of allergens to which the mother is exposed during pregnancy [59]. Cord blood mononuclear cells of all infants produce high levels of the Th2 cytokines IL-4 and IL-5, and low levels of γ-interferon (IFN-γ), upon stimulation of cells by house dust mite allergen. During the first year of life of non-atopic children, there is rapid suppression of these Th2 responses, with skewing towards the Th1 phenotype (high expression of IFN-γ and low expression of IL-4 and IL-5) [60]. However, in potentially atopic children, Th2 responses are consolidated, which appears to be associated with a defective neonatal IFN-γ response [60]. During this postnatal period, environmental exposures appear to be important. Exposure to high levels of microbial products reduces the risk for atopy and asthma [61]. Furthermore, exposure to dietary allergens in early childhood leads to negative regulation of Th responses via

T-cell anergy and/or deletion [57]. In contrast, postnatal exposure to inhalant allergens results in redirection towards the Th1 profile in non-atopics or in further boosting of the fetally primed Th2 response in potential atopic children [57].

Still, only a subset of subjects who are sensitized during childhood develop severe long-term sequelae [62]. An important feature appears to be the (dysregulation of) Th1–Th2 cell balance [63]. Recently, it has been shown that atopic asthmatic patients with severe persistent disease have a reduced allergen-induced Th1 response, whereas those subjects with resolved asthma do not. On the other hand, subjects with a history of asthma have increased house dust mite induced Th2 cytokine responses, irrespective of the presence or absence of ongoing asthma. These observations suggest that impaired house dust mite induced IFN-γ production might be an important factor contributing to ongoing severe asthma, whereas increased IL-5 and IL-13 production by Th2 cells upon allergen stimulation reflects the presence of the atopic state per se rather than being specifically linked to ongoing asthma [63]. In other words, this may imply that an exaggerated Th2 response induces atopy, whereas impairment in the Th1 response contributes to the severity of the disease.

Once high levels of Th2-mediated inflammation are manifest, airway remodelling may occur [57,58]. In atopic asthmatic subjects, the 'inappropriate' Th2 response may cause pulmonary inflammation, airway eosinophilia, mucus hypersecretion and airways hyperresponsiveness to a variety of specific and non-specific stimuli, and together result in the symptoms of asthma [64]. Notably, when considering those patients with early-onset asthma, the earlier in life sensitization develops, the more likely they are to have persistent wheeze at an adult age [65], and the more severe are the long-term consequences including wheeze [66,67] and bronchial hyperresponsiveness [67]. Nevertheless, overall, patients with late-onset asthma have more severe asthma than those with early-onset disease.

A central part in the transition from atopy to allergic asthma appears to be played by the airway epithelium, which is in a key position to translate gene–environment interactions [68]. It has been postulated that, in asthma, the airway epithelium has enhanced susceptibility to injury or an inadequate repair response, or a combination of both. As a consequence, the epithelium maintains a 'repair phenotype', which is responsible for increased production of pro-inflammatory mediators and pro-fibrinogenic growth factors [68]. For instance, activated epithelium releases transforming growth factor β2 (TGF-β2), which activates myofibroblasts under the epithelium to secrete matrix proteins, and smooth muscle and vascular mitogens [69]. Together, these processes may result in the airway remodelling that is characteristic in asthma and involves epithelial shedding, sub-basement membrane thickening, smooth muscle hyperplasia and an increase in nerves and blood vessels [70].

Pathophysiology

What are the consequences of inflammation and airway remodelling on airway physiology? The two predominant manifestations of disordered lung function in asthma are airways hyperresponsiveness and airflow limitation [4].

Subjects with asthma can have an exaggerated bronchoconstrictor response to a wide variety of stimuli such as allergen, exercise, cold air, fumes and chemicals [4]. Typically, in subjects with asthma, the dose–response curve to bronchoconstrictor stimuli is characterized by increased sensitivity, reactivity and maximal response plateau [71]. Several factors may contribute to the development and/or worsening of hyperresponsiveness. As such, reduced airway calibre, increased smooth muscle contractility, dysfunctional neural regulation, altered permeability of the bronchial mucosa, pro-inflammatory humoral and cellular mediators, and cytokines including granulocyte–macrophage colony-stimulating factor (GM-CSF) and tumour necrosis factor α (TNF-α) have been discussed as critical for bronchial hyperresponsiveness [70].

Many factors contribute to airway narrowing in asthma, including contraction of airway smooth muscle, swelling of the airways as a result of oedema, mucus plug formation and airway wall remodelling [4]. In most subjects with asthma, these features appear to be variable, as reflected in day-to-day variation in lung function which is reversible either spontaneously or upon treatment with bronchodilators and/or anti-inflammatory agents [4,70]. In some subjects, the airflow limitation is not reversible, which seems more prominent in patients with severe asthma [72].

In addition to hyperresponsiveness and airflow limitation, it has been hypothesized that destruction and subsequent remodelling of the airways in asthma is also associated with an accelerated decline in lung function. Accelerated decline in lung function is an important feature of COPD, again underlining the parallels between the two diseases. Interestingly, in patients with persistent asthma followed prospectively, the number of CD8+ T lymphocytes in the lamina propria of bronchial biopsies is associated with the subsequent decline in FEV_1 [73]. This is of interest because CD8+ T lymphocytes were thought to be important, particularly in COPD patients. Furthermore, it has been demonstrated that subjects with self-reported asthma have a greater decline in FEV_1 over time than those without asthma [74]. Risk factors that further seem to worsen the yearly decline in FEV_1 are airflow limitation [75], bronchial hyperresponsiveness [74,76] and adult-onset asthma [77].

It should not be forgotten that in patients with asthma, smoking is a risk factor for an increased decline in lung function [74], as is the case in COPD. The influence of atopy on the rate of decline in FEV_1 is unclear, as some studies have shown no effect of atopic status [75,76], while others report a steeper decline in atopics [78], or a steeper decline in non-atopic asthmatics [77,79].

A new concept in the understanding of airway narrowing and bronchial hyperresponsiveness is perturbed myosin binding within airway smooth muscle [80,81]. According to this concept, the binding of myosin to actin, within the smooth muscle cell, is perturbed with each breath in healthy individuals. As a consequence, the number of bridges between actin and myosin are low, and the rate of turnover of actin–myosin bridges is high. In subjects with asthma, the cytokine-driven thickening of the airway wall that is associated with remodelling is thought to uncouple the load fluctuations of each breath from the muscle [82]. This allows an unperturbed binding equilibrium of myosin to actin. In this state, there are many links between myosin and actin that cycle very slowly, resulting in a static condition of the smooth muscle, also called latch [80,81]. The unperturbed myosin-binding concept can be used to explain the airways obstruction, excessive airway narrowing and bronchial hyperresponsiveness as is seen in clinical asthma.

Relations between airway inflammation and severity of asthma

It is evident that airways inflammation has a central role in asthma. Several studies have demonstrated that the severity of asthma is related to the degree of airways inflammation. Eosinophil and neutrophil numbers in sputum increase significantly over the spectrum from intermittent to severe persistent asthma [54,83,84]. Fibroblast accumulation and airway smooth muscle hypertrophy are specific characteristics of severe asthma, as opposed to mild asthma [85]. In particular, airways hyperresponsiveness is associated with the cellular infiltrate; with mast cells, CD8[+] T lymphocytes and eosinophils within the lamina propria [86], but also eosinophil numbers in sputum [87,88] showing an inverse correlation with PC_{20}. Furthermore, increased sputum eosinophils are also associated with more pronounced exercise-induced bronchoconstriction [89] and lower lung function [87]. In patients with persistent asthma, the level of airflow limitation is inversely related to the number of eosinophils [35] and neutrophils in induced sputum [90]. Finally, exacerbations of asthma are associated with a further increase in eosinophils [91] and/or neutrophils in sputum [92] and sputum eosinophils can even be predictive of an exacerbation [93–95].

The associations between degree of inflammation and severity of asthma are usually weak and show a large variation. Nevertheless, these associations indicate that patients with more severe or unstable asthma, as characterized by increased bronchial hyperresponsiveness to various stimuli, airflow limitation and/or exacerbations, have more pronounced airway inflammation.

Different phenotypes of asthma

Clearly, asthma is a heterogeneous disease and different phenotypes within this disease have been recognized. Important and distinct phenotypes of asthma that may have an important role in the differential diagnosis of COPD include non-allergic asthma and/or late-onset or adult-onset asthma. These two phenotypes of asthma have an important overlap because the majority of patients with late-onset asthma are non-atopic [33].

Non-allergic patients with asthma have a negative skin prick test and score negative for allergen-specific IgEs in a radioallersorbent test (RAST). Asthma in non-atopic individuals has been associated with risk factors such as older age, female sex, sinonasal polyposis, late onset of asthma, FEV_1 below 80% predicted, lower socioeconomic class, smoking, urban location [96–98] and with a polymorphism in the RANTES gene promoter region [99].

In non-allergic subjects with asthma, a steeper decline in FEV_1 has been described [77,100], which seems associated with a (history of a) high degree of reversibility in FEV_1 [100]. As such, non-atopic asthma seems distinctly different from atopic asthma, because in atopics not reversibility in FEV_1 but rather the degree of airways obstruction (FEV_1 : FVC) together with need for treatment with oral corticosteroids are associated with a more pronounced and progressive decline in FEV_1 [100]. Again, these studies underline that those patients with non-allergic asthma are the most difficult to distinguish from COPD.

In addition to this, the pathology in the airways is different between allergic and non-allergic asthmatics: eosinophil and mast cell numbers in the lamina propria of bronchial biopsies are increased both in atopic and non-atopic asthmatics, although eosinophil numbers are significantly more increased in atopic asthmatics. Furthermore, neutrophil numbers are increased in non-atopic asthmatics whereas CD3, CD4, CD8 and CD25 positive T lymphocytes are increased in biopsy specimens from atopic asthmatics only [101]. Also, cytokine expression is different between the two phenotypes, with IL-4 and IL-5 being expressed in airway tissue from atopic asthmatics and IL-8 in non-atopic patients with asthma [101]. The mechanism by which T cells are activated in non-atopic asthma, where no causative antigen is identified, is not fully understood.

Recently, an *ex vivo* study demonstrated that T cells infiltrating in the lower airways of non-atopic patients with asthma recognize relatively limited epitopes of antigens and are clonally expanded by antigen-driven stimulation [102], which may, at least in part, explain cellular activation pathways in non-atopic asthma.

Asthma as risk factor for COPD

Recent studies show that asthma, in some patients, is a risk factor for the development of COPD [103]. In addition, the presence of 'asthmatic features', including bronchial hyperresponsiveness and IgE, are significant predictors of the rate of FEV_1 decline in patients with COPD [104]. These studies are in line with the 'Dutch Hypothesis' from the early 1960s, stating that asthma and COPD should be considered as different expressions of one disease entity, in which both endogenous (host) and exogenous (environmental) factors have a role in the pathogenesis [105]. According to this hypothesis, the phenotype of the patient (i.e. clinical expression of asthma or COPD) is the result of a combination of genetic and environmental factors, modulated by age and sex.

Primary prevention

In view of the increasing prevalence of asthma and allergic diseases, primary prevention in at-risk infants is a public health priority. Several risk factors have been identified with potential for primary prevention of asthma, of which the most important is indoor allergen avoidance [106]. Recently, it was shown by Koopman *et al.* [107] that when house dust mite impermeable mattress encasings are applied to the beds of atopic, expecting parents and of the infant, there is a 35% risk reduction for cough at night at the age of 2 years. When indoor allergen avoidance measures are extended (the combination of mattress and pillow encasings, use of high filtration vacuum cleaner, removing wall-to-wall carpets from the bedroom, and chemical cleaning of carpets and soft furnishings), there is a 50–80% risk reduction for the infant to wheeze at the age of 1 year [108]. Interestingly, in genetically at-risk children, such interventions, when combined with breastfeeding during infancy, may reduce the risk for current wheeze, nocturnal cough, asthma and atopy by approximately 80% [109]. Further follow-up of these cohorts of children is needed to determine the effect of the interventions on the development of atopic disease, including asthma.

Several reports have suggested that exposure to environmental endotoxin might prevent the development of atopy and asthma [61,110,111]. Remarkably, in farm children who are frequently exposed to dust in stables and consume raw milk, both of which contain high levels of endotoxin, there is a very low prevalence of asthma, hay fever and atopic sensitization [61,110]. This may be explained by the fact that endotoxins reduce IgE production, Th2 cytokine production and airway eosinophilia [112].

A number of other environmental factors are known to be associated with a lower incidence of allergic diseases early in life. Oral supplementation with *Lactobacillus rhamnosus* (probiotics) during pregnancy and breastfeeding [113,114], the presence, from birth onward, of a furred pet in the home [115], and attendance at day care during the first year of life [116] are all environmental factors that protect against the development of allergies and asthma in childhood. Furthermore, active immunoprophylaxis [114,117,118] and anthroposophic lifestyle [119] have been associated with lower prevalence of allergies and asthma.

The role of breastfeeding in the prevention of atopy and asthma is controversial. Some studies show a protective effect of exclusive breastfeeding during the first 4 months of life for atopy and asthma during childhood [120], while this is associated with an increased risk for allergies and asthma during adulthood [121]. A suggested explanation for this complex relation might be that breastfeeding reduces the effect of bacteria and endotoxins on the immune system, either by direct reduction of exposure or by passive transfer of immune responses from the mother. This may lead to incomplete development of mature immune response mechanisms in the infant, resulting in a lower prevalence of atopy and asthma early in life, and a reversed trend in adulthood [121].

In addition to these issues, smoking (during pregnancy) clearly has an effect on fetal growth and preterm delivery [122]. More importantly, a lower birth weight is associated with worse lung function at adult age, and with death from chronic obstructive airways disease [123]. Furthermore, smoking has been identified as a risk factor for the development of persistent asthma later in life [124]. As such, cessation of smoking by pregnant mothers should be considered as primary prevention of both asthma and COPD.

Current treatment

Treatment of asthma consists of two parts: first, avoidance of the sensitizing trigger and, secondly, pharmacological treatment.

Avoidance of allergen exposure is an integral part of the management of atopic asthmatic patients [4,125]. Effectiveness of avoidance measures was first demonstrated in patients with atopic asthma moving to a low allergenic environment at high altitude, resulting in large improvements in clinical outcomes [126–128]. Measures aimed at reducing indoor allergen levels, including house dust mite impermeable mattress and/or pillow covers, and chemical approaches, are much more practical. However, conflicting data on the effectiveness of such allergen avoidance have been reported [129,130].

At present, pharmacological treatment of asthma aims at reducing symptoms and optimizing lung function [4]. In most patients, daily treatment with inhaled corticosteroids with or without the addition of long- and/or short-acting β_2-agonists is sufficient to obtain control of asthma [4,125].

In asthmatic patients, treatment with inhaled corticosteroids improves lung function and bronchial hyperresponsiveness, and reduces eosinophil numbers in induced sputum [131–133], even at very low doses of inhaled steroids [134]. Furthermore, the exacerbation rate is reduced during treatment with inhaled corticosteroid treatment [135]. These changes are accompanied by a decrease in mucosal mast cells, eosinophils and T lymphocytes [136], a reduction in reticular layer thickness [137] and in submucosal vascularity [138]. During treatment with long-acting bronchodilators alone, lung function improves, but inflammatory parameters in sputum remain unchanged [139]. However, the combination of inhaled steroids with long-acting bronchodilators is very effective and widely recommended for treatment of persistent asthma [4].

Patients at the severe end of the spectrum may still have recurrent exacerbations and non-optimal control of their disease, despite treatment with inhaled steroids and (long-acting) bronchodilators. Addition of theophylline, oral corticosteroids and/or leukotriene receptor antagonists is optional and may improve disease outcomes in these patients [4]. Nevertheless, novel treatments are needed for the management of severe disease. At present, many different specific anticytokine treatments are being developed for the indication of persistent asthma [140,141], but these seem to have limited clinical effect. Among the few effective novel therapies for severe allergic asthma is treatment with antibodies directed against IgE [142].

Finally, an integral part of the treatment of persistent asthma (as in COPD) should always be smoking cessation. Several studies have demonstrated that smokers with chronic asthma have a reduced response to corticosteroid therapy [143,144], requiring higher doses of corticosteroids to obtain clinical control. Patients with COPD show a form of steroid resistance, which appears to be caused by decreased histone deacetylase activity [145]. Such a decrease in histone deacetylase activity allows a pro-inflammatory state, as is seen in COPD. It has been hypothesized that histone deacetylase activity in COPD is impaired by cigarette smoking and oxidative stress, and that this leads to a pronounced reduction in the responsiveness to corticosteroids [146]. This mechanism may also have a role in steroid insensitivity in smoking asthmatics. Together,

this underlines the importance of smoking cessation in both asthma and COPD.

Limitations of current treatment

Surveys investigating clinical management of asthma globally have shown that asthma control is suboptimal for many patients despite the availability of effective therapies [147]. In part, this is because of lack of compliance to prescribed therapy [148], which in turn may be caused by lack of patient education [148] and difficulties with inhaler devices [4]. An additional finding of these surveys was that education of treating physicians may be suboptimal and could be improved [149].

Current guidelines state that treatment of patients should be aimed at reducing symptoms and optimizing lung function [4]. However, in patients with 'controlled' asthma, the disease management can be improved if treatment is aimed at additional outcomes. For instance, when reducing airways hyperresponsiveness is included in the treatment algorithm, patients have fewer exacerbations of asthma, better FEV_1, and a reduction in mast cell numbers and reticular layer thickness in bronchial biopsies when compared with the patients who are treated by the conventional treatment strategy [150]. In addition, inclusion of normalizing sputum eosinophilia in the treatment algorithm results in a reduction in sputum eosinophil count and bronchial hyperresponsiveness, together with a 70% reduction in exacerbation rate [151]. Together, this suggests that monitoring of (markers of) inflammation, in addition to symptoms and lung function, improves the long-term management and control of asthma. More importantly, these studies imply that the current treatment regimens are far from optimal, leaving room for further clinical improvement. In COPD, studies aiming treatment at outcomes other than those conventionally included (symptoms and lung function) has not yet been performed and, intuitively, seem more difficult.

Asthma versus COPD

As reflected in this and previous chapters, both asthma and COPD can (in general) be described as airways diseases that are characterized by airflow limitation and chronic persistent airways inflammation [1,4]. Otherwise, however, the two airways diseases are distinctly different (Table 14.1). The main cause of asthma is atopic sensitization to (inhalant) allergens, while that in COPD is tobacco smoking [152], although a sizable proportion of asthmatics are non-atopic and smoke. Both diseases have a genetic component, albeit at different genetic locations [153]. The pathological findings implicated in asthma consist of increased influx of eosinophils, mast cells and CD4$^+$ T lymphocytes, whereas

Table 14.1 Similarities and differences between asthma and COPD.

	Asthma	**COPD**
Aetiology		
Environmental	Atopic sensitization	Tobacco smoke
Genetic	+	+
Symptoms	Episodic wheeze	Dyspnoea upon exertion
	Breathlessness	Sputum production
	Chest tightness	Cough
	Cough	
Airflow limitation	+	+
Bronchodilator response	+	−
Bronchial hyperresponsiveness	+	+/−
Airways inflammation	+	+
Biopsies	Eosinophils	Macrophages
	Mast cells	Mast cells
	CD4$^+$ T lymphocytes	CD8$^+$ T lymphocytes
Sputum	Eosinophils	Neutrophils
Exacerbation	Neutrophils	Eosinophils
Restructuring airways	+	+
Destruction parenchyma	−	+
Steroid responsiveness	+	−
Main limits of current treatment	Severe asthma	Across all severity groups

in COPD this is characterized by macrophages, mast cells and CD8$^+$ T lymphocytes [154,155]. During stable disease, the sputum of patients with asthma is characterized by eosinophilia, with an additional increase in neutrophils during exacerbation of the disease. COPD is characterized by massive influx of neutrophils within the airway lumen [156]. The physiological abnormalities seen in asthma are bronchial hyperresponsiveness and reversible airflow limitation as opposed to the progressive, irreversible airflow limitation seen in patients with COPD [1]. Furthermore, the mechanisms underlying airflow limitation are different for asthma and COPD. Primary prevention can be achieved in both diseases by avoidance of the trigger: sensitizing allergens in asthma, tobacco smoke in COPD [1]. At present, treatment of both asthma and COPD consists of trigger avoidance and pharmacological intervention. Patients with asthma can achieve trigger avoidance mainly by reducing the indoor allergen load; in patients with COPD this is smoking cessation [1,157]. However, in patients with asthma, smoking cessation is also an important issue. Pharmacological options of asthma and COPD are essentially the same. All interventions aim at reducing or preventing symptoms and consist of inhaled bronchodilators in combination with corticosteroids [1]. However, for milder forms of disease the approaches are markedly different: a patient with asthma who has few symptoms may be of particular concern as symptoms may be underestimated. On the other hand, the current concept for COPD would suggest that a patient with this disease and no symptoms

should not be treated at all. Furthermore, the benefits of treatments, for example with the combination of inhaled steroids and bronchodilators, are markedly different for asthma and COPD. Following inhalation of bronchodilators, a bronchodilator response can be demonstrated in patients with asthma, which is usually absent in patients with COPD. Furthermore, lung function, bronchial hyperresponsiveness and eosinophilia improve upon inhaled corticosteroid therapy in asthmatics. In contrast, neither lung function [158–160] nor airway inflammation [161–163] is affected by inhaled corticosteroid therapy in patients with COPD.

Conclusions

Given the increasing prevalence of and morbidity from asthma and COPD, and the increasing costs of treatment, it is becoming more important to tailor treatment to individuals. In patients with asthma, current pharmacological treatment in general is effective, but there is room for improvement in the subset of patients who suffer from severe asthma and in those who do not use or receive adequate treatment. However, current pharmacological treatments have real but limited benefits in patients with COPD and none of the drugs available influence the accelerated loss of lung function observed in these patients. Novel drugs are needed for the treatment of patients with severe asthma and patients with COPD, in order to improve the long-term outcome of disease in these patients. Finally, physicians need to differentiate, wherever possible, between asthma and COPD in order to tailor treatment more accurately. This is more difficult in more advanced forms of asthma and COPD.

References

1 Global Initiative for Chronic Obstructive Lung Disease. Global strategy for the diagnosis, management, and prevention of chronic obstructive pulmonary disease. NHLBI/WHO Workshop Report. NIH Publication Number 2701, 2001. (www.goldcopd.com)

2 Fabbri LM, Romagnoli M, Corbetta L et al. Differences in airway inflammation in patients with fixed airflow obstruction due to asthma or chronic obstructive pulmonary disease. *Am J Respir Crit Care Med* 2003;**167**:418–24.

3 Vonk JM, Jongepier H, Panhuysen CI et al. Risk factors associated with the presence of irreversible airflow limitation and reduced transfer coefficient in patients with asthma after 26 years of follow up. *Thorax* 2003;**58**:322–7.

4 Global Initiative for Asthma. Global strategy for asthma management and prevention. NHLBI/WHO Workshop Report. NIH Publication Number 02-3659, 2002. Revised version. (www.ginasthma.com)

5 Quanjer P, Tammeling GJ, Cotes JE et al. Lung volumes and forced ventilatory flows. *Eur Respir J* 1993;**6**(Suppl 16):5–40.

6 Sterk PJ, Fabbri LM, Quanjer P et al. Airway responsiveness: standardized challenge testing with pharmacological, physical and sensitizing stimuli in adults. *Eur Respir J* 1993;**6** (Suppl 16):53–83.

7 Grootendorst DC, Rabe KF. Mechanisms of bronchial hyperreactivity in asthma and chronic obstructive pulmonary disease. *Proc Am Thorac Soc* 2004;**1**:77–87.

8 Janson C, Anto J, Burney P et al. The European Community Respiratory Health Survey: what are the main results so far? European Community Respiratory Health Survey II. *Eur Respir J* 2001;**18**:598–611.

9 Pearce N, Sunyer J, Cheng S et al. Comparison of asthma prevalence in the ISAAC and the ECRHS. ISAAC Steering Committee and the European Community Respiratory Health Survey. International Study of Asthma and Allergies in Childhood. *Eur Respir J* 2000;**16**:420–6.

10 Beasley R, Crane J, Lai CK, Pearce N. Prevalence and etiology of asthma. *J Allergy Clin Immunol* 2000;**105**:S466–72.

11 Wieringa MH, Vermeire PA, Brunekreef B, Weyler JJ. Increased occurrence of asthma and allergy: critical appraisal of studies using allergic sensitization, bronchial hyper-responsiveness and lung function measurements. *Clin Exp Allergy* 2001;**31**:1553–63.

12 Toelle BG, Ng K, Belousova E et al. Prevalence of asthma and allergy in schoolchildren in Belmont, Australia: three cross-sectional surveys over 20 years. *BMJ* 2004;**328**:386–7.

13 Pearce N, Pekkanen J, Beasley R. How much asthma is really attributable to atopy? *Thorax* 1999;**54**:268–72.

14 Warner JO, Naspitz CK, Cropp G. Third international pediatric consensus statement on the management of childhood asthma. *Pediatr Pulmonol* 1998;**25**:1–17.

15 Sporik R, Holgate ST, Platts-Mills T, Cogswell JJ. Exposure to house-dust mite allergen (Der p I) and the development of asthma in childhood: a prospective study. *N Engl J Med* 1990;**323**:502–7.

16 Halonen M, Stern DA, Wright AL, Taussig LM, Martinez FD. *Alternaria* as a major allergen for asthma in children raised in a desert environment. *Am J Respir Crit Care Med* 1997; **155**:1356–61.

17 Rosenstreich DL, Eggleston P, Kattan M et al. The role of cockroach allergy and exposure to cockroach allergen in causing morbidity among inner-city children with asthma. *N Engl J Med* 1997;**336**:1356–63.

18 Peat JK, Tovey E, Toelle BG et al. House dust mite allergens: a major risk factor for childhood asthma in Australia. *Am J Respir Crit Care Med* 1996;**153**:141–6.

19 Lau S, Illi S, Sommerfeld C et al. Early exposure to house-dust mite and cat allergens and development of childhood asthma: a cohort study. Multicentre Allergy Study Group. *Lancet* 2000;**356**:1392–7.

20 Perzanowski MS, Ronmark E, Platts-Mills TA, Lundback B. Effect of cat and dog ownership on sensitization and development of asthma among preteenage children. *Am J Respir Crit Care Med* 2002;**166**:696–702.

21 Custovic A, Taggert S, Francis HC, Chapman MD, Woodcock A. Exposure to house dust mite allergens and the clinical activity of asthma. *J Allergy Clin Immunol* 1996;**98**:64–72.

22 Langley SJ, Goldthorpe S, Craven M et al. Exposure and sensitization to indoor allergens: association with lung function, bronchial reactivity, and exhaled nitric oxide measures in asthma. *J Allergy Clin Immunol* 2003;**112**:362–8.

23 Zureik M, Neukirch C, Leynaert B et al. Sensitisation to airborne moulds and severity of asthma: cross-sectional study from European Community respiratory health survey. *BMJ* 2002;**325**:411.

24 Meijer GG, Postma DS, van der Heide S et al. Seasonal variations in house dust mite influence the circadian peak expiratory flow amplitude. *Am J Respir Crit Care Med* 1996; **154**:881–4.

25 van der Heide S, De Monchy J, de Vries K, Bruggink TM, Kauffman HF. Seasonal variation in airway hyperresponsiveness and natural exposure to house dust mite allergens in patients with asthma. *J Allergy Clin Immunol* 1994;**93**: 470–5.

26 London SJ, James GW, Avol E, Rappaport EB, Peters JM. Family history and the risk of early-onset persistent, early-onset transient, and late-onset asthma. *Epidemiology* 2001; **12**:577–83.

27 Xuan W, Marks GB, Toelle BG et al. Risk factors for onset and remission of atopy, wheeze, and airway hyperresponsiveness. *Thorax* 2002;**57**:104–9.

28 Hakonarson H, Wjst M. Current concepts on the genetics of asthma. *Curr Opin Pediatr* 2001;**13**:267–77.

29 Van Eerdewegh P, Little RD, Dupuis J et al. Association of the ADAM33 gene with asthma and bronchial hyper-responsiveness. *Nature* 2002;**418**:426–30.

30 Celedon JC, Litonjua AA, Ryan L et al. Exposure to cat allergen, maternal history of asthma, and wheezing in first 5 years of life. *Lancet* 2002;**360**:781–2.

31 Poyser MA, Nelson H, Ehrlich RI et al. Socioeconomic

deprivation and asthma prevalence and severity in young adolescents. *Eur Respir J* 2002;**19**:892–8.

32 Segala C, Priol G, Soussan D *et al.* Asthma in adults: comparison of adult-onset asthma with childhood-onset asthma relapsing in adulthood. *Allergy* 2000;**55**:634–40.

33 Burrows B, Martinez FD, Halonen M, Barbee RA, Cline MG. Association of asthma with serum IgE levels and skin-test reactivity to allergens. *N Engl J Med* 1989;**320**:271–7.

34 Rackemann FM. A working classification of asthma. *Am J Med* 1947;**3**:601–6.

35 ten Brinke A, Zwinderman AH, Sterk PJ, Rabe KF, Bel EH. Factors associated with persistent airflow limitation in severe asthma. *Am J Respir Crit Care Med* 2001;**164**:744–8.

36 Samter M, Beers RF Jr. Intolerance to aspirin: clinical studies and consideration of its pathogenesis. *Ann Intern Med* 1968;**68**:975–83.

37 Guerra S, Sherrill DL, Martinez FD, Barbee RA. Rhinitis as an independent risk factor for adult-onset asthma. *J Allergy Clin Immunol* 2002;**109**:419–25.

38 Malo JL, Chan-Yeung M. Occupational asthma. *J Allergy Clin Immunol* 2001;**108**:317–28.

39 Ward GW Jr, Karlsson G, Rose G, Platts-Mills TA. *Trichophyton* asthma: sensitisation of bronchi and upper airways to dermatophyte antigen. *Lancet* 1989;**1**:859–62.

40 Hahn DL. *Chlamydia pneumoniae*, asthma, and COPD: what is the evidence? *Ann Allergy Asthma Immunol* 1999;**83**:271–88, 291.

41 Holgate ST. The cellular and mediator basis of asthma in relation to natural history. *Lancet* 1997;**350**(Suppl 2):SII5–9.

42 Hogg JC. Pathophysiology of airflow limitation in chronic obstructive pulmonary disease. *Lancet* 2004;**364**:709–21.

43 Ollerenshaw SL, Woolcock AJ. Characteristics of the inflammation in biopsies from large airways of subjects with asthma and subjects with chronic airflow limitation. *Am Rev Respir Dis* 1992;**145**:922–7.

44 Laitinen LA, Laitinen A, Haahtela T. Airway mucosal inflammation even in patients with newly diagnosed asthma. *Am Rev Respir Dis* 1993;**147**:697–704.

45 Miranda C, Busacker A, Balzar S, Trudeau J, Wenzel SE. Distinguishing severe asthma phenotypes: role of age at onset and eosinophilic inflammation. *J Allergy Clin Immunol* 2004;**113**:101–8.

46 Wenzel SE, Schwartz LB, Langmack EL *et al.* Evidence that severe asthma can be divided pathologically into two inflammatory subtypes with distinct physiologic and clinical characteristics. *Am J Respir Crit Care Med* 1999;**160**:1001–8.

47 Sur S, Crotty TB, Kephart GM *et al.* Sudden-onset fatal asthma: a distinct entity with few eosinophils and relatively more neutrophils in the airway submucosa? *Am Rev Respir Dis* 1993;**148**:713–9.

48 Jeffery PK, Wardlaw AJ, Nelson FC, Collins JV, Kay AB. Bronchial biopsies in asthma: an ultrastructural, quantitative study and correlation with hyperreactivity. *Am Rev Respir Dis* 1989;**140**:1745–53.

49 Hirst SJ, Walker TR, Chilvers ER. Phenotypic diversity and molecular mechanisms of airway smooth muscle proliferation in asthma. *Eur Respir J* 2000;**16**:159–77.

50 McDonald DM. Angiogenesis and remodeling of airway vasculature in chronic inflammation. *Am J Respir Crit Care Med* 2001;**164**:S39–45.

51 Vignola AM, Chanez P, Campbell AM *et al.* Airway inflammation in mild intermittent and in persistent asthma. *Am J Respir Crit Care Med* 1998;**157**:403–9.

52 Wardlaw AJ, Dunnette S, Gleich GJ, Collins JV, Kay AB. Eosinophils and mast cells in bronchoalveolar lavage in subjects with mild asthma: relationship to bronchial hyperreactivity. *Am Rev Respir Dis* 1988;**137**:62–9.

53 Pin I, Gibson PG, Kolendowicz R *et al.* Use of induced sputum cell counts to investigate airway inflammation in asthma. *Thorax* 1992;**47**:25–9.

54 Jatakanon A, Uasuf C, Maziak W *et al.* Neutrophilic inflammation in severe persistent asthma. *Am J Respir Crit Care Med* 1999;**160**:1532–9.

55 in't Veen J, De Gouw H, Smits HH *et al.* Repeatability of cellular and soluble markers in induced sputum from patients with asthma. *Eur Respir J* 1996;**9**:2441–7.

56 Fahy JV, Liu J, Wong H, Boushey HA. Cellular and biochemical analysis of induced sputum from asthmatic and from healthy subjects. *Am Rev Respir Dis* 1993;**147**:1126–31.

57 Holt PG, Macaubas C, Stumbles PA, Sly PD. The role of allergy in the development of asthma. *Nature* 1999;**402**:B12–7.

58 Holt PG, Sly PD. Interactions between respiratory tract infections and atopy in the aetiology of asthma. *Eur Respir J* 2002;**19**:538–45.

59 Prescott SL, Macaubas C, Holt BJ *et al.* Transplacental priming of the human immune system to environmental allergens: universal skewing of initial T cell responses toward the Th2 cytokine profile. *J Immunol* 1998;**160**:4730–7.

60 Prescott SL, Macaubas C, Smallacombe T *et al.* Development of allergen-specific T-cell memory in atopic and normal children. *Lancet* 1999;**353**:196–200.

61 Braun-Fahrlander C, Riedler J, Herz U *et al.* Environmental exposure to endotoxin and its relation to asthma in school-age children. *N Engl J Med* 2002;**347**:869–77.

62 Woolcock AJ, Peat JK, Trevillion LM. Is the increase in asthma prevalence linked to increase in allergen load? *Allergy* 1995;**50**:935–40.

63 Smart JM, Horak E, Kemp AS, Robertson CF, Tang ML. Polyclonal and allergen-induced cytokine responses in adults with asthma: resolution of asthma is associated with normalization of IFN-γ responses. *J Allergy Clin Immunol* 2002;**110**:450–6.

64 Umetsu DT, McIntire JJ, Akbari O, Macaubas C, DeKruyff RH. Asthma: an epidemic of dysregulated immunity. *Nat Immunol* 2002;**3**:715–20.

65 Sears MR, Greene JM, Willan AR *et al.* A longitudinal, population-based, cohort study of childhood asthma followed to adulthood. *N Engl J Med* 2003;**349**:1414–22.

66 Sherrill D, Stein R, Kurzius-Spencer M, Martinez F. On early sensitization to allergens and development of respiratory symptoms. *Clin Exp Allergy* 1999;**29**:905–11.

67 Peat JK, Salome CM, Woolcock AJ. Longitudinal changes in atopy during a 4-year period: relation to bronchial hyper-responsiveness and respiratory symptoms in a population sample of Australian schoolchildren. *J Allergy Clin Immunol* 1990;**85**:65–74.

68 Davies DE. The bronchial epithelium: translating gene and environment interactions in asthma. *Curr Opin Allergy Clin Immunol* 2001;**1**:67–71.

69 Richter A, Puddicombe SM, Lordan JL *et al*. The contribution of interleukin (IL)-4 and IL-13 to the epithelial-mesenchymal trophic unit in asthma. *Am J Respir Cell Mol Biol* 2001;**25**:385–91.

70 Bousquet J, Jeffery PK, Busse WW, Johnson M, Vignola AM. Asthma: from bronchoconstriction to airways inflammation and remodeling. *Am J Respir Crit Care Med* 2000;**161**: 1720–45.

71 Sterk PJ, Bel EH. The shape of the dose–response curve to inhaled bronchoconstrictor agents in asthma and in chronic obstructive pulmonary disease. *Am Rev Respir Dis* 1991;**143**: 1433–7.

72 Hudon C, Turcotte H, Laviolette M, Carrier G, Boulet LP. Charactcristics of bronchial asthma with incomplete reversibility of airflow obstruction. *Ann Allergy Asthma Immunol* 1997;**78**:195–202.

73 van Rensen EL, Sont JK, Evertse CE *et al*. Bronchial CD8 cell infiltrate and lung function decline in asthma. *Am J Respir Crit Care Med* 2005;**172**:837–41.

74 Lange P, Parner J, Vestbo J, Schnohr P, Jensen G. A 15-year follow-up study of ventilatory function in adults with asthma. *N Engl J Med* 1998;**339**:1194–200.

75 Peat JK, Woolcock AJ, Cullen K. Rate of decline of lung function in subjects with asthma. *Eur J Respir Dis* 1987;**70**: 171–9.

76 Van Schayck CP, Dompeling E, Van Herwaarden CL, Wever AM, van Weel C. Interacting effects of atopy and bronchial hyperresponsiveness on the annual decline in lung function and the exacerbation rate in asthma. *Am Rev Respir Dis* 1991;**144**:1297–301.

77 ten Brinke A, van Dissel JT, Sterk PJ *et al*. Persistent airflow limitation in adult-onset non-atopic asthma is associated with serologic evidence of *Chlamydia pneumoniae* infection. *J Allergy Clin Immunol* 2001;**107**:449–54.

78 Jaakkola MS, Jaakkola JJ, Ernst P, Becklake MR. Respiratory symptoms in young adults should not be overlooked. *Am Rev Respir Dis* 1993;**147**:359–66.

79 Ulrik CS, Backer V, Dirksen A. Mortality and decline in lung function in 213 adults with bronchial asthma: a ten-year follow up. *J Asthma* 1992;**29**:29–38.

80 Fredberg JJ. Frozen objects: small airways, big breaths, and asthma. *J Allergy Clin Immunol* 2000;**106**:615–24.

81 Fredberg JJ. Airway smooth muscle in asthma: perturbed equilibria of myosin binding. *Am J Respir Crit Care Med* 2000;**161**:S158–60.

82 Macklem PT. A theoretical analysis of the effect of airway smooth muscle load on airway narrowing. *Am J Respir Crit Care Med* 1996;**153**:83–9.

83 Louis R, Lau LC, Bron AO *et al*. The relationship between airways inflammation and asthma severity. *Am J Respir Crit Care Med* 2000;**161**:9–16.

84 Gibson PG, Simpson JL, Hankin R, Powell H, Henry RL. Relationship between induced sputum eosinophils and the clinical pattern of childhood asthma. *Thorax* 2003;**58**: 116–21.

85 Benayoun L, Druilhe A, Dombret MC, Aubier M, Pretolani M. Airway structural alterations selectively associated with severe asthma. *Am J Respir Crit Care Med* 2003;**167**:1360–8.

86 Sont JK, van Krieken J, Evertse CE *et al*. Relationship between the inflammatory infiltrate in bronchial biopsy specimens and clinical severity of asthma in patients treated with inhaled steroids. *Thorax* 1996;**51**:496–502.

87 Ronchi MC, Piragino C, Rosi E *et al*. Role of sputum differential cell count in detecting airway inflammation in patients with chronic bronchial asthma or COPD. *Thorax* 1996;**51**: 1000–4.

88 Louis R, Sele J, Henket M *et al*. Sputum eosinophil count in a large population of patients with mild to moderate steroid-naive asthma: distribution and relationship with methacholine bronchial hyperresponsiveness. *Allergy* 2002;**57**: 907–12.

89 Yoshikawa T, Shoji S, Fujii T *et al*. Severity of exercise-induced bronchoconstriction is related to airway eosinophilic inflammation in patients with asthma. *Eur Respir J* 1998; **12**:879–84.

90 Little SA, MacLeod KJ, Chalmers GW *et al*. Association of forced expiratory volume with disease duration and sputum neutrophils in chronic asthma. *Am J Med* 2002;**112**:446–52.

91 in't Veen JC, Smits HH, Hiemstra PS *et al*. Lung function and sputum characteristics of patients with severe asthma during an induced exacerbation by double-blind steroid withdrawal. *Am J Respir Crit Care Med* 1999;**160**:93–9.

92 Fahy JV, Woo Kim K, Liu J, Boushey HA. Prominent neutrophilic inflammation in sputum from subjects with asthma exacerbation. *J Allergy Clin Immunol* 1995;**95**: 843–52.

93 Jatakanon A, Lim S, Barnes PJ. Changes in sputum eosinophils predict loss of asthma control. *Am J Respir Crit Care Med* 2000;**161**:64–72.

94 Leuppi JD, Salome CM, Jenkins CR *et al*. Predictive markers of asthma exacerbation during stepwise dose reduction of inhaled corticosteroids. *Am J Respir Crit Care Med* 2001;**163**: 406–12.

95 Pizzichini M, Pizzichini E, Clelland L *et al*. Sputum in severe exacerbations of asthma: kinetics of inflammatory indices after prednisone treatment. *Am J Respir Crit Care Med* 1997;**155**:1501–8.

96 Court CS, Cook DG, Strachan DP. Comparative epidemiology of atopic and non-atopic wheeze and diagnosed asthma in a national sample of English adults. *Thorax* 2002;**57**:951–7.

97 Romanet-Manent S, Charpin D, Magnan A, Lanteaume A, Vervloet D. Allergic vs non-allergic asthma: what makes the difference? *Allergy* 2002;**57**:607–13.

98 Inouye T, Tarlo S, Broder I *et al*. Severity of asthma in skin test-negative and skin test-positive patients. *J Allergy Clin Immunol* 1985;**75**:313–9.

99 Hizawa N, Yamaguchi E, Konno S *et al*. A functional polymorphism in the RANTES gene promoter is associated with the development of late-onset asthma. *Am J Respir Crit Care Med* 2002;**166**:686–90.

100 Ulrik CS, Backer V, Dirksen A. A 10 year follow up of 180 adults with bronchial asthma: factors important for the decline in lung function. *Thorax* 1992;**47**:14–8.

101 Amin K, Ludviksdottir D, Janson C *et al*. Inflammation and structural changes in the airways of patients with atopic and non-atopic asthma. BHR Group. *Am J Respir Crit Care Med* 2000;**162**:2295–301.

102 Umibe T, Kita Y, Nakao A *et al*. Clonal expansion of T cells infiltrating in the airways of non-atopic asthmatics. *Clin Exp Immunol* 2000;**119**:390–7.

103 Silva GE, Sherrill DL, Guerra S, Barbee RA. Asthma as a risk factor for COPD in a longitudinal study. *Chest* 2004;**126**: 59–65.

104 Tashkin DP, Altose MD, Connett JE *et al*. Methacholine reactivity predicts changes in lung function over time in smokers with early chronic obstructive pulmonary disease. The Lung Health Study Research Group. *Am J Respir Crit Care Med* 1996;**153**:1802–11.

105 Sluiter HJ, Koeter GH, de Monchy JG *et al*. The Dutch hypothesis (chronic non-specific lung disease) revisited. *Eur Respir J* 1991;**4**:479–89.

106 Peat JK, Li J. Reversing the trend: reducing the prevalence of asthma. *J Allergy Clin Immunol* 1999;**103**:1–10.

107 Koopman LP, van Strien RT, Kerkhof M *et al*. Placebo-controlled trial of house dust mite-impermeable mattress covers: effect on symptoms in early childhood. *Am J Respir Crit Care Med* 2002;**166**:307–13.

108 Custovic A, Simpson BM, Simpson A, Kissen P, Woodcock A. Effect of environmental manipulation in pregnancy and early life on respiratory symptoms and atopy during first year of life: a randomised trial. *Lancet* 2001;**358**:188–93.

109 Arshad SH, Bateman B, Matthews SM. Primary prevention of asthma and atopy during childhood by allergen avoidance in infancy: a randomised controlled study. *Thorax* 2003;**58**:489–93.

110 Riedler J, Braun-Fahrlander C, Eder W *et al*. Exposure to farming in early life and development of asthma and allergy: a cross-sectional survey. *Lancet* 2001;**358**:1129–33.

111 Gereda JE, Leung DY, Thatayatikom A *et al*. Relation between house-dust endotoxin exposure, type 1 T-cell development, and allergen sensitisation in infants at high risk of asthma. *Lancet* 2000;**355**:1680–3.

112 Gerhold K, Blumchen K, Bock A *et al*. Endotoxins prevent murine IgE production, T$_H$2 immune responses, and development of airway eosinophilia but not airway hyper-reactivity. *J Allergy Clin Immunol* 2002;**110**:110–6.

113 Kalliomaki M, Salminen S, Arvilommi H *et al*. Probiotics in primary prevention of atopic disease: a randomised placebo-controlled trial. *Lancet* 2001;**357**:1076–9.

114 Rautava S, Kalliomaki M, Isolauri E. Probiotics during pregnancy and breast-feeding might confer immunomodulatory protection against atopic disease in the infant. *J Allergy Clin Immunol* 2002;**109**:119–21.

115 Reijonen TM, Kotaniemi-Syrjanen A, Korhonen K, Korppi M. Predictors of asthma three years after hospital admission for wheezing in infancy. *Pediatrics* 2000;**106**:1406–12.

116 Celedon JC, Litonjua AA, Ryan L, Weiss ST, Gold DR. Day care attendance, respiratory tract illnesses, wheezing, asthma, and total serum IgE level in early childhood. *Arch Pediatr Adolesc Med* 2002;**156**:241–5.

117 Holt PG. A potential vaccine strategy for asthma and allied atopic diseases during early childhood. *Lancet* 1994;**344**: 456–8.

118 Oddy WH, Peat JK, De Klerk NH. Maternal asthma, infant feeding, and the risk of asthma in childhood. *J Allergy Clin Immunol* 2002;**110**:65–7.

119 Alm JS, Swartz J, Lilja G, Scheynius A, Pershagen G. Atopy in children of families with an anthroposophic lifestyle. *Lancet* 1999;**353**:1485–8.

120 Gdalevich M, Mimouni D, Mimouni M. Breast-feeding and the risk of bronchial asthma in childhood: a systematic review with meta-analysis of prospective studies. *J Pediatr* 2001;**139**:261–6.

121 Sears MR, Greene JM, Willan AR *et al*. Long-term relation between breastfeeding and development of atopy and asthma in children and young adults: a longitudinal study. *Lancet* 2002;**360**:901–7.

122 Li YF, Langholz B, Salam MT, Gilliland FD. Maternal and grandmaternal smoking patterns are associated with early childhood asthma. *Chest* 2005;**127**:1232–41.

123 Barker DJ, Godfrey KM, Fall C *et al*. Relation of birth weight and childhood respiratory infection to adult lung function and death from chronic obstructive airways disease. *BMJ* 1991;**303**:671–5.

124 Hammoud AO, Bujold E, Sorokin Y *et al*. Smoking in pregnancy revisited: findings from a large population-based study. *Am J Obstet Gynecol* 2005;**192**:1856–62.

125 The British guidelines on asthma management 1995 review and position statement. *Thorax* 1997;**52**(Suppl 1):S1–21.

126 Benckhuijsen J, van den Bos JW, van Velzen E, ve Bruijn R, Aalbers R. Differences in the effect of allergen avoidance on bronchial hyperresponsiveness as measured by methacholine, adenosine 5′-monophosphate, and exercise in asthmatic children. *Pediatr Pulmonol* 1996;**22**:147–53.

127 van Velzen E, van den Bos JW, Benckhuijsen J, van Essel T, de Bruijn R, Aalbers R. Effect of allergen avoidance at high altitude on direct and indirect bronchial hyperresponsiveness and markers of inflammation in children with allergic asthma. *Thorax* 1996;**51**:582–4.

128 Boner AL, Niero E, Antolini I, Valletta EA, Gaburro D. Pulmonary function and bronchial hyperreactivity in asthmatic children with house dust mite allergy during prolonged stay in the Italian Alps (Misurina, 1756 m). *Ann Allergy* 1985;**54**:42–5.

129 Gotzsche PC, Hammarquist C, Burr M. House dust mite control measures in the management of asthma: meta-analysis. *BMJ* 1998;**317**:1105–10.

130 Custovic A, Simpson A, Chapman MD, Woodcock A. Allergen avoidance in the treatment of asthma and atopic disorders. *Thorax* 1998;**53**:63–72.

131 Jatakanon A, Lim S, Chung KF, Barnes PJ. An inhaled steroid improves markers of airway inflammation in patients with mild asthma. *Eur Respir J* 1998;**12**:1084–8.

132 Lim S, Jatakanon A, John M *et al*. Effect of inhaled budesonide on lung function and airway inflammation: assessment by various inflammatory markers in mild asthma. *Am J Respir Crit Care Med* 1999;**159**:22–30.

133 van Rensen EL, Straathof KC, Veselic-Charvat MA *et al*. Effect of inhaled steroids on airway hyperresponsiveness,

sputum eosinophils, and exhaled nitric oxide levels in patients with asthma. *Thorax* 1999;**54**:403–8.

134 Gershman NH, Wong HH, Liu JT, Fahy JV. Low- and high-dose fluticasone propionate in asthma: effects during and after treatment. *Eur Respir J* 2000;**15**:11–8.

135 Pauwels RA, Lofdahl CG, Postma DS *et al.* and Formoterol and Corticosteroids Establishing Therapy (FACET) International Study Group. Effect of inhaled formoterol and budesonide on exacerbations of asthma. *N Engl J Med* 1997;**337**:1405–11.

136 Djukanovic R, Wilson JW, Britten KM *et al.* Effect of an inhaled corticosteroid on airway inflammation and symptoms in asthma. *Am Rev Respir Dis* 1992;**145**:669–74.

137 Trigg, CJ, Manolitsas ND, Wang J *et al.* Placebo-controlled immunopathologic study of four months of inhaled corticosteroids in asthma. *Am J Respir Crit Care Med* 1994;**150**:17–22.

138 Chetta A, Zanini A, Foresi A *et al.* Vascular component of airway remodeling in asthma is reduced by high dose of fluticasone. *Am J Respir Crit Care Med* 2003;**167**:751–7.

139 Bacci E, Di Franco A, Bartoli ML *et al.* Comparison of anti-inflammatory and clinical effects of beclomethasone dipropionate and salmeterol in moderate asthma. *Eur Respir J* 2002;**20**:66–72.

140 Holgate ST. Cytokine and anti-cytokine therapy for the treatment of asthma and allergic disease. *Cytokine* 2004;**28**:152–7.

141 Barnes PJ. New drugs for asthma. *Nat Rev Drug Discov* 2004;**3**:831–44.

142 Holgate S, Casale T, Wenzel S *et al.* The anti-inflammatory effects of omalizumab confirm the central role of IgE in allergic inflammation. *J Allergy Clin Immunol* 2005;**115**:459–65.

143 Thomson NC, Spears M. The influence of smoking on the treatment response in patients with asthma. *Curr Opin Allergy Clin Immunol* 2005;**5**:57–63.

144 Livingston E, Thomson NC, Chalmers GW. Impact of smoking on asthma therapy: a critical review of clinical evidence. *Drugs* 2005;**65**:1521–36.

145 Ito K, Ito M, Elliott WM *et al.* Decreased histone deacetylase activity in chronic obstructive pulmonary disease. *N Engl J Med* 2005;**352**:1967–76.

146 Barnes PJ, Ito K, Adcock IM. Corticosteroid resistance in chronic obstructive pulmonary disease: inactivation of histone deacetylase. *Lancet* 2004;**363**:731–3.

147 Rabe KF, Adachi M, Lai CK *et al.* Worldwide severity and control of asthma in children and adults: the global asthma insights and reality surveys. *J Allergy Clin Immunol* 2004;**114**:40–7.

148 Cerveri I, Locatelli F, Zoia MC *et al.* International variations in asthma treatment compliance: the results of the European Community Respiratory Health Survey (ECRHS). *Eur Respir J* 1999;**14**:288–94.

149 Rabe KF, Vermeire PA, Soriano JB, Maier WC. Clinical management of asthma in 1999: the Asthma Insights and Reality in Europe (AIRE) study. *Eur Respir J* 2000;**16**:802–7.

150 Sont JK, Willems LN, Bel EH *et al.* Clinical control and histopathologic outcome of asthma when using airway hyperresponsiveness as an additional guide to long-term treatment. The AMPUL Study Group. *Am J Respir Crit Care Med* 1999;**159**:1043–51.

151 Green RH, Brightling CE, Mckenna S *et al.* Asthma exacerbations and sputum eosinophil counts: a randomised controlled trial. *Lancet* 2002;**360**:1715–21.

152 Donato F, Pasini GF, Buizza MA *et al.* Tobacco smoking, occupational exposure and chronic respiratory disease in an Italian industrial area. *Monaldi Arch Chest Dis* 2000;**55**:194–200.

153 Prescott E, Vestbo J. Socioeconomic status and chronic obstructive pulmonary disease. *Thorax* 1999;**54**:737–41.

154 Grashoff WF, Sont JK, Sterk PJ *et al.* Chronic obstructive pulmonary disease: role of bronchiolar mast cells and macrophages. *Am J Pathol* 1997;**151**:1785–90.

155 O'Shaughnessy TC, Ansari TQ, Barnes NC, Jeffery PK. Inflammation in bronchial biopsies of subjects with chronic bronchitis: inverse relationship of CD8[+] T lymphocytes with FEV_1. *Am J Respir Crit Care Med* 1997;**155**:852–7.

156 Keatings VM, Barnes PJ. Granulocyte activation markers in induced sputum: comparison between chronic obstructive pulmonary disease, asthma, and normal subjects. *Am J Respir Crit Care Med* 1997;**155**:449–53.

157 Anthonisen NR, Connett JE, Murray RP. Smoking and lung function of lung health study participants after 11 years. *Am J Respir Crit Care Med* 2002;**166**:675–9.

158 Pauwels RA, Löfdahl C-G, Laitinen LA *et al.* and for the European Respiratory Society Study on Chronic Obstructive Pulmonary Disease. Long-term treatment with inhaled budesonide in persons with mild chronic obstructive pulmonary disease who continue smoking. *N Engl J Med* 1999;**340**:1948–53.

159 Vestbo J, Sorensen T, Lange P *et al.* Long-term effect of inhaled budesonide in mild and moderate chronic obstructive pulmonary disease: a randomised controlled trial. *Lancet* 1999;**353**:1819–23.

160 The Lung Health Study Research Group. Effect of inhaled triamcinolone on the decline in pulmonary function in chronic obstructive pulmonary disease. *N Engl J Med* 2000;**343**:1902–9.

161 Keatings VM, Jatakanon A, Worsdell YM, Barnes PJ. Effects of inhaled and oral glucocorticoids on inflammatory indices in asthma and COPD. *Am J Respir Crit Care Med* 1997;**155**:542–8.

162 Culpitt SV, Maziak W, Loukidis S *et al.* Effect of high dose inhaled steroid on cells, cytokines, and proteases in induced sputum in chronic obstructive pulmonary disease. *Am J Respir Crit Care Med* 1999;**160**:1635–9.

163 Hattotuwa KL, Gizycki MJ, Ansari TW, Jeffery PK, Barnes NC. The effects of inhaled fluticasone on airway inflammation in chronic obstructive pulmonary disease: a double-blind, placebo-controlled biopsy study. *Am J Respir Crit Care Med* 2002;**165**:1592–6.

164 Soriano JB, Davis KJ, Coleman B *et al.* The proportional Venn diagram of obstructive lung disease: two approximations from the United States and the United Kingdom. *Chest* 2003;**124**:474–81.

CHAPTER 15

COPD: clinical presentation and evaluation

Bartolome R. Celli

The American Thoracic Society and the European Respiratory Society (ATS/ERS) [1] have recently defined chronic obstructive pulmonary disease (COPD) as a preventable and treatable disease state characterized by airflow limitation that is not fully reversible.

The airflow limitation is usually progressive and associated with an abnormal inflammatory response of the lungs to noxious particles or gases, primarily caused by cigarette smoking. In some areas of the world where biomass fuel is used as a source of energy primarily for cooking, persons exposed to the particles can develop airflow obstruction that is indistinguishable from that characteristic of COPD [2].

Although COPD primarily affects the lungs, it also produces significant systemic consequences which are very important because their presence is associated with significant morbidity and mortality and also because some of them are amenable to therapy. Indeed, as detailed elsewhere in this book, oxygen therapy, an intervention that does not reverse airflow limitation, has been shown to prolong survival [3,4].

Clinical manifestations

The clinical evaluation is based on a medical history and physical examination. Although a complete examination is indicated for all patients, there are specifically important elements for patients with suspected COPD. These elements include specific symptoms and signs that relate to the respiratory system and the presence of certain risk factors.

Symptoms

Several symptoms should alert the clinician to the possible presence of COPD. Although not pathognomonic for the disease, they are intimately associated with the exposure to the risk factor and the manifestations of COPD. They include cough, sputum and dyspnoea.

Cough

The cough may initially be intermittent (early morning), progressively becoming present throughout the day, but is seldom entirely nocturnal [1,2,5]. Once it becomes chronic, the cough is usually productive and is very often discounted by the patient as being an expected consequence of smoking. Thus, the patient may not offer the information and the astute clinician should always ask for its presence and its specific characteristics. If the cough is severe and persistent, syncope or cough rib fractures may occur.

Sputum

The presence of sputum is associated and usually follows the development of progressive cough. It initially occurs in the morning but later may be present throughout the day. It is usually tenacious and mucoid in small quantities [5]. The production of sputum for ≥ 3 months in 2 consecutive years is the epidemiological definition of chronic bronchitis [1,2]. This definition has been useful to attempt to characterize the phenotypical presentation of certain patients with COPD. A change in sputum colour (purulent) or volume suggests an infectious exacerbation [6].

Dyspnoea

Perhaps the most alarming symptom of COPD is the presence of dyspnoea. It is usually progressive and becomes persistent over time. At the onset it occurs during exercise (climbing up stairs, walking up hills) and may by avoided entirely by appropriate behavioural changes (e.g. using a lift or avoiding exercise or physical effort). However, as the disease progresses dyspnoea is elicited even during minimal exertion or at rest.

A quantification of dyspnoea using the Modified Medical Research Council scale is indicated. This simple scale

Table 15.1 Modified Medical Research Council scale recommended to evaluate grade of functional dyspnoea.

0 Not troubled with breathlessness except with strenuous exercise
1 Troubled by shortness of breath when hurrying or walking up a slight hill
2 Walks slower than people of the same age because of breathlessness or has to stop for breath when walking at own pace on the level
3 Stops for breath after walking approximately 100 m or after a few minutes on the level
4 Too breathless to leave the house or breathless when dressing or undressing

(Table 15.1) objectively grades the level of functional dyspnoea and should become part of the evaluation of all patients with COPD because it predicts quality of life and survival independent of the degree of physiological airflow limitation [7,8]. Furthermore, the evaluation of functional dyspnoea may be the single most helpful way to evaluate the effect of therapy [1,2].

Dyspnoea with activities can also be objectively evaluated with the use of scales such as the visual analogue scale (VAS) or the modified Borg dyspnoea scale (Fig. 15.1a,b) [9]. These scales are simple and provide information regarding the level of dyspnoea perceived by the patient, for example with a known exercise load. These scales have been very useful in evaluating the beneficial effect of therapy using cardiopulmonary exercise testing or timed walked distance as the load.

Although there is some correlation between the degree of airflow limitation and dyspnoea, this correlation is weak at best [8,9]. The same can be said for the correlation between arterial blood gas abnormality and the presence and degree of dyspnoea [9]. These findings are best explained by the fact that dyspnoea is a very complex symptom where several factors interact. There is evidence that the intrinsic response of the central controller [10], the dissociation between the demand to breath and the mechanical response [11], the action of the respiratory muscles [12] and the nature of the mechanical load and the final output can all relate to the genesis of dyspnoea. However, independent of the mechanism, the presence of dyspnoea with previously well-tolerated activities or, worse yet, with daily activities, should alert the clinician to the possible presence of COPD.

Other symptoms

Patients may report the presence of wheeze, especially during episodes of respiratory tract infection or heavy exercise. Similarly, some patients may complain of chest pain associated with cough or increased activity. This may be caused by increased respiratory muscle effort or stress on ribs or vertebrae.

The development of leg oedema could indicate development of right-side heart failure cor pulmonale. In such cases, the possibility of associated sleep apnoea should also be explored as the coexistence of two highly prevalent diseases is very common [13].

In more advanced disease, the development of weight loss and skeletal muscle wasting should be cause for concern. Indeed, a low body mass index (BMI < 21 kg/m²) is an independent predictor of mortality [14,15]. This has led to the recommendation that all patients with COPD should have their weight and height determined and the BMI calculated using the simple formula:

BMI = weight in kilograms/height in metres squared.

Many patients with COPD complain of fatigue and are often depressed. The latter may be manifested by the presence of its characteristic complaints of malaise, change in appetite, lack of interest in life, sleepiness and insomnia. Clinicians should be aware of this problem because treatment of depression may become a therapeutic goal in itself.

The development of haemoptysis is unusual in COPD and should raise the possibility of lung cancer. Seasonal exacerbation during spring or summer, or the development of symptoms with exposure to specific agents, suggests

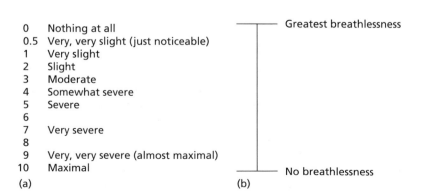

0	Nothing at all
0.5	Very, very slight (just noticeable)
1	Very slight
2	Slight
3	Moderate
4	Somewhat severe
5	Severe
6	
7	Very severe
8	
9	Very, very severe (almost maximal)
10	Maximal

(a)

(b)

Greatest breathlessness

No breathlessness

Figure 15.1 The Borg (a) and the visual analogue scale (b) are validated scales that can be used to estimate the perception of dyspnoea during activities.

asthma. The presence of large amounts of purulent sputum is more consistent with bronchiectasis. The presence of chest pain can also be caused by concomitant coronary artery disease or pulmonary embolism.

Presence of risk factors

A history of exposure to risk factors, such as smoking, or occupational or environmental noxious agents, should be noted. A detailed smoking history is essential. A useful tool to express the exposure to cigarettes is the calculation of pack-years. This is obtained by multiplying the number of pack equivalents smoked every day by the total number of years; thus, 20 pack-years can result from smoking one pack per day for 20 years. The number of pack-years calculated in this way correlates well with objective determination of cigarette exposure [16]. The possibility of passive smoking should also be ascertained, with special emphasis on early exposure to smoking parents, a factor that has been shown to relate to early development of lung disease [17].

In patients from areas of the world where biomass fuel is used as a source of energy or heat, the history of closed environment exposure (i.e. cooking with wood) should also raise the possibility of COPD [18].

In addition to exposure, other risk factors known to be associated with COPD should be investigated. The most important is the presence of a family history of COPD, with α_1-antitrypsin as the main risk [19,20].

Signs

As part of the vital signs, all patients should have their respiratory rate measured, weight and height determined, and their BMI calculated. A normal physical examination is frequent in early COPD [1,2]. As the disease progresses some signs become apparent and in the advanced stages many are almost pathognomonic.

The examination should be aimed at eliciting the presence of the respiratory and systemic effects of COPD. On inspection, check for barrel chest deformity, pursed lips breathing, chest or abdominal wall paradoxical movements and use of accessory respiratory muscles. All these are signs of severe airflow limitation, hyperinflation and impairment of the mechanics of breathing [21].

Percussion can reveal decreased motion of the diaphragm and tympanic sounds resulting from hyperinflation or bullae; in addition, the liver becomes easily palpable. During auscultation, a forced expiratory manoeuvre that is unduly prolonged (> 6 s) suggests significant airflow limitation. Adventitious rhonchi and wheezing may help differentiate COPD from congestive heart failure or pulmonary fibrosis, which are often associated with rales. The heart sounds

may be distant as a result of hyperinflation. However, with advanced disease they may show signs of cor pulmonale, such as split of second sound (pulmonic), murmurs of pulmonic or tricuspid insufficiency. In addition, atrial arrhythmias such as fibrillation and flutter may be detected in patients with significant compromise. Cyanosis or bluish colour of the mucosal membranes may indicate hypoxaemia. Clubbing is not a usual feature of COPD and its presence should direct the physician to evaluate other possible explanations such as the presence of lung cancer, idiopathic pulmonary fibrosis or bronchiectasis.

Laboratory tests

The suspected clinical diagnosis of COPD needs to be confirmed with the rational use of laboratory testing. Mandatory tests for all patients include spirometry using the forced vital capacity (*FVC*) manoeuvre and the chest roentgenogram [1,2]. Other tests that can complement and help in a more comprehensive evaluation of a particular patient are listed as optional.

All patients

Spirometry

Spirometry should be performed in all patients suspected of COPD. This is necessary for diagnosis [22], assessment of the severity of the disease [23] and for following the progress of the disease [24]. Without spirometry, the diagnosis of persistent and partially reversible airflow limitation cannot be confirmed. Spirometry should include an evaluation of bronchodilator reversibility using an inhaled bronchodilator. This should be performed at least once to exclude asthma, to establish the best lung function for the individual patient and, to a lesser degree, to estimate the prognosis. The increase in forced expiratory volume in 1 s (*FEV*$_1$) should be expressed as a percentage of the predicted value which is less dependent on the baseline *FEV*$_1$. Although some bronchodilation may be present in some patients with COPD, a large increase in postbronchodilator *FEV*$_1$ supports the diagnosis of asthma [23].

A typical spirogram of a patient with COPD is shown in Figure 15.2. The *FEV*$_1$ and its ratio to the *FVC* remain as the gold standard to diagnosis and follow-up in patients with COPD. The *FEV*$_1$ should also be expressed as a percentage of the predicted values obtained from population studies of non-smokers without lung disease. The factors known to determine lung function include gender, age, height and race. After the diagnosis is established, the exact frequency and timing of repeat spirometry has not been determined. However, it is advisable to repeat the test 2–4 weeks after initiation of therapy, whenever the patient reports changes

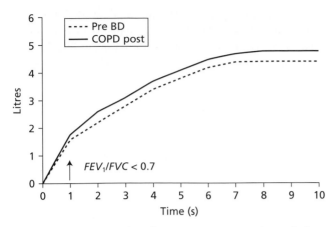

Figure 15.2 The forced vital capacity manoeuvre is needed to confirm the diagnosis of airflow limitation, as shown in this tracing. The small increment in postbronchodilator FEV_1 confirms poor reversibility characteristic of COPD. BD, bronchodilator; FEV_1, forced expiratory volume in 1 s; FVC, functional residual capacity.

in symptoms or at least every year. The advent of portable and reliable pneumotacograph-based spirometers should make testing easier and more widely available [25].

Chest roentgenography

Chest radiography [1,2,26] should be obtained in all patients. It is not used for the diagnosis, but is helpful in excluding other diseases (pneumonia, cancer, congestive heart failure, pleural effusions and pneumothorax). It is also of value to detect bullous disease. Common but not specific signs of emphysema are (Fig. 15.3): flattening of the diaphragm, irregular lung radiolucency and reduction or absence of vasculature (rapid tapering). The presence of cardiomegaly with encroachment of the cardiac silhouette on the retrosternal space and increased width of the

descending branch of the right pulmonary artery (> 20 mm) suggests the diagnosis of cor pulmonale. The presence of other abnormalities, such as infiltrates, hilar node enlargement, parenchymal nodules and interstitial infiltrates, should suggest an alternative diagnosis.

Selected patients

Lung volumes

The measurement of static lung volumes is useful in the evaluation of patients because the level of hyperinflation helps to determine the degree of air trapping and loss of lung elastic recoil [21,27]. Lung volumes are best measured using body plethysmography. This method is more precise than the simpler method of gas dilution because with increasing disease severity, the amount of non-communicating portions of the lung results in an underestimation of air-trapping by dilution methods [28]. The total lung capacity (TLC), residual volume (RV), functional residual capacity and the ratio RV/TLC are all characteristically increased in advanced COPD. The increase in TLC is the consequence of loss of lung elastic recoil, which allows the inspiratory muscles to stretch the lungs to a greater volume. The increase in RV occurs because of premature closure of narrowed airways at higher lung volumes. Usually, the increase in RV is greater than the change in TLC and therefore the RV/TLC increases. The most important lung volumes are shown in Figure 15.4.

The evaluation of the degree of hyperinflation has gained popularity because it has been related to the development of dynamic hyperinflation with increased ventilatory demand, such as during exercise [29–31]. A good index of hyperinflation is the measure of the inspiratory capacity, which in essence represents the mirror image of the end-expiratory lung volume (EELV). Figure 15.5(a,b) represents the inspiratory capacity as determined during flow

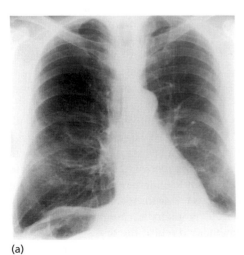

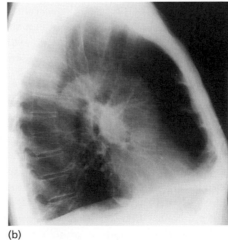

Figure 15.3 (a,b) The chest roentgenograms of patients with severe COPD characteristically show hyperlucent fields, flattened diaphragm and increased retrosternal and retrocardiac air space.

(a)

(b)

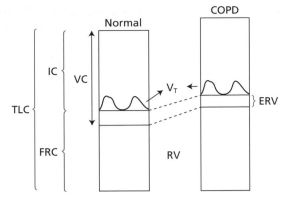

Figure 15.4 The lung volumes are useful in determining degree of inflation. The most important lung volumes are: total lung capacity (TLC), inspiratory capacity (IC), functional residual capacity (FRC), vital capacity (VC), residual volume (RV), end-expiratory reserve (ERV) and tidal volume (V_T). All except VC increase in COPD, especially in patients with predominant emphysema. However, because RV increases more than TLC, the ratio of RV/TLC decreases as the disease progresses.

volume manoeuvres at rest and during exercise in a patient with COPD who does not hyperinflate with exercise and that of a patient with COPD who develops significant air trapping during exercise. The importance of this measurement stems from the fact that the degree of dynamic hyperinflation relates better to the degree of dyspnoea measured with increased ventilatory demand than more conventional measurements of lung function such as the

FEV_1. Further, lesser increases in EELV have been associated with the symptomatic benefit observed after bronchodilators [30,31]. Indeed, measurements of static lung volume and lung volume response to exercise have become important physiological independent outcomes after interventions [31,32]. Finally, the determination of lung volumes is useful in patients with advanced disease who are being considered for surgery [33,34] (see Chapter 55).

Diffusing capacity for carbon monoxide

Transfer factor of the lung for carbon monoxide (TLCO) is usually reduced in COPD, particularly in emphysema [35] because of the destruction of alveolar and capillary beds. The TLCO is interchangeable with the term diffusing capacity for carbon monoxide (DLCO) as used in North America. The term is very indicative of the test itself. In essence, it provides information regarding the ease of transfer of CO molecules from alveolar gas to pulmonary capillary haemoglobin. The diffusion capacity for CO is low in smokers compared with non-smokers even in the absence of spirometric abnormality. Of interest, if DLCO is reduced, asthma can be excluded. The measurement of DLCO is important in the evaluation of patients being considered for lung volume reduction surgery because values lower than 20% of predicted implies undue risk of poor outcome [34].

Arterial blood gases

As COPD progresses, there is development of progressive ventilation/perfusion mismatch. This results in hypoxaemia

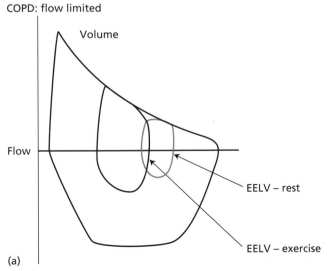

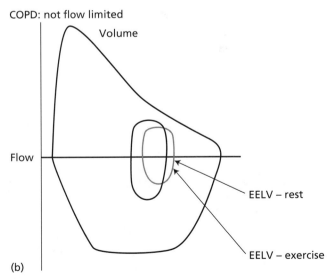

Figure 15.5 The two flow–volume loops shown correspond to those of two patients with COPD. (a) The patient is flow-limited so that increase in ventilatory demand (as during exercise) results in air-trapping and an increase in end-expiratory lung volume (EELV). Because total lung capacity (TLC) does not change, the inspiratory capacity decreases. These changes have been shown to relate to degree of breathlessness during exercise. (b) The other patient has no flow limitation, the EELV does not increase during exercise and inspiratory capacity remains unchanged.

easily shown while the patient breathes room air. The hypoxaemia may determine compensatory hyperventilation, which, at least at the beginning, may cause mild hypocarbia. As the disease progresses and hypoventilation becomes more manifest, hypercapnia may be seen. Hypoxaemia and hypercapnia are independent predictors of morbidity and mortality [36]. As a consequence of the progressive increase in $Paco_2$, there is compensatory bicarbonate retention and the serum bicarbonate may be elevated (respiratory acidosis with compensatory metabolic alkalosis).

In stable patients, the measurement of arterial blood gases while the patient breathes room air is recommended in moderate and severe stages of the disease. The documentation of hypoxaemia ($Pao_2 < 55$ mmHg) indicates the need to consider long-term oxygen therapy (LTOT) because it reverses hypoxaemia and has been shown to improve life expectancy [3,4].

In some patients with low but not critical hypoxaemia ($Pao_2 > 60$ mmHg), the Pao_2 usually worsens during exacerbations and may reach levels consistent with respiratory failure [37]. Indeed, arterial blood gases should be obtained during exacerbations as the level of Pao_2 should be used to guide oxygen treatment. In addition, arterial blood gases provide the level of $Paco_2$, which, in combination with the degree of acidosis, determines the need for non-invasive or invasive mechanical ventilation [38,39].

The determination of oxygen saturation is very helpful in clinical practice [40]. Non-invasive pulse oximetry Spo_2 is useful for assessing changes in Sao_2 as well as adjusting oxygen flow settings; it is less reliable in exercise studies than at rest (although newer pulse oximeters may be less sensitive to movement artefact and may be more accurate during exercise). Patients with values < 94% at sea level breathing room air suggests the need for blood gases. However, a word of caution must be raised. Some patients may manifest borderline oxygen desaturation easily correctible with supplemental oxygen. This correction may hide the development of hypercapnia [41]. Therefore, arterial blood gases should be obtained in patients with low oxygen saturation requiring progressive oxygen supplementation to maintain the targeted oxygen saturation.

Assessment for air travel

Commercial airliners can cruise at altitudes over 40 000 feet (12 000 m) with cabins pressurized from 6000 to 8000 feet (from 1800 to 2400 m). This is equivalent to an inspired O_2 concentration at sea level of approximately 15%. Patients with severe COPD experience falls in Pao_2 that average 25 mmHg but may be more than 30 mmHg at 8000 feet (2400 m) during this exposure to hypobaric hypoxia. Because their sea level Pao_2 values are on the steep part of the

oxygenhaemoglobin dissociation curve, the fall in Sao_2 with falls in Pao_2 may be quite sharp [42].

The preflight assessment should incorporate the following steps:
1 Estimate the expected degree of hypoxaemia at altitude;
2 Identify comorbid disease conditions;
3 Prescribe oxygen if necessary [43].
Counselling the patient and documenting recent clinical condition and laboratory tests are also desirable elements of preflight patient care, particularly if the patient is travelling abroad. Most national and international airlines will provide supplemental oxygen on request.

Exercise tests

Exercise testing is of practical value in patients with a disproportional degree of dyspnoea to FEV_1 because it may help establish the physiological cause of dyspnoea [44,45]. Exercise tests can also help in the evaluation of candidates who are not hypoxaemic at rest for oxygen therapy. In addition, an increasing body of evidence has shown that exercise capacity is a predictor of mortality [46,47] independent of the FEV_1. There are several exercise protocols. For simplicity they can be classified as laboratory tests (the cardiopulmonary exercise test) and field tests (timed walked distance and the shuttle walk test).

Cardiopulmonary exercise test

The cardiopulmonary exercise test (CPET) can be performed on a cycle or treadmill ergometer. The CPET provides very accurate information regarding the physiological response to exercise [48]. The variables measured include: mechanical work performed, oxygen consumption ($\dot{V}o_2$), carbon dioxide output ($\dot{V}co_2$) and ventilatory response with its components (minute ventilation [$\dot{V}_E$], tidal volume [V_T] and respiratory rate). In addition, continuous monitoring of the cardiac rhythm and electrocardiography as well as blood pressure allows an accurate evaluation of the cardiac response to exercise. The measurement of blood gases at rest and at peak exercise provides information related to gas exchange, dead space and alveolar ventilation. Finally, the measurement of dyspnoea using the VAS or Borg scale at intervals during the test and at its end, add very important information. Indeed, the systematic evaluation of dyspnoea during exercise has helped to explain the mechanisms underlying the genesis of dyspnoea and the effect of bronchodilators on this symptom. Recent evidence indicates that peak exercise $\dot{V}o_2$ is an excellent predictor of long-term survival [46] and also helps in the prognosis of postoperative outcome in patients being considered for lung resection [49]. The response to a cardiopulmonary exercise test also helps to plan the exercise intensity to be used in pulmonary rehabilitation [50]. The use of CPET should be encouraged because the completeness of information obtained from its performance compensates for the need for special equipment and resources.

Field exercise tests

Field exercise testing should be available to everyone. These tests are becoming increasingly popular because they not only provide information of functional capacity, but the 6-minute walk distance has also been shown to be an independent predictor of mortality in COPD [47,51] and of morbidity and mortality after lung volume reduction [52].

Six-minute walk test

This test has recently been standardized by the ATS [53]. In summary, the test should be performed in a corridor 30–40 m long. The patient is instructed to walk as far as possible at his or her own pace for a total of 6 minutes. The dyspnoea induced by the exercise is scored using the VAS or modified Borg scale. The distance walked over that time is measured and reported. Two tests performed at least 30 minutes apart are recommended because more than two tests do not provide additional information. Two recent studies have provided values from control subjects which can be used to normalize the results [54,55]. The predictive formulas are summarized in Table 15.2. They are very helpful because the distance walked is influenced by gender, age and height, and the formulas help to correct for these differences. The 6-minute walk test is highly reproducible, simple and easy to administer. It represents the functional capacity of patients very well and is an excellent predictor of mortality [47]. There is increasing support for the inclusion of the 6-minute walk test in the routine evaluation of patients with moderate to severe COPD.

Incremental shuttle walk test

Although it is a field test, the incremental shuttle walk test truly represents an intermediate test between the CPET and the 6-minute walk test. It is easy to conduct in a monitored setting and involves walking at ever faster speed around cones placed 10 m apart [56]. Increasing speed is encouraged by the use of an audio signal from a tape cassette. In essence, it is a symptom-limited maximal performance test. Indeed, the values of oxygen uptake measured during this test approximate those achieved during a formal CPET [57]. Thus, the maximum heart rate, oxygen uptake and ventilatory demands are higher than those seen during the 6-minute walk test.

Stair climbing

Walking up stairs is a less explored test that correlates very well with cycle ergometry [58]. It is more demanding than walking but it has not been compared with the shuttle walk test. However, it has recently proven very useful in predicting postoperative pulmonary complications [59]. Like the incremental shuttle walk test, its applicability remains to be more widely explored.

Respiratory muscle testing

The function of the respiratory muscles is invariable affected in patients with COPD. With disease progression there is flattening of the diaphragm which results in the incapacity of this muscle to generate adequate inspiratory pressure [60]. The diaphragm adapts by shortening the number of sarcomeres and adopting a new optimal length–tension relationship [61]. Indeed, studies from biopsies of patients with severe COPD have revealed an increase in the proportion of fatigue-resistant muscle fibres type IA and a reduction of the less fatigue-resistant muscle fibres type II [62]. In order to maintain appropriate ventilation, especially in situations of increased ventilatory demand, the accessory muscles increase their participation in pressure generation. This results in the frequent observation of accessory muscle recruitment during tidal breathing in patients with severe COPD.

The tests used to evaluate respiratory muscle function have been recently updated by the ATS/ERS [63] and include tests of strength and endurance. In general, respiratory muscle function should be tested in patients with evidence of poor nutrition or with suspected myopathy, including that induced by continuous use of corticosteroids. In addition, one should consider testing respiratory muscle function if dyspnoea or hypercapnia is disproportionally increased with respect to FEV_1.

The maximum inspiratory pressure is impaired usually because of hyperinflation or abnormal mechanics of breathing. In contrast, a reduction in maximum expiratory pressure could be attributed to muscle weakness (see Chapter 3).

Pulmonary vasculature and heart function

Pulmonary vascular pressure and right ventricular function

Table 15.2 Spirometric classification of severity of COPD.

Severity	Postbronchodilator FEV_1/FVC	FEV_1 (% predicted)
At risk	> 0.7	≥ 80
Mild COPD	≤ 0.7	≥ 80
Moderate COPD	≤ 0.7	50–80
Severe COPD	≤ 0.7	30–50
Very severe COPD	≤ 0.7	< 30

FEV_1, forced expiratory volume in 1 s; FVC, functional residual capacity.

can be assessed using non-invasive methods, such as two-dimensional and Doppler echocardiography [64,65]. Left ventricular function is usually normal in patients with COPD. However, in patients with a significant degree of emphysema it may be technically difficult to obtain adequate imaging because of the greater distance between the probe and the heart resulting from the hyperinflation. In these patients, transoesophageal echocardiography appears to offer an advantage and can provide information not otherwise routinely obtainable. The most frequent echocardiographical findings in patients with cor pulmonale include: increased right ventricular size, moderate to severe tricuspid regurgitation with widened right ventricular to right atrial pressure drop, and a delayed onset of right ventricular filling. However, the gold standard method of measuring pulmonary hypertension and its possible response to therapy remains right heart catheterization.

Electrocardiography

Frequently performed in all patients needing medical services, the electrocardiogram (ECG) is not a good tool to detect the cardiac consequences of pulmonary disease. The ECG is relatively insensitive to detect pulmonary hypertension and right ventricular enlargement. However, it is very good in diagnosing and helping to monitor the presence of arrhythmias, such as atrial fibrillation and flutter, frequently found in patients with COPD. The ECG finding of an R or R′ inflection greater or equal to the S wave in V_1, the presence of an R wave smaller than the S wave in V_6, or right axis deviation greater than 110° without right bundle branch block are all supportive of the presence of coexisting cor pulmonale [66].

Computed tomography

Computed tomography (CT) should be recommended if the diagnosis is in doubt or for preoperative assessment for bullectomy or lung volume reduction surgery. However, as this relatively new and ever-expanding technology is increasingly used, more indications are found for its use [67–70].

High-resolution CT is defined as thin section images (1–2 mm collimation scans). Spiral CT provides continuous scanning as the patient is moved through the scanner. High-resolution CT has helped to visualize early interstitial and vascular disease, as well as help in diagnosing bronchiectasis and detecting small lesions [71]. Experimentally, it has been used to detect and follow-up emphysematous changes as well as attempt to quantify bronchial size and infer the degree of bronchitis [71,72]. There are recent reports of the capacity of CT to detect emphysematous changes in patients with α_1-antitrypsin deficiency earlier than the development of pulmonary function

Table 15.3 Current indications for computerized tomography (CT) in patients with COPD.

1 Evaluation for surgery
  bullectomy
  lung volume reduction
  transplant
  lung resection
2 Consideration of pulmonary embolism (spiral CT with contrast)
3 Suspicion of bronchiectasis

changes [73]. Spiral CT with the use of intravenous contrast is very good at detecting pulmonary embolism, a diagnosis frequently suspected in patients with COPD who develop worsening dyspnoea.

The use of CT in the evaluation of patients with moderate to severe COPD has been expanded with the results of the National Emphysema Therapy Trial (NETT), which studied the value of lung volume reduction surgery compared with pulmonary rehabilitation and optimal medical care [34]. The results of NETT, conducted in 1277 patients, showed CT to be instrumental in the selection of candidates who may benefit from surgery as well as those for whom surgery may confer a poor outcome. Indeed, the most important factor to predict outcome was the tomographical distribution of emphysematous lesions. The presence of inhomogeneous lesions of upper lobe predominance indicates a good prognosis after surgery while the converse, the presence of homogeneous distribution with non-upper lobe predominance was indicative of a poor outcome. Table 15.3 shows the indications for CT scans based on current available information. With the expansion of its use, this list is likely to increase.

Blood tests

Haemography

The effects of hypoxaemia on compensatory erythrocytosis have been well studied [74]. However, the red blood cell line response of patients with COPD to the effects of hypoxaemia is less well characterized. Indeed, normal, decreased or increased responses have all been documented. This may in part be caused by the difficulty in studying patients with 'pure' COPD and also to the multiple factors influencing the red cell life cycle. There is evidence of erythrocytosis in smokers and also increased red cells in patients with sleep apnoea and associated hypoxia. However, many patients with COPD have normal values, especially if receiving supplemental oxygen, and others may present with anaemia. However, severe anaemia (haemoglobin values < 10 g/dL) should alert the clinician to the possible presence of coexisting disease.

Smokers without airflow obstruction also have an increased number of peripheral neutrophils, which is also present in patients with COPD even after having stopped smoking [75]. The actual reason for this and its pathophysiological implications are under investigation. Elevation of white blood cell counts during exacerbations should suggest the presence of bacterial infection of the respiratory tract, especially if there is coexisting fever and purulent sputum.

α₁-Antitrypsin

The $α_1$-antitrypsin levels should be measured in young patients (< 45 years) who develop COPD, especially if the disease predominantly affects the lower lobes [1,2]. The diagnosis is even more likely if there is an associated strong family history. A serum value of $α_1$-antitrypsin < 15–20% of the normal limits is highly suggestive of homozygous $α_1$-antitrypsin deficiency. If the diagnosis is confirmed, it may be followed by a family screening. A deficiency of the ZZ allele is the best documented genetic factor for COPD. This recessive trait may lead to emphysema even if the person has never smoked and certainly accelerates the development of COPD in patients with the deficiency who smoke. Heterozygotes usually have intermediate levels of the inhibitor and are therefore more susceptible to the development of emphysema than normal subjects without the trait [76–78].

Sputum examination

In spite of providing information on the functional dynamic of the airways and the lungs, the routine analysis of the sputum has not gained wide acceptance in clinical practice. Present in patients whose main expression of the disease is that of chronic bronchitis, it is often contaminated by mouth secretions, thereby rendering any finding somewhat difficult to interpret. In the stable state, the sputum should be mucoid and if examined under the microscope it usually shows a predominance of macrophages with neutrophils and in some cases bacteria. The presence of the same bacteria in cultures of the sputum suggests chronic colonization. Recent evidence indicates that mutations in the typing of the same bacteria may be associated with exacerbations of COPD [79]. During exacerbations, the sputum becomes purulent, changing its colour and viscosity. The most frequent bacteria associated with exacerbations include *Streptococcus pneumoniae*, *Haemophilus influenzae* and *Moraxella catarrhalis*. Using polymerase chain reaction (PCR) techniques, careful evaluation of sputum from patients during exacerbations has documented a significant proportion of them to be caused by viruses, which apparently confer a slower recovery [80].

There is new interest in attempting to standardize the appropriate collection, examination and interpretation of sputum [81–83]. Indeed, because many patients produce it in significant amounts and sputum induction using nebulized hypertonic saline is safe and effective, there is reason to expect that more use of this technique will be made in future.

Bronchoalveolar lavage and biopsy

These techniques have proven useful in providing new insights into the inflammatory nature of COPD. Indeed, results from such studies have shown that in COPD the inflammation is primarily characterized by the presence of CD4 lymphocytes, neutrophils and macrophages. In addition, the effect of therapy on the type and number of cells has also been explored using this technique [84–86]. The possibility that lung volume reduction could be accomplished with the insertion of one-way valves or airway sealing material via the bronchoscope will probably accelerate the use of these techniques in the management of COPD.

Exhaled breath

This is a recently applied technique that is finding its true role in the evaluation of patients with COPD. A number of substances can be identified and their presence and levels measured [87]. These substances include: leukotrienes, prostaglandins, cytokines, isoprostanes, products of lipid peroxidase, ethane and, most frequently, nitric oxide (NO). There have been problems with standardization and reliability; however, its simplicity and the fact that exhaled breath could provide a window to metabolic lung function make this a very attractive tool. Of all of the substances reported, NO is the one that has been most consistently detected [88]. The findings suggest that the levels of NO are lower in smokers and patients with COPD than in normal individuals [89]. In contrast, the levels appear elevated in patients with asthma [90]. Although it may be premature to use the levels as a specific disease marker, it is possible to conceive that a high level of NO in a patient suspected of COPD could actually represent an overlapping case of asthma and may suggest a possible reason for the use of corticosteroids. There have already been studies reporting increased levels of interleukin-6 (IL-6) and leukotriene B_4 (LTB$_4$) in patients with COPD.

Sleep studies

Sleep has effects on breathing, which include changes in central respiratory control, airways resistance and muscle contractility. These do not have an adverse effect in healthy individuals but may cause problems in patients with COPD [91]. The sleep-related disturbances in gas exchange in COPD are a consequence of the disease itself, and are different from sleep apnoea. Sleep-related hypoxaemia and hypercapnia in COPD are most pronounced during rapid eye movement (REM) sleep. Oxygen desaturation in COPD is considerably greater during sleep than during maximum exercise [92] and predisposes to nocturnal cardiac arrhythmias [93], pulmonary hypertension and possibly death during acute exacerbations [94].

Patients with COPD have a higher prevalence of insomnia, fragmentation with frequent arousals, nightmares and daytime sleepiness than the general population, with close to 50% of patients reporting significant disturbance in sleep quality. Sleep disturbance probably contributes to the non-specific daytime symptoms of chronic fatigue, lethargy and overall impairment in quality of life [95].

Disturbances of breathing during sleep are highly prevalent in the population at large and increase with increasing age. This makes the possible coexistence of sleep apnoea in patients with COPD a frequent problem. A polysomnogram is indicated in these patients. Treatment of the apnoea and the COPD can lead to improvement above and beyond that expected from the treatment of the hypoxaemia or airflow limitation [96].

Classification of severity and staging of COPD

COPD is characterized by poorly reversible airflow limitation [1]. Since it was first described by Fletcher *et al.* [97], the rate of decline of lung function has become the hallmark of the progression of COPD. This is expressed in a modified version in Figure 15.6 which not only shows the change in FEV_1 over time, but also adds the theoretical change brought about by early smoking and also the effect of smoking cessation on that rate of decline. It is interesting that therapy has been directed at reversing what has been

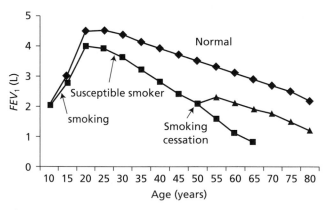

Figure 15.6 The forced expiratory volume in 1 s (FEV_1) increases from birth until about age 21 years and then progressively decreases with age. In patients susceptible to the effects of cigarette smoke, the decline is steeper so patients become symptomatic by the 5th or 6th decade. Notice that smoking cessation results in an early increase in FEV_1 and, very importantly, a normalization of the rate of decline, which tends to return to that of non-smokers of similar age.

defined as being irreversible and to altering the accelerated rate of decline of the FEV_1 in patients with the disease. So far, only smoking cessation [98] has been shown to reduce the rate of lung function, as shown in Figure 15.6. However, supplemental oxygen in hypoxaemic patients [3,4], lung volume reduction surgery in patients with non-homogeneous emphysema of upper lobe predominance [34], and non-invasive ventilation during acute on chronic respiratory failure [99] have all been proven to increase survival in patients with COPD.

Unfortunately, the fact that several trials of medication failed to show any effect on the rate of lung function decline [100,101] has led to a dangerously nihilistic attitude towards the disease. Traditionally, the severity of COPD has been graded using a single physiological variable, the FEV_1 [1,2]. However, COPD is associated with systemic consequences such as dyspnoea and exercise limitation [102], pulmonary hypertension [103], peripheral muscle weakness [104] and malnutrition [105]. Furthermore, the FEV_1 is not the only predictor of mortality in COPD. Several studies have identified other risk factors such as hypoxaemia or hypercapnia [106], the timed walk distance [47,51], degree of functional breathlessness [107] and a low BMI [108]. Therefore, grading COPD solely on the FEV_1 does not adequately reflect the clinical manifestations of the disease and its ultimate prognosis. The ATS recently expressed the need for a multicomponent staging system that in addition to the degree of impairment could express the heterogeneous manifestations of COPD.

Using the FEV_1, the disease has been classified arbitrarily in five stages (see Table 15.2). This classification has proven useful in epidemiological and large group and drug studies, but the simple grading by spirometry fails to fully represent the different dimensions that are affected by the disease. COPD could be represented as a pulmonary disease that affects several domains: the respiratory, systemic and perceptive. All of these domains can be evaluated with relatively simple tools (Fig. 15.7) and provide important prognostic information. Indeed, the measurement of dyspnoea with the Medical Reseach Council (MRC) scale [107], of exercise capacity with the cardiopulmonary exercise test or the 6-minute walk distance [47] and the BMI [108] have been shown independently to predict survival. We have expanded this concept to develop a grading system that includes all of these domains in a single index, the BODE index (body mass index, airflow obstruction, dyspnoea, exercise performance). The BODE index proved to be a better predictor of all cause and disease-specific mortality than the FEV_1 [109]. The measurement of outcomes different from the FEV_1 is important because it changes the way in which we interpret the course of the disease. Based on this concept, several medical therapies that failed to show changes in FEV_1 have been deemed ineffective [100,101]. However, the same studies demonstrated improvement

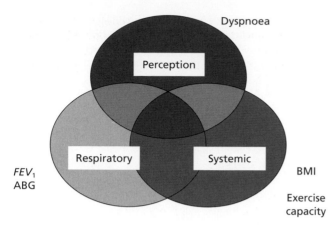

Figure 15.7 The patients with COPD may be affected in several domains. Although primarily a disease of airways and thus leading to respiratory impairment, COPD can also result in changes in perception and alterations in other non-pulmonary areas (systemic effects). This is represented in this schema with the details of simple tests that can help measure the affection in each one of the domains. An integrative score of these domains helps provide a better assessment of patient's outcomes. ABG, arterial blood gas; BMI, body mass index; FEV_1, forced expiratory volume in 1 s.

in other outcomes such as rate of exacerbation, dyspnoea and health status, all of which are of extreme importance to patients with COPD. These contradictory findings can be reconciled by acknowledging that COPD is not just a pulmonary disease and is therefore incompletely described by the FEV_1.

Prognosis

The disease has been termed progressive and irreversible. However, this is not so and therapeutic interventions such as smoking cessation, supplemental oxygen for hypoxaemic patients, non-invasive ventilation in patients with acute on chronic respiratory failure and lung volume reduction surgery in selected patients with inhomogeneous emphysema have all been shown to prolong survival. In addition, pharmacological therapy and pulmonary rehabilitation improve dyspnoea, exercise capacity and health status. Finally, preventive measures such as vaccination have decreased the rate of complications and, more specifically, the dreaded exacerbations. Perhaps the most important problem facing this disease is its lack of recognition and the lack of use of spirometry [110]. Currently, patients who are diagnosed at an early stage have a very good prognosis. Once symptomatic, treatment is very effective in improving symptoms and smoking cessation usually helps to reverse the progression of the disease. In more severe disease, which unfortunately represents most of the patients who are seen by specialists, there are many therapeutic tools

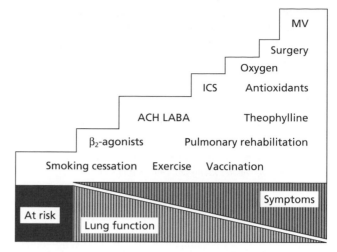

Figure 15.8 There are many available therapeutic options for patients with COPD. A nihilistic attitude is not justified. ACH, anticholinergics; ICS, inhaled corticosteroids; LABA, long acting β-agonists; MV, mechanical ventilation.

that can help patients to maintain a productive life. Figure 15.8 represents the therapeutic options that are available to patients with COPD. With these tools at hand, a negative attitude is not justified.

References

1 Celli B, McNee W. Standards for the diagnosis and treatment of patients with chronic obstructive pulmonary disease. *Eur Respir J* 2004;**23**:841–5.

2 Pauwels RA, Buist AS, Calverley PM, Jenkins CR, Hurd SS, the GOLD Scientific Committee. Global strategy for the diagnosis, management, and prevention of chronic obstructive pulmonary disease. NHLBI/WHO Global Initiative for Chronic Obstructive Lung Disease (GOLD) Workshop summary. *Am J Respir Crit Care Med* 2001;**163**:1256–76.

3 Report of the Medical Research Council Working Party. Long-term domiciliary oxygen therapy in chronic hypoxic cor pulmonale complicating chronic bronchitis and emphysema. *Lancet* 1981;**1**:681–5.

4 Nocturnal Oxygen Therapy Trial Group. Continuous or nocturnal oxygen therapy in hypoxemic chronic obstructive lung disease. *Ann Intern Med* 1980;**93**:391–8.

5 Georgopoulos D, Anthonisen NR. Symptoms and signs of COPD. In: Cherniack NS, ed. *Chronic Obstructive Pulmonary Disease*. Toronto: WB Saunders, 1991: 357–63.

6 Stockley R, O'Brien C, Pye A, Hill S. Relationship of sputum color to nature and outpatient management of COPD. *Chest* 2000;**117**;1638–45.

7 Nishimura K, Izumi T, Tsukino M, Oga T. Dyspnoea is a better predictor of 5-year survival than airway obstruction in patients with COPD. *Chest* 2002;**121**:1434–40.

8 Hajiro T, Nishimura K, Tsukino M *et al.* Comparison of discriminative properties among disease-specific questionnaires for measuring health-related quality of life in patients

with chronic obstructive pulmonary disease. *Am J Respir Crit Care Med* 1998;**157**:785–90.

9 Mahler DA, Weinberg DH, Wells CK *et al*. The measurement of dyspnoea: contents, interobserver agreement, and physiologic correlates of two new clinical indexes. *Chest* 1984;**85**: 751–8.

10 Marin J, Montes De Oca M, Rassulo J, Celli BR. Ventilatory drive at rest and perception of exertional dyspnoea in severe COPD. *Chest* 1999;**115**:1293–300.

11 O'Donnell D, Kebb K. Exertional breathlessness in patients with chronic airflow limitation: the role of lung hyperinflation. *Am Rev Respir Dis* 1993;**148**:1351–7.

12 Breslin EH, Garroutte BC, Carrieri VK, Celli BR. Correlations between dyspnoea, diaphragm and sternomastoid recruitment during inspiratory resistance breathing in normal subjects. *Chest* 1990;**98**:298–302.

13 Chaouat A, Weitzenbum E, Krieger J *et al*. Association of chronic obstructive pulmonary disease and sleep apnoea syndrome. *Am J Respir Crit Care Med* 1995;**151**:82–6.

14 Schols AMWJ, Soeters PB, Dingemans AMC *et al*. Prevalence and characteristics of nutritional depletion in patients with stable COPD eligible for pulmonary rehabilitation. *Am Rev Respir Dis* 1993;**147**:1151–6.

15 Landbo C, Prescott E, Lange P, Vestbo J, Almdal TP. Prognostic value of nutritional status in chronic obstructive pulmonary disease. *Am J Respir Crit Care Med* 1999;**160**: 1856–61.

16 Bernaards C, Twisk J, Snel J, Van Mechelen W, Kemper H. Is calculating pack-years retrospectively a valid method to estimate life-time tobacco smoking? A comparison between prospectively calculated pack-years and retrospectively calculated pack-years. *Addiction* 2001;**96**:1653–61.

17 Gold DR, Wang X, Wipyj D *et al*. Effects of cigarette smoking on lung function in adolescent boys and girls. *N Engl J Med* 1996;**335**:931–7.

18 Dennis R, Maldonado D, Norman S, Baena E, Martinez G. Woodsmoke exposure and risk for obstructive airways disease in women. *Chest* 1996;**109**:115–9.

19 Sandford AJ, Weir TD, Pare P. Genetic risk factors for chronic obstructive pulmonary disease. *Eur Respir J* 1997; **10**:1380–91.

20 Silverman EK, Speizer FE. Risk factors for the development of chronic obstructive pulmonary disease. *Med Clin North Am* 1996;**80**:501–22.

21 Martinez F, Couser J, Celli BR. Factors that determine ventilatory muscle recruitment in patients with chronic airflow obstruction. *Am Rev Respir Dis* 1990;**142**:276–82.

22 Celli B, Halbert R, Isonaka S, Schau B. Population impact of different definitions of airway obstruction. *Eur Respir J* 2003;**22**:268–73.

23 Hansen E, Phanareth K, Laursen L, Kok-Jensen A, Dirksen A. Reversible and irreversible airflow obstruction as predictor of overall mortality in asthma and chronic obstructive pulmonary disease. *Am J Respir Crit Care Med* 1999;**159**: 1267–71.

24 Burrows B, Earle R. Course and prognosis of chronic obstructive lung disease: a prospective study of 200 patients. *N Engl J Med* 1969;**280**:397–404.

25 Rebuck D, Hanania N, D'Urzo A, Chapman K. The accuracy of a handheld portable spirometer. *Chest* 1996;**109**:152–7.

26 Gibson GJ, MacNee W. Chronic obstructive pulmonary disease: investigations and assessment of severity. *Eur Respir Mon* 1998;**7**:25–40.

27 Newton M, O'Donnell D, Forkert L. Response of lung volumes to inhaled salbutamol in a large population of patients with severe hyperinflation. *Chest* 2002;**121**:1042–50.

28 Bates D. *Respiratory Function in Disease*. Philadelphia: WB Saunders, 1989: 158–69.

29 Marin J, Carrizo S, Gascon M *et al*. Inspiratory capacity, dynamic hyperinflation, breathlessness and exercise performance during the 6-minute walk test in chronic obstructive pulmonary disease. *Am J Respir Crit Care Med* 2001;**163**: 1395–400.

30 Belman M, Botnick W, Shin J. Inhaled bronchodilators reduce dynamic hyperinflation during exercise in patients with obstructive lung disease *Am J Respir Crit Care Med* 1996;**153**:967–75.

31 O'Donnell D, Lam M, Webb K. Spirometric correlates of improvement in exercise performance after anticholinergic therapy in chronic obstructive pulmonary disease. *Am J Respir Crit Care Med* 1999;**160**:542–9.

32 Martinez F, Montes de Oca M, Whyte R *et al*. Lung-volume reduction surgery improves dyspnoea, dynamic hyperinflation and respiratory muscle function. *Am J Respir Crit Care Med* 1997;**155**:2018–23.

33 Bolliger CT, Perruchoud AP. Functional evaluation of the lung resection candidate. *Eur Respir J* 1998;**11**:198–212.

34 National Emphysema Treatment Trial Research Group. A randomized trial comparing lung-volume-reduction surgery with medical therapy for severe emphysema. *N Engl J Med* 2003;**348**:2059–73.

35 Hughes J. Diffusing capacity (transfer factor) for carbon monoxide. In: Hughes J, Pride N, eds. *Lung Function Tests, Physiology, Principles and Clinical Applications*. London: WB Saunders, 1999: 93–106.

36 Anthonisen N, Wright E, Hodgkin J. Prognosis in chronic obstructive pulmonary disease. *Am Rev Respir Dis* 1986; **133**:14–20.

37 Zielinski J, Tobiasz M, Hawrylkiewicz I, Sliwinksi P, Palasiewicz G. Effects of long-term oxygen therapy on pulmonary hemodynamics in COPD patients: a 6-year prospective study. *Chest* 1998;**113**:65–70.

38 International Consensus Conferences in Intensive Care Medicine: non-invasive positive pressure ventilation in acute respiratory failure. *Am J Respir Crit Care Med* 2001;**163**: 283–91.

39 Lightowler JV, Wedzicha JA, Elliot M, Ram SF. Non-invasive positive pressure ventilation to treat respiratory failure resulting from exacerbations of chronic obstructive pulmonary disease: Cochrane systematic review and meta-analysis. *BMJ* 2003;**326**:185–9.

40 Tiep BL, Barnett J, Schiffman G, Sanchez O, Carter R. Maintaining oxygenation via demand oxygen delivery during rest and exercise. *Respir Care* 2002;**47**:887–92.

41 Aubier M, Murciano D, Milic-Emili M *et al*. Effects of the administration of oxygen therapy on ventilation and blood

gases in patients with chronic obstructive pulmonary disease during acute respiratory failure. *Am Rev Respir Dis* 1980;**122**: 747–54.

42 Christensen CC, Ryg M, Refvem OK *et al*. Development of severe hypoxaemia in chronic obstructive pulmonary disease patients at 2438 m (8000 ft) altitude. *Eur Respir J* 2000;**15**:635–9.

43 Berg BW, Dillard TA, Rajagopal KR, Mehm WJ. Oxygen supplementation during air travel in patients with chronic obstructive pulmonary disease. *Chest* 1992;**101**:638–41.

44 Martinez FJ, Stanopolous I, Acero R *et al*. Graded comprehensive cardiopulmonary exercise testing in the evaluation of dyspnoea unexplained by routine evaluation. *Chest* 1994; **105**:168–74.

45 Weissman I, Zeballos J. Clinical exercise testing. *Clin Chest Med* 2001;**22**:679–703.

46 Oga T, Nishimura K, Tsukino M, Sato S, Hajiro T. Analysis of the factors related to mortality in chronic obstructive pulmonary disease: role of exercise capacity and health status. *Am J Respir Crit Care Med* 2002;**167**:544–9.

47 Pinto-Plata V, Cote C, Cabral H, Taylor J, Celli B. The six-minute walk distance: change over time and its value as predictor of survival. *Eur Respir J* 2004;**23**:28–33.

48 Jones NL, Killian KJ. Exercise limitation in health and disease. *N Engl J Med* 2000;**343**:632–41.

49 Bolliger CT, Jordan P, Soler M *et al*. Pulmonary function and exercise capacity after lung resection. *Eur Respir J* 1996;**9**: 415–21.

50 ATS statement: pulmonary rehabilitation. *Am J Respir Crit Care Med* 1999;**159**:1666–82.

51 Gerardi DA, Lovett L, Benoit-Connors ML, Reardon JZ, ZuWallack RL. Variables related to increased mortality following out-patient pulmonary rehabilitation. *Eur Respir J* 1996;**9**:431–5.

52 Szekely L, Oelberg D, Wrinight C *et al*. Preoperative predictors of operative mortality in COPD patients undergoing bilateral lung volume reduction surgery. *Chest* 1997;**111**: 550–8.

53 ATS statement: guidelines for the six-minute walk test. *Am J Respir Crit Care Med* 2002;**166**:111–7.

54 Troosters T, Gosselink R, Decramer M. Six minute walking distance in health elderly subjects. *Eur Respir J* 1999;**14**: 270–4.

55 Enright P, Sherrill D. Reference equations for the six-minute walk in healthy adults. *Am J Respir Crit Care Med* 1998;**158**:1384–7.

56 Singh S, Morgan M, Scott S, Walters D, Hardman A. Development of a shuttle walk test of disability in patients with chronic airways obstruction. *Thorax* 1992;**47**:1019–24.

57 Singer S, Morgan M, Hardman A. Comparison of oxygen uptake during a conventional treadmill test and the shuttle walking test in chronic airflow limitation. *Eur Respir J* 1994;**7**:2016–20.

58 Pollock M, Roa J, Benditt J, Celli BR. Estimation of ventilatory reserve by stair climbing: a study in patients with chronic airflow obstruction. *Chest* 1993;**104**:1378–83.

59 Girish M, Trayner E, Dammann O, Pinto-Plata V, Celli B. Symptom-limited stair climbing as a predictor of post-operative cardiopulmonary complications after high-risk surgery. *Chest* 2001;**120**:1147–51.

60 Roussos CH, Macklem PT. The respiratory muscles. *N Engl J Med* 1982;**307**:786–97.

61 Supinsky GS, Kelsen S. Effect of elastase-induced emphysema on the force-generating ability of the diaphragm. *J Clin Invest* 1982;**70**:978–88.

62 Levine S, Kaiser L, Leferovich J, Tikunov B. Cellular adaptations in the diaphragm in chronic obstructive pulmonary disease. *N Engl J Med* 1997;**337**:1799–806.

63 ATS/ERS statement: respiratory muscle testing. *Am J Respir Crit Care Med* 2002;**166**:518–624.

64 Dabestani A, Mahan G, Gardin J *et al*. Evaluation of pulmonary artery pressure and resistance by pulsed Doppler echocardiography. *Am J Cardiol* 1987;**59**:662–8.

65 MacNee W. Pathophysiology of cor pulmonale in chronic obstructive pulmonary disease. *Am J Respir Crit Care Med* 1994;**150**:833–52 (Part 1); 1158–68 (Part 2).

66 Mittal S, Jain S, Sharma S. The role of electrocardiographic criteria for the diagnosis of right ventricular hypertrophy in chronic obstructive pulmonary disease. *Int J Cardiol* 1986; **11**:165–73.

67 Cosio M, Snider GL. Chest computerized tomography: is it ready for major studies of chronic obstructive pulmonary disease? *Eur Respir J* 2001;**17**:162–4.

68 Ferreti G, Bricault I, Coulomb M. Virtual tools for imaging of the thorax. *Eur Respir J* 2001;**18**:381–92.

69 Remy-Jardin M, Edme J, Boulenguez C *et al*. Longitudinal follow-up study of smoker's lung with thin-section CT in correlation with pulmonary function tests. *Radiology* 2002; **222**:261–70.

70 Muller N, Coxson H. Chronic obstructive pulmonary disease: imaging the lungs in patients with COPD. *Thorax* 2002;**57**:982–5.

71 Hansell D. Small airways diseases: detection and insights with computed tomography. *Eur Respir J* 2001;**17**:1294–313.

72 Soejima K, Yamaguchi K, Kohda E *et al*. Longitudinal follow-up study of smoking-induced lung density changes by high-resolution computed tomography. *Am J Respir Crit Care Med* 2000;**161**:1264–73.

73 Dowson L, Guest P, Stockley R. Longitudinal changes in physiological, radiological, and health status measurement in α_1-antitrypsin deficiency and factors associated with decline. *Am J Respir Crit Care Med* 2001;**164**:1805–9.

74 Wedzicha J, Coates P, Empey D *et al*. Serum reactive erythropoietin in hypoxic lung disease with and without polycythemia. *Clin Sci* 1985;**69**:413–22.

75 Pesci A, Majori M, Cuomo A *et al*. Neutrophils infiltrating bronchial epithelium in chronic obstructive pulmonary disease. *Respir Med* 1998;**92**:863–70.

76 Laurell C, Erikson S. The electrophoretic α_1-globulin pattern in serum in α_1-antitrypsin deficiency. *Scand J Clin Lab Invest* 1963;**15**:132–40.

77 Sandford A, Weir T, Spinelli J, Pare P. Z and S mutations of the α_1-antitrypsin gene and the risk of chronic obstructive pulmonary disease. *Am J Respir Cell Mol Biol* 1999;**20**:287–91.

78 Tarjan E, Magyar P, Vaczi Z, Lantos A, Vaszar L. Longitudinal lung function study in heterozygous PiMZ phenotypes subjects. *Eur Respir J* 1994;**7**:2199–204.

79 Sethi S, Evans N, Grant B, Murphy T. New strains of bacteria and exacerbations of chronic obstructive pulmonary disease. *N Engl J Med* 2002;**347**:465–71.

80 Seemungal TA, Donaldson GC, Bhowmik A, Jeffries DJ, Wedzicha JA. Time course and recovery of exacerbations in patients with chronic obstructive pulmonary disease. *Am J Respir Crit Care Med* 2000;**161**:1608–13.

81 Keatings V, Collins P, Scott D, Barnes P. Differences in interleukin-8 and tumor necrosis factor-alpha in induced sputum from patients with chronic obstructive pulmonary disease or asthma. *Am J Respir Crit Care Med* 1996;**153**:530–4.

82 Vlachos-Mayer H, Leigh R, Sharon R, Hussack P, Hargreave F. Success and safety of sputum induction in the clinical setting. *Eur Respir J* 2000;**16**:997–1000.

83 European Respiratory Society Task Force. Standardized methodology of sputum induction and processing. *Eur Respir J* 2002;**20**:1–55S.

84 O'Shaughnessy TC, Ansari TW, Barnes NC, Jeffery PK. Inflammation in bronchial biopsies of subjects with chronic bronchitis: inverse relationship of CD8$^+$ T lymphocytes with FEV_1. *Am J Respir Crit Care Med* 1997;**155**:852–7.

85 Saetta M, Di Stefano A, Maestrelli P *et al*. Activated T-lymphocytes and macrophages in bronchial mucosa of subjects with chronic bronchitis. *Am Rev Respir Dis* 1993;**147**:301–6.

86 Hattotuwa K, Gizycki M, Ansari T, Jeffery P, Barnes N. The effects of inhaled fluticasone on airways inflammation in chronic obstructive pulmonary disease: a double blind placebo controlled biopsy study. *Am J Respi Crit Care Med* 2002;**165**:1592–6.

87 Kharinotov S, Barnes P. Exhaled markers of pulmonary disease. *Am J Respir Crit Care Med* 2001;**163**:1693–722.

88 Papi A, Romagnoli M, Baraldo S *et al*. Partial reversibility of airflow limitation and increased NO and sputum eosinophilia in chronic obstructive pulmonary disease. *Am J Respir Crit Care Med* 2000;**162**:1773–7.

89 Campagnano G, Kharitonov S, Foschino-Barbaro M *et al*. Increased inflammatory markers in the exhaled breath condensate of cigarette smokers. *Eur Respir J* 2003;**21**:589–93.

90 Maziak W, Loukides S, Culpitt S *et al*. Exhaled nitric oxide in chronic obstructive pulmonary disease. *Am J Respir Crit Care Med* 1998;**157**:998–1002.

91 Klink M, Quan S. Prevalence of reported sleep disturbances in a general population and their relationship to obstructive airways diseases. *Chest* 1987;**91**:540–6.

92 Mulloy E, McNicholas WT. Ventilation and gas exchange during sleep and exercise in patients with severe COPD. *Chest* 1996;**109**:387–94.

93 Tirlapur VG, Mir MA. Nocturnal hypoxemia and associated electrocardiographic changes in patients with chronic obstructive airways disease. *N Engl J Med* 1982;**306**:125–30.

94 McNicholas WT, FitzGerald MX. Nocturnal death among patients with chronic bronchitis and emphysema. *BMJ* 1984;**289**:878.

95 Cormick W, Olson LG, Hensley MJ, Saunders NA. Nocturnal hypoxemia and quality of sleep in patients with chronic obstructive lung disease. *Thorax* 1986;**41**:846–54.

96 Martin RJ, Bucher BL, Smith P *et al*. Effect of ipratropium bromide treatment on oxygen saturation and sleep quality in COPD. *Chest* 1999;**115**:1338–45.

97 Fletcher C, Peto R, Tinker C, Speizer F. *The Natural History of Chronic Bronchitis and Emphysema*. New York: Oxford University Press, 1976.

98 Anthonisen NR, Connett JE, Kiley JP *et al*. Effects of smoking intervention and the use of an inhaled anticholinergic bronchodilator on the rate of decline of FEV_1. *JAMA* 1994;**272**:1497–505.

99 Mehta S, Hill NS. Non-invasive ventilation: state of the art. *Am J Respir Crit Care Med* 2001;**163**:540–77; 751–8.

100 Burge PS, Calverley PM, Jones PW *et al*. Randomised, double blind, placebo controlled study of fluticasone propionate in patients with moderate to severe chronic obstructive pulmonary disease: the ISOLDE trial. *BMJ* 2000;**320**:1297–303.

101 The Lung Health Study Research Group. Effect of inhaled triamcinolone on the decline in pulmonary function in chronic obstructive pulmonary disease. *N Engl J Med* 2000;**343**:1902–9.

102 Hay JG, Stone P, Carter J *et al*. Bronchodilator reversibility, exercise performance and breathlessness in stable chronic obstructive pulmonary disease. *Eur Respir J* 1992;**5**:659–64.

103 France AJ, Prescott RJ, Biernacki W, Muir AL, MacNee W. Does right ventricular function predict survival in patients with chronic obstructive lung disease? *Thorax* 1988;**43**:621–6.

104 Decramer M, Gosselink R, Troosters T, Verschueren M, Evers G. Muscle weakness is related to utilization of health care resources in COPD patients. *Eur Respir J* 1997;**10**:417–23.

105 Schols AM, Slangen J, Volovics L, Wouters EF. Weight loss is a reversible factor in the prognosis of chronic obstructive pulmonary disease. *Am J Respir Crit Care Med* 1998;**157**:1791–7.

106 Anthonisen NR, Wright EC, Hodgkin JE, the IPPB Trial Group. Prognosis in chronic obstructive pulmonary disease. *Am Rev Respir Dis* 1986;**133**:14–20.

107 Nishimura K, Izumi T, Tsukino M, Oga T. Dyspnoea is a better predictor of 5-year survival than airway obstruction in patients with COPD. *Chest* 2002;**121**:1434–40.

108 Schols AM, Slangen J, Volovics L, Wouters EF. Weight loss is a reversible factor in the prognosis of chronic obstructive pulmonary disease. *Am J Respir Crit Care Med* 1998;**157**:1791–7.

109 Celli B, Cote CG, Marin J *et al*. The body mass index, airflow obstruction, dyspnoea, exercise performance (BODE) index in chronic obstructive pulmonary disease. *N Engl J Med* 2004;**23**:932–46.

110 Mannino DM, Homa DM, Akinbami LJ, Ford ES, Reed SC. Chronic obstructive pulmonary disease surveillance – United States, 1971–2000. *MMWR* 2002;**51**:1–16.

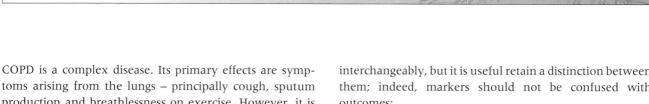

CHAPTER 16
Monitoring and outcomes

Paul W. Jones

COPD is a complex disease. Its primary effects are symptoms arising from the lungs – principally cough, sputum production and breathlessness on exercise. However, it is now clear that there are major secondary effects on other organs. The impact of pulmonary hypertension and chronic hypoxia on right ventricular function has been recognized for a long time, but there is now good evidence, discussed elsewhere in this book, concerning the link between the lungs, skeletal muscle and lean body mass. While breathlessness is recognized universally to be important in COPD, the impact of fatigue is less well known, although it has been described as a major factor in COPD for a long time [1,2]. Mechanisms responsible for fatigue are almost completely unknown, but progress is being made, because recent studies have shown that quadriceps strength is linked to circulating proinflammatory cytokines, which rise during an exacerbation [3]. Sleep disturbance resulting from respiratory symptoms is a common feature of COPD, affecting half of patients [4], and disturbances of mood state occur [5].

Put together, a picture emerges of a disease affecting many organ systems through many different mechanisms. Specific measurements are available for many of the effects of COPD: physiological tests including lung function, exercise capacity and muscle strength; psychophysiological tests of breathlessness and fatigue during exercise; diary cards for symptoms; questionnaires for disability and mood. While all of these build up a picture of the components of the disease and their effects, they do not provide a measure of the overall impact of COPD on the patient. This can only be achieved through formal measurement of health status.

Outcomes and markers

Two general terms are used when discussing the effects of a disease: outcomes and markers. They are often used interchangeably, but it is useful retain a distinction between them; indeed, markers should not be confused with outcomes:
• *Outcome:* consequence of the disease, as experienced by the patient.
• *Marker:* disease-related factor known to be associated with a clinical outcome.

Examples of outcomes in COPD include: symptoms, weight loss, exercise intolerance, disability, exacerbations, impaired health-related quality of life (HRQoL), increased health resource use and death. Quantification is important in medicine, both for routine care and research, so outcomes should be measured, but many patient-experienced outcomes are difficult to quantify in a standardized manner. By contrast, a marker should be a standardized measurement. For example, exercise intolerance in daily life is an outcome resulting from COPD, but it is difficult to quantify each patient's unique and subjective experience of his or her exercise intolerance. Exercise capacity, on the other hand, is a standardized measurement obtained in the laboratory. It can be used as a marker of exercise intolerance because there is good evidence that exercise capacity correlates with patients' reports of the effect of exercise limitation on their daily physical activity (reviewed in [6]).

The distinction between an outcome and its associated markers is also important when considering the impact of disease on the patient's quality of life. A number of terms are used in this setting, often interchangeably: 'health status', 'functional status', 'well-being', 'quality of life' and 'health-related quality of life'. Well-being is usually reserved for subjective perceptions, but may include symptoms as well as global evaluations of health status. The concept of quality of life is much broader than health status, because it includes aspects of the patient's environment that may not be affected by health or treatment. Because there are so many other influences on a patient's quality of life, the term health-related quality of life (HRQoL)

181

was coined to indicate that the measurement is focused on the specific effects of health conditions. Unfortunately, it has also come to be used loosely as a synonym for all self-reported health status measures. The factors that determine an individual's quality of life are unique to that person, so the quality of life effects of disease will also be unique to each patient. Methods of measuring individual HRQoL have been developed [7], but they are difficult to standardize. Nearly all so-called HRQoL questionnaires are standardized and treat each patient as if they were a 'typical' patient. As a result, the capacity for a patient to express the individuality of their experience is very limited. For that reason these questionnaires should be called health status instruments. Health status scores provide a marker of the patient's HRQoL – which is an outcome that is currently not measurable.

The term 'surrogate' is used often in the context of outcomes and markers. In one respect this is quite appropriate because a marker is measured when it is not possible to measure its associated outcome, but in medicine the term 'surrogate marker' takes on a specific meaning where one marker is used in place of the marker of interest. A good example is emphysema – which is difficult to measure directly *in vivo*, so diffusing capacity is often used in practice as a surrogate. Another term in wide use is biomarker, which is a characteristic that is objectively measured and evaluated as an indicator of normal biological processes, pathogenic processes or pharmacological responses to therapeutic interventions. An example in COPD is exhaled nitric oxide (NO), when used as a biomarker for an inflammatory process in the airways.

An important feature of markers is that there should be a known and well-characterized relationship between the marker and its outcome. It is important to appreciate that this relationship may be modified by other factors, and those factors may change. These modifiers may be internal to the patient (e.g. presence of comorbidities) or external (e.g. level of family or social support). The influence of modifiers is yet another reason why it is important to maintain a clear distinction between markers and outcome. The relationship between the two is probabilistic. For example, a low forced expiratory volume in 1 s (FEV_1) is a marker for an increased risk of exacerbations (an outcome), but that does not mean that all patients with low FEV_1 have many exacerbations, or that patients with relatively well-preserved FEV_1 may not also have frequent exacerbations [8].

Use of markers

Markers are used for different purposes and the same variable can be used as a different type of marker, depending upon the application.

Diagnostic marker

In this context, markers are used mainly as a dichotomous variable (i.e. it is either present or absent). This does not mean that the marker has to be measured on a dichotomous scale, but that the measured value is assigned to one of two states (normal or disease), based on ranges defined from experience (e.g. α_1-antitrypsin level, or FEV_1, when used for COPD diagnosis).

Measure of disease severity

A marker may be used to define different levels of disease severity, or stage. When used in this way, measured values for the marker are categorized into predefined ranges. The chosen ranges for these categories may or may not be evidence based. Examples include: body mass index (BMI), or FEV_1 – as used in ERS and Global Initiative for Chronic Obstructive Lung Disease (GOLD) staging.

Marker of disease progression

In this application, the marker is used as a derived parameter, usually as a value per year (e.g. exacerbation rate, decline of FEV_1 or deterioration of health status score).

Marker of treatment effect

These are the familiar markers used to measure response to treatment (e.g. dyspnoea score, lean body mass, exercise capacity, health status, FEV_1). Confusion around terminology can arise in this setting, because in clinical trials these markers are often termed 'outcome variables'. They are, of course, outcomes for the trial, not clinical outcomes.

Patient-reported outcomes

This term has come into use to describe outcomes that depend on the patient's self-report or self-assessment. This dependence is entirely appropriate, although the terminology is slightly tautologous, because outcomes are consequences of disease experienced by the patient. The remainder of this chapter discusses outcomes concerned with symptomatic well-being and what used to be termed impairment, disability and handicap. The concept of disability has changed over time and in some respects has become quite complex. The current World Health Organization (WHO) definition uses the word as an umbrella to include impairment, activity limitation and participation restriction:
• *Impairments:* include problems in body function (e.g. lung function or exercise capacity).

- *Activity limitations:* difficulties an individual may have in executing activities (such as mobility or self-care).
- *Participation restrictions:* problems an individual may experience in involvement in life (what an individual does in his or her current environment).

Impairments and activity limitations can usually be measured as markers, whereas participation restriction is an outcome that is difficult to assess in a standardized way.

Measures of activity limitations

Scales used to quantify limitation of activity in daily life in COPD come under a number of labels.

Dyspnoea scales

Breathlessness can be measured directly using the Visual Analogue and Borg Scales during laboratory exercise tests. Unfortunately, the term 'breathlessness measurement' is also used to describe methods of recording patients' self-report of activities that cause them breathlessness, or more usually are limited by breathlessness. The most widely used example is the Medical Research Council (MRC) Dyspnoea Scale (Table 16.1). Although described as a dyspnoea scale, this is really a scale of activity limitation resulting from breathlessness. It is simple to use and can be translated into different languages with little ambiguity. Its principal application is as a marker of severity, because it categorizes patients into five levels of breathlessness-associated disability. A recent validation in COPD patients has shown that it discriminates between different levels of disability, at least in the three most severe grades [9]. However, it has two minor weaknesses. The first is that its simplicity is achieved at the cost of precision. The five-point scale is adequate for assessing severity, but is too coarse for measuring treatment effects or disease progression. The second weakness arises

Table 16.1 Medical Research Council (MRC) Dyspnoea Scale.

MRC breathlessness questionnaire
I only get breathless with strenuous exercise
I get short of breath when hurrying on the level of walking up a slight hill
I walk slower than people of the same age on the level because of breathlessness, or I have to stop for breath when walking at my own pace on the level
I stop for breath after walking about 100 yards or after a few minutes on the level
I am too breathless to leave the house or I am breathless when dressing or undressing

from the combination of two activity limitations within one grade (e.g. grade 5: difficulty dressing and leaving the house). Using factor analysis of a range of activities limited by breathlessness, we found that these limitations were highly correlated (P.W. Jones, unpublished observations), but no formal analysis has ever been published of the validity of combining these different aspects of dyspnoea-induced disability. When using this scale, it is important to be aware of the existence of two methods of scoring: 0–4 (widely used in the USA) and 1–5 (used in the USA, UK and elsewhere). Whenever the MRC grade is reported, the scale must also be clarified. Despite these minor deficiencies, this questionnaire is a very good marker of disability in chronic lung disease.

A more sophisticated measure of disability resulting from breathlessness is the Baseline Dyspnea Index (BDI) [10]. It provides an index of functional impairment by addressing the magnitude of the task and the magnitude of effort associated with it. Unlike the other instruments described in this chapter, it is currently only available as a clinician-administered instrument. The BDI could be used as a marker of severity, but does not appear to be used in this way very often. Its usual application is to provide a baseline for the Transition Dyspnea Index (TDI) which quantifies the change in breathlessness. Like the BDI, this is clinician administered, but a computerized patient self-administration method has been developed. The TDI was developed as a marker of treatment efficacy and has been shown to be responsive in a number of studies [11,12]. It is not yet clear whether it has properties that make it suitable for use as a marker of disease progression.

The UCSD Shortness of Breath Questionnaire is a comprehensive 24-item dyspnoea questionnaire that measures disability resulting from breathlessness [13]. It has good reliability and validity and has found application in trials of pulmonary rehabilitation [14].

Functional limitation questionnaires

These questionnaires record limitations of function, not necessarily limited to physical activity. They are used as markers of treatment efficacy. The most comprehensive is the Sickness Impact Profile (SIP) [15]. It has 136 items and is often also classified as a general health measure because it covers a wide range of functions, both physical and psychosocial. It was widely used in COPD studies in the past [16], but has been abandoned, largely because of its size and the fact that its content results in low severity scores even in patients with severe disease.

There are two comprehensive function limitation questionnaires, developed specifically for COPD, the modified Pulmonary Functional Status and Dyspnea Questionnaire (PFSDQ-M) [17] and the Pulmonary Functional Status

Scale (PFSS) [18]. These cover physical functions and are used most widely in the context of pulmonary rehabilitation, especially in the USA.

Activity of daily living scales

Activity of daily living (ADL) scales are usually restricted to basic self-care and mobility around the home, so questionnaires of this type tend to be more suitable for patients with severe COPD. The Nottingham Extended Activity of Daily Living Scale, developed for patients with stroke, has been shown have validity in COPD [19] and a new ADL questionnaire specifically for COPD has also been described [20].

Health status questionnaires

Health status questionnaires cover a wider range of effects of disease than measures of activity limitation and include well-being. They fall into two types: generic and disease-specific. The most widely used general health status measure is the SF-36 (www.sf-36.org). This questionnaire is a population-based marker of disease severity. It is used as a marker of treatment efficacy in COPD, and can be used as a marker of disease progression [21], but is not consistently responsive to effective treatments for COPD [22–24].

The two most widely used disease-specific health status measures for COPD are the CRQ [25] and St George's Respiratory Questionnaire (SGRQ) [26,27]. They differ a little in content, but more significantly in their design philosophy and scoring systems. The CRQ was designed as an evaluative instrument (i.e. as a marker of therapeutic outcome). The SGRQ was designed not only as a marker of outcome, but also to have discriminative properties so that it could be a marker of disease severity. It was developed to be suitable for long-term trials and be used as a marker of disease progression. These different design considerations led to the use of different methods of collecting responses to the constituent items and for scoring the instrument. The CRQ uses Lickert scales that offer seven severity response categories to each item. The SGRQ uses mainly dichotomous (yes/no or true/false) responses, and each response in the questionnaire has an empirically derived weight. The SGRQ falls very clearly into the category of a health status measure, but the CRQ has one element that permitted it to be designated as an HRQoL instrument. As originally designed, the dyspnoea component of the CRQ required the patient to identify activities restricted by breathlessness that are important to them (i.e. a component of quality of life). More recently, a standardized and self-administered version has been developed and validated [28,29], although this means loss of its HRQoL designation. Direct compar-

ison of the sensitivity of the two instruments in rehabilitation studies is now possible. Overall, they appear to have similar levels of sensitivity and responsiveness [23,24,30]. Direct comparisons of the two instruments in pharmacological studies have not been made. There have also been few long-term comparisons, but in a large 1-year follow-up of patients in a rehabilitation trial, differences between treatment and control arms of the study were more apparent with the SGRQ than the CRQ [23].

The CRQ and SGRQ are complex instruments, but the development of the standardized self-complete version of the CRQ should make it easier to apply. To improve ease of scoring of the SGRQ, a Microsoft Excel-based scoring system has been available for users of paper-based questionnaires for some time, but the development and validation of a computerized patient-entered and scored system is a significant step forward. The advantage of computer systems for patient questionnaire completion is that data capture is always 'clean' with no missed responses. Both are available from the author (pjones@sghms.ac.uk). Other shorter questionnaires have become available, but there are fewer data about them than the two more established instruments. One is the Quality-of-life for Respiratory Illness Questionnaire (QOLRIQ), developed originally in Dutch, but available in English [31]. Two other questionnaires are the Breathing Problems Questionnaire (BPQ) [32] and the AQ20. The latter has been validated in COPD in Japan and in the USA [33,34]. A UK study concluded that the BPQ provided more valid assessments of health status than the CRQ [35], although a Japanese group found that the CRQ and SGRQ discriminated between patients with different degrees of severity better than the BPQ [36]. There is one report that the BPQ was not as sensitive as the CRQ in detecting change following a pulmonary rehabilitation programme, but the AQ20 did discriminate between patients as well as the CRQ and SGRQ and was also responsive to changes following pulmonary rehabilitation [33].

Health status as a marker of disease severity

The standard method of assessing and categorizing COPD severity is through the FEV_1, but COPD is characterized by disability that results, not only from breathlessness, but also through secondary effects on other organs such as musculoskeletal function. For that reason, the association between FEV_1 and health status is weak. Within each GOLD category of COPD severity, there is a very wide range of health impairment (Fig. 16.1). Quite clearly these two measurements provide complementary information. This has been confirmed by the demonstration that health status scores, when measured using the SGRQ or the SF-36

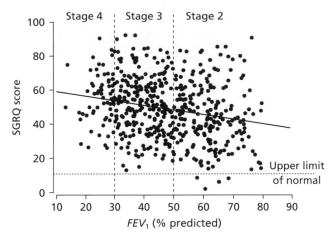

Figure 16.1 Correlation between forced expiratory volume in 1 s (FEV_1) and St George's Respiratory Questionnaire (SGRQ) score. High SGRQ score indicates poor health. Global Initiative for Chronic Obstructive Lung Disease (GOLD) categories for COPD severity are superimposed. (Data derived from Burge *et al.* [46].)

predicted death in patients with COPD independently of age, FEV_1 and BMI [37]. A similar observation was made in another study, in which exercise capacity appeared to be the key determinant of health status (measured using the SGRQ) that linked it to risk of death [38]. It should be noted that these authors found that the CRQ did not predict COPD mortality [39].

Health status as a marker of treatment efficacy

These questionnaires are designed to provide a measure of the overall impact of COPD on patients' health and an overall measure of treatment efficacy. This requires an estimate of the threshold for clinical significance. Such estimates are available for both the CRQ and the SGRQ. Issues around the development of these thresholds are too complex to be addressed here, but they have been reviewed recently [40]. The first demonstration that health status measurement can make a major contribution to trials of pharmacological therapy in COPD was the demonstration that clinically worthwhile improvements in health could be obtained with salmeterol in COPD, despite only modest improvements in FEV_1 [22]. Since then, health status measurements have been incorporated into nearly all major trials in COPD. In addition to providing estimates of the overall efficacy of the treatment, these trials have provided new insights into COPD. This is illustrated well in a comparison of the long-acting bronchodilator tiotropium compared with regular ipratropium (Fig. 16.2). The benefit of the

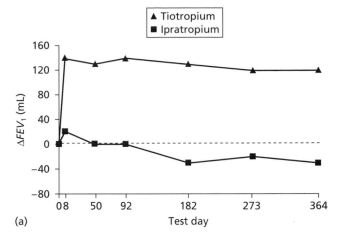

(a)

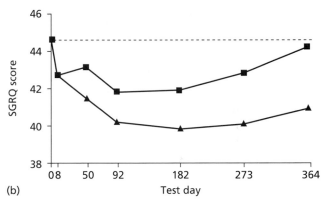

(b)

Figure 16.2 Changes in (a) trough (morning pre-dose) forced expiratory volume in 1 s (FEV_1) and (b) St George's Respiratory Questionnaire (SGRQ) score with tiotropium and four times daily ipratropium in COPD. A fall in SGRQ score indicates improved health. The difference in FEV_1 and differences in SGRQ score at day 50 and day 182 onwards were significant at $P < 0.05$. (From Casaburi *et al.* [42] with permission.)

long-acting drug on trough FEV_1 over the short-acting agent was apparent within a few days, but there was little further change during the following year. By contrast, the improvements in SGRQ score continued to improve over the next 6 months and the difference between treatment arms increased throughout the study [41]. A very similar pattern was seen when tiotropium was compared with placebo [42]. The different time course of response is almost certainly caused by different mechanisms of action of the drug. Exercise capacity with tiotropium improved over 6 weeks of treatment [43]. Thereafter, the accumulating benefit may be a result of the reduction in exacerbations that occurs with this drug [41], because there is evidence that the effect of inhaled corticosteroid on health status in COPD is attributable to a reduction in exacerbations [44]. Demonstration that the benefit of modern therapies for COPD increases progressively over time is a major

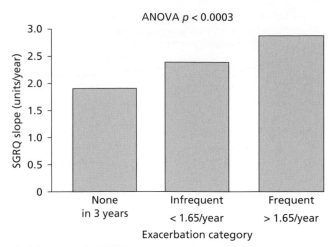

Figure 16.3 Rate of deterioration in St George's Respiratory Questionnaire (SGRQ) score (higher score indicates faster deterioration) in patients who had no exacerbations over a 3-year period and patients split into those with infrequent and frequent exacerbations. (From Spencer *et al.* [44] with permission.)

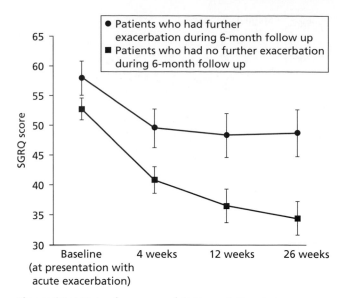

Figure 16.4 Rate of recovery of St George's Respiratory Questionnaire (SGRQ) score following an Anthonisen type 1 acute exacerbation of COPD. Error bars are 95% confidence intervals.

contribution of health status markers to current understanding of the disease.

Health status as a marker of disease progression

COPD is a progressive disease. The rate of deterioration in health is quantifiable with use of appropriate questionnaires, such as the SGRQ and SF-36 [21], although it has proved difficult to detect longitudinal changes with the CRQ [45]. Mechanisms responsible for the deterioration include decline in FEV_1 and exacerbation rate (Fig. 16.3), but these explain only part of the deterioration [44]. There is evidence from the ISOLDE study [46], that reducing exacerbations with fluticasone reduces the rate of deterioration in health status.

Use of health status measurement has forced a re-evaluation of the importance of acute exacerbations of COPD. Using standard clinical criteria for treatment success following an Anthonisen type 1 exacerbation of COPD, in a recent trial of antibiotics 85% of patients were judged cured or improved 2 weeks after the start of treatment [47]. In a similar study, measurements using the SGRQ showed that it took much longer for health to recover [48]. The improvement between 4 and 12 weeks after the exacerbation was greater than the threshold for a clinically significant improvement and even between 12 and 26 weeks there was a further small but statistically significant improvement (Fig. 16.4). Equally important was the observation that patients who had a further exacerbation within 6 months of

the first had a much smaller improvement in health. Early pulmonary rehabilitation greatly improved the degree of recovery of health following hospital admission for a COPD exacerbation [24].

Measurements of health status in routine practice

Assessment of health status clearly has an important role in COPD that complements spirometry. Reliance on the FEV_1 would fail to identify the true impact of the disease in many patients with COPD, as shown in Figure 16.1. It is clear that simple markers of the severity of health status impairment are needed for use in routine practice. Most of the available questionnaires are still too complex for everyday practice, but the MRC Dyspnoea Scale is easy to use, standardized and can be used in any clinical setting whether primary care or specialist clinic. It correlates well with health status measured using the SGRQ (Fig. 16.5). The development of health status questionnaires for use as markers of treatment efficacy in individual patients provides a complex challenge. There are many technical issues concerning methodology that have to be resolved before practical and reliable methods can be applied in routine practice. There is, however, good evidence that patients' retrospective estimates of overall treatment efficacy correlate with assessment made prospectively using the SGRQ [22]. An assessment that the treatment was effective was associated with a clinically significant change in SGRQ score.

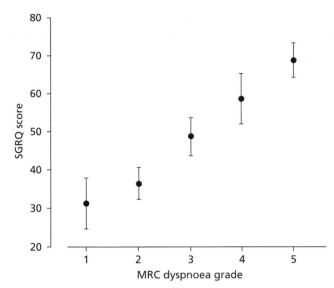

Figure 16.5 Relationship between Medical Research Council (MRC) dyspnoea grade and St George's Respiratory Questionnaire (SGRQ) score. Error bars are 95% confidence intervals. (Data from Jones *et al.* [27].)

Conclusions

Health status measurement provides an important marker of COPD severity and complements spirometry. Measurements made with well-validated questionnaires can now provide reliable markers of treatment efficacy and disease progression. In recent years they have provided major insights into COPD, but they still remain largely research tools, except in rehabilitation where they are often used to monitor a programme's effectiveness. In routine practice, the MRC Dyspnoea Scale provides a reliable marker of impaired health, but for the foreseeable future the patient's global estimate of treatment efficacy will remain the only practical marker of treatment efficacy in individual patients.

References

1 Guyatt GH, Townsend M, Berman LB, Pugsley SO. Quality of life in patients with chronic airflow limitation. *Br J Dis Chest* 1987;**81**:45–54.

2 Killian KJ, Leblanc P, Martin DH *et al.* Exercise capacity and ventilatory, circulatory and symptom limitation in patients with chronic airflow limitation. *Am Rev Respir Dis* 1992;**146**: 935–40.

3 Spruit MA, Gosselink R, Troosters T *et al.* Muscle force during an acute exacerbation in hospitalised patients with COPD and its relationship with CXCL8 and IGF-1. *Thorax* 2003;**58**: 752–6.

4 British Lung Foundation. *Living with Chronic Obstructive Pulmonary Disease*. London: British Lung Foundation, 2000.

5 Janssens JP, Rochat T, Frey JG *et al.* Health-related quality of life in patients under long-term oxygen therapy: a home-based descriptive study. *Respir Med* 1997;**91**:592–602.

6 Jones PW. Health status measurement in chronic obstructive pulmonary disease. *Thorax* 2001;**56**:880–7.

7 Hickey AM, Bury G, O'Boyle CA *et al.* A new short form individual quality of life measure (SEIQoL-DW): application in a cohort of individuals with HIV/AIDS. *BMJ* 1996;**313**:29–33.

8 Jones PW, Willits LR, Burge PS, Calverley PMA. Disease severity and the effect of fluticasone proprionate on chronic obstructive pulmonary disease exacerbations. *Eur Respir J* 2003;**21**:1–6.

9 Bestall JC, Paul EA, Garrod R *et al.* Usefulness of the Medical Research Council (MRC) Dyspnoea Scale as a measure of disability in patients with chronic obstructive pulmonary disease. *Thorax* 1999;**54**:581–6.

10 Mahler DA, Weinberg DH, Wells CK, Feinstein AR. Measurements of dyspnea: contents, interobserver correlates of two new clinical indices. *Chest* 1984;**85**:751–8.

11 Mahler DA, Donohue JF, Barbee RA *et al.* Efficacy of salmeterol xinafoate in the treatment of COPD. *Chest* 1999;**115**: 957–65.

12 Mahler DA, Wire P, Horstman D *et al.* Effectiveness of fluticsone proprionate and salmeterol combination delivered via the diskus device in the treatment of chronic obstructive pulmonary disease. *Am J Respir Crit Care Med* 2002;**166**: 1084–91.

13 Eakin EG, Resnikoff PM, Prewitt LM, Ries AL, Kaplan RM. Validation of a new dyspnea measure. *Chest* 1998;**113**:619–24.

14 Ries AL, Kaplan RM, Myers R, Prewitt LM. Maintenance after pulmonary rehabilitation in chronic lung disease: a randomized trial. *Am J Respir Crit Care Med* 2003;**167**:880–8.

15 Bergner M. The sickness impact profile. In: Walker SR, Rosser RM, eds. *Quality of Life: Assessment and Application*. Boston: MTP, 1987: 79–94.

16 Jones PW. Quality of life measurement for patients with diseases of the airways. *Thorax* 1991;**46**:676–82.

17 Lareau SC, Breslin EH, Meek PM. Functional status instruments: outcome measure in the evaluation of patients with chronic obstructive pulmonary disease. *Heart Lung* 1996;**25**: 212–24.

18 Weaver TE, Narsavage GL, Guilfoyle MJ. The development and psychometric evaluation of the Pulmonary Functional Status Scale: an instrument to assess functional status in pulmonary disease. *J Cardiopulm Rehabil* 1998;**18**:105–11.

19 Okubadejo AA, O'Shea L, Jones PW, Wedzicha JA. Home assessment of activities of daily living in patients with severe chronic obstructive pulmonary disease on long-term oxygen. *Eur Respir J* 1997;**10**:1572–5.

20 Garrod JC, Bestall EA, Paul EA, Wedzicha JA, Jones PW. Development and validation of a standardized measure of activity of daily living in patients with severe COPD: the London Chest Activity of Daily Living Scale (LCADL). *Respir Med* 2000;**2000**:589–96.

21 Spencer S, Calverley PMA, Burge PS, Jones PW. Health status deterioration in patients with chronic obstructive pulmonary disease. *Am J Respir Crit Care Med* 2001;**163**:122–8.

22 Jones PW, Bosh TK. Changes in quality of life in COPD patients treated with salmeterol. *Am J Respir Crit Care Med* 1997;**155**:1283–9.

23 Griffiths TL, Burr ML, Campbell IA *et al.* Results at 1 year of outpatient multidisciplinary pulmonary rehabilitation: a randomised controlled trial. *Lancet* 2000;**355**:362–8.

24 Man WD-C, Polkey MI, Donaldson N, Gray BJ, Moxham J. Community pulmonary rehabilitation after hospitalisation for acute exacerbations of chronic obstructive pulmonary disease: randomised controlled study. *BMJ* 2004;**329**:1209–11.

25 Guyatt GH, Berman LB, Townsend M, Pugsley SO, Chambers LW. A measure of quality of life for clinical trials in chronic lung disease. *Thorax* 1987;**42**:773–8.

26 Jones PW, Quirk FH, Baveystock CM. The St George's Respiratory Questionnaire. *Respir Med* 1991;**85**(Suppl B):25–31.

27 Jones PW, Quirk FH, Baveystock CM, Littlejohns P. A self-complete measure for chronic airflow limitation: the St George's Respiratory Questionnaire. *Am Rev Respir Dis* 1992;**145**:1321–7.

28 Puhan MA, Behnke M, Laschke M *et al.* Self-administration and standardisation of the chronic respiratory questionnaire: a randomised trial in three German-speaking countries. *Respir Med* 2004;**98**:342–50.

29 Schunemann HJ, Griffith L, Jaeschke R *et al.* A comparison of the original chronic respiratory questionnaire with a standardized version. *Chest* 2003;**124**:1421–9.

30 Wedzicha JA, Bestall JC, Garrod R *et al.* Randomized controlled trial of pulmonary rehabilitation in severe chronic obstructive pulmonary disease patients, stratified with the MRC dyspnoea scale. *Eur Respir J* 1998;**12**:363–9.

31 Maille AR, Koning CJ, Zwinderman AH *et al.* The development of the 'Quality-of-life for Respiratory Illness Questionnaire (QOL-RIQ)': a disease-specific quality-of-life questionnaire for patients with mild to moderate chronic non-specific lung disease. *Respir Med* 1997;**91**:297–309.

32 Hyland ME, Singh SJ, Sodergren SC, Morgan MP. Development of a shortened version of the Breathing Problems Questionnaire suitable for use in a pulmonary rehabilitation clinic: a purpose-specific, disease-specific questionnaire. *Qual Life Res* 1998;**7**:227–33.

33 Hajiro T, Nishimura K, Jones PW *et al.* A novel, short and simple questionnaire to measure health-related quality of life in patients with chronic obstructive pulmonary disease. *Am J Respir Crit Care Med* 1999;**159**:1874–8.

34 Alemayehu B, Aubert RE, Feifer RA, Paul LD. Comparative analysis of two quality-of-life instruments for patients with chronic obstructive pulmonary disease. *Value Health* 2002;**5**:436–41.

35 Yohannes AM, Roomi J, Waters K, Connolly MJ. Quality of life in elderly patients with COPD: measurement and predictive factors. *Respir Med* 1998;**92**:1231–6.

36 Hajiro T, Nishimura K, Tsukino M *et al.* Comparison of discriminative properties among disease-specific questionnaires for measuring health-related quality of life in patients with chronic obstructive pulmonary disease. *Am J Respir Crit Care Med* 1998;**157**:785–90.

37 Domingo-Salvany A, Lamarca R, Ferrer M *et al.* Health-related quality of life and mortality in male patients with chronic obstructive pulmonary disease. *Am J Respir Crit Care Med* 2002;**166**:680–5.

38 Oga T, Nishimura K, Tsukino M, Sato S, Hajiro T. Analysis of the factors related to mortality in chronic obstructive pulmonary disease. *Am J Respir Crit Care Med* 2003;**167**:544–9.

39 Oga T, Nishimura K, Tsukino M *et al.* Health status measured with the CRQ does not predict mortality in COPD. *Eur Respir J* 2002;**20**:1147–51.

40 Jones PW. Interpreting thresholds for a clinically significant changes in health status in asthma and COPD. *Eur Respir J* 2002;**19**:398–404.

41 Vincken W, van Noord JA, Greefhorst AP *et al.*, Dutch/Belgian Tiotropium Study Group. Improved health outcomes in patients with COPD during 1 year's treatment with tiotropium. *Eur Respir J* 2002;**19**:209–16.

42 Casaburi R, Mahler DA, Jones PW *et al.* A long-term evaluation of once daily inhaled tiotropium in chronic obstructive pulmonary disease. *Eur Respir J* 2002;**19**:209–16.

43 O'Donnell DE, Fluge T, Gerken F *et al.* Effects of tiotropium on lung hyperinflation, dyspnoea and exercise tolerance in COPD. *Eur Respir J* 2004;**23**:832–40.

44 Spencer S, Calverley PMA, Burge PS, Jones PW. Impact of preventing exacerbations on deterioration of health status in COPD. *Eur Respir J* 2004;**23**:1–5.

45 Oga T, Nishimura K, Tsukino M *et al.* Longitudinal changes in health status using the chronic respiratory disease questionnaire and pulmonary function in patients with stable chronic obstructive pulmonary disease. *Qual Life Res* 2004;**13**:1109–16.

46 Burge PS, Calverley PM, Jones PW *et al.* Randomised, double blind, placebo controlled study of fluticasone propionate in patients with moderate to severe chronic obstructive pulmonary disease: the ISOLDE trial. *BMJ* 2000;**320**:1297–303.

47 Wilson R, Allegra L, Huchon G *et al.*, Mosaic Study Group. Short-term and long-term outcomes of moxifloxacin compared to standard antibiotic treatment in acute exacerbations of chronic bronchitis. *Chest* 2004;**125**:953–64.

48 Spencer S, Jones PW. Time course of recovery of health status following an infective exacerbation of chronic bronchitis. *Thorax* 2003;**58**:589–93.

SECTION 3
Host defences and inflammation

CHAPTER 17
Mucociliary clearance

Souheil El-Chemaly, Adam Wanner and Matthias Salathe

The lungs fulfil the unique task of gas exchange, requiring a human body to ventilate approximately 20 000 L of air during quiet breathing every day. This task exposes the conducting airways and the alveoli to a significant burden of organic and inorganic particulate and gaseous material that must be either prevented from entering or, if it has entered, be constantly removed from the airways. An initial mechanical barrier at the entrance of the nose, nasal hair, serves as a coarse filter. Turbulent flow in the nose, pharynx and larynx causes larger particles to settle before they can enter the trachea. Furthermore, turbulent flow in large airways also enhances the deposition of particles onto the liquid/mucus blanket covering the epithelium. At locations of extreme turbulent flow, such as airway bifurcations, particle deposition rate is enhanced and reaches values that are approximately 100 times higher than elsewhere [1]. While the body has developed multiple mechanisms to prevent growth of organic infectious materials that have been deposited onto the airway surface (be it in the nose or lower airways), these organisms still need to be removed from these sites together with inorganic substances before they can cause harm, a task handled by the mucociliary transport system. Like other transport mechanisms, this system contains a motor for propulsion provided by cilia beating in the periciliary fluid layer on the airway surface and a vehicle provided by a mucus layer which is transported out of the airways by cilia. When this system fails, regardless of the underlying mechanism, respiratory secretions accumulate in the airways, leading to airflow obstruction and an increased susceptibility to bacterial colonization of normally sterile airways.

This chapter reviews the main concepts of mucociliary clearance, focusing on ciliary function and the collective clearance mechanism.

Cilia

Each human airway cilium is approximately 6 μm long and 0.3 μm in diameter and contains an array of microtubules in the classic '9 + 2' configuration (the detergent-resistant structure called axoneme). This morphological configuration is a hallmark of almost all motile cilia (with the exception of cilia in the embryonic node, which are motile despite their '9 + 0' structure [2]), indicative of their structural preservation throughout evolution [3]. The microtubules are constructed primarily from heterodimers of α- and β-tubulin and dynein, but more than 200 other proteins are associated with a variety of circumferential, spoke and radial linkages which serve to maintain the axonemal structure and play a part in the control of ciliary movement [3–5]. Bridges between the ciliary membrane and the outer nine doublet microtubules along the length of the cilium seem to participate in the regulation of ciliary beating [6,]. Along the entire axonemal length (except for the tip region and the base), the doublet is a repetitive structure with a unit length of 96 nm consisting of four outer dynein arms, three to four inner dynein arms, one spoke group (three radial spokes) and one pair of interdoublet links [3]. The outer arm dynein from mammalian tracheal cilia is a two-headed bouquet-like molecule with a molecular size of 1–2 million daltons (MDa) [8]. Each head contains a heavy chain ATPase of 400 000–500 000 Da.

During ciliary movement, dynein arms originating from outer microtubule doublets interact transiently with adjacent microtubules and undergo a conformational change using energy from ATP hydrolysis. This conformational change causes microtubules to slide relative to each other [9]. To date, several distinctly different axonemal dynein genes have been cloned; for instance, seven cDNAs were cloned from rat airway epithelium [10]. Although it seems logical that this dynein variety has biological consequences, the exact location of assembly of the different dynein isoforms is not known. *In vitro* data, however, suggest that at least the inner and outer dynein arms are functionally distinct [11], a finding confirmed in *Chlamydomonas* mutants where outer arm dynein was found to be responsible for ciliary beat frequency (CBF) regulation and inner arm dynein for bend formation and beating form [12,13]. The correlation between outer dynein arm and CBF regulation seems to hold true in humans based on evidence from subjects with primary ciliary dyskinesia [14].

The beating of airway cilia has been adjusted to the unique task of mucus transportation [15,16]. The cycle consists of a resting state as well as effective and recovery strokes. Through its recovery stroke, the cilium swings almost 180° backwards close to the cell surface. The ability of the cilium to do so in a watery environment (i.e. within the periciliary fluid level) is critical for adequate mucociliary clearance (see below). After the recovery stroke, the cilium fully extends and goes directly through its effective stroke in a plane perpendicular to the cell surface, reaching a maximal velocity of 1 mm/s at its tip. The extended cilium engages the overlying mucus describing an arc of approximately 110°. This engagement has been thought to be critical for adequate mucociliary clearance; however, recent data have challenged this concept (see below). After completion of the effective stroke, the cilium rests shortly and then resumes its recovery and effective strokes. Distal to the larynx, the effective stroke has a cephalad orientation and is about two to three times faster than the recovery stroke [17,18]. When CBF increases, all three phases of the beat cycle are shortened, but the resting period is most markedly affected [17]. The power that the cilium produces is related to the number of dynein–microtubule interactions [19,20] and can be, at least partially, adjusted to different loads of varying viscosity [21]. Ciliary beating in the airways seems coordinated (i.e. cilia beat as part of a metachronal wave). As cilia are densely packed onto the airway epithelial surface, significant hydrodynamic forces exist between single cilia. These hydrodynamic interactions are likely the most important factor for ciliary coordination [22] and may explain why the lengths of metachronal waves are limited, restricting the field of metachrony [16,23].

Human cilia beat at approximately 12–15 Hz at body temperature when measured *in vitro*. CBF is adjusted by the regulation of dynein–microtubule interactions, but the cellular and molecular mechanism by which this is accomplished is incompletely understood. Evidence has been accumulated showing that mammalian CBF changes in response to changes in the phosphorylation state of ciliary targets (mainly through cyclic adenosine monophosphate [cAMP]-dependent phosphorylation) and to changes in cytoplasmic calcium ($[Ca^{2+}]_i$).

Many different experimental methods have been used to increase cAMP levels inside cells, and all have been shown to increase human, bovine, ovine and rabbit CBF. Manipulations of cAMP were achieved with β-adrenergic agonists that stimulate transmembrane adenylyl cyclases (tmAC) [24–29], forskolin that directly activates tmAC, and membrane-permeable cAMP analogues. CBF increases upon cAMP rise were blockable by non-specific protein kinase inhibitors, implicating a role for cAMP-dependent protein kinase (PKA) [27,30–32]. The molecular mechanism by which PKA increases mammalian CBF is likely analogous to the stimulation of *Paramecium* ciliary activity by PKA. Hamasaki *et al.* [33] showed that a ciliary PKA phosphorylation target of 29 kDa in *Paramecium* was an outer dynein arm light chain [34] and that the phosphorylation of this light chain was sufficient to increase the velocity of microtubule gliding across dynein-coated surfaces *in vitro* and the swimming speed *in vivo* [34]. Since then, mammalian respiratory axonemal targets of PKA with similar molecular weights have been identified by their cAMP-dependent phosphorylation [35–37]. It is also clear that a ciliary PKA is localized to mammalian axonemes [35–37], a fact supported by the presence of a specific A-kinase anchoring protein in human airway cilia [35].

cGMP-dependent protein kinase (PKG) has also been shown to be involved in the regulation of CBF in certain mammalian species [27,38,39]. There is controversy whether or not a combined signalling by $[Ca^{2+}]_i$ is required [38,39] and some experiments suggest that PKG may act through PKA to stimulate CBF [27].

The intracellular calcium concentration ($[Ca^{2+}]_i$) has a crucial role in the regulation of CBF but the mechanism by which calcium influences frequency seems to differ between unicellular organisms and mammals. In *Paramecium*, rising $[Ca^{2+}]_i$ slows CBF to the point where the beat direction is reversed [40]. Mammalian cilia, on the other hand, never reverse their beating direction and elevations of $[Ca^{2+}]_i$ increase CBF [24,25,41–46] whereas decreases in $[Ca^{2+}]_i$ below baseline decrease CBF [43]. Some reports, using inhibitors of calmodulin, have suggested that $[Ca^{2+}]_i$ may act through calmodulin via Ca^{2+}/calmodulin-dependent kinase (CaM kinase) [41,47] and ciliary targets of CaM kinase have been described at least in *Tetrahymena* [48]. However, some of these calmodulin inhibitors are ciliotoxic and CaM kinase targets were not found in mammalian cilia [49]. More recent evidence suggests that Ca^{2+} in mammalian cells acts directly on the axoneme, presumably on a Ca^{2+}-binding protein that is not calmodulin [50], to change CBF [39,51–53]. However, increases in intracellular calcium may also rise cAMP [54,55] and potentially cGMP via an NO pathway to activate PKG inside cilia that modulates CBF as well [56]. This complicates interpretation of the calcium-related CBF increase. Whether or not an elevation of cyclic nucleotides is required for calcium to change CBF is currently under intense investigation [38,39,57].

The cAMP and Ca^{2+} pathways have been shown to interact at several levels with respect to ciliary function. β-Adrenergic agonists, for instance, have been shown to stimulate CBF not only through a cAMP-dependent pathway, but also through an initial calcium-coupled mechanism [25,30]. Furthermore, Smith *et al*. [58] reported that CBF of human nasal cells was rendered insensitive to $[Ca^{2+}]_i$ changes upon continued exposure to increased intracellular cAMP levels and that the cAMP-mediated changes of the CBF sensitivity to $[Ca^{2+}]_i$ were dependent on PKA activation.

A large body of literature has been published on mediator- and drug-induced changes of ciliary beating. It is beyond the scope of this chapter to discuss all these publications (reviewed in [59]). However, under normal conditions, paracrine actions of secreted adenosine triphosphate (ATP), primarily via $[Ca^{2+}]_i$ and secondarily via cAMP, have been identified to be crucial in regulating CBF [54,55,60,61]. There is also some evidence that acetylcholine, made within the airway epithelium itself, may be used in a paracrine fashion to stimulate M3 receptors [56,62,63]; however, there seems to be a vast difference in the importance of this pathway between different mammalian species.

It is interesting that many inflammatory mediators stimulate ciliary beating *in vitro* [64–67], although mucociliary transport velocity is usually decreased during established airway inflammation, including COPD (see below). Exceptions are platelet-activating factor [68,69] and major basic protein of eosinophils which accumulates in the sputum of asthmatic patients [70]. Furthermore, serum proteins released into the airway lumen during inflammation [71,72], leucocyte elastase [73,74], and neutral protease are cilioinhibitory [75]. The latter mediators of inflammation are especially relevant in COPD.

Periciliary fluid

The periciliary fluid is a watery environment allowing the cilia to beat without interacting with mucus at all times. In the presence of mucus, the fluid depth is approximately equal to the extended cilium in length [76]. The height of this fluid above the airway epithelial cells is tightly regulated, as recently shown in cell culture systems [77–79]. The regulation mechanisms are still poorly understood but are related to the ion transport characteristics of airway epithelial cells [80]. A small osmiophilic film is present on the luminal surface of the periciliary fluid layer and represents surfactant [81], likely produced locally by epithelial cells rather than stemming from the alveoli [82–84].

For a long time, it was assumed that ciliary tips could not interact with mucus if the periciliary fluid level was too high and thus mucus could not be moved under these conditions. However, this concept has been challenged by showing that the whole periciliary fluid layer actually moves in a cephalad direction together with the mucus blanket (but only if mucus is present [85]), suggesting that cilia may not need to interact directly with the mucus blanket. In support of this hypothesis, it has been found that patients with a genetic defect in an apical sodium channel, resulting in increased water amounts in the airways, actually have significantly increased mucociliary transport, again suggesting that an excess of apical water is not deleterious, but in fact beneficial to mucociliary transport [86].

On the other hand, if the periciliary fluid level is too low, the mucus blanket itself impedes ciliary beating by interacting with cilia during the recovery stroke. That this mechanism truly impedes mucus transport has been shown in culture models of cystic fibrosis [80]. Restoring appropriate depth of the periciliary fluid level in these models restores mucociliary transport [87].

The periciliary space is not only filled with electrolyte solution; close to the apical surface of the epithelium, high molecular weight structures such as glycosaminoglycans and membrane-bound mucins can be found. These structures fulfil their own functions on the apical surface. Glycosaminoglycans, for instance, immobilize host defence molecules at the surface thereby protecting them from clearance [88]. The glycocalyx also prevents viruses from infecting ciliated cells [89]. Many of these functions have not been examined in detail but are currently under investigation.

Mucus

Mucus is mandatory for mucociliary transport; if no mucus is present the system fails [85,90]. Mucus is a mixture of glycoproteins, proteoglycans, lipids, other proteins, and sometimes DNA. Mucus contains secretory IgA immunoglobulins that form an immunological barrier against bacterial colonization, lysozyme that is bactericidal, and lactoferrin that scavenges oxygen radicals and traps iron ions, thereby preventing biofilm formation [91]. Multiple other innate host defence molecules such as defensins [92–94] and the lactoperoxidase system can be found in mucus and the periciliary fluid [95–97].

Gel-forming mucins form the basic polymer structure of mucus. The gel phase is initially formed by rapid hydration of mucins secreted from vesicles where they are stored in a condensed form. Secretion of mucus from these granules has been has been compared to a 'jack-in-the-box' mechanism [98]. To stay in a condensed form inside the cell, the charges of the mucin polyions are rendered neutral by acidic pH and counterion shielding, achieved by high $[Ca^{2+}]$ inside the vesicles [98]. Upon secretion, the condensed mucus undergoes a polymer phase transition by hydration according to Tanaka's [99] polymer gel theory. This hydration is aided by an exchange of calcium in the vesicles with sodium ions which are weaker supporters of the condensed phase form. Thus, hydration of mucus results in rapid expansion of the gel with a volume increase of several hundred-fold in only a few seconds.

The rheological properties of mucus, a non-Newtonian fluid, are expressed by its viscosity and elasticity; these are mainly determined by the mucin tangle density in the gel [100], which decreases during mucus hydration. Thus, one of the most critical factors regarding mucus rheology is mucus hydration (another would be mucin molecule length), a fact shown by the inability of cilia to move mucus with high solute concentrations [87]. The ability of cilia to transport mucus is indirectly proportional to viscosity and directly proportional to elasticity [101]. Other physical properties of mucus such as adhesivity, cohesitivity and wettability [102] are also important in particle–mucus interactions and mucus transportability, but are less well defined.

Multiple substances have been shown to stimulate mucus or glycoconjugate secretion from goblet cells or submucosal glands. Physiologically, purinergic agonists released from the airway epithelium as well as from goblet cell granules [103] have a major role in releasing mucus [104–106]. Cholinergic input also stimulates mucus secretion (reviewed in [107]). Controversy exists, however, on whether or not human airways secrete mucus upon β-agonist stimulation. While human tissues mounted in Ussing chambers revealed increased glycoprotein release in one study upon salbutamol stimulation [108], isoproterenol did not elicit radiolabelled glycoconjugate release in human preparations [109,110]. In addition, mucus secretion by human bronchial epithelial cell xenograft cultures was non-responsive to membrane-permeable cAMP analogues while ATP stimulated it (C. William Davis, University of North Carolina Chapel Hill, personal communication). Thus, β-agonist stimulation of mucus secretion in humans is likely not very relevant. Mediators that stimulate mucus secretion or production in disease are discussed below.

Mucociliary clearance

Mucociliary transport velocity and mucociliary clearance rates have been assessed by several methods *in vivo*. Using a fibreoptic bronchoscope to measure the motion of small Teflon discs insufflated into the trachea, the tracheal transport rate was estimated at approximately 20 mm/min [111]. Using a radiographical technique to assess the motion of bronchoscopically insufflated bismuth-coated Teflon discs in the trachea, tracheal transport rates were estimated at approximately 10 mm/min [112]. Finally,

using a radioaerosol bolus technique and radiolabelled microspheres inhaled with adjusted flows to enhance central deposition, tracheal transport rates are estimated at 4–5 mm/min [113]. These rates decrease towards the periphery of the lung; they reach the lowest value in the bronchioles with rates of less than 0.4 mm/min. Transport rates also decrease with age.

Radiolabelled particle techniques can also be used to assess overall mucociliary clearance of the lung [114,115]. An initial exponentially decreasing phase with a half-life of approximately 4 h represents mucociliary clearance in the tracheobronchial tree. A much slower phase with a half-life of several weeks to months represents clearance from alveoli by mechanisms unrelated to mucociliary transport. As initial particle deposition influences measured overall clearance rates (differences of transport rates in the periphery of the lung and the central airways), it is critical to match particle deposition in all subjects by altering breathing patterns during inspiration if necessary. This is especially important when studying older subjects, smokers, or subjects with airflow obstruction where central deposition of particles is enhanced [116]. If assessed correctly, mucociliary clearance is reduced in the elderly, in chronic smokers (even if they are asymptomatic) and in chronic obstructive lung diseases such as chronic bronchitis, bronchiectasis, bronchial asthma and cystic fibrosis [116–118].

Mucociliary dysfunction

Mucociliary function can be disturbed by inappropriate mucus rheology and amount or decreased ciliary activity. Because rheology mainly depends on hydration, breathing air with a relative humidity of less than 30% through the mouth produces transport stasis in the trachea [119]. Dehydration of mucus may not be the only problem in this situation as low temperatures also decrease CBF. Because humans normally breathe through the nose (a highly efficient air conditioner), this issue only has a role in patients who bypass nose breathing (e.g. in patients with tracheostomies).

Exogenous pollutants such as cigarette smoke and SO_2 or NO_2 as well as anaesthetic gases, high inspiratory oxygen concentrations, and inhalations of platelet-activating factor decrease transport rates [120], at least in part through reduction of CBF [68,121].

Drug effects on mucociliary clearance

Cholinergic agonists stimulate mucociliary clearance, possibly by increasing CBF, at least in some species, although this effect is not certain in humans (see above and [63]), and by optimizing mucus hydration through increased fluid secretion from submucosal glands [122,123], if glycoprotein release does not overwhelm fluid secretion. Locally produced acetylcholine may act as a paracrine signalling molecule under physiological conditions, but cholinergic agonists cannot not be used therapeutically in a patient with mucociliary dysfunction because of their bronchoconstrictive effects. Atropine, a tertiary ammonium compound and anticholinergic drug, decreases mucociliary clearance [124,125], possibly because of decreased hydration of mucus. However, ipratropium bromide, a quaternary ammonium compound, has no effect on mucus clearance [126].

α-Adrenergic agonists have little or no influence on the mucociliary clearance rate in the lower airways. β-Adrenergic agonists including the long-acting salmeterol on the other hand increase CBF in a variety of mammalian airway epithelial cells [24–27,30,127–136]. However, β-agonists have a relatively small effect on overall ion and water transport, as originally evaluated in excised human bronchi [123], they do not seem to significantly stimulate secretion from submucosal glands in humans [122] and do not seem to stimulate mucus release. Thus, the general increase in transport and clearance rates seen in most healthy individuals and patients upon β-agonist administration (at least in the trachea [137–141]) is likely because of their effect on ciliary beating.

Chronic bronchitis and COPD

Mucociliary clearance is dysfunctional in chronic bronchitis [139,142–144] and COPD [145,146]; however, cough clearance may be able to compensate for some of the loss of ciliary clearance [147]. The fact that cough is effective in these patients may indicate that abnormally high mucus production may be present, a hypothesis supported by a study that did not find mucociliary dysfunction in pure emphysema in patients with α_1-antitryspin deficiency but no airways disease or mucus hypersecretion [148].

In chronic bronchitis, lower clearance is present in patients with a high neutrophil count in their sputum compared with patients without purulent sputum [149]. This finding indicates that infections, frequently encountered by patients with chronic bronchitis and COPD, may play an important part in decreasing mucociliary clearance. In support of this hypothesis, several lines of evidence link products from neutrophils and bacteria to mucociliary dysfunction. For instance, neutrophil elastase, a potent mucus secretagogue [150–152] and inducer of mucin gene expression [153], also causes abnormal ciliary function, possibly by disruption of epithelial barriers [73–75]. The combined effect of these changes results in mucociliary dysfunction [154].

Bacterial colonization of airways, seen in patients with COPD [155], can also contribute to mucociliary dysfunction. Bacteria have been shown to release proteases that cause human nasal epithelial disruption as well as CBF slowing *in vitro* [73,156]. Bacterial products such as hydroxyphenazine, pyocyanin and a rhamnolipid as well as bacterial culture supernatants have been shown to decrease CBF [157–161] and mucus clearance [162,163]. In addition, *Haemophilus influenzae*, a bacterium commonly encountered in chronic bronchitis, can induce epithelial cell damage [164] and ciliary dysfunction [157], thereby leading to a decrease in mucociliary clearance. Extensive destruction of the epithelium during infections with *Mycoplasma pneumoniae* [165], viruses especially from the influenza group [166] and after aspiration of gastric acid [167] decreases mucociliary transport rate if the epithelial cell destruction includes more than 50% of ciliated cells even if the remaining cilia beat normally [168]. Finally, airway inflammation can cause acquired ciliary disorders including misalignments of the central microtubules between adjacent cilia, compound cilia, supernumerary microtubules and other malformations [169], all of which may contribute to mucociliary dysfunction.

Conclusions

Mucociliary clearance is an important host defence mechanism. Mucociliary transport is tightly regulated. Effective mucociliary clearance depends on ciliary beating as well as appropriate rheology and amount of mucus. This chapter reviews basic regulatory mechanisms of ciliary beating, the effects of mucus secretion and hydration on mucociliary transport, as well as scenarios in which mucociliary clearance fails. Possible treatments for mucociliary dysfunction in these diseases are reviewed in Chapters 57–62. It is hoped that with a better understanding of the fundamental mechanisms that make mucociliary clearance efficient, more effective treatment strategies can be developed to prevent or treat mucociliary dysfunction in airways diseases, including COPD.

References

1 Schlesinger RB, Gurman JL, Lippmann M. Particle deposition within bronchial airways: comparison using constant and cyclic inspiratory flow. *Ann Occup Hyg* 1982;**26**:47–64.
2 Nonaka S, Tanaka Y, Okada Y *et al.* Randomization of left–right asymmetry due to loss of nodal cilia generating leftward flow of extraembryonic fluid in mice lacking KIF3B motor protein. *Cell* 1998;**95**:829–37.

3 Satir P, Sleigh MA. The physiology of cilia and mucociliary interactions. *Annu Rev Physiol* 1990;**52**:137–55.

4 Afzelius B. Electron microscopy of the sperm tail: results obtained with a new fixative. *J Biophys Biochem Cytol* 1959;**5**: 269–78.

5 Fawcett DW, Porter KW. A study of the fine structure of ciliated epithelia. *J Morphol* 1954;**94**:221–81.

6 Dentler WL, Pratt MM, Stephens RE. Microtubule–membrane interactions in cilia. II. Photochemical cross-linking of bridge structures and the identification of a membrane-associated dynein-like ATPase. *J Cell Biol* 1980;**84**:381–403.

7 Dentler WL. Microtubule–membrane interactions in cilia and flagella. *Int Rev Cytol* 1981;**72**:1–47.

8 Hastie AT, Marchese-Ragona SP, Johnson KA, Wall JS. Structure and mass of mammalian respiratory ciliary outer arm 19S dynein. *Cell Motil Cytoskeleton* 1988;**11**:157–66.

9 Gibbons IR. Chemical dissection of cilia. *Arch Biol (Liège)* 1965;**76**:317–52.

10 Andrews KL, Nettesheim P, Asai DJ, Ostrowski LE. Identification of seven rat axonemal dynein heavy chain genes: expression during ciliated cell differentiation. *Mol Biol Cell* 1996;**7**:71–9.

11 Hard R, Blaustein K, Scarcello L. Reactivation of outer-arm-depleted lung axonemes: evidence for functional differences between inner and outer dynein arms *in situ*. *Cell Motil Cytoskeleton* 1992;**21**:199–209.

12 Brokaw CJ, Kamiya R. Bending patterns of *Chlamydomonas* flagella: IV. Mutants with defects in inner and outer dynein arms indicate differences in dynein arm function. *Cell Motil Cytoskeleton* 1987;**8**:68–75.

13 Brokaw CJ. Control of flagellar bending: a new agenda based on dynein diversity. *Cell Motil Cytoskeleton* 1994;**28**:199–204.

14 de Iongh RU, Rutland J. Ciliary defects in healthy subjects, bronchiectasis, and primary ciliary dyskinesia. *Am J Respir Crit Care Med* 1995;**151**:1559–67.

15 Marino MR, Aiello E. Cinemicrographic analysis of beat dynamics of human respiratory cilia. *Cell Motil* 1982;**1** (Suppl):35–9.

16 Sanderson MJ, Sleigh MA. Ciliary activity of cultured rabbit tracheal epithelium: beat pattern and metachrony. *J Cell Sci* 1981;**47**:331–47.

17 Sanderson MJ, Dirksen ER. A versatile and quantitative computer-assisted photoelectronic technique used for the analysis of ciliary beat cycles. *Cell Motil* 1985;**5**:267–92.

18 Wilson GB, Jahn TL, Fonseca JR. Studies on ciliary beating of frog pharyngeal epithelium *in vitro*. I. Isolation and ciliary beat of single cells. *Trans Am Microsc Soc* 1975;**94**:43–57.

19 Gibbons BH, Gibbons IR. Flagellar movement and adenosine triphosphatase activity in sea urchin sperm extracted with Triton X-100. *J Cell Biol* 1972;**54**:75–97.

20 Holwill ME. Dynein motor activity during ciliary beating. In: Salathe M, ed. *Cilia and Mucus: From Development to Respiratory Disease.* New York: Marcel Dekker, 2001: 19–25.

21 Johnson NT, Villalon M, Royce FH, Hard R, Verdugo P. Autoregulation of beat frequency in respiratory ciliated cells: demonstration by viscous loading. *Am Rev Respir Dis* 1991;**144**:1091–4.

22 Gheber L, Korngreen A, Priel Z. Effect of viscosity on metachrony in mucus propelling cilia. *Cell Motil Cytoskeleton* 1998;**39**:9–20.

23 Gheber L, Priel Z. Synchronization between beating cilia. *Biophys J* 1989;**55**:183–91.

24 Sanderson MJ, Dirksen ER. Mechanosensitive and β-adrenergic control of the ciliary beat frequency of mammalian respiratory tract cells in culture. *Am Rev Respir Dis* 1989;**139**:432–40.

25 Lansley AB, Sanderson MJ, Dirksen ER. Control of the beat cycle of respiratory tract cilia by Ca^{2+} and cAMP. *Am J Physiol* 1992;**263**:L232–42.

26 Verdugo P, Johnson NT, Tam PY. Beta-adrenergic stimulation of respiratory ciliary activity. *J Appl Physiol* 1980;**48**: 868–71.

27 Wyatt TA, Spurzem JR, May K, Sisson JH. Regulation of ciliary beat frequency by both PKA and PKG in bovine airway epithelial cells. *Am J Physiol* 1998;**275**(4 Pt 1):L827–35.

28 Tamaoki J, Kondo M, Takizawa T. Effect of cyclic AMP on ciliary function in rabbit tracheal epithelial cells. *J Appl Physiol* 1989;**66**:1035–9.

29 Di Benedetto G, Manara-Shediac FS, Mehta A. Effect of cyclic AMP on ciliary activity of human respiratory epithelium. *Eur Respir J* 1991;**4**:789–95.

30 Frohock JI, Wijkstrom-Frei C, Salathe M. Effects of albuterol enantiomers on ciliary beat frequency in ovine tracheal epithelial cells. *J Appl Physiol* 2002;**92**:2396–402.

31 Salathe M, Lieb T, Bookman RJ. Lack of nitric oxide involvement in cholinergic modulation of ovine ciliary beat frequency. *J Aerosol Med* 2000;**13**:219–29.

32 Yang B, Schlosser RJ, McCaffrey TV. Dual signal transduction mechanisms modulate ciliary beat frequency in upper airway epithelium. *Am J Physiol* 1996;**14**:L745–51.

33 Hamasaki T, Murtaugh TJ, Satir BH, Satir P. *In vitro* phosphorylation of *Paramecium axonemes* and permeabilized cells. *Cell Motil Cytoskeleton* 1989;**12**:1–11.

34 Hamasaki T, Barkalow K, Richmond J, Satir P. cAMP-stimulated phosphorylation of an axonemal polypeptide that copurifies with the 22S dynein arm regulates microtubule translocation velocity and swimming speed in *Paramecium*. *Proc Nat Acad Sci U S A* 1991;**88**:7918–22.

35 Kultgen PL, Byrd SK, Ostrowski LE, Milgram SL. Characterization of an a-kinase anchoring protein in human ciliary axonemes. *Mol Biol Cell* 2002;**13**:4156–66.

36 Salathe M, Pratt MM, Wanner A. Cyclic AMP-dependent phosphorylation of a 26 kDa axonemal protein in ovine cilia isolated from small tissue pieces. *Am J Respir Cell Mol Biol* 1993;**9**:306–14.

37 Sisson JH, Mommsen J, Spurzem JR, Wyatt TA. Localization of PKA and PKG in bovine bronchial epithelial cells and axonemes. *Am J Respir Crit Care Med* 2000;**161**:A449.

38 Uzlaner N, Priel Z. Interplay between the NO pathway and elevated $[Ca^{2+}]_i$ enhances ciliary activity in rabbit trachea. *J Physiol* 1999;**516**:179–90.

39 Zhang L, Sanderson MJ. The role of cGMP in the regulation of rabbit airway ciliary beat frequency. *J Physiol* 2003;**551**: 765–76.

40 Naitoh Y, Kaneko H. Reactivated triton-extracted models of

Paramecium: modification of ciliary movement by calcium ions. *Science* 1972;**176**:523–4.

41 Di Benedetto G, Magnus CJ, Gray PTA, Mehta A. Calcium regulation of ciliary beat frequency in human respiratory epithelium *in vitro*. *J Physiol* 1991;**439**:103–13.

42 Girard PG, Kennedy JR. Calcium regulation of ciliary activity in rabbit tracheal explants and outgrowth. *Eur J Cell Biol* 1986;**40**:203–9.

43 Salathe M, Bookman RJ. Coupling of $[Ca^{2+}]_i$ and ciliary beating in cultured tracheal epithelial cells. *J Cell Sci* 1995;**108**:431–40.

44 Sanderson MJ, Charles AC, Dirksen ER. Mechanical stimulation and intercellular communication increase intracellular calcium in epithelial cells. *Cell Regul* 1990;**1**:585–96.

45 Verdugo P. Calcium-dependent hormonal stimulation of ciliary activity. *Nature* 1980;**283**:764–5.

46 Villalon M, Hinds TR, Verdugo P. Stimulus-response coupling in mammalian ciliated cells: demonstration of two mechanisms of control for cytosolic $[Ca^{2+}]$. *Biophys J* 1989;**56**:1255–8.

47 Verdugo P, Raess BV, Villalon M. The role of calmodulin in the regulation of ciliary movement in mammalian epithelial cilia. *J Submicrosc Cytol* 1983;**15**:95–6.

48 Hirano-Ohnishi J, Watanabe Y. Target molecules of calmodulin on microtubules of *Tetrahymena* cilia. *Exp Cell Res* 1988;**178**:18–24.

49 Salathe M, Pratt MM, Wanner A. Protein kinase C-dependent phosphorylation of a ciliary membrane protein and inhibition of ciliary beating. *J Cell Sci* 1993;**106**:1211–20.

50 Kakuta Y, Kanno T, Sasaki H, Takishima T. Effect of Ca^{2+} on the ciliary beat frequency of skinned dog tracheal epithelium. *Respir Physiol* 1985;**60**:9–19.

51 Lansley AB, Sanderson MJ. Regulation of airway ciliary activity by Ca^{2+}: simultaneous measurement of beat frequency and intracellular Ca^{2+}. *Biophys J* 1999;**77**:629–38.

52 Zhang L, Sanderson MJ. Oscillations in ciliary beat frequency and intracellular calcium concentration in rabbit tracheal epithelial cells induced by ATP. *J Physiol* 2003;**546**:733–49.

53 Salathe M, Bookman RJ. Mode of Ca^{2+} action on ciliary beat frequency in single ovine airway epithelial cells. *J Physiol* 1999;**520**:851–65.

54 Morse DM, Smullen JL, Davis CW. Differential effects of UTP, ATP, and adenosine on ciliary activity of human nasal epithelial cells. *Am J Physiol* 2001;**280**:C1485–97.

55 Lieb T, Wijkstrom Frei C et al. Prolonged increase in ciliary beat frequency after short-term purinergic stimulation in human airway epithelial cells. *J Physiol* 2002;**538**:633–46.

56 Gertsberg I, Hellman V, Fainshtein M. et al. Intracellular Ca^{2+} regulates the phosphorylation and the dephosphorylation of ciliary proteins via the NO pathway. *J Gen Physiol* 2004;**124**:527–40.

57 Ma W, Silberberg SD, Priel Z. Distinct axonemal processes underlie spontaneous and stimulated airway ciliary activity. *J Gen Physiol* 2002;**120**:875–85.

58 Smith RP, Shellard R, Dhillon DP, Winter J, Mehta A. Asymmetric interactions between phosphorylation pathways regulating ciliary beat frequency in human nasal respiratory epithelium *in vitro*. *J Physiol* 1996;**496**:883–9.

59 Wanner A, Salathe M, O'Riordan TG. State of the art: mucociliary clearance in the airways. *Am J Respir Crit Care Med* 1996;**154**:1868–902.

60 Wong LB, Yeates DB. Luminal purinergic regulatory mechanisms of tracheal ciliary beat frequency. *Am J Respir Cell Mol Biol* 1992;**7**:447–54.

61 Korngreen A, Priel Z. Purinergic stimulation of rabbit ciliated airway epithelia: control by multiple calcium sources. *J Physiol* 1996;**497**:53–66.

62 Reinheimer T, Bernedo P, Klapproth H et al. Acetylcholine in isolated airways of rat, guinea pig, and human: species differences in role of airway mucosa. *Am J Physiol* 1996;**270**:L722–8.

63 Salathe M, Lipson E, Ivonnet PI, Bookman RJ. Muscarinic signal transduction in tracheal epithelial cells: effects of acetylcholine on intracellular Ca^{2+} and ciliary beating. *Am J Physiol* 1997;**272**:L301–10.

64 Maurer DR, Sielczak M, Oliver W Jr, Abraham WM, Wanner A. Role of ciliary motility in allergic mucociliary dysfunction. *J Appl Physiol* 1982;**52**:1018–23.

65 Maurer DR, Schor J, Sielczak M, Wanner A, Abraham WM. Ciliary motility in airway anaphylaxis. *Prog Clin Biol Res* 1982;**80**:67–70.

66 Wanner A, Maurer DR, Abraham WM, Szepfalusi Z, Sielczak M. Effects of chemical mediators of anaphylaxis on ciliary function. *J Allergy Clin Immunol* 1983;**72**:663–7.

67 Wanner A, Sielczak M, Mella JF, Abraham WM. Ciliary responsiveness in allergic and non-allergic airways. *J Appl Physiol* 1986;**60**:1967–71.

68 Ganbo T, Hisamatsu K, Nakazawa T, Kamijo A, Murakami Y. Platelet activating factor (PAF) effects on ciliary activity of human paranasal sinus mucosa *in vitro*. *Rhinology* 1991;**29**:231–7.

69 Seybold ZV, Mariassy AT, Stroh D et al. Mucociliary interaction *in vitro*: effects of physiological and inflammatory stimuli. *J Appl Physiol* 1990;**68**:1421–6.

70 Frigas E, Loegering DA, Gleich GJ. Cytotoxic effects of the guinea pig eosinophil major basic protein on tracheal epithelium. *Lab Invest* 1980;**42**:35–43.

71 Kennedy JR, Lin KD, Duckett KE. Serum complement (C3a and C5)-induced inhibition of rabbit tracheal cilia. *Prog Clin Biol Res* 1982;**80**:71–5.

72 Sanderson MJ, Sleigh MA. Serum proteins agglutinate cilia and modify ciliary coordination. *Pediatr Res* 1981;**15**:219–28.

73 Amitani R, Wilson R, Rutman A et al. Effects of human neutrophil elastase and *Pseudomonas aeruginosa* proteinases on human respiratory epithelium. *Am J Respir Cell Mol Biol* 1991;**4**:26–32.

74 Smallman LA, Hill SL, Stockley RA. Reduction of ciliary beat frequency *in vitro* by sputum from patients with bronchiectasis: a serine proteinase effect. *Thorax* 1984;**39**:663–7.

75 Tegner H, Ohlsson K, Toremalm NG, von Mecklenburg C. Effect of human leukocyte enzymes on tracheal mucosa and its mucociliary activity. *Rhinology* 1979;**17**:199–206.

76 Hulbert WC, Forster BB, Laird W, Lihl CE, Walker DC. An improved method for fixation of the respiratory epithelial surface with the mucous and surfactant layers. *Lab Invest* 1982;**47**:354–63.

77 Tarran R, Grubb BR, Gatzy JT, Davis CW, Boucher RC. The relative roles of passive surface forces and active ion transport in the modulation of airway surface liquid volume and composition. *J Gen Physiol* 2001;**118**:223–36.

78 Tarran R, Loewen ME, Paradiso AM *et al*. Regulation of murine airway surface liquid volume by CFTR and Ca^{2+}-activated Cl^- conductances. *J Gen Physiol* 2002;**120**:407–18.

79 Tarran R, Boucher RC. Thin-film measurements of airway surface liquid volume/composition and mucus transport rates *in vitro*. *Methods Mol Med* 2002;**70**:479–92.

80 Matsui H, Grubb BR, Tarran R *et al*. Evidence for periciliary liquid layer depletion, not abnormal ion composition, in the pathogenesis of cystic fibrosis airways disease. *Cell* 1998;**95**:1005–15.

81 Geiser M, Bastian S. The surface-lining layer of airways in cystic fibrosis mice. *Am J Physiol Lung Cell Mol Physiol* 2003;**285**:L1277–85.

82 Auten RL, Watkins RH, Shapiro DL, Horowitz S. Surfactant apoprotein A (SP-A) is synthesized in airway cells. *Am J Respir Cell Mol Biol* 1990;**3**:491–6.

83 Phelps DS, Floros J. Localization of surfactant protein synthesis in human lung by *in situ* hybridization. *Am Rev Respir Dis* 1988;**137**:939–42.

84 Phelps DS, Floros J. Localization of pulmonary surfactant proteins using immunohistochemistry and tissue *in situ* hybridization. *Exp Lung Res* 1991;**17**:985–95.

85 Matsui H, Randell SH, Peretti SW, Davis CW, Boucher RC. Coordinated clearance of periciliary liquid and mucus from airway surfaces. *J Clin Invest* 1998;**102**:1125–31.

86 Kerem E, Bistritzer T, Hanukoglu A *et al*. Pulmonary epithelial sodium-channel dysfunction and excess airway liquid in pseudohypoaldosteronism. *N Engl J Med* 1999;**341**:156–62.

87 Tarran R, Grubb BR, Parsons D *et al*. The CF salt controversy: *in vivo* observations and therapeutic approaches. *Mol Cell* 2001;**8**:149–58.

88 Forteza R, Lieb T, Aoki T *et al*. Hyaluronan serves a novel role in airway mucosal host defense. *FASEB J* 2001;**15**:2179–86.

89 Pickles RJ, Fahrner JA, Petrella JM, Boucher RC, Bergelson JM. Retargeting the coxsackievirus and adenovirus receptor to the apical surface of polarized epithelial cells reveals the glycocalyx as a barrier to adenovirus-mediated gene transfer. *J Virol* 2000;**74**:6050–7.

90 Sade J, Eliezer N, Silberberg A, Nevo AC. The role of mucus in transport by cilia. *Am Rev Respir Dis* 1970;**102**:48–52.

91 Singh PK, Parsek MR, Greenberg EP, Welsh MJ. A component of innate immunity prevents bacterial biofilm development. *Nature* 2002;**417**:552–5.

92 Smith JJ, Travis SM, Greenberg EP, Welsh MJ. Cystic fibrosis airway epithelia fail to kill bacteria because of abnormal airway surface fluid. *Cell* 1996;**85**:229–36.

93 Goldman MJ, Anderson GM, Stolzenberg ED *et al*. Human beta-defensin-1 is a salt-sensitive antibiotic in lung that is inactivated in cystic fibrosis. *Cell* 1997;**88**:553–60.

94 Cole AM, Dewan P, Ganz T. Innate antimicrobial activity of nasal secretions. *Infect Immun* 1999;**67**:3267–75.

95 Salathe M, Holderby M, Forteza R *et al*. Isolation and characterization of a peroxidase from the airway. *Am J Respir Cell Mol Biol* 1997;**17**:97–105.

96 Gerson C, Sabater J, Scuri M *et al*. The lactoperoxidase system functions in bacterial clearance of airways. *Am J Respir Cell Mol Biol* 2000;**22**:665–71.

97 Wijkstrom-Frei C, El-Chemaly S, Ali-Rachedi R *et al*. Lactoperoxidase and human airway host defense. *Am J Respir Cell Mol Biol* 2003;**29**:206–12.

98 Verdugo P. Mucin exocytosis. *Am Rev Respir Dis* 1991;**144**(Suppl):S33–7.

99 Tanaka T. Gels. *Sci Am* 1981;**244**:124–38.

100 Edwards SF. The theory of macromolecular networks. *Biorheology* 1986;**23**:589–603.

101 Ross SM, Corrsin S. Results of an analytical model of mucociliary pumping. *J Appl Physiol* 1974;**37**:333–40.

102 Puchelle E, Zahm JM, Duvivier C. Spinability of bronchial mucus: relationship with viscoelasticity and mucous transport properties. *Biorheology* 1983;**20**:239–49.

103 Lazarowski ER, Boucher RC, Harden TK. Constitutive release of ATP and evidence for major contribution of ecto-nucleotide pyrophosphatase and nucleoside diphosphokinase to extracellular nucleotide concentrations. *J Biol Chem* 2000;**275**:31061–8.

104 Kim KC, Lee BC. P_2 purinoceptor regulation of mucin release by airway goblet cells in primary culture. *Br J Pharmacol* 1991;**103**:1053–6.

105 Davis CW, Dowell ML, Lethem MI, Van Scott M. Goblet cell degranulation in isolated canine tracheal epithelium: response to exogenous ATP, ADP, and adenosine. *Am J Physiol* 1992;**262**:C1313–23.

106 Abdullah LH, Conway JD, Cohn JA, Davis CW. Protein kinase C and Ca^{2+} activation of mucin secretion in airway goblet cells. *Am J Physiol* 1997;**273**:L201–10.

107 Rogers DF. Motor control of airway goblet cells and glands. *Respir Physiol* 2001;**125**:129–44.

108 Phipps RJ, Williams IP, Richardson PS *et al*. Sympathomimetic drugs stimulate the output of secretory glycoproteins from human bronchi *in vitro*. *Clin Sci (Lond)* 1982;**63**:23–8.

109 Boat TF, Kleinerman JI. Human respiratory tract secretions. II. Effect of cholinergic and adrenergic agents on *in vitro* release of protein and mucous glycoprotein. *Chest* 1975;**67**(2 Suppl):32S–34S.

110 Shelhamer JH, Marom Z, Kaliner M. Immunologic and neuropharmacologic stimulation of mucous glycoprotein release from human airways *in vitro*. *J Clin Invest* 1980;**66**:1400–8.

111 Sackner MA, Rosen MJ, Wanner A. Estimation of tracheal mucus velocity by bronchofiberoscopy. *J Appl Physiol* 1973;**34**:495–9.

112 Friedman MF, Scott D, Poole DO *et al*. A new roentgenographic method for estimating mucous velocity in airways. *Am Rev Respir Dis* 1977;**115**:67–76.

113 Yeates DB, Aspin N, Levison H, Jones MT, Bryan AC. Mucociliary tracheal transport rates in man. *J Appl Physiol* 1975;**30**:487–95.

114 Albert RE, Lippmann M, Peterson HT Jr *et al*. Bronchial deposition and clearance of aerosols. *Arch Intern Med* 1973;**131**:115–27.

115 Albert RE, Arnett LC. Clearance of radioactive dust from the lung. *AMA Arch Ind Health* 1955;**12**:99–106.

116 Del Donno M, Pavia D, Agnew JE, Lopez-Vidriero MT, Clarke SW. Variability and reproducibility in the measurement of tracheobronchial clearance in healthy subjects and patients with different obstructive lung diseases. *Eur Respir J* 1988;**1**:613–20.

117 Goodman RM, Yergin BM, Landa JF, Golivanux MH, Sackner MA. Relationship of smoking history and pulmonary function tests to tracheal mucous velocity in non-smokers, young smokers, ex-smokers, and patients with chronic bronchitis. *Am Rev Respir Dis* 1978;**117**:205–14.

118 Puchelle E, Zahm JM, Bertrand A. Influence of age on bronchial mucociliary transport. *Scand J Respir Dis* 1979;**60**: 307–13.

119 Hirsch JA, Tokayer JL, Robinson MJ, Sackner MA. Effects of dry air and subsequent humidification on tracheal mucous velocity in dogs. *J Appl Physiol* 1975;**39**:242–6.

120 Nieminen MM, Moilanen EK, Nyholm JEJ *et al.* Platelet-activating factor impairs mucociliary transport and increase plasma leukotriene B$_4$ in man. *Eur Respir J* 1991;**4**:551–60.

121 Klettke U, Luck W, Wahn U, Niggemann B. Platelet-activating factor inhibits ciliary beat frequency of human bronchial epithelial cells. *Allergy Asthma Proc* 1999;**20**:115–8.

122 Joo NS, Irokawa T, Wu JV *et al.* Absent secretion to vasoactive intestinal peptide in cystic fibrosis airway glands. *J Biol Chem* 2002;**277**:50 710–5.

123 Knowles M, Murray G, Shallal J *et al.* Bioelectrical properties and ion flow across excised human bronchi. *J Appl Physiol* 1984;**56**:868–77.

124 Gallagher JT, Kent PW, Passatore M, Phipps RJ, Richardson PS. The composition of tracheal mucus and the nervous control of its secretion in the cat. *Proc R Soc Lond B Biol Sci* 1975;**192**:49–76.

125 Corssen G. Eine Methode zur Testung toxischer Eigenschaften von Lokalanaesthetika unter Verwendung von Flimmerepithel des menschlichen Respirationstraktes in Gewebekultur. *Anaesthetist* 1958;**7**:309.

126 Wanner A. Effect of ipratropium bromide on airway mucociliary function. *Am J Med* 1986;**81**(Suppl 5A):23–7.

127 Yanaura S, Imamura N, Misawa M. Effects of beta-adrenoceptor stimulants on the canine tracheal ciliated cells. *Jpn J Pharmacol* 1981;**31**:951–6.

128 Lopez-Vidriero MT, Jacobs M, Clarke SW. The effect of isoprenaline on the ciliary activity of an *in vitro* preparation of rat trachea. *Eur J Pharmacol* 1985;**112**:429–32.

129 Ingels KJ, Meeuwsen F, Graamans K, Huizing EH. Influence of sympathetic and parasympathetic substances in clinical concentrations on human nasal ciliary beat. *Rhinology* 1992;**30**:149–59.

130 Agu RU, Jorissen M, Willems T *et al.* Effects of pharmaceutical compounds on ciliary beating in human nasal epithelial cells: a comparative study of cell culture models. *Pharm Res* 1999;**16**:1380–5.

131 Jain B, Rubinstein I, Robbins RA, Leise KL, Sisson JH. Modulation of airway epithelial cell ciliary beat frequency by nitric oxide. *Biochem Biophys Res Commun* 1993;**191**:83–8.

132 Wong LB, Miller IF, Yeates DB. Regulation of ciliary beat frequency by autonomic mechanisms: *in vitro*. *J Appl Physiol* 1988;**65**:1895–901.

133 Wong LB, Miller IF, Yeates DB. Stimulation of ciliary beat frequency by autonomic agonists: *in vivo*. *J Appl Physiol* 1988;**65**:971–81.

134 Chandra T, Yeates DB, Miller IF, Wong LB. Stationary and non-stationary correlation-frequency analysis of heterodyne mode laser light scattering: magnitude and periodicity of canine tracheal ciliary beat frequency *in vivo*. *Biophys J* 1994;**66**(3 Pt 1):878–90.

135 Devalia JL, Sapsford RJ, Rusznak C, Toumbis MJ, Davies RJ. The effects of salmeterol and salbutamol on ciliary beat frequency of cultured human bronchial epithelial cells, *in vitro*. *Pulm Pharmacol* 1992;**5**:257–63.

136 Tamaoki J, Chiyotani A, Sakai N, Konno K. Stimulation of ciliary motility mediated by atypical beta-adrenoceptor in canine bronchial epithelium. *Life Sci* 1993;**53**:1509–15.

137 Bennett WD. Effect of beta-adrenergic agonists on mucociliary clearance. *J Allergy Clin Immunol* 2002;**110**(6 Suppl): S291–7.

138 Foster WM, Bergofsky EH, Bohning DE, Lippmann M, Albert RE. Effect of adrenergic agents and their mode of action on mucociliary clearance in man. *J Appl Physiol* 1976; **41**:146–52.

139 Mossberg B, Strandberg K, Philipson K, Camner P. Tracheobronchial clearance and beta-adrenoceptor stimulation in patients with chronic bronchitis. *Scand J Respir Dis* 1976;**57**:281–9.

140 Mossberg B, Strandberg K, Philipson K, Camner P. Tracheobronchial clearance in bronchial asthma: response to beta-adrenoceptor stimulation. *Scand J Respir Dis* 1976; **57**:119–28.

141 Wood RE, Wanner A, Hirsch J, Di Sant'Agnese A. Tracheal mucociliary transport in patients with cystic fibrosis and its stimulation by terbutaline. *Am Rev Respir Dis* 1975;**111**: 733–8.

142 Svartengren K, Ericsson CH, Svartengren M *et al.* Deposition and clearance in large and small airways in chronic bronchitis. *Exp Lung Res* 1996;**22**:555–76.

143 Dirksen H, Hermansen F, Groth S, Molgaard F. Mucociliary clearance in early simple chronic bronchitis. *Eur J Respir Dis Suppl* 1987;**153**:145–9.

144 Vastag E, Matthys H, Kohler D, Gronbeck L, Daikeler G. Mucociliary clearance and airways obstruction in smokers, ex-smokers and normal subjects who never smoked. *Eur J Respir Dis Suppl* 1985;**139**:93–100.

145 Smaldone GC, Foster WM, O'Riordan TG *et al.* Regional impairment of mucociliary clearance in chronic obstructive pulmonary disease. *Chest* 1993;**103**:1390–6.

146 Camner P, Mossberg B, Philipson K. Tracheobronchial clearance and chronic obstructive lung disease. *Scand J Respir Dis* 1973;**54**:272–81.

147 Ericsson CH, Svartengren K, Svartengren M *et al.* Repeatability of airway deposition and tracheobronchial clearance rate over three days in chronic bronchitis. *Eur Respir J* 1995;**8**:1886–93.

148 Mossberg B, Philipson K, Camner P. Tracheobronchial clearance in patients with emphysema associated with α$_1$-antitrypsin deficiency. *Scand J Respir Dis* 1978;**59**:1–7.

149 Puchelle E, Zahm JM, Girard F *et al.* Mucociliary transport

in vivo and *in vitro*: relations to sputum properties in chronic bronchitis. *Eur J Respir Dis* 1980;**61**:254–64.

150 Fahy JV, Schuster A, Ueki I, Boushey HA, Nadel JA. Mucus hypersecretion in bronchiectasis the role of neutrophil proteases. *Am Rev Respir Dis* 1992;**146**:1430–3.

151 Maizieres M, Kaplan H, Millot JM *et al*. Neutrophil elastase promotes rapid exocytosis in human airway gland cells by producing cytosolic Ca^{2+} oscillations. *Am J Respir Cell Mol Biol* 1998;**18**:32–42.

152 Sommerhoff CP, Nadel JA, Basbaum CB, Caughey GH. Neutrophil elastase and cathepsin G stimulate secretion from cultured bovine airway gland serous cells. *J Clin Invest* 1990;**85**:682–9.

153 Fischer BM, Voynow JA. Neutrophil elastase induces *MUC5AC* gene expression in airway epithelium via a pathway involving reactive oxygen species. *Am J Respir Cell Mol Biol* 2002;**26**:447–52.

154 O'Riordan TG, Otero R, Mao YM, Lauredo I, Abraham WM. Elastase contributes to antigen-induced mucociliary dysfunction in ovine airways. *Am J Respir Crit Care Med* 1997;**155**:1522–8.

155 Cabello H, Torres A, Celis R *et al*. Bacterial colonization of distal airways in healthy subjects and chronic lung disease: a bronchoscopic study. *Eur Respir J* 1997;**10**:1137–44.

156 Hingley ST, Hastie AT, Kueppers F, Higgins ML. Disruption of respiratory cilia by proteases including those of *Pseudomonas aeruginosa*. *Infect Immun* 1986;**54**:379–85.

157 Wilson R, Roberts D, Cole P. Effect of bacterial products on human ciliary function *in vitro*. *Thorax* 1985;**40**:125–31.

158 Jackowski JT, Szepfalusi ZS, Wanner DA *et al*. Effects of *P. aeruginosa*-derived bacterial products on tracheal ciliary function: role of O$_2$ radicals. *Am J Physiol* 1991;**260**:L61–7.

159 Wilson R, Pitt T, Taylor G *et al*. Pyocyanin and 1-hydroxyphenazine produced by *Pseudomonas aeruginosa* inhibit the beating of human respiratory cilia *in vitro*. *J Clin Invest* 1987;**79**:221–9.

160 Hingley ST, Hastie AT, Kueppers F *et al*. Effect of ciliostatic factors from *Pseudomonas aeruginosa* on rabbit respiratory cilia. *Infect Immun* 1986;**51**:254–62.

161 Kanthakumar K, Taylor G, Tsang KW *et al*. Mechanisms of action of *Pseudomonas aeruginosa* pyocyanin on human ciliary beat *in vitro*. *Infect Immun* 1993;**61**:2848–53.

162 Munro NC, Barker A, Rutman A *et al*. Effect of pyocyanin and 1-hydroxyphenazine on *in vivo* tracheal mucus velocity. *J Appl Physiol* 1989;**67**:316–23.

163 Seybold ZV, Abraham WM, Gazeroglu H, Wanner A. Impairment of airway mucociliary transport by *Pseudomonas aeruginosa* products: role of oxygen radicals. *Am Rev Respir Dis* 1992;**146**(5 Pt 1):1173–6.

164 Dowling RB, Johnson M, Cole PJ, Wilson R. Effect of salmeterol on *Haemophilus influenzae* infection of respiratory mucosa *in vitro*. *Eur Respir J* 1998;**11**:86–90.

165 Biberfeld C, Biberfeld P. Ultrastructural features of *Mycoplasma pneumoniae*. *J Bacteriol* 1970;**102**:855–61.

166 Camner P, Jarstrand C, Philipson K. Tracheobronchial clearance in patients with influenza. *Am Rev Respir Dis* 1973;**108**:69–76.

167 Wynne JW, Ramphal R, Hood CI. Tracheal mucosal damage after aspiration. *Am Rev Respir Dis* 1981;**124**:728–32.

168 Battista SP, Denine EP, Kensler CJ. Restoration of tracheal mucosa and ciliary particle transport activity after mechanical denudation in the chicken. *J Toxicol Appl Pharmacol* 1972;**22**:56–69.

169 Afzelius BA, Camner P, Mossberg B. Acquired ciliary defects compared to those seen in the immotile-cilia syndrome. *Eur J Respir Dis* 1983;**64**(Suppl 127):5–10.

CHAPTER 18
Mucosal immunity

Hugues Chanteux, Charles Pilette and Yves Sibille

The mucosal surface, in particular in the gut and the respiratory tract, represents by far the largest interface of the host with its environment and therefore requires efficient protective mechanisms against potentially noxious agents. Thus, the epithelial monolayer represents a filter between the environment and the mucosa that is able to prevent or facilitate the passage of molecules from the lumen to the submucosa and vice versa. Specifically, the mucosal epithelium regulates the active transport of immunoglobulins A and M (IgA and IgM) produced in the lamina propria, into mucosal secretions, as a major component of mucosal immunity. This suggests a key role for secretory (S) immunoglobulins, mostly SIgA in both innate and specific immunity [1].

Although the respiratory tract shares many characteristics including defence mechanisms with other mucosae, the airways also exhibit some properties specific for the tracheobronchial tree. In particular, mechanical functions such as sneeze, cough and the mucociliary escalator represent major defence mechanisms to eliminate exogenous material reaching the upper and lower airways (Table 18.1).

The respiratory epithelium is divided into two compartments with different functions: the airways and the lung parenchyma. While the conducting airways (from the nose to membranous bronchioles) exhibit a typical mucosal epithelium (ciliated brushes, mucus secretion, secretory Igs production), the lung (from distal respiratory bronchioles to the alveoli) differs considerably from mucosal including bronchial surfaces, with a charasteristic epithelial profile; mostly flat, non-ciliated, type I epithelial cells and a few cuboidal type II epithelial cells, the latter accounting for the production of surfactant. This relates clearly to the different functions of the bronchial tree as compared to the lungs. The airways only conduct the inhaled and exhaled air, eventually trapping particulate material to prevent its deposition in the alveolar space. By contrast, the alveoli represent the unit controlling gas exchange between

Table 18.1 Defence mechanisms of the respiratory tract. (Adapted from Pilette *et al.* [1,99].)

First-line defence mechanisms
Airways
• Mechanical: nasal hairs, sneezing, cough, bronchial branching, mucociliary clearance
• Epithelial cell-derived products: mucus, lactoferrin, defensins, lysozyme, lectins, Clara cell protein
• Innate immunity: SIgA, complement, proteases
• γδ Intraepithelial T cells

Alveoli
• Alveolar macrophages: phagocytosis, oxygen and nitrogen metabolites, lysozyme, hydrolases
• Surfactant (SP-A, SP-B, SP-D)

Second-line defence mechanisms
• Alveolar macrophages and epithelial cells-derived product: cytokines and chemokines
• Recruited granulocytes (mostly neutrophils): phagocytosis, oxygen and nitrogen metabolites, cytokines, chemokines, antimicrobial products (defensins, natural antibiotics), proteolytic enzymes
• Adaptive immunity: antigen-presenting cells, αβ T cells, B cells (production of antigen-specific immunoglobulins)

airspace and the pulmonary capillary bed. Therefore, impairments in defence mechanisms have a completely different impact in the airways than in the alveoli, explaining the heterogeneous pattern of disorders affecting the airways and lungs.

In normal conditions, defence mechanisms aim at preventing inflammatory and immune reactions in the airways and alveoli. Little is known about the mechanisms underlying this relative tolerance but mechanical filters in the upper airways and mucociliary clearance are likely to have crucial roles. Thus, only few leucocytes can be observed in the respiratory tract lumen and the bronchial-associated lymphoid tissue (BALT) is virtually absent in healthy humans. By contrast, in pathological conditions, especially during infections, both inflammatory and immune cells can be easily, rapidly and often massively recruited [2,3]. The regulatory mechanisms involved in this recruitment are now better understood, providing potential new therapeutic targets.

Lymphocyte trafficking to the respiratory mucosa

Orchestration and memory of immune responses mounted at mucosal surfaces depend on the presence of T and B lymphocytes within mucosal tissues. The distribution of lymphocytes around the airways is organized differently according to the level of the respiratory tract. In the upper airways, most lymphocytes are located within the surface mucosa, in the lamina propria and in epithelium-associated lymphoid structures referred to as nasal associated lymphoid tissues (NALT). Lymphocytes are normally only rarely observed within the bronchial mucosa, peribronchial lymph nodes containing most mononuclear cells. Thus, primary immune responses require an efficient system to recruit selectively lymphocytes to the airways.

Several molecular mechanisms underlying the recruitment of lymphocytes to mucosal tissues have been unravelled in recent studies. Naive lymphocytes continously recirculate through lymph nodes using L-selectin, the peripheral lymph node addressin PNAd [4] and corresponding chemokines. In contrast, tissue-specific migration of memory/activated lymphocytes to mucosal tissues use different addressin/homing receptor pairs and chemokines, with differences between T cells, B cells and IgA$^+$ cells. Traffic of T and IgA$^+$ B cells committed to populate the intestinal mucosa depends primarily on the $\alpha_4\beta_7$ integrin–mucosal addressin cellular adhesion molecule 1 (MadCAM-1) (mucosal homing receptor) interaction occuring in gut venules, and thereafter on CCR9/CCL25 (TECK) [5,6]. The selective pathway(s) related to trafficking to the respiratory mucosa remain(s) so far elusive. The β_7 integrin and MadCAM-1 molecules are weakly expressed in the lung and therefore other mechanisms should take place to direct immune cells toward the airway mucosae.

While $\alpha_4\beta_7^+$ CCR9$^+$ blood T cells are committed to the gut, cutaneous lymphocyte antigen (CLA)$^+$ CCR4^{high} population traffic to the skin [7]. The $\alpha_4\beta_7^-$ CLA$^-$ CCR4$^+$ blood subpopulation has been suggested to target the airways, but BALT cells seem to express low levels of CCR4 and poorly respond to CCR4 chemokine ligands [7]. CCR10 is expressed by circulating IgA plasmablasts and IgA-secreting

plasma cells in various intestinal and non-intestinal mucosal tissues [8,9]; mucosal epithelial cells producing the CCR10 ligand, CCL28 (MEC). Recently, it was shown that L-selectin$^+$ $\alpha_4\beta_1^+$ memory T cells traffic to BALT, through recognition of PNAd and vascular cell adhesion molecule 1 (VCAM-1) in the bronchial mucosa microvessels [10]. $\alpha_4\beta_1^{high}$–VCAM-1 interaction, followed by activation of CCR10 by CCL28, could thus be involved in trafficking of lymphocytes, including IgA$^+$ B cells to the respiratory mucosa.

Once B cells have been primed by mucosal T cells, they recirculate and migrate to the primary mucosal site of antigen exposure and elsewhere; a phenomenon referred to as 'cross-dissemination' in the so-called common mucosal immune system [11]. Thus, immunization through the upper airway (intranasal or intratonsillar) activates local B cells that can reach remote sites such as the urinogenital tract [12], but without affinity for the gastrointestinal tract, suggesting a regional compartimentalization within mucosal immunity. The bronchi and the gut appear segregated in terms of humoral immune responses generating secretory antibodies [13]. Similarly, intranasal immunization evokes an antibody response in the nasopharyngeal tonsil but not in the palatine tonsil [14]. Once in the effector site, activated B cells undergo several functional changes related to terminal differentiation: class switching, clonal proliferation and somatic hypermutation of variable regions. Class switch from Cμ to Cα depends on the local expression of transforming growth factor β (TGF-β) [15], probably provided by epithelial cells under normal conditions or by macrophages during inflammatory responses. Interleukin 10 (IL-10), along with IL-2, IL-5 and IL-6, promotes the clonal proliferation of antigen-specific IgA-committed B cells [16].

It has been recently shown that the terminal B-cell differentiation occurs only in organized mucosal associated lymphoid tissue (MALT), and not in the diffuse lamina propria of mucosal effector sites [17]. This observation is of importance because a true BALT organization is only observed in humans in pathological conditions, such as in diffuse bronchiolitis or rheumatoid arthritis [18]. In contrast, NALT, consisting of the Waldeyer ring (lingual, nasopharyngeal and palatine tonsils) and lymphoepithelial structures (lymphoid aggregates, microfold cells) within the nasal mucosa, are much more developed than in lower airways and share features with the Peyer patches in the gut (GALT). Thus, under normal circumstances, mucosal immune responses to inhaled antigens are triggered in the nose, whereas immunity to inhaled microparticles that reach the bronchial mucosa rely on the peribronchial glands and thereby on systemic immunity to elicit primary specific immune responses. Interestingly, the presence of lymphoid follicles has been recently observed around small airways of patients with COPD [19].

IgA transcytosis

Located in the underlying mucosal epithelium, plasma cells secrete IgA mainly in its dimeric form. Dimeric IgA contains two conventional immunoglobulin subunits and an intersubunit joining (J) chain. The incorporation of this J chain into polymeric IgA endows these antibodies with high affinity for the polymeric immunoglobulin receptor (pIgR) [20]. The pIgR is a transmembrane protein with an external IgA-binding domain, a transmembranous domain and a cytoplasmic tail that contains cellular sorting signals. The extracellular region of pIgR is divided into the leader peptide and five Ig-like domains (D1–D5) [21,22]. A sixth non-Ig-like domain connects the extracellular domain to the transmembrane region. The pIgR is crucial for the generation of SIgA because it mediates transport of pIgA to mucosal secretions. Polymeric IgA binds efficiently to pIgR on the basolateral surface of epithelial cells. The pIgA–pIgR complex is then endocytosed from the basolateral pole and translocated by vesicular transport to the apical surface of the epithelium. At the apical surface, proteolytic cleavage splits the external domain of the pIgR (termed the secretory component, SC) from its membrane-spanning domain; this releases the dimeric IgA–SC complex, known as SIgA, into the mucosal secretions.

Mucosal immunity (SIgA and SC) in defence of respiratory tract

Secretory IgA participates in the first line of specific immune defence that protects the mucous membranes from inhaled pathogens. The mucosae largely rely on this mucosal immune system because it is continuously exposed to airborne agents that are potentially harmful. In recent years, it became obvious that beyond its well-recognized activity in scavenging particles and microorganisms at the mucosal surface, IgA has additional roles in mucosal defence. This is particularly evident at the level of the epithelial barrier [23] and of the regulation of phagocyte functions (Fig. 18.1) [24].

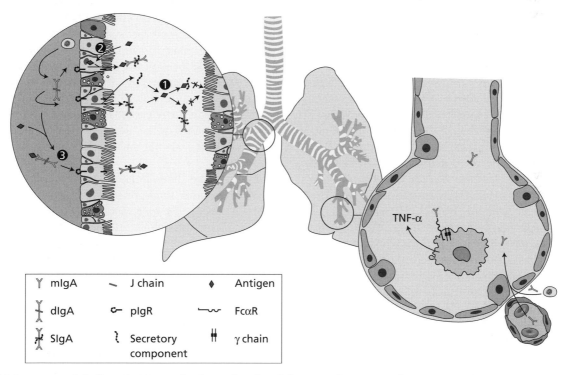

Figure 18.1 Immunoglobulin A (IgA) contribution to first-line defence mechanisms in the airways and alveoli. In upper conducting airways, IgA is produced by plasma cells as J chain-containing polymeric IgA (pIgA) and is transported across the airway epithelium through the pIgR into the mucosal lumen where it can synergize with the mucociliary system to clear inhaled antigens ❶. IgA can also interact with antigens within the epithelial cell ❷ and in the lamina propria ❸. In distal airways and alveoli, IgA mainly arises as monomeric IgA from plasma exudation and possibly from local synthesis by infiltrating plasma cells. Both monomeric IgA and SIgA (originating from proximal airways) can interact with the alveolar macrophage, the resident phagocyte of the lung which expresses a spliced variant of FcαR (CD89). FcαR triggering by IgA on macrophages may modulate the release of proinflammatory mediators such as tumour necrosis factor-α (TNF-α).

Immune exclusion in the lumen

The first role recognized for SIgA in the lumen is to neutralize bacteria by interfering with their motility and by competing for epithelial adhesion sites [25]. The ability of IgA to agglutinate microbes and to interfere with the action of their flagella renders them less motile and thereby more susceptible to be cleared by respiratory ciliary movements. As bacterial adhesion may operate through lectins, the oligosaccharides in the constant region of IgA may bind and therefore compete with carbohydrate moieties on epithelial cells that act as receptors for pathogens [26]. These two properties of IgA have a major role in protecting airway mucosal surfaces against colonization and invasion by pathogenic microorganisms. This so-called immune exclusion has been extended to viruses, parasites and bacterial toxins [27,28].

Intraepithelial neutralization

It is generally believed that all antibody classes are only active against the extracellular form of pathogens. Once a pathogen enters the cell and is sheltered intracellularly, it is considered to be inaccessible and protected from the actions of antibodies. Phagocyte-mediated immunity is thought to be the only immune system to fight these intracellular infections. However, recent studies have shown that intracellular pathogens such as viruses may be neutralized by IgA antibodies within epithelial cells during their assembly [29,30]. This particular property of IgA is possible through its mucosal transport mechanism; pIgA binds to pIgR on the basolateral surface of epithelial cells and the pIgA–pIgR complex is then transcytosed to the apical surface where a proteolytic cleavage leads to the release of pIgA–SC (SIgA) [31]. During this transport, IgA, in transit in the epithelial cell, could interact with the antigens of a virus infecting that cell. Both *in vitro* and *in vivo* experiments showed that IgA antibodies are able to neutralize intracellular viruses with different degrees of effectiveness according to the reactivity to the epitope. The capacity of neutralizing viruses is not only dependent on intrinsic properties of IgA, but also on the chance that IgA meets viral proteins during the virus' life cycle.

This virus neutralization by IgA appears as a compensation system within the epithelium which can trap antigens missed by the initial SIgA barrier ('immune exclusion') in the lumen.

A recent study has shown another role for intracellular IgA, demonstrating that pIgA transcytosed through the pIgR has the ability to down-regulate lipopolysaccharide (LPS) induced inflammation within epithelial cells [32]. This anti-inflammatory role for intracellular pIgA represents an additional protective mechanism contributing to IgA-mediated protection of the host.

Excretory immune function

In addition to these two properties in the lumen and within the epithelium, IgA has also a role in lamina propria. Indeed, pIgA binds to pIgR by its Fc region and this allows epithelial cells to transport not only free IgA but also IgA complexes [33]. The transcellular route for IgA immune complexes and for free IgA appears to be identical, in that everything is transported intact into secretions, with no major diversion to an intracellular degradation pathway. Such mechanism leads to the removal of antigens and pathogens out of the underlying lamina propria.

In most cases, this excretory function of IgA is beneficial for the host. However, in certain situations the IgA transcellular routing could be misused by pathogens and thereby become detrimental. In particular, after initial pharyngitis, it was shown that Epstein–Barr virus (EBV) spreads to regional lymph nodes where lymphoid cells are chronically infected. When the virus is released from this region, it forms a complex with IgA which can therefore be excreted in the mucosal lumen. However, EBV is the most important identified aetiological factor for nasopharyngeal cancer. Recent studies have shown that a specific mutation in the gene encoding for pIgR is associated with a higher risk of nasopharyngeal cancer [34]. This mutation could involve a failure in the transcytosis of EBV–IgA complex, leading to an alteration of the release of this complex in the secretion and consequently to an increase in susceptibility in the population of endemic areas to develop nasopharyngeal cancer.

Other studies have implicated the pIgR transcytosis in promoting rather than preventing invasion by pathogens. Thus, *Streptococcus pneumoniae*, one of the most common pathogens in respiratory infections, frequently colonizes the nasopharynx. This property reflects the capacity of *S. pneumoniae* to resist host immunity by expressing a polysaccharide capsule and to adhere to mucosal epithelia. Several surface-associated molecules of *S. pneumoniae* have been identified as contributing to pneumococcal adhesion to respiratory epithelia. Among them, choline binding protein A (CbpA) has been shown by mutagenesis studies to be required for pneumococcal nasal colonization [35,36] and lung infection [37,38]. This protein exhibits a specific binding with free SC or the SC portion of SIgA and pIgR [39]. This interaction is of pathogenic significance because it provides a mechanism of adherence of pneumococci to nasopharyngeal pIgR-expressing cells. Recent studies have identified D3 and D4 regions of pIgR as the binding sites for CbpA providing a mechanism for colonization [40,41].

However, three factors normally prevent pIgR-mediated internalization of pneumococci:

1 cleavage of pIgR from the apical surface;

2 the relative inefficiency of apical–basolateral transcytosis; and

3 the presence of free SC and SIgA antibodies in the respiratory secretions.

Nevertheless, an imbalance in any of these factors, or an overwhelming infection with pneumococci, could tip the scales in favour of invasion.

Constant pIgR transcytosis could occur efficiently with unoccupied receptors leading to the release of free SC at the apical surface of mucosal epithelial cell [42]. The amount of free SC in the respiratory secretions is relatively abundant (up to 60% of the total SC) [43], suggesting that this product of pIgR transcytosis may serve biological functions distinct from its association with IgA.

For decades, the main role attributed to SC has been to protect IgA from proteolytic degradation [44]. Recently, improved pIgA–antibody stability on SC binding was demonstrated in the oral cavity [45]. Moreover, free SC can also neutralize bacterial toxins and act as a non-specific microbial scavenger by binding to fimbriae colonization factor and preventing bacterial adhesion [46,47]. However, its susceptibility to proteolytic degradation limits its efficacy. This means that on association with specific IgA, SC can add to the capacity of SIgA to intercept and clear pathogens. SC has also been shown to bind to and inhibit the chemotactic activity of IL-8, a potent neutrophil chemoattractant [48], which is critical for the recruitment of neutrophils to sites of infection but also contributes to the persistence of the chronic inflammatory response in COPD or cystic fibrosis airways [49]. In cystic fibrosis, the binding of IL-8 to SC is reduced, probably because of an overglycosylation of free SC [50].

A new role for SC has been described recently. It has been shown that SC contributes to efficient IgA-mediated protection by ensuring, through its carbohydrate residues, the appropriate localization of the antibody molecules, which therefore results in optimal prevention of infection of mucosal surfaces by immune exclusion [51].

Because inflammation is not triggered via the three mechanisms described above, IgA is considered as a non-inflammatory antibody. This was further suggested by the fact that IgA is a poor activator of complement. Although IgA has been shown to be capable of triggering the alternative complement pathway (via C3b binding), IgA complexes fail to activate the classical pathway [52].

However, IgA may also bind to its receptor present on the surface of leucocytes and trigger cell activation through the Fcα receptor (CD89).

Although the main role of IgA is to scavenge bacteria in mucosal lumen through its Fab fragment, its immunomodulatory function appears relevant to the inflammatory response triggered by infectious, toxic or allergic stimuli. Indeed, bacterial exoenzyme, exotoxins, LPS, lipoteichoic acid released by bacteria exhibit a strong proinflammatory activity affecting the immune system [53], mainly by triggering the complex cytokine network. Therefore, the modulation of inflammation appears critical because the role of cytokines and chemokines in the severity of the disease, or even death resulting from infection is evident [54]. FcαR expression is restricted to cells of the myeloid lineage including neutrophils, eosinophils, most of monocytes–macrophages including alveolar macrophages [55–58]. Under normal conditions, mucosal secretions of the upper airways contain only few leucocytes, in contrast to distal airways occupied by resident alveolar macrophages. However, in the presence of inflammation, granulocytes and mononuclear cells are recruited to the airways and participate in SIgA-mediated immune response through their Fcα receptor (FcαR). FcαR participates in many aspects of host defence through engagement with antibodies complexed to antigens, initiating several biological processes including phagocytosis, antigen presentation, antibody-dependent cell-mediated cytotoxicity (ADCC), superoxide generation and release of cytokines and inflammatory mediators [24]. The cellular functions triggered by IgA binding to FcαR depend mostly on its association or not with the FcR γ-chain [59]. Indeed, the FcR γ-chain is essential for antigen presentation [60] and cytokine production but not for endocytosis [61]. It contains a so-called ITAM (immunoreceptor tyrosine-based activation motif) signalling motif [62], which is phosphorylated after IgA binding and triggers phosphorylation of several tyrosine kinases and mitogen-activated protein (MAP) kinases [63]. In monocytes, this activation leads to the production of several cytokines (IL-6, TNF-α, IL-1β, IL-8) [64,65] as well as superoxide release [66]. Similarly, pIgA and SIgA trigger a respiratory burst inducing superoxide release in neutrophils as well as in alveolar macrophages [63,67].

Although γ-less FcαR represents the majority of cell surface receptors, they seem unable to mediate downstream functions. They recycle internalized IgA complexes and protect them from degradation, putatively playing a role in serum IgA homoeostasis [61].

Another function initiated by FcαR is ADCC. Cells primed by IgA antibodies mediate lysis of target cells such as bacteria and erythrocytes, as well as tumour cells [68].

In addition to FcαR, eosinophils, unlike neutrophils, express a receptor specific for SC [69]. This receptor, which has not yet been characterized, is able to bind SC and SIgA but not serum, monomeric IgA and triggers the degranulation of eosinophils [70].

Exogenous compounds could also have an important

role in the regulation of airways inflammation. It is now largely accepted that some classes of antibiotics are endowed with anti-inflammatory properties in addition to their antimicrobial activities. Among them, macrolides and quinolones are the most studied. This is of particular interest considering the use of antibiotics in respiratory disorders including COPD [71]. Macrolide antibiotics, 14- and 15-membered ring compounds, exhibit immunomodulatory functions that are distinct from their anti-infective properties. Several *in vitro* studies have shown that erythromycin reduced IL-6, IL-8 and ICAM-1 levels [72,73]. In addition, treatment with macrolides reduces neutrophil influx to the airways [74] and sputum production in patients with mucus hypersecretion [75]. The molecular target of these effects seems to be nuclear factor κB (NF-κB), as recently shown for clarithromycin [76]. Indeed, it inhibits NF-κB activation in pulmonary epithelial cells and in peripheral blood monocytes, as observed with erythromycin [77]. These studies have led to the evaluation of long-term treatment with macrolides in inflammatory respiratory disease such as diffuse panbronchiolitis, cystic fibrosis, asthma, chronic rhinosinusitis and COPD, with some promising results because both symptoms and airways function were improved by macrolides [78,79]. Telithromycin, a ketolide derived from clarithromycin, was also reported to have immunomodulatory activity because it down-regulates IL-1α and tumour necrosis factor α (TNF-α) production by human monocytes [80]. However, no clinical studies are yet available.

Clinical studies showing the beneficial immunomodulatory effects of quinolones are not available. However, several *in vitro* data indicate that most fluoroquinolones derivatives, while inducing IL-2 synthesis [81,82], inhibit the synthesis of IL-1, TNF-α [83–85] and IL-8 [86]. Quinolones increase the cellular level of cyclic adenosine monophosphate (cAMP), probably through the inhibition of phosphodiesterase [87,88]. The accumulation of cAMP increases protein kinase A (PKA) activity, which is known to suppress the expression of TNF-α [89]. Quinolones may also exert their effects through modulation of nuclear transcription factors. The inhibition of TNF-α, IL-1 and IL-8 are associated with inhibition of NF-κB activation, resulting most likely from the inhibition of IκB degradation, while the induction of IL-2 is associated with increased AP1 activation [90]. Although progress has been made in understanding the mechanisms involved in the effects of fluoroquinolones, in-depth research is required to fully identify host targets of quinolones. Moreover, well-designed clinical studies should be performed to assess the potential immunomodulating effects of quinolones *in vivo*.

Both macrolides and fluoroquinolones are promised a successful future and it appears likely that a better understanding of the mechanisms of interplay between the host, pathogens and inflammatory cells will provide potential targets for the use of drugs, including antibiotics, in chronic inflammatory disease of the airways.

Mucosal immunity in obstructive airways disease

IgA production in COPD

IgA levels have been determined in bronchoalveolar lavage (BAL) fluid and sputum of smokers with and without COPD [91–94], but these studies are difficult to compare because of the different methods used and the different patient populations assessed. Despite this limitation, standard techniques used to distinguish between the molecular forms of IgA, as well as the correction of IgA levels for albumin exudation, suggested that the local bronchial production of IgA is decreased in patients with COPD [93,94]. In contrast, systemic antibody responses do not seem to be affected in COPD [95,96]. A decrease in pIgR expression in the bronchial epithelium was proposed as the underlying mechanism accounting for impaired local IgA responses in patients with COPD [97]. The decrease in pIgR content in COPD airways appears closely related to proteinases (elastase, proteinase-3) released by activated neutrophils, which can degrade this receptor and its soluble form, SC [98]. Impaired IgA responses within the airways can contribute to further enhance neutrophil infiltration through several mechanisms [99] and to disease pathogenesis, as supported by the relationship between pIgR expression and lung function tests of airways obstruction in patients with severe COPD [97]. The hypothesis that pIgR deficiency could reflect the epithelial impairment associated with an increased risk of COPD will be tested by assessing pIgR knockout mice for their susceptibility to develop COPD when exposed to smoke-related toxics.

IgA response in asthma and allergy

Allergen-specific IgA antibodies have been detected in the airways of patients with allergic rhinitis and/or asthma to dust mite or pollens [100,101], and display different epitope specificities as compared with IgE [101]. It has been suggested that IgA contributes to eosinophil activation during allergic reactions in the airways. Thus, IgA represents a highly potent stimulus for eosinophil degranulation *in vitro* [70,102], and correlation between the IgA response and markers of eosinophil activation has been observed *in vivo* in several studies of patients with allergic rhinitis or asthma. In addition, SIgA complexes can inhibit the release of γ-interferon (IFN-γ) by eosinophils triggered through CD28 [103], thereby promoting a Th2 profile.

Despite these data suggesting IgA as a pathogenic factor

Table 18.2 Main changes in defence mechanisms associated with asthma and COPD. First-line defence mechanisms are profoundly affected in both diseases, whereas adaptive immune response to inhaled antigens is only documented in asthma and different effector cells are involved.

	Asthma	COPD
First-line defence		
Mucociliary clearance	Decreased	Decreased
Secretory IgA	?	Decreased*
Epithelium	Denudated and activated	Hyperplasia
Adaptive immunity		
T-cell activation	Th2 cytokines	IFN-γ, CD8$^+$ T cells?
Antibody response	IgE	?
Effector cells	Eosinophils, mast cells	Neutrophils, macrophages

* May be increased during exacerbations of mild COPD patients.
IFN-γ, γ-interferon; IgA, immunoglobulin A; IgE, immunoglobulin E.

during allergic responses, several observations indicate that IgA can have protective roles against the development of allergic diseases:

1 selective IgA deficiency or delayed IgA production in childhood is a risk factor for atopy [104];

2 unlike IgE, allergen-specific IgA is detected in BAL from healthy subjects;

3 epidemiological evidence suggests a protective role of mucosal gut IgA production against cow's milk allergy [105,106];

4 intranasal treatment of mice with antigen-specific monoclonal IgA antibody prevented increases in bronchial hyperresponsiveness, tissue eosinophilia, and IL-4 and IL-5 production after allergen challenge [107];

5 increases in serum IgA is observed during high-dose allergen immunotherapy, along with IgG4, probably as a result of the induction of TGF-β and IL-10-producing regulatory T cells and monocytes [108] as observed in healthy subjects exposed to very high levels of allergen such as bee keepers.

The IgA response could therefore be part of the normal mucosal immune response to allergens.

Impaired first-line defence

The increased susceptibility of COPD patients to airways colonization and infection is probably multifactorial, and probably mainly relates to epithelial changes. First, mucociliary clearance is impaired in COPD [109], probably as a consequence of neutrophilic inflammation which increases mucus production (mucins MUC5AC and 5B) but reduces ciliary beating [110] and viscoelastic properties [111]. Activated neutrophils can also degrade both IgA and the epithelial pIgR [98], leading to impaired secretory IgA immunity. IgA normally acts within mucosal secretions by inhibiting adherence of microbes to the epithelium and thereby potentiates their clearance through the mucociliary mechanisms. Mucosal IgA deficiency in COPD could thus

favour the chronic presence of pathogens at the level of the bronchial tract. In addition, bacterial enzymes can also cleave IgA (classically the IgA1 subclass), leading to a vicious circle of impaired mucosal immunity and exaggerated inflammatory response, underlying the airway damage associated with COPD.

In asthma, mucociliary clearance is also impaired [112], both in large and small airways, and correlates with airflow limitation. Although mucus overproduction is observed in asthma, the epithelial changes are quite different than those observed in COPD. Mucous metaplasia (and hyperplasia) is a classical pathological feature in COPD, reflecting usual clinical symptoms, while epithelial denudation and/or shedding characterizes asthma, particularly severe stages of the disease (Table 18.2) [113].

Role of the bronchial epithelium

Beyond its role in mucociliary clearance and IgA transport, the bronchial epithelium can actively participate in the response to inhaled antigens and toxics through the production of cytokines and chemokines. After appropriate stimulation, epithelial cells can release molecules involved in the regulation of trafficking and activation of neutrophils (IL-8), eosinophils (IL-5, eotaxins), lymphocytes (IL-16, TARC/CCL17) and IgA$^+$ B cells (TECK/CCL25). In asthma, the production of the T-cell chemokine IL-16 mainly arises from the bronchial epithelium [114]. TARC/CCL17, along with MDC/CCL22, is induced after segmental allergen challenge [115] and selectively attracts Th2 cells expressing CCR4. The role of the epithelium in first-line defence mechanisms of the airways has been further illustrated in the recent study by Zhu *et al.* [116]. They showed that asthma epithelial cells, along with alveolar macrophages, produce acidic chitinases putatively targeting chitin-containing allergenic organisms such as house dust mite, cockroaches and fungi [116]. Beyond inhibition of the growth of chitin-containing organisms, the epithelial production of chitinases (which depends on IL-13) could potentiate the release of chemokines (MCP-1, eotaxin-1) involved in the recruitment of mononuclear cells and eosinophils. However, the relevance of chitinases to asthma pathogenesis requires further investigation. Also it remains poorly understood in COPD and asthma whether epithelial changes represent intrinsic changes or consequences of the ongoing airway inflammation. It has been recently shown that C/EBP-α deficiency characterizes asthmatic airway smooth muscle cells [117] and may underlie increased proliferative capacity [118] and shortening velocity. Interestingly, the increased proliferative capacity of airway smooth muscle cells in asthma appears intrinsic, as the phenotype was maintained through multiple passages in culture [118] – long after any inflammatory mediators present in the tissue would have been washed away. It would be of great interest to assess potential intrinsic changes of epithelial cells in COPD and asthma, and determine to what extent these changes relate to cell exposure to cigarette smoke or allergens in susceptible individuals.

References

1 Pilette C, Ouadrhiri Y, Godding V, Vaerman JP, Sibille Y. Lung mucosal immunity: immunoglobulin-A revisited. *Eur Respir J* 2001;**18**:571–88.

2 Sibille Y, Marchandise FX. Pulmonary immune cells in health and disease: polymorphonuclear neutrophils. *Eur Respir J* 1993;**6**:1529–43.

3 Sibille Y, Reynolds HY. Macrophages and polymorphonuclear neutrophils in lung defense and injury. *Am Rev Respir Dis* 1990;**141**:471–501.

4 Butcher EC, Williams M, Youngman K, Rott L, Briskin M. Lymphocyte trafficking and regional immunity. *Adv Immunol* 1999;**72**:209–53.

5 Zabel BA, Agace WW, Campbell JJ et al. Human G protein-coupled receptor GPR-9-6/CC chemokine receptor 9 is selectively expressed on intestinal homing T lymphocytes, mucosal lymphocytes, and thymocytes and is required for thymus-expressed chemokine-mediated chemotaxis. *J Exp Med* 1999;**190**:1241–56.

6 Bowman EP, Kuklin NA, Youngman KR et al. The intestinal chemokine thymus-expressed chemokine (CCL25) attracts IgA antibody-secreting cells. *J Exp Med* 2002;**195**:269–75.

7 Campbell DJ, Butcher EC. Rapid acquisition of tissue-specific homing phenotypes by CD4+ T cells activated in cutaneous or mucosal lymphoid tissues. *J Exp Med* 2002;**195**:135–41.

8 Kunkel EJ, Kim CH, Lazarus NH et al. CCR10 expression is a common feature of circulating and mucosal epithelial tissue IgA Ab-secreting cells. *J Clin Invest* 2003;**111**:1001–10.

9 Hieshima K, Kawasaki Y, Hanamoto H et al. CC chemokine ligands 25 and 28 play essential roles in intestinal extravasation of IgA antibody-secreting cells. *J Immunol* 2004;**173**:3668–75.

10 Xu B, Wagner N, Pham LN et al. Lymphocyte homing to bronchus-associated lymphoid tissue (BALT) is mediated by L-selectin/PNAd, α4β1 integrin/VCAM-1, and LFA-1 adhesion pathways. *J Exp Med* 2003;**197**:1255–67.

11 Wu HY, Russell MW. Nasal lymphoid tissue, intranasal immunization, and compartmentalization of the common mucosal immune system. *Immunol Res* 1997;**16**:187–201.

12 Czerkinsky C, Holmgren J. Exploration of mucosal immunity in humans: relevance to vaccine development. *Cell Mol Biol (Noisy-le-grand)* 1994;**40**(Suppl 1):37–44.

13 Nadal D, Albini B, Chen CY et al. Distribution and engraftment patterns of human tonsillar mononuclear cells and immunoglobulin-secreting cells in mice with severe combined immunodeficiency: role of the Epstein–Barr virus. *Int Arch Allergy Appl Immunol* 1991;**95**:341–51.

14 Quiding-Jarbrink M, Granstrom G, Nordstrom I, Holmgren J, Czerkinsky C. Induction of compartmentalized B-cell responses in human tonsils. *Infect Immun* 1995;**63**:853–7.

15 Coffman RL, Lebman DA, Shrader B. Transforming growth factor β specifically enhances IgA production by lipopolysaccharide-stimulated murine B lymphocytes. *J Exp Med* 1989;**170**:1039–44.

16 Fayette J, Dubois B, Vandenabeele S et al. Human dendritic cells skew isotype switching of CD40-activated naive B cells towards IgA1 and IgA2. *J Exp Med* 1997;**185**:1909–18.

17 Shikina T, Hiroi T, Iwatani K et al. IgA class switch occurs in the organized nasopharynx- and gut-associated lymphoid tissue, but not in the diffuse lamina propria of airways and gut. *J Immunol* 2004;**172**:6259–64.

18 Sato A, Hayakawa H, Uchiyama H, Chida K. Cellular distribution of bronchus-associated lymphoid tissue in rheumatoid arthritis. *Am J Respir Crit Care Med* 1996;**154**(6 Pt 1):1903–7.

19 Hogg JC, Chu F, Utokaparch S et al. The nature of small-airway obstruction in chronic obstructive pulmonary disease. *N Engl J Med* 2004;**350**:2645–53.

20 Brandtzaeg P, Prydz H. Direct evidence for an integrated function of J chain and secretory component in epithelial transport of immunoglobulins. *Nature* 1984;**311**:71–3.

21 Mostov KE, Friedlander M, Blobel G. The receptor for transepithelial transport of IgA and IgM contains multiple immunoglobulin-like domains. *Nature* 1984;**308**:37–43.

22 Piskurich JF, Blanchard MH, Youngman KR, France JA, Kaetzel CS. Molecular cloning of the mouse polymeric Ig receptor: functional regions of the molecule are conserved among five mammalian species. *J Immunol* 1995;**154**:1735–47.

23 Mazanec MB, Nedrud JG, Kaetzel CS, Lamm ME. A three-tiered view of the role of IgA in mucosal defense. *Immunol Today* 1993;**14**:430–5.

24 Monteiro RC, Van De Winkel JG. IgA Fc receptors. *Annu Rev Immunol* 2003;**21**:177–204.

25 Williams RC, Gibbons RJ. Inhibition of bacterial adherence by secretory immunoglobulin A: a mechanism of antigen disposal. *Science* 1972;**177**:697–9.

26 Wold AE, Mestecky J, Tomana M et al. Secretory immunoglobulin A carries oligosaccharide receptors for *Escherichia coli* type 1 fimbrial lectin. *Infect Immun* 1990;**58**:3073–7.

27 Gilbert JV, Plaut AG, Longmaid B, Lamm ME. Inhibition of

microbial IgA proteases by human secretory IgA and serum. *Mol Immunol* 1983;**20**:1039–49.

28 Outlaw MC, Dimmock NJ. Mechanisms of neutralization of influenza virus on mouse tracheal epithelial cells by mouse monoclonal polymeric IgA and polyclonal IgM directed against the viral haemagglutinin. *J Gen Virol* 1990;**71**(Pt 1):69–76.

29 Mazanec MB, Coudret CL, Fletcher DR. Intracellular neutralization of influenza virus by immunoglobulin A anti-hemagglutinin monoclonal antibodies. *J Virol* 1995;**69**:1339–43.

30 Mazanec MB, Kaetzel CS, Lamm ME, Fletcher D, Nedrud JG. Intracellular neutralization of virus by immunoglobulin A antibodies. *Proc Natl Acad Sci U S A* 1992;**89**:6901–5.

31 Solari R, Kraehenbuhl JP. Biosynthesis of the IgA antibody receptor: a model for the transepithelial sorting of a membrane glycoprotein. *Cell* 1984;**36**:61–71.

32 Fernandez MI, Pedron T, Tournebize R *et al.* Anti-inflammatory role for intracellular dimeric immunoglobulin a by neutralization of lipopolysaccharide in epithelial cells. *Immunity* 2003;**18**:739–49.

33 Kaetzel CS, Robinson JK, Chintalacharuvu KR, Vaerman JP, Lamm ME. The polymeric immunoglobulin receptor (secretory component) mediates transport of immune complexes across epithelial cells: a local defense function for IgA. *Proc Natl Acad Sci U S A* 1991;**88**:8796–800.

34 Hirunsatit R, Kongruttanachok N, Shotelersuk K *et al.* Polymeric immunoglobulin receptor polymorphisms and risk of nasopharyngeal cancer. *BMC Genet* 2003;**4**:3.

35 Balachandran P, Brooks-Walter A, Virolainen-Julkunen A, Hollingshead SK, Briles DE. Role of pneumococcal surface protein C in nasopharyngeal carriage and pneumonia and its ability to elicit protection against carriage of *Streptococcus pneumoniae*. *Infect Immun* 2002;**70**:2526–34.

36 Rosenow C, Ryan P, Weiser JN *et al.* Contribution of novel choline-binding proteins to adherence, colonization and immunogenicity of *Streptococcus pneumoniae*. *Mol Microbiol* 1997;**25**:819–29.

37 Hava DL, Camilli A. Large-scale identification of serotype 4 *Streptococcus pneumoniae* virulence factors. *Mol Microbiol* 2002;**45**:1389–406.

38 Lau GW, Haataja S, Lonetto M *et al.* A functional genomic analysis of type 3 *Streptococcus pneumoniae* virulence. *Mol Microbiol* 2001;**40**:555–71.

39 Hammerschmidt S, Talay SR, Brandtzaeg P, Chhatwal GS. SpsA, a novel pneumococcal surface protein with specific binding to secretory immunoglobulin A and secretory component. *Mol Microbiol* 1997;**25**:1113–24.

40 Elm C, Braathen R, Bergmann S *et al.* Ectodomains 3 and 4 of human polymeric immunoglobulin receptor (hpIgR) mediate invasion of *Streptococcus pneumoniae* into the epithelium. *J Biol Chem* 2004;**279**:6296–304.

41 Lu L, Lamm ME, Li H, Corthesy B, Zhang JR. The human polymeric immunoglobulin receptor binds to *Streptococcus pneumoniae* via domains 3 and 4. *J Biol Chem* 2003;**278**:48178–87.

42 Mostov KE. Transepithelial transport of immunoglobulins. *Annu Rev Immunol* 1994;**12**:63–84.

43 Brandtzaeg P. Structure, synthesis and external transfer of mucosal immunoglobulins. *Ann Immunol (Paris)* 1973;**124**:417–38.

44 Lindh E. Increased risistance of immunoglobulin A dimers to proteolytic degradation after binding of secretory component. *J Immunol* 1975;**114**(1 Pt 2):284–6.

45 Ma JK, Hikmat BY, Wycoff K *et al.* Characterization of a recombinant plant monoclonal secretory antibody and preventive immunotherapy in humans. *Nat Med* 1998;**4**:601–6.

46 Boren T, Falk P, Roth KA, Larson G, Normark S. Attachment of *Helicobacter pylori* to human gastric epithelium mediated by blood group antigens. *Science* 1993;**262**:1892–5.

47 Dallas SD, Rolfe RD. Binding of *Clostridium difficile* toxin A to human milk secretory component. *J Med Microbiol* 1998;**47**:879–88.

48 Marshall LJ, Perks B, Ferkol T, Shute JK. IL-8 released constitutively by primary bronchial epithelial cells in culture forms an inactive complex with secretory component. *J Immunol* 2001;**167**:2816–23.

49 Davis PB, Drumm M, Konstan MW. Cystic fibrosis. *Am J Respir Crit Care Med* 1996;**154**:1229–56.

50 Marshall LJ, Perks B, Bodey K *et al.* Free secretory component from cystic fibrosis sputa displays the cystic fibrosis glycosylation phenotype. *Am J Respir Crit Care Med* 2004;**169**:399–406.

51 Phalipon A, Cardona A, Kraehenbuhl JP *et al.* Secretory component: a new role in secretory IgA-mediated immune exclusion *in vivo*. *Immunity* 2002;**17**:107–15.

52 Pfaffenbach G, Lamm ME, Gigli I. Activation of the guinea pig alternative complement pathway by mouse IgA immune complexes. *J Exp Med* 1982;**155**:231–47.

53 Nau R, Eiffert H. Modulation of release of pro-inflammatory bacterial compounds by antibacterials: potential impact on course of inflammation and outcome in sepsis and meningitis. *Clin Microbiol Rev* 2002;**15**:95–110.

54 Cohen J, Abraham E. Microbiologic findings and correlations with serum tumor necrosis factor-α in patients with severe sepsis and septic shock. *J Infect Dis* 1999;**180**:116–21.

55 Geissmann F, Launay P, Pasquier B *et al.* A subset of human dendritic cells expresses IgA Fc receptor (CD89), which mediates internalization and activation upon cross-linking by IgA complexes. *J Immunol* 2001;**166**:346–52.

56 van Egmond M, van Garderen E, van Spriel AB *et al.* FcαRI-positive liver Kupffer cells: reappraisal of the function of immunoglobulin A in immunity. *Nat Med* 2000;**6**:680–5.

57 Monteiro RC, Cooper MD, Kubagawa H. Molecular heterogeneity of Fcα receptors detected by receptor-specific monoclonal antibodies. *J Immunol* 1992;**148**:1764–70.

58 Sibille Y, Chatelain B, Staquet P *et al.* Surface IgA and Fc-α receptors on human alveolar macrophages from normal subjects and from patients with sarcoidosis. *Am Rev Respir Dis* 1989;**139**:740–7.

59 Pfefferkorn LC, Yeaman GR. Association of IgA-Fc receptors (FcαR) with FcεRI γ2 subunits in U937 cells: aggregation induces the tyrosine phosphorylation of γ2. *J Immunol* 1994;**153**:3228–36.

60 Shen L, van Egmond M, Siemasko K *et al.* Presentation of ovalbumin internalized via the immunoglobulin-A Fc

receptor is enhanced through Fc receptor γ-chain signaling. *Blood* 2001;**97**:205–13.

61 Launay P, Patry C, Lehuen A *et al.* Alternative endocytic pathway for immunoglobulin A Fc receptors (CD89) depends on the lack of FcRγ association and protects against degradation of bound ligand. *J Biol Chem* 1999;**274**:7216–25.

62 Reth M. Antigen receptor tail clue. *Nature* 1989;**338**:383–4.

63 Ouadrhiri Y, Pilette C, Monteiro RC, Vaerman JP, Sibille Y. Effect of IgA on respiratory burst and cytokine release by human alveolar macrophages: role of ERK1/2 mitogen-activated protein kinases and NF-κB. *Am J Respir Cell Mol Biol* 2002;**26**:315–32.

64 Patry C, Herbelin A, Lehuen A, Bach JF, Monteiro RC. Fcα receptors mediate release of tumour necrosis factor-α and interleukin-6 by human monocytes following receptor aggregation. *Immunology* 1995;**86**:1–5.

65 Foreback JL, Remick DG, Crockett-Torabi E, Ward PA. Cytokine responses of human blood monocytes stimulated with IgS. *Inflammation* 1997;**21**:501–17.

66 Shen L, Collins J. Monocyte superoxide secretion triggered by human IgA. *Immunology* 1989;**68**:491–6.

67 Mackenzie SJ, Kerr MA. IgM monoclonal antibodies recognizing FcαR but not FcγRIII trigger a respiratory burst in neutrophils although both trigger an increase in intracellular calcium levels and degranulation. *Biochem J* 1995;**306**(Pt 2):519–23.

68 van Egmond M, van Spriel AB, Vermeulen H *et al.* Enhancement of polymorphonuclear cell-mediated tumor cell killing on simultaneous engagement of FcγRI (CD64) and FcαRI (CD89). *Cancer Res* 2001;**61**:4055–60.

69 Lamkhioued B, Gounni AS, Gruart V *et al.* Human eosinophils express a receptor for secretory component: role in secretory IgA-dependent activation. *Eur J Immunol* 1995;**25**:117–25.

70 Abu-Ghazaleh RI, Fujisawa T, Mestecky J, Kyle RA, Gleich GJ. IgA-induced eosinophil degranulation. *J Immunol* 1989;**142**:2393–400.

71 Sohy C, Pilette C, Niederman MS, Sibille Y. Acute exacerbation of chronic obstructive pulmonary disease and antibiotics: what studies are still needed? *Eur Respir J* 2002;**19**:966–75.

72 Takizawa H, Desaki M, Ohtoshi T *et al.* Erythromycin modulates IL-8 expression in normal and inflamed human bronchial epithelial cells. *Am J Respir Crit Care Med* 1997;**156**:266–71.

73 Khair OA, Devalia JL, Abdelaziz MM, Sapsford RJ, Davies RJ. Effect of erythromycin on *Haemophilus influenzae* endotoxin-induced release of IL-6, IL-8 and sICAM-1 by cultured human bronchial epithelial cells. *Eur Respir J* 1995;**8**:1451–7.

74 Sakito O, Kadota J, Kohno S *et al.* Interleukin 1β, tumor necrosis factor α, and interleukin 8 in bronchoalveolar lavage fluid of patients with diffuse panbronchiolitis: a potential mechanism of macrolide therapy. *Respiration* 1996;**63**:42–8.

75 Tamaoki J, Takeyama K, Tagaya E, Konno K. Effect of clarithromycin on sputum production and its rheological properties in chronic respiratory tract infections. *Antimicrob Agents Chemother* 1995;**39**:1688–90.

76 Ichiyama T, Nishikawa M, Yoshitomi T *et al.* Clarithromycin inhibits NF-κB activation in human peripheral blood mononuclear cells and pulmonary epithelial cells. *Antimicrob Agents Chemother* 2001;**45**:44–7.

77 Aoki Y, Kao PN. Erythromycin inhibits transcriptional activation of NF-κB, but not NFAT, through calcineurin-independent signaling in T cells. *Antimicrob Agents Chemother* 1999;**43**:2678–84.

78 Gotfried MH. Macrolides for the treatment of chronic sinusitis, asthma, and COPD. *Chest* 2004;**125**:52S–60S; quiz 60S–61S.

79 Rubin BK, Henke MO. Immunomodulatory activity and effectiveness of macrolides in chronic airway disease. *Chest* 2004;**125**:70S–8S.

80 Araujo FG, Slifer TL, Remington JS. Inhibition of secretion of interleukin-1α and tumor necrosis factor α by the ketolide antibiotic telithromycin. *Antimicrob Agents Chemother* 2002;**46**:3327–30.

81 Yoshimura T, Kurita C, Usami E *et al.* Immunomodulatory action of levofloxacin on cytokine production by human peripheral blood mononuclear cells. *Chemotherapy* 1996;**42**:459–64.

82 Dalhoff A, Shalit I. Immunomodulatory effects of quinolones. *Lancet Infect Dis* 2003;**3**:359–71.

83 Khan AA, Slifer TR, Remington JS. Effect of trovafloxacin on production of cytokines by human monocytes. *Antimicrob Agents Chemother* 1998;**42**:1713–7.

84 Ono Y, Ohmoto Y, Ono K, Sakata Y, Murata K. Effect of grepafloxacin on cytokine production *in vitro*. *J Antimicrob Chemother* 2000;**46**:91–4.

85 Araujo FG, Slifer TL, Remington JS. Effect of moxifloxacin on secretion of cytokines by human monocytes stimulated with lipopolysaccharide. *Clin Microbiol Infect* 2002;**8**:26–30.

86 Williams AC, Galley HF, Webster NR. The effect of moxifloxacin on release of interleukin-8 from human neutrophils. *Br J Anaesth* 2001;**87**:671–2.

87 Blaine TA, Pollice PF, Rosier RN *et al.* Modulation of the production of cytokines in titanium-stimulated human peripheral blood monocytes by pharmacological agents: the role of cAMP-mediated signaling mechanisms. *J Bone Joint Surg Am* 1997;**79**:1519–28.

88 Bailly S, Fay M, Roche Y, Gougerot-Pocidalo MA. Effects of quinolones on tumor necrosis factor production by human monocytes. *Int J Immunopharmacol* 1990;**12**:31–6.

89 Ollivier V, Parry GC, Cobb RR, de Prost D, Mackman N. Elevated cyclic AMP inhibits NF-κB-mediated transcription in human monocytic cells and endothelial cells. *J Biol Chem* 1996;**271**:20828–35.

90 Riesbeck K, Forsgren A, Henriksson A, Bredberg A. Ciprofloxacin induces an immunomodulatory stress response in human T lymphocytes. *Antimicrob Agents Chemother* 1998;**42**:1923–30.

91 Merrill WW, Naegel GP, Olchowski JJ, Reynolds HY. Immunoglobulin G subclass proteins in serum and lavage fluid of normal subjects: quantitation and comparison with immunoglobulins A and E. *Am Rev Respir Dis* 1985;**131**:584–7.

92 Ablin RJ. The elevation of serum IgA in emphysema. *Am Rev Respir Dis* 1972;**106**:283–4.

93 Stockley RA, Burnett D. Local IgA production in patients with chronic bronchitis: effect of acute respiratory infection. *Thorax* 1980;**35**:202–6.

94 Atis S, Tutluoglu B, Salepci B, Ocal Z. Serum IgA and secretory IgA levels in bronchial lavages from patients with a variety of respiratory diseases. *J Invest Aller Clin Immunol* 2001;**11**:112–7.

95 Von Hertzen L, Alakarppa H, Koskinen R *et al*. *Chlamydia pneumoniae* infection in patients with chronic obstructive pulmonary disease. *Epidemiol Infect* 1997;**118**:155–64.

96 Qvarfordt I, Riise GC, Andersson BA, Larsson S. IgG subclasses in smokers with chronic bronchitis and recurrent exacerbations. *Thorax* 2001;**56**:445–9.

97 Pilette C, Godding V, Kiss R *et al*. Reduced epithelial expression of secretory component in small airways correlates with airflow obstruction in chronic obstructive pulmonary disease. *Am J Respir Crit Care Med* 2001;**163**:185–94.

98 Pilette C, Ouadrhiri Y, Dimanche F, Vaerman JP, Sibille Y. Secretory component is cleaved by neutrophil serine proteinases but its epithelial production is increased by neutrophils through NF-κB- and p38 mitogen-activated protein kinase-dependent mechanisms. *Am J Respir Cell Mol Biol* 2003;**28**:485–98.

99 Pilette C, Durham SR, Vaerman JP, Sibille Y. Mucosal immunity in asthma and chronic obstructive pulmonary disease: a role for immunoglobulin A? *Proc Am Thorac Soc* 2004;**1**:125–35.

100 Nahm DH, Kim HY, Park HS. Elevation of specific immunoglobulin A antibodies to both allergen and bacterial antigen in induced sputum from asthmatics. *Eur Respir J* 1998;**12**:540–5.

101 Aghayan-Ugurluoglu R, Ball T, Vrtala S *et al*. Dissociation of allergen-specific IgE and IgA responses in sera and tears of pollen-allergic patients: a study performed with purified recombinant pollen allergens. *J Allergy Clin Immunol* 2000;**105**:803–13.

102 Dubucquoi S, Desreumaux P, Janin A *et al*. Interleukin 5 synthesis by eosinophils: association with granules and immunoglobulin-dependent secretion. *J Exp Med* 1994;**179**:703–8.

103 Woerly G, Roger N, Loiseau S *et al*. Expression of CD28 and CD86 by human eosinophils and role in the secretion of type 1 cytokines (interleukin 2 and interferon γ): inhibition by immunoglobulin A complexes. *J Exp Med* 1999;**190**:487–95.

104 Ludviksson BR, Eiriksson TH, Ardal B, Sigfusson A, Valdimarsson H. Correlation between serum immunoglobulin A concentrations and allergic manifestations in infants. *J Pediatr* 1992;**121**:23–7.

105 Hidvegi E, Cserhati E, Kereki E, Savilahti E, Arato A. Serum immunoglobulin E, IgA, and IgG antibodies to different cow's milk proteins in children with cow's milk allergy: association with prognosis and clinical manifestations. *Pediatr Allergy Immunol* 2002;**13**:255–61.

106 Saarinen KM, Vaarala O, Klemetti P, Savilahti E. Transforming growth factor-β1 in mothers' colostrum and immune responses to cows' milk proteins in infants with cows' milk allergy. *J Allergy Clin Immunol* 1999;**104**:1093–8.

107 Schwarze J, Cieslewicz G, Joetham A *et al*. Antigen-specific immunoglobulin-A prevents increased airway responsiveness and lung eosinophilia after airway challenge in sensitized mice. *Am J Respir Crit Care Med* 1998;**158**:519–25.

108 Jutel M, Akdis M, Budak F *et al*. IL-10 and TGF-β cooperate in the regulatory T cell response to mucosal allergens in normal immunity and specific immunotherapy. *Eur J Immunol* 2003;**33**:1205–14.

109 Smaldone GC, Foster WM, O'Riordan TG *et al*. Regional impairment of mucociliary clearance in chronic obstructive pulmonary disease. *Chest* 1993;**103**:1390–6.

110 Stockley RA. Role of inflammation in respiratory tract infections. *Am J Med* 1995;**99**:8S–13S.

111 Puchelle E, Zahm JM, Girard F *et al*. Mucociliary transport *in vivo* and *in vitro*: relations to sputum properties in chronic bronchitis. *Eur J Respir Dis* 1980;**61**:254–64.

112 O'Riordan TG, Zwang J, Smaldone GC. Mucociliary clearance in adult asthma. *Am Rev Respir Dis* 1992;**146**:598–603.

113 Jeffery PK. Remodeling in asthma and chronic obstructive lung disease. *Am J Respir Crit Care Med* 2001;**164**(10 Pt 2):S28–38.

114 Laberge S, Pinsonneault S, Varga EM *et al*. Increased expression of IL-16 immunoreactivity in bronchial mucosa after segmental allergen challenge in patients with asthma. *J Allergy Clin Immunol* 2000;**106**:293–301.

115 Pilette C, Francis JN, Till SJ, Durham SR. CCR4 ligands are up-regulated in the airways of atopic asthmatics after segmental allergen challenge. *Eur Respir J* 2004;**23**:876–84.

116 Zhu Z, Zheng T, Homer RJ *et al*. Acidic mammalian chitinase in asthmatic Th2 inflammation and IL-13 pathway activation. *Science* 2004;**304**:1678–82.

117 Roth M, Johnson PR, Borger P *et al*. Dysfunctional interaction of C/EBPα and the glucocorticoid receptor in asthmatic bronchial smooth-muscle cells. *N Engl J Med* 2004;**351**:560–74.

118 Johnson PR, Roth M, Tamm M *et al*. Airway smooth muscle cell proliferation is increased in asthma. *Am J Respir Crit Care Med* 2001;**164**:474–7.

CHAPTER 19

COPD and pulmonary surfactant

Carola Seifart and Bernd Muller

Composition, structure and function of the surfactant system

Normal lung function and effective gas exchange is strictly related to an essential lung structure termed 'pulmonary surfactant'. This phospholipid–protein rich material lines the inner surface of the alveoli as well as the terminal bronchioles. Its clinical importance became obvious when neonatal infants died from the infant respiratory distress syndrome (IRDS), which occurs when there is a lack of surfactant. In the acute respiratory distress syndrome (ARDS) in adults, surfactant exists but is severely impaired in structure and function [1]. Apart from these acutely life-threatening situations, there are inflammatory diseases in which pulmonary surfactant is structurally and functionally impaired [2]. This chapter summarizes the current knowledge of surfactant structure and function and its potential role in COPD.

Composition and structure of pulmonary surfactant

Pulmonary surfactant is synthesized in the alveoli by type II pneumocytes, which make up only 4% of alveolar cells. After synthesis, surfactant is secreted into the alveolar lumen [3]. Surfactant is harvested from patients by lung lavage procedures. Subsequent procedures exhibit its complex composition of lipids and proteins. The main portion (80.7%) consists of several species of phospholipids, which contain 76% phosphatidylcholine. Other components are cholesterol (5.6%), glycerol (6.7%), free fatty acids (1.6%) and surfactant associated proteins (5.4%) (Fig. 19.1). The proteins found in pulmonary surfactant are hydrophilic (surfactant proteins A and D, SP-A, SP-D) and hydrophobic (surfactant proteins B and C, SP-B, SP-C).

The structure of surfactant varies. Within type II cells pulmonary surfactant occurs as a lamellated structure (lamellar bodies). Upon its secretion into the hypophase of the alveolar lumen the structure is converted into tubular myelin and finally into a monolayer at the air–liquid interface (Fig. 19.2). Only correct composition and structure guarantees normal function in the lung.

Biophysical function and homoeostasis of surfactant

The most prominent surfactant function became obvious from studies of neonates with IRDS, who lack surfactant and as consequence show atelectasis. This observation was followed by biophysical studies revealing the potential of surfactants to prevent the distal lung from collapse. However, a prerequisite for this is normal surfactant composition and the ability to adsorb at the air–liquid interface of the alveoli. This is achieved by the hydrophobicity of the phospholipids and their interaction with SP-B and SP-C. Once the surfactant film is formed it reduces surface tension and prevents collapse of the alveoli and distal airways, keeping the lung open at low lung volume and preserves bronchiolar patency during normal and forced respiration [4].

From the hydrophilic surfactant proteins, SP-A is considered to be a modulator of surfactant homoeostasis. After its secretion from type II pneumocytes it prevents these cells, at least *in vitro*, from secreting surfactant phospholipids. It also stimulates type II cells to internalize phospholipids from the alveolar space. These functions regulate the amount of alveolar surfactant [5].

Surfactant in pulmonary defence

In the last decade, SP-A and SP-D became of interest for lung innate immunobiology [6]. Both hydrophilic proteins are multimeric complexes belonging to type C lectins (*syn.*

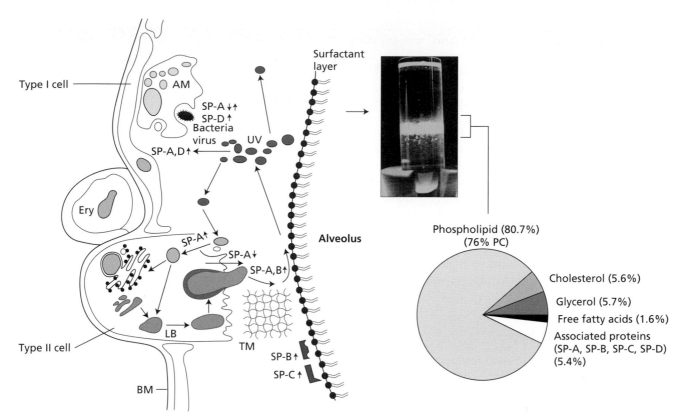

Figure 19.1 Surfactant structures and functions. When lamellar bodies (LB) containing surfactant are secreted into the alveoli they appear as lamellar structure, as tubular myelin (TM) and the surfactant layer. For this structural conversion surfactant proteins SP-A, SP-B and SP-C are necessary. In addition, SP-A and SP-D participate in the innate immunity modulating phagocytosis and killing pathogens by alveolar macrophages (AM). After brochoalveolar lavage, surfactant appears as a distinct band after centrifugation and sedimentation, containing surfactant proteins and several classes of lipids.

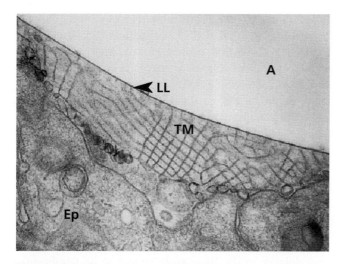

Figure 19.2 Microscopic graph of surfactant secreted from epithelial type II cells (Ep) showing lamellated strucure, tubular myelin (TM) and at the air (A)–liquid interface as lining layer (LL). (Picture courtesy of Professor H. Fehrenbach, University of Marburg.)

collectins). Of all structural elements the carbohydrate recognition domain (CRD) is the most important because of its binding to carbohydrate residues of pathogens and allergens.

It was seen from *in vitro* studies that SP-A is involved in innate immunity. It was shown that SP-A stimulated phagocytosis of alveolar macrophages and accelerated superoxide anion production. Additionally, SP-A opsonized a number of pathogens. These data clearly suggest the involvement of SP-A in first-line defence of the lung. SP-D is involved in stimulation of phagocytosis and respiratory burst, and serves as opsonin for several pathogens. Recently, the antimicrobial capacity of both collectins was described [7]. A number of *in vitro* data were confirmed by *in vivo* studies using surfactant protein knockout mice. It was shown that individuals lacking SP-A and SP-D had a higher risk of infection, whereby the immune reaction depends on the type of pathogen [8]. However, surfactant has a role in general immunomodulatory mechanisms of the lung. Inflammatory cytokines that are involved in airway inflammation, such as tumour necrosis factor α

(TNF-α) and interleukin 1β (IL-1β), are capable of inducing nuclear factor-κB (NF-κB), a ubiquitous transcription factor. By suppressing the activity of NF-κB, surfactant provides inhibitory effects on pro-inflammatory cytokine production, a mechanism that is important in disease pathogenesis of inflammatory airway diseases such as asthma and COPD [9].

There are an increasing number of studies on SP-A and SP-D that suggest the involvement of these collectins in acquired immunity of the lung [10–15]. So far, known functions in acquired immunity are binding to pollen and allergens, suppression of histamine release and suppression of T-cell proliferation and immune reaction after allergen challenge. Whereas expression of the collectins in immune response to allergens from pathogenic microorganisms show both increased and reduced levels of SP-A and SP-D, there is an increase of both proteins after ovalbumin challenge.

Surfactant in lung injury

Data on surfactant structure and function in injured lungs have mostly been obtained from inhalation studies with oxidants. Influx of inflammatory cells into the alveolar lumen is a general observation. In addition, the alveoli are flooded with serum proteins that inactivate the surface activity of surfactant. Lung injury caused by inhalation of deleterious agents can also directly impair the surfactant components such as phospholipids and proteins. The underlying mechanism is mostly oxidation of the components, resulting in reduced surface tension lowering capacity.

Pathophysiology, alteration and importance of the surfactant system in COPD

In addition to other physiological functions that may be of importance in airway obstruction (Fig. 19.3), pulmonary surfactant is essential for normal lung function. Surfactant proteins are part of the innate and adaptive immune system of the lung. Thus, the surfactant system may be involved in the regulation of inflammation in the lung and in the development and progression of COPD. However, current knowledge of the biology, function, potential dysfunction and alteration of the surfactant system in COPD are limited.

Cigarette smoke-induced alteration of the surfactant system

Cigarette smoking is the main single risk factor for the development of COPD. Therefore, the influence of cigarette smoke on the surfactant system was evaluated in order to

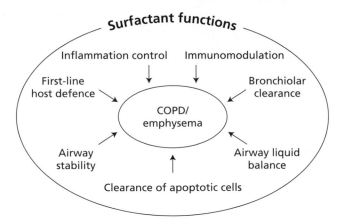

Figure 19.3 Physiological functions of the surfactant system of potential importance in the development and progression of COPD.

establish the potential importance of surfactant in the development or progression of COPD. Several studies provided evidence for a disturbed surfactant system in smoking individuals, as cigarette smoke was demonstrated to alter surfactant composition and activity, as well as reduce the elastic recoil pressure of the lungs [16–18].

Early in surfactant research, a rise of surface tension was observed in endobronchial washings of long-term cigarette smokers [19], and in human emphysematous lung tissue specimens [20]. Nevertheless, conflicting data exist with regard to the content of phospholipids in bronchoalveolar lavage (BAL) from smokers, the main component of pulmonary surfactant that provides surface tension lowering properties. In some studies, no differences in total phospholipid content in BAL between smokers and non-smokers were found [21–23], while others described significantly reduced [24,25] or increased phospholipid content [26] in BAL of smokers. However, there are consistent findings concerning altered phospholipid composition in BAL of smokers [22,26–28]. Furthermore, cigarette smoke-treated medium inhibited stimulated phospholipid secretion in a dose- and time-dependent fashion in cultured type II pneumocytes, while basal secretion remained unaffected [29]. Figure 19.4 summarizes the known effects induced by cigarette smoke on the surfactant system.

Additionally, studies of surfactant-specific protein content emphasize the role of surfactant in the pathogenesis of cigarette smoke-related disease. The content of SP-A and SP-D, both important components of the first-line host defence of the lung, were shown to be significantly decreased in BAL of smokers [21,23]. SP-B, an important modulator of physical surfactant function, was also shown to be significantly reduced in BAL of rats chronically exposed to cigarette smoke, while SP-A and SP-B lung tissue protein and mRNA levels remained unchanged [30].

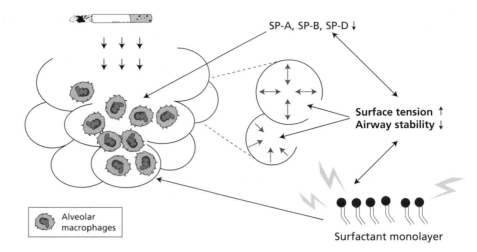

Figure 19.4 Influence of cigarette smoke on the surfactant system: surfactant composition is altered, surfactant specific proteins are reduced and surface tension is increased with lower airway stability.

The underlying mechanisms resulting in altered (reduced?) surfactant phospholipid and protein content in BAL of smokers have not yet been clarified, but may be related to the increased number of alveolar macrophages in smokers' lung tissue and consecutive increased phagocytosis of surfactant material [24,31] and/or alveolocapillary leakage induced by cigarette smoke.

Interestingly, in a model analysing the influence of surface tension and intraluminal fluid on the mechanics of small airways, the area of air–liquid interface decreased if the amount of intraluminal fluid was > 2%, whereby surface tension contributed to airway compression [32]. It was concluded that instability of small airways is correlated to intraluminal fluid and surface tension.

Pulmonary surfactant in emphysema

Pulmonary emphysema is a feature of COPD showing progressive destruction of alveolar structures. An imbalance of proteases (e.g. neutrophil elastase) and antiproteases seem to be of distinct importance in disease pathogenesis. On the one hand, neutrophil elastase is capable of cleaving surfactant specific proteins, the modulators of surfactant homoeostasis. These altered surfactant proteins have been shown to affect surfactant function by reducing the adsorption rate of surfactant lipids at the air–liquid interface [33]. On the other hand, protective effects of exogenous surfactant with respect to elastase-induced emphysema *in vivo* were demonstrated, as administration of surfactant in the first 4 days after elastase instillation resulted in significantly reduced enlargement of airspace [34].

Additionally, morphological studies indicate a role for pulmonary surfactant in emphysema. Synthesis and secretion of surfactant is a main function of type II pneumocytes. The number of these cells is significantly reduced in patients with emphysema [35]. As the evaluated patients had

already been diagnosed with established disease, it is not clear if the limited number of type II cells could also be observed early in the disease process. Nevertheless, it was postulated that the reduced number of type II cells may result in decreased surfactant synthesis or secretion. This could be of distinct importance under certain circumstances, such as in chronic cigarette smoke exposure known to induce increased elastase activity in lung tissue, where undisturbed surfactant function and composition are needed to serve as a protective screen.

Lessons learned from gene-targeted mice

Direct evidence for the hypothesis that the surfactant system is relevant for the development of COPD has been obtained in studies of gene-targeted mice. Targeted ablation of SP-D in mice resulted in chronic inflammation, emphysema and fibrosis of the lungs (Fig. 19.5) [36]. Homozygous SP-D knockout mice exhibit increased metalloproteinase (MMP) activity in BAL (MMP-2 and MMP-9) and in alveolar macrophages (MMP-9 and MMP-12). Furthermore, hydrogen peroxide production by isolated alveolar macrophages was significantly increased.

Cigarette smoke induces alveolar macrophage apoptosis *in vitro* [37] and *in vivo* [38] in a dose-dependent fashion, in particular in smokers with emphysema [39]. As apoptotic cells lining the airways may promote ongoing airway inflammation and lung tissue destruction, accumulation of apoptotic macrophages and consecutive enhanced alveolar wall cell turnover were postulated to be of distinct importance in COPD and emphysema [39,40]. Necrotic and apoptotic alveolar macrophages were five- to 10-fold increased in SP-D deficient mice. Treatment with recombinant SP-D resulted in reduced accumulation of apoptotic macrophages, suggesting a specific role for SP-D in promoting clearance of apoptotic cells from the lungs [41].

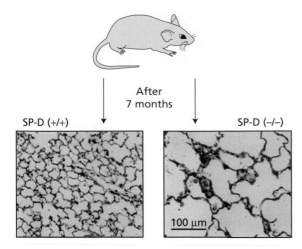

Figure 19.5 Spontaneous emphysema is observed in 7-month-old SP-D (–/–) knockout mice compared with wild type mice [36].

Gene-targeted mice of both SP-A and SP-B show pathophysiological alterations similar to those observed in patients with COPD. SP-A is involved in immunomodulation and inflammation control of the lung. SP-A knockout mice are deficient in clearing bacteria from their lungs [42]; thus, it was postulated that SP-A deficiency correlates with a higher risk for pulmonary infections. SP-B is essential for maintaining undisturbed physical function of the surfactant system [43] and normal lung function. Homozygous SP-B (–/–) knockout mice [44] die shortly after birth and heterozygous SP-B (+/–) mice exhibit decreased lung compliance and increased residual lung volume [45], as well as higher susceptibility to oxidant lung injury [46]. Currently, the exact correlation between surfactant specific proteins and COPD disease development or progression needs to be further elucidated. However, the data suggest that SP-A, SP-B and especially SP-D are relevant for the development and progression of COPD.

Genetic background

Current studies concerning the genetic background of patients with COPD provide novel insights and emphasize a potential correlation of altered surfactant composition and function with the disease. Genetic heterogeneity of the surfactant protein genes could result in different concentrations of surfactant proteins in the lung [47], directly influencing protein and surfactant functions. In the gene–environment context of the disease, the surfactant protein genotype may influence airway defence systems, resulting in altered risk to developing respiratory infections, and in turn to different susceptibility to COPD, or be correlated to other mechanisms associated with higher susceptibility to COPD.

The SP-A and SP-D genes have been mapped to human chromosome 10q21-q24. Two functional genes, *SP-A1* and *SP-A2*, have been described, with four *SP-A1* (6A, 6A², 6A³, 6A⁴) and six *SP-A2* (1A, 1A⁰, 1A¹, 1A², 1A³, 1A⁵) alleles found in more than 1% in the population and several others in less than 1% (6A⁶⁻⁸, 6A¹⁰, 6A¹²⁻¹⁵; 1A⁶, 1A⁹, 1A¹⁰, 1A¹², 1A¹⁴, 1A¹⁵). Functional human SP-A consists of products of both SP-A genes at a ratio of 2 : 1 (*SP-A1* : *SP-A2*). Quantitative and functional differences of the SP-A alleles have been demonstrated, such as different carbohydrate-binding characteristics and TNF stimulatory capacities [48,49].

For SP-D, three biallelic polymorphisms are known. Each one is localized in the amino-terminal part (Met11Thr), in the collagenous domain (Ala160Thr) and in the carbohydrate recognition domain (Ser270Thr). Four polymorphisms in the SP-B gene (−18(A/C), 1013 (A/C), 1580 (C/T) and 9306 (A/G)) and one large intron variation had been described.

Several studies show associations of these surfactant protein polymorphisms with pulmonary disease. Associations with infectious diseases were demonstrated for *SP-A2* : *1A3*, *SP-A1* : *6A4* and *SP-D 11_C*, which seems to be associated with higher risk for tuberculosis in a Mexican population [50]. *SP-A2* : *1A3*, SNP AA223_A and SP-D 11_T were significantly increased, while *SP-A2* : *1A* seemed to be protective in infants with severe respiratory syncytial virus (RSV) infection [51]. In COPD patients from Mexico, several surfactant protein polymorphisms have been found, with significantly higher frequencies in the COPD group compared with healthy smokers: one SP-A (*AA62_A*) and two SP-B alleles (*B1580_C/D2S3388_5*) [52]. The association of the *SP-I3* polymorphism B158Ø-C (SFTPBThrl3lSie) with the presence of COPD was replicated in the Boston Early-Onset Study [53]. Another large SP-B gene variation was associated with acute respiratory failure in COPD [54].

Exogenous surfactant application in COPD

Exogenous surfactant application is used routinely and successful in IRDS. However, data concerning surfactant application in patients with COPD are rare. One clinical surfactant treatment study suggests that aerosolized surfactant may improve mucociliary clearance and lung function in patients with stable chronic bronchitis [55]. In two studies, patients with acute asthma attacks and mild airflow limitation, respectively, were treated. These revealed an improvement of lung function parameters (*FEV*₁, *FVC*, Pao₂) in acute asthma, but not in patients with mild airflow limitation [56,57]. One case report describes successful surfactant application in a patient with severe exacerbation in COPD requiring mechanical ventilation [58].

Recombinant surfactant protein D therapy has recently become available. Interestingly, nasal application of recombinant SP-D was shown to reduce chronic inflammation and accumulation of apoptotic macrophages in SP-D deficient mice [41].

Conclusions

Pulmonary surfactant lines the inner surface of the lung and is essential for normal lung function, airway stability, airway inflammation control and in first-line host defence of the lungs. Several studies emphasize the potential importance of pulmonary surfactant in smoking-related diseases, such as COPD. Direct evidence for a relation between disturbed surfactant and COPD comes from studies evaluating gene-targeted mice.

It is known that disturbed surfactant function or composition contribute to small airway closure, as well as to an increased risk for recurrent and prolonged airway infections and altered mucociliary clearance; mechanisms that are thought to be of central importance for the development and progression of COPD. Nonetheless, many questions remain, including the usefulness of surfactant application in severe COPD, the significance of genetic heterogeneity of the surfactant system and the importance of surfactant components in host defence and repair mechanisms.

References

1 Poynter SE, LeVine AM. Surfactant biology and clinical application. *Crit Care Clin* 2003;**19**:459–72.

2 Meyer KC, Zimmerman JJ. Inflammation and surfactant. *Paediatr Respir Rev* 2002;**3**:308–14.

3 Dobbs LG. Pulmonary surfactant. *Annu Rev Med* 1989;**40**:431–46.

4 Goerke J. Pulmonary surfactant: functions and molecular composition. *Biochim Biophys Acta* 1998;**19**:79–89.

5 McCormack FX. Functional mapping of surfactant protein A. *Pediatr Pathol Mol Med* 2001;**20**:293–318.

6 McCormack FX, Whitsett JA. The pulmonary collectins, SP-A and SP-D, orchestrate innate immunity in the lung. *J Clin Invest* 2002;**109**:707–12.

7 Wu H, Kuzmenko A, Wan S *et al.* Surfactant protein A and D inhibit growth of gram-negative bacteria by increasing membrane permeability. *J Clin Invest* 2003;**111**:1589–97.

8 LeVine AM, Whitsett JA, Gwozdz JA *et al.* Distinct effects of surfactant protein A or D deficiency during bacterial infection on the lung. *J Immunol* 2000;**165**:3934–40.

9 Antal JM, Divis LT, Erzurum SC, Wiedemann HP, Thomassen MJ. Surfactant surpresses NF-κB activation in human monocytic cells. *Am J Respir Cell Mol Biol* 1996;**14**:374–9.

10 Madan T, Kishore U, Singh M *et al.* Surfactant proteins A and D protect mice against pulmonary hypersensitivity by *Aspergillus fumigatus* antigens and allergens. *J Clin Invest* 2001;**107**:467–75.

11 Wang JY, Shieh CC, Yu CK, Lei HY. Allergen-induced bronchial inflammation is associated with decreased levels of surfactant proteins A and D in a murine model of asthma. *Clin Exp Allergy* 2001;**31**:652–62.

12 Haley KJ, Ciota A, Contreras JP *et al.* Alterations in lung collectins in an adaptive allergic immune response. *Am J Physiol Lung Cell Mol Physiol* 2001;**282**:L573–84.

13 Atochina E, Beers MF, Tomer, Y *et al.* Attenuated allergic airway hyperresponsiveness in C57BL/6 mice is associated with enhanced surfactant protein (SP)-D production following allergic sensitisation. *Respir Res* 2003;**4**:15–27.

14 Hohlfeld JM, Erpenbeck VJ, Krug N. Surfactant proteins SP-A and SP-D as modulators of the allergic inflammation in asthma. *Pathobiology* 2002;**70**:287–92.

15 Wright JR. Host defence functions of pulmonary surfactant. *Biol Neonate* 2004;**85**:326–32.

16 Miller D, Bondurant S. Effects of cigarette smoke on the surface characteristics of lung extracts. *Am Rev Respir Dis* 1962;**85**:682–92.

17 Higenbottam T. Pulmonary surfactant and chronic lung disease. *Eur J Respir Dis* 1987;**71**(Suppl 153):222–8.

18 Schmekel B, Bos JA, Khan AR *et al.* Integrity of the alveolar–capillary barrier and alveolar surfactant system in smokers. *Thorax* 1992;**47**:603–8.

19 Cook WD, Webb DR. Surfactant in chronic smokers. *Ann Thorac Surg* 1966;**2**:327–33.

20 Thomas PA. Diagnostic lung biopsy: a correlative determination of histopathology and pulmonary surfactant. *Am Rev Respir Dis* 1967;**96**:1222–8.

21 Low RB, Davis GS, Giancola MS. Biochemical analyses of bronchoalveolar lavage fluids of healthy human volunteer smokers and non-smokers. *Am Rev Respir Dis* 1978;**118**:863–75.

22 Mancini NM, Bene MC, Gerard H *et al.* Early effects of short-time cigarette smoking on the human lung: a study of bronchoalveolar lavage fluids. *Lung* 1993;**171**:277–91.

23 Honda Y, Takahashi H, Kuroki Y, Akino T, Abe S. Decreased contents of surfactant proteins A and D in BAL fluids of healthy smokers. *Chest* 1996;**109**:1006–9.

24 Finley TN, Ladman AJ. Low yield of pulmonary surfactant in cigarette smokers. *N Engl J Med* 1972;**286**:223–7.

25 Lusuardi M, Capelli A, Carli S *et al.* Role of surfactant in chronic obstructive pulmonary disease: therapeutic implications. *Respiration* 1992;**59**(Suppl 1):28–32.

26 Hughes DA, Haslam PL. Effect of smoking on the lipid composition of lung lining fluid and relationship between immunostimulatory lipids, inflammatory cells and foamy macrophages in extrinsic allergic alveolitis. *Eur Respir J* 1990;**3**:1128–39.

27 Meyer W, Burkhardt A, Klenke B *et al.* Lung phospholipid metabolism after smoke exposure in rabbits *Prog Respir Res* 1981;**15**:141–7.

28 Lundgren R, Soderberg M, Horstedt P, Stenling R. Morphological studies of bronchial mucosal biopsies from asthmatics before and after 10 years of treatment with inhaled steroids. *Eur Respir J* 1988;**1**:883–9.

29 Wirtz HR, Schmidt M. Acute influence of cigarette smoke on secretion of pulmonary surfactant in rat alveolar type II cells in culture. *Eur Respir J* 1996;**9**:24–32.

30 Subramanian S, Whitsett JA, Hull W, Gairola CG. Alteration of pulmonary surfactant proteins in rats chronically exposed to cigarette smoke. *Toxicol Appl Pharmacol* 1996;**140**:274–80.

31 Giammona ST, Tocci P, Webb WB. Effects of cigarette smoke on incorporation of radioisotopically labelled palmitic acid into pulmonary surfactant and on surface activity of canine lung extracts. *Am Rev Respir Dis* 1971;**104**:358–67.

32 Hill MJ, Wilson TA, Lambert RK. Effects of surface tension and intraluminal fluid on mechanics of small airways. *J Appl Physiol* 1997;**82**:233–9.

33 Pison U, Tam EK, Caughey GH, Hawgood S. Proteolytic inactivation of dog lung surfactant-associated proteins by neutrophil elastase. *Biochem Biophys Acta* 1989;**992**:251–7.

34 Otto-Verbene CJM, Ten Have-Opbroek AAW, Franken C, Hermans J, Dijkman JH. Protective effect of pulmonary surfactant on elastase induced emphysema in mice. *Eur Respir J* 1992;**5**:1223–30.

35 Otto-Verbene CJM, Ten Have-Opbroek AAW, Willems LNA *et al.* Lack of type II cells and emphysema in human lungs. *Eur Respir J* 1991;**4**:316–23.

36 Wert SE, Yoshida M, LeVine AM *et al.* Increased metalloproteinase activity, oxidant production, and emphysema in surfactant protein D gene-inactivated mice. *Proc Natl Acad Sci U S A* 2000;**97**:5972–7.

37 Aoshiba K, Tamaoki J, Nagai A. Acute cigarette smoke exposure induces apoptosis of alveolar macrophages. *Am J Physiol Lung Cell Mol Physiol* 2001;**281**:L1392–401.

38 D'Agostini F, Balansky RM, Izzotti A *et al.* Modulation of apoptosis by cigarette smoke and cancer chemopreventive agents in the respiratory tract of rats. *Carcinogenesis* 2001;**22**:375–80.

39 Majo J, Ghezzo H, Cosio MG. Lymphozyte population and apoptosis in the lungs of smokers and their relation to emphysema. *Eur Respir J* 2001;**17**:946–53.

40 Yokohori N, Aoshiba K, Nagai A, Respiratory Failure Research Group in Japan. Increased level of cell death and proliferation in alveolar wall cells in patients with pulmonary emphysema. *Chest* 2004;**125**:626–32.

41 Clark H, Palaniyar N, Hawgood S, Reid KBM. A recombinant fragment of human surfactant protein D reduces alveolar macrophage apoptosis and pro-inflammatory cytokines in mice developing pulmonary emphysema. *Ann N Y Acad Sci* 2003;**1010**:113–6.

42 LeVine AM, Kurak KE, Bruno MD *et al.* Surfactant protein-A-deficient mice are susceptible to *Pseudomonas aeruginosa* infection. *Am J Respir Cell Mol Biol* 1998;**19**:700–8.

43 Schürch S, Green FHY, Bachofen H. Formation and structure of surface films: captive bubble surfactometry. *Biophy Biochem Acta* 1998;**1408**:180–202.

44 Clark JC, Wert SE, Bachurski CJ *et al.* Targeted disruption ot the surfactant protein B gene disrupts surfactant homeostasis, causing respiratory failure in newborn mice. *Proc Natl Acad Sci USA* 1995;**92**:7794–8.

45 Clark JC, Weaver TE, Iwamoto HS *et al.* Decreased lung compliance and airtrapping in heterozygous SP-B deficient mice. *Am J Respir Cell Mol Biol* 1997;**16**:46–52.

46 Tokieda K, Iwamoto HS, Bachurski C *et al.* Surfactant protein-B deficient mice are susceptible to hyperoxic lung injury. *Am J Respir Cell Mol Biol* 1999;**21**:449–50.

47 Karinch AM, deMello DE, Floros J. Effect of genotype on the levels of surfactant protein A mRNA and on the SP-A2 splice variants in adult humans. *Biochem J* 1997;**32**:39–47.

48 Wang G, Phelps DS, Umstead TM, Floros J. Human SP-A protein variants derived from one or both genes stimulate TNF-α production in the THP-1 cell line. *Am J Physiol Lung Cell Mol Physiol* 2000;**278**:L946–54.

49 Oberley RE, Snyder JM. Recombinant human SP-A1 and SP-A2 proteins have different carbohydrate-binding characteristics. *Am J Physiol Lung Cell Mol Physiol* 2003;**284**:L871–81.

50 Floros J, Lin HM, Garcia A *et al.* Surfactant protein genetic marker alleles identify a subgroup of tuberculosis in a Mexican population. *J Infect Dis* 2000;**182**:1473–8.

51 Lofgren J, Ramet M, Renko M, Marttila R, Hallman M. Association between surfactant protein A gene locus and severe respiratory syncytical virus infection in infants. *J Infect Dis* 2002;**185**:283–9.

52 Guo X, Lin HM, Lin Z *et al.* Surfactant protein gene A, B, D marker alleles in chronic obstructive pulmonary disease of a Mexican population. *Eur Respir J* 2001;**18**:482–90.

53 Hersh CP, Demeo DL, Lange C *et al.* Attempted replication of reported chronic obstructive pulmonary disease candidate gene associations. *Am J Respir Cell Mol Biol* 2005;**33**(4):71–8.

54 Seifart C, Plagens A, Brodje D *et al.* Surfactant protein B intron 4 variation in German patients with COPD and acute respiratory failure. *Dis Markers* 2002;**18**:1–8.

55 Anzueto A, Jubran A, Ohar JA *et al.* Effects of aerolized surfactant in patients with stable chronic bronchitis. *JAMA* 1997;**17**:1426–31.

56 Kurashima K, Ogawa H, Ohka T *et al.* A pilot study of surfactant inhalation in the treatment of asthmatic attack. *Aerugi (Jpn J Allergol)* 1991;**40**:160–3.

57 Oetomo SB, Dorrepaal C, Bos H *et al.* Surfactant nebulization does not alter airflow obstruction and bronchial responsiveness to histamine in asthmatic children. *Am J Respir Crit Care Med* 1996;**153**:1148–52.

58 Wirtz H, Habscheid W, Ertl G, Schmidt M, Kochsiek K. Exogenous surfactant application in respiratory failure due to chronic obstructive pulmonary disease. *Respiration* 1995;**62**:157–9.

CHAPTER 20

The macrophage and its role in the pathogenesis of COPD

Kellie R. Jones and Jordan P. Metcalf

Through its release of elastase and destruction of connective tissue, the neutrophil has traditionally been viewed as the principal inflammatory cell involved in the pathogenesis of chronic obstructive pulmonary disease (COPD). However, a series of elegant studies involving clinical science, cell biology and genetic manipulations have broadened the narrow and simplistic view of this complex disorder. Through these investigations, it is now understood that the action of many cells, including cells of the haematopoietic system as well as those of other origins, likely have a role in the development of COPD. With regards to haematopoietic cells, there is overwhelming evidence that the macrophage both directly and indirectly participates in disordered inflammation, which leads to the tissue destruction seen in patients with emphysema.

The purpose of this chapter is to familiarize the reader with the macrophage and its role in the pathogenesis of COPD. Although other types of lung macrophages are discussed, the focus is on the alveolar macrophage. This is partially of necessity, as the limits of technology have made the cell most accessible to the bronchoscope, the alveolar macrophage, the one for which the most data exists. First, the phylogeny of the lung macrophage is discussed. The increased density of macrophages in patients with the clinical diagnosis of COPD and in healthy smokers is the simplest evidence of the importance of this cell type. The data demonstrating this increased density and the mechanisms responsible for this finding is reviewed. Then, information demonstrating the importance of elastolytic products of the macrophage in COPD is covered. Finally, evidence demonstrating macrophage activation in COPD results in oxidant production and release of cytokines is discussed.

Origin and classification of the lung macrophage

The cellular origin of alveolar macrophage precursors is ultimately pluripotent stem cells residing in the bone marrow. This is supported by the demonstration of donor macrophages repopulating the alveoli in bone marrow transplant recipients [1]. Landmark studies from the 1970s confirmed that a large component of the stable alveolar macrophage population originates directly from infiltrating bone marrow-derived monocyte/macrophages [2]. More recent studies have shown that a small proportion of alveolar macrophages do not arise directly from the peripheral blood monocytes, but instead are the result of replication of a local population of more mature cells of monocyte/macrophage lineage. In leukaemic patients with prolonged monocytopenia, normal numbers of alveolar macrophages are present [3]. Approximately 0.5% of macrophages from normal subjects can synthesize DNA, and presumably can replicate. This amount can increase fourfold in patients who smoke or have pulmonary inflammatory conditions [4].

The pluripotent stem cell becomes committed to the monoblast cell line, with the final step of differentiation resulting in the macrophage (Fig. 20.1) [5,6]. The macrophage reaches the lung through the blood stream, and then migrates to various lung compartments. Approximately 15% of monocytes in the circulation ultimately become pulmonary macrophages. Pulmonary macrophages consist of three types: airway, interstitial and alveolar.

An additional cell considered to be related to the macrophage, although it appears to branch early from the monocyte differentiation pathway, is the dendritic cell. This cell resides in many of the same regions as the macrophage, as well as the bronchial-associated lymphoid tissue and the mediastinal lymph nodes. When found in the alveolar

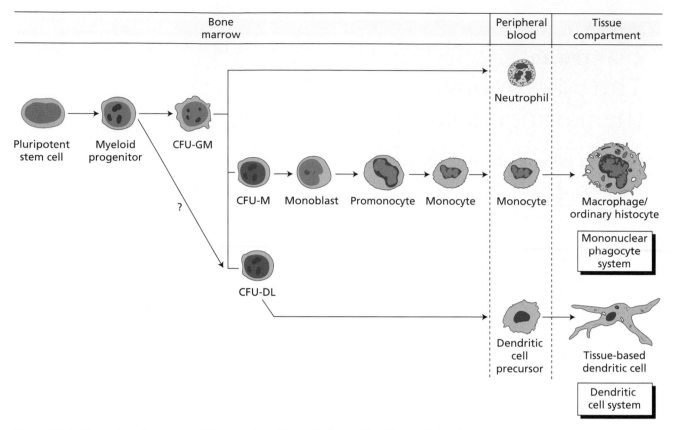

Figure 20.1 Macrophage/monocyte differentiation. (From Hoffman [5] with permission.)

compartment, these cells reside at or below the epithelium. Relative to macrophages, these cells are more effective at antigen presentation, but less effective at phagocytosis [2,7,8]. Thus, they appear to potentiate T-cell activation in the lung, playing a part in the connection between the innate and the adaptive immune systems. In terms of their role in innate immunity, dendritic cells, as well as alveolar macrophages and polymorphonuclear leukocytes (PMNs), have pattern-recognition receptors. These receptors bind to molecular structures that are basic to different microbes, in order to provide an immediate cellular response. This allows the cells of the innate immune system to begin phagocytosis, release cytokines or upregulate cell receptors, depending on which cellular signalling is activated [9]. The dendritic cell is not discussed in further depth in this chapter.

Another potential macrophage population is the pulmonary intravascular macrophage (PIM). Although plentiful in lower animals, in the normal human lung there are likely few PIMs but increasing evidence suggests that they are induced during inflammation [10].

With regards to macrophages that reside in the tracheobronchial tree, the alveolar macrophage dwells at the surface of the alveoli, while airway macrophages are in the final generations of respiratory bronchioles [6]. For all

practical purposes, there are no absolute physiological differences in the function of airway and alveolar macrophages. Alveolar macrophages are most often investigated in the role of emphysema. There is evidence of relative differences between these populations as the initial aliquots of bronchoalveolar fluid, which should be enriched for airway macrophages, contain larger and less active macrophages than subsequent aliquots. It would be expected that these later aliquots should consist of primarily alveolar macrophages [11]. This finding, of two distinct lavage macrophage populations, has been contested [12]. Because of their more proximal anatomical location, airway macrophages may be more important than alveolar macrophages in killing of bacteria and reaction to other foreign materials that are inhaled or aspirated. Also, the airway macrophage is an intrinsic part of the mucociliary transport system, a process, which when disrupted, may have a role in the pathogenesis of COPD [4].

The alveolar macrophage (Fig. 20.2 [13]) originates directly from either local proliferation of pulmonary macrophages or from differentiation of infiltrating bone-marrow-derived blood monocytes [14–19]. Typical bronchoalveolar lavage (BAL) from non-smokers recovers 1×10^7 total cells [20]. These cells are predominantly macrophages, typically

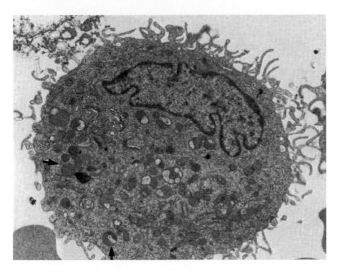

Figure 20.2 The alveolar macrophage. (From Fraser [13] with permission.) Lysosomes denoted by arrows (×8500).

90–95% of the total cell number. Animal models have revealed a life span of the alveolar macrophage of approximately 3–4 weeks [21]. From work carried out on human bone marrow transplant recipients, the life span appears to be between 27 days [2] and several months [1]. Within an alveolus of the normal lung, there exists approximately 50–70 inflammatory cells. Approximately 80% of these cells are macrophages [22].

Interstitial macrophages are monocyte-derived cells that reside between the pulmonary vasculature and the airway. They are viewed as precursors to the alveolar macrophage, but differ in some respects from their alveolar counterparts. These cells are somewhat difficult to study, because they require special techniques to harvest, and because preparations are frequently contaminated by residual alveolar macrophages. Likely because of these problems, estimates of relative number of interstitial macrophages to alveolar macrophages range widely, even within studies [23,24]. Recent studies in animals and human tissue show interstitial macrophages are smaller than alveolar macrophages and are not as proficient at phagocytosis or oxidant production [23,25,26]. In contrast, these cells are better at antigen presentation than alveolar macrophages [27]. As precursors to alveolar macrophages, and in their role in antigen presentation, they likely play a similar part in the pathogenesis of COPD, although this has not been thoroughly studied.

Increased macrophage density in the lung in COPD

The simplest and earliest evidence suggesting the role of the macrophage in the pathophysiology of COPD was the consistent finding that macrophage numbers are increased in the lower respiratory tract of smokers and patients with COPD. The following section attempts to review these data. The mechanisms for the increased macrophage density in COPD is also discussed.

There are several methods to investigate the cellular composition of the lung parenchyma, including the alveolus. The most frequently used means have been bronchoalveolar lavage, transbronchial biopsies and sputum (induced or spontaneous).

The primary technique to quantify cellularity in the distal airways is BAL. In normal BAL specimens, macrophages are the predominant cells [20]. In an early study to evaluate BAL as a means of comparison of controls with affected patients, a series of non-smokers were evaluated by Merchant *et al.* [28]. The lower respiratory tract cellularity of 111 volunteers who had never smoked and who had no evidence of respiratory disease or significant toxin exposure was compared by BAL. All of the lavage cell counts revealed a majority of macrophages, with only 3.6% of patients having less than 80% macrophages [28]. In an additional group of 19 healthy smokers, total cell counts, as well as the percentage of macrophages and lymphocytes, were increased when compared with the non-smokers [28].

In an additional study by Thompson *et al.* [29], both the initial lavage aliquots and distal aliquots, representing bronchial and distal airway samples respectively, were compared in patients with chronic bronchitis with a history of smoking, asymptomatic smokers and controls. Concentrations of cells in the lavage aliquots was also adjusted to estimate their actual concentration in the fluid lining the airways (epithelial lining fluid, ELF) using lavage urea level to correct for sample dilution. Subjects with chronic bronchitis had significantly greater numbers and concentration of cells in the bronchial BAL fluid and estimated bronchial ELF when compared with the other patient populations. There was no increase in the bronchial lavage or bronchial ELF macrophage concentrations, although neutrophil concentrations were increased. In the alveolar sample, only asymptomatic smokers had increased concentrations of macrophages in the raw lavage samples, but both smoking groups had increased macrophage concentrations as determined in the ELF [29]. Thus, both studies suggest that, at least in the distal airway, macrophage density is increased in smokers.

Bronchial biopsies have also been used to evaluate lower respiratory tract cellularity. In a study comparing 10 smokers with chronic bronchitis with six non-smokers, macrophages and T lymphocytes were significantly increased in the patients with chronic bronchitis. Cells that indicated lymphocytic activation (CD25+ cells) were also increased in the affected patients, although it could not be determined that this increased lymphocyte number and activation status was attributable to macrophages. CD4 and CD8 cells were not significantly different between the patient groups [30].

Evaluation of sputum has also been used to evaluated lung cellularity in patients with COPD. In patients with COPD, Domagala-Kulawik *et al.* [31] compared sputum samples from current smokers with those from a group of patients who had quit smoking for at least 1 year. There was no difference in cell count, including macrophage quantity, in the two patient sets. The macrophages present were subjected to further scrutiny, with subtypes expressing CD11b, CD14, CD54 and CD71 identified. This confirmed that the cells present in induced sputum were of similar phenotype to macrophages recovered in other studies by BAL. The distribution of these macrophage subtypes was also studied and revealed no difference between current and former smokers [31]. These data indicate that smoking cessation does not rapidly normalize cellular constituents in induced sputum samples.

Mechanisms responsible for increased macrophage density in the lung in COPD

Healthy smokers, smokers with COPD and ex-smokers with COPD have increased numbers of macrophages in the lower respiratory tract. There are three likely mechanisms that could be responsible for this phenomenon. First, increased numbers of macrophage precursors could be recruited to the lung. Second, local proliferation of macrophage precursors could be increased. Finally, the life span of terminally differentiated macrophages already present in the lung could be increased. A discussion follows of how each of these mechanisms contributes to the increased density in the lower respiratory tract of patients with COPD.

Enhanced recruitment of macrophages in COPD

Recruitment of macrophages is generally thought to be the primary mechanism responsible for increased macrophage density in the lung. Recruitment occurs through a subset of cytokines known as chemotactic cytokines or chemokines. Generally, cytokines in the lung are important mediators of cellular signalling. They are also referred to as peptide growth factors or biological response modifiers [32]. These proteins typically affect cells in close proximity, at relatively low concentrations.

There is evidence that enhanced recruitment of monocytes contributes to the increased macrophage density in the lung of patients with COPD. Koyama *et al.* [33] compared the monocyte chemotactic activity in BAL fluid (BALF) from 15 smokers with 16 non-smokers. They found enhanced monocyte chemotactic activity in the BALF of smokers. This activity correlated with BALF macrophage

numbers and several physiological markers of lung function decline including forced expiratory volume in 1 s (FEV_1) and diffusion capacity for carbon monoxide (DLCO) [33]. Hoogsteden *et al.* [34] showed that BALF from smokers has higher percentages of alveolar macrophages with monocyte-like morphology, which suggests recent recruitment. There are several cytokines with known monocyte chemotactic activity including tumour necrosis factor α (TNF-α), transforming growth factor β (TGF-β) and monocyte chemoattractant protein-1 (MCP-1) that are increased in tissue or BALF of smokers or patients with COPD [35–38].

These data are supported by *in vitro* studies. Smoke extract stimulates both lung fibroblasts and bronchial epithelial cells to release monocyte chemotaxins in response to cigarette smoke extract [39,40]. Furthermore, degradation products of the basement-membrane proteins collagen and elastin, which are formed during the lung destruction seen in emphysema, are chemotactic for monocytes and macrophages [41,42].

Increased macrophage replication in COPD

In the normal lung, the replication of the macrophage is nominal. In experiments with alveolar macrophages labelled with ^{3}H-thymidine, the pulmonary alveolar macrophage was found to have minimal division. This supported the theory that, in the steady state of the normal lung, maintenance of the alveolar macrophage population is by cellular migration from peripheral blood [2].

In contrast, inflammation clearly alters macrophage kinetics. One of the first studies showing this occurred was carried out by van Oud Alblas *et al.* [14], who demonstrated that exposure of mice to bacillus Calmette–Guerin (BCG) increased the replicating macrophage population to six times the usual number, with peak induction at 72 h after exposure. Of specific relevance to the current discussion, in a human study comparing non-smokers with both smokers and patients with chronic inflammatory lung disease, macrophage replication was quadrupled in smokers, and further increased in the subset of patients with inflammatory lung disease. Interestingly, only 5 pack-years of cigarette smoke exposure was required to cause significant elevation in the actively dividing macrophage population [4]. The division of macrophages serves to continue increasing the total number of macrophages after the initial influx triggered by cytokines. Thus, increased macrophage replication from both resident and recruited macrophages contributes to the increased macrophage density seen in COPD.

Increased macrophage survival in COPD

Macrophage half-life is limited by programmed cell death,

or apoptosis. There is evidence that this process is inhibited in patients with COPD. This prolongs macrophage survival, which at baseline is already longer than other inflammatory cells such as neutrophils and eosinophils. In smokers, the antiapoptotic protein Bcl-Xl is increased, potentially delaying the turnover of macrophages in the alveoli [43]. Additionally, interleukin 4 (IL-4), which is increased in smokers, significantly decreases the amount of TNF-α induced apoptosis in the monocyte/macrophage [44]. Another cytokine upregulated in COPD, macrophage-inhibiting factor, also delays apoptosis [45]. This occurs by suppression of p53 dependent apoptosis.

Thus, many different mediators are likely to be responsible for delaying macrophage death in smokers and patients with COPD. The net effect contributes to the increased macrophage burden in the lower respiratory tract in patients with this disorder.

Macrophage activation in COPD

Alveolar macrophages are the most numerous resident phagocytic cells in the lower respiratory tract in normal adults, and these cells have a variety of responses to infectious pathogens and foreign materials. Not only do macrophages remove soluble materials from the lung via fluid-phase pinocytosis, they also engulf infectious agents and particulate debris by phagocytosis. In their housekeeping role, they are armed with various elastases to facilitate breakdown of tissue debris. They also respond to stimuli by producing oxidants that interfere with infecting organisms, and cytokines to activate other components of the immune system.

Although these products are designed primarily to deal with pathogens, toxins or damaged tissue, they may, of course, damage normal lung components, and participate in the pathogenesis of emphysema.

Elastases

Elastin is usually a relatively insoluble protein component of the infrastructure of the lung. The idea that emphysema was caused by proteolysis was confirmed by induction of pathology by various proteases in animal models. Previously, several theories had been proposed to explain the pathogenesis of emphysema. These included the mechanical theory, which explains the airway damage as being caused by expiratory obstruction. The expiratory obstruction was explained by air trapping during bronchiole obstruction, leading to overdistention. The ischaemic explanation attempted to explain the disappearance of lung capillaries [46]. These theories have become less popular with the discovery that direct application of elastases to the lung causes emphysema. Animals that received papain (a plant protease with elastolytic action) intratracheally uniformly develop emphysema. The effect of papain on the development of experimental emphysema is specifically caused by its elastolytic properties, as other proteases such as collagenase and trypsin have not been shown to induce emphysema [47].

Another protease with elastolytic properties, pancreatic elastase, has also been demonstrated to cause emphysema in animal models. When pancreatic elastase was administered to hamsters, the animals were found to have a reduction of total elastin by two-thirds. New connective tissue was synthesized, and the elastin and collagen amounts normalized within weeks [45]. When living alveolar macrophages were cultured with elastin, the macrophages demonstrated significant elastolytic properties within 24 h of culture. The elastolytic process could also be predominantly inhibited by the addition of cysteine proteinase inhibitors, and therefore was likely a result of the cysteine proteases cathepsin G and L [48]. Proteases may interact, as when trypsin or chymotrypsin was given 24 h after pancreatic elastase; the resultant emphysema was more severe than in animals receiving elastase alone [49]. In additional studies, both activated and inactivated radio-labelled porcine pancreatic elastase was administered intratracheally to hamsters. Only the animals that received the activated enzyme were found to have emphysema [50], showing that active protease activity was necessary for the development of emphysema.

A human phenotypic correlate for the elastase–antielastase theory was found when it was discovered that some patients with premature emphysema had decreased serum levels of α_1-antitrypsin [51]. Subsequent studies supported the role of this protein in maintenance of the elastase–antielastase balance in the lung. Furthermore, data now suggest that a subset of patients with mild COPD and α_1-antitrypsin deficiency benefits from supplementation [52]. This is the ultimate proof-of-concept model for the elastase–antielastase theory.

Historically, the focus on elastolytic enzymes in COPD has been on elastolytic products of the neutrophil, and thus neutrophils were viewed as the 'first responder' in COPD. This view was supported by animal studies showing that neutrophil elastase induced emphysema, and human studies showing, for example, correlation of neutrophil number in BALF with the amount of airway obstruction and smoking history [29].

In contrast, for many years the role of the macrophage in disrupting normal lung architecture through digestion of elastin was questioned. More recently, however, through the work of Shapiro and others, the macrophage is now recognized as an important source of enzymes involved in the pathogenesis of emphysema.

Table 20.1 Matrix metalloprotease nomenclature. (From Kadoglou and Liapis [53] with permission.)

MMPs	Enzyme	Substrates
Collagenases		
MMP-1	Collagenase-1 (interstitial collagenase)	Collagens (I, II, III, VII, VIII, X), gelatin, proteoglycans, MMP-2, MMP-9
MMP-8	Collagenase-2 (neutrophil collagenase)	Collagens (I, II, III, V, VII, VIII, X), gelatin, proteoglycans
MMP-13	Collagenase-3	Collagens (I, II, III, IV, IX, X, XIV), gelatin, MMP-9
MMP-18	Collagenase-4 (*Xenopus* collagenase)	Not determined
Gelatinases		
MMP-2	Gelatinase A	Gelatin, collagens (I, IV, V, VII, X, XI, XIV), elastin, fibronectin, laminin, MMP-1, MMP-9, MMP-13
MMP-9	Gelatinase B	Gelatin, collagens (IV, V, VII, X, XIV), elastin, fibronectin, plasminogen
Stromelysins		
MMP-3	Stromelysin-1	Collagens (III, IV, V, IX, X), gelatin, fibronectin, laminin, MMP-1, MMP-7, MMP-8, MMP-9, MMP-13
MMP-10	Stromelysin-2	Collagens (III, IV, V), gelatin, casein, MMP-1, MMP-8
MMP-11	Stromelysin-3	Gelatin, collagen IV, fibronectin, casein, proteoglycans
Matrilysins		
MMP-7	Matrilysin-1	Collagens (IV, X), gelatin, fibronectin, laminin, MMP-1, MMP-2, MMP-9, MMP-9/TIMP-1 complex
MMP-26	Matrilysin-2	Collagen IV, fibronectin, gelatin, proMMP-9, fibrinogen
Membrane type		
MMP-14	MT1-MMP	Collagens (I, II, III), gelatin, casein, elastin, fibronectin, laminin, MMP-2, MMP-13
MMP-15	MT2-MMP	Gelatin, fibronectin, laminin, MMP-2
MMP-16	MT3-MMP	Collagen III, gelatin, casein, fibronectin, MMP-2
MMP-17	MT4-MMP	Gelatin, proMMP-2
MMP-24	MT5-MMP	Proteoglycans, proMMP-2, collagen I, gelatin, fibronectin, laminin
MMP-25	MT6-MMP	Collagen IV, proMMP-8, proMMP-9
Other MMPs		
MMP-12	Macrophage metalloelastase	Collagen IV, gelatin, elastin, fibronectin, casein, fibrinogen, plasminogen, MMP-2
MMP-19, 20	–	Aggrecan, cartilage oligomeric matrix protein

MMP, matrix metalloproteinases; MT, membrane type; TIMP, tissue inhibitor of metalloproteinase.

Products of the macrophage that are thought to participate in the pathogenesis of emphysema include the matrix metalloproteinases (Table 20.1 [53]) and tissue inhibitors of metalloproteinases (TIMPs). The first indication that an enzyme with elastolytic properties existed in macrophages were experiments by Werb and Gordon [54] demonstrating elastin degradation by mouse macrophage-conditioned media. Inhibition of this activity by chelators showed that it was caused by a metalloproteinase. The proteinase was first isolated in mice [55], and a human homologue was shown to be capable of degrading elastin as well as all basement-membrane components [56].

This human analogue of the mouse macrophage elastase, also termed matrix metalloproteinase-12 (MMP-12) has very similar biochemical properties, and was sequenced in 1993 [56]. Human MMP-12 is produced as a 54-kDa proenzyme which is activated by amino terminal cleavage and by COOH-terminal domain processing to a 22-kDa mature species. The COOH terminal domain appears to be important for substrate binding with the inhibitors. This complex processing creates an active elastolytic product, and a site for regulation of the elastolytic process by binding of inhibitors [56].

The matrix metalloproteinases are an ever-expanding family of active enzymes, with currently 20 recognized members. Prior to identification and classification of the numerous MMPs, knockout mice were created that did not have macrophage elastase (MMP-12). In normal MMP-12 +/+ mice, exposure of mice to 6 months of cigarette smoke resulted in emphysematous changes similar to that seen in mice with pulmonary instillation with neutrophil elastase. Smoke exposure also caused upregulation of MMP-12 in alveolar macrophages as determined by immunohisto-chemistry. Despite chronic exposure to cigarette smoke, the MMP-12 −/− animals did not develop emphysema. Even when MCP-1, a monocyte chemoattractant, was introduced to equalize the number of macrophages present in both control and MMP-12 −/− mice, MMP-12 −/− mice did not development emphysema. On the other hand, treatment of MMP-12 +/+ smoke-exposed mice with MCP-1 further enhanced the development of emphysema [57].

There are additional MMPs produced by macrophages that may contribute to the pathogenesis of emphysema. The presence and activity of gelatinase A (MMP-2) and gelatinase B (MMP-9) are significantly increased in patients with COPD (as defined by spirometry) [58]. Macrophages from patients with emphysema, suggested by pulmonary function tests (PFTs) and further confirmed by computed tomography (CT), have higher mRNA levels of MMP-1 (collagenase) and MMP-9 than controls [59]. The MMPs gelatinase and collagenase are also significantly elevated in the BALF of patients with the diagnosis of COPD [59].

Production of MMPs by macrophages is also regulated by other cells of the immune system. IL-13 is a Th2 cytokine thought to be important in the pathogenesis of asthma. However, when IL-13 is overexpressed in mice, the result-ant lung pathology is very similar to that of human emphysema. Physiologically, these animals also had enhanced pulmonary compliance as one would expect with COPD with emphysema [60]. These changes were accompanied by induction of MMP-2, -9, -12, -13 and -14. The primary source of the MMP-12 was, as expected, the macrophage. Further studies with MMP-9 and -12 knockout mice in the setting of IL-13 overexpression have shown decreased amounts of alveolar enlargement, compliance changes and death when compared with controls. The roles of the two MMPs studied appeared to be quite different, with MMP-9 being linked to inhibition of neutrophils recovered in BAL, while MMP-12 deficient mice had reduced numbers of eosinophils and macrophages in their respective BALs [61]. This further implicates both the macrophage and its prod-ucts in the pathogenesis of COPD.

There are additional data implicating these enzymes in the pathogenesis of COPD. During the maturation pro-cess of macrophages, there is a shift in metalloproteinase species produced towards MMP-2 and -9. Since MMP-9 has emerged as an enzyme in the forefront of elastin degrada-tion, its production in different patient populations has been evaluated. When patients with COPD were compared with healthy smokers and non-smokers, the patients with COPD released greater amounts of MMP-9. The MMP-9 released in the COPD patients was more biologically active. Another important observation in the same study was that non-smokers produced greater amounts of tissue inhibitor of MMP (TIMP-1, specifically) than their smoking counter-parts, regardless of whether or not the smokers had been diagnosed with COPD [62]. This suggests that not only is macrophage elastase production and activity enhanced in smokers, but the ability of the lung to protect itself with antielastases is also inhibited by tobacco smoke.

Macrophage elastase (MMP-12) may be the final medi-ator of emphysema induced by alteration of other structural molecules such as integrins. The αv-β6 integrin binds and activates TGF-β. Knockout mice (Itgb6−) deficient in expression of the β6 integrin subunit express 200 times the mRNA of MMP-12 than that of their Itgb6+ counterparts. Furthermore, while Itgb6+ had no pulmonary histological changes suggestive of emphysema, the mice deficient in this integrin subunit had progressive spontaneous age-related emphysema that was comparable to that seen in humans [63]. This, together with the finding that MMP-12 knockout mice do not become emphysematous, even with long-term smoke exposure [57], and do not have an influx of macrophages with cigarette smoke exposure implicates this macrophage-produced elastase in the pathogenesis of emphysema. One explanation for these findings is that MMP-12 mice do not degrade elastin, so lung architecture is preserved, and elastin fragments, which are chemotactic for macrophages, are not produced [42,64]. Also, active MMP-12 appears to be important in the release of pro-inflammatory cytokines [65].

Oxidants

Alterations in the elastase–antielastase balance in the lung have a clear role in the pathogenesis of COPD. Less well understood is the role of alterations in oxidant–antioxidant balance in this disease state. There are two types of oxidant species generally relevant to this discussion, reactive oxidant species (ROS) and reactive nitrogen species (RNS). Cigarette smoke contains more than 10^{14} free radicals of both species per puff [66]. As the focus of the chapter is on the macrophage, this section briefly discusses the evidence that these species are harmful to the lung, and then discusses in more detail the production of oxidants by macrophages in relevant laboratory and clinical studies.

The oxidants produced by macrophages in response to stimuli include the ROS superoxide, hydrogen peroxide and hydroxyl radicals [67]. Hypohalides, while made by neutrophils, do not appear to be generated by macrophages [68]. The RNS nitric oxide is also produced by these cells. It is generally recognized that exposure to these products from external sources or from inflammatory cells has a role in the pathogenesis of COPD.

Exposure of rats to hyperoxic conditions where ROS would be expected to predominate induces mild emphysema [69]. This effect seems to be because of an alteration in the protease–antiprotease balance as protease inhibitors prevent collagen degradation in hyperoxic conditions [70]. The mechanism for this alteration is caused by inactivation of α_1-antitrypsin. Hydrogen peroxide directly oxidizes the methionine residues 351 and 358 of α_1-antitrypsin, which then loses the ability to inhibit neutrophil elastase [71].

RNS also damage the lung. The most direct evidence of this is that exposure of rats and hamsters to nitrogen dioxide causes bronchial inflammation and emphysema [72,73]. In hamsters, focal areas of pigmented macrophages mark the areas of pathological alteration [72]. Occupational exposure to nitrogen dioxide has also been implicated in lung function decline [74].

The macrophage produces the ROS superoxide through the action of a multicomponent enzyme complex of nicotinamide adenine dinucleotide phosphate (NADPH). The assembly of both cytoplasmic and membrane-bound components is necessary for activation, and is primarily designed to produce toxic oxygen products for destruction of phagocytosed pathogens [75]. Superoxide is then converted to hydrogen peroxide through the action of myeloperoxidase in immature monocytes, or through other means including superoxide dismutase in mature alveolar macrophages [76,77]. It may be significant that mature macrophages, while lacking myeloperoxidase, engulfs this enzyme from the environment. This engulfed enzyme retains its activity for several hours, and its presence may be necessary for macrophages to inactivate α_1-antitrypsin [78,79]. Although oxidative enzymes are primarily designed for use in the internalized surface membrane, which becomes the phagosome, these species are highly toxic to cell membranes, and inactivate α_1-antitrypsin [71]. Iron is also present in the cell surface of macrophages, and can be sequestered by macrophages [80]. Iron is increased in the lower respiratory tract of smokers with and without COPD [81]. This is significant because the interaction of iron with ROS is important in the generation of hydroxyl radicals through the Fenton reaction [82].

There is specific evidence that the production of ROS is augmented in smokers and patients with COPD. In a study by Baughman *et al.* [83], alveolar macrophages from 21 of 24 smokers, but none of six non-smokers, spontaneously released hydrogen peroxide. In addition, exhaled breath condensate of asymptomatic cigarette smokers contains five times the amount of hydrogen peroxide than non-smokers, the major source of which is presumed to be alveolar macrophages [84]. These amounts are also signi-

ficantly increased during COPD exacerbations. Alveolar macrophages of young and elderly smokers, in comparison to age-matched non-smokers, have increased production of superoxide, and the older smokers have decreased anti-oxidant enzyme activity [85,86]. Phorbol myristate acetate (PMA) or platelet-activating factor (PAF) stimulated super-oxide production is also increased in alveolar macrophages from tobacco smokers [87].

Macrophage/monocytes from animal models and from humans also are stimulated to release ROS in response to tobacco. Components of tobacco smoke increase rat alveolar macrophage oxygen consumption and superoxide release [88]. Lavaged cells, which are mainly macrophages, from rats exposed to cigarette smoke also have enhanced phagocytic-induced superoxide production [89]. Isolated human precursors of alveolar macrophages and peripheral blood monocytes increase superoxide production in response to tobacco smoke [90]. Enhanced oxidant production is not a uniform finding in smoke-exposed animal models. Chronic tobacco smoke exposure inhibits unstimulated oxidant production while causing emphysema in a mouse model [91].

There is evidence that RNS are increased in patients with COPD. Nitrogen dioxide is clearly harmful to the lung. It is produced from nitric oxide through an intermediate, nitrite, by the action of peroxidases, including myeloperoxidase [92]. For the most part, exhaled nitric oxide has been shown to be increased and may also correlate with FEV_1 decline in patients with COPD [93–95]. However, there are some studies that contest this finding [96]. This may be because of consumption of the nitric oxide by reaction with local substrate prior to exhalation [97].

It is less well established whether macrophages participate in the production of RNS in humans. Some authors have argued that neutrophils are the source, as neutrophilia in sputum appears to correlate with exhaled nitric oxide levels [95]. Furthermore, human alveolar macrophage nitric oxide synthesis appears to be less than that of lower animals *in vitro* [98]. However, macrophages in patients with COPD contain inducible nitric oxide synthase, which could be responsible for the increased levels seen in exhaled breath or indirectly determined in lung tissue [97,99].

Cytokines

Chemotactic cytokines that have a role in increasing the macrophage burden in the lung have already been discussed. This section discusses cytokines produced by macrophages that are important in the pathogenesis of COPD through other mechanisms (Table 20.2).

A number of different cytokines are increased in lavage fluids, sputum samples or tissue samples from patients with COPD. Sputum samples from patients with COPD have

Table 20.2 Macrophage cytokines.

Macrophage/monocyte mediators in COPD	
Mediator	**Function in COPD**
Tumor necrosis factor-α	↑ MMP, ↑ oxidant burst, ↑ cytokine release, ↑ monocyte chemotactic activity
Interleukin-1β	↑ Neutrophil degranulation, ↑ MMP, ↑ TIMP, ↑ cytokine release
Interleukin-4	↓ TNF-α induced apoptosis
Interleukin-6	↑ Correlates with COPD exacerbations
Interleukin-8	Major neutrophil chemotactic factor, ↑ neutrophil degranulation, ↑ respiratory burst, ↑ LTB4
Monocyte chemotactic protein-1	↑ Monocyte chemotaxis

MMP, matrix metalloproteinases; LTB4, leukotriene B_4; TIMP, tissue inhibitor of metalloproteinase; TNF-α, tumour necrosis factor α.

increased levels of TNF-α, IL-1β, IL-6, IL-8, growth-related oncogene-α (GROα) and monocyte chemoattractant protein-1 (MCP-1) [35,36]. Bronchoalveolar lavage has also revealed elevated levels of these cytokines in smokers, or patients with COPD [100–102]. Current smokers with emphysema by high-resolution CAT scan have three times the IL-8 BAL levels of smokers without these changes [103]. Furthermore, sputum levels of IL-6 and IL-8 correlate with the number of exacerbations in COPD patients [104], and sputum IL-6 levels are increased during exacerbations [104]. Sputum IL-8 and TNF-α levels are also increased in exacerbations associated with bacterial infections [105].

There is both *in vitro* and *in vivo* evidence that activated macrophages contribute to the burden of inflammatory mediators in COPD. Peripheral lung tissue of patients with COPD shows MCP-1 and IL-8 are expressed in macrophages as well as other cells [37].

The physiological role of these cytokines in the pathogenesis of COPD is apparent from their biological activity in overexpression mouse models or their behaviour *in vitro*. For example, stimulation of neutrophil chemotaxin release from lung cells by infectious agents known to be associated with COPD exacerbations provides a presumptive role for this chemotaxin in exacerbations of COPD.

TNF-α, originally described as a mediator of haemor-rhagic tumour necrosis in mice injected with BCG and endotoxin [106], is a major proinflammatory cytokine that is clearly important in the pathogenesis of COPD. TNF-α release is increased in macrophages exposed to a variety of stimuli, including bacterial cell wall components [107]. It enhances macrophage and neutrophil oxidant burst, matrix metalloprotease production and stimulation of cytokine release from macrophages [108–110]. Arguing against the role of TNF in the pathogenesis of COPD is the finding that alveolar macrophage TNF-α release appears to be inhibited in smokers or with acute exposure to cigarette smoke [111–113]. However, cigarette smoke exposure enhances whole lung TNF-α levels and alveolar macrophage TNF-α secretion in animal models, which is dependent on MMP-12 [65]. Also, overexpression of TNF-α in mouse lungs causes chronic inflammation and emphysema-like pathology and decreased elastic recoil [114]. Further evidence that TNF-α is, in fact, important in smoke-induced lung destruction comes from a TNF-α receptor knockout mouse model. These mice have no cytokine response and no increase in lavage neutrophil or macrophage counts or markers of elastolysis when exposed to cigarette smoke compared with controls, which have both a cytokine response and evidence of elastin degradation [115]. The TNF-α receptor knockout mice also have markedly reduced emphysema in response to intratracheal pancreatic elastase [116].

IL-1β also is a potent mediator of inflammation, partly through stimulation of release of cytokines from macrophages [117]. Alveolar macrophages release this cytokine in response to a variety of stimuli including bacterial cell wall components, although this effect is less than that of its monocyte precursors [118]. Chronic smoking stimulates IL-1β release from alveolar macrophages in some, but not all studies [119–123]. IL-1β stimulates release of MMP-9 and TIMP-1 from alveolar macrophages [62]. The most convincing evidence that IL-1β is involved in the pathogenesis of lung destruction that occurs in COPD is the fact that knockout of the IL-1 receptor in mice prevents emphysema induced by intratracheal administration of pancreatic elastase [116].

IL-8 has been described as the major neutrophil chemotactic factor in the lung [124]. Its release from macrophages is stimulated by numerous stimuli, including bacterial agents [125]. A major source of this chemokine is the macrophage, and one of its original names was 'monocyte-derived neutrophil chemotactic factor'. Although it is a potent chemokine, it is also a potent proinflammatory cytokine. It stimulates numerous activities of neutrophils including degranulation and respiratory burst [126,127]. It also stimulates release of the lipid mediator and neutrophil chemotaxin leukotriene B_4 (LTB4) from neutrophils [128]. Although BALF levels of IL-8 have been reported to be elevated in smokers, spontaneous or lipopolysaccharide (LPS)-induced secretion from alveolar macrophages may be lower in smokers [129]. There are several reasons why it is presumed that much of the neutrophil accumulation in COPD is a result of IL-8. Most of the neutrophil chemotactic activity in sputum from COPD patients is neutralized by IL-8 antibody [130]. Inhibition of IL-8 induction by macrophages in cigarette smoke exposed animals prevents neutrophil accumulation in the airways [131]. Finally, many forms of neutrophilic lung inflammation are inhibited by neutralizing antibody to IL-8 or animal homologues [132–134].

Conclusions

The macrophage, once thought to be an innocent bystander in the pathophysiology of COPD, is now accepted as a central figure in this disorder. It produces enzymes, which degrade lung tissue components *in vitro*. It produces numerous modulators of the inflammatory response, both by recruiting additional cells of the immune system, and by amplifying these cells' activity. *In vivo* studies using genetic knockouts have presented clear and convincing evidence that these macrophage products are important in the pathogenesis of COPD. Perhaps because they are not directly targeted at pathophysiological causes of COPD, current therapies have not yet demonstrated the ability to change the natural history of this disorder. Future therapies, which will likely be directly aimed at modulating the function of the lung macrophage or its products, may finally achieve this goal.

References

1 Thomas ED, Ramberg RE, Sale GE, Sparkes RS, Golde DW. Direct evidence for a bone marrow origin of the alveolar macrophage in man. *Science* 1976;**192**:1016–8.

2 van oud Alblas AB, van Furth R. Origin, kinetics, and characteristics of pulmonary macrophages in the normal steady state. *J Exp Med* 1979;**149**:1504–18.

3 Golde DW, Finley TN, Cline MJ. The pulmonary macrophage in acute leukemia. *N Engl J Med* 1974;**290**:875–8.

4 Bitterman PB, Saltzman LE, Adelberg S, Ferrans VJ, Crystal RG. Alveolar macrophage replication: one mechanism for the expansion of the mononuclear phagocyte population in the chronically inflamed lung. *J Clin Invest* 1984;**74**:460–9.

5 Hoffman R. *Hematology, Basic Principles and Practice*. Philadelphia: Churchill Livingstone, 1999.

6 Holian A, Scheule RK. Alveolar macrophage biology. *Hosp Pract* 1990;**25**:53–62.

7 Holt PG, Schon-Hegrad MA, Phillips MJ, McMenamin PG. Ia-positive dendritic cells form a tightly meshed network within the human airway epithelium. *Clin Exp Allergy* 1989;**19**:597–601.

8 Hance AJ. Pulmonary immune cells in health and disease: dendritic cells and Langerhans' cells. *Eur Respir J* 1993;**6**: 1213–20.

9 Welsh DA, Mason CM. Host defense in respiratory infections. *Med Clin North Am* 2001;**85**:1329.

10 Warner AE, Brain JD. The cell biology and pathogenic role of pulmonary intravascular macrophages. *Am J Physiol* 1990;**258**:L1.

11 Kelly CA, Ward C, Stenton SC, Hendrick DJ, Walters EH. Assessment of pulmonary macrophage and neutrophil function in sequential bronchoalveolar lavage aspirates in sarcoidosis. *Thorax* 1988;**43**:787–91.

12 Lehnert BE, Morrow PE. Size, adherence, and phagocytic characteristics of alveolar macrophages harvested 'early' and 'later' during bronchoalveolar lavage. *J Immunol Methods* 1984;**73**:329–35.

13 Fraser RG. *Diagnosis of Diseases of the Chest*. Philadelphia: WB Saunders, 1990.

14 van Oud Alblas BA, van der Linden-Schrever B, van Furth R. Origin and kinetics of pulmonary macrophages during an inflammatory reaction induced by intravenous administration of heat-killed bacillus Calmette–Guérin. *J Exp Med* 1981;**154**:235–52.

15 van Oud Alblas AB, van der Linden-Schrever B, van Furth R. Origin and kinetics of pulmonary macrophages during an inflammatory reaction induced by intra-alveolar administration of aerosolized heat-killed BCG. *Am Rev Respir Dis* 1983;**128**:276–81.

16 van Furth R, Diesselhoff-den Dulk MC, Mattie H. Quantitative study on the production and kinetics of mononuclear phagocytes during an acute inflammatory reaction. *J Exp Med* 1973;**138**:1314–30.

17 Lin HS, Kuhn C III, Chen DM. Effects of hydrocortisone acetate on pulmonary alveolar macrophage colony-forming cells. *Am Rev Respir Dis* 1982;**125**:712–5.

18 Tarling JD, Coggle JE. Evidence for the pulmonary origin of alveolar macrophages. *Cell Tissue Kinet* 1982;**15**:577–84.

19 Coggle JE, Tarling JD. The proliferation kinetics of pulmonary alveolar macrophages. *J Leukoc Biol* 1984;**35**:317–27.

20 Reynolds HY, Newball HH. Analysis of proteins and respiratory cells obtained from human lungs by bronchial lavage. *J Lab Clin Med* 1974;**84**:559–73.

21 Adamson IY, Bowden DH. Role of monocytes and interstitial cells in the generation of alveolar macrophages. II. Kinetic studies after carbon loading. *Lab Invest* 1980;**42**:518–24.

22 Saltini C, Hance AJ, Ferrans VJ *et al.* Accurate quantification of cells recovered by bronchoalveolar lavage. *Am Rev Respir Dis* 1984;**130**:650–8.

23 Fathi M, Johansson A, Lundborg M *et al.* Functional and morphological differences between human alveolar and interstitial macrophages. *Exp Mol Pathol* 2001;**70**:77–82.

24 Crowell RE, Heaphy E, Valdez YE, Mold C, Lehnert BE. Alveolar and interstitial macrophage populations in the murine lung. *Exp Lung Res* 1992;**18**:435–46.

25 Prokhorova S, Lavnikova N, Laskin DL. Functional characterization of interstitial macrophages and subpopulations of alveolar macrophages from rat lung. *J Leukoc Biol* 1994; **55**:141–6.

26 Franke-Ullmann G, Pfortner C, Walter P *et al*. Characterization of murine lung interstitial macrophages in comparison with alveolar macrophages *in vitro*. *J Immunol* 1996;**157**: 3097–104.

27 Masten BJ, Yates JL, Pollard Koga AM, Lipscomb MF. Characterization of accessory molecules in murine lung dendritic cell function: roles for CD80, CD86, CD54, and CD40L. *Am J Respir Cell Mol Biol* 1997;**16**:335–42.

28 Merchant RK, Schwartz DA, Helmers RA, Dayton CS, Hunninghake GW. Bronchoalveolar lavage cellularity: the distribution in normal volunteers. *Am Rev Respir Dis* 1992; **146**:448–53.

29 Thompson AB, Daughton D, Robbins RA *et al*. Intraluminal airway inflammation in chronic bronchitis: characterization and correlation with clinical parameters. *Am Rev Respir Dis* 1989;**140**:1527–37.

30 Saetta M, Di Stefano A, Maestrelli P *et al*. Activated T-lymphocytes and macrophages in bronchial mucosa of subjects with chronic bronchitis. *Am Rev Respir Dis* 1993; **147**:301–6.

31 Domagala-Kulawik J, Maskey-Warzechowska M, Kraszewska I, Chazan R. The cellular composition and macrophage phenotype in induced sputum in smokers and ex-smokers with COPD. *Chest* 2003;**123**:1054–9.

32 Kelley J. Cytokines of the lung. *Am Rev Respir Dis* 1990; **141**:765–88.

33 Koyama S, Rennard SI, Daughton D, Shoji S, Robbins RA. Bronchoalveolar lavage fluid obtained from smokers exhibits increased monocyte chemokinetic activity. *J Appl Physiol* 1991;**70**:1208–14.

34 Hoogsteden HC, van Hal PT, Wijkhuijs JM *et al*. Expression of the CD11/CD18 cell surface adhesion glycoprotein family on alveolar macrophages in smokers and non-smokers. *Chest* 1991;**100**:1567–71.

35 Keatings VM, Collins PD, Scott DM, Barnes PJ. Differences in interleukin-8 and tumor necrosis factor-alpha in induced sputum from patients with chronic obstructive pulmonary disease or asthma. *Am J Respir Crit Care Med* 1996;**153**:530–4.

36 Traves SL, Culpitt SV, Russell RE, Barnes PJ, Donnelly LE. Increased levels of the chemokines GROα and MCP-1 in sputum samples from patients with COPD. *Thorax* 2002;**57**: 590–5.

37 de Boer WI, Sont JK, van Schadewijk A *et al*. Monocyte chemoattractant protein 1, interleukin 8, and chronic airways inflammation in COPD. *J Pathol* 2000;**190**:619–26.

38 de Boer WI, van Schadewijk A, Sont JK *et al*. Transforming growth factor β1 and recruitment of macrophages and mast cells in airways in chronic obstructive pulmonary disease. *Am J Respir Crit Care Med* 1998;**158**:1951–7.

39 Sato E, Koyama S, Takamizawa A *et al*. Smoke extract stimulates lung fibroblasts to release neutrophil and monocyte chemotactic activities. *Am J Physiol* 1999;**277**(6 Pt 1): L1149–57.

40 Koyama S, Rennard SI, Leikauf GD, Robbins RA. Bronchial epithelial cells release monocyte chemotactic activity in response to smoke and endotoxin. *J Immunol* 1991;**147**: 972–9.

41 Laskin DL, Soltys RA, Berg RA, Riley DJ. Activation of alveolar macrophages by native and synthetic collagen-like polypeptides. *Am J Respir Cell Mol Biol* 1994;**10**:58–64.

42 Hunninghake GW, Davidson JM, Rennard S *et al*. Elastin fragments attract macrophage precursors to diseased sites in pulmonary emphysema. *Science* 1981;**212**:925–7.

43 Tomita K, Caramori G, Lim S *et al*. Increased p21(CIP1/WAF1) and B cell lymphoma leukemia-x(L) expression and reduced apoptosis in alveolar macrophages from smokers. *Am J Respir Crit Care Med* 2002;**166**:724–31.

44 Brodbeck WG, Shive MS, Colton E, Ziats NP, Anderson JM. Interleukin-4 inhibits tumor necrosis factor-α-induced and spontaneous apoptosis of biomaterial-adherent macrophages. *J Lab Clin Med* 2002;**139**:90–100.

45 Bucala R. Signal transduction: a most interesting factor. *Nature* 2000;**408**:146–7.

46 Snider GL. Emphysema: the first two centuries – and beyond. A historical overview, with suggestions for future research: Part 2. *Am Rev Respir Dis* 1992;**146**:1615–22.

47 Karlinsky JB, Snider GL. Animal models of emphysema. *Am Rev Respir Dis* 1978;**117**:1109–33.

48 Shapiro SD. The pathogenesis of emphysema: the elastase–antielastase hypothesis 30 years later. *Proc Assoc Am Physicians* 1995;**107**:346.

49 Osman M, Keller S, Hosannah Y *et al*. Impairment of elastin resynthesis in the lungs of hamsters with experimental emphysema induced by sequential administration of elastase and trypsin. *J Lab Clin Med* 1985;**105**:254–8.

50 Stone PJ, Calore JD, Snider GL, Franzblau C. The dose-dependent fate of enzymatically active and inactivated tritiated methylated pancreatic elastase administered intratracheally in the hamster. *Am Rev Respir Dis* 1979;**120**: 577–87.

51 Laurell CB. The electrophoretic α_1-globulin pattern of serum in α_1-antitrypsin deficiency. *Scand J Clin Lab Invest* 1963;**15**: 132–40.

52 The α_1-Antitrypsin Deficiency Registry Study Group. Survival and *FEV*$_1$ decline in individuals with severe deficiency of α_1-antitrypsin. *Am J Respir Crit Care Med* 1998;**158**:49–59.

53 Kadoglou NP, Liapis CD. Matrix metalloproteinases: contribution to pathogenesis, diagnosis, surveillance and treatment of abdominal aortic aneurysms. *Curr Med Res Opin* 2004;**20**:419–32.

54 Werb Z, Gordon S. Secretion of a specific collagenase by stimulated macrophages. *J Exp Med* 1975;**142**:346–60.

55 Banda MJ, Werb Z. Mouse macrophage elastase: purification and characterization as a metalloproteinase. *Biochem J* 1981;**193**:589–605.

56 Shapiro SD, Kobayashi DK, Ley TJ. Cloning and characterization of a unique elastolytic metalloproteinase produced by human alveolar macrophages. *J Biol Chem* 1993;**268**: 23824–9.

57 Hautamaki RD, Kobayashi DK, Senior RM, Shapiro SD. Requirement for macrophage elastase for cigarette smoke-induced emphysema in mice. *Science* 1997;**277**:2002–4.

58 Russell RE, Thorley A, Culpitt SV *et al*. Alveolar macrophage-mediated elastolysis: roles of matrix metalloproteinases, cysteine, and serine proteases. *Am J Physiol Lung Cell Mol Physiol* 2002;**283**:L867–73.

59 Finlay GA, O'Driscoll LR, Russell KJ *et al.* Matrix metalloproteinase expression and production by alveolar macrophages in emphysema. *Am J Respir Crit Care Med* 1997;**156**:240–7.

60 Zheng T, Zhu Z, Wang Z *et al.* Inducible targeting of IL-13 to the adult lung causes matrix metalloproteinase- and cathepsin-dependent emphysema. *J Clin Invest* 2000;**106**:1081–93.

61 Lanone S, Zheng T, Zhu Z *et al.* Overlapping and enzyme-specific contributions of matrix metalloproteinases-9 and -12 in IL-13-induced inflammation and remodeling. *J Clin Invest* 2002;**110**:463–74.

62 Russell RE, Culpitt SV, DeMatos C *et al.* Release and activity of matrix metalloproteinase-9 and tissue inhibitor of metalloproteinase-1 by alveolar macrophages from patients with chronic obstructive pulmonary disease. *Am J Respir Cell Mol Biol* 2002;**26**:602–9.

63 Morris DG, Huang X, Kaminski N *et al.* Loss of integrin α(v)β6-mediated TGF-β activation causes MMP12-dependent emphysema. *Nature* 2003;**422**:169–73.

64 Senior RM, Griffin GL, Mecham RP. Chemotactic activity of elastin-derived peptides. *J Clin Invest* 1980;**66**:859–62.

65 Churg A, Wang RD, Tai H *et al.* Macrophage metalloelastase mediates acute cigarette smoke-induced inflammation via tumor necrosis factor-α release. *Am J Respir Crit Care Med* 2003;**167**:1083–9.

66 Pryor WA, Prier DG, Church DF. Electron-spin resonance study of mainstream and sidestream cigarette smoke: nature of the free radicals in gas-phase smoke and in cigarette tar. *Environ Health Perspect* 1983;**47**:345–55.

67 Iles KE, Forman HJ. Macrophage signaling and respiratory burst. *Immunol Res* 2002;**26**:95–105.

68 Wang JF, Komarov P, de Groot H. Luminol chemiluminescence in rat macrophages and granulocytes: the role of NO, O_2^-/H_2O_2, and HOCl. *Arch Biochem Biophys* 1993;**304**:189–96.

69 Riley DJ, Kerr JS. Oxidant injury of the extracellular matrix: potential role in the pathogenesis of pulmonary emphysema. *Lung* 1985;**163**:1–13.

70 Kerr JS, Chae CU, Nagase H, Berg RA, Riley DJ. Degradation of collagen in lung tissue slices exposed to hyperoxia. *Am Rev Respir Dis* 1987;**135**:1334–9.

71 Taggart C, Cervantes-Laurean D, Kim G *et al.* Oxidation of either methionine 351 or methionine 358 in α$_1$-antitrypsin causes loss of antineutrophil elastase activity. *J Biol Chem* 2000;**275**:27258–65.

72 Kleinerman J. Some effects of nitrogen dioxide on the lung. *Fed Proc* 1977;**36**:1714–8.

73 Blank J, Glasgow JE, Pietra GG, Burdette L, Weinbaum G. Nitrogen-dioxide-induced emphysema in rats: lack of worsening by β-aminopropionitrile treatment. *Am Rev Respir Dis* 1988;**137**:376–9.

74 Johns R. Chronic occupational exposure to nitrogen dioxide is associated with decline in lung function. *Thorax* 2004;**59**:420.

75 Yagisawa M, Yuo A, Yonemaru M *et al.* Superoxide release and NADPH oxidase components in mature human phago-cytes: correlation between functional capacity and amount of functional proteins. *Biochem Biophys Res Commun* 1996;**228**:510–6.

76 Weissler JC, Lipscomb MF, Lem VM, Toews GB. Tumor killing by human alveolar macrophages and blood monocytes: decreased cytotoxicity of human alveolar macrophages. *Am Rev Respir Dis* 1986;**134**:532–7.

77 Fridovich I. The biology of oxygen radicals. *Science* 1978;**201**:875–80.

78 Shepherd VL, Hoidal JR. Clearance of neutrophil-derived myeloperoxidase by the macrophage mannose receptor. *Am J Respir Cell Mol Biol* 1990;**2**:335–40.

79 Wallaert B, Gressier B, Aerts C *et al.* Oxidative inactivation of α$_1$-proteinase inhibitor by alveolar macrophages from healthy smokers requires the presence of myeloperoxidase. *Am J Respir Cell Mol Biol* 1991;**5**:437–44.

80 Olakanmi O, McGowan SE, Hayek MB, Britigan BE. Iron sequestration by macrophages decreases the potential for extracellular hydroxyl radical formation. *J Clin Invest* 1993;**91**:889–99.

81 Thompson AB, Bohling T, Heires A, Linder J, Rennard SI. Lower respiratory tract iron burden is increased in association with cigarette smoking. *J Lab Clin Med* 1991;**117**:493–9.

82 Rojanasakul Y, Wang L, Hoffman AH *et al.* Mechanisms of hydroxyl free radical-induced cellular injury and calcium overloading in alveolar macrophages. *Am J Respir Cell Mol Biol* 1993;**8**:377–83.

83 Baughman RP, Corser BC, Strohofer S, Hendricks D. Spontaneous hydrogen peroxide release from alveolar macrophages of some cigarette smokers. *J Lab Clin Med* 1986;**107**:233–7.

84 Nowak D, Antczak A, Krol M *et al.* Increased content of hydrogen peroxide in the expired breath of cigarette smokers. *Eur Respir J* 1996;**9**:652–7.

85 Hoidal JR, Fox RB, LeMarbe PA, Perri R, Repine JE. Altered oxidative metabolic responses *in vitro* of alveolar macrophages from asymptomatic cigarette smokers. *Am Rev Respir Dis* 1981;**123**:85–9.

86 Kondo T, Tagami S, Yoshioka A, Nishimura M, Kawakami Y. Current smoking of elderly men reduces antioxidants in alveolar macrophages. *Am J Respir Crit Care Med* 1994;**149**:178–82.

87 Sherman MP, Campbell LA, Gong H Jr, Roth MD, Tashkin DP. Antimicrobial and respiratory burst characteristics of pulmonary alveolar macrophages recovered from smokers of marijuana alone, smokers of tobacco alone, smokers of marijuana and tobacco, and non-smokers. *Am Rev Respir Dis* 1991;**144**:1351–6.

88 Drath DB, Shorey JM, Huber GL. Functional and metabolic properties of alveolar macrophages in response to the gas phase of tobacco smoke. *Infect Immun* 1981;**34**:11–5.

89 Gairola CG. Cadmium-enriched cigarette smoke-induced cytological and biochemical alterations in rat lungs. *J Toxicol Environ Health* 1989;**27**:317–29.

90 Pinot F, Bachelet M, Francois D, Polla BS, Walti H. Modified natural porcine surfactant modulates tobacco smoke-induced stress response in human monocytes. *Life Sci* 1999;**64**:125–34.

91 March TH, Barr EB, Finch GL, Nikula KJ, Seagrave JC. Effects of concurrent ozone exposure on the pathogenesis of cigarette smoke-induced emphysema in B6C3F1 mice. *Inhal Toxicol* 2002;**14**:1187–213.

92 Eiserich JP, Hristova M, Cross CE *et al.* Formation of nitric oxide-derived inflammatory oxidants by myeloperoxidase in neutrophils. *Nature* 1998;**391**:393–7.

93 Paredi P, Kharitonov SA, Leak D *et al.* Exhaled ethane, a marker of lipid peroxidation, is elevated in chronic obstructive pulmonary disease. *Am J Respir Crit Care Med* 2000;**162**(2 Pt 1):369–73.

94 Ansarin K, Chatkin JM, Ferreira IM *et al.* Exhaled nitric oxide in chronic obstructive pulmonary disease: relationship to pulmonary function. *Eur Respir J* 2001;**17**:934–8.

95 Silkoff PE, Martin D, Pak J, Westcott JY, Martin RJ. Exhaled nitric oxide correlated with induced sputum findings in COPD. *Chest* 2001;**119**:1049–55.

96 Rutgers SR, van der Mark TW, Coers W *et al.* Markers of nitric oxide metabolism in sputum and exhaled air are not increased in chronic obstructive pulmonary disease. *Thorax* 1999;**54**:576–80.

97 Ichinose M, Sugiura H, Yamagata S, Koarai A, Shirato K. Increase in reactive nitrogen species production in chronic obstructive pulmonary disease airways. *Am J Respir Crit Care Med* 2000;**162**(2 Pt 1):701–6.

98 Muijsers RB, ten Hacken NH, Van Ark I *et al.* L-Arginine is not the limiting factor for nitric oxide synthesis by human alveolar macrophages *in vitro. Eur Respir J* 2001;**18**:667–71.

99 van Straaten JF, Postma DS, Coers W *et al.* Macrophages in lung tissue from patients with pulmonary emphysema express both inducible and endothelial nitric oxide synthase. *Mod Pathol* 1998;**11**:648–55.

100 Soler N, Ewig S, Torres A *et al.* Airway inflammation and bronchial microbial patterns in patients with stable chronic obstructive pulmonary disease. *Eur Respir J* 1999;**14**:1015–22.

101 Kuschner WG, D'Alessandro A, Wong H, Blanc PD. Dose-dependent cigarette smoking-related inflammatory responses in healthy adults. *Eur Respir J* 1996;**9**:1989–94.

102 Riise GC, Ahlstedt S, Larsson S *et al.* Bronchial inflammation in chronic bronchitis assessed by measurement of cell products in bronchial lavage fluid. *Thorax* 1995;**50**:360–5.

103 Tanino M, Betsuyaku T, Takeyabu K *et al.* Increased levels of interleukin-8 in BAL fluid from smokers susceptible to pulmonary emphysema. *Thorax* 2002;**57**:405–11.

104 Bhowmik A, Seemungal TA, Sapsford RJ, Wedzicha JA. Relation of sputum inflammatory markers to symptoms and lung function changes in COPD exacerbations. *Thorax* 2000;**55**:114–20.

105 Sethi S, Muscarella K, Evans N *et al.* Airway inflammation and etiology of acute exacerbations of chronic bronchitis. *Chest* 2000;**118**:1557–65.

106 Carswell EA, Old LJ, Kassel RL *et al.* An endotoxin-induced serum factor that causes necrosis of tumors. *Proc Natl Acad Sci U S A* 1975;**72**:3666–70.

107 Rich EA, Panuska JR, Wallis RS *et al.* Dyscoordinate expression of tumor necrosis factor-α by human blood monocytes and alveolar macrophages. *Am Rev Respir Dis* 1989;**139**:1010–6.

108 Nelson S, Summer WR. Innate immunity, cytokines, and pulmonary host defense. *Infect Dis Clin North Am* 1998;**12**:555–67, vii.

109 Mayer AM, Pittner RA, Lipscomb GE, Spitzer JA. Effect of *in vivo* TNF administration on superoxide production and PKC activity of rat alveolar macrophages. *Am J Physiol* 1993;**264**(1 Pt 1):L43–52.

110 Bajaj MS, Kew RR, Webster RO, Hyers TM. Priming of human neutrophil functions by tumor necrosis factor: enhancement of superoxide anion generation, degranulation, and chemotaxis to chemoattractants C5a and F-Met-Leu-Phe. *Inflammation* 1992;**16**:241–50.

111 Dandrea T, Tu B, Blomberg A *et al.* Differential inhibition of inflammatory cytokine release from cultured alveolar macrophages from smokers and non-smokers by NO$_2$. *Hum Exp Toxicol* 1997;**16**:577–88.

112 McCrea KA, Ensor JE, Nall K, Bleecker ER, Hasday JD. Altered cytokine regulation in the lungs of cigarette smokers. *Am J Respir Crit Care Med* 1994;**150**:696–703.

113 Dubar V, Gosset P, Aerts C *et al. In vitro* acute effects of tobacco smoke on tumor necrosis factor α and interleukin-6 production by alveolar macrophages. *Exp Lung Res* 1993;**19**:345–59.

114 Fujita M, Shannon JM, Irvin CG *et al.* Overexpression of tumor necrosis factor-α produces an increase in lung volumes and pulmonary hypertension. *Am J Physiol Lung Cell Mol Physiol* 2001;**280**:L39–49.

115 Churg A, Dai J, Tai H, Xie C, Wright JL. Tumor necrosis factor-α is central to acute cigarette smoke-induced inflammation and connective tissue breakdown. *Am J Respir Crit Care Med* 2002;**166**:849–54.

116 Lucey EC, Keane J, Kuang PP, Snider GL, Goldstein RH. Severity of elastase-induced emphysema is decreased in tumor necrosis factor-α and interleukin-1β receptor-deficient mice. *Lab Invest* 2002;**82**:79–85.

117 Terui T, Kato T, Suzuki R, Kumagai K, Tagami H. Effect of interleukin 1 on chemotaxis and chemiluminescence of human neutrophils. *Tohoku J Exp Med* 1986;**149**:317–22.

118 Bernaudin JF, Yamauchi K, Wewers MD *et al.* Demonstration by *in situ* hybridization of dissimilar IL-1β gene expression in human alveolar macrophages and blood monocytes in response to lipopolysaccharide. *J Immunol* 1988;**140**:3822–9.

119 Morimoto Y, Tsuda T, Hori H *et al.* Combined effect of cigarette smoke and mineral fibers on the gene expression of cytokine mRNA. *Environ Health Perspect* 1999;**107**:495–500.

120 Renoux M, Lemarie E, Renoux G. Interleukin-1 secretion by lipopolysaccharide-stimulated alveolar macrophages: relationships to cell numbers – influence of smoking habits. *Respiration* 1989;**55**:158–68.

121 Nagai S, Takeuchi M, Watanabe K, Aung H, Izumi T. Smoking and interleukin-1 activity released from human alveolar macrophages in healthy subjects. *Chest* 1988;**94**:694–700.

122 Brown GP, Iwamoto GK, Monick MM, Hunninghake GW. Cigarette smoking decreases interleukin 1 release by human alveolar macrophages. *Am J Physiol* 1989;**256**(2 Pt 1): C260–4.

123 Mikuniya T, Nagai S, Tsutsumi T *et al.* Proinflammatory or regulatory cytokines released from BALF macrophages of healthy smokers. *Respiration* 1999;**66**:419–26.

124 Kunkel SL, Standiford T, Kasahara K, Strieter RM. Interleukin-8 (IL-8): the major neutrophil chemotactic factor in the lung. *Exp Lung Res* 1991;**17**:17–23.

125 Larsson BM, Larsson K, Malmberg P, Palmberg L. Gram positive bacteria induce IL-6 and IL-8 production in human alveolar macrophages and epithelial cells. *Inflammation* 1999;**23**:217–30.

126 Walz A, Meloni F, Clark-Lewis I, von Tscharner V, Baggiolini M. [Ca^{2+}]$_i$ changes and respiratory burst in human neutrophils and monocytes induced by NAP-1/interleukin-8, NAP-2, and gro/MGSA. *J Leukoc Biol* 1991; **50**:279–86.

127 Willems J, Joniau M, Cinque S, van Damme J. Human granulocyte chemotactic peptide (IL-8) as a specific neutrophil degranulator: comparison with other monokines. *Immunology* 1989;**67**:540–2.

128 Schroder JM. The monocyte-derived neutrophil activating peptide (NAP/interleukin 8) stimulates human neutrophil arachidonate-5-lipoxygenase, but not the release of cellular arachidonate. *J Exp Med* 1989;**170**:847–63.

129 Ohta T, Yamashita N, Maruyama M, Sugiyama E, Kobayashi M. Cigarette smoking decreases interleukin-8 secretion by human alveolar macrophages. *Respir Med* 1998;**92**:922–7.

130 Richman-Eisenstat JB, Jorens PG, Hebert CA, Ueki I, Nadel JA. Interleukin-8: an important chemoattractant in sputum of patients with chronic inflammatory airway diseases. *Am J Physiol* 1993;**264**(4 Pt 1):L413–8.

131 Nishikawa M, Kakemizu N, Ito T *et al.* Superoxide mediates cigarette smoke-induced infiltration of neutrophils into the airways through nuclear factor-κB activation and IL-8 mRNA expression in guinea pigs *in vivo. Am J Respir Cell Mol Biol* 1999;**20**:189–98.

132 Matsumoto T, Yokoi K, Mukaida N *et al.* Pivotal role of interleukin-8 in the acute respiratory distress syndrome and cerebral reperfusion injury. *J Leukoc Biol* 1997;**62**:581–7.

133 Folkesson HG, Matthay MA, Hebert CA, Broaddus VC. Acid aspiration-induced lung injury in rabbits is mediated by interleukin-8-dependent mechanisms. *J Clin Invest* 1995;**96**: 107–16.

134 Frevert CW, Huang S, Danaee H, Paulauskis JD, Kobzik L. Functional characterization of the rat chemokine KC and its importance in neutrophil recruitment in a rat model of pulmonary inflammation. *J Immunol* 1995;**154**:335–44.

CHAPTER 21
Eosinophils and COPD

Andrew J. Wardlaw

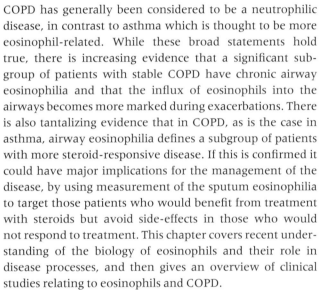

COPD has generally been considered to be a neutrophilic disease, in contrast to asthma which is thought to be more eosinophil-related. While these broad statements hold true, there is increasing evidence that a significant subgroup of patients with stable COPD have chronic airway eosinophilia and that the influx of eosinophils into the airways becomes more marked during exacerbations. There is also tantalizing evidence that in COPD, as is the case in asthma, airway eosinophilia defines a subgroup of patients with more steroid-responsive disease. If this is confirmed it could have major implications for the management of the disease, by using measurement of the sputum eosinophilia to target those patients who would benefit from treatment with steroids but avoid side-effects in those who would not respond to treatment. This chapter covers recent understanding of the biology of eosinophils and their role in disease processes, and then gives an overview of clinical studies relating to eosinophils and COPD.

Eosinophils are end-stage granulocytes which are usually present in relatively small numbers in peripheral blood and, in health, are scanty in tissues other than the intestine. Eosinophils are closely associated with helminthic parasite infections where they are considered to play in important part in host defence. In industrialized countries, the most usual cause of a peripheral blood and tissue eosinophilia is an allergic disease such as asthma, rhinitis or atopic dermatitis. There is an extensive literature detailing the, albeit circumstantial, evidence for a proinflammatory role for eosinophils in asthma and other allergic diseases [1]. This is based on three lines of evidence: the close relationship between clinical evidence of asthma and the presence of eosinophils in the bronchial mucosa; the relevance of eosinophil-derived mediators to the pathophysiology of asthma; and the intimate association between the beneficial effects of glucocorticoids in asthma and their anti-eosinophilic properties. Eosinophils are closely associated with immune responses caused by the activation of Th2

lymphocytes through the production of eosinophilic-specific growth factors such as interleukin 5 (IL-5) and the generation of IL-4 and IL-13, which promote selective trafficking of eosinophils to tissue [2]. Activation of Th2 lymphocytes is associated with specific T-cell responses to allergens, which for the most part are otherwise harmless foreign proteins derived from foods, plants, fungi, and animal and insect excreta and fur delivered to the mucosal surfaces of the gut and respiratory tract. Generally, although not invariably, these Th2-associated eosinophilic responses are associated with production of specific immunoglobulin E (IgE).

It is common practice to compare and contrast asthma and COPD (by which is meant smoking-related obstructive airways disease) as two sides of the same coin in which asthma is caused by antigen-specific Th2 responses characterized by eosinophilia, and COPD is associated with neutrophil-associated innate responses to the toxic effects of cigarette smoke complicated by Th1-associated immune responses to repeated respiratory tract infections [3]. However, just as some studies have suggested a role for the neutrophil in asthma [4], others have demonstrated the presence of eosinophils in the airways for patients with COPD [5], which has blurred the demarcation between these two conditions. This cross-over is mirrored by those patients with COPD who present with clinical and physiological features more suggestive of asthma. There is an unresolved debate as to whether such patients should be labelled as having asthma or COPD, or both. Understanding the mechanism of the eosinophilia in some patients with COPD and the extent to which this relates to the clinical and physiological presentation may shed light on this question.

Another ongoing debate in asthma that is relevant to the role of eosinophils in COPD is the extent to which this cell type has a proinflammatory as opposed to a bystander or even ameliorative function. This debate has been informed by the use of an anti-IL-5 antibody in clinical trials.

This antibody profoundly inhibited the blood and tissue eosinophilia but had no effect on the early or late phase response to allergen challenge [6]. In addition, it had no effect on symptoms or lung function in an as yet unpublished clinical study. However, the antibody had a much less marked effect on tissue eosinophils, reducing numbers by only approximately 50% so that the interpretation of the effects of this antibody have been less conclusive than originally thought [7].

In this chapter, eosinophil biology is reviewed, focusing on more recent insights relevant to airway inflammatory disease and then evidence for a potential role for eosinophils in the pathogenesis of COPD is discussed. The biology of eosinophils has been extensively reviewed over the years [8–11] and this chapter focuses on those aspects that either offer new insights into their function or are directly relevant to their role in COPD.

Eosinophil biology

Causes of eosinophilia

The normal eosinophil count, which is best expressed as total numbers rather than a percentage, is less than 0.4×10^6/mL. Moderate eosinophil counts of up to 1.5×10^6 mL are found in a number of conditions, in particular the atopic diseases of asthma, rhinitis and atopic dermatitis. A more dramatic eosinophilia is uncommon and associated with severe asthma syndromes, drug reactions, pulmonary eosinophilia and hypereosinophilic syndromes [12]. The peripheral blood eosinophil count reflects a balance between the rate of egress of eosinophils from the bone marrow (which itself depends on the rate of eosinophil production and the rate of migration through bone marrow sinus endothelium) and the rate of entry into tissues, which is dependent on signals associated with organ-specific inflammation. There is therefore an inconstant relationship between peripheral blood eosinophil count and tissue eosinophilia. Although generally speaking there is a correlation between the two measurements, it is far from uncommon for a dramatic tissue eosinophilia (e.g. in diseases such as eosinophilic oesophagitis and chronic pulmonary eosinophilia) to be associated with only a modest elevation in the eosinophil count. Similarly, in some patients with hypereosinophilic syndrome (HES), the tissue eosinophilia is not prominent. Although a raised blood eosinophil count therefore alerts the physician to a possible eosinophilic-related disease, it is the tissue eosinophilia that is usually more relevant to what is happening in disease.

It has been known for many years that in most cases where it has been studied, an eosinophilia is T-cell dependent. In the 1970s, Basten and Beeson [13] established

that T-cell depletion abrogated the eosinophilic response to parasite infection. It was subsequently shown that T-cell-derived supernatants contained growth factors for eosinophils and this led to the characterization of IL-5 and awareness of the pivotal role that this cytokine has in eosinophil development [14]. IL-5 seems to be a rate-limiting step for eosinophil production in that administration of IL-5 either exogenously or through transgenic manipulation in mice results in a marked eosinophilia [15] and anti-IL-5 in humans dramatically diminishes the peripheral blood eosinophil count [6]. Increased eosinophilopoiesis as a result of increased IL-5 synthesis appears to be a feature of a number of diseases including parasitic and allergic diseases. For example, pulmonary eosinophilia resulting from *Necator americanus* infection in mice was IL-5-dependent [16], and both the eosinophilia and host defence to filiriasis and *Trichinella spiralis* was markedly impaired in IL-5-deficient mice [17]. In asthma, IL-5 mRNA can be detected in increased amounts in the airways as well as the serum of steroid-dependent asthmatics [18,19]. However, IL-5 gene deleted mice still have a baseline eosinophilia and can develop pulmonary eosinophilia after infection with paramyxovirus, demonstrating that cytokines other than IL-5 can cause late differentiation [20]. It is therefore an accepted paradigm that a blood and tissue eosinophilia in IgE-mediated diseases such as atopic asthma and helminthic parasite infections are caused by antigen-dependent activation of Th2 cells, leading to IL-5 production and increased eosinophilopoiesis and tissue recruitment of eosinophils. The control of Th2 and Th1 cell development is beyond the scope of this chapter but the current understanding has recently been reviewed [21]. However, many eosinophilic diseases, including many cases of pulmonary eosinophilia, are not associated with atopy and IgE production and therefore do not entirely fit with the Th2-driven eosinophilic paradigm. Intrinsic asthma is generally assumed to associated with IL-5-producing T cells; however, the evidence for this is limited. One model for non-IgE-associated eosinophilic disease is those cases of eosinophilic oesophagitis caused by a defined food allergen in which there is no specific IgE [22]. In some of these cases, the patients are patch test positive to the food allergen concerned, which raises the possibility of a Th2 type IV cell-mediated immunity, but this is still unexplored.

There is increasing interest in the role of T-regulatory cells (Tr) in controlling inappropriate immune responses including those associated with Th2 cell activation. Tr were first identified as mediating some aspects of immune tolerance and were then found to have an important role in suppressing immunomediated inflammatory bowel disease in mice. This is a rapidly developing area and the exact identity of Tr is still unclear. However, three types of Tr cells have been identified: CD4+/CD25+ cells, which require direct contact to mediate their immunosuppressive effects; Tr cells producing transforming growth factor β (TGF-β); and Tr cells producing IL-10 [23–25]. Increasing understanding of the pivotal role that Tr have in controlling immune responses has led to the interesting refinement of the 'hygiene hypothesis', which suggests that the increase in allergic disease – which is also paralleled by an increase in autoimmune disease – is not caused by a Th1 to Th2 switch as a result of lack of immune stimulation in infancy but by a failure to develop Tr responses, which leads to enhancement of both Th1 and Th2 immunity [26,27]. IL-10-producing Tr are of particular interest in the context of pulmonary eosinophilia because of evidence that immunotherapy works by inducing expansion of antigen-specific IL-10 producing Tr cells [28]. In addition, regulatory T cells were able to suppress ovalbumin-induced pulmonary eosinophilia in mice [29,30].

Eosinophil morphology and receptor phenotype

Eosinophils are 8-μm end-stage non-dividing leucocytes derived from the bone marrow under the influence of granulocyte–macrophage colony-stimulating factor (GM-CSF), IL-3 and IL-5. The electron microscopic (EM) morphology of the mature eosinophil has been well described (Fig. 21.1) [31,32]. The relatively specific features that distinguish the eosinophil from other leucocytes are the bilobed nucleus, the 20 or so specific granules with their electron-dense core, the paucity of mitochondria (approximately 20 per cell) and endoplasmic reticulum, and the dense network of cytoplasmic tubulovesicular structures or secretory vesicles which contain albumin and cytochrome b558 and are

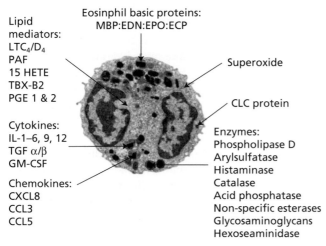

Lipid mediators:
LTC$_4$/D$_4$
PAF
15 HETE
TBX-B2
PGE 1 & 2

Cytokines:
IL-1–6, 9, 12
TGF α/β
GM-CSF

Chemokines:
CXCL8
CCL3
CCL5

Eosinphil basic proteins:
MBP:EDN:EPO:ECP

Superoxide

CLC protein

Enzymes:
Phospholipase D
Arylsulfatase
Histaminase
Catalase
Acid phosphatase
Non-specific esterases
Glycosaminoglycans
Hexoseaminidase

Figure 21.1 Electron microscope view of an eosinophil (courtesy of Ann Dewar) showing the characteristic morphology; in particular the specific granules with an electron dense core. The major mediator classes produced by the eosinophil are listed.

therefore thought to be involved in superoxide production. Eosinophils also contain approximately five lipid bodies, which are the major site of eicosanoid synthesis, primary granules and small granules. Small granules are particularly prominent in tissue eosinophils and contain arylsulphatase B, acid phosphatase and catalase. They may be derived from specific granules and act as a lysosomal compartment especially as specific granules have been shown to express lysosome-associated membrane proteins 1 and 2 (LAMP1/2) as well as lysosome integral membrane protein 1 (LIMP-1: CD63) [33]. Eosinophils also contain multilaminar bodies that contain TGF-α. Eosinophil precursors derived from cord blood can be first identified morphologically when specific core-containing granules appear, although expression of Charcot Leyden Crystal (CLC) protein and the basic granules proteins can be detected by immunohistochemistry or mRNA expression at the promyelocyte stage where they are found in the endoplasmic reticulum (ER), golgi apparatus and large round coreless granules, most of which develop into specific granules. EM can clearly distinguish activated from resting peripheral blood eosinophils by the increased number of lipid bodies, primary and small granules, secretory vesicles and endoplasmic reticulum. Cytoplasmic crystals of CLC protein may also be present. Activated eosinophils are also often less dense than resting cells although, with the advent of immunomagnetic selection rather than density gradients to purify eosinophils, density is less often used as a marker of activation [34]. Eosinophils are thought to be relatively poorly phagocytic although they can ingest opsonized zymosan, which gets taken up into phagolysosomes formed in part by fusion with specific granules. The eosinophil also degranulates onto large opsonized surfaces such as a sephadex bead or parasitic larvae in the process of 'frustrated phagocytosis'.

The ultrastructure of *in vitro* activated and tissue-infiltrating eosinophils has suggested three potential mechanisms of degranulation: necrosis or cytolytic degranulation, exocytosis or 'classical degranulation', and piecemeal degranulation [35]. Cytolytic degranulation is associated with loss of eosinophil plasma membrane integrity and results in the release of clusters of free membrane-bound granules (termed Cfegs). This is commonly observed in eosinophilic inflammation, being particularly marked in severe disease such as asthma deaths where large quantities of basic proteins can be detected in the tissue by immunohistochemistry, often with relatively few intact eosinophils [36]. This type of degranulation is also a feature of milder disease such as allergic rhinitis [37,38] as well as Fc-mediated degranulation *in vitro* [39]. Exocytosis or classic degranulation occurs in mast cells and basophils after cross-linking of IgE receptors. It describes a process whereby granules migrate to the plasma membrane and fuse with it, leading to the extrusion of membrane-free granule contents. This has been described in the gut, but not in airway mucosa. Piecemeal degranulation was described in cord blood derived eosinophils by Dvorak *et al.* [40]. This term describes the appearance of empty or partially empty granules, which retain their structure, together with small granule protein-containing vesicles in the cytoplasm which transport the granule proteins to the cell surface where they are released [41]. These appearances are common in tissue eosinophils in asthma and other allergic diseases.

Many studies have used a mouse model involving ovalbumin challenge to generate a lung eosinophilia and increased airway hyperresponsiveness (AHR). An interesting and striking feature of this model is that the lung eosinophils do not have the appearance of having undergone degranulation either by cytolysis or piecemeal degranulation [42]. Immunostaining of the mouse lung in this model locates all the basic proteins within intact eosinophils and bronchoalveolar lavage (BAL) contains no free major basic protein (MBP) [43,44]. This is quite unlike human disease where cell free basic proteins can be readily detected in both tissue and BAL. Consistent with this observation, mice in which the gene for eosinophil peroxidase (EPO) or MBP has been deleted had the same phenotype as wild type mice in this model [45]. This observation may explain, in part, the paucity of epithelial damage seen in the mouse asthma model. It also further calls into question the physiological relevance of this type of experiment as well as emphasizing the complex and poorly understood relationship between eosinophil recruitment and degranulation.

Apoptotic eosinophils are small cells with a shrunken nucleus and condensed chromatin but an intact plasma membrane [46]. They are readily identifiable in aged cell populations *in vitro* and in cells from the airway lumen such as sputum, but are more difficult to identify in tissue. This has led some investigators to argue that the majority of airway eosinophils, at least in asthma and rhinitis, are removed through lumenal entry rather than by undergoing apoptosis in tissue [35].

Like all leucocytes, eosinophils express a large number of membrane receptors which allow them to interact with the extracellular environment. These include receptors required for locomotion, activation, growth and mediator release. Most of the receptors are shared to some extent with other leucocytes but some have a degree of specificity in terms of level of expression and function. An important feature of tissue eosinophils is that they express a different pattern of receptors to peripheral blood eosinophils consistent with a more activated phenotype. This includes induction of expression of CD69, intercellular adhesion molecule-1 (ICAM-1) and FcγR1 and increased expression of HLA-DR and Mac-1. Changes in expression can be induced *in vitro* by culture with cytokines such as IL-5, but also occur to some extent as the result of transmigration

through endothelium [47]. A major difference between eosinophils and neutrophils, which has been exploited to purify eosinophils by immunomagnetic selectin, is the expression of CD16 by neutrophils but not eosinophils. Another important difference is the expression of VLA-4 by eosinophils but not to any great extent by neutrophils. Most recently, Siglec 8 has been identified as a receptor expressed only by eosinophils, mast cells and basophils [48–50]. Siglecs are sialic acid-recognizing animal lectins of the immunoglobulin superfamily. Eosinophils, as well as monocytes and a subset of dendritic cells, also express Siglec 10 [51]. In contrast, neutrophils express Siglec 9 [52]. The function of the Siglec 8 on eosinophils remains uncertain but may be involved in triggering apoptosis [53].

Eosinophil trafficking and tissue accumulation

Eosinophils are not normally found in tissues other than the gut, and the appearance of increased numbers of these cells can be a notable feature of the pathology of a number of diseases. The normal pattern of gut homing of eosinophils is mediated by eotaxin, which is constitutively expressed in the gut, and the integrin α4β7 binding to MAdCAM-1 which is selectively expressed in the intestine [54]. Although an eosinophilia can accompany a general inflammatory response, as for example in fibrosing tissue alveolitis where increased numbers of eosinophils and neutrophils can be seen in BAL fluid, it often occurs without a marked increase in other leucocytes so raising the question of the mechanism behind the specific tissue accumulation of these picturesque leucocytes. Selective eosinophil accumulation occurs as a result of the coordinated effect of a number of adhesion, chemotactic and growth/survival orientated signals at each stage in the life cycle of the cell. Generally speaking, these events are controlled by mediators released by Th2 cells, in particular the cytokines IL-4, IL-5, IL-13, possibly IL-9 and most recently IL-25. This latter cytokine appears to act through an intermediate cell type to produce IL-5 and IL-13 dependent effects [55].

Eosinophil trafficking has been extensively investigated in recent years [56–58], and will only be briefly reviewed here. As well being crucial for differentiation, IL-5 is also important in promoting emigration from the bone marrow. In particular, it acts as a priming factor for specific chemoattractants such as eotaxin [59]. Eosinophil emigration from the bone marrow in guinea pigs is inhibited by blocking anti-CD18 antibodies, but interestingly IL-5-dependent emigration is promoted by blocking anti-VLA-4 antibodies [60]. One explanation for this finding is that VLA-4/ VCAM-1 is responsible for eosinophil precursors binding to bone marrow stromal cells as has been shown for a range of cell types, although it has not been formally demonstrated in eosinophils. The interesting observation that eotaxin decreased adhesion to VCAM-1 while increasing adhesion to the CD18 ligand BSA may be a mechanism for promoting egress from the bone marrow [61]. A localized inflammatory response causing systemic effects has been demonstrated after allergen challenge in mice in which IL-5-producing cells (both T cells and non-T cells) increased in the bone marrow [62,62].

Accumulation of leucocytes in tissue is a highly regulated process with the aim of being able to respond effectively to noxious insults without causing an inappropriate inflammatory response. An obligate step in the migration of all leucocytes from the systemic circulation into tissue is their capture by endothelium as they flow at high shear rates through the postcapillary endothelium. A key receptor mediating eosinophil capture is P-selectin whose low level surface expression is selectively induced on endothelium by IL-4 and IL-13. Eosinophils express higher levels of PSGL-1 (the primary receptor for P-selectin) than other leucocytes and this results in increased avidity for P-selectin compared with neutrophils, especially at the low levels of expression induced by Th2 cytokines [64]. Increased expression of PSGL-1 leading to enhanced recruitment has also been reported in allergic disease [65]. IL-4 and IL-13 can also induce low levels of VCAM-1 expression which can bind eosinophils through VLA-4 and also capture flowing cells, albeit at lower shear stresses. VLA-4/VCAM-1 and PSGL-1/P-selectin cooperate as a major endothelial control point for selective eosinophil migration [66]. Once captured, eosinophils roll along the surface of the blood vessel until they are activated, which allows the CD18 integrins binding to ICAM-1 and ICAM-2 to non-selectively promote transmigration, although VLA-4/VCAM-1 can also exert selective pressure at this stage.

The activation step mediated by chemoattractants expressed on the endothelial surface is another potential point of eosinophil selection as shown by the effect of exogenously added chemoattractants such as eotaxin, but the identity of the endogenous chemoattractant involved and the extent to which it is selectively expressed in eosinophilic inflammation remains to be resolved [67].

The blood supply to the bronchi via the bronchial arteries is part of the high flow systemic circulation. In contrast, cell migration into the alveoli and interstitium of the lung occurs through the low-pressure pulmonary circulation including the pulmonary capillaries. In this low sheer circulation, selectins are not necessary to mediate the capture step and consistent with this neither E- or P-selectin are expressed on pulmonary capillaries, whereas P-selectin is very well expressed in the bronchial circulation [68,69]. In some inflammatory insults in mice, such as *Streptococcus pneumoniae* infection, CD18 and VLA-4 integrins are also not required for neutrophils to migrate into the alveolar bed [70].

Once the eosinophil has transmigrated through the endothelium it has to migrate through the basement membrane and into the tissue. Interestingly, in a mouse model in which CCR3, the major chemokine receptor on eosinophils, had been deleted the cells appeared to be able to migrate through the endothelium, suggesting that CCR3-binding chemokines such as eotaxin were not essential for the activation step, but not through the basement membrane either because they lacked a chemotactic signal or were unable to digest the extracellular matrix [71]. Once in the tissue, the eosinophil has a number of potential fates: it can remain within the bronchial mucosa where it may become associated with one of several mesenchymal structures such as nerves or mucous glands; it can migrate into the lumen, undergo apoptosis and be expectorated; or, in some circumstances, it may migrate via the efferent lymphatics to the regional lymph nodes [72]. If it remains in the tissue it may undergo apoptosis and be engulfed by macrophages or undergo cytolytic degranulation.

Apoptosis is the universal mechanism by which cells undergo cell senescence in a manner that allows them to be removed efficiently by macrophages without inducing an inflammatory response. Erjefalt and Persson [35], based on morphological observations, have argued persuasively that eosinophil apoptosis is an unusual event in tissue and that most eosinophils either die by cytolysis or migrate into the lumen where they become apoptotic [73]. A slow rate of apoptosis in tissues is consistent with the survival signals delivered to eosinophils by the extracellular matrix as part of normal homoeostasis as well as increased production of eosinophil growth factors during Th2-mediated inflammation [74,75]. The importance of prolonged survival of eosinophils in tissue as a mechanism for selective accumulation has been emphasized by the studies using anti-IL-5 which effectively inhibits blood and sputum eosinophil numbers but has a much less marked effect on tissue eosinophils [7]. Glucocorticoids (GC) directly enhance the rate of eosinophil apoptosis through an unknown mechanism, unlike neutrophils where they prolong survival [76]. It is tempting to suggest that the dramatic effect of GC in resolving eosinophilic inflammation (e.g. in simple pulmonary eosinophilia) is a result of this direct effect. However, GC only induce eosinophil apoptosis at high concentrations and the effect is modest over and above the spontaneous rate of apoptosis. It is more likely that GC are working by inhibiting the production of eosinophil growth factors such as IL-5, IL-3 and GM-CSF generated both in an autocrine fashion by eosinophils in response to matrix signal and as part of the inflammatory process [77]. Recently, TRAIL, another family of survival modulating mediators related to TNF, has been reported as prolonging eosinophil survival both *in vitro* and *ex vivo* after allergen challenge [78].

The biochemical mechanism by which growth factors mediate eosinophil survival is still poorly understood. The effect is dependent on both new protein synthesis and phosphorylation events. The survival effects of IL-5 are dependent on activation of the Ras-Raf-MEC pathway and the Jak-2 Stat 1 and 5 pathway and involve lyn kinase which binds to the IL5-R alpha chain [79]. The roles of p38 and PI3 kinase are less clear and in our hands wortmannin, which blocks PI3 kinase, had no effect on eosinophil apoptosis although it did inhibit IL-5 enhancement of adhesion to fibrinogen. Eosinophils express significant amounts of the pro-apoptotic Bax and the antiapoptotic Bcl-xl but very little Bad or Bcl-2 [80]. As in other cell types, both spontaneous and Fas-induced eosinophil apoptosis is associated with the migration of Bax into the mitochondria. This led to loss of mitochondrial membrane potential, cytochrome c release and activation of downstream caspases. These events were inhibited by IL-5, demonstrating that IL-5 works by blocking Bax translocation [81,82]. Treatment of eosinophils with dexamethasone also leads to loss of mitochondrial permeability [83].

A recent study used a gene microarray approach to identify genes whose expression is modulated by IL-5 [84]. *Pim-1* was one of the genes up-regulated by IL-5 both in human peripheral blood eosinophils and an IL-5-dependent cell line. *Pim-1* was also found to be relatively highly expressed in human eosinophils. *Pim-1* is a serine/threonine kinase that was first identified as a putative lymphoma-associated oncogene. Expression of *Pim-1* in a myeloid leukaemia cell line was found to be closely linked to IL-3 and GM-CSF stimulation [85]. Subsequently, *Pim-1* was shown to be involved in IL-3-mediated survival, although not proliferation, of bone marrow derived mouse mast cells downstream of Jak2 and Stat 5 signalling [86]. In an IL-3-dependent murine cell line, ectopic *Pim-1* expression was able to replace the survival prolonging effects of IL-3 and was also able to counteract the effects of overexpression of Bax on apoptosis [87]. *Pim-1* is therefore a good candidate signalling molecule mediating the downstream effects of IL-5 and related growth factors on eosinophil survival.

Another potential mechanism involved in eosinophil tissue accumulation is *in situ* differentiation from eosinophil precursors. Eosinophil precursors can be identified in an IL-5Rα⁺ CD34⁺ population in peripheral blood, which are increased after allergen challenge and in atopic disease. These cells have also been found in asthmatic airways [88].

Of equal importance as endothelial interactions to the kinetics of eosinophil migration are the factors controlling the fate of the eosinophil once it enters the tissue. There are three possible outcomes. The eosinophil can remain in the tissue interacting with matrix proteins, other leucocytes or structural cells such as in the bronchial mucosa, the epithelium, airway smooth muscle, mucous glands and nerves; alternatively, the cell can migrate into the lumen of the gut or airway where it is likely to undergo apoptosis and be removed; or it can return to the circulation via the lymphatics. There is limited evidence that eosinophils can recirculate although they have been reported to be present in lymph nodes where it has been speculated that they are involved in antigen presentation [89]. The length of time that eosinophils remain in tissue before migrating into the lumen is unclear as there are virtually no studies of the kinetics of eosinophil migration *in vivo* in humans. However, studies using anti-IL-5 in which there remained a significant tissue eosinophilia even after the blood eosinophilia was almost completely inhibited would suggest that eosinophils can remain in the tissue for at least 12 weeks [7]. Anti-IL-5 also completely inhibited migration into the lumen, which suggests that transepithelial migration is IL-5 dependent. It is of interest that in the mouse model of asthma, eosinophil migration into the lumen did not occur in the MMP-2 gene deleted mouse which caused the animals to asphyxiate [90]. IL-5 may therefore be important in activating the eosinophils to digest the epithelial basement membrane in an MMP-2 dependent manner [91]. It is interesting to speculate that, as has been shown with senescent neutrophils, when tissue eosinophils become senescent they start to alter their receptor phenotype in a way that inhibits tissue retention and promotes migration into the lumen [92]. The factors controlling the retention and survival of eosinophils in tissue are likely to involve the integration of chemoattractant, adhesive and survival signals delivered by interactions with matrix proteins and structural cells.

There are very few kinetic studies to provide a basis on which to calculate which of the various mechanisms described above make the largest contribution to eosinophil accumulation in tissues. In the mouse, after allergen challenge, 80% of the eosinophils appeared to be newly arrived from the bone marrow [62]. In contrast, the anti-IL-5 study by Flood-Page *et al.* [7] suggested that prolonged survival in tissues is of central importance. It is likely that each pathway contributes, with the emphasis varying between individuals and over time within one individual.

Animal models of eosinophilic lung disease

Animal models, particularly the mouse model of ovalbumin challenge, which results in a selective and marked pulmonary eosinophilia, have been used extensively to analyse the molecular basis of eosinophil trafficking to the lung and the pathological consequences of this. The combination of transgenic, gene deletion and antibody-based manipulations in the mouse make this a powerful tool for analysing the biology of eosinophil migration, although the relevance of the findings to human disease must always be treated with caution, particularly as the eosinophils do not appear to be particularly activated when they migrate into the tissue [42]. Generally speaking, these studies have supported the concept of eosinophil migration as being the result of a series of interlinked and obligate steps with IL-5 necessary for providing a pool of circulating eosinophils, priming eosinophils for chemotactic responsiveness and prolonging eosinophil survival, and IL-4 and IL-13 controlling adhesion-related events in the endothelium and enhancing the release of eosinophil chemoattractants, particularly CCR3-binding chemokines from mesenchymal cells within the airway [93]. However, there are a number of other studies that challenge this neat concept, by looking at other aspects of the immune response, in particular showing potential roles for innate immunity as well as other inflammatory mediators such as platelet-activating factor (PAF), tryptase and prostaglandin D_2 (PGD2).

Eosinophil functions

The eosinophil exerts its effects largely through its mediators (see Fig. 21.1). These are either newly generated, as is the case with leukotrienes and other lipid mediators, or stored preformed in various compartments within the cytoplasm and released when the eosinophil receives a degranulating stimulus. The eosinophil is relatively biosynthetically inactive and, although new protein synthesis does occur, the majority of its protein mediators are stored. Although the eosinophil can phagocytose particles, its interactions with larval forms of helminthic parasites have formed the model by which eosinophil function has been described.

In this situation, the eosinophil adheres tightly to the organism and releases its granule contents in high local concentrations onto the surface in a process described as frustrated phagocytosis. The paradigm of eosinophil effector function in host defence was developed from the observation that the basic granule proteins in particular were highly toxic for larval parasites, and was extended to include a pro-inflammatory role when they were also shown to be toxic for bronchial epithelium and therefore associated with the epithelial desquamation that is a well-established feature of severe asthma. In recent years, it has been demonstrated that eosinophils can also release a plethora of cytokines and chemokines although many of these are generated in low amounts compared with other cells and the extent to which they are important in eosinophil function is not clear [94]. The eosinophil has also been shown to have the capacity to present antigen to T cells, although how efficient they are compared to professional antigen-presenting cells is uncertain [89]. Eosinophils can release a number of lipid mediators and are one of the relatively few sources of sulphidopeptide leukotrienes although they release approximately 10-fold less per cell than mast cells and basophils. Eosinophils certainly release significant amounts of TGF-β and TGF-α and this has stimulated interest in a potential role in causing

structural changes in the lung that come under the heading of airway remodelling. There is evidence that TGF-β released by eosinophils can promote the generation of fibromyocytes and anti-IL-5 reduced the amount of tenascin in the reticular subepithelial membrane [95,96]. Certainly, thickening of this membrane is closely associated with eosinophilic airway inflammation although not with airway hyperresponsiveness or airflow obstruction [97]. Airway remodelling is also a feature of COPD, although this is more often described as a destructive process involving loss of the alveolar wall in emphysema and obliteration of the small airways. A BAL eosinophilia in cryptogenic fibrosing alveolitis (CFA) has been shown to be associated with more rapid progression of fibrosis in idiopathic pulmonary fibrosis (IPF) [98].

Eosinophils in COPD

The idea that eosinophils have an effector role in asthma is based on evidence of increased numbers of eosinophils in asthmatic airways, a correlation between severity of asthma and eosinophils especially in severe exacerbations [99], a link with responsiveness to corticosteroids and the relevance of eosinophil-derived mediators to the pathophysiology of the disease. To what extent do these tenets hold true for COPD? Three types of studies have been performed: those involving lung resection specimens from patients with lung cancer, bronchoscopy studies and studies of induced sputum. The first has the advantage of sampling the small airways where much of the disease is thought to occur; the second has the advantage of combining pathology with accurate and detailed physiology; and the third has the potential advantage of allowing sampling of larger numbers of subjects on more than one occasion.

Lung resection studies

Saetta *et al.* [100] examined the alveolar walls of patients undergoing lung resection and found increased numbers of CD8+ tissue lymphocytes, which appears to be a reasonably consistent finding in COPD, but no increase in eosinophils (or neutrophils) in smokers with COPD versus smokers without COPD. However, Lams *et al.* [101] investigated the immunopathology of small airways disease in patients undergoing lung resection comparing current with ex-smokers or non-smokers, and patients with and without airflow obstruction. Increased numbers of eosinophils were found in current smokers although there was no correlation with airflow obstruction. However, there was a correlation between lung function and the numbers of neutrophils, which were increased in smokers compared with lifelong non-smokers. Grashoff *et al.* [102] found increased numbers of mast cells and macrophages in the epithelium but not the submucosa in the small airways of patients with COPD undergoing lung resection compared with those without. No differences in T cells were found and eosinophils were generally very scanty.

Bronchoscopy studies

Lacoste et al. [103] investigated patients with asthma, chronic bronchitis and COPD and compared findings with normal controls by bronchial biopsy and BAL. They found increased numbers of eosinophils in all the patient groups with no difference between asthmatics and patients with COPD. They did observe that the eosinophils in asthma but not COPD appeared degranulated, and unlike asthma there was no increase in eosinophil cationic protein (ECP) in BAL in COPD compared with normal controls. In contrast there was no increase in neutrophils in the submucosa of patients with COPD but there was an increase in neutrophils and elastase in BAL [103]. However, O'Shaughnessy et al. [104] found no increase in the number of eosinophils (or neutrophils) in the submucosa of patients with COPD compared with normal controls although they did find an increase in CD8$^+$ cells. Pesci et al. [105] found an increase in the number of eosinophils and ECP in BAL in patients with COPD compared with non-smoking normal subjects (1.6% vs 0.15% and 21.5 µg/L vs 2 µg/L) as well as neutrophils and MBP. Rutgers et al. [106], in a study of patients with COPD who were current non-smokers, found evidence of ongoing inflammation compared with normal controls with increased numbers of eosinophils ($P < 0.49$) in the submucosa and eosinophils, ECP and neutrophils in BAL. There was an increase in CD4$^+$ but not CD8$^+$ cells. This does raise the question as to whether these patients were the same as those with raised CD8$^+$ T-cell numbers [107]. In a study comparing asthmatics with fixed airflow obstruction to patients with COPD, the asthmatics had significantly more eosinophils and CD4 cells and less neutrophils than patients with COPD [108].

Sputum studies

Ronchi et al. [109] compared the sputum (a mixture of induced and spontaneous) differential cell count between patients with asthma and COPD and found that neutrophils predominated in the sputum of patients with COPD and eosinophils in asthma. Similarly, Balzano et al. [110] found that eosinophils were markedly raised in the sputum of asthmatics (22%) but only slightly raised in COPD (0.7% vs 0.2% in controls), whereas neutrophils were more raised in COPD. ECP was raised in both groups but concentrations correlated with eosinophil counts. Some patients with COPD exhibit features of asthma with greater bronchodilator reversibility and steroid responsiveness. The possibility that

this subgroup also has a more asthmatic inflammatory pattern with an airway eosinophilia was supported by the study of Papi et al. [111] who found that only patients with COPD with significant reversibility had increased numbers of eosinophils compared to normal controls. Similarly Rutgers et al. [112] found that patients with COPD who were hyperresponsive to adenosine 5'-monophosphate had increased numbers of airway eosinophils compared with those without. Eosinophilic inflammation is a feature of induced sputum in asymptomatic smokers where 14 out of 34 had increased numbers compared with controls and these subjects had a lower forced expiratory flow (*FEF*) 25–75% and increased number of pack-years smoking history [113]. Most studies have been undertaken in patients with stable disease; however, more striking increases in eosinophils have been seen in sputum during exacerbations of the disease [114].

COPD, eosinophils and corticosteroids

The evidence that corticosteroids are beneficial in COPD is mixed, with apparently only minor benefits of inhaled steroids in preventing exacerbations and slowing the rate of decline in lung function, and limited evidence that oral steroids are beneficial in acute exacerbations as they clearly are in asthma [115]. There is no good evidence that steroids prevent deaths from COPD or alter the natural history of the disease in any major way. Nonetheless, anecdotally it is clear that some patients with COPD benefit from oral corticosteroids. Some of these patients have other features suggestive of asthma and probably represent an overlap syndrome, but others appear to have otherwise typical COPD. There is increasing evidence that steroid responsiveness to COPD is seen in a subgroup of patients with an airway eosinophilia [116]. In an open uncontrolled study of the effects of prednisolone on lung function, Chanez et al. [117] found that 12 of 25 patients had a greater than 200 mL increase in *FEV*$_1$ after a 2-week course of steroids and that these patients had more eosinophils and ECP in the BAL and increased thickness of the reticular basement membrane than non-responders. No difference in eosinophils was seen, however, in bronchial biopsies. In a randomized controlled trial of a course of oral prednisolone for 2 weeks in patients with stable clinically typical irreversible COPD, Brightling et al. [118] found that approximately one-third of patients had a sputum eosinophilia of greater than 3% and that this subgroup of patients had a significant improvement in *FEV*$_1$, quality of life score and exercise tolerance, which was not seen in the patients with a normal sputum eosinophil count. This study adds further weight to the hypothesis that there is a subgroup of patients with COPD who have more eosinophilic disease and that the benefit of steroids is confined to this group.

Conclusions

Although broadly speaking the general paradigm that asthma is an eosinophilic disease and COPD a neutrophilic disease holds true, it is an oversimplification of a complex picture. Just as there appear to be a subset of asthmatics with non-eosinophilic disease, there is a subset of patients with COPD who have a significant airway eosinophilia most clearly seen in the lumenal compartment sampled by BAL or sputum. The discrepancies between the various studies highlighted above are presumably a result of different compartments being sampled or patient selection. For example, most studies have involved non-atopic patients. It would seem that up to one-third of COPD patients with stable disease have a significant airway eosinophilia and this finding could have major implications for targeting corticosteroid treatment to this subgroup. There is little information on why some patients with COPD should have an airway eosinophilia. The large amount of data investigating Th2-mediated mechanisms involved in recruiting eosinophils into the airways in asthma has not been extensively replicated in COPD, although it is likely that many of the mechanisms are similar. However, Th1 inflammatory stimuli can also recruit eosinophils in a non-selective way and it is possible that the eosinophilia in COPD, which is generally modest in degree, represents a non-specific inflammatory process particularly in exacerbations of the disease. The evidence for a role for specific eosinophil mediators in COPD is limited. The function of the eosinophil basic proteins and bronchoconstricting mediators such as the sulphidopeptide leukotrienes appear more relevant to asthma than COPD. Important eosinophil-derived cytokines such as TGF-β and TGF-α are more related to fibrotic than destructive processes. Interestingly, there are very few data on eosinophil proteases that could be responsible for the development of emphysema, although eosinophils are potent producers of superoxide ions, which have been strongly implicated in the pathogenesis of COPD [119]. What could be triggering eosinophil mediator release in COPD is also not clear. Nonetheless, the link between corticosteroid responsiveness and eosinophils discussed above does suggest that in some patients at least they may be playing a pathogenic part. More studies of the natural history and treatment response of this eosinophilic subgroup are required.

References

1 Wardlaw AJ, Brightling C, Green R, Woltmann G, Pavord I. Eosinophils in asthma and other allergic diseases. *Br Med Bull* 2000;**56**:985–1003.

2 Kay AB. T cells as orchestrators of the asthmatic response. *Ciba Found Symp* 1997;**206**:56–67.

3 Jeffery PK. Differences and similarities between chronic obstructive pulmonary disease and asthma. *Clin Exp Allergy* 1999;**29**(Suppl 2):14–26.

4 Green RH, Brightling CE, Woltmann G et al. Analysis of induced sputum in adults with asthma: identification of subgroup with isolated sputum neutrophilia and poor response to inhaled corticosteroids. *Thorax* 2002;**57**:875–9.

5 Saetta M, Di Stefano A, Maestrelli P et al. Airway eosinophilia in chronic bronchitis during exacerbations. *Am J Respir Crit Care Med* 1994;**150**:1646–52.

6 Leckie MJ, ten Brinke A, Khan J et al. Effects of an interleukin-5 blocking monoclonal antibody on eosinophils, airway hyper-responsiveness, and the late asthmatic response. *Lancet* 2000;**356**:2144–8.

7 Flood-Page PT, Menzies-Gow AN, Kay B, Robinson DS. Anti-IL-5 (mepolizumab) only partially depletes eosinophils from asthmatic airway tissue. *Am J Respir Crit Care Med* 2003;**167**:199–204.

8 Gleich GJ, Adolphson CR, Leiferman KM. The biology of the eosinophilic leukocyte. *Annu Rev Med* 1993;**44**:85–101.

9 Wardlaw AJ, Moqbel R, Kay AB. Eosinophils: biology and role in disease. *Adv Immunol* 1995;**60**:151.

10 Seminario MC, Gleich GJ. The role of eosinophils in the pathogenesis of asthma. *Curr Opin Immunol* 1994;**6**:860–4.

11 Weller PF. Human eosinophils. *J Allergy Clin Immunol* 1997;**100**:283–7.

12 Wardlaw A, Kay AB. Eosinophils and their disorders. In: Beutler E, Lichtman MA, Coller BS et al. eds. *Williams Hematology*, 7th edn. USA: McGraw Hill, 2006: 863–78.

13 Basten A, Beeson PB. Mechanisms of eosinophilia. II. Role of lymphocyte. *J Exp Med* 1970;**131**:1288–305.

14 Sanderson CJ. Interleukin-5, eosinophils, and disease. *Blood* 1992;**79**:3101–9.

15 Van Rensen EL, Stirling RG, Scheerens J et al. Evidence for systemic rather than pulmonary effects of interleukin-5 administration in asthma. *Thorax* 2001;**166**:935–40.

16 Culley FJ, Brown A, Girod N, Pritchard DI, Williams TJ. Innate and cognate mechanisms of pulmonary eosinophilia in helminth infection. *Eur J Immunol* 2002;**32**:1376–85.

17 Martin C, Al-Qaoud KM, Ungeheuer MN et al. IL-5 is essential for vaccine-induced protection and for resolution of primary infection in murine filariasis. *Med Microbiol Immunol* 2000;**189**:67–74.

18 Humbert M, Corrigan CJ, Kimmitt P et al. Relationship between IL-4 and IL-5 mRNA expression and disease severity in atopic asthma. *Am J Respir Crit Care Med* 1997;**156**:704.

19 Alexander AG, Barkans J, Moqbel R et al. Serum interleukin 5 concentrations in atopic and non-atopic patients with glucocorticoid-dependent chronic severe asthma. *Thorax* 1994;**49**:1231.

20 Domachowske JB, Bonville CA, Easton AJ, Rosenberg HF. Pulmonary eosinophilia in mice devoid of interleukin-5. *J Leukoc Biol* 2002;**71**:966.

21 Neurath MF, Finotto S, Glimcher LH. The role of Th1/Th2 polarization in mucosal immunity. *Nat Med* 2002;**8**:567–73.

22 Rothenberg ME, Mishra A, Collins MH, Putnam PE. Pathogenesis and clinical features of eosinophilic esophagitis. *J Allergy Clin Immunol* 2001;**108**:891–4.

23 McHugh RS, Shevach EM. The role of suppressor T cells in regulation of immune responses. *J Allergy Clin Immunol* 2002;**110**:693–702.

24 Levings MK, Sangregorio R, Sartirana C *et al*. Human CD25⁺ CD4⁺ T suppressor cell clones produce transforming growth factor beta, but not interleukin 10, and are distinct from type 1 T regulatory cells. *J Exp Med* 2002;**196**:1335–46.

25 Curotto de Lafaille MA, Lafaille JJ. CD4⁺ regulatory T cells in autoimmunity and allergy. *Curr Opin Immunol* 2002;**14**:771–8.

26 Yazdanbakhsh M, Kremsner PG, van Ree R. Allergy, parasites, and the hygiene hypothesis. *Science* 2002;**296**:490–4.

27 Wills-Karp M, Santeliz J, Karp CL. The germless theory of allergic disease: revisiting the hygiene hypothesis. *Nat Rev Immunol* 2001;**1**:69–75.

28 Akdis CA, Blaser K. Mechanisms of interleukin-10-mediated immune suppression. *Immunology* 2001;**103**:131–6.

29 Zuany-Amorim C, Sawicka E, Manlius C *et al*. Suppression of airway eosinophilia by killed *Mycobacterium vaccae*-induced allergen-specific regulatory T-cells. *Nat Med* 2002;**8**:625–9.

30 Suto A, Nakajima H, Kagami SI *et al*. Role of CD4⁺ CD25⁺ regulatory T cells in T helper 2 cell-mediated allergic inflammation in the airways. *Am J Respir Crit Care Med* 2001; **164**:680–7.

31 Egesten A, Calafat J, Janssen H *et al*. Granules of human eosinophilic leucocytes and their mobilization. *Clin Exp Allergy* 2001;**31**:1173–88.

32 Dvorak AM, Weller PF. Ultrastructural analysis of human eosinophils. *Chem Immunol* 2000;**76**:1–28.

33 Persson T, Calafat J, Janssen H *et al*. Specific granules of human eosinophils have lysosomal characteristics: presence of lysosome-associated membrane proteins and acidification upon cellular activation. *Biochem Biophys Res Commun* 2002;**291**:844–54.

34 Wardlaw A. Eosinophil density: what does it mean? *Clin Exp Allergy* 1995;**25**:1145–9.

35 Erjefalt JS, Persson CG. New aspects of degranulation and fates of airway mucosal eosinophils. *Am J Respir Crit Care Med* 2000;**161**:2074–85.

36 Filley WV, Holley KE, Kephart GM, Gleich GJ. Identification by immunofluorescence of eosinophil granule major basic protein in lung tissues of patients with bronchial asthma. *Lancet* 1982;**2**:11–6.

37 Erjefalt JS, Greiff L, Andersson M *et al*. Allergen-induced eosinophil cytolysis is a primary mechanism for granule protein release in human upper airways. *Am J Respir Crit Care Med* 1999;**160**:304–12.

38 Erjefalt JS, Greiff L, Andersson M *et al*. Degranulation patterns of eosinophil granulocytes as determinants of eosinophil driven disease. *Thorax* 2001;**56**:341–4.

39 Weiler CR, Kita H, Hukee M, Gleich GJ. Eosinophil viability during immunoglobulin-induced degranulation. *J Leukoc Biol* 1996;**60**:493–501.

40 Dvorak AM, Furitsu T, Letourneau L, Ishizaka T, Ackerman SJ. Mature eosinophils stimulated to develop in human cord blood mononuclear cell cultures supplemented with recombinant human interleukin-5. I. Piecemeal degranulation of specific granules and distribution of Charcot–Leyden crystal protein. *Am J Pathol* 1991;**138**:69–82.

41 Dvorak AM, Ackerman SJ, Furitsu T *et al*. Mature eosinophils stimulated to develop in human-cord blood mononuclear cell cultures supplemented with recombinant human interleukin-5. II. Vesicular transport of specific granule matrix peroxidase, a mechanism for effecting piecemeal degranulation. *Am J Pathol* 1992;**140**:795–807.

42 Malm-Erjefalt M, Persson CG, Erjefalt JS. Degranulation status of airway tissue eosinophils in mouse models of allergic airway inflammation. *Am J Respir Cell Mol Biol* 2001; **24**:352–9.

43 Denzler KL, Borchers MT, Crosby JR *et al*. Extensive eosinophil degranulation and peroxidase-mediated oxidation of airway proteins do not occur in a mouse ovalbumin-challenge model of pulmonary inflammation. *J Immunol* 2001;**167**:1672–82.

44 Stelts D, Egan RW, Falcone A *et al*. Eosinophils retain their granule major basic protein in a murine model of allergic pulmonary inflammation. *Am J Respir Cell Mol Biol* 1998; **18**:463–70.

45 Denzler KL, Farmer SC, Crosby JR *et al*. Eosinophil major basic protein-1 does not contribute to allergen-induced airway pathologies in mouse models of asthma. *J Immunol* 2000;**165**:5509–17.

46 Dvorak AM. Images in clinical medicine: an apoptotic eosinophil. *N Engl J Med* 1999;**340**:437.

47 Yamamoto H, Sedgwick JB, Vrtis RF, Busse WW. The effect of transendothelial migration on eosinophil function. *Am J Respir Cell Mol Biol* 2000;**23**:379–88.

48 Aizawa H, Plitt J, Bochner BS. Human eosinophils express two Siglec-8 splice variants. *J Allergy* 2002;**109**:176–80.

49 Kikly KK, Bochner BS, Freeman SD *et al*. Identification of SAF-2, a novel siglec expressed on eosinophils, mast cells, and basophils. *J Allergy Clin Immunol* 2000;**105**:1093–1100.

50 Floyd H, Ni J, Cornish AL *et al*. Siglec-8: a novel eosinophil specific member of the immunoglobulin superfamily. *J Biol Chem* 2000;**275**:861–6.

51 Munday J, Kerr S, Ni J *et al*. Identification, characterisation and leucocyte expression of Siglec-10, a novel human sialic acid-binding receptor. *Biochem J* 2001;**355**:489–97.

52 Zhang JQ, Nicoll G, Jones C, Crocker PR. Siglec-9, a novel sialic acid binding member of the immunoglobulin superfamily expressed broadly on human blood leukocytes. *J Biol Chem* 2000;**275**:22 121–6.

53 Nutku E, Aizawa H, Hudson SA, Bochner BS. Ligation of Siglec-8: a selective mechanism for induction of human eosinophil apoptosis. *Blood* 2003;**101**:5014–20.

54 Mishra A, Hogan SP, Brandt EB *et al*. Enterocyte expression of the eotaxin and interleukin-5 transgenes induces compartmetalized dysregulation of eosinophil trafficking. *J Biol Chem* 2002;**277**:4406–12.

55 Hurst SD, Muchamuel T, Gorman DM *et al*. New IL-17 family members promote Th1 or Th2 responses in the lung: *in vivo* function of the novel cytokine IL-25. *J Immunol* 2002;**169**: 443–53.

56 Bochner BS. Road signs guiding leukocytes along the inflammation superhighway. *J Allergy Clin Immunol* 2000; **106**:817–28.

57 Wardlaw AJ. Molecular basis for selective eosinophil trafficking in asthma: a multistep paradigm. *J Allergy Clin Immunol* 1999;**104**:917–26.

58 Rothenberg ME. Eosinophilia. *N Engl J Med* 1998;**338**:1592–600.

59 Palframan RT, Collins PD, Williams TJ, Rankin SM. Eotaxin induces a rapid release of eosinophils and their progenitors from the bone marrow. *Blood* 1998;**91**:2240–8.

60 Palframan RT, Collins PD, Severs NJ *et al*. Mechanisms of acute eosinophil mobilization from the bone marrow stimulated by interleukin 5: the role of specific adhesion molecules and phosphatidylinositol 3-kinase. *J Exp Med* 1998;**188**:1621–32.

61 Tachimoto H, Burdick MM, Hudson SA *et al*. CCR3-active chemokines promote rapid detachment of eosinophils from VCAM-1 *in vitro*. *J Immunol* 2000;**165**:2748–54.

62 Tomaki M, Zhao LL, Lundahl J *et al*. Eosinophilopoiesis in a murine model of allergic airway eosinophilia: involvement of bone marrow IL-5 and IL-5 receptor alpha. *J Immunol* 2000;**165**:4040–50.

63 Inman MD. Bone marrow events in animal models of allergic inflammation and hyperresponsiveness. *J Allergy Clin Immunol* 2000;**106**:S235–41.

64 Edwards BS, Curry MS, Tsuji H *et al*. Expression of P-selectin at low site density promotes selective attachment of eosinophils over neutrophils. *J Immunol* 2000;**165**:404–10.

65 Dang B, Wiehler S, Patel KD. Increased PSGL-1 expression on granulocytes from allergic-asthmatic subjects results in enhanced leukocyte recruitment under flow conditions. *J Leukoc Biol* 2002;**72**:702–10.

66 Woltmann G, McNulty CA, Dewson G, Symon FA, Wardlaw AJ. Interleukin-13 induces PSGL-1/P-selectin-dependent adhesion of eosinophils, but not neutrophils, to human umbilical vein endothelial cells under flow. *Blood* 2000;**95**:3146–52.

67 Kitayama, J, Mackay CR, Ponath PD, Springer TA. The C-C chemokine receptor CCR3 participates in stimulation of eosinophil arrest on inflammatory endothelium in shear flow. *J Clin Invest* 1998;**101**:2017–24.

68 Ainslie MP, McNulty CA, Huynh T, Symon FA, Wardlaw AJ. Characterisation of adhesion receptors mediating lymphocyte adhesion to bronchial endothelium provides evidence for a distinct lung homing pathway. *Thorax* 2002;**57**:1054–9.

69 Doerschuk CM. Leukocyte trafficking in alveoli and airway passages. *Respir Res* 2000;**1**:136.

70 Doerschuk CM. Mechanisms of leukocyte sequestration in inflamed lungs. *Microcirculation* 2001;**2001**:71–88.

71 Humbles AA, Lu B, Friend DS *et al*. The murine CCR3 receptor regulates both the role of eosinophils and mast cells in allergen-induced airway inflammation and hyperresponsiveness. *Proc Natl Acad Sci U S A* 2002;**99**:1479–84.

72 Shi HZ, Humbles A, Gerard C, Jin Z, Weller PF. Lymph node trafficking and antigen presentation by endobronchial eosinophils. *J Clin Invest* 2000;**105**:945–53.

73 Woolley KL, Gibson PG, Carty K *et al*. Eosinophil apoptosis and the resolution of airway inflammation in asthma. *Am J Respir Crit Care Med* 1996;**154**:237–43.

74 Simon HU, Yousefi S, Schranz C *et al*. Direct demonstration of delayed eosinophil apoptosis as a mechanism causing tissue eosinophilia. *J Immunol* 1997;**158**:3902–8.

75 Anwar AR, Moqbel R, Walsh GM, Kay AB, Wardlaw AJ. Adhesion to fibronectin prolongs eosinophil survival. *J Exp Med* 1993;**177**:839–43.

76 Meagher LC, Cousin JM, Seckl JR, Haslett C. Opposing effects of glucocorticoids on the rate of apoptosis in neutrophilic and eosinophilic granulocytes. *J Immunol* 1996;**156**:4422–8.

77 Walsh GM, Wardlaw AJ. Dexamethasone inhibits prolonged survival and autocrine granulocyte-macrophage colony-stimulating factor production by human eosinophils cultured on laminin or tissue fibronectin. *J Allergy Clin Immunol* 1997;**100**:208–15.

78 Robertson NM, Zangrilli JG, Steplewski A *et al*. Differential expression of TRAIL and TRAIL receptors in allergic asthmatics following segmental antigen challenge: evidence for a role of TRAIL in eosinophil survival. *J Immunol* 2002;**169**:5986–96.

79 Adachi T, Alam R. The mechanism of IL-5 signal transduction. *Am J Physiol* 1998;**275**:C623–33.

80 Dewson G, Walsh GM, Wardlaw AJ. Expression of Bcl-2 and its homologues in human eosinophils: modulation by interleukin-5. *Am J Respir Cell Mol Biol* 1999;**20**:720–8.

81 Dewson G, Cohen GM, Wardlaw AJ. Interleukin-5 inhibits translocation of Bax to the mitochondria, cytochrome c release, and activation of caspases in human eosinophils. *Blood* 2001;**98**:2239–47.

82 Letuve S, Druilhe A, Grandsaigne M, Aubier M, Pretolani M. Involvement of caspases and of mitochondria in Fas ligation-induced eosinophil apoptosis: modulation by interleukin-5 and interferon-gamma. *J Leukoc Biol* 2001;**70**:767–75.

83 Letuve S, Druilhe A, Grandsaigne M, Aubier M, Pretolani M. Critical role of mitochondria, but not caspases, during glucocorticosteroid-induced human eosinophil apoptosis. *Am J Respir Cell Mol Biol* 2002;**26**:565–71.

84 Temple R, Allen E, Fordham J *et al*. Microarray analysis of eosinophils reveals a number of candidate survival and apoptosis genes. *Am J Respir Cell Mol Biol* 2001;**25**:425–33.

85 Lilly M, Le T, Holland P, Hendrickson SL. Sustained expression of the pim-1 kinase is specifically induced in myeloid cells by cytokines whose receptors are structurally related. *Oncogene* 1992;**7**:727–32.

86 O'Farrell AM, Ichihara M, Mui AL, Miyajima A. Signaling pathways activated in a unique mast cell line where interleukin-3 supports survival and stem cell factor is required for a proliferative response. *Blood* 1996;**87**:3655–68.

87 Lilly M, Sandholm J, Cooper JJ, Koskinen PJ, Kraft A. The PIM-1 serine kinase prolongs survival and inhibits apoptosis-related mitochondrial dysfunction in part through a bcl-2-dependent pathway. *Oncogene* 1999;**18**:4022–31.

88 Robinson DS, Damia R, Zeibecoglou K *et al*. CD34⁺/interleukin-5Rα messenger RNA+ cells in the bronchial mucosa in asthma: potential airway eosinophil progenitors. *Am J Respir Cell Mol Biol* 1999;**20**:9–13.

89 Shi HZ, Humbles A, Gerard C, Jin Z, Weller P. Lymph node trafficking and antigen presentation by endobronchial eosinophils. *J Clin Invest* 2000;**105**:945–53.

90 Corry DB, Rishi K, Kanellis J *et al*. Decreased allergic lung inflammatory cell egression and increased susceptibility to asphyxiation in MMP-2 deficiency. *Nat Immunol* 2002; **3**:347–53.

91 Okada S, Kita H, George TJ, Gleich GJ, Leiferman KM. Transmigration of eosinophils through basement membrane components *in vitro*: synergistic effects of platelet-activating factor and eosinophil-active cytokines. *Am J Respir Cell Mol Biol* 1997;**6**:455–63.

92 Martin C, Burdon PC, Bridger G *et al*. Chemokines acting via CXCR2 and CXCR4 control the release of neutrophils from the bone marrow and their return following senescence. *Immunity* 2003;**19**:583–93.

93 Foster PS, Mould AW, Yang M *et al*. Elemental signals regulating eosinophil accumulation in the lung. *Immunol Rev* 2001;**179**:173–81.

94 Lacy P, Moqbel R. Eosinophil cytokines. *Chem Immunol* 2000;**76**:134–55.

95 Flood-Page P, Menzies-Gow A, Phipps S *et al*. Anti-IL-5 treatment reduces deposition of ECM proteins in the bronchial subepithelial basement membrane of mild atopic asthmatics. *J Clin Invest* 2003;**112**:1029–36.

96 Phipps S, Ying S, Wangoo A *et al*. The relationship between allergen-induced tissue eosinophilia and markers of repair and remodeling in human atopic skin. *J Immunol* 2002;**169**: 4604–12.

97 Brightling CE, Bradding P, Symon FA *et al*. Mast-cell infiltration of airway smooth muscle in asthma. *N Engl J Med* 2002; **346**:1699–75.

98 Rudd RM, Haslam PL, Turner-Warwick M. Cryptogenic fibrosing aleolitis: relationship of pulmonary physiology and bronchoalveolar lavage to response to treatment and prognosis. *Am Rev Respir Dis* 1981;**124**:1–8.

99 Green RH, Brightling CE, McKenna S *et al*. Asthma exacerbations and sputum eosinophil counts: a randomised controlled trial. *Lancet* 2002;**360**:1715–21.

100 Saetta M, Baraldo S, Corbino L *et al*. CD8[+] cells in the lungs of smokers with chronic obstructive pulmonary disease. *Am J Respir Crit Care Med* 1999;**160**:711–7.

101 Lams BE, Sousa AR, Rees PJ, Lee TH. Immunopathology of the small-airway submucosa in smokers with and without chronic obstructive pulmonary disease. *Am J Respir Crit Care Med* 1998;**158**:1518–23.

102 Grashoff WF, Sont JK, Sterk PJ *et al*. Chronic obstructive pulmonary disease: role of bronchiolar mast cells and macrophages. *Am J Pathol* 1997;**151**:1785–90.

103 Lacoste JY, Bousquet J, Chanez P *et al*. Eosinophilic and neutrophilic inflammation in asthma, chronic bronchitis, and chronic obstructive pulmonary disease. *J Allergy Clin Immunol* 1993;**92**:537–48.

104 O'Shaughnessy TC, Ansari TW, Barnes NC, Jeffery PK. Inflammation in bronchial biopsies of subjects with chronic bronchitis: inverse relationship of CD8[+] T lymphocytes with FEV_1. *Am J Respir Crit Care Med* 1997;**55**:852–7.

105 Pesci A, Balbi B, Majori M *et al*. Inflammatory cells and mediators in bronchial lavage of patients with chronic obstructive pulmonary disease. *Eur Respir J* 1998;**12**:380–6.

106 Rutgers SR, Postma DS, ten Hacken NH *et al*. Ongoing airway inflammation in patients with COPD who do not currently smoke. *Thorax* 2000;**55**:12–8.

107 Lams BE, Sousa AR, Rees PJ, Lee TH. Subepithelial immunopathology of the large airways in smokers with and without chronic obstructive pulmonary disease. *Eur Respir J* 2000;**2000**:512–6.

108 Fabbri LM, Romagnoli M, Corbetta L *et al*. Differences in airway inflammation in patients with fixed airflow obstruction due to asthma or chronic obstructive pulmonary disease. *Am J Respir Crit Care Med* 2003;**167**:418–24.

109 Ronchi MC, Piragino C, Rosi E *et al*. Role of sputum differential cell count in detecting airway inflammation in patients with chronic bronchial asthma or COPD. *Thorax* 1996;**51**:1000–4.

110 Balzano G, Stefanelli F, Iorio C *et al*. Eosinophilic inflammation in stable chronic obstructive pulmonary disease: relationship with neutrophils and airway function. *Am J Respir Crit Care Med* 1999;**160**:1486–92.

111 Papi A, Romagnoli M, Baraldo S *et al*. Partial reversibility of airflow limitation and increased exhaled NO and sputum eosinophilia in chronic obstructive pulmonary disease. *Am J Respir Crit Care Med* 2000;**162**:1773–7.

112 Rutgers SR, Timens W, Tzanakis N *et al*. Airway inflammation and hyperresponsiveness to adenosine 5′-monophosphate in chronic obstructive pulmonary disease. *Clin Exp Allergy* 2000;**30**:657–62.

113 Dippolito A, Foresi A, Chetta A *et al*. Eosinophils in induced sputum from asymptomatic smokers with normal lung function. *Respir Med* 2001;**95**:969–74.

114 Delmastro M, Balbi B. Acute exacerbations of COPD: is inflammation central to prevention and treatment strategies. *Monaldi Arch Chest Dis* 2002;**57**:293–6.

115 Sutherland ER, Allmers H, Ayas NT, Venn AJ, Martin RJ. Inhaled corticosteroids reduce the progression of airflow limitation in chronic obstructive pulmonary disease: a meta-analysis. *Thorax* 2003;**58**:937–41.

116 Fujimoto K, Kubo K, Yamamoto H, Yamaguchi S, Matsuzawa Y. Eosinophilic inflammation in the airways is related to glucocorticoid reversibility in patients with pulmonary emphysema. *Chest* 1999;**115**:697–702.

117 Chanez P, Vignola AM, O'Shaugnessy T *et al*. Corticosteroids reversibility in COPD is related to features of asthma. *Am J Respir Crit Care Med* 1997;**155**:1529–34.

118 Brightling CE, Monteiro W, Ward R *et al*. Sputum eosinophilia and short-term response to prednisolone in chronic obstructive pulmonary disease: a randomised controlled trial. *Lancet* 2000;**356**:1480–5.

119 MacNee W, Donaldson K. Pathogenesis of chronic obstructive pulmonary disease. In: Wardlaw AJ, Hamid Q, eds. *Respiratory Cell and Molecular Biology*. London: Martin Dunitz, 2002: 99–127.

CHAPTER 22
Airway epithelial defence, repair and regeneration

Christelle Coraux, Jean-Marie Tournier, Jean-Marie Zahm and Edith Puchelle

Airway epithelial cells: mechanisms of defence and injury

Defence mechanisms

The airway epithelium represents the first line of lung defence. The diversity of the cells lining the airways is adapted to airway mucosa protection through a variety of defence mechanisms that act together in order to protect the airway epithelium from injury. The airway surface liquid covering the mucociliary epithelium contains critical molecules for innate airway defence which maintain the sterility of the airways. The integrity of the fluid balance and optimal physical and biochemical properties of the airway secretions allow the mucociliary clearance of inhaled particles and create a protective interface between the external environment and the underlying epithelial cells. In the upper (nasal), lower (bronchi) and distal airways (bronchioles), several epithelial cell types contribute to the defence functions of the airway epithelium:
- Brush border cells (in the upper airways).
- Ciliated cells along the surface epithelium from the upper up to the distal airways, including the bronchioles.
- Secretory cells: mucous (goblet) cells in the surface epithelium and serous and mucous glandular cells in the submucosa.
- Clara cells in the distal bronchioles.
- Basal cells in the upper, lower and non-terminal distal airways (bronchioles).

The first protection barrier of the airways is the airway surface liquid and mucus, which form a continuous filter at the cell–air interface and serve as a physical barrier to noxious particles and bacteria [1]. Ciliated cells are not only involved in the mechanical mucous transport function, but also contribute to the regulation of ion and water content in the airway lining fluid through chloride channel activity

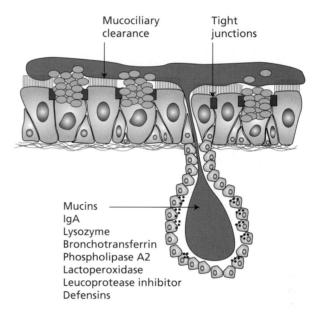

Figure 22.1 Schematic representation of airway epithelium defence mechanisms. IgA, immunoglobulin A.

[2,3]. The biochemical constituents of the airway surface liquids are numerous, and actively participate to the antibacterial, antioxidant and antiprotease defence of the epithelium (Fig. 22.1) [4]. Mucin glycoproteins directly interfere in the protective role of mucociliary clearance. The heterogeneity of their glycan chains represents a mosaic of receptors allowing the recognition and adhesion of bacteria to mucus, then eliminated from the airways by the ciliary transport mechanism, therefore avoiding the microorganisms being recognized and adhering to the surface of the underlying epithelial cells [5]. Several other proteins possess antibacterial properties: secretory immunoglobulin A (IgA), lysozyme, bronchotransferrin, secretory phospholipase A_2, lactoperoxidase and secretory leucoprotease inhibitor [6]. These molecules exhibit

microbicidal activity and are mainly produced by the serous cells of airway glands. Other molecules such as defensin peptides are also involved in the defence of the airway epithelium. It has been recently reported that the human cathelicidin antimicrobial peptide has a central role in innate immunity by linking host defence and inflammation with angiogenesis and arteriogenesis [7,8]. Surfactant proteins (SP-A, SP-B, SP-D), also called collectins, have an important role in the defence of the epithelium [9]. These human lung collectins are synthesized by alveolar epithelial cells, non-ciliated bronchiolar cells and some epithelial cells lining the larger airways and airway glands. At bronchiolar level, the Clara cell secretory protein (CCSP), also called CC16, CC10 or uteroglobin, is able to modulate lung inflammatory and immune response [10,11].

In response to reactive oxygen and nitrogen molecules induced by the inhalation of pollutants and generated by phagocytes, glutathione peroxidase is synthesized by the airway epithelial cells. Glutathione acts as a first line of defence against inhaled reactive oxygen and nitrogen species [12].

Unlike most of the matrix metalloproteinases (MMPs) synthesized and released by epithelial cells following injury, MMP-7 (matrilysin) may serve as a defence MMP and is constitutively expressed by the airway epithelium of peribronchial glands and conducting airways. Matrilysin also functions in host defence by activating the latent form of the defensin antimicrobial peptides [13].

The airway epithelial cells can rapidly alter their structure and functions, either to adapt to changes in the local environment or to repair the epithelium following injury. The 'plasticity' or remodelling of the airway epithelium has been described after irritation or injury which leads to increased cell proliferation and changes in the proportion of specific cell types. Whether the cellular changes observed reflect a response to injury or a normal repair process is not clearly defined.

At the cellular level, the tight junction (TJ) proteins play a central part in epithelial cytoprotection by maintaining a physical selective barrier between external and internal environments. Apart from their barrier function, the TJ intercellular proteins (ZO-1, claudin, occludin) interact with actin filaments and actively participate in epithelial signalling. The TJs are highly labile structures whose formation and structure may be very rapidly altered following injury. Their function may be perturbed by airway inflammation. Coyne *et al.* [14] have shown that TJ proteins are regulated by pro-inflammatory cytokines on primary cultures of airway epithelial cells and that the combined exposure to tumour necrosis factor (TNF) and γ-interferon (IFN-γ) induces drastic effects on TJ expression and barrier functions with significant alterations in the epithelial permeability.

Apart from inflammatory cytokines, bacterial toxins are also able to induce TJ degradation and to alter the epithelial integrity [15]. The disruption of TJ in bronchial biopsies from asthmatics described by Elias [16] has been reported to be associated with extensive epithelial damage. In infected airways, the neutrophil products may decrease the transepithelial resistance with a reduced number and width of TJ strands.

Main sources of airway epithelial injury

Infectious as well as non-infectious agents may significantly alter the integrity of the epithelial barrier. Bacteria interfere with the airway mucociliary transport by disorganizing or slowing ciliary activity. Microorganisms, such as *Haemophilus influenzae*, *Streptococcus pneumoniae*, *Staphylococcus aureus* and *Pseudomonas aeruginosa* are responsible for inducing hypersecretion of mucus, slowing of ciliary beating and epithelial shedding. Non-infectious agents, such as inhaled oxidants (NO_2, SO_2, O_3), may exert a toxic effect on airway epithelium, the gravity of the injury being dependent on the physicochemical characteristics of the inhaled gas, its concentration, solubility and the duration of exposure. Whatever the source, the response of the airway surface epithelium to an acute injury includes a succession of cellular events, varying from the loss of surface epithelial impermeability to the shedding of the epithelium (only basal cells still being attached to the basal lamina), or to a complete denudation of the basement membrane (Fig. 22.2).

Epithelial shedding, even to the point of airway denudation, has already been described as a common and unifying feature of asthma. However, the capacity of basal cells to take over the barrier properties of the epithelium after a selective loss of columnar cells was described more recently [17]. Very few studies have been devoted to the relationship between airway epithelial damage and inflammation in patients with recurrent bronchitis and frequent exacerbation episodes. In most cases in children with recurrent

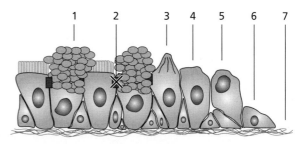

Figure 22.2 Chronology of the different steps of airway epithelium injury. Mucus release (1), loss of junctional integrity (2), compound cilia (3), loss of cilia (4), loss of polarity (5), epithelium shedding (6) and basement membrane denudation (7).

bronchitis outside of recent acute infections, bronchial biopsies showed extensive epithelial damage and a significant correlation between the degree of shedding and oedema of the airway mucosa [18].

In vivo and *in vitro* models of airway epithelial repair and regeneration

Animal models of airway epithelium regeneration

Different sources of injury (oxidants, cigarette smoke, mechanical injury, and viral or bacterial infections) have been analysed using a variety of animal models including dogs, rabbits, guinea pigs, hamsters, rats and mice. These models of airway epithelium injury and repair demonstrate progressive restoration of TJs, premitosis dedifferentiation followed by squamous metaplasia, active mitosis leading to basal and mucous cell hyperplasia and progressive redifferentiation with emergence of 'preciliated' cells (a mixed phenotype of ciliated and mucous cells) and ciliogenesis allowing the regeneration of a functional mucociliary epithelium [19].

Regeneration of the hamster tracheal epithelium after mechanical injury has demonstrated rapid re-epithelialization of the denuded basement membrane and has shown that cell migration, rather than cell proliferation, occurs first [20]. Epithelial cells at the border of the wounded area are able to dedifferentiate, spread and migrate over the denuded basement membrane to cover the de-epithelialized area. Ramphal *et al.* [21] have shown that, after influenza virus infection, complete desquamation of the epithelium occurs within 3 days, then regeneration begins within 5 days and is completed after 2 weeks.

In vivo studies in animal models suggest that several categories of stem cells and progenitor cells, including columnar, basal and ciliated duct cells, can participate in airway epithelium regeneration and renewal [22–25]. Nevertheless, histological differences exist between human airways and those of other animal species. Mouse tracheal epithelium is composed mainly of ciliated and Clara cells, the latter being present only in human distal airways and only a few submucosal gland cells are identified at the upper tracheal level in mice.

Human airway xenografts in tolerant mice

We explored regeneration and maturation of the adult human airway epithelium [26], adapting the tracheal xenografts in nude mice initially developed by Engelhardt *et al.* [27]. Epithelial cells dissociated from human nasal polyps were seeded into the lumen of rat tracheas denuded of their own epithelium by successive cycles of freezing and thawing. The rat tracheas, tied at their distal end to sterile polyethylene tubing, were inoculated with the human adult epithelial cells and implanted subcutaneously into the flanks of recipient nude mice. We analysed, in terms of cell proliferation, differentiation and integrity of the epithelial barrier, the sequence of events involved in the regeneration of the human airway epithelium, which were partly similar to those described in epithelial regeneration *in vivo* after airway injury. At 3 days after implantation in nude mice, tracheas were partly repopulated with a flattened, non-ciliated and poorly differentiated untight epithelium. By the end of the first week, cell proliferation produced a squamous-type epithelium on the entire surface of the host rat trachea which was stratified into multiple layers and tightly sealed. This squamous epithelium phenotype, which represents a highly protective phenotype, previously described after injury, reflects a protective dynamic regenerative process. During the following weeks, cell proliferation decreased markedly and the epithelium became progressively columnar, secretory and ciliated but was still partly untight, although already polarized. After 4–6 weeks, the regenerated airway epithelium was well differentiated and pseudostratified (Fig. 22.3; see also Plate 22.1; colour plate section falls between pp. 354 and 355). This chimeric model has the main advantage of reconstituting a human adult airway epithelium exposed to the air environment in the same way as in adult human airways. Pharmacological application of this air-opened humanized airway graft has been successfully assayed with an anti-inflammatory molecule in cystic fibrosis (CF) [28]. Other important applications of this model will be to identify molecules able to activate epithelial regeneration in respiratory diseases such as chronic bronchitis, asthma and CF. Ultimately, this xenochimera may be very useful to analyse the capacity of recombinant viral vectors to target progenitor cells for surface epithelium [29].

A model of human airway development *in vivo* relying on the transplantation of embryonic and fetal lung rudiments into xenotolerant severe combined immunodeficient (SCID) mice has been described [30,31]. Proximal or distal airway primordia grew rapidly in SCID mice and differentiated after 6–12 weeks into tracheal or pulmonary structures, including a pseudostratified ciliated and secretory surface epithelium, submucosal glands and cartilage rings as well as alveolar structures and interstitium. Irrespective of initial stages of development, fragments of human fetal tracheas implanted subcutaneously into SCID mice developed as closed fluid-filled xenografts, lined on their whole inner surface with a pseudostratified and secretory epithelium. The presence of airway fluid inside the lumen of these tracheal grafts resulted from surface cell and submucosal gland secretion and from transepithelial active transport of

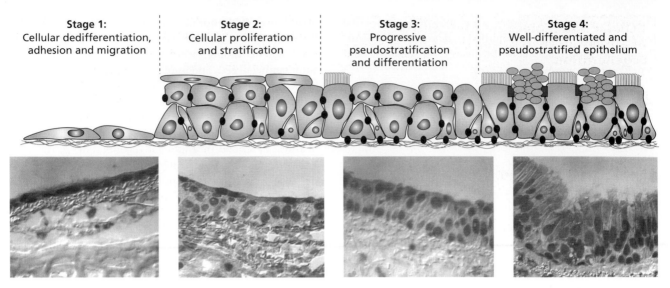

Stage 1:
Cellular dedifferentiation, adhesion and migration

Stage 2:
Cellular proliferation and stratification

Stage 3:
Progressive pseudostratification and differentiation

Stage 4:
Well-differentiated and pseudostratified epithelium

Figure 22.3 Sequence of events in the regeneration of airway epithelium. See also Plate 22.1; colour plate section falls between pp. 354 and 355. (From Dupuit *et al.* [26] with permission.)

ions and water. The bioelectric properties of these human tracheal grafts implanted in SCID mice were stable over several months and showed that the mature and well-differentiated lining epithelium acted as a selective barrier to ion transport [32]. Xenografts were similar to postnatal normal airways with respect to transepithelial potential difference, short-circuit current and transepithelial resistance as well as to responses to amiloride, forskolin and extracellular adenosine triphosphate (ATP). A lower baseline electrogenic ion transport activity, similar to that described in CF postnatal airways, was observed in CF fetal grafts. A limitation of this model is that the xenograft is not exposed to air and probably mimics the prenatal rather than the postnatal human airway environment.

In vitro and *ex vivo* models of airway epithelial repair and regeneration

Several assays have been described to analyse *in vitro* the wound repair following airway cell culture damage. After bronchial or alveolar cell culture at confluence, the cell layer is mechanically damaged by gently scraping the epithelium, and the area of denuded epithelium is quantified over 24 h at regular time intervals.

Chemical injury has been also used for inducing a wound [33]. Primary cultures of confluent airway cells were injured by depositing a 1 μL drop of 1 mol/L sodium hydroxide rapidly neutralized with phosphate buffer saline at the centre of the culture. The advantage of this technique is that the wound surface is well standardized. Evolution of the remaining surface of the wound area can be examined using a videocamera connected to a microscope and the corresponding wound surface is calculated. A cell migration assay was also developed in parallel to analyse the migra-

tion speed of the airway cells in culture after injury. After wound induction, cell nuclei were stained with a fluorescent dye and the wounded culture was placed in a small transparent culture chamber of an inverted microscope. Images of the cell nuclei are digitized and cell migration is quantified through the detection of cell nuclei, the computation of the trajectories of these nuclei and the analysis of these trajectories. From each nucleus trajectory, the computer calculated the cell migration speed.

In order to analyse the molecular mechanisms involved in airway epithelial repair, it is of major interest to create a wound where only surface epithelial cells are damaged without any alteration of the underlying extracellular matrix molecules. Freshly collected human bronchial tissues can be locally injured using a small metallic probe frozen with liquid nitrogen and applied for 10 s to the tissue sample with a calibrated pressure. Under these conditions, only cells of the surface epithelium are eliminated, but the underlying extracellular matrix is not altered [34].

Another *in vitro* model of three-dimensional culture of human airway epithelial cells in suspension has been developed that allows the analysis of the regeneration of nasal epithelium [35]. Using this three-dimensional airway spheroid culture model, the kinetics of differentiation, polarization and ciliated and secretory epithelial regeneration have been analysed [36]. After complete dissociation of human airway epithelial cells, the expression of apical membrane proteins disappears and the re-establishment of cell–cell junctionality, polarity and differentiation observed after approximately 1 month of culture is associated with the apical plasma membrane localization of cystic fibrosis transmembrane conductance regulator (CFTR) and of associated proteins such as ezrin and a glycophosphatidyl-inositol-anchored protein: CD59.

Cellular and molecular mechanisms of airway epithelial repair and regeneration

The cellular and molecular factors involved in the repair and regeneration of airway epithelium are numerous and closely interact. Early repair events have been examined in detail by Erjefält et al. [37] who have shown that, immediately after epithelial denudation without any damage to the basement membrane, the epithelial cells from the wound border dedifferentiate into 'repair cells' that migrate rapidly to recover the wounded area.

Cell migration involves protrusion of the plasma membrane (lamellipodium extension) at the leading edge of the cell which implies cytoskeleton reorganization. Cell movement also implies the formation of new sites of adhesion to the extracellular matrix at the front of the wound but also the release of adhesion sites at the back of the cells. This necessarily implies a coordinated sequence of events involving contraction of the actin and actomyosin cytoskeleton, interaction with extracellular matrix proteins (ECM) and MMPs, with regulation between MMPs and their inhibitors. Furthermore, production of ECM by the airway epithelial cells during the migration process requires signalling pathways through specific receptors on the airway cell surface.

In the in vivo situation, such as in asthma, chronic obstructive pulmonary diseases (COPD) and CF or in in vivo experimental models where the host-tissue responses are preserved (such as in human airway xenografts), there is a rapid increased plasma exudation associated with a deposition of fibrin and plasma-derived proteins on the denuded plasma membrane and an efflux of plasma-derived growth factors, cytokines, MMPs, associated with recruitment of leucocytes, as well as proliferation of fibroblasts and myofibroblasts, which may contribute to the initiation of the repair process. In normal conditions, this inflammatory host-tissue response progressively decreases in order to allow the reparative processes to occur (wound closure, redifferentiation and regeneration of the airway epithelium). To accomplish successful wound repair and tissue regeneration, the inflammation response must be tightly regulated in vivo. Among the regulatory cytokines, it can be expected that, as in cutaneous wound healing, IL-10 has a major role in suppressing the inflammatory response and inhibiting the synthesis of proinflammatory cytokines observed at the onset of wound repair [38].

Role of matrix metalloproteinases in the repair and regeneration of airway epithelium

During spreading and migration, cells adhere to the ECM molecules through focal and primordial contacts that enable the anchorage by which the cells can exert traction on the matrix. These contacts are transient structures that are required for traction but have to be rapidly cleaved during migration. MMPs are directly involved in airway epithelial wound repair, especially in the remodelling of the provisional matrix on which the epithelial cells migrate. Buisson et al. [39] have shown, using the in vitro model of airway epithelium wound repair, that MMP-9 and MMP-3 (stromelysin-1) are strongly expressed by the repairing airway cells. Furthermore, a MMP-9 antibody, known to inhibit MMP-9 activation, resulted in a dose-dependent decrease of the wound repair speed. These observations suggest that MMP-9 acts at the interface between repairing epithelial cells and the ECM and is involved in the remodelling of the newly synthesized ECM. According to Planus et al. [40], MMPs play a major part in tissue repair by several mechanisms: first by remodelling ECM but also by releasing growth factors such as vascular endothelial growth factor (VEGF), transforming growth factor β (TGF-β) or basic fibroblast growth factor (bFGF) from the proteoglycans were they are stored, or by cleaving some growth factor receptors such as FGF receptor. MMPs could also facilitate de-adhesion during the cell migration process, as suggested by the fact that alveolar cell migration on type I collagen is promoted by collagenases. Matrilysin (MMP-7) is an important MMP that functions in defence and repair as well as in inflammation. MMP-7 is expressed in migrating epithelium in injured airway [41]. In matrilysin null mice airway tissues, tracheal wound does not repair, whereas it repairs rapidly in tracheas of wild-type mice. Moreover, it has been recently shown that matrilysin shedding of syndecan-1 regulates chemokine mobilization and confines neutrophil influx to sites of injury [42]. Both collagen IV and MMP-9 are involved in airway epithelial cell migration. Legrand et al. [34] have shown that when cell–collagen IV interaction is blocked, cells spread slightly but do not migrate and when MMP-9 activation is prevented, cells remain fixed on primordial contacts and do not migrate. These observations suggest that MMP-9 controls cell migration by remodelling the provisional ECM implicated in primordial contacts. MMP-7 and MMP-9 act also as modulators of airway epithelial differentiation. It was recently demonstrated in the nude-mice xenograft model that incubation of the epithelial cells with MMP inhibitors in the course of epithelial regeneration led to an abnormal epithelial differentiation attested by immature and mature squamous metaplasia with areas of basal cell hyperplasia [43].

Role of cytokines and growth factors in airway epithelial repair

Cytokines represent a large group of heterogeneous proteins with diverse biological activities. These polypeptide mediators include chemokines, interleukins, tumour necrosis factors, growth factors and colony-stimulating factors. During airway inflammation, great attention has been devoted to the mediators involved in the early inflammatory and chemotactic response and in the resolution of inflammation. Less information is available on the cytokines such as growth factors that are involved in airway epithelial wound repair and regeneration. These growth factors are mainly secreted by mesenchymal cells and macrophages but also by epithelial cells. The incubation of wounded human airway epithelial cell cultures with recombinant epidermal growth factor (EGF) increases significantly the wound closure rate [44]. EGF stimulates migration and wound repair of guinea pig airway epithelial cells [45]. Other growth factors, such as insulin-like growth factor 1 (IGF-1), platelet-derived growth factor (PDGF), TGF-β or keratinocyte growth factor (KGF) can enhance the wound repair by acting as chemotactic or growth-stimulating factors, stimulating the synthesis of ECM and interacting with MMPs through specific cell receptors.

Airway epithelial migration is induced by several 'motogen' peptides including insulin, insulin-like growth factors (IGF), calcitonin gene-related peptide (CGRP) and EGF. Another group of peptides, the trefoil factor family (TFF) has been shown to promote migration and repair in the gastrointestinal tract and, more recently, in wounded airway epithelial cell cultures where they exhibit a synergistic effect with EGF [46]. TFF peptides would act as motogens in the human respiratory epithelium, triggering rapid repair of damaged mucosa in the course of airway diseases such as asthma.

Extracellular matrix proteins, integrin and non-integrin receptors

Cell–cell and cell–extracellular matrix interactions represent vital aspects of the repair mechanisms. These cellular processes are mediated by the ECM constituents that represent ligands for specific transmembrane cellular receptors, the integrins. Each integrin consists of two subunits, α and β, and the resulting heterodimer mediates cell adhesion to one or more matrix proteins such as collagen, laminin, fibrinogen or fibronectin [47]. The migrating cells attach to a provisional matrix that includes the inflammatory glycoproteins fibronectin and vitronectin as well as components of basement membrane, laminin and type IV collagen. It has been shown that the matrix proteins themselves can serve as stimuli for migration of bronchial epithelial cells *in vitro* [48]. Among the ECM proteins, fibronectin appears to have a key role in airway epithelium repair. By immunocytochemistry, Hérard *et al.* [49] have shown that fibronectin is deposited at the airway cell–matrix interface during the wound repair process. In addition, the incubation of wounded cultures with antifibronectin antibody partially inhibits the wound closure. In association with the deposition of fibronectin, they also observed that the $\alpha_5\beta_1$-integrin, which is one of the fibronectin cellular receptors, was up-regulated in the migrating cells of the repairing area. Using an *in vivo* human/SCID mouse chimeric model of airway repair, Pilewski *et al.* [50] reported a similar induction of the $\alpha_5\beta_1$-integrin during wound repair. Airway epithelial cells may use other matrix receptors such as α-dystroglycan (a non-integrin laminin receptor) to facilitate spreading and migration during repair [51].

Non-integrin receptors such as CD44 and the receptor for hyaluronic acid mediated-mobility [52] may be also implicated in respiratory injury and repair. CD44 is responsible for binding to hyaluronic acid that serves as an anchor for secreted proteins and could possibly retain mitogenic and motogenic molecules involved in airway epithelial repair.

Apart from its functional role in cell adhesion via integrin receptors, cell surface glycosylation may mediate repair of human airway epithelial cells [53].

Airway stem cells and progenitor cells

The repair of injured airway epithelium involves stem cells and progenitor cells. Much evidence supports the presence of stem and or progenitor cells in the airways. Although the proliferation index is less than 0.2% in healthy bronchial epithelium [54], tissue homoeostasis exists, and denuded-graft experiments have shown the ability of airway epithelial cells to reform a complete array of tracheal and bronchial epithelial cells. For example, epithelial cells from human undifferentiated fetal trachea rudiments seeded on denuded human fetal tracheas and grafted on the back of tolerant mice are able to reform a fully differentiated airway epithelium [31]. In the same way, the presence of stem or progenitor cells in adult human bronchi [55] and adult human nasal polyps [26] has been suggested. Despite these results, the exact identity of airway stem cells remains to be determined.

The airways are classically subdivided in large cartilage-containing airways (trachea and bronchi) and small airways without cartilage (bronchioles). Although the concept of a single stem cell common to the epithelium of the whole respiratory organ has been proposed (for review, see Emura [56]), it is now accepted that each subdivision of the lung possesses its own stem cell.

Stem cells are quiescent undifferentiated cells able to divide slowly but indefinitely under particular conditions such as injury, to self-renew for their entire life span and to give rise to less proliferative committed daughter cells, called transient amplifying cells or progenitor cells [57]. Stem cells differentiate to form all the cell types of the tissue [58,59] and are therefore multipotent.

Tracheal and bronchial airway stem/progenitor cells

In order to determine the identity of stem cells in the tracheal and bronchial epithelium, metabolic labelling or Ki67 antigen immunodetection has been used to study the epithelial cell kinetics. The proliferation capacity of basal and secretory cells suggested that these cells were good candidates for stem or progenitor cell status [60–62]. In animals, the differentiation potential of purified subpopulations of airway epithelial cells has also been investigated by using xenograft models. After an initial step of cell separation based on elutriation or cell sorting, basal or secretory epithelial cells were seeded on tracheas depleted of their own epithelium and then transplanted. Authors reported the capacity of both basal and secretory cells to dedifferentiate into a similar highly proliferative phenotype called 'poorly differentiated cells' and then to redifferentiate and regenerate after 3–4 weeks of engraftment a pseudostratified mucociliary airway epithelium [63–65] with a respiratory gland network [66]. Based on evidence of stem cell niches in many organs such as intestine or skin, Borthwick *et al.* [24] have reported the existence of stem cell niches in airways characterized by slow-cycling cells able to retain the nucleotide analogue BrdU in their genomic DNA for long periods of time. These stem cell niches were principally localized in the gland ducts in the upper trachea of mice.

Bronchiolar stem cells

As in large cartilage-containing airways, the nature of proliferative cells in bronchioles has been investigated using Ki67 antigen immunodetection. In the terminal bronchioles of normal human airways, 15% of proliferating airway epithelial cells were Clara cells, and this percentage increased up to 44% in the respiratory bronchioles [67]. In the airways depleted of Clara cells, a normal epithelium could not be regenerated [68]. In rabbits, Clara cells separated by elutriation following Percoll density centrifugation and inoculated into denuded rat trachea were able to regenerate a cuboidal epithelium resembling that seen in normal bronchioles [69]. These data favour the concept that the Clara cells represent stem or progenitor cells of the bronchioles.

Bone-marrow-derived airway stem cells

It was previously thought that stem cells were tissue-specific but in the last decade, a number of studies has demonstrated that stem cells from one organ can differentiate into cells of another, and this is particularly true for bone-marrow-derived stem cells. This notion of 'cell plasticity' in the airways has primarily been reported by Krause *et al.* [70]. This group showed that a single stem cell from the bone marrow could not only repopulate an irradiated host, but was also able to generate cells found in several tissues. In the bronchi, these cells represented 3.7% of the total tissue cells. In humans, Kleeberger *et al.* [71] reported approximately 10% integration of recipient-derived cells in the bronchial epithelium for the patients with lung allograft, with a markedly high degree of chimerism (24%) in structures displaying signs of chronic injury. However, these exciting results apparently contradict the data of Davies *et al.* [72] who did not observe any differentiation of airway cells from bone marrow cells into the upper airway respiratory epithelium in the absence of infection and inflammation. These data suggest that airway injury is a prerequisite to the differentiation of bone-marrow cells into airway epithelial cells.

Although airway stem cell research extensively progressed during this last decade, the precise identity of human airway stem cells remains to be elucidated.

Strategies for future therapy of airway cytoprotection, repair and regeneration

Repair of the airway epithelium after injury is critical for the maintenance of the barrier function and the limitation of airway hyperreactivity. Future therapy of airway epithelial injury and repair should aim to improve the protection of airway epithelium against injury. In the case of severe injury, these therapies should enhance wound repair and epithelial function regeneration.

Based on *in vitro* and *in vivo* studies, growth factors have been shown to be able to stimulate cell proliferation and differentiation after injury. Among the different growth factors, EGF has been shown to promote wound repair almost *in vitro* [73]. Moreover, EGF enhances the number of β_2-adrenergic receptors (β_2-AR) [74]. The increase in β_2-AR could improve the effect of β_2-AR agonists such as salmeterol, which has been shown to protect the airway epithelial integrity via an increase in the TJ protein ZO-1 [75]. Recombinant EGF and β_2-AR agonists could therefore prevent the airway epithelium from deleterious insults and accelerate the re-epithelialization of wounded epithelia, which frequently occurs in viral and bacterial pathologies. Among the proteins able to limit airway epithelial injury, recombinant CC10 (rh CC10) protein has been reported to inhibit phospholipase A_2 and to possess anti-inflammatory properties. We can speculate that rh CC10 could represent a promising therapy not only for the prevention of lung therapy in preterm infants [76], but also for the prevention of airway and lung epithelial injury.

Other growth factors such as KGF have been reported to enhance alveolar epithelial repair by non-mitogenic mechanisms. Atabai *et al.* [77] have shown in rats that administration of KGF markedly improves the epithelial repair by altering cellular adherence, spreading and migration through stimulation of the EGF receptors. KGF is also able to accelerate wound closure in airway epithelium during cyclic mechanical strain and to protect from oxidant injury [78,79].

Apart from growth factors, antibiotics such as tetracyclins and cefazolin [80] have been shown to increase cell proliferation and differentiation and be helpful in protecting from cell damage and augmenting the healing of acute airway epithelial injury [79]. Future drugs should also include molecules that are capable to increase wound closure and to induce a completely reconstituted and regenerated functional airway epithelium.

In the long term, future therapy of repair and regeneration should be orientated toward the development of pharmacological molecules active on airway epithelial progenitor and stem cells. The identification of these cells represents a major challenge in the perspective of a reparative therapeutic approach to airway epithelium.

References

1 Jeffery PK. Microscopic structure of the lung. In: Gibson GJ, Geddes DM, Costabel U, Sterk P, Corrin B, eds. *Respiratory Medicine*. Saunders, 2003: 34–50.

2 Smith JJ. Fluid and electrolytic transport by cultured human airway epithelia. *J Clin Invest* 1993;**91**:1590–7.

3 Puchelle E, Gaillard D, Ploton D *et al.* Differential localization of the CFTR in normal and cystic fibrosis airway epithelium. *Am J Respir Cell Mol Biol* 1992;**7**:485–91.

4 Puchelle E, de Bentzmann S, Zahm JM *et al.* Defense properties of airway surface liquid. In: Gibson GJ, Geddes DM, Costabel U, Sterk P, Corrin B, eds. *Respiratory Medicine.* Saunders, 2003: 194–204.

5 Lamblin G, Aubert JP, Perini JM *et al.* Human respiratory mucins. *Eur Respir J* 1992;**5**:196–200.

6 Nelson S, Summer WR. Innate immunity, cytokines and pulmonary host defense. *Infect Dis Clin North Am* 1998;**12**: 555–67.

7 Koczulla R, von Degenfeld G, Kuppatt C *et al.* An angiogenic role for the human peptide LL-37/hCAP-1. *J Clin Invest* 2003; **111**:177–201.

8 Bals R, Wang X, Zasloff M *et al.* The peptide antibiotic LL-37/h CAP-18 is expressed in epithelia of the human lung where it has broad antimicrobial activity at the airway surface. *Proc Natl Acad Sci U S A* 1998;**95**:9541–6.

9 Crouch EC. Collectins and pulmonary host defense. *Am J Respir Cell Mol Biol* 1998;**19**:177–201.

10 Miele L. Antiflammins: bioactive peptides derived from uteroglobin. *Ann NY Acad Sci* 2000;**923**:128–40.

11 Wang SZ, Rosenberger CL, Bao YX *et al.* Clara cell secretory protein modulates lung inflammatory and immune responses to respiratory syncytial virus infection. *J Immunol* 2003;**171**: 1051–60.

12 Rahmzin I, MacNee W. Oxidative stress and regulation of glutathione in lung inflammation. *Eur Respir J* 2000;**16**:534.

13 Parks WC, Lopez-Boado YS, Wilson CL. Matrilysin in epithelial repair and defense. *Chest* 2001;**120**:36–41S.

14 Coyne CB, Vanhook MK, Gambling TM *et al.* Regulation of airway tight junctions by pro-inflammatory cytokines. *Mol Biol Cell* 2002;**13**:3218–34.

15 Azghani AO. *Pseudomonas aeruginosa* and epithelial permeability: role of virulence factors elastase and exotoxin A. *Am J Respir Cell Mol Biol* 1996;**15**:132–40.

16 Elias JA. Airway remodeling in asthma: unanswered questions. *Am J Respir Crit Care Med* 2000;**161**:S168–71.

17 Erjefält JS, Persson CGA. Airway epithelial repair: breathtakingly quick and multipotentially pathogenic. *Thorax* 1997;**52**: 1010–2.

18 Gaillard D, Jouet JB, Egreteau L *et al.* Airway epithelial damage and inflammation in children with recurrent bronchitis. *Am J Respir Crit Care Med* 1994;**150**:810–7.

19 Puchelle E, Zahm JM. Repair processes of the airway epithelium. In: Chretien J, Dusser D, eds. *Environmental Impact of Airways: From Injury to Repair*. New York: Dekker, 1996: 157–82.

20 Keenan KP, Combs JW, McDowell EM. Regeneration of hamster tracheal epithelium after mechanical injury. *Virchows Arch B Cell Pathol* 1982;**41**:193–214.

21 Ramphal R, Small PM, Shands JW *et al.* Adherence of *Pseudomonas aeruginosa* to tracheal cells injured by influenza infection or by endotracheal incubation. *Infect Immun* 1990; **27**:614–9.

22 Johnson NF, Hubbs AF. Epithelial progenitor cells in the rat trachea. *Am J Respir Cell Mol Biol* 1990;**3**:579–85.

23 Shimizu T, Nettesheim P, Ramaekers FC. Expression of 'cell-type-specific markers' during rat tracheal epithelial regeneration. *Am J Respir Cell Mol Biol* 1992;**7**:30–41.

24 Borthwick DW, Shabazian M, Krantz QT *et al.* Evidence for stem cell niches in the tracheal epithelium. *Am J Respir Cell Mol Biol* 2001;**24**:662–70.

25 Puchelle E, Peault B. Human airway xenograft models of epithelial cell regeneration. *Respir Med* 2002;**1**:125–8.

26 Dupuit F, Gaillard D, Hinnrasky J *et al.* Differentiated and functional human airway epithelium regeneration in tracheal xenografts. *Am J Physiol Lung Cell Mol Physiol* 2000;**278**: L165–76.

27 Engelhardt JF, Yankaskas JR, Wilson JM. *In vivo* retroviral gene transfer into human bronchial epithelia of xenografts. *J Clin Invest* 1992;**90**:2598–607.

28 Escotte S, Danel C, Gaillard D *et al.* Fluticasone propionate inhibits lipopolysaccharide-induced pro-inflammatory response in human cystic fibrosis airway grafts. *J Pharmacol Exp Ther* 2002;**302**:1151–7.

29 Lim FY, Kobinger GP, Weiner DJ *et al.* Human fetal trachea-SCID-mouse xenograft: efficacy of vesicular stomatis virus-G pseudotyped lentiviral-mediated gene transfer. *J Pediatr Surg* 2003;**38**:834–9.

30 Peault B, Tirouvanziam R, Sombardier MN *et al.* Gene transfer to human fetal pulmonary tissue developed in immunodeficient SCID mice. *Hum Gene Ther* 1994;**5**:1131–7.

31 Delplanque A, Coraux C, Tirouvanziam R *et al.* Epithelial

stem cell-mediated development of the human respiratory mucosa in SCID mice. *J Cell Sci* 2000;**113**:767–78.

32 Tirouvanziam R, Desternes A, Saari A *et al.* Bioelectric properties of human cystic fibrosis and non-cystic fibrosis fetal tracheal xenografts in SCID mice. *Am J Physiol* 1998;**274**:875–82.

33 Zahm JM, Kaplan H, Hérard AL *et al.* Cell migration and proliferation during the *in vitro* wound repair of the respiratory epithelium. *Cell Motil Cytoskeleton* 1997;**37**:33–43.

34 Legrand C, Gilles SC, Zahm JM. Airway epithelial cell migration dynamics: MM.9 role in cell–extracellular matrix remodeling. *J Cell Biol* 2000;**146**:517–29.

35 Jorissen M, Van der Schueren B, Van der Berghe H *et al.* The preservation and regeneration of cilia on human nasal epithelial cells cultured *in vitro.* *Arch Otorhinolaryngol* 1989; **246**:308–14.

36 Castillon N, Hinnrasky J, Zahm JM *et al.* Polarized expression of cystic fibrosis transmembrane conductance regulator and associated epithelial proteins during the regeneration of human airway surface epithelium in three-dimensional culture. *Lab Invest* 2002;**82**:989–98.

37 Erjefält JS, Korsgren M, Nilsson MC *et al.* Prompt epithelial damage and restitution processes in allergen challenged guinea-pig trachea. *Clin Exp Allergy* 1997;**27**:1344–55.

38 Sato Y, Ohshima T, Kondo T. Regulatory role of endogenous interleukin-10 in cutaneous inflammatory response of murine wound healing. *Biochem Biophys Res Commun* 1999;**265**:104–99.

39 Buisson AC, Zahm JM, Polette M. Gelatinase B is involved in the *in vitro* wound repair of human respiratory epithelium. *J Cell Physiol* 1996;**166**:413–26.

40 Planus E, Galliacy S, Matthay M. Role of collagenase in mediating *in vitro* alveolar epithelial wound repair. *J Cell Sci* 1999;**112**:243–52.

41 Dunsmore SE, Saarialho-Kere UK, Roby JD *et al.* Matrilysin expression and function in airway epithelium. *J Clin Invest* 1998;**102**:1321–31.

42 McGuire JK, Li Q, Parks WC. Matrilysin (matrix metalloproteinase-7) mediates E-cadherin ectodomain shedding in injured lung epithelium. *Am J Pathol* 2003;**162**:1831–43.

43 Coraux C, Martinella-Catusse C, Nawrocki-Raby B *et al.* Differential expression of matrix metalloproteinases and interleukin-8 during regeneration of human airway epithelium *in vivo.* *J Pathol* 2005;**206**:160–9.

44 Zahm JM, Pierrot D, Puchelle E. Epidermal growth factor promotes wound repair of human respiratory epithelium. *Wound Repair Regen* 1993;**1**:175–80.

45 Kim JS, McKinnis VS, Nawrocki A *et al.* Stimulation of migration and wound repair regeneration of guinea-pig airway epithelial cells in response to epidermal growth factor. *Am J Respir Cell Mol Biol* 1998;**18**:66–74.

46 Oertel M, Graness A, Thim L *et al.* Trefoil factor family-peptides promote migration of human bronchial epithelial cells: synergic effect with epidermal growth factor. *Am J Respir Cell Mol Biol* 2001;**25**:418–24.

47 Albeda SM. Endothelial and epithelial cell adhesion molecules. *Am J Respir Cell Mol Biol* 1991;**4**:195–203.

48 Rickard KA, Taylor J, Rennard SI *et al.* Migration of bovine bronchial epithelial cells to extracellular matrix components. *Am J Respir Cell Mol Biol* 1993;**8**:63–8.

49 Hérard AL, Zahm JM, Pierrot D. Epithelial barrier integrity during *in vitro* wound repair of the airway epithelium. *Am J Respir Cell Mol Biol* 1996;**15**:624–32.

50 Pilewski J, Latoche JD, Arcasoy SM *et al.* Expression of integrin cell adhesion receptors during human airway epithelial repair *in vivo.* *Am J Physiol Lung Cell Mol Physiol* 1997;**17**:L256–63.

51 White SR, Wojcik KR, Gruenert D *et al.* Airway epithelial cell wound repair mediated by alpha-dystroglycan. *Am J Respir Cell Mol Biol* 2001;**24**:179–86.

52 Cheung WF, Cruz TF, Turley EA. Receptor for hyaluronan-mediated motility (RHAMM) a hyaladerin that regulated cell response to growth factors. *Biochem Soc Trans* 1999;**27**: 135–42.

53 Dorscheid DR, Wojcik KR, Yule K *et al.* Role of cell surface glycosylation in mediating repair of human airway epithelial cell monolayers. *Am J Physiol Lung Cell Mol Physiol* 2001;**28**: L982–91.

54 Leigh MW, Kylander JE, Yankaskas JR *et al.* Cell proliferation in bronchial epithelium and submucosal glands of cystic fibrosis patients. *Am J Respir Cell Mol Biol* 1995;**12**:605–12.

55 Zepeda ML, Chinoy MR, Wilson JM. Characterization of stem cells in human airway capable of reconstituting a fully differentiated bronchial epithelium. *Somat Cell Mol Genet* 1995;**21**:61–73.

56 Emura M. Stem cells of the respiratory epithelium and their *in vitro* cultivation. *In Vitro Cell Dev Biol Anim* 1997;**33**:3–14.

57 Lajtha LG. Stem cell concepts. *Differentiation* 1979;**14**:23–34.

58 Slack JMW. Stem cells in epithelial tissues. *Science* 2000;**287**: 1431–3.

59 Hall PA, Watt FM. Stem cells: the generation and maintenance of cellular diversity. *Development* 1989;**106**:619–33.

60 Boers JE, Ambergen AW, Thunnissen FBJM. Number and proliferation of Clara cells in normal human airway epithelium. *Am J Respir Crit Care Med* 1999;**159**:1585–91.

61 Breuer R, Zajicek G, Christensen TG *et al.* Cell kinetics of normal hamster bronchial epithelium in the steady state. *Am J Respir Cell Mol Biol* 1990;**2**:51–8.

62 Evans MJ, Shami SG, Cabral-Anderson LJ *et al.* Role of non-ciliated cells in renewal of the bronchial epithelium of rats exposed to NO_2. *Am J Pathol* 1986;**123**:126–33.

63 Liu JY, Nettesheim P, Randell SH. Growth and differentiation of tracheal progenitor cells. *Am J Physiol Lung Cell Mol Physiol* 1994;**266**:L296–307.

64 Randell SH, Comment CE, Ramaekers FCS *et al.* Properties of rat tracheal epithelial cells separated based on expression of cell surface α-galactosyl end groups. *Am J Respir Cell Mol Biol* 1991;**4**:544–54.

65 Inayama Y, Hook GER, Brody AR *et al.* The differentiation potential of tracheal basal cells. *Lab Invest* 1988;**58**:706–17.

66 Engelhardt JF, Schlossberg H, Yankaskas JR *et al.* Progenitor cells of the adult human airway involved in submucosal gland development. *Development* 1995;**121**:2031–46.

67 Boers JE, Ambergen AW, Thunnissen FBJM. Number and proliferation of basal and parabasal cells in normal human airway epithelium. *Am J Respir Crit Care Med* 1998;**157**:2000–6.

68 Hong KU, Reynolds SD, Giangreco A *et al.* Clara cell secretory protein-expressing cells of the airway neuroepithelial body microenvironment include a label-retaining subset and are

critical for epithelial renewal after progenitor cell depletion. *Am J Respir Cell Mol Biol* 2001;**24**:671–81.

69 Brody AR, Hook GE, Cameron GS *et al.* The differentiation capacity of Clara cells isolated from the lungs of rabbits. *Lab Invest* 1987;**57**:219–29.

70 Krause DS, Theise ND, Collector MI. Multi-organ, multi-lineage engraftment by a single bone marrow-derived stem cell. *Cell* 2001;**105**:369–77.

71 Kleeberger W, Versmold A, Rothamel T. Increased chimerism of bronchial and alveolar epithelium in human lung allografts undergoing chronic injury. *Am J Pathol* 2003;**162**:1487–94.

72 Davies JC, Potter M, Bush A *et al.* Bone marrow stem cells do not repopulate the healthy upper respiratory tract. *Pediatr Pulmonol* 2002;**34**:251–6.

73 Barrow RE, Wang CZ, Evans MJ *et al.* Growth factors accelerate epithelial repair in sheep trachea. *Lung* 1993;**171**:335–44.

74 Yeh CK, Hymer TK, Sousa AL *et al.* Epidermal growth factor upregulates β-adrenergic receptor signaling in a human salivary cell line. *Am J Physiol Cell Physiol* 2003;**284**:C1164–75.

75 Coraux C, Kileztky C, Polette M *et al.* Airway epithelial integrity is protected by a long-acting β$_2$-adrenergic receptor agonist. *Am J Respir Cell Mol Biol* 2004;**30**:605–12.

76 Chandra S, Davis JM, Drexler S *et al.* Safety and efficacy of intratracheal recombinant human Clara cell protein in a newborn piglet model of acute lung injury. *Pediatr Res* 2003;**54**:509–15.

77 Atabai K, Ishigaki M, Geiser T *et al.* Keratinocyte growth factor can enhance alveolar epithelial repair by non-mitogenic mechanisms. *Am J Physiol Lung Cell Mol Physiol* 2002;**283**:L163–9.

78 Waters CM, Savla U. Keratinocyte growth factor accelerates wound closure in airway epithelium during cyclic mechanical strain. *J Cell Physiol* 1999;**181**:424–32.

79 Chapman KE. Continuous exposure of airway epithelial cells to hydrogen peroxide: protection by KGF. *J Cell Physiol* 2002;**192**:71–80.

80 Barrow RE. Efficacy of cefazolin in promoting ovine tracheal epithelial repair. *Respiration* 1993;**171**:335–44.

CHAPTER 23
The role of the neutrophil in the pathogenesis of COPD

Ian S. Woolhouse and Robert A. Stockley

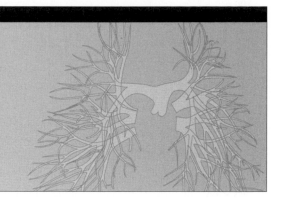

The neutrophil is the most abundant circulating leucocyte. It is derived from pluripotential stem cells in the bone marrow and is characterized by the presence of a multilobed nucleus and cytoplasmic granules. The primary, or azurophilic granules contain many of the important proteins required in host defence, including the proteinases (elastase, proteinase-3 and cathepsin G), antibacterial proteins (such as the defensins, lysozyme and azurocidin) and the enzyme myeloperoxidase. However, the capacity of the neutrophil and its products for bacterial killing carries with it an implicit capacity for host tissue destruction.

The neutrophil has been implicated in the pathogenesis of chronic lung disease for over 30 years. The association dates back to an observation in 1963 that severe early-onset emphysema was associated with deficiency of α_1-antitrypsin, the serum inhibitor of the proteolytic enzyme neutrophil elastase [1]. This led to the proteinase–antiproteinase theory of the pathogenesis of emphysema and subsequent studies, both in animal models and human subjects, have led to this theory being widely accepted as a key mechanism of disease development.

This chapter reviews the data implicating the neutrophil in the pathogenesis of COPD, summarizes the process of neutrophil recruitment to the lungs from bone marrow production through to migration into the airways, outlines the mechanisms of neutrophil-mediated connective tissue destruction and, finally, discusses the neutrophil as a target for anti-inflammatory therapy in COPD.

Evidence for the role of the neutrophil in the pathogenesis of COPD

Animal models

Animal studies have been critical in understanding the role of the neutrophil and its products in the pathogenesis of

COPD. Early studies using intrapulmonary challenges demonstrated that proteinases, including human neutrophil elastase, can lead to the development of emphysema, when instilled into the lungs of experimental animals [2,3], as a result of elastin degradation. Subsequent studies confirmed that neutrophil elastase is also able to induce other features of COPD, including mucous gland hyperplasia, excessive mucus secretion, bronchial hyperresponsiveness and tissue damage a short time after instillation into the airways [4–6].

However, recently it has been shown that a variety of metalloproteinases can also degrade elastin and that mice lacking macrophage metalloelastase 12 (MMP-12) do not develop smoke-induced emphysema [7,8]. These findings led to an alternative hypothesis in which macrophages and macrophage-derived metalloproteases were thought to be responsible for the development of emphysema. However, new studies have re-emphasized the importance of neutrophil-derived proteases and their inhibitor α_1-antitrypsin. Using a mouse model, Dhami *et al.* [9] and Churg *et al.* [10] have demonstrated that both MMP-12 and neutrophils are required for acute smoke-induced matrix breakdown, the precursor of emphysema. This process appears to be mediated by MMP-12 induced release of tumour necrosis factor-α from alveolar macrophages, with subsequent endothelial activation, neutrophil influx and connective tissue destruction by neutrophil-derived proteases [11]. In addition, the same group has demonstrated that exogenous administration of α_1-antitrypsin ameliorates both the acute and chronic connective tissue destruction seen in this mouse model of cigarette smoke-induced emphysema [9,12], providing further evidence for the role of neutrophil-derived proteases in the pathogenesis of COPD.

Human studies

Early studies on patients with chronic bronchitis

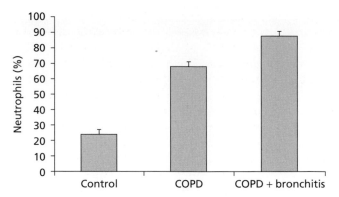

Figure 23.1 The proportion of neutrophils identified in induced sputum samples is shown for healthy control subjects and subjects with COPD. In addition, the proportion of neutrophils is shown for COPD patients who have chronic cough and sputum expectoration.

demonstrated an increased percentage of neutrophils in bronchoalveolar lavage fluid compared with asymptomatic smokers, which was greater the worse the airflow obstruction [13–15]. In addition to greater numbers of neutrophils in the bronchoalveolar fluid from patients with COPD, subsequent studies also demonstrated the presence of increased markers of neutrophil activation, in particular myeloperoxidase and interleukin 8 (IL-8) [16,17].

These results have been reproduced in studies examining neutrophil counts and markers of neutrophil activation in sputum from patients with COPD, confirming the presence of neutrophilic inflammation in the larger airways, as well the peripheral airways of smokers with COPD (Fig. 23.1) [18–20]. Furthermore, the observed association between neutrophilic airway inflammation and the severity and rapidity of airflow obstruction [20,21] provides further support for the role of the neutrophil in the progression of the disease.

Although the airway lumen in smokers with COPD displays a neutrophilic inflammation, studies of tissue inflammatory cell response in these patients have produced conflicting results. Saetta *et al.* [22] and Di Stefano *et al.* [23] have demonstrated increased numbers of neutrophils in the bronchial glands of smokers with chronic bronchitis and in the bronchial subepithelium of smokers with severe airflow obstruction. However, the same group found that numbers of CD8+ lymphocytes, not neutrophils, were increased in the peripheral airways epithelium and alveolar walls of smokers with COPD, compared with smokers without airflow obstruction [24,25]. Other histological studies have confirmed increased numbers of CD8+ lymphocytes in the alveolar walls of smokers with emphysema [26], although patients with severe airflow obstruction also had significantly increased numbers of neutrophils [27]. The

precise role of the lymphocyte in the pathogenesis of COPD remains unclear and the discrepancy between the increased presence of neutrophils in the airway but not tissues may be explained by selective passage of neutrophils across the epithelium into the airway lumen.

During exacerbations of COPD there is a further increase in the number of airway neutrophils [28], although the role of the neutrophil in exacerbations is uncertain. Many of these episodes are related to bacterial infection, therefore the neutrophil response is likely to represent an important component of secondary host responses. However, the recruitment of neutrophils during exacerbations is also associated with a rise in neutrophil activation markers, in particular neutrophil elastase, myeloperoxidase (MPO), leukotriene (LT) B$_4$ and (in severe episodes) IL-8 [29–31], all of which have the potential to perpetuate the inflammatory process and hence lead to further bronchial damage. Studies of bronchial neutrophilic inflammation during exacerbations show resolution usually within 5 days following treatment, and this parallels clinical recovery [30].

Neutrophil differentiation and maturation

Neutrophil differentiation occurs entirely within the bone marrow, where several distinct stages can be recognized. In the first stage, which takes 5–7 days, the cells divide and differentiate from myeloblasts to form promyelocytes. During this period the primary, or azurophilic, granules, which contain the proteinases elastase, proteinase-3 and cathepsin G, antibacterial proteins such as the defensins, lysozyme and azurocidin and the enzyme myeloperoxidase are produced. The secondary, or specific granules, which contain collagenase, lactoferrin and gelatinase, among other proteins, are formed as the cell proceeds to the metamyelocytic stage. Cell divisions ensure that all cells contain a full complement of primary and secondary granules. From the metamyelocyte stage onwards the cells no longer undergo division but mature through a recognized band cell stage to form adult neutrophils. At maturity, neutrophils develop highly mobilizable secretory granules with adhesion molecules and cytochrome b_{558} on their surface. This whole process takes approximately 2 weeks, with the mature cells remaining in the bone marrow for a further 2 days before being released into the circulation, where they have a half-life of 8 h [32].

A number of studies have demonstrated that cigarette smoke exposure has a stimulatory effect on this process within the bone marrow causing peripheral blood leucocytosis and neutrophilia [33,34]. In addition, total peripheral blood leucocyte count has been found to correlate inversely with absolute forced expiratory volume in 1 s (FEV_1) values [35,36]. These observations are consistent with the hypothesis that the neutrophil is of major importance in the pathogenesis of COPD, and higher numbers of this cell within peripheral blood (resulting from increased bone marrow production) may be related to the severity of airflow obstruction, as increased numbers of neutrophils are available for recruitment to the airways which would lead to increased elastase-mediated connective tissue destruction.

Neutrophil recruitment to the lungs

The walls of the bronchi and bronchioles are supplied with systemic blood through the bronchial arteries, which are derived from the descending aorta and the intercostal and internal mammary arteries [37]. Microvascular injection techniques demonstrate an extremely rich vascular network supplying the airway wall [38]. The alveoli receive their blood supply from the pulmonary circulation via branches of the pulmonary artery, which divides to form a meshwork of short capillary segments in close contact with the alveolar space.

The relative contribution of the bronchial and pulmonary circulation to the blood supply of human lungs is not know. Although studies in dogs using fluorescent microspheres have demonstrated that 97% of the blood supply to the intraparenchymal airways down to 1 mm in diameter comes from the bronchial circulation [39], whether this is the same in humans remains unknown and very little is known of the relative contributions of the two circulations to neutrophil recruitment in COPD. In healthy sheep, 50–60% of radiolabelled neutrophils in the bronchial vasculature are retained, compared with 80% of those in the pulmonary circulation being retained [40]. Given the presence of neutrophils and their products at bronchial and alveolar level in patients with COPD, one may assume that neutrophil migration occurs from both the bronchial and pulmonary circulations. The mechanisms of neutrophil recruitment to the lung are thought to differ according to the site of migration, which may have implications in terms of the pathological features of COPD and potential new therapies.

Neutrophil migration in the bronchial circulation

Neutrophil traffic into the bronchial submucosa occurs via the bronchial circulation and is assumed to follow the complex multistep process seen elsewhere in the systemic circulation (i.e. cell capture, rolling, activation and arrest) [41,42].

Initiation of migration begins with capture of neutrophils from flowing blood and subsequent rolling along the endothelial surface in postcapillary venules, which is a normal feature of circulating neutrophils. This process is mediated through reversible binding of a group of transmembrane glycoprotein adhesion molecules known as the selectins. Leucocyte (L) selectin is constitutively expressed on projecting microvilli of circulating neutrophils. It is responsible for early, rapid and short-lived binding to an endothelial ligand that has yet to be fully characterized, but is thought to be a fucosylated variant of CD34, a member of a group of sialomucin oligosaccharides that share affinity for selectins [43–45]. Platelet (P) selectin, which is stored intracellularly in Weibel–Palade bodies of endothelial cells, is mobilized to the endothelial surface within minutes of exposure to inflammatory mediators such as histamine, thrombin and various cytokines [46,47]. The neutrophil counterligand for P-selectin is glycoprotein ligand-1, and binding to this receptor results in slower rolling velocities and eventual tethering of the neutrophil to the vessel surface [48]. Endothelial (E) selectin can also support rolling and tethering of neutrophils in a similar fashion to P-selectin [49]. The ligand for E-selectin has not yet been fully characterized; however, it may be a uniquely modified mucin known as E-selectin ligand-1 [50]. E-selectin, unlike P-selectin, is not stored intracellularly and therefore peak expression is not seen until 4–6 h after exposure to pro-inflammatory cytokines [51]. Thus, the role of E-selectin may be to maintain neutrophil rolling after P-selectin has been down-regulated [52].

The next step in transendothelial migration is the transition from neutrophil rolling to firm adhesion to the vessel wall. The initiating signal for this may be either a receptor-mediated response to endothelial presented cytokine [53,54] or an event propagated by selectin activation [55], leading to up-regulation of a group of heterodimeric transmembrane glycoproteins on the neutrophil surface known as integrins. Neutrophil binding to activated endothelium is mediated primarily by two integrins that consist of β_2 (CD18) subunits. These are lymphocyte-associated function antigen-1 (LFA-1; CD11a/CD18) and macrophage antigen-1 (Mac-1; CD11b/CD18). A third CD18 integrin, p150,95 (CD11c/CD18) can also promote neutrophil trafficking; however, Mac-1 has emerged as the critical CD18 integrin in many models of neutrophil migration [56,57]. Preformed Mac-1 is stored within neutrophil granules [58] and can be rapidly mobilized to the neutrophil surface after exposure to stimuli such as bacterial peptides including formyl-methionyl-leucyl-phenylalanine (fMLP), LTB_4 and the CXC chemokines such as IL-8 [54,59]. β_2-Integrins, and especially Mac-1, have high affinity for intercellular adhesion molecule-1 (ICAM-1) [56], an immunoglobulin-like molecule expressed constitutively in low levels on endothelial cell membranes and rapidly up-regulated following exposure to inflammatory cytokines such as tumour necrosis factor α (TNF-α) and IL-1β [51,60].

The final step of neutrophil recruitment from the blood stream into the lungs is transendothelial migration; however, the mechanisms of neutrophil extravasation are incompletely understood. Transmigration through endothelial cell monolayers *in vitro* occurs preferentially at tricellular junctions [61] and the immunoglobulin G (IgG) type adhesion molecule, platelet–endothelial cell adhesion molecule-1 (PECAM-1; CD31) appears to be critical [62]. PECAM-1 is found on neutrophils and endothelial cells, where it is concentrated at intercellular junctions [63]. Treatment of neutrophils or endothelial monolayers with antibodies to PECAM-1 can block transmigration [64].

Even less is known of the mechanisms of migration through the subendothelial matrix. Adhesion and migration is accompanied by release of neutrophil-derived proteases [65] and both chemotaxis and migration through artificial substances can be inhibited by antiproteases [66]. However, protease inhibitors appear to have no effect on neutrophil migration through intact endothelial cell monolayers [67].

In COPD, studies examining the expression of the adhesion molecule thought to be important in neutrophil migration from the bronchial circulation have produced conflicting results. Noguera *et al.* [68] demonstrated increased surface expression of Mac-1 (CD11b) in smokers with COPD compared with those with normal lung function. However, Gonzalez *et al.* [69] found similar levels of neutrophil adhesion molecule expression in lungs resected from smokers with and without airflow obstruction, although neutrophil activation during the migration process may have affected these results. Similarly, conflicting evidence exists for the expression of the endothelial ligands for neutrophils in COPD. In one study, increased plasma levels of the soluble adhesion molecules ICAM-1 and E-selectin were demonstrated in COPD patients with chronic bronchitis [70], whereas another found that levels of soluble ICAM-1 were lower in the COPD group compared with healthy controls [71].

Nevertheless, neutrophils from patients with chronic bronchitis and emphysema do demonstrate enhanced chemotaxis across an inert membrane [72] and data from our laboratory show that neutrophil endothelial interactions under flow are increased in smokers with COPD compared with smokers without the disease (Fig. 23.2) [73]. This was associated with increased expression of Mac-1 upon neutrophil stimulation, suggesting that the up-regulation of this molecule is responsible for the enhanced endothelial interactions seen in COPD.

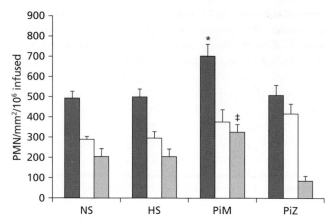

Figure 23.2 The adhesive and migratory response of purified neutrophils from never smokers (NS), healthy smokers (HS), COPD patients with normal levels of α_1-AT (PiM) and COPD patients with α_1-AT deficiency (PiZ). Data are mean ± SE. Black bars indicate total neutrophil–endothelial interactions, open bars indicate adherent neutrophils and light grey bars indicate migrated neutrophils. * $P < 0.05$.
‡ $P = 0.001$ vs NS, HS and PiZ. PMN, neutrophils.

Neutrophil migration in the pulmonary circulation

The basic mechanisms of neutrophil trafficking in the pulmonary circulation are far less well understood but there appear to be differences compared with the systemic circulation.

In normal lungs, the pulmonary capillary bed contains a large pool of marginated neutrophils [74], and in animal models of acute pulmonary inflammation neutrophil sequestration occurs from the pulmonary capillary bed, not from the postcapillary venules [75,76], with no requirement for conventional adhesion molecules [77,78].

Human studies examining the passage of radiolabelled autologous neutrophils through the pulmonary vasculature in patients with stable COPD and in resected lung specimens confirmed slower neutrophil transit times (relative to red blood cells) but no difference in sequestration compared with disease-free controls [79,80]. The exception were neutrophils from COPD patients experiencing an acute exacerbations, where sequestration in the pulmonary vasculature was increased. The clinical relevance of this observation is not clear given that the neutrophilic inflammation seen during exacerbations of COPD occurs predominantly at the bronchial level [81].

The increased transit time and sequestration of neutrophils in the capillary bed is thought to be a result of the need for neutrophils to deform to an oblong shape to pass through the 40–60% of pulmonary capillary segments that are narrower than spherical neutrophils [82]. This delayed passage of neutrophils through the relatively narrow vessels may be increased further during acute inflammatory responses, as neutrophils become less deformable upon activation [83,84].

Once sequestered in the pulmonary capillaries, neutrophil transmigration can occur through at least two pathways: one that uses the adhesion molecule CD11/CD18 and one that does not. The pathway selected appears to depend upon the stimulus and the level of neutrophil activation. In animal models, stimuli that can induce CD11/CD18-independent neutrophil emigration include *Streptococcus pneumoniae, Staphylococcus aureus* and hydrochloric acid. In humans, CD11/CD18-independent neutrophil migration has been demonstrated towards the host-derived chemoattractants IL-8 and LTB$_4$ but not towards the bacterial-derived peptide fMLP [85,86]. The mechanisms of CD11/CD18-independent migration are not understood; however, γ-interferon might be an important regulator of the response [41].

The only study examining the role of CD18 in transendothelial migration of neutrophils from patients with chronic pulmonary inflammation, including those with COPD, found that the requirement for this adhesion molecule did not differ from control neutrophils [87]. However, these studies were performed using static transwell assays with pulmonary artery endothelium, which has a different adhesion molecule profile to pulmonary microvascular endothelium. This may explain the surprising observation of a higher percentage of migrated neutrophils in the control group compared with both the acute and chronic pulmonary inflammation groups in this study.

Soluble mediators of neutrophil migration

Pro-migratory stimuli for neutrophils can be classified generally as either non-chemotactic cytokines, chemoattractants or chemotactic cytokines (chemokines).

Two of the most important pro-adhesive cytokines that are present in most inflammatory responses are TNF-α and IL-1β. The macrophage–monocyte is the primary cellular source of TNF-α and IL-1β, but these cytokines are also produced by airway epithelium, endothelial cells and mast cells [88,89]. Both neutrophils and endothelial cells possess receptors for TNF-α and IL1-β. Neutrophils respond to TNF-α and IL-1β by activating and expressing integrins, and likewise, endothelial cells mobilize selectins and up-regulate ICAM-1 [51,90]. Thus, the early appearance of TNF-α and IL-1β in plasma during inflammation is likely to be critical for the capture and firm adhesion of neutrophils to vascular endothelium. Although TNF-α and IL-1β are not themselves chemotactic for neutrophils, their exposure to endothelial cells can elicit transendothelial migration through production of endothelial-derived chemoattractants [91].

Sputum levels of TNF-α are increased in smokers with COPD, both in the stable clinical state and during exacerbations [31,92,93]. Similarly, alveolar macrophage release of IL-1β is increased in COPD [94] and in one study the concentration of IL-1β in the sputum of patients with chronic bronchitis and bronchiectasis was an order of magnitude higher than TNF-α [95], suggesting an important role for IL-1β, in conjunction with TNF-α, in the pathogenesis of COPD.

In addition to non-chemotactic cytokine receptors, neutrophils have at least five different receptors for chemotactic stimuli. A number of chemotactic stimuli have been implicated in the pathogenesis of COPD, in particular the potent neutrophil chemoattractant LTB$_4$ and the chemokine IL-8.

Leukotriene B$_4$ is produced from arachidonic acid, a major component of cell membranes [96], mainly by monocytes, alveolar macrophages and activated neutrophils. The release of LTB$_4$ can be stimulated by a number of other inflammatory mediators, including complement factor C5a, IL-1β, TNF-α, granulocyte–macrophage colony-stimulating factor (GM-CSF), platelet-activating factor (PAF), neutrophil elastase and LTB$_4$ itself [97,98]. As well as being an important and potent neutrophil chemoattractant, LTB$_4$ also increases aggregation and chemokinesis of these cells [99]. Its activity is mediated by two sets of neutrophil surface receptors. Low-affinity receptors mediate degranulation and increased oxidative metabolism and their high-affinity counterparts influence aggregation, chemokinesis and increased adherence, via the neutrophil adhesion molecule Mac-1 [59]. LTB$_4$ can also promote neutrophil transendothelial migration *in vitro* by directly activating endothelial cell monolayers, although the mechanism underlying this observation remains unclear [100].

Interleukin-8 is a 16-kDa protein that is produced by endothelial cells, bronchial epithelial cells, monocytes, macrophages and activated neutrophils [54,101]. It is a potent neutrophil chemoattractant and activator, resulting in up-regulation of the adhesion molecule Mac-1 [59,102]. Production of IL-8 can be stimulated by exposure to IL-1β and TNF-α [103], cigarette smoke extract [104], bacterial endotoxin [105] and possibly neutrophil elastase [106]. Thus, IL-8 is involved in both the neutrophil adhesive process within the vessel, via its endothelial production and presentation following cytokine stimulation, and chemotaxis into the airway, via the directional gradient found across the bronchial wall resulting from the production of IL-8 by activated epithelial cells, macrophages and neutrophils.

In COPD, a number of studies have demonstrated increased sputum levels of LTB$_4$ and IL-8 [92,107]. In addition, the concentrations of LTB$_4$ and IL-8 correlate with markers of neutrophil activation and elastase activity [20] in these patients. Taking these data together suggests an important role for these two chemoattractants in the neutrophil recruitment seen in COPD. This has been confirmed in two recent studies with an LTB_4 receptor antagonist and mouse anti-IL-8 antibody. Both studies demonstrated that approximately 50% of the chemotactic activity of sputum in COPD is accounted for by LTB_4 and 30% by IL-8 [108,109]. In addition, Woolhouse *et al.* [108] found that sputum concentration of LTB_4, but not IL-8, correlated with overall chemotactic activity, suggesting that LTB_4 is of particular importance with respect to sputum chemotactic activity in the stable clinical state, and may be central to the increased neutrophil recruitment seen in COPD patients (Fig. 23.3).

The remaining sputum neutrophil chemotactic activity, unaccounted for by LTB_4 or IL-8, could come from other chemoattractants such as the chemokines $GRO\alpha$ and ENA-78, which are known to be present in the bronchial secretions of patients with COPD [110,111]. Other chemotactic agents that could have a role in the airways include C5a [112]; elastase–inhibitor complexes [113]; protein and peptide components of damaged extracellular matrix such as collagen [114], elastin [115] and laminin [116]; α_1-antitrypsin polymers [117] and bacterial products such as fMLP [118]. However, to date there are no studies examining the contribution of these chemoattractants in the secretions of patients with COPD.

Neutrophil effector function in COPD

Once the neutrophil has passed from the blood stream into the interstitium and then the airways, there are a number of mechanisms through which it can cause the pathological features seen in COPD.

The first and, as discussed above, probably the most important mechanism is via the release of the serine proteinases from the azurophil granules, in particular neutrophil elastase, which leads to the breakdown of connective tissue and subsequent airflow obstruction. The mechanisms by which neutrophils degranulate are not completely understood, but studies have shown that granule release is dependent either on protein kinase C and/or on cyclic guanosine 3′,5′-monophosphate-dependent kinase activation [119,120].

It has been known for some time that neutrophils from patients with COPD exhibit greater extracellular proteolysis when compared with those from smokers without the disease [72]; however, it is only relatively recently that studies have helped to explain how neutrophil elastase causes connective tissue damage in patients with COPD, despite normal serum and lung levels of the antiprotease α_1-AT [121].

Neutrophil elastase is stored within the azurophil granules at a concentration of approximately 5 mmol. Following neutrophil activation, the granules undergo exocytosis and as the enzyme diffuses away from the granule, its concentration decreases. Antiproteases, such as α_1-AT, inactivate neutrophil elastase on a 1 : 1 molecule : molecule basis. The concentration of α_1-AT in the interstitium is unknown; however, albumin (which is the same molecular size as α_1-AT) is thought to be present in the interstitium at approximately 80% of the concentration in the serum [122]. Because the serum concentration of α_1-AT in healthy subjects is approximately 30 μmol, the predicted concentration of α_1-AT in the lung interstitium of healthy subjects should be approximately 24 μmol, which is 200 times lower than the concentration of elastase in the azurophil granule. Thus, active neutrophil elastase diffuses away from the granule until the concentration has fallen sufficiently for the enzyme to be completely inactivated by the local

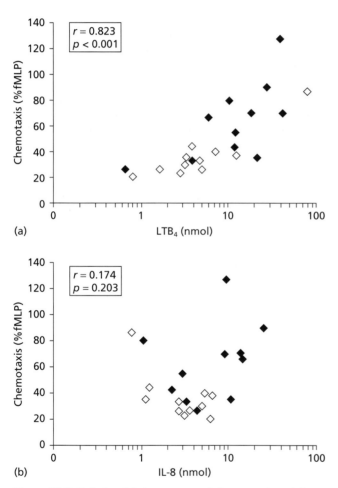

Figure 23.3 Relationship between total chemotactic activity and the contribution made by: (a) LTB_4; and (b) IL-8 in COPD patients with and without α_1-AT deficiency. Closed symbols indicate patients with α_1-AT deficiency (PiZ) and open symbols indicate patients with normal α_1-AT levels (PiM). Correlation coefficients (*r*) and significance (*p*) for all data are shown. fMLP, formyl-methionyl-leucyl-phenylalanine; IL-8, interleukin 8; LTB_4, leukotriene B_4.

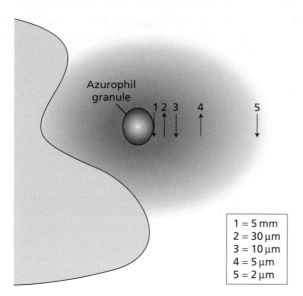

| 1 = 5 mm |
| 2 = 30 μm |
| 3 = 10 μm |
| 4 = 5 μm |
| 5 = 2 μm |

Figure 23.4 Diagrammatic representation of the mechanism involved in neutrophil elastase (NE) release from a neutrophil azurophil granule. Once the granule undergoes exocytosis from the neutrophil, elastase diffuses away. The high intrinsic concentration rapidly decreases initially and subsequently decreases more slowly. The individual arrows on the figure indicate representative concentrations at given distances from the granule. Note: in patients with normal levels of α_1-AT, the enzyme activity would be completely blocked at a distance away from the granule when the concentration falls to less than 30 μmol. On the other hand, in patients with α_1-AT deficiency, the enzyme activity would not be inhibited until it is diffused far enough away for the concentration to fall to 5 μmol.

concentration of α_1-AT, allowing a degree of tissue damage to occur within the immediate vicinity of the degranulating neutrophil. This theoretical relationship, in conjunction with the increased neutrophilic burden seen within the lungs of patients with COPD, may explain the elastase induced connective tissue destruction that occurs, even in the absence of α_1-AT deficiency. This process is summarized in Figure 23.4.

The second mechanism of neutrophil-mediated lung destruction in COPD is via the release of oxidative molecules following the neutrophil respiratory burst. The neutrophil respiratory burst results in the release of oxidative molecules, originating from the membrane-bound nicotinamide adenine dinucleotide phosphate (NADPH) oxidase system. Superoxide production starts with the reduction of oxygen by NADPH to form the superoxide radical (O_2^-). These radicals either react spontaneously with water to produce molecular oxygen and hydrogen peroxide, or the process can by catalysed by the enzyme superoxide dismutase. The reduction of hydrogen peroxide to water, or to the highly reactive hyperchlorous acid in

the presence of chloride, is catalysed by myeloperoxidase present in the azurophil granules. These products are usually released into the phagolysosome, where they destroy ingested bacteria. However, the neutrophil products of the respiratory burst also have the ability to damage normal cells directly resulting in cell death [123]. In health, the potential damaging effects of these oxidants are controlled by antioxidants [124]; however, there is evidence of oxidative stress in smoking-related lung disease with reduced plasma antioxidant capacity and increased lipid peroxidation [125]. Furthermore, neutrophils from patients with COPD demonstrate enhanced respiratory burst compared with smokers with normal lung function [68]. In addition, oxidants themselves can be proinflammatory [126,127], hence amplifying the inflammatory process and potential tissue damage.

A schematic summary of the cells and stages thought to be involved in the process of neutrophil recruitment and subsequent inflammation and tissue damage in COPD are shown in Figure 23.5.

The neutrophil as a target for anti-inflammatory therapy

Increasing our understanding of the processes of neutrophil recruitment and activation within the lung during the development and progression of COPD has allowed the identification of a number of potential therapeutic targets. These therapeutic strategies can act at a variety of stages along the pathogenic pathway, including the processes of neutrophil activation, adhesion, transmigration and proteolytic tissue damage.

Cytokine–chemoattractant antagonists

Blockade of cytokines produced early in the inflammatory cascade, such as IL-1β, TNF-α and PAF, would be expected to abrogate subsequent events including neutrophil adhesion, migration and activation. Humanized TNF-α antibodies have been found to be effective in chronic inflammatory conditions such as rheumatoid arthritis and Crohn disease [128,129], and this approach may be effective in COPD.

Blocking the effects of more distal mediators, such as IL-8, might regulate neutrophilic inflammation more specifically and antibodies directed against IL-8 have been shown to block neutrophil-mediated tissue injury in animal models [130]. Another approach would be to block binding of IL-8 to its neutrophil receptors (CXCR1 and CXCR2) via disruption to the transmembrane spanning structures common to these receptors. Peptides have been developed to prevent the receptor binding of IL-8 [131], although the long-term safety and efficacy of these drugs has yet to be assessed.

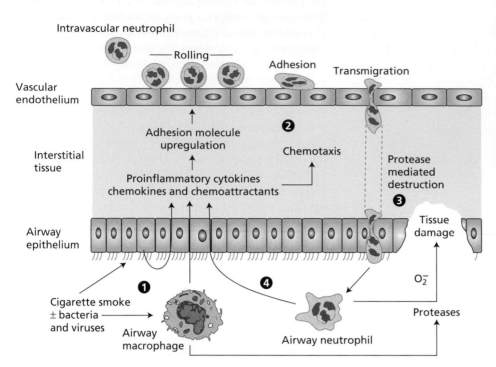

Figure 23.5 Schematic summary of the cells and inflammatory mediators involved in the pathogenesis of COPD. Activation of airway macrophages and epithelial cells causes the release of proinflammatory mediators ❶ which leads to adhesion molecule upregulation on the endothelial surface and subsequent neutrophil capture (in the bronchial circulation), firm adhesion and transmigration ❷. As the neutrophil migrates though the interstitium and into the airway the release of proteases and oxygen free radicals (O_2^-), leads to connective tissue and epithelial cell damage ❸. The inflammatory cycle is perpetuated by the further release of proinflammatory mediators by activated neutrophils within the airway ❹.

The potent neutrophil chemoattractant LTB_4 is another distal mediator with potential as a therapeutic target in COPD. Indeed, a recent randomized placebo-controlled trial of the LTB_4 synthesis inhibitor BAYx1005 demonstrated modest reductions in some measures of neutrophilic bronchial inflammation in patients with COPD [132]. Potent selective LTB_4 receptor antagonists have now been developed that may prove to be more effective.

Neutrophil adhesion molecule antagonists

Glycomimetics with structural similarities to the saccharide residues on endogenous ligands for L- and P-selectin, such as fucoidan and sialyl-Lewis$_x$, have been shown to block selectin binding *in vitro* and have been used effectively in a variety of pulmonary disease and injury models [133–135]. Newer generations of glycomimetics are being developed with structural modifications that increase specificity for individual selectins, which may therefore limit inflammation with less potential to disrupt the immune system or repair processes [136], and such an approach may prove to be of benefit in chronic pulmonary diseases such as COPD.

For instance, leumedins are a class of small molecular weight drugs that inhibit CD18-dependent neutrophil adhesion [137] and can block pulmonary leucocyte recruitment in a number of acute inflammatory and allergic conditions [138,139]. The mechanism of action of leumedins is not completely understood, but appears not to be specific to integrin-mediated adhesion [140].

Antiproteases

Given that the final common pathway in the pathogenesis of COPD is thought to be lung destruction by neutrophil elastase, a logical form of therapy would be to supplement or enhance the protective antiprotease screen within the lung. Indeed, this approach has already been taken in patients with α_1-AT deficiency, and augmentation therapy has proved to be safe [141], although there has yet to be a significantly powered, controlled study to prove that is effective. Synthetic inhibitors of neutrophil elastase have also been developed that inhibit elastase-mediated lung injury in experimental animals [142] and inhibit elastase-induced mucus secretion *in vitro* [143]. There are few clinical studies of such inhibitors in COPD, although one short study showed no overall effect on plasma levels of elastin-derived peptides or urinary levels of desmosine, which are markers of lung elastin destruction [144].

Corticosteroids

The effects of corticosteroids are multicellular, limiting both the production of inflammatory mediators by leucocytes and the response to those mediators by target cells (e.g. other leucocytes, endothelial and parenchymal cells). Glucocorticoids modulate the function of nuclear factor κB (NF-κB) [145], a transcription factor associated with the regulation of an array of genes that code for cytokines and other inflammatory mediators. NF-κB is also involved in the regulation of the expression of endothelial and leuco-cyte adhesion molecules [146,147]. In COPD, corticosteroids can reduce the neutrophil chemotactic activity of sputum [148], but neither inhaled nor oral steroids have been shown to have any effect on sputum neutrophil counts, granule proteins or inflammatory cytokines in induced sputum [149,150]. This is consistent with the lack of effect seen with inhaled corticosteroids on disease progression [151], although corticosteroids are effective in preventing and treating acute exacerbations in COPD [152], presumably via some as yet undetermined anti-inflammatory effect.

Non-steroidal anti-inflammatory drugs

The effects of non-steroidal anti-inflammatory drugs (NSAIDs) are most often attributed to their ability to inhibit the inducible form of cyclo-oxygenase-2 (COX-2), which mediates the conversion of arachidonic acid to prostaglandins, thromboxanes and other lipid mediators involved in inflammation and normal physiological responses. Inhibition of the adhesive and migratory processes between neutrophils and endothelial cells can occur after treatment *in vitro* with NSAIDs such as aspirin [153]. *In vivo*, 14 days treatment with the NSAID indometacin can change the population of circulating neutrophils, resulting in reduced chemotaxis and decreased potential to destroy connective tissue [154]. Clinical trials of indometacin in chronic bronchitis have demonstrated reductions in airway prostaglandins, sputum volume and dyspnoea [155]; however, there are currently no published data demonstrating a beneficial effect on disease progression in COPD.

Neutrophil inhibitors

Inhibition of phosphodiesterases (PDE) increases the cyclic adenosine monophosphate (AMP) content of neutrophils and reduces chemotaxis, activation, degranulation and adherence [156–159]. Theophylline is a weak and non-selective PDE inhibitor that has inhibitory effects on neutrophil function *in vitro* [156], and one study has demonstrated reduced sputum neutrophil counts following treatment *in vivo* [160]. The predominant PDE isoenzyme in neutrophils is PDE4 and several selective PDE4 inhibitors have now been developed that that may be effective at reducing neutrophil influx and subsequent inflammation in COPD [161–163].

Other neutrophil inhibitors include colchicine, which potently inhibits neutrophil activation, enzyme release and chemotaxis by disrupting cytoskeletal microtubule structure [164]. A controlled trial of colchicine in COPD showed some reduction in neutrophil elastase activity and in an observational study, smokers who were treated with colchicine had a lower annual decline in lung function than untreated smokers [165]. Macrolide antibiotics, such as erythromycin, also have inhibitory effects on neutrophil function that are independent of their antibiotic actions [166]. These drugs have been shown to be effective in panbronchiolitis [167]; however, there are currently no published data showing efficacy of these agents as anti-neutrophil drugs in COPD.

Conclusions

In conclusion, there is substantial evidence that the neutrophil is central to the pathogenesis of COPD. The neutrophil is the only cell that contains the products that have been shown directly to cause all the pathological features of COPD. It is likely therefore, that even in the absence of α_1-antitrypsin deficiency, the size, site and extent of neutrophil traffic is of major pathogenic importance. Understanding the mechanisms involved should lead to the identification of potential therapeutic targets and thus amelioration of the neutrophil-mediated inflammatory process.

References

1 Laurell CB, Eriksson S. The electrophoretic α_1-globulin pattern of serum in α_1-antitrypsin deficiency. *Scand J Clin Lab Invest* 1963;**15**:132–40.

2 Gross P, Pfitzer EA, Tolker E. Experimental emphysema: its production with papain in normal and silicotic rats. *Arch Environ Health* 1965;**11**:50–8.

3 Kuhn C, Yu SY, Chraplyvy M, Linder HE, Senior RM. The induction of emphysema with elastase. II. Changes in connective tissue. *Lab Invest* 1976;**34**:372–80.

4 Suzuki T, Wang W, Lin JT *et al.* Aerosolized human neutrophil elastase induces airway constriction and hyperresponsiveness with protection by intravenous pretreatment with half-length secretory leukoprotease inhibitor. *Am J Respir Crit Care Med* 1996;**153**:1405–11.

5 Lucey EC, Stone PJ, Breuer R *et al.* Effect of combined human neutrophil cathepsin G and elastase on induction of secretory cell metaplasia and emphysema in hamsters, with *in vitro* observations on elastolysis by these enzymes. *Am Rev Respir Dis* 1985;**132**:362–6.

6 Sommerhoff CP, Nadel JA, Basbaum CB, Caughey GH. Neutrophil elastase and cathepsin G stimulate secretion from cultured bovine airway gland serous cells. *J Clin Invest* 1990;**85**:682–9.

7 Sansores RH, Abboud RT, Becerril C *et al.* Effect of exposure of guinea pigs to cigarette smoke on elastolytic activity of pulmonary macrophages. *Chest* 1997;**112**:214–9.

8 Hautamaki RD, Kobayashi DK, Senior RM, Shapiro SD. Requirement for macrophage elastase for cigarette smoke-induced emphysema in mice. *Science* 1997;**277**:2002–4.

9 Dhami R, Gilks B, Xie C *et al*. Acute cigarette smoke-induced connective tissue breakdown is mediated by neutrophils and prevented by α_1-antitrypsin. *Am J Respir Cell Mol Biol* 2000;**22**:244–52.

10 Churg A, Zay K, Shay S *et al*. Acute cigarette smoke-induced connective tissue breakdown requires both neutrophils and macrophage metalloelastase in mice. *Am J Respir Cell Mol Biol* 2002;**27**:368–74.

11 Churg A, Wang RD, Tai H *et al*. Macrophage metalloelastase mediates acute cigarette smoke-induced inflammation via tumor necrosis factor-alpha release. *Am J Respir Crit Care Med* 2003;**167**:1083–9.

12 Churg A, Wang RD, Xie C, Wright JL. α_1-Antitrypsin ameliorates cigarette smoke-induced emphysema in the mouse. *Am J Respir Crit Care Med* 2003;**168**:199–207.

13 Martin TR, Raghu G, Maunder RJ, Springmeyer SC. The effects of chronic bronchitis and chronic air-flow obstruction on lung cell populations recovered by bronchoalveolar lavage. *Am Rev Respir Dis* 1985;**132**:254–60.

14 Thompson AB, Daughton D, Robbins RA *et al*. Intraluminal airway inflammation in chronic bronchitis: characterization and correlation with clinical parameters. *Am Rev Respir Dis* 1989;**140**:1527–37.

15 Lacoste JY, Bousquet J, Chanez P *et al*. Eosinophilic and neutrophilic inflammation in asthma, chronic bronchitis, and chronic obstructive pulmonary disease. *J Allergy Clin Immunol* 1993;**92**:537–48.

16 Riise GC, Ahlstedt S, Larsson S *et al*. Bronchial inflammation in chronic bronchitis assessed by measurement of cell products in bronchial lavage fluid. *Thorax* 1995;**50**:360–5.

17 Pesci A, Balbi B, Majori M *et al*. Inflammatory cells and mediators in bronchial lavage of patients with chronic obstructive pulmonary disease. *Eur Respir J* 1998;**12**:380–6.

18 Stockley RA. Neutrophils and the pathogenesis of COPD. *Chest* 2002;**121**:151S–5S.

19 Keatings VM, Barnes PJ. Granulocyte activation markers in induced sputum: comparison between chronic obstructive pulmonary disease, asthma, and normal subjects. *Am J Respir Crit Care Med* 1997;**155**:449–53.

20 Hill AT, Bayley D, Stockley RA. The interrelationship of sputum inflammatory markers in patients with chronic bronchitis. *Am J Respir Crit Care Med* 1999;**160**:893–8.

21 Stanescu D, Sanna A, Veriter C *et al*. Airways obstruction, chronic expectoration, and rapid decline of FEV_1 in smokers are associated with increased levels of sputum neutrophils. *Thorax* 1996;**51**:267–71.

22 Saetta M, Turato G, Facchini FM *et al*. Inflammatory cells in the bronchial glands of smokers with chronic bronchitis. *Am J Respir Crit Care Med* 1997;**156**:1633–9.

23 Di Stefano A, Capelli A, Lusuardi M *et al*. Severity of airflow limitation is associated with severity of airway inflammation in smokers. *Am J Respir Crit Care Med* 1998;**158**:1277–85.

24 Saetta M, Baraldo S, Corbino L *et al*. CD8+ cells in the lungs of smokers with chronic obstructive pulmonary disease. *Am J Respir Crit Care Med* 1999;**160**:711–7.

25 Saetta M, Turato G, Baraldo S *et al*. Goblet cell hyperplasia and epithelial inflammation in peripheral airways of smokers with both symptoms of chronic bronchitis and chronic airflow limitation. *Am J Respir Crit Care Med* 2000;**161**:1016–21.

26 Majo J, Ghezzo H, Cosio MG. Lymphocyte population and apoptosis in the lungs of smokers and their relation to emphysema. *Eur Respir J* 2001;**17**:946–53.

27 Retamales I, Elliot MW, Meshi B *et al*. Amplification of inflammation in emphysema and its association with latent adenoviral infection. *Am J Respir Crit Care Med* 2001;**164**:469–73.

28 Balbi B, Bason C, Balleari E *et al*. Increased bronchoalveolar granulocytes and granulocyte–macrophage colony-stimulating factor during exacerbations of chronic bronchitis. *Eur Respir J* 1997;**10**:846–50.

29 Crooks SW, Bayley DL, Hill SL, Stockley RA. Bronchial inflammation in acute bacterial exacerbations of chronic bronchitis: the role of leukotriene B_4. *Eur Respir J* 2000;**15**:274–80.

30 Gompertz S, O'Brien C, Bayley DL, Hill SL, Stockley RA. Changes in bronchial inflammation during acute exacerbations of chronic bronchitis. *Eur Respir J* 2001;**17**:1112–9.

31 Aaron SD, Angel JB, Lunau M *et al*. Granulocyte inflammatory markers and airway infection during acute exacerbation of chronic obstructive pulmonary disease. *Am J Respir Crit Care Med* 2001;**163**:349–55.

32 Burnett D. Neutrophils. In: Stockley RA, ed. *Pulmonary Defences*. Chichester: Wiley, 1997: 113–26.

33 Corre F, Lellouch J, Schwartz D. Smoking and leucocyte-counts: results of an epidemiological survey. *Lancet* 1971;**2**:632–4.

34 Van Eeden SF, Hogg JC. The response of human bone marrow to chronic cigarette smoking. *Eur Respir J* 2000;**15**:915–21.

35 Yeung MC, Buncio AD. Leukocyte count, smoking, and lung function. *Am J Med* 1984;**76**:31–7.

36 Sparrow D, Glynn RJ, Cohen M, Weiss ST. The relationship of the peripheral leukocyte count and cigarette smoking to pulmonary function among adult men. *Chest* 1984;**86**:383–6.

37 Deffebach ME, Charan NB, Lakshminarayan S, Butler J. The bronchial circulation: small, but a vital attribute of the lung. *Am Rev Respir Dis* 1987;**135**:463–81.

38 Laitinen LA, Laitinen A, Widdicombe J. Effects of inflammatory and other mediators on airway vascular beds. *Am Rev Respir Dis* 1987;**135**:S67–S70.

39 Bernard SL, Glenny RW, Polissar NL, Luchtel DL, Lakshminarayan S. Distribution of pulmonary and bronchial blood supply to airways measured by fluorescent microspheres. *J Appl Physiol* 1996;**80**:430–6.

40 Baile EM, Pare PD, Ernest D, Dodek PM. Distribution of blood flow and neutrophil kinetics in bronchial vasculature of sheep. *J Appl Physiol* 1997;**82**:1466–71.

41 Doerschuk CM. Leukocyte trafficking in alveoli and airway passages. *Respir Res* 2000;**1**:136–40.

42 Springer TA. Traffic signals for lymphocyte recirculation and leukocyte emigration: the multistep paradigm. *Cell* 1994;**76**:301–14.

43 Spertini O, Luscinskas FW, Kansas GS *et al*. Leukocyte

adhesion molecule-1 (LAM-1, L-selectin) interacts with an inducible endothelial cell ligand to support leukocyte adhesion. *J Immunol* 1991;**147**:2565–73.

44 Krause DS, Fackler MJ, Civin CI, May WS. CD34: structure, biology, and clinical utility. *Blood* 1996;**87**:1–13.

45 Varki A. Selectin ligands: will the real ones please stand up? *J Clin Invest* 1997;**100**:S31–5.

46 Hattori R, Hamilton KK, Fugate RD, McEver RP, Sims PJ. Stimulated secretion of endothelial von Willebrand factor is accompanied by rapid redistribution to the cell surface of the intracellular granule membrane protein GMP-140. *J Biol Chem* 1989;**264**:7768–71.

47 Bahra P, Rainger GE, Wautier JL, Nguyet-Thin L, Nash GB. Each step during transendothelial migration of flowing neutrophils is regulated by the stimulatory concentration of tumour necrosis factor-alpha. *Cell Adhes Commun* 1998;**6**: 491–501.

48 Davenpeck KL, Steeber DA, Tedder TF, Bochner BS. P- and L-selectin mediate distinct but overlapping functions in endotoxin-induced leukocyte-endothelial interactions in the rat mesenteric microcirculation. *J Immunol* 1997;**159**: 1977–86.

49 Lawrence MB, Springer TA. Neutrophils roll on E-selectin. *J Immunol* 1993;**151**:6338–46.

50 Steegmaier M, Levinovitz A, Isenmann S *et al*. The E-selectin-ligand ESL-1 is a variant of a receptor for fibroblast growth factor. *Nature* 1995;**373**:615–20.

51 Scholz D, Devaux B, Hirche A *et al*. Expression of adhesion molecules is specific and time-dependent in cytokine-stimulated endothelial cells in culture. *Cell Tissue Res* 1996; **284**:415–23.

52 Malik AB, Lo SK. Vascular endothelial adhesion molecules and tissue inflammation. *Pharmacol Rev* 1996;**48**:213–29.

53 Tanaka Y, Adams DH, Shaw S. Proteoglycans on endothelial cells present adhesion-inducing cytokines to leukocytes. *Immunol Today* 1993;**14**:111–5.

54 Huber AR, Kunkel SL, Todd RF III, Weiss SJ. Regulation of transendothelial neutrophil migration by endogenous interleukin-8. *Science* 1991;**254**:99–102.

55 Gopalan PK, Smith CW, Lu H *et al*. Neutrophil CD18-dependent arrest on intercellular adhesion molecule 1 (ICAM-1) in shear flow can be activated through L-selectin. *J Immunol* 1997;**158**:367–75.

56 Diamond MS, Staunton DE, de Fougerolles AR *et al*. ICAM-1 (CD54): a counter-receptor for Mac-1 (CD11b/CD18). *J Cell Biol* 1990;**111**:3129–39.

57 Rainger GE, Buckley C, Simmons DL, Nash GB. Cross-talk between cell adhesion molecules regulates the migration velocity of neutrophils. *Curr Biol* 1997;**7**:316–25.

58 Borregaard N, Cowland JB. Granules of the human neutrophilic polymorphonuclear leukocyte. *Blood* 1997;**89**: 3503–21.

59 Tonnesen MG, Anderson DC, Springer TA *et al*. Adherence of neutrophils to cultured human microvascular endothelial cells: stimulation by chemotactic peptides and lipid mediators and dependence upon the Mac-1, LFA-1, p150,95 glycoprotein family. *J Clin Invest* 1989;**83**:637–46.

60 Klein CL, Bittinger F, Kohler H *et al*. Comparative studies on vascular endothelium *in vitro*. III. Effects of cytokines on the expression of E-selectin, ICAM-1 and VCAM-1 by cultured human endothelial cells obtained from different passages. *Pathobiology* 1995;**63**:83–92.

61 Burns AR, Walker DC, Brown ES *et al*. Neutrophil transendothelial migration is independent of tight junctions and occurs preferentially at tricellular corners. *J Immunol* 1997;**159**:2893–903.

62 Vaporciyan AA, DeLisser HM, Yan HC *et al*. Involvement of platelet-endothelial cell adhesion molecule-1 in neutrophil recruitment *in vivo*. *Science* 1993;**262**:1580–2.

63 Newman PJ. The biology of PECAM-1. *J Clin Invest* 1997; **100**:S25–9.

64 Muller WA, Weigl SA, Deng X, Phillips DM. PECAM-1 is required for transendothelial migration of leukocytes. *J Exp Med* 1993;**178**:449–60.

65 Wright DG, Gallin JI. Secretory responses of human neutrophils: exocytosis of specific (secondary) granules by human neutrophils during adherence *in vitro* and during exudation *in vivo*. *J Immunol* 1979;**123**:285–94.

66 Lomas DA, Stone SR, Llewellyn-Jones C *et al*. The control of neutrophil chemotaxis by inhibitors of cathepsin G and chymotrypsin. *J Biol Chem* 1995;**270**:23437–43.

67 Mackarel AJ, Cottell DC, Russell KJ, FitzGerald MX, O'Connor CM. Migration of neutrophils across human pulmonary endothelial cells is not blocked by matrix metalloproteinase or serine protease inhibitors. *Am J Respir Cell Mol Biol* 1999;**20**:1209–19.

68 Noguera A, Batle S, Miralles C *et al*. Enhanced neutrophil response in chronic obstructive pulmonary disease. *Thorax* 2001;**56**:432–7.

69 Gonzalez S, Hards J, Van Eeden S, Hogg JC. The expression of adhesion molecules in cigarette smoke-induced airways obstruction. *Eur Respir J* 1996;**9**:1995–2001.

70 Riise GC, Larsson S, Lofdahl CG, Andersson BA. Circulating cell adhesion molecules in bronchial lavage and serum in COPD patients with chronic bronchitis. *Eur Respir J* 1994;**7**: 1673–7.

71 Noguera A, Busquets X, Sauleda J *et al*. Expression of adhesion molecules and G proteins in circulating neutrophils in chronic obstructive pulmonary disease. *Am J Respir Crit Care Med* 1998;**158**:1664–8.

72 Burnett D, Chamba A, Hill SL, Stockley RA. Neutrophils from subjects with chronic obstructive lung disease show enhanced chemotaxis and extracellular proteolysis. *Lancet* 1987;**2**:1043–6.

73 Woolhouse IS, Bayley D, Lalor P, Adams DH, Stockley RA. Endothelial interactions of neutrophils under flow in chronic obstructive pulmonary disease. *Eur Respir J* 2005; **25**:612–7,

74 Lien DC, Wagner WW Jr, Capen RL *et al*. Physiological neutrophil sequestration in the lung: visual evidence for localization in capillaries. *J Appl Physiol* 1987;**62**:1236–43.

75 Doerschuk CM, Allard MF, Hogg JC. Neutrophil kinetics in rabbits during infusion of zymosan-activated plasma. *J Appl Physiol* 1989;**67**:88–95.

76 Downey GP, Worthen GS, Henson PM, Hyde DM. Neutrophil sequestration and migration in localized pulmonary

inflammation: capillary localization and migration across the interalveolar septum. *Am Rev Respir Dis* 1993;**147**: 168–76.

77 Doerschuk CM. The role of CD18-mediated adhesion in neutrophil sequestration induced by infusion of activated plasma in rabbits. *Am J Respir Cell Mol Biol* 1992;**7**:140–8.

78 Kubo H, Doyle NA, Graham L *et al*. L- and P-selectin and CD11/CD18 in intracapillary neutrophil sequestration in rabbit lungs. *Am J Respir Crit Care Med* 1999;**159**:267–74.

79 Selby C, Drost E, Lannan S, Wraith PK, MacNee W. Neutrophil retention in the lungs of patients with chronic obstructive pulmonary disease. *Am Rev Respir Dis* 1991;**143**: 1359–64.

80 Selby C, Drost E, Gillooly M *et al*. Neutrophil sequestration in lungs removed at surgery: the effect of microscopic emphysema. *Am J Respir Crit Care Med* 1994;**149**:1526–33.

81 White AJ, Gompertz S, Stockley RA. Chronic obstructive pulmonary disease 6: The aetiology of exacerbations of chronic obstructive pulmonary disease. *Thorax* 2003;**58**: 73–80.

82 Doerschuk CM, Beyers N, Coxson HO, Wiggs B, Hogg JC. Comparison of neutrophil and capillary diameters and their relation to neutrophil sequestration in the lung. *J Appl Physiol* 1993;**74**:3040–5.

83 Worthen GS, Schwab B III, Elson EL, Downey GP. Mechanics of stimulated neutrophils: cell stiffening induces retention in capillaries. *Science* 1989;**245**:183–6.

84 Motosugi H, Graham L, Noblitt TW *et al*. Changes in neutrophil actin and shape during sequestration induced by complement fragments in rabbits. *Am J Pathol* 1996;**149**: 963–73.

85 Mackarel AJ, Russell KJ, Brady CS, FitzGerald MX, O'Connor CM. Interleukin-8 and leukotriene-B$_4$, but not formylmethionyl leucylphenylalanine, stimulate CD18-independent migration of neutrophils across human pulmonary endothelial cells *in vitro*. *Am J Respir Cell Mol Biol* 2000;**23**:154–61.

86 Morland CM, Morland BJ, Darbyshire PJ, Stockley RA. Migration of CD18-deficient neutrophils *in vitro*: evidence for a CD18-independent pathway induced by IL-8. *Biochim Biophys Acta* 2000;**1500**:70–6.

87 Mackarel AJ, Russell KJ, Ryan CM *et al*. CD18 dependency of transendothelial neutrophil migration differs during acute pulmonary inflammation. *J Immunol* 2001;**167**:2839–46.

88 Le J, Vilcek J. Tumor necrosis factor and interleukin 1: cytokines with multiple overlapping biological activities. *Lab Invest* 1987;**56**:234–48.

89 Abdelaziz MM, Devalia JL, Khair OA *et al*. The effect of conditioned medium from cultured human bronchial epithelial cells on eosinophil and neutrophil chemotaxis and adherence *in vitro*. *Am J Respir Cell Mol Biol* 1995;**13**:728–37.

90 Burke-Gaffney A, Hellewell PG. Tumour necrosis factor-alpha-induced ICAM-1 expression in human vascular endothelial and lung epithelial cells: modulation by tyrosine kinase inhibitors. *Br J Pharmacol* 1996;**119**:1149–58.

91 Smart SJ, Casale TB. TNF-alpha-induced transendothelial neutrophil migration is IL-8 dependent. *Am J Physiol* 1994; **266**:L238–45.

92 Keatings VM, Collins PD, Scott DM, Barnes PJ. Differences in interleukin-8 and tumor necrosis factor-alpha in induced sputum from patients with chronic obstructive pulmonary disease or asthma. *Am J Respir Crit Care Med* 1996;**153**:530–4.

93 Bresser P, Out TA, van Alphen L, Jansen HM, Lutter R. Airway inflammation in non-obstructive and obstructive chronic bronchitis with chronic *Haemophilus influenzae* airway infection: comparison with non-infected patients with chronic obstructive pulmonary disease. *Am J Respir Crit Care Med* 2000;**162**:947–52.

94 Chung KF. Cytokines in chronic obstructive pulmonary disease. *Eur Respir J Suppl*. 2001;**34**:50S–9S.

95 Woolhouse IS, Bayley DL, Stockley RA. Effect of sputum processing with dithiothreitol on the detection of inflammatory mediators in chronic bronchitis and bronchiectasis. *Thorax* 2002;**57**:667–71.

96 Henderson WR. The role of leukotrienes in inflammation. *Ann Intern Med* 1994;**121**:684–97.

97 Crooks SW, Stockley RA. Leukotriene B$_4$. *Int J Biochem Cell Biol* 1998;**30**:173–8.

98 Borgeat PE, Krump E, Palmantier R *et al*. The synthesis of leukotrienes by the human neutrophil. In: Holgate S, Dahlen SE, eds. *SRS-A to Leukotrienes: The Dawning of a New Treatment*. Oxford: Blackwell Scientific Publications, 1997: 69–84.

99 Ford-Hutchinson AW, Bray MA, Doig MV, Shipley ME, Smith MJ. Leukotriene B, a potent chemokinetic and aggregating substance released from polymorphonuclear leukocytes. *Nature* 1980;**286**:264–5.

100 Nohgawa M, Sasada M, Maeda A *et al*. Leukotriene B$_4$-activated human endothelial cells promote transendothelial neutrophil migration. *J Leukoc Biol* 1997;**62**:203–9.

101 Pang G, Ortega M, Zighang R, Reeves G, Clancy R. Autocrine modulation of IL-8 production by sputum neutrophils in chronic bronchial sepsis. *Am J Respir Crit Care Med* 1997; **155**:726–31.

102 Smith WB, Gamble JR, Clark-Lewis I, Vadas MA. Interleukin-8 induces neutrophil transendothelial migration. *Immunology* 1991;**72**:65–72.

103 Cromwell O, Hamid Q, Corrigan CJ *et al*. Expression and generation of interleukin-8, IL-6 and granulocyte–macrophage colony-stimulating factor by bronchial epithelial cells and enhancement by IL-1β and tumour necrosis factor-α. *Immunology* 1992;**77**:330–7.

104 Mio T, Romberger DJ, Thompson AB *et al*. Cigarette smoke induces interleukin-8 release from human bronchial epithelial cells. *Am J Respir Crit Care Med* 1997;**155**:1770–6.

105 Khair OA, Devalia JL, Abdelaziz MM *et al*. Effect of *Haemophilus influenzae* endotoxin on the synthesis of IL-6, IL-8, TNF-α and expression of ICAM-1 in cultured human bronchial epithelial cells. *Eur Respir J* 1994;**7**:2109–16.

106 Nakamura H, Yoshimura K, McElvaney NG, Crystal RG. Neutrophil elastase in respiratory epithelial lining fluid of individuals with cystic fibrosis induces interleukin-8 gene expression in a human bronchial epithelial cell line. *J Clin Invest* 1992;**89**:1478–84.

107 Hill AT, Bayley DL, Campbell EJ, Hill SL, Stockley RA. Airways inflammation in chronic bronchitis: the effects of

smoking and α_1-antitrypsin deficiency. *Eur Respir J* 2000;**15**: 886–90.

108 Woolhouse IS, Bayley DL, Stockley RA. Sputum chemotactic activity in chronic obstructive pulmonary disease: effect of α_1-antitrypsin deficiency and the role of leukotriene B_4 and interleukin 8. *Thorax* 2002;**57**:709–14.

109 Beeh KM, Kornmann O, Buhl R *et al.* Neutrophil chemotactic activity of sputum from patients with COPD: role of interleukin 8 and leukotriene B_4. *Chest* 2003;**123**:1240–7.

110 Traves SL, Culpitt SV, Russell RE, Barnes PJ, Donnelly LE. Increased levels of the chemokines GROα and MCP-1 in sputum samples from patients with COPD. *Thorax* 2002;**57**: 590–5.

111 Morrison D, Strieter RM, Donnelly SC *et al.* Neutrophil chemokines in bronchoalveolar lavage fluid and leukocyte-conditioned medium from non-smokers and smokers. *Eur Respir J* 1998;**12**:1067–72.

112 Fick RB Jr, Robbins RA, Squier SU, Schoderbek WE, Russ WD. Complement activation in cystic fibrosis respiratory fluids: *in vivo* and *in vitro* generation of C5a and chemotactic activity. *Pediatr Res* 1986;**20**:1258–68.

113 Banda MJ, Rice AG, Griffin GL, Senior RM. The inhibitory complex of human alpha 1-proteinase inhibitor and human leukocyte elastase is a neutrophil chemoattractant. *J Exp Med* 1988;**167**:1608–15.

114 Senior RM, Hinek A, Griffin GL *et al.* Neutrophils show chemotaxis to type IV collagen and its 7S domain and contain a 67 kD type IV collagen binding protein with lectin properties. *Am J Respir Cell Mol Biol* 1989;**1**:479–87.

115 Senior RM, Griffin GL, Mecham RP. Chemotactic activity of elastin-derived peptides. *J Clin Invest* 1980;**66**:859–62.

116 Bryant G, Rao CN, Brentani M *et al.* A role for the laminin receptor in leukocyte chemotaxis. *J Leukoc Biol* 1987;**41**: 220–7.

117 Parmar JS, Mahadeva R, Reed BJ *et al.* Polymers of α_1-antitrypsin are chemotactic for human neutrophils: a new paradigm for the pathogenesis of emphysema. *Am J Respir Cell Mol Biol* 2002;**26**:723–30.

118 Casale TB, Abbas MK, Carolan EJ. Degree of neutrophil chemotaxis is dependent upon the chemoattractant and barrier. *Am J Respir Cell Mol Biol* 1992;**7**:112–7.

119 Abdullah LH, Conway JD, Cohn JA, Davis CW. Protein kinase C and Ca^{2+} activation of mucin secretion in airway goblet cells. *Am J Physiol* 1997;**273**:L201–10.

120 Ko KH, Jo M, McCracken K, Kim KC. ATP-induced mucin release from cultured airway goblet cells involves, in part, activation of protein kinase C. *Am J Respir Cell Mol Biol* 1997;**16**:194–8.

121 Liou TG, Campbell EJ. Quantum proteolysis resulting from release of single granules by human neutrophils: a novel, non-oxidative mechanism of extracellular proteolytic activity. *J Immunol* 1996;**157**:2624–31.

122 Gorin AB, Stewart PA. Differential permeability of endothelial and epithelial barriers to albumin flux. *J Appl Physiol* 1979;**47**:1315–24.

123 Weiss SJ, Young J, LoBuglio AF, Slivka A, Nimeh NF. Role of hydrogen peroxide in neutrophil-mediated destruction of cultured endothelial cells. *J Clin Invest* 1981;**68**:714–21.

124 MacNee W. Oxidants/antioxidants and COPD. *Chest* 2000; **117**:303S–17S.

125 Rahman I, Morrison D, Donaldson K, MacNee W. Systemic oxidative stress in asthma, COPD, and smokers. *Am J Respir Crit Care Med* 1996;**154**:1055–60.

126 Antonicelli F, Parmentier M, Drost EM *et al.* Nacystelyn inhibits oxidant-mediated interleukin-8 expression and NF-κB nuclear binding in alveolar epithelial cells. *Free Radic Biol Med* 2002;**32**:492–502.

127 Rahman I, Gilmour PS, Jimenez LA, MacNee W. Oxidative stress and TNF-α induce histone acetylation and NF-κB/AP-1 activation in alveolar epithelial cells: potential mechanism in gene transcription in lung inflammation. *Mol Cell Biochem* 2002;**234/235**:239–248.

128 Elliott MJ, Maini RN, Feldmann M *et al.* Repeated therapy with monoclonal antibody to tumour necrosis factor alpha (cA2) in patients with rheumatoid arthritis. *Lancet* 1994; **344**:1125–7.

129 Hanauer SB, Feagan BG, Lichtenstein GR *et al.* Maintenance infliximab for Crohn's disease: the ACCENT I randomised trial. *Lancet* 2002;**359**:1541–9.

130 Sekido N, Mukaida N, Harada A *et al.* Prevention of lung reperfusion injury in rabbits by a monoclonal antibody against interleukin-8. *Nature* 1993;**365**:654–7.

131 Hayashi S, Kurdowska A, Miller EJ *et al.* Synthetic hexa- and heptapeptides that inhibit IL-8 from binding to and activating human blood neutrophils. *J Immunol* 1995;**154**: 814–24.

132 Gompertz S, Stockley RA. A randomized, placebo-controlled trial of a leukotriene synthesis inhibitor in patients with COPD. *Chest* 2002;**122**:289–94.

133 Shimaoka M, Ikeda M, Iida T *et al.* Fucoidin, a potent inhibitor of leukocyte rolling, prevents neutrophil influx into phorbol-ester-induced inflammatory sites in rabbit lungs. *Am J Respir Crit Care Med* 1996;**153**:307–11.

134 Reignier J, Sellak H, Lemoine R *et al.* Prevention of ischemia-reperfusion lung injury by sulfated Lewis(a) pentasaccharide. The Paris-Sud University Lung Transplantation Group. *J Appl Physiol* 1997;**82**:1058–63.

135 Mulligan MS, Warner RL, Lowe JB *et al. In vitro* and *in vivo* selectin-blocking activities of sulfated lipids and sulfated sialyl compounds. *Int Immunol* 1998;**10**:569–75.

136 Jenison RD, Jennings SD, Walker DW, Bargatze RF, Parma D. Oligonucleotide inhibitors of P-selectin-dependent neutrophil-platelet adhesion. *Antisense Nucleic Acid Drug Dev* 1998;**8**:265–79.

137 Endemann G, Abe Y, Bryant CM *et al.* Novel anti-inflammatory compounds induce shedding of L-selectin and block primary capture of neutrophils under flow conditions. *J Immunol* 1997;**158**:4879–85.

138 Jorens PG, Richman-Eisenstat JB, Housset BP *et al. Pseudomonas*-induced neutrophil recruitment in the dog airway *in vivo* is mediated in part by IL-8 and inhibited by a leumedin. *Eur Respir J* 1994;**7**:1925–31.

139 Kaneko T, Jorens PG, Richman-Eisenstat JB, Dazin PF, Nadel JA. Leumedin NPC 15669 inhibits antigen-induced recruitment of inflammatory cells into the canine airways. *Am J Physiol* 1994;**267**:L250–5.

140 Endemann G, Feng Y, Bryant CM *et al.* Novel anti-inflammatory compounds prevent CD11b/CD18, alpha M beta 2 (Mac-1)-dependent neutrophil adhesion without blocking activation-induced changes in Mac-1. *J Pharmacol Exp Ther* 1996;**276**:5–12.

141 Seersholm N, Wencker M, Banik N *et al.* Does α_1-antitrypsin augmentation therapy slow the annual decline in FEV_1 in patients with severe hereditary α_1-antitrypsin deficiency? Wissenschaftliche Arbeitsgemeinschaft zur Therapie von Lungenerkrankungen (WATL) α_1-AT study group. *Eur Respir J* 1997;**10**:2260–3.

142 Williams JC, Falcone RC, Knee C *et al.* Biologic character-ization of ICI 200,880 and ICI 200,355, novel inhibitors of human neutrophil elastase. *Am Rev Respir Dis* 1991;**144**:875–83.

143 Sommerhoff CP, Krell RD, Williams JL *et al.* Inhibition of human neutrophil elastase by ICI 200,355. *Eur J Pharmacol* 1991;**193**:153–8.

144 Luisetti M, Sturani C, Sella D *et al.* MR889, a neutrophil elastase inhibitor, in patients with chronic obstructive pulmonary disease: a double-blind, randomized, placebo-controlled clinical trial. *Eur Respir J* 1996;**9**:1482–6.

145 Wissink S, van Heerde EC, vand der BB, van der Saag PT. A dual mechanism mediates repression of NF-κB activity by glucocorticoids. *Mol Endocrinol* 1998;**12**:355–63.

146 Lee DH, Tam SS, Wang E *et al.* The NF-κB inhibitor, tepo-xalin, suppresses surface expression of the cell adhesion molecules CD62E, CD11b/CD18 and CD106. *Immunol Lett* 1996;**53**:109–13.

147 Brostjan C, Anrather J, Csizmadia V, Natarajan G, Winkler H. Glucocorticoids inhibit E-selectin expression by targeting NF-κB and not ATF/c-Jun. *J Immunol* 1997;**158**:3836–44.

148 Llewellyn-Jones CG, Harris TA, Stockley RA. Effect of fluticasone propionate on sputum of patients with chronic bronchitis and emphysema. *Am J Respir Crit Care Med* 1996;**153**:616–21.

149 Keatings VM, Jatakanon A, Worsdell YM, Barnes PJ. Effects of inhaled and oral glucocorticoids on inflammatory indices in asthma and COPD. *Am J Respir Crit Care Med* 1997;**155**:542–8.

150 Culpitt SV, Maziak W, Loukidis S *et al.* Effect of high dose inhaled steroid on cells, cytokines, and proteases in induced sputum in chronic obstructive pulmonary disease. *Am J Respir Crit Care Med* 1999;**160**:1635–9.

151 Burge PS, Calverley PM, Jones PW *et al.* Randomised, double blind, placebo controlled study of fluticasone propionate in patients with moderate to severe chronic obstructive pulmonary disease: the ISOLDE trial. *BMJ* 2000;**320**:1297–303.

152 Davies L, Angus RM, Calverley PM. Oral corticosteroids in patients admitted to hospital with exacerbations of chronic obstructive pulmonary disease: a prospective randomised controlled trial. *Lancet* 1999;**354**:456–60.

153 Pierce JW, Read MA, Ding H, Luscinskas FW, Collins T. Salicylates inhibit I kappa B-alpha phosphorylation, endothelial-leukocyte adhesion molecule expression, and neutrophil transmigration. *J Immunol* 1996;**156**:3961–9.

154 Ip M, Lomas DA, Shaw J, Burnett D, Stockley RA. Effect of non-steroidal anti-inflammatory drugs on neutrophil chemotaxis: an *in vitro* and *in vivo* study. *Br J Rheumatol* 1990;**29**:363–7.

155 Tamaoki J, Chiyotani A, Kobayashi K *et al.* Effect of indomethacin on bronchorrhea in patients with chronic bronchitis, diffuse panbronchiolitis, or bronchiectasis. *Am Rev Respir Dis* 1992;**145**:548–52.

156 Nielson CP, Vestal RE, Sturm RJ, Heaslip R. Effects of select-ive phosphodiesterase inhibitors on the polymorphonuclear leukocyte respiratory burst. *J Allergy Clin Immunol* 1990;**86**:801–8.

157 Schudt C, Winder S, Forderkunz S, Hatzelmann A, Ullrich V. Influence of selective phosphodiesterase inhibitors on human neutrophil functions and levels of cAMP and Cai. *Naunyn Schmiedebergs Arch Pharmacol* 1991;**344**:682–90.

158 Llewellyn-Jones CG, Stockley RA. The effects of beta 2-agonists and methylxanthines on neutrophil function *in vitro*. *Eur Respir J* 1994;**7**:1460–6.

159 Bloemen PG, van den Tweel MC, Henricks PA *et al.* Increased cAMP levels in stimulated neutrophils inhibit their adhesion to human bronchial epithelial cells. *Am J Physiol* 1997;**272**:L580–7.

160 Culpitt SV, De Matos C, Russell RE *et al.* Effect of theo-phylline on induced sputum inflammatory indices and neutrophil chemotaxis in chronic obstructive pulmonary disease. *Am J Respir Crit Care Med* 2002;**165**:1371–6.

161 Sturton G, Fitzgerald M. Phosphodiesterase 4 inhibitors for the treatment of COPD. *Chest* 2002;**121**:192S–6S.

162 Profita M, Chiappara G, Mirabella F *et al.* Effect of cilomilast (Ariflo) on TNF-α, IL-8, and GM-CSF release by airway cells of patients with COPD. *Thorax* 2003;**58**:573–9.

163 Gamble E, Grootendorst DC, Brightling CE *et al.* Anti-inflammatory effects of the phosphodiesterase 4 inhibitor cilomilast (Ariflo) in COPD. *Am J Respir Crit Care Med* 2003;**168**:976–82.

164 Molad Y. Update on colchicine and its mechanism of action. *Curr Rheumatol Rep* 2002;**4**:252–6.

165 Cohen AB, Girard W, Mclarty J *et al.* A controlled trial of colchicine to reduce the elastase load in the lungs of cigarette smokers with chronic obstructive pulmonary disease. *Am Rev Respir Dis* 1990;**142**:63–72.

166 Anderson R, Theron AJ, Feldman C. Membrane-stabilizing, anti-inflammatory interactions of macrolides with human neutrophils. *Inflammation* 1996;**20**:693–705.

167 Ichikawa Y, Ninomiya H, Koga H *et al.* Erythromycin reduces neutrophils and neutrophil-derived elastolytic-like activity in the lower respiratory tract of bronchiolitis patients. *Am Rev Respir Dis* 1992;**146**:196–203.

CHAPTER 24
Lymphocytes

Simonetta Baraldo, Maria Elena Zanin, Renzo Zuin and Marina Saetta

According to the most recent guidelines, COPD is a preventable and treatable disease state characterized by airflow limitation that is not fully reversible. The airflow limitation is usually progressive and is associated with an abnormal inflammatory response of the lungs to noxious particles or gases, primarily caused by cigarette smoking. Although COPD affects the lungs, it also produces significant systemic consequences [1,2]. A number of studies in recent years demonstrated that, in patients with COPD, a chronic inflammation is present throughout the airways, lung parenchyma and pulmonary vasculature and extends even outside the lung, involving lymph nodes, eventually reaching the systemic circulation [3–7]. The most recent definitions of COPD introduced the concept that inflammation is a key event in the pathogenesis of the disease, highlighting the need for a better knowledge of the mechanisms involved in the perpetuation of the inflammatory response.

It has long been recognized that smoking is the most important risk factor for the development of COPD and that exposure to cigarette smoke can elicit an exaggerated inflammatory response [8,9]. However, only a minority of cigarette smokers develop overt airflow obstruction and the pathogenetic mechanisms are still poorly understood. The aim of this chapter is to review the present knowledge of the inflammatory response in smokers with COPD, with a special focus on lymphocytes. In particular, we first describe how these cells are recruited to the lung in physiological conditions. We then discuss how lymphocytes could be involved in the development of structural alterations in the airways and lung parenchyma, thus promoting the establishment of airflow limitation. Finally, we consider how these events evolve when COPD progresses towards its most severe stages.

Lymphocytes in immune responses

The physiological function of the immune system is defence against infectious organisms and potentially harmful foreign substances. The pulmonary immune system is continuously exposed to pathogens and foreign antigens within inhaled air. It is therefore essential that cells orchestrating immune responses within the lung can correctly determine whether an antigenic molecule is potentially dangerous and can build an appropriate defence. The immune system can be thought of as having two lines of defence: the first represents a non-specific (no memory) response to antigens (the innate immune system); and the second displays a high degree of memory and specificity (the adaptive immune system). The innate immune system is based on the cooperation of several cell types and proteins, including epithelial cells, macrophages, neutrophils, dendritic cells, natural killer (NK) cells and complement. As the innate system represents the first line of defence to an intruding pathogen, the response evolved has to be extremely rapid. However, the innate system is unable to memorize the same pathogen, should the body be exposed to it in the future. Conversely, adaptive immune responses, which require activation of lymphocytes, have evolved to provide a more versatile mean of defence. The adaptive immune system has much slower temporary dynamics, but it possesses a high degree of specificity and evokes a more potent response to a secondary exposure to the pathogen [10].

In normal conditions, most infectious agents or foreign antigenic material may be removed by the innate immune system without requiring an inflammatory response. By contrast, when antigenic molecules are recognized as dangerous, antigen-presenting cells in the lung initiate the adaptive inflammatory response displaying the antigen to

T lymphocytes. Moreover, by releasing chemokines and cytokines, they trigger the expansion of antigen-specific B and T cells in the secondary lymphoid tissues or within the alveolar spaces [11]. Antigen-specific lymphocytes have evolved a number of effector mechanisms to fight foreign antigens, including direct cytotoxicity and secretion of lymphokines that can activate themselves or other pulmonary immunocompetent cells.

As pointed out by Cosio [12], it is important to highlight that the innate and the adaptive immune responses are not completely isolated from each other, but act as an integrated system of host defence in which numerous cells and molecules function cooperatively. Two important links exist between innate and adaptive immunity. First, the innate response to pathogens stimulates adaptive immune responses and influences their nature. Secondly, the adaptive immune response uses many of the effector mechanisms of innate immunity to eliminate microbes or other antigenic substances, enhancing the antimicrobic activity of the innate immunity system.

To have a clear view of mechanisms leading to lymphocyte accumulation and activation in COPD, it is important to review how these cells are recruited to the lung in physiological conditions. According to their specific properties and functions, human lymphocytes are functionally compartmentalized in the lung. Lung lymphoid tissue includes the bronchus-associated lymphoid tissue (BALT) as well as lymph nodes that receive drainage from the nose or lung [13]. In addition, lymphoid follicles are located throughout the bronchial tree as far down as the small bronchioles and are constituted by B-cell germinal centres surrounded by T cells, macrophages and dendritic cells (DC). Naive B and T cells keep moving continuously in the lymphoid tissue until they respond to their cognate antigen, proliferate and differentiate in memory and effector lymphocytes. Moreover, the activation of T cells after antigen presentation results in up-modulation of several adhesion molecules and homing receptors, which are necessary for migration of T cells to different compartments in the lung.

Lymphocytes in COPD

The inflammatory cells of the adaptive immune response (mainly T and B lymphocytes), which have evolved to protect individuals from infection and eliminate foreign substances, should be promptly removed as soon as the originating stimulus disappears. However, in some situations, as in COPD, the inflammatory response may persist and cause tissue injury and disease. We describe below the mechanisms through which lymphocytes may promote structural changes in the airways, lung parenchyma and pulmonary arteries of smokers with COPD.

Central and peripheral airways

To understand the immune reaction to cigarette-smoke exposure, it is important to realize that innate and adaptive immune responses are components of an integrated system. Cigarette smoke produces a clear innate immune response, as elegantly shown by Niewoehner *et al.* [14], who demonstrated that an inflammatory reaction is already present in the peripheral airways of young smokers who experienced sudden death outside of the hospital setting. Early lesions already present in young smokers included an inflammatory infiltrate in the airway wall consisting predominantly of mononuclear cells and clusters of macrophages in the respiratory bronchioles. Interestingly, the authors reported that these lesions were present in the absence of noteworthy tissue destruction and fibrosis, and suggested that this stage of the disease could still be largely reversible. Therefore, the great majority of smokers develop a chronic non-specific inflammation that should be interpreted as the innate immune response to cigarette smoke damage. In those smokers who develop COPD, beside the innate immune response, the adaptive immune response involving B and T cells becomes activated. These same smokers would also develop structural abnormalities in peripheral airways and parenchyma, which contribute to airflow limitation by increasing peripheral airway resistance and decreasing the elastic recoil of the lung. The susceptibility factors determining those smokers who would develop COPD are still poorly understood. These may involve several components, such as genetic predisposition (i.e. genetic control of the balance of helper and cytotoxic T lymphocytes, polymorphisms of cytokines and growth factors) or environmental conditions triggering or maintaining the disease (i.e. viral or bacterial infections and pollutants). It has been proposed that perpetuation of the inflammation initiated by cigarette smoke and its shift toward an adaptive response may lead to the development of structural changes in the lung, which in turn may promote the establishment of airflow limitation and its subsequent progression [15].

In central airways, the development of airflow obstruction is associated with an increase of macrophages and T lymphocytes in the airway wall and a specific recruitment of neutrophils in the airway lumen and glands [16–18]. Because the adhesion molecules E-selectin and ICAM-1 are up-regulated on submucosal vessels and on bronchial epithelium of smokers with COPD [19], these molecules seem to be important for neutrophil recruitment. Interestingly, mediators released by neutrophils may stimulate the activity of mucus-secreting cells as neutrophil elastase, which is a remarkably potent secretagogue. It is therefore conceivable that neutrophils could be crucial for the development of mucus hypersecretion in central airways, which are indeed the main site responsible for mucus production expressed clinically as chronic bronchitis.

Conversely, peripheral airways are the major site of increased resistance in smokers, as elegantly shown by the pioneering work of Hogg *et al.* [20], who proposed that peripheral airways (less than 2 mm in diameter) represent the lungs 'quiet zone' where disease can accumulate for many years before becoming clinically relevant.

The main pathological lesions associated with the development of COPD in peripheral airways include structural changes, such as epithelial metaplasia, airway wall fibrosis, smooth muscle hypertrophy and inflammatory changes, mainly increased numbers of CD8$^+$ T and B lymphocytes [3,5,21,22] (see Plate 24.1; colour plate section falls between pp. 354 and 355).

Inflammation, fibrosis and smooth muscle hypertrophy, by increasing the thickness of the airway wall, may facilitate uncoupling between airways and parenchyma, therefore promoting airway closure. In addition, airway wall inflammation could contribute to the destruction of alveolar attachments (i.e. the alveolar walls directly attached to the airway wall), allowing the airway wall to deform and thus narrowing the airway lumen. This hypothesis is supported by the observation that, in smokers, the destruction of alveolar attachments is correlated with the degree of inflammation in peripheral airways [23]. This finding suggests a pathogenetic role for airway inflammation in inducing destruction of alveolar attachments. It is possible that mediators released by inflammatory cells may weaken the alveolar tissue and facilitate its rupture, particularly at the point where the attachments join the airway wall, where the mechanical stress is maximal.

CD8$^+$ T lymphocytes, which are increased not only in peripheral but also in central airways and in lung parenchyma [5,6,24], seem to have a crucial role in the pathophysiology of COPD. Traditionally, the major activity of CD8$^+$ cytotoxic T lymphocytes has been considered the rapid resolution of acute viral infections, and viral infections are a frequent occurrence in patients with COPD. The observation that people with frequent respiratory infections in childhood are more prone to develop COPD supports the role of viral infections in this disease [25]. It is conceivable that, in response to repeated viral infections, an excessive recruitment of CD8$^+$ T lymphocytes may occur and damage the lung in susceptible smokers, possibly through the release of tumour necrosis factor α (TNF-α) and perforins [26]. On the other hand, it is also possible that CD8$^+$ T lymphocytes are able to damage the lung even in the absence of a stimulus such as viral infection, as shown by Enelow *et al.* [27], who clearly demonstrated that recognition of a lung 'autoantigen' by cytotoxic T cell may directly produce a marked lung injury. Taking into account these findings, it can be hypothesized that the

CD8$^+$ cytotoxic T-cell accumulation observed in COPD could be a response to an 'autoantigenic' stimulus induced by cigarette smoking [12] (see Plate 24.2; colour plate section falls between pp. 354 and 355).

To better characterize the nature of the inflammatory response present in COPD, the pattern of cytokine profile and chemokine receptor expression has been recently investigated. A current paradigm in immunology is that the nature of an immune response to an antigenic stimulus is determined largely by the pattern of cytokines produced by activated T cells. Type 1 T cells express cytokines, such as γ-interferon (IFN-γ), crucial in the activation of macrophages and in the response to viral and bacterial infections, whereas type 2 T cells express cytokines, such as interleukin 4 (IL-4) and IL-5, involved in immunoglobulin E (IgE) mediated responses and eosinophilia characteristic of allergic diseases. It has recently been shown that the CD8$^+$ T cells infiltrating the peripheral airways in COPD produce IFN-γ and express CXCR3 [28], a chemokine receptor that is known to be preferentially expressed on type 1 cells. Moreover, CXCR3 expression is parallelled by a strong epithelial expression of its ligand CXCL10, suggesting that the CXCR3–CXCL10 axis may be involved in the recruitment of type 1 cells in peripheral airways of smokers with COPD. Recently, Grumelli *et al.* [29] confirmed the presence of CXCR3 on lymphocytes isolated from smokers with COPD. Moreover, they extended those findings by showing that the interaction of CXCL10 with CXCR3 drives the release of matrix metalloproteinase 12 (MMP-12) by macrophages. Because MMP-12 is a potent enzyme which degrades elastin and can cause lung tissue destruction, these data suggest a possible mechanism through which Th1 lymphocytes can drive the progression of emphysema, thus relating the inflammation in peripheral airways to the alveolar wall destruction.

Lung parenchyma and pulmonary arteries

Emphysema is one of the most important pathological hallmarks of COPD, defined anatomically as a condition of the lung characterized by permanent abnormal enlargement of the respiratory airspaces, accompanied by destruction of their walls without obvious fibrosis. Although emphysema has long been recognized as a key component of COPD, the pathogenesis of parenchymal destruction remains enigmatic. The most widely accepted hypothesis relates emphysema to an imbalance of the lung protease–antiprotease system. This hypothesis is based on the observation that activated inflammatory cells release proteases that, overwhelming local antiprotease activity, can destroy lung parenchyma. In particular, neutrophils and macrophages, which are activated by cigarette smoking, are potential sources of proteases such as leucocyte elastase and MMPs, which can damage lung cells and degrade the interstitium (e.g. elastin, collagen, proteoglycans). However, because many cigarette smokers and patients with other inflammatory lung diseases (pneumonia and acute respiratory distress syndrome, ARDS) do not develop significant lung destruction despite a striking inflammatory process, this hypothesis may not fully explain the loss of lung tissue in cigarette smoking-induced emphysema.

There is recent evidence that parenchymal destruction is associated with the presence of an inflammatory process in the alveolar walls [30–32], consisting predominantly of CD8+ T lymphocytes [5]. The observation that these cells are increased in the lung parenchyma of smokers with COPD and show a significant correlation with the degree of airflow obstruction is intriguing and supports the notion that tissue injury may be dependent on T-cell activity. One of the most important consequences of the effects of cytotoxic CD8+ T lymphocytes is the apoptosis of target cells, and it would not be surprising that apoptosis has a role in the destruction of lung tissue in patients with emphysema [32]. Majo et al. [31] have reported that, in smokers with emphysema, both the degree of apoptosis and the number of CD8+ T cells in the alveolar walls increased in parallel with the amount of cigarette smoke inhaled. It can therefore be hypothesized that the proliferation of cytotoxic CD8+ T lymphocytes observed in smokers with COPD may promote lung destruction by inducing apoptosis of alveolar wall cells.

The structural changes occurring in the lungs of patients with COPD may have an important effect on the pulmonary circulation. Indeed, pulmonary hypertension and cor pulmonale are common sequelae to chronic airflow obstruction, but the precise mechanisms of increased vascular resistance are unclear. Potential causes of pulmonary hypertension in COPD include emphysematous destruction of the capillary bed, remodelling of pulmonary vessels and hypoxic pulmonary vasoconstriction [3].

In the pulmonary arteries of subjects with COPD, the most consistent morphological change is the thickening of the intimal layer [33,34], produced by the proliferation of smooth muscle cells and by the deposition of both elastic and collagen fibres. Less frequently, some authors reported a moderate degree of muscular hypertrophy [35]. Endothelium has a crucial role in the regulation of vascular cell growth and tone, through the release of endothelium-derived relaxing factors [36]. Endothelial dysfunction, which results in an impaired release of these factors, has been shown in patients with COPD, even in the absence of hypoxaemia [37]. These functional and structural changes in pulmonary arteries are associated with the infiltration of inflammatory cells, mainly CD8 T lymphocytes, in the adventitial layer [5,38]. This observation supports a possible role for these cells in inducing the vascular alterations in patients with COPD. As pointed out by Barbera et al. [33], it is possible that endothelial damage by cigarette smoke components is the first vascular alteration occurring in COPD. This early alteration may predispose smokers to develop further vascular damage as a result of additional factors, such as hypoxia and inflammation, ultimately leading to pulmonary hypertension.

Lymphocytes in severe COPD

COPD is a progressive disease that, in a minority of subjects, may worsen toward a very severe stage. It has been shown that, in COPD patients, the inflammatory response in the lung enhances as airflow obstruction progressively worsens. Two pioneering studies examined the lung pathology in patients with severe COPD undergoing lung volume reduction surgery [39,40]. Retamales et al. [39] demonstrated that there is an increase in the intensity of the inflammatory response in the alveolar walls and alveolar spaces of these patients, suggesting that the lung inflammation induced by cigarette smoking is amplified in severe emphysema. In a subsequent study, we extended those findings by demonstrating that in severe stages of COPD there is an amplification of the inflammatory response even in the peripheral airways. This enhanced airway inflammatory process correlated with the degrees of airflow limitation, lung hyperinflation, CO diffusion impairment and radiological emphysema, suggesting that the inflammatory response could have a crucial role in the clinical progression of the disease [40]. More recently, Hogg et al. [22] examined lung specimens from a large population of smokers, evaluating the evolution of pathological changes as airflow obstruction progressively worsened. The authors elegantly showed that the progression of COPD (from GOLD stage 0 to GOLD stage 4) [2] was associated with increased mucus production in peripheral airways, thickening of the airway wall and amplification of the inflammatory response, mainly because of an increase in CD8+ T and B cells. Moreover, they showed that, in patients with the most severe stages of COPD, inflammatory cells in the airway wall organize into lymphoid follicles to facilitate antigen presentation to the cells of the adaptive immune response. The authors suggested that these follicles represent an adaptive immune response, which may develop in relation to microbial colonization and infection occurring in the later stages of COPD.

Subjects with severe COPD are notoriously prone to develop exacerbations of the disease, which are a major cause of morbidity and mortality, being associated with a significant health and economic burden through hospital admission and absenteeism from work [2]. Although exacerbations typically punctuate the progression of COPD, their role was underestimated until the study by Donaldson *et al.* [41] demonstrated that the frequency of acute exacerbations contributes to long-term decline in lung function. The authors showed that patients with COPD who suffered frequent exacerbations experienced a significantly greater decline in forced expiratory volume in 1 s (FEV_1) than patients who had infrequent exacerbations. The aetiology of COPD exacerbations has not been established, although there is increased evidence that both bacterial and viral infections may have a role [42,43]. The precise mechanism by which these respiratory infections may induce COPD exacerbations are poorly understood. Examination of patients during exacerbations of COPD by collecting bronchial biopsies, bronchoalveolar lavage and, more recently, spontaneous or induced sputum showed increased airway inflammation and elevated levels of airway inflammatory cytokines [44–46]. In particular, exacerbations are characterized by a marked recruitment of neutrophils, which is associated with an increased expression of IL-8, mieloperoxidase and TNF-α, suggesting a pathogenetic role for bacterial infection. In mild exacerbations of COPD, neutrophilia is parallelled by a marked eosinophilia, which is associated with up-regulation of the eosinophil chemoattractants eotaxin and RANTES [46,47]. Viral infections are the most likely causes of this eosinophilia, because respiratory viruses are able to stimulate the production of both eotaxin and RANTES. There is also evidence that RANTES may act synergistically with CD8$^+$ cells to enhance apoptosis of virally infected cells. As suggested by Zhu *et al.* [47], when CD8$^+$ cells predominate, as in stable COPD, the increase in RANTES occurring during exacerbations may promote tissue damage mediated by CD8$^+$ cells, encouraging the development of emphysema. In this way, repeated exacerbations resulting from viral infections may accelerate the lung function decline in smokers whose CD8$^+$ T-cell numbers are already increased. This hypothesis is supported by the recent observation that, as mentioned above, exacerbation frequency is an important determinant of lung function decline in COPD [41].

Finally, it is important to highlight the need for a better understanding of the mechanisms regulating the interaction between the acute inflammation activated during exacerbations and the underlying inflammatory response in patients with COPD. This is a critical issue when considering that hospital admission for severe exacerbations of COPD is associated with a mortality rate of 49% at 2 years, a dramatic figure resembling that of lung cancer [48]. This knowledge could help to prevent or treat exacerbations and hopefully to improve the otherwise inexorable clinical outcome of these patients.

References

1 Celli BR, MacNee W. ATS/ERS Task Force: Standards for the diagnosis and treatment of patients with COPD: a summary of the ATS/ERS position paper. *Eur Respir J* 2004;**23**:932–46.

2 Pawels RA, Buist AS, Calverley PM, Jenkins CR, Hurd SS. GOLD Scientific Committee: Global strategy for the diagnosis, management and prevention of chronic obstructive pulmonary disease. NHLBI/WHO Global Initiative for Chronic Obstructive Lung Disease (GOLD) Workshop summary. *Am J Respir Crit Care Med* 2001;**163**:1256–76.

3 Saetta M, Turato G, Maestrelli P, Mapp CE, Fabbri LM. Cellular and structural bases of chronic ostructive pulmonary disease. *Am J Respir Crit Care Med* 2001;**163**:1304–9.

4 O'Shaughnessy TC, Ansari TW, Barnes NC, Jeffery PK. Inflammation in bronchial biopsies of subjects with chronic bronchitis: inverse relationship of CD8$^+$ T lymphocytes with FEV_1. *Am J Respir Crit Care Med* 1997;**155**:852–7.

5 Saetta M, Di Stefano A, Turato G *et al.* CD8$^+$ T-lymphocytes in peripheral airways of smokers with chronic obstructive pulmonary disease. *Am J Respir Crit Care Med* 1998;**157**:822–6.

6 Saetta M, Baraldo S, Corbino L *et al.* CD8$^+$ cells in the lungs of smokers with chronic obstructive pulmonary disease. *Am J Respir Crit Care Med* 1999;**160**:711–7.

7 Saetta M, Baraldo S, Turato G *et al.* Increased proportion of CD8$^+$ T lymphocytes in the paratracheal lymph nodes of smokers with mild COPD. *Sarcoidosis Vasc Diffuse Lung Dis* 2003;**20**:28–32.

8 Miller LG, Goldstein G, Murphy M, Ginns LC. Reversible alterations in immunoregulatory T cells in smoking: analysis by monoclonal antibodies and flow cytometry. *Chest* 1982; **82**:526–9.

9 Costabel U, Bross KJ, Reuter C, Ruhle KH, Matthys H. Alterations in immunoregulatory T-cell subsets in cigarette smokers: a phenotypic analysis of bronchoalveolar and blood lymphocytes. *Chest* 1986;**90**:39–44.

10 Janeway CA Jr, Travers P. Principles of innate and adaptive immunity. In: Janeway CA Jr, Travers P, eds. *Immunobiology: the Immune System in Health and Disease*, 3rd edn. London: Current Biology/New York: Garland Publishing, 1996: 1:11–1:20.

11 Jahnsen FL, Brandtzaeg P. Antigen presentation and stimulation of the immune system in human airways. *Allergy* 1999; **54**(Suppl 57):37–49.

12 Cosio MG. T lymphocytes. In: Barnes P, ed. *Chronic Obstructive Pulmonary Disease*. New York: Marcel Dekker, 2005.

13 Pabst R, Schuster M, Tschernig T. Lymphocyte dynamics in the pulmonary microenvironment: implications for the pathophysiology of pulmonary sarcoidosis. *Sarcoidosis Vasc Diffuse Lung Dis* 1999;**16**:197–202.

14 Niewoehner DE, Klienerman J, Rice D. Pathological changes in the peripheral airways of young cigarette smokers. *N Engl J Med* 1974;**291**:755–8.

15 Barnes PJ. Small airways in COPD. *N Engl J Med* 2004;**350**: 2635–7.

16 Di Stefano A, Turato G, Maestrelli P *et al.* Airflow limitation in

chronic bronchitis is associated with T-lymphocyte and macrophage infiltration of the bronchial mucosa. *Am J Respir Crit Care Med* 1996;**153**:629–32.

17 Saetta M, Turato G, Facchini FM *et al.* Inflammatory cells in the bronchial glands of smokers with chronic bronchitis. *Am J Respir Crit Care Med* 1997;**156**:1633–9.

18 Keatings VM, Collins PD, Scott DM, Barnes PJ. Differences in interleukin-8 and tumor necrosis factor-alpha in induced sputum from patients with chronic obstructive pulmonary disease or asthma. *Am J Respir Crit Care Med* 1996;**153**:530–4.

19 Di Stefano A, Maestrelli P, Roggeri A *et al.* Upregulation of adhesion molecules in the bronchial mucosa of subjects with chronic obstructive bronchitis. *Am J Respir Crit Care Med* 1994;**149**:803–10.

20 Hogg JC, Macklem PT, Thurlbeck WM. Site and nature of airway obstruction in chronic obstructive lung disease. *N Engl J Med* 1968;**278**:1355–60.

21 Bosken CH, Hards J, Gatter K, Hogg JC. Characterization of the inflammatory reaction in the peripheral airways of cigarette smokers using immunohistochemistry. *Am Rev Respir Dis* 1992;**145**:911–7.

22 Hogg JC, Chu F, Utokaparch S *et al.* The nature of small-airway obstruction in chronic obstructive pulmonary disease. *N Engl J Med* 2004;**350**:2645–53.

23 Saetta M, Ghezzo H, Kim WD *et al.* Loss of alveolar attachments in smokers: an early morphometric correlate of lung function impairment. *Am Rev Respir Dis* 1985;**132**:894–900.

24 O'Shaughnessy TC, Ansari TW, Barnes NC, Jeffery PK. Inflammation in bronchial biopsies of subjects with chronic bronchitis: inverse relationship of CD8+ T lymphocytes with FEV_1. *Am J Respir Crit Care Med* 1997;**155**:852–7.

25 Paoletti P, Prediletto R, Carrozzi L *et al.* Effects of childhood and adolescence–adulthood respiratory infections in a general population. *Eur Respir J* 1989;**2**:428–36.

26 Liu AN, Mohammed AZ, Rice WR *et al.* Perforin-independent CD8+ T-cell-mediated cytotoxicity of alveolar epithelial cells is preferentially mediated by tumor necrosis factor-alpha: relative insensitivity to Fas ligand. *Am J Respir Cell Mol Biol* 1999;**20**:849–58.

27 Enelow RI, Mohammed AZ, Stoler MH *et al.* Structural and functional consequences of alveolar cell recognition by CD8+ T lymphocytes in experimental lung disease. *J Clin Invest* 1998;**102**:1653–61.

28 Saetta M, Mariani M, Panina-Bordignon P *et al.* Increased expression of the chemokine receptor CXCR3 and its ligand CXCL10 in peripheral airways of smokers with chronic obstructive pulmonary disease. *Am J Respir Crit Care Med* 2002;**165**:1404–9.

29 Grumelli S, Corry D, Song LZ *et al.* An immune basis for lung parenchymal destruction in chronic obstructive pulmonary disease and emphysema. *PLoS Med* 2004;**1**:75–83.

30 Finkelstein R, Fraser RS, Ghezzo H, Cosio MG. Alveolar inflammation and its relation to emphysema in smokers. *Am J Respir Crit Care Med* 1995;**152**:1666–72.

31 Majo J, Ghezzo H, Cosio MG. Lymphocyte population and apoptosis in the lungs of smokers and their relationship with emphysema. *Eur Respir J* 2001;**17**:946–53.

32 Calabrese F, Giacometti C, Beghe B *et al.* Marked alveolar apoptosis/proliferation imbalance in end-stage emphysema. *Respir Res* 2005;**6**:14.

33 Barberà JA, Riverola A, Roca J *et al.* Pulmonary vascular abnormalities and ventilation–perfusion relationship in mild chronic obstructive pulmonary disease. *Am J Respir Crit Care Med* 1994;**149**:423–9.

34 Wright JL, Lawson L, Parè PD *et al.* The structure and function of the pulmonary vasculature in mild chronic obstructive pulmonary disease. *Am Rev Respir Dis* 1983;**128**:702–7.

35 Hale KA, Ewing SL, Gusmell BA, Niewoehner DE. Lung disease in long-term cigarette smokers with and without chronic airflow obstruction. *Am Rev Respir Dis* 1984;**130**:716–21.

36 Dinh-Xuan AT, Higenbottam T, Clelland C *et al.* Impairment of endothelium-dependent pulmonary-artery relaxation in chronic obstructive pulmonary disease. *N Engl J Med* 1991;**324**:1539–47.

37 Peinado VI, Barbcrà JA, Ramircz J *et al.* Endothelial dysfunction in pulmonary arteries of patients with mild COPD. *Am J Physiol* 1998;**274**:L908–13.

38 Peinado VI, Barberà JA, Abate P *et al.* Inflammatory reaction in pulmonary muscular arteries of patients with mild chronic obstructive pulmonary disease. *Am J Respir Crit Care Med* 1999;**159**:1605–11.

39 Retamales I, Elliott WM, Meshi B *et al.* Amplification of inflammation in emphysema and its association with latent adenoviral infection. *Am J Respir Crit Care Med* 2001;**164**:469–73.

40 Turato G, Zuin R, Miniati M *et al.* Airway inflammation in severe chronic obstructive pulmonary disease: relationship with lung function and radiologic emphysema. *Am J Respir Crit Care Med* 2002;**166**:105–10.

41 Donaldson GC, Seemungal TA, Bhowmik A, Wedzicha JA. Relationship between exacerbation frequency and lung function decline in chronic obstructive pulmonary disease. *Thorax* 2002;**57**:847–52.

42 Patel IS, Seemungal TA, Wilks M *et al.* Relationship between bacterial colonisation and the frequency, character, and severity of COPD exacerbations. *Thorax* 2002;**57**:759–64.

43 Seemungal T, Harper-Owen R, Bhowmik A *et al.* Respiratory viruses, symptoms, and inflammatory markers in acute exacerbations and stable chronic obstructive pulmonary disease. *Am J Respir Crit Care Med* 2001;**164**:1618–23.

44 Crooks SW, Bayley DL, Hill SL, Stockley RA. Bronchial inflammation in acute bacterial exacerbations of chronic bronchitis: the role of leukotriene B_4. *Eur Respir J* 2000;**15**:274–80.

45 Aaron SD, Angel JB, Lunau M *et al.* Granulocyte inflammatory markers and airway infection during acute exacerbation of chronic obstructive pulmonary disease. *Am J Respir Crit Care Med* 2001;**163**:349–55.

46 Saetta M, Di Stefano A, Maestrelli P *et al.* Airway eosinophilia in chronic bronchitis during exacerbations. *Am J Respir Crit Care Med* 1994;**150**:1646–52.

47 Zhu J, Qui YS, Majumdar S *et al.* Exacerbations of bronchitis: bronchial eosinophilia and gene expression for interleukin-4, interleukin-5, and eosinophil chemoattractants. *Am J Respir Crit Care Med* 2001;**164**:109–16.

48 Connors FA, Dawson NV, Thomas C *et al.* Outcomes following acute exacerbation of severe chronic obstructive lung disease. *Am J Respir Crit Care Med* 1996;**154**:959–67.

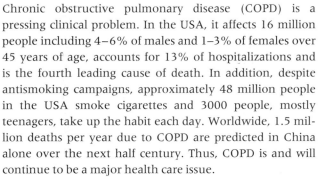

CHAPTER 25
Cytokines

Jack A. Elias and Robert J. Homer

Chronic obstructive pulmonary disease (COPD) is a pressing clinical problem. In the USA, it affects 16 million people including 4–6% of males and 1–3% of females over 45 years of age, accounts for 13% of hospitalizations and is the fourth leading cause of death. In addition, despite antismoking campaigns, approximately 48 million people in the USA smoke cigarettes and 3000 people, mostly teenagers, take up the habit each day. Worldwide, 1.5 million deaths per year due to COPD are predicted in China alone over the next half century. Thus, COPD is and will continue to be a major health care issue.

The GOLD guidelines recognize COPD for the first time to be a chronic inflammatory condition [1]. Cytokines are extracellular signalling peptides critically important in the regulation of inflammation as well as having important effector functions of their own. Cytokines generally are produced in patterns characteristic of a particular disease. A description of the cytokines involved in COPD would not only further our understanding of the basic biology of the process, but would also shed light on clinical subgroups of patients and would provide novel targets for therapeutic intervention.

A basic understanding of cytokine biology is needed before discussing their role in COPD [2]. Cytokines can be divided into several subgroups including inflammatory cytokines, immune cytokines, chemokines and anti-inflammatory cytokines. Inflammatory cytokines include tumour necrosis factor α (TNF-α) and interleukin 1β (IL-1β). These cytokines are characterized by participation in virtually any non-specific inflammatory process. They are made by a wide variety of cells, although IL-1β and TNF are principally made by macrophages. They induce a variety of acute phase reactions including fever, leucocytosis, production of other cytokines from a variety of cells, and expression of adhesion molecules on endothelium. Chemokines are important chemoattractants and growth factors. Biochemically they are generally in the 8–10 kDa range and can be subclassified into four different structural families. The two most important subfamilies are the CC and the CXC families based on the presence of two cysteine residues either adjacent to each other (CC family) or separated by another amino acid (CXC family). The CC chemokines including eotaxin, RANTES and macrophage chemotactic protein-1 (MCP-1) are involved in chemoattraction of eosinophils, monocytes and T cells and function through the CCR family of receptors. The CXC chemokines including IL-8, GRO-α, and ENA-78 are involved in the recruitment and activation of neutrophils and function through the CXCR family of receptors. Immune cytokines include interleukin-4 (IL-4), IL-13 and γ-interferon (IFN-γ). These cytokines are produced predominantly, although not exclusively, by T cells and are generally thought to reflect specialized differentiation of T cells into Th1 (IFN-γ) and Th2 (IL-4, IL-13) subsets. Th1 T cells are thought to be critically important in resistance to intracellular infections such as tuberculosis while Th2 T cells are thought to be critically important in parasitic infections and allergy. Cytolytic T cells may have similar divisions into Tc1 and Tc2 cells. Cytokines such as IL-10 and transforming growth factor β (TGF-β) one are generally considered anti-inflammatory and may be critically important in so-called regulatory T cells.

Expression in human disease

Investigators have attempted to define the inflammatory profile of COPD by examining the inflammatory cell and cytokine pattern seen in these patients. The interpretation is complex because the function of each cytokine depends on the overall inflammatory context (e.g. the presence of other cytokines). Neutrophils, T cells, macrophages and eosinophils are involved in the inflammatory response in patients with COPD. However, the importance of each is difficult to ascertain because of confounding influences relating to methods of assessment (sputum vs bronchoalveolar lavage [BAL] vs biopsy), site of assessment (central vs peripheral airway vs parenchyma) and the compartmentalization of the inflammation in these patients [3]. As a result of the latter, neutrophils are more readily appreciated in sputum and BAL than biopsies, eosinophils are seen with equal efficacy in all assessments and lymphocytes are predominantly noted in tissues [3–5].

It is not known whether this reflects differences in transit time in tissue or transit from other anatomical sites, such as from airway rather than parenchyma. Another major problem is interpreting the results with appropriate control groups. Many studies have attempted to include patients with COPD, 'healthy' smokers and non-smokers. However, because all studies to date have been cross-sectional rather than longitudinal, it is not clear whether some of the 'healthy' smokers simply were identified early in their disease progression and ultimately will become 'unhealthy' smokers. Finally, because of COPD clinical heterogeneity, it is hard to know how comparable different patient groups are among different studies.

Studies using BAL have demonstrated at least a fivefold increase in cell recovery with 95% or more of these cells being macrophages. Increases in neutrophil recovery have also been noted [3]. Comparisons of central airway biopsies from smokers and non-smokers demonstrate increased numbers of macrophages and T lymphocytes, without significant differences in neutrophils, eosinophils or mast cell [3,6]. In addition, a number of studies have demonstrated that eosinophilia is a prominent finding in sputum, BAL and tissues from patients with COPD during exacerbations [3,7] and that eosinophilia can be seen in the submucosa of bronchioles from smokers [8]. Eosinophils may be present in some patients, which may correlate with corticosteroid responsiveness [7]. Eosinophil degradation products are found in virtually all COPD patients, however, in levels higher than in asthmatics [9]. It has been suggested that the discrepancy between the number of cells vs cell products is caused by increased cell death, possibly because of concurrent presence of neutrophils. In patients with exacerbations of COPD or severe COPD, increases in neutrophils have been noted [3].

A mononuclear inflammatory response has also been noted in biopsies from the peripheral airways and parenchyma of smokers [10,11]. Even after smoking has ceased, the inflammatory response continues [12]. Importantly, comparisons of tissues from smokers with and without COPD demonstrated that many of the lymphocytes in COPD tissues are CD8$^+$ cells [11]. At present it is not clear if these CD8$^+$ cells are the result of the recurrent viral infections experienced by these patients [11] or perhaps associated with an occult viral infection. One group has long proposed that occult adenoviral infection is related to COPD and has shown that there is a correlation of number of CD8 cells and of number of epithelial cells expressing adenoviral E1A protein [13]. Experimentally, coinfection with adenovirus increases CD8 cells in a smoking model [14]. CD8$^+$ cell number correlates directly with the number of pack-years of cigarette smoke exposure [11].

In an attempt to understand the importance of these cell populations, investigators have looked for correlations between their presence and number, and disease severity. Lymphocyte counts correlate directly with indices of alveolar destruction [15] and the number of CD8$^+$ cells correlates with the degree of airflow limitation [6,11]. The importance of neutrophils is less clear with correlations between neutrophil number and airflow limitation [3], and neutrophil number and integrity of pulmonary function being reported [15]. In the latter study, it was proposed that, as long as the inflammatory response was composed of granulocytes, there was no destruction of the lung.

The lymphocytes express CXCR3, a chemokine receptor preferentially expressed on Th1 lymphocytes [16,17]. The number of CXCR3$^+$ cells in the epithelium and submucosa is increased in smokers with COPD compared with non-smoking subjects, but not compared with smokers with normal lung function. Immunoreactivity for IP10, the ligand for CXCR3, is present in the bronchiolar epithelium of smokers with COPD but not in the bronchiolar epithelium of smoking and non-smoking control subjects. Most CXCR3$^+$ cells coexpressed CD8 and produced IFN-γ [16,17]. The Th1 cells also show evidence of activation with increased expression of the transcription factor STAT-4 [18]. This is consistent with the demonstration that the adoptive transfer of Th1 cells to the lung elicits a neutrophilic inflammatory response [19]. A Th1 predominance can also be seen in peripheral blood [20]. Experimentally, IFN induces emphysema by itself (see below). CD8 T cells also make granzyme and perforins which may injure the lung. Finally, these cells may either make cytokines, which recruit other inflammatory cells that injure the lung, or they may induce parenchymal cells to produce such signals [21].

Concentrations of TNF-α, IL-1β, IL-6, IL-8 and MCP-1 are elevated in the lungs of smokers [22–24]. Furthermore, IL-1β and IL-8 are elevated in a cigarette dose-dependent manner and TNF-α and IL-8 are elevated in the patients with COPD compared with the smoking and non-smoking control subjects [22,23]. TNF is particularly important as it activates macrophages to produce proteases ([25] and see below). IL-8 may be the most significant of the neutrophilic chemokines. Significant correlation was found in lavage fluid of COPD patients between IL-8 and neutrophils [4]. Of five chemoattractants examined in one study (IL-8, ENA-78, leukotriene B$_4$ which are primarily chemotactic for neutrophils; MCP-1 and macrophage inflammatory protein-1α [MIP-1α] which are predominantly chemotactic for mononuclear leucocytes) only the level of IL-8 in BAL fluid clearly distinguished between subjects with and without emphysema among current smokers [26]. Both GRO-α and MCP-1 are also overexpressed in patients with COPD but not healthy smokers or controls [27].

Not only are there increased amounts of cytokines in COPD lungs at baseline, but lung macrophages from patients with COPD can be stimulated to produce enhanced amount of IL-8, TNF and IL-10 [25]. Other CXC chemokines (GRO-α, ENA-78) also show enhanced release [28]. *In vitro*, cigarette smoke causes increased expression of IL-8 and G-CSF (neutrophilic activity) and MCP-1 (monocytic activity) by bronchial epithelial cells, and TNF and IL-6 by alveolar macrophages [29–31]. Not only does smoke cause enhanced release of cytokines from COPD macrophages, but IL-10 inhibits release of proteases in macrophages from controls but not smokers [25].

COPD is characterized by recurrent exacerbations during which there is an acute decline in respiratory function. During these exacerbations, eosinophils and T lymphocytes represent common features in the airways. Despite the presence of eosinophils, no increased IL-5 is seen in tissue [32]. Results have differed among groups concerning other products known to regulate eosinophils, with either eotaxin or RANTES correlating with pulmonary eosinophilia [33–35]. All of the IL-4 and IL-5 positive T cells were CD4 and none were CD8.

Recently, it has been recognized that systemic effects are commonly seen in patients with COPD. These effects are clinically relevant because they modify and can help in the classification and management of the disease [36]. These include affective disorders, cardiovascular and musculoskeletal abnormalities, and metabolic and nutritional disturbances. At least some of these may be caused by systemic levels of cytokines produced in the lung. It is known that patients with COPD have increased skeletal muscle atrophy and apoptosis [37]. Circulating levels of TNF-α may cause increased apoptosis of skeletal muscle as well as weight loss [38–41]. Some authors have associated hypoxia per se with production of TNF-α or associated greater energy expenditure to TNF-α levels [42–45].

Another approach to determine the role of cytokines in COPD is to look at genetic polymorphisms that alter expression or activity of these products [46]. TNF-α polymorphisms have attracted considerable attention [47–55]. Unfortunately, no consensus is apparent, with some papers strongly supporting a claim of association and others opposing one. Fewer papers have examined other cytokines. Polymorphism in the *IL4RA* gene has been associated with accelerated decline in lung function [56]. In this study, association with IL-13 was much weaker. Other studies have shown a stronger association with IL-13 polymorphism [57]. The redundancy of the cytokine or inflammatory system may make it impossible to see any but the strongest effects unless enormous populations are examined.

Experimental models of emphysema

It is crucial to have a theoretical understanding of the biology of emphysema in order to interpret the results of necessarily descriptive human data and to guide future human experimentation. This requires intensive analysis of animal models. Groups have taken a variety of approaches to this problem [58]. The most straightforward approach is simply to expose an appropriate animal to cigarette smoke. This model has the advantage of being perhaps the most relevant but is very slow and the effects are relatively small. Some groups still use intratracheal applications of protease, because it is more rapid than cigarette smoke exposure and effects are large. The most recent approach involves genetic modification of mice, either through transgenic overexpression or knockout of specific genes. A potential drawback of genetic manipulation of mice is that development-dependent phenotypes must be distinguished from acquired adult-onset phenotypes more relevant to human COPD. One group has approached this problem by use of tightly controlled externally regulated promoters [59]. Other groups have simply ensured that any effect is not apparent until adulthood. We discuss only those models most relevant to the role of cytokines in COPD.

Any description of COPD ultimately requires an understanding of the relationship of proteases, inflammation and cytokines. The current dominant model in emphysema is the so-called protease–antiprotease hypothesis [60]. In this concept, the normal lung is believed to be protected by an antiprotease 'shield' which negates the function of proteolytic enzymes that are released into the airway or parenchyma. The increase in proteinase burden is thought to derive from inflammatory cells which are recruited to the lung in response to cigarette smoke and possibly other agents. Ineffective or disordered repair of elastic fibres and or collagen and oxidant-induced injury may also contribute to the pathogenesis of these disorders [61].

This classic model suggests that proteases work primarily via proteolytic digestion of the extracellular matrix, particularly elastin. This theory has been challenged recently by the concept of lung apoptosis or vascular insufficiency as a major source of lung parenchymal loss [62,63]. The two approaches may be reconciled because it is possible that proteases may contribute to tissue destruction by promoting apoptosis [64,65]. Direct experimental evidence also suggests that proteases are upstream from at least a portion of the inflammatory response [66,67].

The specific proteases and antiproteases involved in COPD are still unclear [60]. Candidate proteases include members of the serine protease family (e.g. neutrophil elastase [NE]), cysteine protease family (e.g. cathepsin B) and the matrix metalloproteinase family (MMPs, e.g. MMP-12) [68]. The MMPs have attracted considerable attention because expression of various MMPs are seen in smokers' lungs but not in controls, genetic polymorphisms of MMPs have been implicated in human emphysema and overexpression of MMP-1 in the murine lung leads to acquired adult-onset emphysema [58,69–74]. Numerous antiproteases have also been implicated in the control of pulmonary proteolysis. They include α_1-antitrypsin, secretory leucocyte protease inhibitor (SLPI) and elafin (inhibitors of various serine proteinases), α_2-macroglobulin (a broad-spectrum protease inhibitor) and the tissue inhibitors of metalloproteinases (TIMPs). Members of the cystatin superfamily may also be important [60]. Mice deficient in TIMP-3 develop spontaneous air space enlargement in the lung which is evident at 2 weeks after birth and progresses with the age of the animal [75].

IL-13 and IFN-γ

Although cigarette smoke exposure is the single most important predictor of the development of COPD after age 35, it is important to appreciate the complex nature of the relationship between COPD and cigarette smoke. Population-based studies such as the Lung Health Study, Normative Aging Study and epidemiological studies from the Netherlands have demonstrated that asthma and airways hyperresponsiveness (AHR) are independent risk factors for the development of COPD and for a COPD phenotype characterized by the accelerated loss of pulmonary function [76–79]. Rapid loss of lung function is also seen in asthmatic patients who smoke. The forced expiratory volume in 1 s (FEV_1) decline experienced by these patients is greater than that in non-asthmatic smokers or asthmatic non-smokers [7,80]. Smokers can also have elevated immunoglobulin E (IgE) levels and elevated levels of circulating eosinophils. In these studies, eosinophilia correlates inversely with pulmonary function, highlighting a group of patients that experience a rapid loss of pulmonary function [79]. These sorts of observations led, in 1961, to the formulation of the 'Dutch hypothesis', which proposes that the distinctions between COPD and asthma are not absolute and that some of the mechanisms that are responsible for asthma are also important in the pathogenesis of COPD. This hypothesis points to endogenous factors including AHR and atopy as markers of a basic disturbance or constitution that predisposes to the development of chronic non-specific obstructive lung disease. This contrasts with the 'British hypothesis', which focuses strictly on exogenous factors such as exposure to cigarette smoke and postulated that recurrent airway infections are responsible for the generation of chronic airflow limitation in COPD.

IL-13 is a 12-kDa protein product of a gene on chromosome 5 at q31 which is produced in large quantities by activated Th2 cells and is thought to be critically important in allergic responses including asthma [81]. It has also been demonstrated in the airways of patients with COPD with mucus hypersecretion [82]. In light of the Dutch hypothesis, which suggests a role for allergy in COPD, studies were undertaken to define the chronic *in vivo* effector functions of IL-13 in the airway [83]. An externally regulated system was used to overexpress IL-13 in lung. These mice showed a significant increase in induced IL-13 protein production within 48 h and steady state levels of IL-13 (0.5–1.5 ng/mL in BAL fluid) within 96 h. The animals' lungs developed an inflammatory infiltrate over approximately 2–3 weeks, which was characterized by increased numbers of macrophages, lymphocytes and eosinophils (see Plate 25.1; colour plate section falls between pp. 354 and 355). During this interval, massive alveolar septal destruction and alveolar enlargement also occurred as shown by both casual inspection and morphometry. Alveolar enlargement could be appreciated within 48 h, was prominent within 7 days and continued to progress for at least 1 month. Furthermore, comparable to human COPD in which total lung capacity is increased, the transgenic mice showed a two- to threefold increase in lung volume. The overinflation was accompanied by enhanced pulmonary compliance, again as seen in human disease. Airway changes included fibrosis and mucus metaplasia. Similar to some patients with COPD, these mice had marked airway hyperresponsiveness.

To begin to understand the mechanism(s) of IL-13-induced emphysema, studies were undertaken to determine if IL-13 altered the levels of, and/or bioactivities of, a variety of proteases (Table 25.1). By a variety of techniques, IL-13 was a potent stimulator of MMP-2, -9, -12, -13 and -14. The alterations in MMP-9 and MMP-12 were quite prominent. In contrast, IL-13-induced alterations in the levels of mRNA encoding MMP-7 were not detected. Interestingly, immunohistochemistry (IHC) demonstrated that MMP-12 was most prominent in alveolar macrophages, while MMP-9 staining was most prominent in epithelial and other stromal cells. Increases in the levels of mRNA encoding cathepsin B, K and L and lesser increases in S were also seen. Antiproteases were also affected, because α_1-antitrypsin was significantly reduced and TIMP-1 was increased, while TIMP-2, TIMP-3, SLPI and cystatin C were not significantly altered.

To further understand the importance of these pathways, specific protease inhibitors were given to the animals. Both the specific MMP inhibitor GM6001 and the cystein protease inhibitors E-64 or leupeptin caused an approximately 70% decrease in the IL-13-induced increase in lung volume and chord length and a > 90% decrease in BAL cellularity with a > 95% decrease in eosinophil influx and lymphocyte accumulation. Neither inhibitor affected mucus metaplasia or the levels of BAL IL-13.

To further characterize the role of these proteases, the

Table 25.1 Comparison of effects of murine lung overexpression of interleukin 13 and γ-interferon.

Protease/ antiprotease/mucus	IL-13 mice	Interferon mice
Proteases		
MMP-2, -9, -13, -14	Increased	Unchanged
MMP-12	Increased	Increased
Cathepsin B, H, S	Increased	Increased
Cathepsin D	Unchanged	Increased
Cathepsin K	Increased	Unchanged
Antiproteases		
SLPI		Decreased
TIMP-1	Increased	Unchanged
α_1-antitrypsin	Decreased	Unchanged
Mucus	Increased	No change

IL-13, interleukin 13; MMP, matrix metalloproteinase; SLPI, secretory leucocyte protease inhibitor; TIMP-1, tissue inhibitor of metalloproteinase-1.

IL-13 mice were bred with mice specifically deficient in MMP-9 and MMP-12, which have been heavily implicated in murine and human emphysema. In both cases, the emphysema as measured by chord length, compliance and lung size was markedly reduced, showing that both enzymes are specifically required [84]. The induction of MMP-2, -9, -13 and -14 was at least partially dependent on MMP-12 because IL-13 overexpressing mice deficient in MMP-12 showed reduced induction of those enzymes. The MMP-12 deficient mice also showed a reduction in recovery of total leucocytes, eosinophils and macrophages, but not lymphocytes or neutrophils. On the other hand, loss of MMP-9 from the IL-13 overexpressing mice had no effect on induction of MMP-2, -12, -13 and -14 and did not alter eosinophil, macrophage or lymphocyte recovery, but increased the recovery of total leucocytes and neutrophils in BAL fluids. This suggests that MMP-9 is downstream in the effector cascade from MMP-12.

The role of chemokines in the development in the IL-13 phenotype was also examined [85]. IL-13 stimulates expression of a large number of CC chemokines including MCP-1, -2, -3 and -5, macrophage inflammatory protein 1α (MIP-1α), MIP-1β, MIP-2, MIP-3α, thymus- and activation-regulated chemokine, thymus-expressed chemokine, eotaxin, eotaxin 2, macrophage-derived chemokines, and C10. The role of the CC chemokine receptor CCR2 in mediating the effects of IL-13 was then examined by breeding CCR2 knockout mice with the IL-13 mice. The CCR2 knockout mice showed reduced lung size, alveolar size and lung compliance with reduced inflammation. However, CCR2

deficiency did not decrease the basal or IL-13-stimulated expression of target matrix MMPs or cathepsins but did increase the levels of mRNA encoding α_1-antitrypsin, tissue inhibitor of MMP-1, -2 and -4, and SLPI. These studies demonstrate that IL-13 is a potent stimulator of MCPs and other CC chemokines and document the importance of MCP–CCR2 signalling in the pathogenesis of the IL-13-induced pulmonary phenotype.

CD8+ lymphocytes have been identified to be in excess in lungs of patients with COPD and are thought to produce IFN-γ. In order to examine the role of IFN-γ directly, mice that overexpress IFN-γ in the lung were examined [86]. These mice also developed emphysema, but there were striking differences from the IL-13 mice (see Plate 25.1; colour plate section falls between pp. 354 and 355). There was only a mild tissue inflammatory response made up of mononuclear cells and occasional granulocytes. BAL revealed an approximately threefold increase in cell recovery, with 18% neutrophils and the remainder macrophages and lymphocytes. In contrast to the IL-13 animals, no mucus was seen. In fact, IFN-γ is known to inhibit mucus production [87].

Proteases were also evaluated in these mice (see Table 25.1). IFN-γ enhanced the levels of mRNA encoding MMP-12 and cathepsins S, H and D. Lesser increases in cathepsin B were noted. Alterations in MMP-9, MMP-13 or cathepsin K were not appreciated. Zymography and Western blot confirmed the selective induction of MMP-12 and E-64 active site probe analysis confirmed the induction of cathepsins S, H and B. In contrast, IFN-γ was a potent inhibitor of the levels of SLPI mRNA and otherwise had no effect on antiproteases. Protease inhibitors prevented emphysema in these mice. In addition, the IFN-γ mice showed increased epithelial cell apoptosis. Interestingly, inhibition of either cathepsin S or caspases reduced apoptosis, inflammation and emphysema indicated that these three features are closely interrelated [88].

The data noted above demonstrate that IL-13 and IFN-γ both cause emphysema when targeted to the adult murine lung. IL-13 caused mucus metaplasia while IFN-γ did not. In addition, emphysema induced by IL-13 was associated with an inflammatory response made up of macrophages, eosinophils and lymphocytes while that caused by IFN-γ was associated with macrophages and granulocytes. The mechanisms of these emphysematous responses also appeared to differ because IL-13 and IFN-γ caused different patterns of MMP and cathepsin activation and only IFN-γ decreased SLPI expression (see Table 25.1). These similarities and differences are intriguing when one compares them with the different clinical presentations seen in patients with COPD. In many ways, the IFN-γ mice have a phenotype that is similar to patients who are commonly encountered clinically as having COPD associated with BAL neutrophilia. In contrast, the IL-13 mice may model patients with asthma, eosinophilia or AHR who manifest accelerated rates of loss of lung function after exposure to cigarette smoke. In many ways, the IL-13 mouse is the transgenic substantiation of aspects of the Dutch hypothesis because these mice show that genes that are strongly implicated in the asthmatic diathesis can have a key role in the generation of emphysema.

Vascular endothelial growth factor and apoptosis

A striking series of experiments have shown that continuous stimulation with vascular endothelial growth factor (VEGF, a trophic and survival factor for endothelial cells), which is normally highly expressed in the lung, is required for prevention of emphysema in the rat [89,90]. Chronic treatment of rats with a VEGF receptor antagonist led to enlargement of the air spaces, indicative of emphysema. Viewed by angiography, these rat lungs showed a pruning of the pulmonary arterial tree as well as increased alveolar septal cell apoptosis. Treatment with a caspase inhibitor prevented VEGF antagonist induced septal cell apoptosis and emphysema. There was no lung infiltration by inflammatory cells. When oxidative injury, which is known to be elevated in lungs of smokers, was blocked, emphysema lessened. In support of the VEGF hypothesis, VEGF, VEGF R2 protein and mRNA expression are significantly reduced in emphysema [62,91]. Given the current clinical interest in VEGF antagonists for therapy of malignancies and the possible need to give these reagents for long periods of time, the role of VEGF in human disease is a critical issue. However, regardless of the ultimate role of VEGF in human disease, these studies established the critical concept that proteolytic matrix degradation does not need to be the primary event in the development of emphysema. The presence of apoptosis of septal cells in human disease was supported by two subsequent studies, which included multiple apoptosis assays including TUNEL, single-stranded DNA staining, caspase 3 immunohistochemistry, a DNA ligase assay and DNA laddering [62,63].

Cigarette smoke, MMP-12 and TNF-α

Mice with a targeted disruption of MMP-12 are resistant to cigarette smoke-induced emphysema [92]. Interestingly, MMP-12 deficiency also decreased cigarette smoke-induced pulmonary inflammation. RS113456, a metalloprotease inhibitor, also prevented neutrophil influx and connective tissue breakdown. Thus, acute smoke-induced connective tissue breakdown, the precursor to emphysema, requires MMP-12 and the neutrophil influx appears to be secondary

to macrophage activation [93]. Similar results are obtained with a synthetic serine elastase inhibitor or with α_1-antitrypsin. Some proteases are therefore upstream of the inflammatory response and not simply an effector mechanism [94,95]. Both wild type (MMP-12 +/+) mice and mice lacking MMP-12 (MMP-12 −/−) demonstrated rapid increases in whole-lung nuclear factor-κB activation and gene expression of pro-inflammatory cytokines after cigarette smoke exposure, indicating that a lack of MMP-12 does not produce a global failure to up-regulate inflammatory mediators. However, only MMP-12 +/+ mice demonstrated increased whole-lung TNF-α protein or release of TNF-α from cultured alveolar macrophages exposed to smoke *in vitro*. Levels of whole-lung E-selectin, an endothelial activation marker, were increased only in MMP-12 +/+ mice. These findings suggest that, acutely, MMP-12 mediates smoke-induced inflammation by releasing TNF-α from macrophages, with subsequent endothelial activation, neutrophil influx and proteolytic matrix breakdown caused by neutrophil-derived proteases [96]. Furthermore, mice deficient in both TNF-α receptor subunits (p55 and p75) show no increase in gene expression of TNF-α, neutrophil chemoattractant, MIP-2 and MCP-1 due to cigarette smoke. At 24 h, control mice demonstrated increases in lavage neutrophils, macrophages, desmosine (a measure of elastin breakdown) and hydroxyproline (a measure of collagen breakdown), whereas TNF-α receptor knockout mice did not [67].

Additional evidence that proteases can be upstream from the inflammatory process rather than function only as effector molecules is provided by studies with mice deficient in TNF-α receptor exposed to an exogenous protease. A single intratracheal dose of porcine pancreatic elastase, which is cleared from the lung by 24 h, was administered to wild type IL-1β type 1 receptor-deficient, double TNF-α (type 1 and type 2) receptor-deficient, and combined TNF-α (type 1 receptor) plus IL-1β receptor-deficient mice. There was marked reduction in the development of emphysema in the combined knockout mice and moderate reduction in the TNF-α receptor knockout mice. The level of apoptosis assessed by a TUNEL assay was increased at 5 days after elastase treatment and was markedly and similarly attenuated in the IL-1β, the double TNF-α and the combined receptor-deficient mice [66]. This shows that the injury induced by exogenous elastase requires amplification via induction of endogenous mediators.

TGF-β1

TGF-β1 is a member of the TGF-β superfamily with complex effector functions. It is produced by all leucocytes and some stromal cells. It is best known for its anti-inflammatory and profibrotic activity, although in appropriate settings it can induce inflammation and cell death, and inhibit wound healing. TGF-β1 is secreted in an inactive form and requires extracellular activation. A number of activation pathways for TGF-β1 have been identified, including interaction with the epithelial-restricted integrin αvβ6. In mice deficient in this integrin, MMP-12 was seen to be markedly up-regulated [97]. These mice consequently develop age-related emphysema. This emphysema is completely abrogated either by transgenic expression of versions of the β6 integrin subunit that support TGF-β activation, the loss of MMP-12 or simultaneous transgenic expression of active TGF-β1. TGF-β1 suppresses MMP-12 production by macrophages directly. This implies a role for TGF-β1 in preventing emphysema. Defects in fibrillin and TGF-β latent binding protein-4 also lead to reduced TGF-β activity and adult-onset emphysma [98,99]. The relevance of these findings to human disease is not clear, especially because the role of MMP-12 in human as opposed to murine emphysema has been strongly questioned [68]. Furthermore, TGF-β is overexpressed in COPD, not underexpressed [100]. It is also not clear from these results if MMP-12 is acting via matrix proteolysis directly or if it is inducing alveolar cell apoptosis.

Conclusions

A number of novel experimental findings have changed the paradigm of COPD research. The ability of IL-13 to induce COPD was unexpected and raised the issue of the relation of COPD and asthma. The significance of CD8 T cells in human COPD is enhanced by the experimental data that IFN-γ can produce emphysma. The difference in protease and antiprotease expression of those two models reinforces

the notion of COPD heterogeneity. The data on apoptosis and COPD raised an entirely new hypothesis about the pathogenesis of this disease and suggests a new relationship of proteases, inflammation and lung destruction. Our understanding of the biology of this disease is just beginning, however. For example, IL-13 induces both VEGF and TGF-β1 [101,102]. Clearly, the presence of these mediators in the IL-13 mice does not provide complete protection from emphysema in this model. Whether these products are providing partial protection in this model is not known.

A model incorporating these newer data is shown in Figure 25.1. The canonical smoking–inflammation–protease pathway is shown in the middle. Question marks are indicated next to areas of uncertainty. It is not known how and if IL-13 and IFN-γ boxes are produced in human smokers' lungs. The presence of MMP-12 in human lungs is similarly controversial. While cigarette smoke reduces VEGF, which may lead to apoptosis, the ability of cigarette smoke to increase free radicals is well known, which may also directly lead to apoptosis independent of VEGF deficiency. TGF-β is included as a negative regulator of MMP-12, thus potentially preventing emphysema despite evidence that TGF-β is overexpressed in human emphysma.

The human data show a large number of mediators expressed but does not address the significance of any one mediator. In order to do so, clinical trials of various inhibitors will be required. TNF and IL-1β antagonists are possible but not exclusive choices because they are already in clinical use for other indications. It seems likely that many of these mediators will be important in specific subsets of patients. Data correlating expression with specific clinical phenotypes will therefore be critical in order to direct therapeutic trials.

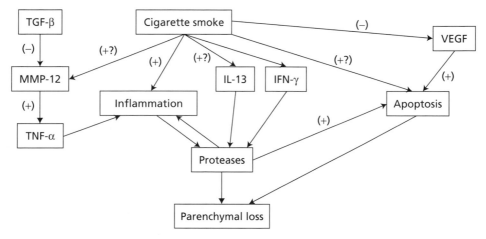

Figure 25.1 Model of human COPD. Canonical model of inflammation leading to elastolytic proteases is shown in the centre. Note that data now show that some elastases require induction of additional inflammation to induce parenchymal loss. In addition, it is known that proteases can lead to an alternative mode of parenchymal loss, namely apoptosis (see text for discussion). IFN-γ, γ-interferon; IL-13, interleukin 13; MMP-12, metalloproteinase 12; TGF-β, transforming growth factor β; TNF-α, tumour necrosis factor α; VEGF, vascular endothelial growth factor.

References

1 National Institutes of Health, National Heart, Lung, and Blood Institute. *Global Initiative for Chronic Obstructive Lung Disease. Global Strategy for the Diagnosis, Management, and Prevention of Chronic Obstructive Pulmonary Disease.* NHLBI/WHO Workshop Report. Publication no. 2701, 2001.

2 Chung KF. Cytokines in chronic obstructive pulmonary disease. *Eur Respir J Suppl* 2001;**34**:50S–9S.

3 Saetta M, Turato G, Maestrelli P, Mapp CE, Fabbri LM. Cellular and structural bases of chronic obstructive pulmonary disease. *Am J Respir Crit Care Med* 2001;**163**:1304–9.

4 Pesci A, Balbi B, Majori M *et al.* Inflammatory cells and mediators in bronchial lavage of patients with chronic obstructive pulmonary disease. *Eur Respir J* 1998;**12**:380–6.

5 Rutgers SR, Timens W, Kaufmann HF *et al.* Comparison of induced sputum with bronchial wash, bronchoalveolar lavage and bronchial biopsies in COPD. *Eur Respir J* 2000;**15**:109–15.

6 O'Shaughnessy TC, Ansari TW, Barnes NC, Jeffery PK. Inflammation in bronchial biopsies of subjects with chronic bronchitis: inverse relationship of CD8$^+$ T lymphocytes with FEV_1. *Am J Respir Crit Care Med* 1997;**155**:852–7.

7 Boushey HA. Glucocorticoid therapy for chronic obstructive pulmonary disease. *N Engl J Med* 1999;**340**:1990–1.

8 Lams BE, Sousa AR, Rees PJ, Lee TH. Subepithelial immunopathology of the large airways in smokers with and without chronic obstructive pulmonary disease. *Eur Respir J* 2000;**15**:512–6.

9 Barnes PJ. New concepts in chronic obstructive pulmonary disease. *Annu Rev Med* 2003;**54**:113–29.

10 Saetta M, Di Stefano A, Turato G *et al.* CD8$^+$ T-lymphocytes in peripheral airways of smokers with chronic obstructive pulmonary disease. *Am J Respir Crit Care Med* 1998;**157**:822–6.

11 Saetta M, Baraldo S, Corbino L *et al.* CD8$^+$ cells in the lungs of smokers with chronic obstructive pulmonary disease. *Am J Respir Crit Care Med* 1999;**160**:711–7.

12 Rutgers SR, Postma DS, ten Hacken NH *et al.* Ongoing airway inflammation in patients with COPD who do not currently smoke. *Thorax* 2000;**55**:12–8.

13 Retamales I, Elliott WM, Meshi B *et al.* Amplification of inflammation in emphysema and its association with latent adenoviral infection. *Am J Respir Crit Care Med* 2001;**164**:469–73.

14 Meshi B, Vitalis TZ, Ionescu D *et al.* Emphysematous lung destruction by cigarette smoke: the effects of latent adenoviral infection on the lung inflammatory response. *Am J Respir Cell Mol Biol* 2002;**26**:52–7.

15 Finkelstein R, Fraser RS, Ghezzo H, Cosio MG. Alveolar inflammation and its relation to emphysema in smokers. *Am J Respir Crit Care Med* 1995;**152**:1666–72.

16 Saetta M, Mariani M, Panina-Bordignon P *et al.* Increased expression of the chemokine receptor CXCR3 and its ligand CXCL10 in peripheral airways of smokers with chronic obstructive pulmonary disease. *Am J Respir Crit Care Med* 2002;**165**:1404–9.

17 Grumelli S, Corry DB, Song LZ *et al.* An immune basis for lung parenchymal destruction in chronic obstructive pulmonary disease and emphysema. *PLoS Med* 2004;**1**:e8.

18 Di Stefano A, Caramori G, Capelli A *et al.* STAT4 activation in smokers and patients with chronic obstructive pulmonary disease. *Eur Respir J* 2004;**24**:78–85.

19 Cohn L, Homer RJ, Marinov A, Rankin J, Bottomly K. Induction of airway mucus production by T helper 2 (Th2) cells: a critical role for interleukin 4 in cell recruitment but not mucus production. *J Exp Med* 1997;**186**:1737–47.

20 Majori M, Corradi M, Caminati A *et al.* Predominant Th1 cytokine pattern in peripheral blood from subjects with chronic obstructive pulmonary disease. *J Allergy Clin Immunol* 1999;**103**:458–62.

21 Zhao MQ, Amir MK, Rice WR, Enelow RI. Type II pneumocyte-CD8$^+$ T-cell interactions: relationship between target cell cytotoxicity and activation. *Am J Respir Cell Mol Biol* 2001;**25**:362–9.

22 Keatings VM, Collins PD, Scott DM, Barnes PJ. Differences in interleukin-8 and tumor necrosis factor-α in induced sputum from patients with chronic obstructive pulmonary disease or asthma. *Am J Respir Crit Care Med* 1996;**153**:530–4.

23 Kuschner WG, D'Alessandro A, Wong H, Blanc PD. Dose-dependent cigarette smoking-related inflammatory responses in healthy adults. *Eur Respir J* 1996;**9**:1989–94.

24 de Boer WI, Sont JK, van Schadewijk A *et al.* Monocyte chemoattractant protein 1, interleukin 8, and chronic airways inflammation in COPD. *J Pathol* 2000;**190**:619–26.

25 Lim S, Roche N, Oliver BG *et al.* Balance of matrix metalloprotease-9 and tissue inhibitor of metalloprotease-1 from alveolar macrophages in cigarette smokers: regulation by interleukin-10. *Am J Respir Crit Care Med* 2000;**162**:1355–60.

26 Tanino M, Betsuyaku T, Takeyabu K *et al.* Increased levels of interleukin-8 in BAL fluid from smokers susceptible to pulmonary emphysema. *Thorax* 2002;**57**:405–11.

27 Traves SL, Culpitt SV, Russell RE, Barnes PJ, Donnelly LE. Increased levels of the chemokines GROα and MCP-1 in sputum samples from patients with COPD. *Thorax* 2002;**57**:590–5.

28 Morrison D, Strieter RM, Donnelly SC *et al.* Neutrophil chemokines in bronchoalveolar lavage fluid and leukocyte-conditioned medium from non-smokers and smokers. *Eur Respir J* 1998;**12**:1067–72.

29 Masubuchi T, Koyama S, Sato E *et al.* Smoke extract stimulates lung epithelial cells to release neutrophil and monocyte chemotactic activity. *Am J Pathol* 1998;**153**:1903–12.

30 Mio T, Romberger DJ, Thompson AB *et al.* Cigarette smoke induces interleukin-8 release from human bronchial epithelial cells. *Am J Respir Crit Care Med* 1997;**155**:1770–6.

31 Dubar V, Gosset P, Aerts C *et al. In vitro* acute effects of tobacco smoke on tumor necrosis factor alpha and interleukin-6 production by alveolar macrophages. *Exp Lung Res* 1993;**19**:345–59.

32 Saetta M, Di Stefano A, Maestrelli P *et al.* Airway eosinophilia and expression of interleukin-5 protein in asthma and in exacerbations of chronic bronchitis. *Clin Exp Allergy* 1996;**26**:766–74.

33 Bocchino V, Bertorelli G, Bertrand CP *et al.* Eotaxin and CCR3 are up-regulated in exacerbations of chronic bronchitis. *Allergy* 2002;**57**:17–22.

34 Zhu J, Majumdar S, Qiu Y *et al.* Interleukin-4 and interleukin-5 gene expression and inflammation in the mucus-secreting

glands and subepithelial tissue of smokers with chronic bronchitis: lack of relationship with CD8$^+$ cells. *Am J Respir Crit Care Med* 2001;**164**:2220–8.

35 Zhu J, Qiu YS, Majumdar S *et al.* Exacerbations of bronchitis: bronchial eosinophilia and gene expression for interleukin-4, interleukin-5, and eosinophil chemoattractants. *Am J Respir Crit Care Med* 2001;**164**:109–16.

36 Agusti AG, Noguera A, Sauleda J *et al.* Systemic effects of chronic obstructive pulmonary disease. *Eur Respir J* 2003;**21**: 347–60.

37 Agusti AG, Sauleda J, Miralles C *et al.* Skeletal muscle apoptosis and weight loss in chronic obstructive pulmonary disease. *Am J Respir Crit Care Med* 2002;**166**:485–9.

38 Gosker HR, Wouters EF, van der Vusse GJ, Schols AM. Skeletal muscle dysfunction in chronic obstructive pulmonary disease and chronic heart failure: underlying mechanisms and therapy perspectives. *Am J Clin Nutr* 2000;**71**:1033–47.

39 Eid AA, Ionescu AA, Nixon LS *et al.* Inflammatory response and body composition in chronic obstructive pulmonary disease. *Am J Respir Crit Care Med* 2001;**164**:1414–8.

40 Yasuda N, Gotoh K, Minatoguchi S *et al.* An increase of soluble Fas, an inhibitor of apoptosis, associated with progression of COPD. *Respir Med* 1998;**92**:993–9.

41 Pitsiou G, Kyriazis G, Hatzizisi O *et al.* Tumor necrosis factor-α serum levels, weight loss and tissue oxygenation in chronic obstructive pulmonary disease. *Respir Med* 2002;**96**:594–8.

42 Takabatake N, Nakamura H, Abe S *et al.* The relationship between chronic hypoxemia and activation of the tumor necrosis factor-α system in patients with chronic obstructive pulmonary disease. *Am J Respir Crit Care Med* 2000;**161**: 1179–84.

43 Nguyen LT, Bedu M, Caillaud D *et al.* Increased resting energy expenditure is related to plasma TNF-α concentration in stable COPD patients. *Clin Nutr* 1999;**18**:269–74.

44 de Godoy I, Donahoe M, Calhoun WJ, Mancino J, Rogers RM. Elevated TNF-α production by peripheral blood monocytes of weight-losing COPD patients. *Am J Respir Crit Care Med* 1996;**153**:633–7.

45 Di Francia M, Barbier D, Mege JL, Orehek J. Tumor necrosis factor-α levels and weight loss in chronic obstructive pulmonary disease. *Am J Respir Crit Care Med* 1994;**150**:1453–5.

46 Sandford AJ, Silverman EK. Chronic obstructive pulmonary disease. I. Susceptibility factors for COPD the genotype–environment interaction. *Thorax* 2002;**57**:736–41.

47 Kucukaycan M, Van Krugten M, Pennings HJ *et al.* Tumor necrosis factor-α +489G/A gene polymorphism is associated with chronic obstructive pulmonary disease. *Respir Res* 2002; **3**:29.

48 Sakao S, Tatsumi K, Igari H *et al.* Association of tumor necrosis factor-α gene promoter polymorphism with low attenuation areas on high-resolution CT in patients with COPD. *Chest* 2002;**122**:416–20.

49 Sandford AJ, Chagani T, Weir TD *et al.* Susceptibility genes for rapid decline of lung function in the lung health study. *Am J Respir Crit Care Med* 2001;**163**:469–73.

50 Sakao S, Tatsumi K, Igari H *et al.* Association of tumor necrosis factor α gene promoter polymorphism with the presence of chronic obstructive pulmonary disease. *Am J Respir Crit Care Med* 2001;**163**:420–2.

51 Teramoto S, Ishii T. No association of tumor necrosis factor-α gene polymorphism and COPD in Caucasian smokers and Japanese smokers. *Chest* 2001;**119**:315–6.

52 Keatings VM, Cave SJ, Henry MJ *et al.* A polymorphism in the tumor necrosis factor-α gene promoter region may predispose to a poor prognosis in COPD. *Chest* 2000;**118**:971–5.

53 Ishii T, Matsuse T, Teramoto S *et al.* Neither IL-1β, IL-1 receptor antagonist, nor TNF-α polymorphisms are associated with susceptibility to COPD. *Respir Med* 2000;**94**:847–51.

54 Patuzzo C, Gile LS, Zorzetto M *et al.* Tumor necrosis factor gene complex in COPD and disseminated bronchiectasis. *Chest* 2000;**117**:1353–8.

55 Higham MA, Pride NB, Alikhan A, Morrell NW. Tumour necrosis factor-α gene promoter polymorphism in chronic obstructive pulmonary disease. *Eur Respir J* 2000;**15**:281–4.

56 He JQ, Connett JE, Anthonisen NR, Sandford AJ. Polymorphisms in the IL13, IL13RA1, and IL4RA genes and rate of decline in lung function in smokers. *Am J Respir Cell Mol Biol* 2003;**28**:379–85.

57 Van Der Pouw Kraan TC, Kucukaycan M, Bakker AM *et al.* Chronic obstructive pulmonary disease is associated with the -1055 IL-13 promoter polymorphism. *Genes Immun* 2002;**3**: 436–9.

58 Mahadeva R, Shapiro SD. Chronic obstructive pulmonary disease. III. Experimental animal models of pulmonary emphysema. *Thorax* 2002;**57**:908–14.

59 Zhu Z, Zheng T, Lee CG, Homer RJ, Elias JA. Tetracycline-controlled transcriptional regulation systems: advances and application in transgenic animal modeling. *Semin Cell Dev Biol* 2002;**13**:121–8.

60 Chapman HA Jr, Shi GP. Protease injury in the development of COPD: Thomas A. Neff Lecture. *Chest* 2000;**117**(Suppl 1): 295S–9S.

61 Wright JL, Churg A. Smoke-induced emphysema in guinea pigs is associated with morphometric evidence of collagen breakdown and repair. *Am J Physiol* 1995;**268**:L17–20.

62 Kasahara Y, Tuder RM, Cool CD *et al.* Endothelial cell death and decreased expression of vascular endothelial growth factor and vascular endothelial growth factor receptor 2 in emphysema. *Am J Respir Crit Care Med* 2001;**163**:737–44.

63 Segura-Valdez L, Pardo A, Gaxiola M *et al.* Upregulation of gelatinases A and B, collagenases 1 and 2, and increased parenchymal cell death in COPD. *Chest* 2000;**117**:684–94.

64 Aoshiba K, Rennard SI, Spurzem JR. Cell–matrix and cell–cell interactions modulate apoptosis of bronchial epithelial cells. *Am J Physiol* 1997;**272**:L28–37.

65 Giancotti FG, Ruoslahti E. Integrin signaling. *Science* 1999; **285**:1028–32.

66 Lucey EC, Keane J, Kuang PP, Snider GL, Goldstein RH. Severity of elastase-induced emphysema is decreased in tumor necrosis factor-α and interleukin-1β receptor-deficient mice. *Lab Invest* 2002;**82**:79–85.

67 Churg A, Dai J, Tai H, Xie C, Wright JL. Tumor necrosis factor-α is central to acute cigarette smoke-induced inflammation and connective tissue breakdown. *Am J Respir Crit Care Med* 2002;**166**:849–54.

68 Hogg JC, Senior RM. Chronic obstructive pulmonary disease. II. Pathology and biochemistry of emphysema. *Thorax* 2002;**57**:830–4.

69 Wallace AM, Sandford AJ. Genetic polymorphisms of matrix metalloproteinases: functional importance in the development of chronic obstructive pulmonary disease? *Am J Pharmacogenomics* 2002;**2**:167–75.

70 Joos L, He JQ, Shepherdson MB *et al*. The role of matrix metalloproteinase polymorphisms in the rate of decline in lung function. *Hum Mol Genet* 2002;**11**:569–76.

71 Foronjy RF, Okada Y, Cole R, D'Armiento J. Progressive adult-onset emphysema in transgenic mice expressing human MMP-1 in the lung. *Am J Physiol Lung Cell Mol Physiol* 2003;**284**:L727–37.

72 Ohnishi K, Takagi M, Kurokawa Y, Satomi S, Konttinen YT. Matrix metalloproteinase-mediated extracellular matrix protein degradation in human pulmonary emphysema. *Lab Invest* 1998;**78**:1077–87.

73 Finlay GA, O'Driscoll LR, Russell KJ *et al*. Matrix metalloproteinase expression and production by alveolar macrophages in emphysema. *Am J Respir Crit Care Med* 1997;**156**: 240–7.

74 Finlay GA, Russell KJ, McMahon KJ *et al*. Elevated levels of matrix metalloproteinases in bronchoalveolar lavage fluid of emphysematous patients. *Thorax* 1997;**52**:502–6.

75 Leco KJ, Waterhouse P, Sanchez OH *et al*. Spontaneous air space enlargement in the lungs of mice lacking tissue inhibitor of metalloproteinases-3 (TIMP-3). *J Clin Invest* 2001; **108**: 817–29.

76 Rijcken B, Weiss ST. Longitudinal analyses of airway responsiveness and pulmonary function decline. *Am J Respir Crit Care Med* 1996;**154**:S246–9.

77 Rijcken B, Schouten JP, Xu X, Rosner B, Weiss ST. Airway hyperresponsiveness to histamine associated with accelerated decline in *FEV*$_1$. *Am J Respir Crit Care Med* 1995;**151**:1377–82.

78 Tashkin DP, Altose MD, Connett JE *et al*. Methacholine reactivity predicts changes in lung function over time in smokers with early chronic obstructive pulmonary disease. The Lung Health Study Research Group. *Am J Respir Crit Care Med* 1996; **153**:1802–11.

79 Weiss ST. Atopy as a risk factor for chronic obstructive pulmonary disease: epidemiological evidence. *Am J Respir Crit Care Med* 2000;**162**:S134–6.

80 Lange P, Parner J, Vestbo J, Schnohr P, Jensen G. A 15-year follow-up study of ventilatory function in adults with asthma. *N Engl J Med* 1998;**339**:1194–200.

81 Elias JA, Zheng T, Lee CG *et al*. Transgenic modeling of interleukin-13 in the lung. *Chest* 2003;**123**(3 Suppl):339S–45S.

82 Miotto D, Ruggieri MP, Boschetto P *et al*. Interleukin-13 and -4 expression in the central airways of smokers with chronic bronchitis. *Eur Respir J* 2003;**22**:602–8.

83 Zheng T, Zhu Z, Wang Z *et al*. Inducible targeting of IL-13 to the adult lung causes matrix metalloproteinase- and cathepsin-dependent emphysema. *J Clin Invest* 2000;**106**:1081–93.

84 Lanone S, Zheng T, Zhu Z *et al*. Overlapping and enzyme-specific contributions of matrix metalloproteinases-9 and -12 in IL-13-induced inflammation and remodeling. *J Clin Invest* 2002;**110**:463–74.

85 Zhu Z, Ma B, Zheng T *et al*. IL-13-induced chemokine responses in the lung: role of CCR2 in the pathogenesis of IL-13-induced inflammation and remodeling. *J Immunol* 2002;**168**:2953–62.

86 Wang Z, Zheng T, Zhu Z *et al*. Interferon gamma induction of pulmonary emphysema in the adult murine lung. *J Exp Med* 2000;**192**:1587–600.

87 Cohn L, Herrick C, Niu N, Homer R, Bottomly K. IL-4 promotes airway eosinophilia by suppressing IFN-γ production: defining a novel role for IFN-γ in the regulation of allergic airway inflammation. *J Immunol* 2001;**166**:2760–7.

88 Zheng T, Kang MJ, Crothers K *et al*. Role of cathepsin S-dependent epithelial cell apoptosis in IFN-gamma-induced alveolar remodeling and pulmonary emphysema. *J Immunol* 2005;**174**:8106–15.

89 Kasahara Y, Tuder RM, Taraseviciene-Stewart L *et al*. Inhibition of VEGF receptors causes lung cell apoptosis and emphysema. *J Clin Invest* 2000;**106**:1311–9.

90 Tuder RM, Zhen L, Cho CY *et al*. Oxidative stress and apoptosis interact and cause emphysema due to VEGF receptor blockade. *Am J Respir Cell Mol Biol* 2003;**31**:31.

91 Koyama S, Sato E, Haniuda M *et al*. Decreased level of vascular endothelial growth factor in bronchoalveolar lavage fluid of normal smokers and patients with pulmonary fibrosis. *Am J Respir Crit Care Med* 2002;**166**:382–5.

92 Hautamaki RD, Kobayashi DK, Senior RM, Shapiro SD. Requirement for macrophage elastase for cigarette smoke-induced emphysema in mice. *Science* 1997;**277**:2002–4.

93 Churg A, Zay K, Shay S *et al*. Acute cigarette smoke-induced connective tissue breakdown requires both neutrophils and macrophage metalloelastase in mice. *Am J Respir Cell Mol Biol* 2002;**27**:368–74.

94 Churg A, Wang RD, Xie C, Wright JL. α$_1$-Antitrypsin ameliorates cigarette smoke-induced emphysema in the mouse. *Am J Respir Crit Care Med* 2003;**10**:10.

95 Wright JL, Farmer SG, Churg A. Synthetic serine elastase inhibitor reduces cigarette smoke-induced emphysema in guinea pigs. *Am J Respir Crit Care Med* 2002;**166**:954–60.

96 Churg A, Wang RD, Tai H *et al*. Macrophage metalloelastase mediates acute cigarette smoke-induced inflammation via tumor necrosis factor-α release. *Am J Respir Crit Care Med* 2003;**167**:1083–9.

97 Morris DG, Huang X, Kaminski N *et al*. Loss of integrin α(v)β6-mediated TGF-β activation causes MMP12-dependent emphysema. *Nature* 2003;**422**:169–73.

98 Neptune ER, Frischmeyer PA, Arking DE *et al*. Dysregulation of TGF-β activation contributes to pathogenesis in Marfan syndrome. *Nat Genet* 2003;**33**:407–11.

99 Sterner-Kock A, Thorey IS, Koli K *et al*. Disruption of the gene encoding the latent transforming growth factor-β binding protein 4 (LTBP-4) causes abnormal lung development, cardiomyopathy, and colorectal cancer. *Genes Dev* 2002;**16**: 2264–73.

100 de Boer WI, van Schadewijk A, Sont JK *et al*. Transforming growth factor β1 and recruitment of macrophages and mast cells in airways in chronic obstructive pulmonary disease. *Am J Respir Crit Care Med* 1998;**158**:1951–7.

101 Corne J, Chupp G, Lee CG *et al*. IL-13 stimulates vascular endothelial cell growth factor and protects against hyperoxic acute lung injury. *J Clin Invest* 2000;**106**:783–91.

102 Lee CG, Homer RJ, Zhu Z *et al*. Interleukin-13 induces tissue fibrosis by selectively stimulating and activating transforming growth factor β1. *J Exp Med* 2001;**194**:809–22.

CHAPTER 26

Leukotrienes in COPD: the unexploited potential

Sven-Erik Dahlén

Although leukotrienes, prostaglandins and other eicosanoids are ubiquitous signalling molecules with a diverse number of biological activities, their role in COPD remains to be explained. There are few clinical studies that have directly addressed the potential functions of leukotrienes or prostaglandins in the symptomatology or pathophysiology of COPD. This is somewhat surprising in view of the established role of leukotrienes as mediators of the airway obstruction and inflammation in asthma and the use of prostaglandins in the treatment of pulmonary hypertension. In fact, the lung was one of the first organs where prostaglandins were discovered and their biological activities investigated [1]. The formation of eicosanoids in different cells within the lung is extensive [2], but their possible contribution to COPD has not received much attention. In part influenced by the 'Dutch hypothesis', this account focuses on the experience with antileukotrienes in the treatment of asthmatic airway disease, with the deliberate hope this may stimulate further studies to evaluate the role of leukotrienes and other eicosanoids in COPD. After an outline of the biosynthetic pathways for formation of leukotrienes and other eicosanoids, the focus is on the the biological effects of leukotrienes that may be relevant for treatment of COPD.

Biosynthesis, receptors and metabolism

Leukotrienes constitute a class of potent biological lipid mediators derived from arachidonic acid [3]. However, leukotrienes are not to be found in a resting cell. Biosynthesis of leukotrienes requires a cellular activation, such as cross-binding of the immunoglobulin E (IgE) receptor on the mast cell surface, to stimulate cellular conversion of the substrate arachidonic acid into biologically active messenger products. Arachidonic acid is normally esterified to membrane phospholipids. The release of arachidonic

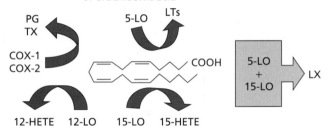

Figure 26.1 Main mammalian transformations of arachidonic acid (eicosa-5,8,11,14-tetraenoic acid) indicating the position of oxygenations in the different pathways (carbon 1 being the carboxyl end). COX, cyclo-oxygenase; HETE, hydroxy-ETA; LO, lipoxygenase; LT, leukotriene; LX, lipoxin; PG, prostaglandin; TX, thromboxane.

acid is predominantly controlled by the action of different phospholipase A_2 enzymes, all of which cleave arachidonic acid from membrane phospholipids. The liberated arachidonic acid can be metabolized to prostaglandins, thromboxane A_2 (TXA_2) or leukotrienes, as well as a great number of other molecules collectively named eicosanoids (Fig. 26.1).

The name eicosanoids is derived from the Greek prefix *eicosa* (εικοσι, twenty) and refers to the number of carbon atoms in the substrate arachidonic acid. As indicated in Figure 26.1, oxygenation of different carbon atoms in arachidonic acid initiates different pathways. Although not covered in this chapter, it should be recognized that different lipoxygenation and p450 derived hydroxyacids and downstream metabolites make up a major proportion of arachidonic acid metabolites in human lung tissue, with 15(S)-hydroxy-eicosatetraenoic acid being predominant [2]. Recent attention has focused on the potential of lipoxins as anti-inflammatory regulators of inflammation and remodelling [4].

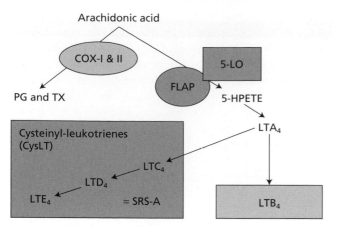

Figure 26.2 5-Lipoxygenase (5-LO) and cyclo-oxygenase pathways. Cyclo-oxygenase (COX, two isoenzymes COX-1 and COX-2) catalyse the formation of prostaglandins (PG) and thromboxane (TX). The biosynthesis of leukotrienes (LT) is catalysed by 5-LO in cooperation with FLAP (five lipoxygenase activating protein). The primary leukotriene intermediate LTA_4 is metabolized to LTB_4 or the cysteinyl-leukotrienes LTC_4, LTD_4 and LTE_4, that made up the biological activity previously known as slow reacting substance of anaphylaxis (SRS-A).

The initating enzyme in leukotriene synthesis is 5-lipoxygenase (5-LO). The enzyme has two catalytic activities: the conversion of arachidonic acid to 5-hydroperoxy-eicosatetraenoic acid (5-HPETE) and the subsequent formation of leukotriene A_4 (LTA_4) (Fig. 26.2). LTA_4 is a short-lived compound that can be further metabolized to LTB_4 or LTC_4, in reactions catalysed by LTA_4 hydrolase (LTA-H) and LTC_4 synthase (LTC-S), respectively. LTC_4 and its metabolites, LTD_4 and LTE_4, are collectively designated cysteinyl-leukotrienes (CysLT) because of the common constituent cysteine in the side-chain.

In contrast, prostaglandin H synthase (PGHS) initiates the metabolism of arachidonic acid to prostaglandins and TXA_2 (see Fig. 26.2). PGHS is, as 5-LO, a dual enzyme catalysing two coupled reactions: an initial cyclo-oxygenation and an a subsequent hydroperoxidase reaction. However, as drugs that inhibit prostaglandin formation usually inhibit the first cyclo-oxygenase reaction, PGHS is usually functionally and pharmacologically described as the prostaglandin cyclo-oxygenase (COX). Two forms of the enzyme exist: COX-1, which is constitutively expressed in many cells and believed to be mainly involved in the production of prostanoids in physiological reactions; and COX-2, which is often induced in cells during inflammation and therefore considered primarily involved in pathological states [5]. As illustrated by the recently documented cardiovascular side-effects of selective COX-2 inhibitors [6], there are several important exceptions to the general dogma of COX-2 as an inducible and exclusively proinflammatory enzyme.

5-LO is restrictively expressed in the human body and predominantly found in myeloid cells such as granulocytes, monocytes, macrophages, mast cells and B-lymphocytes [3]. The human 5-LO gene is located on chromosome 10 [7] and the protein has a molecular weight of 78 kDa. Some mutations in the 5-LO promoter region have been reported [8]. However, it remains unclear if enzyme polymorphisms have relevance for the enhanced biosynthesis of leukotrienes found in certain patients with asthma. The cellular biosynthesis of leukotrienes involves a 18-kDa membrane-bound protein named FLAP (five-lipoxygenase activating protein). It is an arachidonate-binding protein, which stimulates the conversion of cellular arachidonic acid by 5-LO [9–11]. The human gene is located on chromosome 13q12. The FLAP protein was discovered because some inhibitors of leukotriene formation such as MK-886, MK-591 and BAYx1005 bind to this protein and thereby inhibit leukotriene biosynthesis.

LTA_4 hydrolase (LTA-H) is a cytosolic 69-kDa enzyme that catalyses the conversion of LTA_4 to LTB_4 (reviewed in Haeggstrom [12]). The enzyme is a zinc metalloenzyme which also exhibits aminopeptidase activity with unknown physiological relevance. The gene is on region 12q of chromosome 22. In contrast to 5-LO, LTA-H is widely distributed and has been found in almost all mammalian cells. One possible explanation for this discrepancy would be that LTA-H is primarily involved in leukotriene synthesis in cells expressing 5-LO, whereas aminopeptide activity occurs in cells that do not produce leukotrienes. Alternatively, LTA-H might have a role in the transcellular metabolism of leukotrienes (see below).

LTC_4 synthase (LTC_4-S) is an integral membrane 18-kDa protein, catalysing the final step in LTC_4 formation (reviewed in Lam and Austen [13]. The enzyme catalyses the conjugation of glutathione with LTA_4 and is active as a homodimer. Expression of LTC_4-S is high in cells with an established role in the biosynthesis of CysLT such as mast cells and eosinophils. LTC_4-S activity is also detected in cells that apparently do not express 5-LO such as endothelial cells and platelets. Overexpression of LTC_4-S was reported in bronchial biopsies from aspirin-intolerant asthmatic patients [14]. LTC-S is a member of the MAPEG (membrane-associated proteins in eicosanoid and glutathione metabolism) family of proteins that also includes FLAP, microsomal prostaglandin E synthase (mPGES) and several microsomal glutathione S-transferases (reviewed in Jakobsson *et al.* [15]). The gene for LTC_4-S is on the 35q region of chromosome 5, close to the locus for genes encoding pro-inflammatory cytokines and growth factor receptors.

The mechanisms involved in the cellular biosynthesis of leukotrienes are still incompletely understood [3]. The physiological relevance of the localization of the 5-LO and FLAP to the nuclear envelope is not known, but it is possible that 5-LO products also have a function in transcriptional regulation of genes.

Eosinophils and mast cells have high capacity to generate LTC_4, from the endogenous pool of arachidonic acid. However, several lines of evidence suggests that CysLT as well as LTB_4 can also be produced in the lung through interaction between structural and infiltrating inflammatory cells. Such transcellular metabolism means that stimulated leucocytes, and in particular neutrophils, can release LTA_4 which then can be further metabolized by other surrounding cells into LTB_4 or LTC_4 (reviewed in Lindgren and Edenius [16]). This means that cells without the initial 5-LO but with expression of distal enzymes permitting further metabolism of LTA_4 nevertheless may form the biologically active leukotrienes in such interactions. Activated myeloid cells may release LTA_4 which is subsequently metabolized by endothelial cells and platelets to LTC_4. Likewise, LTA_4 produced by neutrophils may be accepted by endothelials cells and form LTB_4, despite lack of 5-LO in the endothelial cells. Transcellular metabolism of LTA_4 in arterosclerotic plaques has recently gained considerable interest as a critical event in vascular inflammation, and altered expression of the receptors for LTB_4 seem to be involved [17].

After intracellular formation of LTC_4, the compound is released to the extracellular space. Export of LTC_4 has been demonstrated in many cells to be carried out by the multidrug-resistence protein (MRP) [3]. Mice lacking MRP have a decreased export of LTC_4 and an attenuated response to inflammatory stimuli [18]. After the carrier-mediated export of LTC_4, metabolism of LTC_4 provides the extracellular LTD_4 and LTE_4. Intracellular LTB_4 is also secreted via a specific transporter [19]. These carrier proteins are a potential future target for antileukotriene drugs.

There are four G-protein-coupled receptors that have been identified for leukotrienes (reviewed in Brink *et al.* [20]). For the cysteinyl-leukotrienes $CysLT_1$ and $CysLT_2$, and for LTB_4 BLT_1 and BLT_2 (see Fig. 26.2). There is pharmacological evidence suggesting the presence of a third receptor for CysLT, as the response to LTC_4 in the human pulmonary artery is resistant to all currently available antagonists [21,22]. Current evidence suggests that most, if not all, effects of leukotrienes with relevance to asthma are mediated by activation of the $CysLT_1$ receptor. For example, it was recently established that bronchoconstriction as well as ventilation–perfusion mismatch in subjects with asthma challenged with inhaled LTD_4 was completely blocked by montelukast [23]. However, with regard to events of relevance to COPD, much less is known about the involvement of leukotriene receptors. In animal models of lung fibrosis, there appears to be opposing effects of $CysLT_1$ and $CysLT_2$ receptors [24,25].

Our understanding is as yet limited with regard to how different enzymes, receptors and transporters in the leukotriene pathway are regulated in health and disease. With airway inflammation, it must be taken into account that changes in the expression of a particular enzyme in a particular cell is only one part of the events that occur. Diseases or drugs may change the number and composition of cells in the airway tissue with dramatic effects *in vivo* on the profile and amounts of compounds formed. Therefore, *in vivo* measurements of eicosanoids are generally most conclusive regarding the amounts and profile of products formed in a particular situation.

The circulating levels of any of the CysLT are below the detection limits of immunoassays but the endogenous formation may be followed by collection of sputum, nasal or bronchioalveolar lavage fluids or by measurement of the stable urinary end product LTE_4 [26]. There are recent indications that exhaled breath condensates (EBC) may be used to measure CysLT [27], but there remain questions about the identity and source of CysLT immunoreactivity in EBC.

Measurement of urinary LTE_4 is thus a validated and sensitive method to monitor whole body production of CysLT [26]. It has been used to provide mechanistic information about the response to different bronchoprovocations. Urinary LTE_4 is typically increased following most indirect bronchprovocations studied. This has been made possible because of the rapid excretion of CysLT into the urine. Following inhalation of LTD_4, there is a significant increase in urinary LTE_4 within 30–60 min. Likewise, allergen-induced bronchoconstriction is followed by increased urinary LTE_4 within an hour. This means that this measure may be more reflective of acute episodes of airway obstruction than chronic inflammatory changes. However, subjects with aspirin-intolerant asthma have generally, on the population level, been found to have increased urinary LTE_4 [26,28]. There are currently no definitive data on urinary LTE_4 in COPD.

In the case of LTB_4, the methods for *in vivo* measurement are even more limited. As for CysLT, the circulating blood levels are below the detection limit of reliable assays. When very high doses of LTB_4 were injected in volunteers, it was possible to measure some metabolites in urine [29]. Normally, physiological concentrations of LTB_4 are completely metabolized into water and carbon dioxide [30]. For LTB_4, we are therefore currently limited to measurements in different body fluids where the problems of erroneous formation during sampling become significant. A common approach has been to estimate the ability of blood cells *ex vivo* to generate leukotrienes [31]. The method involves normal collection of blood and subsequent stimulation of whole blood, neutrophils or any other cell of interest with, for example, calcium ionophore for a defined time period, followed by measurement of LTB_4 in the sample. However, it is not conclusively established to what extent this measure of capacity to generate LTB_4 in the test tube reflects *in vivo* propensity to form leukotrienes.

Biological actions of leukotrienes with relevance to the respiratory system

Soon after their discovery, it was documented that LTC_4 and LTD_4 were potent inducers of bronchoconstriction in guinea-pig airways *in vitro* and *in vivo* [32,33] and caused contractions of isolated human bronchi [34–36] (Fig. 26.3). Local injection of these two CysLT also increased accumulation of intravenous injected Evans blue in the skin [32,33], suggesting an increase in microvascular permeability. In the hamster cheek pouch, it could be established that LTC_4 and LTD_4 caused exudation of plasma proteins in postcapillary venules [37]. In the guinea-pig, it was shown that LTC_4, LTD_4 and LTE_4 were capable of plasma protein extravasation in all segments of the airways [38].

The biological effects of LTE_4 have been less studied, perhaps because this leukotriene was found to be an incomplete and less potent agonist than LTC_4 and LTD_4 in some standard bioassays such as the guinea-pig ileum [39–41]. However, LTE_4 has been documented to possess a bronchoconstrictor activity *in vitro* and *in vivo* that is closely similar to that of LTC_4 and LTD_4 [42,43]. It has also been observed that prolonged exposure to LTE_4 may produce enhancement of the responsiveness of smooth muscle to histamine [44,45]. Moreover, LTE_4 is a full agonist for contraction of human bronchi *in vitro* [46], and its potency is similar to that of LTC_4 and LTD_4.

Of particular relevance to COPD, it has been observed that LTC_4 and LTD_4 may stimulate mucus secretion in isolated animal and human airways [47–49]. Additional effects with relevance to the role of CysLT in pulmonary inflammation have been reported. Thus, increased infiltration of eosinophils into the airway mucosa of asthmatics was observed following inhalation of LTE_4 [50], and

inhalation of LTD_4 increased the number of eosinophils in induced sputum samples from asthmatics [51,52]. However, it has been overlooked that inhalation of LTE_4 also increased the number of neutrophils in the airways [50]. The capacity of CysLT to promote eosinophil recruitment has been studied in experimental models [53,54], although the mechanisms involved remain undefined. There is also experimental data *in vitro* [55–58] and *in vivo* [59] supporting the view that CysLT may be involved in airway smooth muscle proliferation and remodelling.

The exquisite spasmogenic potency of CysLT on isolated human bronchi has been confirmed in bronchoprovocation studies of control subjects [60–62]. The CysLT are the most potent endogenous bronchoconstrictors known so far. Accordingly, CysLT have generally been found to produce bronchoconstriction in doses that were 100–10 000 times lower than those required with histamine or methacholine. Asthmatics have also been found to be hyperresponsive to inhalation of LTC_4, LTD_4 and LTE_4 [63–65]. There are indications that LTD_4 may cause greater airway narrowing than methacholine [66]. On the other hand, at least for LTC_4 and LTD_4, there are observations indicating that the hyperresponsiveness of asthmatics to these leukotrienes relative to methacholine was less than in controls [31,64,67]. This raises the interesting hypothesis that chronically elevated production of leukotrienes in the airways induces adaptive changes in the effector cells or at the receptor level [68]. However, concerning LTE_4, the opposite finding has been reported, namely that asthmatics were especially hyperresponsive to this particular leukotriene [69]. Altogether, the studies where bronchial challenge with CysLT have been performed are relatively few and more work is needed. In this context, there are also indications that repeated challenge with CysLT is associated with tachyphylaxis mediated by local generation of a prostanoid, and presumably PGE_2 [70].

LTB_4 has been found to have primarily leucocytes as targets for its biological activity (see Fig. 26.3). Thus, it is a potent stimulus for activation of leucocytes, eliciting chemokinetic and chemotactic responses *in vitro* [71]. *In vivo*, LTB_4 increases leucocyte rolling and adhesion to the venular endothelium [37], followed by their emigration into the extravascular space. During a short-lasting exposure to LTB_4, polymorphonuclear leucocytes are mainly recruited. With prolonged exposure to LTB_4, as presumably occurs when LTB_4 is formed *in vivo*, other granulucytes, including eosinophils, are found in tissues or exudates after challenge with LTB_4 [72]. More recently, the effects of LTB_4 on T-lymphocyte migration in the lung has attracted attention [73]. Altogether, it is an attractive hypothesis that LTB_4 contributes to the neutrophilic inflammation in COPD. Indeed, there are studies where altered levels or changed responsiveness to LTB_4 have been reported in

Cysteinyl-leukotrienes (CysLT) = LTC_4 + LTD_4 + LTE_4	LTB_4
Bronchoconstriction Plasma exudation (oedema) Mucus secretion	Neutrophil chemotaxis
Blood flow changes Cell infiltration	Activation and recruitment of inflammatory cells
Smooth muscle proliferation	Vasoconstriction
Remodelling Receptors: $CysLT_1$ & $CysLT_2$	T-lymphocyte migration Receptors: BLT_1 & BLT_2

Figure 26.3 Biological effects of leukotrienes and receptors (see text for explanations).

sputum from patients with COPD [74], but the studies are limited and confirmation is required.

In addition to effects on leucocyte adhesion and migration, LTB_4, as other secretagogues, stimulates secretion of superoxide anion and release of different granular constituents from leucocytes [75,76]. Possibly relating to effects of LTB_4 on B-cells, it has been established that sensitized 5-LO-deficient mice produced lower levels of IgG and IgE upon ovalbumin challenge than wild-type mice [77]. Furthermore, it has been reported that LTB_4, similar to many other eicosanoids, is an agonist for the nuclear transcription factor peroxisome proliferator-activated receptor α (PPARα) [78]. The finding may implicate a role for LTB_4 in the control of central events in lipid metabolism and inflammation, but also the possibility that LTB_4 has intracellular and nuclear targets, which may participate in long-term control of gene expression. It is noteworthy though that there have been few new publications to follow-up on the original observations.

With respect to effects of LTB_4 on the lung, it is established that LTB_4 has contractile activity in the guinea-pig lung parenchyma [79–82]. The response is indirect, involving release of TXA_2 and histamine, possible from pulmonary mast cells. It has been established that the effect in the lung parenchyma is a result of activation of the pulmonary blood vessels rather than the airway elements [83]. This particular response to LTB_4 has been confirmed in the human pulmonary artery but not in other non-vascular smooth muscle, including human bronchi.

In a dog model, LTB_4 was found to increase airway reactivity to acetylcholine [84], whereas among non-asthmatic humans there was no change in bronchial hyperresponsiveness to histamine following the inhalation of LTB_4, alone or in combination with PGD_2 [85]. Nor was there any direct bronchoconstrictor effect of inhaled LTB_4 [86]. A subsequent study observed that inhalation of LTB_4 by healthy human volunteers was followed by distinct cellular changes in the airways, and possibly also some plasma exudation [87]. In a study where LTB_4 was inhaled by a group of asthmatics, the lack of immediate bronchoconstrictive properties was confirmed as well as prominent acute effects on leucocyte traffic in the lung and blood [88].

As COPD is a disease with many systemic and metabolic consequences, it is of interest that there are suggestions of leukotrienes as mediators in chronic inflammation in general, and cardiovascular diseases in particular. For example, there is a case for LTB_4 in artherosclerotic inflammation [17]. Thus, treatment with a leukotriene biosynthesis inhibitor has been reported to have a beneficial effect on a surrogate marker of ischaemic heart disease in a group of subjects with a particular polymorphism in 5-LO and altered capacity to biosynthesize LTB_4 [89]. Another genetic population study has suggested that certain polymorphisms

in 5-LO carry risk odd ratios of similar magnitude as diabetes or smoking [90]. However, CysLT may also be much involved in cardiovascular events. For example, experiments in isolated perfused hearts disclosed a depressive effect of CysLT on cardiac contractility [91,92]. The effect correlated with coronary vasoconstriction [93], but a direct negative inotropic effect on the myocardium may also be involved [92,94]. Such effects may be of relevance to the comorbidity between ischaemic heart disease and COPD.

There is recent experimental evidence that leukotrienes have important functions in innate immunity [95] and immunological responses including lung fibrosis [96], actions that may have bearing on the pathophysiology of COPD. There may also be intricate feedback mechanisms within the eicosanoid family as, for example, 15-HETE has been reported to inhibit LTB_4 production in sputum of patients with COPD [97].

Pharmacology of antileukotrienes

The inhibition of the leukotriene pathway may be directed towards their formation or actions (see Figs 26.2 and 26.3). The leukotriene biosynthesis inhibitors result in inhibition of both LTB_4 and CysLT, whereas $CysLT_1$-antagonists selectively inhibit the action of CysLT at one of their receptors.

The 5-LO inhibitor zileuton was the first antileukotriene compound to be approved for treatment of asthma in the USA, but has not been registered for use in Europe [98]. Zileuton is an N-hydroxyurea derivative, and its mechanism of action is likely to involve chelation of iron at the active site of 5-LO, thereby blocking the redox potential of the enzyme. Among drugs that inhibit leukotriene biosynthesis, the FLAP-antagonists MK-886 [99], MK-591 [100] and BAYx1005 [101] have been documented to be potent inhibitors of leukotriene formation when given to humans *in vivo*, but none have been taken into final clinical development.

It would seem straightforward to establish the effective dose of a 5-LO inhibitor by measuring the degree by which it inhibits endogenous leukotriene formation. During the development of 5-LO inhibitors, measurements of *ex vivo* formation of LTB_4 in ionophore stimulated blood has generally been used to assess the degree of 5-LO inhibition [102]. This measure correlates well with plasma drug level, but it might have overestimated the degree of tissue inhibition of leukotriene formation [26]. For LTB_4, there is no indicator metabolite that can be measured in urine or blood [26]. For CysLT, measurements of urinary excretion of the end product LTE_4 is currently the most reliable estimate of the degree of inhibition of endogenous whole body bio-synthesis [26].

It is worth noting that the level of inhibition of urinary LTE_4 has been consistently less than 50% in the studies where significant effects on clinical outcome variables have been established [86,103,104]. This may indicate either that this level of inhibition is sufficient to obtain maximal clinical efficacy, or that the clinical efficacy can be increased further if the inhibition of leukotriene formation is increased. The latter possibility gains some support from the results of the only allergen challenge study performed with the highest dose of BAYx1005 so far tested [101]. There was more than 80% inhibition of allergen-induced urinary excretion of LTE_4 and more than 75% inhibition of bronchconstriction, which incidentally is the greatest degree of inhibition reported for this particular outcome variable by any antileukotriene drug. The phase II treatment trials with BAYx1005 were subsequently performed at a lower dose level and ambiguous results led to the discontinuation of further development of this particular drug for treatment of respiratory diseases, whereas its potential for treatment of artherosclerosis continues to be explored [89].

The other main strategy, to develop leukotriene receptor antagonists, is completely dominated by the $CysLT_1$ antagonists, although there are BLT antagonists that have been tested in humans [105]. A number of potent and selective $CysLT_1$ antagonists have been developed. The compounds are administered orally, and have been found to cause significant shifts (25- to 1000-fold) in the dose–response relation for inhaled LTD_4 in control subjects or asthmatics [106–109]. Although a great number of $CysLT_1$ antagonists have been developed, only three have reached the market: montelukast (Singulair®), pranlukast (Onon™) and zafirlukast (Accolate®). Montelukast and pranlukast are also registered for treatment of rhinitis. With regard to $CysLT_2$ antagonists, there are only early preclinical candidate substances [20], and it is unclear if the $CysLT_2$ receptor is an interesting target for the treatment of asthma. However, it remains possible that the pathophysiology of COPD may have significant $CysLT_2$ components. For example, the structure–activity relations for the effects of CysLT on mucous secretion are different from those normally exhibited at the $CysLT_1$ receptor [48].

Some selective and relatively potent antagonists of LTB_4 have been developed [105]. A few compounds have entered into early clinical testing in humans. The compound LY-293,111 (VML 295) was found to inhibit LTB_4-induced neutrophil responses *in vivo* and allergen-induced neutrophil activation, but it had no effect on allergen-induced early or late phase airway obstruction in asthmatics [105]. The results with LY-293,111 in asthmatics argue against an important role for LTB_4 as a mediator of antigen-induced bronchoconstriction, but do not exclude the possibility that LTB_4 may be involved in other manifestations of chronic asthma, such as increased bronchial responsiveness, or in other lung diseases. For example, there is a case for LTB_4 in innate immunity [95], and it would seem particularly

important to assess the effects of potent 5-LO inhibitors in clinical COPD or on surrogate markers of airway inflammation in COPD. There is one pilot study of the ability of the 5-LO inhibitor BAYx1005 to inhibit leukotriene production and inflammatory markers of patients with COPD [110].

Lessons to be learned from the effects of antileukotrienes in the treatment of asthma: questions for COPD research

A number of studies of different antileukotrienes have established that leukotrienes mediate significant components of bronchoconstriction evoked by common triggers of airway obstruction (Fig. 26.4). This has been demonstrated both with different inhibitors of the biosynthesis such as zileuton and the FLAP antagonists MK-886, MK-591 and BAYx1005, and with different $CysLT_1$ antagonists such as MK-571, MK-679, montelukast, pranlukast, pobilukast and zafirlukast. The beneficial effects of 5-LO inhibitors and the $CysLT_1$ antagonists were rather similar in the challenge models and in short-term treatment studies. This led to the reasonable conclusion that it was principally the CysLT antagonists that mediated reactions with relevance to asthma, and further clinical development has been dominated by the receptor antagonists. However, the dismissal of a role for LTB_4 in airway obstruction and inflammation may be premature. In particular, studies are required where long-term effects of potent 5-LO inhibitors are compared with selective $CysLT_1$ antagonists. There are at least three areas where LTB_4 may be more important than previously thought. First, one of the hallmarks of asthma, bronchial

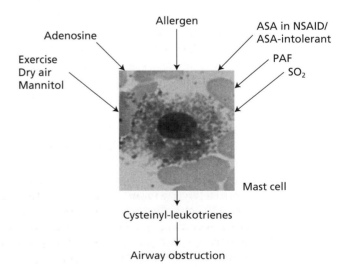

Figure 26.4 Leukotrienes as a final common path for different trigger factors causing airway obstruction. The mast cell is often a main effector cell in the responses.

hyperresponsiveness (BHR) is not extensively modified by $CysLT_1$ antagonists, whereas there seem to be such effects after 5-LO inhibition [86,111]. Secondly, LTB_4 is the main leukotriene formed in the nasal mucosa [112], and the 5-LO inhibitor zileuton had a striking effect on nasal symptoms in aspirin-intolerant asthma [86]. It would be of interest to investigate the effects of 5-LO inhibitors more aggressively in rhinitis and rhinopolyposis where again provocation studies support potential for this class of compounds. Thirdly, there are several indications that LTB_4 may have important effects on lymphocyte trafficking and homing in the lung [73].

Antileukotrienes do not cause relaxation of airways per se. Thus, they have no direct bronchodilatory effects on airway smooth muscle nor inhibitory effects on the bronchoconstrictor response evoked by methacholine or histamine in subjects with mild asthma. However, administration of antileukotrienes has consistently been observed to produce variable degrees of acute bronchodilatation when given to subjects with chronic asthma and baseline airway obstruction [86,113–115]. This is explained by the mode of action to inhibit the action or formation of leukotrienes in the airways. It can be shown also in an *in vitro* model of increased baseline tone that there is a component of spontaneous muscle tone that is mediated by CysLT [116]. Presumably the contribution of leukotrienes to the airflow limitation in asthma is increased because of increased production of leukotrienes in asthmatic airway inflammation. There are studies supporting that the acute bronchodilatation in response to antileukotrienes is greater in studies of subjects with more severe depression of lung function at baseline [114] or more severe disease severity [117]. The bronchodilatory effect of antileukotrienes is also present after treatment with glucocorticosteroids [113,115]. There are indications of a synergy between beta-stimulants and antileukotrienes [113,114] but this requires further studies. Interestingly, there are two preliminary studies suggesting that airway obstruction in COPD is sensitive to treatment with a $CysLT_1$ antagonist [118,119]. It appears highly warranted to investigate systematically the effects of 5-LO inhibitors and $CysLT_1$ antagonists on airway function in COPD.

One of the most well-documented effects of antileukotrienes is to protect against bronchoconstriction induced by different trigger factors. This includes the response to allergen-induced airway obstruction [99–101,120–123] as well as all other trigger factors examined (see Fig. 26.4). Both early and the late asthmatic reactions have major leukotriene-dependent components [123,124]. This supports the hypothesis that antileukotrienes protect against bronchospasm as well as oedema and cellular response that are part of the antigen-induced airway reactions. One of the first proof of concept studies was in exercise-induced bronchoconstriction (EIB) [125]. It has subsequently been thoroughly documented that antileukotrienes have significant protective effects in that particular model, and in other models of bronchoconstriction that are considered to be 'exercise-mimetics', such as eucapnic hyperpnoea [126], cold air [127] or mannitol inhalation [128]. Although SO_2-induced bronchoconstriction is considered to primarily activate sensory nerves in the airways, the reflex apparently involves CysLT as zafirlukast was able to partially inhibit the response [129]. Adenosine-induced bronchoconstriction appears to activate mast cells in the airways [130], and this is supported by the protective effect of antileukotrienes in adenosine bronchial challenge [131].

All in all, the most likely explanation of the broad bronchoprotective effects of antileukotrienes in indirect bronchial challenges is that release of CysLT is a final common response to mast cell activation despite the particular route that is used to activate the mast cell (e.g. IgE, hyperosmolarity in EIB, COX-1 inhibition in NSAID-intolerant asthma) (see Fig. 26.4). The hypothesis is supported by the documentation of increased *in vivo* release of the sensitive mast cells marker $9\alpha,11\beta$-PGF_2 in conjunction with these bronchoconstrictive responses [132]. Another example is aspirin-induced bronchoconstriction in aspirin-intolerant asthma where mast cell activation can be shown [133] and the protective effects of antileukotrienes have been established [105,134,135]. It has been observed that patients with COPD bronchoconstrict in response to inhalation of hypertonic saline. As this particular response is inhibited both by montelukast and cetirazine [136,137], it seems reasonable to assume that mast cell dependent bronchoconstriction may be generating symptoms also in COPD, and hence serve as a target for treatment. It has been proposed that increased responsiveness of peripheral airways is an important aspect in COPD [138].

The introduction of antileukotrienes as new asthma treatment obviously followed a conventional clinical development where the potential new medications were documented to have beneficial effects on asthma outcomes that were superior to placebo. This included treatments for a duration of weeks to months with registration of endpoints such as pulmonary function, asthma symptoms, use of bronchodilators, asthma exacerbations and asthma-specific quality of life [139–143]. A comprehensive account of the development of each individual drug can be found in Drazen *et al.* [144]. In addition, the protective effects in EIB were extensively documented both in adults and children [145,146]. There are studies that have documented that the clinically beneficial effects of antileukotrienes are associated with inhibition of inflammatory cell reactions in, for example, blood, sputum and bronchial biopsies [147,148]. When comparing different treatments in asthma, it seems that montelukast in ordinary doses (10 mg once daily) in steroid-naive subjects provides improved asthma control more promptly (i.e. within a few days after start of treatment), compared with low doses of inhaled steroid. After a few weeks of therapy, the group mean effect of the steroid is larger than for montelukast [149]. However, there were large variations in therapeutic response, not only to montelukast but also to the steroid treatment in this particular investigation. From studies in children, it has recently been shown that montelukast decreases the number of viral-induced exacerbations [150]. Neither inhaled [151] nor oral steroids [152] have particularly significant prophylactic effects in similar populations of children between the ages of 2 and 5 years. There are also indications that LTB_4 may have a role in the bacterial inflammation of COPD exacerbations [153], again supporting the relevance of thoroughly testing 5-LO inhibition of the disease.

A relatively recent study has compared the effects of addition of a long-acting beta-agonist, salmeterol, or montelukast, to patients not controlled on inhaled fluticasone alone. The investigation included 1490 patients with asthma treated with a constant dosage of 100 µg/day fluticasone. During 1 year, a double-blind placebo-controlled comparison of daily addition of 10 mg montelukast or 200 µg salmeterol was made [154]. For the primary endpoint, the number of asthma worsenings during the study year, there was no significant difference between the two treatments. This was achieved despite that salmeterol was significantly better as a bronchodilator, and that montelukast, in contrast to salmeterol, displayed anti-inflammatory effects. The study illustrates that the same overall therapeutic response can be obtained with two strategies that have completely different modes of action. This type of study needs to be repeated with different outcomes but, mechanistically, it illustrates that several different targets may be useful in the treatment of asthma. Perhaps a future strategy would be to combine drugs with different modes of action to an even greater extent.

The current documentation of add-on effects of antileukotrienes [155–157] in the treatment of subjects not sufficiently controlled by glucocorticosteroids has mechanistic implications. The previous textbook knowledge was that glucocorticosteroids inhibit leukotriene biosynthesis by virtue of inhibition of the phospholipase step that is required for liberation of arachidonic acid from its esterified state in the cellular membranes. However, a number of studies have established that this is not the case in humans *in vivo* [158–161]. Leukotriene biosynthesis remains unaffected by inhaled or oral glucocorticosteroids. There is even *in vitro* evidence that certain enzymes in the leukotriene cascade are up-regulated by glucocorticosteroids [162]. Irrespective of the relevance of that particular *in vitro* study,

the relative steroid resistance of the leukotriene pathway is the mechanistic explanation of why the addition of antileukotrienes for patients not sufficiently controlled by steroids has been found to be effective. In practical terms, leukotriene biosynthesis is one aspect of airway inflammation that is steroid resistant. Again, this aspect should be another impetus for evaluating the effects of antileukotriene drugs in COPD.

In the treatment of subjects with more severe varities of asthma, it might also be of interest that addition of antileukotrienes allow for reduction of the dosage of inhaled glucocorticosteroids with maintained therapeutic response [163,164]. Such steroid tapering may be of particular interest in children with severe asthma for whom the side-effects of glucocorticosteroids become an issue. In the case of insufficient asthma control with inhaled glucocorticosteroid alone, there are observations suggesting that the addition of montelukast may provide the same therapeutic response as doubling of the dose of the current inhalation steroid [165].

The side-effects that have been observed during treatment with antileukotrienes have generally been modest, such as headache and intestinal troubles. In most clinical trials, these effects have not been different between active treatment and placebo. The low incidence of side-effects has been one reason that antileukotrienes can be administered by the oral route. The problem with reversible elevations of liver enzymes during treatment with zileuton has been discussed. The most serious suspicion of significant side-effects with antileukotrienes was reported after a few years' use of this new class of drugs in the USA. There seemed to be an aggregation of new cases with the severe vasculitic disease Churg–Strauss syndrome (CSS) [166]. However, independent panels reviewing the cases concluded that the reported cases not were directly related to the specific class of drugs but a consequence of steroid tapering in subjects with hidden CSS [167,168]. Similar episodes of CSS exacerbations have been reported also after withdrawal of oral prednisone in patients given inhalation therapy with glucocorticosteroids.

Conclusions and perspective

Approximately 25 years after the discovery of leukotrienes and the elucidation of the structure of slow reacting substance of anaphylaxis (SRS-A) [169], antileukotrienes are now established as a treatment for asthma and rhinitis. However, the cumulated clinical experience with this class of drugs is less than 10 years and in most countries of the world limited to the $CysLT_1$ receptor antagonists montelukast and pranlukast. It is clearly documented that antileukotrienes have anti-inflammatory and bronchoprotective effects that alleviate symptoms in adults and children with asthma and rhinitis. Antileukotrienes may be used as monotherapy or added to inhaled glucocorticosteroids. Published studies support the use of antileukotrienes at all levels of asthma therapy, from very mild cases to treatment of subjects with very severe asthma; in the mild cases as monotherapy, in the more severe cases as combination therapy with glucocorticosteroids. The first-line therapy option dominates in the USA, whereas usage in Europe is as an add-on to inhaled steroids or prophylaxis against EIB.

One area for future research is to identify subjects with leukotriene-dependent asthma. So far, this has largely been unsuccessful, and no baseline variable including urinary levels of LTE_4 have been found to predict the therapeutic response to montelukast or zileuton. A few relatively limited studies using $CysLT_1$ antagonists [170] or 5-LO inhibitors [171] have suggested relations between therapeutic response to these particular drugs and genetic polymorphisms in the LTC_4-S and 5-LO, respectively. The effects are not very large and currently not of such a magnitude that a certain genetic profile can predict the therapeutic response to antileukotrienes. A recent study in subjects with asthma failed to identify biochemical factors relating to the capacity for leukotriene biosynthesis that could predict the airway responsiveness to inhaled leukotrienes [31]. Studies in subjects with aspirin-intolerant asthma [86,156] have been taken as evidence of a particularly favourable response in this peculiar subgroup of subjects, but it has been overlooked that these patients received antileukotrienes not as single therapy but as add-on to both inhaled and oral glucocorticosteroids. The remarkable therapeutic responses in these two studies may rather support that patients with more severe asthma improve further when an antileukotriene is added to baseline treatment with glucocorticosteroids. There are studies in aspirin-tolerant subjects with severe asthma that also report striking therapeutic responses after addition of pranlukast [163] or zafirlukast [155].

In conclusion, a particular challenge for clinical COPD research is now to build on the experiences with antileukotrienes in asthma and perform studies that can assess whether antileukotrienes have value in the treatment of COPD, or may contribute to the systemic and metabolic components of COPD. The research must be unbiased and not governed by today's dogmas concerning mechanisms and strategies. An additional and related challenge is to characterize the role of other eicosanoids in COPD, where a number of proinflammatory (e.g. COX-2 derived PGE_2) and anti-inflammatory molecules (e.g. lipoxins and COX-1-derived PGE_2) deserve attention.

Acknowledgements

The author's main funding is by Karolinska Institute, the Swedish Heart Lung Foundation and the Swedish MRC.

References

1 von Euler US. Weitere Untersuchungen über Prostaglandin, die physiologisch aktive Substanz gewisser Genitaldrüsen. *Skand Arch Physiol* (now *Acta Physiol Scand*) 1939;**81**:65–80.

2 Dahlén S-E, Hansson G, Hedqvist P *et al*. Allergen challenge of lung tissue from asthmatics elicits bronchial contraction that correlates with the release of leukotrienes C_4, D_4 and E_4. *Proc Natl Acad Sci U S A* 1983;**80**:1712–6.

3 Funk CD. Prostaglandins and leukotrienes: advances in eicosanoid biology. *Science* 2001;**294**:1871–5.

4 Serhan CN, Savill J. Resolution of inflammation: the beginning programs the end. *Nat Immunol* 2005;**6**:1191–7.

5 FitzGerald GA. COX-2 and beyond: approaches to prostaglandin inhibition in human disease. *Nat Rev Drug Discov* 2003;**2**:879–90.

6 Fitzgerald GA. Coxibs and cardiovascular disease. *N Engl J Med* 2004;**351**:1709–11.

7 Funk CD, Hoshiko S, Matsumoto T, Rådmark O, Samuelsson B. Characterization of the human 5-lipoxygenase gene. *Proc Natl Acad Sci U S A* 1989;**86**:2587–91.

8 In KH, Asano K, Beier D *et al*. Naturally occurring mutations in the human 5-lipoxygenase gene promoter that modify transcription factor binding and reporter gene transcription. *J Clin Invest* 1997;**99**:1130–7.

9 Miller DK, Gillard JW, Vickers PJ *et al*. Identification and isolation of a membrane protein necessary for leukotriene production. *Nature* 1990;**343**:278–81.

10 Dixon RAF, Diehl RE, Opas E *et al*. Requirement of a 5-lipoxygenase-activating protein for leukotriene synthesis. *Nature* 1990;**343**:282–4.

11 Abramovitz M, Wong E, Cox ME *et al*. 5-lipoxygenase-activating protein stimulates the utilization of arachidonic acid by 5-lipoxygenase. *Eur J Biochem* 1993;**215**:105–11.

12 Haeggstrom JZ. Leukotriene A_4 hydrolase/aminopeptidase, the gatekeeper of chemotactic leukotriene B_4 biosynthesis. *J Biol Chem* 2004;**279**:50639–42.

13 Lam BK, Austen KF. Leukotriene C_4 synthase: a pivotal enzyme in cellular biosynthesis of the cysteinyl leukotrienes. *Prostaglandins Other Lipid Mediat* 2002;**68–69**:511–20.

14 Cowburn AS, Sladek K, Soja J *et al*. Overexpression of leukotriene C_4 synthase in bronchial biopsies from patients with aspirin-intolerant asthma. *J Clin Invest* 1998;**101**:834–46.

15 Jakobsson PJ, Morgenstern R, Mancini J, Ford-Hutchinson A, Persson B. Membrane-associated proteins in eicosanoid and glutathione metabolism (MAPEG): a widespread protein superfamily. *Am J Respir Crit Care Med* 2000;**161**(2 Pt 2): S20–4.

16 Lindgren JÅ, Edenius C. Transcellular biosynthesis of leukotrienes and lipoxins via leukotriene A$_4$ transfer. *Trends Pharmacol Sci* 1993;**14**:351–4.

17 Bäck M, Bu D, Bränström R *et al*. Leukotriene B$_4$ signaling trough NF-κB-dependent BLT1 receptors on vascular smooth muscle cells in atherosclerosis and intimal hyperplasia. *Proc Natl Acad Sci U S A* 2005;**102**:17501–6.

18 Wijnholds J, Evers R, Vanleusden MR *et al*. Increased sensitivity to anticancer drugs and decreased inflammatory response in mice lacking the multidrug resistance-associated protein. *Nat Med* 1997;**3**:1275–9.

19 Lam BK, Gagnon L, Austen KF, Soberman RJ. The mechanism of leukotriene B$_4$ export from human polymorphonuclear leukocytes. *J Biol Chem* 1990;**265**:13438–41.

20 Brink C, Dahlén S-E, Drazen J *et al*. International Union of Pharmacology XXXVII. Nomenclature for leukotriene and lipoxin receptors. *Pharmacol Rev* 2003;**55**:195–227.

21 Bäck M, Norel X, Walch L *et al*. Prostacyclin modulation of contractions of the human pulmonary artery by cysteinyl-leukotrienes. *Eur J Pharmacol* 2000;**401**:389–95.

22 Walch L, Norel X, Bäck M *et al*. Pharmacologic evidence for a novel cysteinyl-leukotriene receptor subtype in human pulmonary artery smooth muscle. *Br J Pharmacol* 2002;**137**:1339–45.

23 Casas A, Gomez FP, Dahlén B *et al*. Leukotriene D$_4$-induced hypoxaemia in asthma is mediated by the cys-leukotriene1 receptor. *Eur Respir J* 2005;**26**:442–8.

24 Beller TC, Friend DS, Maekawa A *et al*. Cysteinyl leukotriene 1 receptor controls the severity of chronic pulmonary inflammation and fibrosis. *Proc Natl Acad Sci U S A* 2004;**101**:3047–52.

25 Beller TC, Maekawa A, Friend DS, Austen KF, Kanaoka Y. Targeted gene disruption reveals the role of the cysteinyl leukotriene 2 receptor in increased vascular permeability and in bleomycin-induced pulmonary fibrosis in mice. *J Biol Chem* 2004;**279**:46 129–34.

26 Kumlin M. Measurement of leukotrienes in humans. *Am J Respir Crit Care Med* 2000;**161**:S102–6.

27 Horvath I, Hunt J, Barnes PJ *et al*. ATS/ERS TaskForce on Exhaled Breath Condensate. Exhaled breath condensate: methodological recommendations and unresolved questions. *Eur Respir J* 2005;**26**:523–48.

28 Higashi N, Taniguchi M, Mita H *et al*. Clinical features of asthmatic patients with increased urinary leukotriene E$_4$ excretion (hyperleukotrienuria): involvement of chronic hyperplastic rhinosinusitis with nasal polyposis. *J Allergy Clin Immunol* 2004;**113**:277–83.

29 Berry KA, Borgeat P, Gosselin J, Flamand L, Murphy RC. Urinary metabolites of leukotriene B$_4$ in the human subject. *J Biol Chem* 2003;**278**:24449–60.

30 Serafin WE, Oates JA, Hubbard WC. Metabolism of leukotriene B$_4$ in the monkey: identification of the principal nonvolatile metabolite in the urine. *Prostaglandins* 1984;**27**:899–911.

31 Gyllfors P, Kumlin M, Dahlen SE *et al*. Relation between bronchial responsiveness to inhaled leukotriene D$_4$ and markers of leukotriene biosythesis. *Thorax* 2005;**60**:902–8.

32 Hedqvist P, Dahlén S-E, Gustafsson LE, Hammarström S, Samuelsson B. Biological profile of leukotrienes C$_4$ and D$_4$. *Acta Physiol Scand* 1980;**110**:331–3.

33 Drazen JM, Austen KF, Lewis RA *et al*. Comparative airway and vascular activities of leukotrienes C-1 and D *in vivo* and *in vitro*. *Proc Natl Acad Sci U S A* 1980;**77**:4354–8.

34 Dahlén S-E, Hedqvist P, Hammarström S, Samuelsson B. Leukotrienes are potent constrictors of human bronchi. *Nature* 1980;**288**:484–6.

35 Hanna CJ, Bach MK, Pare PD, Schellenberg RR. Slow reacting substances (leukotrienes) contract human airway and pulmonary vascular smooth muscle. *Nature* 1981;**290**:343–4.

36 Jones TR, Davies C, Daniel EE. Pharmacological study of the contractile activity of leukotriene C$_4$ and D$_4$ on isolated human airway smooth muscle. *Can J Physiol Pharmacol* 1982;**60**:638–43.

37 Dahlén S-E, Björk J, Hedqvist P *et al*. Leukotrienes promote plasma leakage and leukocyte adhesion in postcapillry venules: *in vivo* effects with relevance to the acute inflammatory response. *Proc Natl Acad Sci U S A* 1981;**78**:3887–91.

38 Hua X-Y, Dahlén S-E, Lundberg JM, Hammarström S, Hedqvist P. Leukotrienes C$_4$, D$_4$ and E$_4$ cause extensive and widespread plasma extravasation in the guinea pig. *Naunyn-Schmiedebergk's Arch Pharmacol* 1985;**330**:136–41.

39 Drazen JM, Lewis RA, Austen KF *et al*. Contractile activities of structural analogs of leukotrienes C and D: necessity of a hydrophobic region. *Proc Natl Acad Sci U S A* 1981;**78**:3195–8.

40 Lewis RA, Drazen JM, Austen KF *et al*. Contractile activities of structural analogs of leukotrienes C and D: role of the polar substituents. *Proc Natl Acad Sci U S A* 1981;**78**:4579–83.

41 Gardiner PJ, Abram TS, Cuthbert NJ. Evidence for two leukotriene receptor types in the guinea-pig isolated ileum. *Eur J Pharmacol* 1990;**182**:291–9.

42 Buckner CK, Fedyna JS, Robertson JL *et al*. Examination of the influence of the epithelium on contractile responses to peptidoleukotrienes and blockade by ICI 204,219 in isolated guinea-pig trachea and human intralobar airways. *J Pharm Exp Ther* 1990;**252**:77–85.

43 Weichman BM, Muccitelli Rm, Osborn RR *et al*. In vitro and *in vivo* mechanisms of leukotriene-mediated bronchoconstriction in the guinea pig. *J Pharm Exp Ther* 1982;**222**:202–8.

44 Lee TH, Austen KF, Corey EJ, Drazen JM. LTE$_4$-induced airway hyperresponsiveness of guinea pig tracheal smooth muscle to histamine and evidence for three separate sulfidopeptide receptors. *Proc Natl Acad Sci U S A* 1984;**81**:4922–5.

45 Jaques CAJ, Spur BW, Johnson M, Lee TH. The mechanism of LTE$_4$-induced histamine hyperresponsiveness in guinea-pig tracheal and human bronchial smooth muscle *in vitro*. *Br J Pharmacol* 1991;**104**:859–66.

46 Buckner CK, Fedyna JS, Robertson JL *et al*. Examination of the influence of the epithelium on contractile responses to peptidoleukotrienes and blockade by ICI 204,219 in isolated guinea-pig trachea and human intralobar airways. *J Pharm Exp Ther* 1990;**252**:77–85.

47 Coles SJ, Neill KH, Reid LM *et al*. Effects of leukotrienes C$_4$

and D_4 on glycoprotein and lysozyme secretion by human bronchial mucosa. *Prostaglandins* 1982;**25**:155–70.

48 Marom Z, Shelhamer JH, Bach MK, Morton DR, Kaliner M. Slow reacting substances, leukotrienes C_4 and D_4, increase the release of mucus from human airways *in vitro*. *Am Rev Respir Dis* 1982;**126**:449–51.

49 Peatfield AC, Piper PJ, Richardson PS. The effects of leukotriene C_4 on mucin release into the cat trachea *in vivo* and *in vitro*. *Br J Pharmacol* 1982;**77**:391–3.

50 Laitinen L, Laitinen A, Haahtela T *et al.* Leukotriene E_4 causes granulocyte infiltration into asthmatic airways. *Lancet* 1993;**341**:989–90.

51 Diamant Z, Hiltermann JT, van Rensen EL *et al.* The effect of inhaled leukotriene D_4 and methacholine on sputum cell differentials in asthma. *Am J Respir Crit Care Med* 1977;**155**: 1247–53.

52 Echazarreta AL, Dahlén B, García G *et al.* Pulmonary gas exchange and sputum cellular responses to inhaled leukotriene D_4 in asthma. *Am J Respir Crit Care Med* 2001; **164**:202–6.

53 Underwood DC, Osborn RR, Newsholme SJ, Torphy TJ, Hay DWP. Persistent airway eosinophilia after leukotriene (LT) D_4 administration in the guinea-pig: modulation by the LTD_4 receptor antagonist pranlukast or an interleukin-5 monoclonal antibody. *Am J Repir Crit Care Med* 1996;**154**: 850–7.

54 Munoz NM, Douglas I, Mayer I *et al.* Eosinophil chemotaxis inhibited by 5-lipoxygenase blockade and leukotriene receptor antagonism. *Am J Respir Crit Care Med* 1997;**155**: 1398–403.

55 Palmberg L, Claesson H-E, Thyberg J. Leuktrienes stimulate initiation of DNA synthesis in cultured arterial smooth muscle cells. *J Cell Sci* 1987;**88**:151–9.

56 Palmberg L, Lindgren J-Å, Thyberg J, Claesson H-E. On the mechanism of induction of DNA synthesis in cultured arterial smooth muscle cells by leukotrienes. Possible role of prostaglandin endoperoxide synthase products and platelet-derived growth factor. *J Cell Sci* 1991;**98**:141–9.

57 Peppelenbosch MP, Teretoolen LGJ, Hage WJ, de Laat SW. Epidermal growth factor-induced actin remodeling is regulated by 5-lipoxygenase and cyclooxygenase products. *Cell* 1993;**74**:565–75.

58 Rajah R, Nunn SE, Herrick DJ, Grunstein MM, Cohen P. Leukotriene D_4 induces MMP-1, which functions as an IGFBP protease in human airway smooth muscle cells. *Am J Physiol* 1996;**271**:L1014–22.

59 Wang CG, Du T, Xu LJ, Martin JG. Role of leukotriene D_4 in allergen-induced increases in airway smooth muscle in the rat. *Am Rev Respir Dis* 1993;**148**:413–7.

60 Holroyde MC, Altounyan REC, Cole M, Dixon M, Elliott EV. Bronchoconstriction produced in man by leukotrienes C & D. *Lancet* 1981;**6**:17–8.

61 Weiss JW, Drazen JM, Coles N *et al.* Bronchoconstrictor effects of leukotriene C in humans. *Science* 1982;**216**:196–8.

62 Barnes NC, Piper PJ, Costello JF. Comparative effects of inhaled leukotriene C_4 and D_4 in normal human subjects. *Thorax* 1984;**39**:500–4.

63 Griffin M, Weiss JW, Leitch AG *et al.* Effects of leukotriene D on the airways in asthma. *N Engl J Med* 1983;**308**:436–9.

64 Ädelroth E, Morris MM, Hargreave FE, O'Byrne PM. Airway responsiveness to leukotrienes C_4 and D_4 and to methacholine in patients with asthma and normal controls. *N Engl J Med* 1986;**315**:480–4.

65 O'Hickey SP, Arm JP, Rees PJ, Spur PJ, Lee TH. The relative responsiveness to inhaled leukotriene E_4, metacholine and histamine in normal and asthmatic subjects. *Eur Repir J* 1988;**1**:913–7.

66 Bel EH, Van Der Veen H, Kramps JA, Dijkman JH, Sterk PJ. Maximal airway narrowing to inhaled leukotriene D_4 in normal subjects. *Am Rev Respir Dis* 1987;**136**:979–84.

67 Davidson AB, Lee TH, Scanlon PD, Solway J, McFadden ER. Bronchhoconstrictor effects of leukotriene E_4 in normal and asthmatic subjects. *Am Rev Respir Dis* 1987;**135**:333–7.

68 Ketchell RI, D'Amato M, Jensen MW, O'Connor BJ. Contrasting effects of allergen challenge on airway responsiveness to cysteinyl leukotriene D_4 and methacholine in mild asthma. *Thorax* 2002;**57**:575–80.

69 Arm JP, O'Hickey SP, Hawksworth RJ *et al.* Asthmatic airways have a disproportionate hyperresponsiveness to LTE_4, as compared with normal airways, but not to LTC_4, LTD_4 methacholine, and histamine. *Am Rev Respir Dis* 1990;**142**: 1112–8.

70 Manning PJ, Watson RW, O'Byrne PM. Exercise-induced refractoriness in asthmatic subjects involves leukotriene and prostaglandin interdependent mechanisms. *Am Rev Respir Dis* 1993;**148**:950–4.

71 Ford-Hutchinson AW, Bray MA, Doig MV, Shipley ME, Smith MJH. Leukotriene B_4, a potent chemokinetic and aggregating substance released from polymorphonuclear leukocytes. *Nature* 1980;**286**:264–5.

72 Bray MA, Ford-Hutchinson AW, Smith MJH. Leukotriene B_4: an inflammatory mediator *in vivo*. *Prostaglandins* 1981; **22**:213–22.

73 Ott VL, Cambier JC, Kappler J, Marrack P, Swanson BJ. Mast cell-dependent migration of effector CD8+ T cells through production of leukotriene B4. *Nat Immunol* 2003;**4**: 974–81.

74 Beeh KM, Kornmann O, Buhl R *et al.* Neutrophil chemotactic activity of sputum from patients with COPD: role of interleukin 8 and leukotriene B_4. *Chest* 2003;**123**:1240–7.

75 Hafström I, Palmblad J, Malmsten C, Rådmark O, Samuelsson B. Leukotriene B_4 – a stereospecific stimulator for release of lysosomal enzymes from neutrophils. *FEBS Lett* 1981;**130**:14–7.

76 Rae SA, Smith MJH. The stimulation of lysosomal enzyme secretion from human polymorphonuclear leukocytes by leukotriene B_4. *J Pharm Pharmacol* 1981;**33**:616–8.

77 Irvin CG, Tu YP, Sheller JR, Funk CD. 5-lipoxygenase products are necessary for ovalbumin-induced airway responsiveness in mice. *Am J Physiol* 1997;**16**:L1053–8.

78 Devchand PR, Keller H, Peters JM *et al.* The $PPAR_\alpha$-leukotriene B_4 pathway to inflammation control. *Nature* 1996;**384**:39–43.

79 Hansson G, Lindgren JÅ, Dahlén S-E, Hedqvist P,

Samuelsson B. Identification and biological activity of novel x-oxidized metabolites of leukotriene B_4 from human leukocytes. *FEBS Lett* 1981;**130**:107–12.

80 Piper PJ, Samhoun MN. Stimulation of arachidonic acid metabolism and generation of thromboxane A_2 by leukotrienes B_4, C_4 and D_4 in guinea-pig lung *in vitro*. *Br J Pharmacol* 1982;**77**:267–75.

81 Sirois P, Roy S, Borgeat P, Picard S, Vallerand P. Evidence for a mediator role of thromboxane A_2 in the myotropic action of leukotriene B_4 (LTB_4) on the guinea-pig lung. *Prostaglandins Leukot Med* 1982;**8**:157–70.

82 Dahlén S-E, Hedqvist P, Westlund P *et al.* Mechanisms for leukotriene-induced contractions of guinea pig airways: leukotriene C_4 has a potent direct action whereas leukotriene B_4 acts indirectly. *Acta Physiol Scand* 1983;**118**: 393–403.

83 Sakata K, Dahlén S-E, Bäck M. The contractile action of leukotriene B_4 in the guinea-pig lung involves a vascular component. *Br J Pharmacol* 2004;**141**:449–56.

84 O'Byrne PM, Leikauf GD, Aizawa H *et al.* Leukotriene B_4 induces airway hyperresponsiveness in dogs. *J Appl Physiol* 1985;**59**:1941–6.

85 Black PN, Fuller RW, Taylor GW, Barnes PJ, Dollery CT. Effect of inhaled leukotriene B_4 alone and in combination with prostaglandin D_2 on bronchial responsiveness to histamine in normal subjects. *Thorax* 1989;**44**:491–5.

86 Dahlén B, Nizankowska E, Szczeklik A *et al.* Benefits from adding the 5-lipoxygenase inhibitor zileuton to conventional therapy in aspirin-intolerant asthmatics. *Am J Respir Crit Care Med* 1998;**157**:1187–94.

87 Martin TR, Pistorese BP, Chi EY, Goodman RB, Matthay MA. Effects of leukotriene B_4 in the human lung. *J Clin Invest* 1989;**94**:1609–19.

88 Sampson SE, Costello JF, Sampson AP. The effect of inhaled leukotriene B_4 in normal and asthmatic subjects. *Am J Respir Crit Care Med* 1997;**155**:1789–92.

89 Hakonarson H, Thorvaldsson S, Helgadottir A *et al.* Effects of a 5-lipoxygenase-activating protein inhibitor on biomarkers associated with risk of myocardial infarction: a randomized trial. *JAMA* 2005;**293**:2245–56.

90 Dwyer JH, Allayee H, Dwyer KM *et al.* Arachidonate 5-lipoxygenase promoter genotype, dietary arachidonic acid, and atherosclerosis. *N Engl J Med* 2004;**350**:29–37.

91 Terashita ZI, Fuki H, Hirata M *et al.* Coronary vasoconstriction and PGI_2 release by leukotrienes in isolated guinea pig hearts. *Eur J Pharmacol* 1981;**73**:357–61.

92 Letts LG, Piper PJ. The actions of leukotrienes C_4 and D_4 on guinea-pig isolated hearts. *Br J Pharmacol* 1982;**76**:169–76.

93 Michelassi F, Landa L, Hill RD *et al.* Leukotriene D_4: a potent coronary artery vasoconstrictor associated with impaired ventricular contraction. *Science* 1982;**217**:841–3.

94 Burke JA, Levi R, Guo Z-G, Corey EJ. Leukotrienes C_4, D_4 and E_4: effects on human and guinea-pig cardiac preparations *in vitro*. *J Pharm Exp Ther* 1982;**221**:235–41.

95 Peters-Golden M, Canetti C, Mancuso P, Coffey MJ. Leukotrienes: underappreciated mediators of innate immune responses. *J Immunol* 2005;**174**:589–94.

96 Charbeneau RP, Peters-Golden M. Eicosanoids: mediators and therapeutic targets in fibrotic lung disease. *Clin Sci* 2005;**108**:479–91.

97 Profita M, Sala A, Riccobono L *et al.* 15(S)-HETE modulates LTB_4 production and neutrophil chemotaxis in chronic bronchitis. *Am J Physiol Cell Physiol* 2000;**279**:C1249–58.

98 McGill KA, Busse WW. Zileuton. *Lancet* 1996;**348**:519–24.

99 Friedman BS, Bel EH, Buntinx A *et al.* Oral leukotriene inhibitor (MK-886) blocks allergen-induced airway responses. *Am Rev Respir Dis* 1993;**147**:839–44.

100 Diamant Z, Timmers MC, van der Veen H *et al.* The effect of MK-0591, a novel 5-lipoxygenase activating protein inhibitor, on leukotriene biosynthesis and allergen-induced airway responses in asthmatic subjects *in vivo*. *J Allergy Clin Immunol* 1995;**95**:42–51.

101 Dahlén B, Kumlin M, Ihré E, Zetterström O, Dahlén S-E. Inhibition of allergen-induced airway obstruction and leukotriene generation in atopic asthmatics by the leukotriene-biosynthesis inhibitor BAY x1005. *Thorax* 1997;**52**:342–7.

102 Wong SL, Locke C, Dubé LM, Granneman GR, Awni WM. Meta-analysis of the pharmcodynamic relationship between the *ex vivo* LTB_4 inhibition in whole blood and zileuton plasma concentrations from Phase I studies in normal volunteers using NONMEM approach. *Pharm Res* 1994;**11**(Suppl 10):434.

103 Israel E, Fischer AR, Rosenberg MA *et al.* The pivotal role of 5-lipoxygenase products in the reaction of aspirin-sensitive asthmatics to aspirin. *Am Rev Respir Dis* 1993;**148**: 1447–51.

104 Israel E, Rubin P, Kemp JP *et al.* The effect of inhibition of 5-lipoxygenase by Zileuton in mild-to-moderate asthma. *Ann Intern Med* 1993;**119**:1059–66.

105 Evans DJ, Barnes PJ, Spaethe SM *et al.* Effects of a leukotriene B_4 receptor antagonist, LY293111, on allergen-induced responses in asthma. *Thorax* 1996;**51**:1178–84.

106 Smith LJ, Geller S, Ebright L, Glass M, Thyrum PT. Inhibition of leukotriene D_4-induced bronchoconstriction in normal subjects by the oral leukotriene D_4 antagonist ICI-204,219. *Am Rev Respir Dis* 1990;**141**:988–92.

107 Smith LJ, Glass M, Minkwitz MC. Inhibition of leukotriene D_4-induced bronchoconstriction in subjects with asthma: a concentration-effect study of ICI 204,219. *Clin Pharmacol Ther* 1993;**54**:430–6.

108 O'Shaughnessy TC, Georgiou P, Howland K *et al.* The effect of pranlukast, an oral leukotriene D_4 antagonist, on leukotriene D_4 (LTD_4) challenge in normal volunteers. *Thorax* 1997;**52**:524–7.

109 De Lepeleire I, Reiss TF, Rochette F *et al.* Montelukast causes prolonged, potent leukotriene D_4-receptor antagonism in the airways of patients with asthma. *Clin Pharmacol Ther* 1997;**61**:83–92.

110 Gompertz S, Stockley RA. A randomized, placebo-controlled trial of a leukotriene synthesis inhibitor in patients with COPD. *Chest* 2002;**122**:289–94.

111 Fischer AR, McFadden CA, Frantz R *et al.* Effect of chronic 5-lipoxygenase inhibition on airway hyperresponsiveness

in asthmatic subjects. *Am J Respir Crit Care Med* 1995;**152**: 1203–7.

112 Miadonna A, Tedeschi A, Leggieri E *et al.* Behavior and clinical relevance of histamine and leukotrienes C_4 and B_4 in grass pollen-induced rhinitis. *Am Rev Respir Dis* 1987;**136**: 357–62.

113 Hui KP, Barnes NC. Lung function improvement in asthma with a cysteinyl-leukotriene receptor antagonist. *Lancet* 1991;**337**:1062–3.

114 Gaddy JN, Margolskee DJ, Bush RK, Williams VC, Busse WW. Bronchodilation with a potent and selective leukotriene D_4 (LTD_4) receptor antagonist (MK-571) in asthma patients. *Am Rev Respir Dis* 1992;**146**:358–63.

115 Reiss TF, Sorkness CA, Stricker W *et al.* Effects of montelukast (MK-0476), a potent cysteinyl-leukotriene receptor antagonist, on bronchodilation in asthmatic subjects treated with and without inhaled corticosteroids. *Thorax* 1997;**52**:45–8.

116 Watson N, Magnussen H, Rabe KF. Inherent tone of human bronchus: role of eicosanoids and epithelium. *Br J Pharmacol* 1997;**121**:1099–104.

117 Dahlén B, Margolskee DJ, Zetterström O, Dahlén S-E. Effect of the leukotriene-antagonist MK-0679 on baseline pulmonary function in aspirin-sensitive asthmatics. *Thorax* 1993;**48**:1205–10.

118 Nannini LJ Jr, Flores DM. Bronchodilator effect of zafirlukast in subjects with chronic obstructive pulmonary disease. *Pulm Pharmacol Ther* 2003;**16**:307–11.

119 Cazzola M, Boveri B, Carlucci P *et al.* Lung function improvement in smokers suffering from COPD with zafirlukast, a $CysLT_1$-receptor antagonist. *Pulm Pharmacol Ther* 2000;**13**:301–5.

120 Taylor IK, O'Shaoughnessy KM, Fuller RW, Dollery CT. Effect of cysteinyl-leukotriene receptor antagonist ICI 204,219 on allergen-induced bronchoconstriction and airway hyperreactivity in atopic subjects. *Lancet* 1991;**337**: 690–4.

121 Hamilton AL, Watson RM, Wyile G, O'Byrne PM. Attenuation of early and late phase allergen-induced bronchoconstriction in asthmatic subjects by a 5-lipoxygenase activating protein antagonist, BAY x1005. *Thorax* 1997;**52**: 348–54.

122 Diamant Z, Grootendorst DC, Veselic-Charvat M *et al.* The effect of montelukast (MK-0476), a cysteinyl leukotriene receptor antagonist, on allergen-induced airway responses and sputum cell counts in asthma. *Clin Exp Allergy* 1999; **29**:42–51.

123 Roquet A, Dahlén B, Kumlin M *et al.* Combined antagonism of leukotrienes and histamine produces predominant inhibition of allergen-induced early and late phase airway obstruction in asthmatics. *Am J Respir Crit Care Med* 1997; **155**:1856–63.

124 Leigh R, Vethanayagam D, Yoshida M *et al.* Effects of montelukast and budesonide on airway responses and airway inflammation in asthma. *Am J Respir Crit Care Med* 2002;**166**: 1212–7.

125 Manning PJ, Watson RM, Margolskee DJ *et al.* Inhibition of

exercise-induced bronchoconstriction by MK-571: a potent leukotriene D_4 receptor antagonist. *N Engl J Med* 1990;**323**: 1736–9.

126 Rundell KW, Spiering BA, Baumann JM, Evans TM. Effects of montelukast on airway narrowing from eucapnic voluntary hyperventilation and cold air exercise. *Br J Sports Med* 2005;**39**:232–6.

127 Israel E, Dermarkarian R, Rosenberg M *et al.* The effects of a 5-lipoxygenase inhibitor on asthma induced by cold, dry air. *N Engl J Med* 1990;**323**:1740–4.

128 Brannan JD, Anderson SD, Gomes K *et al.* Fexofenadine decreses sensitivity to and montelukast improves recovery from inhaled mannitol. *Am J Respir Crit Care Med* 2001;**163**: 1420–5.

129 Lazarus SC, Lavins BJ, Wong HH, Watts MJ, Minkwitz MC. Effect of oral zafirlukast on sulphur dioxide (SO_2)-induced bronchoconstriction in patients with asthma. *Am J Respir Crit Care Med* 1997;**156**:1725–30.

130 Björck T, Gustafsson LE, Dahlén S-E: Isolated bronchi of asthmatics are hyperresponsive to adenosine which apparently acts indirectly by liberation of leukotrienes and histamine. *Am Rev Respir Dis* 1992;**145**:1087–91.

131 Rorke S, Jennison S, Jeffs JA *et al.* Role of cysteinyl leukotrienes in adenosine 5'-momophosphate induced bronchoconstriction in asthma. *Thorax* 2002;**57**:323–7.

132 O'Sullivan S, Roquet A, Dahlén B, Kumlin M, Dahlén S-E. Urinary excretion of inflammatory mediators during allergen-induced early and late phase asthmatic reactions. *Clin Exp Allergy* 1998;**28**:1332–9.

133 O'Sullivan S, Dahlén B, Dahlén S-E, Kumlin M. Increased urinary excretion of the prostaglandin D_2 metabolite $9\alpha,11\beta$-PGF_2 following aspirin challenge supports mast cell activation in aspirin-induced airway obstruction. *J Allergy Clin Immunol* 1996;**98**:421–32.

134 Israel E, Fischer AR, Rosenberg MA *et al.* The pivotal role of 5-lipoxygenase products in the reaction of aspirin-sensitive asthmatics to aspirin. *Am Rev Respir Dis* 1993;**148**: 1447–51.

135 Dahlén B, Kumlin M, Margolskee DJ *et al.* The leukotriene-receptor antagonist MK-0679 blocks airway obstruction induced by inhaled lysine-aspirin in aspirin-sensitive asthmatics. *Eur Respir J* 1993;**6**:1018–26.

136 Zuhlke IE, Kanniess F, Richter K *et al.* Montelukast attenuates the airway response to hypertonic saline in moderate-to-severe COPD. *Eur Respir J* 2003;**22**:926–30.

137 Gronke L, Schlenker J, Holz O *et al.* Effect of cetirizine dihydrochloride on the airway response to hypertonic saline aerosol in patients with chronic obstructive pulmonary disease (COPD). *Respir Med* 2005;**99**:1241–8.

138 DeJongste JC, Mons H, Block R *et al.* Increased *in vitro* histamine responses in human small airways smooth muscle from patients with chronic obstructive pulmonary disease. *Am Rev Respir Dis* 1987;**135**:549–53.

139 Israel E, Rubin P, Kemp JP *et al.* The effect of inhibition of 5-lipoxygenase by Zileuton in mild-to-moderate asthma. *Ann Intern Med* 1993;**119**:1059–66.

140 Spector LS, Miller CJ, Glass M and the Accolate study

group. Effects of six weeks therapy with oral doses of ICI 204,219, a leukotriene D_4 receptor antagonist, in subjects with bronchial asthma. *Am J Respir Crit Care Med* 1995;**150**: 618–23.

141 Liu MC, Dubé LM, Lancaster J and the Zileuton Clinical Trial Group. Acute and chronic effects of a 5-lipoxygenase inhibitor in asthma: a 6-month randomized multicenter-trial. *J Allergy Clin Immunol* 1996;**98**:859–71.

142 Reiss TF, Altman LC, Chervinsky P *et al.* Effects of montelukast (MK-0476), a new potent cysteinyl-leukotriene (LTD_4) receptor antagonist, in patients with chronic asthma. *J Allergy Clin Immunol* 1996;**98**:528–34.

143 Barnes NC, Pujet J-C. Pranlukast, a novel leukotriene receptor antagonist: results of the first European, placebo conrolled, multicentre clinical study in asthma. *Thorax* 1997;**52**:523–7.

144 Drazen JM, Dahlén S-E, Lee TH. Five-lipoxygenase products in asthma. In: *Lung Biology in Health and Disease*, vol. 120. New York: Marcel Dekker, 1998.

145 Leff JA, Busse WW, Pearlman D *et al.* Montelukast, a leukotriene-receptor antagonist, for the treatment of mild asthma and exercise-induced bronchoconstriction. *N Engl J Med* 1998;**339**:147–52.

146 Kemp JP, Dockhorn RJ, Shapiro GG *et al.* Montelukast once daily inhibits exercise-induced bronchoconstriction in 6- to 14-year-old children with asthma. *J Pediatr* 1998;**133**: 424–8.

147 Kane GC, Pollice M, Kim C-J *et al.* A controlled trial of the effect of the 5-lipoxygenase inhibitor, zileuton, on lung inflammation produced by segmental antigen challenge in human beings. *J Allergy Clin Immunol* 1996;**97**:646–54.

148 Pizzichini E, Leff JA, Reiss TF *et al.* Montelukast reduces airway eosinophilic inflammation in asthma: a randomized, controlled trial. *Eur Respir J* 1999;**14**:12–8.

149 Malmstrom K, Rodriguez-Gomez G, Guerra J *et al.* Oral montelukast, inhaled beclomethasone, and placebo for chronic asthma: a randomized, controlled trial. Montelukast / Beclomethasone Study Group. *Ann Intern Med* 1999;**130**: 487–95.

150 Bisgaard H, Zielen S, Garcia-Garcia ML *et al.* Montelukast reduces asthma exacerbations in 2- to 5-year-old children with intermittent asthma. *Am J Respir Crit Care Med* 2005; **171**:315–22.

151 Doull IJ, Lampe FC, Smith S *et al.* Effect of inhaled corticosteroids on episodes of wheezing associated with viral infections in school age childred: randomized double blind placebo controlled trial. *BMJ* 1997;**315**:858–62.

152 Oommen A, Lambert PC, Grigg J. Efficacy of a short course of parent-initiated oral prednisolone for viral wheeze in children aged 1–5 years: randomised controlled trial. *Lancet* 2003;**362**:1433–8.

153 Crooks SW, Baykey DL, Hill SL, Stockley RA. Bronchial inflammation in acute bacterial exacerbations of chronic bronchitis: the role of leukotriene B_4. *Eur Respir J* 2000; **15**:274–80.

154 Bjermer L, Bisgaard H, Bousquet J *et al.* Montelukast and fluticasone compared with salmeterol and fluticasone in protecting against asthma exacerbation in adults: one year, double blind, randomised, comparative trial. *BMJ* 2003;**327**:891–7.

155 Virchow JC Jr, Prasse A, Naya I, Summerton L, Harris A. Zafirlukast improves asthma control in patients receiving high-dose inhaled corticosteroids. *Am J Respir Crit Care Med* 2000;**162**:578–85.

156 Dahlén S-E, Malmström K, Nizankowska E *et al.* Improvement of aspirin-intolerant asthma by montelukast, a leukotriene antagonist: a randomized, double-blind, placebo-controlled trial. *Am J Respir Crit Care Med* 2002;**165**:9–14.

157 Laviolette M, Malmström K, Lu S *et al.* Montelukast added to inhaled beclomethasone in treatment of asthma. Montelukast/Beclomethasone Additivity Group. *Am J Respir Crit Care Med* 1999;**160**:1862–8.

158 Sebaldt RJ, Sheller JR, Oates JA, Roberts LJ, FitzGerald GA. Inhibition of eicosanoid biosynthesis by glucocorticoids in humans. *Proc Natl Acad Sci U S A* 1990;**87**:6974–8.

159 Manso G, Baker AJ, Taylor IK, Fuller RW. *In vivo* and *in vitro* effects of glucocorticoids on arachidonic acid metabolism and monocyte function in humans. *Eur Respir J* 1992;**5**: 712–6.

160 O'Shaughnessy KM, Wellings R, Gillies B, Fuller RW. Differential effects of fluticasone proprionate on allergen-evoked bronchoconstriction and increased urinary leukotriene E_4 excretion. *Am Rev Respir Dis* 1993;**147**:1472–6.

161 Dworski R, FitzGerald GA, Oates JA, Sheller JR. Effect of oral prednisone on airway inflammatory mediators in atopic asthma. *Am J Respir Crit Care Med* 1994;**149**:953–9.

162 Riddick CA, Ring WL, Baker JR, Hodulik CR, Bigby TD. Dexamethasone increases expression of 5-lipoxygenase and its activating protein in human monocytes and THP-1 cells. *Eur J Biochem* 1997;**146**:112–8.

163 Tamaoki J, Kondo M, Sakai N *et al.* Leukotriene antagonist prevents exacerbation of asthma during reduction of high-dose inhaled corticosteroid. *Am J Respir Crit Care Med* 1997; **155**:1235–40.

164 Löfdahl CG, Reiss TF, Leff JA *et al.* Randomised, placebo controlled trial of effect of a leukotriene receptor antagonist, montelukast, on tapering inhaled corticosteroids in asthmatic patients. *BMJ* 1999;**319**:87–90.

165 Price DB, Hernandez D, Magyar P *et al.* Clinical Outcomes with Montelukast as a Partner Agent to Corticosteroid Therapy (COMPACT) International Study Group. Randomised controlled trial of montelukast plus inhaled budesonide versus double dose inhaled budesonide in adult patients with asthma. *Thorax* 2003;**58**:211–6.

166 Wechsler ME, Garpestad E, Flier SR *et al.* Pulmonary infiltrates, eosinophilia, and cardiomyopathy following corticosteroid withdrawal in patients with asthma receiving zafirlukast. *JAMA* 1998;**279**:455–7.

167 Wechsler ME, Finn D, Gunawardena D *et al.* Churg–Strauss syndrome in patients receiving montelukast as treatment for asthma. *Chest* 2000;**117**:708–13.

168 Martin RM, Wilton LV, Mann RD. Prevalence of Churg–Strauss syndrome, vasculitis, eosinophilia and associated

conditions: retrospective analysis of 58 prescription-event monitoring cohort studies. *Pharmacoepidemiol Drug Saf* 1999; **8**:179–89.

169 Murphy RC, Hammarström S, Samuelsson B. Leukotriene C: a slow reacting substance from murine mastocytoma cells. *Proc Natl Acad Sci U S A* 1979;**76**:4275–9.

170 Sampson AP, Siddiqui S, Buchanan D *et al*. Variant LTC_4 synthase allele modifies cysteinyl leukotriene synthesis in eosinophils and predicts clinical response to zafirlukast. *Thorax* 2000;**55**(Suppl 2):S28–31.

171 Drazen JM, Yandava CN, Dube L *et al*. Pharmacogenetic association between ALOX5 promoter genotype and the response to anti-asthma treatment. *Nat Genet* 1999;**22**: 168–70.

CHAPTER 27

Cigarette smoking, emphysema and lung endothelium

Stephanie A. Nonas, Irina Petrache and Joe G. N. Garcia

Pulmonary emphysema, characterized by alveolar wall destruction and permanent enlargement of the airways distal to terminal bronchioles, is the fourth leading cause of death (along with chronic bronchitis) in the USA, with a rising incidence and prevalence. Despite the clear observation that the vast majority of emphysema is associated with chronic cigarette smoking, the complete pathogenesis of emphysema remains unclear. Historically held concepts of the biochemical and molecular basis of emphysema have highlighted the obvious critical role of tobacco smoke exposure as well as the importance of effector cells, such as inflammatory leukocytes, which target tissues such as the bronchial and alveolar epithelium (see Chapters 17 & 22). However, the increasing knowledge of complex cell biologic processes and cellular homeostasis has led to paradigm-shifting hypotheses and the identification of previously unappreciated pathogenic mechanisms in COPD development. In concert with this explosion of information in the post-genome era, attention has shifted in recent years to include the potential for the meaningful contribution of vascular components in the complex pathophysiology associated with chronic airflow obstruction.

Endothelial cell barrier function in lung inflammation

The pulmonary circulation has a number of important functions including a critical role in gas exchange. Microvessels exchange solutes and water, and the mechanisms regulating the balance of fluid and solutes in extravascular spaces of the lung are central to understanding the pathophysiology of inflammatory pulmonary conditions such as acute respiratory distress syndrome (ARDS) and sepsis where increases in vascular permeability contribute to profound pulmonary oedema and physiologic derangements. Because of the enormous surface area of

the pulmonary vasculature, the pulmonary endothelium, a multidimensional tissue lining the entire vasculature, serves a specialized function as a semi-permeable barrier between the vascular space and the interstitium. The barrier function of lung endothelial cells is actively regulated. While the integrity of the endothelial cell monolayer is a critical requirement for preservation of pulmonary function, disruption of the endothelial barrier is now recognized as a cardinal feature of inflammation (Fig. 27.1). Endothelial barrier properties are not uniform throughout the pulmonary vasculature. There is greater macromolecule diffusion in postcapillary venules compared with pulmonary arterioles in whole lung models, and microvascular endothelium exhibits 10-fold higher barrier properties than macrovascular endothelium *in vitro* [1]. Although the precise mechanisms that regulate this variability in segmental barrier function are unknown, barrier regulatory components such as Ca^{2+} signalling pathways and differences in content and regulation of barrier protective cyclic adenosine monophosphate (cAMP) are likely involved [2].

The contribution of increased vascular permeability to acute inflammatory processes is much better defined than its role in chronic inflammatory disorders such as COPD, although loss of barrier integrity may be an important component of the acute exacerbation of chronic bronchitis. It remains well appreciated, however, that the pulmonary vascular endothelial barrier also actively participates in regulating cell trafficking across the vessel wall (see Fig. 27.1) and thus is essential to the entire spectrum of COPD from chronic bronchitis to emphysema. In its highly advantageous spatial locale, the endothelium serves as an integral member of both innate immunity and adaptive immunity response with highly specialized and complex signalling and regulatory pathways, which are selective for the type of inflammatory and immune effectors cells allowed entry into lung tissues. The narrow dimensions of the lung capillary lumen (less than 10 μm diameter) implicate an

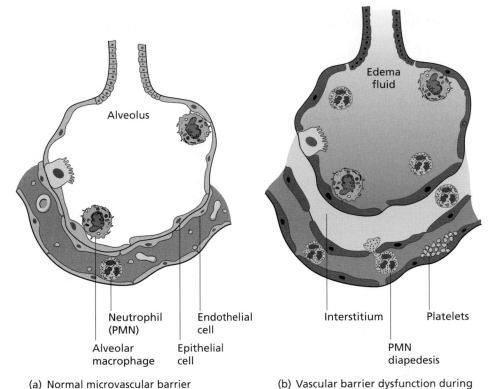

Figure 27.1 Pulmonary microcirculation in health and disease. (a) In the normal alveolar septum, the endothelial layer is intact and in close apposition with the alveolar epithelium, facilitating gas exchange while maintaining a tight barrier. (b) In disease states, endothelial perturbation leads to loss of barrier function with interstitial oedema and tissue inflammation. PMN, polymorphonuclear leucocyte.

Alveolus

Neutrophil (PMN)
Endothelial cell
Alveolar macrophage
Epithelial cell

(a) Normal microvascular barrier

Edema fluid

Interstitium
Platelets
PMN diapedesis

(b) Vascular barrier dysfunction during severe inflammation

intimate involvement of biophysical properties of both leukocytes as well as the mechanically challenged lung endothelium in regulating diapedesis [3,4]. In the context of the chronic low-level inflammatory status of lungs from both cigarette smokers and patients with emphysema, this leucocyte gatekeeper function of the endothelium becomes relevant to the development of irreversible lung disease.

Endothelial cell paracrine and cell survival function in lung homeostasis

In addition to serving as gatekeeper to circulating inflammatory and immune effector cells, the pulmonary vascular endothelium has an active role in maintaining both systemic and local (paracrine) feedback systems, by active processing of signalling mediators. In the lungs, alveolar septae (comprising endothelium, epithelium and a thin interstitium) form the air–blood barrier through which gas is exchanged. The endothelial and epithelial basement membranes appear to be fused for a length expanding over half of the capillary perimeter, creating the alveolar–capillary septum, an ideal site for gas transfer because of the maximal surface area available for gas exchange and minimal diffusion distance. Endothelium-dependent growth of

pulmonary vascular structures (vasculogenesis) occurs during early development and is crucial to the development of lung structures, specifically functional alveoli, and inhibition of vasculogenesis/angiogenesis decreases alveolarization of the developing lung [5]. Because of the intimate contact between septal components, mature endothelial cells continue to interact with neighboring epithelial cells in maintaining alveolar structures. One key mediator of this cell–cell cross-talk involved in septal homeostasis is vascular endothelial growth factor (VEGF), a potent mitogen and angiogenic factor involved in the development and maintenance of vascular endothelial cells as well as vascular permeability and vasodilatation. Expressed in nearly all tissues, VEGF acts as a potent survival factor for endothelial cells, inhibiting apoptosis both *in vitro* and *in vivo* [6–11]. VEGF has two major receptor tyrosine kinases, VEGFR-1 (Flt1) and VEGFR-2 (KDR/Flk1), which are expressed on vascular endothelial cells and hematopoietic cells, with VEGFR-2 responsible for the majority of the mitogenic, angiogenic and permeability enhancing properties of VEGF [7]. VEGF is abundantly expressed in normal lung tissues, where it is localized mainly to alveolar epithelial cells with receptors present on adjacent endothelial cells [12–16]. During development, expression of VEGF by mesenchymal and epithelial cells in branching airways guide endothelial cell differentiation and angiogenesis, and inhibition of

VEGF in the lungs leads to pulmonary endothelial cell death [17–19]. This key confluence of spatial localization, cell–cell cross-talk and intercellular survival dependency has led to the development of novel concepts in the pathogenesis of emphysema and airspace enlargement.

Endothelial cells in emphysema development: a historical perspective

Until recently, the pathogenic schemes of emphysema development have not incorporated an active participation of the pulmonary endothelium. The prevailing concept for the alveolar destruction characteristic of anatomic emphysema invoked a protease–antiprotease imbalance in which an excess of proteases digest the parenchymal extracellular matrix connective tissue, altering alveolar architecture [20,21]. In this model, chronic exposure to cigarette smoke leads to invasion of inflammatory cells into airspaces with release of large quantities of proteases in excess of antiproteases, leading to tissue destruction and airspace enlargement. However, this current model of inflammation and excessive proteolysis does not fully explain why alveolar cells and wall structures are lost.

In the early 1950s, researchers studying other potential contributors to the pathogenesis of emphysema first appreciated a pruning of the arterial tree in pathologic specimens from patients with emphysema [22,23]. Noting a lack of vascularity in the lungs of patients with emphysema on pathology and the presence of enlarged, almost avascular alveoli, Liebow [23] postulated that alveolar thinning might be the result of a reduction in blood supply and put forth the first hypothesis of vascular atrophy as a model for emphysema. Research into the possible vascular contribution to the pathogenesis of emphysema remained dormant until recent findings that operate entirely outside of the concept of inflammatory alveolar destruction led to a major re-evaluation of the current conceptual framework of emphysema development.

Endothelium in airspace enlargement: role of endothelial growth factors

The prominent expression of VEGFR-2 on alveolar septal endothelial cells suggested to insightful investigators that airway epithelial cells may have a significant role in regulating the maintenance of vascular structure and function, as well as repair and remodelling of alveolar structures through VEGF expression [15,16]. VEGF acts as a potent survival factor for endothelial cells, inhibiting apoptosis both *in vitro* and *in vivo* [6–11]. A seminal paper by the Tuder and Voelkel laboratories contains the series of experiments that revisited the vascular atrophy model of emphysema using entirely novel approaches [24]. These scientists postulated that endothelial cell apoptosis, induced by antagonizing the survival signalling of VEGF, may produce decreased vascularity, induce alveolar cell apoptosis and result in the airspace enlargement characteristic of emphysema. Chronic *in vivo* blockade of VEGF receptors (with the pharmacologic specific VEGF receptor inhibitor SU5416) in rats for just 3 weeks produced alveolar wall cell death, airspace enlargement and pruning of the pulmonary vascular tree – all in the notable absence of inflammation or fibrosis (see Plate 27.1; colour plate section falls between pp. 354 and 355). Furthermore, the alveolar septal destruction caused by VEGF receptor blockade was the result of increased alveolar cell apoptosis and not of inhibited normal cellular proliferation. In these studies, the development of apoptosis preceded airspace enlargement and its inhibition with a caspase inhibitor prevented both alveolar cell apoptosis and the development of emphysematous airspace enlargement (see Plate 27.1; colour plate section falls between pp. 354 and 355). These landmark studies demonstrated that emphysema could be caused by a non-inflammatory insult and that chronic blockade of VEGF receptors causes lung endothelial cell apoptosis and the development of emphysema.

The remarkable findings of Tuder *et al.* have been confirmed in other experimental animal models. Gerber *et al.* [25] found that treatment of mice with a soluble VEGFR2 chimeric protein effectively neutralizes VEGF and results in airspace enlargement, while Tang *et al.* [26] found that lung-targeted ablation of VEGF in mice (using a Cre-Lox transfection strategy) resulted in decreased levels of both VEGF and VEGFR2 and concomitant alveolar septal destruction and loss of elastic recoil. Taken together, these studies suggest that VEGF signalling is required for the maintenance of alveolar structures, and that blockade of this important factor leads to disruption and endothelial cell death by apoptosis, and ultimately to parenchymal destruction and emphysema.

What relevance does this have for human emphysema? Following up on these animal studies, several groups have examined VEGF expression in patients with emphysema. Postulating that decreased expression of VEGF and/or VEGFR2 were involved in human emphysema, Kasahara *et al.* [27] compared lung tissue from patients with emphysema with tissue from healthy smoking and non-smoking controls, and found decreased expression of mRNA and protein of both VEGF and VEGFR2 in emphysematous lungs compared with either smoking or non-smoking controls. They also found a marked increase in apoptosis of both epithelial and endothelial alveolar septal cells in emphysematous lungs compared with controls (Fig. 27.2). Notably, as in the VEGF-blockade experimental rat

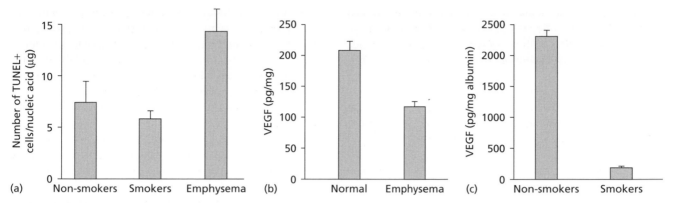

Figure 27.2 Apoptosis and vascular endothelial growth factor (VEGF) levels in non-smoking controls, healthy smokers and patients with emphysema. (a) Comparison of apoptotic cells (measured by terminal deoxynuclotidyltransferase-mediated UTP end labelling, TUNEL) in the alveolar septae of non-smokers, smokers and patients with emphysema. There are significantly more TUNEL+ cells in the emphysema lungs when compared with the lungs from non-smokers and healthy smokers. (b) Lung tissue VEGF. VEGF protein expression is significantly reduced in emphysema compared with controls. (c) Bronchoalveolar lavage fluid (BALF) VEGF in normal volunteers and healthy smokers. There is significantly less VEGF in the BALF from smokers compared with controls, even in the absence of emphysema. All data are expressed as mean ± SEM. (Modified from Kasahara *et al.* [24] and Koyama *et al.* [30].)

model, the increased apoptosis seen in emphysematous lungs was not accompanied by a significant increase in inflammation.

In a parallel study, investigators comparing VEGF levels, spirometry and gas transfer in patients with pulmonary disease (emphysema, asthma, chronic bronchitis and healthy controls) found decreased levels of VEGF in induced sputum from patients with emphysema compared with controls, in marked contrast to patients with asthma or chronic bronchitis in whom VEGF levels were actually increased [28,29]. Furthermore, the decrease in VEGF in patients with emphysema correlated with the severity of airflow obstruction (measured by forced expiratory volume in 1 s, FEV_1) and gas transfer defect (measured by DLCO). Further studies comparing VEGF levels in the bronchoalveolar lavage fluid (BALF) of patients with pulmonary disease and healthy controls noted a marked decrease in VEGF expression both in patients with pulmonary disease and in healthy smokers compared with healthy non-smokers [30]. In fact, while healthy non-smokers had robust expression of VEGF, there was a nearly 10-fold decrease in VEGF expression in smokers, even in the absence of known pulmonary disease, suggesting that the decrease in VEGF precedes the development of emphysema in smokers (see Fig. 27.2).

The presence of apoptotic alveolar septal cells in emphysema is emerging as a key finding in experimental models beyond the VEGFR blockade model, including *in vitro* studies and traditional elastase-induced animal models of emphysema [31,32]. In addition, follow-up human studies have confirmed the presence of apoptosis of both epithelial and endothelial cells in the alveolar septae of patients with emphysema, correlating the degree of apoptosis with the severity of disease [27,33–37]. Furthermore, studies comparing lung apoptosis rates among healthy controls, healthy smokers and emphysematous patients have shown an increase in lung cell apoptosis in chronic smokers preceding the development of clinical emphysema, with a further increase in apoptosis seen in smokers with overt emphysema [27,37].

To further explore the role of apoptosis in the pathogenesis of emphysema, Aoshiba *et al.* [38] performed a series of *in vivo* and *in vitro* experiments using active caspase-3, a direct apoptotic agent, and nodularin, a serine/threonine kinase inhibitor that induces caspase-dependent apoptosis. Although direct instillation of active caspase-3 had no effect, both instillation of nodularin and transfection of airspace epithelial cells with even a single dose of active caspase-3 caused alveolar cell apoptosis and airspace enlargement as early as 2 h after administration, with effects lasting up to 15 days, notably in the absence of inflammation or fibrosis. Using *in situ* elastin zymography, these investigators found an increase in elastolytic activity in the BALF of animals as early as 1 h after treatment that was localized to apoptotic epithelial cells. Both transfection of active caspase-3 and instillation of nodularin led to the loss of alveolar wall elastin as early as 6 h after treatment with a concomitant increase in soluble elastin products in BALF. These studies are the first to provide direct evidence that alveolar cell apoptosis, in the absence of inflammation, can trigger significant release of elastases sufficient to cause elastin destruction and emphysematous changes.

Cigarette smoke and the role of oxidative stress in endothelial dysfunction and emphysema development

However, how do we integrate these new findings in a disease that is overwhelmingly associated with cigarette smoking (Fig. 27.3)? Cigarette smoke contains more than 5000 chemical compounds and more than 10^{15} free radical molecules per puff. *In vivo*, chronic cigarette smoke causes dose-dependent increases in apoptosis of endothelial cells, bronchial and alveolar epithelial cells, and alveolar macrophages [39,40]. *In vitro*, smoke extract activates caspase-3 and induces apoptosis in cultured human umbilical and pulmonary endothelial cells as well as airway epithelial cells [41–43]. Cigarette smoke triggers apoptosis in cells through multiple pathways including direct oxidative stress, survival factor signalling, mitochondrial and nuclear DNA damage, and lymphocyte-dependent or TNF-receptor signalling. Long known to have a role in apoptosis and implicated in the development of emphysema, oxidative stress has a key role in normal cell maintenance [44]. As oxidants are known to not only cause cell damage and death, but to modulate the type of death: apoptotic versus necrotic, oxidative stress seems a likely participant in cigarette smoke-induced apoptosis and the subsequent development of emphysema. Already exposed to the highest oxygen environment of any organ in the body, the lungs of smokers are further exposed to cigarette smoke each puff of which exposes the lungs directly to,

in addition to oxidant molecules, many elements, including nicotine, which indirectly induce oxidative stress [44–48]. More recently, *in vivo* studies revealed evidence of oxidative stress, measured by markers of lipid peroxidation, including thiobarbituric acid-reactive substrates and 4-hydroxy-2-nonenal (4-HNE), in the lungs of smokers with emphysema, with levels inversely correlating with the severity of disease measured by FEV_1 [49,50]. In fact, markers of lipid peroxidation, DNA oxidation and protein oxidation have been shown to be increased in the BALF and lung tissue of smokers even in the absence of emphysema [50–54].

Using their original model, Tuder *et al.* postulated that oxidative stress was required for endothelial cell apoptosis and the development of emphysema with VEGFR blockade and demonstrated that a superoxide dismutase mimetic inhibited lung expression of markers of oxidative stress and blocked subsequent alveolar septal cell apoptosis and emphysematous changes induced by VEGFR blockade [24]. Caspase inhibition – already known to block apoptosis and emphysema in this model – also reduced lung expression of markers of oxidative stress, introducing the possibility that apoptosis itself contributes to the oxidative stress seen in these patients, creating a positive feedback loop in which oxidative stress causes apoptosis which in turn further increases the oxidative stress. The intricate link of cigarette smoke-induced oxidative stress and endothelial cell apoptosis is clearly emphasized in studies of mice in which enhanced susceptibility to oxidative stress by genetic deletion of Nrf2, a transcription factor that regulates

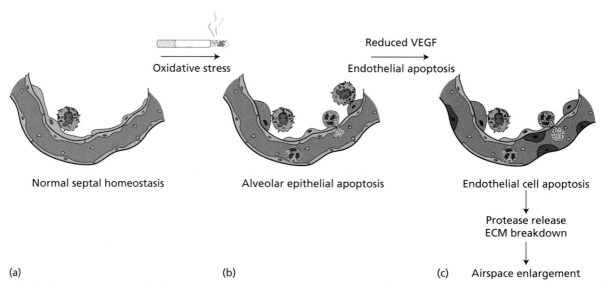

Figure 27.3 Cigarette smoke, oxidative stress and apoptosis in the pathogenesis of COPD. Oxidative stress from cigarette smoke leads to alveolar epithelial cell apoptosis and decreased vascular endothelial growth factor (VEGF) expression. This in turn induces alveolar septal endothelial cell apoptosis with release of proteases, destruction of the extracellular matrix (ECM) and eventual loss of the alveolar unit.

antioxidant enzymes, increases the risk of cigarette smoke-induced apoptosis and emphysema [55].

Direct oxidative stress does not represent the sole link between cigarette smoke and apoptosis. Cigarette smoke also down-regulates expression of the VEGF receptor, reduces VEGF expression by epithelial cells and endothelial cells, and inhibits the VEGF-dependent survival of endothelial cells in culture [56,57]. The induction of mitochondrial and DNA damage by cigarette smoke exposure also induces apoptosis of epithelial and endothelial alveolar cells. Finally, cigarette smoke evokes alveolar inflammation with the release of cytokines such as tumour necrosis factor α (TNF-α), interleukin 1B (IL-1B), IL-8, leukotriene B_4 (LTB$_4$) and transforming growth factor β (TGF-β), which have been shown to contribute to elastolytic damage in pulmonary emphysema [58].

These developments in the understanding of the mechanisms of lung destruction in emphysema highlight the presence of positive feedback mechanisms engaging apoptosis, oxidative stress and matrix proteolysis, which together with inflammatory mediators overwhelm the defense or maintenance mechanisms of endothelial alveolar cells [59]. Ongoing studies are identifying potentially critical mediators that link and amplify these destructive processes, and may emerge as key targets of therapeutic interventions in emphysema. A potentially central relay of endothelial cell apoptosis linked to inflammatory mediator signalling (TNF-α) and oxidative stress generation is ceramide, a signalling sphingolipid and known mediator of apoptosis and tissue injury in different organs which has been shown to mediate VEGF receptor blockade-induced emphysema and oxidative stress in both mice and rats [60,61].

Conclusions

Despite a notable hiatus from being considered as an effector or target in the pathogenesis of chronic airflow obstruction, the pulmonary endothelium has now assumed a potentially major role in the development of emphysema. Current models of apoptosis-induced emphysema are notable for lack of inflammation – a mainstay of the current protease–antiprotease theory of emphysema. These findings do not necessarily directly refute the importance of the protease–antiprotease imbalance in emphysema, but instead offer an alternative paradigm in which chronic cigarette smoke causes oxidative stress and alveolar epithelial cell apoptosis, which in turn disrupts the normal VEGF-dependent maintenance of alveolar capillary endothelial cell health. These recent studies do imply, however, that alveolar apoptosis, in addition to inflammation, constitutes a primary event leading to the release of elastolytic enzymes and alveolar wall destruction. The endothelium-dependent models of emphysema have provided us with a new conceptual framework in which to study the links between inflammation, protease–antiprotease imbalance, oxidative stress and alveolar septal cell destruction. The finding of decreased VEGF levels in smokers, both with and without emphysema, is particularly interesting as a variety of stimuli (chronic hypoxia, TNF-α, IL-1β, neutrophil elastase) stimulate VEGF expression and secretion by epithelial cells [16,30], resulting in an expected preservation or increase in VEGF expression in smokers. The fact that decreased VEGF levels in healthy smokers precedes the development of apoptosis and airspace enlargement suggests that a breakdown in the normal maintenance of alveolar vascular structures may be a key step in the development of COPD. Future research will explore the roles of VEGF, apoptosis and oxidative stress in human emphysema and likely identify novel endothelial cell targets for the prevention or treatment of this devastating disease.

References

1 Garcia JGN, Malik AB. The pulmonary circulation and lung fluid exchange. In: Murray JF and Nadel JA. *Textbook of Respiratory Medicine*, 3rd edn. Philadelphia: Saunders, 2000.

2 Dudek SM, Garcia JG. Cytoskeletal regulation of pulmonary vascular permeability. *J Appl Physiol* 2001;**91**:1487–500.

3 Birukov KG, Csortos C, Marzilli L *et al.* Differential regulation of alternatively spliced endothelial cell myosin light chain kinase isoforms by p60(Src). *J Biol Chem* 2001;**276**:8567–73.

4 Birukov KG, Leitinger N, Bochkov VN, Garcia JG. Signal transduction pathways activated in human pulmonary endothelial cells by OxPAPC, a bioactive component of oxidized lipoproteins. *Microvasc Res* 2004;**67**:18–28.

5 Jakkula M, Le Cras TD, Gebb S *et al.* Inhibition of angiogenesis decreases alveolarization in the developing rat lung. *Am J Physiol Lung Cell Mol Physiol* 2000;**279**:L600–7.

6 Alon T, Hemo I, Itin A *et al.* Vascular endothelial growth factor acts as a survival factor for newly formed retinal vessels and has implications for retinopathy of prematurity. *Nat Med* 1995;**1**:1024–8.

7 Ferrara N, Gerber HP, LeCouter J. The biology of VEGF and its receptors. *Nat Med* 2003;**9**:669–76.

8 Yuan F, Chen Y, Dellian M *et al.* Time-dependent vascular regression and permeability changes in established human tumor xenografts induced by an anti-vascular endothelial growth factor/vascular permeability factor antibody. *Proc Natl Acad Sci U S A* 1996;**93**:14765–70.

9 Gerber HP, McMurtey A, Kowalski J *et al.* Vascular endothelial growth factor regulates endothelial cell survival through the phosphatidylinositol 3'-kinase/Akt signal transduction pathway: requirement for Flk-1/KDR activation. *J Biol Chem* 1998;**273**:30336–43.

10 Gerber HP, Dixit V, Ferrara N. Vascular endothelial growth factor induces expression of the antiapoptotic proteins Bcl-2

and A1 in vascular endothelial cells. *J Biol Chem* 1998;**273**: 13313–6.

11 Benjamin LE, Golijanin D, Itin A, Pode D, Keshet E. Selective ablation of immature blood vessels in established human tumors follows vascular endothelial growth factor withdrawal. *J Clin Invest* 1999;**103**:159–65.

12 Monacci WT, Merrill MJ, Oldfield EH. Expression of vascular permeability factor/vascular endothelial growth factor in normal rat tissues. *Am J Physiol* 1993;**264**:C995–1002.

13 Berse B, Brown LF, Van de Water L, Dvorak HF, Senger DR. Vascular permeability factor (vascular endothelial growth factor) gene is expressed differentially in normal tissues, macrophages, and tumors. *Mol Biol Cell* 1992;**3**:211–20.

14 Claffey KP, Wilkison WO, Spiegelman BM. Vascular endothelial growth factor: regulation by cell differentiation and activated second messenger pathways. *J Biol Chem* 1992;**267**: 16317–22.

15 Tuder RM, Flook B, Voelkel NF. Increased gene expression for VEGF and the VEGF receptors KDR/Flk and Flt in lungs exposed to acute or to chronic hypoxia: modulation of gene expression by nitric oxide. *J Clin Invest* 1995;**95**: 1798–807.

16 Koyama S, Sato E, Tsukadaira A *et al.* Vascular endothelial growth factor mRNA and protein expression in airway epithelial cell lines *in vitro*. *Eur Respir J* 2002;**20**:1449–56.

17 Taraseviciene-Stewart L, Kasahara Y, Alger L *et al.* Inhibition of the VEGF receptor 2 combined with chronic hypoxia causes cell death-dependent pulmonary endothelial cell proliferation and severe pulmonary hypertension. *FASEB J* 2001;**15**:427–38.

18 Shaheen RM, Davis D, Liu W *et al.* Antiangiogenic therapy targeting the tyrosine kinase receptor for vascular endothelial growth factor receptor inhibits the growth of colon cancer liver metastasis and induces tumor and endothelial cell apoptosis. *Cancer Res* 1999;**59**:5412–6.

19 Maeda S, Kanematsu M, Kondo H *et al.* Analysis of intrapulmonary vessels and epithelial–endothelial interactions in the human developing lung. *Lab Invest* 2002;**82**:293–301.

20 Laurell CB, Eriksson S. The serum alpha-l-antitrypsin in families with hypo-alpha-l-antitrypsinemia. *Clin Chim Acta* 1965;**11**:395–8.

21 Gross P, Pfitzer EA, Tolker E, Babyak MA, Kaschak M. Experimental emphysema: its production with papain in normal and silicotic rats. *Arch Environ Health* 1965;**11**:50–8.

22 Cudkowicz L, Armstrong JB. The bronchial arteries in pulmonary emphysema. *Thorax* 1953;**8**:46–58.

23 Liebow A. The bronchopulmonary venous collateral circulation with special reference to emphysema. *Am J Pathol* 1953; **29**:251–89.

24 Kasahara Y, Tuder RM, Taraseviciene-Stewart L *et al.* Inhibition of VEGF receptors causes lung cell apoptosis and emphysema. *J Clin Invest* 2000;**106**:1311–9.

25 Gerber HP, Hillan KJ, Ryan AM *et al.* VEGF is required for growth and survival in neonatal mice. *Development* 1999;**126**: 1149–59.

26 Tang K, Rossiter HB, Wagner PD, Breen EC. Lung-targeted VEGF inactivation leads to an emphysema phenotype in mice. *J Appl Physiol* 2004;**97**:1559–66; discussion 1549.

27 Kasahara Y, Tuder RM, Cool CD *et al.* Endothelial cell death and decreased expression of vascular endothelial growth factor and vascular endothelial growth factor receptor 2 in emphysema. *Am J Respir Crit Care Med* 2001;**163**:737–44.

28 Kanazawa H, Asai K, Hirata K, Yoshikawa J. Possible effects of vascular endothelial growth factor in the pathogenesis of chronic obstructive pulmonary disease. *Am J Med* 2003; **114**:354–8.

29 Kanazawa H, Hirata K, Yoshikawa J. Imbalance between vascular endothelial growth factor and endostatin in emphysema. *Eur Respir J* 2003;**22**:609–12.

30 Koyama S, Sato E, Haniuda M *et al.* Decreased level of vascular endothelial growth factor in bronchoalveolar lavage fluid of normal smokers and patients with pulmonary fibrosis. *Am J Respir Crit Care Med* 2002;**166**:382–5.

31 Lucey EC, Keane J, Kuang PP, Snider GL, Goldstein RH. Severity of elastase-induced emphysema is decreased in tumor necrosis factor-alpha and interleukin-1beta receptor-deficient mice. *Lab Invest* 2002;**82**:79–85.

32 Nakajoh M, Fukushima T, Suzuki T *et al.* Retinoic acid inhibits elastase-induced injury in human lung epithelial cell lines. *Am J Respir Cell Mol Biol* 2003;**28**:296–304.

33 Majo J, Ghezzo H, Cosio MG. Lymphocyte population and apoptosis in the lungs of smokers and their relation to emphysema. *Eur Respir J* 2001;**1**:946–53.

34 Segura-Valdez L, Pardo A, Gaxiola M *et al.* Upregulation of gelatinases A and B, collagenases 1 and 2, and increased parenchymal cell death in COPD. *Chest* 2000;**117**:684–94.

35 Imai K, D'Armiento J. Differential gene expression of sFRP-1 and apoptosis in pulmonary emphysema. *Chest* 2002;**121** (3 Suppl):7S.

36 Kasahara Y, Tuder RM, Cool CD, Voelkel NF. Expression of 15-lipoxygenase and evidence for apoptosis in the lungs from patients with COPD. *Chest* 2000;**117**(5 Suppl 1):260S.

37 Yokohori N, Aoshiba K, Nagai A. Increased levels of cell death and proliferation in alveolar wall cells in patients with pulmonary emphysema. *Chest* 2004;**125**:626–32.

38 Aoshiba K, Yokohori N, Nagai A. Alveolar wall apoptosis causes lung destruction and emphysematous changes. *Am J Respir Cell Mol Biol* 2003;**28**:555–62.

39 Jung M, Davis WP, Taatjes DJ, Churg A, Mossman BT. Asbestos and cigarette smoke cause increased DNA strand breaks and necrosis in bronchiolar epithelial cells *in vivo*. *Free Radic Biol Med* 2000;**28**:1295–9.

40 Aoshiba K, Tamaoki J, Nagai A. Acute cigarette smoke exposure induces apoptosis of alveolar macrophages. *Am J Physiol Lung Cell Mol Physiol* 2001;**281**:L1392–401.

41 Wang J, Wilcken DE, Wang XL. Cigarette smoke activates caspase-3 to induce apoptosis of human umbilical venous endothelial cells. *Mol Genet Metab* 2001;**72**:82–8.

42 Tuder RM, Wood K, Taraseviciene L, Flores SC, Voelkel NF. Cigarette smoke extract decreases the expression of vascular endothelial growth factor by cultured cells and triggers apoptosis of pulmonary endothelial cells. *Chest* 2000;**117** (5 Suppl 1):241S–2S.

43 Hoshino Y, Mio T, Nagai S *et al.* Cytotoxic effects of cigarette smoke extract on an alveolar type II cell-derived cell line. *Am J Physiol Lung Cell Mol Physiol* 2001;**281**:L509–16.

44 Crowley-Weber CL, Dvorakova K, Crowley C *et al*. Nicotine increases oxidative stress, activates NF-κB and GRP78, induces apoptosis and sensitizes cells to genotoxic/xenobiotic stresses by a multiple stress inducer, deoxycholate: relevance to colon carcinogenesis. *Chem Biol Interact* 2003;**145**:53–66.

45 Tuder RM, Zhen L, Cho CY *et al*. Oxidative stress and apoptosis interact and cause emphysema due to vascular endothelial growth factor receptor blockade. *Am J Respir Cell Mol Biol* 2003;**29**:88–97.

46 Macnee W, Rahman I. Oxidants and antioxidants as therapeutic targets in chronic obstructive pulmonary disease. *Am J Respir Crit Care Med* 1999;**160**(5 Pt 2):S58–65.

47 Noronha-Dutra AA, Epperlein MM, Woolf N. Effect of cigarette smoking on cultured human endothelial cells. *Cardiovasc Res* 1993;**27**:774–8.

48 van der Vaart H, Postma DS, Timens W, ten Hacken NH. Acute effects of cigarette smoke on inflammation and oxidative stress: a review. *Thorax* 2004;**59**:713–21.

49 Rahman I, van Schadewijk AA, Crowther AJ *et al*. 4-Hydroxy-2-nonenal, a specific lipid peroxidation product, is elevated in lungs of patients with chronic obstructive pulmonary disease. *Am J Respir Crit Care Med* 2002;**166**:490–5.

50 Repine JE, Bast A, Lankhorst I. Oxidative stress in chronic obstructive pulmonary disease. Oxidative Stress Study Group. *Am J Respir Crit Care Med* 1997;**156**(2 Pt 1):341–57.

51 Rahman I, MacNee W. Lung glutathione and oxidative stress: implications in cigarette smoke-induced airway disease. *Am J Physiol* 1999;**277**(6 Pt 1):L1067–88.

52 Nadiger HA, Mathew CA, Sadasivudu B. Serum malanodialdehyde (TBA reactive substance) levels in cigarette smokers. *Atherosclerosis* 1987;**64**:71–3.

53 Morrison D, Rahman I, Lannan S, MacNee W. Epithelial permeability, inflammation, and oxidant stress in the air spaces of smokers. *Am J Respir Crit Care Med* 1999;**159**:473–9.

54 Asami S, Manabe H, Miyake J *et al*. Cigarette smoking induces an increase in oxidative DNA damage, 8-hydroxydeoxyguanosine, in a central site of the human lung. *Carcinogenesis* 1997;**18**:1763–6.

55 Rangasamy T, Cho CY, Thimmulappa RK *et al*. Genetic ablation of Nrf2 enhances susceptibility to cigarette smoke-induced emphysema in mice. *J Clin Invest* 2004;**114**:1248–59.

56 Michaud SE, Menard C, Guy LG, Gennaro G, Rivard A. Inhibition of hypoxia-induced angiogenesis by cigarette smoke exposure: impairment of the HIF-1alpha/VEGF pathway. *FASEB J* 2003;**17**:1150–2.

57 Belgore FM, Lip GY, Blann AD. Vascular endothelial growth factor and its receptor, Flt-1, in smokers and non-smokers. *Br J Biomed Sci* 2000;**57**:207–13.

58 Moodie FM, Marwick JA, Anderson CS *et al*. Oxidative stress and cigarette smoke alter chromatin remodeling but differentially regulate NF-κB activation and proinflammatory cytokine release in alveolar epithelial cells. *FASEB J* 2004;**18**:1897–9.

59 Tuder RM, Petrache I, Elias JA, Voelkel NF, Henson PM. Apoptosis and emphysema: the missing link. *Am J Respir Cell Mol Biol* 2003;**28**:551–4.

60 Petrache I, Natarajan V, Zhen L, Medler TR, Tuder RM. Ceramide upregulation is necessary for the development of rat emphysema induced by inhibition of the vascular endothelial growth factor receptors (VEGF-R). *Am J Respir Crit Care Med* 2004;**169**:A831.

61 Petrache I, Zhen L, Medler TR, Tuder RM. Intra-tracheal instillation of ceramide causes alveolar cell apoptosis and murine emphysema. *Am J Respir Crit Care Med* 2004;**169**:A206.

CHAPTER 28
Mesenchymal cells of the lung

Stephen I. Rennard and J. Graham Sharp

Mesenchymal cells are a diverse class of highly specialized cells that produce and remodel extracellular matrix, modulate tissue development and epithelial differentiation, and regulate inflammatory responses. Mesenchymal cells have key roles both in normal tissue function and in the pathophysiology of many diseases including chronic obstructive pulmonary disease (COPD). Unfortunately, understanding of mesenchymal cell classification and ontogeny is incomplete. This stems in part from the lack of unique biochemical and histological markers for specific mesenchymal cells, and in part from the structural and functional plasticity of these cells. In addition, mesenchymal cells can be readily cultured *in vitro*. This has resulted in a rich investigative literature. However, because the *in vitro* culture of mesenchymal cells alters cellular phenotype, the *in vivo* significance of *in vitro* studies is not always readily apparent. Nevertheless, it is becoming clear that mesenchymal cells contribute to the pathogenesis of COPD, are attractive targets for future therapeutic interventions and may be vehicles to mediate novel therapeutic strategies such as gene-based treatments. This chapter provides an overview of mesenchymal cells, particularly as they relate to COPD. For a more comprehensive review of COPD pathophysiology, see Section 4.

Origins of mesenchymal cells

All complex multicellular organisms contain sheets of epithelial cells [1]. These cells adhere to each other through several types of junctions and rest on a specialized extracellular matrix, the basement membrane. Epithelial cells often demonstrate marked structural and functional polarity, with marked differences between the apical and the basal portions of cells. The simplest of multicellular organisms consist of a single layer of epithelial cells. More complex organisms generate multiple epithelial layers by differentiation, indentation and folding of the epithelial surface. By this mechanism, the outer epithelial layer (ectoderm) and an inner epithelial layer (endoderm) are generated. By further folding, intermediate layers of epithelial cells (mesoderm) can also be generated. Mesenchymal cells arise by a different mechanism. (See Hay [1] for a detailed discussion of the origin of mesenchymal cells in embryology.)

In the formation of mesenchymal cells, epithelial cells undergo a pronounced morphological and functional shift, the epithelial–mesenchymal transition (EMT) [1,2]. In this process, cells detach from their neighbours, assume an elongated shape, separate from and invade the subjacent basement membrane and migrate through the connective tissue beneath the epithelium. In complex organisms, therefore, mesenchymal cells are present in the mesoderm. However, 'mesodermal' and 'mesenchymal' are not synonymous. Mesodermal structures, for example, can include epithelia. Conversely, some mesodermal organisms, such as the protochordate Amphioxus, lack mesenchyme. Characteristically, these organisms remain small and are structurally simple. Mesenchymal cells are key to the development of structural complexity. Specifically, mesenchymal cells migrate through the mesoderm, condense and differentiate into the cartilage and bone required to form the vertebral column. By an analogous process of migration, condensation and differentiation, mesenchymal cells contribute to the formation of somites, the extremities and parenchymal organs. A large number of differentiated mesenchymal cell types result from these processes.

The molecular events that control the EMT process are incompletely delineated. However, a key feature of epithelial cells is the expression of the adhesion molecule E-cadherin [3]. This molecule participates in the organization of the adherens junctions that characterize epithelia. It also binds and segregates free β-catenin [1]. If present, free β-catenin can bind to and activate the transcription factor LEF-1 which activates genes causing epithelial cells to lose epithelial features and acquire a mesenchymal phenotype.

Interestingly, in epithelial cells transfected with a LEF-1 expressing adenoviral vector, which induces EMT, this process is reversible with loss of the lymphocyte effector function-1 (LEF-1) activity, suggesting plasticity between epithelial and mesenchymal cells [4]. A variety of other factors including transforming growth factor β (TGF-β), Wnt, Hedgehog and Notch can also modulate EMT, possibly via their interaction with β-catenin and modulation of LEF-1 activity.

Mesenchymal cells express a number of characteristic genes including vimentin, several forms of actin and produce fibronectin. However, none of these are specific for mesenchymal cells. A consensus conference therefore, has suggested a definition of a mesenchymal cell (in the context of the EMT) that includes:

1 front–back end polarity;
2 elongate morphology;
3 filopodia; and
4 invasive motility (reviewed by Hay [1]).

As pointed out in the same review, a frequently used definition of myofibroblasts, the presence of stress fibres, is not appropriate because stress fibres are often an artefact that results from *in vitro* adhesion of mesenchymal cells to rigid substrates [1]. The difficulties with this definition is confounded by artefacts generated by *in vitro* studies recapitulated in attempts to define subsets of mesenchymal cells, particularly fibroblasts and myofibroblasts, cells likely to have important roles in COPD pathogenesis (see below). The lack of definitive biochemical and histochemical markers has also confounded studies of mesenchymal cell ontogeny.

All mesenchymal cells originate from primitive epithelia. However, it is likely that there are specific populations of mesenchymal cell stem precursors/stem cells that maintain mesenchymal cell populations. In this context, a stem cell is a cell that has the capability of dividing to maintain its own population (i.e. self-renewal) and of forming at least one type of differentiated cell. If a stem cell can give rise to several cell types it is pluripotent. If it can give rise to all cell types including whole organisms (i.e. it has all the capability of a fertilized egg) it is totipotent. For a variety of reasons, mesenchymal stem cells (MSCs) have attracted much recent interest [5].

MSCs have been isolated and defined based on *in vitro* characteristics [5]. For example, when bone marrow cells are isolated and plated on a rigid surface, a subpopulation of cells will adhere and proliferate to form colonies of spindle-shaped fibroblast-like cells. When subcultured under various specific conditions, these cells can differentiate into a number of lineages. The cells present in the original marrow isolate that formed the original colonies have been defined as MSCs. Unfortunately, no unique markers have been established that specifically identify MSCs, although they characteristically express the surface markers STRO-1,

SH2, SH3 and SH4 and lack the haematopoietic markers CD45, CD34 and CD14. It is likely, moreover, that MSCs are heterogeneous. In this context, a number of methods have been developed to isolate and culture MSCs. These have resulted in varied results together with a number of sometimes confusing names [5–7]. It seems quite likely that the differences among studies are in part caused by isolation of subpopulations of cells from within the MSC population [8].

MSCs have been reported to lack telomerase and to have a considerable, but limited, potential for self-renewal. However, subpopulations of cells from the MSC population have been reported to undergo more extensive population doublings [7]. Similarly, the addition of specific growth factors (e.g. fibroblast growth factor 2 (FGF2)) can result in extended population doublings [9], consistent with the selective expansion of a subpopulation of cells from within the MSC population.

MSCs have the potential to differentiate into a number of cell types. This includes a variety of mesenchymal cell types: cartilage, bone, adipocytes, smooth muscle, cardiac muscle [10], skeletal muscle [11] and stromal cells [5]. In addition, MSCs have been reported to give rise to neural cells [12] and epithelial cells [13]. On the other hand, isolated clones of MSCs have been reported to have limited potential for differentiation. Thus, some clones can give rise chondrocytes, bone cells and adipocytes, while other clones can give rise to only two types or one type of cell, supporting the concept of heterogeneity in the MSC population [5]. These findings are also consistent with a model in which MSC 'differentiation' is accompanied by a progressive restriction in self-renewal and differentiation potential. However, Song and Tuan [14] have reported that differentiated cells derived from MSCs can be induced to dedifferentiate, replicate and subsequently redifferentiate into other types of cells. This 'trans-differentiation' suggests considerable plasticity exists within mesenchymal cell populations.

In addition to bone marrow, cells with the functional characteristics of MSCs have been isolated from many other tissues [5]. However, neither the *in vivo* role of MSCs, nor even their location within tissues has been defined. Nevertheless, it is clear that populations of cells are present within many tissues that have considerable potential for proliferation and differentiation. Interestingly, circulating pools of stem/precursor cells are also present. A population of circulating mononuclear cells that express collagen type I and can form fibroblast-like cells, termed fibrocytes, has been suggested to be a precursor for mesenchymal cells and to participate in wound healing [15]. These cells have been suggested to contribute to myofibroblast populations in the airway in asthma [16], to the development of pulmonary fibrosis [17] and may contribute to vascular remodelling in pulmonary hypertension [18].

At the present time, the precursor–progeny relationship among the various mesenchymal cell populations in the lung remains undefined. Similarly, it is unclear what the roles of the various potential precursor/stem cell populations are *in vivo*. However, as methods for tracking cell lineages advance, and as methods for identifying differentiated cell populations improve, enhanced understanding of mesenchymal cell lineages and of the molecular events that control differentiation and proliferation of specific cell types can be anticipated.

Cell types

Chondrocytes

Chondrocytes are present in the bronchial cartilages where they produce the collagenous and proteoglycan components of cartilage [19]. Like other cartilage, it is likely that airway cartilage responds to mechanical stimuli [20,21], a feature that is characteristic of other mesenchymal cells (see below). Abnormalities in bronchial cartilage are present in airway disease. Degeneration of bronchial cartilage occurs in COPD, particularly when chronic bronchitis is present, and in asthma [22,23]. Perichondrial fibrosis and neutrophilic inflammation are often associated with this degeneration. Interestingly, evidence of chondrocyte activation is also often present, suggesting that chondrocytes may contribute to cartilage degeneration, perhaps by producing MMPs. Functional alterations in airway cartilage may contribute to abnormalities in the trachea and large airways, such as collapse during cough or forced exhalations and to the structural alterations present in 'saber sheath trachea' [24].

Smooth muscle cells

In the lung, smooth muscle cells (SMC) are present in the airways, and in the arterial, venous and lymphatic vessels. SMC are elongated, surrounded by a basement membrane and are connected to each other by gap junctions. They characteristically contain desmin, smooth muscle myosin and α-smooth muscle actin (α-SMA) [25]. Because these markers may also be present in myofibroblasts, they are not specific markers for SMCs. Smoothelin, however, is a cytoskeletal protein that may be specific for SMCs [26]. Because SMCs can reversibly contract in response to a number of stimuli, they are crucial in regulating the luminal diameter of the vessels they surround.

SMCs from different sites vary in important ways; for example, in their response to contractile and relaxant stimuli and in their response to growth factors. Qualitative and quantitative alterations in SMCs have key roles in many lung diseases including asthma [27], pulmonary hypertension [28,29] and lymphangioleiomyomatosis [30]. It is likely that alterations in airway and vascular smooth muscle also contribute to the pathogenesis of COPD. Recognition of the role of the *TSC2* gene in lymphangioleiomyomatosis [31] and of the bone morphogenic protein receptor 2 gene in primary pulmonary hypertension [32] has not only aided understanding of these diseases, but promises to clarify the mechanisms that control SMC biology in general.

Pericytes

Pericytes are smooth muscle like cells that partially surround the endothelial cells of small vessels. They are present in the lung in postcapillary venules and in alveolar capillaries. They are surrounded by a basement membrane that fuses with that of the vascular endothelial cell. Pericytes, which express α-SMA and are assumed to be contractile, have been suggested to regulate alveolar capillary blood flow [25]. Mice deficient in platelet derived growth factor-B (PDGF-B) fail to develop pericytes and develop microaneurysms, suggesting a role for pericytes in maintenance of microvascular structure [33]. MSCs from bone marrow appear to be closely related to pericytes [34].

Fibroblasts and myofibroblasts

Fibroblasts and myofibroblasts are spindle-shaped interstitial cells that are believed to be the major cells responsible for the synthesis and organization of structural extracellular matrix macromolecules, including collagen and elastin [25,35]. These two types of cells are themselves heterogeneous. For example, the dense collagen bundles present in tendon are believed to be synthesized and organized by highly specialized fibroblasts [36,37]. Similarly, the loose but highly organized extracellular matrix of organs such as the lung is believed to be synthesized primarily by local fibroblasts [38]. The observation that fibroblasts cultured from different tissues are functionally distinct supports the concept that fibroblasts in different tissues represent committed populations of distinct differentiated cells [39–42]. Even within a tissue, it is likely that myofibroblasts and fibroblasts at different sites can be functionally different. In the gut, for example, two morphologically distinct types of myofibroblasts are present [43,44]. These cells differ in their responses to cytokines and in their ability to induce responses in gut epithelial cells.

Myofibroblasts are distinguished from fibroblasts in having more highly developed cytoskeletal structures together with gap junctions [25,35]. This suggests coordinated contractile function for myofibroblasts, making them a cell intermediate between a fibroblast and an SMC. The most commonly used feature to characterize myofibroblasts is the presence of α-SMA. However, expression of α-SMA is not a universal feature of myofibroblasts. A more characteristic feature that can distinguish myofibroblasts from fibroblasts is the presence of stress fibres. These are intracellular bundles of actin together with other contractile proteins. They insert into the cell membrane at the fibronexus, a specialized structure that links the intracellular fibre bundle with cell surface integrins and through this structure with extracellular matrix fibres. The fibronexus can mediate both outside-in and inside-out signalling. Thus, the fibronexus is believed to provide a means for the cell to exert mechanical force on the components of the surrounding matrix and to respond to external mechanical stress. While fibroblasts may express stress fibres when cultured *in vitro*, this is believed to be an artefact of the culture conditions [1,35]. *In vivo*, fibroblasts are thought to lack well-defined stress fibres. Myofibroblasts, in contrast, contain stress fibres. Consistent with this, they respond to mechanical loading and are thought to generate tension within tissue.

The distinction between fibroblasts and myofibroblasts is complicated by the fact that a large and rapidly expanding group of mediators can induce α-SMA expression in fibroblasts. This has often been used as a demonstration of myofibroblast differentiation from fibroblasts. TGF-β, for example, is a particularly effective inducer of this phenotype in fibroblasts [45]. Together with the acquisition of α-SMA expression, TGF-β induces fibroblasts to produce more collagen and fibronectin and to more vigorously contract three-dimensional collagen gels. After removal of the TGF-β, however, the original functional phenotype is gradually restored [46]. Thus, is it unclear if TGF-β induces a 'differentiation' of fibroblasts or causes a change in functional status.

TGF-β induction of α-SMA and collagen type I expression in fibroblasts, but not of plasminogen activator-1 expression, is dependent on extracellular fibronectin containing the ED-A splice variant [47]. This is also induced by TGF-β, but indicates that the differentiation (or functional regulation) of fibroblasts into myofibroblasts requires a set of signals that include specific signals from the extracellular matrix. In contrast, α-SMA expression by rat myofibroblasts does not depend on CaRG elements [48], unlike murine smooth muscle cells where these elements are required [49]. Although species differences may account for this difference, the results are also consistent with distinct regulatory pathways acting to control similar phenotypes in different populations of mesenchymal cells and therefore support the functional heterogeneity of these cells.

Fibroblasts and myofibroblasts also have key roles in embryologic development and in the regulation of other cells within tissues. The development of many-branched parenchymal organs, including the lung, liver, pancreas, salivary gland and kidney, depends on interactions between the epithelial cells and the subjacent mesenchymal cells (epithelial–mesenchymal interactions) [50–54]. In addition, in the lung, a specialized population of lipid-containing fibroblasts has been described that has been suggested to play a key part in alveolar wall formation [55]. The signals that provide specificity for the site and structure of these organs during embryogenesis are, in large part, a function of the mesenchymal cells. Mesenchymal stromal cells also have a critical role in the maintenance of haematopoietic stem cells [56–58] and mesenchymal cell derived niches are likely important in supporting other stem/progenitor cells as well [59–63]. In the crypt of the small intestine, for example, bone marrow derived subepithelial fibroblasts have been shown to have a regulatory role over epithelial stem cells [64,65]. Whether fibroblasts or myofibroblasts provide similar regulatory functions in the stem cell niches present in the lung remains to be defined.

The ability of fibroblasts and myofibroblasts to provide regulatory functions likely extends beyond the role in development and in maintaining stem cell niches. These cells are active producers of inflammatory mediators, as are SMC [66]. It is likely, therefore, that mesenchymal cells play an active part in driving inflammatory processes in the lung and in modulating their resolution.

Alveolar myofibroblasts are specialized cells that differ from many other myofibroblasts in lacking α-SMA [1,35]. Alveolar myofibroblasts are relatively numerous, with up to 20 surrounding an alveolus. The nuclei are generally located at the junction of three alveolar septa into which the cell extends processes. Alveolar myofibroblasts are distinguished from pericytes by lack of a basement membrane and lack of α-SMA expression. However, like other myofibroblasts, they have gap junctions and stress fibres and are believed to account for the contractility of excised lung parenchyma. It has been suggested that the alveolar myofibroblasts, by virtue of their contractile function, have an important role in normal lung physiology [25]. Specifically, the contraction of these cells can be modified by a variety of factors including hypoxia [67], supporting a role in ventilation–perfusion matching. A role for these cells in the altered physiology of COPD, particularly altered lung volumes, is appealing.

Myofibroblasts are also thought to have key roles in the pathophysiology of several lung diseases. The cells that accumulate in fibroblastic foci and adjacent areas of fibrosis in idiopathic pulmonary fibrosis (IPF) are α-SMA positive myofibroblasts [68,69]. Similar cells are present in Masson bodies at sites of fibrosis in bronchiolitis obliterans [68] and are present in animal models of fibrosis induced by bleomycin [70]. Myofibroblasts are increased in the airway wall in asthma [71], where the number of myofibroblasts is related to the thickness of the basal lamina [72], consistent with a role in airway wall remodelling. These disease-related myofibroblasts could potentially be derived locally, for example from TGF-β induced differentiation of resident fibroblasts. Alternatively, cells with the features of circulating fibrocytes have been described in the airway wall in asthma, suggesting a role for circulating precursors [16]. A circulating source has been suggested for the myofibroblasts present in the pulmonary parenchyma in lung fibrosis [17,73]. Similarly, a circulating source has been suggested to contribute to the remodelling that occurs in pulmonary vascular disease [18]. These studies have used different species and different experimental models and the phenotype of the circulating mesenchymal cell precursors has shown some differences. Whether these represent true heterogeneity or reflects species differences remains to be determined.

A role for myofibroblasts in the peribronchial fibrosis that characterizes many patients with COPD is appealing [74,75]. However, the precise origin and functional contribution of these cells to COPD pathogenesis remains to be determined. Experimental evidence suggests alveolar myofibroblasts, or rather their lack, can contribute to the development of emphysema. Mice that are deficient for PDGF-A fail to develop alveolar myofibroblasts and also develop emphysema, likely because of failed development of alveolar wall [76]. Whether a similar process contributes to human emphysema is not defined.

Altered populations of cells versus altered functional states

A major unanswered question is to what degree the alterations in mesenchymal cells present in COPD represent changes in populations of differentiated cells or changes in the functional state of cells in response to the cytokines and mediators present in the local milieu. This is an important issue, as the two different models should lead to different therapeutic approaches. While the latter would suggest pharmacotherapy to block specific mediator pathways, the former would require treatments that would alter structural cell populations.

Fibroblasts from different tissues are functionally distinct. These differences are preserved during extended *in vitro* cultures, suggesting they represent a true differentiated commitment rather than a response to a local mediator. This supports the concept of distinct populations of mesenchymal cells. Similarly, cells cultured from the lungs of patients with IPF show a persistently abnormal phenotype, including altered growth characteristics, increased expression of α-SMA, increased production of TGF-β1, increased

contractility and reduced production of prostaglandin E_2 (PGE_2) [77,78]. The persistence of similar abnormalities in culture is also observed in fibroblasts cultured from other fibrotic tissues [79–81] and in animal models of lung fibrosis [82,83]. These observations support the concept that the fibroblasts in fibrotic lung tissue represent a unique, distinct, differentiated phenotype, different from that of fibroblasts present in normal lung.

Consistent with this concept, mesenchymal cells cultured from the airways of asthmatics show persistent differences from normal cells in culture including increased contraction of collagen gels [84], increased production of the protease matrix metalloprotease-2 (MMP-2) [85] and increased cytokine responsiveness [86]. These observations, together with the persistence of structural abnormalities in the airway, despite adequate anti-inflammatory therapy [87,88], have suggested the possibility that a primary abnormality of structural cells may be present in asthma [89].

Mesenchymal cells cultured from the lungs of COPD patients have also been assessed. Holz *et al.* [90] have reported reduced proliferation of fibroblasts derived from emphysematous tissues. Noordhoek *et al.* [91], however, found no difference in proliferation under 'control' conditions, but found altered response to interleukin 1 (IL-1) and TGF-β. Nobukuni *et al.* [92] also found reduced proliferation of emphysema fibroblasts and noted that they were more inhibited than control fibroblasts by cigarette smoke. It is unclear if differences in methodology or if heterogeneity in the patient populations studied contribute to these experimental differences. Nevertheless, while the properties of mesenchymal cells cultured from the lungs in emphysema remain to be fully delineated, a functional alteration consistent with a change in the differentiated population is possible.

The deficient proliferation observed in mesenchymal cells cultured from emphysematous lung suggests deficient repair function and contrasts markedly with the augmented function discussed above for fibroblasts isolated from fibrotic tissues. In this context, deficient repair could lead to net loss of lung tissue and could be a mechanism for the development of emphysema [93]. Interestingly, fibroblasts from aged animals have a phenotype characterized by deficient 'repair' type functions including migration [94], cytoskeletal organization, integrin expression [95] and proliferation [96,97]. This could provide a mechanism for the development of senile emphysema.

Mesenchymal cells may also be targets for cigarette smoke toxicity that leads to COPD. In this context, *in vitro* cigarette smoke can inhibit lung fibroblast chemotaxis, proliferation [98], production of extracellular matrix and contraction of three-dimensional collagen gels [99]. Inhibition of these 'repair' functions could contribute to the development of emphysema. Inhibition of collagen gel contraction is mediated by smoke-induced inhibition of fibronectin production and can be reversed by the addition of exogenous fibronectin [99]. This effect, however, is observed in cells cultured at low density. In high-density cultures, smoke can cause activation of TGF-β and can augment gel contraction [100]. This variability with cell density suggests that the *in vivo* effect of cigarette smoke on mesenchymal cell repair functions may vary with local conditions.

Therapeutic implications

Mesenchymal cells are already major targets for therapeutic intervention in lung disease. Inhibition of airway smooth muscle contraction by anticholinergic drugs that block contraction and by β-adrenergic agonists that directly relax smooth muscle are mainstays in the treatment of COPD and asthma. Similarly, the vasodilator effects of prostacyclin and its analogues and of endothelin antagonists on vascular smooth muscle are key in treating pulmonary hypertension. A greatly expanded role for mesenchymal cells in the treatment of lung diseases in general and COPD specifically seems likely in the future for several reasons.

First, mesenchymal cells, particularly alveolar myofibroblasts, may be key in regulating ventilation–perfusion matching [25]. The ability of these cells to modulate alveolar volume offers an opportunity to alter the hyperinflation that compromises function in COPD at rest and with exercise [101].

Secondly, COPD is characterized by structural alterations of the lung that result, likely in large part, from the activity of mesenchymal cells [74,75]. It is reasonable therefore that therapy directed at mesenchymal cells could prevent or, possibly, reverse these changes.

Thirdly, several lines of evidence suggest that the lung, like many tissues, can substantially repair following injury. Retinoic acid, for example, has been demonstrated to facilitate regeneration of alveolar wall in rodent lungs following the development of emphysema [102]. Collaborative interactions among a variety of cell types, including mesenchymal cells, are required for alveolar wall formation, It is likely therefore that mesenchymal cells could be targets of treatments designed to restore lung structure.

Finally, it is possible that therapy designed to restore lung function will require replacing a population of cells. In this context, engraftment of circulating stem/precursor cells may not only contribute to disease, but could also be therapeutic. Ortiz *et al.* [103], for example, were able to block the development of bleomycin-induced fibrosis in a sensitive animal by transplanting cells from a resistant strain. This occurred even though a very small number of donor cells were engrafted, consistent with a regulatory role for the transplanted mesenchymal cells.

MSCs, and a number of similarly derived cells, which can be expanded *in vitro*, infused into living recipients and subsequently differentiate into functional tissues are being widely investigated for a variety of therapeutic applications [5]. Interestingly, MSCs appear to have a low risk for inducing graft-versus-host disease (GVHD) and may actually suppress active GVHD [104,105]. These characteristics have suggested that MSCs may be ideal carriers to introduce novel genetic material for gene-based therapy.

Conclusions

Mesenchymal cells are a heterogeneous population of cells that mediate a diverse set of functions in the lung. These include lung development, responses to injury and regulation of functions of the normal lung. As understanding of the part that mesenchymal cells play in health and disease advances, these cells are likely to become increasingly important in the therapy of lung diseases including COPD.

References

1 Hay ED. The mesenchymal cell, its role in the embryo, and the remarkable signaling mechanisms that create it. *Dev Dyn* 2005;**233**:706–20.

2 Thiery JP. Epithelial–mesenchymal transitions in tumour progression. *Nat Rev Cancer* 2002;**2**:442–54.

3 Savagner P, Yamada KM, Thiery JP. The zinc-finger protein slug causes desmosome dissociation, an initial and necessary step for growth factor-induced epithelial–mesenchymal transition. *J Cell Biol* 1997;**137**:1403–19.

4 Kim K, Lu Z, Hay ED. Direct evidence for a role of beta-catenin/LEF-1 signaling pathway in induction of EMT. *Cell Biol Int* 2002;**26**:463–76.

5 Baksh D, Song L, Tuan RS. Adult mesenchymal stem cells: characterization, differentiation, and application in cell and gene therapy. *J Cell Mol Med* 2004;**8**:301–16.

6 Castro-Malaspina H, Gay RE, Resnick G *et al.* Characterization of human bone marrow fibroblast colony-forming cells (CFU-F) and their progeny. *Blood* 1980;**56**:289–301.

7 Reyes M, Lund T, Lenvik T *et al.* 2001. Purification and *ex vivo* expansion of postnatal human marrow mesodermal progenitor cells. *Blood* **98**(9):2615–25.

8 Horwitz EM, Le Blanc K, Dominici M *et al.* Clarification of the nomenclature for MSC: the International Society for Cellular Therapy position statement. *Cytotherapy* 2005;**7**: 393–5.

9 Bianchi G, Banfi A, Mastrogiacomo M *et al.* *Ex vivo* enrichment of mesenchymal cell progenitors by fibroblast growth factor 2. *Exp Cell Res* 2003;**287**:98–105.

10 Toma C, Pittenger MF, Cahill KS, Byrne BJ, Kessler PD. Human mesenchymal stem cells differentiate to a cardiomyocyte phenotype in the adult murine heart. *Circulation* 2002;**105**:93–8.

11 Ferrari G, Cusella-De Angelis G, Coletta M *et al.* Muscle regeneration by bone marrow-derived myogenic progenitors. *Science* 1998;**279**:1528–30.

12 Zhao LR, Duan WM, Reyes M *et al.* Human bone marrow stem cells exhibit neural phenotypes and ameliorate neurological deficits after grafting into the ischemic brain of rats. *Exp Neurol* 2002;**174**:11–20.

13 Lange C, Bassler P, Lioznov MV *et al.* Hepatocytic gene expression in cultured rat mesenchymal stem cells. *Transplant Proc* 2005;**37**:276–9.

14 Song L, Tuan RS. Transdifferentiation potential of human mesenchymal stem cells derived from bone marrow. *FASEB J* 2004;**18**:980–2.

15 Abe R, Donnelly SC, Peng T, Bucala R, Metz CN. Peripheral blood fibrocytes: differentiation pathway and migration to wound sites. *J Immunol* 2001;**166**:7556–62.

16 Schmidt M, Sun G, Stacey MA, Mori L, Mattoli S. Identification of circulating fibrocytes as precursors of bronchial myofibroblasts in asthma. *J Immunol* 2003;**171**:380–9.

17 Phillips RJ, Burdick MD, Hong K *et al.* Circulating fibrocytes traffic to the lungs in response to CXCL12 and mediate fibrosis. *J Clin Invest* 2004;**114**:438–46.

18 Stenmark KR, Davie NJ, Reeves JT, Frid MG. Hypoxia, leukocytes, and the pulmonary circulation. *J Appl Physiol* 2005;**98**:715–21.

19 Muir H. The chondrocyte, architect of cartilage: biomechanics, structure, function and molecular biology of cartilage matrix macromolecules. *Bioessays* 1995;**17**:1039–48.

20 Gray ML, Pizzanelli AM, Lee RC, Grodzinsky AJ, Swann DA. Kinetics of the chondrocyte biosynthetic response to compressive load and release. *Biochim Biophys Acta* 1989;**991**:415–25.

21 Bonassar LJ, Grodzinsky AJ, Frank EH *et al.* The effect of dynamic compression on the response of articular cartilage to insulin-like growth factor-I. *J Orthop Res* 2001;**19**:11–7.

22 Haraguchi M, Shimura S, Shirato K. Morphometric analysis of bronchial cartilage in chronic obstructive pulmonary disease and bronchial asthma. *Am J Respir Crit Care Med* 1999;**159**:1005–13.

23 Tetlow LC, Freemont AJ, Woolley DE. Bronchial cartilage atrophy in chronic bronchitis: observations on chondrolytic processes. *Pathobiology* 1999;**67**:196–201.

24 Callan E, Karandy EJ, Hilsinger RL Jr. 'Saber-sheath' trachea. *Ann Otol Rhinol Laryngol* 1988;**97**:512–5.

25 Kapanci Y, Gabbiani G. Contractile cells in pulmonary alveolar tissue. In: Crystal RG, West JB, Weibel ER, Barnes PJ, eds. *The Lung: Scientific Foundations.* Philadelphia: Lippincott-Raven, 1997: 697–707.

26 van der Loop FT, Schaart G, Timmer ED, Ramaekers FC, van Eys GJ. Smoothelin, a novel cytoskeletal protein specific for smooth muscle cells. *J Cell Biol* 1996;**134**:401–11.

27 Lazaar AL. Airway smooth muscle: new targets for asthma pharmacotherapy. *Expert Opin Ther Targets* 2002;**6**:447–59.

28 Humbert M, Morrell NW, Archer SL *et al.* Cellular and molecular pathobiology of pulmonary arterial hypertension. *J Am Coll Cardiol* 2004;**43**(12 Suppl S):13S–24S.

29 Mandegar M, Fung YC, Huang W *et al.* Cellular and molecular mechanisms of pulmonary vascular remodeling: role in the development of pulmonary hypertension. *Microvasc Res* 2004;**68**:75–103.

30 Glassberg MK. Lymphangioleiomyomatosis. *Clin Chest Med* 2004;**25**:573–82; vii.

31 Carsillo T, Astrinidis A, Henske EP. Mutations in the tuberous sclerosis complex gene TSC2 are a cause of sporadic pulmonary lymphangioleiomyomatosis. *Proc Natl Acad Sci U S A* 2000;**97**:6085–90.

32 Lane KB, Machado RD, Pauciulo MW *et al.* Heterozygous germline mutations in BMPR2, encoding a TGF-beta receptor, cause familial primary pulmonary hypertension. The International PPH Consortium. *Nat Genet* 2000;**26**:81–4.

33 Lindahl P, Johansson BR, Leveen P, Betsholtz C. Pericyte loss and microaneurysm formation in PDGF-B-deficient mice. *Science* 1997;**277**:242–5.

34 Muguruma Y, Yahata T, Miyatake H *et al.* Reconstitution of the functional human hematopoietic microenvironment derived from human mesenchymal stem cells in the murine bone marrow compartment. *Blood* 2006;**107**:1878–87.

35 Tomasek JJ, Gabbiani G, Hinz B, Chaponnier C, Brown RA. Myofibroblasts and mechano-regulation of connective tissue remodelling. *Nat Rev Mol Cell Biol* 2002;**3**:349–63.

36 Banes AJ, Donlon K, Link GW *et al.* Cell populations of tendon: a simplified method for isolation of synovial cells and internal fibroblasts: confirmation of origin and biologic properties. *J Orthop Res* 1988;**6**:83–94.

37 Birk DE, Trelstad RL. Fibroblasts create compartments in the extracellular space where collagen polymerizes into fibrils and fibrils associate into bundles. *Ann N Y Acad Sci* 1985;**460**:258–66.

38 Bienkowski RS, Gotkin MG. Control of collagen deposition in mammalian lung. *Proc Soc Exp Biol Med* 1995;**209**:118–40.

39 Webster DF, Burry HC. The effects of hypoxia on human skin, lung and tendon cells in vitro. *Br J Exp Pathol* 1982;**63**:50–5.

40 Mollenhauer J, Bayreuther K. Donor-age-related changes in the morphology, growth potential, and collagen biosynthesis in rat fibroblast subpopulations *in vitro. Differentiation* 1986;**32**:165–72.

41 Westergren-Thorsson G. TGF-β enhances the production of hyaluronan in human lung but not in skin fibroblasts. *Exp Cell Res* 1990;**186**:192–5.

42 Fries KM, Blieden T, Looney RJ *et al.* Evidence of fibroblast heterogeneity and the role of fibroblast subpopulations in fibrosis. *Clin Immunol Immunopathol* 1994;**72**:283–92.

43 Powell DW, Mifflin RC, Valentich JD *et al.* Myofibroblasts. I. Paracrine cells important in health and disease. *Am J Physiol* 1999;**277**:C1–9.

44 Powell DW, Mifflin RC, Valentich JD *et al.* Myofibroblasts. II. Intestinal subepithelial myofibroblasts. *Am J Physiol* 1999;**277**:C183–201.

45 Vaughan MB, Howard EW, Tomasek JJ. Transforming growth factor-beta1 promotes the morphological and functional differentiation of the myofibroblast. *Exp Cell Res* 2000;**257**:180–9.

46 Liu XD, Umino T, Ertl R *et al.* Persistence of TGF-beta1 induction of increased fibroblast contractility. *In Vitro Cell Dev Biol Anim* 2001;**37**:193–201.

47 Serini G, Bochaton-Piallat ML, Ropraz P *et al*. The fibronectin domain ED-A is crucial for myofibroblastic phenotype induction by transforming growth factor-beta1. *J Cell Biol* 1998;**142**:873–81.

48 Roy SG, Nozaki Y, Phan SH. Regulation of alpha-smooth muscle actin gene expression in myofibroblast differentiation from rat lung fibroblasts. *Int J Biochem Cell Biol* 2001;**33**:723–34.

49 Mack CP, Owens GK. Regulation of smooth muscle alpha-actin expression *in vivo* is dependent on CArG elements within the 5′ and first intron promoter regions. *Circ Res* 1999;**84**:852–61.

50 Cunha GR. Role of mesenchymal–epithelial interactions in normal and abnormal development of the mammary gland and prostate. *Cancer* 1994;**74**(3 Suppl):1030–44.

51 Hieda Y, Nakanishi Y. Epithelial morphogenesis in mouse embryonic submandibular gland: its relationships to the tissue organization of epithelium and mesenchyme. *Dev Growth Differ* 1997;**39**:1–8.

52 Warburton D, Schwarz M, Tefft D *et al*. The molecular basis of lung morphogenesis. *Mech Dev* 2000;**92**:55–81.

53 Cardoso WV. Lung morphogenesis revisited: old facts, current ideas. *Dev Dyn* 2000;**219**:121–30.

54 Kedinger M, Duluc I, Fritsch C *et al*. Intestinal epithelial–mesenchymal cell interactions. *Ann N Y Acad Sci* 1998;**859**:1–17.

55 McGowan SE, Torday JS. The pulmonary lipofibroblast (lipid interstitial cell) and its contributions to alveolar development. *Annu Rev Physiol* 1997;**59**:43–62.

56 Morrison SJ, Uchida N, Weissman IL. The biology of hematopoietic stem cells. *Annu Rev Cell Dev Biol* 1995;**11**:35–71.

57 Allen TD, Dexter TM. The essential cells of the hemopoietic microenvironment. *Exp Hematol* 1984;**12**:517–21.

58 Dexter TM, Coutinho LH, Spooncer E *et al*. Stromal cells in haemopoiesis. *Ciba Found Symp* 1990;**148**:76–86.

59 Watt FM, Hogan BL. Out of Eden: stem cells and their niches. *Science* 2000;**287**:1427–30.

60 Spradling A, Drummond-Barbosa D, Kai T. Stem cells find their niche. *Nature* 2001;**414**:98–104.

61 Borthwick DW, Shahbazian M, Krantz QT, Dorin JR, Randell SH. Evidence for stem-cell niches in the tracheal epithelium. *Am J Respir Cell Mol Biol* 2001;**24**:662–70.

62 Giangreco A, Reynolds SD, Stripp BR. Terminal bronchioles harbor a unique airway stem cell population that localizes to the bronchoalveolar duct junction. *Am J Pathol* 2002;**161**:173–82.

63 Engelhardt JF. Stem cell niches in the mouse airway. *Am J Respir Cell Mol Biol* 2001;**24**:649–52.

64 Haffen K, Kedinger M, Simon-Assmann P. Mesenchyme-dependent differentiation of epithelial progenitor cells in the gut. *J Pediatr Gastroenterol Nutr* 1987;**6**:14–23.

65 Brittan M, Hunt T, Jeffery R *et al*. Bone marrow derivation of pericryptal myofibroblasts in the mouse and human small intestine and colon. *Gut* 2002;**50**:752–7.

66 Panettieri RA Jr. Airway smooth muscle: an immuno-modulatory cell. *J Allergy Clin Immunol* 2002;**110**(Suppl):S269–74.

67 Kapanci Y, Baud M, Mo Costabella P. Alveolar contractile interstitial cells: their morphology and reactions to hypoxia and to epinephrine stimulation. *Curr Probl Clin Biochem* 1983;**13**:134–41.

68 Kuhn C, McDonald JA. The roles of the myofibroblast in idiopathic pulmonary fibrosis. *Am J Pathol* 1991;**138**:1257–65.

69 Kapanci Y, Desmouliere A, Pache JC, Redard M, Gabbiani G. Cytoskeletal protein modulation in pulmonary alveolar myofibroblasts during idiopathic pulmonary fibrosis: possible role of transforming growth factor beta and tumor necrosis factor alpha. *Am J Respir Crit Care Med* 1995;**152**:2163–9.

70 Mitchell J, Woodcock-Mitchell J, Reynolds S *et al*. Alpha-smooth muscle actin in parenchymal cells of bleomycin-injured rat lung. *Lab Invest* 1989;**60**:643–50.

71 Gizycki MJ, Adelroth E, Rogers AV, O'Byrne PM, Jeffery PK. Myofibroblast involvement in the allergen-induced late response in mild atopic asthma. *Am J Respir Cell Mol Biol* 1997;**16**:664–73.

72 Roche WR, Beasley R, Williams JH, Holgate ST. Sub-epithelial fibrosis in the bronchi of asthmatics. *Lancet* 1989;**i**:520–4.

73 Hashimoto N, Jin H, Liu T, Chensue SW, Phan SH. Bone marrow-derived progenitor cells in pulmonary fibrosis. *J Clin Invest* 2004;**113**:243–52.

74 Cosio M, Ghezzo H, Hogg JC *et al*. The relations between structural changes in small airways and pulmonary function tests. *N Engl J Med* 1978;**298**:1277–81.

75 Hogg JC, Chu F, Utokaparch S *et al*. The nature of small-airway obstruction in chronic obstructive pulmonary disease. *N Engl J Med* 2004;**350**:2645–53.

76 Bostrom H, Willetts K, Pekny M *et al*. PDGF-A signaling is a critical event in lung alveolar myofibroblast development and alveogenesis. *Cell* 1996;**85**:863–73.

77 Torry DJ, Richards CD, Podor TJ, Gauldie J. Anchorage-independent colony growth of pulmonary fibroblasts derived from fibrotic human lung tissue. *J Clin Invest* 1994;**93**:1525–32.

78 Miki H, Mio T, Nagai S *et al*. Fibroblast contractility: usual interstitial pneumonia and nonspecific interstitial pneumonia. *Am J Respir Crit Care Med* 2000;**162**:2259–64.

79 Botstein GR, Sherer GK, Leroy EC. Fibroblast selection in scleroderma. *Arthritis Rheum* 1982;**25**:189–95.

80 Galambos JT, Hollingsworth MA Jr, Falek A *et al*. The rate of synthesis of glycosaminoglycans and collagen by fibroblasts cultured from adult human liver biopsies. *J Clin Invest* 1977;**60**:107–14.

81 Knittel T, Kobold D, Saile B *et al*. Rat liver myofibroblasts and hepatic stellate cells: different cell populations of the fibroblast lineage with fibrogenic potential. *Gastroenterology* 1999;**117**:1205–21.

82 Ogushi F, Endo T, Tani K *et al*. Decreased prostaglandin E2 synthesis by lung fibroblasts isolated from rats with bleomycin-induced lung fibrosis. *Int J Exp Pathol* 1999;**80**:41–9.

83 Zhang HY, Gharaee-Kermani M, Zhang K, Karmiol S, Phan SH. Lung fibroblast alpha-smooth muscle actin expression

and contractile phenotype in bleomycin-induced pulmonary fibrosis. *Am J Pathol* 1996;**148**:527–37.

84 Goulet F, Boulet L, Chakir J *et al.* Morphologic and functional properties of bronchial cells isolated from normal and asthmatic subjects. *Am J Respir Cell Mol Biol* 1996;**15**:312–8.

85 Laliberte R, Rouabhia M, Bosse M, Chakir J. Decreased capacity of asthmatic bronchial fibroblasts to degrade collagen. *Matrix Biol* 2001;**19**:743–53.

86 Burgess JK, Johnson PR, Ge Q *et al.* Expression of connective tissue growth factor in asthmatic airway smooth muscle cells. *Am J Respir Crit Care Med* 2003;**167**:71–7.

87 Ward C, Pais M, Bish R *et al.* Airway inflammation, basement membrane thickening and bronchial hyperresponsiveness in asthma. *Thorax* 2002;**57**:309–16.

88 Jeffery PK, Godfrey RW, Adelroth E *et al.* Effects of treatment on airway inflammation and thickening of basement membrane reticular collagen in asthma: a quantitative light and electron microscopic study. *Am Rev Respir Dis* 1992; **145**:890–9.

89 Black JL, Johnson PR. Factors controlling smooth muscle proliferation and airway remodelling. *Curr Opin Allergy Clin Immunol* 2002;**2**:47–51.

90 Holz O, Zuhlke I, Jaksztat E *et al.* Lung fibroblasts from patients with emphysema show a reduced proliferation rate in culture. *Eur Respir J* 2004;**24**:575–9.

91 Noordhoek JA, Postma DS, Chong LL *et al.* Different proliferative capacity of lung fibroblasts obtained from control subjects and patients with emphysema. *Exp Lung Res* 2003; **29**:291–302.

92 Nobukuni S, Watanabe K, Inoue J *et al.* Cigarette smoke inhibits the growth of lung fibroblasts from patients with pulmonary emphysema. *Respirology* 2002;**7**:217–23.

93 Rennard S. Defective repair in COPD: the American hypothesis. In: Pauwels RA, Postma DS, eds. *Long-Term Intervention in Chronic Obstructive Pulmonary Disease.* New York: Marcel Dekker, 2004: 165–200.

94 Albini A, Pontz B, Pulz M *et al.* Decline of fibroblast chemotaxis with age of donor and cell passage number. *Collagen Rel Res* 1988;**1**:23–37.

95 Reed MJ, Ferara NS, Vernon RB. Impaired migration, integrin function, and actin cytoskeletal organization in dermal fibroblasts from a subset of aged human donors. *Mech Ageing Dev* 2001;**122**:1203–20.

96 Shiraha H, Gupta K, Drabik K, Wells A. Aging fibroblasts present reduced epidermal growth factor (EGF) responsiveness due to preferential loss of EGF receptors. *J Biol Chem* 2000;**275**:19343–51.

97 Pendergrass WR, Lane MA, Bodkin NL *et al.* Cellular proliferation potential during aging and caloric restriction in rhesus monkeys (*Macaca mulatta*). *J Cell Physiol* 1999;**180**:123–30.

98 Nakamura Y, Romberger DJ, Tate L *et al.* Cigarette smoke inhibits lung fibroblast proliferation and chemotaxis. *Am J Respir Crit Care Med* 1995;**151**:1497–503.

99 Carnevali S, Nakamura Y, Mio T *et al.* Cigarette smoke extract inhibits fibroblast-mediated collagen gel contraction. *Am J Physiol Lung Cell Mol Physiol* 1998;**274**:L591–8.

100 Wang H, Liu X, Umino T *et al.* Effect of cigarette smoke on fibroblast-mediated gel contraction is dependent on cell density. *Am J Physiol Lung Cell Mol Physiol* 2003;**284**:L205–13.

101 O'Donnell DE, Revill SM, Webb KA. Dynamic hyperinflation and exercise intolerance in chronic obstructive pulmonary disease. *Am J Respir Crit Care Med* 2001;**164**: 770–7.

102 Massaro G, Massaro D. Retinoic acid treatment abrogates elastase-induced pulmonary emphysema in rats. *Nat Med* 1997;**3**:675–7.

103 Ortiz LA, Gambelli F, McBride C *et al.* Mesenchymal stem cell engraftment in lung is enhanced in response to bleomycin exposure and ameliorates its fibrotic effects. *Proc Natl Acad Sci U S A* 2003;**100**:8407–11.

104 Aggarwal S, Pittenger MF. Human mesenchymal stem cells modulate allogeneic immune cell responses. *Blood* 2005;**105**: 1815–22.

105 Le Blanc K, Rasmusson I, Sundberg B *et al.* Treatment of severe acute graft-versus-host disease with third party haploidentical mesenchymal stem cells. *Lancet* 2004;**363**: 1439–41.

Pathogenesis

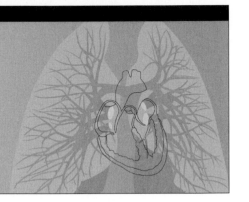

CHAPTER 29
Lung development

Cheng Chen, David Warburton and Wei Shi

Lung developmental process

The functional mammalian lung has a honeycomb-like structure, containing extensively branched, perfectly matched conduits for air and blood. This configuration maximizes the gas exchange surface area, supports effective gas ventilation and exchange between air and blood, and facilitates maximally efficient packing within the chest cavity. In humans, the gas exchange membrane (approximately 0.1 μm thick) consists of alveolar epithelial cells, basement membrane and endothelial cells, and the total surface area is approximately 70 m². This complex structure is developed sequentially by early epithelial tube branching and by late septation of terminal air sacs. Perturbation of this developmental process results in abnormal lung structure and hence deficiency of respiratory gas exchange function. Therefore fundamental knowledge about this basic developmental process and the underlying molecular regulatory mechanisms that drive it is essential to understand the pathogenesis of many respiratory diseases and, more importantly, to design novel therapeutic strategies to prevent and treat related pulmonary diseases, such as bronchopulmonary dysplasia, and their chronic sequelae.

The origin of lung

The lung originates from the ventral surface of the primitive foregut at 5 weeks' gestation in humans. The lung anlage emerges as the laryngo-tracheal groove, located in the ventral foregut endoderm, which invaginates into the surrounding splanchnic mesenchyme (Fig. 29.1). A pair of primary buds then evaginate from the laryngo-tracheal groove and the respiratory tree develops by branching morphogenesis, in which reiterated outgrowth, elongation and subdivision of epithelial buds occurs in a bilaterally asymmetrical pattern. Three lobes on the right side and two lobes on the left side are formed in human lung. There are 23 generations of airway branching in humans. The first 16 generations branching is stereotypically reproducible and is completed by 16 weeks, while the remaining seven generations are random and are completed by approximately 24 weeks. Alveolization begins at around 20 weeks' gestation in the human lung, and is completed postnatally at approximately 7 years of age.

Lung organogenesis is under the control of many gene products that act cooperatively to define precisely the location of the laryngo-tracheal groove formation and specify proximal–distal, dorsal–ventral and left–right axes of the developing lung. The earliest endodermal signal essential for gut morphogenesis are the GATA (zinc finger proteins that recognize GATA DNA sequence) and hepatocyte nuclear factor (HNF) transcription factors. GATA-6 is required for activation of the lung developmental programme in the foregut endoderm. *Hnf-3β* is a survival factor for the endoderm, and expression of *Hnf-3β* is induced by Sonic Hedgehog (*Shh*) signalling. Also, *Tbx4* can induce ectopic bud formation in the oesophagus by activating the expression of *Fgf10* [1]. In addition, left–right asymmetry is controlled by several gene products, including *nodal*, *Lefty-1,2* and *Pitx-2*. For example, single-lobed lungs are found bilaterally in *Lefty-1* mice, and isomerism of lung is found in *Pitx-2* null mutants. The exact molecular mechanisms responsible for primary lung bud induction are as yet only incompletely understood.

Histology and cytology of lung development

Histological stages of lung development

Histologically, lung development and maturation has been divided into four stages: the pseudoglandular stage, the canalicular stage, the terminal sac stage and the alveolar stage (see Plate 29.1; colour plate section falls between pp. 354 and 355).

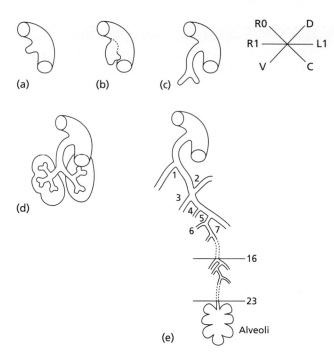

Figure 29.1 Diagrams showing key events in human lung morphogenesis. (a) The primitive lung anlage emerging as the laryngo-tracheal groove from the ventral surface of the primitive foregut at 5 weeks' gestation in humans. (b) The primitive trachea separating dorso-ventrally from the primitive oesophagus as the two primary bronchial branches arise from the lateral aspects of the laryngo-tracheal groove at 5 ± 6 weeks' gestation in humans. (c) The embryonic larynx and trachea with the two primary bronchial branches separated dorso-ventrally from the embryonic oesophagus at 6 weeks' gestation in humans. (d) The primitive lobar bronchi branching from the primary bronchi at 7 weeks' gestation in humans. (e) A schematic rendering of the term fetal airway in humans. The stereotypically reproducible first 16 airway generations are complete by 16 weeks' gestation in humans. Between 16 and 23 weeks, the branching pattern is random and this is completed by approximately 24 weeks in humans. Alveolization begins after about 28 ± 30 weeks in humans and is complete by 7 years of age at the earliest.

Pseudoglandular stage (5–17 weeks' human gestation, E9.5–16.6 days in mouse embryo)
This is the earliest stage of lung development, in which the embryonic lung undergoes branching morphogenesis, developing epithelial tubular structures with lining cuboidal epithelial cells that resemble an exocrine gland. This fluid containing respiratory tree structure cannot support gas exchange.

Canalicular stage (16–25 weeks' human gestation, E16.6–17.4 days in mouse embryo)
The cranial part of the lung develops relatively faster than the caudal part, resulting in partial overlap between this stage and the previous stage. During the canalicular stage, the respiratory tree is further expanded in diameter and length, accompanied by vascularization and angiogenesis along the airway. A massive increase in the number of capillaries occurs. The terminal bronchioles are then divided into respiratory bronchioles and alveolar ducts, and the airway epithelial cells are differentiated into peripheral squamous cells and proximal cuboidal cells.

Terminal sac stage (24 weeks' to late fetal period in humans, E17.4 to postnatal day 5 (P5) in mouse)
There is substantial thinning of the interstitium during the terminal sac stage. This results from apoptosis as well as ongoing differentiation of mesenchymal cells [2,3]. Additionally, at this stage, the alveolar epithelial cells are more clearly differentiated into mature squamous type I pneumocytes and secretory rounded type II pneumocytes. The capillaries also grow rapidly in the mesenchyme surrounding the alveoli to form a complex network. The lymphatic network in lung tissue becomes well developed during this stage. Towards the end of this stage, the fetal lung can support gas exchange to maintain the life of prematurely born neonates. Although human premature infants can breathe with the lung that has developed towards the end of terminal sac stage, the immature lung is nevertheless vulnerable to hyperoxic injury and barotrauma, resulting in the alveolar hypoplasia phenotypes progressing toward bronchopulmonary dysplasia. Maturation of surfactant synthesis and secretion is a key factor in determining whether the newborn lung can sustain gas exchange without collapsing. Another key factor is the rapid switch from chloride ion driven fluid secretion into the airway to sodium driven uptake of fluid out of the airway. This latter is driven by the response of the adrenergic system to cord cutting at birth.

How lung development is controlled at this stage is still incompletely known. The hydrostatic pressure inside the lumen of the airway, which results from chloride ion and hence liquid secretion from epithelium in the developing lung [4–6], integrated with chemotactic signals from the mesenchyme such as FGF10 have important roles in forming terminal sacs. Mechanical factors also play an important part. Diaphragm muscle in *MyoD*(–/–) mice is significantly thinned and cannot support fetal breathing movements. As a result, lung is hypoplastic, and the number of proliferating lung cells is decreased in *MyoD*(–/–) lungs at E18.5. Therefore, mechanical forces generated by contractile activity of the diaphragm muscle have an important role in normal lung growth at this stage [7].

Alveolar stage (late fetal period to childhood in humans, P5–P30 in mouse)
Alveolization is the last step of lung development. The

majority of the gas exchange surface is formed during this stage. Alveolarization can be positively and negatively influenced by many exogenous factors including oxygen concentration, stretch in fetal airway, dexamethasone and retinoic acid.

Forming new septa within terminal sacs is the key step for differentiation of the saccule into alveoli. This involves a complex interaction between myofibroblasts in the mesenchyme, adjacent airway epithelial cells and vascular endothelial cells. Controlled multiplication and differentiation as well as migration of the myofibroblast progenitors cells within terminal sac walls are important for new septa formation. Myofibroblasts, smooth muscle precursor cells having the morphology of fibroblasts, migrate to the proper position within nascent alveolar septa, and synthesize and deposit elastin [8,9]. This is the first step of new secondary septa development [9]. PDGF-A and its receptor PDGF-α have important roles in forming new septa. $Pdgf$-A(−/−) or $Pdgf$-$α$(−/−) show a phenotype comprising loss of alveolar myofibroblasts and elastin, failure of alveolar septation, and this develops into emphysema resulting from alveolar hypoplasia [8,10]. Besides PDGF-A, there are other key proteins that mediate cell–cell interaction within terminal sac walls. For example, Roundabout (ROBO) is a receptor known to be involved in repellent signalling controlling axonal extension in the developing neuronal system. ROBO and its ligand SLIT are also involved in the regulation of non-neuronal cell migration [11]. In E18, 1 day before birth, $Slit$-2 is expressed in the saccular mesenchyme surrounding the airways. At the same time, $Robo$ is expressed on the apical aspects of the airway epithelium adjacent to the ligand $Slit$-2, suggesting interactive roles in pulmonary bronchiolar development [12]. A $Robo$ knockout mouse has been shown to have loss of septation and thickened mesenchyme [13].

Two additional processes are necessary in septum differentiation to form a septum with final mature morphology and function: the thinning out of the septal mesenchyme and maturation of the capillary bed. Thinning of the mesenchymal tissue involves apoptosis of 'unwanted' cells in the postnatal lung. There is a substantial reduction in the number of interstitial myofibroblasts resulting from increased apoptosis during this phase of rapid alveolarization [14,15]. The immature lung contains at least two morphologically distinct fibroblast populations: lipid-filled interstitial fibroblasts (LFIF) and non-LIF (NLFIF). After alveolarization, apoptosis occurs preferentially in only one of these fibroblast populations, the LFIF. Apoptosis was correlated with down-regulation of insulin-like growth factor I receptor (Igf-IR) mRNA and cell surface protein expression [16]. This thinning of the previously thickened immature interstitium occurs simultaneously with the ongoing expansion of the epithelial, blood vessel and airspace compartments in the rapidly developing septa. A mature capillary bed is also vital for the proper function of alveoli, but the mechanism is still incompletely known. In developing lungs, vascular endothelial growth factor (VEGF) isoforms and its receptors have been identified as being important for endothelial survival and proliferation in the alveolar wall. Inhibition of VEGF signalling results in abnormal lung vascular growth and reduced alveolarization [17]. Finally, the new septum differentiates into a functional respiratory membrane that consists of type I alveolar epithelial cells, basement membrane and capillary endothelial cells. The respiratory membrane provides a short distance for gas diffusion and thus facilitates optimal gas exchange. It is estimated that approximtaely 50 million alveoli are present in neonatal human lung. However, by age 7–8 years, when alveolarization is substantially complete, the number of alveolar units in the human lung has grown about six times to approximately 300 million alveoli.

Retinoid acid (RA) has been shown to increase the number of alveoli [18] and partially rescue a block in alveolar formation induced by dexamethasone [19]. In adult rats, RA has also been reported to reverse the anatomical features of elastase-induced emphysema in which there is destruction of septa [18]. In the RAR-$γ$ gene deletion mouse, there is a developmental defect in alveolar formation most consistent with a defect in elastin deposition. The additional deletion of one retinoid X receptor (RXR-$α$) allele results in a decrease in alveolar surface area and alveolar number [20]. Retinoids affect multiple cellular functions that are involved in alveolar septal formation such as proliferation, migration and temporal differentiation of cells [21]. RA is an active metabolite of vitamin A. Vitamin A deficiency has long been known to injure lung and impair function of rat type II pneumocytes [20]. Taken together, the evidence suggests that RA may have an important role in alveolar development.

Specific cell types in lung

More than 40 specific types of cells are differentiated during embryonic lung development. The epithelial cell lineages are arranged in a distinct proximal–distal spatial pattern in the airways.

Cartilage lies outside the submucosa and decreases in amount as the calibre of the bronchi decreases. Cartilage is present in the bronchi, but is not present in the bronchioles. Two major cell components of the proximal bronchial epithelium are identified: pseudostratified ciliated columnar cells and mucous (goblet) cells. Both of them may derive from basal cells, but ciliated cells predominate in number. Goblet cells release mucus granules into the bronchial lumen to prevent drying of the walls and trap particulate matter. Mucous cells begin to mature around 13 weeks' gestation in humans, when the mature ciliated columnar cells are already present. The most widey used molecular markers for mucous cells are mucins (MUC5B, -5A, -5C). The beating of cilia results in a cephalad movement of the mucus blanket, thereby cleaning and protecting the airway. In the case of cystic fibrosis, cilia movement is disabled because of the thick mucous layer that is caused by mutation of *CFTR* gene, which encodes a transmembrane Na^+ ion transporter protein. This phenotype also makes the airway surface vulnerable to microbial infection. In chronic airway injury, repair or experimental exposure of the epithelium to cytokines can result in goblet cell hyperplasia. Exposure to interleukin 9 (IL-9) resulted in increased lysozyme and mucus production by the epithelia [22]. IL-4, IL-13 and allergens enhance the release of transforming growth factor α (TGF-α), which is a ligand for the epidermal growth factor receptor that also stimulates fibroblast proliferation and goblet cell differentiation [23].

There are three different types of cells in bronchial submucosal glands: myoepithelial cells surround the gland, while mucous cells (pale cytoplasm) and serous cells (basophilic cytoplasm) produce mucins. These secreted mucins mix with lysozyme and immunoglobulin A (IgA) on the airway surface.

Kulchitsky cells are also found on the airway surface next to bronchial glands. Their finger-like cytoplasmic extensions usually reach the airway lumen. Their precise function is unclear. It is believed that they are pulmonary neuroendocrine cells (PNEC) that produce a variety of peptide hormones such as serotonin and calcitonin. PNEC differentiate by 10 weeks' gestation in humans. Kulchitsky cells expressing the markers gastrin-related peptide (GRP), calcitonin gene-related peptide (CGRP) and chromogranin may be related to certain lung neoplasms (i.e. small cell carcinoma and carcinoid tumours).

Clara cells are found in the distal bronchiolar airway epithelium which normally lacks mucous cells. They produce a mucus-poor, watery proteinaceous secretion. They assist with clearance and detoxification, as well as reduction of surface tension in small airways. The most important cellular marker of Clara cell is Clara cell-specific protein (CCSP). Cytochrome p450 reductase and uteroglobulin can also be used as cellular markers for Clara cells. Clara cells begin to mature during the 19th week in humans.

The majority of the alveolar surface is normally covered by type I epithelial cells. These flat cells are believed to be terminally differentiated cells, expressing several specific molecular markers, such as T1α and aquaporin 5. T1α is a differentiation marker gene of lung alveolar epithelial type I cells. It is developmentally regulated and encodes an apical membrane protein of unknown function. In the absence of T1α protein, type I cell differentiation is blocked. Homozygous T1α null mice die at birth of respiratory failure, and their lungs cannot be inflated to normal volumes [24]. Aquaporin 5 is a water channel in type I epithelial cells.

Type I epithelial cells only account for 40% of the total airway epithelial cells, even though 95% of the surface area of the alveolar wall is covered by this type of cells. The other 60% of the epithelial cells, named type II pneumocytes, are rounded cells that cover only 3% of the alveolar surface. Type II pneumocytes are plump or cubical and have a finely stippled cytoplasm and surface microvilli. They manufacture surfactant phospholipids and proteins that reduce the surface tension in the lung. This equalizes pressures, stabilizes and maintains all the alveoli in an open position despite variations in alveolar size. Type II cells are capable of regeneration and replacement of type I cells after injury. A commonly used cellular marker of type II cell is surfactant protein C (SPC).

Alveolar macrophages constitute a small percentage of the cells in alveoli, but they represent a major cellular sentinel of the host defence mechanism in the alveolar space. They are part of the mononuclear phagocyte system and are derived primarily from blood monocytes.

Stem and progenitor cells in the respiratory system

Respiratory stem and progenitor cells have important functions in repairing damaged trachea, bronchi, bronchioles or alveoli. However, the precise identification of lung stem or progenitor cells remains uncertain. The large surface area and highly branched and folded geography of the lung dictates that there must be several kinds of stem or progenitor cells in the respiratory system. In the trachea and bronchi, certain basal cells and mucus-gland duct cells are believed to be stem or progenitor cells. Clara-like cells and type II pneumocytes are also thought to function as stem/progenitor cells in bronchioles and alveoli, respectively.

It has recently been reported that bone marrow derived mesenchymal stem cells can differentiate into airway epithelial cells in airway and type I pneumocytes in alveoli, particularly following injury. In contrast, *in vitro* cell culture indicates that Syrian hamster fetal lung epithelial M3E3/C3 cells can differentiate into Clara cells and type II pneumocytes under different culture conditions. Whether CCSP-expressing cells with pre-Clara cell phenotypes are stem cells for the entire respiratory tract remains to be determined. In addition, the concept of a pluripotent stem cell for the whole lung needs to be further investigated because of the great differences between identified stem cell or progenitor candidates in proximal bronchi and distal alveoli. Recently, we have discovered that lung contains a population of cells with stem or progenitor cell characteristics that can be sorted by fluorescence-activated cell sorting (FACS) from adult rat lung. This population is relatively resistant to apoptosis and may possibly be responsible for repopulation of the damaged alveolar surface. Another such population of stem or progenitor cells sorted as 'side cells' on FACS has been identified to possibly repopulate several different tissues, including the bone marrow. Research on both systemically derived as well as resident lung stem or progenitor cells may hold the key to understanding lung morphogenesis, lung regeneration and pathogenesis of lung cancer.

Molecular mechanisms of lung development

Normal embryonic lung development is controlled by many coordinated factors, including:

1 Transcription factors that directly modulate gene expression in the cell nucleus.

2 Peptide growth factors and cytokines as well as their related intracellular signalling components that mediate cell–cell interaction.

3 Extracellular matrix that provides important environmental cues for developing lung cells to differentiate.

The specific integrated regulatory mechanisms are still largely unknown, but the interaction between epithelial and mesenchymal compartments has long been known to have a critical role during airway branching morphogenesis and lung maturation.

Transcription factors

Lung growth is initiated and developed through changes in specific gene expression. The activity and expression level of the relevant transcription factors determines gene expression profiles in the developing lung, and consequently the morphogenetic process in a particular temporospatial manner. Recent advances in mouse genetic technology allow us to evaluate each factor by either overexpressing or knocking out a specific gene [25]. Some of the pulmonary phenotypes in mice that resulted from a loss or gain of gene function are listed in Table 29.1 [25–63]. Therefore, three groups of transcription factors, forkhead box transcription factors, Nkx homoeodomain transcription factors, and *Gli*, have important roles in ciliated epithelial cell differentiation and airway branching.

Forkhead box transcription factor family

Many members of the forkhead box family transcription factors, such as HNF-3α, HNF-3β, HFH8 and HFH4, are important regulatory factors involved in lung development. These transcription factors share homology in the winged helix DNA binding domain, and have important roles in pulmonary cellular proliferation and differentiation.

HNF-3α (*Foxa1*) and HNF-3β (*Foxa2*) share 93% homology in their amino acid sequences, and were first identified as essential factors in hepatocyte differentiation [64]. However, *Hnf-3β* is also expressed in developing lung, with higher levels in proximal airway lining epithelial cells and lower levels in the distal type II epithelial cells [65]. Overexpression of *Hnf-3β* under the control of the lung epithelial specific *SP-C* promoter *in vivo* inhibits lung branching morphogenesis and vasculogenesis [35]. Also, HNF-3α and HNF-3β have important functions in regulating expression of CCSP as well as surfactant proteins in both bronchiolar and type II epithelial cells [66–68]. *Hnf-3β* is inducible by interferon, and regulates in turn the expression of the *Nkx* homoeodomain transcription factor *Nkx2.1* (also termed *Ttf-1* and *Cebp1*), which in turn regulates transcription of the surfactant protein genes in lung peripheral epithelium [69,70].

HFH8 is another important member of this family of proteins that contribute to lung development. At E9.5, *Hfh-8* expression is restricted to the splanchnic mesoderm contacting the embryonic gut and presumptive lung bud, suggesting that *Hfh-8* may participate in the mesenchymal–epithelial induction of lung and gut morphogenesis. *Hfh-8* expression continues in lateral mesoderm-derived tissue during development. By day E18.5, *Hfh-8* expression is restricted to the distal lung mesenchyme and the muscular layer of the bronchi [71]. One important regulated target of *Hfh-8* is *Pdgf* receptor that is also expressed in mesenchyme [8,72,73]. The level of *Hfh-8* expression is important for normal lung development, as an alveolar hemorrhage phenotype is observed in *Hfh-8*(+/−) mice, while *Hfh-8*(−/−) mice died *in utero*. In addition, reduction of *Hfh-8* expression in *Hfh-8*(+/−) mutants is accompanied by decreased expression of VEGF and its receptor 2 (Flk-1), bone morphogenetic protein 4 (BMP-4), and the transcription factors of the Brachyury T-Box family (Tbx2–Tbx5) and lung Kruppel-like factor [74]. HFH-8 binding sites are also found in the promoter region of genes, such as *Bmp4*, *Hgf* and *Hoxa5* which are very important in controlling lung morphogenesis [75,76].

Hfh-4 (*Foxj1*) is the key factor controlling ciliated epithelial cell differentiation. *Hfh-4* is expressed in E15.5 airway epithelium just before the appearance of ciliated epithelial cells [77]. Defective ciliogenesis in airway epithelial cells and randomized left–right asymmetry are observed in *Hfh-4*(−/−) null mutant mice, mimicking Kartagener syndrome in humans. This congenital syndrome can result in perinatal lethality, but in low penetrance gives rise to situs inversus, sinusitis, bronchiectasis and sterlity, all resulting from defects in ciliary beat [28,29]. Interestingly, in mesenchyme-free airway epithelial culture, inhibition of endogenous BMP-4 signalling by adding exogenous BMP antagonist Noggin results in increased expression of the proximal lung markers CCSP and HFH-4 [78].

Foxp1, *Foxp2* and *Foxp3* are newly discovered members of the forkhead box family of transcription factors that are expressed at a high level in mouse lung and gut tissues. All

Table 29.1 Pulmonary phenotypes of mice with a specific gene null mutation or with a transgenic (TG) overexpression in lungs.

Gene	Pulmonary phenotype	Reference
Transcription factors		
Gli2(–/–) mice	Perinatal lethal phenotypes with severe skeletal and neuronal defects, and hypoplastic trachea and oesophagus are observed in *Gli2* knockout fetuses. Also, only one right lung lobe instead of the normal four lobes is formed in the knockout mice. Other *Shh* signalling pathway components, such as *Patch* and *Gli1*, less expressed in the knockout lungs	25
Gli2(–/–), *Gli3*(–/–) mice	Complete absence of lung, trachea and oesophagus is observed in this double knockout	26,27
Gli2(–/–), *Gli3*(+/–) mice	Oesophageal atresia with tracheoesophageal fistula and a severe lung phenotype occur in this mutant mouse. A single tracheoesophageal tube connects pharynx to the stomach. Hypoplastic embryonic lung fails to separate into left and right lobes	25
Hfh4(–/–) mice	Loss of *Hfh4* function results in retarded growth and perinatal lethality, as well as randomized left–right asymmetry of internal organs (50% situs inversus). Defective ciliogenesis in airway epithelial cells and absence of left–right dynein expression in the embryonic lungs are observed in *Hfh4* null mutant lung. Motile cilia (9 + 2 microtubules) are absent	28,29
Hoxa5(–/–) mice	Homozygous *Hoxa5* knockout mice die during perinatal stages with improper tracheal and lung morphogenesis leading to tracheal occlusion and diminished surfactant expression. Reduction in lung branching morphogenesis and thickening of the alveolar walls, as well as disorganization of proximal and distal respiratory airways are observed in *Hoxa5* null mutants. Reduced expression of surfactant protein, TTF-1, HNF-3β and c-Myc was detected in the knockout lungs	30,31
Pod1(–/–) mice	Lung branching morphogenesis and alveolarization are dramatically reduced. Airway epithelial cell differentiation is perturbed as shown by abnormal *SP-C* and *CCSP* expression pattern	32
Smad3(–/–) mice	*Smad3*(–/–) mice exhibit centrilobular emphysema-like pathology	33
SP-C-driven *Hfh4* TG mice	Overexpression of *Hfh4* in lung epithelial cells results in abnormal lung development with altered epithelial cell differentiation and inhibited branching morphogenesis. Atypical cuboidal or columnar epithelial cells line the lung periphery of *SP-C/Hfh-4* transgenic mice. These atypical cells express *Ttf1* and *Hnf3β*, as well as ciliated cell marker *β-tubulin IV*, but not *SP-B*, *SP-C* and *CCSP*	34
SP-C-driven *Hnf3β* TG mice	Overexpression of *Hnf3β (Foxa2)* in lung epithelial cells arrests distal airway epithelial cell differentiation in the early pseudoglandular stage. Branching morphogenesis and vasculogenesis were markedly disrupted in association with decreased E-cadherin and vascular endothelial growth factor expression	35
Ttf1(–/–) mice	Null mutant mice of *Ttf1* are perinatal lethal with abnormal lung branching morphogenesis and missing thymus and pituitary gland. Failure in septum formation between trachea and the oesophagus in the knockout fetuses mimics the pathology of tracheo-oesophageal fistula. Furthermore, peripheral lung development is arrested at early pseudoglandular stage with a large airway sac, in which distal airway epithelial cells fail to express surfactant proteins and CCSP	36–38
Growth factors and their signalling pathways		
β-catenin (conditional knockout)	When β-catenin was conditionally excised in epithelial cells of the developing mouse lung prior to E14.5, the proximal lung tubules grew and differentiated appropriately. The mice died at birth because of respiratory failure. Lungs were composed primarily of proximal airways	39

(Continued . . .)

Table 29.1 (*Continued . . .*)

Gene	Pulmonary phenotype	Reference
Egfr(–/–) mice	*Egfr*(–/–) mice show abnormal branching and poor alveolization of lung. The severity of phenotypes depend on genetic background	40–42
Fgf10(–/–) mice	Tracheal development is present, but main-stem bronchial formation and all subsequent pulmonary branching morphogenesis, as well as vasculogenesis are completely disrupted	43,44
Fgf9(–/–) mice	*Fgf9*(–/–) mice die in the early postnatal period as a result of lung hypoplasia, particularly in mesenchyme. Lung branching morphogenesis is also inhibited, but proximal and distal airway cell differentiation is normal	45
Fgfr2(IIIb)(–/–) mice	Lung agenesis as in *Fgf10* null mutant	44,46
Igfr(–/–) mice	Severe growth deficiency and died at birth with respiratory failure	47
Pdgf-A(–/–) mice	*Pdgf-A*(–/–) mice survive postnatally, but develop lung emphysema secondary to the failure of alveolar septation	8
Pdgfr-α(–/–) mice	Failure of alveolar septation in postnatal lungs results in development of emphysema	10
Doxycycline-inducible SP-C-driven *mSpry4* TG mice	Continuous expression of *Spry4* caused severe lung hypoplasia. Expression of *Spry4* from E16.5 to 18.5 reduced lung growth and resulted in perinatal death from respiratory failure. Expression of *Spry4* from E18.5 to postnatal day 21, caused mild emphysema	48
Shh(–/–) mice	In *Shh* null mutant mice, embryo trachea and oesophagus do not separate properly and the lungs form a rudimentary sac because of failure of branching and growth after formation of the primary lung buds, but normal proximo-distal differentiation of the airway epithelium occurred	49–51
TGF-β1(–/–) mice	Develop normally but die within the first 2 months as a result of aggressive pulmonary inflammation. When raised under strict condition, they do not develop lung inflammation	52
TGF-β2(–/–) mice	Lung of E18.5 *TGF-β2*(–/–) mice shows dilated conducting airways and collapsed terminal and respiratory bronchioles	53,54
TGF-β3(–/–) mice	The hypoplastic lungs have thick mesenchyme between terminal airspaces. The number of C-positive cells is decreased and certain extracellular matrix protein expression is also reduced in TGF-β3-null mutant lungs	55,56
Extracellular matrix and others Elastin(–/–) mice	Terminal airway development is arrested, resulting in fewer and dilated distal air sac formation at birth	57
Fibrillin(–/–) mice	Lung abnormalities are evident in the immediate postnatal period and manifest as a developmental impairment of distal alveolar septation. Emphysema-like phenotype occurs in aged mice	58
Integrin *β6*(–/–) mice	Spontaneous, progressive pulmonary emphysema is developed in the adult null mutant mice, attributed to failure of activation of TGF-β1	59
LTBP4	Mice with homozygous disruption of *LTBP4* gene develop severe pulmonary emphysema with abnormal elastic fibre structure and reduced deposition of TGF-β in the extracellular space	60
SP-D(–/–) mice	Progressive development of pulmonary emphysema occurs from 3 weeks of age	61
TACE(–/–) mice	Lungs fail to form normal saccular structure with deficient sepatation and thick mesenchyme	62
TIMP3(–/–) mice	Progressive airspace enlargement is observed at 2 weeks. Aged animals have enhanced collagen degradation in the peribronchiolar space, and disorganization of collagen fibris in the alveolar interstitium	63

three proteins are expressed in lung epithelium. *Foxp1* and *Foxp4* are expressed in both proximal and distal airway epithelium while *Foxp2* is expressed primarily in distal epithelium. Foxp1 protein expression is also observed in the mesenchyme and vascular endothelial cells of the lung [3].

Nkx and Hox homoeodomain transcription factors

One of the most important homeodomain transcription factors in lung development is NKX2.1, also called TTF-1 (thyroid-specific transcription factor) or CEBP-1. *Nkx2.1* is expressed in foregut endoderm-derived epithelial cells including developing lungs, thyroid and pituitary, as well as in some restricted regions of fetal brain [79,80]. *Nkx2.1*(−/−) mice suffer severe impairment in branching morphogenesis of the lung and tracheo-oesophageal septum formation. The distal airway branches are totally absent, while only the two main bronchial stems are formed in *Nkx2.1* knockout mice, which indicates that lung development is arrested at a very early stage [36,37]. In developing mouse lung, *Nkx2.1* is expressed in the proximal and distal airway epithelia and, at later stages of lung development, in the distal alveolar epithelial cells [65]. *Nkx2.1* expression is strictly controlled, and increased expression of *Nkx2.1* causes dose-dependent morphological alterations in postnatal lung. Modest over-expression of *Nkx2.1* causes type II pneumocyte hyperplasia and increased levels of SP-B. Higher expression level of *Nkx2.1* disrupts alveolar septation, causing emphysema brought about by alveolar hypoplasia. The highest over-expression of *Nkx2.1* in transgenic mice causes severe pulmonary inflammation, fibrosis and respiratory failure, associated with eosinophil infiltration as well as increased expression of eotaxin and IL-6 [81]. Nkx2.1 is critical for surfactant protein, *T1α*, and *CCSP* gene expression [79,82–87]. *Nkx2.1*-deficient pulmonary epithelial cells fail to express non-ciliated marker genes, including differentiated *SP-B*, *SP-C* and *CCSP*. *Bmp4* expression in these cells is also reduced. Phosphorylation of NKX2.1 is important. Mice with point mutation of seven serine phosphorylation sites of NKX2.1 died immediately following birth with malformation of acinar tubules and pulmonary hypoplasia. Meanwhile, expression of surfactant proteins, secretoglobulin 1A, and VEGF was decreased [88]. *Nkx2.1* expression can be activated by HNF-3β [69] and GATA-6 [89] transcription factors during lung morphogenesis.

The expression of Hox transcription factors shows a proximal to distal polarity in developing lung. *Hoxa5*, *Hoxb2* and *Hoxb5* expression is restricted to distal lung mesenchyme. *Hoxb3* and *Hoxb4* genes are expressed in the mesenchyme of both proximal airway and distal lung [30,90,91]. The importance of these genes during lung development is well illustrated in gene targeting experiments in mice.

Hoxa5(−/−) null mutant mice display defects of tracheal formation and impaired lung branching morphogenesis, with tracheal occlusions, diminished surfactant protein expression and thickening of alveolar walls [30].

GLI family of zinc finger transcription factors

GLI 1–3 are very important zinc finger transcription factors, which are activated by the SHH pathway. All of them are expressed in lung mesoderm rather than endoderm, particularly in the distal portion [92]. Null mutation of *Gli2* plus *Gli3* genes results in total absence of lung. Mice with *Gli3* single deficiency are viable, but the size of the lung is smaller and the shape of the lung is also altered [92]. In *Gli2*(−/−) null mutant mice, the right and left lung are not separated but exist as a single lobe with a reduced size, and the primary branching in the right lung is defective. Also, both the trachea and oesophagus are hypoplastic, although they are separated from each other. However, proximal–distal differentiation is normal [27]. Therefore, *Gli2* has an important role in the asymmetric patterning of the lung.

Peptide growth factors that mediate cell–cell interaction

E11 mouse embryo lung can grow and branch spontaneously in serum-free medium *in vitro*. A variety of growth factors added into the culture medium can influence lung growth in the culture system [93,94]. Such experiments indicate that the embryonic lung mesenchymal and epithelial cells can communicate through autocrine or paracrine factors. In this way, different signalling pathways are coordinated to control lung growth at the right time and right place. Many of those factors are peptide growth factors, including FGF, EGF, TGF, IGF, PDGF and SHH. The expression and modification of these proteins and their downstream signalling components are strictly controlled during normal lung development. Loss of these gene function perturb normal lung development and function in mice (see Table 29.1).

FGF

FGF family members can be found in all vertebrate and invertebrate animals. Their regulatory functions during respiratory organogenesis are very well conserved from *Drosophila* [95,96] to mammals. Based on their protein sequence homology, FGFs have been divided into several subgroups. Similarly, their cognate transmembrane protein tyrosine kinase receptors are classified into several different types, contributing to the specificity of FGF ligand binding [97]. Heparin or heparan sulphate proteoglycan, an extracellular matrix protein, has been reported to be essential for FGF ligand–receptor binding and activation

[98–100]. FGFs have important roles in cell proliferation, migration and differentiation during embryo development. Inhibition of fibroblast growth factor receptor (FGFR) signalling at different stages of embryo development shows that FGF signalling is required for branching morphogenesis early in lung development. Later inhibition of FGFR signalling in E14.5 lung decreased lung tubule formation before birth and caused severe emphysema at maturity. In E16.5, FGFR inhibition caused mild focal emphysema. Inhibition of FGFR signalling after birth did not alter alveolarization [101].

One of the best-studied FGF family members during embryonic lung development is FGF10. Despite the formation of larynx and trachea, the distal embryonic lung is completely missing in *Fgf10(−/−)* null mice [43]. *Fgf10* is expressed in the mesenchyme of E11–12 mouse lungs, adjacent to distal epithelial tubules. These sites of expression change dynamically in a pattern that is compatible with the idea that FGF10 appears in the mesenchyme at prospective sites of bud formation [102]. Culture experiments have shown that FGF10 has a chemotactic effect on nearby epithelium, so that the nearby epithelial tips proliferate and migrate toward FGF10 expressing mesenchyme or FGF10 beads [103,104]. FGF10 also controls the differentiation of the epithelium by inducing *SP-C* expression and by down-regulating the expression of *Bmp4* [78]. Several other regulatory molecules such as SHH, BMP and TGF-β may cross-talk with FGF10 to coordinate control of embryonic lung morphogenesis. These interactions will be further discussed below.

FGF7 (KGF) is found in the developing lung mesenchyme during late stages [105]. In early cultured mouse embryonic lung, addition of FGF7 promotes epithelium growth, and formation of a cyst-like structure with extensive cell proliferation. FGF7 can also contribute to distal airway epithelial cell differentiation [106,107]. *Erm* and *Pea3* are ETS domain transcription factors known to be downstream of FGF signalling. FGF7 can induce *Erm/Pea3* expression more effectively than FGF10. *Erm* is transcribed exclusively in the epithelium, while *Pea3* is expressed in both epithelium and mesenchyme. When examined at E18.5, transgenic expression of a repressor form of *Erm* specifically in the embryonic lung epithelium shows that the distal epithelium of *SP-C–Erm* transgenic lungs is composed predominantly of immature type II cells, while no mature type I cells are observed. In contrast, the differentiation of proximal epithelial cells, including ciliated cells and Clara cells, appears to be unaffected [108,109]. FGF7 does not seem to protect against hyperoxic inhibition of normal postnatal alveoli formation and early pulmonary fibrosis, but FGF7 consistently had a significant protective and/or preventive effect against the development of pulmonary

hypertension during hyperoxia [110]. However, *Fgf7(−/−)* mutant mice have apparently no gross abnormalities in the lung [111], suggesting a redundant function of FGF7 with other factors during lung development.

Another FGF family member, FGF9, also regulates branching morphogenesis. In E10.5 lung, *Fgf9* is expressed in the visceral pleura lining the outside of the lung bud as well as in the epithelium of the developing bronchi. At E12.5 and E14.5, *Fgf9* expression persists in the mesothelium of the visceral pleura, but is no longer detected in airway epithelium [112]. *Fgf9* null mice exhibit reduced mesenchyme and decreased branching of the airways, but show significant distal airspace formation and pneumocyte differentiation. The reduction in the amount of mesenchyme in *Fgf9(−/−)* lungs limits expression of mesenchymal *Fgf10* [44]. Recombinant FGF9 protein inhibits the differentiation response of the mesenchyme to N-SHH, but does not affect proliferation [113].

The signalling cascade activated by FGF10 and FGF9 involves Raf, MAP ERK kinase (MEK), and extracellular-regulated kinases (ERK) 1 and 2 as signal transducers. MEK inhibition has been shown to reduce lung branching and epithelial cell proliferation, but to increase mesenchymal cell apoptosis in fetal lung explants [6]. FGF signalling is regulated at several levels. One of the key negative regulators is the sprouty family. There are four sprouty (*Spry*) genes in mouse (*mSpry1–4*) and human (*hSpry1–4*). Murine *Spry2* is expressed in the distal tip of embryonic lung epithelial branches, but is down-regulated between the sites of new bud formation. Murine *Spry4* is predominantly expressed in the distal mesenchyme of the embryonic lung [114], and may play a part in branching morphogenesis. Sprouties (SPRY1, -2, -4) act as suppressors of Ras-MAP kinase signalling [115–117]. Overexpression of *mSpry2* or *mSpry4* can inhibit lung branching morphogenesis through reducing epithelial cell proliferation [48,118,119]. SPRED-1 and SPRED-2 are two sprouty-related proteins, which contain EVH-1 domains. *Spreds* are predominantly expressed in mesenchymal cells. Expression of *Spreds* is especially strong in the peripheral mesenchyme and epithelium of new bud formation. After birth, *Spreds* expression decreases, while the expression of *Sprouties* expression is still high. Both *Sprouties* and *spreds* have important roles in mesenchyme–epithelium interaction during lung development [2].

TGF-β family growth factor

The transforming growth factor-β (TGF-β) superfamily comprises a large number of structurally related polypeptide growth factors including TGF-β, bone morphogenetic protein (BMP) and activin subfamilies. TGF-β ligands bind to their cognate receptors on the cell surface, and activate downstream Smad proteins, which translocate into the nucleus and modulate target gene expression [120,121].

TGF-β subfamily

TGF-β is well known for its inhibitory effects on embryonic lung branching morphogenesis. There are distinct expression patterns for the three isoforms of TGF-β: TGF-β1–3. In early mouse embryonic lung (E11.5), TGF-β1 is expressed in the mesenchyme, particularly in the mesenchyme underlying distal epithelial branching points, while TGF-β2 is localized in distal epithelium. TGF-β3 is mainly expressed in proximal mesenchyme and mesothelium [122–126]. Each isoform of TGF-β plays a unique and non-redundant role during embryonic development. Mice lacking TGF-β1 develop normally but die within the first 2 months of life as a result of aggressive pulmonary inflammation [52]. A TGF-β2(–/–) null mutation results in embryonic lethality around E14.5 in mice, and one of the abnormally developed organs is lung [53]. TGF-β3(–/–) null mutant mice display cleft palate, retarded lung development and neonatal lethality [55,56]. Misexpression of TGF-β1, leading to excessive TGF-β1 activation, always results in an adverse phenotype, which depends on the developmental stages at which TGF-β1 is expressed. Overexpression of TGF-β1 in early mouse embryonic lung epithelium inhibits lung branching morphogenesis *in vitro* [127], while misexpression of *SP-C* promoter controlled TGF-β1 in embryonic lung epithelium results in arrest of embryonic lung growth and epithelial cell differentiation, as well as inhibition of pulmonary vasculogenesis [128,129]. Clinically, the presence of excess TGF-β1 activity in tracheal aspirates of human premature infants who develop more severe bronchopulmonary dysplasia (BPD) suggests a crucial role for TGF-β1 in lung maturation [130,131]. On the other hand, misexpression of TGF-β1 in adult rats results in a chronic, progressive interstitial pulmonary fibrosis with increased proliferation and matrix secretion by the mesenchyme [132,133]. Misexpression of TGF-β1 in neonatal rat lung using recombinant adenoviral vectors results in neonatal alveolar hypoplasia and interstitial fibrosis that phenocopies BPD [134]. In addition, TGF-β1 may be one of the most important factors involved in the pulmonary inflammation response to exogenous factors, such as infection, bleomycin or endotoxin. Blockade of the TGF-β–Smad3 pathway in Smad3(–/–) null mutant mice strongly attenuates bleomycin-induced pulmonary fibrosis [133]. TGF-β activated kinase-1 binding protein-1 (TAB1) was identified as a molecule that activates TGF-β activated kinase-1 (TAK1). *Tab1* mutant embryonic fibroblast cells displayed drastically reduced TAK1 kinase activities and decreased sensitivity to TGF-β stimulation. *Tab1* mutant mice died due to cardiovascular and lung dysmorphogenesis [135].

The activity of TGF-β signalling can be regulated precisely at multiple levels. For example, β6 integrin, LTBPs and thrombospondin are involved in regulating the release of TGF-β mature peptide, while betaglycan, endoglin or decorin influence the affinity of TGF-β receptor binding. Mutation of the above genes displays phenotypes related to malfunction of TGF-β. For example, loss of function mutation both in the human and mouse endoglin gene, whose protein product binds to both TGF-β ligand and its type I receptor (Alk1), causes hereditary haemorrhagic telangiectasia [136–139].

BMP

Expression of *Bmp3, 4, 5* and *7* are detected in embryonic lung [140–142]. The expression of *Bmp5* and *Bmp7* has been detected in the mesenchyme and endoderm of developing embryonic lung, respectively, while *Bmp4* is expressed in a dynamic pattern that is restricted to the distal epithelial cells at high levels and adjacent mesenchyme at low level [140,141]. Misexpression of *Bmp4* under the control of the *SP-C* promoter in transgenic mice results in lungs that are smaller than normal with grossly dilated terminal sacs, which do not support gas exchange at birth [140]. BMP signalling also regulates proximal–distal differentiation of endoderm in mouse lung development. Inhibiting BMP signalling with BMP antagonist Xnoggin or overexpressed negative BMP receptor results in a severe reduction in distal epithelial cell types and a concurrent increase in proximal cell types [76]. The effect of BMP4 on embryonic lung development is still unclear. Addition of exogenous BMP4 into whole lung explant culture stimulates lung branching morphogenesis, while addition of BMP4 into isolated lung epithelial culture inhibits FGF10-induced epithelial growth [104,122,143]. In addition, BMP signalling is also important in lung vacuologenesis and angiogenesis. Mutations of BMP type II receptor (BMPRII) are associated with primary pulmonary hypertension (PPH) [144].

Sonic hedgehog (Shh) pathway

Sonic hedgehog is a vertebrate homologue of *hedgehog* (Hh) that patterns the segment, leg, wing, eye and brain in *Drosophila*. Hh binds to patched (Ptc), a transmembrane protein, and releases its inhibitory effect on downstream smoothened (Smo), which is a G protein-coupled 7-span transmembrane protein. This leads to the activation of cubitus interruptus (Ci), a 155-kD transcription factor that is usually cleaved to form a 75-kD transcription inhibitor in the cytosol. Elements of the *Drosophila* Hh signalling pathway and their general functions in the pathway are highly conserved in vertebrates, albeit with increased levels of complexity. Gli1, -2 and -3 are the three vertebrate Ci gene orthologues [145].

The SHH signal transduction pathway has important

roles in mesenchyme–epithelium interaction, which is very important in morphogenesis. In developing mouse lung, *Shh* is detected in the tracheal diverticulum, the oesophagus and later in the trachea and lung endoderm. *Shh* is expressed at low levels throughout the epithelium, while at higher level in the growing distal buds [146,147]. Null mutation of *Shh* produces profound hypoplasia of the lung and failure of trachea–oesophageal septation. Mesenchymal expression of *Ptc*, *Gli1* and *Gli3* is down-regulated. However, proximal–distal differentiation of epithelial airway is preserved [50,51]. Also, *Fgf10* expression is widespread in the epithelium in *Shh* null mutant lung, instead of the precisely location-restricted expression seen in wild-type controls. Lung-specific *Shh* overexpression results in severe alveolar hypoplasia and a significant increase in interstitial tissue caused by an increased proliferation of epithelium and mesenchyme [146]. Defective hedgehog signalling may lead to oesophageal atresia and tracheoesophageal fistula [148].

HIP1, a membrane-bound protein, directly binds all mammalian Hedgehog (HH) proteins and attenuates HH signalling [149]. *Hip1* is transcriptionally activated in response to Hh signalling, overlapping the expression domains of *Ptc1* [149,150]. Targeted disruption of *Hip1* results in neonatal lethality with respiratory failure. Although asymmetry in their growth was conserved, the initial stereotyped branching from the two primary buds was absent in *Hip1*(–/–) lungs. Hedgehog signalling is up-regulated in *Hip1* mutants. *Fgf10* expression was slightly down-regulated at the distal tips of the primary lung buds in *Hip1*(–/–) lungs at E10.5, but completely absent from the mesenchyme where secondary branching normally initiates [150]. Attenuated PTC1 activity in a *Hip1*(–/–) mutant lungs leads to an accelerated lethality. *Hip1* and *Ptc1* have redundant roles in lung branching control [150]. Both of them can attenuate SHH signal in lung and pancreas development [150,151].

Wnt–β-catenin pathway

Wnt signals are transduced through seven transmembrane-type Wnt receptors encoded by *Frizzled* (*Fzd*) genes to activate the β-catenin–TCF pathway, the JNK pathway or the Ca^{2+}-releasing pathway. The Wnt–β-catenin pathway has a critical role in many developmental and tumorigenesis processes. Following Wnt binding to the receptor, β-catenin is dephosphorylated and translocates to the nucleus to activate downstream gene expression [152].

Interestingly, all members of *Fzd* gene family are expressed in embryonic and neonatal lung, albeit at different levels. *Fzd* genes are differentially expressed in the epithelium and mesenchyme. Expression of *Fzd2*, *Fzd5*, *Fzd6* and *Fzd8* was observed predominantly in the epithelium, while *Fzd4* and *Fzd10* were expressed in the

mesenchyme. Expression of *Fzd1* and *Fzd7* was observed both in the epithelium and mesenchyme, while *Fzd3* and *Fzd9* were only marginally expressed. This spatial distribution suggests differential roles for different *Fzd* receptor genes in the Wnt signalling pathway during the development of the lung [39].

In mouse lung development, between embryonic days 10.5 and 17.5 (E10.5–E17.5), β-catenin was localized in the cytoplasm, and often also in the nucleus of the undifferentiated primordial epithelium, differentiating alveolar epithelium, and adjacent mesenchyme. Other Wnt–β-catenin pathway members, *Tcf1*, *Lef1*, *Tcf3*, *Tcf4*, *sFrp1*, *sFrp2* and *sFrp4*, are also expressed in the primordial epithelium, alveolar epithelium and adjacent mesenchyme in specific spatiotemporal patterns [153]. In human fetal lung, nuclear β-catenin is present in pulmonary acinar buds [154]. Null mutation of β-catenin in mice results in abnormal, cystic structure formation in the lung and prenatal lethality. Based on molecular marker detection, the lungs are composed primarily of proximal airways, suggesting that β-catenin is one of the essential components to specify proximal–distal axis of the lung [39].

EGF family growth factors

EGF, transforming growth factor-α (TGF-α) and amphiregulin are all epidermal growth factor receptor (EGFR) ligands. Loss or gain of function experiments in mice, rat or other animal models proves that EGF ligands can positively modulate early mouse embryonic lung branching morphogenesis and cytodifferentiation through EGFR [94,155, 156]. EGF is also expressed in mature alveolar epithelial cells and regulates type II cell proliferation through an autocrine mechanism both *in vitro* and *in vivo* [157]. However, respiratory epithelial cell overexpression of TGF-α under the control of the *SP-C* promoter of transgenic mice induces postnatal lung fibrosis [158]. Overexpression of TGF-α caused severe pulmonary vascular disease, which was mediated through EGFR signalling in distal epithelial cells. Reductions in VEGF may contribute to the pathogenesis of pulmonary vascular disease in TGF-α overexpressing mice [159].

EGFR is a tyrosine kinase receptor that transfers EGF signals into the cell. Abnormal branching and poor alveolization are observed in mice deficient in epidermal growth factor receptor (*Egfr*(–/–)). Mechanical stretch stimulated EGFR phosphorylation at least in part, induces differentiation of fetal epithelial cells via EGFR activation of the ERK pathway. Blockade of the EGFR or ERK pathway by specific inhibitors decreased stretch-inducible *SP-C* mRNA expression, suggesting EGFR may be part of a mechanical stimulus signal sensor during fetal lung development [160]. Aberrant expression of matrix metaloprotease proteins (MMPs) is also detected in *Egfr*(–/–) null mutant mice, which suggests MMPs may be involved in EGFR-regulated lung growth [40].

Tumour necrosis factor-α converting enzyme (TACE) is a transmembrane metalloprotease-disintegrin that functions as a membrane sheddase to release the ectodomain portions of many transmembrane proteins, including the precursors of TNF-α and several other cytokines, as well as the receptors for TNF-α, and neuregulin (ErbB4) [161]. Neonatal TACE-deficient mice had visible respiratory distress and their lungs failed to form normal saccular structures resulting in a reduction of normal air exchange surface. In mouse embryonic lung explant cultures, TGF-α and EGF can rescue lung development in the presence of TACE deficiency [62].

PDGF

There are four types of PDGF peptides. PDGF-A and PDGF-B can form homodimers (AA or BB) or heterodimers (AB). Two types of PDGF receptors, α and β, are present in embryonic mouse lung, and are differentially regulated in fetal rat lung epithelial cells and fibroblasts [162]. PDGF-A regulates both DNA synthesis and early branching in early mouse embryonic lung epithelium *in vitro* [163]. *Pdgf-A* homozygous null mutant mice die perinatally. The pulmonary phenotypes include lack of lung alveolar smooth muscle cells (SMC), reduced deposition of elastin fibres in the lung parenchyma, and development of lung emphysema because of complete failure of alveogenesis [8,10]. Abrogation of PDGF-B chain expression with antisense oligodeoxynucleotides reduces the size of the epithelial component of early embryonic mouse lung explants, but does not reduce the number of branches [164]. PDGF-B and its receptor are crucial for vascular growth and integrity during the alveolar phase [9]. PDGF-C and PDGF-D also dimerize and bind to PDGF α or β receptor [165,166]. PDGF-C mRNA expression shows a significant increase in lung fibrosis induced by bleomycin [167].

IGF

The insulin-like growth factors (IGFs) and their receptors are expressed in both rodent and human fetal lung [168–172]. Null mutant mice for the cognate type 1 IGF receptor (*Igf1r*) gene always die at birth with respiratory failure and severe growth deficiency (45% of normal birth weight). Dwarfism is further exacerbated (70% of size reduction) in either *Igf1* and *Igf2* double null mutants or in *Igf1r* and *Igf2* double null mutants. There does not appear to be a gross defect in primary branching morphogenesis per se; the lungs merely appear hypoplastic [47]. IGF signalling may have a role in facilitating other peptide growth factor pathways during lung morphogenesis. IGF1R signalling function is required for both the mitogenic and transforming activities of the EGF receptor [173]. The lungs display reduced airspace in *Igf1*-deficient embryos and neonates,

and the phenotype is exacerbated in additionally leukaemia inhibitory factor (*Lif*) null mutant mice, which showed abnormal epithelial cells and decreased SP-B expression. In addition, *Nkx2.1* and *SP-B* expression is reduced in the lung of these double null mutant neonates. Thus, LIF and IGF-I have cooperative and distinct tissue functions during lung development [174]. IGF1 is also a potent trophic factor for fetal lung endothelial cells. In human fetal lung explants, inactivation of IGF-IR results in a loss of endothelial cells, attenuates time-dependent increase in budding of distal airway and increases mesenchymal cell apoptosis [175].

VEGF isoforms and cognate receptors

Lung development must form a fine alignment between the alveolar surface and the surrounding pulmonary capillary system for effective gas exchange. Vascular endothelial growth factors (VEGF) are potent effectors of vascular development in lung morphogenesis. VEGF signals through the cognate receptors Flk-1 (fetal liver kinase-1, VEGFR2) and Flt-1 (fetal liver tyrosinase-1, VEGFR1) [176]. VEGF is diffusely distributed in pulmonary epithelial and mesenchymal cells, and is involved in controlling endothelial proliferation and the maintenance of vascular structure [177]. VEGF can be regulated by hypoxia-inducible transcription factor-2α [178].

Vasculogenesis is initiated as soon as the lung evaginates from the foregut epithelium [179]. Development of the vascular system influences branching morphogenesis of the airway as well as alveolarization. In transgenic mice, where the *Vegf* transgene is misexpressed under the control of the *SP-C* promoter, gross abnormalities in lung morphogenesis are associated with a decrease in acinar tubules and mesenchyme [180]. VEGF has also been demonstrated to have a role in maintaining alveolar structure [17]. Lungs from newborn mice treated with antibodies to Flt-1 were reduced in size and displayed significant immaturity with a less complex alveolar pattern [181].

Extracellular matrix and lung development

The protein components of extracellular basement membrane, laminins, entactin/nidogen, type IV collagen, perlecan, SPARC and fibromodulin, are important in mediating cell–cell and cell–extracellular matrix (ECM) interaction during fetal lung morphogenesis. Basement membrane components are differentially expressed, and have a specific cell distribution during lung morphogenesis. ECM components may not only provide the support for tissue architecture, but may also have an active role in modulation of cell proliferation and differentiation [182]. For example, basement membrane components may serve as a barrier and reservoir of growth factors, which in turn regulate epithelial and mesenchymal cell proliferation.

Absence or inhibition of the interaction of epithelial cells with the basement membrane results in failure of normal lung development [183,184].

Laminins (LNs) are glycoproteins involved in cell adhesion, migration, proliferation and differentiation during tissue development and remodelling. LNs are composed of three chains, one central (α) and two laterals (β and γ) that are linked by disulphide bonds to form a cross-shaped molecule [185]. To date, five α, three β and three γ chain isoforms have been identified, which suggests that their combination can lead to approximately 30 variants of LN [186–195]. The α1 chain has been found principally localized in the basement membrane at the epithelial–mesenchymal interface, with a predominant distribution in specific zones. The LN α1 chain has also been identified around some mesenchymal cells. Molecular analysis dissecting the α1 chain isoform has shown that a domain in the cross-region of the α1 chain is involved in the regulation of lung epithelial cell proliferation [196]. The α4 chain, found in LN8 and LN9 variants, has been reported to be highly expressed in lung and heart tissues during mouse development [189–191,197]. The LN α4 chain, localized principally around vessels in fetal lung, may have a role in the organization of lung mesenchyme [194,198]. The α5 chain, found in LN10 and LN11, has been found to be abundantly expressed during fetal lung morphogenesis [194,199,200]. Mouse embryos bearing mutated LN α5 chain isoform display poor lobar septation and bronchiolar branching, suggesting that the LN α5 chain isoform might be the most indispensable LN variant for lung branching morphogenesis.

A constant expression of β1 and γ1 is observed during fetal lung development [201]. These two chains also have a role in cell adhesion. The globular domains near the N-terminal of B1 and γ1 chains participate in the regulation of cell polarization [202,203]. Immunohistochemistry studies have demonstrated that the LN β2 chain isoform is localized in the basement membrane of prealveolar ducts, airways, smooth muscle cells of airways, and arterial blood vessels, as well as type II pneumocytes.

Nidogen (150 kDa) is a constituent of the basement membranes. Nidogen binds to the γ1 and γ3 chains of LN, and forms a link between LN and collagen IV [193, 204,205]. Nidogen is actively synthesized by mesenchymal cells during fetal lung development, which suggests that nidogen has a key role in the organization of the basement membrane during lung morphogenesis [206]. Blocking the interaction of nidogen with LN affects the progression of lung development [204,206,207]. Susceptibility of nidogen to degradation by matrix metalloproteinases may contribute to the remodelling and degradation of the basement membrane [208].

Proteoglycans (PGs) contain a core protein with sulphated carbohydrate side chains. They function as flexible structures in the organization of the basement membrane and may also have an important role as a reservoir for growth factors, water and ions. Perlecan is a predominant proteoglycan in the basement membrane. It is composed of an approximately 450-kDa core protein with three heparan sulphate chains. Perlecan is involved in the control of smooth cell proliferation and differentiation because increased cell proliferation of fetal lung smooth muscle cells is accompanied by a highly increased synthesis of perlecan [209]. Growth and branching of E13 mouse lung explants can be disrupted by inhibiting PG sulphation. The migration of epithelial cells towards invading lung mesenchyme as well as towards beads soaked in FGF10 is inhibited and branching morphogenesis in lung mesenchymal and epithelial tissue recombinants is severely decreased when PG sulphation is inhibited by chlorate.

Fibronectin also has an important role in lung development. In branching morphogenesis, repetitive epithelial cleft and bud formation creates the complex three-dimensional branching structure characteristic of many organs. Fibronectin is essential for cleft formation during the initiation of epithelial branching in salivary gland. Immunofluorescence comparisons of fibronectin localization during early branching of lung and kidney also showed an accumulation of fibronectin at sites of epithelial constriction and indentation [210], supporting a possible role for fibronectin in branching morphogenesis of the lung [211]. Direct tests for the role of fibronectin, by treatment of developing lung rudiments with antifibronectin antibody or siRNA, inhibited branching morphogenesis, while fibronectin supplementation promoted branching of lung [210]. The EIIIA segment of fibronectin is one of the major alternatively spliced segments and modulates the cell proliferative potential of fibronectin *in vitro*. The EIIIA-containing fibronectin isoform localized in both the epithelial cells and the mesenchyme. Its expression gradually decreased from the pseudoglandular stage to the saccular stage and then slightly increased from the saccular stage to the alveolar stage. This change in expression pattern of EIIIA-containing fibronectin seemed to be in accord with the change in the number of proliferating cell nuclear antigen (PCNA)-positive cells in the distal pulmonary cells throughout lung development [212].

Extracellular matrix is under dynamic control during lung development. The matrix metalloproteinases (MMPs) are a large family of ECM-degrading enzymes. They are inhibited by the family of tissue inhibitors of metalloproteinases (TIMPs). Activity of MMPs may be required during development and normal physiology in several ways:

1 to degrade ECM molecules and allow cell migration;

2 to alter the ECM microenvironment and result in alteration in cellular behaviour;

3 to modulate the activity of biologically active molecules by direct cleavage, release from bound stores, or by modulating of activity of their inhibitors [213].

In *Timp3* null mutant mouse lung, airway branching is inhibited. Compared with wild type, in the *Timp3* null mouse the number of bronchioles is reduced and alveologenesis is attenuated [214]. The *Timp3* null animals spontaneously develop progressive alveolar airspace enlargement similar to that seen in human emphysema [215]. Early postnatal exposure to dexamethasone (Dex) influences MMP2 and MMP9, as well as their tissue inhibitors (TIMP1 and TIMP2) in the developing rat lung; the expression of *Timp2* is reduced and *Mmp9* expression increases. These changes may be responsible, in part, for some of the known adverse maturational effects of steroids on lung structure in the newborn [216]. MT1-MMP, which acts as a potent activator of MMP2, is a major downstream target of EGFR signalling in lung. *Egfr*(–/–) mice had low expression of *MT1-Mmp*. Extracts from lungs of *Egfr*(–/–) mice showed a 10-fold reduction in active MMP-2. At birth, the abnormal lung alveolization phenotype of *Mmp2*(–/–) mice is similar to that of *Egfr*(–/–) mice, albeit somewhat less severe [40]. The balance between the activity of MMPs and TIMPs is important to normal lung development.

Retinoic acid and lung morphogenesis

Retinoids (all-*trans*, 9-*cis*, 13-*cis*) are fundamental for normal development and homoeostasis of a number of biological systems including the lung. There is a precisely controlled RA synthesis and degradation system in mammals [217]. Retinaldehyde dehydrogenase-2 (RALDH-2) has a prominent role in generating RA during organogenesis [218–220]. RA signalling is mediated by its nuclear receptors of the steroid hormone receptor superfamily: RAR (α, β, γ) and retinoid RXR (α, β, γ), [217]. RAR/RXR heterodimers have also been shown to transduce RA signalling *in vivo* [221]. Within the E13.5 lung, *Rarβ* isoform transcripts are specifically localized to the proximal airway epithelium and immediately adjacent mesenchyme, whereas *Rarα1*, *Rarα2* and *Rarγ2* isoforms are ubiquitously expressed [222].

RA signalling is required for lung bud initiation. Acute vitamin A deprivation in pregnant rats at the onset of lung development results in blunt-end tracheae and lung agenesis in some embryos, which is similar to *Fgf10*(–/–) null mutant mice [223,224]. Disruption of RA signalling in *Rarα/β2* knockout mice leads to agenesis of the left lung and hypoplasia of the right lung [225]. Interestingly, lung branching morphogenesis is characterized by a dramatic down-regulation of RA signalling in the lung. Treating embryonic lung explants with high concentrations of RA (10^{-6}–10^{-5} mol) results in dramatic disruption of distal budding and formation of proximal-like immature airways

[226,227]. Continued RA activation by overexpression of constitutively activated *Rarα* chimeric receptors also resulted in lung immaturity, and lungs did not expand to form saccules or morphologically identifiable type I cells. High levels of *SP-C*, *Nkx2.1* and *Gata6*, but not *SP-A* or *SP-B*, in the epithelium at birth suggested that in these lungs differentiation was arrested at an early stage. Downregulation of RA signalling, however, is required to allow completion of later steps of this differentiation programme that ultimately forms mature type I and II cells [228]. RA inhibits expression and alters distribution of *Fgf10* and *Bmp4*, which are required for distal lung formation [226,227]. Pan-RAR antagonism alters the expression of *Tgf-β3*, *Hnf-3β* and *Cftr* in proximal tubules and alters expression of *Bmp4*, *Fgf10* and *Shh* within the distal buds [222].

It is also noteworthy that during early stages of lung branching (days 11–12.5), *Raldh-2* expression is concentrated in trachea (mesenchyme) and proximal lung (mesothelium) at sites of low branching activity. The *Raldh-2* pattern is not overlapping with that of *Fgf10*, supporting the idea that RA signalling restricts *Fgf10* expression and helps to define the proximal–distal axis of the developing lung. However, during later postnatal stages of lung development, RA has been shown to increase the number of alveoli and therefore partially rescue dexamethasone-induced suppression of alveolarization. In adult rats, RA has also been reported to reverse the anatomical features of elastase-induced emphysema in which there is destruction of septal structures [18,19,229]. In the *Rarγ* gene deletion mouse, there is a developmental defect in alveolar formation, consistent with a defect in elastin deposition [21]. This combined evidence suggests that RA may have an important but rather complex role in alveolar development during late lung development.

Lung development and COPD

Chronic obstructive pulmonary disease (COPD) is defined as airflow obstruction that does not change appreciably over a period of several months. It is a syndrome comprised of chronic bronchitis, small airways disease (bronchiolitis) and emphysema, which vary in proportion between affected individuals [230]. There is some structural remodelling inappropriate to maintaining normal lung function, and chronic inflammation characterized by infiltration of airways, pulmonary vessels and lung parenchyma by CD8[+] T-cytotoxic lymphocytes. Small airways mucous metaplasia, increased small airways smooth muscle mass, airway wall fibrosis, and emphysema are specific features of structural remodelling in COPD [231].

COPD results from a complex interaction between

genetic and environmental factors. The normal interactions between mesenchymal and epithelial cells that maintains proper structure and function of the airways and gas exchange surface, as described herein, are dramatically perturbed. The structural damage of lung in COPD cannot be repaired or regenerated properly, suggesting that stem or progenitor cell reparative functions are overwhelmed and some important signal transduction pathways that control lung development have been perturbed, leading to abnormal airway remodelling in COPD. It is likely that developmental processes have a role in abnormal tissue remodelling in COPD. For example, *Shh* is up-regulated in epithelial cells at sites of fibrotic disease and the Shh receptor Patched was detected in infiltrating mononuclear cells and alveolar macrophages, as well as normal resting peripheral blood T lymphocytes [232]. On the other hand, RA, which has an important role in lung morphogenesis and alveolarization, can induce the complete regeneration of alveoli that have been destroyed by various noxious treatments in some experimental systems [229]. Therefore, continued elucidation of the molecular mechanisms of lung development may identify novel rationally based therapeutic targets in the quest to prevent and even cure COPD.

References

1 Sakiyama J, Yamagishi A, Kuroiwa A. Tbx4-Fgf10 system controls lung bud formation during chicken embryonic development. *Development* 2003;**130**:1225–34.

2 Hashimoto S, Nakano H, Singh G, Katyal S. Expression of Spred and Sprouty in developing rat lung. *Mech Dev* 2002; **119**(Suppl 1):S303–9.

3 Lu MM, Li S, Yang H, Morrisey EE. Foxp4: a novel member of the Foxp subfamily of winged-helix genes co-expressed with Foxp1 and Foxp2 in pulmonary and gut tissues. *Mech Dev* 2002;**119**(Suppl 1):S197–202.

4 Blewett CJ, Zgleszewski SE, Chinoy MR, Krummel TM, Cilley RE. Bronchial ligation enhances murine fetal lung development in whole-organ culture. *J Pediatr Surg* 1996; **31**:869–77.

5 Kitano Y, Yang EY, von Allmen D *et al.* Tracheal occlusion in the fetal rat: a new experimental model for the study of accelerated lung growth. *J Pediatr Surg* 1998;**33**:1741–4.

6 Papadakis K, Luks FI, De Paepe ME, Piasecki GJ, Wesselhoeft CW Jr. Fetal lung growth after tracheal ligation is not solely a pressure phenomenon. *J Pediatr Surg* 1997; **32**:347–51.

7 Inanlou MR, Kablar B. Abnormal development of the diaphragm in mdx:MyoD–/–(9th) embryos leads to pulmonary hypoplasia. *Int J Dev Biol* 2003;**47**:363–71.

8 Bostrom H, Willetts K, Pekny M *et al.* PDGF-A signalling is a critical event in lung alveolar myofibroblast development and alveogenesis. *Cell* 1996;**85**:863–73.

9 Lindahl P, Karlsson L, Hellstrom M *et al.* Alveogenesis failure in PDGF-A-deficient mice is coupled to lack of distal spreading of alveolar smooth muscle cell progenitors during lung development. *Development* 1997;**124**:3943–53.

10 Bostrom H, Gritli-Linde A, Betsholtz C. PDGF-A/PDGF alpha-receptor signalling is required for lung growth and the formation of alveoli but not for early lung branching morphogenesis. *Dev Dyn* 2002;**223**:155–62.

11 Wu JY, Feng L, Park HT *et al.* The neuronal repellent Slit inhibits leukocyte chemotaxis induced by chemotactic factors. *Nature* 2001;**410**:948–52.

12 Anselmo MA, Dalvin S, Prodhan P *et al.* Slit and robo: expression patterns in lung development. *Gene Expr Patterns* 2003;**3**:13–9.

13 Xian J, Clark KJ, Fordham R *et al.* Inadequate lung development and bronchial hyperplasia in mice with a targeted deletion in the *Dutt1/Robo1* gene. *Proc Natl Acad Sci U S A* 2001;**98**:15 062–6.

14 Awonusonu F, Srinivasan S, Strange J, Al Jumaily W, Bruce MC. Developmental shift in the relative percentages of lung fibroblast subsets: role of apoptosis postseptation. *Am J Physiol* 1999;**277**:L848–59.

15 Schittny JC, Djonov V, Fine A, Burri PH. Programmed cell death contributes to postnatal lung development. *Am J Respir Cell Mol Biol* 1998;**18**:786–93.

16 Srinivasan S, Strange J, Awonusonu F, Bruce MC. Insulin-like growth factor I receptor is downregulated after alveolarization in an apoptotic fibroblast subset. *Am J Physiol Lung Cell Mol Physiol* 2002;**282**:L457–67.

17 Kasahara Y, Tuder RM, Taraseviciene-Stewart L *et al.* Inhibition of VEGF receptors causes lung cell apoptosis and emphysema. *J Clin Invest* 2000;**106**:1311–9.

18 Massaro GD, Massaro D. Postnatal treatment with retinoic acid increases the number of pulmonary alveoli in rats. *Am J Physiol* 1996;**270**:L305–10.

19 Massaro GD, Massaro D. Retinoic acid treatment partially rescues failed septation in rats and in mice. *Am J Physiol Lung Cell Mol Physiol* 2000;**278**:L955–60.

20 McGowan S, Jackson SK, Jenkins-Moore M *et al.* Mice bearing deletions of retinoic acid receptors demonstrate reduced lung elastin and alveolar numbers. *Am J Respir Cell Mol Biol* 2000;**23**:162–7.

21 Chytil F. Retinoids in lung development. *FASEB J* 1996; **10**:986–92.

22 Vermeer PD, Harson R, Einwalter LA, Moninger T, Zabner J. Interleukin-9 induces goblet cell hyperplasia during repair of human airway epithelia. *Am J Respir Cell Mol Biol* 2003;**28**: 286–95.

23 Lordan JL, Bucchieri F, Richter A *et al.* Cooperative effects of Th2 cytokines and allergen on normal and asthmatic bronchial epithelial cells. *J Immunol* 2002;**169**:407–14.

24 Ramirez MI, Millien G, Hinds A *et al.* T1α, a lung type I cell differentiation gene, is required for normal lung cell proliferation and alveolus formation at birth. *Dev Biol* 2003;**256**: 61–72.

25 Costa RH, Kalinichenko VV, Lim L. Transcription factors in mouse lung development and function. *Am J Physiol Lung Cell Mol Physiol* 2001;**280**:L823–38.

26 Mo R, Freer AM, Zinyk DL *et al.* Specific and redundant functions of Gli2 and Gli3 zinc finger genes in skeletal patterning and development. *Development* 1997;**124**:113–23.

27 Motoyama J, Liu J, Mo R *et al*. Essential function of Gli2 and Gli3 in the formation of lung, trachea and oesophagus. *Nat Genet* 1998;**20**:54–7.

28 Brody SL, Yan XH, Wuerffel MK, Song SK, Shapiro SD. Ciliogenesis and left–right axis defects in forkhead factor HFH-4-null mice. *Am J Respir Cell Mol Biol* 2000;**23**:45–51.

29 Chen J, Knowles HJ, Hebert JL, Hackett BP. Mutation of the mouse hepatocyte nuclear factor/forkhead homologue 4 gene results in an absence of cilia and random left–right asymmetry. *J Clin Invest* 1998;**102**:1077–82.

30 Aubin J, Lemieux M, Tremblay M, Berard J, Jeannotte L. Early postnatal lethality in *Hoxa-5* mutant mice is attributable to respiratory tract defects. *Dev Biol* 1997;**192**:432–45.

31 Aubin J, Chailler P, Menard D, Jeannotte L. Loss of *Hoxa5* gene function in mice perturbs intestinal maturation. *Am J Physiol* 1999;**277**:C965–73.

32 Quaggin SE, Schwartz L, Cui S *et al*. The basic-helix-loop-helix protein pod1 is critically important for kidney and lung organogenesis. *Development* 1999;**126**:5771–83.

33 Chen H, Sun J, Buckley S *et al*. Abnormal mouse lung alveolarization caused by Smad3 deficiency is a developmental antecedent of centrilobular emphysema. *Am J Physiol Lung Cell Mol Physiol* 2005;**288**(4):L683–91.

34 Tichelaar JW, Lim L, Costa RH, Whitsett JA. HNF-3/forkhead homologue-4 influences lung morphogenesis and respiratory epithelial cell differentiation *in vivo*. *Dev Biol* 1999;**213**:405–17.

35 Zhou L, Dey CR, Wert SE *et al*. Hepatocyte nuclear factor-3β limits cellular diversity in the developing respiratory epithelium and alters lung morphogenesis *in vivo*. *Dev Dyn* 1997;**210**:305–14.

36 Kimura S, Hara Y, Pineau T *et al*. The T/ebp null mouse: thyroid-specific enhancer-binding protein is essential for the organogenesis of the thyroid, lung, ventral forebrain, and pituitary. *Genes Dev* 1996;**10**:60–9.

37 Minoo P, Su G, Drum H, Bringas P, Kimura S. Defects in tracheoesophageal and lung morphogenesis in Nkx2.1(–/–) mouse embryos. *Dev Biol* 1999;**209**:60–71.

38 Yuan B, Li C, Kimura S *et al*. Inhibition of distal lung morphogenesis in Nkx2.1(–/–) embryos. *Dev Dyn* 2000;**217**:180–90.

39 Mucenski ML, Wert SE, Nation JM *et al*. β-Catenin is required for specification of proximal/distal cell fate during lung morphogenesis. *J Biol Chem* 2003;**278**:40231–8.

40 Kheradmand F, Rishi K, Werb Z. Signalling through the EGF receptor controls lung morphogenesis in part by regulating MT1-MMP-mediated activation of gelatinase A/MMP2. *J Cell Sci* 2002;**115**:839–48.

41 Miettinen PJ, Berger JE, Meneses J *et al*. Epithelial immaturity and multiorgan failure in mice lacking epidermal growth factor receptor. *Nature* 1995;**376**:337–41.

42 Threadgill DW, Dlugosz AA, Hansen LA *et al*. Targeted disruption of mouse EGF receptor: effect of genetic background on mutant phenotype. *Science* 1995;**269**:230–4.

43 Min H, Danilenko DM, Scully SA *et al*. Fgf-10 is required for both limb and lung development and exhibits striking functional similarity to *Drosophila* branchless. *Genes Dev* 1998;**12**:3156–61.

44 Ohuchi H, Hori Y, Yamasaki M *et al*. FGF10 acts as a major ligand for FGF receptor 2 IIIb in mouse multi-organ development. *Biochem Biophys Res Commun* 2000;**277**:643–9.

45 Colvin JS, White AC, Pratt SJ, Ornitz DM. Lung hypoplasia and neonatal death in Fgf9-null mice identify this gene as an essential regulator of lung mesenchyme. *Development* 2001;**128**:2095–106.

46 De Moerlooze L, Spencer-Dene B, Revest J *et al*. An important role for the IIIb isoform of fibroblast growth factor receptor 2 (FGFR2) in mesenchymal–epithelial signalling during mouse organogenesis. *Development* 2000;**127**:483–92.

47 Liu JP, Baker J, Perkins AS, Robertson EJ, Efstratiadis A. Mice carrying null mutations of the genes encoding insulin-like growth factor I (Igf-1) and type 1 IGF receptor (Igf1r). *Cell* 1993;**75**:59–72.

48 Perl AK, Hokuto I, Impagnatiello MA, Christofori G, Whitsett JA. Temporal effects of Sprouty on lung morphogenesis. *Dev Biol* 2003;**258**:154–68.

49 Chiang C, Litingtung Y, Lee E *et al*. Cyclopia and defective axial patterning in mice lacking Sonic hedgehog gene function. *Nature* 1996;**383**:407–13.

50 Litingtung Y, Lei L, Westphal H, Chiang C. Sonic hedgehog is essential to foregut development. *Nat Genet* 1998;**20**:58–61.

51 Pepicelli CV, Lewis PM, McMahon AP. Sonic hedgehog regulates branching morphogenesis in the mammalian lung. *Curr Biol* 1998;**8**:1083–6.

52 McLennan IS, Poussart Y, Koishi K. Development of skeletal muscles in transforming growth factor-beta 1 (TGF-β1) null-mutant mice. *Dev Dyn* 2000;**217**:250–6.

53 Bartram U, Molin DG, Wisse LJ *et al*. Double-outlet right ventricle and overriding tricuspid valve reflect disturbances of looping, myocardialization, endocardial cushion differentiation, and apoptosis in TGF-β(2)-knockout mice. *Circulation* 2001;**103**:2745–52.

54 Sanford LP, Ormsby I, Gittenberger-de Groot AC *et al*. TGFβ2 knockout mice have multiple developmental defects that are non-overlapping with other TGFβ knockout phenotypes. *Development* 1997;**124**:2659–70.

55 Kaartinen V, Voncken JW, Shuler C *et al*. Abnormal lung development and cleft palate in mice lacking TGF-β3 indicates defects of epithelial–mesenchymal interaction. *Nat Genet* 1995;**11**:415–21.

56 Shi W, Heisterkamp N, Groffen J *et al*. TGFβ3-null mutation does not abrogate fetal lung maturation *in vivo* by glucocorticoids. *Am J Physiol* 1999;**277**:L1205–13.

57 Wendel DP, Taylor DG, Albertine KH, Keating MT, Li DY. Impaired distal airway development in mice lacking elastin. *Am J Respir Cell Mol Biol* 2000;**23**:320–6.

58 Neptune ER, Frischmeyer PA, Arking DE *et al*. Dysregulation of TGFβ activation contributes to pathogenesis in Marfan syndrome. *Nat Genet* 2003;**33**:407–11.

59 Morris DG, Huang X, Kaminski N *et al*. Loss of integrin α(v)β6-mediated TGFβ activation causes MMP12-dependent emphysema. *Nature* 2003;**422**:169–73.

60 Sterner-Kock A, Thorey IS, Koli K *et al*. Disruption of the gene encoding the latent transforming growth factor-β

binding protein 4 (LTBP-4) causes abnormal lung development, cardiomyopathy, and colorectal cancer. *Genes Dev* 2002;**16**:2264–73.

61 Yoshida M, Korfhagen TR, Whitsett JA. Surfactant protein D regulates NF-κB and matrix metalloproteinase production in alveolar macrophages via oxidant-sensitive pathways. *J Immunol* 2001;**166**:7514–9.

62 Zhao J, Chen H, Peschon JJ *et al*. Pulmonary hypoplasia in mice lacking tumor necrosis factor-α converting enzyme indicates an indispensable role for cell surface protein shedding during embryonic lung branching morphogenesis. *Dev Biol* 2001;**232**:204–18.

63 Leco KJ, Waterhouse P, Sanchez OH *et al*. Spontaneous air space enlargement in the lungs of mice lacking tissue inhibitor of metalloproteinases-3 (TIMP-3). *J Clin Invest* 2001;**108**:817–29.

64 Qian X, Costa RH. Analysis of hepatocyte nuclear factor-3β protein domains required for transcriptional activation and nuclear targeting. *Nucleic Acids Res* 1995;**23**:1184–91.

65 Zhou L, Lim L, Costa RH, Whitsett JA. Thyroid transcription factor-1, hepatocyte nuclear factor-3β, surfactant protein B, C, and Clara cell secretory protein in developing mouse lung. *J Histochem Cytochem* 1996;**44**:1183–93.

66 Bingle CD, Hackett BP, Moxley M, Longmore W, Gitlin JD. Role of hepatocyte nuclear factor-3α and hepatocyte nuclear factor-3β in Clara cell secretory protein gene expression in the bronchiolar epithelium. *Biochem J* 1995;**308**:197–202.

67 Bohinski RJ, Di Lauro R, Whitsett JA. The lung-specific surfactant protein B gene promoter is a target for thyroid transcription factor 1 and hepatocyte nuclear factor 3, indicating common factors for organ-specific gene expression along the foregut axis. *Mol Cell Biol* 1994;**14**:5671–81.

68 He Y, Crouch EC, Rust K, Spaite E, Brody SL. Proximal promoter of the surfactant protein D gene: regulatory roles of AP-1, forkhead box, and GT box binding proteins. *J Biol Chem* 2000;**275**:31051–60.

69 Ikeda K, Shaw-White JR, Wert SE, Whitsett JA. Hepatocyte nuclear factor 3 activates transcription of thyroid transcription factor 1 in respiratory epithelial cells. *Mol Cell Biol* 1996;**16**:3626–36.

70 Samadani U, Porcella A, Pani L *et al*. Cytokine regulation of the liver transcription factor hepatocyte nuclear factor-3β is mediated by the C/EBP family and interferon regulatory factor 1. *Cell Growth Differ* 1995;**6**:879–90.

71 Peterson RS, Lim L, Ye H *et al*. The winged helix transcriptional activator HFH-8 is expressed in the mesoderm of the primitive streak stage of mouse embryos and its cellular derivatives. *Mech Dev* 1997;**69**:53–69.

72 Shinbrot E, Peters KG, Williams LT. Expression of the platelet-derived growth factor beta receptor during organogenesis and tissue differentiation in the mouse embryo. *Dev Dyn* 1994;**199**:169–75.

73 Souza P, Tanswell AK, Post M. Different roles for PDGF-α and -β receptors in embryonic lung development. *Am J Respir Cell Mol Biol* 1996;**15**:551–62.

74 Kalinichenko VV, Lim L, Stolz DB *et al*. Defects in pulmonary vasculature and perinatal lung hemorrhage in mice

heterozygous null for the Forkhead Box f1 transcription factor. *Dev Biol* 2001;**235**:489–506.

75 Ohmichi H, Koshimizu U, Matsumoto K, Nakamura T. Hepatocyte growth factor (HGF) acts as a mesenchyme-derived morphogenic factor during fetal lung development. *Development* 1998;**125**:1315–24.

76 Weaver M, Yingling JM, Dunn NR, Bellusci S, Hogan BL. Bmp signalling regulates proximal–distal differentiation of endoderm in mouse lung development. *Development* 1999; **126**:4005–15.

77 Hackett BP, Brody SL, Liang M *et al*. Primary structure of hepatocyte nuclear factor/forkhead homologue 4 and characterization of gene expression in the developing respiratory and reproductive epithelium. *Proc Natl Acad Sci U S A* 1995;**92**:4249–53.

78 Hyatt BA, Shangguan X, Shannon JM. BMP4 modulates fibroblast growth factor-mediated induction of proximal and distal lung differentiation in mouse embryonic tracheal epithelium in mesenchyme-free culture. *Dev Dyn* 2002;**225**: 153–65.

79 Guazzi S, Price M, De Felice M *et al*. Thyroid nuclear factor 1 (TTF-1) contains a homeodomain and displays a novel DNA binding specificity. *EMBO J* 1990;**9**:3631–9.

80 Lazzaro D, Price M, De Felice M, Di Lauro R. The transcription factor TTF-1 is expressed at the onset of thyroid and lung morphogenesis and in restricted regions of the foetal brain. *Development* 1991;**113**:1093–104.

81 Wert SE, Dey CR, Blair PA, Kimura S, Whitsett JA. Increased expression of thyroid transcription factor-1 (TTF-1) in respiratory epithelial cells inhibits alveolarization and causes pulmonary inflammation. *Dev Biol* 2002;**242**:75–87.

82 Boggaram V. Regulation of lung surfactant protein gene expression. *Front Biosci* 2003;**8**:D751–64.

83 Bruno MD, Bohinski RJ, Huelsman KM, Whitsett JA, Korfhagen TR. Lung cell-specific expression of the murine surfactant protein A (SP-A) gene is mediated by interactions between the SP-A promoter and thyroid transcription factor-1. *J Biol Chem* 1995;**270**:6531–6.

84 Ramirez MI, Rishi AK, Cao YX, Williams MC. TGT3, thyroid transcription factor I, and Sp1 elements regulate transcriptional activity of the 1.3-kilobase pair promoter of T1α, a lung alveolar type I cell gene. *J Biol Chem* 1997;**272**:26285–94.

85 Whitsett JA, Glasser SW. Regulation of surfactant protein gene transcription. *Biochim Biophys Acta* 1998;**1408**:303–11.

86 Yan C, Sever Z, Whitsett JA. Upstream enhancer activity in the human surfactant protein B gene is mediated by thyroid transcription factor 1. *J Biol Chem* 1995;**270**:24 852–7.

87 Zhang L, Whitsett JA, Stripp BR. Regulation of Clara cell secretory protein gene transcription by thyroid transcription factor-1. *Biochim Biophys Acta* 1997;**1350**:359–67.

88 DeFelice M, Silberschmidt D, DiLauro R *et al*. TTF-1 phosphorylation is required for peripheral lung morphogenesis, perinatal survival, and tissue-specific gene expression. *J Biol Chem* 2003;**278**:35 574–83.

89 Shaw-White JR, Bruno MD, Whitsett JA. GATA-6 activates transcription of thyroid transcription factor-1. *J Biol Chem* 1999;**274**:2658–64.

90 Bogue CW, Lou LJ, Vasavada H, Wilson CM, Jacobs HC.

Expression of Hoxb genes in the developing mouse foregut and lung. *Am J Respir Cell Mol Biol* 1996;**15**:163–71.

91 Volpe MV, Martin A, Vosatka RJ, Mazzoni CL, Nielsen HC. Hoxb-5 expression in the developing mouse lung suggests a role in branching morphogenesis and epithelial cell fate. *Histochem Cell Biol* 1997;**108**:495–504.

92 Grindley JC, Bellusci S, Perkins D, Hogan BL. Evidence for the involvement of the Gli gene family in embryonic mouse lung development. *Dev Biol* 1997;**188**:337–48.

93 Jaskoll TF, Don-Wheeler G, Johnson R, Slavkin HC. Embryonic mouse lung morphogenesis and type II cyto-differentiation in serumless, chemically defined medium using prolonged *in vitro* cultures. *Cell Differ* 1988;**24**:105–17.

94 Warburton D, Seth R, Shum L *et al.* Epigenetic role of epidermal growth factor expression and signalling in embryonic mouse lung morphogenesis. *Dev Biol* 1992;**149**:123–33.

95 Glazer L, Shilo BZ. The *Drosophila* FGF-R homolog is expressed in the embryonic tracheal system and appears to be required for directed tracheal cell extension. *Genes Dev* 1991;**5**:697–705.

96 Sutherland D, Samakovlis C, Krasnow MA. Branchless encodes a *Drosophila* FGF homolog that controls tracheal cell migration and the pattern of branching. *Cell* 1996;**87**:1091–101.

97 Ornitz DM, Itoh N. Fibroblast growth factors. *Genome Biol* 2001;**2**:Reviews 3005.

98 Izvolsky KI, Zhong L, Wei L *et al.* Heparan sulfates expressed in the distal lung are required for Fgf10 binding to the epithelium and for airway branching. *Am J Physiol Lung Cell Mol Physiol* 2003;**285**:L838–46.

99 Izvolsky KI, Shoykhet D, Yang Y *et al.* Heparan sulfate–FGF10 interactions during lung morphogenesis. *Dev Biol* 2003;**258**:185–200.

100 Lin X, Buff EM, Perrimon N, Michelson AM. Heparan sulfate proteoglycans are essential for FGF receptor signalling during *Drosophila* embryonic development. *Development* 1999;**126**:3715–23.

101 Hokuto I, Perl AK, Whitsett JA. Prenatal, but not postnatal, inhibition of fibroblast growth factor receptor signalling causes emphysema. *J Biol Chem* 2003;**278**:415–21.

102 Bellusci S, Grindley J, Emoto H, Itoh N, Hogan BL. Fibroblast growth factor 10 (FGF10) and branching morphogenesis in the embryonic mouse lung. *Development* 1997;**124**:4867–78.

103 Park WY, Miranda B, Lebeche D, Hashimoto G, Cardoso WV. FGF-10 is a chemotactic factor for distal epithelial buds during lung development. *Dev Biol* 1998;**201**:125–34.

104 Weaver M, Dunn NR, Hogan BL. Bmp4 and Fgf10 play opposing roles during lung bud morphogenesis. *Development* 2000;**127**:2695–704.

105 Post M, Souza P, Liu J *et al.* Keratinocyte growth factor and its receptor are involved in regulating early lung branching. *Development* 1996;**122**:3107–15.

106 Cardoso WV, Itoh A, Nogawa H, Mason I, Brody JS. FGF-1 and FGF-7 induce distinct patterns of growth and differentiation in embryonic lung epithelium. *Dev Dyn* 1997;**208**:398–405.

107 Deterding RR, Jacoby CR, Shannon JM. Acidic fibroblast growth factor and keratinocyte growth factor stimulate fetal rat pulmonary epithelial growth. *Am J Physiol* 1996;**271**:L495–505.

108 Liu Y, Jiang H, Crawford HC, Hogan BL. Role for ETS domain transcription factors Pea3/Erm in mouse lung development. *Dev Biol* 2003;**261**:10–24.

109 Liu Y, Hogan BL. Differential gene expression in the distal tip endoderm of the embryonic mouse lung. *Gene Expr Patterns* 2002;**2**:229–33.

110 Frank L. Protective effect of keratinocyte growth factor against lung abnormalities associated with hyperoxia in prematurely born rats. *Biol Neonate* 2003;**83**:263–72.

111 Guo L, Degenstein L, Fuchs E. Keratinocyte growth factor is required for hair development but not for wound healing. *Genes Dev* 1996;**10**:165–75.

112 Colvin JS, Feldman B, Nadeau JH, Goldfarb M, Ornitz DM. Genomic organization and embryonic expression of the mouse fibroblast growth factor 9 gene. *Dev Dyn* 1999;**216**:72–88.

113 Weaver M, Batts L, Hogan BL. Tissue interactions pattern the mesenchyme of the embryonic mouse lung. *Dev Biol* 2003;**258**:169–84.

114 Mailleux AA, Tefft D, Ndiaye D *et al.* Evidence that SPROUTY2 functions as an inhibitor of mouse embryonic lung growth and morphogenesis. *Mech Dev* 2001;**102**:81–94.

115 Hacohen N, Kramer S, Sutherland D, Hiromi Y, Krasnow MA. Sprouty encodes a novel antagonist of FGF signalling that patterns apical branching of the *Drosophila* airways. *Cell* 1998;**92**:253–63.

116 Kramer S, Okabe M, Hacohen N, Krasnow MA, Hiromi Y. Sprouty: a common antagonist of FGF and EGF signalling pathways in *Drosophila*. *Development* 1999;**126**:2515–25.

117 Reich A, Sapir A, Shilo B. Sprouty is a general inhibitor of receptor tyrosine kinase signalling. *Development* 1999;**126**:4139–47.

118 Hadari YR, Kouhara H, Lax I, Schlessinger J. Binding of Shp2 tyrosine phosphatase to FRS2 is essential for fibroblast growth factor-induced PC12 cell differentiation. *Mol Cell Biol* 1998;**18**:3966–73.

119 Tefft D, Lee M, Smith S *et al.* mSprouty2 inhibits FGF10-activated MAP kinase by differentially binding to upstream target proteins. *Am J Physiol Lung Cell Mol Physiol* 2002;**283**:L700–6.

120 Massague J. TGF-β signal transduction. *Annu Rev Biochem* 1998;**67**:753–91.

121 Shi Y, Massague J. Mechanisms of TGF-β signalling from cell membrane to the nucleus. *Cell* 2003;**113**:685–700.

122 Bragg AD, Moses HL, Serra R. Signalling to the epithelium is not sufficient to mediate all of the effects of transforming growth factor beta and bone morphogenetic protein 4 on murine embryonic lung development. *Mech Dev* 2001;**109**:13–26.

123 Millan FA, Denhez F, Kondaiah P, Akhurst RJ. Embryonic gene expression patterns of TGFβ1, β2 and β3 suggest different developmental functions *in vivo*. *Development* 1991;**111**:131–43.

124 Pelton RW, Saxena B, Jones M, Moses HL, Gold LI. Immunohistochemical localization of TGFβ1, TGFβ2, and

TGFβ3 in the mouse embryo: expression patterns suggest multiple roles during embryonic development. *J Cell Biol* 1991;**115**:1091–105.

125 Pelton RW, Johnson MD, Perkett EA, Gold LI, Moses HL. Expression of transforming growth factor-β1, -β2, and -β3 mRNA and protein in the murine lung. *Am J Respir Cell Mol Biol* 1991;**5**:522–30.

126 Schmid P, Cox D, Bilbe G, Maier R, McMaster GK. Differential expression of TGFβ1, β2 and β3 genes during mouse embryogenesis. *Development* 1991;**111**:117–30.

127 Zhao J, Sime PJ, Bringas P Jr *et al.* Spatial-specific TGF-β1 adenoviral expression determines morphogenetic phenotypes in embryonic mouse lung. *Eur J Cell Biol* 1999;**78**:715–25.

128 Zeng X, Gray M, Stahlman MT, Whitsett JA. TGF-β1 perturbs vascular development and inhibits epithelial differentiation in fetal lung *in vivo. Dev Dyn* 2001;**221**:289–301.

129 Zhou L, Dey CR, Wert SE, Whitsett JA. Arrested lung morphogenesis in transgenic mice bearing an SP-C-TGFβ1 chimeric gene. *Dev Biol* 1996;**175**:227–38.

130 Lecart C, Cayabyab R, Buckley S *et al.* Bioactive transforming growth factor-beta in the lungs of extremely low birthweight neonates predicts the need for home oxygen supplementation. *Biol Neonate* 2000;**77**:217–23.

131 Toti P, Buonocore G, Tanganelli P *et al.* Bronchopulmonary dysplasia of the premature baby: an immunohistochemical study. *Pediatr Pulmonol* 1997;**24**:22–8.

132 Sime PJ, Xing Z, Graham FL, Csaky KG, Gauldie J. Adenovector-mediated gene transfer of active transforming growth factor-β1 induces prolonged severe fibrosis in rat lung. *J Clin Invest* 1997;**100**:768–76.

133 Zhao J, Shi W, Wang YL *et al.* Smad3 deficiency attenuates bleomycin-induced pulmonary fibrosis in mice. *Am J Physiol Lung Cell Mol Physiol* 2002;**282**:L585–93.

134 Gauldie J, Galt T, Bonniaud P *et al.* Transfer of the active form of transforming growth factor-beta1 gene to newborn rat lung induces changes consistent with bronchopulmonary dysplasia. *Am J Pathol* 2003;**163**(6):2575–84.

135 Komatsu Y, Shibuya H, Takeda N *et al.* Targeted disruption of the *Tab1* gene causes embryonic lethality and defects in cardiovascular and lung morphogenesis. *Mech Dev* 2002;**119**:239–49.

136 Li DY, Sorensen LK, Brooke BS *et al.* Defective angiogenesis in mice lacking endoglin. *Science* 1999;**284**:1534–7.

137 Massague J. How cells read TGF-β signals. *Nat Rev Mol Cell Biol* 2000;**1**:169–78.

138 McAllister KA, Grogg KM, Johnson DW *et al.* Endoglin, a TGF-β binding protein of endothelial cells, is the gene for hereditary haemorrhagic telangiectasia type 1. *Nat Genet* 1994;**8**:345–51.

139 Urness LD, Sorensen LK, Li DY. Arteriovenous malformations in mice lacking activin receptor-like kinase-1. *Nat Genet* 2000;**26**:328–31.

140 Bellusci S, Henderson R, Winnier G, Oikawa T, Hogan BL. Evidence from normal expression and targeted misexpression that bone morphogenetic protein (Bmp-4) plays a role in mouse embryonic lung morphogenesis. *Development* 1996;**22**:1693–702.

141 King JA, Marker PC, Seung KJ, Kingsley DM. BMP5 and the molecular, skeletal, and soft-tissue alterations in short ear mice. *Dev Biol* 1994;**166**:112–22.

142 Takahashi H, Ikeda T. Transcripts for two members of the transforming growth factor-beta superfamily BMP-3 and BMP-7 are expressed in developing rat embryos. *Dev Dyn* 1996;**207**:439–49.

143 Shi W, Zhao J, Anderson KD, Warburton D. Gremlin negatively modulates BMP-4 induction of embryonic mouse lung branching morphogenesis. *Am J Physiol Lung Cell Mol Physiol* 2001;**280**:L1030–9.

144 Lane KB, Machado RD, Pauciulo MW *et al.* Heterozygous germline mutations in BMPR2, encoding a TGF-β receptor, cause familial primary pulmonary hypertension. The International PPH Consortium. *Nat Genet* 2000;**26**:81–4.

145 van Tuyl M, Post M. From fruitflies to mammals: mechanisms of signalling via the Sonic hedgehog pathway in lung development. *Respir Res* 2000;**1**:30–5.

146 Bellusci S, Furuta Y, Rush MG *et al.* Involvement of Sonic hedgehog (Shh) in mouse embryonic lung growth and morphogenesis. *Development* 1997;**124**:53–63.

147 Urase K, Mukasa T, Igarashi H *et al.* Spatial expression of Sonic hedgehog in the lung epithelium during branching morphogenesis. *Biochem Biophys Res Commun* 1996;**225**:161–6.

148 Spilde TL, Bhatia AM, Mehta S *et al.* Defective sonic hedgehog signalling in esophageal atresia with tracheoesophageal fistula. *Surgery* 2003;**134**:345–50.

149 Chuang PT, McMahon AP. Vertebrate Hedgehog signalling modulated by induction of a Hedgehog-binding protein. *Nature* 1999;**397**:617–21.

150 Goodrich LV, Johnson RL, Milenkovic L, McMahon JA, Scott MP. Conservation of the hedgehog/patched signalling pathway from flies to mice: induction of a mouse patched gene by Hedgehog. *Genes Dev* 1996;**10**:301–12.

151 Kawahira H, Ma NH, Tzanakakis ES *et al.* Combined activities of hedgehog signalling inhibitors regulate pancreas development. *Development* 2003;**130**:4871–9.

152 Wodarz A, Nusse R. Mechanisms of Wnt signalling in development. *Annu Rev Cell Dev Biol* 1998;**14**:59–88.

153 Tebar M, Destree O, de Vree WJ, Have-Opbroek AA. Expression of Tcf/Lef and sFrp and localization of β-catenin in the developing mouse lung. *Mech Dev* 2001;**109**:437–40.

154 Eberhart CG, Argani P. Wnt signalling in human development: β-catenin nuclear translocation in fetal lung, kidney, placenta, capillaries, adrenal, and cartilage. *Pediatr Dev Pathol* 2001;**4**:351–7.

155 Schuger L, Johnson GR, Gilbride K, Plowman GD, Mandel R. Amphiregulin in lung branching morphogenesis: interaction with heparan sulfate proteoglycan modulates cell proliferation. *Development* 1996;**122**:1759–67.

156 Seth R, Shum L, Wu F *et al.* Role of epidermal growth factor expression in early mouse embryo lung branching morphogenesis in culture: antisense oligodeoxynucleotide inhibitory strategy. *Dev Biol* 1993;**158**:555–9.

157 Raaberg L, Nexo E, Buckley S *et al.* Epidermal growth factor transcription, translation, and signal transduction by rat type II pneumocytes in culture. *Am J Respir Cell Mol Biol* 1992;**6**:44–9.

158 Korfhagen TR, Swantz RJ, Wert SE *et al.* Respiratory epithelial cell expression of human transforming growth factor-alpha induces lung fibrosis in transgenic mice. *J Clin Invest* 1994; **93**:1691–9.

159 Le Cras TD, Hardie WD, Fagan K, Whitsett JA, Korfhagen TR. Disrupted pulmonary vascular development and pulmonary hypertension in transgenic mice overexpressing transforming growth factor-α. *Am J Physiol Lung Cell Mol Physiol* 2003;**285**:L1046–54.

160 Sanchez-Esteban J, Wang Y, Gruppuso PA, Rubin LP. Mechanical stretch induces fetal type II cell differentiation via an EGFR-ERK signalling pathway. *Am J Respir Cell Mol Biol* 2004;**30**:76–83.

161 Shi W, Chen H, Sun J *et al.* TACE is required for fetal murine cardiac development and modeling. *Dev Biol* 2003;**261**: 371–80.

162 Buch S, Jassal D, Cannigia I *et al.* Ontogeny and regulation of platelet-derived growth factor gene expression in distal fetal rat lung epithelial cells. *Am J Respir Cell Mol Biol* 1994;**11**:251–61.

163 Souza P, Kuliszewski M, Wang J *et al.* PDGF-AA and its receptor influence early lung branching via an epithelial–mesenchymal interaction. *Development* 1995;**121**:2559–67.

164 Souza P, Sedlackova L, Kuliszewski M *et al.* Antisense oligodeoxynucleotides targeting PDGF-B mRNA inhibit cell proliferation during embryonic rat lung development. *Development* 1994;**120**:2163–73.

165 LaRochelle WJ, Jeffers M, McDonald WF *et al.* PDGF-D, a new protease-activated growth factor. *Nat Cell Biol* 2001; **3**:517–21.

166 Li X, Ponten A, Aase K *et al.* PDGF-C is a new protease-activated ligand for the PDGF alpha-receptor. *Nat Cell Biol* 2000;**2**:302–9.

167 Zhuo Y, Zhang J, Laboy M, Lasky JA. Modulation of PDGF-C and PDGF-D expression during bleomycin-induced lung fibrosis. *Am J Physiol Lung Cell Mol Physiol* 2004;**286**:L182–8.

168 Batchelor DC, Hutchins AM, Klempt M, Skinner SJ. Developmental changes in the expression patterns of IGFs, type 1 IGF receptor and IGF-binding proteins-2 and -4 in perinatal rat lung. *J Mol Endocrinol* 1995;**15**:105–15.

169 Lallemand AV, Ruocco SM, Joly PM, Gaillard DA. *In vivo* localization of the insulin-like growth factors I and II (IGF I and IGF II) gene expression during human lung development. *Int J Dev Biol* 1995;**39**:529–37.

170 Maitre B, Clement A, Williams MC, Brody JS. Expression of insulin-like growth factor receptors 1 and 2 in the developing lung and their relation to epithelial cell differentiation. *Am J Respir Cell Mol Biol* 1995;**13**:262–70.

171 Retsch-Bogart GZ, Moats-Staats BM, Howard K, D'Ercole AJ, Stiles AD. Cellular localization of messenger RNAs for insulin-like growth factors (IGFs), their receptors and binding proteins during fetal rat lung development. *Am J Respir Cell Mol Biol* 1996;**14**:61–9.

172 Schuller AG, van Neck JW, Beukenholdt RW, Zwarthoff EC, Drop SL. IGF, type I IGF receptor and IGF-binding protein mRNA expression in the developing mouse lung. *J Mol Endocrinol* 1995;**14**:349–55.

173 Coppola D, Ferber A, Miura M *et al.* A functional insulin-like growth factor I receptor is required for the mitogenic and transforming activities of the epidermal growth factor receptor. *Mol Cell Biol* 1994;**14**:4588–95.

174 Pichel JG, Fernandez-Moreno C, Vicario-Abejon C *et al.* Developmental cooperation of leukemia inhibitory factor and insulin-like growth factor I in mice is tissue-specific and essential for lung maturation involving the transcription factors Sp3 and TTF-1. *Mech Dev* 2003;**120**:349–61.

175 Han RN, Post M, Tanswell AK, Lye SJ. Insulin-like growth factor-I receptor-mediated vasculogenesis/angiogenesis in human lung development. *Am J Respir Cell Mol Biol* 2003; **28**:159–69.

176 Larrivee B, Karsan A. Signalling pathways induced by vascular endothelial growth factor (review). *Int J Mol Med* 2000;**5**:447–56.

177 Acarregui MJ, Penisten ST, Goss KL, Ramirez K, Snyder JM. Vascular endothelial growth factor gene expression in human fetal lung *in vitro*. *Am J Respir Cell Mol Biol* 1999; **20**:14–23.

178 Compernolle V, Brusselmans K, Acker T *et al.* Loss of HIF-2α and inhibition of VEGF impair fetal lung maturation, whereas treatment with VEGF prevents fatal respiratory distress in premature mice. *Nat Med* 2002;**8**:702–10.

179 Gebb SA, Shannon JM. Tissue interactions mediate early events in pulmonary vasculogenesis. *Dev Dyn* 2000;**217**: 159–69.

180 Zeng X, Wert SE, Federici R, Peters KG, Whitsett JA. VEGF enhances pulmonary vasculogenesis and disrupts lung morphogenesis *in vivo*. *Dev Dyn* 1998;**211**:215–27.

181 Gerber HP, Hillan KJ, Ryan AM *et al.* VEGF is required for growth and survival in neonatal mice. *Development* 1999; **126**:1149–59.

182 Lwebuga-Mukasa JS. Matrix-driven pneumocyte differentiation. *Am Rev Respir Dis* 1991;**144**:452–7.

183 Hilfer SR. Morphogenesis of the lung: control of embryonic and fetal branching. *Annu Rev Physiol* 1996;**58**:93–113.

184 Minoo P, King RJ. Epithelial–mesenchymal interactions in lung development. *Annu Rev Physiol* 1994;**56**:13–45.

185 Burgeson RE, Chiquet M, Deutzmann R *et al.* A new nomenclature for the laminins. *Matrix Biol* 1994;**14**:209–11.

186 Bernier SM, Utani A, Sugiyama S *et al.* Cloning and expression of laminin alpha 2 chain (M-chain) in the mouse. *Matrix Biol* 1995;**14**:447–55.

187 Ehrig K, Leivo I, Argraves WS, Ruoslahti E, Engvall E. Merosin, a tissue-specific basement membrane protein, is a laminin-like protein. *Proc Natl Acad Sci U S A* 1990;**87**:3264–8.

188 Galliano MF, Aberdam D, Aguzzi A, Ortonne JP, Meneguzzi G. Cloning and complete primary structure of the mouse laminin alpha 3 chain: distinct expression pattern of the laminin alpha 3A and alpha 3B chain isoforms. *J Biol Chem* 1995;**270**:21 820–6.

189 Iivanainen A, Sainio K, Sariola H, Tryggvason K. Primary structure and expression of a novel human laminin alpha 4 chain. *FEBS Lett* 1995;**365**:183–8.

190 Iivanainen A, Vuolteenaho R, Sainio K *et al.* The human laminin beta 2 chain (S-laminin): structure, expression in

fetal tissues and chromosomal assignment of the *LAMB2* gene. *Matrix Biol* 1995;**14**:489–97.

191 Iivanainen A, Kortesmaa J, Sahlberg C *et al.* Primary structure, developmental expression, and immunolocalization of the murine laminin α4 chain. *J Biol Chem* 1997;**272**:27 862–8.

192 Iivanainen A, Morita T, Tryggvason K. Molecular cloning and tissue-specific expression of a novel murine laminin γ3 chain. *J Biol Chem* 1999;**274**:14 107–11.

193 Koch M, Olson PF, Albus A *et al.* Characterization and expression of the laminin γ3 chain: a novel, non-basement membrane-associated, laminin chain. *J Cell Biol* 1999;**145**: 605–18.

194 Pierce RA, Griffin GL, Mudd MS *et al.* Expression of laminin α3, α4, and α5 chains by alveolar epithelial cells and fibroblasts. *Am J Respir Cell Mol Biol* 1998;**19**:237–44.

195 Vuolteenaho R, Nissinen M, Sainio K *et al.* Human laminin M chain (merosin): complete primary structure, chromosomal assignment, and expression of the M and A chain in human fetal tissues. *J Cell Biol* 1994;**124**:381–94.

196 Schuger L, Varani J, Killen PD, Skubitz AP, Gilbride K. Laminin expression in the mouse lung increases with development and stimulates spontaneous organotypic rearrangement of mixed lung cells. *Dev Dyn* 1992;**195**:43–54.

197 Frieser M, Nockel H, Pausch F *et al.* Cloning of the mouse laminin α4 cDNA: expression in a subset of endothelium. *Eur J Biochem* 1997;**246**:727–35.

198 Miner JH, Patton BL, Lentz SI *et al.* The laminin alpha chains: expression, developmental transitions, and chromosomal locations of α1–5, identification of heterotrimeric laminins 8–11, and cloning of a novel α3 isoform. *J Cell Biol* 1997;**137**:685–701.

199 Miner JH, Lewis RM, Sanes JR. Molecular cloning of a novel laminin chain, α5, and widespread expression in adult mouse tissues. *J Biol Chem* 1995;**270**:28523–6.

200 Miner JH, Cunningham J, Sanes JR. Roles for laminin in embryogenesis: exencephaly, syndactyly, and placentopathy in mice lacking the laminin α5 chain. *J Cell Biol* 1998; **143**:1713–23.

201 Durham PL, Snyder JM. Characterization of α1, β1, and γ1 laminin subunits during rabbit fetal lung development. *Dev Dyn* 1995;**203**:408–21.

202 Schuger L, Skubitz AP, de las Morenas A, Gilbride K. Two separate domains of laminin promote lung organogenesis by different mechanisms of action. *Dev Biol* 1995;**169**: 520–32.

203 Schuger L, Skubitz AP, Gilbride K, Mandel R, He L. Laminin and heparan sulfate proteoglycan mediate epithelial cell polarization in organotypic cultures of embryonic lung cells: evidence implicating involvement of the inner globular region of laminin β1 chain and the heparan sulfate groups of heparan sulfate proteoglycan. *Dev Biol* 1996;**179**:264–73.

204 Dziadek M. Role of laminin–nidogen complexes in basement membrane formation during embryonic development. *Experientia* 1995;**51**:901–13.

205 Reinhardt D, Mann K, Nischt R *et al.* Mapping of nidogen binding sites for collagen type IV, heparan sulfate proteoglycan, and zinc. *J Biol Chem* 1993;**268**:10 881–7.

206 Senior RM, Griffin GL, Mudd MS *et al.* Entactin expression by rat lung and rat alveolar epithelial cells. *Am J Respir Cell Mol Biol* 1996;**14**:239–47.

207 Ekblom P, Ekblom M, Fecker L *et al.* Role of mesenchymal nidogen for epithelial morphogenesis *in vitro*. *Development* 1994;**120**:2003–14.

208 Mayer U, Mann K, Timpl R, Murphy G. Sites of nidogen cleavage by proteases involved in tissue homeostasis and remodelling. *Eur J Biochem* 1993;**217**:877–84.

209 Belknap JK, Weiser-Evans MC, Grieshaber SS, Majack RA, Stenmark KR. Relationship between perlecan and tropoelastin gene expression and cell replication in the developing rat pulmonary vasculature. *Am J Respir Cell Mol Biol* 1999;**20**: 24–34.

210 Sakai T, Larsen M, Yamada KM. Fibronectin requirement in branching morphogenesis. *Nature* 2003;**423**:876–81.

211 Roman J. Fibronectin and fibronectin receptors in lung development. *Exp Lung Res* 1997;**23**:147–59.

212 Kikuchi W, Arai H, Ishida A, Takahashi Y, Takada G. Distal pulmonary cell proliferation is associated with the expression of EIIIA+ fibronectin in the developing rat lung. *Exp Lung Res* 2003;**29**:135–47.

213 Vu TH, Werb Z. Matrix metalloproteinases: effectors of development and normal physiology. *Genes Dev* 2000;**14**: 2123–33.

214 Gill SE, Pape MC, Khokha R, Watson AJ, Leco KJ. A null mutation for tissue inhibitor of metalloproteinases-3 (TIMP-3) impairs murine bronchiole branching morphogenesis. *Dev Biol* 2003;**261**:313–23.

215 Leco KJ, Waterhouse P, Sanchez OH *et al.* Spontaneous air space enlargement in the lungs of mice lacking tissue inhibitor of metalloproteinases-3 (TIMP-3). *J Clin Invest* 2001;**108**:817–29.

216 Valencia AM, Beharry KD, Ang JG *et al.* Early postnatal dexamethasone influences matrix metalloproteinase-2 and -9, and their tissue inhibitors in the developing rat lung. *Pediatr Pulmonol* 2003;**35**:456–62.

217 Chambon P. A decade of molecular biology of retinoic acid receptors. *FASEB J* 1996;**10**:940–54.

218 Niederreither K, McCaffery P, Drager UC, Chambon P, Dolle P. Restricted expression and retinoic acid-induced down-regulation of the retinaldehyde dehydrogenase type 2 (*RALDH-2*) gene during mouse development. *Mech Dev* 1997;**62**:67–78.

219 Niederreither K, Subbarayan V, Dolle P, Chambon P. Embryonic retinoic acid synthesis is essential for early mouse post-implantation development. *Nat Genet* 1999;**21**:444–8.

220 Ulven SM, Gundersen TE, Weedon MS *et al.* Identification of endogenous retinoids, enzymes, binding proteins, and receptors during early postimplantation development in mouse: important role of retinal dehydrogenase type 2 in synthesis of all-*trans*-retinoic acid. *Dev Biol* 2000;**220**: 379–91.

221 Kastner P, Mark M, Ghyselinck N *et al.* Genetic evidence that the retinoid signal is transduced by heterodimeric RXR/RAR functional units during mouse development. *Development* 1997;**124**:313–26.

222 Chazaud C, Dolle P, Rossant J, Mollard R. Retinoic acid signalling regulates murine bronchial tubule formation. *Mech Dev* 2003;**120**:691–700.

223 Dickman ED, Thaller C, Smith SM. Temporally-regulated retinoic acid depletion produces specific neural crest, ocular and nervous system defects. *Development* 1997;**124**:3111–21.

224 Sekine K, Ohuchi H, Fujiwara M *et al.* Fgf10 is essential for limb and lung formation. *Nat Genet* 1999;**21**:138–41.

225 Mendelsohn C, Lohnes D, Decimo D *et al.* Function of the retinoic acid receptors (RARs) during development. II. Multiple abnormalities at various stages of organogenesis in RAR double mutants. *Development* 1994;**120**:2749–71.

226 Cardoso WV, Williams MC, Mitsialis SA *et al.* Retinoic acid induces changes in the pattern of airway branching and alters epithelial cell differentiation in the developing lung *in vitro*. *Am J Respir Cell Mol Biol* 1995;**12**:464–76.

227 Malpel S, Mendelsohn C, Cardoso WV. Regulation of retinoic acid signalling during lung morphogenesis. *Development* 2000;**127**:3057–67.

228 Wongtrakool C, Malpel S, Gorenstein J *et al.* Down-regulation of retinoic acid receptor alpha signalling is required for sacculation and type 1 cell formation in the developing lung. *J Biol Chem* 2003;**278**:46911–8.

229 Maden M, Hind M. Retinoic acid: a regeneration-inducing molecule. *Dev Dyn* 2003;**226**:237–44.

230 Lomas DA, Silverman EK. The genetics of chronic obstructive pulmonary disease. *Respir Res* 2001;**2**:20–6.

231 Jeffery PK. Remodeling in asthma and chronic obstructive lung disease. *Am J Respir Crit Care Med* 2001;**164**:S28–38.

232 Stewart GA, Hoyne GF, Ahmad SA *et al.* Expression of the developmental Sonic hedgehog (Shh) signalling pathway is up-regulated in chronic lung fibrosis and the Shh receptor patched 1 is present in circulating T lymphocytes. *J Pathol* 2003;**199**:488–95.

CHAPTER 30
Animal models

Piero A. Martorana, Monica Lucattelli, Barbara Bartalesi and Giuseppe Lungarella

The main purpose of studying animal models of human disease is to gain insight into the underlying mechanisms of the disease. The recognition that chronic obstructive pulmonary disease (COPD) is a global health problem with no effective treatment has resulted in recent years in an explosion of new animal models of emphysema, a major component of COPD. Bronchial pathological changes were also described in some of these models. A very comprehensive review of these models has recently been published [1].

This chapter reviews some selected animal models developed in recent years that, in the eyes of the authors, may provide new insight into the pathogenesis of emphysema and COPD.

Genetic models

Strains of mice that spontaneously develop emphysema have been reported. Here we present only those strains of mice where the genetic mutation has been described and/or the mechanism leading to the lung changes investigated. Strains with developmental lung changes (i.e. a defect in alveolar formation) are not presented.

Tight-skin mouse

This mutant is commercially available on a C57Bl/6J background. The tight-skin (*Tsk*) gene on chromosome 2 is associated with a tandem duplication of the fibrillin-1 gene, which results in a larger-than-normal protein [2]. A potential effect of the incorporation of Tsk fibrillin-1 into microfibrils is increased proteolytic susceptibility.

In these mice, massive emphysema develops early, at approximately 2–4 weeks of age, and progresses thereafter [3]. Biochemical analysis reveals a decrease in lung elastin content that coincides in time with parenchymal destruction [4]. In fact, these mice also have abnormally high levels of elastase and cathepsin G in their neutrophils, coupled with low serum α_1-antitrypsin (AAT) levels and serum elastase inhibitory capacity (EIC) [5].

This is, to our knowledge, the only strain of mice with spontaneous emphysema in which the development of the lung disease is followed by the development of right-ventricular hypertrophy. This begins between 8 and 16 months of age and progresses thereafter [6].

Pallid mouse

This is commercially available on a C57Bl/6J background. The pallid (*pa*) gene is situated on chromosome 2 and encodes a novel syntaxin-13-interacting protein [7].

The serum of pallid mice has lower AAT levels (−55%) and EIC values (−71%) than those of other strains and spontaneous emphysema develops late in life between 8 and 12 months of age [8]. This is the first animal model in which emphysema has been shown to develop as a result of the following sequence of events [5,9]:
- deficient activity of serum antielastase screen;
- increased lung elastase burden; and
- decreased lung elastin content.
These results give an experimental basis for the protease–antiprotease theory of emphysema and indicate the pallid mouse as the mouse counterpart of the human AAT-deficient MZ phenotype.

Klotho mouse

This is a mutant that resulted as a consequence of a transgenic experiment. Insertion-mutation of several copies of the transgene in the 5′-flanking region of the *klotho* gene yielded a null mutation in the klotho mouse. The *klotho* gene encodes a membrane protein homologous to β-glucosidase enzymes.

In *klotho*(−/−) mice, emphysema starts to develop at 4 weeks of age with a gradual progression with increasing age. The heterozygous (+/−) mutant develops emphysema late in life at approximately 120 weeks of age. The *klotho* gene may be important for maintaining pulmonary integrity [10].

Models of cytokine expression

Some cytokines that are known to orchestrate the inflammatory response in asthma and in other inflammatory diseases may also have a major role in the pathogenesis of COPD. Transgenic and gene deletion technology has been used to explore the temporal role of cytokines in the development of COPD animal models. Models with developmental defects are not presented.

γ-Interferon

When γ-interferon (IFN-γ) is targeted in a transgenic fashion to the adult murine lung using the reverse tetracycline transactivator system and a promoter active in Clara cells, the response is emphysema and a macrophage- and neutrophil-rich inflammation.

Significant protease and antiprotease alterations are also found, such as:
1 induction and activation of matrix metalloproteinases (MMPs) MMP-12, MMP-9 and cathepsins B, H, D, S; and
2 selective inhibition of secretory leucocyte protease inhibitor (SLPI) [11].

Additionally, it has been found that IFN-γ *in vivo* is a potent stimulator of alveolar epithelial cell apoptosis. This response is associated with both the death receptor and the mitochondrial apoptotic pathways. Treatment with Z-VAD abrogates the apoptotic response and causes an impressive decrease in IFN-γ-induced emphysema. IFN-γ also stimulates the expression of pulmonary cathepsins and treatment with leupeptin or E-64 abrogates IFN-γ-induced apoptosis and emphysema. Cathepsin S (14150) and cathepsin B (CA 074) inhibitors have similar effects. Interestingly, Z-VAD and leupeptin also decrease IFN-γ-induced inflammation and the induction of MMPs and cathepsins. These studies demonstrate that a cathepsin-dependent alveolar apoptotic response is a critical event in the pathogenesis of IFN-γ-induced emphysema. They also highlight a potential positive feedback loop in which IFN-γ-induced apoptosis contributes to local inflammation and tissue protease degradation. These findings integrate existing hypotheses of the pathogenesis of emphysema (see also Models of apoptosis) [12].

Interleukin 13

Overexpression of interleukin 13 (IL-13) in the airway epithelium of adult mice results in emphysema, goblet cell metaplasia and inflammation. MMP-2, -9, -12, -13 and -14 and cathepsin B, S, L, H and K are also induced. Inhibition of MMPs substantially prevents the development of emphysema and reduces the influx of inflammatory cells by more than 90%. Inhibitors of thiol proteinases also reduce emphysema and inflammation. Neither class of proteinase inhibitors blocked goblet cell metaplasia.

Thus, IL-13 is a potent stimulator of MMP- and cathepsin-based proteolytic pathways in the lung and may cause emphysema via an MMP- and cathepsin-dependent mechanism [13].

Tumour necrosis factor-α

Overexpression of tumour necrosis factor-α (TNF-α) in alveolar type II cells of mice under the control of the human surfactant protein C promoter results in bronchiolitis, chronic inflammation and emphysema. Limited fibrosis can be seen only in the subpleural, peribronchial and perivascular regions. Physiological assessment shows an increase in lung volumes and a decrease in elastic recoil. Gelatinase activity is increased in bronchoalveolar lavage (BAL) fluids [14].

Mice with knocked-out TNF-α or IL-1β receptors have significantly less emphysema than wild type mice, following an intratracheal instillation of porcine pancreatic elastase. It was suggested that elastase-induced emphysema might be driven in large measure through ongoing TNF-α and IL-1β-induced inflammation, and possibly through TNF-α and IL-1β-mediated inhibition of elastin and collagen repair (see also Models of cigarette smoke exposure) [15].

Transforming growth factor-β

In an elegant study it has been recently demonstrated that mice lacking the β6 subunit of the integrin αvβ6 (which occurs only in epithelial cells such as those the line the lungs) are protected against pulmonary fibrosis but develop pulmonary emphysema with age.

The mechanism is based on the knowledge that integrin αvβ6 binds and activates latent transforming growth factor-β (TGF-β). In mice lacking the subunit β6, this binding and activation does not take place and results in increased expression of the extracellular macrophage MMP-12 in the lungs and the development with time of spontaneous emphysema. MMP-12 is clearly necessary for disease onset, because mice lacking both MMP-12 and the integrin subunit β6 do not develop emphysema. Also, when β6-deficient mice are genetically manipulated to produce permanently active TGF-β, emphysema does not develop [16]. These results broaden the spectrum of factors involved in emphysema to those that activate latent TGF-β in the lung and, by inference, to TGF-β-triggered signalling molecules.

Models of apoptosis

Recent clinical studies have shown elevated levels of apoptosis in alveolar walls of emphysematous lungs. Accordingly, animal models have been developed in an attempt to investigate if apoptosis may have a role in the mechanism of emphysema. The following is a review of some of these models.

Vascular endothelial growth factor receptor blockade

In rats, chronic inhibition of vascular endothelial growth factor (VEGF) R2, which is responsible for endothelial cell growth, migration and differentiation, by the VEGF receptor blocker and angiogenesis inhibitor SU5416 results in emphysema. The emphysema is characterized by alveolar septal cell death, as assessed by TUNEL, activated caspase-3 immunostaining and DNA oligonucleosomal laddering. There is no lung infiltration by inflammatory cells or fibrosis. Treatment with the caspase inhibitor Z-Asp-CH2 prevents SU5416-induced septal cell apoptosis and emphysema development [17].

Also, when compared with control animals, rats treated with the VEGF receptor blocker show expression of markers of oxidative stress, all of which are prevented by the superoxide dismutase mimetic M40419. The preservation of lung structure in SU5416+M40419-treated lungs is associated with increased septal cell proliferation, and enhanced phosphorylation of the prosurvival and anti-apoptotic Akt, when compared with SU5416-treated lungs. Consistently with a positive feedback interaction between oxidative stress and apoptosis, it was found that apoptosis predominates in areas of oxidative stress, and that apoptosis blockade by a broad-spectrum caspase inhibitor markedly reduces the expression of markers of oxidative stress induced by the SU5416 treatment [18].

Active caspase-3

A single intratracheal instillation of active caspase-3 and Chariot, a new protein transfection reagent, causes alveolar cell apoptosis and significant emphysema. Elastica and van Gieson-stained lung tissue sections demonstrate loss of elastin layers within the alveolar walls. There is no alveolar or airway inflammation or fibrosis. In mice killed at different time points, emphysema is evident as early as 2 h after treatment and is maintained for at least 15 days. However, the increase in mean linear intercept (Lm) is reduced by 60% from 6 h to 15 days, suggesting that the lesion may be partially reversible. In mice instilled with the combination active caspase-3 and Chariot plus the caspase inhibitor DEVD-CHO, the lungs have a normal appearance.

Airspace enlargement, alveolar wall destruction and loss of elastin layers are also noted in lungs of mice instilled with nodularin, a serine/threonine kinase inhibitor that induces caspase-dependent apoptosis [19].

Calorie restriction

In adult mice, calorie restriction (two-thirds reduction for 2 weeks) diminishes alveolar number by 55%, alveolar volume increases 1.9-fold and alveolar surface area decreases by 25%; however, lung volume is not affected. Within 72 h of calorie restriction, alveolar wall cell apoptosis is increased and lung DNA diminished (−20%). Refeeding fully reverses these changes. Thus, according to this study, adult mice have endogenous programmes to destroy (apoptosis) and regenerate alveoli [20].

It may be important to determine if calorie restriction-related alveolar loss and progressive alveolar loss of COPD are mediated by the same signalling pathways. Also, the observation that alveolar cell apoptosis is a major factor in the pathogenesis of emphysema in many different animal models will probably result in the focusing of future research on the molecular and cellular requirements of the alveolar wall for its maintenance throughout a lifetime.

Models of cigarette smoke exposure

Cigarette smoke is the greatest risk factor of COPD. However, only approximately 15–20% of cigarette smokers develop COPD. The fact that these susceptible individuals are generally clustered into families hints that there may be certain genes that predispose people to smoking-induced COPD. In recent years there has been a great effort to develop animal models of cigarette smoke-induced lung lesions with the goal of detecting the mechanism(s) that may be responsible for the greater sensitivity of responders. Both acute and chronic animal models of cigarette smoke exposure have been used. These models are here presented separately.

Acute smoke exposure

Obviously, in the acute animal models the end-points

are not the physiological, biochemical or morphological changes classical of COPD but rather represent changes that reflect the occurrence either of an acute inflammatory process or of an acute oxidative stress. This model is also used to assess the efficacy of compounds on markers of inflammation or oxidation.

Role of an oxidative stress

Acute exposure of C57Bl/6J mice to cigarette smoke causes a significant decrease in total antioxidant capacity (Trolox equivalent antioxidant capacity, TEAC) and significant changes in oxidized glutathione, ascorbic acid, protein thiols and 8-epi-PGF-2α in bronchoalveolar lavage fluids (BALF).

Because the major mouse trypsin inhibitor is not sensitive to oxidation, and the mouse SLPI does not inhibit trypsin while human recombinant (hr) SLPI is sensitive to oxidants and inhibits trypsin, this model has been used to investigate the oxidative inactivation of hrSLPI. Intratracheal hrSLPI significantly increases BALF antitryptic activity *in vivo* in the mouse. Acute cigarette smoke exposure induces a 50% drop in the antitryptic activity of hrSLPI. Pretreatment with *N*-acetylcysteine prevents this fall of activity as well as the decrease of the BALF antioxidant capacity and the elevation of 8-epi-PGF-2α [21]. Thus, this is a model for investigating the effects of cigarette smoke oxidative stress on human protease inhibitors with antitrypsin activity *in vivo*.

In the same model of acute oxidative stress, mice of the inbred strains DBA/2 and C57Bl/6J respond to acute cigarette smoke exposure with a decrease of the TEAC of their BALF, while mice of the strain ICR increase their BALF TEAC. These results may have predictive value on the outcome of chronic exposure to cigarette smoke in these strains of mice [22].

Role of proteases in the acute inflammatory process

In C57Bl/6J mice, acute exposure to cigarette smoke causes a dose–response increase in BALF in neutrophils, desmosine (DES, a marker of elastin breakdown) and hydroxyproline (HP, a marker of collagen breakdown) but not of alveolar macrophages. Pretreatment with an antibody against neutrophils reduces after smoke exposure BALF neutrophils to undetectable levels, prevents increases in BALF DES and HP and does not affect alveolar macrophages. Intraperitoneal injection of human AAT before cigarette smoke exposure increases serum level of AAT threefold and completely abolishes smoke-induced connective tissue breakdown by-products as well as the increase in neutrophils without affecting alveolar macrophages in BALF. These results indicate that in this model, cigarette smoke acutely induces connective tissue break-

down, an effect probably brought about by neutrophil-derived proteases. Exogenous AAT is protective and inhibits both matrix degradation and neutrophil influx [23].

In a subsequent study, macrophage metalloelastase knockout mice (MME(–/–)), as well as MME(+/+) mice, were acutely exposed to cigarette smoke. In MME(+/+) mice, the acute smoke exposure results in an elevation in neutrophils, DES and HP in BALF but no elevation in MME-deficient mice. Both neutrophil influx and increased level of DES and HP are restored by administering alveolar macrophages from MME(+/+) mice to MME(–/–) mice and then exposing them to cigarette smoke.

These studies show that acute smoke-induced connective tissue breakdown, the precursor to emphysema, requires both neutrophils and macrophage metalloelastase (MME or MMP-12) [24]. Thus, these studies together underline the importance of both classes of proteases (serine elastases and MMPs) in the pathogenesis of lung matrix degradation.

Role of TNF-α in the acute inflammatory process

Mice with knocked out p55/p75 TNF-α receptors (TNF-α RKO) and control mice were exposed acutely to cigarette smoke. Two hours after smoke exposure, increases in gene expression of TNF-α, neutrophil chemoattractant macrophage inflammatory protein-2 and macrophage chemoattractant protein-1 are seen in control mice. By 6 h, TNF-α, macrophage inflammatory protein-2 and macrophage chemoattractant protein-1 gene expression levels are back to control values. In TNF-α RKO mice, no changes in gene expression of these mediators are seen at any time. At 24 h, control mice show increases in BALF neutrophils, DES and HP, whereas no elevation in these parameters are seen in TNF-α RKO mice.

In a separate experiment, mice of the strain 129, which produce low levels of TNF-α, show no inflammatory response to smoke either at 24 h or 7 days. These results indicate that TNF-α is central to acute cigarette smoke-induced tissue breakdown [25].

In another study, both mice lacking MMP-12 (MMP-12(–/–)) and wild type mice (MMP-12(+/+)) demonstrate rapid increases in whole-lung nuclear factor-κB activation and gene expression of proinflammatory cytokines after acute cigarette smoke exposure. This indicates that lack of MMP-12 does not produce a global failure to up-regulate inflammatory mediators. However, only MMP-12(+/+) mice demonstrate an increase in whole-lung TNF-α protein. Similarly, levels of whole-lung E-selectin, a marker of endothelial activation, are increased only in MMP-12(+/+) mice. These findings suggest that MMP-12 mediates cigarette smoke-induced inflammation acutely by releasing TNF-α, from macrophages, with subsequent endothelial activation, neutrophil influx and proteolytic matrix breakdown caused by neutrophil-derived proteases.

TNF-α release may be a general mechanism whereby metalloproteases drive cigarette smoke-induced inflammation [26].

Taken together these data support the idea that in humans TNF-α promoter polymorphism may be of importance in determining the individual responders who develop cigarette smoke-induced COPD (see also Models of cytokine expression).

Pharmacological studies

The effects of compounds on markers of inflammation can be investigated in acute models of cigarette smoke exposure. These studies may also serve as a relatively quick test for the activity of these compounds in the lung prior to their investigation in a time-consuming chronic model.

The serine elastase inhibitor ZD0892 (AstraZeneca, Lund, Sweden), an agent that selectively inhibits human neutrophil elastase and has an additional anti-inflammatory activity, was investigated in two acute models: the guinea pig and the mouse.

In the guinea pig model, animals given ZD0892 orally at doses of 10 and 30 mg/kg prior to smoke exposure, lowers the smoke-induced increases in total cell number and neutrophil number, as well as the increases in DES and HP content in BALF compared with untreated animals [27].

In the mouse model, ZD0892 administered orally at a dose of 30 mg/kg before cigarette smoke exposure, reduces the smoke-induced gene expression of macrophage inflammatory protein-2 and macrophage chemoattractant protein-1 in lung tissue but not of TNF-α. However, ZD0892 completely prevents the smoke-induced increase in plasma TNF-α [27].

Thus, compounds with antielastase and anti-inflammatory activities are effective in models of acute exposure to cigarette smoke.

Chronic smoke exposure

These models have been used to investigate the sensitivity of various strains of inbred mice to the effects of chronic smoke exposure, the role played by proteases in causing the lesions, the potentiating effects of viral infections and the potential therapeutic effects of compounds.

Mouse strain sensitivity

As a follow-up to the study of the model of acute smoke exposure, mice of the strains ICR, DBA/2 and C57Bl/6J have been chronically exposed to cigarette smoke for 7 months.

Mice of the strain ICR are not sensitive to oxidants and have normal levels of serum AAT, DBA/2 mice also have normal levels of serum AAT but are sensitive to oxidants while C57Bl/6J mice are both sensitive to oxidant and have a moderate deficit (−25%) of serum AAT. After the chronic exposure to cigarette smoke, ICR mice have normal levels of lung elastin content and no emphysema. On the other hand, both DBA/2 and C57Bl/6J mice show a significant drop in lung elastin content as well as emphysema assessed by three different methods. Histologically, emphysema was patchy and of the panlobular type (Fig. 30.1a,b).

In a separate experiment, pallid mice with a severe serum AAT deficiency and that develop spontaneous emphysema were exposed to cigarette smoke for 4 months. This resulted in an acceleration of the development of spontaneous emphysema assessed by morphometrical and biochemical (lung elastin content) methods [22]. In a recent study it was found that the lack of sensitivity of the ICR mice to the effects of chronic smoke exposure, is probably due to the activation of the nuclear factor erythroid-derived 2, like 2 (Nrf2) in this strain. Nrf2 is a redox-sensitive basic leucine zipper protein transcription factor that is involved in the regulation of many detoxification and antioxidant genes. The disruption of the Nrf2 gene in the ICR mice led to extensive emphysema in these mice following chronic cigarette smoke exposure [28].

Recently, a study was carried out in an attempt to differentiate the pattern of emphysema induced by chronic cigarette smoke exposure in C57Bl/6J and pallid mice. After 6 months of smoking, pallid mice, but not C57Bl/J mice, show a T-cell inflammation in the alveolar wall and an increase in lung compliance. Also, in pallid mice the emphysematous lesion is more diffuse than in C57 mice, affecting all airspaces [29].

These studies together indicate that the response to cigarette smoke exposure in mice is strain-dependent and suggest further investigations of the genetic differences in the susceptibility to cigarette smoke-induced lesions that may have implications for human disease.

Role of MMPs in chronic cigarette smoke exposure

In this study, macrophage elastase deficient mice (MME(−/−)) were subjected to cigarette smoke exposure for 6 months. In contrast to their littermates (MME(+/+)), these mice do not show an increased number of macrophages in their lungs and do not develop emphysema in response to cigarette smoke.

Smoke-exposed MME(−/−) mice that received monthly intratracheal instillations of macrophage chemoattractant protein-1 show accumulation of macrophages but not emphysema [30].

In another study, it was found that the development of emphysema in smoke-exposed guinea pigs correlates with alveolar macrophage numbers and alveolar macrophage-derived proteolytic activity but not with neutrophil numbers [31]. Furthermore, depletion of alveolar macrophages prevents smoke-induced emphysema, whereas depletion of neutrophils is not protective [32].

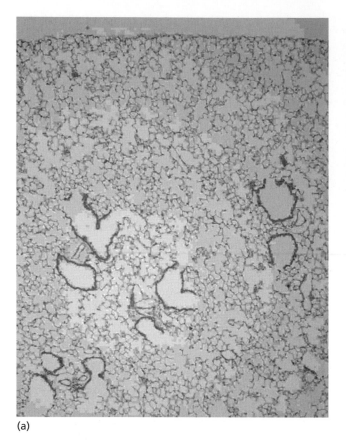
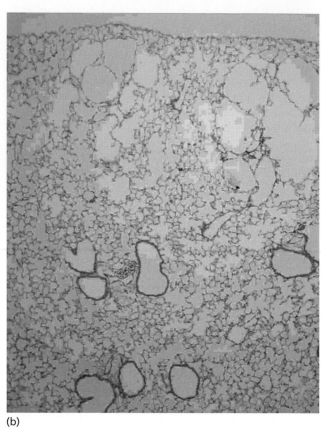

(a) (b)

Figure 30.1 (a) Well-fixed normal lung of a C57B1/6J control mouse exposed to room air for 7 months. (b) Lung of a C57B1/6J mouse exposed to the smoke of three cigarettes/day for 7 months showing emphysematous changes. The emphysema is patchy and of the panlobular type. HE, original magnification × 32.

Thus, these studies taken together indicate that macrophage elastases have an important role in the pathogenesis of chronic cigarette smoke-induced emphysema.

Role of neutrophil elastase in chronic cigarette smoke exposure

Mice lacking neutrophil elastase are approximately 60% protected against cigarette smoke-induced emphysema [33].

In another investigation, groups of mice were exposed daily to cigarette smoke for up to 6 months. One group of mice received human AAT every 48 h. In mice receiving AAT there was an approximately twofold increase in serum AAT levels and elastase inhibitory capacity. Treated mice, contrary to untreated ones, did not show elevations in BALF neutrophil numbers and matrix breakdown products measured from 2 to 30 days of smoke exposure. After 6 months exposure to cigarette smoke the AAT-treated mice show a 63% protection against emphysema and full protection against the smoke-mediated increase in plasma TNF-α.

There is thus direct as well as indirect evidence that neutrophil elastase also has a role in chronic cigarette smoke-induced emphysema. The latter study also suggests an anti-inflammatory activity for AAT [34].

Potentiating effects of viral infections

This study was designed to test the hypothesis that cigarette smoke-induced inflammation and emphysema are amplified by the presence of latent adenoviral infection. The results confirm that in guinea pigs, chronic cigarette-smoke exposure causes lesions similar to human centrilobular emphysema. They also show that latent adenoviral infection combined with cigarette-smoke exposure causes a greater increase in lung volume, air-space volume and lung weight, and a further decrease in surface : volume ratio compared with smoke exposure alone.

Analysis of inflammatory response in parenchymal and airway tissue shows that smoking causes an increase of polymorphonuclear leucocytes, macrophages and CD4 cells and that latent adenoviral infection independently increases polymorphonuclear leukocytes (PMN), macrophages and CD8 cells.

Thus, latent adenoviral infection amplifies the emphysematous lung destruction and increases the inflammatory response produced by cigarette-smoke exposure. In this study, the increase in CD4 is associated with cigarette smoke and the increase in CD8 cells with latent adenoviral infection [35].

Table 30.1 Theories and hypotheses of the pathogenesis of emphysema and/or COPD that have been either confirmed or put forward in animal models.

Theories/hypotheses	Animal model	References
NE/AAT	Pallid mouse, knocked out, acute smoke, chronic smoke	8, 9, 23, 33, 34
MMPs	Acute smoke, knocked out, chronic smoke	24, 30, 31, 32
Apoptosis	Transgenic, specific models, feed restriction	12, 17, 18, 19, 20
IFN-γ	Transgenic	11, 12
TGF-β	Knocked out	16
TNF-α	Transgenic, knocked out, acute smoke	14, 15, 25
Integrative hypothesis:		
CS $\rightarrow$ Mac $\rightarrow$ MMP-12 $\rightarrow$ TNF-α $\rightarrow$ ENDO $\rightarrow$ NE	Acute smoke	26

AAT, alpha-1 antitrypsin; CS, cigarette smoke; ENDO, endothelial activation; IFN-γ, interferon-γ; Mac, macrophage activation; MMP, matrix metalloprotease; NE, neutrophil elastase; TGF-β, transforming growth factor β; TNF-α, tumour necrosis factor α.

Pharmacological studies

The compound ZD0892 was investigated in a model of chronic cigarette smoke exposure in guinea pigs. Long-term (6 months) cigarette smoke exposure results in emphysema, in an increase in neutrophils, DES and HP in BALF, and in an increase in TNF-α in plasma. ZD0892 treatment abolishes the BALF changes, reduces the plasma increase in TNF-α by 30% and emphysema by 45%. Thus, the positive results obtained with ZD0892 in the model of acute smoke exposure have a predictive value for the effects of ZD0892 in the model of chronic smoke exposure [27].

In a recent study groups of C57Bl/6J mice were dosed daily with the phosphodiesterase 4 inhibitor roflumilast at two dose levels (1 and 5 mg/kg p.o.) and were exposed to cigarette smoke for 7 months. In control animals chronic smoke exposure caused a 1.8-fold increase in lung macrophage density, emphysema, an increase of the mean linear intercept (+21%), a decrease of the internal surface area (−13%), and a drop (−13%) in lung desmosine content. The low dose of roflumilast did not have any effect, whereas the high dose prevented the increase in lung macrophage density by 70% and fully prevented the other changes [36]. This study supports the role of an inflammatory process in the development of cigarette smoke-induced matrix destruction and emphysema.

In another study the 3-hydroxy-3-methyl-glutaryl-coenzyme-A reductase inhibitor simvastatin was given daily at the dose of 5 mg/kg p.o. to Sprague–Dawley rats and the animals were exposed to cigarette smoke for 4 months. Simvastatin inhibited lung parenchymal destruction and development of pulmonary hypertension, and also inhibited peribronchial and perivascular infiltration of inflammatory cells and induction of matrix metalloproteinase-9 activity in lung tissue [37]. The amelioration by simvastatin of the structural derangements caused by cigarette smoking was attributed to an anti-inflammatory effect of this compound.

In conclusion, the investigation of novel pharmacological approaches in the amelioration of emphysema in animal models has provided new leads for the treatment of this disease. Additionally, the study of the pathogenesis of emphysema and/or COPD in animal models of this disease has been very intense in recent years and novel hypotheses have been put forward. The theories and hypotheses that have been confirmed in animal models are summarized in Table 30.1.

References

1 Snider GL, Martorana PA, Lucey EC, Lungarella G. Animal models of emphysema. In: Voelkel NF, MacNee W, eds. *Chronic Obstructive Lung Diseases*. Hamilton, BC Decker: 2002, 237–56.

2 Siracusa LD, McGrath R, Ma Q *et al.* A tandem duplication within the fibrillin-1 gene is associated with the mouse tight-skin mutation. *Genome Res* 1996;**6**:300–13.

3 Martorana PA, van Even P, Gardi C, Lungarella G. A 16-month study of the development of genetic emphysema in tight-skin mice. *Am Rev Respir Dis* 1989;**139**:226–32.

4 Gardi C, Martorana PA, de Santi MM, van Even P, Lungarella G. A biochemical and morphological investigation of the early development of genetic emphysema in tight-skin mice. *Exp Mol Pathol* 1989;**50**:398–410.

5 Gardi C, Cavarra E, Calzoni P *et al.* Neutrophil lysosomal dysfunction in mutant C57Bl/6J mice: interstrain variations in content of lysosomal elastase, cathepsin G and their inhibitors. *Biochem J* 1994;**299**:237–45.

6 Martorana PA, Wilkinson M, van Even P, Lungarella G. Tsk mice with genetic emphysema: right ventricular hypertrophy occurs without hypertrophy of muscular pulmonary arteries or muscularization of arterioles. *Am Rev Respir Dis* 1990;**142**:333–7.

7 Huang L, Kuo YM, Gitschier J. The pallid gene encodes a novel, syntaxin13-interacting protein involved in platelet storage pool deficiency. *Nat Genet* 1999;**23**:329–32.

8 Martorana PA, Brand T, Gardi C *et al.* The pallid mouse: a model of genetic α_1-antitrypsin deficiency. *Lab Invest* 1993; **68**:233–41.

9 de Santi MM, Martorana PA, Cavarra E, Lungarella G. Pallid mice with genetic emphysema: neutrophil elastase burden and elastin loss occur without alteration in the bronchoalveolar lavage cell population. *Lab Invest* 1995;**73**:40–7.

10 Suga T, Kurabayashi M, Sando Y *et al.* Disruption of the *klotho* gene causes pulmonary emphysema in mice: defect in maintenance of pulmonary integrity during postnatal life. *Am J Respir Cell Mol Biol* 2000;**22**:26–33.

11 Wang Z, Zheng T, Zhu Z *et al.* Interferon-γ induction of pulmonary emphysema in the adult murine lung. *J Exp Med* 2000;**192**:1587–600.

12 Elias JA. IFN-γ-induced emphysema: a marriage of theories of emphysema pathogenesis. Abstract Book of the 2nd Siena International Conference on Animal Models of COPD, Siena (Italy), Sept. 6–8, 2003.

13 Zheng T, Zhu Z, Wang Z *et al.* Inducible targeting of IL-13 to the adult lung causes matrix metalloproteinase- and cathepsin-dependent emphysema. *J Clin Invest* 2000;**106**:1081–93.

14 Fujita M, Shannon JM, Irvin CG *et al.* Overexpression of tumor necrosis factor-alpha produces an increase in lung volumes and pulmonary hypertension. *Am J Physiol Lung Cell Mol Physiol* 2001;**280**:L39–49.

15 Lucey EC, Keane J, Kuang P-P, Snider GL, Goldstein RH. Severity of elastase-induced emphysema is decreased in tumor necrosis factor-α and interleukin-1β receptor-deficient mice. *Lab Invest* 2002;**82**:79–85.

16 Morris DG, Huang X, Kaminski N *et al.* Loss of integrin $\alpha v\beta 6$-mediated TGF-β activation causes MMP-12-dependent emphysema. *Nature* 2003;**422**:169–73.

17 Kasahara Y, Tuder RM, Taraseviciene-Stewart L *et al.* Inhibition of vascular endothelial growth factor receptors causes lung cell apoptosis and emphysema. *J Clin Invest* 2000;**106**:1311–9.

18 Tuder RM, Zhen L, Cho CY *et al.* Oxidative stress and apoptosis interact and cause emphysema due to vascular endothelial growth factor receptor blockade. *Am J Repir Cell Mol Biol* 2003;**29**:88–97.

19 Aoshiba K, Yokohori N, Nagai A. Alveolar wall apoptosis causes lung destruction and emphysematous changes. *Am J Repir Cell Mol Biol* 2003;**28**:555–62.

20 De Carlo Massaro G, Radaeva S, Biadasz Clerch L, Massaro D. Lung alveoli: endogenous programmed destruction and regeneration. *Am J Physiol Lung Cell Mol Physiol* 2002;**283**:L305–9.

21 Cavarra E, Lucattelli M, Gambelli F *et al.* Human SLPI inactivation after cigarette smoke exposure in a new *in vivo* model of pulmonary oxidative stress. *Am J Physiol Lung Cell Mol Physiol* 2001;**281**:L412–7.

22 Cavarra E, Bartalesi B, Lucattelli M *et al.* Effects of cigarette smoke in mice with different levels of α_1-proteinase inhibitor and sensitivity to oxidants. *Am J Respir Crit Care Med* 2001; **164**:886–90.

23 Dhami R, Gilks B, Xie C *et al.* Acute cigarette smoke-induced connective tissue breakdown is mediated by neutrophils and prevented by α_1-antitrypsin. *Am J Respir Cell Mol Biol* 2000; **22**:244–52.

24 Churg A, Zay K, Shay S *et al.* Acute cigarette smoke-induced connective tissue breakdown requires both neutrophils and macrophage metalloelastase in mice. *Am J Respir Cell Mol Biol* 2002;**27**:368–74.

25 Churg A, Dai J, Tai C, Wright JL. Tumor necrosis factor α is central to acute cigarette smoke-induced inflammation and connective tissue breakdown. *Am J Respir Crit Care Med* 2002;**166**:849–54.

26 Churg A, Wang RD, Tai H *et al.* Macrophage metalloelastase mediates acute cigarette smoke-induced inflammation via tumor necrosis factor-α release. *Am J Respir Crit Care Med* 2003;**167**:1083–9.

27 Wright JL, Farmer SG, Churg A. Synthetic serine elastase inhibitor reduces cigarette smoke-induced emphysema in guinea pigs. *Am J Respir Crit Care Med* 2002;**166**:954–60.

28 Rangasamy T, Cho CY, Thimmulappa RK *et al.* Genetic ablation of Nrf2 enhances susceptibility to cigarette smoke-induced emphysema in mice. *J Clin Invest* 2004;**114**:1248–59.

29 Takubo Y, Guerassimov A, Ghezzo H *et al.* α_1-Antitrypsin determines the pattern of emphysema and function in tobacco smoke-exposed mice: parallel with human disease. *Am J Respir Crit Care Med* 2002;**166**:1596–603.

30 Hautamaki RD, Kobayashi DK, Senior RM, Shapiro SD. Requirement for macrophage elastase for cigarette smoke-induced emphysema in mice. *Science* 1997;**277**:2002–4.

31 Ofulue A, Ko M, Abboud M. Time course of neutrophil and macrophage elastinolytic activities in cigarette smoke-induced emphysema. *Am J Physiol Lung Cell Mol Physiol* 1998;**275**: L1134–44.

32 Ofulue A, Ko M. Effects of depletion of neutrophils or macrophages on the development of cigarette smoke-induced emphysema. *Am J Physiol Lung Cell Mol Physiol* 1999;**277**: L97–105.

33 Shapiro SD, Goldstein NM, Houghton AM *et al.* Neutrophil elastase contributes to cigarette smoke-induced emphysema in mice. *Am J Pathol* 2003;**163**:2329–35.

34 Churg A, Wang RD, Xie C, Wright JL. α_1-Antitrypsin ameliorates cigarette smoke-induced emphysema in the mouse. *Am J Respir Crit Care Med* 2003;**168**:199–207.

35 Meshi B, Vitalis TZ, Ionescu D *et al.* Emphysematous lung destruction by cigarette smoke: the effects of latent adenoviral infection on the lung inflammatory response. *Am J Respir Cell Mol Biol* 2002;**26**:52–7.

36 Martorana PA, Beume R, Lucattelli M, Wollin L, Lungarella G. Roflumilast fully prevents emphysema in mice chronically exposed to cigarette smoke. *Am J Respir Crit Care Med* 2005;**172**:848–53.

37 Lee J-H, Lee D-S, Kim E-K *et al.* Simvastatin inhibits cigarette smoking-induced emphysema and pulmonary hypertension in rat lungs. *Am J Respir Crit Care Med* 2005;**172**:987–93.

CHAPTER 31
Proteinases and COPD

Anita L. Sullivan and Robert A. Stockley

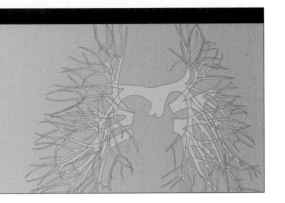

Proteinases are believed to have an important role in the pathogenesis of COPD. The proteinase–antiproteinase hypothesis states that the lung damage of COPD arises when the action of proteinases is no longer controlled by antiproteinases. This may occur when there is a genetic abnormality of antiproteinases, as in α_1-antitrypsin (α_1-AT) deficiency, or a functional loss of antiproteinases through proteolytic or oxidative damage. Alternatively, the same imbalance can arise because of excessive recruitment or activation of proteinases.

Proteinases are classified as serine or cysteine proteinases, depending on the amino acid at their active site, and a third major group, the matrix metalloproteinases (MMPs), which require a metal ion in their structure for their extracellular matrix protein-degrading activity. Proteinases are able to degrade structural lung proteins giving them their capacity as elastases, collagenases or gelatinases (Fig. 31.1 a–c; for c also see Plate 31.1; colour plate section falls between pp. 354 and 355). In addition, many proteinases have roles in post-translational processing of other enzymes, cytokines and receptors. Over the years, a large body of work has accumulated showing important roles for proteinases and antiproteinases from all three of the major groups in the pathogenesis of COPD. However, it is difficult to assess the relative importance of each from the results of studies of individual proteinases, as they are often conflicting. This chapter provides an overview following discussion of the likely contributions from enzymes of each biochemical group.

Serine proteinases

These comprise neutrophil elastase (NE), cathepsin G (CG) and proteinase-3 (PR3), which are stored with myeloperoxidase (MPO) in the azurophil granules of neutrophils [1]. They are made early during neutrophil development

in the bone marrow, with gene expression ceasing at the metamyelocyte stage [2] and are produced as preproenzymes, activated by a lysosomal cysteine proteinase, dipeptidyl peptidase I (cathepsin C) [3]. Although these enzymes are often considered to be neutrophilic in origin, they are also produced by a subgroup of circulating monocytes. Furthermore, these monocytes are also migratory and release the enzymes on activation [4]. The potential importance of these enzymes is underlined by their ability to induce the pathological changes seen in COPD and the increased risk of emphysema in patients deficient in their main inhibitor, α_1-AT [5]. A list of the serine proteinase inhibitors relevant to the lungs is given in Table 31.1.

NE was the first of these enzymes to be shown to produce emphysema in animal models and hence has been the subject of most study. It is believed that the main physiological function of NE is bacterial killing, which takes place after ingestion of opsonized bacteria into a phagosome. Granules are released into a lysosome, which fuses with the phagosome, and the combination of proteinases and oxidants results in bacterial killing [6]. Deficiency of azurophil granule serine proteinases, Chédiak–Higashi syndrome, leads to immunodeficiency [7]. The major role of NE in health is thus probably within the neutrophil.

NE has the capacity to be intensely destructive. It is believed to be a key effector of lung damage in both emphysema and chronic bronchitis [8]. This concept is supported by a number of animal studies, in which instillation of NE and other elastases have reproduced the morphological changes of emphysema and bronchitis (Table 31.2). The development of emphysema is specific to elastase activity [9], and the severity of the ensuing emphysema relates to the elastinolytic potency of the enzyme used [10]. Lung damage by NE can be prevented by specific elastase inhibitors [11,12]. NE can degrade matrix proteins such as elastin, fibronectin [13] and collagen [14], and weakens immunity by attacking immunoglobulins [15]

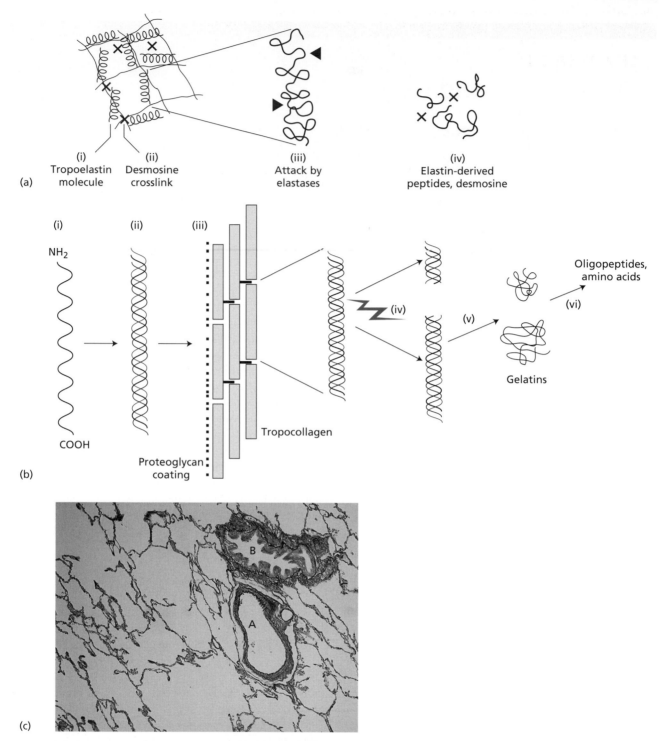

Figure 31.1 (a) Elastin and its degradation. Tropoelastin molecules associate on a framework of fibrillin molecules (i), and are cross-linked between lysine residues. Four lysine residues form a desmosine cross-link (ii). Elastases hydrolyse bonds between amino acids according to their active site specificity (iii), producing characteristic elastin-derived peptides and desmosine cross-links which are specific markers of elastin degradation (iv). (b) The α-helical procollagen strands (i) associate into a triple helix to form a tropocollagen molecule (ii). These molecules then associate into collagen fibres (iii), with cross-links between the telopeptides of each tropocollagen molecule and the hydroxyproline and hydroxylysine residues in the helical area. The fibre is coated with proteoglycans and glycopeptides, which may help to stabilize it or to protect it from collagenolytic attack. Serine and cysteine proteinases can destabilize the fibre by degrading intra- or intertropocollagen bonds, and some can also cleave within the

Table 31.1 Serine proteinase inhibitors in the lungs. Individual references not given for reasons of space.

Inhibitor	Source	Molecular weight (kDa)	Target proteinase	Inhibition
α_1-AT	Serum	54	NE, CG, PR3, mast cell chymase	Irreversible
α_1-ACT	Serum	68	CG, mast cell chymase	Reversible
α_1-M	Serum	725	All classes of proteinase	Irreversible
SLPI	Mucosa	11.7	NE, CG, mast cell chymase and tryptase	Reversible
Elafin	Mucosa	9.9	NE, PR3	Reversible
M-NEI	Neutrophils, monocytes	42	NE, CG, PR3, mast cell chymase	Irreversible

α_1-AT, α_1-antitrypsin; α_1-ACT, α_1-antichymotrypsin; α_2-M, α_2-macroglobulin; CG, cathepsin G; M-NEI, monocyte–neutrophil elastase inhibitor; NE, neutrophil elastase; PR3, proteinase 3; SLPI, secretory leucoproteinase inhibitor.

Table 31.2 Animal experiments using elastases.

Author/year	Animal	Enzyme	Result
Gross et al. 1964 [158]	Rat	Papain (plant elastase)	Demonstrated induction of emphysema using papain
Marco et al. 1971 [159]	Dog	Neutrophil lysates	Demonstrated that neutrophil lysates could induce emphysema
Blackwood et al. 1973 [10]	Rat	Various elastases	Severity of emphysema depends on elastinolytic potency of inducing enzyme
Snider et al. 1974 [9]	Hamster	Various elastases	Ability to induce emphysema depends on elastinolytic activity
Janoff et al. 1977 [160]	Dog	Purified NE	NE can induce emphysema
Senior et al. 1977 [161]	Hamster	Purified NE	NE can induce emphysema
Lucey et al. 1985 [68]	Hamster	Purified NE	NE can also induce secretory cell metaplasia
Kao et al. 1988 [69]	Hamster	Fraction of neutrophil lysate containing PR3	PR3 is as potent as NE in inducing emphysema

NE, neutrophil elastase; PR3, proteinase 3.

and components of the complement system [16,17]. It may also slow wound healing, possibly by its effect on transforming growth factor β [18] or epithelins [19].

In order to reach the lungs, neutrophils must be activated, adhere to endothelium and then migrate through to the airways. Neutrophils may degranulate, releasing enzymes, or may cause tissue damage by close contact with cells and matrix. During neutrophil activation, azurophil granule proteinases are expressed on the neutrophil membrane [20]. In vitro studies have shown that approximately 2% of the azurophil granule proteinases are released into the media on activation of the neutrophil by pro-inflammatory stimuli, the rest remaining associated with the cell by a charge-dependent mechanism [21,22]. While NE bound to the neutrophil membrane exhibits partial resistance to the effects of native inhibitors such as α_1-AT [20], free NE can be readily inhibited by both serum- and tissue-based inhibitors [23], thereby preventing tissue damage at a distance from the cell.

Although the majority of serine proteinase activity remains associated with the neutrophil even after activation, free NE activity can be detected in secretions from

helical region. 'True' collagenases (matrix metalloproteinases [MMPs]-1, -8 and -13) cleave the tropocollagen molecule at three-quarters of the length of the helix, producing characteristic one-quarter and three-quarter length fragments (iv). Collagen fragments spontaneously denature into gelatin at body temperature (v), which can then be further degraded into oligopeptides and amino acids, predominantly hydroxyproline, which thus acts as a marker for collagen breakdown (vi). (c) Section of normal human lung × 100, stained with Elastic van Gieson, which highlights elastic fibres as black (see Plate 31.1; colour plate section falls between pp. 354 and 355). Collagen stains crimson red with this stain (see Plate 31.1; colour plate section falls between pp. 354 and 355). Distinct elastin laminae can be seen within the walls of a bronchiole (B) and its accompanying nutrient artery (A). Collagen is best seen surrounding blood vessels in this photomicrograph (see Plate 31.1; colour plate section falls between pp. 354 and 355). Note the predominance of elastin staining in alveolar tissue. Sections kindly prepared by Dr Simon Trotter, Department of Histopathology, Birmingham Heartlands Hospital, UK.

patients with COPD [24]. This may be the result solely of neutrophil degranulation, but there are several other possibilities. First, when neutrophils die by apoptosis, they are cleared by macrophages [25], which can also scavenge free NE [26], whereas necrotic neutrophils release their contents into the extracellular space [27]. Secondly, the process of phagocytosis may involve release of significant amounts of both NE and PR3 into the media [28]. This might occur when neutrophils attempt to ingest large extracellular structures ('frustrated phagocytosis'), or as a by-product of normal phagocytosis ('sloppy eating'), demonstrated in studies comparing activation by lipopolysaccharide (LPS) alone with ingestion of opsonized yeast cells, which showed that free NE activity was only detected in the media with the latter [29]. Thirdly, studies of macrophages isolated from the lungs of patients with COPD showed that their *in vitro* elastinolytic effect depended largely on serine proteinases within the first 24 h of culture, but MMPs over the next 48 h, suggesting that the early serine proteinase activity was attributable to endocytosed enzymes rather than constitutively secreted enzymes [30]. Earlier studies showed that alveolar macrophages could release active NE that was endocytosed up to 5 days previously [31]. Finally, monocytes can express and secrete serine proteinases, although they lose this capacity on differentiation to macrophages [32].

The majority of NE-related parenchymal tissue destruction may occur in association with the passage of neutrophils from the circulation to the airway. This suggests that NE inhibitors might mediate their protective effect at least in part by reducing neutrophil migration, but studies examining this concept have produced conflicting results. Using the multiple blind well assay system, chemotaxis in response to formyl-methionyl-leucyl-phenylalanine (fMLP) was inhibited by α_1-AT [33], specific antibody against CG and physiological concentrations of mutant forms of α_1-AT and α_1-antichymotrypsin [34]. Synthetic inhibitors of CG were shown to reduce the leading front response in the under agarose assay. Interestingly, the same study suggested that a mutant form of α_1-AT with greater antichymotrypsin activity was effective in reducing migration, implying that CG has a greater role in this activity than NE [34]. Serine proteinase inhibitors have been shown to prevent degradation of basement membrane components by cell-free NE [23]. However, examination of neutrophil migration across fibrinogen or Matrigel barriers has shown conflicting results using NE and MMP-9 inhibitors [23,35,36]. In rats, inhibition of NE could prevent neutrophil migration *in vivo*, but migration across endothelial monolayers *in vitro* was not prevented [37]. Studies using a combination of endothelial cells and basement membrane have consistently shown that proteinase inhibitors do not prevent neutrophil migration [38,39]. Furthermore, *in vitro*

neutrophil migration across endothelium was not impaired in mice deficient in NE or MMP-9 [40]. The variability in the results of these studies demonstrate the difficulties of assessing the importance of proteinases in neutrophil migration, either by using antiproteinases, which may not be able to inhibit cell-associated enzymes in contact with matrix structures, or by eliminating only one proteinase from neutrophils that retain two other potent serine proteinases.

In support of this concept, neutrophils from mice whose genes for NE and CG had been 'knocked out' showed normal migration *in vitro*, and these mice exhibited normal neutrophil infiltration into tissue in response to fungal infection and lipopolysaccharide, although pathogen clearance was severely impaired [41]. In humans, patients with Papillon–Lefèvre syndrome have deficient dipeptidyl peptidase I [42], causing a functional deficiency of NE and CG through impaired processing of the pre-proenzyme, and neutrophil migration is also impaired *in vitro* [43]. The main phenotype, however, is severe periodontitis, with no systemic immunodeficiency – which may imply physiological redundancy, or that another enzyme activates these proteinases after secretion *in vivo*. On the other hand, neutrophils from patients with Chédiak–Higashi syndrome, in which all three neutrophil serine proteinases are deficient, do not migrate towards chemoattractants [44].

Animal studies using proteinase inhibitors often show reduced neutrophil influx to the lungs. For example, studies in guinea pigs demonstrated an acute response to cigarette smoke, consisting of airway neutrophilia and increased connective tissue breakdown products in bronchoalveolar lavage fluid (BALF), which could be inhibited by pre-treatment with a synthetic NE inhibitor [45]. In rats, instillation of NE to the airways induced neutrophil influx, which was inhibited by intratracheal but not intravenous administration of a synthetic NE inhibitor. On the other hand, intratracheal instillation of sputum from cystic fibrosis patients (in whom there is intense neutrophilic inflammation) induced a massive neutrophil influx, which could be prevented by the same inhibitor only when it was administered intravenously rather than intratracheally [46]. This suggests that the effect was related to inhibition of proteinases in the circulation (prior to neutrophil migration) rather than the airway. These studies support the concept that the type of stimulus for neutrophil migration influences the role of proteinases in neutrophil migration, and that the proteinase-dependent process may occur while the neutrophil is still within the circulation.

The mechanisms of neutrophil migration are not well understood. Even if serine proteinases are required, their function is not necessarily degradation of extracellular matrix substrates to allow cell passage, as they may process other important proteins such as adhesion factors [37],

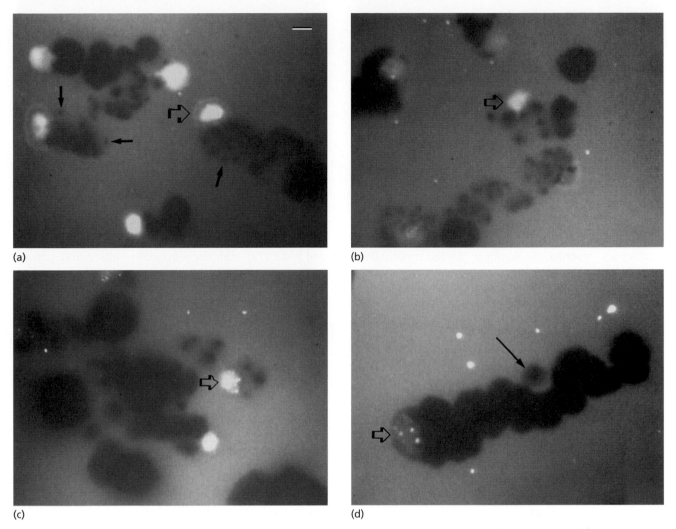

Figure 31.2 Quantum proteolytic events associated with PMNs bathed in serum from donors with various AAT phenotypes. PMNs were allowed to migrate for 30 min at 37°C on opsonized fluoresceinated fibronectin while bathed in serum from phenotypes with (a) Pi M, (b) Pi MZ, (c) Pi SZ and (d) Pi Z. Cells were fixed and then examined by incident-light fluorescence microscopy. Note the discrete, rounded, dark areas associated with migrating cells, which are very localized areas of degraded fibronectin (short arrows in (a) identify selected areas of quantum proteolysis). Note also the coalescent areas of degradation that are related to release of two or more azurophil granules. PMNs remaining on the surface are fluorescent because of ingested fibronectin fragments (broad arrows). The quantum proteolytic events are visually similar in size in a–c. Note also that cell-associated proteolytic events are strikingly larger in cells bathed in Pi Z serum (long arrow in d) when compared with those bathed in serum from the other donors. Scale bar: 10 μm. (From Campbell *et al.* [49] with permission.)

or stimulate intracellular signalling [47]. However, tissue degradation might occur as a side-effect of neutrophil passage without being necessary for migration. The failure of serine proteinase inhibitors to prevent this process might relate to the phenomenon of quantum proteolysis, in which the concentration of NE falls exponentially with the distance from the site of enzyme release [48]. Thus, although the concentration of free NE in the lung is lower than the concentration of its inhibitors, there would be an imbalance between proteinase and inhibitor close to the

site of release of the enzyme, which enables breakdown of elastin to occur. This concept was proved in a series of experiments with serum from patients with normal or deficient α_1-AT (Figure 31.2) [49]. A similar local imbalance, closer in proximity to the neutrophil, could occur without release of free enzyme, as native inhibitors are functionally less effective against membrane-bound proteinases [20]. *In vivo* therefore, neutrophil activation and migration may be sufficient to cause some tissue destruction despite the presence of inhibitors, and the true contribution of serine proteinases to this process may not be determined until development of animal models in which all three enzymes are absent only in the postnatal period.

The mechanism by which neutrophil serine proteinases cause lung damage may be modified by their interaction with proteinase inhibitors, the presence of the neutrophil itself, epithelial cells and the extracellular matrix. For example, NE, once bound to elastin, is poorly inhibited by α_1-AT, while the activity of secretory leucoproteinase inhibitor (SLPI) is unaffected [50]. NE bound to α_2-macroglobulin is prevented from degrading elastin, but can still degrade small substrates [51]. Studies using intratracheal interleukin 8 (IL-8; a neutrophil chemoattractant) in guinea pigs showed that goblet cell degranulation could be prevented by IL-8 blockade or specific inhibitors of NE. Further *in vitro* studies incubating explanted tracheal tissue with neutrophils showed that inhibition of neutrophil adhesion factors also prevented degranulation. The authors speculated that adhesion of neutrophils to goblet cells altered the neutrophil membrane, facilitating release of membrane-bound NE into the intercellular space and triggering goblet cell degranulation [52].

There seems little doubt that NE is the critical proteinase in the mucus hypersecretory phenotype of COPD. Animal models have demonstrated induction of secretory cell metaplasia in direct response to NE (see Table 31.2) and prevention of secretory cell metaplasia with inhibitors of NE [52], while inhibition of other classes of proteinase is not effective [53,54]. The mechanism for these changes is not fully understood, however, and may involve an effect on the epidermal growth factor receptor [55], with NE acting as part of a signalling cascade.

Serine proteinases also have many deleterious effects on respiratory epithelium. In chronic bronchitis, secretions contain a toxic component that influences ciliary beating, which is abrogated by inhibitors of NE [56]. Purified NE *in vitro* reduces ciliary function and damages respiratory epithelial cells [57]. Serine proteinases trigger a state of oxidative stress in respiratory epithelial cells [58], which may contribute to the effect of NE on mucin secretion [59]. NE can also induce the detachment of bronchial epithelial cells from extracellular matrix [60] and apoptosis of epithelial cells [61], while both NE and PR3 induce detachment and apoptosis of endothelial cells [62,63]. This may be important in the pathogenesis of COPD. Serine proteinases, especially NE, are therefore likely to have many effects on the airway epithelium in COPD as well as the connective tissue matrix. Most of this concept, however, has been hypothetical but recent work has shown more clearly that the purulence of sputum relates to the activity of NE in secretions [64], which is in direct contact with the epithelium and results from neutrophil migration. This is particularly important during exacerbations when neutrophil influx and elastase activity increase [64]. The frequency of these episodes relates to the progressive decline in lung function, suggesting a causal relationship [65,66].

The central role of NE in human emphysema has been called into question by animal models showing that NE knockout mice are only partially protected against the development of emphysema [67]. However, these models may be limited by the persisting presence of CG and PR3 in azurophil granules – the former can cause secretory cell metaplasia [68] and the latter can cause both emphysema and secretory cell metaplasia [69]. Nevertheless, indirect data from human studies support the concept that neutrophils and neutrophil enzymes are important in emphysema. Studies have shown that smokers have increased numbers of neutrophils in lung tissue [70], sputum [71,72] and BALF [73], and that neutrophils isolated from patients with emphysema exhibit increased elastinolytic and chemotactic activity compared with those from controls [74], and express more adhesion factors [75]. Even at an early stage with subclinical emphysema on high-resolution CT scan, there is an increase in NE and other neutrophil proteins in BALF [76,77]. Studies on patients with established emphysema indicate that NE activity in BALF correlates with the severity of emphysema in smokers [78] and falls when they stop smoking [79], and cessation of smoking is the only intervention shown to affect progression of COPD to date. On the other hand, although the neutrophil count in lung interstitium correlated with the severity of emphysema in one study [80], it showed an inverse relationship in other studies [81–83]. However, before any conclusions can be drawn from these studies, it should be remembered that the neutrophil is a migratory cell and its residence in the interstitium is short. It is likely that any interstitial damage leading to emphysema relates to the cells that have passed as much as the ones seen while migrating through the tissues.

NE may also have an indirect role as it has the ability to amplify the inflammatory process in the lungs. Leukotriene (LT) B_4 released from lung macrophages is important as a chemoattractant bringing neutrophils to the lungs in COPD [84,85], and release of LTB_4 by macrophages is stimulated by free NE [86]. In addition, NE may stimulate bronchial epithelial cells to release IL-8. Finally, neutrophils themselves release LTB_4 and IL-8, leading to further cell recruitment. In this way, NE released by neutrophils contributes to positive feedback recruiting more neutrophils and amplifying inflammation. This amplification will be greater in patients deficient in α_1-AT, who have greater concentrations of LTB_4 and elastase, and more neutrophilic inflammation in their lung secretions than have non-deficient COPD patients [87].

The overall evidence from *in vitro* work, animal models and human studies suggests that NE is important in

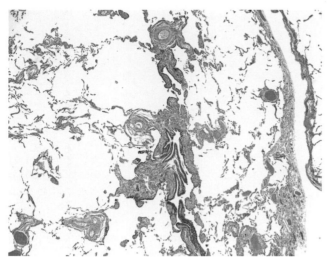

Plate 6.1 Photomicrograph of lung tissue from a patient with endstage COPD/emphysema. This specimen shows the destruction of the alveolar–capillary architecture, highly muscularized arteries and fibrosis around the bronchovascular bundle. The pleura is thickened and hypervascular. (H&E staining, ×200). (Courtesy of Dr Carlyne Cool.)

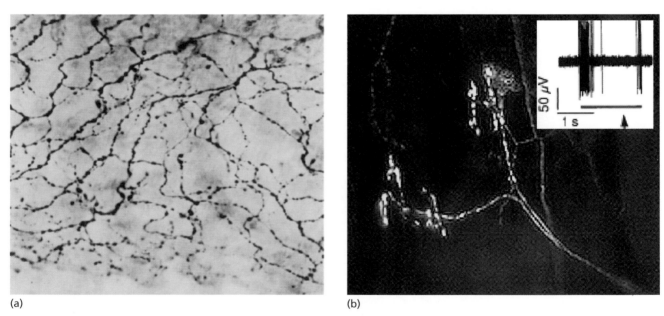

(a)   (b)

Plate 8.1 (a) Photomicrograph of a whole mount preparation of rat tracheal mucosa stained with an antibody against substance P, showing the lattice-like structure of the mucosal C-fibre plexus. To visualize a similar pattern of nerves in human airway mucosa, a non-specific neuronal marker such as PGP 9.5 is required, because only a fraction of the mucosal plexus in humans contains substance P [91]. (From Baluk P, Nadel JA, McDonald DM. Substance P-immunoreactive sensory axons in the rat respiratory tract: a quantitative study of their distribution and role in neurogenic inflammation. *J Comp Neurol* 1992;**319**:586–98 with permission.) (b) Photomicrograph of a mechanosensitive Aδ-fibre stained with the vital dye FM 2-10 in guinea pig trachea. This structure is situated just beneath the basement membrane, and found throughout the trachea and main stem bronchus. The inset shows the rapidly adapting action potential discharge caused by application of a punctate mechanical stimulus (von Frey probe, horizontal bar) to the airway containing this nerve structure (conduction velocity ~4 m/s). Activation of this type of fibre in the guinea pig trachea consistently evokes cough (Courtesy of B. J. Canning.)

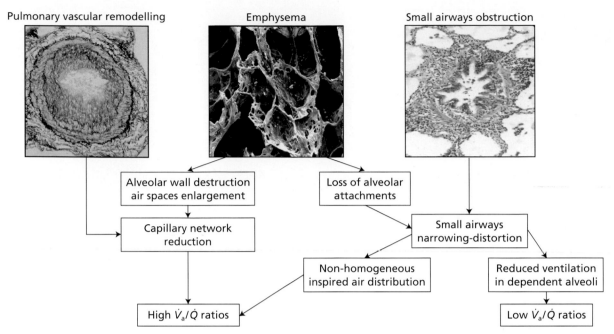

Plate 9.1 Schematic diagram of the correlations between key pathological features of COPD (small airways obstructive, pulmonary emphysema and vascular remodelling) and pulmonary gas exchange state (ventilation/perfusion imbalance) in stable advanced COPD.

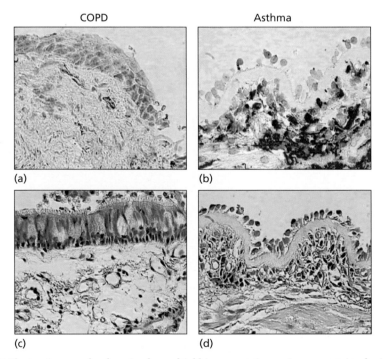

Plate 14.1 (a,b) Photomicrographs showing bronchial biopsy specimens immunostained with anti-EG-2 (eosinophil cationic protein) from: (a) a patient with fixed airflow obstruction and a history of COPD; and (b) a patient with fixed airflow obstruction and a history of asthma. The two patients had a similar degree of fixed airflow obstruction. In (b) there is prominent eosinophilia beneath the destroyed epithelium that is not present in (a). (c,d) Photomicrographs showing bronchial biopsy specimens stained with haematoxylin and eosin (H&E) from: (c) a patient with fixed airflow obstruction and a history of COPD; and (d) a patient with fixed airflow obstruction and a history of asthma. The two patients had a similar degree of airflow obstruction. In (d) there is a thicker reticular layer of the epithelial basement membrane compared with (c). (From Fabbri LM, Romagnoli M, Corbetta L *et al*. Differences in airway inflammation in patients with fixed airflow obstruction due to asthma or chronic obstructive pulmonary disease. *Am J Respir Crit Care Med* 2003;167:418–24 with permission.)

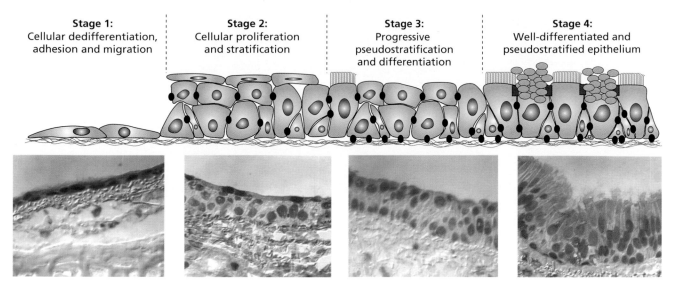

Stage 1: Cellular dedifferentiation, adhesion and migration

Stage 2: Cellular proliferation and stratification

Stage 3: Progressive pseudostratification and differentiation

Stage 4: Well-differentiated and pseudostratified epithelium

Plate 22.1 Sequence of events in the regeneration of airway epithelium. (From Dupuit F, Gaillard D, Hinnrasky J *et al.* Differentiated and functional human airway epithelium regeneration in tracheal xenografts. *Am J Physiol Lung Cell Mol Physiol* 2000;278:L165–76 with permission.)

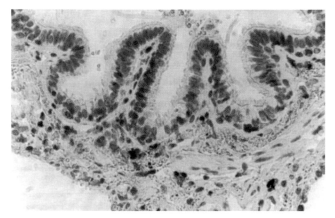

Plate 24.1 Peripheral airway of a smoking subject with COPD showing CD8+ T lymphocyte infiltration in the wall. Immunostaining with anti-CD8 monoclonal antibody. Original magnification: × 200.

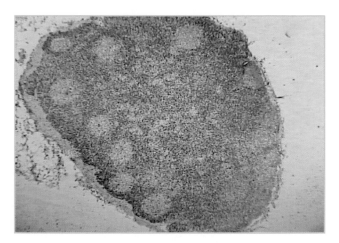

Plate 24.2 Paratracheal lymph node from a smoking subject with COPD. B lymphocytes are organized in lymphoid follicles, surrounded by a paracortical region rich in CD4+ and CD8+ T lymphocytes. Immunostaining with anti-CD8 monoclonal antibody. Original magnification × 50.

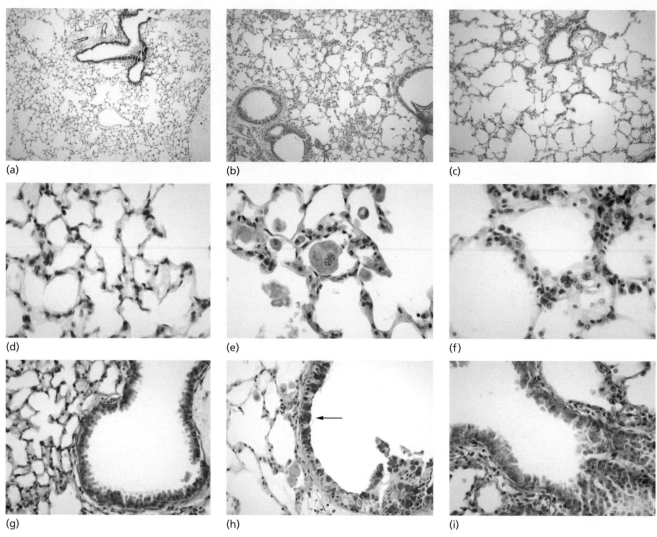

Plate 25.1 Histology of interleukin-13 (IL-13) and γ-interferon-induced emphysema. First column is normal mouse lung, second column is IL-13 overexpressing mouse lung and third column is γ-interferon overexpressing mouse lung. (a–c) Low power, hematoxylin and eosin. Note normal alveolar architecture in wild type mice while both IL-13 and interferon mice show marked alveolar destruction. (d–f) High power hematoxylin and eosin. Note lack of significant infiltrate in normal lung, accumulation of macrophages and eosinophils in IL-13 lung and mononuclear infiltrate in interstitium of interferon lung. (g–i). Periodic Schiff stain. Note mucus accumulation in IL-13 mice (arrow) while no mucus accumulation in normal and interferon expressing mice.

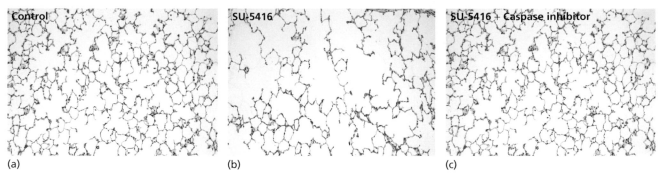

(a)   (b)   (c)

Plate 27.1 Airspace enlargement with VEGF receptor blockade. Hematoxylin-and-eosin staining histology of rat lungs. (a) Section of lung from a control rat showing normal alveolar structure. (b) Section of lung from an SU5416-treated rat showing airspace enlargement. (c) Section of lung from a rat treated with SU5416 plus a caspase inhibitor showing normal alveolar structure. (From Kasahara Y, Tuder RM, Cool CD *et al*. Endothelial cell death and decreased expression of vascular endothelial growth factor and vascular endothelial growth factor receptor 2 in emphysema. *Am J Respir Crit Care Med* 2001;163:737–44 with permission.)

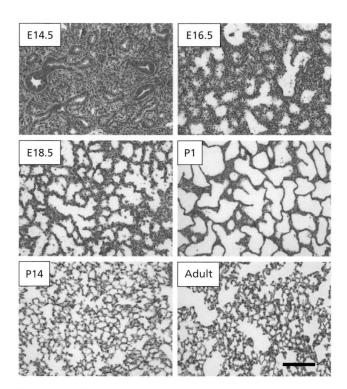

Plate 29.1 Histology of mouse lungs at various stages of development. Embryonic mouse lung develops from early pseudoglandular stage (E14.5), to canalicular stage (E16.5) and further terminal sac stage (E18.5 and P1). Neonatal lungs undergo further alveolarization, resulting in many septa formation (P14). Finally, a mature honeycomb-like structure with normal respiratory function is formed, as observed in adults. Scale bar: 100 μm.

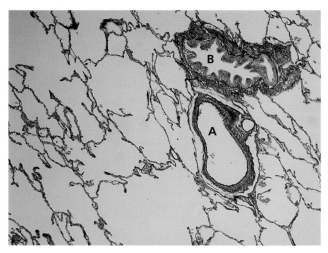

Plate 31.1 Section of normal human lung × 100, stained with Elastic van Gieson, which highlights elastic fibres as black. Collagen stains crimson red with this stain. Distinct elastin laminae can be seen within the walls of a bronchiole (B) and its accompanying nutrient artery (A). Collagen is best seen surrounding blood vessels in this photomicrograph. Note the predominance of elastin staining in alveolar tissue. Sections kindly prepared by Dr Simon Trotter, Department of Histopathology, Birmingham Heartlands Hospital, UK.

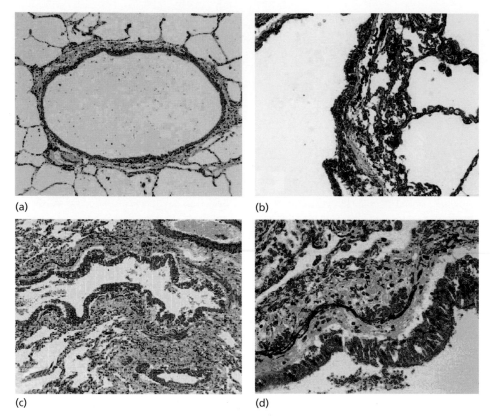

(a)

(b)

(c)

(d)

Plate 34.1 Membranous bronchioles from a lung from Vancouver (a,b) and Mexico City (c,d). Note the greatly thickened airway wall and the marked increase in fibrous tissue and muscle in the Mexico City lung. (a,c) × 50, (b,d) × 200. (From Churg A, Brauer M, del Carmen Avila-Casado M, Fortoul TI, Wright JL. Chronic exposure to high levels of particulate air pollution and small airway remodeling. *Environ Health Perspect* 2003;111:714–8 with permission.)

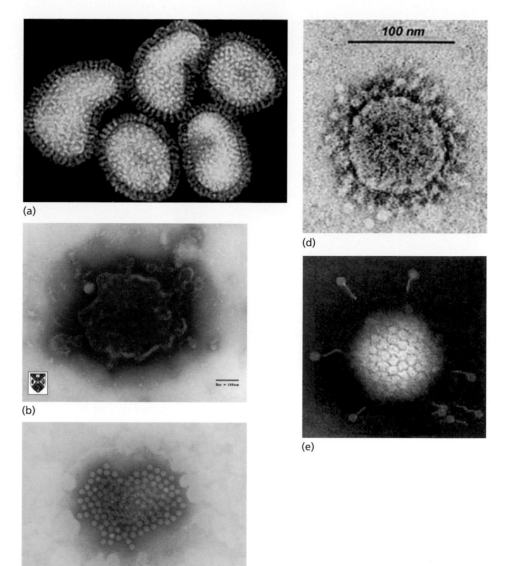

Plate 35.1 Electron microscope images of respiratory viruses common in COPD. (a) Influenza virus. (b) Respiratory syncytial virus (RSV). (c) Human Picornavirus. (d) Severe acute respiratory syndrome (SARS). (e) Adenovirus.

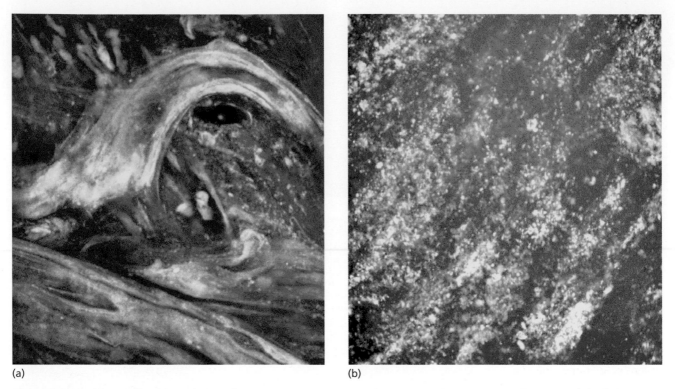

(a)   (b)

Plate 62.1 Peptide mucolytic degradation of DNA. (a) YoYo-1 staining of CF sputum showing DNA polymers, and (b) the same specimen after *in vitro* treatment with rhDNAse.

pathogenesis of COPD and is therefore a potential target for therapeutic intervention. Caution will be needed, however, in suppressing a critical antibacterial defence [88]. Although serine proteinases may have an important role in migration of neutrophils from blood to lung, either they are not essential for this activity, or it is not possible to achieve sufficiently high inhibitor concentrations to inactivate the proteinases in the immediate vicinity of the neutrophil. Reassuringly, studies using LPS as the stimulus for lung damage showed that neutrophil influx was not inhibited by α_1-AT [89], suggesting that the therapeutic use of serine proteinase inhibitors should not affect lung immunity adversely, while limiting the severity of elastase-induced damage.

Animal models have indicated that both synthetic [11] and natural [12,90–92] NE inhibitors are useful when given at the time of administration of the insult causing emphysema. The only animal study examining the effect of NE inhibition on progression of established cigarette smoke-associated disease showed that inflammation and connective tissue breakdown can be reduced by a synthetic NE inhibitor from the time of onset of treatment [45]. More recently, the same group has shown that α_1-AT augmentation has the same effect and prevents the development of emphysema, although this may not be a direct antiproteolytic effect [93]. The relevance of these studies to human disease remains to be determined. Certainly, some animal models have suggested that neutrophil influx is greatest at the onset of lung disease, while macrophage accumulation may be more important later on [94,95]. In human disease, the use of α_1-AT has been confined to patients with deficiency, with some anti-inflammatory effect [96], and indirect studies suggest a reduction in progressive decline in lung function [97,98]. Whether this antiproteinase benefit is of relevance to patients with usual COPD remains unknown.

Other serine proteinases

A subset of mast cells synthesizes cathepsin G together with chymase, while the most important serine proteinase in mast cells as a whole is tryptase. Mast cells may also produce NE and PR3 [99]. There is some evidence that mast cells may be important during exacerbations of COPD [100] and, if so, their proteinases may have a role in tissue damage [101]. Clearly, further studies with these cells are indicated.

Cysteine proteinases

These include cathepsins B, H, K, L and S, inhibited by the cystatins A, C and S and α_2-macroglobulin. This group of proteinases has received less attention, but they have sim-

ilar properties to the serine proteinases and there are imbalances between cysteine proteinases and cystatins in COPD.

Cathepsin B secretion by epithelial cells has been demonstrated *in vitro* [102], but it is not known if this is the major source *in vivo*. This elastinolytic and collagenolytic enzyme is found in sputum from patients with COPD, the amount increases during exacerbations [103] and can be reduced by oral corticosteroids [104]. In patients with bronchiectasis, cathepsin B activity is reduced by antibiotics [104], suggesting it is a feature of inflammation caused by bacteria in this condition. Cathepsin B activity is higher in BALF from smokers than non-smokers [105], although smokers with emphysema had similar cathepsin B levels in BALF to smokers without emphysema [106]. Although cathepsin B is produced by macrophages, not neutrophils [107], its activity in BALF from patients with bronchiectasis correlates with neutrophil but not macrophage counts. Cathepsin B levels also correlate positively with MPO and NE activities, and negatively with cystatin C in these patients [108]. These interrelationships suggest that neutrophilic inflammation and cathepsin B activity are intimately related. It is known that NE generates cathepsin B activity in sputum by activating the pro-enzyme [109]. Cystatin C, which inhibits cathepsin B, is present in mucoid sputum, but in purulent sputum (when NE and cathepsin B activities are detectable), it is only found in a form similar to that produced by NE cleavage *in vitro* [109]. In this form, it inhibits cathepsin B poorly [110]. It therefore seems that NE can play a major part in the activation of cathepsin B, and this may be further amplified because cathepsin B can also inactivate SLPI, the local NE inhibitor (Fig. 31.3) [111]. This amplification and synergy may be of major importance

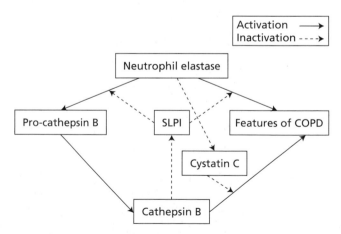

Figure 31.3 Neutrophil elastase (NE) and cathepsin B have synergistic effects. NE can activate pro-cathepsin B while inactivating its inhibitor, cystatin C. Cathepsin B can inactivate an inhibitor of NE, secretory leucoproteinase inhibitor (SLPI), and both NE and cathepsin B degrade connective tissue matrix proteins.

because both NE [68] and cathepsin B [112] can reproduce many of the pathological features of COPD *in vivo*.

Cathepsin K is expressed and synthesized by bronchial and alveolar epithelial cells [113]. It has collagenolytic, gelatinolytic and elastinolytic activity, but its role in the pathogenesis of lung disease is unclear.

Cathepsin L, another elastinolytic proteinase [114], has been studied in COPD, and found in higher concentrations in BALF from smokers with emphysema compared with both non-smokers and smokers without emphysema. Cathepsin L levels did not correlate with NE–α_1-AT complex. In the same study, levels of cystatin C (its natural inhibitor) were found to be elevated in smokers with emphysema [106]. It is unknown whether cathepsin L can directly cause the pathological features of COPD, but it has been shown to degrade α_1-AT *in vitro* [115].

There are few animal models of COPD examining cysteine proteinases and their inhibitors. A study of IL-13-induced emphysema [53] demonstrated an increase in the expression and secretion of cathepsins B, H, K, L and S in the lung. Cysteine proteinase inhibitors E-64 and leupeptin were able to reduce the severity of emphysema by approximately 65% and inflammatory cell infiltrate by approximately 60% when administered alone, and similar results were obtained with a broad-spectrum MMP inhibitor, but even combined administration of both cysteine proteinase and MMP inhibitors did not confer total protection. Interestingly, IL-13 also induced a decrease in pulmonary expression of α_1-AT of approximately 80%, which may induce a critical NE–α_1-AT imbalance.

Matrix metalloproteinases

There has been a major expansion of knowledge of the potential role of MMPs in COPD in recent years. They have important cell signalling functions, as well as the ability to break down extracellular matrix during the remodelling process. They are secreted as pro-enzymes and usually activated by another MMP, often as part of a proteinase cascade. They have the ability to form complexes with inhibitors, dimerize in homologous or heterologous fashion, and remain associated with the cell membrane, sometimes in complexed form. This makes interpretation of activity levels of MMPs in biological fluids difficult. Neutrophils and macrophages each secrete large quantities of MMPs and their inhibitors, the tissue inhibitors of metalloproteinases (TIMPs), although other cells also produce both MMPs and TIMPs in variable amounts.

The potential role of MMPs in COPD is far-reaching, because they not only degrade matrix proteins, but also degrade antiproteinases such as α_1-AT and α_1-antichymotrypsin, activate other enzymes such as those in the clotting cascade, modify cytokines and degrade a number of other miscellaneous proteins such as adhesion factors and substance P. Upwards of 24 mammalian MMPs have now been described, generally grouped as collagenases, gelatinases, etc., according to their primary extracellular matrix (ECM) substrate, but it should be noted that many of these enzymes can degrade all constituents of ECM. Studies in COPD have generally concentrated on those listed in Table 31.3. The main serum inhibitor is α_2-macroglobulin, while all four of the mammalian secreted TIMPs described to date inhibit all of the relevant MMPs (for detailed reviews see [116,117]).

Examination of BALF in patients with emphysema compared with healthy smokers confirmed the presence of metalloelastase activity [118], and studies on isolated macrophages have demonstrated that their elastinolytic activity, while less potent than that of neutrophils, is better preserved in the presence of proteinase inhibitors [119]. The absolute number of macrophages in the lungs of COPD

Table 31.3 Matrix metalloproteinases (MMPs). (Adapted from Sternlicht and Werb [117], additional references not given for reasons of space.)

MMP	Other names	Source	Substrates include
MMP-1	Interstitial collagenase, human collagenase-1	Macrophages, fibroblasts and other stromal cells	Collagens I–III, VII, VIII, X, XI, gelatin
MMP-2	Gelatinase A (72 kDa)	Macrophage, stromal cells	Collagens I, III–V, VII, X, XI, elastin, gelatin
MMP-3	Stromelysin-1	Macrophages, stromal cells	Collagens III–V, VII, IX–XI, elastin, gelatin
MMP-7	Matrilysin	Monocytes	Collagens I, IV, elastin, gelatin
MMP-8	Neutrophil collagenase, collagenase-2	Neutrophils	Collagens I–III
MMP-9	Gelatinase B (92 kDa)	Neutrophils, eosinophils, macrophages, stromal cells	Collagens IV, V, XI, XIV, elastin, gelatin
MMP-12	Macrophage metalloelastase	Macrophages	Collagens I, IV, elastin, gelatin
MMP-13	Collagenase 3	Macrophages, stromal cells	Collagens I–IV, IX, X, XIV
MMP-14	Membrane type (MT) 1-MMP	Macrophages	Collagens I–III, gelatin

patients is always greater than the number of neutrophils, and macrophages are resident cells that have the capacity to continue producing and secreting MMPs throughout their lifetime. For these reasons, it is suspected that they may play a major part in connective tissue degradation in emphysema. Their contribution was demonstrated in histological studies of elastase-induced emphysema in dogs, where alveolar macrophages were seen at the sites of alveolar gaps, although it was unclear whether they had caused the tissue damage, or were part of the repair process [120].

Various studies have produced conflicting results as to the correlation between the numbers of macrophages or neutrophils and the elastinolytic activity in the lung, but it is likely that these cells and the enzymes that they produce also act cooperatively. A number of macrophage enzymes can degrade inhibitors of NE including α_1-AT [121–123] and monocyte–neutrophil elastase inhibitor (M-NEI) [124], and NE degrades TIMPs [125], thereby facilitating MMP activity. Furthermore, NE can activate several of the MMPs [126–128], and MMP-9 is thought to degrade some neutrophil chemoattractants, at least in mice [54], which would potentially decrease PMN recruitment and hence lung NE load. Thus, it is clear that a complex interaction also exists between NE, its inhibitors and the MMPs and TIMPs in a similar way to that for the cysteine proteinases and cystatins. This interaction is evident in animal models of emphysema, which only show partial protection with inhibition of serine, cysteine or MMPs [45,53]. The exceptions to this include the MMP-12 knockout mouse, and the studies by Ofulue *et al.* discussed below.

Animal studies

Macrophage metalloelastase (MMP-12) is the main elastinolytic enzyme of macrophages. A mouse model of cigarette smoke-induced emphysema has demonstrated a critical role for MMP-12 in pathogenesis. Line 129 mice deficient for MMP-12 did not develop emphysema in response to cigarette smoke, and inflammation in the lungs was reduced. The only elastinolytic activity found in whole lung homogenates in wild type mice was derived from MMP-12, and this was absent in the knockout mice. Macrophages from the knockout mice were able to migrate to the lungs in response to instillation of MCP-1, but failed to cause emphysema, while in wild type mice, administration of MCP-1 increased the severity of emphysema [129]. This study suggested that MMP-12 might be the critical proteinase causing lung destruction in emphysema.

Further support for this concept came from studies examining the time course of smoking-induced emphysema in Sprague–Dawley rats over 6 months. While both neutrophil and macrophage numbers increased in response to cigarette smoke, the elevation in neutrophil count and neutrophil elastinolytic activity (defined as that inhibited by a specific NE inhibitor) was greatest in the first month. Connective tissue breakdown and the development of emphysema occurred later, correlating with macrophage count and macrophage elastinolytic activity (defined as that inhibited by ethylenediaminetetraacetic acid [EDTA], i.e. MMP activity), which steadily increased throughout the duration of the study [94]. A second series of studies in the same model examined the effect of depleting either neutrophils or circulating monocytes and macrophages. Monocyte–macrophage depletion was protective against emphysema although the smoke-induced neutrophil influx and associated neutrophil elastinolytic activity was not reduced. Neutrophil depletion was not protective against emphysema, although neutrophil elastinolytic activity was markedly reduced [130]. These studies suggest that macrophages are required for the development of emphysema, while neutrophils play no part. It should be noted, however, that neutrophil versus macrophage elastinolytic activity does not, strictly speaking, equate to serine proteinase versus MMP activity. Neutrophils produce MMP-9, and macrophages can at least take up and release NE, while immature macrophages may not yet have lost their serine proteinase producing capacity, a situation more likely to arise when large numbers of monocytes migrate into the lungs in response to an acute insult.

The role of macrophages and neutrophils was also examined in animal studies using coal and silica to induce lung damage. In C57Bl/6 mice, intratracheal instillation of coal or silica induced early neutrophil influx and an increase in elastase activity and elastin breakdown products at 24 h. Elevation of α_1-AT levels also occurred, although some of the α_1-AT was oxidized or degraded. Macrophage numbers did not rise until 7 days after exposure and, after coal but not silica, the macrophage numbers correlated with collagen breakdown products. Depletion of neutrophils reduced the quantity of elastin breakdown products in BALF at 24 h but not 7 days. The studies showed that mineral dust induces lung damage, which is only driven by neutrophil-derived proteinases in the early stages, and also showed that high levels of α_1-AT do not prevent lung tissue breakdown mediated by neutrophil serine proteinases, supporting the concept of quantum proteolysis [95].

Because this was not an animal model of emphysema, the nature of the challenge and other features of the neutrophilic influx may have influenced the results. The same investigators therefore studied cigarette smoke-induced disease in C57Bl/6 mice, to investigate the mechanisms of damage arising in the first 48 h after smoke inhalation. BALF at 6 and 24 h showed an acute influx of neutrophils with evidence of both elastin and collagen degradation, all related to smoke exposure in a dose-dependent fashion and resolving by 48 h. Macrophage numbers were not affected. Both neutrophil depletion and administration of α_1-AT reduced neutrophilia and release of desmosine and hydroxyproline. Cigarette smoke increased both serine and metalloelastase activity in BALF, but only the former was reduced by α_1-AT. In a model using LPS instead of cigarette smoke, exogenous α_1-AT inhibited elastin breakdown without reducing neutrophil influx, suggesting that it was the direct antiproteolytic effect that was protective [89]. In these studies, progression after 48 h was not assessed, which may explain why the results conflict with the longer-term studies of Ofulue et al. [94,130].

Similar studies in guinea pigs also demonstrated acute responses to cigarette smoke, with neutrophilia and increased desmosine and hydroxyproline in BALF, which could be inhibited by pre-treatment with a synthetic NE inhibitor [45]. In the same study, guinea pigs were exposed to cigarette smoke over 6 months, causing airspace enlargement, elevation of desmosine, hydroxyproline and neutrophil count in BALF, and elevation of tumour necrosis factor α (TNF-α) in plasma. Inhibition of NE reduced plasma TNF-α by 30%, reduced neutrophils, desmosine and hydroxyproline in BALF to control levels, and reduced the severity of emphysema by 45%. This degree of protection is consistent with that found with the NE knockout mouse [67], and suggests that neutrophils and NE have a role in the development of at least some of the emphysema. However, when the NE inhibitor was given after 4 months instead of from the start of the 6 months smoking period, there was no protection against emphysema and TNF-α levels remained elevated, although neutrophils, desmosine and hydroxyproline in BALF were normalized, suggesting that the early changes are critical.

The interaction between TNF-α and neutrophil proteinases was further explored in animal models. A TNF-α receptor knockout mouse was protected against acute neutrophil infiltrate, connective tissue breakdown and up-regulation of neutrophil chemoattractants induced by cigarette smoke. Furthermore, mice from a strain producing lower than usual levels of TNF-α (line 129) were similarly protected [131]. (Because these mice were used to generate the original MMP-12 knockout mouse, this may help to explain why the disease in these mice was predom-inantly macrophage-dependent [129].) Partial protection against elastase-induced emphysema has been shown in mice deficient in the TNF-α receptor or the IL-1β receptor [132] and more detailed studies of the role of TNF-α showed that this cytokine orchestrates up to 70% of the tissue destruction in cigarette smoke-induced emphysema, probably via neutrophil influx [133]. Taken together, these studies suggest that inhibitors of NE may also have an anti-inflammatory effect, possibly by modulating cytokine expression rather than directly preventing neutrophil migration.

Using MMP-12 knockout mice bred back into strain C57Bl/6, the relationship between neutrophils and macrophage proteinases was re-examined. Cigarette smoke induced a neutrophilic infiltrate and the release of desmosine and hydroxyproline in the wild type mice only. Macrophage numbers increased in both, albeit less in the MMP-12 knockout mice. The wild type response to smoke could be reconstituted in the knockout mice by intratracheal instillation of macrophages obtained by lavage in wild type mice. Use of a MMP inhibitor prevented the smoke-induced increase in neutrophils and the release of desmosine and hydroxyproline, while macrophage numbers were unaffected. These studies suggest that MMP-12 is required to elicit the neutrophil response to cigarette smoke. It was noted that α_1-AT increased after smoke, and inhibition of MMPs reduced this effect, suggesting that MMPs do not contribute to NE activity by degradation of α_1-AT in this model [134]. Subsequently the relationship of MMP-12 to TNF-α was examined. Stimulation with cigarette smoke elicited production of TNF-α by alveolar macrophages isolated from wild type mice, but this response was not seen in macrophages from MMP-12 knockout mice, despite normal levels of expression of TNF-α mRNA. It was determined that MMP-12 processes TNF-α after secretion, and without this, expression of endothelial adhesion factors fails, so that neutrophil recruitment does not occur [135].

Gelatinase B (MMP-9) makes up approximately 50% of the elastinolytic activity of macrophages, the rest being attributable to MMP-12 [32]. It is synthesized in neutrophils during maturation [136], stored in the specific and gelatinase granules [137] and released with a proportion bound to neutrophil gelatinase-associated lipocalin (NGAL) [138]. In order to examine the role of MMP-9 in COPD, mice deficient for MMP-9 were exposed to intratracheal LPS. The knockout and wild type mice exhibited the same levels of myeloperoxidase activity (used as a surrogate for neutrophil infiltration) and histological tissue damage, with no difference in the basement membrane breakdown products and total protein in BALF (a surrogate measurement of neutrophil migration) [139]. Other investigators however used a cigarette smoke-induced emphysema model in guinea pigs to examine the effect of a broad-spectrum MMP inhibitor. MMP inhibition reduced the severity of emphysema, inflammatory cell infiltrate and MMP-9 activity in BALF, when measured at 2 or 4 months [140]. An MMP inhibitor was also able to reduce the severity of porcine pancreatic elastase-induced emphysema in hamsters [141], showing that MMPs are involved in the pathological process induced by a serine proteinase.

The complex animal model of emphysema using mice transgenic for human IL-13 was extended to study the role of MMPs [54]. When expression of IL-13 was induced, the animals exhibited infiltration of the lung by macrophages, eosinophils, lymphocytes and neutrophils, and air-space enlargement developed. Combining this model with deletion of the genes for MMP-12 and MMP-9 enabled assessment of the contribution of these MMPs to the pathogenesis of IL-13-induced lung disease in mice. IL-13-mediated secretory cell metaplasia was not inhibited with either cysteine proteinase inhibitors or a broad-spectrum MMP inhibitor, and MMP-9 and MMP-12 knockout mice were not protected either. Furthermore, MMP-9 knockout mice actually exhibited greater neutrophil infiltration, possibly related to the ability of MMP-9 to degrade mouse neutrophil chemoattractants. Airspace enlargement was significantly reduced, but not to control levels, suggesting that the residual tissue damage may be mediated by neutrophil serine proteinases.

Animal models have also been developed to investigate the role of collagenases. Application of the results from these models to human disease should be cautious because there is wide variation in the amount of collagen found in lungs of different species of animals [142]. In a transgenic mouse expressing human MMP-1, enlarged airspaces were seen consistent with emphysema [143]. A developmental abnormality could not be excluded, because the expression of MMP-1 is constitutional. For this reason, further studies were performed [144] which demonstrated that lung histology was normal until expression of the gene was seen. This occurred at variable points after birth in different strains of mice (emphasizing the difficulties of extrapolating results in mouse experiments to humans) and was more severe in homozygous than heterozygous mice. A loss of type III collagen was found, together with deposition of type I collagen, implying increased collagenolysis and increased but disordered collagen deposition, which is consistent with findings in human emphysema [145].

These extensive animal studies suggest a number of conclusions. First, it is difficult to harmonize the conflicting results obtained from different species of animals and even different strains of the same species. The marked disparity between the results of the studies on rats [130] and those on mice and guinea pigs [45,134,140] may indicate an important difference in the pathology of COPD in different species and strains, or simply methodological issues of inhibitors versus cell depletion. Secondly, neutrophil influx appears to be an early event in both single insult and continued insult models, and lavage neutrophils and neutrophil elastinolytic activity relate well to lung damage at this stage. In most models, an acute neutrophil response appears to be the precursor to progressive lung damage. Thirdly, macrophages appear to be necessary, either to initiate the acute neutrophilic response, or to convert acute neutrophil-mediated tissue damage into established progressive emphysema. Fourthly, because these studies generally examine limited exposure to a single type of

insult, they do not enable us to predict the relative importance of individual proteinases once the insult has been withdrawn, as in ex-smokers, or after repeated and varied insults, as in patients having exacerbations of COPD. Fifthly, proteinases have a number of pathological functions beyond destruction of extracellular matrix proteins, and there is a wide functional overlap between proteinases from different biochemical groups and cell populations (Fig. 31.4). Complex interactions between neutrophils, macrophages and their respective proteinase armamentaria may make interpretation of single measurements unreliable or even irrelevant.

Human studies

A number of clinical studies have identified MMPs in patients with COPD, although not consistently. Studies by Segura-Valdez *et al.* [146] showed increased tissue staining for collagenases (MMP-1, MMP-8) and gelatinases (MMP-2, MMP-9) in patients compared with controls. Ohnishi *et al.* [147] found no tissue staining for MMP-1, MMP-8 or MMP-9 protein in emphysematous lung, although mRNA for MMP-1, MMP-2 and MMP-9 was present. MMP-2 and MMP-14 protein were present, and both collagenolytic and gelatinolytic activities were increased in tissue homogenates from patients compared with controls. In this study, neither MMP-12 nor NE-related activity was elevated in patients compared with controls. Another study found MMP-1 mRNA and protein in lung tissue in patients with COPD [146].

Besides these immunohistochemical techniques, cells isolated from patients have been studied. Several studies have shown that macrophages harvested by BAL from COPD patients showed greater expression of MMP-1 and MMP-9 compared with controls [30,149,150]. The study by Finlay *et al.* [150] also showed greater proteinase activity of MMP-1 and MMP-9 associated with these macrophages, and MMP-9 localized on gel electrophoresis at the same place as neutrophil-derived MMP-9 (i.e. complexed with NGAL), suggesting that macrophages from patients with COPD might have internalized either free NGAL or NGAL–MMP-9 complexes, released by neutrophils. Additional NE activity was also detected from macrophages from patients. An alternative explanation to that of internalization is that some of the macrophages in the patients were immature and retained the ability of monocytes to secrete neutrophil enzymes. Interestingly, expression of MMP-2 and MMP-12 was the same in patients and controls, and macrophages did not appear to secrete these enzymes. Collagenase activity was the same in active versus ex-smokers, suggesting that it was a consequence of the emphysematous process rather than an initiating factor [150]. In a study of induced

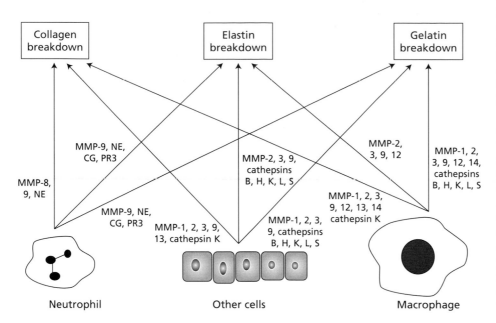

Figure 31.4 This figure demonstrates the overlapping proteinase complement of the cells present in the lung in COPD. Neutrophils produce directly collagenolytic enzymes (matrix metalloproteinase-8 [MMP-8], neutrophil elastase [NE]) and enzymes which can degrade both gelatin and elastin (MMP-9, NE, cathepsin G [CG], proteinase 3 [PR3]). Macrophages produce a large number of proteinases which share collagenolytic and gelatinolytic activities, and in some cases, elastinolytic activity also (MMP-2, MMP-9 and MMP-12). In addition, other cells such as alveolar and bronchial epithelial cells, endothelial cells and fibroblasts between them can produce almost all of the enzymes released by macrophages. Few enzymes are confined to one cell type or one substrate only.

sputum from patients with COPD and healthy smokers, MMP activity was measured according to gelatinase or true collagenase function. Both gelatinase (MMP-9) and collagenase (MMP-8) activity were elevated in COPD compared with controls, and the activity of these two enzymes correlated with each other and with the number of neutrophils, suggesting neutrophilic origin. This was confirmed by immunohistochemistry of sputum cells, showing MMP-8 only in neutrophils, and MMP-9 in both neutrophils and macrophages [151]. In another study, sputum levels of MMP-9 and TIMP-1 were increased in patients with COPD and asthma and correlated with the numbers of neutrophils in sputum [152], while there was no difference in the amount of MMP-9 expressed or secreted by circulating neutrophils from patients or healthy controls [153]. Interestingly, these *in vitro* studies showed release of both the pro-enzyme and the activated form by neutrophils, and the activated form was probably the result of activation of pro-MMP-9 by NE. Thus, it can be predicted that inhibitors of NE may also inhibit MMP-9 activity [36]. In a further study [77], BALF from smokers with emphysema was compared with BALF from healthy smokers. MMP-9 and MMP-8 levels were elevated in emphysema, and MMP-9 was again complexed to NGAL, suggesting neutrophil derivation. NGAL was also elevated in emphysema, although neutrophil numbers were not appreciably increased. Alveolar macrophages were isolated and cultured, but in this study only produced latent MMP-9 with no difference in MMP-9 level between the subjects with

and without emphysema. Finally, induced sputum from patients with COPD has been shown to contain increased MMP-22 activity compared to that from controls [154]. Overall these data indicate that COPD is associated with activation of the MMP class, but this activity appears related to neutrophils rather than macrophages, suggesting that this class of proteinases may be activated as a consequence of neutrophilic inflammation. The contribution of MMPs to the pathology of COPD is likely to be substantial given their broad spectrum of activity. This is supported by genetic studies which have shown that polymorphisms of the MMP-1, MMP-9, MMP-12 and TIMP-2 genes are more common in patients with emphysema [155–157], suggesting their products in some way have a role. However, the effects of these polymorphisms on gene function have yet to be determined.

Conclusions

There is strong evidence linking serine proteinases and matrix metalloproteinases with the pathogenesis of COPD, despite wide discrepancies between studies of individual proteinases. The observation that NE can activate MMPs [36,125] may indicate that NE is an early step in a proteinase cascade that leads to proteinase–antiproteinase imbalance and degradation of lung tissue. Although the absence of α_1-AT in humans predisposes to severe early-onset emphysema, implying a major role for NE in the pathogenesis of emphysema, this could still be a modulatory role rather than as the chief agent of matrix destruction. It seems likely that macrophage-derived MMPs are also critical mediators of lung damage but it is far from clear whether this is related to their ability to break down lung tissue per se, or their other abilities including disordered repair, modulation of cytokine function and degradation of inhibitors of other proteinases.

The therapeutic approach to the role of proteinase inhibitors in COPD should be a pragmatic one. It may be that the critical proteinase in the pathogenic process is not the one causing the tissue destruction, but rather one that activates the destructive enzymes, inactivates endogenous inhibitors or enables recruitment and activation of inflammatory cells. Further complexities that arise when considering the interactions between proteinases and their inhibitors in the lungs include oxidants, which impair the function of inhibitors of NE and activate the inflammatory cascade, and infections. In patients with COPD related to smoking therefore, the proteinase cascade may be different to that arising in patients whose COPD is related to chronic asthma, and different again to that associated with bronchiectasis, where bacterial products can also stimulate neutrophil influx to the lungs, and stimulate a different profile of macrophage cytokine secretion. Equally, smoking-related COPD may have a different proteinase–antiproteinase profile in active smokers versus ex-smokers. Finally, the biochemical and cytokine profile may differ in individuals with advanced disease compared with those with early disease, and in those with pure emphysema versus the bronchiolitis or chronic bronchitis phenotypes. The fact that different rates of progression and different disease phenotypes exist may reflect the polymorphisms of various MMPs and cytokine receptors that have been linked with rate of progression, and this in turn may alter the clinical effect of proteinases and response to proteinase inhibitors. For these reasons, we should continue to try to elucidate the pathogenetic mechanisms related to proteinases, in order to identify patient groups in whom inhibitors can be tested with the best chance of eliciting a clinically significant therapeutic response and thereby clarifying the central processes.

Acknowledgement

Thanks for Dr Anita Pye for her assistance in preparing the figures.

References

1 Ohlsson K, Olsson I, Spitznagel K. Localization of chymotrypsin-like cationic protein, collagenase and elastase in azurophil granules of human neutrophilic polymorphonuclear leukocytes. *Hoppe-Seyler's Z Physiol Chem* 1977; **358**:361–6.

2 Fouret P, du Bois RM, Bernaudin JF *et al.* Expression of the neutrophil elastase gene during human bone marrow cell differentiation. *J Exp Med* 1989;**169**:833–45.

3 Adkison AM, Raptis SZ, Kelley DG, Pham CTN. Dipeptidyl peptidase I activates neutrophil-derived serine proteases and regulates the development of acute experimental arthritis. *J Clin Invest* 2002;**109**:363–71.

4 Owen CA, Campbell MA, Boukedes SS, Stockley RA, Campbell EJ. A discrete subpopulation of human monocytes expresses a neutrophil-like pro-inflammatory (P) phenotype. *Am J Physiol* 1994;**267**:L775–85.

5 Laurell C-B, Eriksson S. The electrophoretic α_1-globulin pattern of serum in α_1-antitrypsin deficiency. *Scand J Clin Lab Invest* 1963;**15**:132–40.

6 Odeberg H, Olsson I. Microbicidal mechanisms of human granulocytes: synergistic effects of granulocyte elastase and myeloperoxidase or chymotrypsin-like cationic protein. *Infect Immun* 1976;**14**:1276–83.

7 Shiflett SL, Kaplan J, Ward DM. Chédiak–Higashi syndrome: a rare disorder of lysosomes and lysosome-related organelles. *Pigment Cell Res* 2002;**15**:251–7.

8 Stockley RA. Neutrophils and the pathogenesis of COPD. *Chest* 2002;**121**:151S–5S.

9 Snider GL, Hayes JA, Franzblau C *et al.* Relationship between elastolytic activity and experimental emphysema inducing properties of papain preparations. *Am Rev Respir Dis* 1974;**110**:254–62.

10 Blackwood CE, Hosannah Y, Perman E, Keller S, Mandl L. Elastolytic titre of inducing enzyme as determinant of the response. *Proc Soc Exp Biol Med* 1973;**144**:450–4.

11 Lucey EC, Stone PJ, Powers JC, Snider GL. Amelioration of human neutrophil elastase-induced emphysema in hamsters by pretreatment with an oligopeptide chloromethyl ketone. *Eur Respir J* 1989;**2**:421–7.

12 Rudolphus A, Kramps JA, Mauve I, Dijkman JH. Intratracheally-instilled antileukoprotease and α_1-proteinase inhibitor: effect on human neutrophil elastase-induced experimental emphysema and pulmonary localization. *Histochem J* 1994;**26**:817–24.

13 Bieth JG. Elastases: catalytic and biological properties. In: Mecham RP, ed. *Biology of Extracellular Matrix: Regulation of Matrix Accumulation.* Orlando FL, Academic, 1986: 217–320.

14 Kafienah W, Buttle DJ, Burnett D, Hollander AP. Cleavage of native type I collagen by human neutrophil elastase. *Biochem J* 1998;**330**:897–902.

15 Niederman MS, Merrill WW, Polomski LM, Reynolds HY, Gee JB. Influence of sputum IgA and elastase on tracheal cell bacterial adherence. *Am Rev Respir Dis* 1986;**133**:255–60.

16 Vogt W. Cleavage of the fifth component of complement and generation of a functionally active C5b6-like complex by human leukocyte elastase. *Immunobiology* 2000;**201**:470–7.

17 Fick RBJ, Robbins RA, Squier SU, Schoderbek WE, Russ WD. Complement activation in cystic fibrosis respiratory fluids: *in vivo* and *in vitro* generation of C5a and chemotactic activity. *Pediatr Res* 1986;**20**:1258–68.

18 Ashcroft GS, Lei K, Jin W *et al*. Secretory leukocyte protease inhibitor mediates non-redundant functions necessary for normal wound healing. *Nat Med* 2000;**6**:1147–53.

19 Zhu J, Nathan C, Jin W *et al*. Conversion of proepithelin to epithelins: roles of SLPI and elastase in host defense and wound repair. *Cell* 2002;**111**:867–78.

20 Owen CA, Campbell MA, Sannes PL, Boukedes SS, Campbell EJ. Cell surface-bound elastase and cathepsin G on human neutrophils: a novel, non-oxidative mechanism by which neutrophils focus and preserve catalytic activity of serine proteinases. *J Cell Biol* 1995;**131**:775–89.

21 Campbell EJ, Campbell MA, Owen CA. Bioactive proteinase 3 on the cell surface of human neutrophils: quantification, catalytic activity, and susceptibility to inhibition. *J Immunol* 2000;**165**:3366–74.

22 Owen CA, Campbell MA, Boukedes SS, Campbell EJ. Cytokines regulate membrane-bound leukocyte elastase on neutrophils: a novel mechanism for effector activity. *Am J Physiol Lung Cell Mol Physiol* 1997;**272**:L385–93.

23 Weitz JI, Huang AJ, Landman SL, Nicholson SC, Silverstein SC. Elastase-mediated fibrinogenolysis by chemoattractant-stimulated neutrophils occurs in the presence of physiologic concentrations of antiproteinases. *J Exp Med* 1987;**166**: 1836–50.

24 Hill AT, Bayley D, Stockley RA. The interrelationship of sputum inflammatory markers in patients with chronic bronchitis. *Am J Respir Crit Care Med* 1999;**160**:893–8.

25 Savill JS, Wyllie AH, Henson JE *et al*. Macrophage phagocytosis of aging neutrophils in inflammation: programmed cell death in the neutrophil leads to its recognition by macrophages. *J Clin Invest* 1989;**83**:865–75.

26 Campbell EJ, White RR, Senior RM, Rodriguez RJ, Kuhn C. Receptor-mediated binding and internalization of leukocyte elastase by alveolar macrophages *in vitro*. *J Clin Invest* 1979; **64**:824–33.

27 Fadok VA, Bratton DL, Guthrie L, Henson PM. Differential effects of apoptotic versus lysed cells on macrophage production of cytokines: role of proteases. *J Immunol* 2001; **166**:6847–54.

28 Bergenfeldt M, Axelsson L, Ohlsson K. Release of neutrophil proteinase 4(3) and leukocyte elastase during phagocytosis and their interaction with proteinase inhibitors. *Scand J Clin Lab Invest* 1992;**52**:823–9.

29 Ohlsson K, Linder C, Lundberg E, Axelsson L. Release of cytokines and proteases from human peripheral blood mononuclear and polymorphonuclear cells following phagocytosis and LPS stimulation. *Scand J Clin Lab Invest* 1996;**56**:461–70.

30 Russell REK, Thorley A, Culpitt SV *et al*. Alveolar macrophage-mediated elastolysis: roles of matrix metalloproteinases, cysteine, and serine proteases. *Am J Physiol Lung Cell Mol Physiol* 2002;**283**:L867–73.

31 Campbell EJ, Wald MS. Fate of human neutrophil elastase following receptor-mediated endocytosis by human alveolar macrophages: implications for connective tissue injury. *J Lab Clin Med* 1983;**101**:527–36.

32 Shapiro SD. Elastolytic metalloproteinases produced by human mononuclear phagocytes: potential roles in destruc-tive lung disease. *Am J Respir Crit Care Med* 1994;**150**: S160–4.

33 Stockley RA, Shaw J, Afford SC, Morrison HM, Burnett D. Effect of α_1-proteinase inhibitor on neutrophil chemotaxis. *Am J Respir Cell Mol Biol* 1990;**2**:163–70.

34 Lomas DA, Stone SR, Llewellyn-Jones C *et al*. The control of neutrophil chemotaxis by inhibitors of cathepsin G and chymotrypsin. *J Biol Chem* 1995;**270**:23437–43.

35 Steadman R, St John PL, Evans RA *et al*. Human neutrophils do not degrade major basement membrane components during chemotactic migration. *Int J Biochem Cell Biol* 1997; **29**:993–1004.

36 Delclaux C, Delacourt C, D'Ortho MP *et al*. Role of gelatinase B and elastase in human polymorphonuclear neutrophil migration across basement membrane. *Am J Respir Cell Mol Biol* 1996;**14**:288–95.

37 Woodman RC, Reinhardt PH, Kanwar S, Johnston FL, Kubes P. Effects of human neutrophil elastase (HNE) on neutrophil function *in vitro* and in inflamed microvessels. *Blood* 1993;**82**:2188–95.

38 Mackarel AJ, Cottell DC, Russell KJ, Fitzgerald MX, O'Connor CM. Migration of neutrophils across human pulmonary endothelial cells is not blocked by matrix metalloproteinases or serine protease inhibitors. *Am J Respir Cell Mol Biol* 1999;**20**:1209–9.

39 Furie MB, Naprstek BL, Silverstein SC. Migration of neutrophils across monolayers of cultured microvascular endothelial cells: an *in vitro* model of leucocyte extravasation. *J Cell Sci* 1987;**88**:161–75.

40 Allport JR, Lim YC, Shipley JM *et al*. Neutrophils from MMP-9 or neutrophil elastase-deficient mice show no defect in transendothelial migration under flow *in vitro*. *J Leukoc Biol* 2002;**71**:821–8.

41 Tkalcevic J, Novelli M, Phylactides M *et al*. Impaired immunity and enhanced resistance to endotoxin in the absence of neutrophil elastase and cathepsin G. *Immunity* 2000;**12**: 201–10.

42 Toomes C, James J, Wood AJ *et al*. Loss-of-function mutations in the cathepsin C gene result in periodontal disease and palmoplantar keratosis. *Nat Genet* 1999;**23**:421–4.

43 Liu R, Cao C, Meng H, Tang Z. Leukocyte functions in 2 cases of Papillon–Lefèvre syndrome. *J Clin Periodontol* 2000;**27**:69–73.

44 Clark RA, Kimball HR. Defective granulocyte chemotaxis in the Chédiak–Higashi syndrome. *J Clin Invest* 1971;**50**: 2645–52.

45 Wright JL, Farmer SG, Churg A. Synthetic serine elastase inhibitor reduces cigarette smoke-induced emphysema in guinea pigs. *Am J Respir Crit Care Med* 2002;**166**:954–60.

46 Delacourt C, Hérigault S, Delclaux C *et al*. Protection against acute lung injury by intravenous or intratracheal pretreatment with EPI-HNE-4, a new potent neutrophil elastase inhibitor. *Am J Respir Cell Mol Biol* 2002;**26**:290–7.

47 Hashimoto S, Maruoka S, Gon Y *et al*. Mitogen-activated protein kinase involves neutrophil elastase-induced morphological changes in human bronchial epithelial cells. *Life Sci* 1999;**64**:1465–71.

48 Liou TG, Campbell EJ. Quantum proteolysis resulting from release of single granules by human neutrophils: a novel,

non-oxidative mechanism of extracellular proteolytic activity. *J Immunol* 1996;**157**:2624–31.

49 Campbell EJ, Campbell MA, Boukedes SS, Owen CA. Quantum proteolysis by neutrophils: implications for pulmonary emphysema in α_1-antitrypsin deficiency. *J Clin Invest* 1999;**104**:337–44.

50 Rice WG, Weiss SJ. Regulation of proteolysis at the neutrophil–substrate interface by secretory leukoprotease inhibitor. *Science* 1990;**249**:178–81.

51 Salvesen GS, Barrett AJ. Covalent binding of proteinases in their reaction with α_1-macroglobulin. *Biochem J* 1980;**187**:695–701.

52 Takeyama K, Agustí C, Ueki IF *et al.* Neutrophil-dependent goblet cell degranulation: role of membrane-bound elastase and adhesion molecules. *Am J Physiol* 1998;**19**:L294–302.

53 Zheng T, Zhu Z, Wang Z *et al.* Inducible targeting of IL-13 to the adult lung causes matrix metalloproteinase- and cathepsin-dependent emphysema. *J Clin Invest* 2000;**106**:1445–6.

54 Lanone S, Zheng T, Zhu Z *et al.* Overlapping and enzyme-specific contributions of matrix metalloproteinases-9 and -12 in IL-13-induced inflammation and remodeling. *J Clin Invest* 2002;**110**:463–74.

55 Shim JJ, Dabbagh K, Ueki IF *et al.* IL-13 induces mucin production by stimulating epidermal growth factor receptors and by activating neutrophils. *Am J Physiol Lung Cell Mol Physiol* 2001;**280**:L134–40.

56 Smallman LA, Hill SL, Stockley RA. Reduction of ciliary beat frequency *in vitro* by sputum from patients with bronchiectasis: a serine proteinase effect. *Thorax* 1984;**39**:663–7.

57 Amitani R, Wilson R, Rutman A *et al.* Effect of human neutrophil elastase and *Pseudomonas aeruginosa* proteinases on human respiratory epithelium. *Am J Respir Cell Mol Biol* 1991;**4**:26–32.

58 Aoshiba K, Yasuda K, Yasui S, Tamaoki J, Nagai A. Serine proteases increase oxidative stress in lung cells. *Am J Physiol Lung Cell Mol Physiol* 2001;**281**:L556–64.

59 Fischer BM, Voynow JA. Neutrophil elastase induces *MUC*5AC gene expression in airway epithelium via a pathway involving reactive oxygen species. *Am J Respir Cell Mol Biol* 2002;**26**:447–52.

60 Rickard KA, Taylor J, Rennard SI. Observations of development of resistance to detachment of cultured bovine bronchial epithelial cells in response to protease treatment. *Am J Respir Cell Mol Biol* 1992;**6**:414–20.

61 Nakajoh M, Fukushima T, Suzuki T *et al.* Retinoic acid inhibits elastase-induced injury in human lung epithelial cell lines. *Am J Respir Cell Mol Biol* 2002;**28**:296–304.

62 Ballieux BE, Hiemstra PS, Klar-Mohamad N *et al.* Detachment and cytolysis of human endothelial cells by proteinase 3. *Eur J Immunol* 1994;**24**:3211–5.

63 Yang JJ, Kettritz R, Falk RJ, Jennette JC, Gaido ML. Apoptosis of endothelial cells induced by the neutrophil serine proteases proteinase 3 and elastase. *Am J Pathol* 1996;**149**:1617–26.

64 Gompertz S, O'Brien C, Bayley DL, Hill SL, Stockley RA. Changes in bronchial inflammation during acute exacerbations of chronic bronchitis. *Eur Respir J* 2001;**17**:1112–9.

65 Dowson LJ, Guest PJ, Stockley RA. Longitudinal changes in

66 Donaldson GC, Seemungal TA, Bhowmik A, Wedzicha JA. Relationship between exacerbation frequency and lung function decline in chronic obstructive pulmonary disease. *Thorax* 2002;**57**:847–52.

67 Shapiro SD. Animal models for COPD. *Chest* 2000;**117**:223S–7S.

68 Lucey EC, Stone PJ, Breuer R *et al.* Effect of combined human neutrophil cathepsin G and elastase on induction of secretory cell metaplasia and emphysema in hamsters, with *in vitro* observations on elastolysis by these enzymes. *Am Rev Respir Dis* 1985;**132**:362–6.

69 Kao RC, Wehner NG, Skubitz KM, Gray BH, Hoidal JR. Proteinase 3: a distinct human polymorphonuclear leukocyte proteinase that produces emphysema in hamsters. *J Clin Invest* 1988;**82**:1963–73.

70 Saetta M, Turato G, Facchini FM *et al.* Inflammatory cells in the bronchial glands of smokers with chronic bronchitis. *Am J Respir Crit Care Med* 1997;**156**:1633–9.

71 Rutgers SR, Timens W, Kaufmann HF *et al.* Comparison of induced sputum with bronchial wash, bronchoalveolar lavage and bronchial biopsies in COPD. *Eur Respir J* 2000;**15**:109–15.

72 Stanescu D, Sanna A, Veriter C *et al.* Airways obstruction, chronic expectoration, and rapid decline of FEV_1 in smokers are associated with increased levels of sputum neutrophils. *Thorax* 1996;**51**:267–71.

73 Martin TR, Raghu G, Maunder RJ, Springmeyer SC. The effects of chronic bronchitis and chronic air-flow obstruction on lung cell populations recovered by bronchoalveolar lavage. *Am Rev Respir Dis* 1985;**132**:254–60.

74 Burnett D, Chamba A, Hill SL, Stockley RA. Neutrophils from subjects with chronic obstructive lung disease show enhanced chemotaxis and extracellular proteolysis. *Lancet* 1987;**2**:1043–6.

75 Noguera A, Busquets X, Sauleda J *et al.* Expression of adhesion molecules and G proteins in circulating neutrophils in chronic obstructive pulmonary disease. *Am J Respir Crit Care Med* 1998;**158**:1664–8.

76 Yoshioka A, Betsuyaku T, Nishimura M *et al.* Excessive neutrophil elastase in bronchoalveolar lavage fluid in subclinical emphysema. *Am J Respir Crit Care Med* 1995;**152**:2127–32.

77 Betsuyaku T, Nishimura M, Takeyabu K *et al.* Neutrophil granule proteins in bronchoalveolar lavage fluid from subjects with subclinical emphysema. *Am J Respir Crit Care Med* 1999;**159**:1985–91.

78 Fujita J, Nelson NL, Daughton DM *et al.* Evaluation of elastase and antielastase balance in patients with chronic bronchitis and pulmonary emphysema. *Am Rev Respir Dis* 1990;**142**:57–62.

79 Finlay GA, Russell KJ, McMahon KJ *et al.* Elevated levels of matrix metalloproteinases in bronchoalveolar lavage fluid of emphysematous patients. *Thorax* 1997;**52**:502–6.

80 Retamales I, Elliott WM, Meshi B *et al.* Amplification of inflammation in emphysema and its association with latent

adenoviral infection. *Am J Respir Crit Care Med* 2001;**164**: 469–73.

81 Eidelman D, Saetta MP, Ghezzo H *et al*. Cellularity of the alveolar walls in smokers and its relation to alveolar destruction: functional implications. *Am Rev Respir Dis* 1990;**141**: 1547–52.

82 Finkelstein R, Fraser RS, Ghezzo H, Cosio MG. Alveolar inflammation and its relation to emphysema in smokers. *Am J Respir Crit Care Med* 1995;**152**:1666–72.

83 Ludwig PW, Schwartz BA, Hoidal JR, Niewoehner DE. Cigarette smoking causes accumulation of polymorphonuclear leukocytes in alveolar septum. *Am Rev Respir Dis* 1985;**131**:828–30.

84 Woolhouse IS, Bayley DL, Stockley RA. Sputum chemotactic activity in chronic obstructive pulmonary disease: effect of α_1-antitrypsin deficiency and the role of leukotriene B_4 and interleukin 8. *Thorax* 2002;**57**:709–14.

85 Crooks SW, Bayley DL, Hill SL, Stockley RA. Bronchial inflammation in acute bacterial exacerbations of chronic bronchitis: the role of leukotriene B_4. *Eur Respir J* 2000; **15**:274–80.

86 Hubbard RC, Fells G, Gadek J *et al*. Neutrophil accumulation in the lung in α_1-antitrypsin deficiency: spontaneous release of leukotriene B_4 by alveolar macrophages. *J Clin Invest* 1991;**88**:891–7.

87 Hill AT, Bayley DL, Campbell EJ, Hill SL, Stockley RA. Airways inflammation in chronic bronchitis: the effects of smoking and α_1-antitrypsin deficiency. *Eur Respir J* 2000; **15**:886–90.

88 Belaaouaj A, McCarthy R, Baumann M *et al*. Mice lacking neutrophil elastase reveal impaired host defence against gram negative bacterial sepsis. *Nat Med* 1998;**4**:615–8.

89 Dhami R, Gilks B, Xie C *et al*. Acute cigarette smoke-induced connective tissue breakdown is mediated by neutrophils and prevented by α_1-antitrypsin. *Am J Respir Cell Mol Biol* 2000;**22**:244–52.

90 Stone PJ, Lucey EC, Virca GD *et al*. α_1-Protease inhibitor moderates human neutrophil elastase-induced emphysema and secretory cell metaplasia in hamsters. *Eur Respir J* 1990;**3**:673–8.

91 Lucey EC, Stone PJ, Ciccolella DE *et al*. Recombinant human secretory leukocyte-protease inhibitor: *in vitro* properties, and amelioration of human neutrophil elastase-induced emphysema and secretory cell metaplasia in the hamster. *J Lab Clin Med* 1990;**115**:224–32.

92 Snider GL, Stone PJ, Lucey EC *et al*. Eglin-c, a polypeptide derived from the medicinal leech, prevents human neutrophil elastase-induced emphysema and bronchial secretory cell metaplasia in the hamster. *Am Rev Respir Dis* 1985;**132**:1155–61.

93 Churg A, Wang RD, Xie C, Wright JL. α_1-Antitrypsin ameliorates cigarette smoke-induced emphysema in the mouse. *Am J Respir Crit Care Med* 2003;**168**:199–207.

94 Ofulue A, Ko M, Abboud R. Time course of neutrophil and macrophage elastinolytic activities in cigarette smoke-induced emphysema. *Am J Physiol Lung Cell Mol Physiol* 1998; **275**:L1134–44.

95 Zay K, Loo S, Xie C *et al*. Role of neutrophils and α_1-

antitrypsin in coal- and silica-induced connective tissue breakdown. *Am J Physiol Lung Cell Mol Physiol* 1999;**276**:L269–79.

96 Stockley RA, Bayley DL, Unsal I, Dowson LJ. The effect of augmentation therapy on bronchial inflammation in α_1-antitrypsin deficiency. *Am J Respir Crit Care Med* 2002;**165**: 1494–8.

97 Seersholm N, Wencker M, Banik N *et al*. Does α_1-antitrypsin augmentation therapy slow the annual decline in FEV_1 in patients with severe hereditary α_1-antitrypsin deficiency. *Eur Respir J* 1997;**10**:2260–3.

98 Wencker M, Fuhrmann B, Banik N, Konietzko N. Longitudinal follow-up of patients with α_1-protease inhibitor deficiency before and during therapy with IV α_1-protease inhibitor. *Chest* 2001;**119**:737–44.

99 Caughey GH. Serine proteinases of mast cell and leukocyte granules. *Am J Respir Crit Care Med* 1994;**150**:S138–42.

100 Hattotuwa KL, Gizycki MJ, Ansari TW, Jeffery PK, Barnes NC. The effects of inhaled fluticasone on airway inflammation in chronic obstructive pulmonary disease: a double-blind, placebo-controlled biopsy study. *Am J Respir Crit Care Med* 2002;**165**:1579–80.

101 Kalenderian R, Raju L, Roth W *et al*. Elevated histamine and tryptase levels in smokers' bronchoalveolar lavage fluid: do lung mast cells contribute to smokers' emphysema? *Chest* 1988;**94**:119–23.

102 Burnett D, Abrahamson M, Devalia JL *et al*. Synthesis and secretion of procathepsin B and cystatin C by human bronchial epithelial cells *in vitro*: modulation of cathepsin B activity by neutrophil elastase. *Arch Biochem Biophys* 1995; **317**:305–10.

103 Burnett D, Crocker J, Stockley RA. Cathepsin B-like cysteine proteinase activity in sputum and immunohistologic identification of cathepsin B in alveolar macrophages. *Am Rev Respir Dis* 1983;**128**:915–9.

104 Burnett D, Stockley RA. Cathepsin B-like cysteine proteinase activity in sputum and bronchoalveolar lavage samples: relationship to inflammatory cells and effects of corticosteroids and antibiotic treatment. *Clin Sci* 1985;**68**:469–74.

105 Chang JC, Lesser M, Yoo OH, Orlowski M. Increased cathepsin B-like activity in alveolar macrophages and bronchoalveolar lavage fluid from smokers. *Am Rev Respir Dis* 1986;**134**:538–41.

106 Takeyabu K, Betsuyaku T, Nishimura M *et al*. Cysteine proteinases and cystatin C in bronchoalveolar lavage fluid from subjects with subclinical emphysema. *Eur Respir J* 1998;**12**: 1033–9.

107 Chapman HAJ, Stone OL. Comparison of live human neutrophil and alveolar macrophage elastolytic activity *in vitro*. *J Clin Invest* 1984;**74**:1693–700.

108 Buttle DJ, Burnett D, Abrahamson M. Levels of neutrophil elastase and cathepsin B activities, and cystatins in human sputum: relationship to inflammation. *Scand J Clin Lab Invest* 1990;**50**:509–16.

109 Buttle DJ, Abrahamson M, Burnett D *et al*. Human sputum cathepsin B degrades proteoglycan, is inhibited by α_2-macroglobulin and is modulated by neutrophil elastase cleavage of cathepsin B precursor and cystatin C. *Biochem J* 1991;**276**:325–31.

110 Abrahamson M, Mason RW, Hansson H *et al.* Human cystatin C: role of the N-terminal segment in the inhibition of human cysteine proteinases and in its inactivation by leucocyte elastase. *Biochem J* 1991;**273**:621–6.

111 Taggart CC, Lowe GJ, Greene CM *et al.* Cathepsin B, L, and S cleave and inactivate secretory leucoprotease inhibitor. *J Biol Chem* 2001;**276**:33345–52.

112 Lesser M, Padilla ML, Cardozo C. Induction of emphysema in hamsters by intratracheal instillation of cathepsin B. *Am Rev Respir Dis* 1992;**145**:661–8.

113 Bühling F, Gerber A, Häckel C *et al.* Expression of cathepsin K in lung epithelial cells. *Am J Respir Cell Mol Biol* 1999;**20**:612–9.

114 Mason RW, Johnson DA, Barrett AJ, Chapman HA. Elastinolytic activity of human cathepsin L. *Biochem J* 1986;**233**:925–7.

115 Johnson DA, Barrett AJ, Mason RW. Cathepsin L inactivates α_1-proteinase inhibitor by cleavage in the reactive site region. *J Biol Chem* 1986;**261**:14748–51.

116 Baker AH, Edwards DR, Murphy G. Metalloproteinase inhibitors: biological actions and therapeutic opportunities. *J Cell Sci* 2002;**115**:3719–27.

117 Sternlicht MD, Werb Z. How matrix metalloproteinases regulate cell behaviour. *Annu Rev Cell Dev Biol* 2001;**17**:463–516.

118 Burnett D, Afford SC, Campbell EJ *et al.* Evidence for lipid-associated serine proteases and metalloproteases in human bronchoalveolar lavage fluid. *Clin Sci (Lond)* 1988;**75**:601–7.

119 Senior RM, Connolly NL, Cury JD, Welgus HG, Campbell EJ. Elastin degradation by human alveolar macrophages: a prominent role of metalloproteinase activity. *Am Rev Respir Dis* 1989;**139**:1251–6.

120 Takaro T, Chapman WE, Burnette R, Cordell S. Acute and subacute effects of injury on the canine alveolar septum. *Chest* 1990;**98**:724–32.

121 Banda MJ, Clark EJ, Werb Z. Limited proteolysis by macrophage elastase inactivates human α_1-proteinase inhibitor. *J Exp Med* 1980;**152**:1563–70.

122 Sires UI, Murphy G, Baragi VM *et al.* Matrilysin is much more efficient than other matrix metalloproteinases in the proteolytic inactivation of α_1-antitrypsin. *Biochem Biophys Res Commun* 1994;**204**:613–20.

123 Liu Z, Zhou X, Shapiro SD *et al.* The serpin α_1-proteinase inhibitor is a critical substrate for gelatinase B/MMP-9 *in vivo. Cell* 2000;**102**:647–55.

124 Cooley J, Takayama TK, Shapiro SD, Schechter NM, Remold-O'Donnell E. The serpin MNEI inhibits elastase-like and chymotrypsin-like serine proteases through efficient reactions at two active sites. *Biochemistry* 2001;**40**:15 762–70.

125 Itoh Y, Nagase H. Preferential inactivation of tissue inhibitor of metalloproteinases-1 that is bound to the precursor of matrix metalloproteinase 9 (progelatinase B) by human neutrophil elastase. *J Biol Chem* 1995;**270**:16 518–21.

126 Rice A, Banda MJ. Neutrophil elastase processing of gelatinase A is mediated by extracellular matrix. *Biochemistry* 1995;**34**:9249–56.

127 Okada Y, Nakanishi I. Activation of matrix metall-

proteinase 3 (stromelysin) and matrix metalloproteinase 2 ('gelatinase') by human neutrophil elastase and cathepsin G. *FEBS Lett* 1989;**249**:353–6.

128 Ferry G, Lonchampt M, Pennel L *et al.* Activation of MMP-9 by neutrophil elastase in an *in vivo* model of acute lung injury. *FEBS Lett* 1997;**402**:111–5.

129 Hautamaki RD, Kobayashi DK, Senior RM, Shapiro SD. Requirement for macrophage elastase for cigarette smoke-induced emphysema in mice. *Science* 1997;**277**:2002–4.

130 Ofulue A, Ko M. Effect of depletion of neutrophils or macrophages on development of cigarette smoke induced emphysema. *Am J Physiol Lung Cell Mol Physiol* 1999;**277**:L97–105.

131 Churg A, Dai J, Tai H, Xie C, Wright JL. Tumor necrosis factor-α is central to acute cigarette smoke-induced inflammation and connective tissue breakdown. *Am J Respir Crit Care Med* 2002;**166**:849–54.

132 Lucey EC, Keane J, Kuang PP, Snider GL, Goldstein RH. Severity of elastase-induced emphysema is decreased in tumor necrosis factor-α and interleukin-1β receptor-deficient mice. *Lab Invest* 2002;**82**:79–85.

133 Churg A, Wang RD, Tai H *et al.* Tumor necrosis factor-α drives 70% of cigarette smoke-induced emphysema in the mouse. *Am J Respir Crit Care Med* 2004;**170**:492–8.

134 Churg A, Zay K, Shay S *et al.* Acute cigarette smoke-induced connective tissue breakdown requires both neutrophils and macrophage metalloelastase in mice. *Am J Respir Cell Mol Biol* 2002;**27**:368–74.

135 Churg A, Wang RD, Tai H *et al.* Macrophage metalloelastase mediates acute cigarette smoke-induced inflammation via TNF-α release. *Am J Respir Crit Care Med* 2003;**167**:1083–9.

136 Borregaard N, Sehested M, Nielsen BS, Sengelov H, Kjeldsen L. Biosynthesis of granule proteins in normal human bone marrow cells: gelatinase is a marker of terminal neutrophil differentiation. *Blood* 1995;**85**:812–7.

137 Borregaard N, Cowland JB. Granules of the human neutrophilic polymorphonuclear leukocyte. *Blood* 1997;**89**:3503–35.

138 Kjeldsen L, Johnsen AH, Sengelov H, Borregaard N. Isolation and primary structure of NGAL, a novel protein associated with human neutrophil gelatinase. *J Biol Chem* 1993;**268**:10 425–32.

139 Betsuyaku T, Shipley JM, Liu Z, Senior RM. Gelatinase B deficiency does not protect against lipopolysaccharide-induced acute lung injury. *Chest* 1999;**116**:17S–8S.

140 Selman M, Cisneros-Lira J, Gaxiola M *et al.* Matrix metalloproteinases inhibition attenuates tobacco smoke-induced emphysema in guinea pigs. *Chest* 2003;**123**:1633–41.

141 Ma D, Jiang Y, Chen F *et al.* Selective inhibition of matrix metalloproteinase isoenzymes and *in vivo* protection against emphysema by substituted g-keto carboxylic acids. *J Med Chem* 2006;**49**:456–8.

142 Rennard SI, Crystal RG. Lung. In: Weiss JB, Jayson MIV, eds. *Collagen in Health and Disease.* Edinburgh: Churchill Livingstone, 1982: 424–44.

143 D'Armiento J, Dalal S, Okada Y, Berg R, Chada K. Collagenase expression in the lung of transgenic mice causes pulmonary emphysema. *Cell* 1992;**71**:955–61.

144 Foronjy RF, Okada Y, Cole R, D'Armiento J. Progressive adult-onset emphysema in transgenic mice expressing human MMP-1 in the lung. *Am J Physiol Lung Cell Mol Physiol* 2003;**284**:L727–37.

145 Finlay GA, O'Donnell MD, O'Connor CM, Hayes JP, Fitzgerald MX. Elastin and collagen remodeling in emphysema: a scanning electron microscopy study. *Am J Pathol* 1996;**149**:1405–15.

146 Segura-Valdez L, Pardo A, Gaxiola M *et al.* Upregulation of gelatinases A and B, collagenases 1 and 2, and increased parenchymal cell death in COPD. *Chest* 2000;**117**:684–94.

147 Ohnishi K, Takagi M, Kurokawa Y, Satomi S, Konttinen YT. Matrix metalloproteinase-mediated extracellular matrix protein degradation in human pulmonary emphysema. *Lab Invest* 1998;**78**:1077–87.

148 Vignola AM, Bonanno A, Mirabella A *et al.* Increased levels of elastase and α_1-antitrypsin in sputum of asthmatic patients. *Am J Respir Crit Care Med* 1998;**157**:505–11.

149 Lim S, Roche N, Oliver BG *et al.* Balance of matrix metalloprotease-9 and tissue inhibitor of metalloprotease-1 from alveolar macrophages in cigarette smokers: regulation by interleukin-10. *Am J Respir Crit Care Med* 2000;**162**:1355–60.

150 Finlay GA, O'Driscoll LR, Russell KJ *et al.* Matrix metalloproteinase expression and production by alveolar macrophages in emphysema. *Am J Respir Crit Care Med* 1997;**156**:240–7.

151 Vernooy JHJ, Lindeman JHN, Jacobs JA *et al.* Increased activity of matrix metalloproteinase-8 and matrix metalloproteinase-9 in induced sputum from patients with COPD. *Chest* 2004;**126**:1802–10.

152 Cataldo D, Munaut C, Noël A *et al.* MMP-2 and MMP-9-linked gelatinolytic activity in the sputum from patients with asthma and chronic obstructive pulmonary disease. *Int Arch Allergy Immunol* 2000;**123**:259–67.

153 Cataldo D, Munaut C, Noël A *et al.* Matrix metalloproteinases and TIMP-1 production by peripheral blood granulocytes from COPD patients and asthmatics. *Allergy* 2001;**56**:145–51.

154 Demedts IK, Morel-Montero A, Lebecque S *et al.* Elevated MMP-12 protein levels in induced sputum from patients with COPD. *Thorax* 2006;**61**:196–201.

155 Minematsu N, Nakamura H, Tateno H, Nakajima T, Yamaguchi K. Genetic polymorphism in matrix metalloproteinase-9 and pulmonary emphysema. *Biochem Biophys Res Commun* 2001;**289**:116–9.

156 Joos L, He JQ, Shepherdson MB *et al.* The role of matrix metalloproteinase polymorphisms in the rate of decline in lung function. *Hum Mol Genet* 2002;**11**:569–76.

157 Hirano K, Sakamoto T, Uchida Y *et al.* Tissue inhibitor of metalloproteinases-2 gene polymorphisms in chronic obstructive pulmonary disease. *Eur Respir J* 2001;**18**:748–52.

158 Gross P, Pfizer EH, Tolker B, Babyok MA, Kaschak M. Experimental emphysema: its production with papain in normal and silicotic rats. *Arch Environ Health* 1964;**11**:50–8.

159 Marco V, Mass B, Meranze DR, Weinbaum G, Kimbel P. Induction of experimental emphysema in dogs using leukocyte homogenates. *Am Rev Respir Dis* 1971;**104**:595–8.

160 Janoff A, Sloan B, Weinbaum G *et al.* Experimental emphysema induced with purified human neutrophil elastase: tissue localization of the instilled protease. *Am Rev Respir Dis* 1977;**115**:461–78.

161 Senior RM, Tegner H, Kuhn C *et al.* The induction of pulmonary emphysema with human leukocyte elastase. *Am Rev Respir Dis* 1977;**116**:469–75.

CHAPTER 32
Oxidants

William MacNee

The toxicity of oxygen in the lungs has been recognized for over 100 years; however, the mechanism of this toxicity was not determined until the importance of oxygen radicals, unstable compounds with an unpaired electron and other non-radical reactive pro-oxidants capable of initiating oxidation, were identified (referred to as reactive oxygen species, ROS). It is now recognized that ROS are not only relevant to oxygen toxicity, but that oxidant reactions occur in a broad spectrum of conditions involving tissue inflammation and injury [1,2]. Every compound, including oxygen, that can accept electrons is an oxidant and a substance that donates electrons is a reductant. A chemical reaction in which a substance gains electrons is defined as a reduction, whereas oxidation is a process in which loss of electrons occurs [2]. Thus, when a reductant donates electrons, it causes another substance to be reduced and, when an oxidant accepts electrons, it causes another substance to be oxidized. Physiologically relevant ROS include superoxide radicals and non-radical pro-oxidants (Table 32.1). To minimize oxidative damage the lungs are equipped with multiple enzymatic and non-enzymatic antioxidant systems (see below).

Reactive oxygen species are found diffusely throughout the lungs and are by-products of normal metabolism. The mitochondria are the largest producers of ROS as a result of the leak of electrons from the electron transfer chain onto oxygen to form superoxide anions [2]. It is estimated that 23% of oxygen produced in cells forms superoxide in this way. Other sources of superoxide include cytosolic xanthine oxidase [3], mitochondrial respiration, membrane nicotinamide adenine dinucleotide phosphate (NADPH) oxidases and the endoplasmic reticulum [4].

Hydrogen peroxide is formed from the dismutation of superoxide, but also by glycolate oxidase in peroxisomes. In the presence of metals, hydrogen peroxide in the Fenton reaction forms the hydroxyl radical. Hydroxy radicals are also produced in the metal-mediated Haber–Weiss reaction in which ferric ions are reduced by superoxide radicals to ferrous ions (Fig. 32.1) [5].

Reactive nitrogen species (RNS) are primarily derived from nitric oxide, which is produced by the action of the three nitric oxide synthases (NOSs) on arginine (Fig. 32.2):
1 constitutive NOS, which is found in respiratory epithelium, blood vessels and nerve endings;
2 inducible NOS, which is found in respiratory epithelium and activated macrophages [6]; and
3 neuronal NOS, which is found in the nerve plexus of the trachea [7].

Antioxidants are the primary defence against ROS/RNS. Antioxidants can be broadly divided into enzymatic or non-enzymatic antioxidants. The antioxidant enzymes include the families of superoxide dismutase (SODs), catalase, glutathione peroxidase, glutathione S-transferase and thiorodoxin (Fig. 32.3) [8,9].

Table 32.1 Radical and non-radical oxygen metabolites.

Name	Symbol
Oxygen radicals	
Oxygen (bi-radical)	O_2
Superoxide	O_2^-
Hydroxyl	OH
Peroxyl	ROO
Alkoxyl	RO
Nitric oxide	NO
Non-radical oxygen derivatives	
Hydrogen peroxide	H_2O_2
Organic peroxide	$ROOH$
Hypochlorous acid	$HOCL$
Ozone	O_3
Aldehydes	$HCOR$
Singlet oxygen	$^1O_2$
Peroxynitrite	$ONOOH$

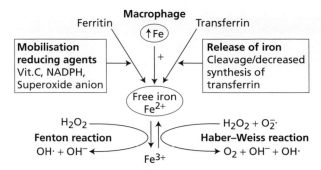

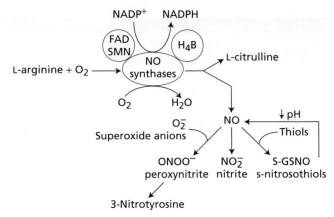

Figure 32.1 The role of iron in oxidant reactions in smokers and COPD patients. Macrophages release more iron which is also mobilized from ferritin by reducing agents and by cleavage and decreased synthesis of transferrin. Free iron in the ferrous form takes part in both the Fenton reaction and Haber–Weiss reaction with H_2O_2 and superoxide anion to produce hydroxyl radicals.

Figure 32.2 Synthesis of nitric oxide (NO) and NO-related products. NO is produced from L-arginine under the influence of NO synthases. NO reacts with thiols to produce nitrosothiols, nitrotyrosine to peroxynitrite. Nitrotyrosine or nitrosothiols can be measured as markers of oxidative stress. FAD, flavin-adenine dinucleotide; FMN, flavin-mononucleotide; H_2O_2, hydrogen peroxide; NADP, the oxidized form of nicotinamide adenine dinucleotide phosphate; NADPH, the reduced form of nicotinamide adenine dinucleotide phosphate; O_2, oxygen; S-GSNO, S nitrosothiols.

The non-enzymatic antioxidants include low molecular weight compounds such as glutathione (GSH), ascorbate, urate, α-tocopherol and bilirubin. Other high molecular weight molecules that might be considered to be antioxidants include proteins that have oxidizable thiol groups such as albumin, or proteins that bind free metals such as transferrin. The concentrations of these antioxidants vary depending on both the anatomical and the subcellular location. For example, GSH is 100-fold more concentrated in airway epithelial lining fluid, compared with plasma, and as such is considered to be a very important antioxidant in the lungs; whereas albumin and transferin are found in high concentrations in serum, but in much lower concentrations in airway epithelial lining fluid [1,10].

Oxidative stress

In the lungs, as in all organs, there is a delicate balance between ROS/RNS and antioxidants. If this balance is in disequilibrium, either because of an excess amount of ROS/RNS and/or depletion of antioxidants, then oxidative stress is said to occur.

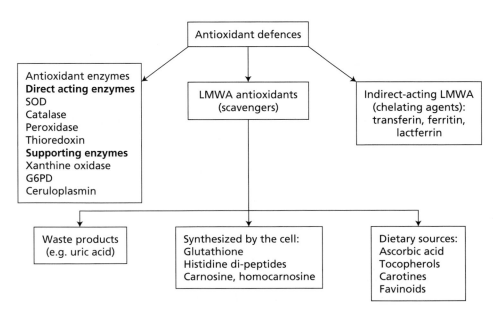

Figure 32.3 Antioxidant defences in the lungs. G6PD, glucose-6-phosphate dehydrogenase; LMWA, low-molecular weight; SOD, superoxide dismutase.

Measuring oxidative stress

Oxidative stress can be assessed by direct measurement of the oxidant burden (e.g. hydrogen peroxide in exhaled breath condensate) or the response to oxidative stress, such as activation of the heme-oxygenase system, assessed by measurements of CO in exhaled breath. Another way to measure oxidative stress is to measure the effects of oxidative stress on target molecules in the lungs, such as the nitration of tyrosine producing nitrotyrosine or the peroxidation of cell membrane lipids which results in products of lipid peroxidation.

Oxidants in cigarette smoke

Cigarette smoke is the main aetiological factor in the pathogenesis of COPD. It is a complex mixture of over 5000 different chemical compounds, including free radicals and other oxidants that are present in high concentrations [11,12]. Both the gas and the tar phase of cigarette smoke contain large amounts of ROS [11]. Each puff of cigarette smoke contains approximately 10^{15} radical molecules, primarily of the alkyl and peroxyl types. Nitric oxide is another oxidant present in the gas phase of cigarette smoke in concentrations of 500–1000 ppm (550–100 mg/L) [12]. The gas phase of cigarette smoke also contains organic carbon and oxygen centred radicals, which can react with unsaturated compounds to form carbon centred organic radicals [12].

In the tar phase of cigarette smoke, there are more stable radicals such as the semi-quinone radical, which can reduce oxygen to produce superoxide anion (O_2^-) and the hydroxyl radical ($\cdot OH$). The tar phase also contains ROS that are not radicals such as hydrogen peroxide (H_2O_2) [12]. The tar from cigarette smoke contains over 5000 different organic compounds from which the water-soluble components, such as aldehydes, catechol and hydroquin-one are extracted out into the epithelial lining fluid [12]. Cigarette smoke condensate, which may form in the epithelial lining fluid, continues to produce ROS for a considerable time.

Cell-derived oxidants

A characteristic feature of COPD is an abnormal inflammatory response in the lungs to inhaled particles or gases [13]. Recent studies, which have characterized the inflammatory response in lung tissue, bronchial biopsies and sputum, have clearly shown increased numbers of leucocytes in the airway and distal airspace walls in patients who develop COPD, compared with smokers with a similar smoking history but who have not developed the disease [14–16].

The increased oxidative burden produced by inhaling cigarette smoke is therefore further enhanced by the release of ROS from inflammatory leucocytes, both neutrophils and macrophages, which migrate in increased numbers

into the lungs of cigarette smokers, particularly in those who develop COPD [17]. In addition, the lungs of smokers who have airway obstruction have more neutrophils than smokers without airway obstruction, with the potential for a further increase in the oxidant burden [18].

Alveolar macrophages from the lungs of smokers are more activated than those from non-smokers [19,20] and release increased amounts of ROS such as O_2^- and H_2O_2, [21–24]. *In vitro* smoke exposure of alveolar macrophages has been shown to increase the oxidative metabolism of alveolar macrophages [25]. Subpopulations of alveolar macrophages with a higher density are more prevalent in the lungs of smokers and are thought to be the source of the increased O_2^- production in smokers [26].

The xanthine/xanthine oxidase (X/XO) system can generate O_2^- and H_2O_2 and XO activity is increased in cell free bronchoalveolar lavage fluid from COPD patients, compared with normal subjects, associated with increased O_2^- and uric acid production [27].

Iron is a critical element in many oxidative reactions [28]. Free iron in the ferrous form catalyses the Fenton reaction and the superoxide-driven Haber–Weiss reaction, which generate the extremely reactive hydroxyl radical (see Fig. 32.1). The lung lining fluid of smokers contains more iron than non-smokers [29,30] and alveolar macrophages from smokers, particularly those who develop chronic bronchitis, both contain [30] and release more iron than those of non-smokers [31,32]. The presence of increased amounts of free iron in the airspaces will therefore enhance the generation of oxidants in the lungs of smokers [33]. Airway epithelial cells are another source of ROS. Type II alveolar epithelial cells can release both H_2O_2 and O_2^- in similar amounts to alveolar macrophages [34] and the release of ROS from these cells is able, in the presence of myeloperoxidase, to inactivate α_1-antitrypsin *in vitro* [35] thereby reducing the protective antiprotease screen.

Tumour necrosis factor α (TNF-α) and lipopolysaccharide (LPS), which are relevant mediators in the inflammatory response in COPD, can stimulate airway epithelial cells to produce increased amounts of ROS and RNS [34]. ROS and RNS can also be generated intracellularly from several sources as described above. Depending on the relative amounts of O_2^- and NO, which are almost invariably produced simultaneously at sites of inflammation, these can react together to produce the powerful oxidant peroxynitrite ($ONOO^-$). Because this reaction occurs at a nearly diffusion-limited rate, it is thought that NO can out-compete SOD for reaction with O_2^- and thus $ONOO^-$ will be generated [1]:

$$O_2^- + NO \rightarrow ONOO^-.$$

Peroxynitrite is directly toxic to cells or may decompose to produce the hydroxyl radical:

$$ONOO^- + H^+ \rightarrow OH\cdot + NO_2.$$

The reaction of free radicals with polyunsaturated fatty acid side-chains in membranes or lipoproteins results in lipid peroxidation. This reaction is self-perpetuating, continuing as a chain reaction [36]. Lipid peroxides also have a role in the signalling events and in the molecular mechanisms involved in inflammation (see below).

Evidence for oxidative stress in COPD

Direct measurements of oxidative stress are difficult as free radicals and ROS are highly reactive and thus short lived. Numerous studies have measured a range of surrogate markers of oxidative stress in smokers and in patients with COPD. These surrogate markers measure oxidants directly (Table 32.2) [37–40], measure the stress responses to an increased oxidant burden or measure the effects of radicals on biomolecules such as lipids, protein or nucleic acids. Measurements of these markers of oxidative stress have been made in blood, exhaled breath or breath condensate and in induced or spontaneously produced sputum. Markers of oxidative stress have also been measured in bronchoalveolar lavage fluid and in lung tissue in patients with COPD.

A valid biomarker of oxidative stress in COPD should be:
1 implicated in the disease;
2 stable;
3 representative of the balance between oxidative damage generation and clearance;
4 determined by an assay that is specific, sensitive, reproducible and robust;
5 free of confounding factors from dietary intake; and
6 present at a detectable level [37–40].

Table 32.2 Measurements of oxidative stress.

Direct measurements of the oxidative burden
Hydrogen peroxide in breath condensate
BAL/peripheral blood leucocyte ROS production
Nitric oxide in exhaled breath

Responses to oxidative stress
CO in breath (haemoxygenase)
Antioxidants, antioxidant enzymes in blood, sputum, BAL and lung tissue

Effects of oxidative stress on target molecules
Nitrotyrosine (peroxinitrite)
Oxidized proteins (orthotyrosine, nitrotyrosine, chlorotyrosine)
Lipid peroxidation products (isoprostanes, 4-hydroxynonenol, hydrocarbons) in breath condensate, sputum, BAL, blood, lung tissue

BAL, bronchoalveolar lavage; CO, carbon monoxide; ROS, reactive oxygen species.

Measurements of oxidative stress in breath, breath condensate and sputum

Exhaled breath condensate is collected by cooling or freezing exhaled air. The content of breath condensate reflects the composition of the airway and airspace epithelial lining fluid, although large molecules may not aerosolize as well as small molecules. Measurement of biomarkers in breath condensate reflects molecules derived from the oral cavity and oral pharynx, tracheal bronchial tree and alveoli. However, their proportional contribution is not fully established. It is assumed that turbulent airflow aerosolizes airway and airspace lining fluid.

Hydrogen peroxide, measured in exhaled breath condensate, is a direct measurement of this oxidant in the airspaces. Smokers and patients with COPD have higher levels of exhaled H_2O_2 than non-smokers [41,42], and levels are even higher during exacerbations of COPD [43]. The source of the increased H_2O_2 is not fully determined but may derive in part from increased release of O_2^- from alveolar macrophages in smokers [44]. However, there is one study that did not show that smoking increased the levels of exhaled H_2O_2 [41], although in this study the levels of exhaled H_2O_2 correlated with the degree of airflow obstruction as measured by forced expiratory volume in 1 s (FEV_1).

Exhaled *nitric oxide* (NO) has been considered to be both a marker of airway inflammation and indirectly as a measure of oxidative stress. Increased levels of NO have been reported in exhaled breath in some studies of patients with COPD [45,46], but not in others [47]. However, the reported levels are not as high in COPD as in asthmatics [48]. Smoking increases NO levels in breath [49], and the reaction of NO with O_2^- and with thiol groups limits the usefulness of this marker in COPD, except perhaps to help to differentiate from asthma [50].

Neutrophils and macrophages are known to migrate in increased numbers into the lungs of cigarette smokers, compared with non-smokers [51]. Moreover, the lungs of smokers with airway obstruction have more neutrophils than smokers without airway obstruction [52]. Neutrophils from cigarette smokers have been shown to have an increased myeloperoxidase content [53] and the levels of myeloperoxidase correlate negatively with the FEV_1 in patients with COPD [43,54], suggesting a role for neutrophil myeloperoxidase-mediated oxidative stress in the pathogenesis of airways obstruction in COPD.

An increased oxidative burden in smokers is also shown by increased release of ROS such as O_2^- and H_2O_2 from smoker's macrophages [55] and peripheral blood neutrophils [56] compared with non-smokers.

Thus, direct measurements of the oxidant burden in the airspaces indicate an enhanced oxidant burden in cigarette

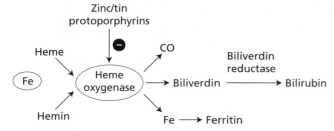

Figure 32.4 The heme-oxygenase system is activated by oxidative stress and converts heme to bilirubin producing carbon monoxide (CO) which can be measured as an indirect marker of oxidative stress. Fe, iron.

smokers in most studies, with even greater oxidant burden in those who have COPD.

Markers of the responses to oxidative stress have also been measured in COPD patients. Carbon monoxide (CO) is produced endogenously as a result of oxidant-mediated induction of the stress protein heme-oxygenase 1 (HO-1) in a variety of cell types [57]. HO-1 converts heme and hemin to biliverdin with the formation of CO (Fig. 32.4). Biliverdin itself is rapidly converted to bilirubin which acts as an antioxidant. Cigarette smoking causes an acute increase in exhaled CO making this measurement less useful in smokers. However, high levels of exhaled CO have been found in ex-smoker COPD patients [57,58]. It is presumed that the high levels of exhaled CO in COPD patients are caused by inflammatory cytokines or ROS inducing HO-1 expression and therefore the high levels of CO may reflect both oxidative stress and inflammation.

A further response to oxidative stress in the lungs is a change in antioxidants. Glutathiane (GSH) is a important antioxidant in lung lining fluids. Reduced GSH is elevated in bronchoalveolar lavage fluid (BALF) in chronic smokers [59–61]. However, the twofold increase in BALF GSH in chronic smokers may be insufficient to deal with the excessive oxidant burden *during* smoking, when acute depletion of GSH may occur [62]. The depletion of GSH in epithelial lining fluid following cigarette smoking is likely to result from direct interaction of GSH with oxidants and electrophilic compounds in cigarette smoke to form oxidized GSH or GSH conjugates [63,64]. The increase in GSH in chronic cigarette smokers is likely a response to oxidative stress by up-regulating γ-glutamylcysteine synthetase, the main synthesizing enzyme for GSH [63,64].

Changes in other antioxidants and antioxidant enzymes in response to cigarette smoke have been variable. Reduced levels of vitamin E have been found in the BALF of smokers compared with non-smokers [65], whereas increased activity of antioxidant enzymes (SOD and catalase) have been reported in alveolar macrophages from young smokers [66]. Others have found that the increased superoxide

generation by alveolar macrophages in elderly smokers compared with non-smokers is associated with decreased antioxidant enzyme activities [67]. There is therefore no consistent change in antioxidant defences in the epithelial lining fluid in smokers and no information in COPD patients.

The effects of oxidative stress on target molecules in the lungs have been assessed. Ethane, pentane and hydrocarbons are released during lipid peroxidation in biological tissues. Ethane derives from the peroxidation of N-6 polyunsaturated acids. Ethane levels in exhaled breath are elevated in COPD patients and correlate with the degree of airflow limitation [68]. Isoprostanes are lipid peroxidation products formed from the peroxidation of arachadonic acid independent of the cyclo-oxygenase enzyme pathway [69,70]. Their presence is therefore an indication not only of oxidative stress, but also that oxidative stress has affected important target molecules to produce a lipid peroxidation product. These compounds may also have an important role in pulmonary pathophysiology [71]. Isoprostanes cause constriction of the pulmonary vasculature and airway smooth muscle cells [72] and have been shown to induce various second messenger systems that result in vaso- and bronchoconstriction [73,74]. Isoprostanes have also been shown to activate inflammatory cells such as neutrophils and to enhance their adhesion [75].

8-Isoprostane levels in exhaled breath condensate are elevated in patients with stable COPD [76,77] and correlate with the degree of airway inflammation as measured by sputum neutrophil numbers [78]. The levels of 8-isoprostane are increased further in exacerbations of COPD [79].

Lipid peroxidation products have been found in increased amounts in lung tissue from cigarette smokers and the levels relate to the length of smoking [80]. BALF from cigarette smokers also contains increased products of lipid peroxidation, such as malondehaldyde [21].

4-hydroxy-2-nonenal (4-HNE) is a highly reactive aldehyde lipid peroxidation product which has been shown to enter cells and activate mitogen-activated protein (MAP) kinase signalling pathways [81]. It also acts as a chemoattractant for neutrophils [81]. Increased levels of 4-HNE-modified proteins have been found in airway, alveolar epithelial cells, endothelial cells and in neutrophils in subjects with airway obstruction compared with subjects without airway obstruction but who have had similar smoking histories. This suggests not only the presence of this lipid peroxidation product but that this product modifies proteins in lung cells to a greater extent in patients with COPD. In addition, the levels of 4-HNE-adducts in alveolar and airway epithelium have been shown to be inversely related to the FEV_1, suggesting a role for 4-HNE in the pathogenesis of COPD (Fig. 32.5) [82].

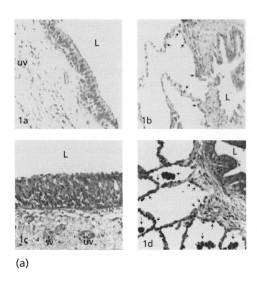

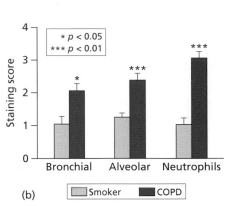

(a)

(b)

Figure 32.5 Immunostaining for 4-hydroxy-2-nonenal adducts in lungs of smokers and COPD patients. (a) Immunostaining in bronchi and alveoli are shown for smokers with the same smoking history as a group of patients with COPD. There is increased immunostaining for 4-hydroxy-2-nonenal in COPD patients. (b) The staining scores for 4-hydroxy-2-nonenal in bronchial and alveolar cells and in neutrophils from both smokers and COPD patients. (From Rahman *et al.* [82] with permission.)

Systemic oxidative stress in COPD

COPD is now considered not only to produce local effects in lungs but also to have systemic manifestations [83,84]. Examples of these systemic effects are the skeletal muscle dysfunction and weight loss that occurs in some patients and are a predictor of reduced survival [85].

There is evidence of an increased systemic oxidative burden in COPD, as shown by the greater ability of circulating neutrophils from patients with COPD to release ROS [56]. The lipid peroxidation products thiobarbituric acid reactive substances have been found in plasma in greater amounts in healthy smokers and in patients with acute exacerbations of COPD, compared with healthy non-smokers [83]. Other products of lipid peroxidation such as conjugated dienes of linoleic acid are also elevated in the plasma in chronic smokers [86]. Similarly, levels of the lipid peroxidation product F_2-isoprostane are elevated in the urine in smokers [87]. Measurements of the antioxidant capacity in the blood can be used as a marker of systemic oxidative stress. Smoking causes a transient decrease in antioxidant capacity which also occurs during exacerbations of COPD [55,83]. The reaction of nitric oxide with superoxide anion leads to the formation of peroxynitrite which has been shown to decrease plasma antioxidant capacity rapidly by oxidation of ascorbic acid, uric acid and plasma sulphydryls [88]. Increased plasma peroxynitrite levels have been demonstrated in cigarette smokers [89] and increased immunoreactivity for nitrotyrosine has been shown in sputum leucocytes in patients with COPD. Nitration of tyrosine residues or proteins in plasma leads to the production of 3-nitrotyrosine. Higher levels of 3-nitrotyrosine have been found in the plasma in smokers compared with non-smokers, which correlated negatively with the plasma antioxidant capacity in smokers [89].

Consequences of oxidative stress in the pathogenesis of COPD

Airspace epithelial injury and permeability

The epithelial surface of the lung airspaces, by virtue of its direct contact with the environment, is particularly vulnerable to the effects of oxidative stress produced by cigarette smoke. Oxidants in cigarette smoke can directly damage components of the lung matrix (such as elastin and collagen) [90]. The synthesis and repair of elastin can also be impaired by cigarette smoke [91], which may augment the proteolytic damage to matrix components and thus enhance the development of emphysema.

One of the earliest injurious events in smokers is increased airspace epithelial permeability [92]. Cigarette smoke produces direct injury to human alveolar epithelial cell monolayers *in vitro* as shown by increased epithelial cell detachment, decreased cell adherence and increased cell lysis [93]. These effects are in part oxidant mediated because they are abrogated by the antioxidant GSH in concentrations (500 µmol/L) that are present in the epithelial lining fluid.

Studies in humans show increased epithelial permeability in chronic smokers compared with non-smokers, as measured by increased [99m]technetium-diethylenetriamine-pentacetate (^{99m}Tc-DTPA) lung clearance, with a further increase in ^{99m}Tc-DTPA clearance following acute smoking [59].

Both extra- and intracellular GSH appear to be critical to the maintenance of epithelial integrity following exposure to cigarette smoke. Studies of increased permeability of epithelial cell monolayers *in vitro* [62,94] and in rat lungs *in vivo* [64] show that smoke exposure is associated with profound changes in the antioxidant GSH. Concentrations of GSH are consistently decreased following smoke exposure, concomitant with a decrease in the activities the enzymes are involved in the GSH redox cycle such as GSH peroxidase and glucose-6-phosphate dehydrogenase. Depletion of lung GSH alone induces increased airspace epithelial permeability both *in vitro* and *in vivo* [64,94,95].

Oxidative stress and apoptosis

Apoptosis or programmed cell death of leucocytes constitutes an important mechanism in the resolution of inflammation [96]. It is now recognized that structural cells in the lungs also undergo apoptosis and oxidant-mediated mechanisms may be involved. Hydrogen peroxide can induce apoptosis in airway epithelial cells [97]. Studies both *in vitro* and *in vivo* in animals and in humans have shown that apoptosis can occur in smoke-exposed macrophages [98]. However, studies *in vitro* in both endothelial cells and airspace epithelial cells indicate that smoke exposure may induce necrosis rather than apoptosis and necrosis itself may be a further stimulus to inflammation in the lungs [99].

It has been suggested that pulmonary capillary epithelial cell apoptosis, induced by cigarette smoking, may be an early event in the process that leads to alveolar wall destruction and emphysema. Studies of human lungs indicate that pulmonary vascular endothelial apoptosis is present in emphysematous lungs [100]. Mechanisms involving transcription factors AP-1 and NF-κB and the down-regulation of the vascular endothelial growth factor receptor KDR (VEGF-KDR) have been proposed as part of the mechanism. Down-regulation of the VEGF-KDR receptor in an animal model can induce both apoptosis and emphysema [101]. It has also been proposed that oxidant-mediated mechanisms are involved in this process, because the apoptosis in emphysematous lungs is also associated with markers of oxidative stress, specifically lipid peroxidation products such as 4-hydroxy-nonenal [102]. Furthermore, the emphysema induced by inhibiting VEGF-KDR can be prevented by antioxidant treatment [102].

Protease–antiprotease imbalance

The development of a proteinase–antiproteinase imbalance in the lungs is thought to be a critical event in the pathogenesis of emphysema. The hypothesis is that increased recruitment of leucocytes to the lungs will increase the protease burden in the lungs and at the same time the antiprotease screen, particularly α_1-antitrypsin (α_1-AT), may be inactivated by oxidation resulting in a relative deficiency of antiproteases in the presence of an excess of proteases, leading to a proteinase–antiproteinase imbalance.

However, this simple hypothesis of an imbalance between an increased elastase burden in the lungs and a functional 'deficiency' of α_1-AT because of its inactivation by oxidants is an oversimplification, not least because

other proteinases and antiproteinases are likely to have a role. Early studies showed that the function of α_1-AT in bronchoalveolar lavage was decreased by approximately 40% in smokers compared with non-smokers [103]. This 'functional α_1-AT deficiency' is thought to be caused by oxidative inactivation by cigarette smoke of the methionine residue of α_1-AT at its active site [104,105]. Oxidation of the methionine residue in α_1-AT has been confirmed in the lungs of healthy smokers [106]. *In vitro* studies show that oxidants [107], including cigarette smoke [108], reduce the inhibitory capacity of α_1-AT. Other studies have shown that macrophages from the lungs of smokers release increased amounts of ROS which can inactivate α_1-AT *in vitro* [105]. However, it has been shown that the α_1-AT in the airspaces in cigarette smokers remains active and is still capable of protecting against the increased protease burden. There are also conflicting data on whether α_1-AT function is altered in cigarette smokers [109], and the original observation that oxidation of α_1-AT occurs in bronchoalveolar lavage in smokers has not been confirmed [110]. Studies of the effects of acute cigarette smoking have only shown a transient but non-significant fall in the antiprotease activity of bronchoalveolar lavage fluid (BALF) 1 h after smoking [111]. Thus, studies assessing the function of α_1-AT in either chronic or acute cigarette smoking have failed to produce a clear picture that oxidative stress inactivates antiproteases.

Neutrophil sequestration and migration in the lungs

The enhanced inflammation that is thought to characterize COPD is associated with the influx of leucocytes of which polymorphonuclear leukocytes are a prominent cell. Neutrophil recruitment into the airspaces is initiated by the sequestration of these cells in the lung microcirculation [112]. Initial sequestration of neutrophils in the pulmonary microcirculation results from the size differential between neutrophils (average diameter 7 μmol) and pulmonary capillary segments (average diameter 5 μmol). Thus, under normal circumstances, a proportion of the circulating neutrophils have to deform in order to negotiate the smaller capillary segments, which delays their transit through the microcirculation. Radiolabelled neutrophil studies in healthy subjects indicate that a proportion of neutrophils are normally delayed in the pulmonary circulation [113]. It has also been shown that there is a correlation between neutrophil deformability measured *in vitro* and the subsequent sequestration of these cells in the pulmonary microcirculation following their re-injection in normal subjects – the less deformable the cells the greater the sequestration of these cells in the pulmonary circulation [112]. Sequestration of neutrophils in the pulmonary capillaries allows time for the neutrophils to interact with the pulmonary capillary endothelium, resulting in their adherence to the endothelium and thereafter their transmigration across the alveolar capillary membrane to the interstitium and airspaces of the lungs in response to inflammation or infection.

Neutrophils in transit in the pulmonary microcirculation neutrophils can be activated by a number of mediators, including cytokines released from alveolar macrophages, epithelial and endothelial cells. Inhaled oxidants such as those contained in cigarette smoke and other air pollutants can influence the transit of cells in the pulmonary capillary bed. Studies using radiolabelled neutrophils and red cells in healthy smokers show a transient increase in neutrophil sequestration in the lungs during smoking [114], which is associated with an acute decrease in cell neutrophil deformability [115,116], an effect that is likely to be oxidant mediated. Support for this comes from *in vitro* studies that show decreased neutrophil deformability induced by cigarette smoke is abolished by antioxidants [115]. There is also evidence of systemic oxidative stress following cigarette smoking, which may affect neutrophils and increase their sequestration in the pulmonary microcirculation [116].

Cigarette smoke has also been shown to cause the release of neutrophils from the bone marrow with decreased deformability, which may preferentially sequester in the pulmonary microcirculation [117]. The mechanism for release of bone marrow neutrophils in response to smoke is as yet unclear, but oxidants may have a role.

Thus, cigarette smoking increases neutrophil sequestration in the pulmonary microcirculation, at least in part, by decreasing neutrophil deformability, an effect that may be oxidant mediated. Once sequestered in the pulmonary microcirculation, components of cigarette smoke can alter neutrophil adhesion to endothelium by up-regulating CD18 integrins [118,119]. Inhalation of cigarette smoke in hamsters increases neutrophil adhesion to the endothelium of both arterioles and venules [118], an event that may be mediated by superoxide anion derived from cigarette smoke, because it is inhibited by pretreatment with CuZn-SOD [118]. Neutrophils sequestered in the pulmonary circulation of the rabbit following cigarette smoke inhalation also show increased expression of CD18 integrins [119].

Oxidant-mediated mechanisms may also result in increased sequestration of neutrophils, which occurs in the pulmonary microcirculation during exacerbations of COPD [55,113]. Studies in animal models of smoke exposure [120] have shown increased neutrophil sequestration in the pulmonary microcirculation, associated with up-regulation of adhesion molecules on the surface of these cells [119]. Activation of neutrophils sequestered in the pulmonary microvasculature could induce the release of reactive oxygen intermediates and proteases within the microenvironment, with limited access for free radical scavengers and antiproteases. Thus, destruction of the alveolar wall, as occurs in emphysema, could result from a proteolytic or oxidant insult from the intravascular space, without the need for the neutrophils to migrate into the airspaces [121].

Mucus hypersecretion

Mucins are complex glycoproteins that are an essential protective mechanism in the upper airways. The regulation of mucus production and clearance is altered in the lungs of COPD patients. The airways of smokers contain more goblet cells than do those of non-smokers and goblet-cell activation results in mucus hypersecretion leading to airway plugging. Cigarette smoke has been shown to activate epidermal growth factor (EGF) receptors, resulting in the induction of mucin (*mucin5ac* gene expression) synthesis in epithelial cells and in lungs *in vitro* and *in vivo* [122]. Oxidants appear to be involved in these events because cigarette smoke-mediated *MUC5ac* gene expression is inhibited by antioxidants [122].

Oxidative stress and muscle dysfunction

COPD is now considered to have important systemic consequences including weight loss and muscle dysfunction. The cause of the muscle dysfunction in COPD is not well understood, but mechanisms involving oxidative stress may be involved. Skeletal muscles can generate ROS at rest and ROS production increases during contractile activity. Increased oxidative stress also occurs in skeletal muscle during skeletal muscle fatigue [123]. This may result from hypoxia, impaired mitochondrial metabolism and increased cytochrome C oxidase activity in skeletal muscle in patients with COPD [124]. Reduced muscle glutamate (a precursor of GSH) occurs in patients with severe COPD, associated with increased muscle glycolytic metabolism [125]. In association with lowered levels of glutamate, GSH levels were also decreased in muscles, suggesting an oxidant–antioxidant imbalance is involved in the skeletal muscle dysfunction in patients with COPD. A causal relationship between abnormally low muscle redox potential at rest and alteration of protein metabolism observed in patients with emphysema has been suggested. This is supported by a study that showed decreased muscle redox capacity, probably as a result of a reduced ability of muscles to synthesize GSH during endurance training in patients with COPD [126]. Several lines of evidence therefore suggest that oxidative stress has a role in mediating muscle mass wasting in susceptible subsets of patients with COPD.

Inflammation, oxidative stress and gene expression

A characteristic feature of COPD is an abnormal inflammatory response in the lungs to inhaled particles or gases [13,127]. The mechanism of this enhanced inflammatory response is the subject of intensive study. Gene expression for many inflammatory mediators, such as those for the cytokines, interleukin 8 (IL-8) and TNF-α, and nitric oxide, are regulated by transcription factors, such as NF-κB. In quiescent cells, NF-κB is present in the cytosol in an inactive form linked to an inhibitory protein IκB. Oxidants are one of the mediators that can activate NF-κB by activating I-κB kinase, which phosphorolates the inhibitory protein IκB resulting in cleaving of IκB from NF-κB and its destruction in the proteosome [128]. Oxidants also activate other signal transduction pathways involved in inflammation, such as the ~ERK and JNK and P_{38} MAP kinase pathways, which may signal through other transcription factors such as C-jun-AP-1. Activation of these transcription factors and their binding to their consensus sites in the nucleus increases transcription of many proinflammatory genes leading to inflammatory cytokine release from lung cells. Inflammation itself will generate further oxidative stress and this may lead to a vicious circle which enhances the inflammatory response (Fig. 32.6).

Studies *in vitro* show that treatment of macrophages, alveolar, bronchial epithelial cells with oxidants result in increased mRNA expression and the release of inflammatory mediators such as IL-8, IL-1 and nitric oxide, associated with increased nuclear binding and activation of NF-κB [129,130]. In addition, a stimulus relevant to exacerbations of COPD, such as particulate air pollution, which has oxidant properties, also activates NF-κB in alveolar epithelial cells and causes the release of IL-8 [131].

Thiol antioxidants such as *N*-acetylcysteine and *N*-acystelyn, which are potential therapies in COPD, have been shown in *in vitro* experiments to block the release of these inflammatory mediators from epithelial cells and macrophages in response to oxidants by a mechanism involving increasing intracellular GSH and decreasing NF-κB activation [129,131]. The intracellular GSH redox status in cells is affected by cigarette smoke and may have a critical role in the regulation of transcription factors such as NF-κB and AP-1 [132–134]. Interaction may also occur between oxidants and TNF, which are both relevant mediators in COPD, producing synergistic activation of NF-κB [135].

A further mechanism that may enhance the inflammatory response in COPD is the remodelling of chromatin which involves histone acetylation–deacetylation [128]. In the nucleus, DNA is normally tightly wound around a core of histone residues. This configuration of the chromatin results in gene silencing by preventing access of transcription factors and RNA polymerase to the transcriptional machinery. Under the influence of enzymes known as histone acetyl transferases (HATs), core histone residues are acetylated, which results in the unwinding of DNA around the core histones and allows access for transcription factors and RNA polymerase to the transcriptional machinery, resulting in transcription. This process is regulated by other enzymes known as histone deacetylases (HDAC), which deacetylate histone residues and cause the rewinding of DNA and gene suppression (Fig. 32.7). Thus, an increase in histone acetylation and/or a decrease in HDAC will alter the balance between acetylation and deacetylation in favour of enhanced gene expression. Oxidants such as H_2O_2 and oxidants derived from cigarette smoke or particulate air pollution alter chromatin remodelling, producing increased acetylation and decreased HDAC expression [136,137]. Cigarette smoke exposure has also been shown to produce decreased HDAC protein expression and increased histone

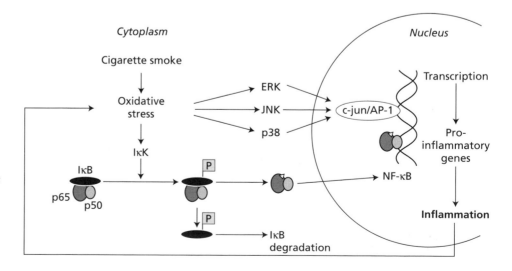

Figure 32.6 Effects of oxidative stress on signalling pathways involving transcription factors NF-κB and AP-1 and the up-regulation of proinflammatory genes.

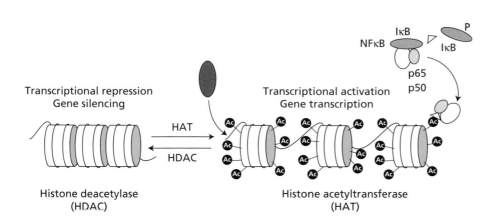

Figure 32.7 Histone acetylation and deacetylation. In resting cells DNA is tightly wound around a core of histones. This configuration results in gene silencing (left). Under the influence of histone acetyl transferase histone residues are acetylated, changing their charge and resulting in unwinding of DNA allowing access for transcription factors such as NF-κB and RNA polymerase II producing increase transcription. The process is reversed by histone deacetylases which deacetylate histone residues and result in the rewinding of DNA and gene silencing.

acetylation in the lungs of animals exposed to cigarette smoke associated with enhanced lung inflammation and increased oxidative stress [138].

Oxidative stress and the development of airways obstruction

Relatively few studies have assessed the relationship between markers of inflammation or oxidative stress and the progression of disease in COPD. The neutrophil appears to be an important cell in the pathogenesis of COPD and one study has shown a relationship between blood neutrophil counts and FEV_1 [139]. Moreover, a relationship has also been shown between the change in peripheral blood neutrophil count and the change in airflow limitation over time [140]. A relationship has also been demonstrated between the release of ROS by neutrophils and measurements of airflow limitation in young cigarette smokers [141]. Neutrophil counts in sputum have also been shown to relate to the decline in FEV_1: the greater the neutrophil count in sputum the more rapid the decline in FEV_1 [142]. Oxidative stress, measured as lipid peroxidation products in plasma, has also been shown to correlate inversely with the percentage predicted FEV_1 in a population study [143], but not in a COPD population [144].

General population studies have shown an association between dietary intake of antioxidant vitamins and lung function. In a population of 2633 subjects, an association was demonstrated between dietary intake of the antioxidant vitamin E and lung function [145], supporting the hypothesis that antioxidants may have a role in protecting against the development of COPD. A further study suggested that antioxidant levels in the diet may explain the differences in COPD mortality in different populations [146]. Dietary polyunsaturated fatty acids have also been suggested as being protective in cigarette smokers against the development of COPD [147,148]. However, intervention studies of dietary antioxidant supplementation have not been able to demonstrate a positive effect in the development of COPD.

Only 15–20% of smokers appear to be very susceptible to the effect of cigarette smoke and have a rapid decline in FEV_1 and develop COPD [149]. There has been considerable interest in identifying those who are susceptible and the mechanisms underlying that susceptibility [149–151] because this would provide an important insight into the pathogenesis of COPD.

Association studies of polymorphisms of various genes have been performed and a number of polymorphisms have been shown to be more prevalent in smokers who develop COPD [150]. Some of these polymorphisms have functional significance, such as the TNF-α gene polymorphism (TNF2), which is associated with increased TNF levels in response to inflammation and the development of chronic bronchitis [152]. Microsomal epoxide hydrolase is an enzyme involved in the metabolism of highly reactive epoxide intermediates which are present in cigarette smoke [153]. The proportion of individuals with slow microsomal epoxide hydrolase activity (homozygotes) is significantly higher in patients with COPD and a subgroup of patients shown to have emphysema (COPD 22%; emphysema 19%), compared with control subjects (6%) [153]. These data, however, have not been reproduced in other patient populations [154]. Although the results of association studies with polymorphisms have shown inconsistent results, there does seem to be more evidence to support abnormal polymorphisms in the oxidant–antioxidant pathways with

Table 32.3 Genetic association studies of COPD and related phenotypes.

Gene categories	Gene/genotype	Phenotype of COPD	Association	Population	Reference
Oxidant/ antioxidant genes	Heme oxygenase 1 (*HMOX1*): GT repeat	Emphysema	Yes	Japanese	154
		Rate of lung function ↓	No	Whites	155
	Microsomal epoxide hydrolase (*mPHX*): 113His/His 39	Emphysema	Yes	Caucasians	156
		COPD	Yes	Caucasians	156
		COPD	No	Koreans	157
		Rate of lung function ↓	Yes	Whites	158
	GSTM1 null	Chronic bronchitis	Yes	Caucasians	159
		Emphysema	Yes	Caucasians	160
		COPD	No	Koreans	157
		Lung function growth	Yes	Whites	161
		Rate of lung function ↓	No	Whites	155
	GSTT1 null	COPD	No	Koreans	157
		Lung function growth	No	Whites	161
		Rate of lung function ↓	No	Whites	155
	GSTP1 105Ile	COPD	Yes	Japanese	162
		COPD	No	Koreans	163
		Rate of lung function ↓	No	Whites	155
		Lung function growth	Yes	Whites	161
	Cytochrome P4501A1:462Val	Emphysema	Yes	Caucasians	164

the development of COPD than with other pathways (Table 32.3) [153–163]. It may be that a panel of 'susceptibility' polymorphisms, of functional significance in enzymes involved in xenobiotic metabolism or antioxidant enzyme genes, may allow individuals to be identified as being susceptible to the effects of cigarette smoke.

Therapy to be targeted at oxidative stress

There is now convincing evidence for an oxidant–antioxidant imbalance in smokers and a probable role for this imbalance in the pathogenesis of COPD. However, proof of concept of the role of oxidative stress in the pathogenesis of COPD will only come with studies of effective antioxidant therapy.

Various approaches have been tried to redress the oxidant–antioxidant imbalance. One approach is to target the inflammatory response by reducing the sequestration or migration of leucocytes from the pulmonary circulation into the airspaces. Possible therapeutic options for this are drugs that alter cell deformability, so preventing neutrophil sequestration or the migration of neutrophils, either by interfering with the adhesion molecules necessary for migration, or preventing the release of inflammatory

cytokines such as IL-8 or leukotriene B_4 which result in neutrophil migration. Agents are available that may in part be effective by preventing activation of leucocytes and in particular the release of ROS. Preliminary results of phosphodiesterase 4 inhibitors have shown some therapeutic benefit in patients with COPD [164]. The mechanism by which such drugs act is by increasing cellular cyclic adenosine monophosphate (cAMP), which decreases neutrophil activation. In particular, the release of ROS by neutrophils may be decreased, because cAMP blocks the assembly of NADPH oxidase [165,166].

Various strategies are available to enhance the lung antioxidant screen in order to quench oxidants. One approach is to use specific spin traps such as α-phenyl-*N*-tert-butyl nitrone to react directly with reactive oxygen and ROS at the site of inflammation. However, considerable work is needed to demonstrate the efficacy of such drugs *in vivo*. Antioxidants that have a double action, such as inhibition of lipid peroxidation and quenching of ROS, may be developed [167]. A further approach might be the manipulation of antioxidant genes, such as GSH peroxidase or the genes involved in the synthesis of GSH, such as γGCS, or by developing molecules with activity similar to these antioxidant enzymes.

Effective oxidant therapy has been shown, at least in animal models, to reduce inflammation. Recombinant

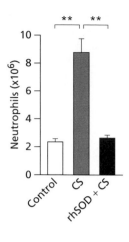
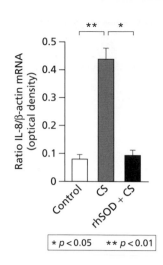
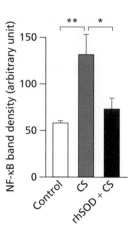

* $p < 0.05$ ** $p < 0.01$

Figure 32.8 The effect of recombinant superoxide dismutase (rhSOD) on cigarette smoke (CS) induced neutrophils, interleukin 8 (IL-8) gene expression and NF-κB binding in guinea pigs lungs. (From Nishikawa *et al.* [168] with permission.)

SOD treatment can prevent neutrophil influx into the airspaces induced by cigarette smoke. IL-8 release from airspace leucocytes induced by cigarette smoking is also decreased by SOD through a mechanism involving down-regulation of NF-κB (Fig. 32.8) [168]. This holds great promise if compounds can be developed with antioxidant enzyme properties that may be able to act as novel anti-inflammatory drugs by regulating the molecular events in lung inflammation.

A further therapeutic approach would be to administer antioxidant agents. This has been attempted in cigarette smokers using various antioxidants such as vitamins C and E. In general, the results have been rather disappointing, although the antioxidant vitamin E has been shown to decrease markers of oxidative stress in patients with COPD [169].

Attempts to supplement lung GSH have been made using GSH or its precursors [170]. GSH itself is not efficiently transported into most animal cells and an excess of GSH may be a source of the thiyl radical under conditions of oxidative stress [171]. Nebulized GSH has also been used therapeutically, but this has been shown to induce bronchial hyperreactivity [172]. The thiol cysteine is the rate-limiting amino acid in GSH synthesis [173]. Cysteine administration is not possible because it is oxidized to cystine, which is neurotoxic. The cysteine-donating compound *N*-acetylcysteine (NAC) acts as a cellular precursor of GSH and is deacetylated in the gut following oral administration to cysteine. This compound reduces disulphide bonds and has the potential to interact directly with oxidants. NAC also has mucolytic properties by reducing disulphide bonds in mucus. The use of NAC in an attempt to enhance GSH in patients with COPD has met with varying success [174,175]. NAC given orally in low doses of 600 mg/day to normal subjects results in very low levels of NAC in the plasma up to 2 h after administration [175].

NAC given in a higher dose of 600 mg three times daily for 5 days produced a significant increase in plasma GSH levels [174]. However, there was no associated significant rise in BAL GSH or in lung tissue [175]. These data may imply that producing a sustained increase in lung GSH is difficult using NAC in subjects who are not already depleted of GSH. In spite of this, several studies have shown that NAC reduces the number of exacerbation days in patients with COPD [176,177], although these results have not been confirmed in all studies [178].

Very recently, preliminary results of a large randomized controlled trial of NAC, 600 mg/day, in patients with COPD has been presented [179]. This study assessed the effect of NAC compared with placebo on the rate of decline in FEV_1, on exacerbation rates and pulmonary function. Unfortunately, the design of this study resulted in a group of patients with mild to moderate COPD being studied with an FEV_1 of approximately 57% predicted. Indeed, 75% of the patients in this study had an FEV_1 greater than 50% predicted. In addition, 75% of the patients were already taking inhaled corticosteroids. The study did not show any significant effect of NAC on the rate of decline in FEV_1, although there were significant improvements in FEV_1, vital capacity and a reduction in functional residual capacity (FRC) as a measure of overinflation in severe COPD patients treated with NAC compared with placebo. There was no overall effect on exacerbation rates when the result of the whole group was analysed. However, in those patients who were not taking inhaled corticosteroids there was a significant fall in exacerbations rates from 1.33 to 0.99 per year (22% reduction), which was similar to the effects of inhaled corticosteroids on exacerbation rates in a moderate to severe group of COPD patients. These data suggest that there may be an effect of NAC on exacerbations rates and pulmonary function, at least in patients with severe COPD who are not already taking inhaled corticosteroids.

Nacystelyn (NAL) is a lysine salt of *N*-acetylinecysteine. It is thiol antioxidant compound and a mucolytic that has a neutral pH in contrast to NAC, which is acidic. NAL can therefore be aerosolized into the lung without causing bronchial hyperreactivity [180]. Studies comparing the effects of NAL and NAC found that both drugs enhanced intracellular GSH in alveolar epithelial cells and inhibited hydrogen peroxide and superoxide anion release from neutrophils harvested from peripheral blood from both smokers and patients with COPD [181].

Molecular regulation of GSH synthesis, by targeting γGCS, has great promise as a means of treating oxidant-mediated injury in the lungs. Recent work has shown that recombinant γGCS in rat hepatoma cells completely protected against the TNF-α-induced activation of NF-κB, AP-1 and apoptosis as well as inflammation [182]. Cellular GSH may be increased by increasing γGCS activity, which may be possible by gene transfer techniques, although this would be an expensive treatment which may not be considered for a condition such as COPD. However, knowledge of how γGCS is regulated may allow the development of other compounds that may act to enhance GSH.

Future perspectives

There is now good evidence for an oxidant–antioxidant imbalance in COPD, and increasing evidence that this imbalance is important in the pathogenesis of this condition. A major effect of oxidative stress is its role in the inflammatory response to cigarette smoke in the lungs through up-regulation of redox-sensitive transcription factors and hence proinflammatory gene expression. Inflammation itself induces oxidative stress in the lungs, and polymorphisms in genes for inflammatory mediators or antioxidant genes may have a role in the susceptibility to the effects of cigarette smoke. Knowledge of the mechanisms of the effects of oxidative stress should allow the development of potent antioxidant therapies which can be used to support the hypothesis that oxidative stress is involved in the pathogenesis of COPD, not only by direct injury to cells, but also as a fundamental factor in the inflammation in smoking-related lung disease.

References

1 van der Vliet A, O'Neill CA, Cross CE *et al.* Determination of low-molecular-mass antioxidant concentrations in human respiratory tract lining fluids. *Am J Physiol* 1999;**276**: L289–96.

2 Halliwell B, Gutteridge JM. *Free Radicals in Biology and Medicine*, 3rd edn. Oxford: Oxford University Press, 1999.

3 Quinlan GJ, Lamb NJ, Tilley R, Evans TW, Gutteridge JM. Plasma hypoxanthine levels in ARDS: implications for oxidative stress, morbidity, and mortality. *Am J Respir Crit Care Med* 1997;**155**:479–84.

4 Goeptar AR, Scheerens H, Vermeulen NP. Oxygen and xenobiotic reductase activities of cytochrome P450. *Crit Rev Toxicol* 1995;**25**:25–65.

5 Merenyi G, Lind J, Goldstein S, Czapski G. Peroxynitrous acid homolyzes into *OH and *NO$_2$ radicals. *Chem Res Toxicol* 1998;**11**:712–3.

6 Kobzik L, Bredt DS, Lowenstein CJ *et al.* Nitric oxide synthase in human and rat lung: immunocytochemical and histochemical localization. *Am J Respir Cell Mol Biol* 1993; **9**:371–7.

7 Guembe L, Villaro AC. Histochemical demonstration of neuronal nitric oxide synthase during development of mouse respiratory tract. *Am J Respir Cell Mol Biol* 1999;**20**: 342–51.

8 Cross CE, van der Vliet A, Louie S, Thiele JJ, Halliwell B. Oxidative stress and antioxidants at biosurfaces: plants, skin, and respiratory tract surfaces. *Environ Health Perspect Suppl* 1998;**106**(Suppl 5):1241–51.

9 Gilbert DL. *Oxygen and Living Processes: An Interdisciplinary Approach.* New York: Springer-Verlag, 1982: 235–49.

10 Reynolds HY, Newball HH. Analysis of proteins and respiratory cells obtained from human lungs by bronchial lavage. *J Lab Clin Med* 1974;**84**:559–73.

11 Church DF, Pryor WA. Free-radical chemistry of cigarette smoke and its toxicological implications. *Environ Health Perspect* 1985;**64**:111–26.

12 Pryor WA, Stone K. Oxidants in cigarette smoke: radicals, hydrogen peroxide, peroxynitrate, and peroxynitrite. *Ann N Y Acad Sci* 1993;**686**:12–27.

13 Pauwels RA, Buist AS, Calverley PM, Jenkins CR, Hurd SS. Global strategy for the diagnosis, management, and prevention of chronic obstructive pulmonary disease. NHLBI/WHO Global Initiative for Chronic Obstructive Lung Disease (GOLD) Workshop summary. *Am J Respir Crit Care Med* 2001;**163**:1256–76.

14 Eidelman D, Saetta MP, Ghezzo H *et al.* Cellularity of the alveolar walls in smokers and its relation to alveolar destruction: functional implications. *Am Rev Respir Dis* 1990;**141**:1547–52.

15 Jeffery PK. Structural and inflammatory changes in COPD: a comparison with asthma. *Thorax* 1998;**53**:129–36.

16 Saetta M, Di Stefano A, Maestrelli P *et al.* Activated T-lymphocytes and macrophages in bronchial mucosa of subjects with chronic bronchitis. *Am Rev Respir Dis* 1993;**147**:301–6.

17 Hunninghake GW, Crystal RG. Cigarette smoking and lung destruction: accumulation of neutrophils in the lungs of cigarette smokers. *Am Rev Respir Dis* 1983;**128**:833–8.

18 Bosken CH, Hards J, Gatter K, Hogg JC. Characterization of the inflammatory reaction in the peripheral airways of cigarette smokers using immunocytochemistry. *Am Rev Respir Dis* 1992;**145**:911–7.

19 Rasp FL, Clawson CC, Hoidal JR, Repine JE. Reversible impairment of the adherence of alveolar macrophages from cigarette smokers. *Am Rev Respir Dis* 1978;**118**:979–86.

20 Costabel U, Guzman J. Effect of smoking on bronchoalveolar lavage constituents. *Eur Respir J* 1992;**5**:776–9.

21 Morrison D, Rahman I, Lannan S, MacNee W. Epithelial permeability, inflammation, and oxidant stress in the air spaces of smokers. *Am J Respir Crit Care Med* 1999;**159**:473–9.

22 Hoidal JR, Fox RB, LeMarbe PA, Perri R, Repine JE. Altered oxidative metabolic responses *in vitro* of alveolar macrophages from asymptomatic cigarette smokers. *Am Rev Respir Dis* 1981;**123**:85–9.

23 Nakashima H, Ando M, Sugimoto M *et al.* Receptor-mediated O_2-release by alveolar macrophages and peripheral blood monocytes from smokers and non-smokers: priming and triggering effects of monomeric IgG, concanavalin A, *N*-formyl-methionyl-leucyl-phenylalanine, phorbol myristate acetate, and cytochalasin D. *Am Rev Respir Dis* 1987;**136**:310–5.

24 Schaberg T, Haller H, Rau M *et al.* Superoxide anion release induced by platelet-activating factor is increased in human alveolar macrophages from smokers. *Eur Respir J* 1992;**5**:387–93.

25 Drath DB, Karnovsky ML, Huber GL. The effects of experimental exposure to tobacco smoke on the oxidative metabolism of alveolar macrophages. *J Reticuloendothel Soc* 1979;**25**:597–604.

26 Schaberg T, Klein U, Rau M, Eller J, Lode H. Subpopulations of alveolar macrophages in smokers and nonsmokers: relation to the expression of CD11/CD18 molecules and superoxide anion production. *Am J Respir Crit Care Med* 1995;**151**:1551–8.

27 Pinamonti S, Muzzoli M, Chicca MC *et al.* Xanthine oxidase activity in bronchoalveolar lavage fluid from patients with chronic obstructive pulmonary disease. *Free Radic Biol Med* 1996;**21**:147–55.

28 Halliwell B, Gutteridge JM. Role of free radicals and catalytic metal ions in human disease: an overview. *Methods Enzymol* 1990;**186**:1–85.

29 Pacht ER, Davis WB. Role of transferrin and ceruloplasmin in antioxidant activity of lung epithelial lining fluid. *J Appl Physiol* 1988;**64**:2092–9.

30 Thompson AB, Bohling T, Heires A, Linder J, Rennard SI. Lower respiratory tract iron burden is increased in association with cigarette smoking. *J Lab Clin Med* 1991;**117**:493–9.

31 Wesselius LJ, Nelson ME, Skikne BS. Increased release of ferritin and iron by iron-loaded alveolar macrophages in cigarette smokers. *Am J Respir Crit Care Med* 1994;**150**:690–5.

32 Mateos F, Brock JH, Perez-Arellano JL. Iron metabolism in the lower respiratory tract. *Thorax* 1998;**53**:594–600.

33 Halliwell B, Gutteridge JM, Cross CE. Free radicals, antioxidants, and human disease: where are we now? *J Lab Clin Med* 1992;**119**:598–620.

34 Rochelle LG, Fischer BM, Adler KB. Concurrent production of reactive oxygen and nitrogen species by airway epithelial cells *in vitro*. *Free Radic Biol Med* 1998;**24**:863–8.

35 Wallaert B, Gressier B, Marquette CH *et al.* Inactivation of α_1-proteinase inhibitor by alveolar inflammatory cells from smoking patients with or without emphysema. *Am Rev Respir Dis* 1993;**147**:1537–43.

36 Gutteridge JM. Lipid peroxidation and antioxidants as biomarkers of tissue damage. *Clin Chem* 1995;**41**:1819–28.

37 Kohen R, Nyska A. Oxidation of biological systems: oxidative stress phenomena, antioxidants, redox reactions, and methods for their quantification. *Toxicol Pathol* 2002;**30**:620–50.

38 Berry EM, Kohen R. Is the biological antioxidant system integrated and regulated? *Med Hypotheses* 1999;**53**:397–401.

39 Griffiths HR, Moller L, Bartosz G *et al.* Biomarkers. *Mol Aspects Med* 2002;**23**:101–208.

40 Wang XL, Rainwater DL, VandeBerg JF, Mitchell BD, Mahaney MC. Genetic contributions to plasma total antioxidant activity. *Arterioscler Thromb Vasc Biol* 2001;**21**:1190–5.

41 Nowak D, Kasielski M, Pietras T, Bialasiewicz P, Antczak A. Cigarette smoking does not increase hydrogen peroxide levels in expired breath condensate of patients with stable COPD. *Monaldi Arch Chest Dis* 1998;**53**:268–73.

42 Nowak D, Antczak A, Krol M *et al.* Increased content of hydrogen peroxide in the expired breath of cigarette smokers. *Eur Respir J* 1996;**9**:652–7.

43 Hill AT, Bayley D, Stockley RA. The interrelationship of sputum inflammatory markers in patients with chronic bronchitis. *Am J Respir Crit Care Med* 1999;**160**:893–8.

44 Dekhuijzen PN, Aben KK, Dekker I *et al.* Increased exhalation of hydrogen peroxide in patients with stable and unstable chronic obstructive pulmonary disease. *Am J Respir Crit Care Med* 1996;**154**:813–6.

45 Maziak W, Loukides S, Culpitt S *et al.* Exhaled nitric oxide in chronic obstructive pulmonary disease. *Am J Respir Crit Care Med* 1998;**157**:998–1002.

46 Corradi M, Majori M, Cacciani GC *et al.* Increased exhaled nitric oxide in patients with stable chronic obstructive pulmonary disease. *Thorax* 1999;**54**:572–5.

47 Rutgers SR, van der Mark TW, Coers W *et al.* Markers of nitric oxide metabolism in sputum and exhaled air are not increased in chronic obstructive pulmonary disease. *Thorax* 1999;**54**:576–80.

48 Kharitonov SA, Barnes PJ. Nitric oxide, nitrotyrosine, and nitric oxide modulators in asthma and chronic obstructive pulmonary disease. *Curr Allergy Asthma Rep* 2003;**3**:121–9.

49 Robbins RA, Millatmal T, Lassi K, Rennard S, Daughton D. Smoking cessation is associated with an increase in exhaled nitric oxide. *Chest* 1997;**112**:313–8.

50 Anonymous. Recommendations for standardized procedures for the online and offline measurement of exhaled lower respiratory nitric oxide and nasal nitric oxide in adults and children, 1999. This offical statement of the American Thoracic Society was adopted by the ATS Board of Directors, July 1999. *Am J Respir Crit Care Med* 1999;**160**:2104–17.

51 Ludwig PW, Schwartz BA, Hoidal JR, Niewoehner DE. Cigarette smoking causes accumulation of polymorphonuclear leukocytes in alveolar septum. *Am Rev Respir Dis* 1985;**131**:828–30.

52 Fiorini G, Crespi S, Rinaldi M *et al.* Serum ECP and MPO are increased during exacerbations of chronic bronchitis with airway obstruction. *Biomed Pharmacother* 2000;**54**:274–8.

53 Fryksmark U. Myeloperoxidase activity in smokers: an

additional factor in the development of pulmonary emphysema. *Eur J Respir Dis* 1985;**67**:81–3.

54 Pesci A, Balbi B, Majori M *et al.* Inflammatory cells and mediators in bronchial lavage of patients with chronic obstructive pulmonary disease. *Eur Respir J* 1998;**12**:380–6.

55 Rahman I, Skwarska E, MacNee W. Attenuation of oxidant/antioxidant imbalance during treatment of exacerbations of chronic obstructive pulmonary disease. *Thorax* 1997;**52**:565–8.

56 Noguera A, Busquets X, Sauleda J *et al.* Expression of adhesion molecules and G proteins in circulating neutrophils in chronic obstructive pulmonary disease. *Am J Respir Crit Care Med* 1998;**158**:1664–8.

57 Slebos DJ, Ryter SW, Choi AM. Heme oxygenase-1 and carbon monoxide in pulmonary medicine. *Respir Res* 2003;**4**:7.

58 Montuschi P, Kharitonov SA, Barnes PJ. Exhaled carbon monoxide and nitric oxide in COPD. *Chest* 2001;**120**:496–501.

59 Morrison D, Lannan S, Langridge A, Rahman I, MacNee W. Effect of acute cigarette smoking on epithelial permeability, inflammation and oxidant status in the airspaces of chronic smokers. *Thorax* 1994;**49**:1077.

60 Cantin AM, North SL, Hubbard RC, Crystal RG. Normal alveolar epithelial lining fluid contains high levels of glutathione. *J Appl Physiol* 1987;**63**:152–7.

61 Linden M, Hakansson L, Ohlsson K *et al.* Glutathione in bronchoalveolar lavage fluid from smokers is related to humoral markers of inflammatory cell activity. *Inflammation* 1989;**13**:651–8.

62 Li XY, Donaldson K, Rahman I, MacNee W. An investigation of the role of glutathione in increased epithelial permeability induced by cigarette smoke *in vivo* and *in vitro*. *Am J Respir Crit Care Med* 1994;**149**:1518–25.

63 Rahman I, Li XY, Donaldson K, Harrison DJ, MacNee W. Glutathione homeostasis in alveolar epithelial cells *in vitro* and lung *in vivo* under oxidative stress. *Am J Physiol* 1995;**269**:L285–92.

64 Rahman I, Li XY, Donaldson K, MacNee W. Cigarette smoke, glutathione metabolism and epithelial permeability in rat lungs. *Biochem Soc Trans* 1995;**23**:235S.

65 Bui MH, Sauty A, Collet F, Leuenberger P. Dietary vitamin C intake and concentrations in the body fluids and cells of male smokers and non-smokers. *J Nutr* 1992;**122**:312–6.

66 McCusker K, Hoidal J. Selective increase of antioxidant enzyme activity in the alveolar macrophages from cigarette smokers and smoke-exposed hamsters. *Am Rev Respir Dis* 1990;**141**:678–82.

67 Kondo T, Tagami S, Yoshioka A, Nishimura M, Kawakami Y. Current smoking of elderly men reduces antioxidants in alveolar macrophages. *Am J Respir Crit Care Med* 1994;**149**:178–82.

68 Paredi P, Kharitonov SA, Leak D *et al.* Exhaled ethane, a marker of lipid peroxidation, is elevated in chronic obstructive pulmonary disease. *Am J Respir Crit Care Med* 2000;**162**:369–73.

69 Morrow JD, Hill KE, Burk RF *et al.* A series of prostaglandin F2-like compounds are produced *in vivo* in humans by a non-cyclooxygenase, free radical-catalyzed mechanism. *Proc Natl Acad Sci U S A* 1990;**87**:9383–7.

70 Liu T, Stern A, Roberts LJ, Morrow JD. The isoprostanes: novel prostaglandin-like products of the free radical-catalyzed peroxidation of arachidonic acid. *J Biomed Sci* 1999;**6**:226–35.

71 Janssen LJ. Isoprostanes: an overview and putative roles in pulmonary pathophysiology. *Am J Physiol* 2001;**280**:L1067–82.

72 Fukunaga M, Makita N, Roberts LJ *et al.* Evidence for the existence of F2-isoprostane receptors on rat vascular smooth muscle cells. *Am J Physiol* 1993;**264**:C1619–24.

73 Fukunaga M, Yura T, Grygorczyk R, Badr KF. Evidence for the distinct nature of F2-isoprostane receptors from those of thromboxane A$_2$. *Am J Physiol* 1997;**272**:F477–83.

74 Fukunaga M, Takahashi K, Badr KF. Vascular smooth muscle actions and receptor interactions of 8-isoprostaglandin E2, an E2-isoprostane. *Biochem Biophys Res Commun* 1993;**195**:507–15.

75 Zahler S, Becker BF. Indirect enhancement of neutrophil activity and adhesion to cultured human umbilical vein endothelial cells by isoprostanes (iPF2α-III and iPE2-III). *Prostaglandins Other Lipid Mediat* 1999;**57**:319–31.

76 Montuschi P, Collins JV, Ciabattoni G *et al.* Exhaled 8-isoprostane as an *in vivo* biomarker of lung oxidative stress in patients with COPD and healthy smokers. *Am J Respir Crit Care Med* 2000;**162**:1175–7.

77 Kostikas K, Papatheodorou G, Psathakis K, Panagou P, Loukides S. Oxidative stress in expired breath condensate of patients with COPD. *Chest* 2003;**124**:1373–80.

78 Frangulyan R, Anderson D, Drost E, Hill A, MacNee W. Exhaled markers of inflammation in breath condensate in patients with bronchiectasis and COPD. *Thorax* 2003;**58**(Suppl 3):S116.

79 Biernacki WA, Kharitonov SA, Barnes PJ. Increased leukotriene B$_4$ and 8-isoprostane in exhaled breath condensate of patients with exacerbations of COPD. *Thorax* 2003;**58**:294–8.

80 Fahn HJ, Wang LS, Kao SH *et al.* Smoking-associated mitochondrial DNA mutations and lipid peroxidation in human lung tissues. *Am J Respir Cell Mol Biol* 1998;**19**:901–9.

81 Leonarduzzi G, Arkan MC, Basaga H *et al.* Lipid oxidation products in cell signaling. *Free Radic Biol Med* 2000;**28**:1370–8.

82 Rahman I, van Schadewijk AA, Crowther AJ *et al.* 4-Hydroxy-2-nonenal, a specific lipid peroxidation product, is elevated in lungs of patients with chronic obstructive pulmonary disease. *Am J Respir Crit Care Med* 2002;**166**:490–5.

83 Rahman I, Morrison D, Donaldson K, MacNee W. Systemic oxidative stress in asthma, COPD, and smokers. *Am J Respir Crit Care Med* 1996;**154**:1055–60.

84 Agusti AG. Systemic effects of chronic obstructive pulmonary disease. *Novartis Found Symp* 2001;**234**:242–9.

85 Schols AM, Slangen J, Volovics L, Wouters EF. Weight loss is a reversible factor in the prognosis of chronic obstructive pulmonary disease. *Am J Respir Crit Care Med* 1998;**157**:1791–7.

86 Duthie GG, Arthur JR, James WP. Effects of smoking and vitamin E on blood antioxidant status. *Am J Clin Nutr* 1991;**53**:1061S–3S.

87 Morrow JD, Frei B, Longmire AW *et al.* Increase in circulating products of lipid peroxidation (F2-isoprostanes) in smokers: smoking as a cause of oxidative damage. *N Engl J Med* 1995;**332**:1198–203.

88 van der Vliet A, Smith D, O'Neill CA *et al.* Interactions of peroxynitrite with human plasma and its constituents: oxidative damage and antioxidant depletion. *Biochem J* 1994;**303**:295–301.

89 Petruzzelli S, Puntoni R, Mimotti P *et al.* Plasma 3-nitrotyrosine in cigarette smokers. *Am J Respir Crit Care Med* 1997;**156**:1902–7.

90 Cantin A, Crystal RG. Oxidants, antioxidants and the pathogenesis of emphysema. *Eur J Respir Dis Suppl* 1985;**139**:7–17.

91 Laurent P, Janoff A, Kagan HM. Cigarette smoke blocks cross-linking of elastin *in vitro*. *Am Rev Respir Dis* 1983;**127**:189–92.

92 Jones JG, Minty BD, Lawler P *et al.* Increased alveolar epithelial permeability in cigarette smokers. *Lancet* 1980;**1**:66–8.

93 Lannan S, Donaldson K, Brown D, MacNee W. Effect of cigarette smoke and its condensates on alveolar epithelial cell injury *in vitro*. *Am J Physiol* 1994;**266**:L92–100.

94 Li XY, Rahman I, Donaldson K, MacNee W. Mechanisms of cigarette smoke induced increased airspace permeability. *Thorax* 1996;**51**:465–71.

95 Li XY, Donaldson K, Brown D, MacNee W. The role of tumor necrosis factor in increased airspace epithelial permeability in acute lung inflammation. *Am J Respir Cell Mol Biol* 1995;**13**:185–95.

96 Rossi AG, Haslett C. Inflammation, cell injury and apoptosis. In: Said SI, ed. *Lung Biology in Health and Disease: Proinflammatory and Antiinflammatory Peptides*. New York: Marcel Dekker, 1998.

97 Nakajima Y, Aoshiba K, Yasui S, Nagai A. H_2O_2 induces apoptosis in bovine tracheal epithelial cells *in vitro*. *Life Sci* 1999;**64**:2489–96.

98 Aoshiba K, Yasui S, Nagai A. Apoptosis of alveolar macrophages by cigarette smoke. *Chest* 2000;**117**(Suppl 1):320S.

99 Wickenden JA, Clarke MC, Rossi AG *et al.* Cigarette smoke prevents apoptosis through inhibition of caspase activation and induces necrosis. *Am J Respir Cell Mol Biol* 2003;**29**:562–70.

100 Kasahara Y, Tuder RM, Cool CD *et al.* Endothelial cell death and decreased expression of vascular endothelial growth factor and vascular endothelial growth factor receptor 2 in emphysema. *Am J Respir Crit Care Med* 2001;**163**:737–44.

101 Kasahara Y, Tuder RM, Taraseviciene-Stewart L *et al.* Inhibition of VEGF receptors causes lung cell apoptosis and emphysema. *J Clin Invest* 2000;**106**:1311–9.

102 Tuder RM, Zhen L, Cho CY *et al.* Oxidative stress and apoptosis interact and cause emphysema due to vascular endothelial growth factor receptor blockade. *Am J Respir Cell Mol Biol* 2003;**29**:88–97.

103 Gadek JE, Fells GA, Crystal RG. Cigarette smoking induces functional antiprotease deficiency in the lower respiratory tract of humans. *Science* 1979;**206**:1315–6.

104 Carp H, Janoff A. Inactivation of bronchial mucous proteinase inhibitor by cigarette smoke and phagocyte-derived oxidants. *Exp Lung Res* 1980;**1**:225–37.

105 Hubbard RC, Ogushi F, Fells GA *et al.* Oxidants spontaneously released by alveolar macrophages of cigarette smokers can inactivate the active site of α_1-antitrypsin, rendering it ineffective as an inhibitor of neutrophil elastase. *J Clin Invest* 1987;**80**:1289–95.

106 Carp H, Miller F, Hoidal JR, Janoff A. Potential mechanism of emphysema: α_1-proteinase inhibitor recovered from lungs of cigarette smokers contains oxidized methionine and has decreased elastase inhibitory capacity. *Proc Natl Acad Sci U S A* 1982;**79**:2041–5.

107 Johnson D, Travis J. The oxidative inactivation of human α_1-proteinase inhibitor: further evidence for methionine at the reactive center. *J Biol Chem* 1979;**254**:4022–6.

108 Carp H, Janoff A. Possible mechanisms of emphysema in smokers: *in vitro* suppression of serum elastase-inhibitory capacity by fresh cigarette smoke and its prevention by antioxidants. *Am Rev Respir Dis* 1978;**118**:617–21.

109 Stone PJ, Calore JD, McGowan SE *et al.* Functional α_1-protease inhibitor in the lower respiratory tract of cigarette smokers is not decreased. *Science* 1983;**221**:1187–9.

110 Boudier C, Pelletier A, Pauli G, Bieth JG. The functional activity of α_1-proteinase inhibitor in bronchoalveolar lavage fluids from healthy human smokers and non-smokers. *Clin Chim Acta* 1983;**132**:309–15.

111 Abboud RT, Fera T, Richter A, Tabona MZ, Johal S. Acute effect of smoking on the functional activity of α_1-protease inhibitor in bronchoalveolar lavage fluid. *Am Rev Respir Dis* 1985;**131**:79–85.

112 Selby C, Drost E, Wraith PK, MacNee W. *In vivo* neutrophil sequestration within lungs of humans is determined by *in vitro* 'filterability'. *J Appl Physiol* 1991;**71**:1996–2003.

113 Selby C, Drost E, Lannan S, Wraith PK, MacNee W. Neutrophil retention in the lungs of patients with chronic obstructive pulmonary disease. *Am Rev Respir Dis* 1991;**143**:1359–64.

114 MacNee W, Wiggs B, Belzberg AS, Hogg JC. The effect of cigarette smoking on neutrophil kinetics in human lungs. *N Engl J Med* 1989;**321**:924–8.

115 Drost EM, Selby C, Lannan S, Lowe GD, MacNee W. Changes in neutrophil deformability following *in vitro* smoke exposure: mechanism and protection. *Am J Respir Cell Mol Biol* 1992;**6**:287–95.

116 Drost EM, Selby C, Bridgeman MM, MacNee W. Decreased leukocyte deformability after acute cigarette smoking in humans. *Am Rev Respir Dis* 1993;**148**:1277–83.

117 Terashima T, Klut ME, English D *et al.* Cigarette smoking causes sequestration of polymorphonuclear leukocytes released from the bone marrow in lung microvessels. *Am J Respir Cell Mol Biol* 1999;**20**:171–7.

118 Lehr HA, Kress E, Menger MD *et al.* Cigarette smoke elicits leukocyte adhesion to endothelium in hamsters: inhibition by CuZn-SOD. *Free Radic Biol Med* 1993;**14**:573–81.

119 Klut ME, Doerschuk CM, van Eeden SF, Burns AR, Hogg JC.

Activation of neutrophils within pulmonary microvessels of rabbits exposed to cigarette smoke. *Am J Respir Cell Mol Biol* 1993;**9**:82–9.

120 Bosken CH, Doerschuk CM, English D, Hogg JC. Neutrophil kinetics during active cigarette smoking in rabbits. *J Appl Physiol* 1991;**71**:630–7.

121 Brumwell ML, MacNee W, Doerschuk CM, Wiggs B, Hogg JC. Neutrophil kinetics in normal and emphysematous regions of human lungs. *Ann N Y Acad Sci* 1991;**624**:30–9.

122 Takeyama K, Jung B, Shim JJ et al. Activation of epidermal growth factor receptors is responsible for mucin synthesis induced by cigarette smoke. *Am J Physiol Lung Cell Mol Physiol* 2001;**280**:L165–72.

123 Rabinovich RA, Ardite E, Troosters T et al. Reduced muscle redox capacity after endurance training in patients with chronic obstructive pulmonary disease. *Am J Respir Crit Care Med* 2001;**164**:1114–8.

124 Sauleda J, Garcia-Palmer FJ, Gonzalez G, Palou A, Agusti AG. The activity of cytochrome oxidase is increased in circulating lymphocytes of patients with chronic obstructive pulmonary disease, asthma, and chronic arthritis. *Am J Respir Crit Care Med* 2000;**161**:32–5.

125 Engelen MP, Schols AM, Does JD, Deutz NE, Wouters EF. Altered glutamate metabolism is associated with reduced muscle glutathione levels in patients with emphysema. *Am J Respir Crit Care Med* 2000;**161**:98–103.

126 Heunks LM, Dekhuijzen PN. Respiratory muscle function and free radicals: from cell to COPD. *Thorax* 2000;**55**:704–16.

127 Keatings VM, Collins PD, Scott DM, Barnes PJ. Differences in interleukin-8 and tumor necrosis factor-α in induced sputum from patients with chronic obstructive pulmonary disease or asthma. *Am J Respir Crit Care Med* 1996;**153**:530–4.

128 Rahman I, MacNee W. Role of transcription factors in inflammatory lung diseases. *Thorax* 1998;**53**:601–12.

129 Parmentier M, Hirani N, Rahman I et al. Regulation of lipopolysaccharide-mediated interleukin-1β release by *N*-acetylcysteine in THP-1 cells. *Eur Respir J* 2000;**16**:933–9.

130 Antonicelli F, Parmentier M, Drost EM et al. Nacystelyn inhibits oxidant-mediated interleukin-8 expression and NF-κB nuclear binding in alveolar epithelial cells. *Free Radic Biol Med* 2002;**32**:492–502.

131 Jimenez LA, Thompson J, Brown DA et al. Activation of NF-κB by PM(10) occurs via an iron-mediated mechanism in the absence of IκB degradation. *Toxicol Appl Pharmacol* 2000;**166**:101–10.

132 Galter D, Mihm S, Droge W. Distinct effects of glutathione disulphide on the nuclear transcription factor κB and the activator protein-1. *Eur J Biochem* 1994;**221**:639–48.

133 Ginn-Pease ME, Whisler RL. Optimal NF-κB mediated transcriptional responses in Jurkat T cells exposed to oxidative stress are dependent on intracellular glutathione and costimulatory signals. *Biochem Biophys Res Commun* 1996;**226**:695–702.

134 Cho S, Urata Y, Iida T et al. Glutathione downregulates the phosphorylation of IκB: autoloop regulation of the NF-κB-mediated expression of NF-κB subunits by TNF-α in mouse vascular endothelial cells. *Biochem Biophys Res Commun* 1998;**253**:104–8.

135 Janssen-Heininger YM, Macara I, Mossman BT. Co-operativity between oxidants and tumor necrosis factor in the activation of nuclear factor (NF)-κB: requirement of Ras/mitogen-activated protein kinases in the activation of NF-κB by oxidants. *Am J Respir Cell Mol Biol* 1999;**20**:942–52.

136 Gilmour PS, Rahman I, Donaldson K, MacNee W. Histone acetylation regulates epithelial IL-8 release mediated by oxidative stress from environmental particles. *Am J Physiol Lung Cell Mol Physiol* 2003;**284**:L533–40.

137 Ito K, Lim S, Caramori G et al. Cigarette smoking reduces histone deacetylase 2 expression, enhances cytokine expression, and inhibits glucocorticoid actions in alveolar macrophages. *FASEB J* 2001;**15**:1110–2.

138 Marwick JA, Kirkham P, Gilmour PS et al. Cigarette smoke-induced oxidative stress and TGF-β1 increase p21waf1/cip1 expression in alveolar epithelial cells. *Ann N Y Acad Sci* 2002;**973**:278–83.

139 Chan-Yeung M, Dybuncio A. Leucocyte count, smoking and lung function. *Am J Med* 1984;**76**:31–7.

140 Chan-Yeung M, Abboud R, Buncio AD, Vedal S. Peripheral leucocyte count and longitudinal decline in lung function. *Thorax* 1988;**43**:462–6.

141 Richards GA, Theron AJ, Van der Merwe CA, Anderson R. Spirometric abnormalities in young smokers correlate with increased chemiluminescence responses of activated blood phagocytes. *Am Rev Respir Dis* 1989;**139**:181–7.

142 Stanescu D, Sanna A, Veriter C et al. Airways obstruction, chronic expectoration, and rapid decline of FEV_1 in smokers are associated with increased levels of sputum neutrophils. *Thorax* 1996;**51**:267–71.

143 Schunemann HJ, Muti P, Freudenheim JL et al. Oxidative stress and lung function. *Am J Epidemiol* 1997;**146**:939–48.

144 Rahman I, Swarska E, Henry M, Stolk J, MacNee W. Is there any relationship between plasma antioxidant capacity and lung function in smokers and in patients with chronic obstructive pulmonary disease? *Thorax* 2000;**55**:189–93.

145 Britton JR, Pavord ID, Richards KA et al. Dietary antioxidant vitamin intake and lung function in the general population. *Am J Respir Crit Care Med* 1995;**151**:1383–7.

146 Grievink L, Smit HA, Ocke MC, van't Veer P, Kromhout D. Dietary intake of antioxidant (pro)-vitamins, respiratory symptoms and pulmonary function: the MORGEN study. *Thorax* 1998;**53**:166–71.

147 Shahar E, Boland LL, Folsom AR et al. Docosahexaenoic acid and smoking-related chronic obstructive pulmonary disease. The Atherosclerosis Risk in Communities Study Investigators. *Am J Respir Crit Care Med* 1999;**159**:1780–5.

148 Shahar E, Folsom AR, Melnick SL et al. Dietary n-3 polyunsaturated fatty acids and smoking-related chronic obstructive pulmonary disease. Atherosclerosis Risk in Communities Study Investigators. *N Engl J Med* 1994;**331**:228–33.

149 Silverman EK, Speizer FE. Risk factors for the development of chronic obstructive pulmonary disease. *Med Clin North Am* 1996;**80**:501–22.

150 Sandford AJ, Weir TD, Pare PD. Genetic risk factors for chronic obstructive pulmonary disease. *Eur Respir J* 1997;**10**:1380–91.

151 Barnes PJ. Genetics and pulmonary medicine. 9. Molecular genetics of chronic obstructive pulmonary disease. *Thorax* 1999;**54**:245–52.

152 Huang SL, Su CH, Chang SC. Tumor necrosis factor-α gene polymorphism in chronic bronchitis. *Am J Respir Crit Care Med* 1997;**156**:1436–9.

153 Smith CA, Harrison DJ. Association between polymorphism in gene for microsomal epoxide hydrolase and susceptibility to emphysema. *Lancet* 1997;**350**:630–3.

154 Yim JJ, Park GY, Lee CT *et al.* Genetic susceptibility to chronic obstructive pulmonary disease in Koreans: combined analysis of polymorphic genotypes for microsomal epoxide hydrolase and glutathione S-transferase M1 and T1. *Thorax* 2000;**55**:121–5.

155 Yamada N, Yamaya M, Okinaga S *et al.* Microsatellite polymorphism in the heme oxygenase-1 gene promoter is associated with susceptibility to emphysema. *Am J Hum Genet* 2000;**66**:187–95.

156 He JQ, Ruan J, Connett JE *et al.* Antioxidant gene polymorphisms and susceptibility to a rapid decline in lung function in smokers. *Am J Respir Crit Care Med* 2002;**166**:323–8.

157 Sandford AJ, Chagani T, Weir TD *et al.* Susceptibility genes for rapid decline of lung function in the lung health study. *Am J Respir Crit Care Med* 2001;**163**:469–73.

158 Baranova H, Perriot J, Albuisson E *et al.* Peculiarities of the GSTM1 0/0 genotype in French heavy smokers with various types of chronic bronchitis. *Hum Genet* 1997;**99**:822–6.

159 Harrison DJ, Cantlay AM, Rae F, Lamb D, Smith CA. Frequency of glutathione S-transferase M1 deletion in smokers with emphysema and lung cancer. *Hum Exp Toxicol* 1997;**16**:356–60.

160 Gilliland FD, Gauderman WJ, Vora H, Rappaport E, Dubeau L. Effects of glutathione-S-transferase M1, T1, and P1 on childhood lung function growth. *Am J Respir Crit Care Med* 2002;**166**:710–6.

161 Ishii T, Matsuse T, Teramoto S *et al.* Glutathione S-transferase P1 (GSTP1) polymorphism in patients with chronic obstructive pulmonary disease. *Thorax* 1999;**54**:693–6.

162 Yim JJ, Yoo CG, Lee CT *et al.* Lack of association between glutathione S-transferase P1 polymorphism and COPD in Koreans. *Lung* 2002;**180**:119–25.

163 Cantlay AM, Lamb D, Gillooly M *et al.* Association between the CYP1A1 gene polymorphism and susceptibility to emphysema and lung cancer. *J Clin Pathol Mol Pathol* 1995;**48**:M210–4.

164 Compton CH, Gubb J, Cedar E *et al.* SB 207499, a second generation oral PDE4 inhibitor, first demonstration of efficacy in patients with COPD. *Eur Respir J* 1999;**14**:281S.

165 Torphy TJ. Phosphodiesterase isozymes: molecular targets for novel antiasthma agents. *Am J Respir Crit Care Med* 1998;**157**:351–70.

166 Drost E, Ouziaux L, Donaldson K, MacNee W. Cilomilast, a second generation phosphodiesterase 4 inhibitor, in combination with PGE2 attenuates fMLP, IL-8 and cigarette smoke-induced effects on the mechanical and functional properties of neutrophils. *Eur Respir J* 2001;**18**(Suppl 33): 161S.

167 Chabrier PE, Auguet M, Spinnewyn B *et al.* BN 80933, a dual inhibitor of neuronal nitric oxide synthase and lipid peroxidation: a promising neuroprotective strategy. *Proc Natl Acad Sci U S A* 1999;**96**:10824–9.

168 Nishikawa M, Kakemizu N, Ito T *et al.* Superoxide mediates cigarette smoke-induced infiltration of neutrophils into the airways through nuclear factor-κB activation and IL-8 mRNA expression in guinea pigs *in vivo. Am J Respir Cell Mol Biol* 1999;**20**:189–98.

169 Steinberg FM, Chait A. Antioxidant vitamin supplementation and lipid peroxidation in smokers. *Am J Clin Nutr* 1998;**68**:319–27.

170 MacNee W, Bridgeman MM, Marsden M *et al.* The effects of *N*-acetylcysteine and glutathione on smoke-induced changes in lung phagocytes and epithelial cells. *Am J Med* 1991;**91**:60S–6S.

171 Ross D, Norbeck K, Moldeus P. The generation and subsequent fate of glutathionyl radicals in biological systems. *J Biol Chem* 1985;**260**:15028–32.

172 Marrades RM, Roca J, Barbera JA *et al.* Nebulized glutathione induces bronchoconstriction in patients with mild asthma. *Am J Respir Crit Care Med* 1997;**156**:425–30.

173 Meister A, Anderson ME. Glutathione. *Annu Rev Biochem* 1983;**52**:711–60.

174 Bridgeman MM, Marsden M, Selby C, Morrison D, MacNee W. Effect of *N*-acetyl cysteine on the concentrations of thiols in plasma, bronchoalveolar lavage fluid, and lung tissue. *Thorax* 1994;**49**:670–5.

175 Bridgeman MM, Marsden M, MacNee W, Flenley DC, Ryle AP. Cysteine and glutathione concentrations in plasma and bronchoalveolar lavage fluid after treatment with *N*-acetylcysteine. *Thorax* 1991;**46**:39–42.

176 Boman G, Backer U, Larsson S, Melander B, Wahlander L. Oral acetylcysteine reduces exacerbation rate in chronic bronchitis: report of a trial organized by the Swedish Society for Pulmonary Diseases. *Eur J Respir Dis* 1983;**64**:405–15.

177 Rasmussen JB, Glennow C. Reduction in days of illness after long-term treatment with *N*-acetylcysteine controlled-release tablets in patients with chronic bronchitis. *Eur Respir J* 1988;**1**:351–5.

178 British Thoracic Society Research Committee. Oral *N*-acetylcysteine and exacerbation rates in patients with chronic bronchitis and severe airways obstruction. *Thorax* 1985;**40**:832–5.

179 Decramer M, Dekhuijzen PN, Troosters T *et al.* The Bronchitis Randomized On NAC Cost-Utility Study (BRONCUS): hypothesis and design. BRONCUS-trial Committee. *Eur Respir J* 2001;**17**:329–36.

180 Gillissen A, Jaworska M, Orth M *et al.* Nacystelyn, a novel lysine salt of *N*-acetylcysteine, to augment cellular antioxidant defence *in vitro. Respir Med* 1997;**91**:159–68.

181 Nagy AM, Vanderbist F, Parij N *et al.* Effect of the mucoactive drug nacystelyn on the respiratory burst of human blood polymorphonuclear neutrophils. *Pulm Pharmacol Ther* 1997;**10**:287–92.

182 Manna SK, Kuo MT, Aggarwal BB. Overexpression of gamma-glutamylcysteine synthetase suppresses tumor necrosis factor-induced apoptosis and activation of nuclear transcription factor-κB and activator protein-1. *Oncogene* 1999;**18**:4371–82.

CHAPTER 33
Cigarette smoke-induced disease

Stephen I. Rennard and Lisa M. Hepp

Cigarette smoking is the major cause of preventable mortality in the developed world, contributing to death from cardiac disease, stroke, pulmonary and extrapulmonary malignancy and chronic obstructive pulmonary disease (COPD) as well as other causes (Table 33.1) [1]. In addition, cigarette smoking contributes to a large number of other disorders that result in significant morbidity (see Table 33.1). Because cigarette smoking is the most important risk factor for the development of COPD, many smokers with COPD suffer from these allied conditions as comorbidities.

The mechanisms by which cigarette smoke causes disease are not fully delineated. It is likely, however, that overlapping mechanisms contribute to the multiple pathologies caused by cigarette smoking. Thus, for example, smokers with COPD are at increased risk for cardiac disease [2] and lung cancer [3] compared with similar smokers without COPD. This suggests a mechanistic connection among these conditions. The current chapter provides an overview of current thinking relating to the mechanisms by which cigarette smoke causes disease.

Cigarette smoke toxins

Several factors contribute to the complex mixture of chemicals present in cigarette smoke including the starting materials, the complex chemistry that results from the burning and heating of the cigarette and the individual way in which each cigarette is smoked [4]. A cigarette contains a blend of tobaccos that are wrapped in a paper. 'American blend' cigarettes include a mixture of burley, flue cured and oriental tobaccos, the composition of which depends on both their source and their processing. In addition, a variety of additives are included that influence the taste, aroma and potentially the delivery of nicotine [5]. When the cigarette is lit, the tip burns at a temperature of approximately 800°C. When air is inhaled through the cigarette the temperature increases by an additional 100–120°C. As the heated air, mixed with the combustion products, is inhaled over the unburned tobacco, it rapidly cools, causing the nicotine and many other substances in the unburned tobacco to volatilize. These substances subsequently condense forming the smoke, which is an aerosol of liquid particles. One millilitre of fresh mainstream smoke contains approximately 4×10^9 particles with a mean diameter of approximately 0.2 µmol [6,7]. For analytical purposes, the components of smoke are divided into the 'particulate phase', which can be retained on a glass fibre filter, and the 'vapour phase', which is not. In general, approximately 90% of the mass of smoke is contained in the vapour phase [8].

The smoke breathed in during active smoking is mainstream smoke. The smoke that is produced by the burning of the cigarette that occurs between puffs is sidestream smoke. The constituents of sidestream smoke are generally similar to that of mainstream smoke, but the relative amounts can differ substantially. Environmental tobacco smoke (ETS) is a mixture of sidestream smoke and the components of mainstream smoke that are exhaled. The composition of ETS will be further modified as the components of smoke age and as they react with other components in the ambient air.

The particles present in mainstream smoke change in size and composition. Coagulation occurs as a function of density and time, resulting in a three- to fourfold increase in diameter over 2 s [4]. In addition, smoke particles can absorb water, resulting in a rapid twofold expansion in size in a completely humid environment. Even with these size increases, however, smoke particles are of the range likely to reach and be deposited in the alveoli [9]. The fraction of the various smoke constituents that is absorbed varies with their chemistry. For example, nicotine, which in the free base form is highly lipophilic, is essentially completely absorbed, while approximately 30% of inhaled solanesol may be exhaled [10].

Table 33.1 Diseases associated with cigarette smoking.

Lung disease
COPD
Emphysema
Chronic bronchitis
Asthma

Other lung diseases
Idiopathic pulmonary fibrosis
Histiocytosis X
Respiratory bronchiolitis
Goodpasture's syndrome
Sleep apnoea
Pneumothorax

Cardiovascular
Atherosclerotic vascular disease
Coronary artery disease
Carotid vascular disease
Mesenteric, renal, iliac
Abdominal aortic aneurysm

Peripheral vascular disease
Thromboangiitis obliterans (Berger's)
Deep venous thrombosis
Pulmonary embolus

Cardiac disease
Angina pectoris
Coronary artery spasm
Arrhythmia

Malignancy
Respiratory tract
Lung cancer
   squamous cell
   adenocarcinoma
   large cell
   small cell
Laryngeal cancer
Oral cancer

Other tissues
Oesophagus
Pancreas
Bladder
Uterine cervix
Kidney
Anus
Penis
Stomach
Liver
Leukaemia

Gastrointestinal disease
Peptic ulcer disease
Gastric
Duodenal

Gastro-oesophageal reflux

Chronic pancreatitis

Crohn's disease

Colonic adenomas

Dermatological disease
Skin wrinkling
Psoriasis

Reproductive disease
Ovarian failure
Pregnancy related
Prematurity
Premature rupture of membranes
Spontaneous abortion

Decreased sperm quality

Fetal effects
Low birthweight
Impaired lung growth
Sudden infant death syndrome

Febrile seizures
Reduced intelligence
Behavioural disorders
Atopic disease/asthma

Effects on children of parental smoking
Asthma
Rhinitis
Otitis
Pneumonia
Increased risk to smoke

Rheumatological disease
Osteoporosis
Rheumatoid arthritis

Psychiatric
Depression
Schizophrenia

Oral disease
Periodontal disease
Loss of taste

Loss of olfaction

Infectious disease
Tuberculosis
Pneumococcal infection
Meningococcal infection

Endocrine disease
Altered hormonal secretion
Graves' disease
Antidiuresis
Goiter

Renal
Glomerulonephritis

Benign prostatic hypertrophy

Cataracts

Smoke contains an estimated 4000–6000 chemical moieties in a large number of chemical classes (Table 33.2). The precise number is difficult to determine, as many of the most reactive, and potentially most toxic, components of cigarette smoke are very short lived. These compounds may be extracted from the unburned tobacco, as nicotine is, or may be generated from the burning of the tobacco, or from reactions that occur in the complex chemical milieu of the hot and cooling smoke. For example, nitric oxide is present in smoke, but quickly reacts to form nitrogen dioxide. These oxides can then react with methanol to form methyl-nitrite, which could be absorbed by a smoker, although it is not a component of 'fresh' mainstream smoke [4].

The compounds present in smoke depend on a large number of factors [11]. The puff volume and intensity [12], which will affect the temperature, the tobacco composition [13], the presence of additives [5] and the deposition of compounds that condense in the unburned tobacco from portions of the cigarette that are previously burned, can all contribute [4]. In addition, many cigarettes, particularly light and ultralight cigarettes, contain a filter with air vents. These air vents, if unblocked, will dilute the smoke stream with air. Partially blocking the vents, which a smoker can easily do by holding the cigarette by the filter, changes the mix and also the yield of compounds [14]. Several standard machine-based smoking methods have been developed to

Table 33.2 Classes of compounds present in fresh tobacco smoke. (From Borgerding & Klus [4] with permission.)

Class	Number
Neutral gases	> 5
Carbon oxides	2
Nitrogen oxides	1 (2)
Amides, imides, lactames	~ 240
Carboxylic acids	~ 230
Lactones	~ 150
Esters	~ 470
Aldehydes	~ 110
Ketones	~ 520
Alcohols	~ 380
Phenols	~ 280
Amines	~ 200
Volatile N-nitrosamines	4
Tobacco specific nitrosamines	4
N-heterocyclics	~ 920
Hydrocarbons, aliphatic, acyclic, aromatic	~ 760
Nitriles	~ 100
Anhydrides	~ 10
Carbohydrates	~ 40
Ethers	~ 310
Nitro-compounds	> 10
Metals	~ 30
Short- and long-living radicals	???

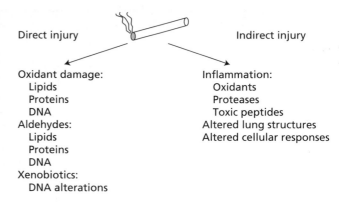

Figure 33.1 Direct and indirect injury due to smoke-derived toxins. Cigarette smoke contains multiple toxins that can directly damage tissues by a variety of mechanisms. Smoke can also activate cells that can result in indirect tissue damage. Mediators produced by inflammatory cells, in particular, are believed to have a major role in causing COPD.

estimate cigarette yields. The Federal Trade Commission (FTC) method, which uses 2-s puffs of 35 mL volume every minute until a final butt length is reached and in which vents are not blocked, has been widely used to estimate yields [15,16]. However, many smokers smoke more intensely and/or block vents, resulting in potentially greater yields. Thus, while standard machine-smoking regimes may have utility for comparing cigarettes, they are limited in providing estimates of exposure for a smoker.

Laboratory methods that attempt to recapitulate 'real' smoking topography are also problematic for several reasons. First, the instruments required to monitor puff behaviour likely change the way smokers smoke. In addition, smokers will vary their smoking behaviour during a single cigarette [17] and from cigarette to cigarette [18]. Because these factors change the composition and yield of smoke constituents, it becomes very difficult to estimate real exposures to smoke. The same issues apply to the smoke used in animal and *in vitro* testing. The lack of standardized and validated smoking regimes complicates comparison of results, as differences in smoking regimes can influence the composition and likely the toxicity of the smoke.

Determining the constituents responsible for the toxicity of cigarette smoke has been a major research goal for

many years. Compounds that have been suggested to contribute are listed (Table 33.3). As additional components are studied, it is likely this list will grow.

Oxidants

Many of the components present in cigarette smoke are potent oxidants, and oxidant injury is believed to be a major mechanism for cigarette smoke-induced toxicity [19]. It has been estimated that cigarette smoke contains approximately 10^{14} free radical oxidants per puff [4]. Most of these are expected to have half-lives of fractions of a second. Despite this, cigarette smoke contains some free radicals that have lifetimes of several minutes [20]. A steady state chemical model, involving the reaction of nitrogen dioxide and polymers containing semi-quinones [21], has been suggested to be responsible for the long-lived oxidants present in smoke. In addition, the inflammatory cells that are recruited and activated by cigarette smoke also produce oxidants [19]. Thus, cigarette smoke may be able to cause oxidant injury both as a direct toxicity and indirectly through the inflammatory response (Fig. 33.1).

It is likely that there are many important targets for oxidant-mediated damage in the lung including lipids, proteins and nucleic acids. Oxidation of arachidonic acid containing lipids, for example, can lead to the generation of isoprostanes that can, in turn, function as proinflammatory molecules [22,23]. Increased levels of isoprostane are present in the urine of smokers and can be reduced by oral antioxidants [24]. Cigarette smoke also can induce oxidation of low-density lipoproteins [25], which is believed to be a major pathogenic mechanism in the development of atherosclerotic vascular disease [26]. Smoke-induced oxidation of methionyl residues in α_1-protease inhibitor can

Table 33.3 Comparison of analytes currently proposed or required in regulatory schema. (After Borgerding & Klus [4] with permission.)

Smoke constituent	Hoffman analytes	Canadian emissions reporting	Massachusetts benchmark study	WHO Study Group on Tobacco Product
Ammonia	×	×	×	
1-aminonaphthalene		×	×	
2-aminonaphthalene	×	×	×	
3-aminobiphenyl		×	×	
4-aminobiphenyl	×	×	×	
Benzo[a]pyrene	×	×	×	×
Formaldehyde	×	×	×	×
Acetaldehyde	×	×	×	×
Acetone		×	×	
Acrolein	×	×	×	
Propionaldehyde		×	×	
Crotonaldehyde	×	×	×	
Butyraldehyde		×	×	
Methyl ethyl ketone			×	
Eugenol		×		
Hydrogen cyanide	×	×	×	×
Mercury	×	×	×	×
Lead	×	×	×	×
Cadmium	×	×	×	×
Nickel	×		×	×
Arsenic	×		×	×
Chromium	×		×	×
Selenium			×	×
Nitric oxide	×	×	×	×
Nox	×	×		
N-nitrosonornicotine	×	×	×	×
4-(*N*-nitrosomethylamino)-1-(3-pyridyl)-1-butanone	×	×	×	×
N-nitrosoanatabine		×	×	×
N-nitrosonanabasine	×	×	×	×
Pyridine	×	×	×	
Quinoline	×	×	×	
Hydroquinone		×	×	
Resorcinol		×	×	
Catechol	×	×	×	
Phenol	×	×	×	
m- + *p*-Cresol		×	×	
o-Cresol		×	×	
1,3-Butadiene	×	×	×	×
Isoprene	×	×	×	
Acrylonitrile	×	×	×	
Benzene	×	×	×	×
Toluene		×	×	
Styrene	×		×	
'Tar'	×	×	×	×
Nicotine	×	×	×	×
Carbon monoxide	×	×	×	

reduce its ability to inhibit neutrophil elastase and could shift the protease–antiprotease balance in favour of tissue destruction [27,28]. In addition, smoke-derived oxidants can activate nuclear factor κβ (NF-κβ) [29] and activator protein-1 (AP-1) [30], thus activating inflammatory pathways. Finally, cigarette smoke-derived oxidants can also lead to DNA damage [31,32].

A variety of oxidants are present in cigarette smoke, and they can react with target molecules in a number of ways. For example, reactive nitrogen species, particularly peroxynitrite, which is formed from nitric oxide and superoxide, can oxidatively nitrate proteins at tyrosine residues [33]. Because tyrosyl residues are important in regulating the function of many proteins, either directly or by serving as substrates for phosphorylation, their nitration is likely to greatly alter function. Consistent with this, reactive nitrogen species inactivation of a variety of proteins has been reported [34,35]. Because oxidants are not the only components in smoke that can damage lipids, proteins and DNA, it is likely that the molecular injury that results from oxidants is compounded and potentially amplified synergistically by other toxins.

Aldehydes

Smoke contains a large number of reactive aldehydes that can also adduct proteins and nucleic acids, thus leading to potentially complex toxicities. For example, both acetaldehyde [36] and acrolein [37] have been demonstrated to have direct genotoxic effects. In addition, acetaldehyde can form adducts with tubulin and dynein and can lead to inactivation of cilia beating in airway epithelial cells [38]. Acetaldehyde can also form adducts with the lipid peroxidation product malondialdehyde leading to complex adducted proteins [39], which can potentiate inflammatory responses through protein kinase C mediated mechanisms [40]. Acrolein, in contrast, has been reported to inhibit inflammatory [41] and immune responses [42]. Finally, both acrolein and acetaldehyde have been reported to inhibit lung fibroblast and airway epithelial cell chemotaxis and proliferation [43–45]. Smoke, which contains relatively large concentrations not only of acetaldehyde and acrolein, but other reactive aldehydes as well, is likely to exert toxic effects through these moieties.

Metals

Smoke contains a number of metals, and it is likely they contribute to smoke-induced disease. Iron contained in smoke, for example, can potentiate the generation of reactive oxygen species by catalysing the Haber–Weiss reaction [46]. Because the availability of iron may be limiting, the increased iron burden that is reported in the lungs of smokers [47] may be a means for persistent generation of excess oxidants.

Among the other metals contained in smoke, evidence supports a role for cadmium in the pathogenesis of COPD. In this context, increased cadmium levels have been associated with reduced lung function in the National Health and Nutrition Examination Survey (NHANES) study [48]. In animal studies, cadmium can cause emphysema [49] and emphysema has been associated with industrial cadmium exposures [50,51]. Although the mechanisms by which cadmium can cause emphysema are undefined, cadmium has been reported to impair several fibroblast-mediated repair responses including proliferation [52], matrix macromolecule production [53] and matrix contraction [54]. Cadmium can activate a number of genes that influence not only inflammation, but potentially repair as well [55]. This suggests that cadmium may cause emphysema, at least in part by altering both tissue injury and repair. An oxidant-dependent mechanism for cadmium toxicity has also been suggested [56], further supporting the notion that cigarette smoke-derived toxins can interact in causing their toxic effects.

Mutagens

Cigarette smoke can also cause a variety of types of DNA damage including point mutations, strand breaks and chromosomal alterations [57]. Smoking is a major cause of cancer, and DNA damage has been most widely studied in the context of carcinogenesis. In this regard, whole smoke and both the particulate and the vapour phases are reported to contribute to carcinogenesis. Smoke, moreover, contains more than 60 compounds that are identified as carcinogens in at least some systems [58]. It is likely that this list will grow as additional compounds are studied. Some, such as the polycyclic aromatic hydrocarbon benzo[a]pyrene (BaP), the tobacco-specific nitrosamine 4-(methylnitrosamino)-1-(3-pyridyl)-1-butanone (NNK) and 1,3-butadiene have been relatively extensively studied. The first two cause lung tumours in rats and mice, but the last in only mice [59]. This difference likely arises from species differences in xenobiotic metabolism and underlies a major issue in the assessment of carcinogens in smoke; metabolic differences greatly influence the carcinogenic potential. This results in marked species differences and likely also contributes to differences in human sensitivity to specific compounds [57].

The mechanisms that lead to DNA mutations are incompletely defined. Oxidants can damage DNA and reactive aldehydes can form adducts with DNA, and both processes can lead to mutations. Many of the other chemical carcinogens are also able to form adducts with DNA [59]. It is likely that formation of chemical adducts leads to activation of

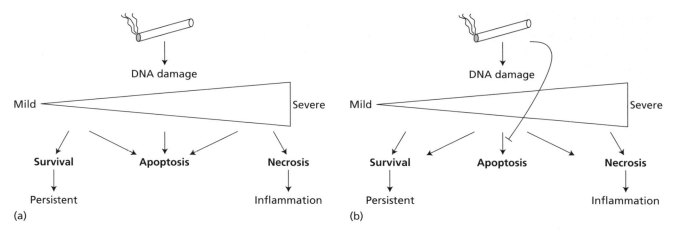

Figure 33.2 Smoke induced DNA damage: consequences. (a) Cigarette smoke can damage DNA by several mechanisms. If mild, this damage can be repaired and cells can survive, although with a risk of persistent DNA mutation. If moderate, apoptotic mechanisms are activated. These lead to cell death, which prevents mutations from persisting and, moreover, results in clearance of the cells without activation of inflammatory mechanisms. If severe, DNA damage can lead to necrosis which can activate inflammation. (b) Smoke also inhibits apoptosis. In so doing, some cells that would have been cleared by apoptosis will survive, leading to persistent mutations. Others will die by necrosis leading to increased inflammation.

DNA repair mechanisms and, if incomplete or incorrect repair results, mutations arise. Specific adducts are thought to lead preferentially to certain specific types of mutations. For example, BaP and NNK produce GC to TA mutations. BaP has been suggested to bind preferentially to sites in the DNA that contain endogenously methylated cytosine-guanine (CpG) dinucleotides [60]. These sites, therefore, represent potential 'hot spots' for BaP-induced mutagenesis. In this context, the *p53* gene is an important regulator of cell survival and replication. It is frequently mutated in lung and other types of cancer. GC to TA mutations are present more commonly in smokers with lung cancer than in non-smokers with lung cancer [57] and these *p53* mutations, moreover, occur selectively at 'hot spots' in the gene that contain methylated CpG sites [60], supporting the concept of sequence sensitivity to individual cigarette smoke component-induced mutagenesis. Interestingly, bladder cancers, which are also associated with cigarette smoking but are believed to result from aromatic amines, are associated with a distinct but different pattern of *p53* mutations, suggesting sequence selectivity in carcinogen induced DNA damage.

Acquired somatic cell mutations, which are likely to occur throughout the lung epithelium, are widely accepted as a likely mechanism for cigarette smoke-induced lung cancer. The suggestion has recently been made that similar somatic cell mutations may also contribute to the pathogenesis of COPD [61]. In support of this concept, microsatellite instability, which is believed to result from mismatch repair, is more frequent in patients with COPD [62]. When DNA damage occurs, repair mechanisms may attempt to correct the defect. Alternatively, in the face of excessive damage, apoptotic mechanisms are activated that lead to cell death, but are thought to protect the genome of the organism. The DNA damage induced by cigarette smoke can, under some conditions, lead to apoptosis [63,64]. However, smoke can also initiate antiapoptotic mechanisms. These may lead to cellular necrosis [65], which could initiate inflammation or, alternatively, may result in DNA repair and cell survival [66,67] (Fig. 33.2). Through such mechanisms, smoke exposure may be a particularly effective means to damage DNA and lead to the subsequent survival of cells with acquired mutations.

Smoke-induced inflammation

Cigarette smokers characteristically have a prominent inflammatory response. This includes the accumulation of pigment-laden macrophages within the lower respiratory tract, a condition termed 'small airways disease' [68,69]. Bronchoalveolar lavage studies reliably demonstrate a marked increase in the number and state of activation of alveolar macrophages obtained from smokers [70,71]. In addition, there are more modest increases in neutrophils in the lower respiratory tract together with an alteration in the distribution of lymphocytes. Specifically, CD8 lymphocytes are increased relative to CD4 lymphocytes, resulting in an increase in the CD8 : CD4 ratio [72]. This alteration resulting from smoking is of particular interest as an increase in CD8 cells is a feature of COPD that increases with disease severity [73,74].

In addition to an inflammatory response in the lung, cigarette smokers have a characteristic systemic inflammatory response. A 20–25% increase in peripheral blood neutrophils is observed in smokers, which correlates with the degree of loss of lung function [75,76]. Activation of the bone marrow leading to increased production of neutrophils has been suggested as a mechanism to account for neutrophilia in smokers [77]. Smoke exposure also leads to neutrophil priming that can occur even at levels encountered with environmental tobacco smoke exposure [78]. Neutrophils of smokers are less deformable than control neutrophils [79] and smoking results in selective retention of neutrophils within the lung where they may cause damage from an intravascular site [80]. Other evidence supporting systemic inflammatory response in smokers includes elevated C-reactive protein and fibrinogen [81] as well as evidence of endothelial cell dysfunction [82]. The ability of cigarette smoke to stimulate local pulmonary and systemic inflammation is believed to be a major pathogenetic mechanism in leading to pulmonary and extrapulmonary disease. Of interest is the fact that the vast majority of smokers have evidence of augmented inflammation although smaller numbers manifest clinically significant disease.

The mechanisms by which cigarette smoke induces inflammation are also multiple (Fig. 33.3). Cigarette smoke can activate complement through the alternate pathway leading to the generation of C5a, which can serve as a chemotactic factor driving the recruitment of inflammatory

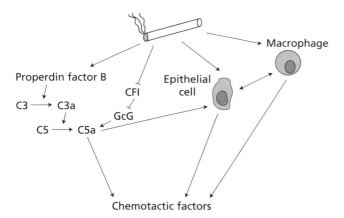

Figure 33.3 Activation of inflammation by cigarette smoke. Cigarette smoke can induce inflammation by a variety of mechanisms. Smoke activates several cells in the lungs. Resident macrophages and epithelial cells are believed to be most prominent as initial responders to smoke. Both can directly release chemotactic factors that can recruit and activate other inflammatory cells. They can also activate each other. Smoke also activates the cell independent complement system. This leads to generation of C5a, which can recruit inflammatory cells and can synergistically augment the activation of epithelial cells. Smoke also blocks part of the down-regulatory mechanisms that serve to control complement activation. (See text for details.)

cells [83]. In addition, the activity of C5a can be potentiated by the vitamin D binding protein Gc globulin, the activity of which can itself be inhibited by a molecule termed chemotactic factor inactivator (CFI) [84]. Cigarette smoke can inactivate CFI, thus leading to potentially augmented activity of C5a [85]. In addition to its direct chemotactic activity, C5a can also interact with receptors located on airway epithelial cells and, by this mechanism, can further potentiate inflammation [86].

Cigarette smoke is also able to directly activate a variety of cells to release proinflammatory molecules. Although it is likely that several mechanisms could account for such activity, evidence has been provided in support of an oxidant-mediated mechanism [87]. Specifically, it has been suggested that cigarette smoke-derived oxidants can activate NF-κβ [88], although the importance of this mechanism has also been questioned [89]. However, the presence of oxidants is thought to lead to or to facilitate the degradation of inhibitor κβ (Iκβ), which ordinarily inhibits the activity of the transcription factor NF-κβ. In the absence of its inhibitor, NF-κβ binds to DNA leading to the activation of a number of proinflammatory genes. Through this mechanism cigarette smoke is believed to induce the production of a variety of proinflammatory molecules including, for example, the chemotactic factor interleukin 8 (IL-8) from airway epithelial cells. Oxidant-dependent activation of AP-1 has also been reported to activate cells to produce proinflammatory mediators [87,90]. Interestingly, C5a interacts synergistically with cigarette smoke in inducing epithelial cell release of IL-8 [91–93]. This suggests that cigarette smoke, by acting through multiple pathways, can lead to dramatically augmented proinflammatory signalling.

Several cell types within the lung can be activated to produce inflammatory mediators in response to cigarette smoke. Smoke can activate both alveolar macrophages and airway epithelial cells [94–96] to release a variety of chemotactic factors and inflammatory mediators. Inhibitory effects of cigarette smoke have also been reported [97,98]. It seems likely that the effects of smoke will depend on the experimental design used and, very likely, on the methods used to prepare the cigarette smoke. As these can vary considerably, depending on methodology, it is not surprising that there are some differences between studies reported. Because differences in smoke composition are likely among smokers, these results suggest that cigarette smoking may lead to heterogeneous inflammatory responses that may depend on differences in specific exposures. Undoubtedly, these variations will be further increased by genetic and other differences among smokers.

The inflammatory cells recruited and activated by cigarette smoke are capable of inducing tissue damage through a number of mechanisms. Inflammatory cells are potent sources of oxidants, and the oxidant burden caused by inflammatory cells can damage protein, lipid and nucleic acid components within the lung. At present, it is difficult to determine if oxidant-induced damage results directly from cigarette smoke-derived oxidants or indirectly from cigarette smoke-induced inflammatory cell generation of oxidants. However, as the capacity of inflammatory cells to produce oxidants greatly exceeds the oxidants contained in cigarette smoke, it is likely that inflammatory cell amplification has a significant role [19].

Inflammatory cells also produce proteases and toxic peptides that can damage cells and tissues within the lung. The production of proteolytic enzymes in excess of the antiprotease defences is believed to have a major role in the pathogenesis of emphysema, the so-called 'protease–antiprotease' hypothesis (see Chapter 31). This concept, which originated with the observations that individuals with deficiency in the α_1-protease inhibitor developed emphysema [99] and that neutrophil elastase, a serine protease inhibited by α_1-protease inhibitor, induced emphysema when instilled in the lungs of animals [100], has now been extended to include a number of other serine, metallo and cysteine proteases and their respective inhibitors [101, 102]. Interestingly, these inhibitors interact in a complex network. Many are released as precursors that can be activated by other proteases. In addition, metalloproteases and serine proteases are capable of inactivating each other's inhibitors. Cigarette smoke can affect this complex network in several ways. By inducing the recruitment in activation of inflammatory cells, the protease burden can be increased. In addition, cigarette smoke can oxidatively inactivate α_1-protease inhibitor resulting in an acquired deficiency of antiprotease [28]. Because α_1-protease inhibitor may also

play a key part in inactivating toxic peptides such as defensins [103], the ability of cigarette smoke to inactivate α_1-protease inhibitor can have several effects leading to augmented tissue damage in the face of an inflammatory burden.

Tissue repair

Cigarette smoke not only leads to tissue damage, but it can also compromise tissue repair mechanisms (Fig. 33.4) [104]. In this context, the lung, like most tissues, has considerable capacity to repair following injury. Mechanical injury of the airways, for example, is followed by migration of epithelial cells to cover the epithelial defect, a process that is initiated within minutes [105,106]. This is followed by an orderly recruitment, proliferation and differentiation of cells within the epithelium. A similar process of recruitment proliferation, production of provisional matrix and eventual resolution takes place in the subjacent mesenchyme [107]. If these processes proceed effectively, tissue structure and function can be completely restored. Cigarette smoke is capable of inhibiting both epithelial cell [45,108] and mesenchymal cell [44] recruitment, proliferation, matrix production, matrix remodelling and apoptosis [66,67]. It is likely therefore that the altered tissue structure that is characteristic of the lungs of smokers results not only from smoke-induced tissue damage, but also from smoke-induced alterations in tissue repair mechanisms. Altered tissue repair likely contributes not only to the lesions present in the airways of smokers, but also to emphysematous changes within alveolar structures and to the vascular changes present within both the pulmonary parenchyma and the airways.

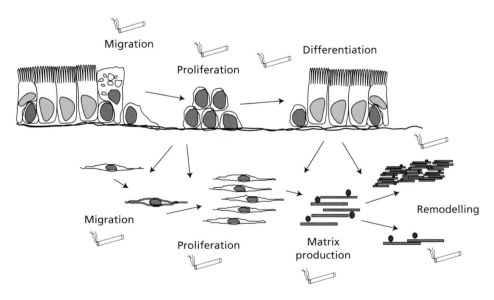

Migration

Proliferation

Differentiation

Migration

Proliferation

Matrix production

Remodelling

Figure 33.4 Injury of the airway epithelium is followed by an orderly sequence of events that can restore structure and function. These include epithelial cell recruitment, proliferation and differentiation. Similar events take place somewhat later in the subjacent mesenchymal tissues. Cigarette smoke has been demonstrated to inhibit many of these processes, indicated by the 'cigarette' in the figure. It is likely that cigarette smoke will alter epithelial cell differentiation as well. By altering repair, smoke could contribute to the structural changes that take place in the airway or in the alveolar walls in COPD. Smoke can also alter vascular repair (not shown).

Conclusions: common disease mechanisms

Cigarette smoke is a major causative factor for many conditions (see Table 33.1). As a result, individuals who have cigarette smoke-induced COPD frequently also have other smoke-related conditions as comorbidities. Individuals with COPD are more likely to have atherosclerotic vascular disease [2], lung cancer [3] and osteoporosis [109] than are individuals with similar smoking histories who do not have COPD. There are a number of mechanisms that could explain the increased comorbidity present in COPD patients. One mechanism is that systemic inflammatory consequences of COPD contribute to these allied conditions. An alternative mechanism is that COPD and its allied conditions result from similar toxic effects of cigarette smoke. As variations in individual susceptibility to the toxic effects of smoke are likely, individuals at increased risk for the development of COPD may also be at increased risk for other conditions. Understanding the mechanisms by which cigarette smoke toxicity leads to the panoply of diseases associated with smoking offers the opportunity to develop new strategies to address these diverse conditions.

References

1 Department of Health and Human Services, Centers for Disease Control and Prevention. *The Health Consequences of Smoking: a Report of the Surgeon General.* Washington, DC: National Center for Chronic Disease Prevention and Health Promotion, Office on Smoking and Health, 2004.

2 Sorlie PD, Kannel WB, O'Connor G. Mortality associated with respiratory function and symptoms in advanced age. The Framingham Study. *Am Rev Respir Dis* 1989;**140**:379–84.

3 Mannino DM, Aguayo SM, Petty TL, Redd SC. Low lung function and incident lung cancer in the United States: data From the First National Health and Nutrition Examination Survey follow-up. *Arch Intern Med* 2003;**163**:1475–80.

4 Borgerding M, Klus H. Analysis of complex mixtures: cigarette smoke. *Exp Toxicol Pathol* 2005;**57**(Suppl 1):43–73.

5 Byrd DM, ed. *The LSRO Report on Review of Ingredients Added to Cigarettes. Phase 1: The Feasibility of Testing Ingredients Added to Cigarettes.* Bethesda, MD: Life Sciences Research Office, 2004: 369.

6 Keith CH. Particle size studies on tobacco smoke. *Beitr Tabakforsch Int* 1982;**11**:123–31.

7 Ceschini P, Lafaye A. Evolution of the gas-vapour phase and the total particulate matter of cigarette smoke in a single puff. *Beitr Tabakforsch* 1976;**8**:378–81.

8 Hoffman D, Brunnemann KD, Prkopczyk B, Djordjevic MV. Tobacco-specific *N*-nitrosamines and Areca-derived *N*-nitrosamines: chemistry, biochemistry, carcinogenicity and relevance to humans. *J Toxicol Environ Health* 1994;**41**:1–52.

9 Afzelius BA. Ciliary dysfunction. In: Crystal RG *et al.*, eds. *The Lung.* Philadelphia: Lippincott-Raven, 1997: 2573–8.

10 Armitage AK, Dixon M, Frost BE, Mariner DC, Sinclair NM. The effect of tobacco blend additives on the retention of nicotine and solanesol in the human respiratory tract and on subsequent plasma nicotine concentrations during cigarette smoking. *Chem Res Toxicol* 2004;**17**:537–44.

11 Norman V. An overview of the vapor phase, semivolatile and novolatile components of cigarette smoke. *Recent Adv Tobacco Sci* 1977;**3**:28–58.

12 Battig K, Buzzi R, Nil R. Smoke yield of cigarettes and puffing behavior in men and women. *Psychopharmacology (Berl)* 1982;**76**:139–48.

13 Harris JE. Smoke yields of tobacco-specific nitrosamines in relation to FTC tar level and cigarette manufacturer: analysis of the Massachusetts Benchmark Study. *Public Health Rep* 2001;**116**:336–43.

14 Zacny JP, Stitzer ML, Yingling JE. Cigarette filter vent blocking: effects on smoking topography and carbon monoxide exposure. *Pharmacol Biochem Behav* 1986;**25**:1245–52.

15 UFT Commission. Cigarettes: testing for tar and nicotine content. *Fed Register* 1967;**32**:11178.

16 UFT Commission. Cigarettes and related matters: carbon monoxide, 'tar' and nicotine content of cigarette smoke: description of new machine and methods to be used in testing. *Fed Regist* 1980;**45**:46 483–7.

17 Guyatt AR, Kirkham AJ, Baldry AG, Dixon M, Cumming G. How does puffing behavior alter during the smoking of a single cigarette? *Pharmacol Biochem Behav* 1989;**33**:189–95.

18 Hatsukami DK, Morgan SF, Pickens RW, Champagne SE. Situational factors in cigarette smoking. *Addict Behav* 1990;**15**:1–12.

19 MacNee W. Oxidants/antioxidants and COPD. *Chest* 2000;**117**(5 Suppl 1):303S–17S.

20 Pryor WA, Tamura M, Church DF. ESR spin trapping study of radicals produced in NO_x/olefin reactions: a mechanism for the production of the apparently long-lived radicals in the gas phase cigarette smoke. *J Am Chem Soc* 1984;**106**:5073–9.

21 Church DF, Pryor WA. Free-radical chemistry of cigarette smoke and its toxicological implications. *Environ Health Perspect* 1985;**64**:111–26.

22 Roberts LJ 2nd, Brame CJ, Chen Y, Morrow JD. Novel eicosanoids: isoprostanes and related compounds. *Methods Mol Biol* 1999;**120**:257–85.

23 Montuschi P, Ciabattoni G, Paredi P *et al.* 8-isoprostane in breath condensate of healthy smokers. *Am J Respir Crit Care Med* 1999;**159**:A887.

24 Dietrich M, Block G, Hudes M *et al.* Antioxidant supplementation decreases lipid peroxidation biomarker F(2)-isoprostanes in plasma of smokers. *Cancer Epidemiol Biomarkers Prev* 2002;**11**:7–13.

25 Santanam N, Sanchez R, Hendler S, Parthasarathy S. Aqueous extracts of cigarette smoke promote the oxidation of low density lipoprotein by peroxidases. *FEBS Lett* 1997;**414**:549–51.

26 Yamaguchi Y, Matsuno S, Kagota S, Haginaka J, Kunitomo M. Oxidants in cigarette smoke extract modify low-density

lipoprotein in the plasma and facilitate atherogenesis in the aorta of Watanabe heritable hyperlipidemic rabbits. *Atherosclerosis* 2001;**156**:109–17.

27 Cohen AB, James HL. Reduction of the elastase inhibitory capacity of alpha 1-antitrypsin by peroxides in cigarette smoke: an analysis of brands and filters. *Am Rev Respir Dis* 1982;**126**:25–30.

28 Janoff A. Reduction of the elastase in inhibitory capacity of alpha-1-antitrypsin by peroxides in cigarette smoke. An analysis of the brands and the filters. *Am Rev Respir Dis* 1982;**126**:25–30.

29 Nishikawa M, Kakemizu N, Ito T *et al.* Superoxide mediates cigarette smoke-induced infiltration of neutrophils into the airways through nuclear factor-κβ activation and IL-8 mRNA expression in guinea pigs *in vivo. Am J Respir Cell Mol Biol* 1999;**20**:189–98.

30 Lavigne MC, Eppihimer MJ. Cigarette smoke condensate induces MMP-12 gene expression in airway-like epithelia. *Biochem Biophys Res Commun* 2005;**330**:194–203.

31 Nakayama T, Kanedo M, Kodama M, Nagata C. Cigarette smoke induces DNA single-strand breaks in human cells. *Nature* 1985;**314**:462–4.

32 Poulsen HE. Oxidative DNA modifications. *Exp Toxicol Pathol* 2005;**57**(Suppl 1):161–9.

33 Yamaguchi Y, Kagota S, Haginaka J, Kunitomo M. Participation of peroxynitrite in oxidative modification of LDL by aqueous extracts of cigarette smoke. *FEBS Lett* 2002;**512**:218–22.

34 Sato E, Koyama S, Camhi SL, Nelson DK, Robbins RA. Reactive oxygen and nitrogen metabolites modulate fibronectin-induced fibroblast migration *in vitro. Free Radic Biol Med* 2001;**30**:22–9.

35 Simmons MS, Connett JE, Nides MA *et al.* Smoking reduction and the rate of decline in FEV_1: results from the Lung Health Study. *Eur Respir J* 2005:**25**:1011–7.

36 Matsuda T, Kawanishi M, Yagi T, Matsui S, Takebe H. Specific tandem GG to TT base substitutions induced by acetaldehyde are due to intra-strand crosslinks between adjacent guanine bases. *Nucleic Acids Res* 1998;**26**:1769–74.

37 Yang Q, Hergenhahn M, Weninger A, Bartsch H. Cigarette smoke induces direct DNA damage in the human B-lymphoid cell line Raji. *Carcinogenesis* 1999;**20**:1769–75.

38 Sisson JH, Tuma DJ, Rennard SI. Acetaldehyde-mediated cilia dysfunction in bovine bronchial epithelial cells. *Am J Physiol* 1991;**260**:L29–L36.

39 Freeman TL, Haver A, Duryee MJ *et al.* Aldehydes in cigarette smoke react with the lipid peroxidation product malonaldehyde to form fluorescent protein adducts on lysines. *Chem Res Toxicol* 2005;**18**:817–24.

40 Wyatt TA, Kharbanda KK, Tuma DJ, Sisson JH. Malondialdehyde-acetaldehyde-adducted bovine serum albumin activates protein kinase C and stimulates interleukin-8 release in bovine bronchial epithelial cells. *Alcohol* 2001;**25**:159–66.

41 Valacchi G, Pagnin E, Phung A *et al.* Inhibition of NFκB activation and IL-8 expression in human bronchial epithelial cells by acrolein. *Antioxid Redox Signal* 2005;**7**:25–31.

42 Lambert C, McCue J, Portas M *et al.* Acrolein in cigarette

smoke inhibits T-cell responses. *J Allergy Clin Immunol* 2005;**116**:916–22.

43 Wang H, Liu X, Umino T *et al.* Cigarette smoke inhibits normal human bronchial epithelial cell chemotaxis and contraction of three dimensional collagen latices. *Am J Respir Crit Care Med* 1999;**159**:A438.

44 Nakamura Y, Romberger DJ, Tate L *et al.* Cigarette smoke inhibits lung fibroblast proliferation and chemotaxis. *Am J Respir Crit Care Med* 1995;**151**:1497–503.

45 Cantral DE, Sisson JH, Veys T, Rennard SI, Spurzem JR. Effects of cigarette smoke extract on bovine bronchial epithelial cell attachment and migration. *Am J Physiol* 1995;**268**:L723–8.

46 Kehrer JP. The Haber–Weiss reaction and mechanisms of toxicity. *Toxicology* 2000;**149**:43–50.

47 Thompson AB, Bohling T, Heires A, Linder J, Rennard SI. Lower respiratory tract iron burden is increased in association with cigarette smoking. *J Lab Clin Med* 1991;**117**:493–9.

48 Mannino DM, Holgium F, Greves HM *et al.* Urinary cadmium levels predict lower lung function in current and former smokers: data from the Third National Health and Nutrition Examination Survey. *Thorax* 2004;**59**:194–8.

49 Snider GL, Hayes JA, Korthy AL, Lewis GP. Centrilobular emphysema experimentally induced by cadmium chloride aerosol. *Am Rev Respir Dis* 1973;**108**:40–8.

50 Lane RE, Campbell ACP. Fatal emphysema in two men making a copper cadmium alloy. *Br J Ind Med* 1954;**11**:118–22.

51 Bonnell JA. Emphysema and proteinuria in men casting copper-cadmium alloys. *Br J Ind Med* 1955;**12**:181–95.

52 Chambers RC, McAnulty RJ, Shock A *et al.* Cadmium selectively inhibits fibroblast procollagen production and proliferation. *Am J Physiol* 1994;**267**:L300–8.

53 Chambers RC, Laurent GJ, Westergren-Thorsson G. Cadmium inhibits proteoglycan and procollagen production by cultured human lung fibroblasts. *Am J Respir Cell Mol Biol* 1998;**19**:498–506.

54 Liu XD, Umino T, Zhu YK *et al.* A study on the effect of cadmium on human lung fibroblasts. *Chest* 2000;**117**(5)(Suppl 1):247S.

55 Shin HJ, Park KK, Lee BH, Moon CK, Lee MO. Identification of genes that are induced after cadmium exposure by suppression subtractive hybridization. *Toxicology* 2003;**191**:121–31.

56 Yang CF, Shen HM, Shen Y, Zhuang ZX, Ong CN. Cadmium-induced oxidative cellular damage in human fetal lung fibroblasts (MRC-5 cells). *Environ Health Perspect* 1997;**105**:712–6.

57 DeMarini DM. Genotoxicity of tobacco smoke and tobacco smoke condensate: a review. *Mutat Res* 2004;**567**:447–74.

58 Hoffmann D, Hoffmann I, El-Bayoumy K. The less harmful cigarette: a controversial issue: a tribute to Ernst L. Wynder. *Chem Res Toxicol* 2001;**14**:767–90.

59 Pfeifer GP, Denissenko MF, Olivier M *et al.* Tobacco smoke carcinogens, DNA damage and *p53* mutations in smoking-associated cancers. *Oncogene* 2002;**21**:7435–51.

60 Yoon JH, Smith LE, Feng Z *et al.* Methylated CpG dinucleotides are the preferential targets for G-to-T transversion

mutations induced by benzo[a]pyrene diol epoxide in mammalian cells: similarities with the *p53* mutation spectrum in smoking-associated lung cancers. *Cancer Res* 2001;**61**: 7110–7.

61 Anderson GP, Bozinovski S. Acquired somatic mutations in the molecular pathogenesis of COPD. *Trends Pharmacol Sci* 2003;**24**:71–6.

62 Siafakas NM, Tzortzaki EG, Sourvinos G *et al.* Microsatellite DNA instability in COPD. *Chest* 1999;**116**:47–51.

63 Carnevali S, Petruzzelli S, Longoni B *et al.* Cigarette smoke extract induces oxidative stress and apoptosis in human lung fibroblasts. *Am J Physiol Lung Cell Mol Physiol* 2003;**284**: L955–63.

64 Wang J, Wilcken DE, Wang XL. Cigarette smoke activates caspase-3 to induce apoptosis of human umbilical venous endothelial cells. *Mol Genet Metab* 2001;**72**:82–8.

65 Wickenden JA, Clarke MC, Rossi AG *et al.* Cigarette smoke prevents apoptosis through inhibition of caspase activation and induces necrosis. *Am J Respir Cell Mol Biol* 2003;**29**: 562–70.

66 Kim H, Liu X, Kobayashi T *et al.* Reversible cigarette smoke extract-induced DNA damage in human lung fibroblasts. *Am J Respir Cell Mol Biol* 2004;**31**:483–90.

67 Liu X, Conner H, Kobayashi T *et al.* Cigarette smoke extract induces DNA damage but not apoptosis in human bronchial epithelial cells. *Am J Respir Cell Mol Biol* 2005;**33**:121–9.

68 Niewoehner DE, Kleinerman J, Rice DB. Pathologic changes in the peripheral airways of young cigarette smokers. *N Engl J Med* 1974;**291**:755–8.

69 Cosio MG, Hale KA, Niewoehner DE. Morphologic and morphometric effects of prolonged cigarette smoking on the small airways. *Am Rev Respir Dis* 1980;**122**:265–71.

70 Reynolds HY. State of the art: bronchoalveolar lavage. *Am Rev Respir Dis* 1987;**135**:250–63.

71 Linder J, Rennard SI. *Atlas of Bronchoalveolar Lavage.* Chicago: American Society of Clinical Pathology Press, 1988: 196.

72 Costabel U, Bross KJ, Reuter C, Ruhle KH, Matthys H. Alterations in immunoregulatory T-cell subsets in cigarette smokers. A phenotypic analysis of bronchoalveolar and blood lymphocytes. *Chest* 1986;**90**:39–44.

73 O'Shaughnessy TC, Ansari TW, Barnes NC, Jeffery PK. Inflammation in bronchial biopsies of subjects with chronic bronchitis: inverse relationship of CD8+ T lymphocytes with FEV_1. *Am J Crit Care Med* 1997;**155**:852–7.

74 Saetta M, Baraldo S, Corbino L *et al.* CD8+ve cells in the lungs of smokers with chronic obstructive pulmonary disease. *Am J Respir Crit Care Med* 1999;**160**:711–7.

75 Corre F, Lellouch J, Schwartz D. Smoking and leucocyte-counts. *Lancet* 1971;**2**:632–4.

76 Chan-Yeung M, Abboud R, Buncio AD, Vedal S. Peripheral leucocyte count and longitudinal decline in lung function. *Thorax* 1988;**43**:462–6.

77 Terashima T, Wiggs B, English D, Hogg JC, van Eeden SF. The effect of cigarette smoking on the bone marrow. *Am J Respir Crit Care Med* 1997;**155**:1021–6.

78 Anderson R, Theron AJ, Richards GA, Myer MS, van Rensburg AJ. Passive smoking by humans sensitizes circulating neutrophils. *Am Rev Respir Dis* 1991;**144**:570–4.

79 Selby C, Drost E, Wraith PK, MacNee W. *In vivo* neutrophil sequestration within lungs of humans is determined by *in vitro* 'filterability'. *J Appl Physiol* 1991;**71**:1996–2003.

80 Terashima T, Klut ME, English D *et al.* Cigarette smoking causes sequestration of polymorphonuclear leukocytes released from the bone marrow in lung microvessels. *Am J Respir Cell Mol Biol* 1999;**20**:171–7.

81 Bazzano LA, He J, Muntner P, Vupputuri S, Whelton PK. Relationship between cigarette smoking and novel risk factors for cardiovascular disease in the United States. *Ann Intern Med* 2003;**138**:891–7.

82 Esen AM, Barutcu I, Acar M *et al.* Effect of smoking on endothelial function and wall thickness of brachial artery. *Circ J* 2004;**68**:1123–6.

83 Robbins RA, Nelson KJ, Gossman GL, Koyama S, Rennard SI. Complement activation by cigarette smoke. *Am J Physiol* 1991;**260**:L254–9.

84 Robbins RA, Hamel FG. Chemotactic factor inactivator interaction with Gc-globulin (vitamin D-binding protein). A mechanism of modulating the chemotactic activity of C5a. *J Immunol* 1990;**144**:2371–6.

85 Robbins RA, Gossman GL, Nelson KJ *et al.* Inactivation of chemotactic factor inactivator by cigarette smoke. A potential mechanism of modulating neutrophil recruitment to the lung. *Am Rev Respir Dis* 1990;**142**:763–8.

86 Floreani AA, Heires AJ, Welniak LA *et al.* Expression of receptors for C5a anaphylatoxin (CD88) on human bronchial epithelial cells: enhancement of C5a mediated release of IL-8 upon exposure to cigarette smoke. *J Immunol* 1998;**160**:5073–81.

87 MacNee W. Oxidants/antioxidants and chronic obstructive pulmonary disease: pathogenesis to therapy. *Novartis Found Symp* 2001;**234**:169–85.

88 Schreck R, Rieber P, Baeuerle PA. Reactive oxygen intermediates as apparently widely used messengers in the activation of the NF-κB transcription factor and HIV-1. *Embo J* 1991;**10**:2247–58.

89 Bowie A, O'Neill LA. Oxidative stress and nuclear factor-kappaB activation: a reassessment of the evidence in the light of recent discoveries. *Biochem Pharmacol*, 2000;**59**:13–23.

90 Walters MJ, Paul-Clark MJ, McMaster SK *et al.* Cigarette smoke activates human monocytes by an oxidant-AP-1 signaling pathway: implications for steroid resistance. *Mol Pharmacol* 2005;**68**:1343–53.

91 Floreani AA, Wyatt TA, Stoner J *et al.* Smoke and C5a induce airway epithelial intercellular adhesion molecule-1 and cell adhesion. *Am J Respir Cell Mol Biol* 2003;**29**:472–82.

92 Hunninghake GW, Gadek JE, Fales HM, Crystal RG. Human alveolar macrophage-derived chemotactic factor for neutrophils: stimuli and partial characterization. *J Clin Invest* 1980;**66**:473–83.

93 Kirkham PA, Spooner G, Ffoulkes-Jones C, Calvez R. Cigarette smoke triggers macrophage adhesion and activation: role of lipid peroxidation products and scavenger receptor. *Free Radic Biol Med* 2003;**35**:697–710.

94 Shoji S, Ertl R, Rennard SI. Cigarette smoke stimulates release of neutrophil chemotactic activity from cultured bronchial epithelial cells. *Clin Res* 1987;**35**:539A.

95 Mio T, Romberger DJ, Thompson AB *et al.* Cigarette smoke induces interleukin-8 release from human bronchial epithelial cells. *Am J Respir Crit Care Med* 1997;**155**:1770–6.

96 Koyama S, Rennard SI, Leikauf GD, Robbins RA. Bronchial epithelial cells release monocyte chemotactic activity in response to smoke and endotoxin. *J Immunol* 1991;**147**: 972–9.

97 Witherden IR, Vanden Bon EJ, Goldstraw P *et al.* Primary human alveolar type II epithelial cell chemokine release: effects of cigarette smoke and neutrophil elastase. *Am J Respir Cell Mol Biol* 2004;**30**:500–9.

98 Laan M, Bozinovski S, Anderson GP. Cigarette smoke inhibits lipopolysaccharide-induced production of inflammatory cytokines by suppressing the activation of activator protein-1 in bronchial epithelial cells. *J Immunol* 2004;**173**: 4164–70.

99 Laurell CB, Eriksson S. The electrophoretic alpha 1-globulin pattern of serum in alpha 1-antitrypsin deficiency. *Scand J Clin Lab Invest* 1963;**15**:132–40.

100 Senior RM, Tegner H, Kuhn C *et al.* The induction of pulmonary emphysema with human leukocyte elastase. *Am Rev Respir Dis* 1977;**116**:469–75.

101 Chapman H, Riese R, Shi G. Emerging roles for cysteine proteases in human biology. *Annu Rev Physiol* 1997;**59**:63–88.

102 Shapiro SD, Senior RM. Matrix metalloproteinases. Matrix degradation and more. *Am J Respir Cell Mol Biol* 1999;**20**: 1100–2.

103 Spencer LT, Paone G, Krein PM *et al.* Role of human neutrophil peptides in lung inflammation associated with alpha1-antitrypsin deficiency. *Am J Physiol Lung Cell Mol Physiol* 2004;**286**:L514–20.

104 Rennard SI. In: Pauwels RA, Postma DS, eds. *Defective Repair in COPD: the American Hypothesis, in Long-Term Intervention in Chronic Obstructive Pulmonary Disease.* New York: Marcel Dekker, 2004: 165–200.

105 Wilhelm DL. Regeneration of tracheal epithelium. *J Pathol Bacteriol* 1953;**55**:543–50.

106 Erjefalt JS, Persson CG. Airway epithelial repair: breath-takingly quick and multipotentially pathogenic. *Thorax* 1997; **52**:1010–2.

107 Erjefalt JS, Erjefalt I, Sundler F, Persson CG. *In vivo* restitution of airway epithelium. *Cell Tissue Res* 1995;**281**:305–16.

108 Wang H, Lui X, Umino T *et al.* Cigarette smoke inhibits human bronchial epithelial cell repair processes. *Am J Respir Cell Mol Biol* 2001;**25**:772–9.

109 Ionescu AA, Schoon E. Osteoporosis in chronic obstructive pulmonary disease. *Eur Respir J Suppl* 2003;**46**:64–75.

CHAPTER 34
COPD and air pollution

Kenneth Donaldson, Andrew Churg and William MacNee

Although cigarette smoking is clearly the major cause of COPD, the lungs of those with COPD are, like everyone's, exposed to such polluting particles and gases as are present in their general environment. There is evidence that levels of harmful air pollutants in the general environment can reach levels high enough to both cause and exacerbate disease, in many instances through mechanisms that are well understood [1]. The predominant mechanism that initiates proinflammatory gene expression in COPD is oxidative stress [2]. The gases and particles in air pollution are also known to cause oxidative stress and inflammation and so some additive impact of air pollution in smokers is to be anticipated. Substantial epidemiologic research has confirmed that there is increased incidence of COPD in more polluted areas, suggesting a chronic effect of pollution. There are clear links between short-term increases in pollution levels and exacerbations of COPD, suggesting an acute effect in some individuals. Air pollution also affects the cardiovascular system in ways that are not well understood, but it has been hypothesized that the mechanisms may involve oxidative stress and inflammation. This chapter outlines the evidence in support of the above, especially relating to the underlying mechanisms.

Air pollutants

The principal types of air pollution found in urban atmospheres are shown in Table 34.1. The impacts of air pollution are best described in conurbations where the levels of air pollutants are higher than in rural settings and where there are more people exposed and so the effects are more likely to be detected.

The major components of modern air pollution monitored by most agencies are particles (PM_{10}), ozone, SO_2 and NO_2, although there are others. Of these, particulate material (PM), and ozone are present at levels where they

Table 34.1 The principal types of air pollution found in urban atmospheres.

Pollutant	Sources
Particles	Motor vehicles, industry, burning of fossil fuels, atmospheric chemistry, biomass cooking
Ozone	Photochemical reaction of nitrogen oxides and hydrocarbons released by motor vehicles and industry
Nitrogen dioxide	Automobile fuel combustion; fossil fuel combustion
Sulphur dioxide	Domestic homes and power stations burning fossil fuels; industry
Other air pollutants less likely to be involved in COPD	Volatile organic compounds, heavy metals, polycyclic aromatic hydrocarbons, fungal products; but note that some of these can be associated with the particle fraction and so may have a role in the effects of PM_{10}

are likely to cause harm as identified in epidemiological and chamber studies, although other components could be relevant in some situations. Both particles and ozone are powerful oxidative stressors although they operate by different pathways to generate harmful free radicals. The other gaseous components of the air pollution mix are also capable of producing oxidative stress either directly or indirectly. PM has received special research attention because of the fact that in several epidemiologic studies there is no threshold for its adverse effects suggesting that, even at the 'normal' levels experienced in cities these adverse effects are occurring. For these reasons and because of the experience of the authors, this review is confined to the effects of PM in COPD. However, the mechanisms described are likely to be relevant to any oxidizing pollutant.

Particulate material

Sources

Particles such as sea salt and windblown and re-entrained dust from natural attrition processes in the Earth's crust arise naturally, and become part of the air pollution particle cloud. Anthropogenic particles, arising from motor vehicles industry and other human activities, add substantially to the concentration of particles in the cloud especially in cities. In addition, complex environmental chemistry gives rise to particles and, no doubt, modifies existing ones. Therefore the ambient particle cloud is a complex mixture comprising organic matter, elemental carbon or soot, metals, chlorides, sulphates, nitrates and geologically derived crustal dust [3]. Particles can be classified as *primary*, formed immediately (e.g. diesel particles), or *secondary*, those particles that form from atmospheric chemistry (e.g. ammonium nitrate) [4]. Not all of the different particles present in the ambient cloud are considered to have equal potency in causing adverse effects. Secondary particles and crustal particles are generally considered to be less potentially harmful than primary combustion-derived particles. Combustion particles, such as diesel particles, can be heterogeneous, with a carbon core plus associated metals and organics derived from the incomplete combustion of fuel or engine oil. Particles may be agglomerated, with individual particles adhering together more or less tightly.

Particle measurement and deposition in the lungs

Particles deposit in the different parts of the bronchial tree depending on their aerodynamic diameter [5] and this forms the basis of health-related size-based sampling of PM in the air, which forms the regulatory basis for control of ambient particles. The PM_{10} sampling convention is a mass measure where particles of 10 μm are collected with 50% efficiency and is increasingly efficient for smaller particles and less efficient for larger particles; it roughly corresponds to the thoracic fraction of particles as defined by the International Organization for Standardization (ISO) [5]. The $PM_{2.5}$ convention captures particles of 2.5 μm with 50% efficiency and roughly corresponds to the respirable fraction of particles as defined by ISO [5]. Therefore, PM_{10} describes the mass of particles that deposit throughout the airways, while $PM_{2.5}$ more accurately describes the mass penetrating beyond the ciliated airways to the sensitive centriacinar region; both conventions are expressed as μg/m³. The European (EC) standard for PM_{10} is currently 50 μg/m³ (24 h daily average) allowing 35 exceedences per year, but is under review. Deposition depends on aerodynamic diameter and is independent of composition, except that it depends on density, but once deposited the fate and effects of the particle depends on its composition. Salts such as nitrates and sulphates may dissolve and be relatively invisible to the lungs, but if the particles, for example, release transition metals that undergo Fenton chemistry, then hydroxyl radicals may be produced. If the ubiquitous bacterial product endotoxin is present in association with the particles, then lung cells may be stimulated to produce inflammation. All of these effects may lead to oxidative stress.

Epidemiologic studies of PM and COPD

PM and the incidence of COPD

There is evidence to suggest that chronic exposure to high levels of PM may not only exacerbate pre-existing COPD, but may also cause chronic airflow obstruction, although the number of reports examining this issue is limited [6]. Abbey *et al.* [7–10] studied a cohort of nearly 4000 non-smoking Seventh Day Adventists in Southern California and found significantly increased risks for the development of new cases of chronic bronchitis and COPD that were associated with increased levels of exposure to ambient PM_{10} and $PM_{2.5}$ [7,8]. Symptom severity correlated with $PM_{2.5}$ and PM_{10} levels. Long-term increases in PM_{10} concentrations were also found to be associated with greater forced expiratory volume in 1 s (FEV_1) decrements [9] as were increases in mortality from non-malignant lung disease [10]. However, one of the peculiarities of these results was that they largely applied to males, with little or no effect observed in females.

Somewhat similar results were obtained in the UCLA-CORD study [11,12], which examined lung function changes over time in three areas of Southern California. In men, FEV_1 declines were found to be significantly greater in both smokers and non-smokers in the region with the highest levels of particulate pollutants (Long Beach), nitrogen oxides and sulphates, but smoking appeared to account for the majority (approximately 70%) of the decline. In women, effects were only seen in never-smokers. Of interest, no chronic effects were seen in the UCLA-CORD study in the region in association with high levels of ozone (Glendora).

A number of other, largely cross-sectional, studies have been performed, consistently reporting that increased levels of air pollutants are associated with greater apparent declines in FEV_1 and/or forced vital capacity (FVC). However, there are differences in the pollutants that seem to be most important; some studies report associations with PM_{10} or total suspended particulates whereas others only find associations with levels of sulphates or acid [6].

All of these studies suffer from a number of methodological

problems [6] and, as noted, there is no consistent correlation with a specific type of pollutant. Nonetheless, there do seem to be reasonably good data to suggest that chronically elevated levels of air pollutants, including PM, can produce COPD.

Similar results have been found in women in developing countries who are exposed to the very high levels of PM emitted from cooking with biomass fuels. Perez-Padilla *et al.* [13] performed a case–control study of Mexican women and reported an increased risk of chronic bronchitis and chronic airflow obstruction associated with cooking with wood; the risk of chronic bronchitis was linearly associated with hours/year of cooking with biomass fuels. Dennis *et al.* [14] came to a similar conclusion examining women in Colombia who cooked with biomass fuels. Cooking with biomass fuels, particularly indoors, produces very high PM exposures [15,16].

PM and COPD mortality

Schwartz [17] noted that the relative risk of death from COPD increased by 1.25 on days when the PM_{10} averaged 141 $\mu g/m^3$ compared with low pollution days when the pollution averaged 47 $\mu g/m^3$. Both PM_{10} and total suspended particulate (TSP) were associated significantly with respiratory mortality, including COPD, in Detroit, Michigan for the 1985–90 period. Relative risk (RR) estimates of 1.123 were reported for PM_{10} and 1.109 for TSP per 5–95th percentile increment [18]. In Barcelona, levels of PM_{10} but not gaseous pollutants were associated with mortality in COPD patients after adjusting for meteorologic variables and influenza epidemics, with an odds ratio of 1.11 for the interquartile difference [6]. The RRs of death in COPD patients in Hong Kong were 1.017 for an increase of 10 $\mu g/m^3$ PM_{10} and 1.034 for ozone and a dose–response effect was evident [19]. In the Netherlands, statistically significant associations between air pollution and mortality in COPD patients were found in the age category of 65 years and above. Significant associations with ozone were found for COPD mortality in those less than 65 years [20].

PM and exacerbations of COPD

Hospital emergency room visits for COPD were studied in Barcelona [21] in relation to temporal trends in air pollution, and a reduction of 50 $\mu g/m^3$ in particles was accompanied by a reduction of approximately 6% in emergency room visits for COPD. Morgan *et al.* [22] studied hospital admissions in Sydney, Australia, 1990–94 and demonstrated that an increase in daily maximum 1-h particulate concentration from 10th to 90th percentile was associated with an increase of 3.01% (95% confidence interval, 0.38–6.52) in COPD admissions. In a prospective study [23], 40 subjects with COPD, who lived within a 5-km radius of the regional council's air pollution monitoring site, com-

pleted symptom diaries twice daily for 3 months during the winter of 1994. Although the pollution levels were low in that year, a rise in the PM_{10} concentration equivalent to the interquartile range was associated with an increase in night-time chest symptoms. The association between air pollution and hospital admissions for COPD was investigated in Minneapolis-St. Paul and Birmingham, Alabama for the period 1986–91 [24]. PM_{10} was associated with hospital admissions but could not be singled out as being more important than SO_2 and NO_2 in this regard.

In the APHEA study [25], admissions for COPD in six European cities were examined. For all ages, the relative risk of admission to hospital for COPD for a 50-$\mu g/m^3$ increase in black smoke was 1.04 (1.01–1.06) and for total suspended particulate was 1.02 (1.00–1.05). Wordley *et al.* [26] reported on hospital admissions in Birmingham, UK in relation to particulate air pollution and described a 10-$\mu g/m^3$ rise in PM_{10} as being associated with a 2.4% increase in respiratory admissions; while low, this risk was linear and without evidence of a threshold. Dab *et al.* [27] reported on the relationship between air pollution and hospital admissions in Paris, 1987–92. PM_{10} and black smoke were associated with hospital admissions for all respiratory causes when the black smoke level exceeded its 5th percentile value by 100 $\mu g/m^3$. Schwartz [28] related hospital admissions for the elderly in Birmingham, Alabama with air pollution levels. Inhalable particles were a risk factor for admission for COPD (RR 1.27; 95% confidence interval, 1.08–1.50). An increase of 25 $\mu g/m^3$ black smoke produced adjusted changes of 6% and 9% in emergency room admissions for COPD in Barcelona during winter, although the change was smaller in the summer [29]. A study was carried out in Delhi, one of the 10 most polluted cities in the world, relating emergency room visits for exacerbations of COPD and air pollution. Over a 2-year period, the daily air pollution often exceeded national air quality standards and emergency room visits for COPD increased by one-quarter when the air pollution was significantly increased. The presence of air conditioning, resulting in lower pollution levels in homes, was reported to be a factor in reducing hospital admissions for COPD in the study of Janssen *et al.* [30].

Inflammatory effects of PM

There are many studies demonstrating acute proinflammatory effects of PM. The initiating mechanism for the proinflammatory effects of PM appears to involve the ability of the particles to generate oxidative stress as a result of various components such as transition metals, particle surfaces and organics. These cellular and molecular mechanisms are detailed in Donaldson *et al.* [31] and examples of the proinflammatory effects of PM are outlined in Table 34.2.

Table 34.2 Proinflammatory effects of particulate material (PM).

Effect	References
PM_{10} particles can generate oxidative stress in cell-free systems	32
PM_{10} causes oxidative stress and activation of oxidative stress-responsive signalling pathways in epithelial cells	33
PM_{10} causes synthesis and release of proinflammatory cytokines	34
PM_{10} causes pulmonary inflammation in laboratory animals	35
PM_{10} causes inflammation in humans exposed to CAPS by inhalation or instilled with soluble components	36

CAPS, concentrated ambient particles.

Mechanism of inflammatory effects

The cellular signalling pathways leading to proinflammatory gene expression that are activated following the encounter between lung target cells and PM are partially understood and involve oxidative-stress responsive mechanisms; these pathways are shown in diagrammatic form in Figure 34.1. There have been a number of studies into the effects of PM_{10} on the mitogen-activated protein kinase (MAPK)

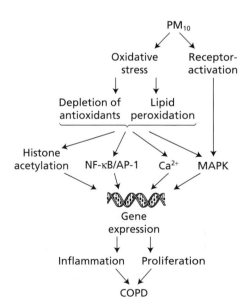

Figure 34.1 Diagrammatic representation of the hypothetical signalling pathways involved in the transcription of proinflammatory genes following exposure to PM_{10}. MAPK, mitogen-activated protein kinase; NF-κB, nuclear factor κB.

pathway. Timblin *et al.* [37] demonstrated increases in Jun N-terminal kinase (JNK) activity in alveolar epithelial cells exposed to PM and this was accompanied by increases in phosphorylated cJun and transcriptional activation of elements of the AP-1 transcription factor complex. These changes were accompanied by increased incorporation of 5'-bromodeoxyuridine, a marker of cell proliferation. Utah Valley PM caused increases in ERK1/2 phosphorylation via activation of the epidermal growth factor receptor (EGFR) [38]. Treatment of alveolar macrophages with residual oil fly ash (ROFA) demonstrated that JNK and p38, but not extracellular signal regulated kinase (ERK), were activated [39] while diesel exhaust particulates (DEP) activated p38 MAPK and induced interleukin 8 (IL-8) production in human bronchial epithelial cells [40]. The importance of transition metals in PM_{10}-induced nuclear factor κB (NF-κB) activation has been demonstrated by Jimenez *et al.* [33], who showed that PM_{10} collected in the UK induced nuclear translocation, DNA-binding and transcriptional activation of NF-κB, which occurred in the absence of IκB degradation in human alveolar epithelial (A549) cells. Treatment of PM_{10} with both deferoxamine and ferrozine, transition metal chelators with high affinities for Fe^{2+} and Fe^{3+}, respectively, completely inhibited NF-κB activation. Furthermore, exposure of A549 cells to soluble fractions from phosphate-buffered saline-treated PM_{10} activated NF-κB, indicating that soluble components such as metals or organic materials present on the surface of PM_{10} are themselves capable of activating NF-κB. Kennedy *et al.* [41] reported that Utah Valley PM_{10} enhanced NF-κB binding to DNA and IL-6 release from the bronchial cell line BEAS 2B by a copper-driven mechanism. Shukla *et al.* [42] reported that inhalation of $PM_{2.5}$ in mice up-regulated several NF-κB-mediated genes including tumour necrosis factor α (TNF-α), IL-6 and transforming growth factor β. $PM_{2.5}$ also enhanced transcriptional activation of a NF-κB-luciferase reporter in murine alveolar type II epithelial cells, which was attenuated in the presence of catalase. In the same study, ultrafine carbon black, a surrogate for the ultrafine fraction of PM_{10} known to cause oxidative stress in lung cells [43] stimulated transcriptional activation of NF-κB.

DEP, an important constituent of air pollution, increased NF-κB activity and caused IκB degradation in human bronchial epithelial (16HBE) cells, responses abrogated by the hydroxyl scavenger dimethyl thiourea [44,45]. Benzene-extracted organic components of DEP and benzo[a]pyrene induced NF-κB activity in BEAS-2B cells concomitant with expression of proinflammatory genes [46].

Quay *et al.* [47], using ROFA, showed a time and dose-dependent increase in IL-6 mRNA which was preceded by NF-κB activation. ROFA particles also induced transcriptional activation of the IL-6 promoter, a response that was attenuated by transition metal chelation. Vanadium, a transition metal component of ROFA, triggered both EGFR activation and Ras-dependent activation of NF-κB [48,49]. In addition, the vanadium-induced NF-κB activation was ameliorated by overexpression of the dominant negative Ras (N17), suggesting that vanadium stimulates NF-κB through cross-talk with the EGFR signalling pathway at the level of Ras.

The AP-1 pathway is also stimulated by PM_{10} via oxidative stress leading to proinflammatory and proliferative gene transcription [34].

We have demonstrated that PM_{10} stimulates the activity of histone acetyltransferase as well as the level of acetylated histone 4 (H4), resulting in chromatin remodelling that allows transcription [50]. The enhanced acetylation of H4 was mediated by oxidative stress as shown by its inhibition with a thiol antioxidant. The acetylation of H4 mediated by PM_{10} was associated with the promoter region of the IL-8 gene. PM_{10}- and trichostatin A (TSA)-mediated increases in IL-8 and histone acetylation were associated with increases in NF-κB activation. These data suggest that the remodelling of chromatin by histone acetylation has a role in the PM_{10}-mediated proinflammatory responses in the lungs [50].

Calcium signalling has been shown to have a role in the activation of epithelial cells in response to nanoparticles [51] and in TNF-α gene expression in macrophages [52].

Taken together, these data imply that transition metals, organics and ultrafine particles are active constituents of particulate air pollution that stimulate intracellular signalling pathways leading to calcium changes, MAPK signalling, NF-κB activation and histone acetylation which combine to cause enhanced transcription of cytokines and other proinflammatory genes through oxidant-mediated mechanisms (see Fig. 34.1).

Chronic PM exposure and changes in airways morphology

In cigarette smokers, COPD is associated with distal airspace enlargement characteristic of emphysema and/or small airway remodelling ('small airways disease') [53]. There are no studies demonstrating PM-induced emphysema, but several studies have looked at pathologic changes in the small airways in individuals chronically exposed to high levels of PM.

Souza et al. [54] evaluated autopsy lungs from forensic (violent death) cases of 34 residents of low PM regions of Brazil, and 50 residents of São Paolo, a region with a mean annual PM_{10} of approximately 80–100 $\mu g/m^3$, 1991–95. The vast majority of the subjects (90%) were males and the mean age at death was approximately 28 years. Approximately 60% were smokers, but the average amount of smoking, 7 pack-years, was low. Souza et al. graded changes in

the small airways in histologic sections and also determined the gland : wall ratio in the large airways. Regardless of smoking status, no differences were seen for gland : wall ratio between high PM and low PM subjects, but anthracosis, inflammation, wall thickness and mucus hypersecretion were generally greater in smokers and somewhat greater in high PM compared with low PM subjects in both the smoking and non-smoking groups. The authors used the anthracosis score as a surrogate of PM exposure, and found that this correlated with airway wall inflammation and airway wall thickness.

The findings of Souza et al. [54] imply that long-term residence in high PM regions leads to the type of small airway remodelling that has been shown to correlate with clinical airflow obstruction in cigarette smokers [53]. However, this study was confounded both by smoking (more than half of the subjects were smokers) and probable occupational dust exposure (again, more than half had occupational dust exposures). Nonetheless, the statistical analysis indicated an effect of PM level after adjustment for these confounders.

Pinkerton et al. [55] also examined forensic death autopsy lungs, in this instance from 42 Hispanic males from the Fresno County Coroner's Office. During the time the samples were collected, mean PM_{10} levels in Fresno were 43.5 $\mu g/m^3$ and mean $PM_{2.5}$ levels were 22 $\mu g/m^3$. The subjects were again relatively young (median age 33 years) and approximately 50% were smokers. Pinkerton et al. found histologic evidence of cigarette smoke injury in the form of chronic bronchitis and more proximal small airway remodelling in about half of the subjects. The larger airways showed few abnormalities, but the distal small airways contained considerable carbonaceous dust and birefringent particles with the highest particle loads in the walls of generation 1 respiratory bronchioles and in membranous bronchioles. Of particular note, the amount of dust (i.e. visible pigment graded on a semi-quantitative scale) correlated with the degree of fibrosis in these airways.

As in the study by Souza et al. [54], occupational dust exposure was a problem because most of these men had worked in local farming operations or in blue collar occupations and farming is known to be a very dusty process in this region. Additionally, smoking produces lesions that are similar in location and appearance to those caused by dusts, and synergistic interactions between smoke and dust may amplify dust effects. Nonetheless, this study lends support to the idea that chronic high level PM can produce small airways abnormalities.

In an attempt to overcome these problems, we (Churg et al. [56]) examined autopsy lungs from a group of women from another high PM region, Mexico City (3-year mean PM_{10} = 66 $\mu g/m^3$) and compared them with lungs of subjects from Vancouver, a city with low PM (1984–93 average

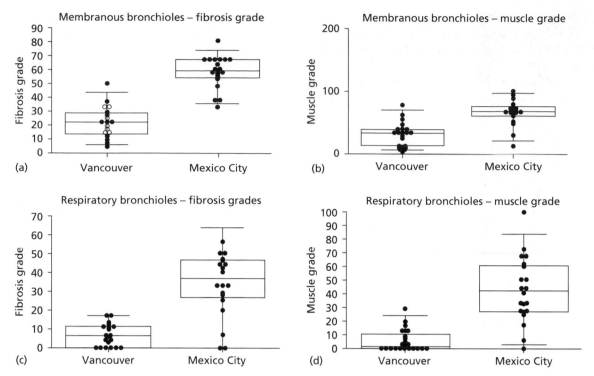

Figure 34.2 (a–d) Box plots showing histologic grades for airway fibrous tissue (a,b) and wall muscle (c,d) in membranous and respiratory bronchioles of autopsy lungs from subjects from Mexico City (high particulate material [PM] area) and Vancouver (low PM area). The bar in the middle of the box is the median and whiskers indicate the 95th and 5th percentiles. For each comparison the measured parameters are significantly greater in the Mexico City lungs.

= 25 μg PM_{10} and 15 μg $PM_{2.5}$) [57]. All subjects were never-smokers, did not have a history of occupational dust exposure and, for the subjects from Mexico City, did not cook with biomass fuels, a process that, as noted above, has been associated with chronic airflow obstruction [13,14]. We carried out a formal grading procedure for amount of muscle and fibrous tissue in the walls of the small airways, and found that the lungs from Mexico City had considerably greater fibrosis and muscle in both the membranous and respiratory bronchioles (Fig. 34.2 and see also Plate 34.1; colour plate section falls between pp. 354 and 355). There was also greater lumenal distortion in the Mexico City lungs. Of particular interest, when we used a microdissection procedure to evaluate particulate content of the airway walls by analytical electron microscopy, we found chained aggregates of carbonaceous spheres with the morphology of DEP.

Thus, our study suggests that, even in the absence of smoking and occupational dust exposure, chronic exposure to high levels of PM leads to small airway remodelling, probably caused by PM particles that enter and are retained in the airway walls. One could argue that our results might also reflect the presence of other types of air pollution, because there are considerably greater concentrations of ozone, NO_2, SO_2 and CO in Mexico City compared with Vancouver. While synergistic interactions are possible, the lesions that we observed are essentially identical to the small airway lesions found in workers occupationally exposed to mineral dusts in the absence of other pollutants [53] and thus we believe that PM are the primary pollutant responsible for these effects.

Taken in aggregate, our data, and the results of Souza *et al.* [54] and Pinkerton *et al.* [55], suggest that chronic exposure to high levels of PM produces distinctly visible small airway lesions, in particular increases in fibrous tissue, muscle and, in the respiratory bronchioles, pigmented dust. These findings thus provide an anatomic basis for the functional abnormalities detected in persons with chronic exposures to elevated PM concentrations.

Experimental studies on PM and airway wall remodelling

Despite the large number of experimental studies demonstrating acute proinflammatory effects of PM outlined in the previous section, relatively little is known about chronic effects.

We have established a tracheal explant system which can be used to examine fibrogenic events in the airway wall.

The model employs small segments of rat trachea which are exposed to dust or PM and then maintained in air organ culture for extended periods, during which time surface particles are taken up by the epithelial cells and eventually transported to the underlying interstitial tissues. Using this system, we showed that amosite asbestos fibres, known fibrogenic agents *in vivo*, produce airway wall remodelling in the form of increased procollagen and hydroxyproline, a measure of collagen content [58]. This process appeared to be driven by active oxygen species (AOS), probably through redox cycling of surface iron on the fibre, because it could be inhibited by deferoxamine and AOS scavengers.

To examine the effects of PM, we employed two different approaches. First, 0.12 μm TiO_2 particles were used as a model of relatively inert fine PM particles [59]. By themselves the TiO_2 particles had no effect in the tracheal explants, but if the particles were first loaded with cationic iron by incubation in an Fe(II)/Fe(III) chloride solution, they caused increased pro-collagen gene expression and increased hydroxyproline in a fashion analogous to asbestos. The hydroxyl radical scavenger tetramethylthiourea (TMTU) and deferoxamine prevented these effects. Fibrogenesis was mediated through NF-κB activation with an unusual pattern of IκBα phosphorylation, because increased levels of both phosphoserine-32/36 and phosphotyrosine were found. These findings suggested that otherwise inert particles that contain bioavailable iron can cause generation of AOS and subsequent fibrogenesis through an NF-κB mediated mechanism involving IκBα degradation, possibly via two different mechanisms in the epithelial and mesenchymal compartments. Of interest, iron loading also lead to an NF-κB dependent increase in gene expression of prolyl-4-hydroxylase, an enzyme crucial to collagen formation, thus providing one mechanism by which AOS may control tissue collagen levels.

To determine whether actual PM could induce airway wall remodelling, explants were exposed to Ottawa Urban Air Particles (EHC93, closely corresponding to PM_{10}) or DEP [60]. After 7 days in air organ culture, both types of PM produced increased procollagen gene expression and increased tissue hydroxyproline, and these effects could be completely blocked by antioxidants and NF-κB inhibitors. Both types of PM also produced increases in gene expression of TGF-β_1, a powerful pro-fibrogenic cytokine. With the Ottawa urban air particles EHC93, TGF-β gene expression operated through an AOS-driven pathway, but for DEP, TGF-β gene expression proceeded through a MAPK pathway. These findings therefore show that PM particles can produce airway wall fibrosis and that a variety of different pathways are involved.

Iron is an important component of many types of PM, and the findings just described correspond in a general way to a considerable number of observations that link PM toxicity to the presence of transition metals, mostly iron, but also vanadium [33,47,61–63]. To further investigate the role of iron, we treated iron-loaded TiO_2 with citrate and then applied the citrate extract to tracheal explants [59]. The extract proved to be an even more powerful inducer of pro-collagen gene expression than was the dust itself. Thus, these results imply that leaching of redox-active iron from PM may be one mechanism behind PM-induced airway wall remodelling, although other mechanisms probably apply to DEP.

Air pollution, COPD and cardiovascular disease

There is now convincing evidence of a link between air pollution, especially particles, and deaths and hospitalizations for cardiovascular disease. In humans, this has been demonstrated epidemiologically as increased cardiovascular deaths [17,64] and hospitalization [65] in relation to increases in PM_{10}. In addition, panel studies have shown increases in PM to be associated with triggering of myocardial infarction [66] and increased dysrhythmia [67]. These effects could be driven by a number of mechanisms including local inflammation in the lungs causing systemic inflammatory effects (reviewed in [68]) that could impact on atherosclerotic plaque stability [69]. Irritative or inflammatory effects of particles could also affect the autonomic nervous system to cause effects on heart rhythm [70].

In COPD there is a two- to threefold increased risk of cardiovascular disease, and ischemic cardiac injury is found in COPD in association with increased acute phase proteins [71]. Systemic inflammation is well-documented in COPD [72] and increases in C-reactive protein [73] and fibrinogen [74] have been reported. Increases in these components of the acute phase response are also related to increases in PM in normal elderly people and are an independent risk factor for acute cardiovascular mortality [75]. Hypertension is also a risk factor for acute cardiovascular death and hypertension is common in COPD [76].

Atheromatous plaques, the inflammatory lesions of coronary artery disease, form in the walls of arteries and typically contain leucocytes, smooth-muscle cells, foam cells and a lipid-rich core capped by a fibrous layer of connective tissue and fibroblasts [77]. The lipid core of the plaque is highly thrombogenic, containing lipid-rich macrophage foam cells. When a plaque ruptures, thrombogenesis can result, leading to an ischemic episode. It is notable that plaque rupture and small areas of denudation and thrombus deposition are a common subclinical finding on the surface of atheromatous plaques at autopsy [78]. These findings suggest that the balance between fibrinogenesis and fibrinolysis is the factor that modifies plaque rupture and dictates whether a thrombus forms or not. Any effect of particle deposition in the lungs that favours clotting would increase the likelihood of thrombus formation in a susceptible individual when a plaque ruptures. Known risk factors include increased plasma fibrinogen, factor VII coagulant activity (factor VIIc), as well as impaired endogenous fibrinolysis. It is the relative balance between the acute local release of tissue plasminogen activator (tPA) and its subsequent inhibition through the formation of complexes with plasminogen activator inhibitor type 1 (PAI-1), which determines the level of endogenous fibrinolytic activity and hence the risk of propagation of subclinical microthrombi on atheromatous plaques, that ultimately lead to coronary arterial occlusion and myocardial ischaemia [29].

In a human *in vivo* model to assess the acute fibrinolytic capacity, the endothelium-dependent vasodilator, substance P can be used to stimulate tPA release in the forearm blood vessels [79]. Acute cigarette smoking has been shown to cause a marked inhibition of both peripheral arterial and coronary arterial substance P-induced tPA release [79,80].

Many of the mechanisms of cigarette smoke induced proinflammatory events are mediated by oxidative stress [81] and similar mechanisms have been invoked for environmental particles [31]. Thus, oxidative stress could be a mechanism for particle-induced changes in fibrinolysis, which may be relevant to thrombosis propagation and coronary artery occlusion in susceptible individuals in response to increased particulate air pollution levels. In COPD, many of the risk factors for sudden cardiovascular death are present: hypertension, acute phase response, oxidative stress, cigarette smoke induced fibrinolytic deficit and all of these are potentially subject to modification by air pollution. Thus, COPD patients can be seen as a particularly susceptible group for the adverse cardiovascular effects of PM.

Conclusions

Epidemiological studies show a clear relationship between increases in air pollution levels and both mortality and morbidity in patients with established COPD. Such studies also suggest that, even in non-smokers, long-term exposure to high levels of ambient pollutants can by itself cause COPD. It is not easy, given the complex nature of air pollution, to ascribe these effects to a single entity, and all of the main gaseous pollution components have proinflammatory effects. However, particles appear to be especially harmful. An accumulating body of experimental evidence suggests that oxidative stress induced by particles, especially those containing transition metals, along with the inflammatory reaction to such particles, are the underlying mechanisms. Chronic inflammatory and fibrogenic responses to the background particle pollution cloud could cause long-term remodelling of airways, while short-term increases in PM_{10} might elicit an additional inflammatory burden on the airways, causing exacerbations. COPD patients are a susceptible group for cardiovascular disease and PM-mediated oxidative stress and inflammation can impact on important coagulation and atherogenic pathways which may explain the increased cardiovascular mortality and morbidity associated with increases in particulate air pollution.

Acknowledgements

A.C. is supported by grants MOP 42539 and 53157 from the Canadian Institutes of Health Research and a grant from the BC Lung Association. K.D. gratefully acknowledges the support of the Colt Foundation.

References

1 MacNee W, Donaldson K. Particulate air pollution: injurious and protective mechanisms in the lungs. In: Holgate ST, Samet JM, Koren HS, Maynard RL, eds. *Air Pollution and Health*. San Diego, CA: Academic Press, 1999: 653–72.

2 Rahman I, MacNee W. Role of oxidants/antioxidants in smoking-induced lung-diseases. *Free Radic Biol Med* 1996;**21**: 669–81.

3 Expert Panel on Air Quality. *Particles*. London: HSO, 1995.

4 Quality of Urban Air Review Group. *Airborne Particulate Matter in the United Kingdom: Third Report of the Quality of Urban Air Review Group*. 1996.

5 International Standards Organization. *Air Quality: Particle Size Fraction Definitions for Health-Related Sampling*. IS 7708. Geneva: ISO, 1994.

6 Sunyer J, Basagana X. Particles, and not gases, are associated with the risk of death in patients with chronic obstructive pulmonary disease. *Int J Epidemiol* 2001;**30**:1138–40.

7 Abbey DE, Mills PK, Petersen FF, Beeson WL. Long-term ambient concentrations of total suspended particulates and oxidants as related to incidence of chronic disease in California Seventh-Day Adventists. *Environ Health Perspect* 1991;**94**:43–50.

8 Abbey DE, Hwang BL, Burchette RJ, Vancuren T, Mills PK. Estimated long-term ambient concentrations of PM_{10} and development of respiratory symptoms in a nonsmoking population. *Arch Environ Health* 1995;**50**:139–52.

9 Abbey DE, Burchette RJ, Knutsen SF *et al*. Long-term particulate and other air pollutants and lung function in nonsmokers. *Am J Respir Crit Care Med* 1998;**158**:289–98.

10 Abbey DE, Nishino N, McDonnell WF *et al*. Long-term inhalable particles and other air pollutants related to mortality in nonsmokers. *Am J Respir Crit Care Med* 1999;**159**:373–82.

11 Detels R, Tashkin DP, Sayre JW *et al*. The UCLA population studies of CORD: X. A cohort study of changes in respiratory function associated with chronic exposure to SOx, NOx, and hydrocarbons. *Am J Public Health* 1991;**81**:350–9.

12 Tashkin DP, Detels R, Simmons M *et al*. The UCLA population studies of chronic obstructive respiratory disease: XI. Impact of air pollution and smoking on annual change in forced expiratory volume in one second. *Am J Respir Crit Care Med* 1994;**149**:1209–17.

13 Perez-Padilla R, Regalado J, Vedal S *et al*. Exposure to biomass smoke and chronic airway disease in Mexican women: a case–control study. *Am J Respir Crit Care Med* 1996;**154**:701–6.

14 Dennis RJ, Maldonado D, Norman S *et al*. Wood smoke exposure and risk for obstructive airways disease among women. *Chest* 1996;**109**:55–6S.

15 Brauer M, Bartlett K, Regalado-Pineda J, Perez-Padilla R. Assessment of particulate concentrations from domestic biomass combustion in rural Mexico. *Environ Sci Technol* 1996;**30**:104–9.

16 Smith K. Fuel combustion, air pollution exposure and health: the situation in developing countries. *Annu Rev Energy Environ* 1993;**18**:529–66.

17 Schwartz J. What are people dying of on high air-pollution days. *Environ Res* 1994;**64**:26–35.

18 Lippmann M, Ito K, Nadas A, Burnett RT. Association of particulate matter components with daily mortality and morbidity in urban populations. *Res Rep Health Eff Inst* 2000;**95**:5–72; discussion 73–82.

19 Wong TW, Tam WS, Yu TS, Wong AH. Associations between daily mortalities from respiratory and cardiovascular diseases and air pollution in Hong Kong, China. *Occup Environ Med* 2002;**59**:30–5.

20 Fischer P, Hoek G, Brunekreef B, Verhoeff A, van Wijnen J. Air pollution and mortality in the Netherlands: are the elderly more at risk? *Eur Respir J Suppl* 2003;**40**:34–38S.

21 Tobias GA, Sunyer DJ, Castellsague PJ, Saez ZM, AntoBoque JM. Impact of air pollution on the mortality and emergencies of chronic obstructive pulmonary disease and asthma in Barcelona. [In Spanish] *Gac Sanit* 1998;**12**:223–30.

22 Morgan G, Corbett S, Wlodarczyk J. Air pollution and hospital admissions in Sydney, Australia, 1990 to 1994. *Am J Public Health* 1998;**88**:1761–6.

23 Harre ES, Price PD, Ayrey RB *et al*. Respiratory effects of air pollution in chronic obstructive pulmonary disease: a three month prospective study. *Thorax* 1997;**52**:1040–4.

24 Moolgavkar SH, Luebeck EG, Anderson EL. Air pollution and hospital admissions for respiratory causes in Minneapolis-St. Paul and Birmingham. *Epidemiology* 1997;**8**:364–70.

25 Anderson HR, Spix C, Medina S *et al*. Air pollution and daily admissions for chronic obstructive pulmonary disease in 6 European cities: results from the APHEA project. *Eur Respir J* 1997;**10**:1064–71.

26 Wordley J, Walters S, Ayres JG. Short term variations in hospital admissions and mortality and particulate air pollution. *Occup Environ Med* 1997;**54**:108–16.

27 Dab W, Medina S, Quenel P *et al*. Short term respiratory health effects of ambient air pollution: results of the APHEA project in Paris. *J Epidemiol Community Health* 1996;**50**(Suppl 1):S42–6.

28 Schwartz J. Air pollution and hospital admissions for the elderly in Birmingham, Alabama. *Am J Epidemiol* 1994;**139**: 589–98.

29 Sunyer J, Saez M, Murillo C *et al*. Air pollution and emergency room admissions for chronic obstructive pulmonary disease: a 5-year study. *Am J Epidemiol* 1993;**137**:701–5.

30 Janssen NA, Schwartz J, Zanobetti A, Suh HH. Air conditioning and source-specific particles as modifiers of the effect of PM_{10} on hospital admissions for heart and lung disease. *Environ Health Perspect* 2002;**110**:43–9.

31 Donaldson K, Stone V, Borm PJ *et al*. Oxidative stress and calcium signaling in the adverse effects of environmental particles (PM_{10}). *Free Radic Biol Med* 2003;**34**:1369–82.

32 Donaldson K, Brown DM, Mitchell C *et al*. Free radical activity of PM_{10}: iron-mediated generation of hydroxyl radicals. *Environ Health Perspect* 1997;**105**:1285–9.

33 Jimenez LA, Thompson J, Brown DA *et al*. Activation of NF-κB by PM_{10} occurs via an iron-mediated mechanism in the absence of IκB degradation. *Toxicol Appl Pharmacol* 2000;**166**: 101–10.

34 Gilmour PS, Rahman I, Hayashi S *et al*. Adenoviral E1A primes alveolar epithelial cells to PM_{10}-induced transcription of interleukin-8. *Am J Physiol Lung Cell Mol Physiol* 2001;**281**: L598–606.

35 Li XY, Gilmour PS, Donaldson K, MacNee W. Free radical activity and pro-inflammatory effects of particulate air pollution (PM_{10}) *in vivo* and *in vitro*. *Thorax* 1996;**51**:1216–22.

36 Ghio AJ, Kim C, Devlin RB. Concentrated ambient air particles induce mild pulmonary inflammation in healthy human volunteers. *Am J Respir Crit Care Med* 2000;**162**: 981–8.

37 Timblin C, BeruBe K, Churg A *et al*. Ambient particulate matter causes activation of the c-jun kinase/stress-activated protein kinase cascade and DNA synthesis in lung epithelial cells. *Cancer Res* 1998;**58**:4543–7.

38 Wu W, Graves LM, Jaspers I *et al*. Activation of the EGF receptor signaling pathway in human airway epithelial cells exposed to metals. *Am J Physiol* 1999;**277**:L924–31.

39 Mondal K, Stephen HJ, Becker S. Adhesion and pollution particle-induced oxidant generation is neither necessary nor sufficient for cytokine induction in human alveolar macrophages. *Am J Respir Cell Mol Biol* 2000;**22**:200–8.

40 Hashimoto S, Gon Y, Takeshita I *et al*. Diesel exhaust particles activate p38 MAP kinase to produce interleukin 8 and RANTES by human bronchial epithelial cells and *N*-acetylcysteine attenuates p38 MAP kinase activation. *Am J Respir Crit Care Med* 2000;**161**:280–5.

41 Kennedy T, Ghio AJ, Reed W *et al*. Copper-dependent inflammation and nuclear factor-κB activation by particulate air pollution. *Am J Respir Cell Mol Biol* 1998;**19**:366–78.

42 Shukla A, Timblin C, BeruBe K *et al*. Inhaled particulate matter causes expression of nuclear factor (NF)-κB-related genes and oxidant-dependent NF-κB activation *in vitro*. *Am J Respir Cell Mol Biol* 2000;**23**:182–7.

43 Stone V, Shaw J, Brown DM *et al*. The role of oxidative stress in the prolonged inhibitory effect of ultrafine carbon black on epithelial cell function. *Toxicol In Vitro* 1998;**12**:649–59.

44 Takizawa H, Ohtoshi T, Kawasaki S *et al*. Diesel exhaust particles induce NF-κB activation in human bronchial epithelial cells *in vitro*: importance in cytokine transcription. *J Immunol* 1999;**162**:4705–11.

45 Bonvallot V, Baeza-Squiban A, Baulig A *et al.* Organic compounds from diesel exhaust particles elicit a proinflammatory response in human airway epithelial cells and induce cytochrome p450 1A1 expression. *Am J Respir Cell Mol Biol* 2001;**25**:515–21.

46 Kawasaki S, Takizawa H, Takami K *et al.* Benzene-extracted components are important for the major activity of diesel exhaust particles: effect on interleukin-8 gene expression in human bronchial epithelial cells. *Am J Respir Cell Mol Biol* 2001;**24**:419–26.

47 Quay JL, Reed W, Samet J, Devlin RB. Air pollution particles induce IL-6 gene expression in human airway epithelial cells via NF-κB activation. *Am J Respir Cell Mol Biol* 1998;**19**: 98–106.

48 Wu W, Jaspers I, Zhang W, Graves LM, Samet JM. Role of Ras in metal-induced EGF receptor signaling and NF-κB activation in human airway epithelial cells. *Am J Physiol Lung Cell Mol Physiol* 2002;**282**:L1040–8.

49 Ghio AJ, Carter JD, Samet JM *et al.* Ferritin expression after *in vitro* exposures of human alveolar macrophages to silica is iron-dependent. *Am J Respir Cell Mol Biol* 1997;**17**:533–40.

50 Gilmour PS, Rahman I, Donaldson K, MacNee W. Histone acetylation regulates epithelial IL-8 release mediated by oxidative stress from environmental particles. *Am J Physiol Lung Cell Mol Physiol* 2003;**284**:L533–40.

51 Stone V, Tuinman M, Vamvakopoulos JE *et al.* Increased calcium influx in a monocytic cell line on exposure to ultrafine carbon black. *Eur Respir J* 2000;**15**:297–303.

52 Brown DM, Donaldson K, Borm PJ, *et al.* Calcium and ROS-mediated activation of transcription factors and TNF-alpha cytokine gene expression in macrophages exposed to ultrafine particles. *Am J Physiol Lung Cell Mol Physiol* 2004;**286**:L344–53.

53 Wright JL, Cagle P, Churg A, Colby TV, Myers J. Diseases of the small airways. *Am Rev Respir Dis* 1992;**146**:240–62.

54 Souza MB, Saldiva PH, Pope CA, Capelozzi VL. Respiratory changes due to long-term exposure to urban levels of air pollution: a histopathologic study in humans. *Chest* 1998; **113**:1312–8.

55 Pinkerton KE, Green FH, Saiki C *et al.* Distribution of particulate matter and tissue remodeling in the human lung. *Environ Health Perspect* 2000;**108**:1063–9.

56 Churg A, Brauer M, del Carmen Avila-Casado M, Fortoul TI, Wright JL. Chronic exposure to high levels of particulate air pollution and small airway remodeling. *Environ Health Perspect* 2003;**111**:714–8.

57 Brook J, Dann TF. The relationship among TSP, PM_{10}, $PM_{2.5}$, and inorganic constituents of atmospheric particulate matter at multiple Canadian locations. *J Air Waste Manag Assoc* 1997; **47**:2–19.

58 Dai J, Churg A. Relationship of fiber surface iron and active oxygen species to expression of procollagen, PDGF-A, and TGF-β_1 in tracheal explants exposed to amosite asbestos. *Am J Respir Cell Mol Biol* 2001;**24**:427–35.

59 Dai J, Xie C, Churg A. Iron loading makes a nonfibrogenic model air pollutant particle fibrogenic in rat tracheal explants. *Am J Respir Cell Mol Biol* 2002;**26**:685–93.

60 Dai J, Xie C, Vincent R, Churg A. Air pollution particles produce airway wall remodeling in rat tracheal explants. *Am J Respir Cell Mol Biol* 2003;**29**:352–8.

61 Costa DL, Dreher KL. Bioavailable transition metals in particulate matter mediate cardiopulmonary injury in healthy and compromised animal models. *Environ Health Perspect* 1997;**105**(Suppl 5):1053–60.

62 Frampton MW, Ghio AJ, Samet JM *et al.* Effects of aqueous extracts of PM_{10} filters from the Utah valley on human airway epithelial cells. *Am J Physiol* 1999;**277**:L960–7.

63 Ghio AJ, Stonehuerner J, Dailey LA, Carter JD. Metals associated with both the water-soluble and insoluble fractions of an ambient air pollution particle catalyze an oxidative stress. *Inhal Toxicol* 1999;**11**:37–49.

64 Hoek G, Schwartz JD, Groot B, Eilers P. Effects of ambient particulate matter and ozone on daily mortality in Rotterdam, the Netherlands. *Arch Environ Health* 1997;**52**:455–63.

65 Poloniecki JD, Atkinson RW, de Leon AP, Anderson HR. Daily time series for cardiovascular hospital admissions and previous day's air pollution in London, UK. *Occup Environ Med* 1997;**54**:535–40.

66 Peters A, Dockery DW, Muller JE, Mittleman MA. Increased particulate air pollution and the triggering of myocardial infarction. *Circulation* 2001;**103**:2810–5.

67 Peters A, Liu E, Verrier RL *et al.* Air pollution and incidence of cardiac arrhythmia. *Epidemiology* 2000;**11**:11–7.

68 Donaldson K, Stone V, Seaton A, MacNee W. Ambient particle inhalation and the cardiovascular system: potential mechanisms. *Environ Health Perspect* 2001;**109**(Suppl 4):523–7.

69 Suwa T, Hogg JC, Quinlan KB *et al.* Particulate air pollution induces progression of atherosclerosis. *J Am Coll Cardiol* 2002; **39**:935–42.

70 Magari SR, Schwartz J, Williams PL *et al.* The association between personal measurements of environmental exposure to particulates and heart rate variability. *Epidemiology* 2002; **13**:305–10.

71 Sin DD, Man SF. Why are patients with chronic obstructive pulmonary disease at increased risk of cardiovascular diseases? The potential role of systemic inflammation in chronic obstructive pulmonary disease. *Circulation* 2003;**107**:1514–9.

72 Agusti AG, Noguera A, Sauleda J *et al.* Systemic effects of chronic obstructive pulmonary disease. *Eur Respir J* 2003;**21**: 347–60.

73 Peters A, Frohlich M, Doring A *et al.* Particulate air pollution is associated with an acute phase response in men; results from the MONICA–Augsburg Study. *Eur Heart J* 2001;**22**: 1198–204.

74 Prescott GJ, Lee RJ, Cohen GR *et al.* Investigation of factors which might indicate susceptibility to particulate air pollution. *Occup Environ Med* 2000;**57**:53–7.

75 Pope CA III. Particulate air pollution, C-reactive protein, and cardiac risk. *Eur Heart J* 2001;**22**:1149–50.

76 Barbera JA, Peinado VI, Santos S. Pulmonary hypertension in COPD: old and new concepts. *Monaldi Arch Chest Dis* 2000; **55**:445–9.

77 Lee RT, Libby P. The unstable atheroma. *Arterioscler Thromb Vasc Biol* 1997;**17**:1859–67.

78 Davies MJ, Woolf N, Rowles PM, Pepper J. Morphology of the endothelium over atherosclerotic plaques in human coronary arteries. *Br Heart J* 1988;**60**:459–64.

79 Newby DE, McLeod AL, Uren NG *et al*. Impaired coronary tissue plasminogen activator release is associated with coronary atherosclerosis and cigarette smoking: direct link between endothelial dysfunction and atherothrombosis. *Circulation* 2001;**103**:1936–41.

80 Newby DE, Wright RA, Labinjoh C *et al*. Endothelial dysfunction, impaired endogenous fibrinolysis, and cigarette smoking: a mechanism for arterial thrombosis and myocardial infarction. *Circulation* 1999;**99**:1411–5.

81 Rahman I, MacNee W. Lung glutathione and oxidative stress: implications in cigarette smoke-induced airway disease. *Am J Physiol* 1999;**277**:L1067–88.

CHAPTER 35

Viruses in COPD

Sam Hibbitts and Colin Gelder

Viruses are comprised of a limited number of proteins and nucleic acid, either in the form of RNA or DNA. They lack the enzymes required for efficient nucleic acid replication and therefore have to subvert the host cell in order to propagate. Viruses vary in complexity from small single-stranded RNA viruses with less than a dozen open reading frames (ORF) (viral equivalent of genes) to large double-stranded DNA viruses containing hundreds of ORF.

The nucleic acid in viruses can be either single or double stranded. Single-stranded RNA viruses can either have their genetic information on one strand or on several short segments of RNA and this nucleic acid can either be the same sense as messenger RNA (positive strand viruses) or as the complementary sense (negative strand). In order to produce mRNA negative strand, viruses have to produce a positive strand template (cRNA).

Viruses are classified as 'lytic' or 'non-lytic' according to whether they destroy the host cell in the process of replication. Much of the pathology seen during a non-lytic viral infection is caused by the host response rather than the virus itself. Some viruses are able to persist after the acute infection either by lying dormant or by integrating part of their genetic information into the host genome. There is currently interest in the possibility that latent adenovirus infection may contribute to the pathogenesis of COPD (see below).

Respiratory viruses typically target the mucosal membrane of the respiratory tract epithelium and cause a localized infection with a short incubation period of 1–3 days. The lung parenchyma may also be targeted as part of a generalized infection. While most respiratory virus infections are self-limiting, the consequences of this acute infection can have longer term complications, and these are discussed below. Electron microscope (EM) images of the different respiratory viruses are illustrated in Plate 35.1 (colour plate section falls between pp. 354 and 355).

Major respiratory viruses

Negative strand RNA viruses

Influenza A and B

Influenza viruses are members of the *Orthomyxoviridae* and are responsible for local outbreaks, epidemics and pandemics of acute respiratory illness. Although influenza infection usually produces a short-lived self-limiting illness, it is associated with complications, including primary viral pneumonia and secondary bacterial infection, and considerable excess morbidity and mortality. Such complications and death are more likely to occur in individuals with chronic respiratory, cardiac or metabolic disease, the immunocompromised and those over the age of 65 years: the high-risk groups.

Influenza viruses are lytic and possess a negative sense segmented single-stranded (ss) RNA genome approximately 10 kb in size. There are three genera (A, B and C), with influenza A and B being the most significant. The viral genome consists of eight fragments that complex with viral proteins to form a helical ribonucleoprotein (RNP). The virions are typically 100–200 nm in size and spherical with spikes projecting from the outer lipid envelope. The surface spike glycoproteins of influenza A are haemagglutinin (HA) and neuraminadase (NA), influenza B has a combined surface coat protein [1,2]. These glycoproteins exhibit regular limited changes in their antigenic structure, termed antigenic drift. This leads to the emergence of new influenza A and B strains and winter outbreaks and epidemics of influenza.

In influenza A, antigenic drift is interspersed by less frequent large changes in structure termed antigenic shift, with different combinations of HA and NA (new subtypes) and these usually cause pandemics of influenza. Such pandemics have occurred in 1890, 1918, 1957, 1968 and 1977. The 1918 pandemic is believed to have killed at least 40 million people [3]. To date, 15 subtypes of haemag-glutinin and nine subtypes of neuraminidase have been described. While only one or two subtypes are found in most mammalian species, all are present in aquatic birds, which are thought to be the original source of the haemag-glutinin and neuraminidase genes found in pandemic influenza A viruses [4] (for further information visit www.cdc.gov/ncidod/diseases/flu/fluvirus.htm).

Respiratory syncytial virus

Respiratory syncytial virus (RSV) is responsible for a range of respiratory illnesses including bronchiolitis in infants, and coryzal illness and tracheobronchitis in adults. In addition, RSV is increasingly recognized to be an important pathogen in COPD (see below). In temperate climates, annual outbreaks of RSV infection occur during the winter season, whereas its incidence in the tropics is during the summer and rainy months. The virus is transmitted through respiratory secretions. During an epidemic, noso-comial infections are common, particularly in hospitals and nurseries, with virus shedding apparent up to 3 weeks after the acute infection.

RSV is a member of the *Paramyxoviridae* family in the *Pneumovirus* genus with a negative sense ssRNA genome and is non-lytic. RSV virions are 120–300 nm in size with a lipid envelope and glycoprotein spikes on their surface. It encodes 10 viral proteins, eight of which are structural and two are non-structural [5]. There are two serological groups, RSV A and RSV B; however, the significance of this strain variation in terms of clinical outcome and epidemiology remains unclear (for further information visit http://www.cdc.gov/ncidod/dvrd/revb/respiratory/rsvfeat.htm).

Metapneumovirus

Human metapneumovirus (hMPV) was first described by van den Hoogen *et al.* [6] who were able to isolate the virus from young children with respiratory tract disease, and demonstrated, by studying old sera, that hMPV has been present in the European community for more than 50 years. The virus causes symptoms that are similar to human RSV and the majority of children appear to have been infected with hMPV by 5 years of age. The virus also impacts upon the elderly and the immunocompromised. Genetically, it is most closely related to type C avian pneu-moviruses (APV; previously termed turkey rhinotracheitis virus, TRTV). The majority of currently published studies have not looked for this virus.

Positive-strand RNA viruses

Picornoviruses

Rhinoviruses are Picornoviruses and are the most common causative agent associated with the common cold. There are at least 100 different serotypes of this virus, which is transmitted through aerosols, infected surfaces and hand-to-hand contact. Rhinoviruses target cells of the upper respiratory tract causing inflammation. Infections occur throughout the year and although the associated illness is mild in healthy individuals, this virus is associated with exacerbations of asthma and COPD (see below).

Rhinoviruses are non-lytic and have a linear positive sense ssRNA genome approximately 8 kb in size with a 5′ protein primer and 3′ poly (A) tail that in itself is infectious. Picornavirus virions are icosahedral, approximately 18–30 nm in diameter, non-enveloped with a protein capsid. The virus particles enter the cell through attachment to intercellular adhesion molecule type 1 (ICAM-1). The viral genome functions as a mRNA for direct translation into a large polyprotein that undergoes a series of cleavages to form the structural and non-structural viral proteins. Cellular mRNA translation is inhibited and virus release involves destruction of the host cell [7].

Rhinoviruses differ from other members of the *Pircornaviridae* family in that they can not withstand acidic environments and have an optimal growth temperature of 33°C. A number of antivirals including interferons have been tested as treatment for the common cold with limited effectivity results and generation of a vaccine has proved difficult because of the numerous rhinovirus serotypes [8].

Coronaviruses

'Usual' coronaviruses

Coronaviruses are the second most common pathogen associated with the common cold (2–10% of cases). There are two known human serotypes (229E and OC43). Replication of these viruses is restricted to the epithelium cells of the upper respiratory tract and in typically healthy individuals only the nasal passages are affected with no fever or sore throat. However, in patients with underlying respiratory disorders including COPD, coronaviruses can exacerbate clinical symptoms (see below).

Coronaviruses have a large RNA genome of approximately 30 kb that is positive sense ssRNA 5′ capped and 3′ polyadenylated and, as with rhinoviruses, the 5′ cap is infectious in its own right. The virions are pleomorphic, ranging in size from 60 to 220 nm, with heavily glycosylated glycoprotein surface spikes. Entry into cells is thought to involve endocytosis and viral RNA translation produces two large polyproteins that, when cleaved, produce an RNA polymerase. This proceeds to transcribe a negative copy of the RNA genome which serves as a template for transcription of a positive copy and subgenomic mRNAs which each encode one of the viral proteins. A lipid envelope is acquired from the host cell and virus release is through fusion of vesicles containing progeny virions with the plasma membrane of the host cell [9,10].

Severe acute respiratory syndrome

The first cases of severe acute respiratory syndrome (SARS) were reported in November 2002 in Guangdong Province, China, with an outbreak of atypical pneumonia affecting 305 people with five deaths. Epidemiological studies identified spread along recognized international air travel routes with reports of cases in Asia, North America and Europe. Health-care workers proved to be at 'high-risk' with potential exposure to a new and readily transmissible disease. By early May 2003 the cumulative number of reported cases exceeded 7000 in 30 countries over six continents with 623 attributable deaths [11].

General symptoms include fever, headache, discomfort and body ache, with some mild respiratory symptoms. Two to seven days following infection air passages may feel blocked and a dry cough can develop. Transmission is via close contact with an infected individual through aerosols and direct contact with infectious material [12].

A previously unrecognized coronavirus has been isolated from patients with SARS and this is thought to be the causative agent [13]. At the time of writing, the initial diagnostic tests for suspected SARS cases include a coronavirus antibody test and reverse transcriptase polymerase chain reaction (RT-PCR). With no vaccine or treatment yet available, control has been via isolation and quarantine with standard, airborne and contact precautions recommended (www.who.int/csr/sars/en/).

DNA viruses

Adenovirus

Adenovirus is a lytic double-stranded DNA virus with more than 40 known serotypes, responsible for a range of human and animal diseases that affect the upper and lower respiratory tract, the eye and the gastrointestinal tract. Adenoviruses are estimated to contribute to 5–10% of respiratory tract infections in children. The replication cycle of adenovirus is initiated when the virus adheres to the host cell receptor followed by internalization via endocytosis. The viral genome is then translocated into the cell nucleus and transcription of both DNA strands occurs using the cellular RNA polymerase II that forms early and late mRNAs encoding the 'early' and 'late' proteins, respectively. The first early gene expressed is E1A which operates in *trans* to activate the host cell transcription machinery. This gene encodes nuclear phosphoproteins that regulate the expression of certain viral and cellular genes. The E1A protein has a number of functions including initiation of cell division, transformation, immunosuppression and influencing cellular transcription by interacting with nuclear regulatory proteins and thus affecting transcription factor DNA binding. There is an overall activation of the cell and the virus in essence takes over its machinery so that the host cell becomes a manufacturer of virus particles [14,15] (for further information visit www.cdc.gov/ncidod/dvrd/revb/respiratory/eadfeat.htm).

Viral detection techniques

Culture

Virus isolation utilizing cell culture remains one of the predominant methods used by clinical laboratories to investigate clinical specimens for potential viral infection. With appropriate samples and cell-lines, this technique remains sensitive and specific for the detection of a range of viruses when there is a visible cytopathic effect (CPE). A positive viral identification indicates viable virus within a sample which can also be used for further investigations. Virus isolation via culture, however, is a slow process which can take up to 7–14 days before a result is obtained, which is often inadequate for appropriate patient management. Primary cell-lines from primates are often required for an accurate result (best yields for influenza and parainfluenza viruses) and their use is becoming increasingly difficult to justify. In addition, culture has been found to be less sensitive than the emerging viral molecular detection methods and inefficient at detecting viruses with limited CPE.

Serology

The humoral response triggered by viral infection forms the basis of serology testing. Typically, during the acute stage of infection an immunoglobulin M (IgM) and IgG antibody response is observed; however, the functional response is variable. Early serology testing did not differentiate between an IgM and IgG response, with diagnosis determined by seroconversion or rise in Ab titre after acute infection. Insensitivity and cross-reactivity with different antigens plus a positive identification only after an acute infection limited its use in a clinical setting. The latest serological tests are based on solid phase linked immunoassays and include:
1 *Indirect assays:* viral Ag fixed onto a solid phase, patient serum added and presence of specific Ab to this Ag detected, with differentiation between IgM and IgG;
2 *Competitive assays:* compete labelled Ab with Ab present in a clinical specimen for binding to a fixed target Ag;
3 *Capture assays:* capture of IgM or IgG species present in a clinical sample to a solid phase followed by addition of target Ag and labelled Ab.
IgM assays give indication of a recent infection and IgG assays indicate prior infection. More recent serology assays are automated and therefore require limited hands-on time. The main drawbacks to serology testing is still possible cross-reactivity and its dependence on an individual mounting an immune response, therefore it is inappropriate for use on immunocompromised patients.

Immunofluoresence

Direct or indirect immunofluorescence (IF) is an effective rapid diagnostic technique. Monoclonal antibodies to a specific pathogen are utilized and this procedure is used routinely for respiratory viral screening of clinical specimens for RSV, parainfluenza, influenza and adenovirus. A range of specimens can be investigated using IF including nasopharyngeal aspirates (NPA), throat and nasal swabs, with results available in a short time frame. The main drawback of the procedure is its requirement for a quality specimen with enough of the viral target cells for a positive identification. Sensitivity of the assay can also vary with virus variants that may possess altered amino acid sequences, envelope or outer capsid proteins and new emerging viral strains would be missed when suitable antibody preparations are not yet available for their detection.

Polymerase chain reaction

To date, molecular amplification procedures mainly use polymerase chain reaction (PCR) amplification for detection and analysis of DNA viral targets and RT-PCR for RNA viruses. PCR requires a pair of primers that each hybridize to one strand of a double-stranded DNA (dsDNA) target across a defined region that becomes exponentially amplified. The hybridized primer acts as a substrate for a DNA polymerase (*Taq*) that creates a complementary strand through addition of deoxynucleotides. The PCR process can be summarized in three steps:

1 dsDNA separation (> 90°C);
2 primer annealing (50–75°C); and
3 polymerization (72–78°C).

The incubation length for each step and the cycling parameters are optimized for each target and require a thermal cycler. Traditional detection of PCR products uses electrophoresis in the presence of ethidium bromide with visualization by illumination with short wave (254 nm) ultraviolet light. 'Nested PCR' is a variant of standard PCR in which a second round of amplification takes place using the product of the first round as the DNA template and a second set of primers specific for regions within this first round amplicon. This technique is extremely sensitive but prone to false-positive reactions unless great care is taken to prevent cross-contamination. The advent of 'real-time' PCR technology reduces the need for post-PCR analysis with fluorogenic labels incorporated onto the probes generating a signal in proportion to the amount of amplification product produced [16].

RT-PCR incorporates the standard PCR technique with an additional pre-PCR-RT step required to produce a DNA copy of an RNA target. This method utilizes random or specific primers to the RNA target and a reverse transcriptase that creates the first strand complementary DNA (cDNA) via addition of deoxynucleotides. Alternative procedures use thermostable polymerases with RT activity or *Taq*/RT mixes for single-tube reverse transcription and amplification.

Nucleic acid sequence based amplification (NASBA)

Nucleic acid sequence based amplification (NASBA) is an alternative procedure for amplification of RNA targets. It amplifies RNA in a manner analogous to the replication of retroviruses (Fig. 35.1) [17,18]. The NASBA reaction contains oligonucleotide primers and three enzymes: avian myeloblastosis virus-reverse transcriptase (AMV-RT), RNase H and T7 RNA polymerase for target specific amplification [19,20]. The reaction occurs at 41°C and results in the exponential amplification of products within 90 min, producing antisense single-stranded RNA as the major amplification product. Detection of NASBA products has been reported using probe-capture hybridization and electrochemiluminescence (ECL) [17,20] and 'real-time' detection using molecular beacons has been described [21,22]. Molecular beacons are hairpin-shaped oligonucleotides with a loop region containing a probe sequence complementary to the target amplicon and a stem with complementary arm sequences located on either end of the probe sequence [23]. A fluorophore is covalently linked to one arm and a quencher to the other, so in the absence of its target amplicon fluorescence is quenched by energy transfer. When the probe hybridizes to its target to form a rigid double helix, a conformational change occurs that separates the quencher from the fluorophore enabling fluorescence to occur.

New molecular technologies (PCR, RT-PCR, NASBA) may give a more accurate reflection of the contribution of respiratory viruses with their increased sensitivity and specificity, plus their ability to identify new emerging

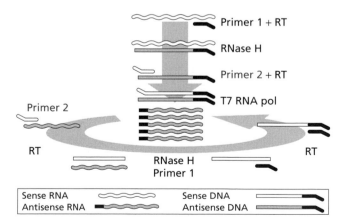

Figure 35.1 Schematic of nucleic acid sequence based amplification (NASBA).

Table 35.1 Comparison of different techniques utilized for viral detection.

Technique	Culture	Serology	Immunofluorescence	PCR	NASBA
Time to result	7–14 days	Variable < 1 day	< 1 day	2–6 h	2–4 h
Cost(s)	Low	Medium	Low–medium	High	High
Assay sensitivity/ assay specificity	Medium–high if there is a visible viral CPE	Medium–high although in some cases cross-reactivity and interference	Variable: high if appropriate Abs available	High	High
Advantages	Viable virus isolated for further study	Speed, numerous sample types can be analysed	Speed, high sensitivity for certain viruses	Speed, possible application to new emerging viruses	Speed, possible application to new emerging viruses
Limitations	Slow and multiple cell-lines required	Some spurious results, inappropriate for immunocompromised patients	High-quality samples for testing required	Cost	Cost
Ease of use	Labour intensive, cell-culture trained staff	Rapid, can be automated	Skilled staff needed	Trained staff required	Trained staff required

CPE, cytopathic effect; NASBA, nucleic acid sequence based amplification; PCR, polymerase chain reaction.

respiratory viruses (e.g. hMPV and SARS) or viruses that grow inadequately in culture and may be missed by traditional procedures. Additional benefits of molecular techniques include fast turn around time for results and use of a range of specimen types even when cell/target copy number is low (e.g. samples from children).

There is a wide variation between the different techniques that have been used to detect respiratory viruses in COPD patients, ranging from traditional culture through to PCR. To elucidate accurately the significance and contribution respiratory viruses have on the pathogenesis of COPD, optimized sensitive and specific viral detection assays should be utilized. Work on this field relying exclusively on culture and/or serology is likely to have underestimated the potential role of viruses. Table 35.1 compares the different techniques currently utilized for viral diagnostics.

Viruses and the development of COPD

Role of childhood infections in later development of COPD

Individuals who develop lower respiratory viral infections in early childhood go on as a group to have reduced lung volume in adulthood [24,25]. The most likely interpretation of these data is that infection of the developing lung in infancy and childhood leads to a reduction in lung growth, although it is possible that individuals with small lungs

as infants who are genetically programmed to have small lungs as adults are more susceptible to lower respiratory tract infection. Viruses are isolated in 20–30% of all cases of respiratory infections in the paediatric setting, and RSV infection is the major cause of bronchiolitis in the first few years of life [26], and has therefore attracted much interest. Indeed, almost 100% of infants are infected with RSV during their early years and of these 66% of infections occur within their first year. Nine studies between 1978 and 2000 studied long-term prognosis of RSV infection with only one studying the control group simultaneously as the RSV-infected hospitalized children [26,27] (study design and results are discussed in more detail later). Study designs varied but all found the post-bronchiolitis group to have increased airway obstructions with diminished lung function that persists for several years (reviewed in [28]). The mechanism by which RSV initiates and induces these changes remains unclear and is likely to involve a number of genetic and environmental factors. However, RSV stimulation of host Th2 immune cells is thought to be a contributing factor.

Strannegard *et al.* [26] studied children hospitalized for RSV-induced bronchiolitis and controls. These children were monitored at 1, 3 and 7 years of age [26,27]. At 1 year, bronchiolitic illness was associated with higher RSV Ab (immune) response and by 3 years allergic sensitization and onset of asthma was more frequent in children with a history of bronchiolitis. Allergic sensitization was elevated in children with higher levels of IgA Ab at 1 year, supporting previous findings that the Th2 response (involved in IgA Ab production) maybe activated by RSV and contribute to subsequent developmental problems in the lung. By 7.5 years of age, bronchial obstructive disease and allergic sensitization (any wheezing) were increased in RSV children, with a higher prevalence of asthma compared with controls. Hereditary and environmental risk factors were also evaluted but RSV bronchiolitis remained the most statistically significant.

A number of studies have investigated potential mechanisms in which RSV can cause dysfunction in the airways. Recent findings suggest that RSV infection may cause changes in both airway and immune function. Kao *et al.* [29] focused on RSV infection of the airway epithelium investigating both *in vitro* and *in vivo* models. Many cell types are thought to be involved in airway injury but the epithelium remains a major target. RSV was found to increase the release of nitric oxide (NO) from epithelial cells and this was dependent upon virus replication and involved Th2 cytokines. NO has numerous functions within the lung and in view of the observed complications associated with RSV infection, may serve as an important signalling molecule for immune cells.

Other groups have shown RSV-induced changes in the autonomic regulation of airway smooth muscle (ASM) and airway hyperresponsiveness (AHR) and sensitization to aeroallergens. Interestingly, early ribavirin treatment of children with RSV bronchiolitis in healthy infants reduced both the incidence and severity of reactive airway disease and hospital admissions for respiratory-related illness [30].

Although many children with RSV-associated wheeze appear to stop wheezing in later childhood, it is not yet known what happens to these individuals in adulthood, and it has been suggested that they might be predisposed to COPD in later life [31].

Adenoviruses and COPD

While cigarette smoking is clearly the major risk factor for the development of COPD, only 10–20% of heavy smokers actually develop significant emphysema and airway obstruction [32]. Thus, other factors including either host genetics and/or environmental exposure must contribute to the pathogenesis of COPD. Latent adenoviral infection has been proposed to contribute to COPD as the production of adenoviral proteins in the absence of viral replication has been demonstrated in an elegant series of studies by Professor J. Hogg *et al.* (see below). Such latent infections are thought to amplify cigarette-induced lung inflammation and contributing to COPD development.

Evidence of persistent adenoviral infection has been reported in the tonsils of children [33], and from PBMCs [34] and lungs [35] of asymptomatic adults [35]. Expression of the E1A protein of adenovirus has been detected in the lung epithelial cells even after the virus has stopped replicating and clinical symptoms have cleared [36]. Studies have reported that the copy number of the E1A gene is found in higher numbers in the lungs of patients with COPD than in matched controls [35].

Animal models with latent adenoviral infection develop an exaggerated inflammatory response and excess emphysema when challenged with cigarette smoke. These studies have supported the hypothesis that cigarette smoke alone results in lung inflammation that is more pronounced when the E1A gene of adenovirus is present. Thus, an excess response to cigarette smoking appears to be linked to latent adenoviral infection.

This has lead to the hypothesisis that the E1A DNA persists after a childhood infection of adenovirus and its gene products contribute to the inflammation process in the lungs of smokers which accounts for why although all smokers display airway inflammation, airway obstruction only occurs in a minority.

A number of groups have attempted to determine the mechanism by which this process of accelerated inflammation in the lung may occur. Keicho *et al.* [32] investigated epithelial lung cells stably transfected with E1A. The inflammatory stimuli lipopolysaccharide (LPS) induced an increase in the surface expression of ICAM-1 and this was mediated by E1A up-regulating IL-8 production (demonstrated at the mRNA and protein level), which was not observed in control cells. The levels of interleukin 1β (IL-1β), IL-6, granulocyte colony-stimulating factor (G-CSF) and granulocyte–macrophage colony-stimulating factor (GM-CSF) were not affected or different between control and transfected cells. Keicho *et al.* [32] speculate that this may be an important mechanism by which amplification of inflammation of the lungs occurs, thereby enhancing its susceptibility to other irritants.

The numbers of neutrophils found in the airways of smokers is proportional to the amount smoked and, interestingly, increased numbers of neutrophils are present in lavage fluid of patients with chronic bronchitis. The role and contribution of neutrophils to airway obstruction is not fully elucidated but is thought to be related to the proteases that they release. However, their presence in the airway would require some form of chemotaxis to enable the observed migration of neutrophils to occur. IL-8 is a potent chemoattractant and activator of neutrophils. In addition, IL-8 levels have been found to be elevated in COPD patients. Taken together, this would suggest that the E1A protein of adenovirus could have a key role in recruiting neutrophils to the airways, thus enhancing the inflammatory response in the lungs that can lead to emphysema.

A study of patients with severe emphysema found the number of different inflammatory cell types to be elevated in the lungs with the exception of B cells [37]. However, there was no significant difference in the smoking history of the patients and control subjects. Interestingly, a fivefold increase in the number of epithelial cells expressing the E1A protein in patients with mild emphysema was observed, which increased to 41-fold in severe cases. The increased levels of E1A were found to be directly proportional to an increased number of inflammatory cells in the tissue and airspaces of the lung. The alveolar type II cells targeted by adenovirus cover 7% of the surface of the lung. Polymorphonuclear cells of the immune system have been found to enter the alveolar space through junctions of type I and II alveolar cells, which would make these cells ideal sites for amplification of inflammatory cell migration. The up-regulation of ICAM-1 and IL-8 by E1A protein that appears to reside in these type II cells long after acute adenovirus infection would increase the number of cells entering the airspace of the lung.

The expression of viral proteins in lung epithelial cells augments the lung inflammatory response via adaptive immune mechanisms. This was demonstrated by a study with transgenic mice expressing influenza viral protein in alveolar epithelial cells. When challenged with CD8+ T cells sensitized to the same viral protein there was an observed epithelial-driven MHC restricted inflammatory response. Thus, there was a specific immune response to the presence of the viral protein in the absence of a lytic infection and this may represent what occurs during a latent infection.

Thus, a number of social, genetic and developmental factors may be required to develop severe infection.

HIV infection and COPD

HIV-1 infects the pulmonary macrophages and lymphocytes of the lung and decreases the numbers of CD4+ T cells. HIV in the lung may also be responsible for the infiltration of cells ('lymphocytic alveolitis') into the alveolar spaces that is observed in all HIV-positive patients [38]. A number of reports have identified a connection between HIV infection and airways disease and emphysema, with an increase in acute bronchitis in HIV-positive patients compared with controls [39]. In addition, HIV is thought to increase susceptibility to smoking-induced emphysema that correlates with increased numbers of CD8+ T-cells as shown in a study comparing lung lymphocyte numbers and physiology between infected and uninfected groups matched by age and smoking history [40].

Viruses and COPD exacerbations

An exacerbation of COPD has been defined as 'a sustained worsening of the patient's condition from the stable state, beyond normal day to day variations, that is acute in onset and necessitates a change in regular medication' [41]. In individuals with mild or moderate disease, an exacerbation may be the first occasion at which they seek medical attention, and is an opportunity for medical intervention and health education [42]. As an individual's lung function slowly declines, the chance that medical care and hospitalization will be required during an exacerbation increases [43,44] and if inpatient care is required it is associated with high treatment cost and considerable mortality (reviewed in [45]).

Individuals with COPD vary considerably in the number of exacerbations they experience. Population-based studies have also established that individuals with chronic lung diseases experience more acute lower respiratory symptoms in association with an upper respiratory tract infection than healthy controls [46,47] and there is evidence that the patients who have the most frequent exacerbations also have the lowest health status [48], and that exacerbation frequency may predict accelerated decline in lung function [49,50], although this is controversial [43,51] and may only relate to current smokers [50]. In addition, while symptoms during an acute exacerbation may be short lived, in a minority of individuals its effects can last for several months [52] possibly because of negative conditioning of skeletal muscles.

Influenza and COPD

Influenza causes regular seasonal outbreaks of acute respiratory illness interspersed by less frequent epidemics and pandemics. During an influenza outbreak there are increases in all cause mortality. Several large epidemiological studies have demonstrated that individuals with chronic illnesses including COPD have an increased risk for respiratory illness-related hospitalization during influenza outbreaks independent of age, and morbidity and mortality in excess of the already high underlying rates associated with old age [53–57].

Influenza vaccines are 70–90% effective in preventing 'flu-like' illness in young fit adults, and approximately 40–60% effective in preventing the symptoms of influenza in individuals over 65 years of age, and have been shown to reduce mortality, hospital admissions and be highly cost effective. These findings lead to the current recommendation that patients with COPD should receive annual influenza vaccinations (ACIP as above). However, while influenza vaccination increases 'herd immunity' it must be emphasized that individuals who have been vaccinated can and do still develop influenza and its complications.

The evidence that viruses have a role in acute exacerbations of COPD

For many years bacterial infection was regarded as the primary cause of acute exacerbations of COPD. However, careful studies have demonstrated that there is no bacteriological evidence of infection in approximately 50% of exacerbations, and that the frequency of isolation of bacteria does not increase during an exacerbation [58,59].

Investigations into the possible role of viruses in exacerbations of COPD can be divided into those employing 'traditional methods' of viral detection including serology and culture, and those using molecular techniques. The advantages and disadvantages of these techniques have already been discussed, the key points being that several viruses, including Rhinoviruses, are difficult to detect by traditional methods, and that the sensitivity of molecular techniques is greater than traditional methods (with the possible exception of immunofluorescence).

Examples of studies using 'traditional methods' include work by Smith *et al.* [47], who detected viruses or *Mycoplasma pneumoniae* infection in 18% of COPD exacerbations and 6% of illness-free periods; Buscho *et al.* [60], who reported viral or *M. pneumoniae* infection in 25% of 166 acute episodes of exacerbation and 14% of 138 remission periods; and Gump *et al.* [61] who reported that one-third of the 116 exacerbations observed could be related to viral infection.

A more detailed study was carried out by Greenberg *et al.* [62] who investigated viral contribution to acute exacerbations of COPD in a longitudinal cohort study, in which they compared patients with COPD with age-matched controls with no previous chronic respiratory disease. Approximately 90% of subjects had received an influenza vaccination. Viral culture and serology were used to provide evidence for viral infection, and exacerbations were considered to be virus-associated if a virus was isolated within 7 days of the onset of symptoms, or if serological evidence of infection was found in consecutive paired samples. There were 221 episodes of respiratory illness in the control group (1.4 per year) compared with 323 in the individuals with COPD (2.4 per year). Within the COPD group, respiratory illness occurred more frequently in individuals with a forced expiratory volume in 1 s (FEV_1) of more than 50% predicted than those with an FEV_1 of less than 50% predicted (3.0 vs 1.8 acute respiratory illnesses per year, respectively). The duration of respiratory illness did not vary significantly between the patients and controls. Viral infections were associated with respiratory symptoms in 39% of the control group and 19% of COPD group, and a similar pattern of viral infection was seen in both groups. In the COPD group, Parainfluenza virus accounted for 29% of exacerbations where a virus was detected, Picornaviruses and Coronaviruses both accounted for 23% (three-quarters of Picornaviruses were Rhinoviruses), influenza A and B viruses (11%), RSV (11%), Adenovirus (1%) and cytomegalovirus (CMV) (1%). No specific viral agent was associated with either mild or severe exacerbations of COPD,

nor was any association found between specific viral pathogens and illness duration.

Walsh *et al.* [63] investigated the impact of respiratory viruses in 134 individuals with COPD or chronic heart disease during two winters. Ninety per cent of these subjects had received influenza vaccination. Nasopharyngeal swabs were taken for viral culture and paired serum samples were examined for serological evidence of viral infection. One hundred and fifty-five illnesses were observed and 36 were probably related to viral infection and five possibly related. The following viruses were associated with exacerbations: influenza A and B (39%), RSV (20%), Rhinovirus (17%), Coronavirus (20%) and Parainfluenza (5%). The clinical symptoms associated with RSV and influenza were the most severe, causing both upper and lower respiratory symptoms, although only the later was associated with fever.

The first study on the role of viruses in acute exacerbations of COPD to use RT-PCR was that of Seemungal *et al.* [48], who investigated a cohort of 83 patients. Respiratory viruses and atypical bacteria were detected by PCR, viral culture and serology. PCR has advantages over traditional culture-based methods for the detection of several respiratory viruses, most notably Rhinovirus. In this study, 64% of exacerbations were associated with a cold up to 18 days before exacerbation. Viruses were detected in 66 of 168 exacerbations (39%). Rhinoviruses accounted for 58% of the viral-associated exacerbations and 16.4% were caused by influenza. Virally associated exacerbations lasted for a longer length of time and occurred more frequently than other exacerbations. Interestingly, in this study, RSV and non-respiratory RSV were detected in 23.5 and 16% of samples taken from patients when stable. This observation needs to be re-examined in future studies, but might indicate a role for RSV in disease pathogenesis, or alternatively that this molecular assay was oversensitive.

The second published study was by Rohde *et al.* [64], who investigated the role of viruses in acute exacerbations of COPD in a case–control study comparing acute exacerbations with stable patients with COPD. Samples from both upper and lower respiratory tract were examined (nasal lavage and induced sputum). Viruses were detected by nested RT-PCR. Respiratory viruses were found more often in respiratory and nasal samples of acute exacerbations of COPD than in stable patients (56 vs 19%), and when the two sets of samples were analysed separately this difference between stable and unwell patents was only seen in the induced sputum samples. The most common viruses detected in this study were Picornaviruses (36%), influenza A (25%) and RSV (22%).

This is a rapidly advancing field: it is important that further studies are conducted, in different populations and with a variety of new molecular techniques including 'real time PCR' and NASBA. Further information is also required on the relative sensitivity and specificity of the molecular assays employed in these studies. In addition, the possibility that the recently discovered metapneumovirus may have a role in COPD exacerbations needs to be examined.

Implications for therapy

The data presented above indicate that viruses can be associated with 30–60% of acute exacerbations of COPD. Current therapy for acute exacerbations relies on bronchodilators, antibiotics and oral corticosteroids. In terms of preventative therapy, all patients with COPD should be advised to have an annual influenza vaccination. To date, attempts to produce a vaccine for RSV and other respiratory viruses have been unsuccessful. Patients should be advised to avoid children (including their own grandchildren) if they are unwell as they are a main source of transmission for many respiratory viruses in the community. In addition, it may not be advisable to bring patients with stable COPD to a general practitioner (GP) or hospital outpatient clinics for review while respiratory viruses are circulating. Staff with acute respiratory symptoms should also avoid contact with individuals with COPD.

Drug therapy for influenza is available in the form of amantadine, and the neuraminidase inhibitors oseltamivir and zanamivir. Studies are required to test the efficacy of these drugs in COPD exacerbations when these viruses are circulating. New therapies for RSV and Rhinovirus infections are coming close to the market and these will need to be rigorously tested in acute exacerbations of COPD.

Overall, there may be a role for the testing of novel antiviral agents in the treatment of COPD exacerbations, through clinical trials supported by viral diagnostics.

References

1 Lamb RA, Krug RM. Orthomyxoviridae: the viruses and their replication. In: Knipe DM, Howley PM, eds. *Fields Virology*, vol. 1, 4th edn. Philadelphia: Lippincott Williams & Wilkins, 2001: 1487.

2 Wright PF, Webster RG. Orthomyxoviruses. In: Knipe DM, Howley PM, eds. *Fields Virology*, vol. 1, 4th edn. Philadelphia: Lippincott Williams & Wilkins, 2001: 1533.

3 Oxford JS. Influenza A pandemics of the 20th century with special reference to 1918: virology, pathology and epidemiology. *Rev Med Virol* 2000;**10**:119–33.

4 Webster RG. The importance of animal influenza for human disease. *Vaccine* 2002;**20**(Suppl 2):S16–20.

5 Collins PL, Chanock RM. Respiratory syncytial virus. In: Knipe DM, Howley PM, eds. *Fields Virology*, vol. 1, 4th edn. Philadelphia: Lippincott Williams & Wilkins, 2001: 1443.

6 van den Hoogen B, de Jong JC, Groen J *et al.* A newly discovered human pneumovirus isolated from young children with respiratory tract disease. *Nat Med* 2001;**7**:19–24.

7 Racaniello VR. Pircornaviridae: the viruses and their replication. In: Knipe DM, Howley PM, eds. *Fields Virology*, vol. 1, 4th edn. Philadelphia: Lippincott Williams & Wilkins, 2001: 685.

8 Couch RB. Rhinoviruses. In: Knipe DM, Howley PM, eds. *Fields Virology*, vol. 1, 4th edn. Philadelphia: Lippincott Williams & Wilkins, 2001: 777.

9 Lai MMC, Holmes KV. Coronaviridae: the viruses and their replication. In: Knipe DM, Howley PM, eds. *Fields Virology*, vol. 1, 4th edn. Philadelphia: Lippincott Williams & Wilkins, 2001: 1163.

10 Holmes KV. Coronaviruses. In: Knipe DM, Howley PM, eds. *Fields Virology*, vol. 1, 4th edn. Philadelphia: Lippincott Williams & Wilkins, 2001: 1187.

11 Drazen JM. SARS: looking back over the first 100 days. *N Engl J Med* 2003;**349**:319–20.

12 Kuiken T, Fouchier RA, Schutten M *et al.* Newly discovered coronavirus as the primary cause of severe acute respiratory syndrome. *Lancet* 2003;**362**:263–70.

13 Ksiazek TG, Erdman D, Goldsmith CS *et al.* SARS Working Group. A novel coronavirus associated with severe acute respiratory syndrome. *N Engl J Med* 2003;**348**:1953–66.

14 Shenk TE. Adenoviridae: the viruses and their replication. In: Knipe DM, Howley PM, eds. *Fields Virology*, vol. 2, 4th edn. Philadelphia: Lippincott Williams & Wilkins, 2001: 2265.

15 Horwitz MS. Adenoviruses. In: Knipe DM, Howley PM, eds. *Fields Virology*, vol. 2, 4th edn. Philadelphia: Lippincott Williams & Wilkins, 2001: 2301.

16 Mackay I, Arden KE, Nitsche A. Real-time PCR in virology. *Nucleic Acids Res* 2002;**30**:1292–305.

17 Guatelli J, Whitfield KM, Kwoh DY *et al.* Isothermal, *in vitro* amplification of nucleic acids by a multienzyme reaction modeled after retroviral replication. *Proc Natl Acad Sci U S A* 1990;**87**:7797.

18 Kievits T, van Gemen B, van Strijp D *et al.* NASBA isothermal enzymatic *in vitro* nucleic acid amplification optimized for the diagnosis of HIV-1 infection. *J Virol Methods* 1991;**35**: 273–86.

19 Fox J, Han S, Samuelson A *et al.* Development and evaluation of nucleic acid sequence based amplification (NASBA) for diagnosis of enterovirus infections using the NucliSens Basic Kit. *J Clin Virol* 2002;**24**:117–30.

20 Chan A, Fox JD. NASBA and other transcription based amplification methods for research and diagnostic microbiology. *Rev Med Micro* 1999;**10**:185–96.

21 Leone G, van Schijndel H, van Gemen B, Kramer FR, Schoen CD. Molecular beacon probes combined with amplification by NASBA enable homogeneous, real-time detection of RNA. *Nucleic Acids Res* 1998;**26**:2150–6.

22 Hibbitts S, Rahman A, John R, Westmoreland D, Fox JD. Development and evaluation of NucliSens basic kit NASBA for diagnosis of parainfluenza virus infection with 'end-point' and 'real-time' detection. *J Virol Methods* 2003;**108**: 145–55.

23 Tyagi S, Kramer FR. Molecular beacons: probes that fluoresce upon hybridization. *Nat Biotechnol* 1996;**14**:303–8.

24 Shaheen S, Barker DJ, Holgate ST. Do lower respiratory tract infections in early childhood cause chronic obstructive pulmonary disease? *Am J Respir Crit Care Med* 1995;**151**:1649–51.

25 Johnston I, Strachan DP, Anderson HR. Effect of pneumonia and whooping cough in childhood on adult lung function. *N Engl J Med* 1998;**338**:581–7.

26 Strannegard O, Cello J, Bjarnason R, Sigurbergsson F, Sigurs N. Association between pronounced IgA response in RSV bronchiolitis and development of allergic sensitization. *Pediatr Allergy Immunol* 1997;**8**:1–6.

27 Sigurs N, Bjarnason R, Sigurbergsson F, Kjellman B. Respiratory syncytial virus bronchiolitis in infancy is an important risk factor for asthma and allergy at age 7. *Am J Respir Crit Care Med* 2000;**161**:1501–7.

28 Sigurs N. Epidemiologic and clinical evidence of a respiratory syncytial virus-reactive airway disease link. *Am J Respir Crit Care Med* 2001;**163**:S2–6.

29 Kao Y, Piedra PA, Larsen GL, Colasurdo GN. Induction and regulation of nitric oxide synthase in airway epithelial cells by respiratory syncytial virus. *Am J Respir Crit Care Med* 2001;**163**:532–9.

30 Edell D, Khoshoo V, Ross G, Salter K. Early ribavarin treatment of bronchiolitis: effect on long-term respiratory morbidity. *Chest* 2002;**122**:935–9.

31 Martinez F. Role of respiratory infection in onset of asthma and chronic obstructive pulmonary disease. *Clin Exp Allergy* 1999;**29**(Suppl 2):53–8.

32 Keicho N, Elliott WM, Hogg JC, Hayashi S. Adenovirus E1A upregulates interleukin-8 expression induced by endotoxin in pulmonary epithelial cells. *Am J Physiol* 1997;**272**: L1046–52.

33 Green M, Wold WS, Mackey JK, Rigden P. Analysis of human tonsil and cancer DNAs and RNAs for DNA sequences of group C (serotypes 1, 2, 5, and 6) human adenoviruses. *Proc Natl Acad Sci U S A* 1979;**76**:6606–10.

34 Horvath J, Palkonyay L, Weber J. Group C adenovirus DNA sequences in human lymphoid cells. *J Virol* 1986;**59**:189–92.

35 Matsuse T, Hayashi S, Kuwano K *et al*. Latent adenoviral infection in the pathogenesis of chronic airways obstruction. *Am Rev Respir Dis* 1992;**146**:177–84.

36 Elliott W, Hayashi S, Hogg JC. Immunodetection of adenoviral E1A proteins in human lung tissue. *Am J Respir Cell Mol Biol* 1995;**12**:642–8.

37 Retamales I, Elliot WM, Meshi B *et al*. Amplification of inflammation in emphysema and its association with latent adenoviral infection. *Am J Respir Crit Care Med* 2001;**164**: 469–73.

38 Beck JM, Rosen MJ, Peavy HH. Pulmonary complications of HIV infection. Report of the Fourth NHLBI Workshop. *Am J Respir Crit Care Med* 2001;**164**:2120–6.

39 Wallace JM, Hansen NI, Lavange L *et al*. Respiratory disease trends in the Pulmonary Complications of HIV Infection Study cohort. Pulmonary Complications of HIV Infection Study Group. *Am J Respir Crit Care Med* 1997;**155**:72–80.

40 Diaz PT, King ER, Wewers MD *et al*. HIV infection increases susceptibility to smoking-induced emphysema. *Chest* 2000; **117**(Suppl 1):285S.

41 Rodriguez-Roisin R. Toward a consensus definition for COPD exacerbations. *Chest* 2000;**117**:398S–401S.

42 Stockley R, O'Brien C, Pye A, Hill SL. Relationship of sputum color to nature and outpatient management of acute exacerbations of COPD. *Chest* 2000;**117**:1638–45.

43 Fletcher C, Peto R. The natural history of chronic airflow obstruction. *BMJ* 1977;**1**:1645–8.

44 Garcia-Aymerich J, Monso E, Marrades RM *et al*. Risk factors for hospitalization for a chronic obstructive pulmonary disease exacerbation. EFRAM study. *Am J Respir Crit Care Med* 2001;**164**:1002–7.

45 Barnes P. Chronic obstructive pulmonary disease. *N Engl J Med* 2000;**343**:269–80.

46 Monto A, Higgins MW, Ross HW. The Tecumseh study of respiratory illness. VIII. Acute infection in chronic respiratory disease and comparison groups. *Am Rev Respir Dis* 1975;**111**: 27–36.

47 Smith C, Golden CA, Kanner RE, Renzetti AD Jr. Association of viral and *Mycoplasma pneumoniae* infections with acute respiratory illness in patients with chronic obstructive pulmonary diseases. *Am Rev Respir Dis* 1980;**121**:225–32.

48 Seemungal T, Harper-Owen R, Bhowmik A *et al*. Respiratory viruses, symptoms, and inflammatory markers in acute exacerbations and stable chronic obstructive pulmonary disease. *Am J Respir Crit Care Med* 2001;**164**:1618–23.

49 Kanner R, Renzetti AD Jr, Klauber MR, Smith CB, Golden CA. Variables associated with changes in spirometry in patients with obstructive lung diseases. *Am J Med* 1979;**67**: 44–50.

50 Kanner R, Anthonisen, NR, Connett, JE. Lower respiratory illnesses promote FEV_1 decline in current smokers but not ex-smokers with mild chronic obstructive pulmonary disease: results from the lung health study. *Am J Respir Crit Care Med* 2001;**164**:358–64.

51 Burrows B, Bloom JW, Traver GA, Cline MG. The course and prognosis of different forms of chronic airways obstruction in a sample from the general population. *N Engl J Med* 1987; **317**:1309–14.

52 Seemungal T, Donaldson GC, Bhowmik A, Jeffries DJ, Wedzicha JA. Time course and recovery of exacerbations in patients with chronic obstructive pulmonary disease. *Am J Respir Crit Care Med* 2000;**161**:1608–13.

53 Listed NA. Prevention and control of influenza. Part I. Vaccines. Recommendations of the Advisory Committee on Immunization Practices (ACIP). *MMWR Recomm Rep* 1993; **42**(RR-6):1–14.

54 Monto A. Influenza: quantifying morbidity and mortality. *Am J Med* 1987;**82**:20–5.

55 Barker W, Mullooly JP. Impact of epidemic type A influenza in a defined adult population. *Am J Epidemiol* 1980;**112**: 798–811.

56 Glezen W, Decker M, Perrotta DM. Survey of underlying conditions of persons hospitalized with acute respiratory disease during influenza epidemics in Houston, 1978–1981. *Am Rev Respir Dis* 1987;**136**:550–5.

57 Foster D, Talsma A, Furumoto-Dawson A *et al*. Influenza vaccine effectiveness in preventing hospitalization for pneumonia in the elderly. *Am J Epidemiol* 1992;**136**:296–307.

58 Sethi S. Infectious etiology of acute exacerbations of chronic bronchitis. *Chest* 2000;**117**(Suppl 2):380S–5S.

59 Hirschmann J. Do bacteria cause exacerbations of COPD? *Chest* 2000;**118**:193–203.

60 Buscho R, Saxtan D, Shultz PS, Finch E, Mufson MA. Infections with viruses and *Mycoplasma pneumoniae* during exacerbations of chronic bronchitis. *J Infect Dis* 1978;**137**:377–83.

61 Gump D, Phillips CA, Forsyth BR *et al*. Role of infection in chronic bronchitis. *Am Rev Respir Dis* 1976;**113**:465–74.

62 Greenberg S, Allen M, Wilson J, Atmar RL. Respiratory viral infections in adults with and without chronic obstructive pulmonary disease. *Am J Respir Crit Care Med* 2000;**162**: 167–73.

63 Walsh E, Falsey AR, Hennessey PA. Respiratory syncytial and other virus infections in persons with chronic cardio pulmonary disease. *Am J Respir Crit Care Med* 1999;**160**: 791–5.

64 Rohde G, Wiethege A, Borg I *et al*. Respiratory viruses in exacerbations of chronic obstructive pulmonary disease requiring hospitalisation: a case–control study. *Thorax* 2003; **58**:37–42.

CHAPTER 36
Bacteria

Sanjay Sethi

Bacterial infection potentially contributes in several ways to the aetiology, pathogenesis and the clinical course of chronic obstructive pulmonary disease (COPD) [1]. However, the precise role of bacterial infection in COPD has been a matter of controversy and debate for several decades [2–5]. Opinion has ranged from a pre-eminent role (along with mucus hypersecretion), as embodied in the British hypothesis, to bacterial infection being regarded as a mere epiphenomenon [2–5]. The last decade has seen a resurgence of interest in this area, with the application of modern research techniques which have significantly increased our understanding of the contribution of bacterial infection to this disease.

Five potential pathways by which bacteria could contribute to the aetiopathogenesis of COPD can be identified:

1 Bacteria cause up to 50% of acute exacerbations of COPD with consequent morbidity and mortality.

2 Chronic colonization of the tracheobronchial tree by bacterial pathogens amplifies the chronic airway inflammation present in COPD and accelerates progressive airway obstruction (vicious circle hypothesis).

3 Invasion and persistence of bacterial pathogens in respiratory tissues alters the host response to noxious stimuli such as tobacco smoke and/or induces a chronic inflammatory response and thus contributes to the pathogenesis of COPD.

4 Patients with COPD develop hypersensitivity to bacterial antigens which enhances airway hyperreactivity and induces eosinophilic inflammation.

5 Acute severe childhood lower respiratory tract bacterial infection damages the immature lung, impairs lung growth resulting in smaller lung volumes in adulthood, thereby predisposing an individual to the development of COPD.

These pathways are used as framework to discuss the potential roles of bacteria in COPD, with an emphasis on typical bacterial pathogens and on information gained from newer research techniques in the last decade. Chronic infection with an atypical bacterial pathogen, *Chlamydia pneumoniae*, which has been a recent focus of investigation in COPD, is also discussed.

Bacterial pathogens as a cause of acute exacerbations of COPD

Both primary bacterial infection of the lower airway and secondary bacterial infection following an antecedent viral infection could cause acute exacerbation [6]. Investigation of bacterial causation of exacerbations in the past relied on sputum culture, serological studies and placebo-controlled antibiotic trials [1]. Because of limitations of the available techniques and study design, the results of these studies have been confusing and contradictory. An understanding of these limitations is important to recognize how more recent investigations with improved methods and design have had different results than these earlier studies.

Sputum cultures

Bacteria are isolated from sputum in 40–60% of acute exacerbations of COPD. Table 36.1 summarizes the sputum bacteriology obtained in 14 recent antibiotic comparison trials in acute exacerbation that enrolled more than 9600 patients [7–20]. Variation in the relative incidence of specific pathogens likely relate to patient inclusion criteria and sputum culture techniques. The three predominant bacterial species isolated are non-typeable *Haemophilus influenzae* (NTHI), *Moraxella catarrhalis* and *Streptococcus pneumoniae*. Other, less frequently isolated, potential pathogens are *Haemophilus parainfluenzae*, *Staphylococcus aureus*, *Pseudomonas aeruginosa* and *Enterobacteriaceae*.

The isolation of a bacterial pathogen from a body site that is normally sterile is strong evidence for a causative role of that pathogen. However, this does not apply to isolation of

Table 36.1 Bacterial pathogens isolated from sputum in recent studies of acute exacerbation of chronic bronchitis. Data is from [7–20]. (From Sethi [114] with permission.)

	No. of patients	% culture Sputum +for PPB	Percentage of total bacterial isolates						
			Non-typeable Haemophilus influenzae	Streptococcus pneumoniae	Moraxella catarrhalis	Enterobacteria	Haemophilus parainfluenzae	Staphylococcus aureus	Pseudomonas aeruginosa
Mean	687	53.7	31.2	14.2	14	11.4	9.4	6.4	5.8
Range	140–2180	28.1–88.6	13–50	7–26	4–21	3–19	0–32	1–20	1–13

PPB, potentially pathogenic bacteria.

bacterial pathogens from sputum in acute exacerbations of COPD. Several longitudinal cohort studies have consistently demonstrated that the incidence of bacterial isolation from sputum was not greater during exacerbations of COPD than during stable disease [21,22].

With increased understanding of bacterial pathogenesis in the past several decades has come the realization that sputum culture, when used alone as a research tool to delineate the cause of exacerbations of COPD, has major limitations. Sputum is invariably contaminated by variable amounts of upper airway secretions that often contain potential pathogens as transient normal flora. This limitation can be overcome when uncontaminated lower respiratory secretions are obtained by bronchoscopy and cultures performed quantitatively, as discussed subsequently. Identification of pathogens as species by sputum culture, in the absence of strain differentiation, does not distinguish between pre-existing colonization and acquisition of a new infecting strain. This limitation can be overcome by strain differentiation with molecular typing of the pathogens recovered from sputum. These new approaches to respiratory sampling and sputum bacteriology, although extremely useful in research settings, because of their complexity are not applicable to everyday clinical practice.

Another important limitation of sputum cultures is sampling error, both within a sputum sample and between sputum samples. Bacterial flora is non-uniformly distributed within a sputum sample, leading to sampling error within a single sample [23]. This error can be reduced by homogenization of sputum and semi-quantitative cultures. Another potential source of error that has not been systematically explored is the sampling error between samples. All studies to date of bacterial causation of exacerbations have utilized a single culture of sputum at the time of presentation. It is quite possible that obtaining multiple sputum cultures during the course of an exacerbation may reveal a larger proportion of possible bacterial aetiology.

Serological studies to bacterial antigens

Development of a host immune response to a microbial pathogen supports a causative role. In the past, this approach was mainly applied to the study of NTHI in exacerbations of COPD, with confusing and contradictory results [1]. A critical analysis of eight of these studies based on current knowledge of bacterial pathogenesis demonstrates their limitations [24–31]. Four of the eight studies compared antibodies in single sera obtained from patients, with sera obtained from healthy controls. Because of wide variability between individuals in such single titres, this approach is not sensitive and could fail to detect significant immune responses [24–27]. In the other four studies with paired sera, the acute sera were obtained at the time of presentation, rather than prior to onset of infection [25–31]. Exacerbations can manifest over days to weeks, therefore a substantial immune response could be present in acute sera obtained at clinical presentation of the exacerbation, which can confound the results. Seven of the eight studies utilized a single or a small panel of laboratory strains of NTHI as an antigen, instead of the strains recovered from sputum during the exacerbations [24–29,31]. Considerable variation exists in the surface antigenic structure among NTHI strains. Therefore, such methodology fails to detect strain-specific immune responses [1]. Furthermore, immunoassays utilized in these seven studies were not specific for antibodies to epitopes exposed on the bacterial surface [24–29,31]. Such potentially protective antibodies often develop against a background of abundant antibodies to non-surface exposed or cross-reactive epitopes, and therefore could easily be missed in such immunoassays.

Recent studies have attempted to address the limitations of previous work and provide a more accurate picture of the immune response to bacterial pathogens following exacerbations. These studies have used the infecting strain as antigen, immunoassays specific for antibodies to surface-exposed epitopes and paired patient serum samples, with the pre-infection samples obtained prior to the exacerbation.

Antibiotic trials

A dramatic benefit of antibiotics over placebo in randomized double blind trials would support the importance of bacteria in acute exacerbations of COPD. However, most placebo-controlled antibiotic trials in acute exacerbations have demonstrated either a small or no benefit with antibiotic therapy [32]. This lack of efficacy of antibiotics has been interpreted as absence of bacterial causation of exacerbations [4]. There are several alternative explanations for trials showing no benefit with antibiotics in acute exacerbations. The expected benefits of antibiotics in a mucosal infection such as exacerbations of COPD primarily are a more rapid resolution of symptoms and prevention of complications. Unfortunately, the speed of resolution of symptoms has not been carefully measured in studies of antibiotics in acute exacerbations. Instead, the primary endpoint in these studies has been resolution or improvement of symptoms 2–3 weeks after the onset of the exacerbation. The systemic immune inflammatory response resolves a large proportion of bacterial exacerbations in this time period, disguising any potential effect of antibiotics. Many of these studies did not enrol sufficient numbers of subjects and are therefore underpowered (type 2 error). This limitation is compounded in studies that included patients with mild impairment of lung function, who are likely to have a low rate of complications. Exacerbations are non-bacterial in 50% of patients, with no expected benefit from antibiotics, again predisposing these studies to a type 2 error. Several of these studies used antibiotics that are not very efficacious against the major respiratory pathogens and may not penetrate well into bronchial tissues and fluids. These factors are likely to diminish the effect of antibiotics in exacerbations and make their effectiveness difficult to discern from placebo.

A meta-analysis of nine trials published in 1995 demonstrated a small but significant beneficial effect of antibiotics over placebo in acute exacerbation [32]. Two more trials have been published since the publication of this meta-analysis. In addition, a trial that was published in Italian in 1991 has been subject to additional analysis and published in English [33–35]. These three trials illustrate the difficulties in interpretation of placebo-controlled antibiotic studies in acute exacerbation. These three trials differ in patient population, antibiotics used, concomitant treatment and endpoints and not surprisingly show different results. Sachs et al. [33] enrolled 71 patients with relatively mild COPD, included patients with asthma and had an 11% incidence of bacterial exacerbations. All

subjects received steroids and were randomized to amoxicillin, co-trimoxazole or placebo. The rate of treatment success in this study was 91.5% and no benefit was seen with antibiotics. Considering the size of the study, the patient population, the aetiology of exacerbation and choice of antibiotics, it would have been surprising to see a benefit with antibiotics.

Nouira et al. [34] enrolled 93 patients with exacerbations of severe underlying COPD requiring ventilatory support in an intensive care unit (ICU) and randomized them to ofloxacin or placebo. No corticosteroids were administered. The tracheobronchial aspirates revealed bacterial pathogens in 61% of the exacerbations. Antibiotics had a dramatic benefit in this study, reducing the risk of mortality and need for additional antibiotics by 17.5-fold and 28.4-fold, respectively.

Allegra et al. [35] compared amoxicillin/clavulanate with placebo in 414 exacerbations in 369 patients with varying severity of underlying COPD. A unique feature of this study was the measurement of primary outcome at 5 days, instead of the traditional 2–3 weeks. Clinical success or improvement was seen with amoxicillin/clavulanate in 86.4% of patients compared with 50.6% of patients with placebo. The difference between antibiotics and placebo was greater with increasing severity of underlying airway obstruction.

Placebo-controlled antibiotic trials demonstrate benefit with antibiotics, especially if patients are enrolled in adequate numbers, have moderate to severe underlying COPD or if the primary endpoint is determined early in the course of the exacerbation [33–35]. Systemic corticosteroids also are of benefit in exacerbations of COPD [36]. Whether the benefit with antibiotics and corticosteroids are independent of each other and therefore additive is an important research question not yet addressed in well-designed and conducted trials. Another important question that needs to be addressed in future antibiotic trials in exacerbations of COPD is whether an antibiotic with greater microbiological efficacy in vitro results in better outcome than an antibiotic with limited microbiological efficacy in vitro.

Taken together, results of sputum culture studies, serological studies and antibiotic trials do not provide conclusive proof for the role of bacteria in exacerbations of COPD. In fact, one interpretation of these observations is that isolation of bacteria from sputum during exacerbations represents chronic colonization: an 'innocent bystander' role [3,4,37,38]. In the last decade, several investigators have revisited the issue of whether bacteria cause acute exacerbations of COPD with either new diagnostic modalities or research techniques, in an attempt to overcome the limitations of previous studies. These investigations provide a more rigorous evaluation of bacteria as a cause of exacerbations.

Table 36.2 Bronchoscopic studies in acute exacerbations of COPD. (From Sethi [114] with permission.)

Study	Subjects	Diagnostic methods	% Bacterial pathogen present	Haemophilus influenzae	Moraxella catarrhalis	Streptococcus pneumoniae	Haemophilus parainfluenzae	Pseudomonas aeruginosa	Other Gram (−)	Other Gram (+)
Fagon et al. [41]	50 ICU patients on ventilator	Protected specimen brush	50*	6	3	7	11	3	5	9
Monso et al. [40]	29 outpatients	Protected specimen brush	51.7	10	2	3		2		
Soler et al. [42]†	50 ICU patients on ventilator	Protected specimen brush Broncho-alveolar lavage Endotracheal aspirate	56	11	4	4		9	6	
Pela et al. [43]	40 outpatients	Protected specimen brush	52.5	1	2	10	1	1	1	7

ICU, intensive care unit.

* $\geq 10^2$ Colony-forming units/mL was used to define a positive culture instead of the usual $\geq 10^3$ colony-forming units/mL.

† Twenty-one patients had antimicrobial therapy in the 24 h prior to admission to the ICU.

Bronchoscopic sampling of lower respiratory tract in exacerbations of COPD

Bronchoscopic samples of tracheobronchial secretions obtained by protected specimen brush (PSB) or by bronchoalveolar lavage (BAL) are uncontaminated by upper respiratory tract secretions and have the additional advantage that bacterial concentrations in these samples above certain thresholds correlate with tissue infection [39]. Studies that have used this methodology in acute exacerbations have consistently shown significant bacterial infection of the distal airways in approximately 50% of patients [40–43]. The bacterial species isolated in these studies are the same spectrum of pathogens usually isolated from sputum during acute exacerbation (Table 36.2).

Chronic colonization of the lower airway remains a potential confounder in these studies. Monso *et al.* [40] addressed this by including a control group of 29 patients with stable COPD for comparison with the patients with exacerbations. Although 25% of patients with stable COPD had bacteria in the lower airways at concentrations of $\geq 10^3$ colony-forming units/mL, exacerbation was associated twice as often with these bacterial concentrations. A higher threshold of $\geq 10^4$ colony-forming units/mL of pathogenic bacteria was seen in 25% with exacerbations and only 5% in stable COPD [40]. Bandi *et al.* [44] utilized bronchoscopy to study infection of the lower airways with NTHI in COPD. Besides sampling the tracheobronchial lumen, bronchial mucosal biopsies were also examined for intracellular NTHI by immunostaining with a monoclonal antibody. Intracellular NTHI was found in 33% of stable subjects and in 87% of exacerbations [44]. The patients with exacerbations were all severely ill, requiring intubation and mechanical ventilatory support.

Bronchoscopic sampling of the tracheobronchial tree provides substantial support for the pathogenic role of bacteria in a proportion of acute exacerbations, in view of the consistent results obtained by different investigators and the increased rate of isolation of pathogenic bacteria in exacerbations than in stable COPD.

Molecular epidemiology of bacterial pathogens

A major controversy in understanding the role of bacteria in exacerbations has been the results of sputum culture studies in cohorts of patients with COPD that included only species identification of the bacterial pathogens isolated. These studies consistently found no difference in the isolation rate of bacterial pathogens during exacerbation and stable COPD [21,22]. An alternative explanation offered for these findings was the 'bacterial load' model of infection in COPD, where an increase in titre of a bacterial species in the airway is responsible for the transition from stable

to exacerbation state [45]. Early studies of bacterial titres in the sputum of patients with COPD did not support this model [21]. However, more recent studies [46,47] have provided evidence that bacterial numbers are increased during acute (purulent) exacerbations compared with the stable clinical state. Recent advances in bacterial pathogenesis have demonstrated considerable genetic diversity between the individual strains of a bacterial species, including alterations in their surface antigenic structure. Such variation in the surface antigenic structure of bacterial pathogens allows bacterial strains to evade pre-existing host immunity and cause recurrent infection. Because the previous cohort studies did not differentiate between the strains of the pathogens isolated from sputum over time in their cohorts, they did not address the possibility that such a mechanism of strain variation could underlie recurrent bacterial exacerbations in COPD.

A recent longitudinal cohort study in COPD combined clinical information, sputum culture and molecular typing of the pathogens isolated from sputum in order to determine whether acquisition of a strain of a pathogen that was new to the patient was associated with the development of an exacerbation [48]. Indeed, the acquisition of a strain that the patient had not been infected with earlier was associated with a 2.15-fold increase in the risk of exacerbation. This increased risk of exacerbation was seen with three of the four major pathogens implicated in acute exacerbation: NTHI, *S. pneumoniae* and *M. catarrhalis* (Table 36.3; Fig. 36.1). *P. aeruginosa* did not demonstrate such an association. These results provide further evidence of the role of bacteria in causing a substantial proportion of exacerbations. Furthermore, they suggest that the mechanism of recurrent exacerbations in these patients is not a periodic increase in bacterial load, but rather infection with a bacterial strain with an antigenic structure new to the host. Such an infection leads to an immune and inflammatory response that presents clinically as an acute exacerbation. Once the

Table 36.3 Isolation of a new strain of bacterial pathogen and the increase in the risk of exacerbation of COPD. (Adapted from Sethi *et al.* [48].)

New strain	Relative risk of exacerbation	95% Confidence interval of relative risk
Any pathogen	2.15*	1.83–2.53
H. influenzae	1.69*	1.37–2.09
M. catarrhalis	2.96*	2.39–3.67
S. pneumoniae	1.77*	1.14–2.75
P. aeruginosa	0.61	0.21–1.82

* Statistically significant increase in risk of exacerbation.

Patient 6: *Haemophilus influenzae*

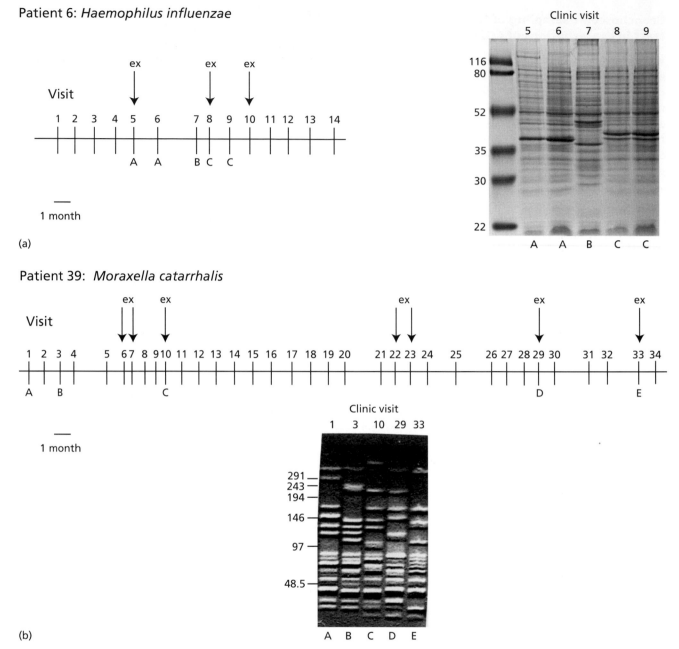

(a)

Patient 39: *Moraxella catarrhalis*

(b)

Figure 36.1 Time lines of patients 6 and 39. Each line with a number on the time lines indicates a clinic visit. The arrows marked 'ex' indicate exacerbations. Isolates of each bacterial species were assigned types based on banding patterns in gels. The first isolate from each patient was assigned the letter A. All subsequent isolates with the identical banding pattern were also assigned the letter A. Subsequent isolates with different banding patterns were assigned consecutive letters B, C, etc. The lettering system is applicable to the individual patient. Therefore, an isolate labelled A in one patient, for example, is not the same strain as an isolate labelled A from another patient. (a) Each letter under the time line represents a positive sputum culture for *Haemophilus influenzae*. Culture results for *H. influenzae* exclusively are shown. The gel on the right is a sodium dodecyl sulphate poyacrylamide gel stained with Coomassie blue showing whole bacterial cell lysates of isolates recovered at visits 5–9. The letters A, B and C indicate the molecular types based on banding patterns. Molecular mass standards are noted on the left of the gel in kilodaltons (kDa). (b) Each letter under the time line represents a positive culture for *Moraxella catarrhalis*. Culture results for *M. catarrhalis* exclusively are shown. The gel below the timeline is a pulsed field gel stained with ethidium bromide showing *Sma*I digested DNA from isolates recovered at clinic visits as noted. The letters A–E represent molecular types based on banding patterns. Molecular mass standards are noted on the left of the gel in kilobases. (From Sethi *et al.* [48] with permission.)

exacerbation is resolved, the strain may be eliminated or may persist in the airways without causing increased symptoms.

In this study, a one-to-one relationship between strain acquisition and development of exacerbation was not demonstrated (i.e. not every exacerbation was associated with acquisition of a new strain and neither was every new strain acquisition associated with an exacerbation) [48]. This is not surprising if one considers the complex biology of the host–pathogen interaction that determines the clinical consequences of a new strain acquisition in a patient with COPD. Strains of bacterial pathogens differ in virulence. Therefore, it is possible that less virulent new strains do not induce enough of a host inflammatory response and therefore symptoms to reach the threshold of a clinical exacerbation. Even when infected with new bacterial strains of comparable virulence, the intensity of the inflammatory response and the threshold of respiratory symptoms at which they perceive the need to be treated may differ among patients with COPD. Adding to the complexity of the situation, strains that were pre-existing in the patient may undergo antigenic variation and the new variant that emerges may evade the host immune response, proliferate and cause increased symptoms [49,50].

Immune responses to bacterial pathogens in acute exacerbations of COPD

Recent investigations have explored the immune response in serum to bacterial pathogens in acute exacerbations of COPD with methods that avoid the pitfalls of earlier studies and are closer to an optimal design. In addition, investigators have started examining other aspects of the immune response to pathogens, such as cell-mediated and mucosal immunity with novel observations. The ability to manipulate bacterial DNA to clone and express recombinant individual bacterial antigens and create bacterial mutants that lack specific antigens has opened up another avenue to investigate the immune response following exacerbations.

Bakri *et al.* [51] have shown that following exacerbations associated with *M. catarrhalis*, new serum immunoglobulin G (IgG) antibodies and/or new sputum IgA antibodies directed at the infecting strain developed in two-thirds of exacerbations. The mucosal and serosal immune response occurred concurrently as well as independently of each other. Outer membrane protein (OMP) CD is a 45-kDa protein, which is a highly conserved surface antigen of *M. catarrhalis* and is a potential vaccine antigen. Approximately 20% of patients with COPD who experience either exacerbation or colonization with *M. catarrhalis* develop new serum IgG to this protein [52].

Several new and exciting observations regarding the immune response to NTHI have also been made recently.

A recent study that characterized the serum antibody response from two adults with exacerbations of COPD resulting from NTHI illustrates that novel findings can be obtained with new investigative techniques [53]. Both patients developed new bactericidal antibodies to their infecting strain. Immunoblot assays with homologous strains revealed antibodies to many antigens, with minimal differences between pre- and postexacerbation sera in spite of development of new bactericidal antibodies (Fig. 36.2).

Immunoblot assays detect antibodies to many epitopes on bacterial OMPs, including those buried within the outer membrane and not available for binding on the intact bacterium. Antibodies to epitopes that are not on the bacterial surface are not likely to be protective. OMPs of NTHI share cross-reactive epitopes with OMPs of many Gram-negative bacteria. Most of the cross-reactive epitopes are buried in the membrane and not on the bacterial surface. In order to detect the meaningful and potentially protective immune response, immunoassays that specifically detect antibodies to epitopes on the bacterial surface should be used. Such assays include whole cell radioimmunoprecipitation assays, flow cytometry and functional assays such as bactericidal and opsonophagocytosis assays. Subjecting the serum in Figure 36.2 to whole cell radioimmunoprecipitation revealed that the patient developed new antibodies to OMP P2 and to higher molecular mass proteins, an observation that was missed by immunoblot assay. Adsorption studies further established that new bactericidal antibodies were directed at strain-specific epitopes on the P2 protein [53]. OMP P2 is strongly immunogenic in experimental animals and humans [54–57]. The surface-exposed loops of the P2 protein are under intense immune selective pressure and show considerable variability among strains of NTHI. The expression of strain-specific immunodominant epitopes represents a mechanism by which the bacterium induces antibodies that will protect against recurrent infection by the homologous strain but will not protect against infection by heterologous strains.

Although most studies of immune response to respiratory pathogens have focused on antibody production, cellular immune responses to these pathogens are also likely to be important. P6 is a highly conserved 16-kDa OMP of NTHI that is immunogenic in animals and humans and is a potential vaccine candidate. Abe *et al.* [58] recently compared blood lymphocyte proliferative response to OMP P6 of NTHI in patients with COPD who had experienced a NTHI exacerbation in the preceding 12 months with patients who had not experienced such an exacerbation and with healthy controls. They demonstrated that susceptibility to NTHI exacerbation was associated with a specific decrease in blood lymphocyte proliferation with OMP P6 (Fig. 36.3). This suggests that failure to recognize OMP P6

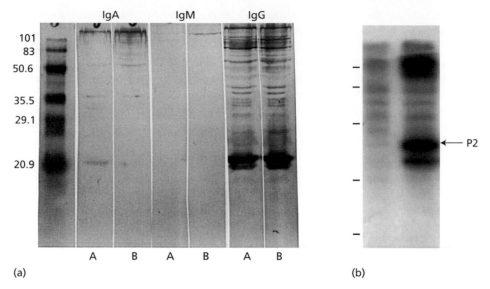

Figure 36.2 Immunoblot assay (a) and whole cell radioimmunoprecipitation assay (b) with pre-exacerbation serum (lanes A) and postexacerbation serum (lanes B) from an adult with COPD who experienced an exacerbation resulting from non-typeable *Haemophilus influenzae*. Assays were performed with the homologous infecting strain. Molecular mass standards are noted in kDa to the left of each panel. Note that immunoblot assays detect antibodies to many bands with minimal difference between pre- and postexacerbation sera. By contrast, whole cell radioimmunoprecipitation assays with the same sera show the development of new antibodies to P2 (arrow) and higher molecular weight proteins following the exacerbation. IgA, immunoglobin A; IgG, immunoglobin G; IgM, immunoglobin M. (From Yi *et al.* [53] with permission.)

as an important antigen may confer susceptibility to NTHI exacerbations in patients with COPD.

King *et al.* [59] compared adaptive immune responses to NTHI in patients with bronchiectasis with chronic NTHI infection with healthy controls and found that while normal controls had a Th1 response, patients with bronchiectasis had a Th2 response. NTHI has the ability to invade cells and persist intracellularly. Therefore, a predominant Th2 response, as seen in patients with bronchiectasis, would not be effective in clearing the NTHI infection. Whether a similar phenomenon is seen in patients with COPD with chronic NTHI infection needs to be investigated.

These studies have demonstrated the development of specific immune responses to infecting strains of NTHI and of *M. catarrhalis* and support the role of bacterial infection in acute exacerbations of COPD. Similar evidence with other bacterial species would help to define their role in acute exacerbations.

Airway inflammation measurement and correlation with bacteriology

An exciting development in airways disease research has been the recognition that sputum measurements of cells and mediators accurately reflect the milieu of the lower airways. Interleukin-8 (IL-8) is the most potent neutrophil chemokine in the lower airways, tumour necrosis factor

α (TNF-α) is important in neutrophil migration in to the airway lumen and neutrophil elastase is released from activated neutrophils and causes matrix degradation. Neutrophilic inflammation is the usual host response to a bacterial infection, therefore bacterial exacerbations should be associated with significantly greater neutrophilic inflammation than non-bacterial exacerbations. Several studies in exacerbations of COPD have systematically examined the effect of bacterial infection on airway inflammation [60–62]. In one such study, bacterial exacerbations were associated with significantly greater IL-8, TNF-α and neutrophil elastase levels in expectorated sputum than non-bacterial exacerbations in the same patients (Fig. 36.4) [60]. Gompertz *et al.* [61] measured markers of neutrophilic inflammation in serial sputum samples obtained from patients experiencing acute exacerbations over 8 weeks and demonstrated that in exacerbations associated with purulent sputum, there is a significant decline in neutrophilic airway inflammation over time. This decline is especially significant in the first 5 days. Contrary to the above studies, Aaron *et al.* [62] were not able to demonstrate a difference in granulocyte inflammatory markers in sputum in bacterial and non-bacterial exacerbations. However, their study was hampered by a small sample size of one bacterial, two viral and 11 exacerbations of unknown aetiology.

This association between pathogen presence and

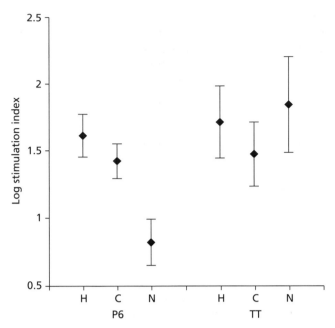

Figure 36.3 Lymphocyte proliferative assays to outer membrane protein P6 of *Haemophilus influenzae*. The three groups of subjects are H, healthy control subjects; C, COPD patients with no exacerbation resulting from *H. influenzae* in the prior year; N, COPD patients with exacerbation resulting from *H. influenzae* in the prior year. The log stimulation index is a measure of lymphocyte proliferation in response to the antigenic stimulus which was either outer membrane protein P6 (P6) or tetanus toxoid (TT). Values shown are log transformed means with standard error bars. (From Abe *et al.* [58] with permission.)

neutrophilic inflammation in the airways strongly supports a bacterial causation of exacerbations. In addition, as neutrophil elastase is a major driver of lung injury, elevated levels of this enzyme seen in bacterial exacerbations could contribute significantly to the loss of lung function seen in COPD.

One can conclude that current evidence indicates that bacterial infection causes approximately 40–50% of acute exacerbations of COPD. The complexity of the host–pathogen interaction that determines the outcome of each encounter between a potential respiratory pathogen and a patient with COPD is being increasingly appreciated.

Vicious circle hypothesis

Because of the wide variety of defence mechanisms, in a healthy lung the tracheobronchial tree is sterile. In patients with COPD, the tracheobronchial tree may be chronically 'colonized' with potential respiratory pathogens, predominantly NTHI, *S. pneumoniae* and *M. catarrhalis* [40,63–66].

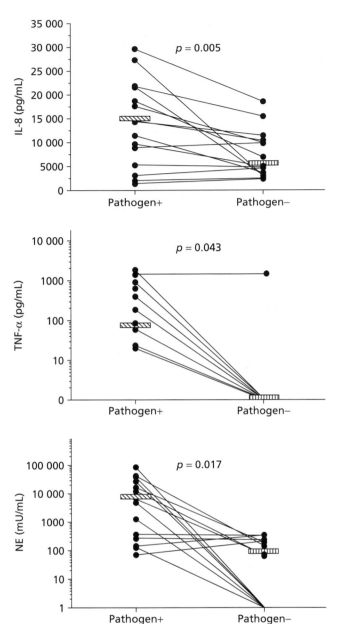

Figure 36.4 Paired comparison of airway inflammation in pathogen-positive exacerbations with pathogen-negative exacerbations. Lines connect the measured values from individual patients. Horizontal bars represent median values. The *p* values obtained with the Wilcoxon signed-rank test are shown. IL-8, interleukin 8; NE, neutrophil elastase; TNF-α, tumour necrosis factor α. (From Sethi *et al.* [60] with permission.)

Although this chronic colonization was recognized several decades ago by bronchoscopic sampling of the respiratory tract, several recent studies have extended those observations [44,65,67–69]. These studies have shown that the incidence of colonization increases with increasing severity

Vicious circle hypothesis

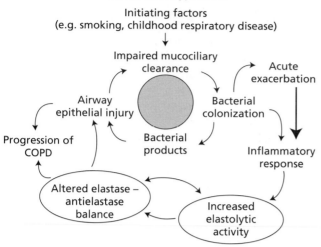

Figure 36.5 Diagrammatic representation of the vicious circle hypothesis. (From Sethi *et al.* [113] with permission.)

of obstructive disease and is more common in current smokers. In one such study, Zalacain *et al.* [65] were able to document colonization by potential respiratory pathogens in 23.1% of mild, 41.7% of moderate and 57.7% of severe cases of COPD. A 'vicious circle hypothesis' explains how chronic bacterial 'colonization' of the lower airways in patients with COPD can perpetuate inflammation and contribute to progression of the disease (Fig. 36.5) [1,70]. There are several reasons to suspect that cofactors besides tobacco smoke contribute to the pathogenesis of COPD. Only approximately 15% of smokers go on to develop COPD. Chronic inflammation persists in the airways and parenchyma in spite of smoking cessation and COPD does develop in non-smokers. The vicious circle hypothesis has been proposed as one such cofactor in the development and the course of COPD. *In vitro* and *in vivo* evidence supporting this hypothesis is discussed below.

Three interlinked components are contained in the vicious circle:

1 Bacteria persist in the lower respiratory tract by impairing mucociliary clearance.
2 Bacterial colonization of the lower respiratory tract is an independent stimulus to airway inflammation with consequent lung damage.
3 Bacterial exacerbations of COPD intermittently further increase airway inflammation and contribute to lung damage and progression of airway obstruction.

Bacterial infection and mucociliary clearance

Excessive or altered mucus production, disruption of normal ciliary activity and airway epithelial injury can contribute to impaired mucociliary clearance. Respiratory tract

pathogens implicated in COPD and their products can cause all of these effects *in vitro*. Cell-free filtrates of broth cultures of some strains of NTHI, *S. pneumoniae* and *P. aeruginosa* stimulate secretion of mucous glycoproteins by explanted guinea pig airway tissue [71]. This stimulation is a true secretory effect and not passive release of preformed intracellular macromolecules resulting from cellular damage. The *Pseudomonas* stimulatory products are 60–100 kDa proteases. The NTHI and pneumococcal stimulatory exoproducts are 50–300 kDa in size and do not possess proteolytic activity. Wang *et al.* [72] have demonstrated that NTHI is a potent stimulator of the mucin gene *MUC5AC* in respiratory epithelial cell lines. Furthermore, cytoplasmic proteins of NTHI were more potent stimulators of *MUC5AC* than whole bacteria and membrane proteins. All 10 clinical isolates tested in this study were capable of *MUC5AC* induction but did differ quantitatively in their mucin inducing capability.

Cell-free supernatants of NTHI and *P. aeruginosa* rapidly inhibit ciliary beat frequency (CBF) of strips of human nasal ciliary epithelium, by inducing ciliary dyskinesia and ciliostasis [73]. Bacterial products may be a potent stimulus for neutrophil migration into the airways, and human neutrophil elastase inhibits ciliary activity and damages respiratory epithelium [74,75]. Therefore, neutrophil elastase released in the airways could act synergistically with bacterial products and cause further inhibition of tracheobronchial ciliary function. NTHI causes airway epithelial injury in an *in vitro* tissue culture model of nasal turbinate epithelium [76]. At 14 h, patchy injury developed to the airway epithelium, with bacterial cells now associating with these damaged epithelial cells but not with intact epithelium. At 24 h, detached epithelial cells with adherent bacteria were seen.

In conclusion, bacteria that colonize and infect the lower respiratory tract in COPD, especially NTHI, are capable of impairing mucociliary clearance by several different mechanisms, which in turn fosters a tracheobronchial milieu in which they can persist, supporting the central tenet of the vicious circle hypothesis (see Fig. 36.5).

Bacterial colonization and airway inflammation

The presence of bacteria in the lower airways in stable COPD has been labelled 'colonization', implying it to be innocuous to the host. Bacteria in the airways are in a constant state of turnover, releasing extracellular products, as well as undergoing lysis with release of a variety of proteins, lipo-oligosaccharide (LOS) and peptidoglycan [77]. LOS is a potent inflammatory stimulus; in fact, repeated instillation of LOS can lead to development of emphysema in hamsters [78]. It is therefore quite likely that this 'colonization' actually is a low-grade smouldering infection that induces chronic airway inflammation. In the large airways, such inflammation would contribute to mucus production and in the small airways it could contribute to respiratory bronchiolitis and progressive airway obstruction [79,80]. Both *in vitro* and *in vivo* studies provide support for these concepts.

Exposure of explant cultures of human bronchial epithelium to LOS from NTHI significantly increases IL-6, IL-8 and TNF-α secretion and intercellular adhesion molecule 1 (ICAM-1) expression in the explanted tissue [81]. The levels of inflammatory mediators attained in the culture medium are adequate to increase neutrophil chemotaxis and adherence *in vitro*. Increased secretion of IL-6, IL-8, TNF-α and monocyte chemoattractant protein-1 (MCP-1) with exposure of a human tracheal epithelial cell-line to whole bacterial cells of NTHI was demonstrated in another recent study [82]. Furthermore, the expression of these pro-inflammatory molecules was only partially accounted for by LOS in the bacterial cell, suggesting that other bacterial components of NTHI also have proinflammatory activity.

An association between bacterial colonization and tracheobronchial inflammation among patients with stable COPD has also been demonstrated in recent studies with both sputum and bronchoscopic samples [83–85]. In the study by Hill *et al.* [83], sputum IL-8, leukotriene B_4 (LTB$_4$), neutrophil elastase and myeloperoxidase activity and albumin leakage from serum to sputum correlated with the bacterial load in the airways determined by quantitative culture of sputum. Soler *et al.* [84] found that isolation of potentially pathogenic bacteria was associated with significantly more polymorphonuclear cells and TNF-α and a trend to higher IL-8 levels in BAL in asymptomatic smokers and patients with COPD. Furthermore, bacterial colonization of the lower respiratory tract occurred not only in 32% of the patients with established COPD, but was also seen in 42% of smokers with normal lung function. Therefore, bacterial colonization of the lower airways appears to be an early phenomenon in the course of COPD. Furthermore, bacterial colonization is an independent stimulus for inflammation in the distal airways and therefore may contribute to the progression of COPD.

Bacterial exacerbations and airway inflammation

Airway inflammation in bacterial exacerbations of COPD is characterized by abundant free neutrophil elastase in the sputum, suggesting that these exacerbations increase the airway elastase burden and could contribute to progressive airway obstruction [60,61]. However, previous epidemiological studies had failed to show a relationship between the number of exacerbations and decline of lung function, which may have been related to limitations of study design [60,86–88]. Two recent longitudinal cohort studies, the Lung Health study in early COPD and the East London study with more advanced COPD, have shown that exacerbations are associated with progressive loss of lung function [89,90]. As the aetiology of exacerbations was not assessed systematically in either of these studies, it is not clear if bacterial and non-bacterial exacerbations contribute equally to progressive airway obstruction.

In conclusion, it is becoming increasingly apparent that the presence of bacteria in the lower airways in patients with COPD, even when they are clinically stable, is not innocuous. Additional airway inflammation secondary to bacterial 'colonization' and infection could contribute to symptoms and progression of airway obstruction in COPD. However, it is possible that this infection-associated inflammation is confined to the larger airways and does not extend to the small airways, which is the predominant site of obstruction in COPD. Thus, this additional inflammation may only contribute to the bronchitic component of COPD with no impact on the more significant obstructive component. Therefore, the vicious circle appears to exist; however, its importance in the natural history of COPD is as yet unknown.

Chronic bacterial infection by respiratory tissues

New, very sensitive and specific detection techniques for determining the presence of bacterial organisms in tissue have produced interesting and somewhat surprising observations regarding the site of NTHI infection in respiratory tissues. *Chlamydia pneumoniae* is an obligate intracellular pathogen that may have a role in the pathogenesis of COPD.

Intracellular and intercellular invasion of non-typeable *H. influenzae*

NTHI has been long regarded as an extracellular pathogen in the respiratory tract. Recent data from several investigators have shown that the organism's niche in the human respiratory tract is not limited to the surface of epithelial cells. Studies utilizing cultures of human lung epithelial cells have revealed that a small percentage of adherent NTHI enter epithelial cells in a process that involves actin filaments and microtubules [91]. In addition, NTHI is capable of paracytosis or passage between cells [92]. NTHI that penetrate the epithelial cell layer are protected from the bactericidal activity of several antibiotics and antibodies [93]. In assays employing primary human airway cultures, NTHI adheres to and enters exclusively non-ciliated cells in the population by the process of macropinocytosis [94]. NTHI has also shown the capability to survive after being phagocytosed by mouse macrophages [95]. In this study, 84% of clinical isolates were able to survive at least 24 h in the mouse macrophages.

In addition to these elegant *in vitro* studies, *in vivo* studies confirm intracellular and intercellular invasion by NTHI of the mucosal surface of the human respiratory tract. Examination of adenoids of children removed at adenoidectomy with *in situ* hybridization and selective cultures for NTHI revealed viable bacteria in macrophage-like cells [96]. In lung explants obtained from patients undergoing lung transplant, NTHI was diffusely present in the epithelium, the submucosa of the bronchi, the bronchioles, the interstitium and the alveolar epithelium as determined by *in situ* hybridization and polymerase chain reaction for OMP P6 [97]. Additional mechanisms that could allow persistence of NTHI in the lower respiratory tract of patients with COPD include the formation of biofilm and the change of host immune response to a Th1 predominance [59,98].

Bacteria in tissues are protected from antibiotics and bactericidal antibodies and may act as reservoirs of infection [93]. Tissue infection by NTHI could also contribute directly or indirectly to the pathogenesis of COPD. Chronic low-grade infection could directly induce a chronic inflammatory response in the lung parenchyma and the airways that could be additive or synergistic to the inflammatory effects of tobacco smoke. Indirectly, such an infection could enhance the damaging effects of tobacco smoke on respiratory tissues. On the other hand, it is possible that this tissue infection is simply a marker of compromised local immunity. The significance of this tissue infection by NTHI in the course of COPD needs to be further investigated.

Chronic *Chlamydia pneumoniae* infection in COPD

Acute *C. pneumoniae* infection can cause bronchitis, pneumonia and acute exacerbations of COPD. Chronic infection with *C. pneumoniae* is being actively investigated as a cause of several systemic diseases, especially coronary artery disease [99]. In a recent study, the incidence of chronic *C. pneumoniae* infection was 71% in patients with severe COPD, 46% in mild–moderate COPD and 0% in the control group [100]. Blasi *et al.* [101] compared COPD patients with and without evidence of chronic infection with *C. pneumoniae* and found more frequent bacterial colonization and more frequent exacerbations in the *C. pneumoniae* positive group. However, the *C. pneumoniae* positive patients had more severe airway obstruction, which confounds the findings ascribed to *C. pneumoniae* infection. A 6-week course of azithromycin in a subset of the *C. pneumoniae* positive patients resulted in a temporary clearance of the infection. Whether chronic infection with *C. pneumoniae* contributes to the pathogenesis of COPD or is a reflection of compromised local immunity warrants further investigation.

Hypersensitivity to bacterial antigens in COPD

Allergic bronchopulmonary aspergillosis is an infectious disease with predominantly allergic manifestations mediated by a Th2 type immune response and characterized by IgE and eosinophil predominance [102]. Persistent infection of the tracheobronchial tree with bacteria is characteristic of COPD, resulting in prolonged contact between the airway lymphoid tissue and bacterial antigens. This could lead to the emergence of IgE antibodies to bacterial antigens, which could induce eosinophil infiltration and mast cell degranulation on repeated exposures to the bacterial antigens. An increased number of eosinophils is a component of airway inflammation in patients with COPD, and tissue and airway lumen eosinophilia becomes more prominent during exacerbations [103].

The ability of bacterial pathogens to induce histamine release, hypersensitivity and IgE-mediated inflammation has been investigated sporadically. Formalin killed suspensions of NTHI and *S. aureus* induced non-IgE-mediated and enhanced IgE-mediated histamine release from human airway mast cells [104]. The enhancement of IgE-mediated histamine release appears to be mediated by the LOS of NTHI [105]. Ahren *et al.* [106] have shown that NTHI interacts with eosinophils through β-glucan receptors and induces an innate inflammatory response.

Patients with acute exacerbations of chronic bronchitis have basophil bound IgE and serum IgE to homologous strains of NTHI and *S. pneumoniae* isolated from sputum with the acute exacerbation [107]. In another study in asthmatics, 29% of patients had serum IgE antibodies to NTHI and/or *S. pneumoniae* [108]. This sensitization to bacterial antigens may contribute to the bronchoconstriction and airway inflammation seen with acute exacerbations of COPD.

These observations regarding histamine release, eosinophil activation and IgE to bacterial antigens suggest that bacterial pathogens, either directly or indirectly via a Th2 type immune response, could contribute to the eosinophilia, airway hyperreactivity and bronchoconstriction seen in patients with COPD.

Childhood lower respiratory tract infection and adult lung function

An association between childhood lower respiratory tract infection and impaired lung function in adulthood was investigated in four studies that reported spirometric lung function in cohorts of adult patients for whom reliable information was available regarding the incidence of lower

Table 36.4 Association of childhood lower respiratory tract infection with lung function in adults. (From Sethi [114] with permission.)

Study	n	Childhood lower respiratory tract infection	Age at follow-up (years)	Effect on FEV_1
Barker *et al.* [109]	639 (all male)	Bronchitis or pneumonia in first year	59–67	↓ 200 mL
Shaheen *et al.* [111]	618	Pneumonia in first 2 years Bronchitis in first 2 years	67–74	↓ 650 mL (in men with pneumonia)
Johnston *et al.* [110]	1392	Pneumonia in first 7 years Whooping cough in first 7 years	34–35	↓ 102 mL (with pneumonia)
Shaheen *et al.* [112]	239	Pneumonia in first 14 years Bronchitis in first 14 years	57.6 ± 4.3	↓ 390 mL (with pneumonia in first 2 years) ↓ 130 mL (with bronchitis in first 2 years)

FEV_1, forced expiratory volume in 1 s.

respiratory tract infection (bronchitis, pneumonia, whooping cough) in childhood (less than 14 years of age) (Table 36.4) [109–112]. All four studies have consistently shown a lower forced expiratory volume in 1 s (FEV_1) and often a lower forced vital capacity (FVC) in association with a history of childhood lower respiratory tract infection, after controlling for confounding factors such as tobacco exposure [109–112]. The magnitude of this defect in FEV_1 tends to be greater in older cohorts but is not large enough to cause symptomatic pulmonary disease on its own. However, this defect in FEV_1 could make the individual susceptible to the effects of additional injurious agents that cause COPD. The defect in lung function is not obstructive but is consistent with 'smaller lungs', suggesting impaired lung growth.

The association between childhood lower respiratory tract infection and impaired lung function in adulthood could stem from damage to a vulnerable lung undergoing rapid postnatal growth and maturation by the infectious process. If this was the case, then the effect of infection on lung function should be seen only in the first 2 years of life, the major period of postnatal lung growth, and not in later childhood (3–14 years). However, this has not been a consistent observation in the studies to date [109–112]. An alternative explanation for the observed association is that an undetermined genetic factor predisposes these individuals to lower respiratory tract infections in childhood as well as a lower FEV_1 in adulthood. This explanation implies that impaired lung growth antedates the respiratory tract infection, with the infectious episode being a marker of the vulnerability of smaller lungs to infection in childhood.

Although a substantial proportion of childhood respiratory infections are viral, bacterial infections, especially with *Streptococcus pneumoniae* and *Haemophilus influenzae*, are common causes of severe pneumonia in children [113]. The aetiology of childhood lower respiratory tract infection was not established in the cohort studies, therefore whether the impact of viral infection differs from bacterial infection is not known. The impact of childhood bacterial lower respiratory tract infection on lung growth and therefore on the development of COPD is likely to be greater in developing countries where such infections are common and often inadequately treated.

Future directions

Substantial new information has emerged regarding the potential pathways by which bacterial infection can contribute to the course of COPD; however, several important questions remain to be answered. The complexity of the host–pathogen interaction that determines the outcome of each encounter between a potential respiratory pathogen and a patient with COPD is being increasingly appreciated. Further studies should try to better understand this interaction. Specifically, the virulence determinants of pathogens that induce host inflammatory responses need to be better understood. There is a large variability in the incidence of exacerbations among patients with COPD. We need to elucidate the host defence factors that protect some of these patients from bacterial exacerbations. In addition, protective host immune response that develops following exacerbations needs to be characterized to facilitate vaccine development. The interplay between different aetiological factors including the environment, viruses, atypical pathogens and bacteria needs to be better understood in order to improve treatment of exacerbations and develop novel preventive strategies.

Whether the vicious circle of bacterial infection leads to progressive airway obstruction or contributes to the symptoms of COPD has not been determined. Whether tissue infection by pathogens such as NTHI and *C. pneumoniae* contributes to progression of disease or is simply a marker of compromised bacterial clearance and local immunity needs investigation.

COPD is a heterogeneous disease and the role of bacteria and the pathways by which infection contributes to its pathogenesis is likely to vary among subsets of patients with COPD. Regarding bacterial infection as the central mechanism of development of all COPD or dismissing it as an epiphenomenon are unlikely to be correct viewpoints. Most likely, in a subset of patients with COPD, bacterial infection contributes substantially to progression of their disease. Identification of this subset of patients could lead to therapeutic interventions to alter the natural history of their disease.

Acknowledgements

This work was supported by the Department of Veterans Affairs and the NHLBI. The author thanks Adeline Thurston for her expertise in preparing the manuscript.

References

1 Murphy TF, Sethi S. Bacterial infection in chronic obstructive pulmonary disease. *Am Rev Respir Dis* 1992;**146**:1067–83.

2 Leeder SR. Role of infection in the cause and course of chronic bronchitis and emphysema. *J Infect Dis* 1975;**131**: 731–42.

3 Tager I, Speizer FE. Role of infection in chronic bronchitis. *N Engl J Med* 1975;**292**:563–71.

4 Hirschmann JV. Do bacteria cause exacerbations of COPD? *Chest* 2000;**118**:193–203.

5 Murphy TF, Sethi S, Niederman MS. The role of bacteria in exacerbations of COPD: a constructive view. *Chest* 2000; **118**:204–9.

6 Smith CB, Golden C, Klauber MR, Kanner R, Renzetti A. Interactions between viruses and bacteria in patients with chronic bronchitis. *J Infect Dis* 1976;**134**:552–61.

7 Allegra L, Konietzko N, Leophonte P *et al.* Comparative safety and efficacy of sparfloxacin in the treatment of acute exacerbations of chronic obstructive pulmonary disease: a double-blind, randomised, parallel, multicentre study. *J Antimicrob Chemother* 1996;**37**(Suppl A):93–104.

8 Anzueto A, Niederman MS, Tillotson GS, Bronchitis Study Group. Etiology, susceptibility, and treatment of acute

bacterial exacerbations of complicated chronic bronchitis in the primary care setting: ciprofloxacin 750 mg bid vs clarithromycin 500 mg bid. *Clin Ther* 1998;**20**:885–900.

9 Chodosh S, Lakshminarayan S, Swarz H, Breisch S. Efficacy and safety of a 10-day course of 400 or 600 milligrams of grepafloxacin once daily for treatment of acute bacterial exacerbations of chronic bronchitis: comparison with a 10-day course of 500 milligrams of ciprofloxacin twice daily. *Antimicrob Agents Chemother* 1998;**42**:114–20.

10 Chodosh S, McCarty J, Farkas S *et al.* Randomized, double-blind study of ciprofloxacin and cefuroxime axetil for treatment of acute bacterial exacerbations of chronic bronchitis. *Clin Infect Dis* 1998;**27**:722–9.

11 Chodosh S, Schreurs JM, Siami G *et al.* Efficacy of oral ciprofloxacin vs clarithromycin for treatment of acute bacterial exacerbations of chronic bronchitis. *Clin Infect Dis* 1998;**27**: 730–8.

12 Davies BI, Maesen FPV. Clinical effectiveness of levofloxacin in patients with acute purulent exacerbations of chronic bronchitis: the relationship with *in vitro* activity. *J Antimicrob Chemother* 1999;**43**(Suppl C):83–90.

13 DeAbate CA, Henry D, Bensch G *et al.* Sparfloxacin vs ofloxacin in the treatment of acute bacterial exacerbations of chronic bronchitis. *Chest* 1998;**114**:20–130.

14 Habib MP, Gentry LO, Rodriguez-Gomez G *et al.* Multicenter, randomized study comparing efficacy and safety of oral levofloxacin and cefaclor in treatment of acute bacterial exacerbations of chronic bronchitis. *Infect Dis Clin Pract* 1998;**7**:101–9.

15 Langan C, Clecner B, Cazzola CM *et al.* Short-course cefuroxime axetil therapy in the treatment of acute exacerbations of chronic bronchitis. *Int J Clin Pract* 1998;**52**:289–97.

16 Langan CE, Cranfield R, Breisch S, Pettit R. Randomized, double-blind study of grepafloxacin versus amoxicillin in patients with acute bacterial exacerbations of chronic bronchitis. *J Antimicrob Chemother* 1997;**40**:63–72.

17 Langan CE, Zuck P, Vogel F *et al.* Randomized, double-blind study of short-course (5 day) grepafloxacin versus 10 day clarithromycin in patients with acute bacterial exacerbations of chronic bronchitis. *J Antimicrob Chemother* 1999;**44**: 515–23.

18 Read RC, Kuss A, Berrisoul F, Torres A, Kubin R. The efficacy and safety of a new ciprofloxacin suspension compared with co-amoxiclav tablets in the treatment of acute exacerbations of chronic bronchitis. *Respir Med* 1999;**93**:252–61.

19 Shah PM, Maesen FPV, Dolmann A *et al.* Levofloxacin versus cefuroxime axetil in the treatment of acute exacerbation of chronic bronchitis: results of a randomized, double-blind study. *J Antimicrob Chemother* 1999;**43**:529–39.

20 Wilson R, Kubin R, Ballin I *et al.* Five day moxifloxacin therapy compared with 7 day clarithromycin therapy for the treatment of acute exacerbations of chronic bronchitis. *J Antimicrob Chemother* 1999;**44**:501–13.

21 Gump DW, Phillips CA, Forsyth BR *et al.* Role of infection in chronic bronchitis. *Am Rev Respir Dis* 1976;**113**:465–73.

22 McHardy VU, Inglis JM, Calder MA, Crofton JW. A study of infective and other factors in exacerbations of chronic bronchitis. *Br J Dis Chest* 1980;**74**:228–38.

23 May JR. The bacteriology of chronic bronchitis. *Lancet* 1953;**ii**:534–7.

24 May JR, Peto R, Tinker CM, Fletcher CM. A study of *Hemophilus influenzae* precipitins in the serum of working men in relation to smoking habits, bronchial infection, and airway obstruction. *Am Rev Respir Dis* 1973;**108**:460–8.

25 Burns MW, May JR. *Haemophilus influenzae* precipitins in the serum of patients with chronic bronchial disorders. *Lancet* 1967;**i**:354–8.

26 Glynn AA. Antibodies to *Haemophilus influenzae* in chronic bronchits. *BMJ* 1959;**2**:911–4.

27 Gump DW, Christmas WA, Forsyth BR, Phillips CA, Stouch WH. Serum and secretory antibodies in patients with chronic bronchitis. *Arch Intern Med* 1973;**132**:847–51.

28 Smith CB, Golden CA, Kanner RE, Renzetti AD. *Haemophilus influenzae* and *Haemophilus parainfluenzae* in chronic obstructive pulmonary disease. *Lancet* 1976;**i**:1253–5.

29 Reichek N, Lewin EB, Rhoden DL, Weaver RR, Crutcher JC. Antibody responses to bacterial antigens during exacerbations of chronic bronchitis. *Am Rev Respir Dis* 1970;**101**: 238–44.

30 Musher DM, Kubitschek KR, Crennan J, Baughn RE. Pneumonia and acute febrile tracheobronchitis due to *Haemophilus influenzae*. *Ann Intern Med* 1983;**99**:444–50.

31 Groeneveld K, Eijk PP, van Alphen L, Jansen HM, Zanen HC. *Haemophilus influenzae* infections in patients with chronic obstructive pulmonary disease despite specific antibodies in serum and sputum. *Am Rev Respir Dis* 1990;**141**:1316–21.

32 Saint S, Bent S, Vittinghoff E, Grady D. Antibiotics in chronic obstructive pulmonary disease exacerbations: a meta-analysis. *JAMA* 1995;**273**:957–60.

33 Sachs APE, Koeter GH, Groenier KH *et al*. Changes in symptoms, peak expiratory flow, and sputum flora during treatment with antibiotics of exacerbations in patients with chronic obstructive pulmonary disease in general practice. *Thorax* 1995;**50**:758–63.

34 Nouira S, Marghli S, Belghith M *et al*. Once daily oral ofloxacin in chronic obstructive pulmonary disease exacerbation requiring mechanical ventilation: a randomised placebo-controlled trial. *Lancet* 2001;**358**:2020–5.

35 Allegra L, Blasi F, de Bernardi B, Cosentini R, Tarsia P. Antibiotic treatment and baseline severity of disease in acute exacerbations of chronic bronchitis: a re-evaluation of previously published data of a placebo-controlled randomized study. *Pulm Pharmacol Ther* 2001;**14**:149–55.

36 Niewoehner DE, Erbland ML, Deupree RH *et al*. Effect of systemic glucocorticoids on exacerbations of chronic obstructive pulmonary disease. *N Engl J Med* 1999;**340**:1941–7.

37 Fagon J-Y, Chastre J. Severe exacerbations of COPD patients: the role of pulmonary infections. *Semin Respir Infect* 1996;**11**:109–18.

38 Nicotra MB, Kronenberg S. Con: antibiotic use in exacerbations of chronic bronchitis. *Semin Respir Infect* 1993;**8**:254–8.

39 Chastre J, Fagon J-Y, Bornet-Lesco M *et al*. Evaluation of bronchoscopic techniques for the diagnosis of nosocomial pneumonia. *Am J Respir Crit Care Med* 1995;**152**:231–40.

40 Monso E, Ruiz J, Rosell A *et al*. Bacterial infection in chronic obstructive pulmonary disease: a study of stable and exacerbated outpatients using the protected specimen brush. *Am J Respir Crit Care Med* 1995;**152**:1316–20.

41 Fagon J-Y, Chastre J, Trouillet J-L *et al*. Characterization of distal bronchial microflora during acute exacerbation of chronic bronchitis. *Am Rev Respir Dis* 1990;**142**:1004–8.

42 Soler N, Torres A, Ewig S *et al*. Bronchial microbial patterns in severe exacerbations of chronic obstructive pulmonary disease (COPD) requiring mechanical ventilation. *Am J Respir Crit Care Med* 1998;**157**:1498–505.

43 Pela R, Marchesani FF, Agostinelli C *et al*. Airways microbial flora in COPD patients in stable clinical conditions and during exacerbations: a bronchoscopic investigation. *Monaldi Arch Chest Dis* 1998;**53**:262–7.

44 Bandi V, Apicella MA, Mason E *et al*. Non-typeable *Haemophilus influenzae* in the lower respiratory tract of patients with chronic bronchitis. *Am J Respir Crit Care Med* 2001;**164**:2114–9.

45 Wilson R. The role of infection in COPD. *Chest* 1998;**113**: 242S–8S.

46 Stockley RA, O'Brien C, Pye A, Hill SL. Relationship of sputum color to nature and outpatient management of acute exacerbations of COPD. *Chest* 2000;**117**(6):1638–45.

47 White AJ, Gompertz S, Bayley DL *et al*. Resolution of bronchial inflammation is related to bacterial eradication following treatment of exacerbations of chronic bronchitis. *Thorax* 2003;**58**(8):680–5.

48 Sethi S, Evans N, Grant BJB, Murphy TF. Acquisition of a new bacterial strain and occurrence of exacerbations of chronic obstructive pulmonary disease. *N Engl J Med* 2002;**347**:465–71.

49 Duim B, van Alphen L, Eijk PP, Jansen HM, Dankert J. Antigenic drift of non-encapsulated *Haemophilus influenzae* major outer membrane protein 2 in patients with chronic bronchitis is caused by point mutations. *Mol Microbiol* 1994;**11**:1181–9.

50 Hiltke TJ, Sethi S, Murphy TF. Sequence stability of the gene encoding outer membrane protein P2 of non-typeable *Haemophilus influenzae* in the human respiratory tract. *J Infect Dis* 2002;**185**:627–31.

51 Bakri F, Brauer AL, Sethi S, Murphy TF. Systemic and mucosal antibody response to *Moraxella catarrhalis* following exacerbations of chronic obstructive pulmonary disease. *J Infect Dis* 2002;**185**:632–40.

52 Murphy TF, Kirkham C, Liu DF, Sethi S. Human immune response to outer membrane protein CD of *Moraxella catarrhalis* in adults with chronic obstructive pulmonary disease. *Infect Immun* 2003;**71**:1288–94.

53 Yi K, Sethi S, Murphy T. Human immune response to non-typeable *Haemophilus influenzae* in chronic bronchitis. *J Infect Dis* 1997;**176**:1247–52.

54 Groeneveld K, van Alphen L, Voorter C *et al*. Antigenic drift of *Haemophilus influenzae* in patients with chronic obstructive pulmonary disease. *Infect Immun* 1989;**57**:3038–44.

55 Murphy TF, Bartos LC. Human bactericidal antibody response to outer membrane protein P2 of non-typeable *Haemophilus influenzae*. *Infect Immun* 1988;**56**:2673–9.

56 Srikumar R, Chin AC, Vachon V *et al*. Monoclonal antibodies specific to porin of *Haemophilus influenzae* type b:

localization of their cognate epitopes and tests of their biological activities. *Mol Microbiol* 1992;**6**:665–76.

57 Yi K, Murphy TF. Importance of an immunodominant surface-exposed loop on outer membrane protein P2 of non-typeable *Haemophilus influenzae*. *Infect Immun* 1997;**65**: 150–5.

58 Abe Y, Murphy TF, Sethi S *et al.* Lymphocyte proliferative response to P6 of *Haemophilus influenzae* is associated with relative protection from exacerbations of chronic obstructive pulmonary disease. *Am J Respir Crit Care Med* 2002;**165**: 967–71.

59 King PT, Hutchinson PE, Johnson PD *et al.* Adaptive immunity to non-typeable *Haemophilus influenzae*. *Am J Respir Crit Care Med* 1915;**167**:587–92.

60 Sethi S, Muscarella K, Evans N *et al.* Airway inflammation and etiology of acute exacerbations of chronic bronchitis. *Chest* 2000;**118**:1557–65.

61 Gompertz S, O'Brien C, Bayley DL, Hill SL, Stockley RA. Changes in bronchial inflammation during acute exacerbations of chronic bronchitis. *Eur Respir J* 2001;**17**:1112–9.

62 Aaron SD, Angel JB, Lunau M *et al.* Granulocyte inflammatory markers and airway infection during acute exacerbation of chronic obstructive pulmonary disease. *Am J Respir Crit Care Med* 2001;**163**:349–55.

63 Haas H, Morris JF, Samson S, Kilbourn JP, Kim PJ. Bacterial flora of the respiratory tract in chronic bronchitis: comparison of transtracheal, fiberbronchoscopic, and oropharyngeal sampling methods. *Am Rev Respir Dis* 1977;**116**:41–7.

64 Laurenzi GA, Potter RT, Kass EH. Bacteriologic flora of the lower respiratory tract. *N Engl J Med* 1961;**265**:1273–8.

65 Zalacain R, Sobradillo V, Amilibia J *et al.* Predisposing factors to bacterial colonization in chronic obstructive pulmonary disease. *Eur Respir J* 1999;**13**:343–8.

66 Theegarten D, Stamatis G, Morgenroth K. The role of persisting infections in the pathogenesis of pulmonary emphysema. *Pathol Res Pract* 1999;**195**:89–92.

67 Monso E, Rosell A, Bonet G *et al.* Risk factors for lower airway bacterial colonization in chronic bronchitis. *Eur Respir J* 1999;**13**:338–42.

68 Qvarfordt I, Riise GC, Andersson BA, Larsson S. Lower airway bacterial colonization in asymptomatic smokers and smokers with chronic bronchitis and recurrent exacerbations. *Respir Med* 2000;**94**:881–7.

69 Cabello H, Torres A, Celis R *et al.* Bacterial colonization of distal airways in healthy subjects and chronic lung disease: a bronchoscopic study. *Eur Respir J* 1997;**10**:1137–44.

70 Cole P. Host–microbe relationships in chronic respiratory infection. *Respiration* 1989;**55**:5–8.

71 Adler KB, Hendley DD, Davis GS. Bacteria associated with obstructive pulmonary disease elaborate extracellular products that stimulate mucin secretion by explants of guinea pig airways. *Am J Pathol* 1986;**125**:514.

72 Wang B, Lim DJ, Han J *et al.* Novel cytoplasmic proteins of non-typeable *Haemophilus influenzae* up-regulate human *MUC5AC* mucin transcription via a positive p38 mitogen-activated protein kinase pathway and a negative phosphoinositide 3-kinase-Akt pathway. *J Biol Chem* 2002;**277**: 949–57.

73 Wilson R, Roberts D, Cole P. Effect of bacterial products on human ciliary function *in vitro*. *Thorax* 1984;**40**:125–31.

74 Amitani R, Wilson R, Rutman A *et al.* Effects of human neutrophil elastase and *Pseudomonas aeruginosa* proteinases on human respiratory epithelium. *Am J Respir Cell Mol Biol* 1991;**4**:26–32.

75 Hiemstra PS, van Wetering S, Stolk J. Neutrophil serine proteinases and defensins in chronic obstructive pulmonary disease: effects on pulmonary epithelium. *Eur Respir J* 1998; **12**:1200–8.

76 Read RC, Wilson R, Rutman A *et al.* Interaction of non-typable *Haemophilus influenzae* with human respiratory mucosa *in vitro*. *J Infect Dis* 1991;**163**:549–58.

77 Gu X-X, Tsai C-M, Apicella MA, Lim DJ. Quantitation and biological properties of released and cell-bound lipooligosaccharides from non-typeable *Haemophilus influenzae*. *Infect Immun* 1995;**63**:4115–20.

78 Stolk J, Rudolphus A, Davies P *et al.* Induction of emphysema and bronchial mucus cell hyperplasia by intratracheal instillation of lipopolysaccharide in the hamster. *J Pathol* 1992;**167**:349–56.

79 Di Stefano A, Capelli A, Lusuardi M *et al.* Severity of airflow limitation is associated with severity of airway inflammation in smokers. *Am J Respir Crit Care Med* 1998;**158**:1277–85.

80 Thompson AB, Daughton D, Robbins RA *et al.* Intraluminal airway inflammation in chronic bronchitis: characterization and correlation with clinical parameters. *Am Rev Respir Dis* 1989;**140**:1527–37.

81 Khair OA, Devalia JL, Abdelaziz MM *et al.* Effect of *Haemophilus influenzae* endotoxin on the synthesis of IL-6, IL-8, TNF-α and expression of ICAM-1. *Eur Respir J* 1994;**7**: 2109–16.

82 Clemans DL, Bauer RJ, Hanson JA *et al.* Induction of proinflammatory cytokines by human respiratory epithelial cells after stimulation by non-typeable *Haemophilus influenzae*. *Infect Immun* 2000;**68**:4430–40.

83 Hill AT, Campbell EJ, Hill SL, Bayley DL, Stockley RA. Association between airway bacterial load and markers of airway inflammation in patients with stable chronic bronchitis. *Am J Med* 2000;**109**:288–95.

84 Soler N, Ewig S, Torres A *et al.* Airway inflammation and bronchial microbial patterns in patients with stable chronic obstructive pulmonary disease. *Eur Respir J* 1999;**14**:1015–22.

85 Bresser P, Out TA, van Alphen L, Jansen HM, Lutter R. Airway inflammation in non-obstructive and obstructive chronic bronchitis with chronic *Haemophilus influenzae* airway infection: comparison with non-infected patients with chronic obstructive pulmonary disease. *Am J Respir Crit Care Med* 2000;**162**:947–52.

86 Howard P. Evolution of the ventilatory capacity in chronic bronchitis. *BMJ* 1967;**3**:392–5.

87 Bates DV. The fate of the chronic bronchitic: a report of the 10-year follow-up in the Canadian Department of Veteran's Affairs coordinated study of chronic bronchitis. *Am Rev Respir Dis* 1973;**108**:1043–65.

88 Fletcher F, Peto R. The natural history of chronic airflow obstruction. *BMJ* 1977;**1**:1645–8.

89 Kanner R, Anthonisen NR, Connett JE, The Lung Health Study Research Group. Lower respiratory illnesses promote *FEV*$_1$ decline in current smokers but not ex-smokers with mild chronic obstructive pulmonary disease: results from the Lung Health Study Research Group. *Am J Respir Crit Care Med* 2001;**164**:358–64.

90 Donaldson GC, Seemungal TA, Bhowmik A, Wedzicha JA. Relationship between exacerbation frequency and lung function decline in chronic obstructive pulmonary disease. *Thorax* 2002;**57**:847–52.

91 St Geme JW III, Falkow S. *Haemophilus influenzae* adheres to and enters cultured human epithelial cells. *Infect Immun* 1990;**58**:4036–44.

92 van Schilfgaarde M, van Alphen L, Eijk PP, Everts V, Dankert J. Paracytosis of *Haemophilus influenzae* through cell layers of NCI-H292 lung epithelial cells. *Infect Immun* 1995;**63**:4729–37.

93 van Schilfgaarde M, Eijk PP, Regelink A *et al.* *Haemophilus influenzae* localized in epithelial cell layers is shielded from antibiotics and antibody-mediated bactericidal activity. *Microb Pathog* 1999;**26**:249–62.

94 Ketterer MR, Shao JQ, Hornick DB *et al.* Infection of primary human bronchial epithelial cells by *Haemophilus influenzae*: macropinocytosis as a mechanisms of airway epithelial cell entry. *Infect Immun* 1999;**67**:4161–70.

95 Craig JE, Cliffe A, Garnett K, High NJ. Survival of non-typeable *Haemophilus influenzae* in macrophages. *FEMS Microbiol Lett* 1911;**203**:55–61.

96 Forsgren J, Samuelson A, Ahlin A *et al.* *Haemophilus influenzae* resides and multiplies intracellularly in human adenoid tissue as demonstrated by *in situ* hybridization and bacterial viability assay. *Infect Immun* 1994;**62**:673–9.

97 Moller LVM, Timens W, van der Bij W *et al.* *Haemophilus influenzae* in lung explants of patients with end-stage pulmonary disease. *Am J Respir Crit Care Med* 1998;**157**:950–6.

98 Murphy TF, Kirkham C. Biofilm formation by non-typeable *Haemophilus influenzae*: strain variability, outer membrane antigen expression and role of pili. *BMC Microbiol* 2002;**2**:7.

99 Linnanmaki E, Leinonen M, Mattila K *et al.* *Chlamydia pneumoniae*: specific circulating immune complexes in patients with chronic coronary heart disease. *Circulation* 1993;**87**:1130–4.

100 von Hertzen L, Alakarppa H, Koskinen R *et al.* *Chlamydia pneumoniae* infection in patients with chronic obstructive pulmonary disease. *Epidemiol Infect* 1997;**118**:155–64.

101 Blasi F, Damato S, Cosentini R *et al.* *Chlamydia pneumoniae* and chronic bronchitis: association with severity and bacterial clearance following treatment. *Thorax* 2002;**57**:672–6.

102 Kauffman HF, Tomee JFC, van der Werf TS, de Monchy JG, Koeter GK. Review of fungus-induced asthmatic reactions. *Am J Respir Crit Care Med* 1995;**151**:2109–16.

103 Saetta M, Di Stefano A, Maestrelli P *et al.* Airway eosinophilia in chronic bronchitis during exacerbations. *Am J Respir Crit Care Med* 1994;**150**:1646–52.

104 Clementsen P, Larsen FO, Milman N, Skov PS, Norn S. *Haemophilus influenzae* release histamine and enhance histamine release from human bronchoalveolar cells. *APMIS* 1995;**103**:806–12.

105 Clementsen P, Milman N, Kilian M *et al.* Endotoxin from *Haemophilus influenzae* enhances IgE-mediated and non-immunological histamine release. *Allergy* 1990;**45**:10–7.

106 Ahren IL, Eriksson E, Egesten A, Riesbeck K. Non-typeable *Haemophilus influenzae* activates human eosinophils through β-glucan receptors. *Am J Respir Cell Mol Biol* 2003;**29**: 598–605.

107 Kjaergard LL, Larsen FO, Norn S *et al.* Basophil-bound IgE and serum IgE directed against *Haemophilus influenzae* and *Streptococcus pneumoniae* in patients with chronic bronchitis during acute exacerbations. *APMIS* 1996;**104**:61–7.

108 Pauwels R, Verschraegen G, van der Straeten M. IgE antibodies to bacteria in patients with bronchial asthma. *Allergy* 1980;**157**:665–9.

109 Barker DJP, Godfrey KM, Fall C *et al.* Relation of birth weight and childhood respiratory infection to adult lung function and death from chronic obstructive airways disease. *BMJ* 1991;**303**:671–5.

110 Johnston IDA, Strachan DP, Anderson HR. Effect of pneumonia and whooping cough in childhood on adult lung function. *N Engl J Med* 1998;**338**:581–7.

111 Shaheen SO, Barker DJP, Shiell AW *et al.* The relationship between pneumonia in early childhood and impaired lung function in late adult life. *Am J Respir Crit Care Med* 1994; **149**:616–9.

112 Shaheen SO, Sterne JAC, Tucker JS, du V Florey C. Birth weight, childhood lower respiratory tract infection, and adult lung function. *Thorax* 1998;**53**:549–53.

113 Vuori E, Peltola H, Kallio MJT, Leinonen M, Hedman K, SE-TU Study Group. Etiology of pneumonia and other common childhood infections requiring hospitalization and parenteral antimicrobial therapy. *Clin Infect Dis* 1998;**27**:566–72.

114 Sethi S. *Bacterial Infection: Chronic Obstructive Lung Diseases.* BC Decker, 2002: 214–26.

CHAPTER 37

Genetic factors

Craig P. Hersh and Edwin K. Silverman

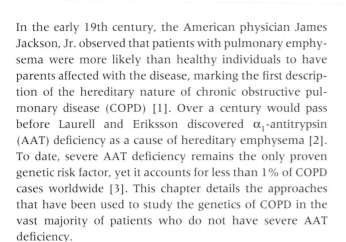

In the early 19th century, the American physician James Jackson, Jr. observed that patients with pulmonary emphysema were more likely than healthy individuals to have parents affected with the disease, marking the first description of the hereditary nature of chronic obstructive pulmonary disease (COPD) [1]. Over a century would pass before Laurell and Eriksson discovered α_1-antitrypsin (AAT) deficiency as a cause of hereditary emphysema [2]. To date, severe AAT deficiency remains the only proven genetic risk factor, yet it accounts for less than 1% of COPD cases worldwide [3]. This chapter details the approaches that have been used to study the genetics of COPD in the vast majority of patients who do not have severe AAT deficiency.

COPD is considered a genetically complex disease; disease inheritance does not follow a simple mendelian pattern. As in other complex diseases, like hypertension and diabetes, family studies have been used to demonstrate familial aggregation of COPD, as well as familial correlations in lung function measures, which are important associated phenotypes. Families have also been used to perform genome-wide linkage analyses, searching for chromosomal regions contributing to COPD and related traits. Finally, case–control studies have examined the association between disease and specific variants in candidate genes.

Similar to other complex human diseases, environmental risk factors have an important role in the development of COPD; these factors are described in Chapters 33 and 34. The critical importance of cigarette smoking as a determinant of COPD requires that any genetic study must consider smoking as a possible modifier of the effects of the genes of interest. The paradigm of gene–environment interaction in COPD, using smoking as a clear and readily quantifiable risk factor, can serve as a model for the study of other complex human diseases, where the environmental exposures may be more difficult to measure.

α_1-Antitrypsin deficiency

Severe AAT deficiency is the only proven genetic risk factor for COPD and is reviewed in detail in Chapter 38. Severe AAT deficiency is usually brought about by homozygosity for the mutant Z allele (protease inhibitor [PI] ZZ), and the development of lung and liver disease appears to follow an autosomal recessive inheritance pattern. There are estimated to be 70 000–100 000 severely AAT-deficient individuals in the USA and a similar number in Europe [4]. Although an important cause of COPD in affected individuals, severe AAT deficiency accounts for only a small fraction of COPD cases worldwide. The risk of COPD in the carriers of a Z allele (e.g. PI MZ) or other variants of the AAT gene is discussed below.

Severe AAT deficiency is classically associated with early-onset COPD, yet many individuals with severe AAT deficiency have normal lung function; the method of subject ascertainment and the history of cigarette smoking can modify the likelihood of COPD development [5]. Severe AAT deficiency provides an instructive model of gene–environment interaction that can be applied to the study of other COPD candidate genes [6]. In addition, other genes are likely to contribute to the development of airflow obstruction in individuals with severe AAT deficiency. Discovery of these modifier genes may lead to insight into the genetics of COPD in the majority of individuals who do not have severe AAT deficiency.

Familial aggregation

The hallmark of any inherited disease is clustering within families, and demonstration of familial aggregation is the necessary first step in the genetic analysis of a complex trait. However, familial similarities may be the result of genetics or shared environmental exposures, or both. Twin studies can be used to separate these two types of effects. If a trait is more correlated within pairs of monozygotic twins, who share all of their genes, than within pairs of dizygotic twins, who usually share a similar environment but only half of their genes, then a genetic influence is likely. Such twin studies have been used to demonstrate a genetic contribution to pulmonary function measures [7,8]. Genetic effects on pulmonary function measures have also been shown in a study of monozygotic twins raised apart, thereby eliminating the shared environment, and in studies of first-degree relatives (nuclear families or sib-pairs); statistical models must be used to estimate familial correlations and to adjust for common environmental exposures in the latter design [9–12].

Familial correlation has been examined for the rate of lung function decline, a different phenotype than the cross-sectional lung function measures, such as forced expiratory volume at 1 s (FEV_1) or forced vital capacity (FVC), that were analysed in previous studies [13]. Gottlieb *et al.* [13] used baseline and follow-up spirometry data from both the original Framingham Heart Study cohort as well as their offspring. They demonstrated significant heritability of the rate of decline in lung function. Genetic factors accounted for 5, 18 and 13% of the population variation in decline in FEV_1, FVC and FEV_1 : FVC ratio, respectively. These heritability estimates were higher in smokers (18, 39 and 14%) suggesting a gene–environment interaction effect.

In the early 1960s, several case reports were published that described families with multiple members affected by COPD [14–16]. Case reports of COPD in twins have been published, but formal twin studies have not been performed [17]. Family studies have shown that both airflow obstruction and chronic bronchitis are more common in first-degree relatives of individuals with COPD than in the general population, even after adjustment for smoking status [18–23].

In the Boston Early-Onset COPD Study, Silverman *et al.* [24] collected data on families ascertained through a proband with severe early-onset COPD, based on the hypothesis that severe early-onset disease is more likely to have genetic influences than later-onset disease. Probands had an FEV_1 less than 40% of predicted, were younger than 53 years old and did not have severe AAT deficiency (e.g. PI Z, PI null–null). All available first-degree relatives, older second-degree relatives (aunts, uncles and grandparents) and spouses were invited to enrol. Participants completed a protocol that included a respiratory questionnaire, spirometry (pre- and postbronchodilator) and a blood draw. Compared with community controls, first-degree relatives of early-onset COPD probands had significantly increased risks of reduced FEV_1 and chronic bronchitis. This was especially prominent in current or ex-smoking first-degree

relatives, with odds ratios (OR) of 4.5 (95% confidence interval [CI], 1.8–11.5) for an FEV_1 of less than 80% predicted and 3.6 (95% CI, 1.1–11.5) for chronic bronchitis [24]. Greater bronchodilator responsiveness was also found in current and ex-smoking first-degree relatives of early-onset COPD probands, compared with current and ex-smoking controls [25]. Further analysis has shown that female first-degree relatives (current and ex-smokers) have an increased risk for reduced FEV_1 and greater bronchodilator responsiveness compared with male first-degree relatives [26].

In a study conducted in the UK, McCloskey *et al.* [27] examined siblings of probands that had been selected with airflow obstruction and a low gas transfer factor, indicative of emphysema. The probands had severe COPD, although the FEV_1 thresholds for inclusion varied by age, from an FEV_1 of less than 60% of predicted for subjects 55 years of age or younger to an FEV_1 of less than 20% of predicted for subjects 61–65 years of age. They found an increased risk of COPD in current or ex-smoking siblings of probands compared with matched controls (OR = 4.7; 95% CI, 2.6–8.4); the odds ratio was even higher in current or ex-smoking siblings with less than a 30 pack-year smoking history. Non-smoking siblings were found to have normal spirometry. The probands recruited by McCloskey *et al.* did not show the female predominance that was seen by Silverman *et al.* [26].

Linkage analysis

In addition to determining familial aggregation of a trait, family studies can be used for linkage analysis. In this method, a panel of DNA-based polymorphic markers, usually consisting of short tandem repeat (STR) markers, is genotyped across the genome in order to determine which chromosomal locations co-segregate with the trait of interest. These markers are usually in non-coding regions, so they do not typically identify specific genes for the disease; rather they mark areas of the genome that are linked to the disease trait. Statistically, this is expressed as a LOD score, which represents the logarithm ($\log_{10}$) of the odds of linkage. Investigators can then focus their search using association studies of biologically plausible genes located in the region of linkage (positional candidate genes) or systematically genotype markers for association at narrow intervals across the linked region (fine mapping).

Using the Boston Early-Onset COPD Study families, Silverman *et al.* [28,29] performed linkage analyses for both qualitative and quantitative COPD-related phenotypes. Using prebronchodilator spirometry, modest evidence for linkage was found on chromosomes 12 and 19 for moderate airflow obstruction (defined as FEV_1 less than 60%

Phenotype	Chromosome	Maximum LOD score*	
		Prebronchodilator	Postbronchodilator
FEV_1	1	1.24	2.24
	8	1.58	3.30
	12	1.66	1.33
	19	1.80	1.94
FEV_1/FVC	1	1.89	2.52
	2	4.05	4.42
	17	2.35	2.44

Table 37.1 Results of linkage analyses of pre- and postbronchodilator spirometry in severe early-onset COPD families [31].

FEV_1, forced expiratory volume in 1 s; FVC, forced vital capacity; LOD, logarithm of the odds. * In extended pedigrees, LOD scores ≥ 1.9 provide evidence of suggestive linkage, and LOD scores ≥ 3.3 provide evidence of significant linkage [30].

predicted with $FEV_1 : FVC$ less than 90% predicted), on chromosomes 8 and 19 for mild airflow obstruction (defined as FEV_1 less than 80% predicted with $FEV_1 : FVC$ less than 90% predicted) and on chromosomes 19 and 22 for chronic bronchitis. Restricting the analysis to smokers only increased the strength of the linkage evidence in several genomic regions. Using quantitative prebronchodilator spirometric phenotypes, more impressive evidence for linkage was demonstrated. Significant evidence for linkage to $FEV_1 : FVC$ was found on chromosome 2q; suggestive evidence for linkage to $FEV_1 : FVC$ on chromosomes 1 and 17 and to FVC on chromosome 1 was also demonstrated [30]. Additional markers were genotyped on chromosome 12p, providing suggestive evidence for linkage of FEV_1 to this region.

In addition, postbronchodilator spirometric measures and bronchodilator responsiveness phenotypes were assessed for linkage [31]. Significant evidence of linkage for postbronchodilator FEV_1 was found on chromosome 8p, with a LOD score of 3.30, which represented a doubling of the LOD score for prebronchodilator FEV_1 (Table 37.1). Significant linkage for postbronchodilator $FEV_1 : FVC$ was found on chromosome 2q (LOD score = 4.42). Regions on chromosomes 3 and 4 showed modest evidence for linkage to measures of bronchodilator responsiveness.

Several linkage studies of pulmonary function measures in non-diseased subjects have been reported. Using families from the Framingham Study, Joost et al. [32] found suggestive evidence for linkage of FEV_1 on chromosome 6 and of FVC on chromosome 21. In a genome scan of families in the National Heart, Lung and Blood Institute Family Heart Study, Wilk et al. [33] found suggestive evidence for linkage of $FEV_1 : FVC$ ratio on chromosome 4 and of both FEV_1 and FVC on two distinct regions on chromosome 18. This study was unable to replicate the findings of Joost et al., but a region of linkage to $FEV_1 : FVC$ ratio on chromosome 1 was

found that was similar to the results in the Boston Early-Onset COPD Study families, although the LOD scores were modest in both studies.

Malhotra et al. [34] analysed 264 members of 26 families in Utah, which had been collected as part of the Centre d'Etude du Polymorphisme Humain (CEPH) genetic mapping project. They found suggestive evidence of linkage for $FEV_1 : FVC$ on chromosome 2 (LOD score = 2.36), which corresponded to the region of significant linkage found by Silverman et al. [29]. Suggestive linkage for $FEV_1 : FVC$ ratio was also seen on chromosome 5 (LOD = 2.23), replicating a result from a previous study by Ober et al. [35] conducted in the isolated population of Hutterites in South Dakota. The validation of previous results in another population by Malhotra et al. marks an important step in the study of the genetics of COPD. However, the varying results of the other previous studies do not necessarily make their results less important. The differences in linkage results could relate to differences in study design and subject ascertainment; Silverman et al. analysed linkage for disease phenotypes, while the other groups examined linkage for lung function in families from the general population.

Association studies

Most studies of the genetic epidemiology of COPD have been association studies. As is the case for many other complex diseases, the majority of association studies in COPD genetics have utilized the case–control design. To perform an association study, a plausible candidate gene is identified, using prior knowledge of the biology of the disease. Genetic variants, usually single nucleotide polymorphisms (SNPs), are genotyped in the candidate gene, and frequencies of these variants are compared with individuals affected by the disease (cases) and unaffected

Table 37.2 Candidate genes that have been associated with COPD or related phenotypes.

Protease–antiprotease
α_1-Antitrypsin
    heterozygotes (Z, S) [21,36–40,43,44]
    3′ region [47,48]
α_1-Antichymotrypsin [51,53]
Matrix metalloproteinases-1, -9, -12 [57,58]
Tissue inhibitor of metalloproteinase-2 [59]

Oxidant–antioxidant
Heme oxygenase-1 [62]
Microsomal epoxide hydrolase-1 [44,65]
Glutathione S-transferase (M1, P1, T1) [70,71,74]

Inflammatory cytokines
Tumour necrosis factor α [78,79]
Interleukin 13 [90]

Others
Vitamin D binding protein (group-specific component)
    [21,91–93]
β_2-Adrenergic receptor [102]
Cystic fibrosis transmembrane conductance regulator [103]
Surfactant proteins A, B, D [104]
Human β defensin-1 [105]
Cytochrome P450 1A1 [106]
Human leucocyte antigen (HLA) [94]
ABO, Lewis blood groups and secretor status [94,107–109]

---

controls. A positive association does not necessarily imply that the variant is functional (i.e. disease-causing); it may be in close genetic proximity (linkage disequilibrium) to the functional variant. Spurious association may also be found because of confounding by ethnic differences between cases and controls, known as population stratification.

Some of the candidate genes that have been associated with COPD in case–control studies are listed in Table 37.2. These candidate genes can be divided into groups, based on pathophysiological mechanisms implicated in COPD [3]. Important pathways include: proteases and protease inhibitors, genes involved in oxidant–antioxidant balance and xenobiotic metabolism, and inflammatory mediators. Association studies of genes in each of these pathways are discussed.

Proteases and antiproteases

α_1-Antitrypsin

Since the discovery of severe AAT deficiency as a rare cause of COPD, many studies have examined the risk associated with the more common heterozygous types. Three different methodologies have been used to assess the risk of COPD in PI MZ heterozygotes, and the results have been inconsistent. Case–control studies have tended to find a moderately increased risk for COPD in PI MZ subjects [21,36–40]. Other investigators have used a population-based design, measuring lung function and AAT type in a community sample. Two large studies of 500 subjects in Rochester, New York and of 2944 subjects in Tucson, Arizona have shown no difference in lung function between PI MZ heterozygotes and normal individuals [41,42].

Several studies have used a longitudinal design to test whether the rate of lung function decline varies across PI phenotypes. In a population-based cohort of over 9000 adults in Copenhagen, Dahl *et al.* [43] found a slightly increased rate of decline in FEV_1 in PI MZ heterozygotes compared with PI MM individuals (25 vs. 21 mL/year; $P = 0.048$).

Sandford *et al.* [44] examined PI MZ heterozygotes in the National Heart, Lung and Blood Institute sponsored Lung Health Study (LHS) population. The LHS recruited 5887 smokers, aged 35–60 years, with mild airflow obstruction on spirometry. They were followed over 5 years to examine the effects of smoking cessation intervention and ipratropium bromide on decline in lung function [45]. From this cohort, Sandford *et al.* [44] identified 283 individuals with rapid decline in lung function ($\Delta FEV_1 = -154 \pm 3$ mL/year) and 308 individuals with no decline ($\Delta FEV_1 = +15 \pm 2$ mL/year); these two groups were used as cases and controls, respectively. Using this approach, they found PI MZ heterozygosity to be more common among the rapid decliners than the non-decliners; the association was stronger in the subjects with a family history of COPD.

Silva *et al.* [46] analysed the relationship between PI phenotype and decline in lung function in a community sample in Tucson. The study included over 2000 randomly sampled white individuals who were followed for an average of 15 years; more than half of the participants were current or former smokers. They found no differences in the rate of decline in FEV_1 between the PI phenotypes. In addition, PI MZ heterozygotes were not found to be more common among individuals with a rapid rate of FEV_1 decline compared with those with a slow decline, categories similar to those used in the Sandford *et al.* [44] paper. The inconsistent results across different studies of PI MZ heterozygotes, which have been performed in different populations and which have employed different study designs, may indicate that only a subgroup of PI MZ individuals are at an increased risk of developing COPD.

A polymorphism in the 3′ region of the PI gene has also been identified; this variant does not appear to affect serum AAT levels. Some studies have found this SNP to be associated with COPD [47,48]; studies in other populations have found no evidence of association [44,49,50].

α_1-Antichymotrypsin

α_1-Antichymotrypsin (AACT) is another serine protease inhibitor, located in close proximity to the AAT gene. Poller *et al.* [51] described one mutation associated with decreased AACT levels (Pro229Ala) and another that caused a dysfunctional protein (Leu55Pro); both of these mutations were associated with COPD. However, these findings could not be replicated in other populations [49,52,53]. Ishii *et al.* [53] found a polymorphism in the signal peptide (Ala-15Thr) to be associated with COPD. As AACT levels were not affected, this is unlikely to be the causative mutation; it may be in linkage disequilibrium with a functional variant. Another study did not find evidence of this association [49].

Matrix metalloproteinases

Mouse models and human experiments have pointed to a role for the matrix metalloproteinases (MMPs) and tissue inhibitors of metalloproteinases (TIMPs) in the development of emphysema [54–56]. A functional polymorphism has been identified in the promoter of MMP-9 (C-1562T) [57]. Among 110 Japanese smokers, the −1562T allele was associated with the presence of emphysema on computed tomography (CT) scan (OR = 2.69; $P = 0.02$) [57]. Joos *et al.* [58] examined MMP polymorphisms in the subjects in the LHS with the fastest and slowest rates of decline in FEV_1. They found the MMP-1 G-1607GG polymorphism to be associated with a fast rate of decline ($P = 0.02$). In addition, haplotypes consisting of the MMP-1 G-1607GG and the MMP-12 Asn357Ser alleles were strongly predictive of rapid decline ($P = 0.0007$). An additional SNP in MMP12 and two MMP-9 polymorphisms were not associated with pulmonary function decline.

Two variants were discovered in tissue inhibitor of metalloproteinases-2 (TIMP-2) in 88 Japanese COPD patients and 40 smoking controls [59]. The allele frequency of a silent variant in exon 3 was significantly higher in COPD cases ($P < 0.0001$). A variant in the promoter region showed a borderline association ($P = 0.049$).

Antioxidants and xenobiotic metabolizing enzymes

Heme oxygenase-1

Cigarette smoke contains reactive oxygen species (ROS) that may contribute to COPD through direct injury to lung tissues, oxidation of antiproteases or up-regulation of inflammatory genes [60]. Heme oxygenase-1 (HMOX1), which degrades heme to biliverdin, is important for protection against heme- and non-heme-mediated oxidant stress in the lung [61]. Yamada *et al.* [62] genotyped a dinucleotide $(GT)_n$ repeat in the promoter region and found a greater number of long repeat alleles in smokers with emphysema compared with smokers without emphysema (OR = 2.4). *In vitro* studies revealed that increased size of the $(GT)_n$ repeat might reduce HMOX1 inducibility by ROS, suggesting a functional mechanism for this polymorphism. However, no association between the number of HMOX1 $(GT)_n$ repeats and rate of decline in lung function was found in the LHS population [63].

Microsomal epoxide hydrolase

Microsomal epoxide hydrolase (EPHX1) is involved in the first-pass metabolism of highly reactive epoxide intermediates, such as those found in cigarette smoke. Polymorphisms in exon 3 (Tyr113His) and exon 4 (His139Arg) have been suggested to decrease (slow allele) or increase (fast allele) enzyme activity, respectively [64]. Smith and Harrison [65] found increased proportions of homozygous slow individuals in groups of patients with clinically diagnosed COPD or pathologically confirmed emphysema compared with control blood donors; however, they also found the fast allele to be more frequent among COPD cases than controls. Sandford *et al.* [44] found a higher frequency of homozygous slow individuals among the rapid decliners compared with the non-decliners in the LHS (OR = 2.4). The effect was stronger in those with a family history of COPD.

In a study of 180 former workers in a Japanese poison gas factory, Yoshikawa *et al.* [66] found no difference in either slow or fast allele EPHX1 frequencies between individuals with and without COPD. However, the slow allele appeared to be associated with the severity of COPD. Studies in two other populations failed to find associations between either EPHX1 polymorphism and the risk of COPD [67,68].

Glutathione S-transferases (M1, P1, T1)

The glutathione S-transferases (GST) are a family of enzymes that are important in the detoxification of hydrophobic and electrophilic compounds, including polycyclic aromatic hydrocarbons found in cigarette smoke. Homozygous deletion of the GST M1 gene can be found in up to 50% of some populations [69]. In a French population, homozygous GST M1 deficiency was more common in individuals with chronic bronchitic with either moderate or severe obstructive lung disease, compared with control smokers [70]. In 168 British patients undergoing surgery for lung cancer, the frequency of GST M1 deletion was higher in those with pathological evidence of emphysema compared with blood donor controls; there was no difference in frequency of the deletion in those with lung cancer only, compared with controls [71]. No association between GST M1 deletion and COPD was found in a Korean population [67].

The GST P1 gene has been found to have greater expression in alveoli, alveolar macrophages and respiratory bronchioles, compared with GST M genes [72]. An exon 5 polymorphism (Ile105Val) in GST P1 has been shown to confer increased activity towards certain substrates [73]. In a study of Japanese men, homozygosity for the wild type GST P1 allele was found more frequently in COPD cases than in smoking controls (OR = 3.5) [74]. This result could not be replicated in a Korean population [75]. In addition, no association was seen between deletion of the GST T1 gene and COPD in the same Korean population [67]. In the LHS subjects, the polymorphisms in GST M1, P1 and T1 were not associated with the rate of lung function decline, when each variant was analysed individually [63]. When all three GST polymorphisms were present, there was a borderline association ($P = 0.03$); the authors note that this may represent type 1 error resulting from the multiple comparisons performed.

Inflammatory cytokines

Tumour necrosis factor α (TNF) is a proinflammatory cytokine that is found in high concentrations in the sputum of COPD patients [76]. A polymorphism at position −308 in the promoter region (TNF1/2) has been described, with increased gene expression *in vitro* resulting from the TNF*2 minor allele [77]. Multiple COPD association studies have been reported, with conflicting results (Table 37.3). Huang *et al.* [78] found a higher frequency of the TNF*2 allele in 42 Taiwanese men with chronic bronchitis compared with matched controls (OR = 11.1) and compared with a second control group that included a population sample of schoolchildren. In a Japanese study, the TNF*2 allele was more frequent in 106 COPD patients than in smoking controls or blood donors [79]. The same authors found a

Table 37.3 Case definitions used in association studies of the tumour necrosis factor α (TNF) −308 polymorphism and COPD [44,78–81,83–86].

Study	Country	Diagnosis	Spirometry	Other criteria
Studies showing evidence of an association				
Huang *et al.* [78]	Taiwan	Chronic bronchitis	$FEV_1 < 80\%$ pred $FEV_1 : FVC < 0.69$	Non-smokers included
Sakao *et al.* [79]	Japan	COPD (ATS)	$FEV_1 < 80\%$ pred $FEV_1 : FVC < 0.7$	Chronic bronchitis excluded Smokers only
Studies without evidence of an association				
Higham *et al.* [81]	UK	COPD (BTS)	$FEV_1 : FVC \leq 80\%$ pred	BD response ≤ 15% Smokers only
Patuzzo *et al.* [83]	Italy	COPD (ATS)	$FEV_1 < 70\%$ pred	BD response < 12% Exclude BHR, wheeze, atopy
Ishii *et al.* [86]	Japan	COPD (ERS)	–	Exclude asthma, AATD, family history of COPD
Sandford *et al.* [44] (Lung Health Study)	USA	Mild COPD	FEV_1 decline ≥ 3%/year	Current smokers
Sakao *et al.* [80]	Japan	COPD (ATS)	$FEV_1 < 80\%$ pred $FEV_1 : FVC < 0.7$	Visual emphysema score on HRCT above/below median
Kucukaycan *et al.* [85]	Netherlands	COPD (ATS)	$FEV_1 < 70\%$ pred	BD response < 10% exclude asthma, AATD
Ferrarotti *et al.* [84]	Italy	COPD (ATS)	$FEV_1 < 50\%$ pred $FEV_1 : FVC < 70\%$ pred	BD response < 12% DLCO < 50% pred

AATD, α_1-antitryspin deficiency; ATS, American Thoracic Society; BD, bronchodilator; BHR, bronchial hyperresponsiveness; BTS, British Thoracic Society; DLCO, carbon monoxide diffusing capacity; ERS, European Respiratory Society; FEV_1, forced expiratory volume in 1 s; FVC, forced vital capacity; HRCT, high-resolution computed tomography; pred, predicted.

trend towards association between the TNF*2 allele and low attenuation areas on high-resolution computed tomography (HRCT) scans of COPD patients [80]. Other studies in Caucasian [81–85] and Japanese [86] populations have failed to observe an association between this TNF promoter polymorphism and COPD. This polymorphism was not associated with lung function decline in the LHS [44]. However, one group did find that COPD patients homozygous for the TNF*2 allele had less reversible airflow obstruction and greater mortality over 2-year follow-up [82]. No associations have been found between a polymorphism in the lymphotoxin-α gene (also known as TNF-β) and COPD or lung function decline [44,83,84].

In a mouse model, inducible overexpression of the cytokine interleukin 13 caused emphysema, mucus metaplasia and inflammation; this phenotype is similar to changes seen in human COPD [87]. Two polymorphisms in IL-13 have been associated with asthma in prior studies [88]. In the LHS population, these two polymorphisms (Arg130Gln, C-1112T) were not associated with rate of lung function decline [89]. However, the IL-13 promoter polymorphism C-1055T (referred to as C-1112T in the previous reference) was found more frequently in COPD patients compared with both smoking ($P = 0.01$) and healthy population ($P = 0.002$) controls in a Dutch study [90].

Other candidate genes

Vitamin D binding protein, also known as group-specific component (GC), has three major serum isotypes (1F, 1S, 2), based on two separate point mutations. It has long been considered a candidate gene for COPD, based on its role in C5a-mediated neutrophil chemotaxis. In 114 matched pairs of COPD patients and controls, Kueppers *et al.* [21] found that homozygosity for Gc-2 allele was protective against COPD ($P = 0.049$). Horne *et al.* [91] observed that even a single Gc-2 allele was protective, and that homozygous Gc-1F individuals were at increased risk of COPD (OR = 7.1). In a study of patients referred for lung cancer surgery, Schellenberg *et al.* [92] found Gc-2 homozygous individuals to be more common among those without airflow obstruction compared with those with obstruction. There was no difference in neutrophil chemotaxis by genotype, suggesting that the protective effect was mediated through a different mechanism. A Japanese study could not replicate the protective effect of the Gc-2 allele, but found the risk of COPD to be increased in Gc-1F homozygotes [93]. However, two other studies failed to find an association between GC variants and lung function [44,94].

Other candidate genes have been shown to be associated with COPD or related phenotypes in single case–control studies (see Table 37.2). It remains to be seen whether these results can be replicated in other populations.

Interpretation of association studies

For most of the candidate gene variants that have been associated with COPD, subsequent studies have often been unable to replicate the positive associations found in the initial study. This lack of consistency is not unique to the study of COPD; it is a problem throughout the field of genetic epidemiology [95,96]. The reasons for this are multiple. One problem is the varied case definitions used in studies of COPD, an inherently heterogeneous disorder. Table 37.3 highlights the different phenotypes used in studies of the TNF −308 polymorphism, as an example. Different authors included or excluded cases with chronic bronchitis or with asthma-related phenotypes, such as bronchodilator responsiveness. If a gene were important in one particular phenotype, such as chronic bronchitis, then this association might be easily missed. In addition, varying thresholds for defining airflow obstruction in COPD cases have been used, which could also contribute to the inconsistent results.

Many of the reported case–control association studies suffer from small sample sizes. High-throughput genotyping technologies have served to reduce costs and should allow for increasingly larger studies [97]. Publication bias is common throughout biomedical research, and it may be even more pronounced in genetic studies [95]. Failure to replicate findings in different studies may also represent true differences in the genetic determinants of disease in different populations, referred to as genetic heterogeneity.

Case–control association studies can be subject to false-positive results because of differences in ethnicity – whether obvious or not – between cases and controls; this is known as population stratification. Statistical techniques are available to test for population stratification in association studies [98], although few authors have performed these tests on a routine basis. Using family-based methods for association studies avoids the potential problem of spurious results brought about by population stratification [99]. Use of this design is increasing in the study of COPD genetics. The potential problems with case–control association studies, as well as a strategy for evaluating these studies, have been reviewed by Silverman and Palmer [100].

Conclusions and future directions

Multiple studies have demonstrated that hereditary factors are important in the development of COPD, but severe AAT deficiency remains the only proven genetic risk factor.

Several interesting associations to biologically plausible candidate genes have been found, but these results have not been consistently replicated in other populations. Family-based linkage studies have identified chromosomal regions where susceptibility genes for COPD are likely to reside, but further work will be necessary to identify the relevant genes, as well as the functional variants within those genes.

Mouse models have been used to identify genes potentially involved in the development of human emphysema, and future animal studies will continue to further our understanding of COPD pathogenesis and uncover candidate genes that can then be studied in human populations. Gene expression profiling using microarray technology is another promising tool in the identification of genetic risk factors for COPD [101]. Clearly, further research is necessary to identify the genetic variants that lead to an increased risk of COPD in the majority of individuals without severe AAT deficiency.

References

1 Knudson RJ. James Jackson, Jr., the young pulmonologist who described familial emphysema: an historical footnote. *Chest* 1985;**87**:673–6.

2 Laurell CB, Eriksson S. The electrophoretic α_1-globulin pattern of serum in α_1-antitrypsin deficiency. *Scand J Clin Invest* 1963;**15**:132–40.

3 Barnes PJ. Chronic obstructive pulmonary disease. *N Engl J Med* 2000;**343**:269–80.

4 de Serres FJ. Worldwide racial and ethnic distribution of α_1-antitrypsin deficiency: summary of an analysis of published genetic epidemiologic surveys. *Chest* 2002;**122**:1818–29.

5 Silverman EK, Pierce JA, Province MA, Rao DC, Campbell EJ. Variability of pulmonary function in α_1-antitrypsin deficiency: clinical correlates. *Ann Intern Med* 1989;**111**:982–91.

6 Silverman EK, Province MA, Campbell EJ, Pierce JA, Rao DC. Family study of α_1-antitrypsin deficiency: effects of cigarette smoking, measured genotype, and their interaction on pulmonary function and biochemical traits. *Genet Epidemiol* 1992;**9**:317–31.

7 Redline S, Tishler PV, Lewitter FI *et al.* Assessment of genetic and non-genetic influences on pulmonary function: a twin study. *Am Rev Respir Dis* 1987;**135**:217–22.

8 Hubert HB, Fabsitz RR, Feinleib M, Gwinn C. Genetic and environmental influences on pulmonary function in adult twins. *Am Rev Respir Dis* 1982;**125**:409–15.

9 Astemborski JA, Beaty TH, Cohen BH. Variance components analysis of forced expiration in families. *Am J Med Genet* 1985;**21**:741–53.

10 Devor EJ, Crawford MH. Family resemblance for normal pulmonary function. *Ann Hum Biol* 1984;**11**:439–48.

11 Lewitter FI, Tager IB, McGue M, Tishler PV, Speizer FE. Genetic and environmental determinants of level of pulmonary function. *Am J Epidemiol* 1984;**120**:518–30.

12 Hankins D, Drage C, Zamel N, Kronenberg R. Pulmonary function in identical twins raised apart. *Am Rev Respir Dis* 1982;**125**:119–21.

13 Gottlieb DJ, Wilk JB, Harmon M *et al.* Heritability of longitudinal change in lung function. The Framingham study. *Am J Respir Crit Care Med* 2001;**164**:1655–9.

14 Wimpfheimer F, Schneider L. Familial emphysema. *Am Rev Respir Dis* 1961;**83**:697–703.

15 Larson RK, Barman ML. The familial occurrence of chronic obstructive pulmonary disease. *Ann Intern Med* 1965;**63**:1001–8.

16 Hole BV, Wasserman K. Familial emphysema. *Ann Intern Med* 1965;**63**:1009–17.

17 Nelson P, Kanner RE. Bullous emphysema in monozygotic twins. *Am Rev Respir Dis* 1989;**140**:1796–9.

18 Larson RK, Barman ML, Kueppers F, Fudenberg HH. Genetic and environmental determinants of chronic obstructive pulmonary disease. *Ann Intern Med* 1970;**72**:627–32.

19 Cohen BH, Ball WC Jr, Bias WB *et al.* A genetic–epidemiologic study of chronic obstructive pulmonary disease. I. Study design and preliminary observations. *Johns Hopkins Med J* 1975;**137**:95–104.

20 Higgins M, Keller J. Familial occurrence of chronic respiratory disease and familial resemblance in ventilatory capacity. *J Chronic Dis* 1975;**28**:239–51.

21 Kueppers F, Miller RD, Gordon H, Hepper NG, Offord K. Familial prevalence of chronic obstructive pulmonary disease in a matched pair study. *Am J Med* 1977;**63**:336–42.

22 Tager I, Tishler PV, Rosner B, Speizer FE, Litt M. Studies of the familial aggregation of chronic bronchitis and obstructive airways disease. *Int J Epidemiol* 1978;**7**:55–62.

23 Khoury MJ, Beaty TH, Tockman MS, Self SG, Cohen BH. Familial aggregation in chronic obstructive pulmonary disease: use of the loglinear model to analyze intermediate environmental and genetic risk factors. *Genet Epidemiol* 1985;**2**:155–66.

24 Silverman EK, Chapman HA, Drazen JM *et al.* Genetic epidemiology of severe, early-onset chronic obstructive pulmonary disease: risk to relatives for airflow obstruction and chronic bronchitis. *Am J Respir Crit Care Med* 1998;**157**:1770–8.

25 Celedon JC, Speizer FE, Drazen JM *et al.* Bronchodilator responsiveness and serum total IgE levels in families of probands with severe early-onset COPD. *Eur Respir J* 1999;**14**:1009–14.

26 Silverman EK, Weiss ST, Drazen JM *et al.* Gender-related differences in severe, early-onset chronic obstructive pulmonary disease. *Am J Respir Crit Care Med* 2000;**162**:2152–8.

27 McCloskey SC, Patel BD, Hinchliffe SJ *et al.* Siblings of patients with severe chronic obstructive pulmonary disease have a significant risk of airflow obstruction. *Am J Respir Crit Care Med* 2001;**164**:1419–24.

28 Silverman EK, Mosley JD, Palmer L *et al.* Genome-wide linkage analysis of severe, early-onset chronic obstructive pulmonary disease: airflow obstruction and chronic bronchitis phenotypes. *Hum Mol Genet* 2002;**11**:623–32.

29 Silverman EK, Palmer LJ, Mosley JD *et al.* Genomewide linkage analysis of quantitative spirometric phenotypes in

severe early-onset chronic obstructive pulmonary disease. *Am J Hum Genet* 2002;**70**:1229–39.

30 Lander E, Kruglyak L. Genetic dissection of complex traits: guidelines for interpreting and reporting linkage results. *Nat Genet* 1995;**11**:241–7.

31 Palmer LJ, Celedon JC, Chapman HA *et al.* Genome-wide linkage analysis of bronchodilator responsiveness and post-bronchodilator spirometric phenotypes in chronic obstructive pulmonary disease. *Hum Mol Genet* 2003;**12**:1199–210.

32 Joost O, Wilk JB, Cupples LA *et al.* Genetic loci influencing lung function: a genome-wide scan in the Framingham Study. *Am J Respir Crit Care Med* 2002;**165**:795–9.

33 Wilk JB, DeStefano AL, Arnett DK *et al.* A genome-wide scan of pulmonary function measures in the National Heart, Lung, and Blood Institute Family Heart Study. *Am J Respir Crit Care Med* 2003;**167**:1528–33.

34 Malhotra A, Peiffer AP, Ryujin DT *et al.* Further evidence for the role of genes on chromosome 2 and chromosome 5 in the inheritance of pulmonary function. *Am J Respir Crit Care Med* 2003;**168**:556–61.

35 Ober C, Abney M, McPeek MS. The genetic dissection of complex traits in a founder population. *Am J Hum Genet* 2001;**69**:1068–79.

36 Barnett TB, Gottovi D, Johnson AM. Protease inhibitors in chronic obstructive pulmonary disease. *Am Rev Respir Dis* 1975;**111**:587–93.

37 Bartmann K, Fooke-Achterrath M, Koch G *et al.* Heterozygosity in the Pi-system as a pathogenetic cofactor in chronic obstructive pulmonary disease (COPD). *Eur J Respir Dis* 1985;**66**:284–96.

38 Shigeoka JW, Hall WJ, Hyde RW *et al.* The prevalence of α-antitrypsin heterozygotes (Pi MZ) in patients with obstructive pulmonary disease. *Am Rev Respir Dis* 1976;**114**:1077–84.

39 Sandford AJ, Weir TD, Spinelli JJ, Pare PD. Z and S mutations of the α_1-antitrypsin gene and the risk of chronic obstructive pulmonary disease. *Am J Respir Cell Mol Biol* 1999;**20**:287–91.

40 Lieberman J, Winter B, Sastre A. α_1-Antitrypsin Pi-types in 965 COPD patients. *Chest* 1986;**89**:370–3.

41 Morse JO, Lebowitz MD, Knudson RJ, Burrows B. Relation of protease inhibitor phenotypes to obstructive lung diseases in a community. *N Engl J Med* 1977;**296**:1190–4.

42 Webb DR, Hyde RW, Schwartz RH *et al.* Serum α_1-antitrypsin variants: prevalence and clinical spirometry. *Am Rev Respir Dis* 1973;**108**:918–25.

43 Dahl M, Tybjaerg-Hansen A, Lange P, Vestbo J, Nordestgaard BG. Change in lung function and morbidity from chronic obstructive pulmonary disease in α_1-antitrypsin MZ heterozygotes: a longitudinal study of the general population. *Ann Intern Med* 2002;**136**:270–9.

44 Sandford AJ, Chagani T, Weir TD *et al.* Susceptibility genes for rapid decline of lung function in the Lung Health Study. *Am J Respir Crit Care Med* 2001;**163**:469–73.

45 Anthonisen NR, Connett JE, Kiley JP *et al.* Effects of smoking intervention and the use of an inhaled anticholinergic bronchodilator on the rate of decline of FEV_1. The Lung Health Study. *JAMA* 1994;**272**:1497–505.

46 Silva GE, Sherrill DL, Guerra S, Barbee RA. A longitudinal study of α_1-antitrypsin phenotypes and decline in FEV_1 in a community population. *Chest* 2003;**123**:1435–40.

47 Poller W, Meisen C, Olek K. DNA polymorphisms of the α_1-antitrypsin gene region in patients with chronic obstructive pulmonary disease. *Eur J Clin Invest* 1990;**20**:1–7.

48 Kalsheker NA, Watkins GL, Hill S *et al.* Independent mutations in the flanking sequence of the α_1-antitrypsin gene are associated with chronic obstructive airways disease. *Dis Markers* 1990;**8**:151–7.

49 Benetazzo MG, Gile LS, Bombieri C *et al.* α_1-Antitrypsin TAQ I polymorphism and α_1-antichymotrypsin mutations in patients with obstructive pulmonary disease. *Respir Med* 1999;**93**:648–54.

50 Sandford AJ, Spinelli JJ, Weir TD, Pare PD. Mutation in the 3′ region of the α_1-antitrypsin gene and chronic obstructive pulmonary disease. *J Med Genet* 1997;**34**:874–5.

51 Poller W, Faber JP, Weidinger S *et al.* A leucine-to-proline substitution causes a defective α_1-antichymotrypsin allele associated with familial obstructive lung disease. *Genomics* 1993;**17**:740–3.

52 Sandford AJ, Chagani T, Weir TD, Pare PD. α_1-Antichymotrypsin mutations in patients with chronic obstructive pulmonary disease. *Dis Markers* 1998;**13**:257–60.

53 Ishii T, Matsuse T, Teramoto S *et al.* Association between α_1-antichymotrypsin polymorphism and susceptibility to chronic obstructive pulmonary disease. *Eur J Clin Invest* 2000;**30**:543–8.

54 Hautamaki RD, Kobayashi DK, Senior RM, Shapiro SD. Requirement for macrophage elastase for cigarette smoke-induced emphysema in mice. *Science* 1997;**277**:2002–4.

55 Mahadeva R, Shapiro SD. Chronic obstructive pulmonary disease 3: Experimental animal models of pulmonary emphysema. *Thorax* 2002;**57**:908–14.

56 Finlay GA, O'Driscoll LR, Russell KJ *et al.* Matrix metalloproteinase expression and production by alveolar macrophages in emphysema. *Am J Respir Crit Care Med* 1997;**156**:240–7.

57 Minematsu N, Nakamura H, Tateno H, Nakajima T, Yamaguchi K. Genetic polymorphism in matrix metalloproteinase-9 and pulmonary emphysema. *Biochem Biophys Res Commun* 2001;**289**:116–9.

58 Joos L, He JQ, Shepherdson MB *et al.* The role of matrix metalloproteinase polymorphisms in the rate of decline in lung function. *Hum Mol Genet* 2002;**11**:569–76.

59 Hirano K, Sakamoto T, Uchida Y *et al.* Tissue inhibitor of metalloproteinases-2 gene polymorphisms in chronic obstructive pulmonary disease. *Eur Respir J* 2001;**18**:748–52.

60 Barnes PJ. New concepts in chronic obstructive pulmonary disease. *Annu Rev Med* 2003;**54**:113–29.

61 Morse D, Choi AM. Heme oxygenase-1: the 'emerging molecule' has arrived. *Am J Respir Cell Mol Biol* 2002;**27**:8–16.

62 Yamada N, Yamaya M, Okinaga S *et al.* Protective effects of heme oxygenase-1 against oxidant-induced injury in the cultured human tracheal epithelium. *Am J Respir Cell Mol Biol* 1999;**21**:428–35.

63 He JQ, Ruan J, Connett JE *et al*. Antioxidant gene polymorphisms and susceptibility to a rapid decline in lung function in smokers. *Am J Respir Crit Care Med* 2002;**166**:323–8.

64 Hassett C, Aicher L, Sidhu JS, Omiecinski CJ. Human microsomal epoxide hydrolase: genetic polymorphism and functional expression *in vitro* of amino acid variants. *Hum Mol Genet* 1994;**3**:421–8.

65 Smith CA, Harrison DJ. Association between polymorphism in gene for microsomal epoxide hydrolase and susceptibility to emphysema. *Lancet* 1997;**350**:630–3.

66 Yoshikawa M, Hiyama K, Ishioka S *et al*. Microsomal epoxide hydrolase genotypes and chronic obstructive pulmonary disease in Japanese. *Int J Mol Med* 2000;**5**:49–53.

67 Yim JJ, Park GY, Lee CT *et al*. Genetic susceptibility to chronic obstructive pulmonary disease in Koreans: combined analysis of polymorphic genotypes for microsomal epoxide hydrolase and glutathione S-transferase M1 and T1. *Thorax* 2000;**55**:121–5.

68 Takeyabu K, Yamaguchi E, Suzuki I *et al*. Gene polymorphism for microsomal epoxide hydrolase and susceptibility to emphysema in a Japanese population. *Eur Respir J* 2000;**15**:891–4.

69 Board P, Coggan M, Johnston P *et al*. Genetic heterogeneity of the human glutathione transferases: a complex of gene families. *Pharmacol Ther* 1990;**48**:357–69.

70 Baranova H, Perriot J, Albuisson E *et al*. Peculiarities of the GSTM1 0/0 genotype in French heavy smokers with various types of chronic bronchitis. *Hum Genet* 1997;**99**:822–6.

71 Harrison DJ, Cantlay AM, Rae F, Lamb D, Smith CA. Frequency of glutathione S-transferase M1 deletion in smokers with emphysema and lung cancer. *Hum Exp Toxicol* 1997;**16**:356–60.

72 Cantlay AM, Smith CA, Wallace WA *et al*. Heterogeneous expression and polymorphic genotype of glutathione S-transferases in human lung. *Thorax* 1994;**49**:1010–4.

73 Sundberg K, Johansson AS, Stenberg G *et al*. Differences in the catalytic efficiencies of allelic variants of glutathione transferase P1-1 towards carcinogenic diol epoxides of polycyclic aromatic hydrocarbons. *Carcinogenesis* 1998;**19**:433–6.

74 Ishii T, Matsuse T, Teramoto S *et al*. Glutathione S-transferase P1 (GSTP1) polymorphism in patients with chronic obstructive pulmonary disease. *Thorax* 1999;**54**:693–6.

75 Yim JJ, Yoo CG, Lee CT *et al*. Lack of association between glutathione S-transferase P1 polymorphism and COPD in Koreans. *Lung* 2002;**180**:119–25.

76 Keatings VM, Collins PD, Scott DM, Barnes PJ. Differences in interleukin-8 and tumor necrosis factor-α in induced sputum from patients with chronic obstructive pulmonary disease or asthma. *Am J Respir Crit Care Med* 1996;**153**:530–4.

77 Wilson AG, Symons JA, McDowell TL, McDevitt HO, Duff GW. Effects of a polymorphism in the human tumor necrosis factor α promoter on transcriptional activation. *Proc Natl Acad Sci U S A* 1997;**94**:3195–9.

78 Huang SL, Su CH, Chang SC. Tumor necrosis factor-α gene polymorphism in chronic bronchitis. *Am J Respir Crit Care Med* 1997;**156**:1436–9.

79 Sakao S, Tatsumi K, Igari H *et al*. Association of tumor necrosis factor α gene promoter polymorphism with the presence of chronic obstructive pulmonary disease. *Am J Respir Crit Care Med* 2001;**163**:420–2.

80 Sakao S, Tatsumi K, Igari H *et al*. Association of tumor necrosis factor-α gene promoter polymorphism with low attenuation areas on high-resolution CT in patients with COPD. *Chest* 2002;**122**:416–20.

81 Higham MA, Pride NB, Alikhan A, Morrell NW. Tumour necrosis factor-α gene promoter polymorphism in chronic obstructive pulmonary disease. *Eur Respir J* 2000;**15**:281–4.

82 Keatings VM, Cave SJ, Henry MJ *et al*. A polymorphism in the tumor necrosis factor-α gene promoter region may predispose to a poor prognosis in COPD. *Chest* 2000;**118**:971–5.

83 Patuzzo C, Gile LS, Zorzetto M *et al*. Tumor necrosis factor gene complex in COPD and disseminated bronchiectasis. *Chest* 2000;**117**:1353–8.

84 Ferrarotti I, Zorzetto M, Beccaria M *et al*. Tumour necrosis factor family genes in a phenotype of COPD associated with emphysema. *Eur Respir J* 2003;**21**:444–9.

85 Kucukaycan M, Van Krugten M, Pennings HJ *et al*. Tumor necrosis factor-α +489G/A gene polymorphism is associated with chronic obstructive pulmonary disease. *Respir Res* 2002;**3**:29.

86 Ishii T, Matsuse T, Teramoto S *et al*. Neither IL-1β, IL-1 receptor antagonist, nor TNF-α polymorphisms are associated with susceptibility to COPD. *Respir Med* 2000;**94**:847–51.

87 Zheng T, Zhu Z, Wang Z *et al*. Inducible targeting of IL-13 to the adult lung causes matrix metalloproteinase- and cathepsin-dependent emphysema. *J Clin Invest* 2000;**106**:1081–93.

88 Wills-Karp M. The gene encoding interleukin-13: a susceptibility locus for asthma and related traits. *Respir Res* 2000;**1**:19–23.

89 He JQ, Connett JE, Anthonisen NR, Sandford AJ. Polymorphisms in the IL13, IL13RA1, and IL4RA genes and rate of decline in lung function in smokers. *Am J Respir Cell Mol Biol* 2003;**28**:379–85.

90 van der Pouw Kraan TC, Kucukaycan M, Bakker AM *et al*. Chronic obstructive pulmonary disease is associated with the -1055 IL-13 promoter polymorphism. *Genes Immun* 2002;**3**:436–9.

91 Horne SL, Cockcroft DW, Dosman JA. Possible protective effect against chronic obstructive airways disease by the GC2 allele. *Hum Hered* 1990;**40**:173–6.

92 Schellenberg D, Pare PD, Weir TD *et al*. Vitamin D binding protein variants and the risk of COPD. *Am J Respir Crit Care Med* 1998;**157**:957–61.

93 Ishii T, Keicho N, Teramoto S *et al*. Association of Gc-globulin variation with susceptibility to COPD and diffuse panbronchiolitis. *Eur Respir J* 2001;**18**:753–7.

94 Kauffmann F, Kleisbauer JP, Cambon-De-Mouzon A *et al*. Genetic markers in chronic air-flow limitation: a genetic epidemiologic study. *Am Rev Respir Dis* 1983;**127**:263–9.

95 Ioannidis JP, Ntzani EE, Trikalinos TA, Contopoulos-Ioannidis DG. Replication validity of genetic association studies. *Nat Genet* 2001;**29**:306–9.

96 Hirschhorn JN, Lohmueller K, Byrne E, Hirschhorn K. A comprehensive review of genetic association studies. *Genet Med* 2002;**4**:45–61.

97 Gray IC, Campbell DA, Spurr NK. Single nucleotide polymorphisms as tools in human genetics. *Hum Mol Genet* 2000; **9**:2403–8.

98 Pritchard JK, Rosenberg NA. Use of unlinked genetic markers to detect population stratification in association studies. *Am J Hum Genet* 1999;**65**:220–8.

99 Schaid DJ. Transmission disequilibrium, family controls, and great expectations. *Am J Hum Genet* 1998;**63**:935–41.

100 Silverman EK, Palmer LJ. Case–control association studies for the genetics of complex respiratory diseases. *Am J Respir Cell Mol Biol* 2000;**22**:645–8.

101 Spira A, Pinto-Plata V, Beane J *et al*. Gene expression profiles in severe emphysema reveal distinct molecular subclasses of disease and may predict outcome after lung volume reduction surgery. *Am J Respir Crit Care Med* 2003;**167**(Suppl):A939.

102 Ho LI, Harn HJ, Chen CJ, Tsai NM. Polymorphism of the β_2-adrenoceptor in COPD in Chinese subjects. *Chest* 2001; **120**:1493–9.

103 Tzetis M, Efthymiadou A, Strofalis S *et al*. CFTR gene mutations – including three novel nucleotide substitutions – and haplotype background in patients with asthma, disseminated bronchiectasis and chronic obstructive pulmonary disease. *Hum Genet* 2001;**108**:216–21.

104 Guo X, Lin HM, Lin Z *et al*. Surfactant protein gene A, B, and D marker alleles in chronic obstructive pulmonary disease of a Mexican population. *Eur Respir J* 2001;**18**: 482–90.

105 Matsushita I, Hasegawa K, Nakata K *et al*. Genetic variants of human β-defensin-1 and chronic obstructive pulmonary disease. *Biochem Biophys Res Commun* 2002;**291**:17–22.

106 Cantlay AM, Lamb D, Gillooly M *et al*. Association between the CYP1A1 gene polymorphism and susceptibility to emphysema and lung cancer. *J Clin Pathol: Mol Pathol* 1995;**48**:210M–4M.

107 Cohen BH, Ball WC Jr, Brashears S *et al*. Risk factors in chronic obstructive pulmonary disease (COPD). *Am J Epidemiol* 1977;**105**:223–32.

108 Cohen BH, Bias WB, Chase GA *et al*. Is ABH non-secretor status a risk factor for obstructive lung disease? *Am J Epidemiol* 1980;**111**:285–91.

109 Kauffmann F, Frette C, Pham QT *et al*. Associations of blood group-related antigens to FEV_1, wheezing, and asthma. *Am J Respir Crit Care Med* 1996;**153**:76–82.

CHAPTER 38
α_1-Antitrypsin deficiency

Loutfi S. Aboussouan and James K. Stoller

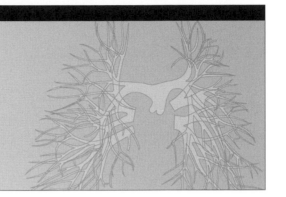

α_1-Antitrypsin (AAT) deficiency is a common but under-recognized condition. In this chapter, we first review the history of AAT deficiency, and then discuss the epidemiology, clinical features and treatment, including augmentation therapy and emerging therapies.

History

AAT deficiency was first described in 1963 when Laurell and Eriksson found that the electrophoretic patterns of stored serum specimens of some patients with emphysema were lacking α_1 bands [1]. Eriksson [2] subsequently described the heritability of emphysema in such individuals in 1964 and some salient clinical features, including bibasilar distribution and premature onset [3].

Significant progress ensued in elucidating the pathogenetic mechanisms of this disease. Experimental emphysema was produced in rats using the plant protease papain [4,5] and Kueppers and Bearn [6] demonstrated the ability of AAT to inhibit proteases. These findings provided an experimental basis for the association between AAT deficiency and the development of emphysema [6], and laid the groundwork for the protease–antiprotease hypothesis of emphysema [7].

The subsequent discovery of neutrophil elastase by Aaron Janoff in 1968 [8] and recognition of the high affinity of neutrophil elastase for AAT [9] established neutrophil elastase rather than trypsin as the natural substrate of AAT. Nevertheless, the original name of AAT deficiency has persisted. Studies by Senior *et al.* [10] in 1977 found that neutrophil elastase could likewise induce emphysema, albeit of a milder form compared with that produced by pancreatic elastase [10,11].

Progress in molecular biology led to key advances, including the sequencing of the AAT protein in 1984 [12], identification of the gene on chromosome 14 [13] and recognition of several clinically relevant variants [13]. While AAT deficiency was recognized in 1969 as a cause of liver storage disease and cirrhosis [14], understanding the mechanism of impaired secretion of the Z-type protein and intrahepatocyte accumulation awaited the elucidation of loop-sheet polymerization by Lomas *et al.* [15] in 1992.

Clinical advances have included the use of purified AAT derived from pooled human plasma for exogenous administration [16], the establishment of important registries, including the National Heart, Lung and Blood Institute (NHLBI) sponsored Registry for Individuals with Severe AAT Deficiency from 1988 to 1996 [17], the patient-sponsored Alpha-1 Foundation Research Registry in 1997 [18], and the Alpha-One International Registry (AIR) in 1996.

Epidemiology of AAT deficiency

A review of the epidemiology of AAT deficiency provides two major insights:
1 AAT deficiency is common; and
2 AAT deficiency is under-recognized by clinicians, causing significant adverse effects.

With regard to the frequency of AAT deficiency, estimates have been undertaken in several ways: an indirect epidemiological approach based on estimates of emphysema prevalence, an indirect analysis of genetic epidemiological surveys and a direct population-based screening approach.

To assess the frequency of AAT deficiency in the USA using indirect means, the National Health Information Survey estimates that 3.2 million Americans have emphysema [19]. Results of a study by Lieberman *et al.* [20] in which 965 patients in the COPD clinic of the Sepulveda Veterans Administration Hospital show that 1.9% had emphysema on the basis of severe deficiency of AAT. Applying this prevalence estimate to the estimated number

Table 38.1 Prevalence estimates of severe α_1-antitrypsin (AAT) deficiency (PI*ZZ and/or PI*Znull) in selected population screening studies.

First author [Ref.]	Years	Location of study	Subject population	Number with severe AAT deficiency/number screened	Prevalence of severe AAT deficiency (%)
Sveger [26]	1972–74	Sweden	Newborns	122/200 000	1/1639 (0.061)
O'Brien [23]	1971–74	Oregon	Newborns	21/107 038	1/5097 (0.0196)
Silverman [24]	1987	St. Louis	Blood donors	7/20 000	1/2857 (0.035)
Spence [25]	1993	New York state	Newborns	3/11 081	1/3694 (0.0271)

of Americans with emphysema suggests that approximately 61 000 Americans have symptomatic COPD on the basis of severe AAT deficiency.

Another approach uses published genetic epidemiological surveys to estimate the PI*Z mean gene frequency in a given population, and then extrapolates to the population at risk for the PI*ZZ allele combination. For the USA, this approach estimates the population at risk for PI*ZZ to be 47 321 [21], although weighed estimates adjusting for the different ethnic subgroups of the US population suggest a higher number of 59 047 [22].

Although derived differently, these estimates agree closely with prevalence estimates that come from direct population-based screening studies. Of the several population-based screening studies performed (Table 38.1) [23–26], the two largest have involved the screening of 200 000 newborns in Sweden [26] and 107 038 newborns in Oregon [23]. In the Swedish screening study, the frequency of PI*Z individuals was found to be 122/200 000, or 1 in 1639. In the Oregon screening experience, the frequency of PI*ZZ individuals was approximately threefold lower at 1 in 5097. Combining the three US studies [23–25] yields a frequency of 1 in 4455. Applying this estimate to the 2000 US population of 281 000 000 [27] suggests that the number of PI*ZZ individuals in the USA today is 63 000, of whom most can be expected to develop emphysema [28–30]. In this regard, the prevalence of severe AAT deficiency approximates that of another common genetic pulmonary condition, cystic fibrosis, the frequency of which has been estimated to be 1 in 11 000 [31].

In the context that AAT deficiency is common, the question naturally arises as to why so few AAT deficient patients are known to the medical community. Indeed, recent estimates of the number of AAT deficient individuals currently receiving intravenous augmentation therapy with pooled human plasma AAT are fewer than 10 000 and large central laboratories for testing for AAT deficiency suggest a ceiling estimate of 14 000 severely deficient individuals (E. Campbell, personal communication).

Studies addressing the frequency of AAT deficient individuals show that individuals with severe AAT deficiency often escape medical detection. For example, in a study of the frequency of severe deficiency of AAT in St. Louis, Silverman *et al.* [24] sampled 20 000 blood specimens donated to the St. Louis blood bank, among which seven individuals with PI*ZZ AAT deficiency were found. Reasoning that blood donation neither selected for nor against having severe AAT deficiency, these investigators suggested that this prevalence among blood donors predicted 700 PI*ZZ individuals in St. Louis with a population of 2 million at the time of the study. Yet, when these investigators attempted to identify all known PI*ZZ individuals by contacting pulmonary physicians in St. Louis, only 28 PI*ZZ patients could be detected (4% of the expected population of 700), suggesting that the majority of AAT deficient individuals in St. Louis at that time were unrecognized by the medical community. Similar findings regarding frequent under-recognition were reported by Tobin *et al.* [30] in a British Thoracic Association survey of all PI*Z samples at two specialized laboratories in England, suggesting that only 4.5% of British PI*Z subjects had been detected by 1980.

Finally, that under-recognition occurs frequently and confers adverse psychological effects has been demonstrated by Stoller *et al.* [32] in a 1992 survey of 300 self-reported PI*ZZ individuals. When given a questionnaire addressing the number of physicians seen for attributable symptoms and the mean interval between the first AAT deficiency-related symptom, the group reported an average delay between first symptom and initial diagnosis of AAT deficiency of 7.2 (± 8.3) years. Furthermore, 44% of these respondents reported having to see at least three physicians with attributable symptoms before the initial diagnosis of severe AAT deficiency was made [32]. More recent estimates confirm this long diagnostic delay and under-recognition. In a survey of 974 individuals mostly receiving augmentation therapy at home, Campos, Sandhaus and Wanner (R.A. Sandhaus, personal communication) observed that the mean interval between first symptom and initial diagnosis was 7.8 ± 9.2 years and that 34.6% reported seeing at least three physicians before the diagnosis of AAT deficiency was made.

That adverse events result from the delayed diagnosis of AAT deficiency has been suggested by Stoller *et al.* [32]. For example, the mean number of adverse psychosocial effects correlated weakly but significantly with the number of doctors seen before initial diagnosis (Spearman's rho = 0.20; *P* = 0.005), although no correlation of adverse effects was observed with the interval between the first attributable symptom and initial diagnosis (Spearman's rho 0.05; *P* = 0.43) [32].

Pathophysiology and genetics of AAT deficiency

Loop-sheet polymerization

AAT is the prototypic member of the *ser*ine *p*rotease *in*hibitor (serpin) superfamily of proteins that have a major role in diverse biological pathways [33]. The characterization of loop-sheet polymerization as the molecular defect underlying AAT deficiency has not only helped clarify the pathogenesis of the associated liver disease, but has also allowed expansion of this model to the pathobiology of other serpinopathies. For instance, mutations and loop-sheet polymerization of other serpins such as antithrombin, C1 inhibitor, and neuroserpins cause thrombosis, angioedema, and inclusion body dementia, respectively [33–35]. This model has been further applied to elucidate other mechanisms of diseases such as Alzheimer's disease, amyloidosis, Huntington's disease and the prion encephalopathies, thereby spanning the gamut of acquired, genetic and 'infectious' diseases [36].

Underlying this susceptibility of serpins to mutations and polymerization is instability of their β-sheet structure

(Fig. 38.1) [37]. In the most common allele associated with severe deficiency, PI*ZZ AAT deficiency, a single substitution of lysine for glutamic acid at position 342 widens the β-sheet and allows partial insertion of the reactive site loop into the gap to create an intermediate and unstable monomeric form (see Fig. 38.1) [38]. The β-sheet can then either accept its own loop and form a latent form, or the loop of an adjacent molecule and form a dimer (see Fig. 38.1) [38]. The dimer stabilizes, increases its β-sheet and proceeds to polymerization in an irreversible process (see Fig. 38.1) [39]. This process is in equilibrium, with approximately 15% of Z antitrypsin secreted into the plasma as monomers [15,33]. Although the Z molecule may polymerize spontaneously, factors that increase the likelihood of polymerization include increase in temperature and in Z antitrypsin concentration [15], and possibly a decrease in pH [39].

Mechanism for the development of emphysema

Neutrophils are present in the lower respiratory tract and provide a chronic low-level burden of neutrophil elastase [40]. Despite its name, AAT reacts with neutrophil elastase much more avidly than with trypsin in a mutually suicidal interaction [41,42]. AAT is produced in the liver and reaches the lungs by diffusion from the circulation and by local production in macrophages and bronchial epithelial cells [33,43]. In the normal state, there is an excess of AAT in the lung, thereby providing an adequate protective screen against the elastolytic effect of neutrophil elastase [28].

In PI*ZZ individuals, the protease–antiprotease concept posits an imbalance between the AAT protective screen and the neutrophil elastase burden, with consequent unchecked proteolytic activity leading to emphysema [7].

Figure 38.1 Structure of α_1-antitrypsin and mechanism of polymerization. A substitution of lysine for glutamic acid at position 342 (arrow) widens the β-sheet A (circle) and results in the formation of an unstable intermediate monomer (M*). The gap in the β-sheet A can either accept its own loop to form a latent conformation (L), or form a dimer by accepting the loop of another α_1-antitrypsin molecule (D). The dimer proceeds to polymerization in an irreversible process (P). (From Lomas and Mahadeva [33] with permission.)

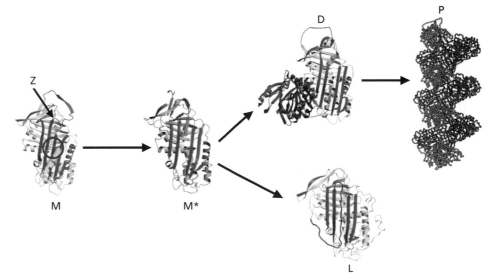

This imbalance results in large part from low serum levels of AAT because of retention of polymers in the endoplasmic reticulum of liver cells [15]. Also, the Z-type antitrypsin is about five times less effective than normal antitrypsin as an inhibitor of neutrophil elastase [44]. Lastly, Z-type antitrypsin has been identified in the lung as loop-sheet polymers that are not only functionally inactive against neutrophil elastase [45], but also chemoattractants for human neutrophils [46].

Indirectly, unchecked neutrophil elastase in AAT deficiency may promote a positive feedback loop by stimulating macrophages to release leukotriene B_4, itself a potential mediator of neutrophil chemotaxis [47,48]. AAT can also act as modulator of the inflammatory response by inhibiting other chemotactic factors such as C3a and C5a [49].

Mechanism of liver disease

Based on the link between temperature and polymerization, febrile episodes were initially proposed as the explanation for the phenotypic variability of liver disease in PI*ZZ individuals [15], although clinical considerations make this is an unlikely mechanism [50]. Rather, a lag in intracellular degradation of Z-type protein correlates with the expression of liver disease in PI*ZZ individuals [51]. Polymers of Z-type protein have been identified on electron microscopy as inclusions within the endoplasmic reticulum of the liver [15], and account for the periodic acid–Schiff stain positivity and diastase-resistant material on liver biopsies of affected individuals. Retention of the mutant Z molecules in the endoplasmic reticulum appears to have a key role in the development of liver disease and may be caused by an impaired interaction between Z-type protein and its molecular chaperone, calnexin [52]. The precise mechanism by which the intrahepatocyte accumulation of unsecreted AAT causes liver disease remains elusive.

Clinical features and diagnosis of AAT deficiency

Lung disease

Emphysema

Although the precise degree of risk is unknown, individuals homozygous for the Z allele are considered to be at high risk for developing emphysema. Differentiating features of this type of emphysema include a more likely occurrence at an early age (i.e. less than 50 years), a panacinar pathology and basilar distribution [53,54]. Studies may be biased towards overestimating the risk of emphysema in AAT deficiency because most patients are ascertained on the basis of pulmonary symptoms. In a survey from the British

Thoracic Association, Tobin *et al.* [30] sought to determine the risk of developing emphysema by identifying PI*ZZ in siblings of their index cases, thereby partially removing the bias of selection based on attendance at a chest clinic. Radiographically confirmed emphysema was present in 87% of all PI*ZZ subjects, 91% of the index cases and 73% of the non-index cases [30]. Ninety per cent of PI*ZZ smokers had emphysema, compared with 65% of non-smokers [30]. Additionally, abnormalities of lung function were reported in the majority of individuals without radiographical changes [30]. These data closely agree with those of the Swedish National Registry, in which only 29% of the participants were identified because of lung disease, indicating that in adult PIZ homozygotes, 29% of never-smokers and 10% of ever-smokers were healthy, with the majority of the remainder identified as having lung disease [28]. Lastly, postmortem series from Malmö General Hospital in Sweden suggest that only 20% of PIZ homozygotes had no chronic obstructive lung disease [28].

Several studies have attempted to further define susceptibility genes for the development of emphysema. Sandford *et al.* [55] have shown that 6% of COPD individuals were heterozygous for the Z allele (PI*MZ) compared with none of the controls, while the S allele was not associated with emphysema. These authors concluded that the Z allele but not the S allele was a risk factor for COPD in the heterozygous state [55]. These observations were supported in other studies by Turino *et al.* [56] and Alvarez-Granda *et al.* [57], who noted that the PI*SZ phenotype confers little or no added risk of developing COPD except in smokers. In a population-based cohort study by Dahl *et al.*, individuals with the MZ genotype had a slightly greater rate of decline of forced expiratory volume in 1 s (FEV_1) were more likely to have airway obstruction, and had a trend towards a higher incidence of hospitalization and mortality from COPD, compared to individuals with the MM genotype [58]. On the other hand, a population study of PI*MZ heterozygotes from the Tucson Epidemiologic Study of Airways Obstructive Diseases failed to show any increased risk of developing airflow obstruction in MZ individuals [59].

Asthma

Several studies have shown a 15–30% prevalence of asthma in patients with AAT deficiency. In 1041 patients from the NHLBI Alpha-One Registry, a self-report of asthma diagnosed by a physician was found in 38% [60]. When asthma was also defined by bronchodilator responsiveness and recurrent wheezing attacks, asthma was diagnosed in 21% and in 12.5% of those with a normal FEV_1 [60]. In another study of 97 young adults (approximately 22 years of age) from an original cohort of 129 PI Z homozygotes identified by neonatal screening, 29% reported recurrent wheezing and 15% carried a diagnosis of asthma despite normal spirometry [61]. The frequency of wheezing in ever-smokers was much higher at 56% [61]. In a study from the Italian Registry, the prevalence of methacholine hyper-responsiveness in 86 individuals with different phenotypes (including MZ, MS, SZ, ZZ) was similar in subjects vs controls (16 vs 11%, respectively; $P = 0.66$), but hyperresponsive subjects demonstrated a positive correlation between AAT blood levels and PD20 FEV_1 values ($r = 0.71$; $P < 0.01$) [62]. In one study of 90 asthmatic patients, plasma elastase inhibitory capacity was markedly reduced in asthmatic subjects compared with controls despite higher plasma α_1-protease inhibitor levels, raising the possibility of a functional AAT deficiency as a component of the inflammatory process of asthma [63].

Recognizing the importance of preventive measures, the World Health Organization has recommended that all patients with COPD and adults and adolescents with asthma be screened for AAT deficiency [64]. Also, a recent international standards document from the American Thoracic Society, European Respiratory Society, American College of Chest Physicians, American Respiratory Care Foundation, and the Alpha-1 Foundation has endorsed diagnostic testing in all symptomatic adults with fixed airflow obstruction [65].

Bronchiectasis

Whether bronchiectasis is associated with severe deficiency of AAT has been the subject of controversy. For example, a computed tomography (CT) study of 117 non-smoking PI*ZZ individuals showed a 26% frequency of bronchiectasis [66], with smaller studies indicating a prevalence as high as 43% [67,68]. However, the distribution of AAT alleles in individuals with bronchiectasis is similar to that of control subjects, suggesting that bronchiectasis develops alongside the emphysema or associated chronic bronchitis rather than as a direct effect of AAT deficiency [69,70]. Moreover, the self-reported prevalence of bronchiectasis from subjects in the NHLBI Registry of Individuals with AAT deficiency was only 2%. This suggests that the high prevalence of bronchiectasis on computed tomography (CT) studies may not carry significant clinical import or that self-reported prevalence represents underdiagnosis [71].

Bronchitis

Chronic sputum expectoration has been found in up to 59% of smokers and 29% of never-smokers with AAT deficiency [30]. Similarly, bronchitis has been found in 33% of individuals enrolled in a patient-organized registry of 712 participants [18]. Also, the odds ratio for developing chronic bronchitis has been reported as 9.6 in PI*ZZ compared with PI*MM individuals [58]. Passive smoking has been proposed as one risk factor associated with the development of chronic bronchitis in AAT deficiency [72]. While

a clinical presentation consistent with chronic bronchitis may simply reflect the underlying pathology of AAT deficiency, a study of non-smoking patients with AAT deficiency suggests that chronic sputum production confers an adverse prognosis with greater impairment in spirometric variables, lower arterial oxygen tension, increased air trapping, inferior health status and an increased number of exacerbations [66].

Liver disease

AAT deficiency is considered the most common genetic cause of liver disease [50]. Although liver dysfunction predominates in the first two decades of life among individuals with the Z allele (and only a few others, e.g. M_{malton}) there is a life-long risk for developing liver disease. For instance, in one large screening study, 22 out of 120 PI Z infants (18%) had some evidence of liver disease, including obstructive jaundice in 14 (12%) and minor abnormalities in eight (7%) [26]. Cirrhosis may develop in 50% of affected children, 25% may die in the first decade of life and 2% present with cirrhosis in later childhood [73]. In a large-scale postmortem study predominantly involving adults, there was a strong link between AAT deficiency in males and the development of cirrhosis (odds ratio 7.8 vs matched controls) and hepatocellular carcinoma (odds ratio 20 vs matched controls) [74].

Panniculitis

Panniculitis is a skin disorder characterized by spontaneous ulceration with clear or serosanguineous drainage and an occasional angioedema-type of presentation [75,76]. It is found in association with several disease entities including lupus, pancreatic fat necrosis, Weber–Christian syndrome, lymphoproliferative disease, erythema nodosum and AAT deficiency [77]. Panniculitis in the setting of AAT deficiency was first described in by Warter et al. [78] in 1972, is uncommon and is associated with a variety of phenotypes, including PI*ZZ [79], PI*SZ [80], PI*SS [81] and, in one report, a PI*MS individual with normal plasma levels [82]. The treatment of choice is augmentation therapy, although dapsone [83] and tetracycline agents have also been used [80,83,84], the latter perhaps because tetracyclines inhibit collagenase activity [84]. The dramatic response of panniculitis to AAT augmentation therapy [85,86] and to liver transplantation [85] suggests that panniculitis, like emphysema, is caused by unopposed proteolytic activity [87].

Other disorders

Several other disorders with common features of either collagen tissue destruction or inflammation have been reported less commonly to be associated with AAT deficiency. Some of these disorders involve impairment of vascular integrity such as dissection of carotid [88], coronary [89] and intracranial [90] arteries, splenic [91], intracranial or abdominal aneurysms [92] and fibromuscular dysplasia [93]. These aneurysms do not appear to develop as a result of a protease–antiprotease imbalance [94], and in one report there was no increased frequency of PI*ZZ AAT deficiency among patients with abdominal aortic aneurysms [95]. Other associations include systemic vasculitis (especially C-ANCA-positive vasculitis) [96], peripheral neuropathy [97], colon cancer [98] and inflammatory bowel disease [99].

Treatment and prevention

Preventive measures

Preventive measures are particularly important because AAT augmentation therapy is not universally available to all the individuals for whom it may be indicated [64]. Reasons for this unavailability include variation between countries on conclusions about whether augmentation therapy is effective and hence approval by regulatory agencies, the cost of augmentation therapy, drug supply constraints and insurance issues.

As with COPD in general, smoking cessation remains the most important initial intervention. For instance, in a long-term follow-up report of PI*ZZ individuals identified in a mass screening programme of newborns in Sweden, although parental rates of smoking were higher than those of a control group when the children were 5–7 years old, the smoking rate of PI*ZZ children at 18–20 years of age was lower than that of age-matched peers [100].

Other preventive measures advocated by the World Health Organization include occupational, environmental, genetic counselling and immunization against influenza and *Pneumococcus* infections [64]. Regarding environmental exposures, kerosene heater use at home and agricultural occupations have been associated with decreased lung function in non-smoking PI*ZZ individuals [72].

Exogenous augmentation therapy

Evidence of biochemical efficacy
Augmentation therapy is the regular administration of purified AAT with the intent of repleting the patient's antielastase capacity. Criteria used to evaluate the efficacy of augmentation therapy have been both biochemical and clinical; the biochemical efficacy criterion is restoring levels of AAT in relevant components (e.g. blood, interstitium) above a so-called 'protective' threshold value, which is the lowest value necessary to eliminate the emphysema risk.

In defining an endpoint for augmentation therapy, a protective serum AAT threshold level of 11 μmol (normal 20–53 μmol) has been established based on the levels separating PI*SZ individuals (levels 8–19 μmol), who have a minimal risk of developing emphysema except in smokers [56], from PI*ZZ individuals (levels 2.5–7 μmol), who have a 65–90% risk of developing emphysema [29,30,101]. Using different preparations of pooled human plasma AAT, Wewers *et al.* [102] and Stoller *et al.* [103] demonstrated that intravenous infusion of AAT at a weekly dose of 60 mg/kg produced serum levels generally exceeding the protective threshold between dosing intervals. Similar results were obtained by Stockley *et al.* [104], who demonstrated a progressively increasing nadir from 10.7 μmol before the second infusion, to 14.4 μmol by the end of the 4th week. Biweekly (120 mg/kg every 14 days) [105] and monthly (250 mg/kg every 28 days) [106,107] schedules for infusion were found to be safe but, in keeping with the 4–5 day serum half-life of exogenous AAT, did not consistently maintain levels above 11 μmol. For instance, serum levels were maintained above this protective threshold for 7–8 days of the biweekly infusion interval [105], and for 23–25 days out of a 28-day infusion interval [106,107]. Currently, the US Food and Drug Administration (FDA) has approved AAT augmentation for weekly administration alone.

A threshold of 1.3 μmol was also suggested for epithelial lining fluid (ELF) levels based on the linear relationship between serum and epithelial lining fluid AAT and by extrapolating from the empirical 11 μmol serum threshold [102]. Studies have shown that weekly administration yielded ELF AAT levels that exceeded the ELF threshold 83% of the time [102]. In the monthly administration regimens, ELF AAT levels averaged 2.35 μmol at day 28 [106]. Moreover, most studies have shown that intravenous augmentation enhances the ability of the lung ELF to inhibit neutrophil elastase [102,103,106].

Overall, the available evidence establishes the biochemical efficacy of augmentation therapy, which was the basis upon which purified pooled human plasma antiprotease was approved by the US FDA in 1988.

Evidence of clinical efficacy
Several studies have addressed the clinical efficacy of augmentation therapy (Table 38.2) [104,107–112] using diverse endpoints of success, including mortality [108], rate of FEV_1 decline [107,108,111,112], rate of elastin degradation based on urinary desmosine [109], loss of lung tissue as assessed by CT scan [107], frequency of lung infections [110] and sputum inflammatory markers [104] (see Table 38.2).

Two observational studies, one comparing treated German patients with untreated Danish patients [111], and one

Table 38.2 Available studies on clinical efficacy of augmentation therapy.

Author(s) [Ref.]	Date	Design	Infusion interval	Outcome measures	Main results
Seersholm et al. [111]	1997	Observational cohort, concurrent controls	Weekly	FEV_1 decline	In patients with FEV_1 31–65% predicted, augmentation slowed the decline of FEV_1 by 21 mL/year ($P = 0.04$)
NHLBI Registry [17]	1998	Observational cohort, concurrent controls	51.3% weekly 25.3% biweekly 21.8% monthly	FEV_1 decline, Survival	In patients with FEV_1 35–49% predicted, augmentation slowed the decline of FEV_1 by 27 mL/year ($P = 0.03$). In the whole group, the risk ratio of death with augmentation was 0.64 compared with non-recipients ($P = 0.02$)
Dirksen et al. [107]	1999	Randomized controlled trial	Every 28 days	FEV_1 decline Lung density (CT)	Loss of lung tissue was 2.6 g/L/year with placebo and 1.5 g/L/year with augmentation ($P = 0.07$). FEV_1 decline was 59 mL/year in the augmentation group and 79 mL/year in the placebo group ($P = 0.25$)
Gottlieb et al. [109]	2000	Descriptive	Weekly	Urinary desmosine	Augmentation did not reduce the rate of elastin degradation
Lieberman [110]	2000	Observational (Web-based survey)	56% weekly 36% biweekly 7% monthly	Frequency of lung infections	The number of lung infections per year decreased from 3–5 pre-augmentation to 0–1 post-augmentation
Wencker et al. [112]	2001	Observational (before–after)	Weekly	FEV_1 decline	Rates of FEV_1 decline pre- and post-augmentation were 49.2 vs 34.2 mL/year, respectively ($P = 0.019$)
Stockley et al. [104]	2002	Descriptive	Weekly	Sputum markers of inflammation	Augmentation reduced sputum leukotriene B_4

CT, computed tomography; FEV_1, forced expiratory volume in 1 s; NHLBI, National Heart, Lung and Blood Institute.

study from the NHLBI Registry [108] comparing treated with untreated patients, both showed that receipt of augmentation therapy was associated with a slowed rate of FEV_1 decline (by more than 20 mL/year in the subset of patient with moderately to severely reduced FEV_1) (see Table 38.2) [108,111]. Similarly, in an observational study by Wencker et al. [112] comparing the rate of decline of FEV_1 before and after weekly augmentation therapy in patients with moderately reduced FEV_1 (mean 41% predicted), the rate of decline was 49 mL/year before augmentation and 34 mL/year after augmentation [112]. In contrast to these observational studies, the single available randomized controlled trial of intravenous augmentation therapy showed no significant difference in the rate of decline of FEV_1 between recipients of placebo and active drug (25.2 vs 26.6 mL/year, respectively) [107]. It is noteworthy that the patients in this randomized trial received monthly instead of weekly augmentation, and that the AAT levels were maintained above the protective threshold for

23–24 days out of the 28-day infusion schedule [107]. At the same time, this trial showed a trend toward a slower loss of lung density among augmentation therapy recipients. Specifically, using CT densitometry as a measure of lung density, augmentation therapy recipients showed a yearly rate of loss of 1.5 vs 2.6 g/L/year in placebo recipients ($P = 0.07$) [107]. This finding has increased enthusiasm to consider CT densitometry as an outcome for assessing emphysema progression in future randomized trials of augmentation therapy [107].

Observational studies have addressed other clinical endpoints of augmentation therapy in patients with AAT deficiency. In a Web-based questionnaire sent to users of an international Internet support group for individuals with AAT deficiency, Lieberman [110] found that the percentage of individuals experiencing two or more lung infections per year was 18% in those receiving augmentation therapy compared with 65% before initiating augmentation ($P < 0.001$) and 55% in those who never received augmentation ($P < 0.001$) compared with augmentation recipients [110].

Finally, Stockley *et al.* [104] treated 12 patients with intravenous augmentation therapy at a dosage of 60 mg/kg weekly for four doses and repeatedly analysed the sputum and serum samples over 8 weeks. The sputum AAT levels were associated with an increase in the ability of secretions to inhibit porcine pancreatic elastase and a significant decrease in sputum leukotriene B$_4$ [104]. This finding is of particular significance in that leukotriene B$_4$ may be the major mediator of neutrophil chemotaxis in AAT deficiency [47,48] and of consequent accelerated lung destruction by neutrophil elastase.

Emerging approaches

In the context that intravenous augmentation poses significant difficulties, there is enthusiasm to develop alternative treatment approaches. Specific examples of the disadvantages of intravenous augmentation therapy are the required frequency of use, the need for intravenous infusion, drug inefficiency and cost [113]. Regarding the efficiency of therapy, only 2–3% of intravenously administered AAT is delivered to the deep lung [114]. Also, in a recent analysis, augmentation therapy with AAT was found to have less cost-effectiveness than other conventional health interventions, with an incremental cost-effectiveness ratio of up to $312 511 per quality-adjusted life-year, indicating a need for more clinically and cost-effective therapy for AAT deficiency [115].

Given these shortcomings of intravenous augmentation therapy, attention has turned to new approaches, including aerosolized AAT with both pooled human plasma antiprotease and recombinant-produced proteins.

Aerosolized AAT

Advantages of replenishing AAT by the aerosol route include enhanced convenience, direct delivery to the target organ and decrease in the amount of drug required. Still, several issues remain to be resolved before this modality becomes available, including bioengineering of the therapeutic aerosol, resolution of patient-dependent variability in delivery technique, documentation of effective alveolar deposition, and demonstration of clinical and biochemical efficacy.

Several clinical studies have addressed the biochemical efficacy of aerosolized AAT. In one study, 29 normal volunteers who inhaled 200 mg of AAT experienced an increase in AAT concentration and antineutrophil activity in bronchoalveolar lavage samples, with a half-time in the lungs for AAT and antineutrophil elastase activity of 69.2 and 53.2 h, respectively [116]. In another study, administering aerosolized recombinant AAT to deficient individuals at single doses ranging from 10 to 200 mg augmented ELF antineutrophil elastase defences in proportion to the dose administered, and was detected in serum, suggesting the protein had crossed the epithelial layer into the interstitium [117]. In one study by Hubbard *et al.* [118], 100 mg of pooled human AAT administered by aerosol every 12 h to 12 patients with AAT deficiency augmented ELF levels to a mean of 5.86 µmol, well above proposed protective levels.

Other studies address factors that affect the alveolar deposition of aerosolized AAT. Kropp *et al.* [114] studied the patterns of deposition of ^{123}I-labelled AAT administered by aerosol to 18 patients with severe AAT deficiency, and found that peripheral deposition was significantly improved in individuals with FEV_1 of more than 40% predicted compared with those with more severe disease. In a study by Brand *et al.* [119], controlled slow and deep inhalation allowed as much as 50% alveolar deposition in 12 patients with moderate to severe AAT deficiency. Other studies suggest that high-intensity nebulization associated with low ventilation enhances drug delivery to the lungs [120].

Gene therapy

Several characteristics of AAT deficiency make it a theoretically attractive target for gene therapy, including the single gene defect, a well-defined molecular biology and encoding by the gene of a secreted product [43]. Additionally, only partial expression of normal AAT may be necessary to address the lung disease, despite persistence of the genetic defect [121]. Studies have usually targeted the lung rather than the liver for transfection with AAT encoded genes for several reasons:

1 the unique susceptibility of the lung to the disease;

2 the alveolo-capillary membrane barrier;

3 the resultant large gradient between serum and ELF AAT levels; and

4 technical limitations in the amount of gene material that can be effectively transferred.

The vectors used to transfect the lung have included recombinant viruses, liposomes and receptor-mediated gene transfer [43,122].

In the one human study to date, plasmid–liposome complexes were used to transfect the nasal epithelium of five AAT deficient individuals with a normal AAT gene, and demonstrated an increase in the concentration of AAT in nasal lavage compared with the control nostril [43]. This study also showed that while nasal lavage AAT levels were much lower than with intravenous augmentation, nasal interleukin 8 concentrations were reduced while the subjects were on gene therapy and not while receiving augmentation. Thus, local expression of AAT, even at subtherapeutic levels, may confer advantages such as the ability to interdict proteolytic activity and reduce markers of inflammation in areas not usually exposed to circulating AAT [43]. Adenoviral vectors have also been shown to be effective in animal models [123].

Disadvantages of these vectors include the paucity of specific cell receptors on the surface of human respiratory epithelium, and their ability to cause an inflammatory response and trigger an immune response [43]. While there are techniques to diminish the side-effects associated with adenoviral vectors, alternatives such as adeno-associated virus vectors have been explored. Nevertheless, use of adeno-associated virus has disadvantages, including impaired transduction to the lungs because of existing airway inflammation and the lack of specific receptors on the apical surface of airway epithelial cells [124].

In another study, transfection of pulmonary macrophages in rats was achieved by targeting mannose receptors to internalize plasmid DNA complexed with a mannose-terminal molecular conjugate [122], suggesting this may be an alternative strategy.

Other emerging approaches

Characterization of AAT deficiency as a conformational disease and better understanding of the mechanisms of its associated liver and lung disease have suggested other new approaches to treatment.

Inhibition of intrahepatic polymerization has been one such approach. In one study, a small peptide homologous to the reactive centre loop was found to selectively bind to the β-sheet of Z AAT and to inhibit polymerization *in vitro* [125]. While this approach may increase secretion, it also inactivates AAT and therefore supplementation may still be necessary for prevention of lung disease. However, it clearly holds promise for treating liver disease [125].

Another study capitalizes on the putative mechanism of retention of polymerized AAT in the endoplasmic reticulum by providing cellular chaperones to reverse the process. Specifically, oral 4-phenylbutyric acid (PBA) administered to mice transgenic for the human AAT gene increased their blood levels of human AAT to 20–50% of normal mouse and human levels [126]. This approach is promising in that PBA has been safely used in children with urea cycle disorders and, if successful, could prevent or treat both liver and lung manifestations of the disease. A pilot study of PBA is currently underway [127].

Recognizing the important role of neutrophil elastase in the pathogenesis of lung disease in AAT deficiency, other inhibitors of this enzyme also have promise. Some of these agents include endogenous low molecular weight inhibitors of neutrophil elastase (such as eglin C) and manufactured compounds such as sivelestat (which has been predominantly studied in acute lung injury) [128] and ONO-6818 [129]. The latter agent was found to inhibit the development of neutrophil elastase-induced emphysema in rats

[129], but human phase II studies in subjects with AAT deficiency were discontinued because of elevation of liver enzymes.

Overall, such emerging approaches offer promise for new and better therapies for severe AAT deficiency.

References

1 Laurell C-B, Eriksson A. The electrophoretic α₁-globulin pattern of serum in α₁-antitrypsin deficiency. *Scand J Clin Lab Invest* 1963;**15**:132–40.

2 Eriksson S. Studies in α₁-antitrypsin deficiency. *Acta Med Scand* 1964;**175**:197–205.

3 Eriksson S. Studies in α₁-antitrypsin deficiency. *Acta Med Scand Suppl* 1965;**432**:1–85.

4 Gross P, Babyak MA, Tolker E, Kaschak M. Enzymatically produced pulmonary emphysema: a preliminary report. *J Occup Med* 1964;**6**:481–4.

5 Gross P, Pfitzer EA, Tolker E, Babyak MA, Kaschak M. Experimental emphysema: its production with papain in normal and silicotic rats. *Arch Environ Health* 1965;**11**:50–8.

6 Kueppers F, Bearn AG. A possible experimental approach to the association of hereditary α₁-antitrypsin deficiency and pulmonary emphysema. *Proc Soc Exp Biol Med* 1966;**121**:1207–9.

7 Janoff A. Elastases and emphysema: current assessment of the protease–antiprotease hypothesis. *Am Rev Respir Dis* 1985;**132**:417–33.

8 Janoff A, Scherer J. Mediators of inflammation in leukocyte lysosomes. IX. Elastinolytic activity in granules of human polymorphonuclear leukocytes. *J Exp Med* 1968;**128**:1137–55.

9 Ohlsson K. Neutral leucocyte proteases and elastase inhibited by plasma α₁-antitrypsin. *Scand J Clin Lab Invest* 1971;**28**:251–3.

10 Senior RM, Tegner H, Kuhn C *et al*. The induction of pulmonary emphysema with human leukocyte elastase. *Am Rev Respir Dis* 1977;**116**:469–75.

11 Hayes JA, Korthy A, Snider GL. The pathology of elastase-induced panacinar emphysema in hamsters. *J Pathol* 1975;**117**:1–14.

12 Long GL, Chandra T, Woo SL, Davie EW, Kurachi K. Complete sequence of the cDNA for human α₁-antitrypsin and the gene for the S variant. *Biochemistry* 1984;**23**:4828–37.

13 Brantly M, Nukiwa T, Crystal RG. Molecular basis of α₁-antitrypsin deficiency. *Am J Med* 1988;**84**:13–31.

14 Sharp HL, Bridges RA, Krivit W, Freier EF. Cirrhosis associated with α₁-antitrypsin deficiency: a previously unrecognized inherited disorder. *J Lab Clin Med* 1969;**73**:934–9.

15 Lomas DA, Evans DL, Finch JT, Carrell RW. The mechanism of Z α₁-antitrypsin accumulation in the liver. *Nature* 1992;**357**:605–7.

16 Hubbard RC, Crystal RG. α₁-Antitrypsin augmentation therapy for α₁-antitrypsin deficiency. *Am J Med* 1988;**84**:52–62.

17 The Alpha-One Antitrypsin Deficiency Registry Study Group. A registry of patients with severe deficiency of α_1-antitrypsin: design and methods. *Chest* 1994;**106**:1223–32.

18 Stoller JK, Brantly M, Fleming LE, Bean JA, Walsh J. Formation and current results of a patient-organized registry for α_1-antitrypsin deficiency. *Chest* 2000;**118**:843–8.

19 Blackwell DL, Collins JG, Coles R. Summary health statistics for US adults: National Health Interview Survey, 1997. National Center for Health Statistics. *Vital Health Stat* 2002; **10**:205.

20 Lieberman J, Winter B, Sastre A. α_1-Antitrypsin Pi-types in 965 COPD patients. *Chest* 1986;**89**:370–3.

21 de Serres FJ. Worldwide racial and ethnic distribution of α_1-antitrypsin deficiency: summary of an analysis of published genetic epidemiologic surveys. *Chest* 2002;**122**:1818–29.

22 de Serres FJ, Blanco I, Fernández-Bustillo E. Genetic epidemiology of α_1-antitrypsin deficiency in North America and Australia/New Zealand: Australia, Canada, New Zealand, and the United States of America. *Clin Genet* 2003;**64**:382–97.

23 O'Brien ML, Buist NR, Murphey WH. Neonatal screening for α_1-antitrypsin deficiency. *J Pediatr* 1978;**92**:1006–10.

24 Silverman EK, Miletich JP, Pierce JA *et al.* α_1-Antitrypsin deficiency: high prevalence in the St. Louis area determined by direct population screening. *Am Rev Respir Dis* 1989;**140**: 961–6.

25 Spence WC, Morris JE, Pass K, Murphy PD. Molecular confirmation of α_1-antitrypsin genotypes in newborn dried blood specimens. *Biochem Med Metab Biol* 1993;**50**:233–40.

26 Sveger T. Liver disease in α_1-antitrypsin deficiency detected by screening of 200 000 infants. *N Engl J Med* 1976;**294**: 1316–21.

27 US Census Bureau. *Census* 2000. 2002.

28 Eriksson S. A 30-year perspective on α_1-antitrypsin deficiency. *Chest* 1996;**110**(Suppl):237S–42S.

29 Gadek JE, Crystal RG. α_1-Antitrypsin deficiency. In: Stanbury JB, Wyngaarden JB, Frederickson DS *et al.*, eds. *The Metabolic Basis of Inherited Disease*. New York: McGraw-Hill, 1983: 1450–67.

30 Tobin MJ, Cook PJ, Hutchison DC. α_1-Antitrypsin deficiency: the clinical and physiological features of pulmonary emphysema in subjects homozygous for Pi type Z. A survey by the British Thoracic Association. *Br J Dis Chest* 1983;**77**:14–27.

31 Genetic testing for cystic fibrosis. NIH Consensus Statement Online 1997 Apr 14–16. 1997;**15**:1–37.

32 Stoller JK, Smith P, Yang P, Spray J. Physical and social impact of α_1-antitrypsin deficiency: results of a survey. *Cleve Clin J Med* 1994;**61**:461–7.

33 Lomas DA, Mahadeva R. α_1-Antitrypsin polymerization and the serpinopathies: pathobiology and prospects for therapy. *J Clin Invest* 2002;**110**:1585–90.

34 Lomas DA, Carrell RW. Serpinopathies and the conformational dementias. *Nat Rev Genet* 2002;**3**:759–68.

35 Davis RL, Shrimpton AE, Holohan PD *et al.* Familial dementia caused by polymerization of mutant neuroserpin. *Nature* 1999;**401**:376–9.

36 Lomas DA, Lourbakos A, Cumming SA, Belorgey D.

Hypersensitive mousetraps, α_1-antitrypsin deficiency and dementia. *Biochem Soc Trans* 2002;**30**:89–92.

37 Kopito RR, Ron D. Conformational disease. *Nat Cell Biol* 2000;**2**:E207–9.

38 Dafforn TR, Mahadeva R, Elliott PR, Sivasothy P, Lomas DA. A kinetic mechanism for the polymerization of α_1-antitrypsin. *J Biol Chem* 1999;**274**:9548–55.

39 Devlin GL, Chow MK, Howlett GJ, Bottomley SP. Acid denaturation of α_1-antitrypsin: characterization of a novel mechanism of serpin polymerization. *J Mol Biol* 2002;**324**: 859–70.

40 Gadek JE, Fells GA, Zimmerman RL, Rennard SI, Crystal RG. Antielastases of the human alveolar structures: implications for the protease–antiprotease theory of emphysema. *J Clin Invest* 1981;**68**:889–98.

41 Beatty K, Bieth J, Travis J. Kinetics of association of serine proteinases with native and oxidized α_1-proteinase inhibitor and α_1-antichymotrypsin. *J Biol Chem* 1980;**255**:3931–4.

42 Crystal RG, Brantly ML, Hubbard RC *et al.* The α_1-antitrypsin gene and its mutations: clinical consequences and strategies for therapy. *Chest* 1989;**95**:196–208.

43 Stecenko AA, Brigham KL. Gene therapy progress and prospects: α_1-antitrypsin. *Gene Ther* 2003;**10**:95–9.

44 Ogushi F, Fells GA, Hubbard RC, Straus SD, Crystal RG. Z-type α_1-antitrypsin is less competent than M1-type α_1-antitrypsin as an inhibitor of neutrophil elastase. *J Clin Invest* 1987;**80**:1366–74.

45 Elliott PR, Bilton D, Lomas DA. Lung polymers in Z α_1-antitrypsin deficiency-related emphysema. *Am J Respir Cell Mol Biol* 1998;**18**:670–4.

46 Parmar JS, Mahadeva R, Reed BJ *et al.* Polymers of α_1-antitrypsin are chemotactic for human neutrophils: a new paradigm for the pathogenesis of emphysema. *Am J Respir Cell Mol Biol* 2002;**26**:723–30.

47 Hill AT, Bayley DL, Campbell EJ, Hill SL, Stockley RA. Airways inflammation in chronic bronchitis: the effects of smoking and α_1-antitrypsin deficiency. *Eur Respir J* 2000;**15**: 886–90.

48 Woolhouse IS, Bayley DL, Stockley RA. Sputum chemotactic activity in chronic obstructive pulmonary disease: effect of α_1-antitrypsin deficiency and the role of leukotriene B4 and interleukin 8. *Thorax* 2002;**57**:709–14.

49 Goetzl EJ. Modulation of human neutrophil polymorphonuclear leucocyte migration by human plasma α-globulin inhibitors and synthetic esterase inhibitors. *Immunology* 1975;**29**:163–74.

50 Perlmutter DH. Liver injury in α_1-antitrypsin deficiency: an aggregated protein induces mitochondrial injury. *J Clin Invest* 2002;**110**:1579–83.

51 Wu SS, de Chadarevian JP, McPhaul L *et al.* Coexpression and accumulation of ubiquitin +1 and ZZ proteins in livers of children with α_1-antitrypsin deficiency. *Pediatr Dev Pathol* 2002;**5**:293–8.

52 Qu D, Teckman JH, Omura S, Perlmutter DH. Degradation of a mutant secretory protein, α_1-antitrypsin Z, in the endoplasmic reticulum requires proteasome activity. *J Biol Chem* 1996;**271**:22791–5.

53 Brantly ML, Paul LD, Miller BH *et al.* Clinical features and history of the destructive lung disease associated with α_1-antitrypsin deficiency of adults with pulmonary symptoms. *Am Rev Respir Dis* 1988;**138**:327–36.

54 Gishen P, Saunders AJ, Tobin MJ, Hutchison DC. α_1-Antitrypsin deficiency: the radiological features of pulmonary emphysema in subjects of Pi type Z and Pi type SZ: a survey by the British Thoracic Association. *Clin Radiol* 1982;**33**:371–7.

55 Sandford AJ, Weir TD, Spinelli JJ, Pare PD. Z and S mutations of the α_1-antitrypsin gene and the risk of chronic obstructive pulmonary disease. *Am J Respir Cell Mol Biol* 1999;**20**:287–91.

56 Turino GM, Barker AF, Brantly ML *et al.* Clinical features of individuals with PI*SZ phenotype of α_1-antitrypsin deficiency. Alpha-One Antitrypsin Deficiency Registry Study Group. *Am J Respir Crit Care Med* 1996;**154**:1718–25.

57 Alvarez-Granda L, Cabero-Perez MJ, Bustamante-Ruiz A *et al.* PI SZ phenotype in chronic obstructive pulmonary disease. *Thorax* 1997;**52**:659–61.

58 Dahl M, Tybjaerg-Hansen A, Lange P, Vestbo J, Nordestgaard BG. Change in lung function and morbidity from chronic obstructive pulmonary disease in α_1-antitrypsin MZ heterozygotes: A longitudinal study of the general population. *Ann Intern Med* 2002;**136**:270–9.

59 Silva GE, Sherrill DL, Guerra S, Barbee RA. A longitudinal study of α_1-antitrypsin phenotypes and decline in FEV_1 in a community population. *Chest* 2003;**123**:1435–40.

60 Eden E, Hammel J, Rouhani FN *et al.* Asthma features in severe α_1-antitrypsin deficiency: experience of the National Heart, Lung, and Blood Institute Registry. *Chest* 2003;**123**:765–71.

61 Piitulainen E, Sveger T. Respiratory symptoms and lung function in young adults with severe α_1-antitrypsin deficiency (PiZZ). *Thorax* 2002;**57**:705–8.

62 Malerba M, Radaeli A, Ceriani L, Tantucci C, Grassi V. Airway hyperresponsiveness in a large group of subjects with α_1-antitrypsin deficiency: a cross-sectional controlled study. *J Intern Med* 2003;**253**:351–8.

63 Gaillard MC, Kilroe-Smith TA, Nogueira C *et al.* α_1-Protease inhibitor in bronchial asthma: phenotypes and biochemical characteristics. *Am Rev Respir Dis* 1992;**145**:1311–5.

64 α_1-Antitrypsin deficiency: memorandum from a WHO meeting. *Bull World Health Organ* 1997;**75**:397–415.

65 Stoller JK, Snider GL, Fallat RA, Stockley RA, Brantly M, for the α_1-antitrypsin Deficiency Task Force. Standards for the diagnosis and management of individuals with α_1-antitrypsin deficiency. *Am J Respir Crit Care Med* 2003;**168**:819–900.

66 Dowson LJ, Guest PJ, Stockley RA. The relationship of chronic sputum expectoration to physiologic, radiologic, and health status characteristics in α_1-antitrypsin deficiency (PiZ). *Chest* 2002;**122**:1247–55.

67 King MA, Stone JA, Diaz PT *et al.* α_1-Antitrypsin deficiency: evaluation of bronchiectasis with CT. *Radiology* 1996;**199**:137–41.

68 Shin MS, Ho KJ. Bronchiectasis in patients with α_1-antitrypsin deficiency: a rare occurrence? *Chest* 1993;**104**:1384–6.

69 Cuvelier A, Muir JF, Hellot MF *et al.* Distribution of α_1-antitrypsin alleles in patients with bronchiectasis. *Chest* 2000;**117**:415–9.

70 Pasteur MC, Helliwell SM, Houghton SJ *et al.* An investigation into causative factors in patients with bronchiectasis. *Am J Respir Crit Care Med* 2000;**162**:1277–84.

71 Fallat RJ. Reactive airways disease and α_1-antitrypsin deficiency. In: Crystal RG, ed. α_1-*Antitrypsin Deficiency: Biology, Pathogenesis, Clinical Manifestations, Therapy.* New York: Marcel Dekker, 1996: 259–79.

72 Piitulainen E, Tornling G, Eriksson S. Environmental correlates of impaired lung function in non-smokers with severe α_1-antitrypsin deficiency (PiZZ). *Thorax* 1998;**53**:939–43.

73 Hussain M, Mieli-Vergani G, Mowat AP. α_1-Antitrypsin deficiency and liver disease: clinical presentation, diagnosis and treatment. *J Inherit Metab Dis* 1991;**14**:497–511.

74 Eriksson S, Carlson J, Velez R. Risk of cirrhosis and primary liver cancer in α_1-antitrypsin deficiency. *N Engl J Med* 1986; **314**:736–9.

75 Balk E, Bronsveld W, Van der Deyl JA, Kwee WS, Thiss LG. α_1-Antitrypsin deficiency with vascular leakage syndrome and panniculitis. *Neth J Med* 1982;**25**:138–41.

76 Furey NL, Golden RS, Potts SR. Treatment of α_1-antitrypsin deficiency, massive edema, and panniculitis with α_1-protease inhibitor. *Ann Intern Med* 1996;**125**:699.

77 Phelps RG, Shoji T. Update on panniculitis. *Mt Sinai J Med* 2001;**68**:262–7.

78 Warter J, Storck D, Grosshans E *et al.* Weber–Christian syndrome associated with an α_1-antitrypsin deficiency: familial investigation. *Ann Med Interne (Paris)* 1972;**123**:877–82.

79 Edmonds BK, Hodge JA, Rietschel RL. α_1-Antitrypsin deficiency-associated panniculitis: case report and review of the literature. *Pediatr Dermatol* 1991;**8**:296–9.

80 Chng WJ, Henderson CA. Suppurative panniculitis associated with α_1-antitrypsin deficiency (PiSZ phenotype) treated with doxycycline. *Br J Dermatol* 2001;**144**:1282–3.

81 Pinto AR, Maciel LS, Carneiro F *et al.* Systemic nodular panniculitis in a patient with α_1-antitrypsin deficiency (PiSS phenotype). *Clin Exp Dermatol* 1993;**18**:154–5.

82 Loche F, Tremeau-Martinage C, Laplanche G, Massip P, Bazex J. Panniculitis revealing qualitative α_1-antitrypsine deficiency (MS variant). *Eur J Dermatol* 1999;**9**:565–7.

83 Ginarte M, Roson E, Peteiro C, Toribio J. Treatment of α_1-antitrypsin-deficiency panniculitis with minocycline. *Cutis* 2001;**68**:86–8.

84 Humbert P, Faivre B, Gibey R, Agache P. Use of anti-collagenase properties of doxycycline in treatment of α_1-antitrypsin deficiency panniculitis. *Acta Derm Venereol* 1991; **71**:189–94.

85 O'Riordan K, Blei A, Rao MS, Abecassis M. α_1-Antitrypsin deficiency-associated panniculitis: resolution with intravenous α_1-antitrypsin administration and liver transplantation. *Transplantation* 1997;**63**:480–2.

86 Chowdhury MM, Williams EJ, Morris JS *et al.* Severe panniculitis caused by homozygous ZZ α_1-antitrypsin deficiency treated successfully with human purified enzyme (Prolastin). *Br J Dermatol* 2002;**147**:1258–61.

87 Filaci G, Contini P, Barbera P, Bernardini L, Indiveri F. Autoantibodies to neutrophilic proteases in a case of panniculitis by deficit of α_1-antitrypsin. *Rheumatology (Oxford)* 2000;**39**:1289–90.

88 Konrad C, Nabavi DG, Junker R *et al*. Spontaneous internal carotid artery dissection and α_1-antitrypsin deficiency. *Acta Neurol Scand* 2003;**107**:233–6.

89 Martin DF, Delgado PM, Garcia RM *et al*. Coronary artery dissection in α_1-antitrypsin deficiency. *Histopathology* 1999;**34**:376–8.

90 Schievink WI, Katzmann JA, Piepgras DG. α_1-Antitrypsin deficiency in spontaneous intracranial arterial dissections. *Cerebrovasc Dis* 1998;**8**:42–4.

91 Gaglio PJ, Regenstein F, Slakey D *et al*. α_1-Antitrypsin deficiency and splenic artery aneurysm rupture: an association? *Am J Gastroenterol* 2000;**95**:1531–4.

92 Cohen JR, Sarfati I, Ratner L, Tilson D. α_1-Antitrypsin phenotypes in patients with abdominal aortic aneurysms. *J Surg Res* 1990;**49**:319–21.

93 Schievink WI, Puumala MR, Meyer FB *et al*. Giant intracranial aneurysm and fibromuscular dysplasia in an adolescent with α_1-antitrypsin deficiency. *J Neurosurg* 1996;**85**:503–6.

94 Sakai N, Nakayama K, Tanabe Y *et al*. Absence of plasma protease–antiprotease imbalance in the formation of saccular cerebral aneurysms. *Neurosurgery* 1999;**45**:34–8.

95 Elzouki AN, Ryden AA, Lanne T, Sonesson B, Eriksson S. Is there a relationship between abdominal aortic aneurysms and α_1-antitrypsin deficiency (PiZ)? *Eur J Vasc Endovasc Surg* 1999;**17**:149–54.

96 Mazodier P, Elzouki AN, Segelmark M, Eriksson S. Systemic necrotizing vasculitides in severe α_1-antitrypsin deficiency. *Q J Med* 1996;**89**:599–611.

97 Frederick WG, Enriquez R, Bookbinder MJ. Peripheral neuropathy associated with α_1-antitrypsin deficiency. *Arch Neurol* 1990;**47**:233–5.

98 Yang P, Cunningham JM, Halling KC *et al*. Higher risk of mismatch repair-deficient colorectal cancer in α_1-antitrypsin deficiency carriers and cigarette smokers. *Mol Genet Metab* 2000;**71**:639–45.

99 Yang P, Tremaine WJ, Meyer RL, Prakash UB. α_1-Antitrypsin deficiency and inflammatory bowel diseases. *Mayo Clin Proc* 2000;**75**:450–5.

100 Thelin T, Sveger T, McNeil TF. Primary prevention in a high-risk group: smoking habits in adolescents with homozygous α_1-antitrypsin deficiency (ATD). *Acta Paediatr* 1996;**85**:1207–12.

101 Guidelines for the approach to the patient with severe hereditary α_1-antitrypsin deficiency. American Thoracic Society. *Am Rev Respir Dis* 1989;**140**:1494–7.

102 Wewers MD, Casolaro MA, Sellers SE *et al*. Replacement therapy for α_1-antitrypsin deficiency associated with emphysema. *N Engl J Med* 1987;**316**:1055–62.

103 Stoller JK, Rouhani F, Brantly M *et al*. Biochemical efficacy and safety of a new pooled human plasma α_1-antitrypsin, Respitin. *Chest* 2002;**122**:66–74.

104 Stockley RA, Bayley DL, Unsal I, Dowson LJ. The effect of augmentation therapy on bronchial inflammation in α_1-antitrypsin deficiency. *Am J Respir Crit Care Med* 2002;**165**:1494–8.

105 Barker AF, Iwata-Morgan I, Oveson L, Roussel R. Pharmacokinetic study of α_1-antitrypsin infusion in α_1-antitrypsin deficiency. *Chest* 1997;**112**:607–13.

106 Hubbard RC, Sellers S, Czerski D, Stephens L, Crystal RG. Biochemical efficacy and safety of monthly augmentation therapy for α_1-antitrypsin deficiency. *JAMA* 1988;**260**:1259–64.

107 Dirksen A, Dijkman JH, Madsen F *et al*. A randomized clinical trial of α_1-antitrypsin augmentation therapy. *Am J Respir Crit Care Med* 1999;**160**:1468–72.

108 The Alpha-1-Antitrypsin Deficiency Registry Study Group. Survival and FEV_1 decline in individuals with severe deficiency of α_1-antitrypsin. *Am J Respir Crit Care Med* 1998;**158**:49–59.

109 Gottlieb DJ, Luisetti M, Stone PJ *et al*. Short-term supplementation therapy does not affect elastin degradation in severe α_1-antitrypsin deficiency. The American–Italian AATD Study Group. *Am J Respir Crit Care Med* 2000;**162**:2069–72.

110 Lieberman J. Augmentation therapy reduces frequency of lung infections in antitrypsin deficiency: a new hypothesis with supporting data. *Chest* 2000;**118**:1480–5.

111 Seersholm N, Wencker M, Banik N *et al*. Does α_1-antitrypsin augmentation therapy slow the annual decline in FEV_1 in patients with severe hereditary α_1-antitrypsin deficiency? Wissenschaftliche Arbeitsgemeinschaft zur Therapie von Lungenerkrankungen (WATL) α_1-AT study group. *Eur Respir J* 1997;**10**:2260–3.

112 Wencker M, Fuhrmann B, Banik N, Konietzko N. Longitudinal follow-up of patients with α_1-protease inhibitor deficiency before and during therapy with IV α_1-protease inhibitor. *Chest* 2001;**119**:737–44.

113 Hubbard RC, Crystal RG. Strategies for aerosol therapy of α_1-antitrypsin deficiency by the aerosol route. *Lung* 1990;**168**(Suppl):565015078.

114 Kropp J, Wencker M, Hotze A *et al*. Inhalation of [^{123}I] α_1-protease inhibitor: toward a new therapeutic concept of α_1-protease inhibitor deficiency? *J Nucl Med* 2001;**42**:744–51.

115 Gildea TR, Shermock KM, Singer ME, Stoller JK. Cost-effectiveness analysis of augmentation therapy for severe α_1-antitrypsin deficiency. *Am J Respir Crit Care Med* 2003;**167**:1387–92.

116 Vogelmeier C, Kirlath I, Warrington S *et al*. The intrapulmonary half-life and safety of aerosolized α_1-protease inhibitor in normal volunteers. *Am J Respir Crit Care Med* 1997;**155**:536–41.

117 Hubbard RC, McElvaney NG, Sellers SE *et al*. Recombinant DNA-produced α_1-antitrypsin administered by aerosol augments lower respiratory tract antineutrophil elastase defenses in individuals with α_1-antitrypsin deficiency. *J Clin Invest* 1989;**84**:1349–54.

118 Hubbard RC, Brantly ML, Sellers SE, Mitchell ME, Crystal RG. Anti-neutrophil-elastase defenses of the lower respiratory tract in α_1-antitrypsin deficiency directly augmented with an aerosol of α_1-antitrypsin. *Ann Intern Med* 1989;**111**:206–12.

119 Brand P, Meyer T, Sommerer K, Weber N, Scheuch G. Alveolar deposition of monodisperse aerosol particles in the lung of patients with chronic obstructive pulmonary disease. *Exp Lung Res* 2002;**28**:39–54.

120 Flament MP, Leterme P, Gayot A. Influence of the technological parameters of ultrasonic nebulisation on the nebulisation quality of α_1-protease inhibitor (α_1-PI). *Int J Pharm* 1999;**189**:197–204.

121 Knoell DL, Wewers MD. Clinical implications of gene therapy for α_1-antitrypsin deficiency. *Chest* 1995;**107**:535–45.

122 Ferkol T, Mularo F, Hilliard J *et al*. Transfer of the human α_1-antitrypsin gene into pulmonary macrophages *in vivo*. *Am J Respir Cell Mol Biol* 1998;**18**:591–601.

123 Rosenfeld MA, Siegfried W, Yoshimura K *et al*. Adenovirus-mediated transfer of a recombinant α_1-antitrypsin gene to the lung epithelium *in vivo*. *Science* 1991;**252**:431–4.

124 Flotte TR. Recombinant adeno-associated virus gene therapy for cystic fibrosis and α_1-antitrypsin deficiency. *Chest* 2002;**121**(3 Suppl):98S–102S.

125 Mahadeva R, Dafforn TR, Carrell RW, Lomas DA. 6-mer peptide selectively anneals to a pathogenic serpin conformation and blocks polymerization: implications for the prevention of Z α_1-antitrypsin-related cirrhosis. *J Biol Chem* 2002;**277**:6771–4.

126 Burrows JA, Willis LK, Perlmutter DH. Chemical chaperones mediate increased secretion of mutant α_1-antitrypsin (α_1-AT) Z: a potential pharmacological strategy for prevention of liver injury and emphysema in α_1-AT deficiency. *Proc Natl Acad Sci U S A* 2000;**97**:1796–801.

127 Bunk S. Chaperones to the rescue. *Scientist* 2002;**16**:21–3.

128 Zeiher BG, Matsuoka S, Kawabata K, Repine JE. Neutrophil elastase and acute lung injury: prospects for sivelestat and other neutrophil elastase inhibitors as therapeutics. *Crit Care Med* 2002;**30**(Suppl):S281–7.

129 Kuraki T, Ishibashi M, Takayama M, Shiraishi M, Yoshida M. A novel oral neutrophil elastase inhibitor (ONO-6818) inhibits human neutrophil elastase-induced emphysema in rats. *Am J Respir Crit Care Med* 2002;**166**:496–500.

CHAPTER 39
Body weight and systemic effects

Emile F. M. Wouters

Chronic obstructive pulmonary disease (COPD) is characterized by the progressive development of airflow limitation that is not fully reversible. The clinical syndrome of COPD encompasses different disease conditions varying from chronic obstructive bronchitis with obstruction of small airways to emphysema characterized by enlargement of airspaces and destruction of lung parenchyma, loss of lung elasticity and closure of small airways. The association of an abnormal inflammatory response of the lungs to noxious particles or gases with airflow limitation in COPD indicates the critical role of the inflammatory process in the pathogenesis of COPD [1].

Besides these primary effects of COPD in the lungs, there is growing evidence in the literature that the clinical syndrome of COPD is often associated with significant extrapulmonary manifestations or systemic effects [2,3]. Weight loss is a phenomenon that has long been recognized in the clinical course of COPD patients. Fowler and Godlee [4] first described this association in patients with emphysema in the late 19th century. Attempts to describe different COPD classifications retained body weight as an important discriminator [5,6]. In the 1960s, several studies reported that low body weight and weight loss are negative predictive factors of survival in COPD [7]. At that time, weight loss was considered to be an integral part of the clinical picture of chronic bronchitis, without adequate analysis of the underlying mechanisms or related functional consequences. Nutritional depletion was considered as an inevitable and irreversible terminal event related to the severity of airflow obstruction. It was even hypothesized that weight loss was an adaptive mechanism to decrease oxygen consumption in these disabled patients.

Based on the emerging public health concern for COPD, there is growing interest in defining treatment and treatment strategies that make a difference in the outcomes of patients. Goals of effective COPD management are widely accepted and are largely related to the experienced symptomatology of patients: relief of symptoms, improvement in exercise capacity, improvement in health status, prevention of exacerbations and complications, prevention of disease progression and reduction of mortality [1]. In a heterogeneous disease condition such as COPD, selection of appropriate outcome measures depends on the aspect of the disease being addressed. This is particularly relevant for COPD, as a variety of non-pharmacological treatment procedures are considered as evidence-based management strategies despite any effect on specific measures such as forced expiratory volume in 1 s (FEV_1). In this paper, body weight will be discussed as part of the multicomponent pathology in COPD patients.

Prevalence of depletion in COPD

If the human body is considered as a single compartment, the measurement of weight and height provides a simple assessment of nutritional status. Generally, the subject's weight is compared with a reference parameter. Actual body weight can be related to the 'ideal body weight' (IBW) as derived from height, sex and frame size, based on the Metropolitan Life insurances tables [8]. Low body weight is generally and arbitrarily defined as body weight less than 90% IBW. Another approach is the use of indices of relative weight such as the body mass index (BMI) or Quetelet index, which is the ratio of body weight divided by height squared.

The US Department of Agriculture and the US Department of Health and Human Services in their 2000 report on 'Nutrition and Your Health' proposed a BMI between 18.5 and 24.9 kg/m^2 as a target for a healthy weight [9]. A BMI lower than 18.5 kg/m^2 is considered underweight, greater than 25 kg/m^2 connotes overweight and a BMI greater than 30 kg/m^2 indicates obesity. However, it was stated in the same report that weights above or below the healthy weight range may actually be healthy and that weights inside the healthy weight range may not be healthy, stressing the assessment of body composition even in normal persons [9]. This is particularly important in clinical conditions where standardization in the nomenclature of body composition in weight loss is important [10]. Roubenoff *et al.* [10] suggested specific definitions for cachexia, wasting and sarcopenia. In cachexia, the loss of body cell mass, the total actively metabolizing and contracting tissue, is greater than the loss of weight. In wasting, the decrease in body cell mass and weight are parallel. Cachexia is always accompanied by wasting, but wasting does not always lead to cachexia. Sarcopenia refers to an involuntary generalized loss of skeletal muscle mass and strength [10].

In the absence of two-compartment analysis of body composition, dividing body weight into a fat and a fat-free compartment, depletion in fat-free mass (FFM) can be masked by an increase in fat mass resulting in a normal body weight, or a low body weight can be present with preservation of FFM [11,12]. Therefore, especially in patients with low body weight, further assessment of body compositional changes has to be advocated.

Presence of low body weight is a frequent finding in COPD patients. Hunter *et al.* [13] reported nutritional depletion in 50% of hospitalized patients with a clinical diagnosis of COPD. Among 779 men included in the National Institutes of Health clinical trial of intermittent positive-pressure breathing, 25% weighed less than 90% IBW: 51% of the more obstructed group (FEV_1 < 35% predicted) and 20% in the less obstructive patients (FEV_1 > 47% predicted) [14].

Schols *et al.* [11] reported data of body weight and body composition in a group of 255 patients with moderate to severe COPD, consecutively admitted to a pulmonary rehabilitation programme. An IBW of less than 90% predicted was found in 27% of patients with a 35% predicted < FEV_1 ≤ 50% predicted, 41% of patients with a FEV_1 less than 35% predicted and even 46% of patients with hypoxaemia (Pao_2 ≤ 7.3 kPa). This study indicates that low body weight commonly occurs in COPD patients eligible for pulmonary rehabilitation and that nutritional depletion significantly contributes to the experienced functional impairment in these patients [11]. Engelen *et al.* [12], studying body composition in relation to respiratory and peripheral skeletal muscle function in a group of COPD outpatients, reported weight loss in 17% of the study group.

Prevalence of malnutrition was studied in a cohort of more than 4000 patients with COPD treated with long-term oxygen therapy [15]. The prevalence of malnutrition, as defined by a BMI of less than 20, was 23% in men and 30% in women. The prevalence of low body weight was reported to be very high in patients with acute respiratory failure and in patients accepted for lung transplantation, with values up to 60% and 72%, respectively [16,17].

Besides measurement of body weight or BMI, nutritional status can be defined by unintentional weight loss. Unintentional weight loss of more than 10% during the past 6 months is categorized as severe malnutrition [18]. A recent prevalence study conducted in the Netherlands of 501 patients admitted to the pulmonary ward for non-oncological illnesses reported more than 10% weight loss in 13% of patients and a 5–10% weight loss in 14% of patients. A weight loss of 5–10% over a 6-month period is considered as a risk for malnutrition. Remarkably, a significant number of patients had manifested unintentional weight loss with BMI values within the normal range [19].

It can be concluded that low body weight and muscle wasting is a common problem in COPD patients. Further studies are needed to illustrate changes in body weight as part of the natural history of the disease.

BMI and the risk for development of COPD

Different studies reported a relationship between low BMI and the risk of COPD. In the Tecumseh Community Health Study it was found that the incidence rate of obstructive airways disease, defined as FEV_1 less than 65% predicted, was highest in lean men and lowest in overweight men [20]. The possibility that subjects who are susceptible to COPD may be leaner than subjects who are not susceptible was also raised by other authors [21]. Chen *et al.* [22] reported that a BMI less than 20 among male subjects and a BMI greater than or equal to 28 among female subjects were associated with an increased prevalence of COPD. In this cross-sectional study, no distinction was made between emphysema and chronic bronchitis. Harik-Khan *et al.* [23], using the Baltimore Longitudinal Study of Aging database, examined if asymptomatic subjects with lower initial body mass were at greater risk of developing COPD during subsequent follow-up. COPD was considered to be present if the participants received any of the following diagnoses during follow-up: emphysema, chronic bronchitis or chronic airway obstruction, or if $FEV_1 : FVC$ was less than 0.7 during follow-up. These authors reported that middle-aged and older men with low body weight, as measured by BMI, were at a substantially higher risk of developing COPD even after adjusting for other potential risk factors, including cigarette smoking, age, FEV_1 percentage of predicted, abdominal obesity and educational status. This inverse association of baseline BMI and subsequent COPD was significant. Guerra *et al.* [24], using a nested case–control study from the longitudinal cohort of the Tucson Epidemiological Study of Airways Obstructive Diseases reported that the association between BMI and COPD is largely affected by the type of diagnosis: emphysema was more associated with low BMI categories and chronic bronchitis with high BMI categories. By combining patients with chronic bronchitis and patients with emphysema in a single COPD category, these authors reported a U-shaped risk trend, meaning that low and high BMIs increase the risk for the disease [24].

The effects of food deprivation on normal lung structure and function have not been well studied in any systematic and detailed manner. One of the earliest pathological studies of human lungs was carried out by Stein and Fenigstein [25] who reported 13.5% of emphysema cases in Warsaw ghetto residents and that these emphysematous lesions were found in all age groups from childhood to senility. Keys et al. [26] described changes in physiology in normal adult men after 24 weeks of semi-starvation. In this study, the vital capacity was progressively diminished, most likely the result of respiratory muscle weakness [26]. Reductions in vital capacity are also described in female patients with anorexia nervosa [27].

Significance of body weight as outcome measure

BMI and disease characterization

In the 1960s, Filley et al. [6] described two contrasting types of patients with chronic airway obstruction based on clinical criteria and body weight: the 'pink puffer' and the 'blue bloater'. The 'pink puffer', the emphysematous patient, was more breathless with marked hyperinflation, thin in appearance with major weight loss. The 'blue bloater' had more severe central cyanosis and was frequently obese; this blue bloating type has often been considered as the chronic bronchitis subtype of COPD [6].

Several authors have attempted to correlate the degree of weight loss with the presence and severity of emphysema. A relationship between the ratio of residual volume to total lung capacity and weight loss had already been reported in the early 1960s [28]. Sukumalchantra and Williams [29] reported that the disease progression in a 5-year follow-up study of patients with severe COPD, as manifested by reduction in maximum mid-expiratory flow rate and increased airway resistance, occurred only in patients who had lost more than 10% of their initial weight; furthermore, the reduction in diffusing capacity was also more severe in patients who had suffered weight loss during the study period. The relationship between nutritional status and COPD subtypes was further evidenced in the paper of Openbrier et al. [30], who demonstrated that patients with emphysema were somatically depleted in comparison with patients with chronic bronchitis. They found that in patients with emphysema a good correlation was present with the degree of airflow limitation as well as with the single-breath

diffusing capacity. Others reported that transfer coefficient of diffusing capacity (Kco) was significantly lower in those COPD patients with FFM depletion vs patients without FFM depletion. Furthermore, 38% of the patients with a Kco less than 60% predicted compared with 5% of the patients with a Kco greater than or equal to 80% were considered depleted [12]. These data indicate that weight loss and nutritional depletion is a particular problem in those patients with impaired diffusing capacity. High-resolution computed tomography (HRCT) is an imaging procedure that allows direct assessment of the presence, extent and severity of emphysema [31]. Engelen et al. [32] analysed body weight and body composition in COPD patients, subdivided into an emphysematous group and a bronchitis group based on HRCT. Body weight and BMI as well as FFM and fat mass were significantly lower in emphysematous patients compared with the bronchitis group.

Remarkably, these data were confirmed by studies focusing on fibre type redistribution in skeletal muscles. Emphysematous patients have a more marked type I–IIX fibre type redistribution in the vastus lateralis than non-emphysematous patients and controls [33]. Further studies are needed to unravel these muscular abnormalities especially in the emphysematous subgroup. At least, these data support evidence for a relationship between COPD subtypes and particular changes in body composition.

Functional performance and health status

Dyspnoea and exercise intolerance are prominent symptoms in COPD patients. In addition to airflow limitation and impaired diffusing capacity, it became evident during last decade that respiratory and skeletal muscle weakness are important determinants of these symptoms [34,35]. Although muscle dysfunction is highly related to muscle wasting [36,37], much of the literature demonstrates that BMI can be considered as an indicator of functional disability. In underweight COPD patients, impaired respiratory muscle strength has been demonstrated [11,38–41]. These data are supported by autopsy data, which demonstrate that body weight and muscularity profoundly affect diaphragm muscle mass [42]. Changes in BMI associated with muscle tissue depletion significantly impairs skeletal muscle strength in COPD patients [37,43].

A close relationship between poor muscle condition, reflected by reduction in percentage ideal body weight or BMI, and maximal aerobic capacity has been observed in several studies [36,44–46]. Furthermore, reduced body mass has an independent negative effect on muscle aerobic capacity in COPD patients, as manifested by a decrease in maximal oxygen consumption, reduction in the lactate threshold and slowing of oxygen consumption kinetics [47]. Data regarding the relationship between walking distance and BMI are rather conflicting. While some authors have reported that in malnourished patients with stable advanced disease the degree of weight loss bears no relation to the work capacity at submaximal levels [44,48], others have demonstrated a significant association between walking distance and body weight [45]. Positive outcomes on peak exercise parameters as well as on walking distance have been reported by nutritional intervention in depleted COPD patients [49].

The functional consequences of being underweight and particularly of FFM depletion have also been reflected as a decreased health status as measured by the St. George Respiratory Questionnaire (SGRQ) [50]. In another study, depletion of FFM had a greater impairment in the activity and impact scores of the SGRQ, irrespective of body weight [51]. Others reported that underweight COPD patients are more dyspnoeic than normal-weight patients, partly as a consequence of decreased respiratory muscle strength [41].

Health care utilization

There is growing evidence in the literature that nutritional depletion in COPD is related to higher health care utilization, especially of inpatient services. In a small group of chronic hypercapnic patients, Vitacca *et al.* [51] reported that basal body weight, the decline in FEV_1 and the rate of deterioration of arterial blood gases were related to the necessity of intensive care unit (ICU) admission. Some years later, the same group reported that underlying general conditions such as malnutrition and a high physiology score (APACHE II) were unfavourable indices of outcome for acute exacerbation of COPD (AECOPD) treated with medical therapy and that flow limitation as assessed by forced expiratory manoeuvres provides additional information. The discriminant analysis showed, in decreasing order of power, that nutritional prognostic index, APACHE II score, FEV_1 : FVC ratio, vital capacity (VC) (% predicted) and FVC (% predicted) provided a significant distinction between patients requiring mechanical ventilation and those who could be treated with medical therapy only [52]. Kessler *et al.* [53] reported that besides gas exchange impairment and pulmonary haemodynamic worsening, the risk of being hospitalized for COPD was significantly increased in patients with a low BMI and patients with a limited 6-minute walking distance [53]. Nutritional depletion also increased the risk of early non-elective readmission in patients previously admitted for an exacerbation [54]. A prospective cohort study of 1016 patients admitted to hospital for AECOPD described that survival time after AECOPD was independently related to severity of illness, BMI, age, prior functional status, Pa_{O_2}, Fi_{O_2}, congestive heart failure, serum albumin and the presence of cor pulmonale [55].

In patients with emphysema undergoing lung volume reduction surgery, a deficient nutritional status identifiable by BMI was found in approximately 50% of patients. This impaired nutritional status was associated with increasing morbidity following lung volume reduction surgery (LVRS), manifested by prolonged ventilatory support and increased length of hospital stay [56]. Similar data were reported in lung transplant candidates: duration of mechanical ventilation and time spent in the ICU was significantly related to initial body composition [17]. Furthermore, it was demonstrated that lung transplant recipients with BMIs lower than the 25th percentile, or less than 80% of the predicted weight for a certain height, and/or those patients with lean body mass depletion have a worse survival rate following lung transplantation [17,57,58]. These findings are confirmed by analysis of the impact of BMI on outcomes in critically ill patients based on a large multi-institutional ICU database. It was found that low BMI was associated with increased mortality and worsened hospital discharge functional status [59]. In patients with severe COPD treated with home long-term oxygen therapy (LTOT), Chailleux *et al.* [15] recently reported that low BMI was the most powerful predictor of duration and rate of hospitalization, independently of blood gas levels and respiratory function. The lowest hospitalization rates were observed in the obese patients in this study.

BMI and COPD-related mortality

The relationship between weight loss and being underweight with mortality has been the subject of investigation since the 1960s. Vandenbergh *et al.* [7] reported a significant association between weight loss and survival in patients with COPD: 5-year mortality was 50% in those losing weight, compared with only 20% in weight-stable patients with COPD. Several retrospective studies using different COPD populations also provided evidence for a relationship between low BMI and mortality, independent of FEV_1 [14,60,61]. Remarkably, a decreased mortality risk was observed in overweight patients with COPD compared with underweight patients and with subjects of normal weight [14,61]. In COPD patients randomly allocated to LTOT or medical treatment, Gorecka *et al.* [62] found that BMI was a significant predictor of survival, independent of FEV_1. In a cohort of more than 4000 patients treated with LTOT, Chailleux *et al.* [15] reported that low body weight was an independent risk factor for mortality: the 5-year survival rates were 24%, 34%, 44% and 59%, respectively, for patients with BMIs of less than 20, 20–24, 25–29 and greater than or equal to 30. The best prognosis again was observed in overweight and obese COPD patients on LTOT. In one study, weight gain after nutritional supplementation was also related to decreased mortality independent of FEV_1, resting arterial blood gases, smoking, age and gender

[61]. Studies describing factors associated with COPD deaths also reported that being underweight is one of the determinants of those patients who died with COPD [63,64]. A Danish population study, including more than 2000 subjects and a 17-year follow-up, confirmed these noted associations between body weight and mortality risk [65]. Using normal-weight subjects (BMI 20.0–24.9 kg/m^2) as reference, the relative risk of death, adjusted for smoking, chronic mucus hypersecretion, FEV_1 and gender was significantly increased in underweight subjects but decreased in overweight and even obese subjects with airflow obstruction. A similar but weaker association was observed in subjects with mild and moderate disease. The specific relationship between FFM and mortality was reported by Marquis et al. [66], demonstrating that midthigh muscle cross-sectional area obtained by CT scan and FEV_1 were found to be the only significant predictors of mortality.

Therefore, it can be concluded that from the point of view that improvement of prognosis is one of the management goals in COPD, assessment of BMI is a good predictor of mortality and outcome in these patients.

Pathogenesis of weight loss

Weight loss, particularly loss of fat mass, occurs if energy expenditure exceeds dietary intake. Muscle wasting is a consequence of an imbalance between synthesis and breakdown of protein. Impairments in total energy balance can occur simultaneously, but these processes can also be dissociated because of altered regulation of substrate metabolism [67]. Several studies have provided evidence for involvement of systemic inflammation in the pathogenesis of tissue depletion in patients with COPD [68–71]. Systemic inflammation could modify energy homoeostasis partly by interaction between cytokines and leptin metabolism. Leptin is synthesized by adipose tissue and is the afferent hormonal signal to the brain regulating fat mass [72,73]. Disturbances in the tightly regulated equilibrium between protein synthesis and breakdown can also be induced by systemic inflammation, at least by activation of the adenosine triphosphate (ATP) dependent ubiquitin–proteasome pathway [74,75]. Direct effects of tumour necrosis factor on differentiated skeletal muscles have been reported. Treatment with this factor reduces the total protein and myosin heavy-chain content in a manner dependent on time and concentration [76]. Muscle wasting might also be the result of a decreased number of fibres, resulting from changes in the regulation of skeletal muscle regeneration or activation of apoptotic pathways [77,78]. New insights into the regulation of the processes of atrophy and hypertrophy could provide opportunities for modulation of these processes in the future [79].

References

1 Pauwels RA, Buist AS, Calverley PM, Jenkins CR, Hurd SS, GOLD Scientific Committee. Global strategy for the diagnosis, management, and prevention of chronic obstructive pulmonary disease. NHLBI/WHO Global Initiative for Chronic Obstructive Lung Disease (GOLD) Workshop summary. *Am J Respir Crit Care Med* 2001;**163**:1256–76.

2 Wouters EFM. Chronic obstructive pulmonary disease. V. Systemic effects of COPD. *Thorax* 2002;**57**:1067–70.

3 Agusti AG, Noguera A, Sauleda J *et al.* Systemic effects of chronic obstructive pulmonary disease. *Eur Respir J* 2003; **21**:347–60.

4 Fowler J, Godlee R. *Emphysema of the Lungs*. London: Longmans, Ed. Green and Co, 1898: 171.

5 Dornhorst A. Respiratory insufficiency. *Lancet* 1955;**268**: 1185–7.

6 Filley GF, Beckwitt HJ, Reeves JT, Mitchell RS. Chronic obstructive bronchopulmonary disease. II. Oxygen transport in two clinical types. *Am J Med* 1968;**44**:26–38.

7 Vandenbergh E, Van de Woestijne KP, Gyselen A. Weight changes in the terminal stages of chronic obstructive pulmonary disease: relation to respiratory function and prognosis. *Am Rev Respir Dis* 1967;**95**:556–66.

8 Metropolitan Life Insurance Company. New weight standards for men and women. *Bull Metropol Life Found* 1983; **64**:1–4.

9 US Department of Agriculture and US Department of Health and Human Services. *Nutrition and Your Health: Dietary Guidelines for Americans*, 5th edn. Home and Garden Bulletin no. 232. Washington, DC: US Government Printing Office, 2000.

10 Roubenoff R, Heymsfield SB, Kehayias JJ, Cannon JG, Rosenberg IH. Standardization of nomenclature of body composition in weight loss. *Am J Clin Nutr* 1997;**66**(1):192–6.

11 Schols AM, Soeters PB, Dingemans AM *et al.* Prevalence and characteristics of nutritional depletion in patients with stable COPD eligible for pulmonary rehabilitation. *Am Rev Respir Dis* 1993;**147**:1151–6.

12 Engelen MP, Schols AM, Baken WC, Wesseling GJ, Wouters EF. Nutritional depletion in relation to respiratory and peripheral skeletal muscle function in out-patients with COPD. *Eur Respir J* 1994;**7**:1793–7.

13 Hunter AM, Carey MA, Larsh HW. The nutritional status of patients with chronic obstructive pulmonary disease. *Am Rev Respir Dis* 1981;**124**:376–81.

14 Wilson DO, Rogers RM, Wright EC, Anthonisen NR. Body weight in chronic obstructive pulmonary disease. The National Institutes of Health Intermittent Positive-Pressure Breathing Trial. *Am Rev Respir Dis* 1989;**139**:1435–8.

15 Chailleux E, Laaban JP, Veale D. Prognostic value of nutritional depletion in patients with COPD treated by long-term oxygen therapy: data from the ANTADIR observatory. *Chest* 2003;**123**:1460–6.

16 Laaban JP, Kouchakji B, Dore MF *et al.* Nutritional status of patients with chronic obstructive pulmonary disease and acute respiratory failure. *Chest* 1993;**103**:1362–8.

17 Schwebel C, Pin I, Barnoud D *et al*. Prevalence and consequences of nutritional depletion in lung transplant candidates. *Eur Respir J* 2000;**16**:1050–5.

18 van Bokhorst DE, van der Schueren MA, van Leeuwen PA *et al*. Assessment of malnutrition parameters in head and neck cancer and their relation to postoperative complications. *Head Neck* 1997;**19**:419–25.

19 Kruizenga HM, Wierdsma NJ, van Bokhorst MA *et al*. Screening of nutritional status in the Netherlands. *Clin Nutr* 2003;**22**:147–52.

20 Higgins MW, Keller JB, Becker M *et al*. An index of risk for obstructive airways disease. *Am Rev Respir Dis* 1982;**125**:144–51.

21 Nemery B, Moavero NE, Brasseur L, Stanescu DC. Smoking, lung function, and body weight. *BMJ* 1983;**286**:249–51.

22 Chen Y, Breithaupt K, Muhajarine N. Occurrence of chronic obstructive pulmonary disease among Canadians and sex-related risk factors. *J Clin Epidemiol* 2000;**53**:755–61.

23 Harik-Khan RI, Fleg JL, Wise RA. Body mass index and the risk of COPD. *Chest* 2002;**121**:370–6.

24 Guerra S, Sherrill DL, Bobadilla A, Martinez FD, Barbee RA. The relation of body mass index to asthma, chronic bronchitis, and emphysema. *Chest* 2002;**122**:1256–63.

25 Stein J, Fenigstein H. Anatomie pathologique de la maladie de famine. In: Apfelbaum E, ed. *Recherches Clinique sur la Famine Executees dan le Chetto de Varsovie en 1942*. Warsaw: American Joint Distribution Committee, 1946: 21–7.

26 Keys A, Brozek J, Henschel A. *Biology of Human Starvation*. Minneapolis: University of Minnesota Press, 1950: 601–6.

27 Cravetto C, Carelli E, Cardellino G, Garbagni R. Osservazioni sulla funzione respiratoria nella anoressia mentale. [Observations on respiratory function in mental anorexia.] *Minerva Med* 1966;**57**:3498–501.

28 Ziegenspeck D, Sundermann A, Roth W. Das Korpergewicht beim Lungenemphysem (eine Klinishstatistische Studie). [The body weight in pulmonary emphysema (a clinical–statistical study).] *Allerg Asthma (Leipz.)* 1963;**31**:233–42.

29 Sukumalchantra Y, Williams MH Jr. Serial studies of pulmonary function in patients with chronic obstructive pulmonary disease. *Am J Med* 1965;**39**:941–5.

30 Openbrier DR, Irwin MM, Rogers RM *et al*. Nutritional status and lung function in patients with emphysema and chronic bronchitis. *Chest* 1983;**83**:17–22.

31 Klein JS, Gamsu G, Webb WR, Golden JA, Muller NL. High-resolution CT diagnosis of emphysema in symptomatic patients with normal chest radiographs and isolated low diffusing capacity. *Radiology* 1992;**182**:817–21.

32 Engelen MP, Schols AM, Lamers RJ, Wouters EF. Different patterns of chronic tissue wasting among patients with chronic obstructive pulmonary disease. *Clin Nutr* 1999;**18**:275–80.

33 Gosker HR, Engelen MP, van Mameren H *et al*. Muscle fiber type IIX atrophy is involved in the loss of fat-free mass in chronic obstructive pulmonary disease. *Am J Clin Nutr* 2002;**76**:113–9.

34 Gosselink R, Troosters T, Decramer M. Peripheral muscle weakness contributes to exercise limitation in COPD. *Am J Respir Crit Care Med* 1996;**153**:976–80.

35 Hamilton AL, Killian KJ, Summers E, Jones NL. Muscle strength, symptom intensity, and exercise capacity in patients with cardiorespiratory disorders. *Am J Respir Crit Care Med* 1995;**152**:2021–31.

36 Baarends EM, Schols AM, Mostert R, Wouters EF. Peak exercise response in relation to tissue depletion in patients with chronic obstructive pulmonary disease. *Eur Respir J* 1997;**10**:2807–13.

37 Gosker HR, Lencer NH, Franssen FM *et al*. Striking similarities in systemic factors contributing to decreased exercise capacity in patients with severe chronic heart failure or COPD. *Chest* 2003;**123**:1416–24.

38 Arora NS, Rochester DF. Respiratory muscle strength and maximal voluntary ventilation in undernourished patients. *Am Rev Respir Dis* 1982;**126**:5–8.

39 Arora NS, Rochester DF. Effect of body weight and muscularity on human diaphragm muscle mass, thickness, and area. *J Appl Physiol* 1982;**52**:64–70.

40 Rochester DF, Arora NS, Braun NM. Maximum contractile force of human diaphragm muscle, determined *in vivo*. *Trans Am Clin Climatol Assoc* 1981;**93**:200–8.

41 Sahebjami H, Sathianpitayakul E. Influence of body weight on the severity of dyspnea in chronic obstructive pulmonary disease. *Am J Respir Crit Care Med* 2000;**161**:886–90.

42 Thurlbeck WM. Diaphragm and body weight in emphysema. *Thorax* 1978;**33**:483–7.

43 Mostert R, Goris A, Weling-Scheepers C, Wouters EF, Schols AM. Tissue depletion and health related quality of life in patients with chronic obstructive pulmonary disease. *Respir Med* 2000;**94**:859–67.

44 Gray-Donald K, Gibbons L, Shapiro SH, Martin JG. Effect of nutritional status on exercise performance in patients with chronic obstructive pulmonary disease. *Am Rev Respir Dis* 1989;**140**:1544–8.

45 Schols AM, Mostert R, Soeters PB, Greve LH, Wouters EF. Nutritional state and exercise performance in patients with chronic obstructive lung disease. *Thorax* 1989;**44**:937–41.

46 Palange P, Forte S, Felli A *et al*. Nutritional state and exercise tolerance in patients with COPD. *Chest* 1995;**107**:1206–12.

47 Palange P, Forte S, Onorati P *et al*. Effect of reduced body weight on muscle aerobic capacity in patients with COPD. *Chest* 1998;**114**:12–8.

48 Efthimiou J, Fleming J, Gomes C, Spiro SG. The effect of supplementary oral nutrition in poorly nourished patients with chronic obstructive pulmonary disease. *Am Rev Respir Dis* 1988;**137**:1075–82.

49 Creutzberg EC, Wouters EF, Mostert R, Weling-Scheepers CA, Schols AM. Efficacy of nutritional supplementation therapy in depleted patients with chronic obstructive pulmonary disease. *Nutrition* 2003;**19**:120–7.

50 Shoup R, Dalsky G, Warner S *et al*. Body composition and health-related quality of life in patients with obstructive airways disease. *Eur Respir J* 1997;**10**:1576–80.

51 Vitacca M, Foglio K, Scalvini S *et al*. Time course of pulmonary function before admission into ICU: a two-year retrospective study of COLD patients with hypercapnia. *Chest* 1992;**102**:1737–41.

52 Vitacca M, Clini E, Porta R, Foglio K, Ambrosino N. Acute

exacerbations in patients with COPD: predictors of need for mechanical ventilation. *Eur Respir J* 1996;**9**:1487–93.

53 Kessler R, Faller M, Fourgaut G, Mennecier B, Weitzenblum E. Predictive factors of hospitalization for acute exacerbation in a series of 64 patients with chronic obstructive pulmonary disease. *Am J Respir Crit Care Med* 1999;**159**:158–64.

54 Pouw EM, Ten Velde GP, Croonen BH *et al*. Early non-elective readmission for chronic obstructive pulmonary disease is associated with weight loss. *Clin Nutr* 2000;**19**:95–9.

55 Connors AF Jr, Dawson NV, Thomas C *et al*. Outcomes following acute exacerbation of severe chronic obstructive lung disease. The SUPPORT investigators (Study to Understand Prognoses and Preferences for Outcomes and Risks of Treatments). *Am J Respir Crit Care Med* 1996;**154**:959–67.

56 Mazolewski P, Turner JF, Baker M, Kurtz T, Little AG. The impact of nutritional status on the outcome of lung volume reduction surgery: a prospective study. *Chest* 1999;**116**:693–6.

57 Sharples L, Hathaway T, Dennis C *et al*. Prognosis of patients with cystic fibrosis awaiting heart and lung transplantation. *J Heart Lung Transplant* 1993;**12**:669–74.

58 Plochl W, Pezawas L, Artemiou O *et al*. Nutritional status, ICU duration and ICU mortality in lung transplant recipients. *Intensive Care Med* 1996;**22**:1179–85.

59 Tremblay A, Bandi V. Impact of body mass index on outcomes following critical care. *Chest* 2003;**123**:1202–7.

60 Gray-Donald K, Gibbons L, Shapiro SH, Macklem PT, Martin JG. Nutritional status and mortality in chronic obstructive pulmonary disease. *Am J Respir Crit Care Med* 1996;**153**:961–6.

61 Schols AM, Slangen J, Volovics L, Wouters EF. Weight loss is a reversible factor in the prognosis of chronic obstructive pulmonary disease. *Am J Respir Crit Care Med* 1998;**157**:1791–7.

62 Gorecka D, Gorzelak K, Sliwinski P, Tobiasz M, Zielinski J. Effect of long-term oxygen therapy on survival in patients with chronic obstructive pulmonary disease with moderate hypoxaemia. *Thorax* 1997;**52**:674–9.

63 Meyer PA, Mannino DM, Redd SC, Olson DR. Characteristics of adults dying with COPD. *Chest* 2002;**122**:2003–8.

64 Domingo-Salvany A, Lamarca R, Ferrer M *et al*. Health-related quality of life and mortality in male patients with chronic obstructive pulmonary disease. *Am J Respir Crit Care Med* 2002;**166**:680–5.

65 Landbo C, Prescott E, Lange P, Vestbo J, Almdal TP. Prognostic value of nutritional status in chronic obstructive pulmonary disease. *Am J Respir Crit Care Med* 1999;**160**:1856–61.

66 Marquis K, Debigare R, Lacasse Y *et al*. Midthigh muscle cross-sectional area is a better predictor of mortality than body mass index in patients with chronic obstructive pulmonary disease. *Am J Respir Crit Care Med* 2002;**166**:809–13.

67 Schols AM, Wouters EF. Nutritional abnormalities and supplementation in chronic obstructive pulmonary disease. *Clin Chest Med* 2000;**21**:753–62.

68 Schols AM, Buurman WA, Staal van den Brekel AJ, Dentener MA, Wouters EF. Evidence for a relation between metabolic derangements and increased levels of inflammatory mediators in a subgroup of patients with chronic obstructive pulmonary disease. *Thorax* 1996;**51**:819–24.

69 Creutzberg EC, Schols AM, Weling Scheepers CA, Buurman WA, Wouters EFM. Characterization of non-response to high caloric oral nutritional therapy in depleted patients with chronic obstructive pulmonary disease. *Am J Respir Crit Care Med* 2000;**161**:745–52.

70 De Godoy I, Donahoe M, Calhoun WJ, Mancino J, Rogers RM. Elevated TNF-α production by peripheral blood monocytes of weight-losing COPD patients. *Am J Respir Crit Care Med* 1996;**153**:633–7.

71 Di Francia M, Barbier D, Mege JL, Orehek J. Tumor necrosis factor alpha levels and weight loss in chronic obstructive pulmonary disease. *Am J Respir Crit Care Med* 1994;**150**:1453–5.

72 Schols AM, Creutzberg EC, Buurman WA *et al*. Plasma leptin is related to proinflamatory status and dietary intake in patients with chronic obstructive pulmonary disease. *Am J Respir Crit Care Med* 1999;**160**:1220–6.

73 Takabatake N, Nakamura H, Abe S *et al*. Circulating leptin in patients with chronic obstructive pulmonary disease. *Am J Respir Crit Care Med* 1999;**159**:1215–9.

74 Mitch WE, Goldberg AL. Mechanisms of muscle wasting: the role of the ubiquitin–proteasome pathway. *N Engl J Med* 1996;**335**:1897–905.

75 Jagoe RT, Goldberg AL. What do we really know about the ubiquitin–proteasome pathway in muscle atrophy? *Curr Opin Clin Nutr Metab Care* 2001;**4**:183–90.

76 Li Y, Schwartz RJ, Waddell ID, Holloway BR, Reid MD. Skeletal muscle myocytes undergo protein loss and reactive oxygen-mediated NFκB activation in response to tumor necrosis factor α. *FASEB J* 1998;**12**:871–80.

77 Langen RC, Schols AM, Kelders MC, Wouters EF, Janssen-Heininger YM. Inflammatory cytokines inhibit myogenic differentiation through activation of nuclear factor-κB. *FASEB J* 2001;**15**:1169–80.

78 Agusti AG, Sauleda J, Miralles C *et al*. Skeletal muscle apoptosis and weight loss in chronic obstructive pulmonary disease. *Am J Respir Crit Care Med* 2002;**166**:485–9.

79 Glass DJ. Signalling pathways that mediate skeletal muscle hypertrophy and atrophy. *Nat Cell Biol* 2003;**5**:87–90.

CHAPTER 40
Lung connective tissue

Sarah E. Dunsmore and Geoffrey J. Laurent

Key concept

The structural integrity of the lung and the biological activity of its resident cells are dependent on a diverse group of connective tissue glycoproteins and proteoglycans.

Fundamental physical properties, such as the intrinsic recoil of the lung, are governed by connective tissue, which consists of cells and extracellular matrix and has the general function of supporting and filling space between organs. In the lung, fibrous connective tissue is found throughout the pulmonary interstitium and large airways. In addition, cartilage, a specialized form of connective tissue, encircles the trachea and large bronchi preventing collapse of these structures. In this chapter, the individual components that confer structure and function to lung connective tissue are described.

Each type of connective tissue is uniquely organized to play a distinct part in normal lung function. Matrix components of lung connective tissue also regulate cell phenotype, gene expression and motility via interactions with integrins and other cell surface receptors (Fig. 40.1). Following a brief discussion of cartilage, this chapter focuses on the cells and matrix proteins found in the pulmonary interstitium. The final section of this chapter provides an introduction to the matrix-related pathology of COPD.

Cartilage

Hyaline cartilage lines the walls of the trachea and large bronchi and is responsible for keeping these airways open despite changes in intrathoracic pressure during breathing.

Figure 40.1 Matrix protein structure and organization. Epithelial cells are linked to connective tissue via a network of matrix proteins. Laminin 5 connects hemidesmosomes on the basal surface of epithelial cells to the type IV collagen network in the lamina densa of the basement membrane. Anchoring fibrils composed of type VII and type XV collagen link the basement membrane to the interstitial matrix where type I collagen, type III collagen and elastic fibres are found. Integrins located on the fibroblast cell surface interact with many matrix proteins including type I collagen. (Reprinted from Gibson *et al.* [225], p. 83, with permission from Elsevier.)

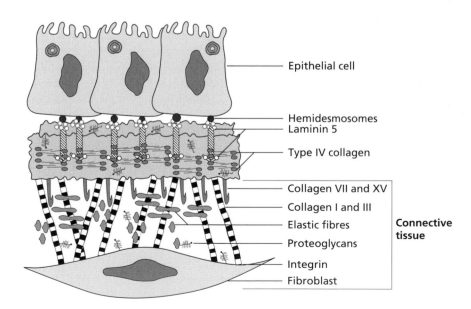

Epithelial cell

Hemidesmosomes
Laminin 5

Type IV collagen

Collagen VII and XV
Collagen I and III
Elastic fibres
Proteoglycans
Integrin
Fibroblast

Connective tissue

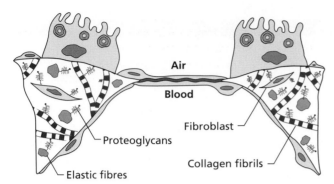

Figure 40.2 Pulmonary interstitium. At the gas exchange interface alveolar capillaries and alveolar type I epithelial cells share a basement membrane. In other portions of the alveolar wall, collagen fibrils and elastic fibres are the major components of the pulmonary interstitium which also contains fibroblasts and proteoglycans (not to scale). (Reprinted from Gibson *et al.* [225], p. 83, with permission from Elsevier.)

Chondroblasts produce the components of the cartilage extracellular matrix: hyaluronan, collagen types II, VI, IX, X, XI and XII, and aggrecan. Mature cartilage consists of chondrocytes embedded in lacunae surrounded by a matrix of proteoglycan aggregates and type II collagen fibres. In one model of cartilage function, collagen fibres in the outer layers oppose tensile forces and proteoglycans in the central zone resist compression forces [1].

The pulmonary interstitium

The connective tissue components of the pulmonary interstitium are key determinants of lung function providing the mechanical scaffold that maintains structural integrity during ventilation. Fibres of the matrix proteins, collagen and elastin, form this scaffold [2–5] (Fig. 40.2). It has long been recognized that devastating consequences result from disruption of pulmonary interstitial matrix homoeostasis [6]. Pulmonary fibrosis is a consequence of increased interstitial matrix deposition, particularly of types I and III collagen. In this disease, gas exchange is adversely affected by the loss of capillary beds and decreased regional compliance resulting from the thickening of the pulmonary interstitium. Conversely, degradation of elastin is a characteristic of pulmonary emphysema [7,8]. The reduction in elastin content of the pulmonary interstitium adversely affects ventilation by decreasing the intrinsic recoil of the lung [9–12].

Cells of the pulmonary interstitium

Fibroblasts are omnipresent in lung connective tissue and are responsible for production of the pulmonary interstitial matrix. Under normal conditions, macrophages are the only other cell type present to an appreciable extent in the pulmonary interstitium. In the inflamed lung, however, leucocytes, lymphocytes and mononuclear cells infiltrate the pulmonary interstitium. In COPD, the normal inflammatory response to cigarette smoke appears to be amplified by oxidative stress [13,14] and/or other mechanisms [15–19] resulting in irreversible elastolysis in the pulmonary interstitium. Much effort is being devoted to the development of novel anti-inflammatory therapies for COPD.

Structure and function of interstitial matrix proteins

Matrix proteins have characteristic structures and functions. Collagens and proteoglycans are ubiquitous components of the extracellular matrix. Elastic fibres, on the other hand, are specialized structures found only in tissues subject to mechanical stress. General aspects of the biology of the major classes of matrix proteins are briefly reviewed in this section.

Collagens

In simple terms, collagens may be thought of as the 'struts' of the lung – rod-like structures that limit lung deformation. Information contained within the collagen amino acid sequence dictates formation of these precisely ordered, rod-like structures. Collagens consist of three polypeptide chains containing the amino acid sequence (Gly-x-y). Gly-x-y sequences associate to form triple helices and, by definition, all collagens contain at least one triple helical region [20]. Although x and y may be any amino acid, proline and hydroxyproline predominate in these positions such that approximately every third x is proline and every third y is hydroxyproline. Hydroxyproline is not unique to collagen; however, concentrations in collagen are much higher than those in other proteins so hydroxyproline can be used as a specific index of collagen synthesis and concentration.

Collagen gene structure and organization

Genetic diversity arose during the metazoan radiation largely as a result of the mechanisms of exon shuffling and gene duplication. Human collagen gene structure reflects these events [21]. A 54 base pair unit that encodes the characteristic Gly-x-y repeat is thought to represent the ancestral collagen gene [22]. Evolution of collagens occurred by deletion, duplication and shuffling of Gly-x-y repeats (i.e. in nine base pair units). Thus, many collagen genes contain exons of 36, 45, 54, 63 and 108 base pairs [23]. Most collagen genes are composed of many exons, with 14 genes consisting of 50 or more exons [23–25]. Five collagen genes contain alternative transcription start sites; 16 are alternatively spliced [23,24,26,27].

The 43 collagen genes are located on 17 different chromosomes [23–27]. Several are found in close proximity on the same chromosome. The genes encoding the six polypeptide chains that are constituents of type IV collagen are clustered head-to-head [28–30] on chromosomes 13 (COL4A1 and COL4A2; 13q34), 2 (COL4A3 and COL4A4; 2q35-q37) and X (COL4A5 and COL4A6; Xq22). Collagen genes are oriented tail-to-tail [31] on chromosomes 2 (COL3A1 and COL5A2; 2q14-q32) and 6 (COL9A1 and COL19A1; 6q12-q14). COL12A1 is also positioned on chromosome 6 [32] slightly over four mega base pairs from COL9A1. Three collagen genes (COL6A1, COL6A2 and COL18A1) map to the same cytogenetic location [33] on chromosome 21 (21q22.3).

Transcription of collagen genes

Binding of a variety of transcription factors [34] to defined motifs in the promoter region of collagen genes [35–53] is the primary determinant of spatial and temporal collagen expression [24,25,27,54–73]. Expression of some collagen genes is also influenced by transcriptional regulatory elements located in introns [74–97] and in 3′ untranslated regions of the genes [98]. Epigenetic mechanisms such as DNA methylation restrict collagen expression to particular cell types [99,100] and to precise developmental stages [101,102]. In the event of tissue injury, cytokines such as transforming growth factor β (TGF-β) and tumour necrosis factor α (TNF-α) can affect collagen transcription by activating signalling pathways that lead to nuclear translocation of DNA binding factors [103–112].

Posttranscriptional regulation of collagen gene expression occurs during the processes of translation initiation and mRNA degradation. An evolutionarily conserved 5′ stem-loop structure which encompasses the AUG start codon inhibits translation of collagen α1(I), α2(I) and α1(III) mRNA transcripts [113]. Interactions of RNA binding proteins with this 5′ stem-loop structure [114,115] and with a 3′ polypyrimidine rich region [116,117] protect collagen α1(I) mRNA from deadenylation-dependent decay. Inhibition of translation initiation which facilitates binding of cytokine-regulated transcription factors [113] and delay of procollagen mRNA degradation may be important mechanisms in the pathogenesis of fibrotic disorders [116].

Procollagen translational modifications

A series of co and posttranslational modifications of collagen polypeptide chains begins with cotranslational cleavage of the signal sequence from preprocollagen. Hydroxylation of proline and lysine residues is required for formation of stable triple helical regions in mature collagen [118–121]. Hydroxylation begins as a cotranslational process and continues posttranslation until triple helix formation is complete. Biochemical reactions are accomplished by three enzymes: procollagenproline dioxy-

genase (EC 1.14.11.2), procollagenproline 3-dioxygenase (EC 1.14.11.7) and procollagen-lysine 5-dioxygenase (EC 1.14.11.4) which recognize specific sequences (X-Pro-Gly, Pro-4Hyp-Gly and X-Lys-Gly, respectively) in procollagen. These enzymes require ferrous iron, 2-oxoglutarate, molecular oxygen and ascorbate for activity.

Collagen triple helical structures are stabilized by glycosylation [122]. Glycosylation of procollagen is a cotranslational event. Two enzymes located on the inner endoplasmic reticulum membrane, procollagen galactosyltransferase (EC 2.4.1.50) and procollagen glucosyltransferase (EC 2.4.1.66), link sugar residues to procollagen hydroxylysines. A lysyl hydrolase isoform (lysyl hydrolase 3) possesses low levels of glucosyltransferase activity [123,124] that appear to be necessary for type IV collagen assembly [125]. Collagen propeptides also contain N-linked oligosaccharides [126–131].

Trimerization of α chains and triple helix propagation

Collagen triple helix formation takes place in the endoplasmic reticulum. Sequences in the C propeptide region of secreted collagens mediate assembly of the appropriate triad of procollagen chains [132,133]. Triple helix assembly is more efficient when inter- [134] and intrachain disulphide bonds [135] are present. Protein disulphide-isomerase (EC 5.3.4.1), one of the most abundant enzymes in the endoplasmic reticulum, catalyses the formation of disulphide bonds in secretory proteins and maintains disulphide isomerase activity [136] when it functions as the β subunit of prolyl 4-hydroxylase [136,137]. Protein disulphide-isomerase also acts as a molecular chaperone by binding to the C propeptide region of monomeric collagen [138] in order to prevent the secretion of unassembled collagen chains [139,140]. Triple helix propagation of secreted collagens proceeds from the C- to the N-terminal [133,141,142]. For transmembrane collagens, triple helix folding appears to be in the more typical N- to C-terminal direction [143,144]. The *cis-trans* isomerization of peptide bonds, which is catalysed by peptidylprolyl isomerase (EC 5.2.1.8), is the rate limiting step in collagen triple helix assembly [141,145–147].

Fibrillogenesis and supramolecular structure assembly

Correctly folded procollagen traffics from the endoplasmic reticulum to the Golgi stacks [148]. A collagen-specific molecular chaperone, HSP47 [149,150], is involved in this process. HSP47 binds to Gly-X-Arg repeats [151–154] in triple helical collagen [154–156] and is necessary for collagen secretion [157] which occurs via cisternal maturation of the Golgi stacks [158]. Collagen function is dependent upon the post-Golgi assembly of procollagen molecules into fibrils and other supramolecular structures (Fig. 40.3).

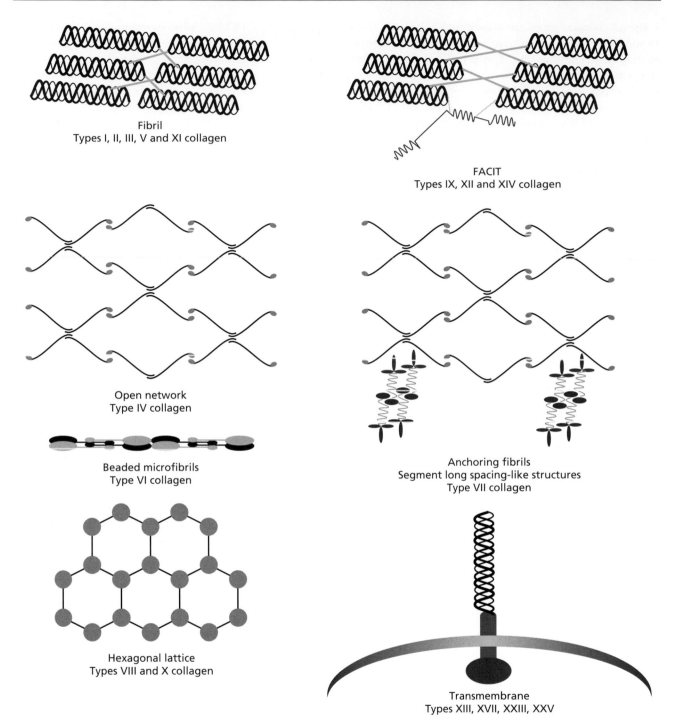

Figure 40.3 Collagen supramolecular structures. (Reprinted from Laurent and Shapiro [226], p. 173, with permission from Elsevier.)

Fibril formation has been well characterized [148,159–163]. Removal of N-terminal telopeptides by procollagen N-endopeptidase (EC 3.4.24.14) and cleavage of C-terminal telopeptide sequences by procollagen C-endopeptidase (EC 3.4.24.19) initiates fibrillogenesis [164–166]. Protein-lysine 6-oxidase (EC 1.4.3.13) cross-links exposed telopep-

tide sequences to stabilize fibril structure. FACIT collagens [167] form bridges between interstitial collagen fibrils.

The macromolecular assembly of the open network structure of type IV collagen, the principal non-fibrillar collagen, has been extensively studied [168]. Anchoring fibrils composed of type VII collagen associate with the type IV collagen network in the cutaneous basement membrane to stabilize the dermal–epidermal boundary [169]. Details of the molecular assembly of other non-fibrillar collagens into beaded microfibrils [170] and hexagonal lattices [168] have been reported. Transmembrane collagens [171] form homotrimers with the collagenous domain extracellularly oriented.

Collagens in the lung

Fibrillar collagens (types I, II, III, V and XI) are the most abundant proteins in the lung accounting for approximately 15–20% of the dry weight of the tissue [172]. Their primary function is to confer tensile strength to all distensible components of the lung such as the large airways, blood vessels and alveolar interstitium. Types I and III collagen (in a ratio of 2 : 1) represent approximately 90% of the collagens in the adult human lung. These collagens are located throughout the alveolar interstitium, in pulmonary blood vessels, the visceral pleura and in the connective tissue sheaths that surround the tracheobronchial tree. Type I collagen confers tensile strength and rigidity to tissues; whereas type III, which forms a more reticular network of fibres, is more important in bestowing compliance. Tensile strength of bronchial and tracheal cartilage is largely determined by types II and XI collagen. Small amounts of type V collagen are present in basement membranes. It is also found in association with type I collagen in the interstitium, alveolar walls and blood vessels.

Type IV collagen is the most abundant non-fibrillar collagen found in the lung, constituting approximately 5% of parenchymal collagen. Instead of forming fibrils, the amino and carboxy terminal regions of the type IV collagen molecule laterally associate to form open network structures which are thought to have a role in the structural and barrier functions of the basement membrane. Type IV collagen is responsible for the tensile strength of the blood–gas barrier and plays a large part in preventing stress failure of the pulmonary capillaries under normal conditions [173].

Many other non-fibrillar collagens are present in the lung. Type VI collagen is found in the pulmonary interstitium and vasculature, as fine filaments associated with types I and III collagen. Pulmonary arterioles and venules contain type VIII collagen. Although information on localization is lacking, expression of types IX and XII collagen in the lung has been documented. Collagen types XV and XVIII, which are also proteoglycans, are components of the lung basement membrane. Although it has been speculated that these other non-fibrillar collagens may have a role in determining tensile strength or in facilitating collagen fibril assembly, their specific functions in the lung are not known.

Elastic fibres

Simplistically, elastic fibres are the springs that snap the lung back to resting volume following inflation. Elastic fibres [174], assembled from fibrillin-rich microfibrils and tropoelastin, are very stable structures; some may last for the life span of the organism [175]. The relative proportion of microfibrils to elastin, however, declines with increasing age. Thus, the scaffold for elastic fibre assembly is only present for a limited period of time, and degradation of elastin in the adult has been believed to lead to irreversible pathology.

In the lung, elastic fibres are predominately found in the parenchyma where, together with collagen fibrils, an integral fibre network that comprises the architectural skeleton of the lung is formed. This fibre network is a key determinant of the mechanical properties of the lung. Elastic fibres encircle respiratory bronchioles and alveolar ducts in a helical fashion and appear as a fine mesh in alveolar walls. In the walls of the pulmonary artery and arterioles, elastic fibres are organized into concentric sheets or lamellae.

Elastin

Elastin is a unique matrix protein that is capable of being stretched several times its resting length under tension with a rapid recovery to its original size when the force is released [176]. It is an insoluble protein composed mainly of hydrophobic amino acids (44%), glycine (33%) and proline (10–13%). Two pentapeptides, Val-Pro-Gly-Val-Gly and Pro-Gly-Val-Gly-Val, repeat frequently in the molecule and are thought to form large spiral regions that contribute to the distensibility of the protein [177]. Phylogenetic analysis indicates that the appearance of elastin in vertebrate species coincides with the development of pulsatile blood flow and closed circulatory systems [178].

Elastin is formed by cross-linking of lysine residues on its soluble precursor, tropoelastin [179]. Tropoelastin is transcribed from a single gene located on chromosome 7 [180,181]. The gene consists of 34 small exons (30–225 base pairs) interspersed between large introns [182,183]. Tropoelastin gene transcription is initiated from three major and four minor sites [182]. Transcripts are subject to alternative splicing particularly in the region encoded by exon 33 [184,185]. Pre and posttranscriptional regulatory mechanisms of tropoelastin gene expression have been described [186–188]. Posttranslational modification of tropoelastin is minimal. Although proline hydroxylation may occur, it is not necessary for tropoelastin secretion [189]. Two molecular chaperones, BiP and FKBP65, are important in the trafficking of tropoelastin from the endoplasmic reticulum to the Golgi apparatus [190]. It has been proposed that a 67-kDa elastin-binding protein functions as an intracellular chaperone to prevent tropoelastin aggregation and degradation [191]. Newly secreted tropoelastin forms globules on the cell surface [192]. These globules then interact with microfibrils via regions in the carboxy terminal of tropoelastin [193]. The process of cross-linking of tropoelastin lysine residues [194], which is catalysed by protein-lysine 6-oxidase (EC 1.4.3.13), begins in the cell surface globules and continues on the elastic fibre [195]. Cross-linking of tropoelastin to fibrillin-1 by protein-glutamine gamma-glutamyltransferase (EC 2.3.2.13) further stabilizes elastic fibre structure [196]. Molecules such as fibulin-5 [197,198], which are found at the interface of cell surface elastin globules and extracellular matrix elastic fibres, are essential for elastogenesis. Impaired elastic fibre assembly may contribute to the pathogenesis of COPD [199].

Proteoglycans

The simplistic analogy for proteoglycans is 'goo'. In the lung and other organs, proteoglycans are the primary 'space-fillers' of connective tissue. Proteoglycans are a diverse family of large molecules in which a core protein is covalently linked to sulphated polysaccharides or glycosaminoglycans (GAGs). GAGs may be divided into three classes: chondroitin sulphate/dermatan sulphate, heparan sulphate/heparin and keratan sulphate; a proteoglycan may be comprised of GAGs from more than one class. Hyaluronan, a non-sulphated GAG, is not a true proteoglycan because of its lack of a core protein. Proteoglycans are synthesized by a variety of cell types and are multifunctional components of most extracellular matrices and plasma membranes. Because of their large hydrodynamic volumes and charge characteristics, hyaluronan and proteoglycans exert a profound influence on lung compliance and fluid balance.

Early studies used cationic dyes, which react with negatively charged regions of carbohydrates and GAGs, to demonstrate the presence of proteoglycans in the lung. More recent studies have utilized antibodies and cDNA probes obtained from molecular cloning of various proteoglycans. These studies have demonstrated that the matrix proteoglycans [200]: versican, perlecan, agrin, decorin, biglycan, PRELP, lumican and fibromodulin are components of the lung extracellular matrix. Versican is a member of the hyalectan gene family which contains proteoglycans that interact with hyaluronan and lectins. In pulmonary fibrotic disorders, versican, a chondroitin/dermatan sulphate proteoglycan, appears to form a provisional matrix in which myofibroblasts synthesize type I collagen [201]. Perlecan and agrin are referred to as basement membrane proteoglycans and are predicted to function in determining the filtration properties of the alveolar basement mem-

brane [202,203]. Both are heparan sulphate proteoglycans and are also likely to function in sequestering growth factors. Agrin, because of its structural similarity to Kazal-type serine protease inhibitors, may have a role in protecting proteins from degradation [204].

Decorin, biglycan, PRELP, lumican and fibromodulin are part of the family of small leucine-rich proteoglycans. This family is divided into three distinct subclasses based on genomic and protein organization. Decorin and biglycan, which contain chondroitin sulphate/dermatan sulphate GAGs, form one subclass. Both are primarily found in the pulmonary interstitium. Levels of decorin and biglycan are increased in pulmonary fibrosis and decreased in pulmonary emphysema [205]. Decorin and biglycan are hypothesized to function by sequestering growth factors and by facilitating collagen fibril assembly. Exogenously administered decorin is antifibrotic. This antifibrotic effect is attributed to binding and inactivation of TGF-β.

PRELP, lumican and fibromodulin, which contain keratan sulphate GAGs, are part of another subclass of the small leucine-rich proteoglycan family. In the lung, PRELP has only been detected at the mRNA level. The walls of the pulmonary vasculature contain lumican. Expression of fibromodulin is observed in animal models of lung injury. Lumican and fibromodulin appear to be important in collagen fibril assembly [206,207]. However, specific functions of these proteoglycans in the lung are not known.

Matrix-related pathology of COPD

Although destruction of elastic fibres in the lung interstitium is regarded as the pathological hallmark of emphysema, it is clear that excess matrix protein deposition or fibrosis often occurs in the airways of the COPD patient. Thus, the response of lung connective tissue to intrinsic and extrinsic factors associated with COPD is not uniform, and this should be taken into account in the design of therapeutic strategies for treatment of this disease.

Airway fibrosis

Deposition of collagenous and non-collagenous matrix proteins in the airways is part of a larger remodelling process that also includes changes in smooth muscle and mucus glands. Persistent inflammation in the small airways leads to subepithelial deposition of fibronectin and tenascin followed by fibroblast activation and production of collagen types I and III. Although the functional consequences of matrix protein deposition in the airways are not completely understood [208], excessive deposition of collagens and other molecules will have profound effects on mechanical properties, metabolism, cell function and transport properties of airways. It is possible that matrix protein deposition in the airways is a teleological response to prevent airway collapse. However, excess matrix protein deposition may contribute to narrowing of the airway lumen and thus, in the long term, limit ventilation.

Emphysema

There are two major forms of emphysema: panacinar and centrilobular. Panacinar emphysema predominates in the lower lung zones and occurs in people deficient in α_1-proteinase inhibitor, the serpin that blocks the activity of neutrophil elastase. Uniform destruction of the alveolar walls and permanent enlargement of the alveoli are observed. As the disease progresses, all respiratory airspaces distal to a terminal bronchiole are affected. Centrilobular emphysema predominates in the upper lung zones and begins with inflammation in the terminal and respiratory bronchioles with subsequent enlargement of the alveoli and more distal respiratory airspaces. It is thought to result as a consequence of prolonged exposure to cigarette smoke.

Treatment of COPD – a matrix perspective

Lung connective tissue is a dynamic structure. Fibroblasts, in particular, are active in synthesis, organization and degradation of extracellular matrix. Some matrix components, such as recently synthesized collagens and proteoglycans, are turned over quite rapidly while other components, such as elastic fibres, are very stable. Initial attempts to understand the role of connective tissue in COPD focused on regulation of matrix turnover and on identification of the enzymes responsible for elastic fibre destruction. Recently, more research effort has been devoted to understanding the process of alveolar regeneration. Thus, from a matrix perspective, emphysema treatment may be viewed as limiting elastic fibre destruction and/or restoring function to damaged alveolar units. Airway fibrosis also is frequently present in COPD patients and may be a major cause of airflow limitation. It remains unclear if specific treatments for airway fibrosis, which remain to be developed, will improve COPD outcome.

Protease inhibition

Since the first association of α_1-antitrypsin deficiency with emphysematous lung disease [209,210], much effort has been focused on the design of neutrophil elastase inhibitors for COPD treatment. Indeed, the elastase–antielastase hypothesis has dominated COPD research for the past 40 years. Although clinical use of neutrophil elastase inhibitors is not common, many compounds have been tested in animal models and in clinical trials [211]. A broad spectrum of extracellular and intracellular proteases, many with elastolytic capacity, is present in the COPD patient [212]. Furthermore, data from animal models [213,214] indicate that other proteases may be important in elastic fibre destruction and COPD pathogenesis. Although it appears that the protease–antiprotease hypothesis may be more extensive than originally envisioned, effective inhibition of elastolytic proteases will continue to be an attractive strategy for attenuating COPD progression.

Alveolar regeneration

To completely restore normal lung function to the COPD patient, repair and regeneration of damaged alveolar units is necessary. Although clinical implementation of regenerative medicine remains a revolutionary and futuristic goal, data from animal studies are providing evidence of some critical components of this process. The complexity of alveolar development is exemplified by the reports of defective alveogenesis in at least eight distinct 'knock-out' mice [215]. Alveolar enlargement in mice deficient in TIMP-3 [216], surfactant protein D [217] and the β_6-integrin subunit [218] underscores the importance of these molecules in regulating alveolar homoeostasis. Models in which emphysema is induced by apoptosis of alveolar endothelial [219] or epithelial cells [220] highlight the role of parenchymal cell turnover in the maintenance of alveolar structure. Perhaps the most promising finding from animal studies is that in elastase-damaged lungs, alveolar function and architecture can be restored by retinoic acid treatment [221]. Translation of these animal studies to clinical practice represents one of the most promising and challenging areas of COPD research.

Conclusions

It has long been recognized that the fundamental physical properties of the lung are determined by connective tissue. More recently, it has been appreciated that matrix proteins interact directly with receptors on the cell surface to initiate signalling cascades with the capacity to regulate the majority of cellular functions including proliferation, migration and differentiation. Despite this knowledge, none of the present clinical strategies for treating COPD directly target matrix proteins. A better understanding of matrix protein biology and new approaches for treating connective tissue disorders are still needed.

One long-term goal is the development of strategies that will enable regeneration of normal lung in damaged areas. The restoration of alveolar architecture in elastase-treated rats by retinoic acid treatment [221] provides evidence that extensive matrix damage can be repaired. Derivation of lung epithelium from embryonic [222] and bone marrow derived stem cells [223,224] implies that various types of precursor cells may be potentially useful in repopulating damaged areas of the lung. Continual application of cutting edge science to current issues in pulmonary medicine is our best hope for development of better treatments for lung disease and eventual realization of the goal of lung regeneration.

Acknowledgement

The authors would like to thank Huw D. Jones, UCL Media Resources, for his help in the preparation of Figures 40.1 and 40.2.

References

1 Roberts CR, Rains JK, Pare PD *et al*. Ultrastructure and tensile properties of human tracheal cartilage. *J Biomech* 1998;**31**:81–6.

2 Matsuda M, Fung YC, Sobin SS. Collagen and elastin fibers in human pulmonary alveolar mouths and ducts. *J Appl Physiol* 1987;**63**:1185–94.

3 Sobin SS, Fung YC, Tremer HM. Collagen and elastin fibers in human pulmonary alveolar walls. *J Appl Physiol* 1988;**64**:1659–75.

4 Mercer RR, Crapo JD. Spatial distribution of collagen and elastin fibers in the lungs. *J Appl Physiol* 1990;**69**:756–65.

5 Weibel ER, Bachofen H. The fiber scaffold of lung parenchyma. In: Crystal RG, West JB, Barnes PJ, Cherniack NA, Weibel ER, eds. *The Lung: Scientific Foundations*. New York: Raven Press, 1991: 787–94.

6 Laurent GJ. Lung collagen: more than scaffolding. *Thorax* 1986;**41**:418–28.

7 Mandl I, Darnule TV, Fierer JA, Keller S, Turino GM. Elastin degradation in human and experimental emphysema. *Adv Exp Med Biol* 1977;**79**:221–31.

8 Barnes PJ. Mediators of chronic obstructive pulmonary disease. *Pharmacol Rev* 2004;**56**:515–48.

9 Christie RV. The elastic properties of the emphysematous lung and their clinical significance. *J Clin Invest* 1934;**13**: 295–321.

10 Stead WW, Fry DL, Ebert RV. The elastic properties of the lung in normal men and in patients with chronic emphysema. *J Lab Clin Med* 1952;**40**:674–81.

11 Mead J, Lindgren I, Gaensler EA. The mechanical properties of the lungs in emphysema. *J Clin Invest* 1955;**34**:1005–16.

12 Cherniack RM. The physical properties of the lung in chronic obstructive pulmonary emphysema. *J Clin Invest* 1956;**35**:394–404.

13 Rahman I. The role of oxidative stress in the pathogenesis of COPD: implications for therapy. *Treat Respir Med* 2005;**4**: 175–200.

14 Rahman I. Oxidative stress in pathogenesis of chronic obstructive pulmonary disease: cellular and molecular mechanisms. *Cell Biochem Biophys* 2005;**43**:167–88.

15 Barnes PJ. Chronic obstructive pulmonary disease. *N Engl J Med* 2000;**343**:269–80.

16 Hogg JC. Role of latent viral infections in chronic obstructive pulmonary disease and asthma. *Am J Respir Crit Care Med* 2001;**164**:S71–5.

17 Anderson GP, Bozinovski S. Acquired somatic mutations in the molecular pathogenesis of COPD. *Trends Pharmacol Sci* 2003;**24**:71–6.

18 Barnes PJ. New concepts in chronic obstructive pulmonary disease. *Annu Rev Med* 2003;**54**:113–29.

19 Barnes PJ, Shapiro SD, Pauwels RA. Chronic obstructive pulmonary disease: molecular and cellular mechanisms. *Eur Respir J* 2003;**22**:672–8.

20 van der Rest M, Garrone R. Collagen family of proteins. *FASEB J* 1991;**5**:2814–23.

21 Exposito JY, Cluzel C, Garrone R, Lethias C. Evolution of collagens. *Anat Rec* 2002;**268**:302–16.

22 Yamada Y, Avvedimento VE, Mudryj M *et al*. The collagen gene: evidence for its evolutionary assembly by amplification of a DNA segment containing an exon of 54 bp. *Cell* 1980; **22**:887–92.

23 Chu M-L, Prockop DJ. Gene structure. In: Royce PM, Steinmann B, eds. *Connective Tissue and Its Heritable Disorders*, 2nd edn. New York: Wiley-Liss, 2002: 223–48.

24 Pace JM, Corrado M, Missero C, Byers PH. Identification, characterization and expression analysis of a new fibrillar collagen gene, COL27A1. *Matrix Biol* 2003;**22**:3–14.

25 Koch M, Schulze J, Hansen U *et al*. A novel marker of tissue junctions, collagen XXII. *J Biol Chem* 2004;**279**:22 514–21.

26 Chou MY, Li HC. Genomic organization and characterization of the human type XXI collagen (COL21A1) gene. *Genomics* 2002;**79**:395–401.

27 Veit G, Kobbe B, Keene DR *et al*. Collagen XXVIII, a novel VWA-domain-containing protein with many imperfections in the collagenous domain. *J Biol Chem* 2006;DOI:10.1074/jbc.M509333200.

28 Poschl E, Pollner R, Kuhn K. The genes for the alpha 1(IV) and alpha 2(IV) chains of human basement membrane collagen type IV are arranged head-to-head and separated by a bidirectional promoter of unique structure. *EMBO J* 1988;**7**:2687–95.

29 Momota R, Sugimoto M, Oohashi T *et al*. Two genes, COL4A3 and COL4A4 coding for the human alpha3(IV) and alpha4(IV) collagen chains are arranged head-to-head on chromosome 2q36. *FEBS Lett* 1998;**424**:11–6.

30 Sugimoto M, Oohashi T, Ninomiya Y. The genes COL4A5 and COL4A6, coding for basement membrane collagen chains alpha 5(IV) and alpha 6(IV), are located head-to-head in close proximity on human chromosome Xq22 and COL4A6 is transcribed from two alternative promoters. *Proc Natl Acad Sci U S A* 1994;**91**:11 679–83.

31 Cutting GR, McGinniss MJ, Kasch LM, Tsipouras P, Antonarakis SE. Physical mapping by PFGE localizes the COL3A1 and COL5A2 genes to a 35-kb region on human chromosome 2. *Genomics* 1990;**8**:407–10.

32 Gerecke DR, Olson PF, Koch M *et al*. Complete primary

structure of two splice variants of collagen XII, and assignment of alpha 1(XII) collagen (COL12A1), alpha 1(IX) collagen (COL9A1), and alpha 1(XIX) collagen (COL19A1) to human chromosome 6q12-q13. *Genomics* 1997;**41**:236–42.

33 Oh SP, Warman ML, Seldin MF *et al.* Cloning of cDNA and genomic DNA encoding human type XVIII collagen and localization of the alpha 1(XVIII) collagen gene to mouse chromosome 10 and human chromosome 21. *Genomics* 1994;**19**:494–9.

34 Ghosh AK. Factors involved in the regulation of type I collagen gene expression: implication in fibrosis. *Exp Biol Med (Maywood)* 2002;**227**:301–14.

35 Rossi P, Karsenty G, Roberts AB *et al.* A nuclear factor 1 binding site mediates the transcriptional activation of a type I collagen promoter by transforming growth factor-beta. *Cell* 1988;**52**:405–14.

36 Ramirez F, Di Liberto M. Complex and diversified regulatory programs control the expression of vertebrate collagen genes. *FASEB J* 1990;**4**:1616–23.

37 Bruggeman LA, Burbelo PD, Yamada Y, Klotman PE. A novel sequence in the type IV collagen promoter binds nuclear proteins from Engelbreth–Holm–Swarm tumor. *Oncogene* 1992;**7**:1497–502.

38 Heikkila P, Soininen R, Tryggvason K. Directional regulatory activity of cis-acting elements in the bidirectional alpha 1(IV) and alpha 2(IV) collagen gene promoter. *J Biol Chem* 1993;**268**:24 677–82.

39 Inagaki Y, Truter S, Ramirez F. Transforming growth factor-beta stimulates alpha 2(I) collagen gene expression through a cis-acting element that contains an Sp1-binding site. *J Biol Chem* 1994;**269**:14 828–34.

40 Karsenty G, Park RW. Regulation of type I collagen genes expression. *Int Rev Immunol* 1995;**12**:177–85.

41 Willimann TE, Maier R, Trueb B. A novel transcription factor and two members of the Sp 1 multigene family regulate the activity of the alpha 2 (VI) collagen promoter. *Matrix Biol* 1995;**14**:653–63.

42 Chung KY, Agarwal A, Uitto J, Mauviel A. An AP-1 binding sequence is essential for regulation of the human alpha2(I) collagen (COL1A2) promoter activity by transforming growth factor-beta. *J Biol Chem* 1996;**271**:3272–8.

43 Mori K, Hatamochi A, Ueki H, Olsen A, Jimenez SA. The transcription of human alpha 1(I) procollagen gene (COL1A1) is suppressed by tumour necrosis factor-alpha through proximal short promoter elements: evidence for suppression mechanisms mediated by two nuclear-factor binding sites. *Biochem J* 1996;**319**:811–6.

44 Higashi K, Kouba DJ, Song YJ, Uitto J, Mauviel A. A proximal element within the human alpha 2(I) collagen (COL1A2) promoter, distinct from the tumor necrosis factor-alpha response element, mediates transcriptional repression by interferon-gamma. *Matrix Biol* 1998;**16**:447–56.

45 Long F, Sonenshein GE, Linsenmayer TF. Multiple transcriptional elements in the avian type X collagen gene: identification of Sp1 family proteins as regulators for high level expression in hypertrophic chondrocytes. *J Biol Chem* 1998;**273**:6542–9.

46 Vindevoghel L, Lechleider RJ, Kon A *et al.* SMAD3/4-dependent transcriptional activation of the human type VII collagen gene (COL7A1) promoter by transforming growth factor beta. *Proc Natl Acad Sci U S A* 1998;**95**:14 769–74.

47 Ritzenthaler JD, Goldstein RH, Fine A *et al.* Transforming-growth-factor-beta activation elements in the distal promoter regions of the rat alpha 1 type I collagen gene. *Biochem J* 1999;**280**:157–62.

48 Chen SJ, Yuan W, Lo S, Trojanowska M, Varga J. Interaction of smad3 with a proximal smad-binding element of the human alpha2(I) procollagen gene promoter required for transcriptional activation by TGF-beta. *J Cell Physiol* 2000;**183**:381–92.

49 Hernandez I, de la Torre P, Rey-Campos J *et al.* Collagen alpha1(I) gene contains an element responsive to tumor necrosis factor-alpha located in the 5' untranslated region of its first exon. *DNA Cell Biol* 2000;**19**:341–52.

50 Norman JT, Lindahl GE, Shakib K *et al.* The Y-box binding protein YB-1 suppresses collagen alpha 1(I) gene transcription via an evolutionarily conserved regulatory element in the proximal promoter. *J Biol Chem* 2001;**276**:29 880–90.

51 Chambers D, Young DA, Howard C *et al.* An enhancer complex confers both high-level and cell-specific expression of the human type X collagen gene. *FEBS Lett* 2002;**531**:505–8.

52 Bridgewater LC, Walker MD, Miller GC *et al.* Adjacent DNA sequences modulate Sox9 transcriptional activation at paired Sox sites in three chondrocyte-specific enhancer elements. *Nucleic Acids Res* 2003;**31**:1541–53.

53 Sakata-Takatani K, Matsuo N, Sumiyoshi H, Tsuda T, Yoshioka H. Identification of a functional CBF-binding CCAAT-like motif in the core promoter of the mouse pro-alpha 1(V) collagen gene (Col5a1). *Matrix Biol* 2004;**23**:87–99.

54 Sakai LY, Keene DR, Morris NP, Burgeson RE. Type VII collagen is a major structural component of anchoring fibrils. *J Cell Biol* 1986;**103**:1577–86.

55 Kapoor R, Sakai LY, Funk S *et al.* Type VIII collagen has a restricted distribution in specialized extracellular matrices. *J Cell Biol* 1988;**107**:721–30.

56 Sage H, Iruela-Arispe ML. Type VIII collagen in murine development: association with capillary formation *in vitro*. *Ann N Y Acad Sci* 1990;**580**:17–31.

57 Ng LJ, Tam PP, Cheah KS. Preferential expression of alternatively spliced mRNAs encoding type II procollagen with a cysteine-rich amino-propeptide in differentiating cartilage and nonchondrogenic tissues during early mouse development. *Dev Biol* 1993;**159**:403–17.

58 Walchli C, Koch M, Chiquet M, Odermatt BF, Trueb B. Tissue-specific expression of the fibril-associated collagens XII and XIV. *J Cell Sci* 1994;**107**:669–81.

59 Miner JH, Sanes JR. Collagen IV alpha 3, alpha 4, and alpha 5 chains in rodent basal laminae: sequence, distribution, association with laminins, and developmental switches. *J Cell Biol* 1994;**127**:879–91.

60 Bohme K, Li Y, Oh PS, Olsen BR. Primary structure of the long and short splice variants of mouse collagen XII and their tissue-specific expression during embryonic development. *Dev Dyn* 1995;**204**:432–45.

61 Niederreither K, D'Souza R, Metsaranta M *et al.* Coordinate patterns of expression of type I and III collagens during mouse development. *Matrix Biol* 1995;**14**:705–13.

62 Lai CH, Chu ML. Tissue distribution and developmental expression of type XVI collagen in the mouse. *Tissue Cell* 1996;**28**:155–64.

63 Marvulli D, Volpin D, Bressan GM. Spatial and temporal changes of type VI collagen expression during mouse development. *Dev Dyn* 1996;**206**:447–54.

64 Pcrala M, Savontaus M, Metsaranta M, Vuorio E. Developmental regulation of mRNA species for types II, IX and XI collagens during mouse embryogenesis. *Biochem J* 1997;**324**:209–16.

65 Sugimoto M, Kimura T, Tsumaki N *et al.* Differential *in situ* expression of alpha2(XI) collagen mRNA isoforms in the developing mouse. *Cell Tissue Res* 1998;**292**:325–32.

66 Saarela J, Rehn M, Oikarinen A, Autio-Harmainen H, Pihlajaniemi T. The short and long forms of type XVIII collagen show clear tissue specificities in their expression and location in basement membrane zones in humans. *Am J Pathol* 1998;**153**:611–26.

67 Aho S, Uitto J. 180-kD bullous pemphigoid antigen/type XVII collagen: tissue-specific expression and molecular interactions with keratin 18. *J Cell Biochem* 1999;**72**:356–67.

68 Sumiyoshi H, Laub F, Yoshioka H, Ramirez F. Embryonic expression of type XIX collagen is transient and confined to muscle cells. *Dev Dyn* 2001;**220**:155–62.

69 Sund M, Vaisanen T, Kaukinen S *et al.* Distinct expression of type XIII collagen in neuronal structures and other tissues during mouse development. *Matrix Biol* 2001;**20**:215–31.

70 Muona A, Eklund L, Vaisanen T, Pihlajaniemi T. Developmentally regulated expression of type XV collagen correlates with abnormalities in Col15a1(–/–) mice. *Matrix Biol* 2002;**21**:89–102.

71 Sato K, Yomogida K, Wada T *et al.* Type XXVI collagen, a new member of the collagen family, is specifically expressed in the testis and ovary. *J Biol Chem* 2002;**277**:37 678–84.

72 Boot-Handford RP, Tuckwell DS, Plumb DA, Rock CF, Poulsom R. A novel and highly conserved collagen (pro(alpha)1(XXVII)) with a unique expression pattern and unusual molecular characteristics establishes a new clade within the vertebrate fibrillar collagen family. *J Biol Chem* 2003;**278**:31 067–77.

73 Koch M, Laub F, Zhou P *et al.* Collagen XXIV, a vertebrate fibrillar collagen with structural features of invertebrate collagens: selective expression in developing cornea and bone. *J Biol Chem* 2003;**278**:43 236–44.

74 Rossi P, de Crombrugghe B. Identification of a cell-specific transcriptional enhancer in the first intron of the mouse alpha 2 (type I) collagen gene. *Proc Natl Acad Sci U S A* 1987;**84**:5590–4.

75 Horton W, Miyashita T, Kohno K, Hassell JR, Yamada Y. Identification of a phenotype-specific enhancer in the first intron of the rat collagen II gene. *Proc Natl Acad Sci U S A* 1987;**84**:8864–8.

76 Killen PD, Burbelo PD, Martin GR, Yamada Y. Characterization of the promoter for the alpha 1 (IV) collagen gene: DNA sequences within the first intron enhance transcription. *J Biol Chem* 1988;**263**:12 310–4.

77 Burbelo PD, Martin GR, Yamada Y. Alpha 1(IV) and alpha 2(IV) collagen genes are regulated by a bidirectional promoter and a shared enhancer. *Proc Natl Acad Sci U S A* 1988;**85**:9679–82.

78 Bennett VD, Adams SL. Identification of a cartilage-specific promoter within intron 2 of the chick alpha 2(I) collagen gene. *J Biol Chem* 1990;**265**:2223–30.

79 Greenspan DS, Lee ST, Lee BS, Hoffman GG. Homology between alpha 2(V) and alpha 1(III) collagen promoters and evidence for negatively acting elements in the alpha 2(V) first intron and 5′ flanking sequences. *Gene Expr* 1991;**1**:29–39.

80 Burbelo PD, Bruggeman LA, Gabriel GC, Klotman PE, Yamada Y. Characterization of a cis-acting element required for efficient transcriptional activation of the collagen IV enhancer. *J Biol Chem* 1991;**266**:22 297–302.

81 Pogulis RJ, Freytag SO. Contribution of specific cis-acting elements to activity of the mouse pro-alpha 2(I) collagen enhancer. *J Biol Chem* 1993;**268**:2493–9.

82 Haniel A, Welge-Lussen U, Kuhn K, Poschl E. Identification and characterization of a novel transcriptional silencer in the human collagen type IV gene COL4A2. *J Biol Chem* 1995;**270**:11 209–15.

83 Krebsbach PH, Nakata K, Bernier SM *et al.* Identification of a minimum enhancer sequence for the type II collagen gene reveals several core sequence motifs in common with the link protein gene. *J Biol Chem* 1996;**271**:4298–303.

84 Bornstein P. Regulation of expression of the alpha 1 (I) collagen gene: a critical appraisal of the role of the first intron. *Matrix Biol* 1996;**15**:3–10.

85 Lefebvre V, Zhou G, Mukhopadhyay K *et al.* An 18-base-pair sequence in the mouse proalpha1(II) collagen gene is sufficient for expression in cartilage and binds nuclear proteins that are selectively expressed in chondrocytes. *Mol Cell Biol* 1996;**16**:4512–23.

86 Bell DM, Leung KK, Wheatley SC *et al.* SOX9 directly regulates the type-II collagen gene. *Nat Genet* 1997;**16**:174–8.

87 Zhang Y, Niu Z, Cohen AJ, Nah HD, Adams SL. The chick type III collagen gene contains two promoters that are preferentially expressed in different cell types and are separated by over 20 kb of DNA containing 23 exons. *Nucleic Acids Res* 1997;**25**:2470–7.

88 Beier F, Vornehm S, Poschl E, von der Mark K, Lammi MJ. Localization of silencer and enhancer elements in the human type X collagen gene. *J Cell Biochem* 1997;**66**:210–8.

89 Hormuzdi SG, Penttinen R, Jaenisch R, Bornstein P. A gene-targeting approach identifies a function for the first intron in expression of the alpha1(I) collagen gene. *Mol Cell Biol* 1998;**18**:3368–75.

90 Leung KK, Ng LJ, Ho KK, Tam PP, Cheah KS. Different cis-regulatory DNA elements mediate developmental stage- and tissue-specific expression of the human COL2A1 gene in transgenic mice. *J Cell Biol* 1998;**141**:1291–300.

91 Zhang Y, Niu Z, Cohen AJ, Adams SL. The internal chondrocyte-specific promoter of the chick type III collagen gene is

activated by AP1 and is repressed in fibroblasts by a complex containing an LBP1-related protein. *Nucleic Acids Res* 1999; **27**:4090–9.

92 Hirata H, Yamamura I, Yasuda K *et al*. Separate cis-acting DNA elements control cell type- and tissue-specific expression of collagen binding molecular chaperone HSP47. *J Biol Chem* 1999;**274**:35 703–10.

93 Liu Y, Li H, Tanaka K, Tsumaki N, Yamada Y. Identification of an enhancer sequence within the first intron required for cartilage-specific transcription of the alpha2(XI) collagen gene. *J Biol Chem* 2000;**275**:12 712–8.

94 Tanaka K, Matsumoto Y, Nakatani F, Iwamoto Y, Yamada Y. A zinc finger transcription factor, alphaA-crystallin binding protein 1, is a negative regulator of the chondrocyte-specific enhancer of the alpha1(II) collagen gene. *Mol Cell Biol* 2000;**20**:4428–35.

95 Ghayor C, Herrouin JF, Chadjichristos C *et al*. Regulation of human COL2A1 gene expression in chondrocytes. Identification of C-Krox-responsive elements and modulation by phenotype alteration. *J Biol Chem* 2000;**275**:27 421–38.

96 Jenkins E, Moss JB, Pace JM, Bridgewater LC. The new collagen gene COL27A1 contains SOX9-responsive enhancer elements. *Matrix Biol* 2005;**24**:177–84.

97 Antoniv TT, Tanaka S, Sudan B *et al*. Identification of a repressor in the first intron of the human alpha2(I) collagen gene (COL1A2). *J Biol Chem* 2005;**280**:35 417–23.

98 Rippe RA, Umezawa A, Kimball JP, Breindl M, Brenner DA. Binding of upstream stimulatory factor to an E-box in the 3′-flanking region stimulates alpha1(I) collagen gene transcription. *J Biol Chem* 1997;**272**:1753–60.

99 Parker MI, Judge K, Gevers W. Loss of type I procollagen gene expression in SV40-transformed human fibroblasts is accompanied by hypermethylation of these genes. *Nucleic Acids Res* 1982;**10**:5879–91.

100 Fernandez MP, Young MF, Sobel ME. Methylation of type II and type I collagen genes in differentiated and dedifferentiated chondrocytes. *J Biol Chem* 1985;**260**:2374–8.

101 Rhodes K, Breindl M. Developmental changes in the methylation status of regulatory elements in the murine alpha 1(I) collagen gene. *Gene Expr* 1992;**2**:59–69.

102 Takatsu M, Uyeno S, Komura J, Watanabe M, Ono T. Age-dependent alterations in mRNA level and promoter methylation of collagen alpha1(I) gene in human periodontal ligament. *Mech Ageing Dev* 1999;**110**:37–48.

103 Vindevoghel L, Kon A, Lechleider RJ *et al*. Smad-dependent transcriptional activation of human type VII collagen gene (COL7A1) promoter by transforming growth factor-beta. *J Biol Chem* 1998;**273**:13 053–7.

104 Chen SJ, Yuan W, Mori Y *et al*. Stimulation of type I collagen transcription in human skin fibroblasts by TGF-beta: involvement of Smad 3. *J Invest Dermatol* 1999;**112**:49–57.

105 Kon A, Vindevoghel L, Kouba DJ *et al*. Cooperation between SMAD and NF-kB in growth factor regulated type VII collagen gene expression. *Oncogene* 1999;**18**:1837–44.

106 Kouba DJ, Chung KY, Nishiyama T *et al*. Nuclear factor-kappa B mediates TNF-alpha inhibitory effect on alpha 2(I) collagen (COL1A2) gene transcription in human dermal fibroblasts. *J Immunol* 1999;**162**:4226–34.

107 Abe H, Matsubara T, Iehara N *et al*. Type IV collagen is transcriptionally regulated by Smad1 under advanced glycation end product (AGE) stimulation. *J Biol Chem* 1999;**279**: 14 201–6.

108 Greenwel P, Tanaka S, Penkov D *et al*. Tumor necrosis factor alpha inhibits type I collagen synthesis through repressive CCAAT/enhancer-binding proteins. *Mol Cell Biol* 2000;**20**: 912–8.

109 Iraburu MJ, Dominguez-Rosales JA, Fontana L *et al*. Tumor necrosis factor alpha down-regulates expression of the alpha1(I) collagen gene in rat hepatic stellate cells through a p20C/EBPbeta- and C/EBPdelta-dependent mechanism. *Hepatology* 2000;**31**:1086–93.

110 Zhang W, Ou J, Inagaki Y, Greenwel P, Ramirez F. Synergistic cooperation between Sp1 and Smad3/Smad4 mediates transforming growth factor beta1 stimulation of alpha 2(I)-collagen (COL1A2) transcription. *J Biol Chem* 2000;**275**:39 237–45.

111 Chadjichristos C, Ghayor C, Herrouin JF *et al*. Down-regulation of human type II collagen gene expression by transforming growth factor-beta 1 (TGF-beta 1) in articular chondrocytes involves SP3/SP1 ratio. *J Biol Chem* 2002;**277**: 43 903–17.

112 Naso M, Uitto J, Klement JF. Transcriptional control of the mouse Col7a1 gene in keratinocytes: basal and transforming growth factor-beta regulated expression. *J Invest Dermatol* 2003;**121**:1469–78.

113 Stefanovic B, Brenner DA. 5′ stem-loop of collagen alpha 1(I) mRNA inhibits translation *in vitro* but is required for triple helical collagen synthesis *in vivo*. *J Biol Chem* 2003; **278**:927–33.

114 Stefanovic B, Hellerbrand C, Brenner DA. Regulatory role of the conserved stem-loop structure at the 5′ end of collagen alpha1(I) mRNA. *Mol Cell Biol* 1999;**19**:4334–42.

115 Stefanovic B, Lindquist J, Brenner DA. The 5′ stem-loop regulates expression of collagen alpha1(I) mRNA in mouse fibroblasts cultured in a three-dimensional matrix. *Nucleic Acids Res* 2000;**28**:641–7.

116 Stefanovic B, Hellerbrand C, Holcik M *et al*. Posttranscriptional regulation of collagen alpha1(I) mRNA in hepatic stellate cells. *Mol Cell Biol* 1997;**17**:5201–9.

117 Lindquist JN, Parsons CJ, Stefanovic B, Brenner DA. Regulation of alpha1(I) collagen messenger RNA decay by interactions with alphaCP at the 3′-untranslated region. *J Biol Chem* 2004;**279**:23 822–9.

118 Berg RA, Prockop DJ. The thermal transition of a non-hydroxylated form of collagen: evidence for a role for hydroxyproline in stabilizing the triple-helix of collagen. *Biochem Biophys Res Commun* 1973;**52**:115–20.

119 Notbohm H, Mosler S, Bodo M *et al*. Comparative study on the thermostability of collagen I of skin and bone: influence of posttranslational hydroxylation of prolyl and lysyl residues. *J Protein Chem* 1992;**11**:635–43.

120 Burjanadze TV, Veis A. A thermodynamic analysis of the contribution of hydroxyproline to the structural stability of the collagen triple helix. *Connect Tissue Res* 1997;**36**:347–65.

121 Jenkins CL, Raines RT. Insights on the conformational stability of collagen. *Nat Prod Rep* 2002;**19**:49–59.

122 Bann JG, Peyton DH, Bachinger HP. Sweet is stable: glycosylation stabilizes collagen. *FEBS Lett* 2000;**473**:237–40.

123 Heikkinen J, Risteli M, Wang C *et al.* Lysyl hydroxylase 3 is a multifunctional protein possessing collagen glucosyltransferase activity. *J Biol Chem* 2000;**275**:36 158–63.

124 Rautavuoma K, Takaluoma K, Passoja K *et al.* Characterization of three fragments that constitute the monomers of the human lysyl hydroxylase isoenzymes 1-3. The 30-kDa N-terminal fragment is not required for lysyl hydroxylase activity. *J Biol Chem* 2002;**277**:23 084 91.

125 Rautavuoma K, Takaluoma K, Sormunen R *et al.* Premature aggregation of type IV collagen and early lethality in lysyl hydroxylase 3 null mice. *Proc Natl Acad Sci U S A* 2004; **101**:14 120–5.

126 Clark CC, Kefalides NA. Carbohydrate moieties of procollagen: incorporation of isotopically labeled mannose and glucosamine into propeptides of procollagen secreted by matrix-free chick embryo tendon cells. *Proc Natl Acad Sci U S A* 1976;**73**:34–8.

127 Olsen BR, Guzman NA, Engel J, Condit C, Aase S. Purification and characterization of a peptide from the carboxy-terminal region of chick tendon procollagen type I. *Biochemistry* 1977;**16**:3030–6.

128 Clark CC. The distribution and initial characterization of oligosaccharide units on the COOH-terminal propeptide extensions of the pro-alpha 1 and pro-alpha 2 chains of type I procollagen. *J Biol Chem* 1979;**254**:10 798–802.

129 Nayak BR, Spiro RG. Localization and structure of the asparagine-linked oligosaccharides of type IV collagen from glomerular basement membrane and lens capsule. *J Biol Chem* 1991;**266**:13 978–87.

130 Fujiwara S, Shinkai H, Timpl R. Structure of N-linked oligosaccharide chains in the triple-helical domains of human type VI and mouse type IV collagen. *Matrix* 1991; **11**:307–12.

131 Lamande SR, Bateman JF. The type I collagen pro alpha 1(I) COOH-terminal propeptide N-linked oligosaccharide: functional analysis by site-directed mutagenesis. *J Biol Chem* 1995;**270**:17 858–65.

132 McLaughlin SH, Bulleid NJ. Molecular recognition in procollagen chain assembly. *Matrix Biol* 1998;**16**:369–77.

133 Soder S, Poschl E. The NC1 domain of human collagen IV is necessary to initiate triple helix formation. *Biochem Biophys Res Commun* 2004;**325**:276–80.

134 Koivu J, Myllyla R. Interchain disulfide bond formation in types I and II procollagen: evidence for a protein disulfide isomerase catalyzing bond formation. *J Biol Chem* 1987;**262**: 6159–64.

135 Gerard S, Puett D, Mitchell WM. Kinetics of collagen fold formation in human type I procollagen and the effect of disulfide bonds. *Biochemistry* 1981;**20**:1857–65.

136 Koivu J, Myllyla R, Helaakoski T *et al.* A single polypeptide acts both as the beta subunit of prolyl 4-hydroxylase and as a protein disulfide-isomerase. *J Biol Chem* 1987;**262**:6447–9.

137 Pihlajaniemi T, Helaakoski T, Tasanen K *et al.* Molecular cloning of the beta-subunit of human prolyl 4-hydroxylase. This subunit and protein disulphide isomerase are products of the same gene. *EMBO J* 1987;**6**:643–9.

138 Wilson R, Lees JF, Bulleid NJ. Protein disulfide isomerase acts as a molecular chaperone during the assembly of procollagen. *J Biol Chem* 1998;**273**:9637–43.

139 Kellokumpu S, Suokas M, Risteli L, Myllyla R. Protein disulfide isomerase and newly synthesized procollagen chains form higher-order structures in the lumen of the endoplasmic reticulum. *J Biol Chem* 1997;**272**:2770–7.

140 Bottomley MJ, Batten MR, Lumb RA, Bulleid NJ. Quality control in the endoplasmic reticulum: PDI mediates the ER retention of unassembled procollagen C-propeptides. *Curr Biol* 2001;**11**:1114–8.

141 Bachinger HP, Bruckner P, Timpl R, Prockop DJ, Engel J. Folding mechanism of the triple helix in type-III collagen and type-III pN-collagen: role of disulfide bridges and peptide bond isomerization. *Eur J Biochem* 1980;**106**:619–32.

142 Dolz R, Engel J, Kuhn K. Folding of collagen IV. *Eur J Biochem* 1988;**178**:357–66.

143 Snellman A, Tu H, Vaisanen T *et al.* A short sequence in the N-terminal region is required for the trimerization of type XIII collagen and is conserved in other collagenous transmembrane proteins. *EMBO J* 2000;**19**:5051–9.

144 Areida SK, Reinhardt DP, Muller PK *et al.* Properties of the collagen type XVII ectodomain: evidence for n- to c-terminal triple helix folding. *J Biol Chem* 2001;**276**:1594–601.

145 Bachinger HP, Bruckner P, Timpl R, Engel J. The role of cis-trans isomerization of peptide bonds in the coil leads to and comes from triple helix conversion of collagen. *Eur J Biochem* 1978;**90**:605–13.

146 Bruckner P, Eikenberry EF. Formation of the triple helix of type I procollagen in cellulo: temperature-dependent kinetics support a model based on cis in equilibrium trans isomerization of peptide bonds. *Eur J Biochem* 1984;**140**:391–5.

147 Davis JM, Boswell BA, Bachinger HP. Thermal stability and folding of type IV procollagen and effect of peptidyl-prolyl cis-trans-isomerase on the folding of the triple helix. *J Biol Chem* 1989;**264**:8956–62.

148 Canty EG, Kadler KE. Procollagen trafficking, processing and fibrillogenesis. *J Cell Sci* 2005;**118**:1341–53.

149 Nagata K. Expression and function of heat shock protein 47: a collagen-specific molecular chaperone in the endoplasmic reticulum. *Matrix Biol* 1998;**16**:379–86.

150 Nagata K. HSP47 as a collagen-specific molecular chaperone: function and expression in normal mouse development. *Semin Cell Dev Biol* 2003;**14**:275–82.

151 Koide T, Asada S, Nagata K. Substrate recognition of collagen-specific molecular chaperone HSP47: structural requirements and binding regulation. *J Biol Chem* 1999;**274**:34 523–6.

152 Koide T, Aso A, Yorihuzi T, Nagata K. Conformational requirements of collagenous peptides for recognition by the chaperone protein HSP47. *J Biol Chem* 2000;**275**:27 957–63.

153 Koide T, Takahara Y, Asada S, Nagata K. Xaa-Arg-Gly triplets in the collagen triple helix are dominant binding sites for the molecular chaperone HSP47. *J Biol Chem* 2002;**277**: 6178–82.

154 Tasab M, Jenkinson L, Bulleid NJ. Sequence-specific recognition of collagen triple helices by the collagen-specific molecular chaperone HSP47. *J Biol Chem* 2002;**277**:35 007–12.

155 Tasab M, Batten MR, Bulleid NJ. Hsp47: a molecular chaperone that interacts with and stabilizes correctly folded procollagen. *EMBO J* 2000;**19**:2204–11.

156 Macdonald JR, Bachinger HP. HSP47 binds cooperatively to triple helical type I collagen but has little effect on the thermal stability or rate of refolding. *J Biol Chem* 2001; **276**:25 399–403.

157 Nagai N, Hosokawa M, Itohara S *et al.* Embryonic lethality of molecular chaperone hsp47 knockout mice is associated with defects in collagen biosynthesis. *J Cell Biol* 2000;**150**: 1499–506.

158 Bonfanti L, Mironov AA Jr, Martinez-Menarguez JA *et al.* Procollagen traverses the Golgi stack without leaving the lumen of cisternae: evidence for cisternal maturation. *Cell* 1998;**95**:993–1003.

159 Kadler KE, Holmes DF, Trotter JA, Chapman JA. Collagen fibril formation. *Biochem J* 1996;**316**:1–11.

160 Kadler KE, Holmes DF, Graham H, Starborg T. Tip-mediated fusion involving unipolar collagen fibrils accounts for rapid fibril elongation, the occurrence of fibrillar branched networks in skin and the paucity of collagen fibril ends in vertebrates. *Matrix Biol* 2000;**19**:359–65.

161 Birk DE. Type V collagen: heterotypic type I/V collagen interactions in the regulation of fibril assembly. *Micron* 2001;**32**:223–37.

162 Hulmes DJ. Building collagen molecules, fibrils, and suprafibrillar structures. *J Struct Biol* 2002;**137**:2–10.

163 Kadler K. Matrix loading: assembly of extracellular matrix collagen fibrils during embryogenesis. *Birth Defects Res Part C Embryo Today* 2004;**72**:1–11.

164 Miyahara M, Njieha FK, Prockop DJ. Formation of collagen fibrils *in vitro* by cleavage of procollagen with procollagen proteinases. *J Biol Chem* 1982;**257**:8442–8.

165 Miyahara M, Hayashi K, Berger J *et al.* Formation of collagen fibrils by enzymic cleavage of precursors of type I collagen *in vitro*. *J Biol Chem* 1984;**259**:9891–8.

166 Kadler KE, Hojima Y, Prockop DJ. Assembly of collagen fibrils *de novo* by cleavage of the type I pC-collagen with procollagen C-proteinase: assay of critical concentration demonstrates that collagen self-assembly is a classical example of an entropy-driven process. *J Biol Chem* 1987; **262**:15 696–701.

167 Shaw LM, Olsen BR. FACIT collagens: diverse molecular bridges in extracellular matrices. *Trends Biochem Sci* 1991; **16**:191–4.

168 Knupp C, Squire JM. Molecular packing in network-forming collagens. *Adv Protein Chem* 2005;**70**:375–403.

169 Burgeson RE. Type VII collagen, anchoring fibrils, and epidermolysis bullosa. *J Invest Dermatol* 1993;**101**:252–5.

170 Baldock C, Sherratt MJ, Shuttleworth CA, Kielty CM. The supramolecular organization of collagen VI microfibrils. *J Mol Biol* 2003;**330**:297–307.

171 Franzke CW, Bruckner P, Bruckner-Tuderman L. Collagenous transmembrane proteins: recent insights into biology and pathology. *J Biol Chem* 2005;**280**:4005–8.

172 Pierce JA, Hocott JB. Studies on the collagen and elastin content of the human lung. *J Clin Invest* 1960;**39**:8–14.

173 West JB, Mathieu-Costello O. Structure, strength, failure, and remodeling of the pulmonary blood–gas barrier. *Annu Rev Physiol* 1999;**61**:543–72.

174 Kielty CM, Sherratt MJ, Shuttleworth CA. Elastic fibres. *J Cell Sci* 2002;**115**:2817–28.

175 Shapiro SD, Endicott SK, Province MA, Pierce JA, Campbell EJ. Marked longevity of human lung parenchymal elastic fibers deduced from prevalence of D-aspartate and nuclear weapons-related radiocarbon. *J Clin Invest* 1991;**87**:1828–34.

176 Mithieux SM, Weiss AS. Elastin. *Adv Protein Chem* 2005; **70**:437–61.

177 Li B, Daggett V. Molecular basis for the extensibility of elastin. *J Muscle Res Cell Motil* 2002;**23**:561–73.

178 Sage H. The evolution of elastin: correlation of functional properties with protein structure and phylogenetic distribution. *Comp Biochem Physiol B* 1983;**74**:373–80.

179 Vrhovski B, Weiss AS. Biochemistry of tropoelastin. *Eur J Biochem* 1998;**258**:1–18.

180 Fazio MJ, Mattei MG, Passage E *et al.* Human elastin gene: new evidence for localization to the long arm of chromosome 7. *Am J Hum Genet* 1991;**48**:696–703.

181 Foster K, Ferrell R, King-Underwood L *et al.* Description of a dinucleotide repeat polymorphism in the human elastin gene and its use to confirm assignment of the gene to chromosome 7. *Ann Hum Genet* 1993;**57**:87–96.

182 Bashir MM, Indik Z, Yeh H *et al.* Characterization of the complete human elastin gene: delineation of unusual features in the 5'-flanking region. *J Biol Chem* 1989;**264**: 8887–91.

183 Tassabehji M, Metcalfe K, Donnai D *et al.* Elastin: genomic structure and point mutations in patients with supravalvular aortic stenosis. *Hum Mol Genet* 1997;**6**:1029–36.

184 Yeh H, Anderson N, Ornstein-Goldstein N *et al.* Structure of the bovine elastin gene and S1 nuclease analysis of alternative splicing of elastin mRNA in the bovine nuchal ligament. *Biochemistry* 1989;**28**:2365–70.

185 Rosenbloom J, Bashir M, Yeh H *et al.* Regulation of elastin gene expression. *Ann N Y Acad Sci* 1991;**624**:116–36.

186 Kahari VM, Fazio MJ, Chen YQ *et al.* Deletion analyses of 5'-flanking region of the human elastin gene: delineation of functional promoter and regulatory cis-elements. *J Biol Chem* 1990;**265**:9485–90.

187 Swee MH, Parks WC, Pierce RA. Developmental regulation of elastin production: expression of tropoelastin pre-mRNA persists after down-regulation of steady-state mRNA levels. *J Biol Chem* 1995;**270**:14 899–906.

188 Parks WC. Posttranscriptional regulation of lung elastin production. *Am J Respir Cell Mol Biol* 1997;**17**:1–2.

189 Rosenbloom J, Cywinski A. Inhibition of proline hydroxylation does not inhibit secretion of tropoelastin by chick aorta cells. *FEBS Lett* 1976;**65**:246–50.

190 Davis EC, Broekelmann TJ, Ozawa Y, Mecham RP. Identification of tropoelastin as a ligand for the 65-kD FK506-binding protein, FKBP65, in the secretory pathway. *J Cell Biol* 1998;**140**:295–303.

191 Hinek A, Rabinovitch M. 67-kD elastin-binding protein is a protective 'companion' of extracellular insoluble elastin and intracellular tropoelastin. *J Cell Biol* 1994;**126**:563–74.

192 Kozel BA, Rongish BJ, Czirok A *et al*. Elastic fiber formation: a dynamic view of extracellular matrix assembly using timer reporters. *J Cell Physiol* 2006;DOI:10.1002/jcp.20546.

193 Kozel BA, Wachi H, Davis EC, Mecham RP. Domains in tropoelastin that mediate elastin deposition *in vitro* and *in vivo*. *J Biol Chem* 2003;**278**:18 491–8.

194 Bedell-Hogan D, Trackman P, Abrams W, Rosenbloom J, Kagan H. Oxidation, cross-linking, and insolubilization of recombinant tropoelastin by purified lysyl oxidase. *J Biol Chem* 1993;**268**:10 345–50.

195 Thomassin L, Werneck CC, Broekelmann TJ *et al*. The Proregions of lysyl oxidase and lysyl oxidase-like 1 are required for deposition onto elastic fibers. *J Biol Chem* 2005; **280**:42 848–55.

196 Rock MJ, Cain SA, Freeman LJ *et al*. Molecular basis of elastic fiber formation: critical interactions and a tropoelastin-fibrillin-1 cross-link. *J Biol Chem* 2004;**279**:23 748–58.

197 Yanagisawa H, Davis EC, Starcher BC *et al*. Fibulin-5 is an elastin-binding protein essential for elastic fibre development *in vivo*. *Nature* 2002;**415**:168–71.

198 Nakamura T, Lozano PR, Ikeda Y *et al*. Fibulin-5/DANCE is essential for elastogenesis *in vivo*. *Nature* 2002;**415**:171–5.

199 Kelleher CM, Silverman EK, Broekelmann T *et al*. A functional mutation in the terminal exon of elastin in severe, early-onset chronic obstructive pulmonary disease. *Am J Respir Cell Mol Biol* 2005;**33**:355–62.

200 Iozzo RV. Matrix proteoglycans: from molecular design to cellular function. *Annu Rev Biochem* 1998;**67**:609–52.

201 Bensadoun ES, Burke AK, Hogg JC, Roberts CR. Proteoglycan deposition in pulmonary fibrosis. *Am J Respir Crit Care Med* 1996;**154**:1819–28.

202 Belknap JK, Weiser-Evans MC, Grieshaber SS, Majack RA, Stenmark KR. Relationship between perlecan and tropoelastin gene expression and cell replication in the developing rat pulmonary vasculature. *Am J Respir Cell Mol Biol* 1999;**20**:24–34.

203 Groffen AJ, Buskens CA, van Kuppevelt TH *et al*. Primary structure and high expression of human agrin in basement membranes of adult lung and kidney. *Eur J Biochem* 1998;**254**:123–8.

204 Verbeek MM, Otte-Holler I, van den Born J *et al*. Agrin is a major heparan sulfate proteoglycan accumulating in Alzheimer's disease brain. *Am J Pathol* 1999;**155**:2115–25.

205 van Straaten JF, Coers W, Noordhoek JA *et al*. Proteoglycan changes in the extracellular matrix of lung tissue from patients with pulmonary emphysema. *Mod Pathol* 1999;**12**: 697–705.

206 Chakravarti S, Magnuson T, Lass JH *et al*. Lumican regulates collagen fibril assembly: skin fragility and corneal opacity in the absence of lumican. *J Cell Biol* 1998;**141**:1277–86.

207 Svensson L, Aszodi A, Reinholt FP *et al*. Fibromodulin-null mice have abnormal collagen fibrils, tissue organization, and altered lumican deposition in tendon. *J Biol Chem* 1999;**274**: 9636–48.

208 Pare OD, Roberts CR, Bai TR, Wiggs BJ. The functional consequences of airway remodeling in asthma. *Monaldi Arch Chest Dis* 1997;**52**:589–96.

209 Laurell C-B, Eriksson S. The electrophoretic a_1-globulin pattern of serum in a_1-antitrypsin deficiency. *Scand J Clin Lab Invest* 1963;**15**:132–40.

210 Eriksson S. Pulmonary emphysema and alpha$_1$-antitrypsin deficiency. *Acta Med Scand* 1964;**175**:197–205.

211 Ohbayashi H. Neutrophil elastase inhibitors as treatment for COPD. *Expert Opin Investig Drugs* 2002;**11**:965–80.

212 Shapiro SD. Proteinases in chronic obstructive pulmonary disease. *Biochem Soc Trans* 2001;**30**:98–102.

213 Hautamaki RD, Kobayashi DK, Senior RM, Shapiro SD. Requirement for macrophage elastase for cigarette smoke-induced emphysema in mice. *Science* 1997;**277**:2002–4.

214 Zheng T, Zhu Z, Wang Z *et al*. Inducible targeting of IL-13 to the adult lung causes matrix metalloproteinase- and cathepsin-dependent emphysema. *J Clin Invest* 2000;**106**:1081–93.

215 Mahadeva R, Shapiro SD. Chronic obstructive pulmonary disease 3: Experimental animal models of pulmonary emphysema. *Thorax* 2002;**57**:908–14.

216 Leco KJ, Waterhouse P, Sanchez OH *et al*. Spontaneous air space enlargement in the lungs of mice lacking tissue inhibitor of metalloproteinases-3 (TIMP-3). *J Clin Invest* 2001;**108**:817–29.

217 Wert SE, Yoshida M, LeVine AM *et al*. Increased metalloproteinase activity, oxidant production, and emphysema in surfactant protein D gene-inactivated mice. *Proc Natl Acad Sci U S A* 2000;**97**:5972–7.

218 Morris DG, Huang X, Kaminski N *et al*. Loss of integrin alpha(v)beta6-mediated TGF-beta activation causes Mmp12-dependent emphysema. *Nature* 2003;**422**:169–73.

219 Kasahara Y, Tuder RM, Taraseviciene-Stewart L *et al*. Inhibition of VEGF receptors causes lung cell apoptosis and emphysema. *J Clin Invest* 2000;**106**:1311–9.

220 Aoshiba K, Yokohori N, Nagai A. Alveolar wall apoptosis causes lung destruction and emphysematous changes. *Am J Respir Cell Mol Biol* 2003;**28**:555–62.

221 Massaro GD, Massaro D. Retinoic acid treatment abrogates elastase-induced pulmonary emphysema in rats. *Nat Med* 1997;**3**:675–7.

222 Ali NN, Edgar AJ, Samadikuchaksaraei A *et al*. Derivation of type II alveolar epithelial cells from murine embryonic stem cells. *Tissue Eng* 2002;**8**:541–50.

223 Krause DS, Theise ND, Collector MI *et al*. Multi-organ, multi-lineage engraftment by a single bone marrow-derived stem cell. *Cell* 2001;**105**:369–77.

224 Kotton DN, Ma BY, Cardoso WV *et al*. Bone marrow-derived cells as progenitors of lung alveolar epithelium. *Development* 2001;**128**:5181–8.

225 Dunsmore SE, Chambers RC, Laurent GJ. Matrix proteins. In: Gibson GJ, Geddes DM, Costabel U, Sterk PJ, Corrin B (eds). *Respiratory Medicine*, 3rd edn. New York: Elsevier, 2003: 83.

226 Dunsmore SE. Collagens. In: Laurent G., Shapiro S., eds. *Encyclopedia of Respiratory Medicine*. New York: Elsevier, 2006: 173.

SECTION 5
Clinical considerations and complications

CHAPTER 41
Aerosols and delivery systems

Stephen P. Newman

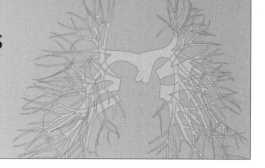

The inhaled drug delivery route is recognized as having a number of advantages over oral and parenteral routes, and these are highly relevant for drug delivery in patients with COPD. These advantages derive from the drug being delivered directly to the site in the body where it is required: the airways of the lungs [1]. Because the drug is targeted direct to the lungs, without having to undergo hepatic first-pass metabolism, it is possible to use a lower dose of inhaled bronchodilator than would be required by the oral route. The onset of drug action is generally relatively rapid, and the incidence of side-effects relatively low.

When drugs are given by inhalation, whether for therapeutic purposes, for bronchial provocation testing or for medical diagnosis, they are delivered as aerosols [2–4]. An aerosol is defined as a stable dispersion or suspension of solid particles or liquid droplets in a gaseous medium [5]. Aerosols vary in size from very small particles such as those in tobacco smoke (sometimes less than 0.1 μm diameter) to fog droplets and pollens exceeding 50 μm diameter, but those aerosols used in the treatment and diagnosis of pulmonary diseases are generally confined to the 0.5–10.0 μm size range.

Aerosol properties

Particle size distributions

Particle or droplet size is the single most important aerosol characteristic, because it is key to determining how much aerosol can enter the patient's lungs, and where within the lungs deposition takes place [6,7]. Two additional properties are also important: density and shape. A particle or droplet with greater than unit density behaves aerodynamically as though it is larger than its physical size, while a particle or droplet with less than unit density behaves aerodynamically as though it is smaller than its physical size [8].

Aerosol particles are seldom perfect spheres; for instance, drug particles delivered from inhaler devices are often micronized crystals of highly irregular shape.

Density and shape are taken into account by defining an aerodynamic diameter (D_a) as

$$D_a = D_p \times \sqrt{\rho},$$

where D_a is the diameter of a spherical unit density (1 g/cm^3) particle or droplet, having the same settling velocity in air as the particle or droplet in question; D_p is the physical diameter of the particle or droplet; and ρ is the specific gravity, i.e. its density relative to that of water.

Aerosol particle or droplet distributions may be termed either monodisperse or heterodisperse. In a monodisperse aerosol, all the particles or droplets are approximately the same size, while in a heterodisperse aerosol, the particles or droplets cover a spectrum of sizes [9]. Virtually all aerosols delivered for the purposes of medical treatment or diagnosis are heterodisperse in character. When considering heterodisperse size distributions, it is important to recognize that the size distribution by number and the size distribution by mass are very different, and that the latter will be more important. Relatively little drug mass is carried by a large number of small particles; for instance, 1000 1-μm particles carry the same amount of drug as a single 10-μm particle.

The particle size spectra of medical aerosols are generally complex, but can often be approximated as log-normal distributions [9]. If the size distribution is plotted cumulatively, then two commonly used parameters may be determined:
1 the mass median aerodynamic diameter (MMAD), which is the size distribution such that half the aerosol mass is contained in smaller droplets and half in larger droplets; and
2 the geometric standard deviation (GSD).
The GSD is dimensionless, one definition being as the ratio of the 84% point on the cumulative distribution to the 50% point (Fig. 41.1). In practice, medical aerosols often have GSDs in the region of 2–3, while a size distribution that is

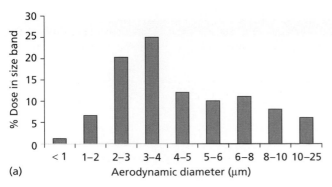
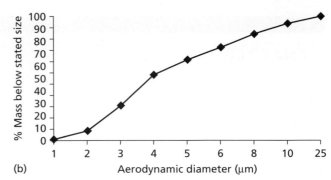

Figure 41.1 Particle size spectrum of a heterodisperse aerosol. (a) Percentage of drug mass plotted versus aerodynamic diameter; and (b) cumulative plot showing percentage of drug mass contained in particles smaller than the stated size. From the cumulative plot, it is possible to determine mass median aerodynamic diameter (MMAD) as the 50% point (3.9 μm), and geometric standard deviation (GSD) as the ratio of 84% to 50% points (7.8 : 3.9 μm, i.e. 2.0).

'acceptably' monodisperse has a GSD less than 1.22 [10]. Monodisperse aerosols can be produced by devices such as the spinning disc generator or condensation aerosol generator [11]. While MMAD is a useful measure of the 'average' particle size, its relevance probably diminishes as the GSD increases [12].

Measuring particle size

The regulatory authorities place great importance upon the particle size distributions of aerosols delivered from inhaler devices, and companies developing new inhaled drug products devote much time and effort to these measurements. Most particle size data are obtained from cascade impactors such as the Andersen Sampler and Multistage Liquid Impinger, in which aerosol particles are collected on a series of stages, according to their aerodynamic sizes [13,14]. In these devices, each stage may be washed with a suitable solvent, so that the mass of drug associated with each size band may be quantified by an appropriate analytical method. The use of simulated breathing patterns [15], or the use of inlets based on models of the human upper airways [16], may improve the precision of impactor measurements. Various optical methods, generally using laser light, may also be used to determine aerosol size distributions [13,17]. While these optical methods may be quick and simple, they measure aerosol particles and droplets irrespective of whether they contain drug, and hence cannot distinguish between drug and carrier particles, or between droplets containing drug and those only containing diluent.

Effects of humidity

Aerosol particles and droplets may be influenced by hygroscopic effects [18]. Some drug and carrier materials are highly water-soluble, and when particles enter the humid environment of the lungs they may absorb moisture and grow rapidly in size [19]. These effects are not confined to solid particles. Liquid aerosols comprising hypertonic droplets may absorb water in the lungs and increase in size, in order to bring the droplets to the same tonicity as the respiratory tract, while hypotonic droplets may shed water and hence reduce in size [20].

Deposition mechanisms

Deposition of aerosols in the human respiratory tract takes place by three main mechanisms: (i) inertial impaction; (ii) gravitational sedimentation; and (iii) Brownian diffusion.

Inertial impaction

Inertial impaction occurs in the upper airways (mouth and pharynx), and at the bifurcations between the larger, more central, airways in the lungs [6]. This process may occur when the airway changes direction; if the aerosol particle has too much inertia, then it may be unable to follow the air-stream and may strike the airway wall where it becomes deposited. The probability of inertial impaction is proportional to the product of $D_a^2 \times Q$, where D_a is the aerodynamic diameter and Q is the linear velocity of air. The product $D_a^2 \times Q$ is sometimes termed the 'impaction parameter' [6]. Experimental studies show upper airway deposition increases in proportion to this parameter [21].

Within the lungs, inertial impaction is confined mostly to the large central airways, because the total airway cross-section increases rapidly after the first few airway generations [22]. Hence, the linear velocity of air (Q in the impaction parameter) is much lower in the more peripheral airways of the lungs. Impaction can occur both during inhalation and exhalation. The effects of impaction may be augmented by the creation of turbulent airflows within the airways; for instance, the passage of air through the larynx creates turbulence and an unstable airflow, which may enhance deposition within the trachea [23].

Gravitational sedimentation

Gravitational sedimentation takes place in the small airways and alveoli, when aerosol particles or droplets fall under gravity onto the airway wall, either during breath-holding, or during slow steady breathing. A particle settling under gravity accelerates to a steady terminal settling velocity, at which the gravitational force is balanced by the resistance of the air through which the particle falls. The terminal settling velocity is directly proportional to the square of the aerodynamic diameter (D_a^2). The product $D_a^2 \times T$, where T is the residence time in the respiratory tract, is sometimes called the 'sedimentation parameter' [6]. In the peripheral regions of the lungs, the linear velocity of air is low and residence times are relatively long. Also, as the lung periphery is approached, diameters of individual airways become narrower, so that particles settling under gravity have a relatively small distance to fall. To give an example, a 5-μm diameter unit density particle sediments at a rate of 0.74 mm/s [24], so that in a 3-s breath-hold pause, the distance fallen is 2 mm; this guarantees that particles of this size will deposit completely in small conducting airways of diameter 2 mm, assuming they are able to penetrate this deeply into the lungs.

Brownian diffusion

Brownian diffusion is a very important deposition mechanism for submicronic particles, especially those less than 0.5 μm diameter, and is confined mostly to the alveoli, although it can occur in other parts of the respiratory tract [24]. Most of the mass of therapeutic aerosols is usually contained in particles more than 1 μm diameter, so that for therapeutic aerosols, Brownian diffusion is generally less important than inertial impaction and gravitational sedimentation.

Electrostatic charge effects

Most aerosol particles and droplets become electrically charged to some degree during their formation process, and may be attracted towards airway surfaces, leading to greater deposition than would be observed for an electrically neutral aerosol [25]. Generally, however, the electrical charging of aerosols appears to have a minor role in determining the probability of aerosol deposition compared with the more probable processes of inertial impaction and gravitational sedimentation. Electrical charges accumulating on inhaler devices may be important, as they may attract aerosol particles onto the walls of the device, reducing the quantity of drug available for inhalation, as will be described subsequently.

Factors determining deposition patterns

The quantity of aerosol deposited in the lungs, and site within the lungs at which deposition occurs, depends on three basic factors: (i) aerodynamic particle size; (ii) inhalation mode; and (iii) airway anatomy.

Effect of particle size

The effect of particle size on deposition in the tracheobronchial and alveolar regions of the lungs, and in the upper airways, has been examined [26] using monodisperse sebacate oil droplets (Fig. 41.2). These data show that as particle size increases, the likelihood of deposition by inertial impaction in the upper airways also increases, which explains why the size band below 5 μm is termed the 'fine particle fraction', or sometimes the 'respirable fraction'. The optimal size for alveolar deposition is smaller than that for tracheobronchial deposition. Total deposition in the airways decreases to reach a minimum around 0.5 μm, but increases below this size as a result of Brownian diffusion. The effect of particle size on distribution of aerosols within the lungs has been shown in calculations [27] of the amount of deposition taking place in different generations of the Weibel model of the lungs [22]. Aerosol particles of 7 μm diameter have their major deposition site in the first few airway generations (by inertial impaction), but particles of 3 μm diameter have their major deposition site in the small conducting airways and alveoli (by gravitational sedimentation).

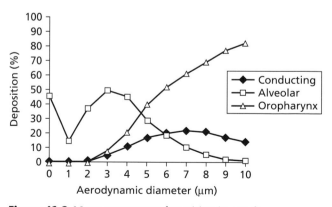

Figure 41.2 Mean percentage deposition in oropharynx, conducting airways of the lungs and alveolated regions of the lungs, of monodisperse particles in healthy subjects, inhaling at 1.5 L tidal volume and a 4-s breathing cycle. (Data from Heyder *et al.* [26].)

Effect of inhalation mode

The inhalation mode is also critically important. Because the nose is a very efficient 'filter' for aerosol particles and droplets, upper airway deposition is higher and lung deposition correspondingly lower, for nose breathing compared with mouth breathing [28]. Hence, inhaled drugs targeted to the lungs should be inhaled via the mouth and not via the nose.

The inhaled flow rate is generally the single most important inhalation parameter, because this determines the likelihood of deposition by inertial impaction in the oropharynx and large central pulmonary airways. Slow inhalation is usually the preferred inhalation technique for therapeutic aerosols in the treatment of COPD patients, because this tends to reduce oropharyngeal deposition and to increase penetration into the lungs [7]. However, inhalation from dry powder inhalers is a major exception to this rule, as is described later. Deep inhalation allows aerosol particles and droplets to penetrate more peripherally into the lungs, where they may undergo gravitational sedimentation. For this reason, a period of breath-holding is generally recommended after inhaling a medical aerosol, and is incorporated into the patient instruction leaflet for many inhaled drug products [29].

Effect of airway anatomy

The airways of the subject inhaling an aerosol are also a critical determinant of the deposition pattern. Even in healthy subjects, there is wide intersubject variability in aerosol deposition patterns, which represents the effect of random variations in airway anatomy [30]. Upper airway anatomy is especially variable, and can be altered at will, for instance by changing the position of the tongue. In addition, there is a more systematic effect in patients with COPD and other obstructive pulmonary conditions, in whom the airways may be narrowed by the presence of oedema, mucus hypersecretion and bronchospasm. Thus, the intrapulmonary deposition pattern is likely to be more 'central' than in healthy subjects [31]. Deposition in large central airways of the lungs results in part from a turbulent airflow, but turbulence can be minimized, and a more peripheral deposition pattern produced, by inhaling drug particles in a helium-oxygen mixture rather than in air [32]. Patients with asthma and COPD may show greater total lung deposition than healthy subjects, because a smaller fraction of the aerosol may be exhaled [33]. Deposition patterns in adolescents broadly resemble those of adults, but younger children would be expected to show lower total lung deposition and a more central deposition pattern within the lungs [34]. These changes result primarily from the airways in children being relatively narrow, but also from differences in breathing patterns between children and adults.

Measuring aerosol deposition

Deposition of medical aerosols can be measured in humans using either radionuclide imaging techniques, or certain pharmacokinetic methods [35,36]. Radionuclide imaging techniques [37,38] consist of the two-dimensional imaging method of gamma scintigraphy, or the three-dimensional methods of single photon emission computed tomography (SPECT) and positron emission tomography (PET). Either the drug formulation, or occasionally the drug molecule itself, is radiolabelled by a gamma-ray-emitting or positron-emitting radionuclide, and the deposition pattern imaged *in vivo* [39–41]. Pharmacokinetic methods are based upon either plasma concentrations or urinary excretion of drug; for instance, utilizing the assumption that drug appearing in the systemic circulation in the first few minutes after inhalation has been absorbed only via the lungs [42–44]. Alternatively, oral charcoal may be used to eliminate drug absorption from the gastrointestinal tract [45]. Pharmacokinetic methods have been made easier by the development of analytical methods capable of quantifying very low concentrations of drug in biological fluids. Taken as a whole, these deposition methods have been used extensively to improve our fundamental understanding of the factors upon which the delivery of medical aerosols depend, and to quantify the deposition of drugs delivered from novel inhaler devices relative to already marketed products. Aerosol deposition patterns have also been predicted in a variety of studies involving mathematical modelling [28,46–48], often showing good agreement with experimental data.

While particle size distributions of medical aerosols are considered excellent laboratory measures of product performance, *in vitro* parameters such as fine particle fraction are not reliable indicators of lung deposition *in vivo* [49]. Fine particle fraction systematically overestimates lung deposition, and may fail to predict accurately the relative performance of two products in clinical practice [50]. Hence, both *in vitro* particle size data and *in vivo* deposition data have important roles in documenting the delivery characteristics of new inhaled drug products. Lung deposition data have been shown to correlate with the clinical effects of drugs used in the treatment of asthma and COPD [51,52].

Aerosol delivery systems

Drugs given by inhalation are delivered as aerosol particles or droplets. If inhalation therapies are to be effective, then the right amount of drug must be delivered to the airways, and inhalation devices that are efficient, reliable and effective are thus required. Pressurized metered dose inhalers (pMDIs) and nebulizers have traditionally been the devices of choice for delivering inhaled drugs to patients with COPD, but these are now being augmented by novel dry powder inhalers (DPIs), and by new 'soft mist inhalers' containing aqueous or ethanolic liquid formulations. The remaining sections of this chapter review the range of inhaler technologies either available now, or likely to be available in the near future. Each type of device has advantages and disadvantages, as set out in Table 41.1.

Pressurized metered dose inhalers

Contents of pressurized metered dose inhalers

The first pMDI was introduced in 1956 by 3M Riker Laboratories [53], initially to deliver non-selective β-agonists such as adrenaline and isoprenaline. Subsequently, they have been used for a range of bronchodilators including

Table 41.1 Advantages and disadvantages of different types of inhaler device.

Device	Advantages	Disadvantages
pMDI	Quick to use Convenient Compact Portable Multidose Cannot contaminate contents Relatively inexpensive	Difficult to use correctly Propellants needed to generate aerosol Delivery of large doses inconvenient Usually low lung deposition/high oropharyngeal deposition Only formulated for limited drug range
pMDI + Spacer	Quick to use Relatively inexpensive Easier to use than pMDI alone Multidose Can be used with facemask by infants Large doses more convenient than by pMDI alone Better lung targeting than for pMDI alone May reduce local and systemic effects for inhaled steroids	More bulky/less convenient than pMDI Propellants needed to generate aerosol Static charge may reduce drug delivery
Nebulizer	Easy to use (relaxed breathing) Suitable for all age groups Suitable in severe COPD Large doses can be given Unusual drugs can be given Oropharyngeal deposition low No propellants needed	Unit-dose Treatments slow Equipment bulky and inconvenient Compressors may be expensive Electricity supply may be needed Easy to contaminate contents Big variations between models
SMIs	Quick to use Generally very high lung deposition Generally compact and portable Multidose No propellants needed	Little experience in clinical practice May be more expensive than pMDI
DPIs	Quick to use Most are breath-actuated No propellants or electricity needed Compact Portable Difficult to contaminate contents	Not all devices are multidose Usually more expensive than pMDI Maximum inspiratory effort usually needed Only formulated for limited drug range Capsule handling problems for elderly

DPI, dry powder inhaler; pMDI: pressurized metered dose inhaler; SMI: soft mist inhaler.

salbutamol, terbutaline, salmeterol, formoterol and ipratropium bromide, together with corticosteroids such as beclometasone dipropionate, budesonide and fluticasone propionate, for use by patients with obstructive airways disease. The drug substance is either a micronized suspension or a solution in propellants, and may be mixed with a surfactant or other excipients [54]. Until recently, all pMDIs contained a mixture of two or three chlorofluorocarbon (CFC) propellants (CFC 12 with CFC 11 and/or CFC 114), often known better by one of their tradenames (Freon). Many pMDIs have now been reformulated with either hydrofluoroalkane (HFA) 134a or HFA 227 (Table 41.2), which do not contain chlorine and hence do not deplete stratospheric ozone [55].

The key component of the pMDI is the metering valve, which allows small quantities (25–100 μL) of the formulation to be dispensed accurately as required. The vapour pressure inside the canister varies from product to product, but is typically 3–4 atmospheres. When the device is fired (actuated), spray formation is a two-step process, consisting of an initial rapid 'flashing' of some of the propellants in the dose, followed by slower evaporation of the remainder [56]. The initial velocity at the actuator nozzle may exceed 30 m/s, and the initial propellant droplet MMAD may exceed 20 μm [57], although rapid decreases in both velocity and particle size occur as the propellants evaporate.

Drug delivery from pressurized metered dose inhalers

The pMDI has many positive features, being compact, portable, convenient and multidose, and these features explain why it has been so successful over almost half a century, despite having changed relatively little (at least prior to the introduction of HFA propellant formulations) during that period [58]. However, the pMDI also has some significant negative features. Most pMDIs are inherently inefficient at delivering drug to the lungs, because the rapid velocity and large size of the propellant droplets will cause most of the dose to deposit by inertial impaction in the oropharynx [59]. No more than approximately 10–20% of the dose actually deposits in the lungs from most pMDIs [60], and this percentage may be further reduced by poor inhaler technique. Some patients cannot co-ordinate actuation with their inhalation [61], and this may result in a reduced amount of drug being deposited in the lungs (or even no drug at all) compared with correct technique. Other patients may exhibit the so-called 'cold Freon' effect, which makes them stop inhaling as the evaporating propellant droplets hit the back of the mouth [62]. If inhalation is resumed quickly, then drug should reach the lungs, but some patients stop inhaling entirely or inhale through the nose [63].

In order to derive optimal benefit from drugs delivered by pMDIs, patients need to use them correctly, and good inhaler technique involves a number of components. Coordination and avoiding 'cold Freon' problems are not the only issues. The dose should be actuated during the course of a slow deep inhalation, and this should be followed by several seconds' breath-holding [64]. This inhalation mode makes sense, because slow deep inhalation allows aerosol particles and droplets the maximum chance of avoiding impaction in the oropharynx, while breath-holding allows particles and droplets to deposit by gravitational sedimentation at their furthest point of penetration into the lungs. Some experts recommend an 'open mouth' inhalation technique, in which the pMDI is held several inches away from the mouth to reduce impaction [60], but placing the mouthpiece of the actuator between closed lips is the method generally adopted. Priming the device (firing doses to waste before use if the pMDI has not been used recently) and shaking the can may also be required in order to assure reproducible dosing. The canister should be held upright with the valve downwards during use, or else the metering chamber will not refill under gravity.

Reformulation with hydrofluoroalkane propellants

Reformulation of drugs for asthma and COPD in HFA propellants is a complex and time-consuming undertaking. HFA 134a has similar thermodynamic properties to CFC 12, but it has not been possible to find direct replacements for CFC 11 or CFC 114 [65], which have higher boiling points and lower vapour pressures (see Table 41.2). Reformulation has required the development of novel surfactants, novel valve components and new filling methods [66], together with conducting clinical studies to demonstrate that these products are safe for administration to humans. To reflect these issues, and in recognition of the importance of pMDIs to the welfare of society, CFCs were granted an exemption under the Montreal Protocol [67], allowing their use in pMDIs to continue temporarily even after other uses had been banned. The introduction of HFA products is proceeding, but is not yet complete, and seems to be most rapid in Europe. It is likely that CFC-based pMDIs will linger on for several more years in some parts of the world. While HFA propellants do not deplete stratospheric ozone, they do have a significant greenhouse warming potential (see Table 41.2).

Some companies have chosen to develop HFA products that directly replace CFC products in equal doses, making a 'seamless transition' [68]. However, other companies have recognized that it is possible, by manipulation of formulation, metering valve and actuator nozzle, to make 'better' pMDIs, which deposit drugs in the more efficiently in the lungs [69], and which are effective in smaller doses [70]. These activities have largely involved reformulation of corticosteroid products in which the drug is in solution, with ethanol as a co-solvent, rather than taking the more

Table 41.2 Properties of propellants used in pressurized metered dose inhalers. (Thermodynamic data from Pischtiak [65].)

Propellant	Structure	ODP	GWP	BP (°C)	VP (bars at 20°C)
CFC 11	CCl_3F	1	1	23.7	0.89
CFC 12	CCl_2F_2	1	3	−29.8	5.66
CFC 114	$C_2Cl_2F_4$	0.7	3.9	3.6	1.82
HFA 134a	$C_2H_2F_4$	0	0.3	−26.1	5.72
HFA 227	C_3HF_7	0	0.7	−15.6	3.90

BP, boiling point; CFC, chlorofluorocarbon; GWP, greenhouse warming potential relative to CFC 11; HFA, hydrofluoroalkane; ODP, ozone depletion potential relative to CFC 11; VP, vapour pressure.

common form of micronized particles. A formulation of beclometasone dipropionate (Qvar®, 3M Healthcare) was the first of these products, and others are under development. They are intended to improve pulmonary targeting of inhaled corticosteroids and to reduce systemic exposure. Irrespective of whether or not their daily drug dose has changed, patients must be educated appropriately when being switched to HFA-based products, and made aware that the spray will probably taste different and may well feel different on the back of the throat [71].

Novel pressurized metered dose inhaler devices

Some recent developments in actuator technology can also help to ensure efficient drug delivery. Breath-actuated pMDIs such as Autohaler [72] and Easi-Breathe [73] fire the spray automatically by a spring mechanism as the patient breathes in, making them potentially very useful for poor coordinators. Another device (Spacehaler) slows down the spray before it leaves the actuator [74]. As well as reducing oropharyngeal deposition and increasing lung deposition, devices like the Spacehaler (now known as Neo-Haler) could also help to ensure drug delivery in patients who experience 'cold Freon' problems.

Pressurized metered dose inhalers with spacer devices

Types of spacer

Spacer devices are attachments or extensions to the mouthpiece of a pMDI, aimed at placing some separation between the pMDI itself and the patient's mouth, so that the likelihood of the spray impacting in the mouth is reduced [75]. The earliest spacer was an elongated mouthpiece on one

model of the original 3M pMDI product [53], followed almost two decades later by much larger homemade spacers or holding chambers constructed from empty plastic bottles [76]. Spacers have been available commercially since the late 1970s, and are essentially of three types:
1 simple tube spacers, which have a volume of 50–200 mL;
2 holding chambers, which also vary in size, often being as large as 750 mL, and generally incorporating a one-way valve in the mouthpiece; and
3 'reverse-flow' devices.
In the last type of device, the pMDI is actuated into the spacer but in the opposite direction to the patient's mouth; on inhalation either the spacer collapses, or vents open so that room air can be entrained via the device.

Drug delivery from spacer devices

The design of spacers (also known as add-on devices, extension devices, chambers, etc.) varies considerably, and hence the drug delivery characteristics of each spacer are probably unique [77]. Nevertheless, they have some common effects on the drug delivery process. Oropharyngeal deposition from pMDIs is always reduced by spacer devices, because the 'ballistic' component of the spray impacts in the device and not in the patient's oropharynx. This may reduce both the systemic side-effects [78] and the local side-effects [79] of inhaled corticosteroids. Lung deposition is often increased, although this is not always the case. The clinical effects of drugs delivered by spacers are likely to be enhanced in patients with poor inhaler technique, but this may not occur in patients with good technique [80], who may already be receiving adequate drug from a pMDI alone. Spacers make pMDIs easier to use, because both coordination and 'cold Freon' problems are reduced. This is especially true for large volume holding chambers such as the Nebuhaler and Volumatic, where the spray may be fired into the spacer, and then inhaled subsequently, but it has also been shown that coordination is less critical when a simple tube spacer is used [81]. Spacer devices appear to be a viable alternative to nebulizers for delivering large doses of inhaled bronchodilators, both to patients with severe acute asthma and to patients with chronic obstructive pulmonary disease [82]. It is possible to use spacers with facemasks, which may be especially valuable in small children [83,84].

Correct use of spacers

While spacers reduce some of the problems of using pMDIs correctly, it is still important that they should be used in the right way. The manufacturer's instructions often recommend inhaling each dose from a spacer in a single deep breath, but a satisfactory clinical response may often be obtained by breathing tidally [85,86]. However, while it

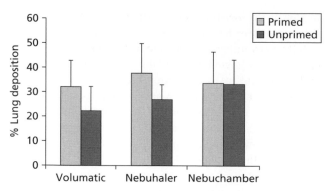

Figure 41.3 Mean (SD) lung deposition (percentage ex-valve dose) from two plastic spacers (Volumatic and Nebuhaler) which were tested both with and without 'priming' to reduce static charge accumulation. The data are compared with those for a metal spacer (Nebuchamber) which had undergone similar treatment. Priming was required to optimize drug delivery from the two plastic spacers, but not from the metal spacer. (Data from Kenyon *et al.* [89].)

is possible to fire multiple doses into spacers and inhale them in a single breath, this will reduce delivery efficiency compared with inhaling the same number of single doses in single breaths [87]. Increasing the delay time between actuation and inhalation also reduces the delivered dose [87]. Perhaps most critically of all, plastic spacers may accumulate static charge during handling, which causes aerosol to be attracted to the walls of the spacer and deposit there prematurely. This may lead to reductions in respirable dose [88], lung deposition [89] and clinical response [90]. In order to reduce static charge build-up, washing a plastic spacer in household detergent and allowing it to air-dry has been recommended [91,92]. A lightweight metal spacer (Nebuchamber) was recently introduced, and drug delivery from this device is not susceptible to static charge effects [89], as shown in Figure 41.3. Plastic spacers that do not require static charge are now available [93].

Nebulizers

Types of nebulizer

Nebulizers convert a drug solution or suspension into a spray. The term 'nebulizer' is usually reserved for unit-dose devices containing liquid volumes between 1 and 5 mL. Novel multidose devices using the same or similar formulations ('soft mist inhalers') are described in the following section of this chapter. Most nebulizers use compressed gas, which passes through a narrow Venturi, to form the spray, and these are known as 'jet' nebulizers [94]. Owing to evaporation, the temperature of the nebulizer solution

decreases, and its concentration increases, during the nebulization process. Ultrasonic nebulizers, in which liquid is atomized as it falls onto a piezoelectric crystal, are now probably less common than a decade ago, partly because sonification has been shown to damage some drug molecules [95]. Some new models of nebulizer are based upon the use of a vibrating mesh of micron-sized holes [96,97]. An aerosol is formed when drug solution passes through the mesh. These devices may overcome some of the limitations of conventional nebulizers, and could replace them in clinical practice in due course.

Advantages and disadvantages of nebulizers

Compared with the pMDI, nebulizers have both advantages and disadvantages. It is easy to use a nebulizer, because the dose can be inhaled by normal relaxed breathing, via either a mouthpiece or a facemask [98], without the need for co-ordination or any specific inhalation manoeuvre. It is possible to deliver very large drug doses if required, for instance up to 1 g of some antibiotics [99]. Nebulizers seem popular with patients, and are often used at home with many hospitals offering a nebulizer service [100]. Because solutions of histamine or methacholine can easily be nebulized, they are the devices of choice in bronchial challenge tests [4].

However, nebulizers have some significant disadvantages or limitations [101]. Only a single dose may be placed in the nebulizer chamber, and treatment times are relatively long, with 10–15 min being needed typically to nebulize several millilitres of solution. Nebulizer apparatus is bulky and inconvenient, because an air compressor or power unit is required, in addition to the nebulizer itself. A range of additives may be included in nebulizer formulations in order to maintain sterility, and the potential of these additives to cause bronchoconstriction should be borne in mind [102]. Nebulizers cannot compete with pMDIs and DPIs in the portable inhaler market, but have their own niche uses, for instance to deliver large doses of inhaled bronchodilators to patients with acute asthma or severe COPD, who might find difficulty using a pMDI successfully, or to deliver less usual drugs such as inhaled antibiotics or inhaled α_1-antitrypsin. However, as has already been described, a pMDI plus spacer device may offer a viable alternative to a nebulizer in some situations [82].

Drug delivery from nebulizers

There are likely to be major differences between nebulizer systems in their output characteristics [103,104] and efficiency of delivery into the lungs [105,106], which should be taken into account when selecting nebulizer equipment. Factors affecting drug delivery from nebulizers include the design and brand of nebulizer, volume fill,

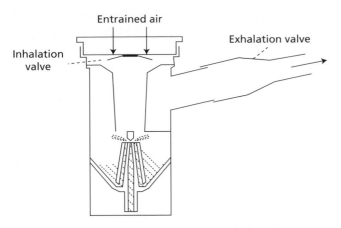

Figure 41.4 Breath-enhanced output jet nebulizer device. (From Knoch and Sommer [107] with permission.)

compressed gas flow rate and whether a solution or suspension is used (solutions are generally easier to nebulize than suspensions). Droplet size of nebulized aerosol decreases as the compressed gas flow rate through the nebulizer is increased. Even when used under optimal conditions, nebulizers are relatively inefficient. The majority of the dose may be retained in the nebulizer as a 'dead volume', lost on connecting tubing or vented during exhalation [106]. The use of 'active Venturi' or 'breath-enhanced output' devices (Fig. 41.4), in which a system of valves is used to control air flow and hence to increase aerosol output during the inhalation phase of breathing, helps to maximize delivery efficiency [107]. Spacer devices attached to nebulizers can be used to store aerosol generated during the exhalation phase of breathing [108], but increase the bulk and complexity of the system. Nebulizers can be placed in ventilator circuits to treat intubated patients [109], but very little of the dose is actually delivered to the lungs [110]. Standards for testing nebulizers in the laboratory [111] have recently been set, and guidelines issued for best nebulizer practice [112].

Novel nebulizer systems

Two recently introduced nebulizer systems have aimed to exert greater control over the particle size and/or patients' breathing patterns. In Adaptive Aerosol Delivery (AAD) devices, a jet nebulizer is equipped with an inhalation monitoring unit, so that the aerosol delivery is continuously adjusted to coincide with the first half of each individual patient's inhalation [113]. This provides a means of controlling more accurately the dose each patient receives, and provides extremely reproducible deposition of drug in the lungs, as well as enhancing patient compliance [114]. In the AKITA system [115], both particle size and breathing pattern are controlled, in order to target drugs as efficiently

as possible to specific lung regions. In one study involving COPD patients, inhaled volume was adjusted for each individual patient, and inhaled flow rate was carefully controlled [116]. AKITA-based devices provided the highest and most reproducible deposition in the peripheral lung, and minimized the time required to deposit a given drug dose. The AKITA system was proposed for delivering inhaled α_1-antitrypsin to patients with emphysema, bearing in mind that it is inherently difficult to achieve high peripheral lung deposition in COPD, owing to the presence of airways obstruction.

Soft mist inhalers

Novel technologies

Multidose inhalers using liquid formulations are a relatively new development in inhaler technology. These devices use formulations similar to those in nebulizers, and yet can compete in the portable inhaler market. They are not true nebulizers, but should be considered as a new category of inhaler device [117,118]. These so-called 'soft mist inhalers' have a variety of operating principles, including forcing liquid through a narrow nozzle or nozzles under pressure [119,120], ultrasonics [121], vibrating meshes [122,123], electrohydrodynamics [124] and thermal inkjet technology [125]. Soft mist inhalers have proved to be amongst the most efficient of inhaler devices [126,127]. They may have their most important roles in the delivery of expensive drug substances [128], targeting drugs intended for systemic delivery via the lungs (such as insulin), and to achieve a reduction in potential systemic side-effects for inhaled corticosteroids.

Respimat® device

One soft mist inhaler (SMI) has particular relevance in the treatment of COPD. Respimat® SMI (Boehringer Ingelheim) is capable of containing more than 100 doses of an aqueous or ethanolic-based formulation, each of which is delivered via a metering valve with a volume as low as 15 µL [129]. The device is actuated by the energy contained in a coiled spring, and the spray is formed by a sophisticated nozzle system (Fig. 41.5). Boehringer have used the opportunity provided by the phasing out of CFC propellants to develop an entirely novel way of delivering inhaled bronchodilators. Compared with a pMDI, the spray velocity from Respimat® SMI is much reduced (hence the term 'soft mist inhaler'), so that less oropharyngeal deposition occurs. The time taken to generate the spray is more than 1 s (compared with approximately 0.2–0.4 s in a pMDI), and it is considered that this combination of factors makes it easier for

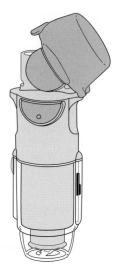

Figure 41.5 Respimat® soft mist inhaler. (Figure kindly supplied by Boehringer Ingelheim Ltd.)

patient to coordinate actuation with their inhalation [130]. Respimat® SMI has been shown to deposit up to 50% of the dose in the lungs (several times greater than that achieved by CFC-based pMDI) [131,127], and clinical trials have confirmed that it is possible to treat asthma and COPD effectively with correspondingly smaller doses [132,133]. Respimat® SMI was the only SMI to have reached the market by the end of 2005.

Dry powder inhalers

Types of dry powder inhaler

The first DPIs to be introduced commercially were the single-dose devices containing drug powder in gelatine capsules. In 1969, Fisons introduced the Spinhaler [134], and this was followed a few years later by the Rotahaler (Glaxo) [135]. Subsequently, inhalers containing multiple doses, either in individual blisters or in a bulk storage reservoir, have become the DPIs of choice for routine use by patients with asthma and COPD [136]. Owing to the cohesive nature of micronized drug particles, most dry powder formulations also contain a carrier substance (usually large lactose particles), which improves the flow properties of the powder [137]. All currently marketed DPIs are 'breath-actuated', using the patient's inhalation to disperse the drug powder, and to deliver it into the lungs [138]. This gives DPIs two inherent advantages over pMDIs:

1 they do not require propellants to form the aerosol cloud; and

2 it is not necessary for patients to 'press and breathe' simultaneously.

Table 41.3 Dry powder inhalers marketed somewhere in the world in 2005.

Single dose (capsules, blisters)
Spinhaler (Fisons, now Sanofi Aventis)
Rotahaler (GlaxoSmithKline)
Aeroliser (Novartis; a.k.a. Cyclohaler, Pharmachemie)
Inhalator (Boehringer Ingelheim)
Handihaler (Boehringer Ingelheim)

Multiple unit dose (multiple capsules, blisters)
Diskhaler (GlaxoSmithKline)
Diskus (GlaxoSmithKline; a.k.a. Accuhaler)
E-haler (Sanofi Aventis)
Inhalator-M (Boehringer Ingelheim)

Multidose (metered from powder reservoir)
Turbuhaler (AstraZeneca)
Easyhaler (Orion)
Novolizer (ASTA Medica, now Viatris)
Pulvinal (Chiesi)
Twisthaler (Schering-Plough)
Clickhaler (Innovata)
Airmax (Ivax)
Jethaler (Ratiopharm)

Several of the pharmaceutical companies most active in inhaled drug delivery for asthma and COPD appear to be prioritizing DPI development over pMDIs at the present time.

By 2005, more than 15 DPIs had been marketed in at least one country, and a number of others were in development (Table 41.3). New single-dose devices are still being introduced, notably the Handihaler DPI for delivery of inhaled tiotropium bromide [139]. However, most new DPIs contain either multiple unit doses or powder reservoirs. Multiple unit dose devices include the Diskus or Accuhaler (GlaxoSmithKline) [140], while reservoir devices include the Turbuhaler (AstraZeneca) [141]. The relative merits of multiple unit dose and reservoir systems have been debated [142]. Multiple unit dose devices have two potential advantages over reservoir devices:

1 it is generally possible to fill individual doses into blisters in the factory more accurately than doses can be dispensed by the patient from a reservoir; and

2 doses contained in blisters should provide better protection for the powder against the effects of moisture.

However, it should be borne in mind that both multiple unit dose and powder reservoir devices have an excellent track record in clinical practice. Combination DPI products containing both a bronchodilator and a corticosteroid are gaining popularity, partly because of increased convenience of giving two drugs concurrently, but also because of possible drug synergies in the combined formulation [143].

Drug delivery from dry powder inhalers

DPIs either deposit drugs in the lungs with similar efficiency to a pMDI, or with greater efficiency [144], thereby allowing lower maintenance doses to be used [145]. However, as in the pMDI, optimal drug delivery depends on inhalation technique. While breath-actuation in DPIs is seen as an advantage, it is linked to a disadvantage, because patients should inhale with maximal inspiratory effort when using most DPIs. Maximal inspiratory effort ensures optimal de-aggregation of drug particles or of drug–lactose complexes, and hence improves fine particle dose and deposition in the lungs. This may appear paradoxical, because increased respiratory effort would be expected to increase particle deposition in the oropharynx, but the effect upon particle deagglomeration seems generally to be greater. To give an example, lung deposition from Turbuhaler DPI averaged 27% and 14% of the dose at a peak inhaled flow rates of 60 and 30 L/min, respectively [146]. Other DPIs may show greater [147] or less [148] dependence of lung deposition on peak inhaled flow rate. Reduction in peak inhaled flow rate through a DPI may lead to a lower clinical response [149]. While achieving a high peak inhaled flow rate through a DPI is important, it is also desirable that the time taken to attain peak inhaled flow rate should be as short as possible [150]. The magnitude of the peak inhaled flow rate associated with maximal inspiratory effort various from device to device. Turbuhaler has a fairly high resistance to airflow, and a peak inhaled flow rate of 60 L/min through this device approximately represents maximal inspiratory effort. Higher flows can be achieved through other DPIs with lower resistances, although there is no clear evidence that devices with low resistance are inherently either superior or inferior to those with high resistance.

In order to minimize the inhaled flow rate dependence of DPIs, novel particle formulations, which can be dispersed easily without using maximal inspiratory effort, have been developed [151,152]. Over 50% of the dose may be deposited in the lungs using these formulations, a much higher percentage than with conventional formulations. Several 'active' DPIs, in which the powder is dispersed by either compressed air [153] or an electric motor [154], have been described. These very sophisticated formulations and devices are likely to be relatively expensive, and may be better suited to delivery of novel therapies such as inhaled peptides and proteins, rather than to daily maintenance therapy of obstructive airways disease.

The need to inhale from most DPI systems with maximal inspiratory effort has raised concerns that some patients with more severe disease might be unable to use them satisfactorily. Recent data suggest that some patients with COPD may have difficulty attaining the required peak inhaled flow rates through Turbuhaler DPI [155], although in another study peak inhaled flow rates were similar in COPD patients to those reported in asthmatic patients [156]. In a recent review, it was concluded that although more data have been obtained in asthmatics than in patients with COPD, the peak inhaled flows attained via DPIs in both asthmatic and COPD patients are probably little different to those obtained in healthy subjects, and that asthmatic children, adults with acute asthma and patients with severe COPD can all use DPIs effectively, and gain good clinical benefit [157]. It has been suggested to use Turbuhaler DPI, rather than a nebulizer, to deliver high-dose domiciliary terbutaline treatment in most patients with severe COPD [158], but this suggestion is controversial.

Conclusions

The range of inhaler devices available is increasing, although the rate of growth of new inhaler technology brought about by the phase-out of CFC propellants now appears to be slowing down. While the proliferation of new inhaler devices with differing instructions for correct use may cause confusion among patients if not carefully managed, patients are now likely to be provided with a range of devices that meet individual needs and preferences. Each category of inhaler has advantages and disadvantages, so that is unlikely that there will ever be a 'perfect' inhaler device appropriate to all patients and to all circumstances.

Recent evidence-based guidelines concluded that while each type of inhaler can be equally effective if used correctly, choice of inhaler should consider a range of factors, including likelihood of correct use, cost and preference [159].

The efficiency with which inhaler devices deposit drug in the lungs has increased dramatically over the last two decades, from approximately 10–20% of the dose for most CFC-based pMDIs and nebulizers, to more than 50% of the dose for some novel devices and formulations. The development of 'formulation integrated dry powder inhalers', combining an efficient inhaler device with an easily dispersible formulation, may lead to further improvements in device efficiency [160]. These technological advances may be of limited value in the maintenance therapy of COPD with inhaled bronchodilators, but are highly relevant for other inhaled therapies in COPD including antibiotics and alpha-1 antitrypsin. Taken as a whole, there is little doubt that the use of inhaled drug therapy will have a major role for the foreseeable future in patients with COPD.

References

1 Labiris NR, Dolovich MB. Pulmonary drug delivery. Part 1: physiological factors affecting therapeutic effectiveness of aerosolised medications. *Br J Clin Pharmacol* 2003;**56**:588–99.

2 Dalby R, Suman J. Inhalation therapy: technological milestones in asthma treatment. *Advanced Drug Delivery Revs* 2003;**55**: 779–91.

3 Lalor CB, Hickey AJ. Generation and characterisation of aerosols for drug delivery to the lungs. In: Adjei AL, Gupta PK, eds. *Inhalation Delivery of Therapeutic Peptides and Proteins.* New York: Marcel Dekker, 1997: 235–76.

4 Anderson SD, Brannan JD, Chan H-K. Use of aerosols for bronchial provocation testing in the laboratory: where we have been and where we are going. *J Aerosol Med* 2002; **15**:313–24.

5 Dolovich MB. Aerosols. In: Barnes PJ, Grunstein MM, Leff AR, Woolcock AJ, eds. *Asthma.* Philadelphia: Lippincott-Raven, 1997: 1349–66.

6 Heyder J, Svartengren MU. Basic principles of particle behavior in the human respiratory tract. In: Bisgaard H, O'Callaghan C, Smaldone GC, eds. *Drug Delivery to the Lung.* New York: Marcel Dekker, 2002: 21–45.

7 Dolovich MB. Influence of inspiratory flow rate, particle size and airway caliber on aerosolized drug delivery to the lung. *Respir Care* 2000;**45**:597–608.

8 Heyder J. Particle transport onto human airway surfaces. *Eur J Respir Dis* 1982;**63**(Suppl 119):29–50.

9 Agnew JE. Physical properties and mechanisms of deposition of aerosols. In: Clarke SW, Pavia D, eds. *Aerosols and the Lung: Clinical and Experimental Aspects.* London: Butterworths, 1984: 49–70.

10 Morrow PE. An evaluation of the physical properties of monodisperse and heterodisperse aerosols used in the treatment of bronchial function. *Chest* 1981;**80**(Suppl):809–13.

11 Mercer TT. Production of therapeutic aerosols: principles and techniques. *Chest* 1981;**80**(Suppl):813–8.

12 Gonda I. Study of the effect of polydispersity of aerosols on regional deposition in the respiratory tract. *J Pharm Pharmacol* 1981;**33**(Suppl):52P.

13 Hallworth GW. Particle size analysis of therapeutic aerosols. In: Morén F, Dolovich MB, Newhouse MT, Newman SP, eds. *Aerosols in Medicine: Principles, Diagnosis and Therapy.* Amsterdam: Elsevier, 1993: 351–74.

14. Mitchell JP, Nagel MW. Cascade impactors for size characterization of aerosols from medical inhalers: their uses and limitations. *J Aerosol Med* 2003;**16**:341–77.

15 Brindley A, Reavill KJ, Sumby BS *et al.* The *in vitro* characterization of inhalation devices using the electronic lung. In: Byron P, Dalby RN, Farr SJ, eds. *Respiratory Drug Delivery IV.* Buffalo Grove: Interpharm Press, 1994: 143–51.

16 Olsson B, Borgström L, Asking L *et al.* Effect of inlet throat on the correlation between measured fine particle dose and lung deposition. In: Dalby RN, Byron PR, Farr SJ, eds. *Respiratory Drug Delivery V.* Buffalo Grove: Interpharm Press, 1996: 273–81.

17 Mitchell JP, Nagel MW. Time-of-flight aerodynamic particle size analysers: their use and limitations for the evaluation of medical aerosols. *J Aerosol Med* 1999;**12**:217–40.

18 Finlay WH, Smaldone GC. Hygroscopic behavior of nebulized aerosols: not as important as we thought? *J Aerosol Med* 1998;**11**:193–95.

19 Hickey AJ, Martonen TB. Behavior of hygroscopic pharmaceutical aerosols and the influence of hydrophobic additives. *Pharm Res* 1993;10:1–7.

20 Phipps PR, Gonda I, Andersen SD *et al.* Regional deposition of saline aerosols of different tonicities in normal and asthmatic subjects. *Eur Respir J* 1994;**7**:1474–82.

21 Lippmann M, Albert RE. The effect of particle size on the regional deposition of inhaled aerosols in the human respiratory tract. *Am Ind Hyg Assoc J* 1969;**30**:257–75.

22 Weibel ER. *Morphometry of the Human Lung.* New York: Academic Press, 1963.

23 Pritchard JN. Particle growth and the influence of airflow. In: Newman SP, Moren F, Crompton GK, eds. *A New Concept in Inhalation Therapy.* Bussum: Medicom, 1987: 3–24.

24 Stuart BO. Deposition of inhaled aerosols. *Arch Intern Med* 1973;**131**:60–73.

25 Bailey AG. Aerosol charge and its influence on particle retention in the lung. In: *Drug Delivery to the Lungs VII.* Bristol: The Aerosol Society, 1996: 5–8.

26 Heyder J, Gebhardt J, Rudolf G *et al.* Deposition of particles in the human respiratory tract in the size range 0.005 to 15 µm. *J Aerosol Sci* 1986;**17**:811–25.

27 Gerrity TR, Lee PS, Hass FJ *et al.* Calculated deposition of inhaled particles in the airway generations of normal subjects. *J Appl Physiol* 1979;**47**:867–73.

28 Brain JD, Blanchard JD. Mechanisms of particle deposition and clearance. In: Morén F, Dolovich MB, Newhouse MT, Newman SP, eds. *Aerosols in Medicine: Principles, Diagnosis and Therapy.* Amsterdam: Elsevier, 1993: 117–56.

29 Hindle M, Newton DAG, Chrystyn H. Investigations of an optimal inhaler technique with the use of urinary salbutamol excretion as a measure of relative bioavailability to the lung. *Thorax* 1993;**48**:607–10.

30 Yu CP, Nicolaides P, Soong TT. Effect of random airway sizes on aerosol deposition. *Am Ind Hyg Assoc J* 1979;**40**:999–1005.

31 Melchor R, Biddiscombe MF, Mak VHF *et al.* Lung deposition patterns of directly labelled salbutamol in normal subjects and in patients with reversible airways obstruction. *Thorax* 1993;**48**:506–11.

32 Anderson M, Svartengren M, Philipson K, *et al.* Deposition in man of particles inhaled in air or in helium-oxygen mixture at different flow rates. *J Aerosol Med* 1990;**3**:209–16.

33 Kim CS, Kang TC. Comparative measurement of lung deposition of inhaled fine particles in normal subjects and patients with obstructive airway disease. *Am J Respir Crit Care Med* 1997;**155**:899–905.

34 Yu CP, Xu GB. Predicted deposition of diesel particles in young humans. *J Aerosol Sci* 1987;**18**:419–29.

35 Snell NJC, Ganderton D. Assessing lung deposition of inhaled medications. *Respir Med* 1999;**93**:123–33.

36 Mobley C, Hochhaus G. Methods used to assess pulmonary deposition and absorption of drugs. *Drug Discov Today* 2001; **6**:367–75.

37 Dolovich MB. Measuring total and regional lung deposition using inhaled radiotracers. *J Aerosol Med* 2001;**14**(Suppl 1): S35–S44.

38 Newman SP, Pitcairn GR, Hirst PH *et al.* Radionuclide imaging technologies and their use in evaluating asthma drug

deposition in the lungs. *Advanced Drug Delivery Revs* 2003;**55**: 851–67.

39 Newman SP. Scintigraphic assessment of therapeutic aerosols. *Crit Rev Ther Drug Carrier Syst* 1993;**10**:65–109.

40 Berridge MS, Lee Z, Heald DL. Regional distribution and kinetics of inhaled pharmaceuticals. *Curr Pharm Des* 2000; **6**:1631–51.

41 Dolovich M, Hahmias C, Coates G. Unleashing the PET: 3D imaging of the lung. In: Dalby RN, Byron PR, Farr SJ, Peart J, eds. *Respiratory Drug Delivery VII*. Raleigh: Serentec Press, 2000: 215–30.

42 Newnham DM, McDevitt DG, Lipworth BJ. Comparison of the extrapulmonary beta-2 adrenoceptor responses and pharmacokinetics of salbutamol metered dose-inhaler and modified actuator device. *Br J Clin Pharmacol* 1993;**36**: 445–50.

43 Chrystyn H. Methods to identify drug deposition in the lungs following inhalation. *Br J Clin Pharmacol* 2001;**51**:289–99.

44 Derendorf H, Hochhaus G, Möllman H. Evaluation of pulmonary absorption using pharmacokinetic methods. *J Aerosol Med* 2001;**14**(Suppl 1):S9–S17.

45 Borgström L, Newman S, Weisz A *et al.* Pulmonary deposition of inhaled terbutaline: comparison of scanning gamma camera and urinary excretion method. *J Pharm Sci* 1992; **81**:753–5.

46 Martonen TB, Musante CJ, Segal RA *et al.* Lung models: strengths and limitations. *Respir Care* 2000;**45**:712–36.

47 Finlay WH, Stapleton KW, Zuberbuhler P. Predicting regional lung dosages of a nebulised suspension: Pulmicort. *Particulate Sci Technol* 1997;**15**:243–51.

48 Clayborough R, Brook BS, Hamill I *et al.* Predictive drug delivery to the respiratory system: the COPHIT approach. In: Dalby RN, Byron PR, Peart J, Farr SF, eds. *Respiratory Drug Delivery VIII*. Raleigh: Davis Horwood, 2002: 351–4.

49 Newman SP. How well do *in vitro* particle size measurements predict drug delivery *in vivo? J Aerosol Med* 1998; **11**(Suppl 1):S97–S104.

50 Farr SJ, Warren SJ, Lloyd P *et al.* Comparison of *in vitro* and *in vivo* efficiencies of a novel unit-dose aerosol generator and a pressurized metered dose inhaler. *Int J Pharm* 2000;**198**: 63–70.

51 Pauwels R, Newman SP, Borgström L. Airway deposition and airway effects of antiasthma drugs delivered from metered dose inhalers. *Eur Respir J* 1997;**10**:2127–38.

52 Laube BL, Edwards AM, Dalby RN *et al.* The efficacy of slow versus faster inhalation of cromolyn sodium in protecting against allergen challenge in patients with asthma. *J Allergy Clin Immunol* 1998;**101**:475–83.

53 Thiel CG. From Susie's question to CFC free: an inventor's perspective on forty years of MDI development and regulation. In: Dalby RN, Byron PR, Farr SJ, eds. *Respiratory Drug Delivery V*. Buffalo Grove: Interpharm Press, 1996: 115–23.

54 Hallworth GW. The formulation and evaluation of pressurised metered dose inhalers. In: Ganderton D, Jones T, eds. *Drug Delivery to the Respiratory Tract*. Chichester: Ellis Horwood, 1987: 87–118.

55 Smith IJ. The challenge of reformulation. *J Aerosol Med* 1995;**8**:S19–S27.

56 Sanders PA. *Principles of Aerosol Technology*. New York: Van Nostrand Reinhold, 1970: 3–7.

57 Clark AR. MDIs: physics of aerosol formation. *J Aerosol Med* 1996;**9**(Suppl 1):S19–S26.

58 Newman SP. Devices for inhaling medications. In: Clark TJH, Lee T, Godfrey S, Thomson NC, eds. *Asthma*, 4th edn. London: Edward Arnold, 2000: 329–54.

59 Spiro SG, Singh CA, Tolfree SEJ *et al.* Direct labelling of ipratropium bromide aerosol and its deposition pattern in normal subjects and patients with chronic bronchitis. *Thorax* 1984;**39**:432–5.

60 Dolovich M, Ruffin RE, Roberts R *et al.* Optimal delivery of aerosols from metered dose inhalers. *Chest* 1981; **80**(Suppl):911–5.

61 Epstein SW, Manning CPR, Ashley MJ *et al.* Survey of the clinical use of pressurized aerosol inhalers. *Can Med Assoc J* 1979;**120**:813–6.

62 Crompton GK. Problems patients have using pressurised aerosol inhalers. *Eur J Respir Dis* 1982;**63**(Suppl 119):57–65.

63 Pedersen S, Frost L Arnfred T. Errors in inhalation technique and efficiency in inhaler use in asthmatic children. *Allergy* 1986;**41**:118–24.

64 Newman SP, Pavia D, Clarke SW. How should a pressurised beta-adrenergic bronchodilator be inhaled? *Eur J Respir Dis* 1981;**62**:3–20.

65 Pischtiak AH. Qualification of HFA 227ea versus HFA 134a for use as a propellant in MDIs. In: Dalby RN, Byron PR, Farr SJ, Peart J, eds. *Respiratory Drug Delivery VII*. Raleigh: Serentec Press, 2000: 519–22.

66 Elvecrog J. Metered dose inhalers in a CFC-free future. *Pharm Tech Eur* 1997;**91**:52–5.

67 McDonald KJ, Martin GP. Transition to CFC-free metered dose inhalers: into the new millennium. *Int J Pharm* 2000;**211**:89–107.

68 Cripps A, Riebe M, Schulze M *et al.* Pharmaceutical transition to non-CFC pressurized metered dose inhalers. *Respir Med* 2000;**94**(Suppl B):S3–S9.

69 Leach CL, Davidson PJ, Boudreau RJ. Improved airway targeting with the CFC-free HFA-beclomethasone metered-dose inhaler compared with CFC-beclomethasone. *Eur Respir J* 1998;**12**:1346–53.

70 Busse WW, Brazinsky S, Jacobson K *et al.* Efficacy response of inhaled beclomethasone dipropionate in asthma is proportional to dose and is improved by formulation with a new propellant. *J Allergy Clin Immunol* 1999;**104**:1215–22.

71 Partridge MR, Woodcock AA, Sheffer AL *et al.* Chlorofluorocarbon-free inhalers: are we ready for the change? *Eur Respir J* 1998;**11**:1006–8.

71 Gabrio BJ, Stein SW, Velasquez DJ. A new method to evaluate plume characteristics of hydrofluoroalkane and chlorofluorocarbon metered dose inhalers. *Int J Pharm* 1999;**186**:3–12.

73 Hardy JG, Jasuja AK, Frier M *et al.* A small volume spacer for use with a breath-operated pressurised metered dose inhaler. *Int J Pharm* 1996;**142**:129–33.

74 Newman SP, Steed KP, Hooper G *et al.* Improved targeting of beclomethasone dipropionate (250 µg metered dose inhaler) to the lungs of asthmatics with the Spacehaler. *Respir Med* 1999;**93**:424–31.

75 Newman SP, Newhouse MT. Effect of add-on devices for aerosol drug delivery: deposition studies and clinical aspects. *J Aerosol Med* 1996;**9**:55–70.

76 Gale AE, Lele V. Beclomethasone dipropionate aerosol. *Med J Aust* 1974;**2**:757.

77 Newman SP. Spacer devices for metered dose inhalers. *Clin Pharmacokinetics* 2004;**43**:349–60.

78 Brown PH, Blundell G, Greening AP *et al.* Do large volume spacers reduce the systemic effects of high dose inhaled corticosteroids? *Thorax* 1990;**45**:736–9.

79 Toogood JH, Baskerville J, Jennings B, Lefcoe NM, Johansson S-A. Use of spacers to facilitate inhaled corticosteroid treatment in asthma. *Am Rev Respir Dis* 1984;**129**:723–9.

80 Lee H, Evans HE. Evaluation of inhalation aids of metered dose inhalers in asthmatic children. *Chest* 1987;**91**:366–9.

81 Bloomfield P, Crompton GK, Winsey NJP. A tube spacer to improve inhalation of drugs from pressurised aerosols. *BMJ* 1979;**2**:1479.

82 Noseda A, Yernault JC. Sympathomimetics in acute severe asthma: inhaled or parenteral, nebuliser or spacer. *Eur Respir J* 1989;**2**:377–82.

83 Bisgaard H, Anhoj J, Wildhaber JH. Spacer devices. In: Bisgaard H, O'Callaghan C, Smaldone GC, eds. *Drug Delivery to the Lung.* New York: Marcel Dekker, 2002: 389–420.

84 Bisgaard H, Munck SL, Nielsen JP *et al.* Inhaled budesonide for treatment of recurrent wheezing in early childhood. *Lancet* 1990;**336**:649–51.

85 Gleeson JGA, Price JF. Nebuhaler technique. *Br J Dis Chest* 1988;**82**:172–74.

86 Green CP, Price JF. Bronchodilator effect of salbutamol via the Volumatic in children. *Respir Med* 1991;**85**:325–6.

87 Barry PW, O'Callaghan C. The effect of delay, multiple actuations and spacer static charge on the *in vitro* delivery of budesonide from the Nebuhaler. *Br J Clin Pharmacol* 1995;**40**:76–8.

88 O'Callaghan C, Lynch J, Cant M *et al.* Improvement in sodium cromoglycate delivery from a spacer device by use of an antistatic lining, immediate inhalation and avoiding multiple actuations of drug. *Thorax* 1993;**48**:603–6.

89 Kenyon CJ, Thorsson L, Borgström L *et al.* The effects of static charge in spacer devices on glucocorticosteroid aerosol deposition in asthmatic patients. *Eur Respir J* 1998;**11**:606–10.

90 Wildhaber JH, Waterer GW, Hall GL *et al.* Reducing electrostatic charge on spacer devices and bronchodilator response. *Br J Clin Pharmacol* 2000;**50**:277–80.

91 Dewsbury NJ, Kenyon CJ, Newman SP. The effect of handling techniques on electrostatic charge on spacer devices: a correlation with *in vitro* particle size analysis. *Int J Pharm* 1996;**137**:261–4.

92 Pierart F, Wildhaber JH, Vrancken I *et al.* Washing plastic spacers in household detergent reduces electrostatic charge and greatly improves delivery. *Eur Respir J* 1999;**13**:673–8.

93 Mitchell J, Morton R, Schmidt J *et al.* Overcoming electrostatic charge retention in a new valved holding chamber (VHC): *in vitro* performance comparison with current devices. In: Dalby RN, Byron PR, Peart J, Suman JD, Farr SJ,

eds. *Respiratory Drug Delivery IX.* River Grove, Illinois: Davis Healthcare International, 2004: 705–7.

94 O'Callaghan C, Barry PW. The science of nebulised drug delivery. *Thorax* 1997;**52**(Suppl 2):S31–S44.

95 Rau JL. Design principles of nebulization devices currently in use. *Respir Care* 2002;**47**:1257–78.

96 Dennis JH, Nerbrink O. New nebulizer technology. In: Bisgaard H, O'Callaghan C, Smaldone GC, eds. *Drug Delivery to the Lung.* New York: Marcel Dekker, 2002: 303–36.

97 Dhand R. Nebulizers that use a vibrating mesh or plate with multiple apertures to generate aerosol. *Respir Care* 2002;**47**: 1406–18.

98 McCallion ONM, Taylor KMG, Bridges PA *et al.* Jet nebulisers for pulmonary drug delivery. *Int J Pharm* 1996;**130**:1–11.

99 Hodson ME, Penketh ARL, Batten JC. Aerosol carbenicillin and gentamicin treatment of *Pseudomonas* infection in patients with cystic fibrosis. *Lancet* 1981;**2**:1137–9.

100 Laroche CM, Harries AVK, Newton RCF *et al.* Domiciliary nebulisers in asthma: a district survey. *BMJ* 1985;**290**: 1611–3.

101 Newman SP. *Nebuliser Therapy: Scientific and Technical Aspects.* Lund: AB Draco, 1989.

102 Snell NJC. Adverse reactions to inhaled drugs. *Respir Med* 1990;**84**:345–8.

103 Newman SP, Pellow PGD, Clay MM *et al.* Evaluation of jet nebulisers for use with gentamicin solution. *Thorax* 1985; **40**:671–6.

104 Kendrick AH, Smith EC, Wilson RSE. Selecting and using nebuliser equipment. *Thorax* 1997;**52**(Suppl 2):S92–S101.

105 Thomas SHL, O'Docherty MJ, Page CJ *et al.* Which apparatus for inhaled pentamidine? A comparison of pulmonary deposition via eight nebulisers. *Eur Respir J* 1991;**4**:616–22.

106 Newman SP. Lung deposition from nebulizers. *Eur Respir Rev* 2000;**10**:224–7.

107 Knoch M, Sommer E. Jet nebulizer design and function. *Eur Respir Rev* 2000;**10**:183–6.

108 Thomas SHL, Langford JA, George RDG *et al.* Improving the efficiency of drug administration with jet nebulisers. *Lancet* 1988;**1**:126.

109 MacIntyre NM, Silver RM, Miller CW *et al.* Aerosol delivery in intubated, mechanically ventilated patients. *Crit Care Med* 1985;**13**:81–4.

110 Fuller HD, Dolovich MB, Posmituck G *et al.* Pressurized aerosol versus jet aerosol delivery to mechanically ventilated patients: comparison of dose to the lungs. *Am Rev Respir Dis* 1990;**141**:440–4.

111 Dennis JH, Pieron CA, Nerbrink O. Standards in assessing *in vitro* nebulizer performance. *Eur Respir Rev* 2000;**10**:178–82.

112 Muers MF, Corris PA. Current best practice for nebuliser treatment. *Thorax* 1997;**52**(Suppl 2):S1–S17.

113 Denyer J, Nikander K, Smith NJ. Adaptive aerosol delivery (AAD) technology. *Expert Opin Drug Deliv* 2004;**1**:165–76.

114 Crockford D, Denyer J. Adaptive aerosol delivery technology: drug delivery technology that adapts to the patient. *Drug Delivery Systems and Sciences* 2002;**2**:110–3.

115 Scheuch G, Brand P, Meyer T *et al.* Regional drug targeting within the lungs by controlled inhalation with the AKITA

inhalation system. In: Dalby RN, Byron PR, Peart J, Farr SF, eds. *Respiratory Drug Delivery VIII*. Raleigh: Davis Horwood, 2002: 471–3.

116 Sommerer K, Meyer T, Brand P *et al*. A strategy to optimize peripheral lung deposition in patients with emphysema. In: Dalby RN, Byron PR, Peart J, Farr SF, eds. *Respiratory Drug Delivery VIII*. Raleigh: Davis Horwood, 2002: 475–8.

117 Dolovich MB. New propellant-free technologies under investigation. *J Aerosol Med* 1999;**12**(Suppl 1):S9–S17.

118 Smart JR. A brief overview of novel liquid-based inhalation technologies. *Drug Deliv Syst Sci* 2002;**2**:67–71.

119 Zierenberg B, Eicher J, Dunne S *et al*. Boehringer Ingelheim nebulizer BINEB. A new approach to inhalation therapy. In: Dalby RN, Byron PR, Farr SJ, eds. *Respiratory Drug Delivery V*. Buffalo Grove: Interpharm Press, 1996: 187–93.

120 Schuster J, Farr SJ, Cipolla D *et al*. Design and performance validation of a highly efficient and reproducible compact aerosol delivery system: AERx. In: Dalby RN, Byron PR, Farr SJ, eds. *Respiratory Drug Delivery VI*. Buffalo Grove: Interpharm Press, 1998: 83–90.

121 Hirst PH, Bacon RE, Newman SP *et al*. Deposition, absorption and bioavailability of aerosolized morphine sulphate delivered by a novel hand-held device, the metered solution inhaler. In: Dalby RN, Byron PR, Farr SJ, Peart J, eds. *Respiratory Drug Delivery VII*. Raleigh: Serentec Press, 2000: 467–9.

122 De Young L, Chambers F, Narayan S *et al*. The Aerodose multidose inhaler device: design and delivery characteristics. In: Dalby RN, Byron PR, Farr SJ, eds. *Respiratory Drug Delivery VI*. Buffalo Grove: Interpharm Press, 1998: 91–5.

123 Stangl R, Luangkhot N, Liening-Ewert R *et al*. Characterising the first prototype of a vibrating menbrane nebuliser. In: Dalby RN, Byron PR, Farr SJ, Peart J, eds. *Respiratory Drug Delivery VII*. Raleigh: Serentec Press, 2000: 455–8.

124 Zimlich WC, Ding JY, Busick DR *et al*. The development of a novel electrohydrodynamic pulmonary drug delivery device. In: Dalby RN, Byron PR, Farr SJ, Peart J, eds. *Respiratory Drug Delivery VII*. Raleigh: Serentec Press, 2000: 241–6.

125 Goodall S, Chew N, Chan H-K *et al*. Aerosolization of protein solutions using thermal inkjet technology. *J Aerosol Med* 2002;**15**:351–7.

126 Farr SJ, Schuster JA, Lloyd P *et al*. AER-X development of a novel liquid aerosol delivery system: concept to clinic. In: Dalby RN, Byron PR, Farr SJ, eds. *Respiratory Drug Delivery V*. Buffalo Grove: Interpharm Press, 1996: 175–85.

127 Newman SP, Brown J, Steed KP *et al*. Lung deposition of fenoterol and flunisolide delivered using a novel device for inhaled medications. *Chest* 1998;**113**:957–63.

128 Clauson PG, Balent B, Brunner GA *et al*. PK-PD of four different doses of pulmonary insulin delivered with the AERx diabetes management system. In: Dalby RN, Byron PR, Farr SJ, Peart J, eds. *Respiratory Drug Delivery VII*. Raleigh: Serentec Press, 2000: 155–61.

129 Zierenberg B. Optimizing the *in vitro* performance of Respimat. *J Aerosol Med* 1999;**12**(Suppl 1):S19–S24.

130 Dalby R, Spallek M, Voshaar T. A review of the development of Respimat soft mist inhaler. *Int J Pharm* 2004;**283**:1–9.

131 Newman SP, Steed KP, Reader SJ *et al*. Efficient delivery to the lungs of flunisolide from a new portable hand-held multidose nebuliser. *J Pharm Sci* 1996;**85**:960–4.

132 Pavia D, Moonen D. Preliminary data from phase II studies with Respimat, a propellant-free soft mist inhaler. *J Aerosol Med* 1999;**12**(Suppl 1):S33–S39.

133 Kilfeather SA, Ponitz HH, Schmidt P *et al*. Improved delivery of ipratropium bromide / fenoterol from Respimat soft mist inhaler in patients with COPD. *Respir Med* 2004;**98**:387–97.

134 Bell JH, Hartley PS, Cox JSG. Dry powder aerosols I: a new powder inhalation device. *J Pharm Sci* 1971;**10**:1559–64.

135 Hallworth GW. An improved design of powder inhaler. *Br J Clin Pharmacol* 1977;**4**:689–90.

136 Newman SP, Busse WW. Evolution of dry powder inhaler design, formulation and performance. *Respir Med* 2002;**96**: 293–304.

137 Ganderton DJ, Kassem NM. Dry powder inhalers. In: Ganderton DJ, Jones T, eds. *Advances in Pharmaceutical Sciences*. London: Academic Press, 1992: 165–91.

138 Smith IJ, Parry-Billings M. The inhalers of the future? A review of dry powder devices on the market today. *Pulmonary Pharmacol and Therapeutics* 2003;**16**:79–95.

139 Hochrainer D, Spallek M. Handihaler: a new powder inhaler for COPD treatment. In: *Drug Delivery to the Lungs XIII*. Bristol: The Aerosol Society, 2002: 140–3.

140 Brindley A, Sumby BS, Smith IJ *et al*. Design, manufacture and dose consistency of the Serevent Diskus Inhaler. *Pharm Tech Eur* 1995;**9**:14–22.

141 Wetterlin K. Turbuhaler: a new powder inhaler for administration of drugs to the airways. *Pharm Res* 1988;**5**:506–8.

142 Prime D, Grant AC, Slater AL *et al*. A critical comparison of the dose delivery characteristics of four alternative inhalation devices delivering salbutamol: pressurized metered dose inhaler, Diskus inhaler, Diskhaler inhaler and Turbuhaler inhaler. *J Aerosol Med* 1999;**12**:75–84.

143 Johnson M. Inhaled corticosteroid – long acting beta-agonist synergism: therapeutic implications in human lung disease. In: Dalby RN, Byron PR, Peart J, Suman JD, Farr SJ, eds. *Respiratory Drug Delivery IX*. River Grove, Illinois: Davis Healthcare International, 2004: 99–108.

144 Newman SP. Dry powder inhalers for optimal drug delivery. *Expert Opinion on Biological Therapy* 2004;**4**:23–33.

145 Bondesson E, Friberg K, Soliman S *et al*. Safety and efficacy of a high cumulative dose of salbutamol inhaled via Turbuhaler or via a pressurised metered dose inhaler in patients with asthma. *Respir Med* 1998;**92**:325–30.

146 Borgström L, Bondesson E, Morén F *et al*. Lung deposition of budesonide inhaled via Turbuhaler: a comparison with terbutaline sulphate in normal subjects. *Eur Respir J* 1994; **7**:69–73.

147 Newman SP, Hollingworth A, Clark AR. Effect of different modes of inhalation on drug delivery from a dry powder inhaler. *Int J Pharm* 1994;**102**:127–32.

148 Hirst PH, Newman SP, Clark DA *et al*. Lung deposition of budesonide from the novel dry powder inhaler Airmax. *Respir Med* 2002;**96**:389–96.

149 Pedersen S. How to use a Rotahaler. *Arch Dis Childhood* 1986; **61**:11–4.

150 Everard ML, Devadson SG, Le Souef PN. Early inspiratory flow determines the aerosol particle size distribution from a Turbuhaler. *Eur Respir J* 1996;**8**(Suppl):204S.

151 Duddu SP, Sisk SA, Walter YH *et al.* Improved lung delivery from a passive dry powder inhaler using an engineered PulmoSphere powder. *Pharm Res* 2002;**19**:689–95.

152 Dunbar C, Scheuch G, Sommerer K *et al. In vitro* and *in vivo* dose delivery characteristics of large porous particles for inhalation. *Int J Pharm* 2002;**245**:179–89.

153 White S, Bennett D, Stevenson C *et al.* Exubera: development of a novel technology solution for pulmonary delivery of insulin. In: Dalby RN, Byron PR, Peart J, Suman JD, eds. *Respiratory Drug Delivery Europe 2005.* River Grove, Illinois: Davis Healthcare International, 2005: 225–7.

154 Labiris NR, Dolovich MB. Pulmonary drug delivery. Part 2: the role of inhalant delivery devices and drug formulations in therapeutic effectiveness of aerosolised medications. *Br J Clin Pharmacol* 2003;**56**:600–12.

155 Nsour W, Alldred A, Corrado OJ *et al.* Measurement of peak inspiration rates with an In-Check meter to identify an elderly patient's ability to use a Turbuhaler. *Respir Med* 2001;**95**:965–8.

156 Dewar M, Jamieson A, McLean A *et al.* Peak inspiratory flow through Turbuhaler in chronic obstructive airways disease. *Respir Med* 1999;**93**:342–4.

157 Borgström L. On the use of dry powder inhalers in situations perceived as constrained. *J Aerosol Med* 2001;**14**:281–7.

158 Hansen NCG, Evald T, Ibsen TB. Terbutaline inhalations by the Turbuhaler as replacement for domiciliary nebulizer therapy in severe chronic obstructive pulmonary disease. *Respir Med* 1994;**88**:267–71.

159 Dolovich MB, Ahrens RC, Hess DR *et al.* Device selection and outcomes of aerosol therapy: evidence-based guidelines. *Chest* 2005;**127**:335–71.

160 Staniforth JN, Braithwaite P, Ganderton D *et al.* Advanced pulmonary systems: a novel high performance formulation-integrated dry powder inhaler for peptide and protein systemic drug delivery. In: *Drug Delivery to the Lungs XII.* Bristol: The Aerosol Society, 2001: 70–3.

CHAPTER 42

Gastro-oesophageal reflux

John K. DiBaise

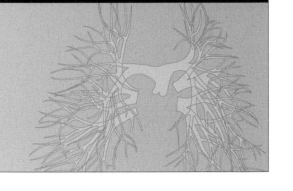

Gastro-oesophageal reflux disease (GERD) reflects a spectrum of disease that is among the most common gastrointestinal conditions seen in a variety of physician practices. Its importance, however, lies not only in its prevalence but also in its diversity of clinical presentations, potential for morbidity and mortality, and high rate of health-care utilization. Much progress has been made in our understanding of the pathophysiology of GERD over the last two decades and the recent introduction of potent antisecretory agents and laparoscopic and endoscopic techniques to treat GERD has resulted in increased interest in this disorder from both lay and scientific communities.

GERD can have a major impact on pulmonary disease. While the association between GERD and pulmonary disease has been best characterized in asthma, GERD has been associated with a variety of other respiratory symptoms and disorders, including chronic obstructive pulmonary disease (COPD). This chapter is intended to provide a general overview of GERD including its prevalence, pathophysiology, presentation, diagnosis and treatment. In the process, a more focused review of the association between GERD and COPD is provided.

Epidemiology and risk factors

Information regarding the prevalence of GERD in the general population has been assessed in a number of epidemiological studies that have typically used the classic symptoms of GERD – heartburn and acid regurgitation – as indicators of the disease. A recent survey of residents from Olmsted County, Minnesota found that the prevalence of heartburn or regurgitation occurring on a yearly, monthly and weekly basis was approximately 60%, 40% and 20%, respectively [1]. In contrast to other studies that suggest an increased prevalence of GERD in males and with increasing age, no significant differences were found relative to gender or age

in this study, although a trend was noted for an inverse association between heartburn and increasing age. The actual prevalence of GERD is probably even higher if those patients with GERD but without heartburn or regurgitation are taken into account. Indeed, patients with so-called 'extraoesophageal' or 'atypical' presentations of GERD are commonly encountered in clinical practice and often do not complain of associated heartburn or regurgitation [2].

GERD is not unique to the USA as similar findings have been reported in Europe [3]. Interestingly, GERD appears to be less common in persons of Asian origin [4], suggesting an influence by cultural factors. Nevertheless, it should be noted that a study from China suggests a prevalence similar to that of Western countries [5]. Certainly, these differences may be explained, at least in part, by differences in the definitions of GERD that were used. Our knowledge of GERD prevalence in minority populations within the USA remains relatively poor.

The role of genetic factors in GERD is unknown. Recently, a gene for severe GERD in children was mapped to chromosome 13q14 [6]. A familial relationship to GERD has been suggested as the prevalence of GERD increases substantially in persons with first-degree relatives with Barrett's oesophagus or oesophageal adenocarcinoma, two complications of GERD [7]. Interestingly, in this study, first-degree relatives of patients with reflux oesophagitis were not more likely to have GERD compared with spouse control relatives, suggesting that there may be genetic predisposition to the development of GERD in families of patients with Barrett's oesophagus and oesophageal adenocarcinoma, but that environmental factors may be more important for uncomplicated reflux. A genetic influence is also supported by a recent report showing an increased concordance for GERD in monozygotic compared with dizygotic twins [8]. It was concluded that genetic influences may account for approximately 31% of the liability to GERD.

Table 42.1 Potential risk factors for developing gastro-oesophageal reflux disease (GERD).

Hiatal hernia
Obesity
Alcohol use
Cigarette smoking
Nasogastric intubation
Medications
Pregnancy
Hypersecretory states
Delayed gastric emptying
Connective tissue diseases
Helicobacter pylori

Table 42.2 Pathophysiology of gastro-oesophageal reflux disease (GERD).

Antireflux barrier
Lower oesophageal sphincter
  increased frequency of tLOSR
  weak resting pressure
Crural diaphragm
Hiatal hernia

Oesophageal factors
Diminished oesophageal clearance
  ineffective peristalsis
  abnormal salivation
Impaired oesophageal mucosal resistance
Altered oesophageal mucosal sensitivity (?)

Gastric factors
Delayed gastric emptying
Production of acid and pepsin
Duodenogastro-oesophageal (non-acid) reflux (?)
Presence of *Helicobacter pylori* (?)

tLOSR, transient lower oesophageal sphincter relaxation.

A number of risk factors for developing GERD have been described (Table 42.1). For several of these putative risk factors the evidence supporting their role is weak, while for others the mechanism(s) by which they act to cause reflux remains unclear [9].

Pathogenesis

The fundamental prerequisite for the development of GERD is movement of the gastric refluxate into the oesophagus. A complete understanding of the pathophysiology of GERD, which is multizfactorial and consists primarily of both oesophageal and gastric factors (Table 42.2), requires consideration of both the determinants of oesophageal acid exposure and the defence mechanisms of the oesophageal epithelium [10]. The major factor responsible for reflux is a defect in the antireflux barrier, which is composed of the lower oesophageal sphincter (LOS), diaphragm and supporting ligaments. The integrity of the antireflux barrier has been attributed to maintenance of intrinsic LOS pressure, contribution by the crural diaphragm to the resting tone of the LOS and its augmentation of this tone during inspiration, preservation of the intra-abdominal location of the LOS, the integrity of the phrenoesophageal ligament, and maintenance of the angle of His which represents the angle of entry of the oesophagus into the stomach. It seems likely that it is an accumulation of abnormalities involving these mechanisms that leads to incompetence of the antireflux barrier and subsequent oesophageal acid exposure.

The occurrence of inappropriate, non-swallow-related LOS relaxation, also known as transient LOS relaxation (tLOSR) rather than a hypotensive LOS or a hiatal hernia is currently believed to be the most common cause of reflux events in both healthy individuals and patients with GERD [11]. Nevertheless, recent evidence suggests that the dominant mechanism may vary depending upon the disease severity, with tLOSR being the main mechanism with mild disease and a hypotensive LOS or hiatal hernia dominating with more severe disease [12]. Major differences between tLOSR and swallow-induced LOS relaxation include that tLOSR occurs without pharyngeal contraction, is not accompanied by oesophageal peristalsis and persists longer. Interestingly, not all tLOSR is accompanied by acid reflux. The major stimulus for tLOSR is gastric distension and it is now clear that tLOSR has a major role in the venting of gas from the stomach (i.e. belching).

A hypotensive LOS may result in either strain-induced reflux or free reflux. Free reflux occurs when the LOS pressure is very low, typically less than 4 mmHg, and is characterized by a fall in intraoesophageal pH without a change in LOS or intragastric pressure. In contrast, strain-induced reflux occurs when a more modestly hypotensive LOS, typically less than 10 mmHg, is overcome by a sudden increase in intra-abdominal pressure. The crural diaphragm has an important role in the competence of the oesophagogastric junction by contributing to the resting tone of the LOS and by augmenting this tone during inspiration [13,14]. A hiatal hernia results in the absence of these additive effects on the LOS and may also impair oesophageal emptying resulting in the re-reflux of hernia contents by permitting retrograde flow of gastric material during LOS relaxation. Recently, it has been shown that the susceptibility to reflux correlates with both weak LOS pressure and with hiatal hernia size [13]; however, a hiatal hernia is neither necessary nor sufficient for the development of reflux oesophagitis.

In addition to the actual occurrence of reflux episodes, oesophageal acid exposure is also related to the process of oesophageal clearance. Therefore, defects in oesophageal clearance mechanisms such as can occur with impaired peristalsis, the presence of a hiatal hernia and impaired salivation increase the susceptibility to GERD. Another oesophageal mechanism that may have a role in the pathogenesis of GERD, particularly as it relates to tissue defence, is altered oesophageal mucosal resistance. This includes luminal factors such as the mucous layer and surface bicarbonate and elements within the epithelium such as the cell membrane and intercellular junctional complex that limit damage during contact of the refluxate with the oesophageal epithelium [15]. Abnormalities in oesophageal epithelial resistance may provide an alternative explanation for the development of GERD in patients with normal oesophageal acid exposure on ambulatory pH testing, as this would seem to imply normally functioning antireflux and clearance mechanisms. Lastly, the contribution of altered mucosal sensitivity to the pathogenesis of GERD remains unclear.

Gastric factors also have a role in the pathogenesis of GERD. The presence of gastric contents such as acid, pepsin, bile salts and pancreatic enzymes in the oesophagus is necessary for oesophageal injury to occur. While acid is clearly important, in the vast majority of GERD patients, there is no evidence of gastric acid hypersecretion. Bile salts and pancreatic enzymes enter the stomach by what is referred to as duodenogastric reflux. While the role of pepsin and bile remains controversial [16], it is currently believed that these substances may contribute to the injury and symptoms that occur as a consequence of gastro-oesophageal reflux, but are unlikely to cause these problems without the aid of acid. The rate of gastric emptying may also be of pathophysiological importance in GERD. Delayed gastric emptying exists commonly in patients with GERD [17] but is suspected to be of pathogenetic importance in only a small proportion. A final gastric factor that has generated considerable interest recently in relation to the pathogenesis of GERD is *Helicobacter pylori*. While there appears to be no excess of *H. pylori* infection in GERD patients when compared with age-matched controls, theory and accumulating circumstantial evidence suggest that this infection may be relatively protective against reflux when it produces gastritis severe enough to cause a major reduction of gastric acid secretion [18,19]. Similarly, when *H. pylori* infection is cured, a significant component of gastritis resolves, acid secretion increases and, theoretically, GERD may be provoked or worsened in the setting of a compromised antireflux barrier [20]. Because of the conflicting data regarding the role of *H. pylori* in GERD, the decision to test for and treat *H. pylori* should be based on other clinical indicators for eradication [21].

Diagnosis and evaluation

GERD is defined as symptoms or tissue injury resulting from exposure of the oesophagus to gastric contents. While a variety of tests are available to aid in the diagnosis of GERD (Table 42.3), there is currently no diagnostic gold standard for reflux disease. In the paragraphs that follow, the tests most clinically useful to diagnose and evaluate GERD are discussed.

The diagnosis of GERD is usually straightforward when classic symptoms are present; however, uncertainty and confusion may result when a patient presents with atypical symptoms as both classic symptoms and oesophagitis are frequently absent [2]. Additionally, not all patients with GERD are symptomatic. For example, the elderly and those with Barrett's oesophagus may be completely asymptomatic until they present with a complication. This may be a consequence of reduced sensitivity to oesophageal acid [22]. Therefore, while symptom evaluation is extremely important for diagnosis of GERD, its sensitivity falls far short of a gold standard [23].

The role of direct visualization of the oesophagus by means of endoscopy in the diagnosis of GERD is also limited because as much as two-thirds of reflux patients, even with classic symptoms, will have a normal endoscopy, both grossly and microscopically [1,24]. Furthermore, symptoms alone cannot reliably distinguish between GERD patients with and without oesophagitis on endoscopy, and the severity of GERD symptoms correlates poorly with endoscopic findings.

Ambulatory oesophageal pH testing, while frequently considered to be the gold standard, is also not so. While pH

Table 42.3 Tests used in the diagnosis of gastro-oesophageal reflux disease (GERD).

Clinically useful
Clinical history
Endoscopy
Ambulatory oesophageal pH test
Empirical trial of medication

Less or not useful
Bernstein test
Standard acid reflux (Tuttle) test
Barium oesophagram
Oesophageal biopsy
Scintigraphy
Oesophageal manometry
Bilirubin monitoring

Usefulness remains to be determined
Combined ambulatory pH-impedance test

testing has many theoretical advantages over other forms of reflux testing, a persistent problem with this technique is that there exists no absolute cut-off value that reliably identifies the presence of GERD [25]. Its use is particularly problematic in patients with atypical symptoms of suspected GERD and endoscopy-negative reflux patients as several studies have demonstrated considerable overlap in oesophageal acid exposure times between asymptomatic controls and patients with these conditions and the documentation of the presence of reflux does not prove causality of symptoms [24].

Recently, an empirical trial of antisecretory therapy has been evaluated as a diagnostic test for GERD [26]. This approach was made available by the introduction of a potent class of antisecretory medications known as proton pump inhibitors which profoundly reduce gastric acid production and the time to heal oesophagitis. With this approach, when symptoms disappear with therapy and return when the medication is stopped, the diagnosis of GERD may be assumed. This approach has been shown to have good sensitivity and specificity in patients presenting with classical reflux symptoms and in patients with suspected reflux-related non-cardiac chest pain [27,28] and has shown economic benefits compared with upfront testing in patients with non-cardiac chest pain and chronic cough [28,29]. Nevertheless, while seemingly more tolerable and cost-effective than ambulatory pH testing or endoscopy, the empirical medication trial approach does not appear to offer any diagnostic superiority. The major disadvantages of this diagnostic approach include false-positive results brought about by a placebo effect from the medication and a lack of direct assessment of either the oesophageal mucosa or oesophageal acid exposure.

The evaluation of GERD depends upon the patient's clinical presentation. Those with classic symptoms and no alarm symptoms usually require no confirmatory testing and should be treated empirically. Further testing should be performed in the following situations: presence of alarm symptoms (Table 42.4), lack of symptom response to medical therapy, need for continuous therapy in a patient at risk for Barrett's oesophagus and prior to antireflux surgery. Additionally, a more aggressive approach in the elderly is

warranted because their disease presentation is typically more severe despite milder symptoms.

A number of tests are available to aid in the evaluation of patients with GERD. These tests should be applied selectively to the individual, based upon the information desired (Table 42.5). The barium oesophagram is useful when evaluating dysphagia, particularly with suspected oropharyngeal or non-obstructive oesophageal (dysmotility)types. It is also more sensitive than endoscopy in detecting subtle mucosal (Schatzki) rings in the distal oesophagus that are associated with GERD and may result in intermittent dysphagia. Suspected obstructive oesophageal dysphagia is better off evaluated initially by endoscopy because, in addition to its overall higher diagnostic sensitivity and ability to biopsy, endoscopy allows therapeutic intervention [30]. The role of endoscopy in GERD patients without alarm symptoms is more controversial. In the era of potent therapeutic options, routine endoscopy is not advocated in all GERD patients prior to treatment and it remains an area of heated debate whether 'once-in-a-lifetime' endoscopy is necessary in patients with GERD symptoms for more than 5 years in order to identify Barrett's oesophagus, an important risk factor for oesophageal adenocarcinoma [31–33].

Oesophageal manometry provides information on the contractile activities of the oesophageal body and the upper and lower oesophageal sphincters both at rest and during swallowing. Oesophageal manometry is most helpful to localize the lower oesophageal sphincter before oesophageal pH testing and, possibly, to evaluate peristalsis prior to

---

Table 42.4 Alarm symptoms suggesting need for further evaluation.

Dysphagia
Odynophagia
Bleeding
Weight loss
Chest pain

Table 42.5 Tests used in the evaluation of gastro-oesophageal reflux disease (GERD).

*To assess suspected oesophageal injury**
Endoscopy
Barium oesophagram

To quantitate reflux†
Ambulatory oesophageal pH test
Combined ambulatory pH–impedance test

To correlate reflux with symptoms†
Ambulatory oesophageal pH test
Combined ambulatory pH–impedance test

To assess peristalsis prior to antireflux surgery
Oesophageal manometry
Combined stationary manometry–impedance test

* Patients with dysphagia or long duration of symptoms and elderly patients.
† Patients with refractory symptoms or atypical presentations and when the diagnosis is in doubt.

antireflux surgery [34], although this latter indication remains controversial [35]. In this regard, the recent introduction of a combined manometry–impedance catheter system to more thoroughly assess oesophageal function holds the potential to improve on our current ability to predict postoperative dysphagia in patients undergoing antireflux surgery [36]. Oesophageal manometry is not useful in the diagnosis of GERD or any of its complications [34].

Similarly, ambulatory oesophageal pH testing is most useful to confirm GERD prior to antireflux surgery in endoscopy-negative patients and to evaluate patients not responding to medical therapy or with recurrent or persistent symptoms after antireflux surgery [25]. An abnormal test while on medical treatment suggests the need for more aggressive therapy, while a normal test points toward an alternative diagnosis. Oesophageal pH testing is not needed in patients with existing or a known history of reflux oesophagitis.

A therapeutic trial with a proton pump inhibitor, as opposed to initial pH testing, seems to be more useful in identifying a causal relationship between reflux and extra-oesophageal or atypical presentations. Ambulatory pH testing while on medical therapy can then be reserved for those patients not responding [37].

The concept that symptoms or complications of GERD may be related to the reflux of non-acid contents has also received recent attention. This is particularly true in the group of patients whose symptoms, whether they are classic or atypical, persist despite aggressive antisecretory therapy or those with symptoms thought to be brought about by reflux but who have a normal pH test. Until recently, there were no sufficiently sensitive tests to detect duodenogastro-oesophageal or non-acid reflux. Two tests are now available that may assist in the detection of non-acid reflux: bilirubin monitoring and combined pH and multichannel intraluminal impedance monitoring.

Bilirubin monitoring is performed much like ambulatory oesophageal pH testing; however, the catheter contains a fibreoptic probe and a spectrophotometer measures the absorption of certain wavelengths in order to detect bilirubin. The presence of bilirubin as a surrogate marker of bile suggests the presence of duodenogastro-oesophageal reflux. Because bilirubin reflux has been found to consistently parallel acid reflux in patients with an intact stomach [38], at the present time, bilirubin monitoring has demonstrated little clinical utility and is used primarily as a research tool.

The combination of standard pH testing with multichannel impedance measurements in the same catheter was recently approved for clinical use. This technique is performed much like pH testing; however, the addition of impedance technology allows for the detection of all types of refluxate within the oesophagus, not just acidic [39–41]. While a promising technique, it remains to be seen whether combined pH–impedance testing will be a clinically useful tool or primarily a research tool.

Clinical presentations and complications

The spectrum of GERD symptoms is diverse and ranges from classic heartburn and acid regurgitation to the less common oesophageal symptoms of dysphagia, odynophagia, water brash, belching, nausea, hiccups and chest pain. In addition, a multitude of extraoesophageal symptoms and conditions that seem to be related to reflux disease are being increasingly recognized (Table 42.6). Given the prevalence of GERD, multiple oesophageal complications of the disease are frequently encountered in clinical practice. The major oesophageal complications of GERD include varying degrees of oesophagitis, peptic stricture and Barrett's oesophagus. Non-cardiac chest pain is also sometimes considered in this category.

The prevalence of oesophagitis seen in patients who undergo endoscopy for reflux symptoms varies considerably; however, it appears to be less than 50%, and probably less than 25% [42]. Presenting symptoms typically include a long history of heartburn and may also include dysphagia, odynophagia, anorexia and chest pain. Reflux oesophagitis is characterized endoscopically by beginning

Table 42.6 Extraoesophageal presentations of gastro-oesophageal reflux disease (GERD).

Pulmonary
Asthma
Chronic cough
Aspiration pneumonia
Obstructive sleep apnoea
Chronic obstructive pulmonary disease
Sudden infant death syndrome

Ear, nose and throat
Hoarseness
Globus sensation
Chronic sinusitis
Pharyngitis
Vocal cord granuloma, ulcer, nodule
Laryngeal, subglottic stenosis
Laryngeal cancer
Otitis media

Oral
Dental erosions
Halitosis
Dysgeusia

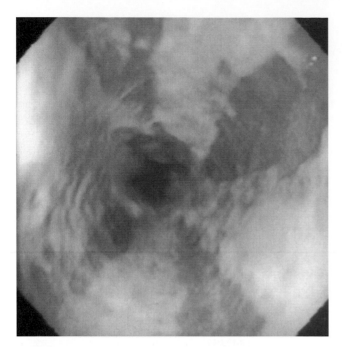

Figure 42.1 Endoscopic photograph of severe reflux oesophagitis. Note the circumferential involvement and several linear erosions with overlying exudate and surrounding erythema extending upward from the gastro-oesophageal junction.

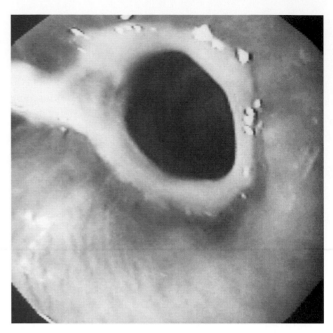

Figure 42.2 Endoscopic photograph of a peptic stricture. Note the circumferential ulceration and narrowing at the gastro-oesophageal junction.

at the oesophagogastric junction and progressing proximally (Fig. 42.1). When severe, oesophagitis can obscure underlying Barrett's oesophagus. The incidence of brisk bleeding as a consequence of oesophagitis, regardless of the severity, is uncommon. It has been suggested that the elderly, those with chronic renal insufficiency and those using anticoagulants or non-steroidal anti-inflammatory drugs (NSAIDs) may be at increased risk of bleeding from oesophagitis [43]. Another obscure and frequently overlooked cause of gastrointestinal bleeding in GERD patients may be seen in those with a large hiatal hernia. Cameron's erosion or ulceration occurs at the diaphragmatic hiatus of a large hiatal hernia and may result in brisk hemorrhage or, more commonly, chronic occult blood loss and iron deficiency anaemia [44].

Peptic strictures (Fig. 42.2) generally occur at the squamocolumnar junction and may occur in up to 10% of patients with GERD who receive medical care and approximately 20% of patients with reflux oesophagitis. While there are currently no reliable risk factors for the development of peptic strictures, the incidence seems to increase with age, those using NSAIDs and in Caucasian men [45–47]. One curious aspect of peptic strictures is that they often develop in patients who have few classic GERD symptoms. This further emphasizes the point that there is little correlation between the severity of GERD symptoms and

severity of findings on endoscopy. Presenting symptoms typically include dysphagia with solids and, less often, odynophagia and food impaction. While either barium oesophagography or endoscopy can be used to diagnose a peptic stricture, endoscopy has the advantage of having both diagnostic and therapeutic capabilities [30]. Barium oesophagography can then be reserved for complex strictures including those that do not allow passage of the endoscope. Peptic strictures can usually be effectively treated and recurrence prevented by aggressive antireflux therapy in the form of a proton pump inhibitor [48] or surgery combined with intermittent dilatation as needed. The need for redilatation varies markedly; some patients will require only a single dilatation while others may need weekly dilatations for several months and still others require less frequent maintenance dilatations to avoid recurrent dysphagia or food impactions. For patients with strictures refractory to repeated dilatation, oesophageal resection may be necessary. For those who are poor surgical candidates, oesophageal stenting has been proposed as an alternative to surgery [49].

Barrett's oesophagus is a condition in which specialized columnar epithelium (with goblet cells), also referred to as intestinal metaplasia, replaces the damaged squamous epithelium in the distal oesophagus (Fig. 42.3). It is now generally accepted that this results from long-standing severe GERD and is the single most important risk factor for oesophageal adenocarcinoma [50,51]. In this regard, it

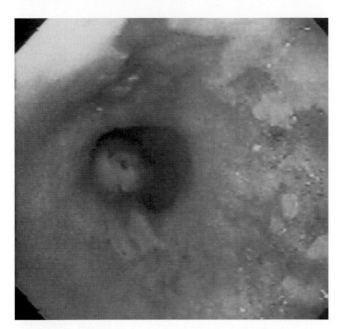

Figure 42.3 Endoscopic photograph of Barrett's oesophagus. Note the mucosa extending upward from the gastro-oesophageal junction.

should be noted that a large case–control study conducted in Sweden recently found that there is a strong and probably causal relationship between GERD and oesophageal adenocarcinoma, independent of the presence of Barrett's oesophagus (odds ratio 43.5; 95% confidence interval [CI], 18.3–103.5) in individuals with long-standing and severe symptoms of reflux [52]. Because of the dramatic increase in the incidence of oesophageal adenocarcinoma, estimated at 300–500% over the last 30–40 years, these data underscore the importance of early recognition and appropriate management of GERD. Nevertheless, in 2002, only half of the 13 100 anticipated oesophageal cancers are expected to be adenocarcinoma. Therefore, despite the increase in incidence, oesophageal adenocarcinoma remains an uncommon tumour and thus represents a small risk for an individual patient [33].

The frequency of Barrett's oesophagus varies depending upon the population studied but usually ranges from 10 to 20% [53]. There is a strong male and Caucasian predominance with an average age at diagnosis of approximately 55 years. The prevalence of adenocarcinoma in Barrett's oesophagus is approximately 10%, while the annual incidence rate in those with known Barrett's undergoing surveillance is approximately 0.5% [54]. Endoscopic surveillance for cancer and dysplasia, the precursor to cancer, is currently considered the standard of care; however, its usefulness and cost-effectiveness remains highly controversial [33]. While surveillance is unlikely to be effective for the GERD population as a whole, endoscopic screening of

all persons with GERD would seem to be infeasible and cost-prohibitive. Nevertheless, a recent cost–utility analysis concluded that screening for Barrett's oesophagus in a high-risk population of 50-year-old white men with symptoms of GERD is cost-effective compared with other accepted medical interventions [55]. Recent recommendations suggest endoscopy for all persons with typical GERD symptoms for at least 5 years, particularly middle-aged Caucasian men, to screen for Barrett's [31]. Alternative methods of screening for Barrett's oesophagus such as cytologic sampling via a transoral balloon-tipped catheter in an unsedated patient, much as is performed in China when screening for squamous cell oesophageal cancer, are currently undergoing investigation in humans [56]. In order to improve our existing screening and surveillance strategies, much investigation is currently being directed at the discovery of biomarkers other than dysplasia that have an improved degree of predictability for the subsequent development of cancer.

The management of patients with Barrett's oesophagus consists of treatment of the associated GERD symptoms, endoscopic surveillance to detect and follow-up dysplasia, and treatment of dysplasia [32]. It remains controversial whether aggressive antireflux therapy, medical or surgical, will lead to regression of Barrett's or dysplasia, or prevent the development of cancer. While techniques exist to ablate the metaplastic and dysplastic epithelium such as photodynamic therapy, argon plasma coagulation and multipolar electrocoagulation, their complication rates are substantial, their overall benefit remains unclear and, as such, these methods are considered investigational [32,33].

The oesophagus may be implicated in almost half of those patients with non-cardiac chest pain. Several mechanisms have been postulated including GERD, dysmotility, ischaemia and abnormal oesophageal sensation or perception. Primary oesophageal motor disorders are very uncommon in these patients [57]. While recent studies suggest that GERD is by far the most common cause of non-cardiac chest pain, opinion seems to be shifting more toward sensory or perception dysfunction. In general, after exclusion of a cardiac source, which is usually not possible based upon historical information alone, it may be reasonable to proceed with an empirical trial of high-dose antisecretory therapy in these patients, particularly if they have typical reflux symptoms [28]. Further evaluation can then be reserved for those without improvement.

Physicians are becoming increasingly aware that GERD may have respiratory and ear, nose and throat manifestations (see Table 42.6). Unfortunately, a direct relationship between GERD and these conditions has been difficult to establish. Other factors contributing to this dilemma include the findings that approximately 40% of these patients will deny any classic reflux symptoms and reflux oesophagitis is generally absent [58,59]. Indeed, the high prevalence of absence of concomitant classical GERD symptoms or oesophagitis in patients with these conditions has led some individuals to refer to this condition not as GERD, but rather as laryngopharyngeal reflux. Two mechanisms have been implicated in the pathogenesis of these extraoesophageal presentations: direct acid contact as a consequence of reflux of gastric contents through the upper oesophageal sphincter (reflux theory) or a vagally mediated reflex initiated by acid exposure in the oesophagus (reflex theory) [60]. Evidence supporting these mechanisms is rather scanty and generally indirect. The degree of importance each of these proposed mechanisms has in causing the various extraoesophageal manifestations remains unclear but probably differs depending upon the condition. Data from our motility laboratory do not support the hypothesis that the nature of the clinical presentation of GERD is related to different patterns of oesophageal acid exposure or oesophageal motility as measured by conventional manometry and dual-channel pH testing [61]. The role of tLOSR in the pathophysiology of extraoesophageal complications of GERD remains unknown at this time.

Ambulatory oesophageal pH testing has been considered to be the best diagnostic tool for identifying extraoesophageal complications of GERD. This technique offers the best opportunity to document the amount and proximal extent of acid reflux. Nevertheless, continuing controversy exists regarding a number of issues related to this technique including the need for single versus multichannel pH monitoring, the optimal position of the proximal probe (pharyngeal versus upper oesophagus) if used, the lack of well-established normal values, poor reproducibility and the occurrence of artefacts involving the proximal pH sensor. There also seems to be a tendency for false-negative tests; thus, a negative test may not confidently exclude the diagnosis. Lastly, and perhaps most importantly, a positive test only confirms that an abnormal amount of gastro-oesophageal reflux is present and does not prove a causal relationship. This can only be assured with confidence when the atypical symptom of suspected GERD shows sustained, dramatic improvement following aggressive treatment of GERD. Therefore, at the present time, there are no sufficiently reliable diagnostic tests that can accurately predict which patients have GERD-related extraoesophageal complications. As a consequence, controlled therapeutic trials may be the only method currently available to answer this question.

GERD and COPD

While there is sufficient evidence showing an association between GERD and chronic cough and asthma [62], GERD may also have a role in many other common pulmonary disorders. The close anatomical relationship and common embryonic origins of the oesophagus and tracheobronchial tree may aid in the explanation of this association. There is a small body of data to suggest a relationship between GERD and COPD. A recent retrospective case–control study from 172 Veterans Administration hospitals involving more than 200 000 discharges found that patients with a diagnosis of oesophagitis or oesophageal stricture had a higher likelihood of having a number of pulmonary diseases than a control group without oesophageal disease, including COPD (odds ratio 1.22; 95% CI, 1.16–1.27) [63]. Another prospective study examined the relationship between hiatal hernia and reflux oesophagitis hospitalization and a subsequent hospitalization with respiratory outcomes in persons free of respiratory disease at baseline and at their first hospitalization [64]. They found odds ratios of 1.8 (95% CI, 1.2–2.7) for chronic bronchitis and 2.9 (95% CI, 1.5–5.5) for emphysema. Similar to the increased prevalence of COPD in patients with GERD, a recent prospective study evaluated the prevalence of GERD in patients with COPD using a validated symptom questionnaire [65]. They found an increased prevalence of frequent heartburn and/or regurgitation (19 vs 0%), dysphagia (17 vs 4%) and antireflux medication use (50 vs 27%) in COPD patients compared with a control group. Therefore, the current evidence suggests that patients with GERD have a higher prevalence of COPD than patients without GERD and patients with COPD have a higher prevalence of GERD than those without COPD.

The role of GERD in the pathogenesis of COPD remains poorly understood. In contrast to asthma patients, oesophageal acid perfusion does not seem to alter airway responsivity in patients with COPD [66,67]. Aspiration related either to GERD [68] or to alterations in oropharyngeal swallowing [69,70] has been suggested as a contributory factor in the pathogenesis of chronic bronchitis. Additional research is needed on oropharyngeal dysfunction in patients with COPD and its relationship with aspiration and COPD exacerbations.

There have been no controlled studies examining the effect of GERD treatment on the pulmonary outcome in patients with COPD. However, a recent study assessed respiratory symptoms in patients with chronic bronchitis treated with either a proton pump inhibitor ($n = 89$) or antireflux surgery ($n = 119$) and found that, although patients treated medically did not experience symptom relief, those who underwent surgery had a pronounced reduction in symptoms [69]. Further research is needed in this area.

Lung transplantation has emerged as a viable treatment option for patients with a variety of end-stage pulmonary disorders, including COPD. Upper gastrointestinal tract dysmotility and GERD appear to occur commonly following lung transplantation [71,72] and GERD-related aspiration has been suggested to be a potential contributing cause of chronic allograft rejection (bronchiolitis obliterans) [73,74]. Antireflux surgery has recently been shown to improve both reflux symptoms and lung function following lung transplantation [75]. The role of antireflux medications in this clinical scenario remains undefined.

Treatment

The major acute and long-term goals of GERD therapy are to relieve symptoms and to heal oesophagitis, thereby preventing complications. The primary treatment options include lifestyle modifications, pharmacological agents and antireflux surgery (Table 42.7). Recently, several endoluminal treatments have also been added to the therapeutic armamentarium (see Table 42.7). The vast majority of reflux patients never seek medical care and instead self-medicate using over-the-counter agents such as antacids, alginate and H_2-receptor antagonists on an as needed basis. For those who do seek medical care, the traditional (step-up) approach has been to start with lifestyle modifications and progress to medications and then surgery for persistent symptoms. A more recent alternative (step-down) approach is to start with the most potent and effective medical therapy and, when symptoms are controlled, to attempt to change therapy to a less potent or less costly agent. The better overall approach remains hotly debated; however, it has been suggested that the step-down approach is more cost-effective [76]. Ultimately, deciding whether a step-up or step-down approach is most appropriate should be based on a case-by-case evaluation.

Lifestyle modifications, which minimize reflux and maximize acid clearance, are listed in Table 42.6. Patient compliance with such changes is often poor. While the scientific evidence supporting these adaptations is generally weak, there may be some patients who benefit and do not require any pharmacological therapy as a result. In addition, many of these measures are useful in treating other diseases and in maintaining overall body health.

A number of pharmacological agents are available to treat GERD (see Table 42.7). In general, the main classes of medications are aimed at either improving the underlying motility disorder (prokinetics) or reducing the noxious effects of the gastric refluxate (antisecretory agents). Mucosal protectants such as sucralfate have demonstrated limited clinical efficacy in GERD and are uncommonly used. Antacids, which briefly neutralize acid, and alginic acid, which mixes with saliva to form a viscous layer that floats on the surface of the gastric pool acting as a mechanical barrier, are useful for treating mild and infrequent reflux symptoms. They do not, however, heal oesophagitis. Nevertheless, a large proportion of GERD patients can be adequately treated with such easily available over-the-counter therapies.

When approved in the late 1970s, H_2-receptor antagonists (H_2RAs) achieved the first real breakthrough in the treatment of GERD [77]. H_2RAs interfere predominantly with the histamine receptor at the level of the parietal and enterochromaffin-like cells, ultimately inhibiting one pathway of parietal cell activation. All four available H_2RAs are equally effective and act to decrease gastric acid production. While symptomatic improvement can be achieved in up to 60% of patients using these agents, healing of oesophagitis occurs less commonly. The over-the-counter doses of H_2RAs, although longer lasting, are generally equivalent to antacids. Higher and more frequent doses of H_2RAs do not seem to be more effective than standard doses in improving severely symptomatic patients [78] and become less cost-effective than a single daily dose proton pump inhibitor. This may be related, at least in part, to the development of tachyphylaxis. In contrast, H_2RAs are highly efficacious in decreasing nocturnal acid secretion and may be the preferred agent in those patients with persistent symptoms despite twice daily proton pump inhibitor therapy and a pH test demonstrating nocturnal acid breakthrough [79].

Prokinetic agents may work by a number of mechanisms which include increasing LOS pressure, reducing tLOSR frequency, improving oesophageal peristalsis, increasing

Table 42.7 Available treatments of gastro-oesophageal reflux disease (GERD).

Lifestyle modifications
Elevate head of bed 10–15 cm (4–6 inches)
Eat smaller meals with less fat content
Avoid recumbency for 3 h after eating
Weight reduction
Avoid smoking and alcohol
Avoid adverse medications and foods
Avoid wearing tight clothing

Pharmacological therapy
Antacids, alginate, over-the-counter H_2-receptor antagonists
H_2-receptor antagonists
Prokinetic agents
Proton pump inhibitors

Surgery
Laparoscopic (or open) fundoplication

Endoscopic/endoluminal therapy
Transoral delivery of radiofrequency energy
Transoral suturing system
Transoral injection of inert substance

salivary flow and improving gastric emptying. In general, the overall efficacy of prokinetic agents has been similar to H_2RAs. A prokinetic agent may be most useful in patients with typical reflux symptoms plus associated bloating and early satiety suggesting dysmotility. The most useful of the prokinetic agents was cisapride, a $5-HT_4$ agonist that exerted its prokinetic action through the indirect release of acetylcholine in the myenteric plexus. Because of concerns over its safety, specifically because of several reports of fatal cardiac dysrhythmias associated with the combination of cisapride and several medications and medical conditions, cisapride was withdrawn from the market in July 2000. As a consequence, there is currently no suitable prokinetic agent available for long-term use. Metoclopramide, a dopamine antagonist, is currently the only prokinetic agent available for use in the USA but has, at best, modest efficacy in relieving symptoms, no proven efficacy in healing oesophagitis and a significant incidence of side-effects. The results of ongoing clinical trials evaluating the efficacy and safety of new prokinetic agents are eagerly awaited.

Proton pump inhibitors (PPIs) profoundly diminish acid secretion by inhibiting the H^+-K^+ ATPase (proton pump), the final step in acid production. Given that the primary determinants of oesophageal healing and symptom relief are the duration of treatment and the proportion of time the intraoesophageal pH is maintained at over 4, it is no wonder that PPIs are more effective than H_2RAs [80]. While some differences exist, the five currently available PPIs seem to be equally effective with regard to symptom improvement and healing of oesophagitis. PPIs have been shown to be highly effective in both symptom reduction and healing rates of oesophagitis (up to 90%). Indeed, they are currently considered first-line treatment in complicated GERD cases. The timing of PPI ingestion seems to be important. These agents seem to be most effective at reducing gastric acid secretion when taken in the morning at least 30 min before breakfast. PPIs do not completely eliminate acid production. Dose escalation is often necessary, particularly in those patients on the more severe end of the GERD spectrum and in those with extraoesophageal complications. When administered twice daily, these drugs should be ingested at least 30 min before the morning and evening meals in order to maximize pump inhibition. Acute side-effects include headache, abdominal cramping and diarrhoea. Side-effects of long-term use are uncommon; concerns over development of gastric carcinoid tumours and atrophic gastritis have not been realized in studies following patients on high-dose omeprazole for over 12 years. Finally, while the use of a prokinetic agent in combination with an H_2RA has recently been shown to have an additive effect on maintenance of healing of reflux oesophagitis, the combination of a prokinetic agent with a PPI does not seem to provide much advantage over a PPI alone [81].

Since the introduction of laparoscopic fundoplication in the early 1990s, there has been renewed interest in antireflux surgery. While PPIs can effectively treat the most severe forms, GERD can only by cured by surgery. With the availability of the laparoscopic approach, the morbidity of antireflux surgery is greatly reduced compared with open fundoplication. The main indications for antireflux surgery include the refractory GERD patient, those who will not or cannot afford to take a daily medication long-term, and the young patient who would otherwise require a very long course of medical treatment. Because the availability of PPIs has made the truly refractory GERD patient rare, a search for an alternative diagnosis in such patients should be entertained prior to proceeding with antireflux surgery. Indeed, it is those patients who respond well to medical therapy who seem to have the best outcome following fundoplication [82]. In experienced hands, laparoscopic fundoplication is safe and highly effective; however, the long-term success rate for the laparoscopic approach is unknown and certain side-effects, such as dysphagia and the gas–bloat syndrome, may be more frequent. Current data suggest that PPI therapy and antireflux surgery are approximately equal for maintaining remission in GERD [83]. Indeed, available evidence suggests that antireflux surgery has no clear advantage over medical therapy for GERD in terms of symptom control, oesophageal healing, efficacy in preventing complications, safety and cost [84]. Ultimately, the decision to undergo surgery should be determined on an individual basis taking into account the goals, expectations and risks involved.

Recognizing the importance of tLOSR in the pathogenesis of GERD, there is now substantial interest in the development of treatments that modulate tLOSR as potential therapy for GERD. Several recent reports indicate that a number of pharmacological agents such as a loxiglumide, baclofen, morphine and atropine can reduce the frequency of tLOSR in healthy individuals and patients with GERD [85]. While none of the agents tested thus far are suitable for long-term clinical use, this remains an intriguing area likely to see major developments in the treatment of GERD.

Three novel transoral endoluminal approaches to the treatment of GERD have recently become available for clinical use. One utilizes a suturing system attached to the tip of the endoscope, the second delivers thermocouple-controlled radiofrequency energy to the region of the gastro-oesophageal junction via a bougie catheter delivery system, and the third method involves the endoscopic implantation of a biocompatible non-biodegradable liquid polymer to the same region. Preliminary studies have demonstrated encouraging results for all three techniques [86–88]. Where these therapies will fit into the overall treatment strategy remains to be determined.

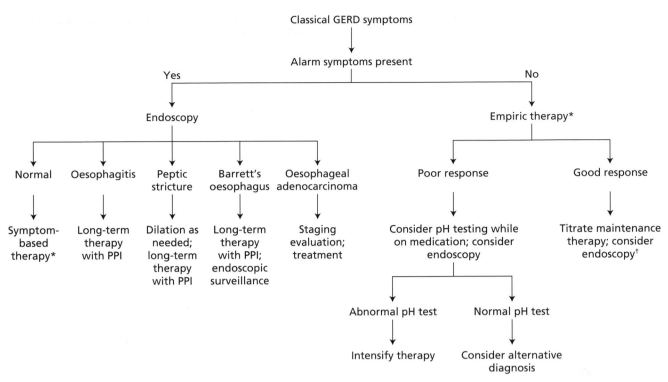

Figure 42.4 Algorithm for the acute and long-term management of the patient with classical gastro-oesophageal reflux disease (GERD) symptoms. Alarm symptoms include dysphagia, odynophagia, weight loss and bleeding. PPI, proton pump inhibitor. * Guided by symptom severity. † To evaluate for Barrett's oesophagus.

Practical approach to evaluation and management

Figure 42.4 illustrates a suggested approach for managing the patient with classic GERD symptoms. Initially, these patients should be evaluated for the presence of alarm symptoms. If present, further diagnostic evaluation, usually endoscopy, is necessary. If absent, empirical therapy guided by symptom severity should be commenced. In those who require long-term therapy for severe symptoms, endoscopy should be considered, even in those with good symptom relief and without alarm symptoms, in order to evaluate for the presence of Barrett's oesophagus. If the patient responds poorly to therapy, further diagnostic testing should be considered. In this setting, endoscopy may be useful to evaluate for other potential aetiologies of the symptoms and oesophageal pH testing, while on therapy, may be useful to assess its adequacy. The management of oesophagitis without Barrett's oesophagus, endoscopy-negative GERD and Barrett's oesophagus is based primarily on symptom relief. Finally, at the present time, patients with Barrett's oesophagus should be enrolled into an endoscopic surveillance programme.

A similar approach to the management of patients with atypical manifestations of GERD, including chest pain, pulmonary and ear, nose and throat symptoms, is illustrated in Figure 42.5. Management of these conditions tends to require higher doses of antisecretory agents for prolonged periods of time [2]. At this time, there are insufficient data to declare any one approach as best. Previously, early oesophageal pH testing, particularly in those patients who did not have concomitant classic GERD symptoms, was recommended as the best initial test for identifying abnormal oesophageal acid exposure and correlating these symptoms with reflux episodes. However, as addressed earlier, several problems arise when oesophageal pH testing is used to identify the potential role of reflux in patients with suspected atypical GERD-related conditions. As a result of the complex relationship of symptoms, presence of GERD and causality, the use of aggressive therapeutic trials, typically with a twice daily PPI, has been advocated to identify patients with true GERD-related atypical symptoms. This approach has been supported by recent reports suggesting that an empirical trial of a twice daily PPI for 2–3 months may be more cost-effective than early testing [29,89]. If no response is seen after this extended therapeutic trial, oesophageal pH testing, while on therapy, is

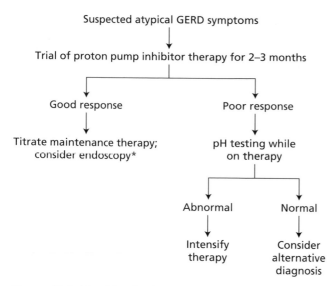

Suspected atypical GERD symptoms

Trial of proton pump inhibitor therapy for 2–3 months

Good response

Poor response

Titrate maintenance therapy; consider endoscopy*

pH testing while on therapy

Abnormal

Normal

Intensify therapy

Consider alternative diagnosis

Figure 42.5 Algorithm for the management of the patient with suspected atypical gastro-oesophageal reflux disease (GERD) symptoms with or without concomitant classical GERD symptoms. * To evaluate for Barrett's oesophagus.

suggested in order to assess its adequacy. For those who do respond, gradual titration of the therapy downward is recommended.

Conclusions

GERD is a common condition with a diversity of clinical presentations, potential for morbidity and mortality, and a high rate of health-care utilization. On the basis of its pathophysiology, GERD is most appropriately considered to be an upper gut motility disorder. Nevertheless, it is acid and possibly other factors present within the gastric refluxate that cause GERD symptoms and oesophageal inflammation. The goals of GERD therapy are to relieve symptoms, heal oesophagitis and prevent complications. Acid suppression is now established as first-line therapy, with antireflux surgery being considered in selected circumstances. While those with classical symptoms and without alarm symptoms may be treated empirically, endoscopy may be useful to identify Barrett's oesophagus even in those who respond well to therapy. Atypical symptoms that fail to respond to PPI therapy and poorly responsive classic symptoms are best evaluated by ambulatory oesophageal pH testing while on therapy. The role of combined multichannel intraluminal impedance testing with oesophageal manometry and pH testing in the evaluation of oesophageal function and non-acid reflux remains to be determined. Further study regarding the optimal cost-effective diagnostic and therapeutic strategies in GERD is needed.

References

1 Locke GR, Talley NJ, Fett SJ, Zinsmeister AR, Melton LJ. Prevalence and clinical spectrum of gastroesophageal reflux: a population-based study in Olmsted County, Minnesota. *Gastroenterology* 1997;**112**:1448–56.

2 Richter JE. Extraoesophageal presentations of gastroesophageal reflux disease. *Semin Gastroenterol Dis* 1997;**8**:75–89.

3 Provenzale D. Epidemiology of gastroesophageal reflux disease. In: Orlando R, ed. *Gastroesophageal Reflux Disease*. New York: Marcel Dekker, 2000: 85–99.

4 Horiki N, Maruyama M, Uchiyama M *et al*. The prevalence of gastroesophageal reflux disease in western and oriental countries. *Gastroenterology* 1999;**116**:A189 (abstract).

5 Chang CS, Poon SK, Lien HC, Chen GH. The incidence of reflux esophagitis among the Chinese. *Am J Gastroenterol* 1997;**92**:668–71.

6 Hu FZ, Preston RA, Post JC *et al*. Mapping of a gene for severe pediatric gastroesophageal reflux to chromosome 13q14. *JAMA* 2000;**284**:325–34.

7 Romero Y, Cameron AJ, Locke GR *et al*. Familial aggregation of gastroesophageal reflux in patients with Barrett's esophagus and esophageal adenocarcinoma. *Gastroenterology* 1997; **113**:1449–56.

8 Cameron AJ, Lagergren J, Henriksson C *et al*. Gastroesophageal reflux disease in monozygotic and dizygotic twins. *Gastroenterology* 2002;**122**:55–9.

9 Horwhat JD, Wong RKH. Risk factors for gastroesophageal reflux disease. In: Orlando R, ed. *Gastroesophageal Reflux Disease*. New York: Marcel Dekker, 2000: 27–83.

10 Kahrilas PJ, Shi G. Pathophysiology of gastroesophageal reflux disease. In: Orlando R, ed. *Gastroesophageal Reflux Disease*. New York: Marcel Dekker, 2000: 137–63.

11 Mittal RK, Holloway RH, Penagini R, Blackshaw LA, Dent J. Transient lower esophageal sphincter relaxation. *Gastroenterology* 1995;**109**:601–10.

12 Barnham CP, Gotley DC, Alderson D. Precipitating causes of acid reflux episodes in ambulant patients with gastro-oesophageal reflux disease. *Gut* 1995;**36**:505–10.

13 Sloan S, Rademaker AW, Kahrilas PJ. Determinants of gastroesophageal junction competence: hiatal hernia, lower esophageal sphincter, or both? *Ann Intern Med* 1992:**117**: 977–82.

14 Mittal RK, Balaban DH. The esophagogastric junction. *N Engl J Med* 1997;**336**:924–32.

15 Orlando RC. Pathophysiology of gastroesophageal reflux disease: esophageal epithelial resistance. In: Castell DO, Richter JE, eds. *The Esophagus*. Philadelphia: Lippincott Williams & Wilkins, 1999: 409–20.

16 Vaezi MF, Singh S, Richter JE. Role of acid and duodenogastric reflux in esophageal mucosal injury: a review of animal and human studies. *Gastroenterology* 1995;**108**:1897–907.

17 McCallum RW, Berkowitz DM, Lerner E. Gastric emptying in patients with gastroesophageal reflux. *Gastroenterology* 1981;**80**:285–91.

18 Csendes A, Smok G, Cerda G *et al*. Prevalence of *Helicobacter pylori* infection in 190 control subjects and in 236 patients

with gastroesophageal reflux, erosive esophagitis or Barrett's esophagus. *Dis Esophagus* 1997;**10**:38–42.

19 Labenz J, Malfertheiner P. *Helicobacter pylori* in gastro-oesophageal reflux disease: causal agent, independent or protective factor? *Gut* 1997;**41**:277–80.

20 Verdú E, Armstrong D, Fraser R *et al.* Effect of *Helicobacter pylori* status on intragastric pH during treatment with omeprazole. *Gut* 1995;**36**:539–43.

21 Vakil N. Gastroesophageal reflux disease and *Helicobacter pylori* infection. *Rev Gastroenterol Disord* 2003;**3**:1–7.

22 Lasch H, Castell DO, Castell JA. Evidence for diminished visceral pain with aging: studies using graded intraesophageal balloon distension. *Am J Physiol* 1997;**272**:G1–3.

23 Klauser AG, Schindlbeck NE, Müller-Lissner SA. Symptoms in gastro-oesophageal reflux disease. *Lancet* 1990;**335**:205–8.

24 Lind T, Havelund T, Carlsson R *et al.* Heartburn without oesophagitis: efficacy of omeprazole therapy and features determining therapeutic response. *Scand J Gastroenterol* 1997;**32**: 974–9.

25 Kahrilas PJ, Quigley EMM. Clinical esophageal pH recording: a technical review for practice guideline development. *Gastroenterology* 1996;**110**:1982–96.

26 Johnsson F, Weywadt L, Solhaug JH, Hernqvist H, Bengtsson L. One week omeprazole treatment in the diagnosis of gastro-oesophageal reflux disease. *Scand J Gastroenterol* 1998;**33**: 15–20.

27 Schindlbeck NE, Klauser AG, Voderholzer WA, Muller-Lissner S. Empiric therapy for gastroesophageal reflux disease. *Arch Intern Med* 1995;**155**:1808–15.

28 Fass R, Fennerty MB, Ofman J. The clinical and economic value of a short course of omeprazole in patients with non-cardiac chest pain. *Gastroenterology* 1998;**115**:42–9.

29 Ours TM, Kavuru MS, Schilz RH, Richter JE. A prospective evaluation of esophageal testing and a double-blind, randomized study of omeprazole in a diagnostic and therapeutic algorithm for chronic cough. *Am J Gastroenterol* 1999;**94**: 3131–8.

30 Esfandyari T, Potter JW, Vaezi MF. Dysphagia: a cost analysis of the diagnostic approach. *Am J Gastroenterol* 2002;**97**:2733–7.

31 Fennerty MB. Barrett's esophagus: what do we really know about this disease? *Am J Gastroenterol* 1997;**92**:1–3.

32 Sampliner RE. Updated guidelines for the diagnosis, surveillance, and therapy of Barrett's esophagus. *Am J Gastroenterol* 2002;**97**:1888–95.

33 Shaheen N, Ransohoff DF. Gastroesophageal reflux, Barrett esophagus, and esophageal cancer: scientific review. *JAMA* 2002;**287**:1972–81.

34 Ergun GA, Kahrilas PJ. Clinical applications of esophageal manometry and pH monitoring. *Am J Gastroenterol* 1996;**91**: 1077–89.

35 Fibbe C, Layer P, Keller J *et al.* Esophageal motility in reflux disease before and after fundoplication: a prospective, randomized, clinical, and manometric study. *Gastroenterology* 2001;**121**:5–14.

36 Srinivasan R, Vela MF, Katz PO *et al.* Esophageal function testing using multichannel intraluminal impedance. *Am J Physiol Gastrointest Liver Physiol* 2001;**280**:G457–62.

37 Katzka DA, Paoletti V, Leite L, Castell DO. Prolonged ambulatory pH monitoring in patients with persistent gastroesophageal reflux symptoms: testing while on therapy identifies the need for more aggressive antireflux therapy. *Am J Gastroenterol* 1996;**91**:2110–3.

38 Vaezi MF, Richter JE. Contribution of acid and duodenogastroesophageal reflux to oesophageal mucosal injury and symptoms in partial gastrectomy patients. *Gut* 1997;**41**:297–302.

39 Sifrim D, Silny J, Holloway R, Janssens J. Patterns of gas and liquid reflux during transient lower oesophageal sphincter relaxation: a study using intraluminal electrical impedance. *Gut* 1999;**44**:47–54.

40 Vela MF, Camacho-Lobato L, Srinivasan R *et al.* Intra-esophageal impedance and pH measurement of acid and non-acid reflux: effect of omeprazole. *Gastroenterology* 2001; **120**:1599–606.

41 Shay S, Bomeli S, Richter J. Multichannel intraluminal impedance accurately detects fasting, recumbent reflux events and their clearing. *Am J Physiol Gastrointest Liver Physiol* 2002;**283**:G376–83.

42 Spechler SJ. Epidemiology and natural history of gastro-oesophageal reflux disease. *Digestion* 1992;**51**(Suppl 1):24–9.

43 Zimmerman J, Shohat V, Tsvang E *et al.* Esophagitis is a major cause of upper gastrointestinal hemorrhage in the elderly. *Scand J Gastroenterol* 1997;**32**:906–9.

44 Cameron AJ, Higgins JA. Linear gastric erosion: a lesion associated with large diaphragmatic hernia and chronic blood loss anemia. *Gastroenterology* 1986;**91**:338–42.

45 Sonnenberg A, Massey T, Jacobsen SJ. Hospital discharges resulting from esophagitis among Medicare beneficiaries. *Dig Dis Sci* 1994;**39**:183–8.

46 Marks RD, Shukla M. Diagnosis and management of peptic esophageal strictures. *Gastroenterologist* 1996;**4**:223–37.

47 El-Serag HB, Sonnenberg A. Association of esophagitis and esophageal strictures with diseases treated with non-steroidal anti-inflammatory drugs. *Am J Gastroenterol* 1997;**92**:52–6.

48 Marks RD, Richter JE, Rizzo J *et al.* Omeprazole versus H$_2$-receptor antagonists in treating patients with peptic stricture and esophagitis. *Gastroenterology* 1994;**106**:907–15.

49 Sheikh RA, Trudeau WL. Expandable metallic stent placement in patients with benign esophageal strictures: results of long-term follow-up. *Gastrointest Endosc* 1998;**48**:227–9.

50 Cameron AJ, Lomboy CT, Pera M, Carpenter HA. Adenocarcinoma of the esophagogastric junction and Barrett's esophagus. *Gastroenterology* 1995;**109**:1541–6.

51 Spechler SJ. Barrett's esophagus. *N Engl J Med* 2002;**346**: 836–42.

52 Lagergren J, Bergstrom R, Lindgren A, Nyren O. Symptomatic gastroesophageal reflux as a risk factor for esophageal adenocarcinoma. *N Engl J Med* 1999;**340**:831.

53 Nandurkar S, Talley NJ. Barrett's esophagus: the long and short of it. *Am J Gastroenterol* 1999;**94**:30–40.

54 Shaheen NJ, Crosby MA, Bozymski EM, Sandler RS. Is there publication bias in the reporting of cancer risk in Barrett's esophagus? *Gastroenterology* 2000;**119**:333–8.

55 Inadomi JM, Sampliner R, Lagergren J *et al.* Screening and surveillance for Barrett esophagus in high-risk groups: a cost–utility analysis. *Ann Intern Med* 2003;**138**:176–86.

56 Falk GW, Chittajallu R, Galdblum JR *et al.* Surveillance of

patients with Barrett's esophagus for dysplasia and cancer with balloon cytology. *Gastroenterology* 1997;**112**:1787–97.

57 Katz PO, Dalton CB, Richter JE, Wu WC, Castell DO. Esophageal testing in patients with non-cardiac chest pain or dysphagia: results of three years experience with 1161 patients. *Ann Intern Med* 1987;**106**:593–7.

58 Richter JE. Typical and atypical presentations of gastroesophageal reflux disease. *Gastroenterol Clin North Am* 1996;**25**:75–102.

59 Koufman JA. The otolaryngeal manifestations of gastroesophageal reflux disease (GERD): a clinical investigation of 225 patients using ambulatory 24-hour pH monitoring and an experimental investigation of the role of acid and pepsin in the development of laryngeal injury. *Laryngoscope* 1991;**101**(Suppl 53):1–78.

60 Harding SM. Pulmonary complications of gastroesophageal reflux disease. In: Castell DO, Richter JE, eds. *The Esophagus*, 3rd edn. Philadelphia: Lippincott Williams & Wilkins, 1999: 493–504.

61 DiBaise JK, Lof J, Quigley EMM. Can symptoms predict esophageal motor function or acid exposure in GERD? A comparison of esophageal manometric and 24-hour pH parameters in typical and extraesophageal GERD. *J Clin Gastroenterol* 2001;**32**:128–32.

62 Harding SM, Richter JE. The role of gastroesophageal reflux in chronic cough and asthma. *Chest* 1997;**111**:1389–402.

63 El-Serag HB, Sonnenberg A. Comorbid occurrence of laryngeal or pulmonary disease with esophagitis in United States military veterans. *Gastroenterology* 1997;**113**:755–60.

64 Ruhl CE, Sonnenberg A, Everhart JE. Hospitalization with respiratory disease following hiatal hernia and reflux esophagitis in a prospective, population-based study. *Ann Epidemiol* 2001;**11**:477–83.

65 Mokhlesi B, Morris AL, Huang C-F *et al.* Increased prevalence of gastroesophageal reflux symptoms in patients with COPD. *Chest* 2001;**119**:1043–8.

66 Orr WC, Shamma-Othman Z, Allen M, Robinson MG. Esophageal function and gastroesophageal reflux during sleep and waking in patients with chronic obstructive pulmonary disease. *Chest* 1992;**101**:1521–5.

67 Ducolone A, Vandevenne A, Jouin H *et al.* Gastroesophageal reflux in patients with asthma and chronic bronchitis. *Am Rev Respir Dis* 1987;**135**:327–32.

68 Crausaz FM, Favez G. Aspiration of solid food particles into the lungs of patients with gastroesophageal reflux and chronic bronchial disease. *Chest* 1988;**93**:376–8.

69 Tibbling L. Wrong-way swallowing as a possible cause of bronchitis in patients with gastroesophageal reflux disease. *Acta Otolaryngol (Stockh)* 1993;**113**:405–8.

70 Mokhlesi B, Logemann JA, Rademaker AW, Stangl CA, Corbridge TC. Oropharyngeal deglutition in stable COPD. *Chest* 2002;**121**:361–9.

71 Berkowitz N, Schulman LL, McGregor C, Markowitz D. Gastroparesis after lung transplantation: potential role in postoperative respiratory complications. *Chest* 1995;**108**:1602–7.

72 Au J, Hawkins T, Venables C *et al.* Upper gastrointestinal dysmotility in heart-lung transplant recipients. *Ann Thorac Surg* 1993;**55**:94–7.

73 Reid KR, McKenzie FN, Menkis AH *et al.* Importance of chronic aspiration in recipients of heart-lung transplants. *Lancet* 1990;**336**:206–8.

74 Rinaldi M, Martinelli L, Volpato G *et al.* Gastro-esophageal reflux as cause of obliterative bronchiolitis: a case report. *Transplant Proc* 1995;**27**:2006–7.

75 Davis RD, Lau CL, Eubanks S *et al.* Improved lung allograft function after fundoplication in patients with gastroesophageal reflux disease undergoing lung transplantation. *J Thorac Cardiovasc Surg* 2003;**125**:533–42.

76 Freston JW, Malagelada JR, Petersen H, McCloy RF. Critical issues in the management of gastroesophageal reflux disease. *Eur J Gastroenterol Hepatol* 1995;**7**:577–86.

77 Brimblecombe RW, Duncan WAM, Durant GJ *et al.* Characterization and development of cimetidine as a histamine H_2-receptor antagonist. *Gastroenterology* 1978;**74**:339–47.

78 Kahrilas PJ, Fennerty MB, Joelsson B. High- versus standard-dose ranitidine for control of heartburn in poorly responsive acid reflux disease: a prospective, controlled trial. *Am J Gastroenterol* 1999;**94**:92–7.

79 Peghini PL, Katz PO, Bracey NA, Castell DO. Nocturnal recovery of gastric acid secretion on thrice-daily proton pump inhibitors. *Am J Gastroenterol* 1998;**93**:763–7.

80 Chiba N, DeGara CJ, Wilkinson JM, Hunt RH. Speed of healing and symptom relief in grade II to IV gastroesophageal reflux disease: a meta-analysis. *Gastroenterology* 1997;**112**: 1798–810.

81 Vigneri S, Termini R, Leandro G *et al.* A comparison of five maintenance therapies for reflux esophagitis. *N Engl J Med* 1995;**333**:1106–10.

82 Muller C, Lissner S. The role of therapeutic trial in the assessment of patients with reflux-like symptoms. In: Lundell L, ed. *Guidelines for Management of Symptomatic Gastroesophageal Reflux Disease*. London: Science Press, 1998: 39–44.

83 Lundell L, Miettinen P, Myrvold HE *et al.* Continued (5-year) follow-up of a randomized clinical study comparing antireflux surgery and omeprazole in gastroesophageal reflux disease. *J Am Coll Surg* 2001;**192**:172–81.

84 Spechler SJ. Medical or invasive therapy for GERD: an acidulous analysis. *Clin Gastroenterol Hepatol* 2003;**1**:81–8.

85 Dent J. Gastro-oesophageal reflux disease. *Digestion* 1998;**59**: 433–45.

86 Triadafilopoulos G, DiBaise JK, Nostrant TT *et al.* Radiofrequency energy delivery to the gastroesophageal junction for the treatment of gastroesophageal reflux disease. *Gastrointest Endosc* 2001;**53**:407–15.

87 Filipi CJ, Lehman GA, Rothstein RI *et al.* Transoral endoscopic suturing for gastroesophageal reflux disease: a multicenter trial. *Gastrointest Endosc* 2001;**53**:416–22.

88 Johnson DA, Ganz R, Aisenberg J *et al.* Endoscopic, deep mural implantation of enteryx for the treatment of GERD: 6-month follow-up of a multicenter trial. *Am J Gastroenterol* 2003;**98**:250–8.

89 O'Connor JFB, Singer ME, Richter JE. The cost-effectiveness of strategies of assessing gastroesophageal reflux as an exacerbating factor in asthma. *Am J Gastroenterol* 1999;**94**: 1472–80.

CHAPTER 43
Upper airway diseases

Maria Rappai and Richard deShazo

Histologically similar respiratory epithelium extends posteriorly from the nasal septum and the lateral walls of the nasal fossa to the nasopharynx, larynx, trachea, bronchi and bronchioles. There is increasing evidence that the nose, sinus and lower airway have similar physiology and function and are indeed, one airway [1]. However, for the purposes of discussion, we will define the upper airway as the nose and sinuses. The clinical relationships between the upper and lower airway will be a theme of this chapter.

Rhinosinusitis and asthma are comorbidities, linked by epidemiological, pathological and physiological characteristics and by a common classification and therapeutic approach. Although not universally accepted, the term 'allergic rhinobronchitis' has been proposed to link the association between allergic asthma and rhinitis. Some have even suggested that asthmatic individuals are a subgroup of the population of patients with rhinitis [2]. Because of the impact of rhinitis on asthma, allergic rhinitis has been reclassified to reflect the classification of asthma (Table 43.1) [3].

Rhinitis is a common condition that may occur on an allergic or non-allergic basis. Of all patients with rhinitis, 43% have allergic rhinitis, 23% have non-allergic rhinitis and 34% have combinations of the two [4]. Allergic rhinitis accounts for at least 2.5% of all physician visits; 2 million lost school days per year, 6 million lost workdays and 28 million restricted workdays per year. Rhinitis occurs in more than 75% of subjects with allergic asthma and 80% of those with non-allergic asthma [5].

Sinusitis is the most common chronic disease in adults in the USA. It results from infectious and non-infectious causes of inflammation and is almost always associated with obstruction of the osteomeatal complex [6]. Rhinosinusitis is a more appropriate term than sinusitis, as sinusitis is inevitably associated with coexistent rhinitis [7].

In this chapter we discuss rhinosinusitis and its relationship to asthma, some other common diseases that involve both the upper and lower airways and newer information on the relationship between the swallowing reflex and obstructive lung disease.

Table 43.1 Classification of allergic rhinitis by frequency and severity.

Frequency		Severity	
Intermittent	Persistent	Mild	Moderate–severe
< 4 days/week < 4 weeks/year	> 4/week > 4 week/year	Absence of disruption of sleep, no impairment of school or work, daily activity, leisure or sport	Sleep disturbance, impairment of daily activity, leisure and/or sport, impairment of school and work Troublesome symptoms

Classification of allergic rhinitis according to frequency and severity of symptoms parallels the classification of asthma. Therefore allergic rhinitis may be mild intermittent, mild persistent, moderate intermittent, moderate persistent, severe intermittent or severe persistent using this classification.

Anatomy and physiology of the nose and sinuses

The nasal cavity is divided into two separate air passages by the nasal septum. The lateral nasal wall has three turbinates: the superior, middle and inferior turbinates (conchae), which divide the nasal cavity into meati. During quiet breathing, the nasal airflow is predominantly directed around the inferior turbinate along the floor of the nasal cavity (Fig. 43.1). The superior meatus drains the posterior ethmoid air cells and the sphenoid sinus. The area under the middle meatus into which the frontal, maxillary and anterior ethmoid drain is the osteomeatal complex. The inferior meatus receives drainage from the nasolacrimal duct (Fig. 43.2).

The biological function of the nose is still debated, but the physiology of the nose has been studied extensively. The nose is lined by pseudostratified epithelium resting on a basement membrane, which separates it from deeper (submucosal) layers. Mast cells are present in both layers. The submucosa contains mucous, seromucous and serous glands [8]. Small arteries, arterioles and arteriovenous anastamoses determine regional blood flow. Capacitance vessels, consisting of veins and cavernous sinusoids, determine nasal patency. The sympathetic nervous system regulates the venous capacitance vessels. The cavernous sinusoids lie beneath the capillaries and venules, are most dense in the inferior and middle turbinates, and contain smooth muscle cells that are also regulated by the sympathetic nervous system. Loss of sympathetic tone or, to a lesser degree, cholinergic stimulation causes this sinusoidal erectile tissue to become engorged and leads to nasal obstruction. Cholinergic stimulation causes arterial dilatation and promotes the passive diffusion of plasma proteins into glands and the active secretion by mucous glands in cells.

The classic mediators of immediate hypersensitivity and novel neurotransmitters, including substance P, calcitonin gene-related peptide and vasointestinal peptide, have been detected in nasal secretions after nasal allergen challenge of patients with allergic rhinitis [9]. Antidromic stimulation of sensory nerve fibres in the nose can release a variety of neurotransmitters including substance P, a mediator of increased vascular permeability. Because neurotransmitters also produce changes in regional blood flow and glandular secretion, their role in rhinitis may be important.

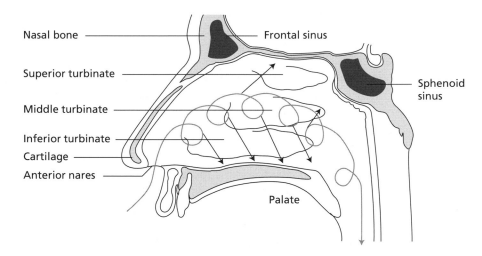

Figure 43.1 Airflow through the nasal air passages. Turbulence of airflow at higher velocities of inspiration leads to impaction of particles in the inspired air on the nasal mucosa. (From Howarth [99], with permission from Elsevier's Health Sciences, Philadelphia.)

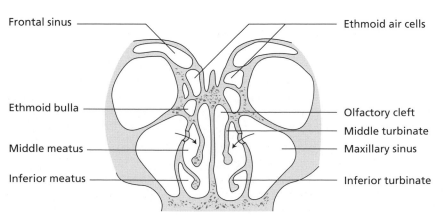

Figure 43.2 The structure of the sinuses.

Mechanisms by which the upper airway influences the lower airway

The upper and lower airway share common features over and above the respiratory epithelium. This includes the ability to entrap particles and irritants in the mucociliary blanket and the nitric oxide system. The nasal airway and sinuses are especially effective in warming and humidification of inspired air and serves a protective function for the protection of the lower airway. For instance, children with mild to moderate asthma had lower decreases in forced expiratory volume in 1 s (FEV_1) while breathing through their nose compared with those breathing orally during exercise [10]. The upper airway influences the lower through the nasobronchial reflex, drainage of inflammatory material and through systemic propagation of mediators of nasal inflammation. The nasobronchial reflex provides a direct pathway for interaction between the upper and lower airway. Animal studies demonstrate reflexes arising from nose and nasopharynx, mediated by the afferent sensory components of the trigeminal and glossopharyngeal nerves and efferent bronchoconstrictor fibres to the vagus nerve. Human studies have shown increased airway resistance after nasal insufflation of silica, an effect prevented by premedication with atropine [11], bronchial hyperresponsiveness after intranasal allergen challenge [12] and significant falls in FEV_1 after nasal insufflation of histamine [13], further supporting the nasobronchial reflex theory. Lower airway remodelling has also been demonstrated in non-asthmatic patients with allergic rhinitis, further supporting the interaction of upper and lower airways [14].

Nitric oxide serves important functions in both the upper and lower airway. These include antiviral and bacteriostatic activity, bronchodilatory effects, vasodilatation, improvement in oxygenation and modulatory effects on lower airway responsiveness [15]. Data on the roll and function of nitric oxide in upper airway inflammation are conflicting. Patients with uncontrolled asthma have increased expiratory nitric oxide [16] concentrations while patients with sinusitis have been reported to have decreased nitric oxide concentrations [17].

Sinobronchial syndromes

The sinobronchial syndromes have simultaneous upper and lower airway involvement and may be classified as congenital or acquired (Table 43.2). The most recently described syndrome is sinobronchial allergic bronchopulmonary mycosis, the SAM syndrome [18]. This syndrome occurs in patients with concomitant allergic fungal sinusitis and allergic bronchopulmonary mycosis.

Table 43.2 Sinobronchial syndromes.

Congenital	Acquired
Cystic fibrosis	Wegener granulomatosis
Kartagener syndrome	Relapsing polychondritis
Immotile cilia syndrome	Sarcoidosis
Young syndrome	Sinobronchial allergic mycosis (SAM)

Allergic fungal sinusitis results from a hypersensitivity response to inhaled fungal allergens in the paranasal sinuses much like allergic bronchopulmonary mycosis. It shares many clinical features with sarcoidosis with concomitant upper and lower airway involvement including chronic sinusitis, nasal polyposis, obstructive airway disease and response to corticosteroids [19]. Both require histopathological evaluation to confirm the diagnosis.

Syndromes of rhinosinusitis

Syndromes of rhinitis may be divided into allergic, infectious, perennial non-allergic and miscellaneous categories (Table 43.3) [20]. Allergic rhinitis should be differentiated from other forms of rhinitis because the approach to management is different. A working knowledge of the aeroallergens present in the patient's geographical location and the allergens in the patient's home and work areas is essential in clinical differentiation of these conditions (Table 43.4).

Allergic rhinitis

Symptoms of allergic rhinitis include paroxysms of itching of the eyes, nose and palate, sneezing, clear rhinorrhoea and nasal obstruction. Postnasal drip, cough, irritability, disordered sleep and fatigue are also common [20–22]. Symptoms develop when persons inhale airborne antigens (allergens) to which they have previously been exposed and against which they have made immunoglobulin E (IgE) antibodies.

Episodic allergic rhinitis results from episodic exposure to inhaled allergens, such as cat dander, that can provoke acute allergic symptoms. If allergen exposure is seasonal, and symptoms are predictable and reproducible, seasonal allergic rhinitis may be diagnosed by the history. Perennial allergic rhinitis is associated with nasal symptoms for more than 2 h/day more than nine months of the year [20]. The latter usually reflects allergy to indoor allergens such as dust mites, cockroaches or animal dander, although aeroallergens may cause perennial rhinitis in tropical or

Table 43.3 Classification of rhinitis.

Allergic rhinitis
    seasonal
    perennial
    occupational
    episodic

Infectious rhinitis
    Acute: viral, bacterial
    Chronic: bacterial, fungal, associated with
      immunodeficiency (antibody deficiency, cystic fibrosis,
      ciliary abnormalities, etc.)

Perennial non-allergic rhinitis
    eosinophilic forms
      non-allergic rhinitis with nasal eosinophilia (NARES)
      non-allergic rhinitis with blood eosinophilia (BENARS)
    non-eosinophilic forms
      Idiopathic: vasomotor rhinitis
      Hormonal: pregnancy, hypothyroidism, oestrogen
        replacement treatment
      Drug-induced: associated with aspirin respiratory
        sensitivity, rhinitis medicamentosa (vasoconstrictor
        nose sprays), antihypertensives, antidepressants
      Food associated: gustatory, immunoglobulin E-mediated
      Atrophic rhinitis (*Klebsiella ozaenae*), post-surgical
      Mechanical: hypertrophied turbinates, deviated nasal
        septum, foreign body, nasal polyps
      Granulomatous: Wegener granulomatosis, sarcoidosis,
        midline granuloma

Table 43.4 Allergens commonly associated with allergic rhinitis.

Allergen	Season	Examples
Seasonal aeroallergens (outdoor)		
Weed pollen	Fall	Ragweed
Grass pollen	Late spring	Rye, Bermuda, Bahia, Johnson
Tree pollen	Spring	Mountain cedar, Elm, Oak, Birch
Mould spores	Spring and summer	*Alternaria, Cladosporium* sp.
Perennial allergens (indoor)		
Insects		
House dust mite		*Dermatophagoides farinae, D. pteronyssinus*
Cockroach		
Pets		Cat saliva, rat urine
Moulds		*Aspergillum* and *Penicillium* sp.
Occupational		
Latex		
Laboratory animals		

subtropical climates. This form is common in subtropical regions with long pollinating seasons and ever-present mould and dust mite allergens, and with occupational allergen exposure [23]. Perennial allergic rhinitis may be difficult to distinguish from non-allergic forms and can require diagnostic testing for accurate diagnosis.

Eleven per cent of patients with rhinitis have seasonal symptoms, 33% have perennial symptoms with seasonal exacerbation and 56% have perennial symptoms alone [24,25]. Seventy eight per cent of patients with seasonal symptoms have an apparent allergic cause, and 68% of patients with perennial symptoms with seasonal exacerbation have a probable allergic cause. Fifty per cent of patients with rhinitis and perennial symptoms alone have allergic rhinitis.

Immunological mechanisms of allergic airways disease

Allergic rhinitis has an autosomal dominant pattern of inheritance with incomplete penetrance. Allergic individuals demonstrate physiological dominance of the Th2 subpopulation of helper T cells in immune responses with the production of interleukin 4 (IL-4), IL-5 and IL-13, and

other cytokines that favour the production of IgE and mast cell dependent, eosinophil-rich, allergic inflammation [9]. Cross-linking of two or more molecules of IgE by allergen on the mast cell surface leads to rapid degranulation and mediator release, which occurs in a calcium-dependent process. The stored (histamine) and generated (leukotrienes and prostaglandins) mast cell derived mediators stimulate epithelial cells, blood vessels, nerves and glands to cause the clinical manifestations of allergic rhinitis and feedback to other elements of the immune system to perpetuate the process. Mast cells release a variety of stored mediators immediately after exposure to allergen within minutes. However, experimental nasal insufflation of histamine reproduces all of the symptoms of acute allergic rhinitis. Generated mediators are released 6–8 h later and produce a second wave of symptoms and an eosinophil-rich inflammatory response called the late phase allergic reaction (Fig. 43.3).

The inflammatory response noted in the mucosa of patients with allergic rhinitis is often present in the sinuses, even when symptoms are not present [9]. The ethmoid sinus appears to have a higher expression of RNA for IL-4 than the maxillary sinus, thus promoting eosinophil infiltration by increased expression of endothelial VCAM-1 in such subjects. The final common pathway by which allergic inflammation causes symptoms of rhinosinusitis is the production of mucosal oedema and hypertrophy and

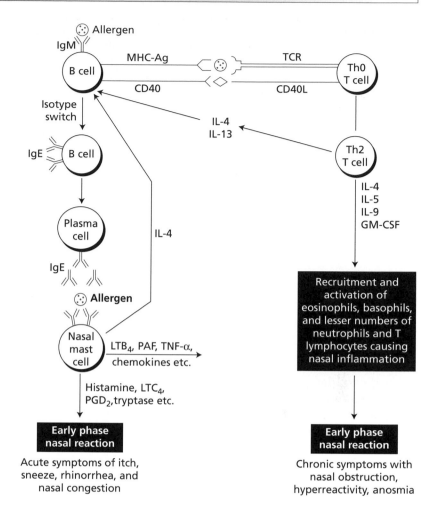

Figure 43.3 Pathophysiology of the allergic rhinitis. GM-CSF, granulocyte-macrophage colony-stimulating factor; IgE, immunoglobulin E; IgM, immunoglobulin M; IL-4, interleukin 4; IL-5, interleukin 5; IL-9, interleukin 9, IL-13, interleukin 13; LTB$_4$, leukotriene B$_4$; LTC$_4$, cysteinyl leukotriene; MHC-Ag, major histocompatibility complex antigen; PAF, platelet activating factor; PGD$_2$, prostaglandin D$_2$; TCR, T-cell receptor; TNF-α, tumour necrosis factor α. (From deShazo [100], with permission from Elsevier's Health Sciences, Philadelphia.)

increased mucous production resulting in obstruction to air flow. In the sinuses, this often obstructs the osteomeatal complex and disables mucociliary clearance mechanisms (Fig. 43.4) and sinusitis occurs.

Risk factors

A host of risk factors for allergic rhinitis have been identified [26]. These include a family history of atopy, male sex, birth during the pollen season, firstborn status, early introduction of formula and food, early use of antibiotics, maternal smoking exposure in the first year of life, exposure to indoor allergens such as animal dander, a serum IgE of more than 100 IU/mL before age 6 and the presence of allergen-specific IgE. Cord blood mononuclear cells of infants who subsequently develop allergic diseases in the first year of life secrete lower levels of γ-interferon, when compared with those who do not. γ-Interferon inhibits the expansion of Th2 lymphocytes and thereby limits production of IgE. There is some evidence that allergic diseases result from specific genetic abnormalities of normal γ-interferon production [27].

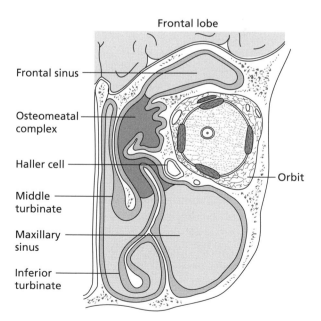

Figure 43.4 The osteomeatal complex. (From Kennedy [101], with permission from Johns Hopkins University, Baltimore.)

Signs and symptoms

Patients with allergic rhinitis most often complain of nasal pruritus and rhinorrhoea while patients with non-allergic rhinitis complain more of nasal obstruction. In univariant statistical analysis, purulent rhinorrhoea, purulent postnasal drip and pain in a maxillary tooth are the only features of the history that have a high sensitivity and specificity for culture-proven rhinosinusitis [28].

In patients with active rhinitis, application of a topical decongestant spray (oxymetazoline) is often required in order to visualize the nasal mucosa well. The pale blue–grey mucosa common in seasonal allergic rhinitis contrasts to the boggy red mucosa often present with non-allergic rhinitis. In patients older than 5 years, flexible fibreoptic rhinoscopy may facilitate examination. It allows inspection of the nasal cavity for septal deviation or other anatomical abnormalities, the inspection of middle meatus to exclude purulent discharge associated with sinusitis, and the detection of polyps, tumours or foreign bodies.

Diagnosis

The diagnosis of allergic rhinitis is made on clinical grounds by the history, the presence of the symptoms and signs and the detection of allergen-specific IgE by skin tests or *in vitro* methods. In the most severe cases, there is intense nasal itching associated with nose rubbing, excoriation of the external nares, pushing the tip of the nose up with the hand (the allergic salute) and a transverse nasal crease [29]. Both infraorbital oedema and darkening resulting from subcutaneous venodilatation (allergic shiners) and accentuated lines or folds below the lower lids (Denie–Morgan lines) suggest concomitant allergic conjunctivitis. While adults and older children frequently blow clear mucus from their noses, young children have persistent rhinorrhoea and often snort, sniff, cough and clear their throats. Some scratch their itchy palates with their tongues producing a clicking sound (palatal click). Clear rhinorrhoea may be visible anteriorly or, with nasal obstruction, dripping down a posterior pharynx that resembles cobblestones and reflects lymphoid hyperplasia. Giemsa or Hansel's stains of these nasal secretions show cell populations to be predominately eosinophils. A highly arched palate, mouth breathing and dental malocclusion are common, especially in children. Symptoms are reproducible on exposure to allergens to which the patient has been sensitized. Most patients have strong family histories of allergic disease.

Allergen-specific IgE may be demonstrated by immediate hypersensitivity skin tests using commercial allergic extracts or *in vitro* assays such as the radioallergoabsorbent test (RAST). Sensitization may occur at allergen levels below those that provoke symptoms. Positive tests indicate sensitization but not necessarily allergy, as symptoms do not always occur on re-exposure to allergens causing sensitization to allergen [20]. For research purposes, allergic rhinitis may be diagnosed with standardized nasal provocation tests using allergen to which the patient has specific IgE. Because such large numbers of patients with allergic rhinitis have an additional non-allergic contribution to their allergic rhinitis (mixed rhinitis), increasing attention has been focused on syndromes of non-allergic rhinitis [30]. Fortunately, topical nasal steroids [31] and topical antihistamines (e.g. azelastine) have been shown to be effective in the treatment of both allergic and perennial non-allergic rhinitis in controlled trials [32]. Thus, a positive response to a therapeutic trial of either does not establish a diagnosis of allergic rhinitis.

Perennial non-allergic rhinitis may be subdivided into eosinophilic and non-eosinophilic forms. Non-allergic rhinitis with nasal eosinophilia syndrome (NARES) occurs in as many as 15% of patients with rhinitis and is characterized by perennial symptoms, an older average age than in patients with allergic rhinitis (39 versus 25 years), and milder symptoms of nasal itching and sneezing [33]. The clear nasal secretions contain more than 25% eosinophils, but the role of eosinophils in the disorder is unclear. Fifty per cent of patients with NARES have sinusitis, 33% have nasal polyps and 14% have asthma. IgE to inhalant allergens is usually absent but anaphylactoid reactions to aspirin may occur. Blood eosinophilia–non-allergic rhinitis syndrome (BENARS) is a variant of NARES [25].

Patients with vasomotor rhinitis complain of chronic nasal congestion intensified by rapid changes in temperature and relative humidity, odours or alcohol. A hypersecretory variant with persistent rhinorrhoea exists [25]. Several lines of evidence suggest that patients have nasal autonomic nervous system dysfunction [34]. They have little nasal itching or sneezing, but headaches, anosmia and sinusitis are common. A family history of allergy or allergic symptom triggers is uncommon. Positive immediate hypersensitivity skin tests to inhalant allergens and nasal eosinophilia are unusual.

Atrophic rhinitis is a syndrome of progressive atrophy of the nasal mucosa in elderly patients who report chronic nasal congestion and constantly perceive a bad odour. Mucosal colonization with *Klebsiella ozaenae* has been associated with this condition. This condition also occurs in patients who have undergone multiple sinus surgeries and lose normal mucosal ciliary function. Rhinitis medicamentosa is a complication of chronic use of vasoconstrictor nasal sprays or intranasal cocaine abuse. Chronic nasal obstruction and nasal inflammation develop and are manifested as swollen, beefy red nasal membranes on physical examination.

Rhinitis of pregnancy and rhinitis associated with birth control pills or hypothyroidism reflect nasal obstruction that occurs because of the influence of hormones. Nasal obstruction may also be a side-effect of antihypertensive drugs. Unilateral rhinitis or nasal polyps are uncommon in uncomplicated allergic rhinitis. Unilateral rhinitis suggests the possibility of nasal obstruction by a foreign body, tumour or polyp.

The presence of nasal polyps suggests NARES, chronic bacterial sinusitis, allergic fungal sinusitis, aspirin hypersensitivity, cystic fibrosis or primary ciliary dyskinesia (immotile cilia syndrome). Prolonged use of neuroleptics, certain antihypertensives including β-blockers, anticonvulsants and some antidepressants may also contribute to rhinitis syndromes.

Sinusitis

Sinusitis is inflammation of one or more of the paranasal sinuses. Acute sinusitis is defined as the presence of symptoms for less than 4 weeks' duration, subacute for 4–12 weeks and chronic as the presence of symptoms for longer than 12 weeks. Recurrent sinusitis refers to repeated episodes of acute sinusitis three times or more per year [35].

Sinusitis remains a clinical diagnosis and there is no consensus on diagnostic criteria, classification or treatment. Sinus aspiration with culture is the gold standard for diagnosis of bacterial sinusitis, but is impractical. Aspiration can be associated with complications and without biopsy, lavage or special culture technique does not exclude viral or non-infectious inflammatory mechanisms such as Wegener granulomatosis. Computed tomography (CT) imaging is useful in following chronic sinusitis, but has a high false-positive rate in acute sinusitis [36]. Rhinoscopy with sterile antral aspiration and culture has promise as a diagnostic technique, but requires further evaluation [37]. Moreover, not all sinusitis is bacterial.

Acute sinusitis is more often associated with purulent nasal discharge or postnasal drip, fever or facial pain. Chronic sinusitis is associated with anosmia, fatigue, facial fullness, persistent halitosis, exacerbation of asthma or no obvious symptoms [38]. Nasal smears show sheets of polymorphonuclear cells and bacteria. When air fluid levels are present (acute sinusitis) or mucosal thickening is greater than 8 mm (chronic sinusitis), plain X-rays of the sinus correlate with antral punctures confirming bacterial infection; sinus opacification is seen with either [39]. This correlation is clinically useful in children over 1 year of age, although less so in adults. Unfortunately, plain X-rays provide little detail of the osteomeatal complex, obstruction of which is usually the root cause of the problem. Limited (coronal) CT studies of the sinuses provide more information, less radiation and generally cost no more than a standard series of plain films [40]. Cautious interpretation of sinus CT is required as temporary opacificiation of the sinuses and obstruction of the osteomeatal complex are common with upper respiratory tract infections (Fig. 43.5) [41].

Most sinusitis, including non-allergic sinusitis, is associated with mucosal eosinophilia of varying degrees. The syndrome of chronic nasal polyposis, aspirin intolerance, asthma and (sinusitis) is called Samter's triad (Tetrad) and usually occurs in individuals with no identifiable allergic sensitivity.

Some investigators have suggested that chronic fungal

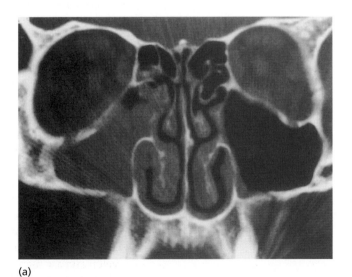

(a)

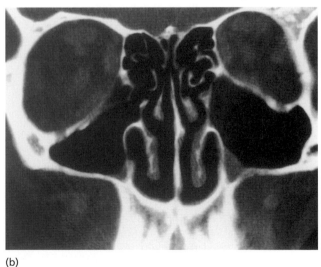

(b)

Figure 43.5 Sinus computed tomography (CT). (a) Coronal CT of the paranasal sinuses in patient with rhinosinusitis demonstrating diffuse mucoperiosteal thickening with opacification of the right maxillary sinus. (b) CT of the same patient after 6-week trial of topical corticosteroids and antihistamines, showing near-complete resolution of the mucoperiosteal thickening. (From Orlandi and Kennedy [102], with permission from Lippincott-Raven Publishers, Philadelphia.)

Table 43.5 Evidence of a causal association for allergic rhinitis asthma.

Observation	References
1 Perennial rhinitis is an epidemiological risk factor for asthma	84,85
2 Increased prevalence of asthma in patients with allergic rhinitis (28–85%)	86–89
3 Increased prevalence of allergic rhinitis in patients with asthma (19–50%)	86–89
4 Increased prevalence of bronchial responsiveness in patients with allergic rhinitis	88,90
Seasonal allergic rhinitis: 11–32% out of season	
48% during season	
Perennial allergic rhinitis: 50%	
5 Nasal allergen challenge increases bronchial hyperresponsiveness	11
6 Treatment of rhinitis with topical nasal steroids decreases bronchial hyperresponsiveness	91–93
7 Bronchial allergen challenge increases nasal inflammation	94
8 Treatment of rhinits with topical nasal steroids or antihistamines in patients with coexistent asthma decreases asthma symptoms	91,93,95–97
9 Treatment of asthma with leukotriene inhibitors decreases symptoms of allergic rhinitis	98

infection may be the underlying cause of all chronic rhinosinusitis, a hypothesis not supported by available data.

Rhinosinusitis and other conditions

Although allergic rhinitis has not been shown to cause asthma, there is evidence for a causal association (Table 43.5). Conditions commonly associated with rhinosinusitis include asthma, nasal polyposis, lower respiratory tract infection, dental malocclusion, sleep disorders [30,42] and anosmia. Allergic rhinitis is strongly associated and is a contributing factor to eustachian tube dysfunction causing concomitant serous and acute otitis media [43]. Allergic rhinitis often occurs concomitantly with other common allergic conditions, including allergic conjunctivitis, allergic asthma and atopic dermatitis (eczema). Twenty-eight to 50% of patients with asthma and up to 30% with eczema have allergic rhinitis. The genetic predisposition to develop these conditions has been termed 'atopy' and patients who have them are often called 'atopic'.

Rhinosinusitis and asthma

Non-specific bronchial hyperreactivity on bronchial challenge with methacholine, histamine or cold air is present in individuals with allergic rhinitis with no symptoms of asthma and normal spirometry. Treatment of asthmatic children treated with topical nasal steroids for perennial rhinitis decreases non-specific bronchial hyperreactivity and nocturnal asthma symptoms [26]. Several mechanisms have been proposed to explain the association between rhinosinusitis and asthma:

1 Nasal inflammation causes bronchospasm via the nasobronchial reflex.

2 Increased expression of intracellular adhesion molecules (ICAM-1) associated with nasal inflammation increases the frequency of viral infections including rhinovirus which binds directly to ICAM-1.

3 Inflammatory nasal cytokines from the nose are aspirated into the lower airway inducing bronchial inflammation.

4 Nasal inflammation contributes to T-cell homing to the lower respiratory tract where these lymphocytes foster inflammation [44].

The persistent inhalation of cold dry air because of mouth breathing may also contribute [20,45].

Acute sinus infection can worsen asthma and therapy for sinus disease can improve asthma when the two conditions coexist. Sinusitis is present in 40–75% of patients with asthma. As in asthma, eosinophilic mucosal infiltration and deposition of major basic protein is present in chronic sinusitis [46] and the same inflammatory mediators identified in allergic rhinitis have been identified in sinusitis. The cultures obtained from the maxillary sinus of asthmatic patients with maxillary sinus radiographical abnormalities often grow no organisms, suggesting that the eosinophilic inflammation present may cause chronic obstruction of the osteomeatal complex without bacterial superinfection. The role of the eosinophil in this process is under intense investigation.

No clear association has been established between sinus disease and chronic obstructive pulmonary disease (COPD).

Management of rhinosinusitis

General

The treatment of rhinosinusitis centres on decreasing nasal inflammation and maintaining patency of the osteomeatal complex [47]. Consensus guidelines have been published for the management of allergic rhinosinusitis [20,48]. The approach to management is based on differentiation of allergic from non-allergic causes of rhinosinusitis. Sinusitis should be suspected in all cases of rhinitis refractory to the usual management. In such cases, rhinoscopy or CT should be considered.

Treatment of non-allergic rhinitis

Because non-allergic rhinitis is usually perennial, the use of topical nasal steroids is the treatment of choice. Although the topical antihistamine Astelin® is effective in the treatment of these conditions, oral antihistamines have little salutory effect. Leukotriene inhibitors often improve symptoms in the subset of patients with nasal polyposis and aspirin hypersensitivity and may inhibit polyp growth.

Treatment of allergic rhinitis

Allergen avoidance
The first step in the treatment of allergic rhinitis is allergen avoidance, when possible and practical. This may be facilitated by maintaining the relative humidity at 50% or less to limit house dust mite and mould growth and avoiding exposure to irritants such as cigarette smoke. Appropriately maintained air conditioners decrease concentrations of pollen, mould and dust mite allergens in indoor air. Removing carpets and furry pets may diminish allergic symptoms to house dust mite faeces. Covering mattresses, box springs and pillows with plastic, and washing bedding in water hotter than 54.4°C (130°F) once weekly may be helpful although the data supporting these are limited and conflicting. Ordinary vacuuming and dusting has little effect, although vacuum cleaners with high-efficiency particulate air (HEPA) filters may be useful [49]. HEPA air cleaners may reduce airborne animal allergen, but are not helpful in the reduction of dust mite allergens, which settle too rapidly for capture.

Pharmacological treatment of allergic rhinitis
If allergen avoidance is not adequate, drug therapy is the next step. Corticosteroids given orally or parenterally abolish symptoms of allergic rhinitis, but are unacceptable for long-term or frequent use. Topical intranasal steroid therapy is the most effective single maintenance therapy and causes few side-effects at recommended doses (Table 43.6). Topical nasal steroids are more effective than cromolyn, second-generation antihistamines and leukotriene inhibitors in treating allergic rhinitis and improve the symptoms of seasonal asthma in patients with concomitant seasonal allergic rhinitis and seasonal allergic asthma [50,51]. Topical nasal corticosteroids are more effective than antihistamines in reducing nasal blockage because of their vasoconstrictor effects but are not effective in reducing symptoms of allergic conjunctivitis.

Antihistamines help control sneezing, rhinorrhoea and itching associated with the early nasal reactions but may not provide adequate relief from nasal obstruction associated with the late phase reaction. First-generation antihistamines commonly produce sedation and other central nervous system symptoms that may adversely affect learning in children and may cause drying of the mouth and urinary hesitancy. Adverse effects on driving include decreased performance on tests of divided attention, working memory, vigilance and speed (Table 43.7). These effects occur less commonly with second-generation antihistamines other than cetirizine and azelastine [52].

Nasal decongestant sprays are not recommended in the treatment of allergic rhinitis as tachyphylaxis develops after 3–7 days and rebound nasal congestion results. Continued use causes rhinitis medicamentosa. They may occasionally be helpful for periods of a week or less when used just prior to the administration of topical nasal steroids for patients with severe nasal obstruction.

Cromolyn and nedocromil decrease allergic inflammation by inhibiting the intermediate conductance chloride channel pathways of mast cells, eosinophils, epithelial and

Table 43.6 Intranasal steroids available in the USA.

Name (Trade name)	Dose approved
Flunisolide (Nasalide, Nasarel)	2 sprays (50 µg) in each nostril b.i.d.–t.i.d.; max 400 µg/day
Beclometasone dipropionate (Beconase, Vancenase, Beconase AQ, Vancenase AQ)	1 spray (42 µg) in each nostril b.i.d.–q.i.d.; max 336 µg/day
Triamcinolone acetonide (Nasacort)	2 sprays (110 µg) in each nostril once a day; max 440 µg/day
Budesonide (Rhinocort)	2 sprays (64 µg) in each nostril once a day; max 256 µg/day
Fluticasone (Flonase)	2 sprays (100 µg) in each nostril once a day; max 200 µg/day
Mometasone furoate monohydrate (Nasonex)	2 sprays (50 µg) in each nostril once a day; max unclear

b.i.d., twice daily; max, maximum; t.i.d., three times daily; q.i.d, four times daily.

Table 43.7 Adverse effects of antihistamines and decongestants.

	Antihistamines	Decongestants
Anticholinergic	Dry mouth and eyes Impotence Urinary hesitancy Glaucoma	Urinary hesitancy Irritability
Central nervous system	Sedation Stimulating rare (children) Confusion and cognitive impairment in older patients	Heachache Insomnia Nervousness Nausea
Miscellaneous	Weight gain Prolonged QT interval Ventricular arrhythmias	
Cardiovascular system		Palpitation Hypertension Tachycardia

endothelial cells, fibroblasts and sensory neurons [53]. They inhibit mast cell mediator release. Cromolyn but not nedocromil is available in the USA.

Ipratropium is more useful in non-allergic rhinitis with predominant rhinorrhea as it does not block sneezing, pruritus or nasal obstruction. The positive effects of ipratropium may be mediated in part by its ability to decrease the release of substance P, a congener of atropine in a 0.03% nasal solution [54].

Antileukotrienes such as montelukast provide effects similar to that of loratadine and has been approved for use in allergic rhinitis. It appears to have additive benefits in the combination with non-sedating antihistamines [55] but the combination appears no more effective than topical nasal steroids alone [56,57].

Allergen immunotherapy

Allergen immunotherapy involves the subcutaneous administration of increasing doses of therapeutic vaccines of allergens to which a patient is known to be allergic. It is maintained at an arbitrary 'maintenance' dose [58]. There is increasing evidence that administration of allergens by the oral route may be effective as well. A number of allergenic vaccines have been standardized and are available in the USA and are dispensed as bioequivalent allergy units (BAU).

Immunotherapy should be considered when avoidance of allergens and pharmacotherapy fail to resolve the symptoms of allergic rhinitis or when pharmacotherapy produces unacceptable side-effects or is not cost effective. High-dose immunotherapy for allergic rhinitis has been shown in controlled studies to relieve symptoms of allergic rhinitis effectively [59]. It should be strongly considered in patients with perennial symptoms, perennial rhinitis with seasonal exacerbations, constitutional symptoms (such as severe fatigue) or in patients with associated sinusitis, allergic conjunctivitis or asthma.

Immunotherapy modulates the immune response to allergen. It decreases IL-4 and IL-5 production by CD4+ T lymphocytes, generates IgE-modulating CD8+ T lymphocytes, increases allergen-blocking IgG antibodies (particularly of the IgG 4 class) and reduces the movement into and the number of mast cells and eosinophils in nasal inflammatory reactions [60]. Immunotherapy blunts the seasonal rise of allergen-specific IgE, decreases up to 75% of the release of mast cell mediators in allergen challenge studies [61] and the expression of messenger RNA for interferon on nasal allergen challenge. These findings reflect a shift away from a Th2 type response associated with allergic inflammation. The clinical result in the inhibition of both the immediate and late nasal allergic response increases [62,63].

Treatment of sinusitis

Treatment studies of sinusitis reflect an empirical diagnosis and empirical treatment based on the most probable infectious agents. *Streptococcus pneumoniae*, *Moraxella catarrhalis* and *Haemophilus influenzae* have been associated with acute sinusitis and most studies and suggest these organisms plus anaerobic bacteria have been implicated in chronic sinusitis [35]. However, the role of antibiotics in the treatment of clinically diagnosed acute sinusitis is not presently evidence-based. The choice of antibiotics is dictated by local patterns of microbial sensitivity because antibiotic resistance to these common microbes is a growing problem.

A course of appropriate antibiotic therapy for 7–10 days for acute and 21 days for chronic allergic sinusitis plus full dose of topical nasal corticosteroids appears appropriate. Three to five days of a topical nasal decongestant to facilitate the entry of corticosteroids into the upper airway is often helpful. Use of oral or nasal antihistamines or oral decongestants may be useful but has not been substantiated. Treatment of sinusitis should be followed by radiological or rhinoscopic studies to establish that the infection has been cleared and the osteomeatal complex is open. Traditionally, patients who fail a single course of treatment have a second prolonged course of appropriate antibiotics and topical nasal steroids. Consultation with an otolaryngologist is appropriate if infection persists. Individuals with recurrent acute sinusitis or chronic sinusitis should receive an allergy evaluation and be considered for immunodeficiency evaluation and allergen immunotherapy.

We feel that treatment of concomitant allergic inflammation in the nose and sinus is essential to successful treatment of sinusitis in allergic individuals. In some individuals, anti-inflammatory treatment alone results in radiologically demonstrable clearing of the sinuses. However, there are limited data to substantiate that treatment of allergic inflammation associated with allergic sinusitis produces a better result than treating the associated infection alone. In a study of patients with allergic rhinosinusitis randomized to treatment with antibiotic for 14 days versus antibiotic with loratadine, oral corticosteroids or placebo for 28 days, patients treated with loratadine had less nasal obstruction and sneezing at day 28 but were otherwise similar [64]. In another study, patients with either acute or chronic sinusitis were treated with 3 weeks of antibiotics plus flunisolide or placebo for 7 weeks. The time to resolution of overall symptoms and normalization of radiological abnormalities in the two groups were similar although patients receiving flunisolide had less nasal obstruction [65].

Results of treatment of coexistent rhinosinusitis and asthma

A number of uncontrolled studies have shown that successful medical treatment of rhinosinusitis in patients with coexistent asthma and rhinosinusitis is associated with improvement of asthma [66]. The uncontrolled studies have reported that surgical treatment of chronic sinusitis by functional endoscopic techniques or sphenoethmoidectomy improves coexistent asthma. In one such study of 79 patients with intractable sinusitis who had functional endoscopic sinus surgery (FESS) procedures, 86% had improvement of rhinosinusitis and 80% had improvement of coexistent asthma [67].

Novel treatments for allergic rhinosinusitis

Theoretically, inhibitors of production or depletion of these cytokines associated with allergic inflammation should improve allergic symptoms. A recent trial of a monoclonal antibody to IL-5 in asthmatic patients resulted in depletion of circulating eosinophils but had no effect on bronchial response to allergic challenge [68]. Recombinant human monoclonal antibody to IgE (rhuMAb-E-25) binds circulating IgE and prevents the interaction of IgE with surface receptors on mast cells. Controlled studies of anti-IgE therapy have been shown to lower IgE levels, decrease early and late phase reactions to allergen challenge, and to improve allergen rhinitis and allergic asthma [69].

Phosphodiesterase-4 (PDE4) inhibitor agents are presently under investigation in both allergic rhinitis and asthma. A recent blinded cross-over study of roflumilast has shown favourable effects in rhinitis. The role of a PDE_4 inhibitor in asthma and COPD is also under investigation [70]. Other therapies under consideration include tryptase inhibitors and chemokine and adhesion receptor inhibitors [71].

Swallowing

The association between pulmonary parenchymal diseases, including COPD, and oropharyngeal function is of increasing interest. Swallowing is a complex physiological process and shares a close anatomical and developmental association with the airway and gastrointestinal tract. The swallowing reflex is co-ordinated by the medulla and involves oral preparation followed by an oral voluntary phase, followed by an involuntary pharyngeal and oesophageal phase [72]. Timing and co-ordination of swallowing is crucial for transfer of food into the oesophagus and for airway protection, and involves complex interactions between various muscles and nerves. Both respiration and swallowing are under complex voluntary and involuntary control. Alterations in the harmonic relationship between respiration and swallowing can result in dysphagia and aspiration. Microaspiration may cause bronchoconstriction or the introduction of bacteria into the upper airway [73].

Techniques for evaluation of swallowing

Many techniques have been used to evaluate swallowing, so many as to suggest that present studies leave much to be desired. The gold standard for evaluation of swallowing is video fluoroscopy. Quantification of pharyngeal contractile forces, incomplete upper oesophageal sphincter (UOS) relaxation and intrabolus pressure during swallowing requires pharyngeal and upper oesophageal manometry. Use of manometry with video fluoroscopy is optimal for a comprehensive approach. Manometry assesses pharyngeal muscle contraction, UOS relaxation and relative timing and coordination of the pharyngeal muscles and UOS relaxation events [74].

Nasal endoscopy visualizes the tongue base, epiglottis, superior pharyngeal wall and the laryngeal vestibule below the epiglottis [73], and can also be used for the evaluation of initiation of pharyngeal swallowing and residue if microaspiration is suspected. Indirect signs of aspiration include accumulated oropharyngeal secretions and dye staining of the subglottic airway [75].

Other techniques that may be useful include:

1 air pulses to assess supraglottic and pharyngeal sensation [76];
2 monitoring of the onset of swallowing with a submental electromyogram (EMG) of the myohyoid–geniohyoid muscle complex;
3 evaluation of chewing with an EMG of the masseter muscle [77]; and
4 oesophageal pressure manometer and inductance plethysmography for evaluation of the relationship of swallowing to respiration and respiratory effort [78].

Table 43.8 Available studies on swallowing in COPD.

Study population	Abnormality	Comments	Reference
Moderate–severe COPD with frequent exacerbations	Dysphagia, GERD, cricopharyngeal dysfunction	Cricopharyngeal myotomy decreased excerbations Medication, sex and age were confounding factors	80
Smokers vs non-smokers	Increased threshold for swallowing initiation in smokers	Overinflation of lungs and laryngeal elevation may have impact on swallowing in COPD	78
COPD vs normal controls	Swallowing is coupled with expiration in normals but altered in COPD during exacerbation	Swallowing co-ordination during exacerbation abnormal	81
COPD vs controls	COPD patients used spontaneous protective manoeuvres during swallowing	No obvious aspiration noted	82

GERD, gastro-oesophageal reflux disease.

Available data on swallowing and COPD

Additional research is required to determine whether COPD is associated with altered function of the oropharynx leads to episodes of microaspiration and if these episodes have a role in COPD exacerbations and lung function decline (Table 43.8). One study demonstrated cricopharyngeal dysfunction in COPD patients with frequent exacerbations and improvement with cricopharyngeal myotomy [79]. Co-ordination of swallowing with the phases of respiration can be altered during exacerbations in COPD patients [80]. Patients with COPD were shown to use spontaneous protective swallowing manoeuvres more frequently than controls, but no increase in aspiration during stable stage of COPD [81] was demonstrated. When present, treatment of hiatal hernia and gastro-oesophageal reflux with fundoplication and diaphragmatic crural repair showed improvement in cough in a group of patients with chronic bronchitis [82]. Smokers have been shown to have an increased threshold volume for the initiating of the pharyngo-UOS contractile reflex. Active smoking results in further increase of the threshold volume although aspiration has not been shown [83].

Key points

1 Inflammation in the upper airway is associated with inflammation in the lower airway and vice versa.
2 Patients with asthma should be evaluated for coexistent rhinosinusitis and, if present, rhinosinusitis should be treated.
3 Topical nasal corticosteroids are the most effective drugs for the treatment of non-infectious rhinosinusitis.

4 A few studies suggest that abnormal oropharyngeal function and swallowing may have a role in COPD.

References

1 Nelson HS. Advances in upper airway diseases and allergen immunotherapy. *J Allergy Clin Immunol* 2003;**111**:S793–8.
2 Tokias A. Rhinitis and asthma: evidence for respiratory system integration. *J Allergy Clin Immunol* 2003;**111**:1171–83.
3 Bousquet J, Cauwenberge P, Khaltaev N. Allergic rhinitis and its impact on asthma. *J Allergy Clin Immunol* 2001;**108**: S147–336.
4 Settipane RA. Demographics and epidemiology of allergic and non-allergic rhinitis. *Allergy Asthma Proc* 2001;**22**:185–9.
5 Sibbald B, Rink E. Epidemiology of seasonal and perennial rhinits: clinical presentation and medical history. *Thorax* 1991;**46**:895–901.
6 Zinreich SJ. Functional anatomy and computed tomography imaging of paranasal sinuses. *Am J Med Sci* 1998;**316**: 2–12.
7 Osguthrope JD, Hadley JA. Rhinosinusitis: current concepts in evaluation and management. *Med Clin N Am* 1999;**83**: 27–41.
8 Ayars G. Non-allergic rhinitis. *Immunol Allergy Clin North Am* 2000;**20**:283–302.
9 Christodoulopoulos P, Cameron L, Duraham S, Hasmid Q. Molecular pathology of allergic disease II. Upper airway disease. *J Allergy Clin Immunol* 2000;**105**:211–23.
10 Shturman-Ellstien R, Zeballos R, Buckley J, Souhrada J. The beneficial effects for nasal breathing on exercise-induced bronchoconstriction. *Am Rev Respir Dis* 1978;**118**:65–73.
11 Kaufman J, Wright G. The effect of nasal and nasopharyngeal irritation on airway resistance in man. *Am Rev Respir Dis* 1969;**100**:626–30.
12 Corren J, Adinoff A, Irvin C. Changes in bronchial

responsiveness following nasal provocation with allergen. *J Allergy Clin Immunol* 1992;**89**:611–8.

13 Yan K, Salome C. The response of the airways to nasal stimulation in asthmatics with rhinitis. *Eur J Respir Dis* 1982;**64**(Suppl 128):105–9.

14 Chakir J, Laviolette M, Boutet M *et al*. Lower airway remodeling in non-asthmatic subjects with allergic rhinitis. *Lab Invest* 1996;**75**:735–44.

15 Hart CM. Nitric oxide in adult lung disease. *Chest* 1999;**115**: 1407–17.

16 Meyts I, Proesmans M, De Boeck K. Exhaled nitric oxide corresponds with office evaluation of asthma control. *Pediatr Pulmonol* 2003;**36**:283–9.

17 Deja M, Busch T, Bachmann S *et al*. Reduced nitric oxide in sinus epithelium of patients with radiologic maxillary sinusitis and sepsis. *Am J Respir Crit Care Med* 2003;**168**: 281–6.

18 Venarske DL, deShazo RD. Sinobronchial allergic mycosis: The SAM syndrome. *Chest* 2002;**121**:1670–6.

19 deShazo RD, O'Brien MM, Justice WK *et al*. Diagnostic criteria for sarcoidosis of the sinuses. *J Allergy Clin Immunol* 1999;**103**:789–95.

20 Dykewicz MS, Fineman S, Skoner DP *et al*. Diagnosis and management of rhinitis: complete guidelines of the Joint Task Force on Practice Paramaters in Allergy, Asthma and Immunology. *Ann Allergy Asthma Immunol* 1998;**81**:478–518.

21 Ng MLS, Wardlow RS, Chrishanthan N *et al*. Preliminary criteria for the definition of allergic rhinitis: a systemic evaluation of clinical parameters in a disease cohort. I. *Clin Exp Allergy* 2000;**30**:1314–31.

22 Ng MLS, Wardlow RS, Chrishanthan N *et al*. Preliminary criteria for the definition of allergic rhinitis: a systemic evaluation of clinical parameters in a disease cohort. II. *Clin Exp Allergy* 2000;**30**:1417–22.

23 Siracusa A, Desrosiers M, Marabini A. Epidemiology of occupational rhinitis: prevalence, aetiology and determinants. *Clin Exp Allergy* 2000;**30**:1519–34.

24 Mullarkey MF, Hill JS, Webb DR. Allergic and non-allergic rhinitis: their characterization with attention to the meaning of nasal eosinophilia. *J Allergy Clin Immunol* 1980;**65**: 122–6.

25 Settipane RA, Lieberman P. Update on non-allergic rhinitis. *Ann Allergy Asthma Immunol* 2001;**86**:494–507.

26 Watson WT, Becker AB, Simons FE. Treatment of allergic rhinitis with intranasal corticosteroids in patients with mild asthma: effect on lower airway responsiveness. *J Allergy Clin Immunol* 1993;**91**:97–101.

27 Schwartz RS. A new element in the mechanism of asthma. *N Engl J Med* 2002;**346**:857–8.

28 Hansen JS, Schimidt H, Rosborg J, Lund E. Predicting acute maxillary sinusitis in a general practice population. *BMJ* 1995;**311**:233–6.

29 Druce HM. Allergic and non-allergic rhinitis In: Middleton E, Reed CE, Ellis EF, eds. *Allergy Principles and Practice*, 5th edn. St. Louis, MO: Mosby Year-Book, 1998; 1007.

30 Craig TJ, Teets S, Lehman EB *et al*. Nasal congestion secondary to allergic rhinitis as a cause of sleep disturbance and

daytime fatigue and the response to topical nasal corticosteroids. *J Allergy Clin Immunol* 1998;**101**:633–7.

31 Wight RG, Jones AS, Beckingham E *et al*. A double blind comparison of intranasal budesonide 400 µg and 800 µg in perennial rhinitis. *Clin Otolaryngol* 1992;**17**:354.

32 Banov C, LaForce C, Lieberman P. Double blind trial of Astelin nasal spray in the treatment of vasomotor rhintis. *Ann Allergy Asthma Immunol* 2000;**84**:138(Abstract).

33 Jacobs RL, Freedman PM, Boswell RN. Non-allergic rhinitis with eosinophilia (NARES syndrome): clinical and immunologic presentations. *J Allergy Clin Immunol* 1981;**67**:253–62.

34 Togias A, Proud D, Kagey-Sobotka A *et al*. Cold dry air (CDA) and histamine (HIST) induce more potent responses in perennial rhinitics compared to normal individuals. *J Allergy Clin Immunol* 1991;**87**:148(Abstract).

35 Antimicrobial treatment guidelines for acute bacterial rhinosinusitis: Sinus and Allergy Health Partnership. *Otolaryngol Head Neck Surg* 2000;**123**: S1–32.

36 Bhattacharyya N, Fried MP. The accuracy of computed tomography in the diagnosis of chronic rhinosinusitis. *Laryngoscope* 2003;**113**:125–9.

37 Vogan JC, Bolger WE, Keyes AS. Endoscopically guided sinonasal cultures: a direct comparison with maxillary sinus aspirate cultures. *Otolaryngol Head Neck Surg* 2000;**122**:470–3.

38 Spector SL, Bernstein IL, Li JT *et al*. Parameters for the diagnosis and management of sinusitis. IV. Complete guidelines and references. *J Allergy Clin Immunol* 1998;**102**(Suppl): S117.

39 Evans FO, Jr, Sydnor JB, Moore WEC *et al*. Sinusitis of the maxillary antrum. *N Engl J Med* 1975;**293**:735–9.

40 Wippold FJ II, Levitt RG, Evens RG *et al*. Limited coronal CT: an alternative screening examination for sinonasal inflammatory disease. *Allergy Proc* 1995;**16**:165–9.

41 Gwaltney JM, Jr, Phillips CD, Miller RD *et al*. Computed tomographic study of the common cold. *N Engl J Med* 1994;**330**:25–30.

42 McColley SA, Carroll JL, Curtis S *et al*. High prevalence of allergic sensitization in children with habitual snoring and obstructive sleep apnea. *Chest* 1997;**111**:170–3.

43 Fireman P. Otitis media and eustachian tube dysfunction: connection to allergic rhinitis. *J Allergy Clin Immunol* 1997; **99**:S787–97.

44 Lack G. Pediatric allergic rhinitis and comorbid disorders. *J Allergy Clin Immunol* 2001;**108**:S9.

45 Mygind N, Dahl R. The nose and paranasal sinuses in asthma. *Allergy* 1999;**54**(Suppl 57):1.

46 Harlin SL, Ansel DG, Lane SR *et al*. A clinical and pathologic study of chronic sinusitis: the role of the eosinophil. *J Allergy Clin Immunol* 1988;**81**:867–75.

47 Berman SZ, Mathison DA, Stevenson DD *et al*. Maxillary sinusitis and bronchial asthma correlation of roentgenograms cultures and thermograms. *J Allergy Clin Immunol* 1974;**53**:311–7.

48 Van Cauwenberge P, Bachert C, Passalacqua G *et al*. Consensus statement on the treatment of allergic rhinitis. Position paper of the European Academy of Allergology and Clinical Immunology. *Allergy* 2000;**55**:116.

49 National Institute of Allergy and Infectious Diseases:

National Institutes of Health. How to create a dust-free bedroom. Fact Sheet. Office of Communication and Public Liaison. June 1997. (Available at http://www.niaid.nih.gov/factsheets/dustfree/htm)

50 Van Bavel J, Findlay SR, Hampel FC, Jr *et al*. Intranasal fluticasone proprionate is more effective than terfenadine tablets for seasonal allergic rhinitis. *Arch Intern Med* 1994; **154**:2699–704.

51 Welsh PW, Sticker WE, Chu CP *et al*. Efficacy of belomethasone nasal solution, flunisolide, and cromolyn in relieving symptoms of ragweed allergy. *Mayo Clin Proc* 1987;**62**:125.

52 Meltzer EO. Performance effects of antihistamines. *J Allergy Clin Immunol* 1990;**86**:613–9.

53 Norris AA, Alton EWFW. Chloride transport and the action of sodium cromoglycate and nedocromil sodium. *Clin Exp Allergy* 1996;**98**:102–6.

54 Milgrom H, Biondi R, Georgitis JW *et al*. Comparison of ipratropium bromide 0.03% with beclomethasone dipropionate in the treatment of perennial rhinitis in children. *Ann Allergy Asthma Immunol* 1999;**83**:105–11.

55 Meltzer EO, Malmstrom K, Lu S *et al*. Concomitant montelukast and loratadine as treatment for seasonal allergic rhinitis: a randomized, placebo-controlled clinical trial. *J Allergy Clin Immunol* 2000;**105**:917–22.

56 Baki HA, Casale TB. The role of leukotrienes in allergic rhinitis: clinical and experimental evidence. *Leukotriene Res Clin Rev* 2001;**2**:4.

57 Israel E. Leukotrienes and rhinitis. *Clin Exp Allergy Rev* 2001;**1**:160.

58 Weber RW. Immunotherapy with allergens. *JAMA* 1997; **278**:1881.

59 Li JT. Immunotherapy for allergic rhinitis. *Immunol Allergy Clin N Am* 2000;**20**:383–400.

60 Akdis CA, Blaser K. Mechanisms of allergen-specific immunotherapy. *Allergy* 2000;**55**:522–30.

61 Hedlin G, Silber G, Naclerio R *et al*. Comparison of the *in vivo* and *in vitro* response to ragweed immunotherapy in children and adults with ragweed-induced rhinitis. *Clin Exp Allergy* 1990;**20**:491–500.

62 Durham SR, Ying S, Varney VA *et al*. Grass pollen immunotherapy inhibits allergen induced infiltration of CD4+ T lymphocytes and eosinophils in the nasal mucosa and increases the number of cells expressing messenger RNA for interferon-γ. *J Allergy Clin Immunol* 1996;**97**:1356–65.

63 Bousquet J, Lockey RF, Malling H-J *et al*. Allergen immunotherapy: therapeutic vaccines for allergic diseases. WHO Position Paper. *Allergy* 1998;**53**:S1.

64 Braun JJ, Alabert JP, Michel FB *et al*. Adjuvant effect of loratadine in the treatment of acute sinusitis in patients with allergic rhinitis. *Allergy* 1997;**52**:650–5.

65 Meltzer EO, Orgel HA, Backhaus JW *et al*. Intranasal flunisolide spray as an adjuvant to oral antibiotic therapy for sinusitis. *J Allergy Clin Immunol* 1993;**92**:812–23.

66 Dykewicz MS. Rhinitis and sinusitis: implications for severe asthma. *Immunol Allergy Clin North Am* 2001;**21**:427.

67 Park AH, Lau J, Stankiewicz J, Chow J. The role of functional endoscopic sinus surgery in asthmatic patients. *J Otolayngol* 1998;**27**:275–80.

68 Leckie MJ, ten Brinke A, Khan Z *et al*. Effects of an interleukin-5 blocking monoclonal antibody on eosinophils, airway hyperresponsiveness, and late asthmatic response. *Lancet* 2000;**356**:2144–8.

69 Casale TB. Experience with monoclonal antibody on allergic mediated disease: seasonal allergic rhinitis. *J Allergy Clin Immunol* 2001;**108**(Suppl):S84–8.

70 Barnet MS. Phoshodiesterase 4 (PDE₄) inhibitors in asthma and chronic obstructive pulmonary disease. *Prog Drug Res* 1999;**168**:981–5.

71 Agosti JM, Sanes-Miller CH. Novel therapeutic approaches for allergic rhinitis. *Immunol Allergy Clin North Am* 2000;**20**: 401.

72 Cook IJ, Kahrilas PJ. AGA technical review on management of oropharyngeal dysphagia. *Gastroenterology* 1999;**116**: 455–78.

73 Kahrilas PJ, Logemann JA, Lin S *et al*. Pharyngeal clearances during swallowing: a combined manometric and video fluoroscopic study. *Gastroenterology* 1992;**103**:128–36.

74 Castell JA, Dalton CB, Castell DO. Pharyngeal and upper esophageal sphincter manometry in humans. *Am J Physiol* 1990;**258**:G173–8.

75 Langmore SE, Schatz K, Olson N. Endoscopic and videofluoroscopic evaluations of swallowing and aspirations. *Ann Otol Rhinol Laryngol* 1991;**100**:678–81.

76 Aviv JE, Martin JH, Keen MS *et al*. Air pulse quantification of supraglottic and pharyngeal sensation: a new technique. *Ann Otol Rhinol Laryngol* 1993;**102**:777–80.

77 Dua KS, Ren J, Bardan E *et al*. Coordination of deglutitive glottal function and pharyngeal bolus transit during normal eating. *Gastroenterology* 1997;**112**:73–83.

78 Sleep-related breathing disorders in adults: recommendations for syndrome definition and measurement technique in clinical research. The Report of an American Academy of Sleep Medicine Task Force. *Sleep* 1999;**22**:667–89.

79 Stein M, Williams AJ, Grossman F *et al*. Cricopharyngeal dysfunction in chronic obstructive pulmonary disease. *Chest* 1990;**97**:347–52.

80 Shaker R, Li Q, Ren J *et al*. Coordination of deglutition and phases of respiration: effect of aging, tachypnea, bolus volume, and chronic obstructive pulmonary disease. *Am J Physiol* 1992;263:G750–5.

81 Mokhlesi B, Logemann JA, Rademaker AW *et al*. Oropharyngeal deglutition in stable COPD. *Chest* 2002; **121**:361–9.

82 Tibbling L. Wrong-way swallowing as a possible cause of bronchitis in patients with gastroesophageal reflux disease. *Acta Otolaryngol* 1993;**113**:405–8.

83 Dua K, Bardan E, Ren J *et al*. Effect of chronic and acute cigarette smoking on the pharyngo-upper esophageal contractile sphincter reflex and reflexive pharyngeal swallow. *Gut* 1998;**43**:537–41.

84 Leynaert B, Bousquet J, Neukirch C *et al*. Perennial rhinitis: an independent risk factor for asthma in nonatopic subjects: results from the European Community Respiratory Health Survey. *J Allergy Clin Immunol* 1999;**104**:301–4.

85 Settipane RJ, Hagy GW, Settipane GA *et al*. Long-term risk factors for developing asthma and allergic rhinitis: a 23-year

follow-up study of college students. *Allergy Proc* 1994;**15**: 21–5.

86 Togias AG. Unique mechanistic features of allergic rhinits. *J Allergy Clin Immunol* 2000;**105**:S599–604.

87 Fireman P. Rhinitis and asthma connection: management of coexisting upper airway allergic diseases and asthma. *Allergy Asthma Proc* 2000;**21**:45–53.

88 Corren J. Allergic rhinitis and asthma: how important is the link? *J Allergy Clin Immunol* 1997;**99**:S781–6.

89 Pedersen PA, Weeke ER. Asthma and allergic rhinitis in the same patients. *Allergy* 1983;**38**:25–9.

90 Madonini E, Briatico-Vangosa G, Pappacoda A *et al.* Seasonal increase of bronchial reactivity in allergic rhinitis. *J Allergy Clin Immunol* 1987;**79**:358–63.

91 Corren J, Adinoff A, Buchmeier A, Irwin C. Nasal beclomethasone prevents the seasonal increase in bronchial responsivenss in the patients with allergic rhinits and asthma. *J Allergy Clin Immunol* 1992;**90**:250–6.

92 Greiff L, Andersson M, Svensson C *et al.* Effects of orally inhaled budesonide in seasonal allergic rhinitis. *Eur Respir J* 1998;**11**:1268–73.

93 Welsh PW, Stricker WE, Chu CP *et al.* Efficacy of beclomethasone nasal solution, flunisolide, and cromolyn in relieving symptoms of ragweed allergy. *Mayo Clin Proc* 1987;**62**:125–34.

94 Braunstahl GJ, Kleinjan A, Overbeek SE *et al.* Segmental bronchial provocation induces nasal inflammation in allergic rhinitis patients. *Am J Respir Crit Care Med* 2000;**161**:2051–7.

95 Henriksen JM, Wenzel A. Effect of an intranasally administered corticosteroid (budesonide) on nasal obstruction, mouth breathing, and asthma. *Am Rev Respir Dis* 1984;**130**: 1014–8.

96 Grant JA, Nicodemus CF, Findlay S *et al.* Cetirizine in patients with seasonal rhinitis and concomitant asthma: prospective, randomized, placebo-controlled trial. *J Allergy Clin Immunol* 1995;**95**:923–32.

97 Corren J, Harris AG, Aaronson D *et al.* Efficacy and safety of loratadine plus pseudoephedrine in patients with seasonal allergic rhinitis and mild asthma. *J Allergy Clin Immunol* 1997;**100**:781–8.

98 Donnelly AL, Glass M, Minkwitz MC *et al.* The leukotriene D$_4$-receptor antagonist, ICI 204,219, relieves symptoms of acute seasonal allergic rhinitis. *Am J Respir Crit Care Med* 1995;**151**:1734–9.

99 Howarth P. Allergic and non-allergic rhinitis. In: Franklin Adkinson N, Jr. *Middleton's Allergy: Principles and* Practice, 6th edn, vol. 2. Philadelphia: Mosby, 2003: 1395.

100 deShazo R. Allergic rhinitis. In: Goldman L, Bennett JC, eds. *Cecil Textbook of Medicine*, 21st edn. Philadelphia: WB Saunders, 2000: 1447.

101 Kennedy DW. Concepts of acute and chronic sinusitis. In: *The Johns Hopkins Medical Grand Rounds*, vol. XVI, program 2, November 1989.

102 Orlandi RR, Kennedy DW. Surgical management of rhinosinusitis. *Am J Med Sci* 1998;**316**:29–38.

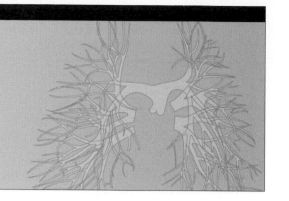

CHAPTER 44
Acute pulmonary embolism

Victor F. Tapson

Venous thromboembolism (VTE) represents the spectrum of disease including deep venous thrombosis (DVT) and pulmonary embolism (PE). While other substances such as tumour cells, fat, air and carbon dioxide can embolize to the lung, our focus is on VTE. Issues involving the interrelationship of VTE and chronic obstructive pulmonary disease (COPD) are emphasized.

Chronic cardiopulmonary disease, including COPD or congestive heart failure, are often present in patients with VTE, and the resulting reduced mobility is very likely a key underlying predisposition. Pulmonary embolism accounts for 100 000–200 000 deaths per year in the USA, but occurs worldwide. Patients often present with fatal PE as the initial presentation, and the poor sensitivity and specificity of the history and physical examination often lead to diagnostic and therapeutic delays. Autopsy studies emphasize the high frequency with which PE has gone unsuspected and thus undetected [1]. Specific risk factors are generally present in patients developing VTE, but the disease may appear to be idiopathic [2–4]. In the latter cases, an underlying thrombophilia may be present, although yet undescribed. Prophylaxis continues to be dramatically underutilized [3].

Pathophysiology

Over 150 years ago, Rudolf Virchow described the triad of stasis, hypercoagulability and intimal injury, and one or more of these is present in most all patients [5]. Deep vein thrombi frequently originate in the calf veins and propagate proximally before embolizing. Emboli may occasionally originate directly from calf vein thrombi, but more than 95% of thrombi that embolize to the lungs detach from a proximal deep vein of the lower extremities (including and above the popliteal veins). Pulmonary embolism may originate from an axillary subclavian source.

When PE occurs, its physiological effect depends upon the embolic load and the resultant cross-sectional area of the pulmonary arterial bed that is occluded. The presence or absence of underlying cardiopulmonary disease also contributes. A patient with COPD and a forced expiratory volume in 1 s (FEV_1) of 30% is less likely to tolerate massive emboli than a patient with milder disease. More than 50% obstruction of the pulmonary arterial bed is usually present before there is substantial elevation of the mean pulmonary artery pressure [6]. When the extent of obstruction of the pulmonary circulation approaches 75%, the right ventricle must generate a systolic pressure in excess of 50 mmHg and a mean pulmonary artery pressure of greater than 40 mmHg to preserve pulmonary perfusion. A normal right ventricle is rarely able to achieve this and hence fails. Death from PE is caused by right ventricular failure.

COPD and pulmonary embolism

COPD is a common comorbidity and/or risk factor for VTE. In DVT-Free, a 5451 patient DVT registry, 668 (12.3%) had COPD as a comorbid condition [3]. The risk of VTE during acute exacerbations of COPD appears to be substantial [7,8]. The DVT rate in 196 COPD patients admitted to a respiratory intensive care unit was 10.7% but it was likely underestimated by the poor sensitivity of ultrasound for asymptomatic DVT. Pulmonary embolism accounts for approximately 10% of deaths in stable COPD patients on chronic oxygen therapy [9]. The frequency of PE during acute COPD exacerbations has not been evaluated by large randomized clinical trials, but it may be as high as 29% [10].

Plasma fibrinogen increases have been reported in COPD exacerbations [11]. The increase compared with baseline has been shown to be significant ($P = 0.001$) and the increased levels of fibrinogen were associated with purulent sputum, increased cough, a higher baseline fibrinogen and age. This correlation is not surprising but the statistical significance does not verify that the demonstrated increase of 0.36 g/L is clinically significant. Of interest, however, is that plasma levels of fibrinogen increased further with exacerbations in association with raised interleukin 6 (IL-6) levels [11]. In view of the procoagulant effect of IL-6, it is possible that this represents an important link to VTE. While it seems possible that elevated levels of fibrinogen may contribute to an increased rate of VTE, the nature of the relationship between smoking and elevated fibrinogen levels appears much clearer. Indeed, it would appear that cigarette smoking is the strongest known environmental influence on plasma fibrinogen concentration and has consistently been linked to elevated plasma fibrinogen levels [12]. A dose–effect relationship between the number of cigarettes smoked per day and plasma fibrinogen concentration has been reported [13]. Conversely, cessation from smoking results in a rapid reduction in plasma fibrinogen [12].

Clinical manifestations of venous thromboembolism

History and physical examination

The history and physical examination are insensitive and non-specific for both DVT and PE, making the clinical diagnosis difficult [14,15]. Patients with lower extremity DVT may not have erythema, warmth, pain, swelling or tenderness. When present, these symptoms are non-specific, but may still merit further evaluation. Pain with dorsiflexion of the foot (Homans' sign) may be present in the setting of DVT but this finding is neither sensitive nor specific. The most common symptom of acute PE is dyspnoea which is often sudden in onset. Pleuritic chest pain and haemoptysis occur more commonly with pulmonary infarction resulting from smaller, peripheral emboli. Palpitations, cough, anxiety and lightheadedness are among the non-specific symptoms of acute PE and may result from a number of other entities, contributing to the difficulty in making the diagnosis. Syncope and/or sudden death may occur with massive PE. Tachypnoea and tachycardia are common signs of pulmonary embolism but are non-specific. Dyspnoea, tachypnoea and hypoxaemia in patients with concomitant cardiopulmonary disease (such as congestive heart failure, pneumonia or COPD) may be caused by the underlying disease or be a result of superimposed acute PE. Symptoms and signs consistent with PE (Tables 44.1 and 44.2) [16] should be particularly heeded in the setting of risk factors for VTE such as reduced mobility [17], the hospitalized medical setting [18], trauma or the postoperative state [19,20], concomitant malignancy [21], recent prolonged travel [22] or pregnancy [23].

Table 44.1 Sympoms of acute pulmonary embolism. The symptoms listed were based upon data from the Prospective Investigation of Pulmonary Embolism Diagnosis (PIOPED) study [14,15] and modified from tables presented in Stein [16].

	All patients (%) ($n = 383$)	No previous cardiopulmonary disease (%) ($n = 117$)
Dyspnoea	78	73
Pleuritic chest pain	59	66
Cough	43	37
Leg pain	27	26
Haemoptysis	16	13
Palpitations	13	10
Wheezing	14	9
Angina-like pain	6	4

Table 44.2 Signs of acute pulmonary embolism. The clinical signs listed were based upon data from the Prospective Investigation of Pulmonary Embolism Diagnosis (PIOPED) study [14,15] and modified from tables presented in Stein [16].

	All patients (%) ($n = 383$)	No previous cardiopulmonary disease (%) ($n = 117$)
Tachypnoea (20/min)	73	70
Crackles	55	51
Tachycardia (> 100/min)	30	30
Leg swelling	31	28
Loud P2	23	23
DVT	15	11
Wheezes	11	5
Diaphoresis	10	11
Temperature (≥ 38.5°C)	7	7
Pleural rub	4	3
Fourth heart sound	–	24
Third heart sound	5	3
Cyanosis	3	1
Homans' sign	3	4
Right ventricular lift	–	4

DVT, deep venous thrombosis; P2, pulmonic component of second heart sound.

Laboratory tests and electrocardiography

Hypoxaemia is common in acute PE. Some individuals, particularly young patients without underlying lung disease, may have a normal arterial oxygen tension (Pao_2) and even rarely a normal alveolar–arterial difference [14,15].

The diagnostic utility of plasma measurements of circulating D-dimer (a specific derivative of cross-linked fibrin) in patients with acute PE has been extensively evaluated [24,25]. A normal enzyme-linked immunosorbent assay (ELISA) appears sensitive in excluding PE, particularly when the clinical suspicion is relatively low. A D-dimer level of 500 µg/L or greater may have a sensitivity for PE as high as 96–98% but the specificity is much lower. A positive D-dimer test means that DVT or PE is possible, but it is by no means proof. Similarly, while a negative D-dimer may strongly suggest that VTE is absent, a high clinical suspicion should not be ignored.

The use of clinical probability scores based upon simple clinical parameters have been used together with a negative D-dimer to help exclude PE. In a recent prospective clinical trial, the SimpliRed D-dimer test (a rapid red blood cell agglutination D-dimer assay) was used together with simple scoring parameters readily available in the emergency department [25]. Of the 437 patients with a negative D-dimer result and low clinical probability in this study, only one developed PE during follow-up (Table 44.3).

Both cardiac troponin T and troponin I levels have been found to be elevated in acute PE [26,27]. This enzyme is specific for cardiac myocyte damage, and the right ventricle appears to be the source of the enzyme elevation in acute PE and, in particular, in more massive embolism in which myocyte injury resulting from right ventricular strain might be expected. Troponin levels cannot, however, be used like D-dimer testing; they are not sensitive enough to rule out PE when clinical suspicion is relatively low without additional diagnostic testing. Brain natriuretic peptide levels may be increased in acute PE. Preliminary data suggest that elevated levels may predict or indicate right ventricular dysfunction in acute PE [28]. While electrocardiographic findings are present in the majority of patients with acute PE, they are non-specific. Only one-third of patients with massive or submassive emboli have manifestations of acute cor pulmonale such as the S1–Q3–T3 pattern, right bundle branch block, P-wave pulmonale or right axis deviation [15].

Chest radiography

The chest radiograph is often abnormal but is nearly always non-specific in acute PE. Atelectasis, pleural effusion, pulmonary infiltrates and mild elevation of a hemidiaphragm may be present [15]. Findings of pulmonary

Table 44.3 Determining pretest probability of acute pulmonary embolism using point system and D-dimer result [25].

Variable	Points
DVT symptoms/signs	3.0
PE as or more likely*	3.0
HR > 100 beats/min	1.5
Immobilization/surgery†	1.5
Previous DVT or PE	1.5
Haemoptysis	1.0
Malignancy	1.0
Total score	*Pretest probability‡*
< 2.0	Low
2.0–6.0	Moderate
> 6.0	High

DVT, deep venous thrombosis; HR, heart rate; PE, pulmonary embolism.
* PE as likely or more likely than an alternative diagnosis. Physicians were told to use clinical information, along with chest radiography, electrocardiography and laboratory tests.
† If in previous 4 weeks.
‡ Of the 437 patients with a negative D-dimer result and low clinical probability, only one developed PE during follow-up; thus, the negative predictive value for the combined strategy of using the clinical model with D-dimer testing in these patients was 99.5%.

infarction such as Hampton's hump or decreased vascularity (Westermark's sign) are suggestive, but uncommon. A normal chest radiograph in the setting of severe dyspnoea and hypoxaemia without evidence of bronchospasm or anatomical cardiac shunt is strongly suggestive of PE. Neither symptoms, signs, radiographical findings, electrocardiography nor the plasma D-dimer measurement can be considered diagnostic of DVT or PE. When suspected, further evaluation is necessary.

Specific radiographical imaging for venous thromboembolism

Deep venous thrombosis

While venography has been the time-honoured gold standard test, ultrasound has a sensitivity of greater than 90% in the setting of symptomatic DVT and is by far the most common technique utilized for suspected DVT. Magnetic resonance imaging (MRI) has proven extremely sensitive for both acute and chronic DVT, although it is generally not necessary [29]. It is very reasonable to consider MRI in the setting of suspected DVT when ultrasound cannot be effectively utilized. A major limitation of ultrasound is its reduced sensitivity in the setting of asymptomatic DVT. Thus, it is not generally used as a screening test.

Pulmonary embolism

The ventilation–perfusion (*V*/*Q*) scan had historically been the most common diagnostic test utilized when PE was suspected. A normal perfusion scan rules out the diagnosis with a high enough degree of certainty that further diagnostic evaluation is almost never necessary [30]. Low or intermediate probability (non-diagnostic) scans are commonly found with PE and in such situations further evaluation with pulmonary arteriography is often appropriate. In the Prospective Investigation of Pulmonary Embolism Diagnosis (PIOPED) when the clinical suspicion of PE was considered very high, it was present in 96% of patients with high probability scans, 66% of patients with intermediate scans and 40% of patients with low probability scans [14]. The diagnosis of PE should be rigorously pursued even when the lung scan is low or intermediate probability if the clinical setting strongly suggests the diagnosis.

Pulmonary arteriography remains the accepted gold standard technique for the diagnosis of acute PE. It is an extremely sensitive, specific and safe test [31]. Complications of pulmonary arteriography among 1111 patients suspected of PE in the PIOPED included death in 0.5% and major non-fatal complications in 1% [14]. It is utilized when PE must be diagnosed or excluded, but preliminary testing has been non-diagnostic. It is being used less frequently as CT has increasingly been employed.

Spiral computed tomography (CT) scanning is replacing *V*/*Q* at many centres. Some clinical trials have suggested very good sensitivity and specificity but others have been less favourable. Retrospective reconstructions can be performed. A contrast bolus is required for imaging of the pulmonary vasculature. A number of clinical trials have been conducted with somewhat variable sensitivity, and a recent large prospective Swiss study revealed a sensitivity of 70%, suggesting that a negative CT scan may not absolutely rule out smaller emboli [32]. Data from a large multicentre trial (PIOPED II) in the USA and Canada comparing CT (chest and legs) with *V*/*Q* scanning is currently being analysed. Spiral CT has the greatest sensitivity for emboli in the main, lobar or segmental pulmonary arteries. For subsegmental emboli, spiral CT appears less accurate. The outcome of selected patients with a negative CT in the setting of suspected PE appears to be good in published trials thus far [33]. An advantage of spiral CT over *V*/*Q* scanning and arteriography includes the ability to define non-vascular structures such as lymphadenopathy, lung tumours, emphysema and other parenchymal abnormalities as well as pleural and pericardial disease. Patients with significant renal insufficiency cannot be scanned without risk of renal failure.

Magnetic resonance imaging has been utilized to evaluate clinically suspected PE but at present the excellent sensitivity and specificity for the diagnosis of DVT is the main advantage of MRI in this disease process [29,34].

Echocardiography in acute pulmonary embolism

Echocardiography can often be obtained more rapidly than other diagnostic tests and may reveal findings that strongly support haemodynamically significant PE [35]. Unfortunately, because these patients often have underlying cardiopulmonary disease such as COPD, neither right ventricular dilatation nor hypokinesis can be reliably used even as indirect evidence of PE in such settings. In the setting of documented acute PE, echocardiographical evidence of right ventricular dysfunction has been suggested as a means by which to determine the need for thrombolytic therapy [36]. Such cases need to be individualized and severe right ventricular dysfunction should lower the threshold for thrombolytic therapy once contraindications have been considered. Intravascular ultrasound imaging has been shown in both the experimental and clinical setting to image large emboli adequately and may be performed at the bedside [37]. Published guidelines are available for the diagnostic approach to acute PE, and these suggest that clinicians need to be given a certain degree of flexibility in this regard [38].

Treatment

Options for therapy of acute DVT and PE have evolved considerably over the past decade. Each approach has specific indications as well as advantages and disadvantages.

Heparin and low molecular weight heparin

Unfractionated heparin and low molecular weight heparin (LMWH) exert a prompt antithrombotic effect by accelerating the action of antithrombin III, preventing thrombus extension. These drugs do not directly lyse thrombus or emboli, but enable the fibrinolytic system to proceed unopposed and more readily reduce the size of the thromboembolic burden. There are substantial advantages of LMWH preparations over unfractionated heparin [39,40] and, because of these, use of the latter has decreased.

When VTE is strongly suspected, anticoagulation should be promptly initiated unless there are contraindications. Confirmatory diagnostic testing should soon follow. When standard unfractionated intravenous heparin is initiated, the activated partial thromboplastin time (APTT) should be followed at 6-h intervals until it is consistently in the therapeutic range of 1.5–2.0 times control values, corresponding to a heparin level of 0.2–0.4 U/mL as measured by protamine sulphate titration. Achieving a therapeutic APTT within 24 h after the onset of treatment of PE has been shown to reduce the recurrence rate. Heparin can be administered as an intravenous bolus of 5000 units followed by a maintenance dose of at least 30 000–40 000 units per 24 h by continuous infusion [41]. The lower dose is administered if the patient is considered at high risk for bleeding. At least 5 days of intravenous heparin or LMWH overlap with warfarin is recommended. Heparin should be maintained at a therapeutic level until two consecutive therapeutic international normalized ratio (INR) values of 2.0–3.0 have been documented at least 24 h apart (Table 44.4).

The LMWH preparations have tremendous advantages over unfractionated heparin and have dramatically changed treatment of thromboembolic disease. Greater bioavailab-

---

Table 44.4 Initiation of low molecular weight heparin for therapy of acute deep venous thrombosis and/or pulmonary embolism.

- Determine appropriateness of outpatient therapy*
- Begin LMWH by subcutaneous administration†
- Determine whether monitoring needed (extremes of weight, renal insufficiency, pregnancy)
- Warfarin from day 1; initial dose 5–10 mg, adjust according to INR
- Check platelet count between days 3 and 5‡
- Stop LMWH after ≥ 5 days of combined therapy, and when INR is ≥ 2.0 for 2 consecutive days
- Anticoagulate with warfarin for ≥ 3 months (goal INR 2.0–3.0)§

DVT, deep venous thrombosis; INR, international normalized ratio; LMWH, low molecular weight heparin; PE, pulmonary embolism.
* Potential outpatients should be medically stable without severely symptomatic DVT. They should be compliant, capable of self-administration (or have a family member or visiting nurse for administration), at low risk of bleeding and reimbursement should be addressed.
† Enoxaparin (Lovenox), tinzaparin (Innohep), and fondaparinux (Arixtra), are US Food and Drug Administration (FDA)-approved for treatment of acute venous thromboembolism. These preparations are often used for acute PE as well as acute DVT, and while clinical trials support these uses, the FDA-approvals read 'established DVT with or without PE' except for fondaparinux which is approved for patients presenting with either.
‡ Heparin-induced thrombocytopenia.
§ The duration of warfarin therapy should be at least 6–12 months in patients with idiopathic venous thromboembolism.

---

ility of the LMWH than standard heparin (with more predictable dosing) [39,40], the lack of need for an intravenous infusion (all indications are once or twice daily by the subcutaneous route) and the lack of need for monitoring of the APTT are among the important differences. The reduced frequency of heparin-induced thrombocytopenia with LMWH relative to unfractionated heparin is a very compelling reason to use LMWH instead of the latter whenever possible. A number of clinical trials as well as meta-analyses have strongly suggested the efficacy and safety of LMWH for treatment of established acute proximal DVT using recurrent symptomatic VTE as the primary outcome measure [42–45]. The incidence of DVT and recurrent bleeding in these trials indicate that LMWH preparations are at least as effective and as safe as unfractionated heparin. Meta-analytic data suggest that the use of LMWH might reduce bleeding as well as mortality compared with unfractionated heparin for treatment of established proximal DVT [44,45].

Anti-factor Xa levels appear reasonable to monitor in certain settings such as in morbidly obese patients, very small patients (less than 40 kg), pregnant patients and those with renal insufficiency. Because these drugs are renally metabolized, monitoring is important, particularly when the creatinine clearance less than 30 mL/min. With severe renal insufficiency, standard heparin should be considered. There is not clear agreement on a weight limit above which LMWH should not be used, but some feel that an upper limit of approximately 120–150 kg is reasonable, with intravenous standard heparin being used in larger patients. It is unnecessary to monitor other patients with anti-factor Xa levels. One LMWH, enoxaparin, now has specific recommendations for therapy when the creatinine clearance is below 30 mL/min. The dose is changed from 1 mg/kg every 12 h to 1 mg/kg once daily. Unfractionated heparin should be used when there are rapid, significant changes in renal function.

In the USA, at the present time, two LMWH preparations (enoxaparin and tinzaparin) are FDA-approved for use to treat patients presenting with DVT with or without acute PE. The most widely used LMWH, enoxaparin, is approved for both inpatient and outpatient use at a dose of 1 mg/kg subcutaneously every 12 h, or at 1.5 mg/kg once daily for inpatient use. Outpatient therapy is increasing and has proven safe in selected patients [46,47]. There is also experience with LMWH for treatment of patients presenting with PE [43]. Recently, the pentasaccharide ('ultra-low molecular weight heparin'), fondaparinux, has been approved for use in patients with acute DVT and PE [48]. It should be noted that the prophylactic doses of these agents differ from the doses used for treating active disease. The characteristics of LMWH compared with standard unfractionated heparin are shown in Table 44.5.

Documented proximal DVT or PE should be treated for 3–6 months. Treatment over a more extended interval

Table 44.5 A comparison of low molecular weight heparin with unfractionated heparin.

Characteristic	UFH	LMWH
Mean molecular weight	12 000–15 000	4000–6000
Protein binding	Substantial	Minimal*
Anti-Xa activity	Substantial	Substantial
Anti-IIa activity	Substantial	Minimal
Administration (treatment)	Intravenous	Subcutaneous
Administration (prophylaxis)	Subcutaneous	Subcutaneous
Monitoring during treatment	aPTT every 6 h	None in most settings†
Outpatient therapy	Difficult	Simplified
Incidence of HIT	3–5%	< 1%
Reversibility with protamine	Complete	Partial

aPTT, activated partial thromboplastin time; HIT, heparin-induced thrombocytopenia; LMWH, low molecular weight heparin; UFH, unfractionated heparin.
* This implies significantly superior bioavailability of LMWH relative to UFH.
† LMWH requires monitoring in renal insufficiency (creatinine clearance < 30 mL/min), significant obesity (> 150 kg), very small patients (< 40 kg), and pregnant patients. Anti-Xa levels are followed, and not the aPTT.

is appropriate when significant risk factors persist, when thromboembolism is idiopathic or when previous episodes of VTE have been documented.

Direct thrombin inhibitors

Unlike heparin and LMWH, which require antithrombin III as a cofactor, direct thrombin inhibitors are efficacious against fibrin-bound thrombin. Ximelagatran, an oral direct thrombin inhibitor, was studied extensively in hopes of simplifying the treatment of acute VTE. The oral delivery, rapid onset, lack of significant drug and food interactions, and lack of need for monitoring were among the advantages over warfarin. It proved effective [49,50] but several issues prevented FDA-approval in the USA. These included abnormal liver function tests resulting from the drug, and an increased incidence of rebound thrombotic events occurring after total joint replacement. Other direct thrombin and direct factor-Xa inhibitors are currently being studied. While ximelagatran is associated with transient elevation in hepatic transaminases between approximately 8 and 12 weeks, this is generally transient and reversible even with continued exposure to the drug. Liver function test monitoring will be recommended, at least temporarily.

The oral delivery, rapid onset, lack of significant drug and food interactions, and lack of need for INR monitoring are among the advantages over warfarin.

Heparin-induced thrombocytopenia (defined as a platelet count less than 150 000/mm^3) typically develops 5 or more days after the initiation of heparin therapy, occurring in approximately 5% of patients [51]. The syndrome is caused by heparin-dependent immunoglobulin G (IgG) antibodies that activate platelets via their Fc receptors. If a patient is placed on heparin for VTE and the platelet count progressively decreases to 150 000 mm^3 or less or to less than 50% of the initial platelet count, heparin-induced thrombocytopenia should be considered. The formation of heparin-dependent IgG antibodies and the risk of thrombocytopenia is lower with LMWH than with standard heparin [52].

Argatroban and lepirudin are FDA-approved for use in the setting of VTE with heparin-induced thrombocytopenia. The half-life of argatroban is prolonged in patients with hepatic dysfunction. Lepirudin is excreted by the kidneys so the dosage must be reduced in renal insufficiency. This drug has a short circulating half-life of 1.3 h in patients with normal renal function but it may be as long as 2 days in patients with advanced renal failure. A detailed discussion of heparin-induced thrombocytopenia is beyond the scope of this chapter.

Vena cava interruption

Inferior vena cava (IVC) filter placement can be performed to prevent lower extremity thrombi from embolizing to the lungs. The primary indications for filter placement include contraindications to anticoagulation, recurrent embolism while on adequate therapy and significant bleeding complications during anticoagulation [52]. Filters are sometimes placed in the setting of massive PE when it is believed that any further emboli might be lethal, particularly if thrombolytic therapy is contraindicated. Filters can be inserted via the jugular or femoral vein. These devices are effective and complications including insertion-related problems and migration are unusual. More recently, temporary filters are being placed in patients in whom the risk of bleeding appears short-term. Most of these devices can be removed up to 2 weeks later, and some may remain in place even longer with subsequent removal.

Thrombolytic therapy

Thrombolytic agents activate plasminogen to form plasmin which then results in fibrinolysis as well as fibrinogenolysis. These agents can dramatically accelerate clot lysis in acute PE (and DVT) clinical trials have culminated in the approval of streptokinase, urokinase and recombinant tissue-type plasminogen activator (t-PA) for the treatment of massive PE [53,54].

The clearly accepted indication for thrombolytic therapy has been PE with haemodynamic instability (hypotension) for the past several decades. Those with severely compromised oxygenation should also be considered. While thrombolytic therapy may result in rapid improvement of right ventricular function in patients with acute PE, there has been controversy as to whether or not patients with echocardiographic right ventricular dysfunction but without hypotension should receive this form of treatment. A recent clinical trial offered further evidence to support this concept, indicating a less frequent need for escalation of treatment when thrombolytic therapy was used in the setting of PE with right ventricular dysfunction [55]. The method of delivery of thrombolytic agents has also been investigated. While standard or low-dose intrapulmonary arterial thrombolytic infusions have been utilized in order to deliver a high concentration of drug in close proximity to the clot, intravenous therapy appears adequate in most cases [56]. More direct techniques, such as catheter-directed administration of intraembolic thrombolytic therapy have been utilized in small clinical studies but the data are inadequate to formulate recommendations [57,58]. Evolution of interventional techniques will encourage additional clinical trials. The use of thrombolytic therapy in patients with proximal occlusive DVT associated with significant swelling and symptoms is increasing. Catheter-directed techniques are often employed [59]. In DVT, such aggressive therapy with thrombolytics may reduce the frequency of postphlebitic syndrome.

Bleeding is the primary concern with thrombolytic therapy. Both lysis of haemostatic fibrin plugs and fibrinogenolysis can lead to bleeding complications which commonly occur at sites of invasive procedures such as pulmonary arteriography or arterial line placement. Invasive procedures should be minimized as much as possible. The most devastating complication associated with thrombolytic therapy is the development of intracranial haemorrhage which occurs in less than 1% of patients. Retroperitoneal haemorrhage may result from a vascular puncture above the inguinal ligament and may be life-threatening. The main contraindications to thrombolytic therapy include active bleeding, surgery within the previous 1–2 weeks (depending on specific procedure), intracranial pathology or previous surgery. When patients appear to be at extraordinary risk of rapid death from PE, clinical judgment should be individualized with regard to contraindications.

Management of unstable haemodynamics in massive PE

Once massive PE associated with hypotension and/or severe hypoxaemia is suspected, supportive treatment is immediately initiated. With hypotension intravenous saline should be infused rapidly but cautiously because right ventricular function is often markedly compromised. Dopamine or noradrenaline (norepinephrine) appear to be the favoured choices of vasoactive therapy in massive PE and should be administered if the blood pressure is not rapidly restored [60]. Because death in this setting results from right ventricular failure, dobutamine may offer benefit. A vasopressor such as noradrenaline combined with dobutamine might offer optimal results and further exploration of such combined therapy would prove enlightening. Oxygen therapy is administered and thrombolytic therapy is considered as described above. Pulmonary embolectomy may be appropriate in patients with massive embolism who cannot receive thrombolytic therapy.

Prognosis

In the International Cooperative Pulmonary Embolism Registry of 2454 patients, all consecutive patients with a diagnosis of PE were included and PE was the principal cause of death [61]. The 3-month mortality was 17.5%. In the PIOPED, the mortality rate was approximately 15% but only 10% of deaths during the first year of follow-up were attributed to PE [14]. Mean 1 month mortality rates of treated and untreated PE have been estimated at 8% and 30%, respectively.

While a small percentage of patients with acute VTE will ultimately develop chronic thromboembolic pulmonary hypertension, most patients who survive the acute episode have no long-term pulmonary sequelae. However, chronic leg pain and swelling from postphlebitic syndrome may cause significant morbidity.

Prevention

Measures to prevent VTE appear to be grossly underutilized [2,3]. A substantial reduction in the incidence of DVT can be achieved when patients at risk receive appropriate prophylaxis. In one of the highest risk settings, total hip or knee replacement, the risk is 50% or greater without prophylaxis. The superiority of LMWH over unfractionated heparin has been demonstrated in these settings, and extending the duration of prophylaxis to approximately 1 month after surgery further reduces the DVT rate in total hip replacement [62]. Unfractionated heparin is not recommended in total joint replacement.

Hospitalized general medical patients are clearly at risk for VTE. Anticoagulant prophylaxis should always be strongly considered as the rate of DVT, based upon a venographic endpoint, is as high as 15% in medical patients receiving placebo [18]. The rate of DVT, including proximal

DVT, is statistically significantly lower when enoxaparin is administered compared with placebo [1]. Low molecular weight heparin (enoxaparin) has been compared directly with subcutaneous standard heparin (5000 units every 8 h) for medical patient prophylaxis and while clear superiority was not proven, VTE rates were lower with enoxaparin [63]. Although 5000 units of heparin every 12 h has been commonly used, there are fewer data to support this preventive regimen in medical patients. Intermittent pneumatic compression devices should be utilized when pharmacological prophylaxis is contraindicated. Both methods combined would be reasonable in patients deemed to be at exceptionally high risk, but an additional reduction in risk in such patients has not been well substantiated.

The efficacy of prophylactic therapy for VTE in COPD exacerbations has been studied, and administration of a LMWH prompted a 45% reduction in the incidence of DVT in acutely decompensated patients compared with placebo in a large prospective randomized trial [64]. Other studies have included large numbers of COPD patients and have confirmed the efficacy of LMWH in preventing VTE in this population [18]. A recent review has characterized the clinical problem of VTE in patients undergoing acute exacerbation of COPD [65].

Each hospitalized patient should be assessed for the need for such prophylactic measures and all hospitals should strongly consider formulating their own written guidelines for each particular clinical setting, based upon the available medical literature [66].

References

1 Lindblad B, Eriksson A, Bergquist D. Autopsy-verified pulmonary embolism in a surgical department: analysis of the period from 1951 to 1988. *Br J Surg* 1991;**78**:849–52.

2 Anderson FA, Wheeler HB. Venous thromboembolism: risk factors and prophylaxis. *Clin Chest Med* 1995;**16**:235–51.

3 Goldhaber SZ, Tapson VF. A prospective registry of 5451 patients with ultrasound confirmed deep vein thrombosis. *Am J Cardiol* 2004;**93**:259–62.

4 Kakkar VV, Howe CT, Nicolaides AN *et al.* Deep vein thrombosis of the legs: is there a 'high risk' group? *Am J Surg* 1970;**120**:527–30.

5 von Virchow R. Weitere Untersuchungen ueber die Verstopfung der Lungenarterien und ihre Folge. *Traube's Beitraege exp path u Physiol, Berlin* 1846;**2**:21–31.

6 McIntyre KM, Sasahara AA. The ratio of pulmonary artery pressure to pulmonary vascular obstruction. *Chest* 1977;**71**:692.

7 Prescott SM, Richards KL, Tikoff G, Armstrong JD, Shigeoka JW. Venous thromboembolism in decompensated chronic obstructive pulmonary disease: a prospective study. *Am Rev Respir Dis* 1981;**123**:32–6.

8 Winter JH, Buckler PW, Bautista AP *et al.* Frequency of venous thrombosis in patients with an exacerbation of chronic obstructive lung disease. *Thorax* 1983;**38**:605–8.

9 Mispelaere D, Glerant JC, Audebert M *et al.* Pulmonary embolism and sibilant types of chronic obstructive pulmonary disease decompensations. *Rev Mal Respir* 2002;**19**:415–23.

10 Schonhofer B, Kohler D. Prevalence of deep-vein thrombosis of the leg in patients with acute exacerbation of chronic obstructive pulmonary disease. *Respiration* 1998;**65**:173–7.

11 Wedzicha JA, Seemungal TA, MacCallum PK *et al.* Acute exacerbations of chronic obstructive pulmonary disease are accompanied by elevations of plasma fibrinogen and serum IL-6 levels. *Thromb Haemost* 2000;**84**:210–5.

12 Tuut M, Hense HW. Smoking, other risk factors and fibrinogen levels: evidence of effect modification. *Ann Epidemiol* 2001;**11**:232–8.

13 Rothwell M, Rampling MW, Cholerton S, Sever PS. Haemorheological changes in the short term after abstention from tobacco by cigarette smokers. *Br J Haematol* 1991;**79**:500–3.

14 The PIOPED investigators. Value of the ventilation/perfusion scan in acute pulmonary embolism: results of the Prospective Investigation of Pulmonary Embolism Diagnosis. *JAMA* 1990;**263**:2753–9.

15 Stein PD, Terrin ML, Hales CA *et al.* Clinical, laboratory, roentgenographic, and electrocardiographic findings in patients with acute pulmonary embolism and no pre-existing cardiac or pulmonary disease. *Chest* 1991;**100**:598–603.

16 Stein PD, ed. *Pulmonary Embolism*. Baltimore: Williams and Wilkins, 1996.

17 Clason S. Three cases of pulmonary embolism following confinement, treated with heparin. *Acta Med Scand* 1941;**107**:131–5.

18 Samama MM, Cohen AT, Darmon J-Y *et al.* A comparison of enoxaparin with placebo for the prevention of venous thromboembolism in acutely ill medical patients. *N Engl J Med* 1999;**341**:793–800.

19 Fitts WT Jr, Lehr HB, Bitner RL *et al.* An analysis of 950 fatal injuries. *Surgery* 1964;**56**:663–8.

20 Clagett GP, Reisch JS. Prevention of venous thromboembolism in general surgical patients: results of a meta-analysis. *Ann Surg* 1988;**208**:227–40.

21 Rickles FR, Edwards RL. Activation of blood coagulation in cancer: Trousseau's syndrome revisited. *Blood* 1983;**62**:14–31.

22 Kraaijenhagen RA, Haverkamp D, Koopman MMW *et al.* Travel and risk of venous thrombosis. *Lancet* 2000;**356**:1492–3.

23 Toglia MR, Weg JG. Current concepts: venous thromboembolism during pregnancy. *N Engl J Med* 1996;**335**:108–14.

24 Bounameaux H, Cirafici P, DeMoerloose P *et al.* Measurement of D-dimer in plasma as diagnostic aid in suspected pulmonary embolism. *Lancet* 1991;**337**:196.

25 Wells PS, Anderson DR, Rodger M *et al.* Excluding pulmonary embolism at the bedside without diagnostic imaging: management of patients with suspected pulmonary embolism presenting to the emergency department by using a simple clinical model and D-dimer. *Ann Intern Med* 2001;**135**:98–107.

26 Douketis JD, Crowther MA, Stanton EB, Ginsberg JS. Elevated cardiac troponin levels in patients with submassive pulmonary embolism. *Arch Intern Med* 2002;**162**:79–81.

27 Tapson VF. Diagnosing and managing acute pulmonary embolism: role of cardiac troponins. *Am Heart J* 2003;**145**: 751–3.

28 Kruger S, Graf J, Merx MW *et al.* Brain natriuretic peptide predicts right heart failure in patients with acute pulmonary embolism. *Am Heart J* 2004;**147**:60–5.

29 Evans AJ, Tapson VF, Sostman HD *et al.* The diagnosis of deep venous thrombosis: a prospective comparison of venography and magnetic resonance imaging. *Chest* 1992;**102**:120S.

30 McNeill BJ, Hessel SJ, Branch WT *et al.* Measures of clinical efficacy. III. The value of the lung scan in the evaluation of young patients with pleuritic chest pain. *J Nucl Med* 1976; **17**:163–4.

31 Stein PD, Athanasoulis C, Alavi A *et al.* Complications and validity of pulmonary angiography in acute pulmonary embolism. *Circulation* 1992;**85**:462–8.

32 Perrier A, Howarth N, Didier D *et al.* Performance of helical computed tomography in unselected outpatients with suspected pulmonary embolism. *Ann Intern Med* 2001;**135**: 88–97.

33 Swensen SJ, Sheedy PF, Ryu JH *et al.* Outcomes after withholding anticoagulation from patients with suspected acute pulmonary embolism and negative computed tomographic findings: a cohort study. *Mayo Clin Proc* 2002;**77**:130–8.

34 Tapson VF. Pulmonary embolism: new diagnostic approaches. *N Engl J Med* 1997;**336**:1449–51.

35 Come PC. Echocardiographic evaluation of pulmonary embolism and its response to therapeutic interventions. *Chest* 1992;**101**:151S–62S.

36 Goldhaber SZ, Haire WD, Feldstein ML *et al.* Alteplase versus heparin in acute pulmonary embolism: randomized trial assessing right ventricular function and pulmonary perfusion. *Lancet* 1993;**341**:507–10.

37 Tapson VF, Davidson CJ, Kisslo KB, Stack RS. Rapid visualization of massive pulmonary emboli utilizing intravascular ultrasound. *Chest* 1994;**105**:888–90.

38 Tapson VF, Carroll BA, Davidson BL *et al.* The diagnostic approach to acute venous thromboembolism. Clinical Practice Guideline. American Thoracic Society. *Am J Respir Crit Care Med* 1999;**160**:1043–66.

39 Tapson VF, Hull R. Management of venous thromboembolic disease: the impact of low-molecular-weight heparin. *Clin Chest Med* 1995;**16**:281–94.

40 Tapson VF. Treatment of acute deep venous thrombosis and pulmonary embolism: use of low molecular weight heparin. *Semin Respir Crit Care Med* 2000;**21**:547–53.

41 Hull R, Raskob G, Rosenbloom D *et al.* Optimal therapeutic level of heparin therapy in patients with venous thrombosis. *Arch Intern Med* 1992;**152**:1589–95.

42 Merli G, Spiro T, Olsson C-G *et al.* Subcutaneous enoxaparin once or twice daily compared with intravenous unfractionated heparin for treatment of venous thromboembolic disease. *Ann Intern Med* 2001;**134**:191–202.

43 Simmoneau G, Sors H, Charbonnier B *et al.* A comparison of low-molecular-weight heparin with unfractionated heparin for acute pulmonary embolism. The THESEE Study Group. *N Engl J Med* 1997;**337**:663–9.

44 Siragusa S, Cosmi B, Piovella F, Hirsh J, Ginsberg JS. Low-molecular-weight heparins and unfractionated heparin in the treatment of patients with acute venous thromboembolism: results of a meta-analysis. *Am J Med* 1996;**100**:269–77.

45 Dolovich LR, Ginsberg JS, Douketis JD *et al.* A meta-analysis comparing low molecular weight heparins with unfractionated heparin in the treatment of venous thromboembolism. *Arch Intern Med* 2000;**160**:181–8.

46 Levine M, Gent M, Hirsh J *et al.* A comparison of low molecular-weight-heparin administered primarily at home with unfractionated heparin administered in the hospital for proximal deep vein thrombosis. *N Engl J Med* 1996;**334**: 677–81.

47 Koopman MM, Prandoni P, Piovella F *et al.* Low molecular-weight-heparin versus heparin for proximal deep vein thrombosis. *N Engl J Med* 1996;**334**:682–7.

48 The Matisse Investigators. Subcutaneous fondaparinux versus intravenous unfractionated heparin in the initial treatment of pulmonary embolism. *N Engl J Med* 2004;**349**:1695–702.

49 Schulman S, Wahlander K, Lundstrom T *et al.* Secondary prevention of venous thromboembolism with the oral direct thrombin inhibitor, ximelagatran. *N Engl J Med* 2003;**349**: 1713–21.

50 Huisman M. Efficacy and safety of the oral direct thrombin inhibitor ximelagatran compared with current standard therapy for acute symptomatic deep vein thrombosis, with or without pulmonary embolism: a randomized, double-blind, multinational study. XIX International Congress. International Society of Thrombosis and Haemostasis, Birmingham, UK 2003. *J Thromb Haemost Suppl* 2003.

51 Warkentin TE, Levine MN, Hirsh J *et al.* Heparin-induced thrombocytopenia in patients treated with low-molecular-weight heparin or unfractionated heparin. *N Engl J Med* 1995;**332**:1330–5.

52 Becker DM, Philbrick JT, Selby JB. Inferior vena cava filters: indications, safety, effectiveness. *Arch Intern Med* 1992;**152**: 1985–94.

53 Symposium: Thrombolytic therapy in thrombosis: a National Institutes of Health Consensus Development Conference. *Ann Intern Med* 1980;**93**:141–3.

54 Goldhaber SZ. Evolving concepts in thrombolytic therapy for pulmonary embolism. *Chest* 1992;**101**(Suppl):183S–5S.

55 Konstantinides S, Geibel A, Huesel G *et al.* Heparin plus alteplase compared with heparin alone in patients with submassive pulmonary embolism. *N Engl J Med* 2002;**347**: 1143–50.

56 Tapson VF, Gurbel PA, Royster R *et al.* Pharmacomechanical thrombolysis of experimental pulmonary emboli: rapid low-dose intraembolic therapy. *Chest* 1994;**106**:1558–62.

57 Verstraete M, Miller GAH, Bounameaux H *et al.* Intravenous and intrapulmonary recombinant tissue-type plasminogen activator in the treatment of acute massive pulmonary embolism. *Circulation* 1988;**77**:353–60.

58 Tapson VF, Witty LA. Massive pulmonary embolism: diagnostic and therapeutic strategies. *Clin Chest Med* 1996;**16**:329.

59 Semba CP, Dake MD. Iliofemoral deep venous thrombosis: aggressive therapy with catheter-directed thrombolysis. *Radiology* 1994;**191**:487–94.

60 Layish DT, Tapson VF. Pharmacologic hemodynamic support in massive pulmonary embolism. *Chest* 1997;**111**:218–24.

61 Goldhaber SZ, Visani L. The International Cooperative Pulmonary Embolism Registry. *Chest* 1995;**108**:302.

62 Comp PC, Spiro T, Friedman RJ *et al.* Prolonged enoxaparin therapy to prevent venous thromboembolism after primary hip or knee replacement. *J Bone Joint Surg* 2001;**83A**:336–45.

63 Kleber F, Witt C, Vogel G *et al.* Randomized comparison of enoxaparin with unfractionated heparin for the prevention of venous thromboembolism in medical patients with heart failure or severe respiratory disease. *Am Heart J* 2003;**145**:614–21.

64 Fraisse F, Holzapfel L, Couland JM *et al.* Nadroparin in the prevention of deep vein thrombosis in acute decompensated COPD. *Am J Respir Crit Care Med* 2000;**161**:1109–14.

65 Ambrosetti M, Ageno W, Spanovello A, Salerno M, Pedretti RFE. Prevalence and prevention of venous thromboembolism in patients with acute exacerbations of COPD. *Thromb Res* 2003;**112**:203–7.

66 Geerts WH, Heit JA, Clagett GP *et al.* Prevention of venous thromboembolism. Sixth American College of Chest Physicians Consensus Conference on Antithrombotic Therapy. *Chest* 2001;**119**(Suppl):132S–75S.

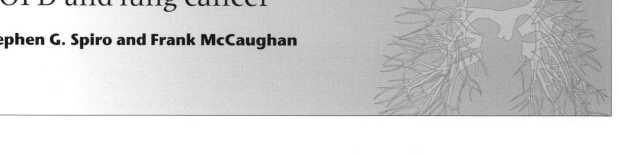

CHAPTER 45
COPD and lung cancer

Stephen G. Spiro and Frank McCaughan

Chronic obstructive pulmonary disease and lung cancer share a common dominant aetiological agent – tobacco smoking. Together they contribute substantially to the burden of lung disease. In this chapter we explore the links between these two important respiratory diseases.

Epidemiology

Lung cancer is now the leading cause of cancer-related mortality in the USA, and it is estimated that it will cause 160 440 deaths in 2004 [1]. This figure amounts to more than the estimated combined total mortality resulting from cancers of the colon, breast, pancreas and prostate. In the European Union (EU), lung cancer accounts for approximately 20% of all cancer deaths [2]. The age-standardized death rate from lung cancer across the EU is 37.6/100 000. There is a marked variation between different countries, with the death rate in the UK approximately double that of Sweden. In the UK, the 1-year survival for males and females with lung cancer is 20% compared with 79% in prostate cancer and 92% in breast cancer. Predictions for the future are also grim as the death rate from lung cancer is predicted to rise significantly worldwide by 2020, particularly in France and Mediterranean countries and it could reach epidemic proportions in China and South-East Asia [2]. The belief that the emergence of low-tar cigarettes would lower the incidence of lung cancer has been discounted [3].

COPD has been identified in a recent EU statement as a major public health issue [4]. Many patients with lung cancer have coexistent COPD and there is increasing evidence that patients with COPD are more likely to develop lung cancer. The number of patients with both these conditions will also rise in forthcoming years.

Prevalence of COPD in patients with lung cancer

There have been a number of observational studies reporting a high prevalence of COPD in patients diagnosed with lung cancer. The criteria for diagnosing COPD have evolved over the years, although recent guidelines have stressed the importance of spirometry and particularly the forced expiratory volume in 1 s (FEV_1) in making the diagnosis [5,6]. In one study, Tockman *et al.* [7] recruited male patients from two major trials: the Intermittent Positive Pressure Breathing (IPPB) Trial which examined the effect of this treatment for COPD and the John Hopkins Lung Project (JHLP) which was a lung cancer screening trial. All patients had a screening chest radiograph at baseline that did not reveal a lung cancer. In the IPPB Trial, 667 men aged 30–74 years were recruited and followed for a mean of 3 years. They all had an FEV_1 of less than 60% predicted and an $FEV_1 : FVC$ ratio of less than 60%. For the JHLP, 3728 men aged 45 years or more with a smoking history of at least 1 pack/day were recruited. They were followed for an average period of 1.2 years only. In total, 41 lung cancers were diagnosed in this group over the follow-up period and of these 66% had an FEV_1 of less than 60% predicted. There are some difficulties with this data. First, the 667 patients from the IPPB trial were already selected as having at least moderate COPD and they contributed 22 of 41 cancers. Secondly, the follow-up period was too short to learn about incidence cancer rates.

In another, much smaller study, Congleton and Muers [8] recorded spirometry in 57 patients who presented with a new diagnosis of lung cancer to a specialist clinic in a single centre in 1 year. They found that 49% of their patients had an FEV_1 of less than 70% predicted. They further prescribed bronchodilators to 15 of their patients with airflow limitation and found that 8/15 had a significant (more than 15%) spirometric response and there was also an improvement in breathlessness scores.

The Copenhagen City Heart Study recruited 13 946 people between 1976 and 1978 and followed them for 10 years on average. In total, 225 developed lung cancer of which only seven were non-smokers. Of the 225, 52% had an FEV_1 recorded at enrolment in the study of less than 80% predicted [9].

In a recent review of these and other relevant studies using the then available methods of defining COPD, the likely prevalence in patients with lung cancer was estimated at between 50% and 64% [10].

Increased risk of lung cancer in patients with COPD

The major risk factors for lung cancer are age, smoking history, social class and FEV_1. The latter has been explored in a number of series that have examined the risk of lung cancer for patients with COPD. They include older series, which used a variety of criteria for diagnosing COPD, and more recent studies which have used spirometric criteria. Although the results are not directly comparable, they consistently report a significantly increased risk of primary lung cancers in patients with COPD.

In a prospective population study in Renfrew and Paisley, Scotland, the investigators enrolled 7058 men and 8353 women aged 45–64 years between 1972 and 1976 and they were followed for at least 15 years [11]. The overall mortality was high in this cohort, mainly as a result of cardiovascular and respiratory disease. Subjects were stratified by FEV_1 into quintiles. The authors reported a significant correlation between a low FEV_1 and death from all causes. With respect to lung cancer, in men in the lowest quintile for relative FEV_1 (which was calculated in this cohort as an FEV_1 of less than 73% predicted), the relative hazards ratio for death from lung cancer compared with those men in the highest FEV_1 quintile was 2.53 (95% confidence interval, 1.69–2.79; $P < 0.001$). Despite correcting for smoking, social class and cardiovascular risk factors, there was a highly significant trend in both sexes for the risk of lung cancer to increase with a lower FEV_1. Furthermore, the absolute number of patients with lung cancer may have been underestimated because subjects dying from other causes may have had synchronous undiagnosed lung cancers.

A more recent study [12] used the new GOLD guidelines to classify patients with COPD in an analysis of participants in the First National Health and Nutrition Examination Survey (NHANES 1). For this survey, 14 407 adults were recruited between 1971 and 1975. The investigators applied the GOLD spirometric criteria to the cohort who had both participated in the cardiorespiratory survey and examination and also had respiratory function tests measured at entry. No subsequent spirometric data were available. Subjects with a history of cancer were excluded. A total of 5402 subjects fulfilled the criteria for entry to the study. (Subjects excluded because of an incomplete dataset tended to be older and were more likely to be non-white in ethnic origin – this group are known to have a higher incidence of lung cancer and this was shown again by subgroup comparison in this study.) The results showed that the presence of moderate or severe airflow obstruction ($FEV_1 : FVC$ less than 70% and FEV_1 less than 80%) in a proportional hazards model adjusted for age, sex, race, education, smoking status and duration and intensity of smoking was associated with a significantly higher risk of incident lung cancer (hazards ratio, 2.8; 95% confidence interval, 1.8–4.4). Furthermore, those subjects with moderate or severe COPD at the initial survey developed lung cancer after a shorter interval (5.3 years) than those without COPD (12.4 years). Interestingly, despite this, the age at which lung cancer was diagnosed was higher in the COPD group.

There are other relevant studies summarized in Table 45.1 [9,13–15], which also confirm that the risk of lung cancer increases in smokers with a lower FEV_1.

There are as yet no data available on whether the COPD phenotype has an influence on the risk of developing lung cancer.

Implications for the early detection of lung cancer

The goal of screening for lung cancer is the detection of cancers at an earlier stage, leading to a curative intervention and therefore improved lung cancer survival. To date, the results of lung cancer randomized screening studies have been disappointing and a recent consensus statement has advised that there is insufficient evidence to recommend screening for lung cancer [16]. This recommendation was based mainly on the trials of the 1970s in which chest radiographs and sputum cytology were used as screening tools, although these trials have been criticized because of methodological flaws. More recently, low-dose spiral CT scanning (LDCT) has been evaluated as a method of detecting early lung cancers [17,18]. These studies were hypothesis generating and produced a prevalence of 1.8–2.8% for lung cancers, almost all being stage 1 and adenocarcinomas. Two large randomized prospective studies are now in progress in the USA:

1 The Prostate, Lung, Colon and Ovary Trial has recruited 155 000 people and divided them into two groups: control

Table 45.1 Summary of studies describing an increased risk of lung cancer in subjects with chronic obstructive airways disease (COPD).

Authors	Year of publication	Reference	Trial summary	RR of lung cancer (95% CI) (adjusted for age and smoking history)
Lange et al.	1990	9	Divided male ($n = 6373$) and female ($n = 7573$) subjects into groups based on percentage predicted FEV_1 : $FEV_1 > 80\%$, 40–79%, < 40% Follow-up: average 10 years	$FEV_1 < 40\%$ RR 3.9 (2.2, 7.2) FEV_1 40–79% RR 2.1 (1.3, 3.4)
Kuller et al.	1990	13	Divided male smokers ($n = 6075$) into quintiles based on FEV_1 (absolute values) Follow-up: average 7.5 years	Lowest vs highest quintile RR 3.57 (0.94, 12.5)
Nomura et al.	1991	14	Divided male subjects ($n = 6317$) into quartiles based on percentage predicted FEV_1 Follow-up: 19 years	Lowest vs highest quartile RR 2.1 (1.3, 3.5)
Islam & Schottenfeld	1994	15	Divided male ($n = 1021$) and female ($n = 714$) smokers into quartiles based on percentage predicted FEV_1 Follow-up: 18–25 years	Lowest vs highest quartile RR 2.7

CI, clearance interval; FEV_1, forced expiratory volume in 1 s; RR, relative risk.

and screened. Those in the screened group had a chest radiograph on entry and then annually for 2 years for non-smokers, 3 years for smokers [19].

2 The National Lung Screening Trial is comparing screening with either LDCT or a chest radiograph in a current or recent ex-smoking population aged between 55 and 74 years with a 30 pack-year smoking history [20].

The epidemiological link between COPD and lung cancer has never been used to set eligibility criteria for a large-scale screening trial. However, the data confirm the increased risk of lung cancer in patients with COPD and that the risk increases with worsening airways obstruction. It has therefore been proposed that screening should be targeted at a high-risk population to include heavy smokers with documented airflow obstruction [21]. One group has published data on screening in such a cohort with COPD and smoking histories of 40 or more pack-years. The authors suggested that a combination of screening modalities including sputum cytology, autofluorescence bronchoscopy and CT scanning could detect lung cancer in up to 4.9% of these high-risk patients [22]. One difficulty with this approach is that patients with severe COPD may not be fit for surgery or radical radiotherapy. However, increasing emphasis is being placed on local lung-sparing endobronchial techniques such as photodynamic therapy and brachytherapy and, secondly, the definition of 'fitness for surgery' with respect to patients with lung cancer and COPD is evolving.

Why is there an increased risk of lung cancer in patients with COPD?

The simple answer is tobacco smoking. However, the biological mechanisms underlying this link are as yet unclear. COPD is an inflammatory process and lung cancer a neoplastic process. Traditionally, these were thought of as distinct entities but it is becoming increasingly clear that there is a link between inflammation and cancer, with examples including Barratt's oesophagus, oesophageal cancer and genitourinary cancers as a result of chronic schistosomiasis infection [23,24]. It is therefore possible that the epidemiological link between COPD and lung cancer may be in part explained by the link between chronic inflammation and neoplastic transformation.

Tobacco smoke contains approximately 4000 separate compounds of which 60 are recognized as carcinogens [25]. A number of carcinogens, notably the polycyclic aromatic hydrocarbons and nitrosamines, have been implicated in the pathogenesis of lung cancer. These compounds can be metabolized to form activated derivatives that bind DNA, forming so-called DNA adducts. Such adducts predispose to mutations if the normal DNA repair mechanisms are evaded. The existing evidence in support of this mechanism has been summarized in a recent comprehensive review [26].

A second possible mechanism of tobacco-related carcinogenesis is oxidative damage where reactive oxygen species are generated as a result of the free radicals present in cigarette smoke. This has been associated both with DNA damage and therefore possible mutagenesis; in addition, tobacco-generated pulmonary and systemic oxidative stress is considered very important in the pathogenesis of COPD [27].

Approximately 11–24% of smokers will develop lung cancer [28] and 15–20% of smokers will develop COPD. The latter statistic is being revised with increasing evidence that 50% of people who smoke for long enough will develop COPD [29]. The determinants of the individual susceptibility of a particular smoker to develop either of these pathologies are unknown. For example α_1-antitrypsin deficiency predisposes to COPD; other associations have been described between particular genes and susceptibility to COPD including glutathione S-transferases and microsomal epoxide hydrolase although results have not been consistent, especially from different populations [29]. Glutathione transferases are involved in detoxification including that of the activated metabolites of polycyclic hydrocarbons responsible for DNA adduct formation. There is also some evidence linking glutathione S-transferase polymorphisms with lung cancer [26]. It may be that for both conditions a polygenic inheritance including multiple susceptible gene polymorphisms will combine to produce a 'susceptible phenotype'.

Management of lung cancer in patients with COPD

A diagnosis of COPD can have a profound effect on the treatment options open to any patient with lung cancer. The primary goal of intervention is cure, but COPD may preclude a patient from a potentially curative treatment such as surgery or radical radiotherapy. Furthermore, performance status, to which COPD can be an important contributing factor, is a key predictor of outcome in lung cancer of any stage.

Preoperative assessment in patients with lung cancer and COPD

Surgery is the treatment modality most likely to cure lung cancer, particularly non-small cell lung cancer (NSCLC). Patients with lung cancer tend to be in their sixties and seventies at diagnosis and often have multiple comorbidities that render surgery hazardous. One of the most important roles of the chest physician, as part of the multidisciplinary team, is to help weigh the operative risk to an individual with operable lung cancer but significant COPD.

Spirometry, and in particular the FEV_1, has been used as a screening test to determine if a patient has airways obstruction severe enough to preclude pulmonary resection. There are more data available on the use of FEV_1 to predict surgical risk than any other test of respiratory physiology [30]. FEV_1 can be measured either in absolute terms or as a percentage of predicted normal. Its use in three retrospective series in the 1970s comprising more than 2000 patients was evaluated by the British Thoracic Society [31]. There was a surgical mortality of less than 5% for a lobectomy or a pneumonectomy if patients had an FEV_1 of more than 1.5 or 2 L, respectively. Therefore, patients whose FEV_1 exceeds this criterion are deemed to be suitable for surgery without requiring further evaluation. Historically, studies have quoted absolute values but it is preferable if the FEV_1 is expressed as a percentage of the predicted value as this takes into account a patient's age, gender and height and allows more standardized comparisons between different cohorts. The accepted recommendation is that if the FEV_1 is more than 80% predicted then a patient is fit for a pneumonectomy [30].

Patients with severe COPD are at greater risk of perioperative morbidity and mortality. In such patients, investigations can be used to predict the postoperative FEV_1 (ppoFEV_1) [30] by attempting to determine what fraction of currently functioning lung will remain after surgery. To do this accurately, detailed respiratory function tests are mandatory in conjunction with further imaging.

The calculation of the ppoFEV_1 can be complicated if a tumour partially or completely obstructs a proximal airway. In such cases, the lung distal to the obstruction will not be contributing to the preoperative FEV_1. However, other patients may have a tumour in a more peripheral location which will not influence the FEV_1 to any great extent. Lung cancer and COPD can both have a profound effect on the relative perfusion of a pulmonary segment, lobe or a lung. Ventilation/perfusion mismatch is well recognized in COPD and it has been shown that obstructing tumours can cause considerable underperfusion of the involved segment [32]. It is useful therefore to attempt to image the relative perfusion to the part of the lung that is earmarked for resection. Postoperatively the cardiac output will be channelled through the remaining pulmonary vasculature, which has implications for ventilation/perfusion matching, particularly in the case of a pneumonectomy when the whole cardiac output suddenly perfuses one lung. This is reflected by the increased KCO (coefficient of transfer of carbon monoxide calculated by dividing the transfer factor of carbon monoxide [DLCO] by the alveolar volume [VA]) postpneumonectomy and can cause pulmonary hypertension and respiratory failure if the pulmonary vasculature bed is not sufficiently compliant.

There are different approaches to calculating the

ppoFEV_1. These utilize ventilation and perfusion scans, quantitative CT scanning and simply counting the number of lung segments that are to be resected as a percentage of the remaining tissues. These methods generally arrive at similar values [33]. The current British Thoracic Society guidelines suggest using a perfusion scan. Recommendations [30,31] are based on the percentage of ppo (%ppo) values for FEV_1 and DLCO rather than absolute values. The commonly used equations for calculating %ppoFEV_1 are documented in Figure 45.1.

These calculations have been validated in some studies but others have noted that there is a tendency for the ppoFEV_1 to underestimate the actual ppoFEV_1 by a factor of up to 10%. Various authorities have advocated different cut-off values below which an operation may be considered high risk. A threshold ppoFEV_1 of 0.8 L was suggested [34] but, as discussed above, it is preferable to consider these issues in terms of %ppoFEV_1. A number of case series have shown that a %ppoFEV_1 of less than 40% can be associated with a poor outcome. Markos *et al.* [35], in a prospective series of 55 patients, reported that three of six patients with a %ppoFEV_1 of less than 40% died, whereas there were no deaths in those with a value greater than 40%. Similar outcomes using this threshold have been reported, but these kinds of results are by no means universal. Other groups have found that some patients with similarly poor respiratory function, if properly selected, can tolerate curative lung cancer resection. Ribas *et al.* [36] described 65 patients who, despite having a ppoFEV_1 of less than 40%, underwent a pneumonectomy (*n* = 21) or a lobectomy/wedge resection (*n* = 44). Despite their significant ventilatory impairment according to the standard criteria, only four subjects died postoperatively (6.2%).

There are therefore some problems associated with using the %ppoFEV_1 as the main criterion for accepting or refusing a patient for surgery. The first is that a diffuse interstitial process may coexist with both COPD and lung cancer so that in the presence of an interstitial infiltrate on a plain chest X-ray, or if there is reported exertional breathlessness inappropriate to the basic spirometric values, a DLCO should be measured. Secondly, there is some evidence to support the use of the DLCO rather than the FEV_1 as the most accurate predictor of postoperative problems. Thirdly, many patients who have survived a lobectomy or pneumonectomy would have been denied surgery on the basis of their %ppoFEV_1.

Ferguson *et al.* [37], who retrospectively reviewed lung function tests on 237 patients undergoing resection, questioned the reliance on basic spirometry. They found that a low preoperative DLCO, expressed as a percentage predicted, was a more accurate predictor of mortality than the percentage predicted FEV_1. They reported a respiratory complication rate of 45% and a mortality of 25% with a DLCO of less than 60% predicted. They extended these observations in an analysis of 376 patients and identified a preoperative DLCO of less than 60% predicted or a %ppoDLCO of less than 50% as the most accurate predictors of postoperative respiratory complications and death [38].

The FEV_1 and DLCO are complementary investigations and should be considered for all candidates for surgical resection of lung cancer. In the patients who are borderline, it is recommended that both the %ppoFEV_1 and the %ppoDLCO are estimated. The British Thoracic Society and the American College of Chest Physicians (ACCP) recommend exercise testing if either of those values are less than 40% predicted, although the evidence for this approach is not strong [30,31]. An algorithm for the consideration of patients with lung cancer for lung resection has been published by the British Thoracic Society and is reproduced in Figure 45.1.

The aim of cardiopulmonary exercise testing (CPET) is to calculate a subject's maximum oxygen uptake or $\dot{V}_{O_{2max}}$. Often this technique is only available in specialized centres. There are a number of studies that have stratified patients according to their $\dot{V}_{O_{2max}}$. It has been shown that those with a value of more than 20 mL/kg/min are not at increased risk of complications or death, whereas the perioperative mortality in those who manage less than 10 mL/kg/min is relatively high [30]. Morice *et al.* [39] showed that a subgroup with a %ppoFEV_1 of less than 33% who managed a $\dot{V}_{O_{2max}}$ of more than 15 mL/kg/min did well. Surrogate exercise tests have been used, with those patients who managed to climb five flights of stairs considered fit enough for a pneumonectomy and this may be considered an alternative to formal exercise testing although it is poorly standardized.

There is no predictive role for routine arterial blood gas analysis in the preoperative assessment.

Combined lung volume reduction surgery and lung cancer resection

There has been renewed interest in lung volume reduction surgery (LVRS) over recent years. This has led to speculation about the role of combined LVRS and surgical resection of lung cancer. It has been suggested that in patients with advanced COPD who previously would not have been considered for curative resection, a combined procedure might be curative with respect to the lung cancer and yield a secondary benefit with both functional and physiological improvements postoperatively. In 2003, the National Emphysema Treatment Trial study [40] reported a significant improvement after lung resection in a highly selected group of patients with heterogeneous emphysema affecting the upper lobes who were severely limited by dyspnoea. McKenna *et al.* [41] have published a series

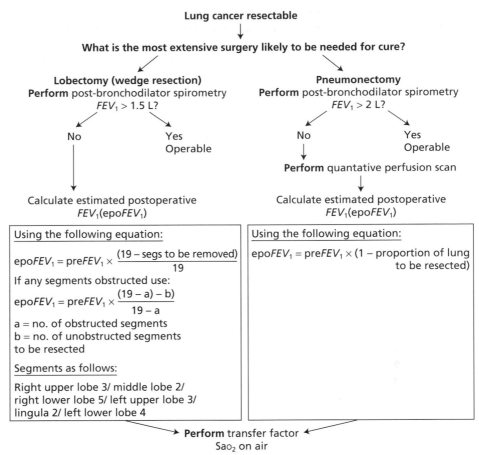

Lung cancer resectable

What is the most extensive surgery likely to be needed for cure?

Lobectomy (wedge resection)
Perform post-bronchodilator spirometry
$FEV_1 > 1.5$ L?

No   Yes
         Operable

Pneumonectomy
Perform post-bronchodilator spirometry
$FEV_1 > 2$ L?

No   Yes
         Operable

Perform quantative perfusion scan

Calculate estimated postoperative
FEV_1(epoFEV_1)

Calculate estimated postoperative
FEV_1(epoFEV_1)

Using the following equation:

$$epoFEV_1 = preFEV_1 \times \frac{(19 - \text{segs to be removed})}{19}$$

If any segments obstructed use:

$$epoFEV_1 = preFEV_1 \times \frac{(19 - a) - b}{19 - a}$$

a = no. of obstructed segments
b = no. of unobstructed segments
to be resected

Segments as follows:

Right upper lobe 3/ middle lobe 2/
right lower lobe 5/ left upper lobe 3/
lingula 2/ left lower lobe 4

Using the following equation:

$$epoFEV_1 = preFEV_1 \times (1 - \text{proportion of lung to be resected})$$

Perform transfer factor
Sao_2 on air

Calculate estimated postoperative T_{LCO} (epoT_{LCO}) using the above formulae

Express absolute epoFEV_1 and epoT_{LCO} as % predicted (from table of normal values)

Allocate to ONE of the following boxes

%ppo$FEV_1 < 40$%
AND
%ppo$T_{LCO} < 40$%

Any other
combination

%ppo$FEV_1 > 40$%
AND
%ppo$T_{LCO} > 40$%
AND
$Sao_2 > 90$% on air

High risk

Exercise testing required*

Average risk (no further
tests required)

Shuttle walk test (best of 2)

< 25 shuttles
or desaturation > 4%

> 25 shuttles
and < 4% desaturation

Full cardiopulmonary exercise test

Peak $\dot{V}o_2 < 15$ mL/kg/min
Refer to high risk box

> 15 mL/kg/min
Average risk

Refer to high risk box

High risk box

Patient is at high risk for the planned
procedure

Consider a less extensive resection

Consider radical radiotherapy

*Note: Ideally, full cardiorespiratory exerise
testing should be performed. Although it
is not available in many district general
hospitals, these facilities are usually available
at cardiothoracic centres. If the facilities
are not readily available, consider a screening
shuttle test

Figure 45.1 Guidelines on the selection of patients with lung cancer for surgery. (From British Thoracic Society and Society of Cardiothoracic Surgeons of Great Britain and Ireland Working Party Writing Group [31] with permission from the BMJ Publishing Group.)

of 325 patients who had LVRS, 51 (16%) of whom had a pulmonary mass in addition to severe emphysema. Of these, 11 (3%) were NSCLCs (seven squamous cell carcinomas, four adenocarcinoma). Three were referred specifically for the combined operation and one was an incidental histopathological diagnosis; therefore seven new cancers were picked up by the preoperative CT scan in this highly selected group. The results were impressive. There was no perioperative mortality and there was no recurrence of lung cancer after a follow-up period of 9 months. Furthermore, average preoperative FEV_1 was 0.65 L (range 12–29% predicted) compared with 1.08 L postoperatively and, of 11 patients, seven improved their dyspnoea score. The patients who benefited the most were the five who had the lung cancer in a lobe already targeted for removal at LVRS. The technique employed to excise the cancer was a wedge resection in eight patients and a formal lobectomy in the others.

The success in selected patients of LVRS indicates that some who were being denied curative surgery for lung cancer on the basis of severe COPD may have derived a physiological and functional benefit. Edwards *et al.* [42] have further explored this concept with the idea of 'lobar volume reduction surgery' to remove a lobe containing a cancer. They stratified patients on the basis of their predicted postoperative FEV_1 expressed as a percentage of their predicted value (%ppoFEV_1). The cut-off chosen was 40% based on earlier work by Markos *et al.* [35] who demonstrated a mortality of 50% in those with a ppoFEV_1 of less than 40%. Edwards *et al.* reported a higher perioperative mortality in the group with a ppoFEV_1 of less than 40%; two of 14 patients died as a result of postoperative pneumonia and empyema. There were no deaths in the other group (ppoFEV_1 of less than 40%). However, at a median follow-up of 12 months there was no difference in mortality between the groups. Furthermore, there was no difference between the pre- and postoperative FEV_1 in the first group; thus, the ppoFEV_1 significantly underestimated the actual postoperative value. The authors concluded that consideration of fitness for surgery in lung cancer should acknowledge the effect of lobar LVRS and that current methods of calculation may underestimate prediction of postoperative respiratory function and should not be clinically binding.

It must be stressed that this dual technique is only appropriate for a few, highly selected patients with COPD and operable lung cancer and that an operation is more likely to be successful if the cancer is in a part of the lung appropriate for LVRS. However, there are reports of successful procedures involving LVRS and an additional wedge resection of a cancer and the indications for surgery in these patients will evolve. It will be necessary to refine current guidelines to acknowledge both the role of surgery in patients with heterogeneous emphysema and lung cancer and that preoperative predictions can underestimate postoperative function. Each patient should be considered carefully with a view to maximizing the number who undergo successful curative resections for lung cancer.

In conclusion, the association of lung cancer and COPD is substantial and their coexistence affects the management of lung cancer in many patients. All possible care should be taken in the evaluation of patients with lung cancer and COPD to offer a potentially curative resection. The association of these two conditions is likely to become more common as COPD is increasingly recognized and as lung cancer rates continue to rise in many countries of the world.

References

1 Jemal A, Tiwari RC, Murray T *et al*. Cancer statistics. *CA Cancer J Clin* 2004;**54**:8–29.

2 Chronic obstructive pulmonary disease. In: *The European Lung White Book*. European Respiratory Society and the European Lung Foundation, 2004: 34–43.

3 Harris JE, Thun MJ, Mondul AM, Calle EE. Cigarette tar yields in relation to mortality from lung cancer in the cancer. *BMJ* 2004;**328**:72–9.

4 Lung cancer. In: *The European Lung White Book*. European Respiratory Society and the European Lung Foundation, 2004: 44–54.

5 Pauwels RA, Buist AS, Calverley PM *et al*. Global strategy for the diagnosis, management, and prevention of chronic obstructive pulmonary disease. NHLBI/WHO Global Initiative for Chronic Obstructive Lung Disease (GOLD) Workshop summary. *Am J Respir Crit Care Med* 2001;**163**:1256–76.

6 National Institute for Clinical Excellence (NICE). Chronic obstructive pulmonary disease: national clinical guideline for management of chronic obstructive pulmonary disease in adults in primary and secondary care. *Thorax* 2004;**59**(Suppl 1).

7 Tockman MS, Anthonisen NR, Wright EC, Donithan MG. Airways obstruction and the risk for lung cancer. *Ann Intern Med* 1987;**106**:512–8.

8 Congleton J, Muers MF. The incidence of airflow obstruction in bronchial carcinoma, its relation to breathlessness, and response to bronchodilator therapy. *Respir Med* 1995;**89**: 291–6.

9 Lange P, Nyboe J, Appleyard M, Jensen G, Schnohr P. Ventilatory function and chronic mucus hypersecretion as predictors of death from lung cancer. *Am Rev Respir Dis* 1990;**141**:613–7.

10 Diez Herranz A. Enfermedad pulmonar obstructiva crónica y cáncer de pulmón: implicaciones prácticas. *Arch Bronconeumol* 2001;**37**:240–7.

11 Hole DJ, Watt GC, Davey-Smith G *et al*. Impaired lung function and mortality risk in men and women: findings from the Renfrew and Paisley prospective population study. *BMJ* 1996;**313**:711–5; discussion 715–6.

12 Mannino DM, Aguayo SM, Petty TL, Redd SC. Low lung function and incident lung cancer in the United States: data from the First National Health and Nutrition Examination Survey Follow-up. *Arch Intern Med* 2003;**163**:1475–80.

13 Kuller LH, Ockene J, Meilahn E, Svendsen KH. Relation of forced expiratory volume in one second (FEV_1) to lung cancer mortality in the Multiple Risk Factor Intervention Trial (MRFIT). *Am J Epidemiol* 1990;**132**:265–74.

14 Nomura A, Stemmermann GN, Chyou PH, Marcus EB, Buist AS. Prospective study of pulmonary function and lung cancer. *Am Rev Respir Dis* 1991;**144**:307–11.

15 Islam SS, Schottenfeld D. Declining FEV_1 and chronic productive cough in cigarette smokers: a 25-year prospective study of lung cancer incidence in Tecumseh, Michigan. *Cancer Epidemiol Biomarkers Prev* 1994;**3**:289–98.

16 Bach PB, Niewoehner DE, Black WC. Screening for lung cancer: the guidelines. *Chest* 2003;**123**:83S–8S.

17 Henschke CI, McCauley DI, Yankelevitz DF *et al.* Early Lung Cancer Action Project: overall design and findings from baseline screening. *Lancet* 1999;**354**:99–105.

18 Sone S, Li F, Yang ZG *et al.* Results of three-year mass screening programme for lung cancer using mobile low-dose spiral computed tomography scanner. *Br J Cancer* 2001;**84**:25–32.

19 http://www3.cancer.gov/prevention/plco/index.html accessed 5 October 2004.

20 http://www3.cancer.gov/prevention/lss/moop2.html#2.3 accessed 5 October 2004.

21 Petty TL. Screening strategies for early detection of lung cancer: the time is now. *JAMA* 2000;**284**:1977–80.

22 Kennedy TC, Miller Y, Prindiville S. Screening for lung cancer revisited and the role of sputum cytology and fluorescence bronchoscopy in a high-risk group. *Chest* 2000;**117**:72S–9S.

23 Balkwill F, Mantovani A. Inflammation and cancer: back to Virchow? *Lancet* 2001;**357**:539–45.

24 Thun MJ, Henley SJ, Gansler T. Inflammation and cancer: an epidemiological perspective. *Novartis Found Symp* 2004;**256**: 6–21; discussion 22–8, 49–52, 266–9.

25 Hecht SS. Tobacco carcinogens, their biomarkers and tobacco-induced cancer. *Nat Rev Cancer* 2003;**3**:733–44.

26 Wiencke JK. DNA adduct burden and tobacco carcinogenesis. *Oncogene* 2002;**21**:7376–91.

27 MacNee W. Oxidants/antioxidants and COPD. *Chest* 2000: **117**;303S–17S.

28 Thun MJ, Henley SJ, Calle EE. Tobacco use and cancer: an epidemiologic perspective for geneticists. *Oncogene* 2002;**21**: 7307–25.

29 Pauwels RA, Rabe KF. Burden and clinical features of chronic obstructive pulmonary disease (COPD). *Lancet* 2004;**364**: 613–20.

30 Beckles MA, Spiro SG, Colice GL, Rudd RM. The physiologic evaluation of patients with lung cancer being considered for resectional surgery. *Chest* 2003;**123**:105S–14S.

31 British Thoracic Society, Society of Cardiothoracic Surgeons of Great Britain, and Ireland Working Party. Guidelines on the selection of patients with lung cancer for surgery. *Thorax* 2001;**56**:89–108.

32 George PJ, Clarke G, Tolfree S, Garrett CP, Hetzel MR. Changes in regional ventilation and perfusion of the lung after endoscopic laser treatment. *Thorax* 1990;**45**:248–53.

33 Wu MT, Pan HB, Chiang AA *et al.* Prediction of postoperative lung function in patients with lung cancer: comparison of quantitative CT with perfusion scintigraphy. *Am J Roentgenol* 2002;**178**:667–72.

34 Olsen GN, Block AJ, Tobias JA. Prediction of postpneumonectomy pulmonary function using quantitative macroaggregate lung scanning. *Chest* 1974;**66**:13–6.

35 Markos J, Mullan BP, Hillman DR *et al.* Preoperative assessment as a predictor of mortality and morbidity after lung resection. *Am Rev Respir Dis* 1989;**139**:902–10.

36 Ribas J, Diaz O, Barbera JA *et al.* Invasive exercise testing in the evaluation of patients at high-risk for lung resection. *Eur Respir J* 1998;**12**:1429–35.

37 Ferguson MK, Little L, Rizzo L *et al.* Diffusing capacity predicts morbidity and mortality after pulmonary resection. *J Thorac Cardiovasc Surg* 1988;**96**:894–900.

38 Wang J, Olak J, Ferguson MK. Diffusing capacity predicts operative mortality but not long-term survival after resection for lung cancer. *J Thorac Cardiovasc Surg* 1999;**117**:581–6; discussion 586–7.

39 Morice RC, Peters EJ, Ryan MB *et al.* Exercise testing in the evaluation of patients at high risk for complications from lung resection. *Chest* 1992;**101**:356–61.

40 Fishman A, Martinez F, Naunheim K *et al.* A randomized trial comparing lung-volume-reduction surgery with medical therapy for severe emphysema. *N Engl J Med* 2003;**348**:2059–73.

41 McKenna RJJ, Fischel RJ, Brenner M, Gelb AF. Combined operations for lung volume reduction surgery and lung cancer. *Chest* 1996;**110**:885–8.

42 Edwards JG, Duthie DJ, Waller DA. Lobar volume reduction surgery: a method of increasing the lung cancer resection rate in patients with emphysema. *Thorax* 2001;**56**:791–5.

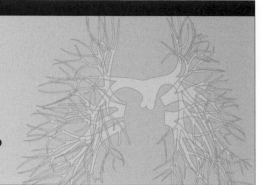

CHAPTER 46
Infection management and airflow obstruction

Alan M. Fein, Jill P. Karpel and Antonio Anzueto

COPD: interaction of infection and obstruction

Progression of COPD: relation to chronic inflammation and exacerbation

Chronic obstructive pulmonary disease (COPD) is a complex multifaceted disease process that continues to increase in incidence. Currently the fourth leading cause of death in the USA, COPD is also increasingly recognized in the developing world [1]. Conceptual definitions relevant to disease development and exacerbation have sought to emphasize three elements: some component of irreversible airflow obstruction; mixed pathology involving variable degrees of emphysema, large and small airway and vascular injury and remodelling; and inflammation encompassing both large and small airways and lung parenchyma [2]. The impact of chronic infection on damage to airways and lung parenchyma is not well defined and it may vary in individual patients. This may, in part, account for the myriad of clinical expressions of COPD.

COPD also has a systemic component that affects the nutritional balance, body habitus, muscle strength, cognition and mood of those affected. Characteristically, during stable periods, mediators of inflammation are increased within the lung as measured in bronchoalveolar lavage and breath condensate, and in the systemic circulation. Even higher levels of these mediators are detectable during acute periods of clinical deterioration termed acute exacerbation of COPD (AECOPD). Based on these findings, current opinion holds that inflammation is the most important contributor to the pathogenesis of COPD.

As COPD progresses, it is often complicated by pulmonary hypertension. Sustained elevation in pulmonary artery pressures is associated with increased mortality although the impact of mild elevations in pulmonary artery

pressures on dyspnoea and exercise performance is not clearly defined.

Cigarette smoking and air pollution, both indoor and outdoor, are recognized as important contributions to COPD. However, sex, bronchial hyperresponsiveness, genetic susceptibility, as observed in α_1-antitrypsin (AAT) deficiency and other polymorphisms identified recently also interact to determine expression of disease. Recent data has suggested that patients who are atopic or have airways hyperresponsiveness experience greater declines in lung function over time [3]. Asthma, particularly when inadequately treated, is associated in some patients with ultimately irreversible lung disease. One study correlated duration of asthma with the degree of airflow limitation and hyperinflation in a cohort of elderly patients [4]. In an advanced clinical state, those problems may be indistinguishable from COPD in individual patients. While smoking contributes to the development of COPD, nearly 10% of patients dying of COPD are reported never to have smoked.

Other contributors thought to facilitate progression of COPD prominently include both viral and bacterial infectious agents (Table 46.1). The role of infection must be considered both from the perspective of disease initiation and modification. This chapter reviews the links between

Table 46.1 Factors resulting in progression of COPD.

1 Cigarette smoke
2 Genetic predisposition: α_1-antitrypsin, possibly other polymorphisms
3 Infection: viral/bacterial – frequency and timing of exacerbations
4 Air pollution: indoor/atmosphere
5 Airway hyperresponsiveness/'asthma'
6 Occupational exposure: total burden of organic and inorganic dusts (asbestos)

infection and COPD progression, the relationship between infection and inflammation, and strategies to prevent and treat infection in COPD patients. The specific contribution of AECOPD to the pathophysiology of COPD and its progression is highlighted.

COPD exacerbation

COPD is characterized by progressive decline in lung function over many years. Although this may be gradual, resulting in cough, dyspnoea, mucus hypersecretion and slowly decreasing health-related quality of life, physiological decline may be subacute, acute or, rarely, precipitous. Until recently, AECOPD has been only loosely defined, reflecting its multiple putative aetiologies. It is the most common cause of hospitalizations in patients with COPD and has been frequently linked to acute airways infection, specifically bacterial tracheobronchitis [5,6]. Many component diseases under the COPD umbrella, including chronic bronchitis, emphysema, asthma and bronchiectasis, are also punctuated by episodic acute deteriorations in pulmonary physiological function. In this scenario, exacerbations are associated with changes in volume and quality of phlegm, as well as dyspnoea and systemic manifestations such as fever and change in mental status. Hypoxaemia, hypercapnoea and altered mental status are associated with severe exacerbations resulting in hospitalization [5–7].

The common clinical symptoms were used by Anthonisen *et al.* [8] to develop the most used clinical classification of AECOPD, the 'Winnipeg Criteria'. Patients were categorized by the presence or absence of the three major clinical symptoms: breathlessness, sputum volume and purulence. Patients with all three symptoms were classified as type I; those with any two as type II; and those with only one symptom as type III. The American Thoracic Society and European consensus conference on standards for COPD management developed the following definition of AECOPD, building on previous concepts: 'An event in the natural course of COPD characterized by a change in baseline dyspnoea, cough and/or sputum beyond day to day variability sufficient to warrant a change in management'. Severity was defined operationally as:
- *Level I:* ambulatory treatment.
- *Level II:* requiring hospitalization.
- *Level III:* acute respiratory failure.

This reflects the broad spectrum of this disease process, from mild episodes that often go unreported to the most severe episodes, where hospitalization and even intensive care may be required (Table 46.2).

In the setting of respiratory failure resulting in hospitalization, mortality rate was 11% while in hospital, 33% at 6 months and 43% at 1 year. In a comprehensive audit of outcomes of AECOPD, 14% of patients died within

Table 46.2 Definitions of COPD exacerbation.

Symptoms	Change	Consequence
Major	Acute	*Level I*
Sputum colour	Sustained	Ambulatory treatment
Sputum volume		
Dyspnoea		*Level II*
		Hospital treatment
Minor		
Fever		*Level III*
Reduced exercise		Respiratory failure
capacity		

3 months of admission. Once a threshold of physiological decline is reached exacerbations occur between two and four times per year. Previous exacerbation, underlying cardiopulmonary disease and mucus hypersecretion are predictive of repeat exacerbations [9,10].

Colonization and infection in the lungs of COPD patients

Again, the underlying cause of AECOPD may be multifactorial, including noxious environmental exposures, and occupational, indoor and outdoor air pollution, as well as structural injury to the lung, as in pneumothorax and pulmonary thromboembolism (Table 46.3). The findings during AECOPD of increasingly purulent sputum, within which are found high concentrations of bacteria, suggests but does not prove bacterial causation. Although respiratory infections are assumed to be mainly responsible for exacerbation of COPD, other considerations are also involved.

Acute viral and bacterial infection, in the setting of airways already colonized with bacteria, is thought to be the predominant mode of initiating an AECOPD. Bacterial

Table 46.3 Contributing factors in acute exacerbation COPD.

1 Viral infection: influenze A & B, rhinovirus, coronavirus, latent adenovirus
2 Bacterial infection: *Haemophilus influenza, Streptococcus pneumoniae, Moraxella catarrhalis,* Gram-negative bacteria, *Pseudomonas aeruginosa,* Enterobacteriaceae
3 Air quality, indoor and outdoor pollution: change in air quality, biomass fuels
4 Heart failure: left ventricular, right ventricular
5 Pulmonary embolism
6 Pneumothorax

colonization of the airways is a dynamic process, which has been correlated with the degree of airflow obstruction and a person's smoking status. A vicious cycle of infection and inflammation develops, causing acute or chronic injury to airways, parenchyma and vessels. Even when the COPD patient is stable, the infection–inflammation cycle may contribute to progressive bronchiolitis and irreversible airflow obstruction. Whether infection is a direct or indirect cause of airway injury or, conversely, is facilitated by an already compromised epithelium is not entirely certain. It is probable that airways already damaged are more easily infected and slower to recover than healthy ones. Bacterial infection promotes mucus hypersecretion and limits mucociliary clearance, an effect demonstrated in animal models of airway injury by *Haemophilus influenzae*, *Streptococcus pneumoniae* and *Pseudomonas aeruginosa*. Similarly, cell-free supernatants, consisting of non-typable *H. influenzae* and *P. aeruginosa*, result in ciliodyskinesia and stasis in isolated airway preparations. The latter may occur directly through the actions of bacteria or indirectly through stimulation of neurophil migration and release of human neutrophil elastase [11].

Bacterial infection itself fosters conditions that favour persistent bacterial growth, termed colonization, and recurrent infection contributes to amplification of inflammation with subsequent airway and vascular remodelling. Neutrophil defensins predispose to enhanced *H. influenzae* adherence. *H. influenzae* has been demonstrated to localize to 'protected' sites within the airway as between cells. Such results make it unlikely that recovered bacteria are merely innocent bystanders in this process. The interrelationship of bacteria and viruses is also complex in the setting of COPD.

Studies utilizing quantitative bacterial cultures during AECOPD are considered most reliable; they have shown that as COPD becomes more advanced, bacteria are usually recovered in sputum, whereas normal airways are usually sterile. The stage in the natural history of COPD when

Table 46.4 Risk factors for bacterial colonization in COPD.

1 Recurrent viral infection, especially influenza
2 Severe COPD
3 Smoking: acuity/quantity
4 Nutritional status
5 Immunosuppression: alcohol, steroids
6 Antibiotic use
7 Hospitalization

bacteria can be recovered consistently, however, is not specifically known. There is a relatively low frequency of persistent colonization with potentially pathogenic bacteria when COPD is only of mild or moderate severity. Rates of colonization rise as disease becomes more severe. In the most compromised patients as measured by pulmonary function, pathogenic Gram-negative organisms are often recovered [11–13].

Risk factors for colonization include heavy smoking (more than 1 pack/day), current smoking, severe airflow limitation and recurrent viral infection. In fact, isolation of viruses, particularly influenza, has been associated with higher rates of recovery of *S. pneumoniae* and *H. influenzae*. Other risk factors associated with colonization include nutritional status, alcohol use, antimicrobial treatment, hospitalizations and steroid use (Table 46.4). In the studies using bacterial cultures, the organisms most commonly isolated from patients with severe obstructive lung disease include Enterobacteriaceae and Pseudomonas sp., *Proteus vulgaris*, *Serratia marcescens*, *Stenotrophomonas maltophilia* and *Escherichia coli*. In contrast, significantly larger numbers of non-pathogenic microorganisms were isolated in the group with forced expiratory volume in 1 s (FEV_1) ≥ 50% (Fig. 46.1). *H. influenzae* was cultured notably more often in patients who were currently smoking and *P. aeruginosa* was cultured more frequently in persons with poor lung

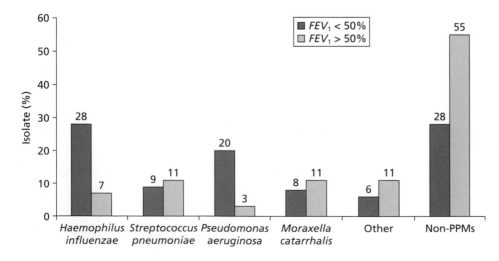

Figure 46.1 The relation of pathogens isolated in patients with COPD and the severity of lung function (forced expiratory volume in 1 s [FEV_1]). (Reprinted from Miravitlles *et al.* [15], with permission.)

function. *S. pneumoniae* is a frequent isolate among groups of all severity [14,15]. In a minority of patients with AECOPD, atypical pathogens such as *Mycoplasma pneumoniae* and *Chlamydia pneumoniae* are recovered. However, because of limitations with serological diagnosis, the true incidence of these organisms in AECOPD is not known. *Chlamydia pneumoniae* can be detected in significant numbers of peripheral blood mononuclear cells in patients with stable COPD [16].

Many asthma exacerbations and approximately one-third of COPD exacerbations are preceded by 'colds', presumably representing recent acquisition of viral infection. Compared with COPD patients with non-viral exacerbations, those with viral exacerbations have higher symptom scores 'especially more fever', at the start of exacerbation and require significantly more time (more than 50%) to resolve. 'Cold' symptoms occurred on average 2–3 weeks prior to exacerbation. Medical resource utilization increased more than twofold in AECOPD associated with viral infection of the airways [16,17].

Respiratory viruses were found in approximately half of COPD exacerbations and in three-quarters of asthmatic exacerbations, with respiratory syncytial virus (RSV), influenza, rhinovirus (RV) and coronavirus accounting for almost all episodes. Coronavirus infection in humans has been associated with wheezing and airways obstruction even in non-asthmatic persons. Patients with COPD are more likely to experience more frequent viral respiratory infections, with RSV, parainfluenza, influenza and coronavirus, which may also predispose them to pneumonia. Some researchers believe that chronic viral infection, particularly with DNA viruses, like adenovirus, may be responsible for inflammatory dysregulation observed in the obstructive airways syndromes [18].

Respiratory viral infection has both systemic and local consequences. Airways are reddened and swollen with injury, and ultimately desquamation of the mucosal epithelial surface occurs. Peripheral airways involvement is evidenced by impaired tests of small airway function and viruses are also linked to chronic excessive sputum production [19–21]. Markers of systemic inflammation like fibrinogen and interleukin 6 (IL-6) have been shown to increase during exacerbation [21]. Acute rhinovirus infection has been demonstrated to increase IL-6 in cell culture and in smokers through an NF-κB dependent pathway. Direct effects on airway smooth muscle have also been demonstrated in association with increased release of IL-5 and IL-1β. Interestingly, chronic viral infection in stable COPD patients has been associated with high circulating levels of plasma fibrinogen and IL-6 and more frequent exacerbations [21]. Because viral infection impairs host defences, colonization becomes more likely, a fact supported by increased recovery of *Haemophilus* and *Pneumococcus*

in sputum or throat cultures. It is likely that acute viral infection adversely affects mucociliary clearance and macrophage function.

Inflammation in asthma and COPD

Asthma and COPD, both diseases of airflow obstruction, cause chronic inflammation that involves both the lung parenchyma and airways. The inflammatory responses of the two diseases, however, differ from each other. Such differences involve the types of inflammatory cells and mediators responsible for the persistent inflammation; the ultimate response to therapy; and permanent changes that occur, notably airway remodelling (Table 46.5).

In allergic triggers of asthma, the sensitizing antigen interacts with mast cell specific immunoglobulin E (IgE) resulting in the release of histamine, leukotrienes, cytokines and granulocyte–macrophage colony-stimulating factor (GM-CSF). Local inflammatory cell recruitment occurs in the airway through interactions between chemokines, adhesion molecules (ICAM-1 and VCAM-1) and eosinophils derived from the bone marrow. Clinically, the increased levels of IgE, cytokines and inflammatory cells (Fig. 46.2) result in bronchial hyperreactivity, airway

Table 46.5 Inflammatory differences between asthma and COPD.

Inflammation	Asthma	COPD
Cells	Eosinophils, CD4$^+$ Mast cells, T lymphocytes Macrophages +	Neutrophils, CD8$^+$ Lymphocytes Macrophages ++ Eosinophils
Mediators	LTB$_4$, histamine IL-4 IL-5, IL-13 Eotaxin, RANTES	LTB$_4$, TNF-α IL-8 Growth-related oncogenes
Oxidative stress	+	+++
Pathobiology	All airways AHR +++ Epithelial shedding Fibrosis + No parenchymal involvement Mucus +	Peripheral airways AHR +/– Epithelial metaplasia Fibrosis ++ Parenchymal destruction Mucus ++
Response to steroids	+++	+/–

IL, interleukin; LTB$_4$, leukotriene B$_4$; TNF-α, tumour necrosis factor α.

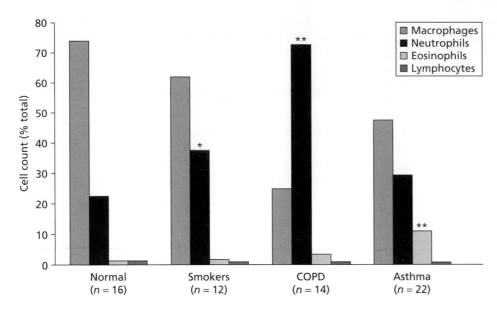

Figure 46.2 Inflammatory cells in induced sputum. A profile of inflammatory cells in induced sputum in normal subjects, cigarette smokers and patients with COPD and asthma is shown. (Adapted from Keatings *et al.* [25], with permission.)

oedema and mucus secretion, all contributing to airways obstruction.

Activated eosinophils are the main cell responsible for the airway inflammation in asthma, and can be demonstrated in bronchial biopsies, bronchoalveolar lavage fluid and induced sputum [22]. The eosinophils do not in general participate in normal airway defence against viral or bacterial infection. Other important cells contributing to asthmatic inflammation include activated CD4+ T lymphocytes (T-helper type 2 cells), macrophages, mast cells, basophils and, to a lesser extent, neutrophils (see Fig. 46.2). These cells release multiple proinflammatory cytokines such as IL-4, IL-5, IL-9, IL-10, IL-13 and IL-25 and GM-CSF, which in turn recruit and activate eosinophils further. Lymphocyte activation also results in the production of chemokines, such as RANTES and exotoxin, which are also important in eosinophil recruitment. This self-perpetuating reaction characterizes chronic inflammation characteristic of asthma. The degree of airway inflammation varies with both the duration and severity of the disease and the response to treatment [23–26].

In general, acute inflammation is thought to be an expected non-specific tissue response to injury that results in repair of normal structure and function. In asthma, chronic inflammation leads to permanent structural and pathological changes, known as airway remodelling in the large and small airways. It is not understood whether such remodelling is the normal response to injury or if the response itself is abnormal. Furthermore, the underlying causes of airway remodelling have not been defined, although both genetic and environmental factors have been implicated. Remodelling includes alteration of the reticular basement membrane, smooth muscle hypertrophy

and hyperplasia, mucous gland metaplasia and increased vascularity [27–30]. These changes occur in children and are present early in the disease process [31,32].

Clinically, airway remodelling results in irreversible airway obstruction and enhances bronchial hyperresponsiveness. Remodelling is diagnosed when pulmonary function remains persistently abnormal, despite optimal therapy.

In contrast to asthma, the neutrophil is the primary affected cell linked to the pathology of COPD. Among the most important initiators of neutrophil-driven injury are infection and cigarette smoke, and neutrophils have been demonstrated to be present in increased numbers in the sputum and lavage fluids of patients with COPD and in smokers. Prominent in the disease process is the role of tumour necrosis factor α (TNF-α) which, when released by macrophages stimulates migration of other macrophages and neutrophils into the airway epithelium. In addition to its inflammatory effects, TNF-α also causes neutrophil degranulation and injures epithelial cells directly. It can also induce airway mucous-cell metaplasia and hypersecretion *in vitro* and *in vivo*, decrease intraepithelial binding, cause cell death *in vitro*, and induce release of other cytokines and chemokines [33].

Interestingly, the eosinophils are also likely to contribute to airway inflammation in COPD. Higher serum eosinophilia in newly diagnosed patients with COPD has been associated with an accelerated decline in FEV_1, especially in smokers. While airway and sputum eosinophilia is not as prominent in COPD as in asthma patients, the number of inflammatory cells in the airways increases during AECOPD. Eosinophilic mediators are capable of injuring the epithelium and interstitium of the lung [21].

Both macrophages and epithelial cells also produce

cytokines, including neutrophil chemotactic factors, such as IL-8 and leukotriene B_4 (LTB_4). These macrophages may recruit other macrophages via chemokines, such as macrophage chemoattractant peptide 1 (MCP-1 and MIP-1α) and growth regulated oncogene-α (GRO-α). IL-8 and GRO-α stimulate further migration of neutrophils and CD8[+] T cells to the airway epithelium. Such migration leads to degranulation of neutrophils and the release of free radicals, which, in turn, causes matrix and epithelial damage.

Additionally, the activated CD8[+] T lymphocytes, epithelial cells and other macrophage mediators also release neutrophilic chemotactic factors. This ultimately causes the release of proteases such as neutrophil elastase and matrix metalloproteinases (MMPs). Both the proteases and free radicals damage the epithelium and underlying basement membrane, resulting in small airways disease (bronchiolitis), chronic bronchitis (mucus hypersecretions) and emphysema (alveolar destruction). Normally, a protective process that includes protease inhibitors such as α-1 antitrypsin and secretory leukoproteases inhibitor (SLP) counterbalances protease activity [33]. In COPD, however, the naturally occurring protective process, or protease–antiprotease balance, is disturbed [34–36]. The result is damage and remodelling of the lung, which may lead to alterations in tissue structure.

Although the relationship between chronic inflammation and remodelling, as well as the relation to infection, is poorly understood in COPD, remodelling is associated with metaplasia of the epithelium of the small airways, increased mucous glands and accompanying hypertrophy, increased smooth muscle mass, airway wall fibrosis, increased vascularity and emphysema. The predominant site of airway obstruction, which varies among individuals, is related to decline in lung function.

The inflammation and airway remodelling in COPD reflect the impact of neutrophilic mediators triggered by the interactions of cigarette smoking, acute and chronic infection, and air pollution. Remodelling and chronic injury to airways disrupt host defences and facilitate chronic growth of bacteria, which in turn amplifies neutrophil-mediated injury. A significant correlation exists between the severity of airflow obstruction and the degree of neutrophilic infiltration and degranulation. High concentrations of neutrophil-derived elastase are detectable in airway secretions during AECOPD.

Infection, inflammation and remodelling

The relationship between infection, inflammation and airway remodelling in both asthma and COPD has not been fully defined. It has been postulated that airway infection may have an important role in the disease process, leading to the decline in lung function. Both lower airway bacterial colonization and chronic viral infection have been implicated as contributory factors.

A proportion of stable patients with advanced COPD (20–40%) experience lower airway bacterial colonization [37–39]. Organisms most commonly cultured include *H. influenzae*, *S. pneumoniae*, *Moraxella catarrhalis* and *P. aeruginosa*. Furthermore, evidence exists that, as well as being present in the airway, *H. influenzae* can be detected in the submucosa and intracellularly, increasing the difficulty of eradicating the organism [40].

Once lower airway colonization occurs it usually persists, especially if lung function is impaired, and leads to increased airway inflammation. Bacteria can affect the inflammatory process by reducing mucociliary clearance, increasing mucus production and damaging airway epithelium [41, 42]. This leads to an influx of neutrophils and the release of neutrophil elastase and other cytokine and chemokines, which further fuels the inflammatory cycle. As bacterial colonization increases so does airway inflammation, an effect that is more pronounced with colonization by *P. aeruginosa* than other bacterial species [42]. A relationship between prognosis and circulating antibodies to *P. aeruginosa* has been specifically demonstrated in bronchiectasis.

Bacterial airway colonization leads to airway inflammation depending on the colonizing load [42]. *H. influenzae* colonization was associated with increased airway inflammatory markers in chronic bronchitis patients who had airflow obstruction compared with those without airflow obstruction [43]. Thus, significant evidence exists that lower airway colonization can lead to chronic inflammation and deterioration in lung function even for stable COPD patients.

COPD exacerbations, which are characterized by increased dyspnoea and increased sputum volume and/or purulence, are also associated with increased airway bacterial loads [44,45]. As with the stable COPD patient, those changes in sputum are associated with increased sputum neutrophils and neutrophilic inflammation, leading to the release of elastase and other proteinases. Such release can result in epithelial damage, reduced mucociliary clearance, increased mucus secretion and increased airway oedema through changes in the bronchial mucosa [46]. LTB_4, however, has a more prominent role than IL-8 in acute exacerbations [45]. Additionally, TNF-α and GM-CSF are also increased in bronchoalveolar lavage fluid during AECOPD. Both of these affect neutrophil and macrophage activation, leading to further inflammation and permanent damage. Resolution of the neutrophilic inflammatory changes has been shown to occur within approximately 5 days of treatment [45].

Interestingly, biopsy studies have also demonstrated increased numbers of both eosinophils and CD4[+] lymphocytes in the airway walls of AECOPD patients [21,47]. This might explain why clinical outcomes are improved in COPD when patients are treated with systemic corticosteroids for exacerbations as opposed to the relative steroid resistance seen in stable patients.

Controversy exists as to whether or not bacteria truly have an important role in AECOPD; however, most studies support the conclusion that they do. Specifically, the proportion of COPD patients with positive bacterial cultures and high bacterial loads during AECOPD are increased in most studies. Previous investigations may not have detected changes in the strain of the same organism, which has been postulated as a cause of acute exacerbations. That possibility is further supported by the fact that treatment with antibiotics appears to improve clinical outcomes during AECOPD. Finally, if one differentiates acute exacerbations associated with purulent sputum from those associated with mucoid sputum, the incidence of positive cultures is markedly different (84 vs 38%) [44].

Most evidence therefore suggests that both chronic lower airway colonization and acute infection contribute significantly to airway inflammation and remodelling in COPD. Clinically, those changes are manifested by deterioration in lung function. Patients with COPD may also be prone to viral respiratory tract infections that, in turn, can lead to ongoing inflammation and lung damage (i.e. alteration of mucociliary clearance, increased mucus). As with bacterial infection, viral infection has been implicated in both chronic and stable COPD, and AECOPD. In addition, viruses can exacerbate COPD by causing increased airway hyperresponsiveness and affecting muscarinic receptors, resulting in bronchoconstriction [47,48]. Viral infection may also predispose patients to secondary bacterial infection.

Hogg *et al.* have postulated that adenovirus can contribute to lung inflammation and emphysema [49–52]. Adenovirus infects lung epithelial cells and remains latent while continuing to produce viral proteins, which cause an increase in $CD8^+$ T cells. The reaction is further exacerbated by cigarettes and is associated with increasing emphysema, findings supported by experiments in the guinea pig demonstrating that latent infection with adenovirus was associated with chronic lung inflammation 7 weeks after inoculation with virus. This inflammatory response was composed of $CD4^+$ and $CD8^+$ T cells, B cells, macrophages and monocytes. When exposed to cigarette smoke, the inflammatory response was heightened and more emphysema was demonstrated in the lungs. The inflammatory response mirrors that seen in humans [53]. These studies suggest that latent adenovirus may have a role in the pathogenesis of COPD.

Some evidence supports the belief that viruses also contribute to AECOPD. Most investigations have used serological conversion at the time of the exacerbation as the basis of establishing infection. The largest study of rhinovirus demonstrated that positive rhinovirus cultures were more commonly associated with exacerbations [54,55].

In summary, infection with bacteria, viruses and atypical organisms may contribute to chronic airway inflammation in COPD and result in progression of the underlying disease process.

Evidence of antibiotic efficacy

While antibiotics are the most commonly prescribed agents in AECOPD and are presumed to have short-term benefit by most clinicians, long-term disease modification has not been proven. The specific aetiology of AECOPD is difficult to determine in an outpatient setting on the basis of symptoms and signs in individual patients. The phenomenon of increasingly purulent sputum observed frequently during AECOPD, within which are found high concentrations of bacteria, suggests but does not prove causation. Although respiratory infections are assumed to be the main perpetuators of exacerbation, other elements are also involved. In addition, routine sputum studies may have significant limitations, including delay in obtaining the results, cost and lack of sensitivity and specificity. As a result of the above considerations, recent treatment guidelines for AECOPD reflect the lack of a high level of evidence to provide specific recommendations for antibiotic use. The GOLD guideline, NHLBI/WHO initiative for COPD [56], recommends antibiotic choices on the basis of local sensitivity patterns of the most common pathogens associated with AECOPD, but do not provide specific guidelines. Another recent guideline also suggested that commonly available inexpensive antibiotics such as amoxicillin are likely to be efficacious in all but the most advanced disease [5].

A number of clinical trials have examined the use of antibiotics in the treatment of AECOPD. Many of the earlier studies showed either no or minimal benefit when antibiotics were prescribed. More recent analysis demonstrated benefit during an acute exacerbation, but not in preventing exacerbations. A landmark study in 1987 utilized a large-scale placebo-controlled trial designed to determine the effectiveness of antibiotics in the treatment of AECOPD [8]. In the investigation, 173 patients with chronic bronchitis were followed for over 3 years. Patients were randomized to either antibiotics or placebo in a double-blind cross-over fashion, and one of three oral antibiotics chosen by the primary physician were used for 10 days: amoxicillin, co-trimoxazole (trimethoprim–sulfamethoxazole) and doxycycline. Approximately 40% of all exacerbations were severe, 40% were moderate and only 20% were mild. Patients with severe exacerbations received a significant benefit from antibiotics, whereas there was no significant difference between antibiotic and placebo in patients with mild exacerbations. Overall, the antibiotic-treated patients

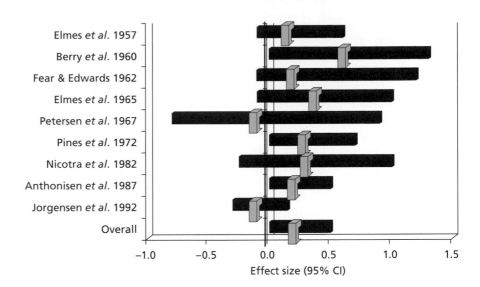

Figure 46.3 Effect sizes (mean differences in outcome divided by the pooled standard deviation) in nine studies of the use of antibiotics for exacerbations of COPD. Horizontal lines denote 95% confidence intervals (CI). The data indicate a significant improvement resulting from antibiotic therapy. (Reprinted from Saint *et al.* [58], with permission.)

showed a more rapid improvement in peak flow, and more overall improvement than those who received placebo. In addition, the length of illness was 2 days shorter for the antibiotic-treated group. However, no microbiology was performed and all antibiotics were assumed to be equivalent.

Allegra and Grassi [57] found significant benefit with the use of amoxicillin-clavulanate acid (Augmentin®) therapy compared with placebo in patients with severe disease. Patients who received this antibiotic exhibited a higher success rate and a lower frequency of recurrent exacerbations. In 1995, the results of a meta-analysis examined the role of antibiotics in the treatment of AECOPD (Fig. 46.3) [58]. The investigators analysed the results of nine randomized placebo-controlled trials published between 1957 and 1992. Comparing outcomes, such as mean number of days of illness, overall symptom score and the changes in peak expiratory flow rate indicated a clinically significant benefit for the antibiotic-treated patients. Analysis of the studies that provided data on expiratory flow rates, for example, noted an improvement of nearly 11 L/min in the antibiotic-treated groups. Antibiotic-associated improvement is likely to be especially relevant to patients who have low baseline peak flow rates and limited respiratory reserve, but the clinical significance of these changes is uncertain in the mildest of cases.

Antibiotic therapy for patients with AECOPD carries additional potential benefits [59]. Antibiotics can reduce the burden of bacteria in the airway. Bronchoscopic studies, using sterile protected specimen brush, have demonstrated that approximately 25% of stable COPD patients are colonized with potentially pathogenic bacteria [60–62]. A much larger percentage of patients with acute exacerbations have potentially pathogenic microorganisms in addition to significantly higher concentrations (frequently $\geq 10^4$ organisms)

of bacteria in the large airways [60–62]. Because treatment with appropriate antibiotics significantly decreases the bacterial burden, and frequently eradicates the organisms, the proper choice of antibiotic will likely reduce the risk of progression to pneumonia. The eradication of bacteria by antibiotics is thought to break the vicious cycle of infection, inflammation potentially leading to progression of the lung disease. In a high-risk group of patients with AECOPD, the antibiotic-treated group had a significantly lower in-hospital mortality rate and significantly reduced length of stay in the hospital compared with the placebo group [63]. In addition, patients receiving ofloxacin were less likely to develop pneumonia than those on placebo, especially during the first week of mechanical ventilation [64]. Patients with AECOPD demonstrating eradication of bacteria from the sputum had a significant improvement in inflammatory profile as exemplified by reduced exhaled NO and IL-8 [65].

Controversy existed as to whether or not the choice of antibiotic is an important determinant of outcome. While a study by Anthonisen *et al.* [8] assumed that all of the antibiotics were equivalent, and that therefore the specific agent prescribed was not important, subsequent evolution of antimicrobial resistance may have invalidated that assumption. As recommended in several clinical practice guidelines, adjusting antibiotic therapy based on local bacterial ecology is most prudent. However, antibiotic trials published more recently compare a new antibiotic with an established compound for the purpose of product registration and licensing. Because equivalence is the desired outcome of such trials, the agent chosen for comparison is not considered important. In addition, such trials frequently include patients with poorly defined disease severity (often without any obstructive lung disease) and acute illness of minor severity.

Another problem with interpreting the literature on AECOPD is the large variation in time frame (from 48 h to 28 days) used to assess either relapse or the resolution of symptoms [66,67]. The former can most clearly be defined as treatment failure necessitating further health-care utilization as the result of persistent or worsening symptoms. Many of these patients experiencing relapse, however, do not seek medical care despite persistent symptoms. The published relapse rates for patients with AECOPD range from 17% to 32%. One recent investigation evaluated the risk factors for therapy failure at 14 days after an acute exacerbation in an elderly cohort of patients with moderate to severe COPD. Most of the patients with severe symptoms received antibiotics, as opposed to only 40% with mild symptoms. The overall relapse rate defined as a return visit with persistent or worsening symptoms within 14 days was 22%. In multivariate analysis, the major risk factor for relapse was lack of antibiotic therapy. The type of antibiotic used was also an important variable associated with the 14-day treatment failure. Patients treated with amoxicillin had a 54% relapse rate compared with only 13% for the other antibiotics. Furthermore, treatment with amoxicillin resulted in a higher incidence of failure, even when compared with those who received no antibiotics. Other variables, such as COPD severity, types of exacerbation, prior or concomitant use of corticosteroids and current use of chronic oxygen therapy were not significantly associated with relapse. The study showed that the use of antibiotics is associated with a significantly lower rate of treatment failure and suggested that antibiotics are beneficial regardless of the severity of COPD. Patients who received antibiotics within 14 days had a significantly higher rate of hospital admissions than those not receiving antibiotics. Evolving resistance is likely to account for variable antibiotic efficacy at this time.

Destache *et al.* [68] reported the impact of antibiotic selection, antimicrobial efficacy and related cost in AECOPD in a retrospective review of 60 outpatients from a pulmonary clinic of a teaching institution who had the diagnoses of COPD and chronic bronchitis. The participants had a total of 224 episodes of AECOPD requiring antibiotic treatment. The antibiotics were arbitrarily divided into three types of agents: first-line (amoxicillin, co-trimoxazole, erythromycin and tetracycline), second-line (cephradine, cefuroxime, cefaclor, cefprozil) and third-line (amoxicillin-clavulanate, azithromycin and ciprofloxacin). The failure rates were significantly higher for the first-line agents compared with the third-line ones. When compared with patients who received the first-line treatment, those treated with the third-line agents doubled the time between exacerbations, had fewer hospitalizations and incurred considerably lower total costs.

Based on widespread reports of increasing antimicrobial resistance to the common pathogens isolated in patients with AECOPD, appropriate antibiotic selection is likely to be important. Conventional endpoints for efficacy of antibiotic treatment in AECOPD include the symptoms and bacteriological resolution measured at 2–3 weeks after the treatment was started. Most of these endpoints rely solely on the subjective report of improvement of symptoms and lack clinical objectivity. Several reports suggest that the infection-free interval, or the time to next episode of AECOPD [69–72], may be a more relevant endpoint. Wilson *et al.* [73] reported that patients with AECOPD treated with gemifloxacin showed a significant increase in the infection-free interval as compared with clarithromycin. This endpoint may reflect the ability of the antibiotic to achieve adequate bacteriological eradication in the airway. Whether or not such improved outcome translates into reduced health-care costs and disease modification is uncertain [74].

An 'ideal' antibiotic for treating patients with AECOPD

Characteristics of the 'ideal' antibiotics that are important to consider when choosing an agent for patients with AECOPD include the following:

1 Significant activity against the most common pathogens isolated in patients with AECOPD and minimizing substantial gaps in the coverage of these organisms [75,76].

2 Adequate coverage of the most likely pathogens in patients with AECOPD based on patient profiles that define the most likely spectrum of causative pathogens. This is especially important in patients with severe underlying obstructive lung disease, who are more commonly infected with Gram-negative organisms than those with mild COPD. Thus, it is important to identify local patterns of colonization and infection. In addition, patients with risk factors for a more complicated course should be prescribed antibiotics with coverage for the pathogens in AECOPD, which may include Gram-negative organisms and methicillin-resistant *Staphylococcus aureus*.

3 Susceptibility of the antimicrobial agent to the likely pathogens in AECOPD. There is an increasing prevalence of *H. influenzae* and *M. catarrhalis*, which produce bacterial enzymes that render traditional β-lactam antibiotics inactive. In addition, a growing number of AECOPD pathogens are resistant to many antibiotics available currently. It is important to know which mechanisms of resistance can affect the treatment of patients with AECOPD. It is also critical to know the local resistance rates of those microorganisms prior to prescribing a specific antibiotic [76].

4 Good penetration into sputum, bronchial mucosa and epithelial lining fluid. The goal of antimicrobial therapy is to deliver the appropriate drug to the specific site of infection.

In AECOPD, the bacteria are found in the airway lumen, along the mucosal cell surfaces and within the mucosal tissue. Various antibiotic classes exhibit markedly different degrees of penetration into the tissues and secretions of the respiratory tract [77].

5 Good therapeutic–toxicity profile. In a 1995 survey of patient attitudes toward antibiotic use, compliance was shown to improve significantly when medications were given at most once or twice a day. In addition, shorter courses of therapy (less than 14 days) were associated with better compliance. Of the patients interviewed, more than 80% stated a preference for once or twice daily dosing and more than 54% admitted to non-compliance with the prescribed regimen [78]. Recent data have supported shorter antibiotic treatment courses in pneumonia. It is likely that shorter durations of treatment will be possible in AECOPD.

6 Cost-effectiveness beyond the initial purchase price of the antibiotics. Several economic considerations should come into play when selecting an antibiotic for patients with AECOPD. In addition to the acquisition outlay, the cost of treatment failures, including the need for further antibiotics and the days of lost work; the resources saved by preventing hospitalization; the duration of disease-free intervals; and the development of antimicrobial resistance must all be accounted for.

Prevention

The two most important measures for preventing AECOPD are smoking cessation and active immunizations, including influenza and pneumococcal vaccinations. Clearly, smoking cessation should be included in the therapy of all patients. The annual rate of decline of the FEV_1 of a smoker is approximately 80 mL/year, compared with a decline in non-smokers of 25–30 mL/year. The Lung Health Study showed that in middle-aged patients with normal or mild lung function impairment, smoking cessation resulted in an improvement in FEV_1 after 1 year. Of the patients who stopped smoking after the first annual visit, 35% registered an increased in mean postbronchodilator decline in FEV_1 compared with those who continue to smoke [79]. It is likely that smoking cessation would have significant effects on bacterial colonization in COPD at all stages. This is not yet supported by empirical data.

Patients who are able to remain smoking quitters experience fewer exacerbations and less profound decrements in pulmonary function. Because of major addictive potential of cigarettes, the vast majority of those who quit smoking relapse within months. Nicotine is the main addictive substance in cigarettes, thus most patients experience severe withdrawal symptoms when they abruptly stop smoking [80]. Nicotine replacement therapy is widely used to overcome the patient's withdrawal symptoms, but such replacement therapy should always include behavioural modification programmes to increase the likelihood of success. Recently, it has been demonstrated that some antidepressants, especially amfebutamone (Zyban®), can be effective in initiating and sustaining quitting. There are several clinical practice guidelines on smoking cessation [81,82].

Viral infection often initiates AECOPD, which may reach epidemic proportions during the winter months. Epidemiological studies have shown that the frequency of lower respiratory infections and their associated morbidity and mortality are markedly reduced with influenza vaccination. In order to define the effects of influenza, and the benefits of influenza vaccination in elderly persons with chronic lung disease, a retrospective multiseason cohort study in a large managed care organization was undertaken. Patient vaccination rates of the organization were greater than 70%. The outcomes in vaccinated and unvaccinated individuals were compared after adjustment for baseline demographics and health characteristics. In unvaccinated persons, the hospitalization rates for pneumonia and influenza were twice as high in the influenza season as they were in the interim non-influenza periods. Vaccinated patients had fewer outpatient visits, fewer hospitalizations and fewer deaths. Influenza vaccine is therefore a cost-effective intervention in patients with COPD [83,84].

The polyvalent pneumococcus vaccine is effective in preventing invasive disease, particularly bacteraemia and meningitis [85]. Whether or not it prevents AECOPD is uncertain. The available 23 serotype vaccine has been shown to have an aggregate efficacy of more than 60%, although efficacy tends to decline with increasing age and immune state [86]. The vaccine is also recommended in patients with COPD. Jackson *et al.* [87] reported the results of a large cohort study of patients over the age of 65 years who were followed for 3 years. Use of the pneumococcal vaccine significantly reduced the incidence of pneumococcal bacteraemia, but did not alter the risk of outpatient community-acquired pneumonia. More recently, the introduction of the protein-polysaccharide conjugated pneumococcal vaccine in children resulted not only in a significant decrease in invasive pneumococcal disease in children, but also an 18% decrease in adults over age the of 65 years [88]. There are no contraindications for use of either pneumococcal or influenza vaccine immediately after an episode of pneumonia or AECOPD, and the vaccines can be given simultaneously without affecting their potency. There are no other vaccines currently available in adults to prevent lower respiratory tract infections. Vaccines intended to prevent infections resulting from non-typable *Haemophilus* sp. or *Pseudomonas* sp. are in development.

Recent studies have suggested a reduction in exacerbation rates when inhaled corticosteroids are used in advanced chronic COPD. This had led to the recommendation that inhaled steroids be incorporated into the routine management of COPD patients who have an FEV_1 of less than 50% and who have more than two exacerbations per year. A recent meta-analysis has suggested that such an approach may limit the decline in lung function as a consequence of AECOPD [56,89,90].

References

1 Anto JM, Vermeire P, Vestbo J, Sunyer J. Epidemiology of chronic obstructive pulmonary disease. *Eur Respir J* 2001;**17**: 982–94.

2 Pietila MP, Thomas CF. Inflammation and infection in exacerbations of chronic obstructive pulmonary disease. *Semin Respir Infect* 2003;**18**:9–16.

3 Hospers JJ, Postma DS, Riijcken B, Weiss ST, Schouten JP. Histamine airway hyper-responsiveness and mortality from chronic obstructive pulmonary disease. *Thorax* 2002;**57**:694–700.

4 Cassino C, Berger KI, Goldring RM *et al.* Duration of asthma and physiologic outcomes in elderly non-smokers. *Am J Respir Crit Care Med* 2000;**162**:1423–8.

5 Bach BP, Brown C, Gelfand SE, McCrory DC. Management of acute exacerbations of chronic obstructive pulmonary disease: a summary and appraisal of published evidence. *Ann Intern Med* 2001;**134**:600–20.

6 White AJ, Gompert S, Stockley RA. Chronic obstructive pulmonary disease. 6. The aetiology of exacerbations of chronic obstructive pulmonary disease. *Thorax* 2003;**58**:73–80.

7 Kidney J, McManus T, Coyle PV. Exacerbations of chronic obstructive pulmonary disease. *Thorax* 2002; **57**:754–6.

8 Anthonisen NR, Manfreda J, Warren CP *et al.* Antibiotic therapy in acute exacerbation of chronic obstructive pulmonary disease. *Ann Intern Med* 1987;**106**:196–204.

9 Roberts CM, Lowe D, Bucknall CE *et al.* Clinical audit indicators of outcome following admission to hospital with acute exacerbation of chronic obstructive pulmonary disease. *Thorax* 2002;**57**:137–41.

10 Almagro P, Calbo E, Ochoa de Echauguen A *et al.* Mortality after hospitalization for COPD. *Chest* 2002;**121**:1441–8.

11 Sethi S, Murphy TF. Bacterial infection in chronic obstructive pulmonary disease in 2000: a state-of-the-art review. *Clin Microbiol Rev* 2001;**14**:336–63.

12 Miravitlles M. Exacerbations of chronic obstructive pulmonary disease: when are bacteria important? *Eur Respir J* 2002;**20**(Suppl 36):9S–19S.

13 Patel IS, Seemungal TAR, Wilks M *et al.* Relationship between bacterial colonization and the frequency, character, and severity of COPD exacerbations. *Thorax* 2002;**57**:759–64.

14 Eller J, Ede A, Schaberg T *et al.* Infective exacerbations of chronic bronchitis: relation between bacteriologic etiology and lung infection. *Chest* 1998;**13**:1542–8.

15 Miravitlles M, Espinosa C, Fernandez-Laso E *et al.* Relationship between bacterial flora in sputum and functional impairment in patients with acute exacerbations of COPD. *Chest* 1999;**116**:40–6.

16 Wedzicha JA. Exacerbations: etiology and pathophysiologic mechanisms. *Chest* 2002;**121**:136S–41S.

17 Seemungal T, Harper-Owen R, Bhowmik A *et al.* Respiratory viruses, symptoms, and inflammatory markers in acute exacerbations and stable chronic obstructive pulmonary disease. *Am J Respir Crit Care Med* 2001;**164**:1618–23.

18 Hayashi S. Latent adenovirus infection in COPD. *Chest* 2002; **121**:183S–7S.

19 Rohde G, Wiethege A, Borg I *et al.* Respiratory viruses in exacerbations of chronic obstructive pulmonary disease requiring hospitalization: a case–control study. *Thorax* 2003; **58**:37–42.

20 Terence AR, Seemungal MRCP, Wedzicha JA. Viral infections in obstructive airway diseases. *Curr Opin Pulm Med* 2003;**9**: 111–6.

21 Barnes PJ, Shapiro SD, Pauwels RA. Chronic obstructive pulmonary disease: molecular and cellular mechanisms. *Eur Respir J* 2003;**22**:672–88.

22 Barnes PJ. Pathophysiology of asthma. *Br J Pharmacol* 1996; **42**:3–10.

23 Jeffrey PK. Structural and inflammatory changes in COPD: a comparison with asthma. *Thorax* 1998:**53**;129–36.

24 Barnes PJ. Mechanisms in COPD differences from asthma. *Chest* 2000;**117**:10S–4S.

25 Keatings VM, Collins PD, Scott DM *et al.* Differences in interleukin-8 and tumor necrosis factor-α induced sputum from patients with chronic obstructive pulmonary disease or asthma. *Am J Respir Crit Care Med* 1996;**153**:530–4.

26 Keatings VN, Barnes PJ. Granulocyte activation markers in induced sputum: comparison between chronic obstructive pulmonary disease, asthma and normal subjects. *Am J Respir Crit Care Med* 1997;**155**:449–53.

27 Howarth PH, Wilson J, Djukanovic R *et al.* Airway inflammation and atopic asthma: a comparative bronchoscopic investigation. *Arch Allergy Appl Immunol* 1991;**94**:266–9.

28 Amin K, Ludviksdottir D, Jansnon C *et al.* Inflammation and structural changes in the airways of patients with atopic and non-atopic asthma. *Am J Respir Crit Care Med* 2000;**163**: 2295–301.

29 O'Shaughnessy TC, Ansari TW, Barnes NC, Jeffery PK. Reticular basement membrane thickness in moderately severe asthma and smoker's chronic bronchitis with and without airflow obstruction. *Am J Respir Crit Care Med* 1996;**153**:A879.

30 Dunnill MS, Massarella GR, Anderson JA. A comparison of the quantitative anatomy of the bronchi in normal subjects, in status asthmaticus, in chronic bronchitis and in emphysema. *Thorax* 1969;**24**:176–9.

31 Beckett PA, Howarth PH. Pharmacotherapy and airway remodeling in asthma? *Thorax* 2003;**58**:163–74.

32 O'Shaughnessy TC, Ansari TW, Barnes NC. Inflammation in bronchial biopsies of subjects with chronic bronchitis: inverse relationship of CD8+ T lymphocytes with FEV_1. *Am J Respir Crit Care Med* 1997;**155**:852–7.

33 De Boer WI. Cytokines and therapy in COPD: a promising combination? *Chest* 2002;**121**:209S–18S.

34 Barnes PJ. Novel approaches and targets for treatment of chronic obstructive pulmonary disease. *Am J Respir Crit Care Med* 1999;**160**:S72–9.

35 Cataldo D, Mumaut C, Frankenne F *et al*. MMP-2 and MMP-9-linked gelatinolytic activity in the sputum from patients with asthma and chronic obstructive pulmonary disease. *Int Arch Allergy Immunol* 2000;**123**:259–67.

36 Stockley RA. Neutrophils and protease–antiprotease imbalance *Am J Respir Crit Care Med* 1999;**160**:S49–52.

37 Monso E, Rose A, Bonet G *et al*. Risk factors for lower airway bacterial colonization in chronic bronchitis. *Eur Resp J* 1999;**13**:338–42.

38 Zalacain R, Sobradillo V, Amilibia J *et al*. Predisposing factors for bacterial colonization in chronic obstructive pulmonary disease. *Eur Respir J* 1999;**13**:343–8.

39 Soler N, Ewig S, Atorres A *et al*. Airway inflammation and bronchial microbial patterns in patients with stable chronic obstructive pulmonary disease. *Eur Respir J* 1999;**14**:1015–22.

40 Wislin R, Sykes D, Rutman A. The effect of *Haemophilus influenzae* lipopolysaccharide on human respiratory epithelium. *Thorax* 1986;**41**:728–9.

41 Khair OA, Devalia JL, Abdelazi MM *et al*. Effect of *Haemophilus influenzae* on the synthesis of IL-6, Il-8, TNF-α, and expression I ICAM-1 in cultured human bronchial epithelial cells. *Eur Respir J* 1994;**7**:2109–16.

42 Hill AT, Cambell EJ, Hill SL, Baykley DL, Stockley RA. Association between airway bacterial load and markers of airway inflammation in patients with stable chronic bronchitis. *Am J Med* 2000;**109**:288–95.

43 Bresser P, Out TA, van Alpen L, Kansen HM, Lutter R. Airway inflammation in non-obstructive and obstructive chronic bronchitis with chronic *Haemophilus influenzae* airway infections. *Am J Respir Crit Care Med* 2000;**162**:947–52.

44 Stockley RA, O'Brien C, Pye A, Hill SL. Relationship of sputum color to nature and outpatient management of acute exacerbations of COPD. *Chest* 2000;**117**:1638–45.

45 Gompertz S, O'Brien C, Bayley DL *et al*. Changes in bronchial inflammation during acute exacerbations of chronic bronchitis. *Eur Respir J* 2001;**17**:1112–9.

46 Zhu JL, Qiu YS, Jamumdar S *et al*. Exacerbations of bronchitis: bronchial eosinophilia and gene expression for interleukin-4, interleukin-5, and eosinophil chemoattractants. *Am J Crit Care Med* 2001;**164**:109–26.

47 Hegele RG, Hayashi S, Hogg J *et al*. Mechanisms of airway narrowing and hyperresponsiveness in viral respiratory tract infections. *Am J Respir Crit Care Med* 1995;**151**:1659–64.

48 Jacoby DB, Fryer D. Interaction of viral infections with muscarinic receptors. *Clin Exp Immunol* 1999;**29**:59–64.

49 Hogg JC. Role of latent viral infections in chronic obstructive pulmonary disease and asthma. *Am J Respir Crit Care Med* 2001;**164**:S71–5.

50 Vitalis TZ, Keocho N, Itabashi S, Hayashi S, Hogg JC. A model of latent adenoviral infection in the guinea pig. *Am J Respir Cell Mol Biol* 1996;**14**:225–31.

51 Vitalis TZ, Kern I, Groom A *et al*. The effect of latent adenovirus 5 infection on cigarette smoke induced lung inflammation. *Eur Respir J* 1998;**11**:662–9.

52 Ratemales I, Elliott WM, Meshi B *et al*. The amplification of inflammation in emphysema and its association with latent adenoviral infection. *Am J Respir Crit Care Med*. 2001;**164**:469–73.

53 Smith CB, Golden C, Klauber MR *et al*. Interactions between viruses and bacteria in patients with chronic bronchitis. *J Infect Dis* 1976;**134**:552–61.

54 Fagon JY, Chastre J. Severe exacerbations of COPD patients; the role of pulmonary infections. *Semin Respir Infect* 1996;**11**:109–18.

55 Seemungal TA, Harper-Owen R, Bhowmik A *et al*. Detection of rhinovirus in induced sputum at exacerbation of chronic obstructive pulmonary disease. *Eur Respir J* 2000;**16**:677–83.

56 Pauwels RA, Buist S, Calvery PMA, Jenkins CR, Hurd SS. Global strategy for the diagnosis, management, and prevention of chronic obstructive pulmonary disease. NHLBI/WHO Global Initiative for Chronic Obstructive Pulmonary Disease (GOLD) Workshop Summary. *Am J Respir Crit Care Med* 2001;**163**:1256–76.

57 Allegra L, Grassi C. Ruolo degli antibiotici nel trattamento delle riacutizza della bronchite cronica. *Ital J Chest Dis* 1991;**45**:138–48.

58 Saint S, Bent S, Vittinghoff E *et al*. Antibiotics in chronic obstructive pulmonary disease exacerbations: a meta-analysis. *JAMA* 1995;**273**:957–60.

59 Sonnesyn SW, Gerdin DN. Antimicrobials for the treatment of respiratory infection. In: Niederman MS, Sarosi GA, Glassroth J, eds. *Respiratory Infections: A Scientific Basis for Management*. Philadelphia: WB Saunders, 1994: 511–37.

60 Cabello H, Torres A, Celis R *et al*. Bacterial colonization of distal airways in healthy subjects and chronic lung disease: a bronchoscopic study. *Eur Respir J* 1997;**10**:1137–44.

61 Fagon JY, Chastre J, Trouillet JL *et al*. Characterization of distal bronchial microflora during acute exacerbation of chronic bronchitis. *Am Rev Respir Dis* 1990;**142**:1004–8.

62 Martinez JA, Rodriguez E, Bastida T *et al*. Quantitative study of the bronchial bacterial flora in acute exacerbations of chronic bronchitis. *Chest* 1994;**105**:976.

63 Nouira S, Marghli S, Belghith M *et al*. Once daily oral ofloxacin in chronic obstructive pulmonary disease exacerbation requiring mechanical ventilation: a randomized placebo-controlled trial. *Lancet* 2001;**358**:2020–5.

64 Murata GH, Gorby MS, Chick TW *et al*. Use of emergency medical services by patients with decompensated obstructive lung disease. *Ann Emerg Med* 1989;**18**:501–6.

65 White AJ, Gompertz S, Bayley DL *et al*. Resolution of bronchial inflammation is related to bacterial eradication following treatment of exacerbations of chronic bronchitis. *Thorax* 2002;**58**:680–5.

66 Murata GH, Gorby MS, Kapsner CO *et al*. A multivariate model for the prediction of relapse after outpatient treatment of decompensated chronic obstructive pulmonary disease. *Arch Intern Med* 1992;**152**:73–7.

67 Adams S, Melo J, Luther M *et al*. Antibiotics are associated with lower relapse rates in outpatients with acute exacerbations of chronic obstructive pulmonary disease. *Chest* 2000;**117**:1345–52.

68 Destache CJ, Dewan N, O'Donohue WJ *et al*. Clinical and economic considerations in the treatment of acute exacerbations of chronic bronchitis. *J Antimicrob Chemother* 1999;**43**(Suppl A):107–13.

69 Ball P. Future antibiotic trials. *Semin Respir Infect* 2000;**15**: 82–9.

70 Anzueto A, Rizzo JA, Grossman RF. The infection-free interval: its use in evaluating antimicrobial treatment in acute exacerbations of chronic bronchitis. *Clin Infect Dis* 1999; **28**:1344–5.

71 Chodosh S, McCarthy J, Farkas S *et al*. Randomized, double-blind study of ciprofloxacin and cefuroxime axetil for treatment of acute exacerbations of chronic bronchitis. *Clin Infect Dis* 1998;**27**:722–9.

72 Chodosh S, Schreurs JM, Siami G *et al*. Efficacy of oral ciprofloxacin vs clarithromycin for treatment of acute exacerbations of chronic bronchitis. *Clin Infect Dis* 1998; **27**:730–8.

73 Wilson R, Schentag JJ, Ball P, Mandell L for the 068 Study Group. A comparison of gemifloxacin and clarithromycin in acute exacerbations of chronic bronchitis and long-term clinical outcomes. *Clin Ther* 2002;**4**:639–52.

74 Niederman MS, McCombs JS, Unger AN *et al*. Treatment cost of acute exacerbations of chronic bronchitis. *Clin Ther* 1999;**21**:576–92.

75 Doern GV, Brueggemann A, Holley HP Jr *et al*. Antimicrobial resistance of *Streptococcus pneumoniae* recovered from outpatients in the United States during the winter months of 1994 to 1995: results of a 30-center national surveillance study. *Antimicrob Agents Chemother* 1996;**40**:1208–13.

76 Doern GV. Antimicrobial resistance with *Streptococcus pneumonia* in the United States. *Semin Respir Crit Care Med* 2000;**21**: 273–84.

77 Nix DE. Intrapulmonary concentrations of antimicrobial agents. *Infect Dis Clin North Am* 1998;**12**:631–46.

78 Gallup Organization. *Consumer Attitudes Toward Antibiotic Use*. New York: American Lung Association, 1995.

79 Anthonisen NR, Connett JE, Kiley JP *et al*. Effect of smoking intervention and the use of an inhaled anticholinergic bronchodilator on the rate of decline of FEV_1. *JAMA* 1994;**272**: 1497–505.

80 Fiore MC, Jorenby DE, Baker TB. Tobacco dependence and the nicotine patch: clinical guidelines for effective use. *JAMA* 1992;**268**:2687–94.

81 Fiose MC, Bailey WC, Cohen SJ *et al*. *Smoking Cessation: Clinical Practice Guidelines*. No. 18. Rockville MD: USD Department of Health and Human Services, Publication No. 96-0692, 1996.

82 Jorenby DE, Leischow SJ, Nides MA *et al*. A controlled trail of sustained-release bupropion, a nicotine patch, or both for smoking cessation. *N Engl J Med* 1999;**340**:685–91.

83 Centers for Disease Control and Prevention. Prevention and control of influenza: recommendations for the Advisory Committee on Immunization practices. *MMWR* 1995;**44**(RR-31):1–22.

84 Nichol KL, Baken L, Nelson A. Relation between influenza vaccination and outpatient visits, hospitalization, and mortality in elderly persons with chronic lung disease. *Ann Intern Med* 1999;**130**:397–403.

85 Centers for Disease Control and Prevention. Update on adult immunization: recommendations of the Immunization Advisory Committee Pneumococcal Disease. *MMWR* 1191; **40**(RR-12):42–4.

86 Butler JC, Breiman RF, Campbell JF *et al*. Pneumococcal polysaccharide vaccine efficacy: an evaluation of current recommendations. *JAMA* 1993;**270**:1826–31.

87 Jackson L, Neuzil KM, Yu O *et al*. Effectiveness of pneumococcal polysaccharide vaccine in older adults. *N Engl J Med* 2003;**348**:1747–55.

88 Whitney C, Farley M, Hadler J *et al*. Decline in invasive pneumococcal disease after the introduction of protein-polysaccharide conjugated vaccine. *N Engl J Med* 2003;**348**:1737–46.

89 Sutherland ER, Allmers H, Ayas Venn AJ, Martin RJ. Chronic obstructive pulmonary disease: inhaled corticosteroids reduce the progression of airflow limitation in chronic obstructive pulmonary disease – a meta-analysis. *Thorax* 2003;**58**:937–41.

90 Burge PS, Lewis SA. Inhaled steroids in COPD: so inhaled steroids slow the rate of decline in FEV_1 in patients with COPD after all? *Thorax* 2003;**58**:911–3.

CHAPTER 47

Mechanical ventilation for exacerbation of COPD

Andrea Rossi, Guido Polese and Lorenzo Appendini

Exacerbations of chronic obstructive pulmonary disease (COPD) may be of differing severity [1]. It ranges from a mild increase of usual symptoms to life-threatening decompensation. In patients with advanced COPD, exacerbations can often be associated with ventilatory failure (a rise in Pa_{CO_2} above 45 mmHg or above baseline), stable hypercapnia if present and respiratory acidosis (pH less than 7.36) [2,3]. In those patients, in addition to optimal medical therapy and adequate oxygenation, mechanical ventilatory assistance may be required if there is evidence of the following:

1 Unbearable breathlessness at rest, often associated with:
- tachypnoea (e.g. more than 30 breaths/min);
- evident use of accessory respiratory muscles; or
- Pradox breathing (i.e. inward movement of the abdomen during inspiration).

2 Arterial pH less than 7.36 and a Pa_{CO_2} of more than 45 mmHg.

3 Pa_{O_2}/Fi_{O_2} less than 300 mmHg.

The aims of mechanical ventilation (MV), independent of the mode and settings selected, are to:
- support the overloaded ventilatory pump;
- improve arterial blood gases and pH;
- relieve dyspnoea and unload the respiratory muscles; and
- 'buy time', to sustain life until the medical therapy controls the event underlying the exacerbation (e.g. respiratory tract infection).

MV can be administered in different modes:

1 Invasive 'conventional' MV through an endotracheal tube bypassing the upper airway.

2 Non-invasive mechanical ventilation (NIMV):
- non-invasive positive pressure ventilation (NPPV); or
- negative pressure ventilation (NPV).

The indications for applying MV and the choice between conventional MV and NIMV, as well as the mode and settings of ventilatory assistance, depends not only upon the severity of the exacerbations and respiratory acidosis, but also on many other factors such as the timing of the intervention, the characteristics of individual patients, the skill of the team and the available monitoring facilities [4,5].

A brief description of the pathophysiology of COPD exacerbations and ventilatory failure will help to elucidate the rationale underlying the need for mechanical ventilatory assistance as well as the choice of ventilatory mode and settings.

Pathophysiology of COPD exacerbations

By definition, COPD is characterized by airflow limitation (i.e. a significant reduction of forced expiratory flow resulting from a loss of lung elastic recoil and abnormal airway resistance) [6]. In many patients with advanced COPD, flow limitation exists even during tidal breathing as documented by the fact that tidal expiratory flow lies below the maximal flow volume envelope. Pulmonary hyperinflation (i.e. an increase of the functional residual capacity [FRC] above the predicted value) is also a common feature in patients with moderate to severe COPD [7].

When an exacerbation occurs, whatever the aetiology, the airway resistance increases and expiratory flow limitation may worsen. In these conditions, the rate of lung emptying is proportionally retarded and the tidal expiration cannot be completed within the time available between two inspiratory efforts (i.e. the next inspiratory effort ensues before the lungs decompress to the elastic equilibrium volume). Because of incomplete expiration, the tidal end-expiratory lung volume is established above the relaxed FRC. This condition is termed dynamic hyperinflation and adds to the existing pulmonary hyperinflation resulting from the loss of lung recoil [8]. The immediate consequence of the incomplete tidal expiration is that the end-expiratory alveolar pressure remains positive. The latter is termed auto- and/or intrinsic positive end-expiratory pressure (PEEPi) in analogy with the positive end-expiratory pressure (PEEP) commonly set by the mechanical ventilator [9] because PEEPi was originally described in mechanically ventilated patients [10].

Low levels of dynamic pulmonary hyperinflation and PEEPi were found also in most patients with severe COPD in a stable condition [7,11]. However, the levels of PEEPi observed during exacerbations and ventilatory failure are much greater than in stable conditions, particularly in COPD patients requiring mechanical ventilation [11]. The first implication of dynamic hyperinflation is that the contracting inspiratory muscles must counterbalance PEEPi in order to create a negative pressure in the central airways and start the inspiratory flow. During exacerbations, the inspiratory threshold load provided by PEEPi can be quite substantial (i.e. more than 10 cm H_2O up to 20–22 cm H_2O) [12].

In patients with exacerbations of COPD, not only the mechanical load upon the ventilatory pump increases because of the higher airway resistance and PEEPi, but also the capacity of the respiratory muscles to generate pressure is diminished because of impaired length–tension relationship and reduced area of apposition, among other factors [8].

The net result of an excessive mechanical load and an impaired respiratory muscle pressure generating capacity creates a significant challenge for the ventilatory pump. Tachypnoea might represent a protective mechanism to prevent excessive work of breathing (WOB) by defending minute ventilation through a reduction in tidal volume and a rise in frequency. However, it is a very poor strategy. In fact, the smaller tidal volume will result in increased Pa_{CO_2} and lower pH, while the shorter expiratory time resulting from the higher frequency of breathing will enhance dynamic hyperinflation and PEEPi, hence further increasing the mechanical load and decreasing the inspiratory muscles' capacity to bear the load. This sort of vicious circle, where the mechanical load progressively rises and the capacity of the respiratory muscles is progressively impaired, may lead to malfunction of the ventilatory pump and impending respiratory arrest [5]. Whether this may be considered 'respiratory muscle fatigue' or not remains a controversial issue which has been extensively reviewed in recent publications [8,12]. However, regardless of the nature of the mechanism leading to its failure, the ventilatory pump must be supported to prevent the ultimate life-threatening exhaustion, severe acidosis and respiratory arrest.

Mechanical ventilation

The widespread and early application of NIMV, not only in the intensive care unit (ICU) but on the medical (pneumological) ward for patients with ventilatory failure and respiratory acidosis resulting from exacerbations of COPD,

should be considered a major advance in clinical medicine. In fact, NIMV accomplishes a key goal in medicine: namely it saves human lives [13–16]. In particular it should be emphasized that among all patients with respiratory failure, those with decompensated COPD obtain the greatest benefit from NIMV [13,14,17]. Despite the widespread use and popularity of NIMV, many COPD patients still need endotracheal intubation and 'conventional' mechanical ventilation.

Invasive mechanical ventilation

For many years, conventional (i.e. 'invasive') MV through an endotracheal tube was the only mode of ventilatory assistance. Nowadays, invasive MV should be considered as the immediate mode of intervention only in some particular conditions, such as in:
- respiratory arrest;
- severe cardiovascular instability (hypotension, arrhythmias, myocardial infarction);
- impaired mental status, somnolence;
- inability to cooperate (e.g. excessive agitation);
- copious and/or viscous bronchial secretions;
- high aspiration risk;
- recent facial or gastroesophageal surgery;
- craniofacial trauma and/or fixed nasopharingeal abnormality;
- extensive burns; and
- extreme obesity.

It is a common experience that many patients with severe exacerbations of COPD arrive at the emergency area either already intubated in the ambulance or urgently requiring intubation [18]. Refractory life-threatening hypoxaemia (Pa_{O_2}/Fi_{O_2} less than 200 mmHg) and/or severe acidosis (pH less than 7.25) could be considered as indications for intubation and conventional MV, depending upon local conditions such as the skill of the team, the facilities available for monitoring, the immediate accessibility of intubation and an ICU [6]. Clearly, intubation must be considered when NIMV fails (i.e. arterial blood gas abnormality and respiratory acidosis persists despite aggressive medical therapy, oxygenation and NIMV).

Controlled mechanical ventilation

In the first hours of critical illness, the patient may need MV in the control mode to provide immediate rest for the respiratory muscles as well as relief of excessive dyspnoea and anxiety. It has been shown that the mechanical properties of the respiratory system are severely abnormal in the first day of ICU admission, such that even assisted ventilation may be problematic because of pathophysiological, clinical and often psychological reasons. In these conditions, a period of controlled mechanical ventilation (CMV) may be warranted to provide adequate rest for the ventilatory pump as well as control of the haemodynamic instability. In some patients, light sedation may help if the level of anxiety does not allow good patient–ventilator interaction, at least in the first hours of MV. Heavy sedation and muscle paralysis should be avoided to prevent the severe complications often associated with those therapies [19]. As soon as the clinical condition of the patient improves, assisted MV can replace the control mode. However, the initial period of CMV, when needed, may be used to take measurements of respiratory mechanics, such as PEEPi, elastance and resistance, which may be helpful in understanding the condition underlying the acute decompensation as well as to plan strategy for ventilator settings, treatment and weaning [20]. Those measurements can be obtained with simple equipment and non-invasive techniques, even on-line [21–24].

In mechanically ventilated COPD patients, a major issue is to avoid, as much as possible, high levels of dynamic hyperinflation resulting from the ventilator settings. Dynamic hyperinflation may impair cardiac function severely [25]. It must be taken into account that high inflation volume and short expiratory duration enhance dynamic hyperinflation and PEEPi. Therefore, the ventilator settings should be adjusted accordingly to minimize dynamic hyperinflation. It has also been suggested that application of PEEP improves gas exchange in COPD patients during CMV [26]. Data from a patient's respiratory mechanics may help to set the ventilator appropriately. It should also be remembered that dynamic hyperinflation can be substantially reduced by aggressive use of bronchodilators, whose effects can be measured and tuned to the targeted objective [27]. The correct ventilator settings and treatment can bring about a rapid transition from CMV to assisted ventilation. The latter is a ventilatory mode in which the patient triggers the ventilator and participates in the act of breathing.

Pressure support ventilation

Pressure support ventilation (PSV) is by far the most widely used mode of assisted ventilation [28] and is also an appropriate technique for weaning [3,4]. However, the level of PSV must be set appropriately to avoid both under- and overassistance, both of which may jeopardize the effectiveness of MV. In fact, over- and underassistance may fail one of the major aims of MV: to rest the overloaded ventilatory pump. With underassistance, the patient's respiratory muscles continue to perform a substantial part of breathing to match the ventilatory demand, because of the insufficient support of the mechanical ventilator [29]. With overassistance, the lack of rest for the respiratory muscles can be the consequence of ineffective effort and patient–ventilator dyssynchrony [29]. A cause of bad patient–ventilator inter-

action is the dissociation between the patient's central drive and the timing of ventilatory assistance. This occurs when the patient's respiratory muscles stop contracting soon after triggering the ventilator, such that the mechanical inspiration is longer than the spontaneous inspiratory effort and the mechanical lung inflation goes into the neural expiration. In other words, the neural inspiration is much shorter than the mechanical inspiration which goes into the neural expiration. Under these circumstances, the patient's inspiratory central control generates inspiratory efforts either during mechanical inflation or during expiration when the elastic recoil is too high to be counterbalanced and expiration proceeds despite the patient's attempt to inspire. The dissociation between central timing and ventilator timing may cause patient–ventilator dyssynchrony and eventually lead to the 'patient fighting the ventilator' [30].

Apart from the unquestionable value of clinical observation and experience, some physiological measurements (e.g. the central drive as expressed by mouth occlusion pressure a 1/100th of a second; $P = 0.1$) may help to adjust the appropriate level of PSV to the individual patient [31].

Proportional assist ventilation

Some years ago, the proportional assist ventilation (PAV), a new mode of partial ventilatory assistance, was introduced to improve patient–ventilator interaction [32,33]. PAV is a patient-guided mode in which the pressure provided by the ventilator is proportional to patient's instantaneous inspiratory effort in terms of both the intensity and the duration of the neuromuscolar drive, such that the end of the effort brings about the end of the ventilatory assistance. However, despite its promising theoretic background and some interesting and favourable clinical studies [33], PAV has not succeeded in entering the real clinical world and it still considered a mode of MV more suitable for clinical research than for routine application.

Positive end-expiratory pressure

PSV is not the only condition in which patient–ventilator dyssynchrony can occur. Assisted controlled ventilation (ACV) and synchronized intermittent mandatory ventilation (SIMV) can be associated with similar events [9]. In addition, there is a condition in which patient–ventilator dyssynchrony may occur regardless the mode of MV (i.e. with high levels of intrinsic PEEP). If the negative intrathoracic pressure generated by the patient's contracting inspiratory muscles is smaller than PEEPi, the effort does not generate sufficient pressure or inspiratory flow in the central airway to trigger the ventilator, remaining 'ineffective'. To be effective for triggering, the negative pressure generated by the inspiratory muscles must be greater than the sum of PEEPi plus the negative triggering pressure [10]. The latter is in general very small, from -0.5 to -2 cm H_2O, whereas the former may be rather substantial, often more than 10 cm H_2O and up to more than 20 cm H_2O [11]. For this reason – the consistent presence of PEEPi – it has been suggested that some levels of PEEP should be set by the ventilator to counterbalance PEEPi and prevent ineffective efforts [29,34,35]. The level of PEEP sufficient to counterbalance most of PEEPi without worsening hyperinflation can be decided either by measuring PEEPi, which might not be easy in an actively breathing patient because it requires the use of the oesophageal balloon technique [29,34,35], or by observing empirically that each patient's effort actually triggers the ventilator. A more detailed discussion on the causes and consequences of PEEPi as well as the technique of adjusting the adequate levels of PEEP may be found elsewhere [10,11,23].

In synthesis, patients with exacerbations of COPD matching the criteria for conventional invasive MV may need a short initial period of CMV. Clearly, heavy sedation and particularly muscle paralysis must be avoided to prevent severe neuromuscular complications [19]. However, that period could be used to obtain some measurements of respiratory mechanics by means of non-invasive techniques [9]. As soon as possible, the patient should be switched to AMV, in general PSV with low levels of PEEP to counterbalance PEEPi. Along these lines, Appendini *et al.* [29] found that the same level of pressure assistance (e.g. 15 cm H_2O) determined a greater reduction of the WOB if PEEP was set (i.e. 5 cm H_2O PEEP + 10 cm H_2O PSV) than ventilation with more than 15 cm H_2O PSV. In addition, they found little advantage in terms of reduction of the inspiratory effort with the increase of PSV from 15 to 25 cm H_2O, either with or without PEEP. These data should call attention to the risk of undue overassistance by setting PSV at excessive levels.

Traditionally, mechanically ventilated patients with exacerbation of COPD present difficulty in weaning and are exposed to the risk of prolonged MV-related complications [36]. Almost half of the time spent by COPD patients on MV is because of the weaning procedure. Furthermore, among patients with difficult weaning, COPD patients represent the clear majority [37]. Weaning from MV is discussed in a separate section.

Non-invasive mechanical ventilation

Currently, invasive MV is applied much less than it used to be in COPD patients, because of the widespread utilization and popularity of NIMV. Recent publications have extensively reviewed this issue [38]. A recent meta-analysis concluded that NIMV should be considered as the first-line treatment for patients with exacerbation of COPD and respiratory acidosis and should be offered to those patients [16] with a favourable cost-effectiveness balance [39].

Several randomized clinical trials, on which high-quality meta-analyses were based [15,40], have shown that the early institution of NIMV when respiratory acidosis is still moderate not only improves arterial blood gases and pH, relieves dyspnoea and unloads the respiratory muscles, but also reduces the rate of intubation, reduces the rate of ventilator-related complications, reduces the length of ICU stay and reduces in-hospital and 1-year mortality.

NPPV is by far the most widely used technique of ventilatory assistance in patients with exacerbations of COPD and moderate respiratory acidosis [4]. However, NPV has been successfully used in some patients by a few well-trained groups that have documented good clinical [41,42] as well as physiological results [43,44]. At present, NPV is still limited to those groups and has not really gained wider popularity. One of the reasons could be that the iron lung, which is the most commonly used equipment to deliver NPV, is cumbersome and makes access to the patient difficult. In addition, the technology of ventilators used to deliver NPPV has improved greatly in recent years. Some latest generation ventilators are very user-friendly and also offer important monitoring facilities and leak compensatory mechanisms [45–47]. The association of positive clinical results and good technology has undoubtly promoted NIMV and particularly NPPV in the real world. In some European countries, NIMV became the key treatment by which pulmonologists gained a reputation in the treatment of critically ill patients and found a role in intensive care medicine [48,49].

Non-invasive positive pressure ventilation

Whereas the role of NPPV in the management of acute respiratory failure remains somehow controversial [17], its role in the treatment of ventilatory failure resulting from exacerbations of COPD seems well established: it may actually represent 'a new gold standard' [50].

NPPV is defined as any form of ventilatory support applied without the use of an endotracheal tube, and it includes:
1 Continuous positive airway pressure (CPAP) with or without:
  • inspiratory pressure support; or
  • proportional assist ventilation.
2 Volume and pressure cycled systems.

The mechanisms through which NPPV improves arterial blood gases and unloads the inspiratory muscles has been carefully investigated in physiological studies [34,51,52].

Physiological basis of NPPV
It has been shown that NPPV improves arterial blood gases through an increase in alveolar ventilation, without significant modifications in the $\dot{V}/\dot{Q}$ mismatching and gas

exchange capability of the lungs [51]. However, NPPV can significantly reduce cardiac output [51], such that the final net effect on Pao_2 depends upon the magnitude of interaction among intrapulmonary ($\dot{V}/\dot{Q}$ mismatching, shunt, diffusing capacity) and extrapulmonary (cardiac output, oxygen consumption, mixed venous Po_2 and minute ventilation) determinants of oxygenation. The decrease in cardiac output reduces mixed venous Po_2 and causes a decrease in Pao_2; on the other hand, the increase in alveolar ventilation reduces $Paco_2$ and improves PAo_2 and hence Pao_2. The available data support the conclusion that the effect of greater alveolar ventilation on Pao_2 is not impaired by the decrease in cardiac output such that NPPV eventually improves Pao_2 [51].

NPPV does not affect passive pulmonary mechanics (i.e. it has a negligible effect on resistance and elastance), although the latter slightly decreases because of the greater tidal volume compared with spontaneous breathing [34]. By contrast, NPPV has a great effect on the respiratory muscles because it substantially reduces the WOB by taking over most of the mechanical load [34]. However, in patients with respiratory acidosis resulting from exacerbations of COPD, elastance and resistance are only a portion of the ventilatory load. PEEPi can contribute considerably to the magnitude of the inspiratory effort, in some studies making up almost half [30]. Not surprisingly, application of CPAP to counterbalance PEEPi significantly improves the effect of NPPV on WOB [34]. There is general agreement that some levels of CPAP should be associated with inspiratory pressure support, not only to reduce the amount of the patient's inspiratory effort, but also to improve patient–ventilator interaction. In fact, the appropriate level of CPAP (i.e. slightly lower than PEEPi) reduces the amount of negative pressure that the patient's inspiratory muscles must create to trigger the ventilator and hence abolishes the ineffective efforts not able to trigger the mechanical breath.

When PEEPi is measured, either non-invasively or by means of the oesophageal balloon technique, it is simple to set the appropriate level of CPAP by establishing a value slightly lower than PEEPi [34]. Without measurement, it is reasonable to observe the patient and to set a level of CPAP sufficient to trigger the ventilator with minimal effort. It has also been suggested that PEEPi may be estimated non-invasively on the basis of clinical observation [53]. However, the validity of this method to set the level of CPAP has not yet been tested on a large group of patients. In common clinical practice, levels of CPAP between 4 and 8 cm H_2O seem appropriate for most patients without the risk of worsening hyperinflation [54].

Clinical studies of NPPV

Almost 100 papers document the wide popularity and success of NIMV since the pioneering work by Meduri *et al.* [55,56]. The majority are observational studies, but some well-conducted prospective randomized clinical trials (RCTs) also confirm that NIMV, and particularly NPPV, is an effective treatment for ventilatory failure resulting from exacerbations of COPD. Good quality meta-analyses on the RCTs further support this conclusion [15–17,40]. However, it should be noted that patients at the two extremes (i.e. either with mild or very severe COPD exacerbations) do not seem to benefit from NPPV [6,15]. In the former group, application of NPPV did not show any advantage compared with standard medical therapy, while in the latter group NPPV may unduly delay intubation. Among observational studies the work by Benhamou *et al.* [57] is worth mentioning because NPPV was successfully administered in very elderly patients.

The published RCTs have three known limitations which, however, do not affect the validity and robustness of the results. First, a placebo was not administered such that it becomes difficult to distinguish between the effect of NPPV itself and that of the greater attention that the caregivers' team might devote to ventilated patients compared with those receiving standard, more conventional treatment. Secondly, patients participating in RCTs are selected according to predetermined criteria and might not be truly representative of the heterogeneous population of COPD patients with exacerbations. Thirdly, the condition of an RCT might not reflect what is happening in actual clinical practice, because the procedures are standardized, the patients are selected, the team is motivated, and so on. Nevertheless, all the studies and meta-analyses provide consistent positive results favouring NPPV, with only patients with mild exacerbations not benefiting [15]. The percentage of NPPV success is consistently in the range 75–80% compared with 40–50% for patients receiving standard medical treatment. The definition of success includes the following:

- The acute episodes resolves without the need for endotracheal intubation.
- Mechanical ventilation can be discontinued.
- The patient is discharged from hospital.

Factors associated with success of NPPV are likely to be:

1 Appropriate selection of patients (see exclusion criteria and/or indications for conventional MV):
  - younger age;
  - ability to cooperate; and
  - lower acuity of illness.
2 Experience of clinicians.
3 Availability of resources.

It is considered that NPPV fails when the patient either needs intubation or dies because intubation is not performed for ethical reasons (e.g. patient's consent, older age, terminal condition) or because it is not available.

Intubation and the institution of conventional MV

should be considered when, after optimization of medical therapy, including MV:

- Arterial blood gases and/or pH do not improve after 4 h or even worsen after 1–2 h [58].
- Other complications either appear or do not resolve (e.g. metabolic abnormalities, sepsis, pneumonia, pulmonary embolism, barotrauma, massive pleural effusion).

Observational studies as well as RCTs on NPPV were performed in different settings. This is important because the availability of monitoring resources as well as the ability of clinicians to bear the workload varies between the general (pneumological or medical) ward and the ICU, and it has been shown that this must be seriously considered [59]. Between the two settings (ward and ICU), some institutions have a level of intermediate care generally referred to as respiratory intermediate care units (RiCU) [48,49], whose specific aim is the treatment of patients with acute (or acute on chronic) respiratory failure without severe multiorgan complications or failure.

In a historical overview of the application of NPPV in exacerbations of COPD, some studies should be mentioned in particular. In 1990, Brochard et al. [60] published a study that was not an RCT, but had a historical control group. Nonetheless, because of the excellent reputation of the group of investigators and the high profile of the journal, this work is commonly considered to be the landmark study that gave NPPV a real scientific role. The same group published a large RCT a few years later [18]. Bott and Carroll [61] performed the first RCT by comparing NPPV with conventional medical therapy in a general ward. More recently, Plant et al. [62] reported a large multicentric trial conducted in the UK in a respiratory ward and not in intensive care areas. That study favoured NPPV over standard medical therapy, documenting that patients receiving NPPV had lower mortality and rate of intubation than controls. The relevance of this study is that it demonstrated that the application of NPPV in patients with moderate acidosis can be performed successfully with little training and outside of special environments such as ICU and RiCU. On the other hand, the study by Conti et al. [63], which is the only RCT comparing conventional MV and NPPV, reported that in an ICU, NPPV could be as successful as conventional MV in terms of treatment of ventilatory failure, but with a significant lower rate of complications, particularly infectious complications. However, the results of that comparison cannot be extrapolated outside of the ICU and could be significantly affected by the extensive experience of that particular team of investigators. Among recent published studies, the one by Thys et al. [64] is noteworthy because it is the only one with a control ventilation to the standard therapy group, suggesting that the success of NPPV was not a result of the greater attention of the team. More recently, Jolliet et al. [65] reported an RCT in which a helium–oxygen ($He-O_2$)

mixture was compared with an air–oxygen mixture for NIMV in decompensated COPD patients. Although $He-O_2$ determined a slightly shorter hospital stay, the rate of intubation did not differ, and the authors concluded that further studies would be needed before recommending $He-O_2$ as a routine NIMV strategy in the ICU.

The physiological study by Vitacca et al. [66] used PAV with low levels of CPAP and showed that, in the short term, arterial blood gases were improved while the inspiratory muscles were significantly unloaded. However, two RCTs comparing PSV and PAV in a heterogeneous group of patients with acute respiratory failure, including COPD, failed to show any significant advantage of the latter over the former, although some patients tolerated PAV better than PSV [67,68]. More recently, Wysocki et al. [68] focused on decompensated COPD patients rather than on the usual heterogeneous group of patients with acute respiratory failure. They failed to observe any significant difference between non-invasive PAV and PSV for any of the physiological variables considered in the study. However, they found that all 12 patients declared feeling more comfortable with PAV than with PSV. At present, the data to support widespread regular use of PAV are scanty.

PSV with low levels of CPAP (e.g. 5 cm H_2O) remains the most popular and widely used mode of delivering NPPV. The individual setting of PSV remains easier than the setting of PAV, which requires the adjustment of two variables, flow and volume, while PSV requires only the setting of pressure. Probably, the additional time-consuming burden for clinicians [46] would need stronger evidence to make PAV preferable to PSV in a routine clinical environment, although repeated reports on greater patient comfort with PAV encourages further clinical studies.

In summary, NPPV can be delivered in different clinical settings:

1 *Medical ward* [61,62]: patients with moderate acidosis (pH < 7.36, > 7.30) and hypercapnia ($Paco_2 > 45$, < 60 mmHg).
2 *Intermediate or high-dependency respiratory unit* [69,70]: patients who present with moderate to severe acidosis (pH < 7.30), the facilities for rapid endotracheal intubation and institution of conventional MV are promptly available.
3 *Intensive care unit* [18]: patients with severe respiratory acidosis (pH < 7.25). In this particular setting, NPPV may be as effective as conventional MV in reversing acute respiratory failure resulting from COPD [63].

Weaning

It is well known that COPD patients belong to the category of difficult-to-wean patients and some may even become ventilator dependent [36]. In this context, it is particularly attractive to consider the use of NPPV to improve weaning and complete discontinuation of MV [71]. Three recent RCTs have shown that the application of NPPV to replace conventional MV after only 24–48 h of intubation resulted in shorter total duration of MV and length of ICU stay, less need for tracheostomy, lower incidence of complications and improved survival [72–74]. In particular, the most recent study by Ferrer *et al.* [74] documented the effectiveness of NPPV to govern the transition from MV to spontaneous breathing in patients with persistent conventional weaning failure. Clearly, many factors are involved in persistent weaning failure and NPPV should not be regarded as the panacea or ultimate solution; however, it provides an additional approach that might be valuable for certain patients [71]. Unfortunately, PAV has not been tested in weaning studies. Theoretically, the greater patient comfort with PAV should favour the transition from MV to spontaneous breathing. In fact, with PAV, it is the patient who adjusts the level and timing of assistance to his or her capacity to sustain the act of breathing completely.

Practical aspects

As in many other fields of respiratory medicine (e.g. asthma, COPD, pneumonia), practice guidelines for the application of NPPV in patients with respiratory failure are available [4,13,14]. There are several clinical choices that must be made when initiating NPPV. Practice guidelines have the intention of facilitating the procedure, particularly in less experienced centres. Key points are as follow:

1 Careful selection of patients:
  • to prevent waste of resources and discomfort in patients with milder exacerbations; and
  • to avoid undue delays in patients in need of intubation.

2 Choice of equipment, ventilator settings and monitoring facilities. When NPPV was first developed it was thought that more sophisticated ICU ventilators would guarantee better success than simpler, more user-friendly, so-called 'home' ventilators, until it was shown that this was not the case [62].

3 Choice of interface (e.g. facial or nasal mask, full face mask, helmet).

4 Motivation of the team, because in the first hours NPPV requires the same workload and degree of attention by clinicians as conventional invasive MV.

5 Some particular issues, such as the use of humidifiers in the ventilator circuits and valves to prevent rebreathing.

These aspects are extremely important to improve the comfort of the patient as much as possible not only to accept, but also to actively cooperate with the NPPV. The patient's collaboration is fundamental for the success of NPPV. In fact, NPPV is generally set 'at patient's comfort' in most studies, to assure a satisfactory patient–ventilator interaction. In this connection it should be noted that NPPV is an evolving technological process and that practice guidelines should also be interpreted as a dynamic tool.

Adverse events

Although some adverse events and complications were reported in patients receiving NPPV, these are much less severe and less common than the well-known complications of conventional MV, in particular barotrauma and infectious complications. Strictly speaking, it cannot be considered a complication or an adverse event, but an inaccurate selection of patients to whom to offer NPPV and an undue delay in intubation might expose the critically ill patient to a life-threatening situation. When applying NPPV, there should always be rapid access to intubation and an ICU, unless NPPV remains the only option (e.g. ICU bed not available). In this circumstance, clinicians should give adequate information to the patient or the next of kin.

The most common complications of NPPV are the following:
• facial skin erythema;
• nasal congestion;
• nasal bridge ulceration;
• sinus/ear pain;
• nasal/oral dryness;
• eye irritation;
• gastric irritationaspiration pneumonia; and
• poor control of secretions.

Despite the lower levels of intrathoracic pressure with NPPV than with conventional MV, cardiac output may be decreased in some patients either in stable [75] or in acute conditions [51]. Although the lower cardiac output could decrease Pao_2, it seems that the rise in alveolar ventilation is sufficient to defend and even increase Pao_2.

Nasal bridge ulcerations are frequent and not only create great discomfort for the patient, but also impair the continuation of NPPV. Lesions are caused by excessive pressure of the nasal/facial mask on the thin nasal skin. The best prevention is to reduce the local pressure of the mask on the nose by accepting some leaks. In fact, modern ventilators have very effective leak compensatory mechanisms such that it is no longer necessary to fix the mask with excessive pressure [47]. Alternatively, full face masks and helmets may be of help, depending on the patient's, and sometimes the clinician's comfort with the interface. It is worth stressing that a comfortable interface is a substantial component in the success of NPPV. The condition of the patient's nose should also be adequately considered [76].

Another unpleasant consequence of NPPV is that of gastric distension, which can impair the inspiratory movements of the patient, at least in part. A decrease in the inflation pressure might help to resolve or reduce the patient's discomfort.

The success of NPPV relies substantially on a good relationship between a cooperative patient and a dedicated caregiver team. First, the ventilator should be set to achieve the best balance between the clinical and physiological targets and the comfort of the patient. Secondly, patients on NPPV must be cared for as the critically ill patients they are. The tendency to consider NPPV as a second-class mode of ventilatory assistance for less severe patients in comparison with the dramatic picture of the intubated, often sedated and paralysed 'really' severely ill patients, should be abandoned. A great amount of effort should be made to obtain success with NPPV because the prevention of intubation substantially reduces endotracheal tube-related infectious complications and mortality.

Chronic home NPPV

This is still a matter of controversy and no definitive conclusions can be presented [77]. Chronic NPPV should not be systematically prescribed for COPD patients with chronic ventilatory failure, although it could produce some benefits in selected patients whose characteristics are not yet clearly defined [78]. A few patients with end-stage COPD undergo tracheostomy and become chronically ventilator dependent [36].

Conclusions

1 NPPV benefits patients with ventilatory failure and respiratory acidosis resulting from exacerbations of COPD. It should be noted that for these patients the evidence is stronger than for other groups of patients with respiratory failure of different aetiology [14,17]. Intubation, mortality and the length of ICU stay are with fewer complications than conventional MV [50].
2 NPPV should be offered early in the course of COPD decompensation, according to locally available monitoring facilities, skill of the team and characteristics of the patient [16].
3 NPPV does not seem to benefit patients with milder exacerbations [15]. On the other hand, patients with more severe acidosis (i.e. pH < 7.25) should be considered for intubation and conventional MV, unless particular local conditions and skills support the use of NPPV [61].
4 NPPV may be valuable for selected patients in the weaning process [71].
5 NPPV is a cost-effective treatment [39], although in the first hours of treatment the load on the clinical team is similar to conventional MV.
6 Careful selection of patients, the skill of the clinical team and availability of monitoring facilities as well as ICU admission are substantial components in the success of NPPV [14].

References

1 Stoller GK. Acute exacerbations of COPD. *N Engl J Med* 2002;**346**;988–94.
2 Barbera JA, Roca J, Ferrer A *et al.* Mechanisms of worsening gas exchange during acute exacerbations of chronic obstructive pulmonary disease. *Eur Respir J* 1997;**10**:1285–91.
3 Schmidt GA, Hall JB. Acute on chronic respiratory failure: assessment and management of patients with COPD in the emergency setting. *JAMA* 1989;**261**:3444–53.
4 BTS Guideline. Non-invasive ventilation in acute respiratory failure. British Thoracic Society Standards of Care Committee. *Thorax* 2002;**57**:192–211.
5 American Thoracic Society. International Consensus Conference in Intensive Care Medicine: Non-invasive positive pressure ventilation in acute respiratory failure. *Am J Respir Crit Care Med* 2001;**163**:283–91.
6 Global Initiative for Chronic Obstructive Lung Disease. *Executive Summary: Global Strategy for the Diagnosis, Management and Prevention of Chronic Obstructive Pulmonary Disease.* Bethesda, MD: National Heart, Lung and Blood Institute, National Institutes of Health, 2001; NIH Publication No 2701A: 1–30.
7 Pride NB, Milic-Emili J. Lung mechanics. In: Calverley P, Pride N, eds. *Chronic Obstructive Pulmonary Disease.* London: Chapman & Hall Medical, 1995: 135–60.
8 Laghi F, Tobin MJ. Disorders of the respiratory muscles. *Am J Respir Crit Care Med* 2003;**168**:10–48.
9 Rossi A, Polese G, Milic-Emili J. Monitoring respiratory mechanics in ventilator-dependent patients. In: Tobin MJ, ed. *Principles and Practice of Intensive Care Monitoring.* New York: McGraw-Hill, 1997: 553–96.
10 Rossi A, Ranieri VM. Positive end-expiratory pressure. In: Tobin MJ, ed. *Principles and Practice of Intensive Care Monitoring.* New York: McGraw-Hill, 1997: 259–303.
11 Rossi A, Polese G. Auto-positive end-expiratory pressure: its clinical significance. In: Roussos C, ed. *Mechanical Ventilation from Intensive Care to Home Care.* European Respiratory Monograph, vol 3, no 8, 1998: 400–29.
12 Tobin J, Brochard L, Rossi A. Assessment of respiratory muscle function in the intensive care unit. *Am J Respir Crit Care Med* 2002;**166**:610–23.
13 Gabrielli A, Caruso LJ, Layon AJ, Antonelli M. Yet another look at non-invasive positive-pressure ventilation. *Chest* 2003;**124**:428–31.
14 Liesching T, Kwok H, Hill NS. Acute applications of non-invasive positive pressure ventilation. *Chest* 2003;**124**:699–713.
15 Keenan SP, Sinuff T, Cook DJ, Hill NS. Which patients with

acute exacerbation of chronic obstructive pulmonary disease benefit from non-invasive positive-pressure ventilation? *Ann Intern Med* 2003;**138**:861–70.

16 Lightowler JV, Wedzicha JA, Elliot M *et al*. Non-invasive positive pressure ventilation to treat respiratory failure resulting from exacerbations of chronic obstructive pulmonary disease: Cochrane systematic review and meta-analysis. *BMJ* 2003; **326**:185–9.

17 Peter JV, Moran JL, Philips-Hughes, Warb D. Non-invasive ventilation in acute respiratory failure: a meta-analysis update. *Crit Care Med* 2002;**30**:555–62.

18 Brochard L, Mancebo J, Wysocki M *et al*. Non-invasive ventilation for acute exacerbations of chronic obstructive pulmonary disease. *N Engl J Med* 1995;**333**:817–22.

19 Anzueto A. Muscle dysfunction in the intensive care unit. *Clin Chest Med* 1999;**20**:435–52.

20 Rossi A, Polese G, Milic-Emili J. Mechanical ventilation in the passive patient. In: Derenne JP, Whitelaw WA, Similowski T, eds. *Acute Respiratory Failure in Chronic Obstructive Pulmonary Disease*. New York: Marcel Dekker, 1996: 709–46.

21 Nucci G, Mergoni M, Bricchi C *et al*. On-line monitoring of intrinsic PEEP in ventilator-dependent patients. *J Appl Physiol* 2000;**89**:985–95.

22 Volta CA, Marangoni E, Alvisi V *et al*. Respiratory mechanics by least squares fitting in mechanically ventilated patients: application on flow-limited COPD patients. *Intensive Care Med* 2002;**28**:48–52.

23 Rossi A, Polese G, Brandi G, Conti G. Intrinsic positive end-expiratory pressure (PEEPi). *Intensive Care Med* 1995;**21**: 522–36.

24 Rossi A, Polese G. As simple as possible, but not simpler. *Intensive Care Med* 2000;**26**:1591–4.

25 Pepe PE, Marini JJ. Occult positive end-expiratory pressure in mechanically ventilated patients with airflow obstruction: the auto-PEEP effect. *Am Rev Respir Dis* 1982;**126**:166–70.

26 Rossi A, Santos C, Roca J *et al*. Effects of positive end-expiratory pressure on pulmonary gas exchange in mechanically ventilated patients with chronic airflow obstruction. *Am J Respir Crit Care Med* 1994;**149**:1077–84.

27 Leatherman JW. Mechanical ventilation in obstructive lung disease. *Clin Chest Med* 1996;**17**:577–602.

28 Brochard L. Pressure support ventilation. In: Tobin MJ, ed. *Principles and Practice of Mechanical Ventilation*. New York: McGraw-Hill, 1994: 239–58.

29 Appendini L, Purro A, Patessio A *et al*. Partitioning of inspiratory muscle workload and pressure assistance in ventilator-dependent COPD patients. *Am J Respir Crit Care Med* 1996; **154**:1301–9.

30 Rossi A, Appendini L. Wasted efforts and dyssynchrony: the patient–ventilator battle is back? *Intensive Care Med* 1995; **21**:867–70.

31 Alberti A, Gallo F, Fongaro A, Valenti S, Rossi A. P 0.1 is a useful measurement for individual setting of pressure support ventilation. *Intensive Care Med* 1995;**21**:547–53.

32 Younes M. Proportional assist ventilation (PAV). In: Tobin MJ, ed. *Principles and Practice of Mechanical Ventilation*. New York: McGraw-Hill, 1994: 349–70.

33 Ambrosino N, Rossi A. Proportional assist ventilation (PAV): a significant advance or a futile struggle between logic and practice. *Thorax* 2002;**57**:272–6.

34 Appendini L, Patessio A, Zanaboni S *et al*. Physiologic effects of positive end-expiratory pressure mask pressure support during exacerbations of chronic obstructive pulmonary disease. *Am J Respir Crit Care Med* 1994;**149**:1069–76.

35 Appendini L, Purro A, Gudjonsdottir M *et al*. Physiologic response of ventilator-dependent patients with chronic obstructive pulmonary disease to proportional assist ventilation and continuous positive airway pressure. *Am J Respir Crit Care Med* 1999;**159**:1510–7.

36 Purro A, Appendini L, De Gaetano A *et al*. Physiologic determinants of ventilator dependance in long-term mechanically ventilated patients. *Am J Respir Crit Care Med* 2000;**161**: 1115–23.

37 Brochard L, Lessard LJ. Weaning from ventilatory support. *Clin Chest Med* 1996;**17**:475–89.

38 Muir JF, Ambrosino N, Simonds AK. *Non-invasive Mechanical Ventilation*. European Respiratory Monograph, vol 6, Monograph 16, 2001.

39 Plant PK, Owen JL, Parrott S, Elliot MW. Cost effectiveness of ward based non-invasive ventilation for acute exacerbatoins of chronic obstructive pulmonary disease: economic analysis of randomised controlled trial. *BMJ* 2003;**326**:1–5.

40 Keenan SP, Kernermann PD, Cook DJ *et al*. Effect of non-invasive positive pressure ventilation on mortality in patients admitted with acute respiratory failure: a meta-analysis. *Crit Care Med* 1997;**25**:1685–92.

41 Corrado A, Confalonieri M, Marchese S *et al*. Iron lung vs mask ventilation in the treatment of acute on chronic respiratory failure in COPD patients. *Chest* 2002;**121**:189–95.

42 Corrado A, Gorini M. Negative pressure ventilation: is there still a role? *Eur Respir J* 2002;**20**:187–97.

43 Gorini M, Corrado A, Aito S *et al*. Ventilatory and respiratory muscle responses to hypercapnia in patients with paraplegia. *Am J Respir Crit Care Med* 2000;**162**:203–8.

44 Gorini M, Villella G, Giananni R *et al*. Effect of assist negative pressure by microprocessor based iron lung on breathing effort. *Thorax* 2002;**57**:258–62.

45 Polese G, Vitacca M, Bianchi L, Rossi A, Ambrosino N. Nasal proportional assist ventilation unloads the inspiratory muscles of stable patients with hypercapnia due to COPD. *Eur Respir J* 2000;**16**:491–8.

46 Porta R, Appendini L, Vitacca M *et al*. Mask proportional assist vs pressure support ventilation in patients in clinically stable condition with chronic ventilatory failure. *Chest* 2002; **122**:479–88.

47 Serra A, Polese G, Braggion C, Rossi A. Non-invasive proportional assist and pressure support ventilation in patients with cystic fibrosis and chronic respiratory failure. *Thorax* 2002; **57**:50–4.

48 Confalonieri M, Gorini M, Ambrosino N, Mollica C, Corrado A. Respiratory intensive care units in Italy: a national census and prospective cohort study. *Thorax* 2001;**56**: 373–8.

49 Corrado A, Roussos C, Ambrosino N *et al*. Respiratory

intermediate care units: a European survey. *Eur Respir J* 2002;**20**:1343–50.

50 Elliott MV. Non-invasive ventilation in acute exacerbations of chronic obstructive pulmonary disease: a new gold standard? *Intensive Care Med* 2002;**28**:1691–4.

51 Diaz O, Iglesia R, Ferrer M *et al*. Effects of non-invasive ventilation on pulmonary gas exchange and hemodynamics during acute hypercapnic exacerbations of chronic obstructive pulmonary disease. *Am J Respir Crit Care Med* 1997;**156**: 1840–5.

52 Rossi A, Appendini L, Roca J. Physiological aspects of non-invasive positive pressure ventilation. *Eur Respir Mon* 2001; **16**:1–10.

53 Kress JP, O'Connor MF, Schmidt GA. Clinical examination reliably detects intrinsic positive end-expiratory pressure in critically ill, mechanically ventilated patients. *Am J Respir Crit Care Med* 1999;**159**:290–4.

54 Rossi A, Appendini L, Ranieri MV. PEEP and CPAP in severe airflow obstruction. In: Marini JJ, Slutsky AS, eds. *Physiological Basis of Ventilatory Support*. New York: Marcel Dekker, 1998: 847–72.

55 Meduri GU, Conoscenti CC, Menashe P *et al*. Non-invasive face mask ventilation in patients with acute respiratory failure. *Chest* 1989;**95**:865–70.

56 Meduri GU, Abou-Shala N, Fox RC *et al*. Non-invasive face mask mechanical ventilation in patients with acute hypercapnic respiratory failure. *Chest* 1991;**100**:445–54.

57 Benhamou D, Girault C, Faure C, Portier F, Muir JF. Nasal mask ventilation in acute respiratory failure: experience in elderly patients. *Chest* 1992;**102**:912–7.

58 Anton A, Guell R, Tarrega J, Sanchis J, Nash EF. Non-invasive ventilation. *Thorax* 2002;**57**:919–20.

59 Tarnow-Mordi WO, Hau C, Warden A, Shearer AJ. Hospital mortality in relation to staff workload: a 4-year study in an adult intensive-care unit. *Lancet* 2000;**356**:185–9.

60 Brochard L, Isabey D, Piquet J *et al*. Reversal of acute exacerbations of chronic obstructive lung disease by inspiratory assistance with a face mask. *N Engl J Med* 1990;**323**: 1523–30.

61 Bott J, Carroll TH. Randomized controlled trial of nasal ventilation in acute ventilatory failure due to chronic obstructive airways disease. *Lancet* 1993;**341**:1555–7.

62 Plant PK, Owen JL, Elliott MW. Early use of non-invasive ventilation for acute exacerbations of COPD in general respiratory wards: a multicenter randomised controlled trial. *Lancet* 2000;**355**:1931–5.

63 Conti G, Antonelli M, Navalesi P *et al*. Non-invasive vs conventional mechanical ventilation in patients with chronic obstructive pulmonary disease after failure of medical treatment in the ward: a randomized trial. *Intensive Care Med* 2002;**28**:1701–7.

64 Thys F, Roeseler J, Reynaert M, Liistro G, Rodenstein DO. Non-invasive ventilation for acute respiratory failure: a prospective randomised placebo-controlled study. *Eur Respir J* 2002;**20**:545–55.

65 Jolliet P, Tasseaux D, Roeseler J *et al*. Helium-oxygen versus air-oxygen non-invasive pressure support in decompensated chronic obstructive disease: a prospective, multicenter study. *Crit Care Med* 2003;**31**:878–84.

66 Vitacca M, Clini E, Pagani M *et al*. Physiologic effects of early administered mask proportional assist ventilation in patients with chronic obstructive pulmonary disease and acute respiratory failure. *Crit Care Med* 2000;**28**:1791–7.

67 Gay PC, Hess DR, Hill NS. Non-invasive proportional assist ventilation for acute respiratory insufficiency. *Am J Respir Crit Care Med* 2001;**164**:1606–11.

68 Wysocki M, Richard JC, Meshaka P. Non-invasive proportional assist ventilation compared with non-invasive pressure support ventilation in hypercapnic acute respiratory failure. *Crit Care Med* 2002;**30**:323–9.

69 Kramer N, Meyer TJ, Meharg J, Cece RD, Hill NS. Randomized, prospective trial of non-invasive positive pressure ventilation in acute respiratory failure. *Am J Respir Crit Care Med* 1995;**151**:1799–806.

70 Celikel T, Sungur M, Ceyahan B, Karakurt S. Comparison of non-invasive positive pressure ventilation with standard medical therapy in hypercapnic acute respiratory failure. *Chest* 1998;**114**:1636–42.

71 Navalesi P. Weaning and non-invasive ventilation. *Am J Respir Crit Care Med* 2003;**163**:5–6.

72 Nava S, Ambrosino N, Clini E *et al*. Non-invasive mechanical ventilation in the weaning of patients with respiratory failure due to chronic obstructive pulmonary disease: a randomized controlled trial. *Ann Intern Med* 1998;**128**:721–8.

73 Girault C, Daudenthun I, Chevron V *et al*. Non-invasive ventilation as a systematic extubation and weaning technique in acute-on-chronic respiratory failure: a prospective, randomized controlled study. *Am J Respir Crit Care Med* 1999;**160**: 86–92.

74 Ferrer M, Esquinas A, Arancibia F *et al*. Non-invasive ventilation during persistent weaning failure. *Am J Respir Crit Care Med* 2003;**168**:70–6.

75 Ambrosino N, Nava S, Torbicki A *et al*. Hemodynamic effects of pressure support and PEEP ventilation by nasal in patients with stable COPD. *Thorax* 1993;**48**:523–8.

76 Lorino AM, Lofaso F, Dahan E *et al*. Combined effects of a mechanical nasal dilator and a topical decongestant on nasal airflow resistance. *Chest* 1999;**115**:1514–8.

77 Clinical indications for non-invasive positive pressure ventilation in chronic respiratory failure due to restrictive lung disease, COPD, and nocturnal hypoventilation: a consensus conference report. *Chest* 1999;**116**: 521–34.

78 Clini E, Sturani C, Biaggi S *et al*. on behalf of Rehabilitation and Chronic Care Study Group AIPO. The Italian multicenter study of non-invasive nocturnal pressure support ventilation (NPSV) in COPD patients. *Eur Respir J* 2002;**20**:529–38.

CHAPTER 48

Comorbidity

Martin Sevenoaks and Robert A. Stockley

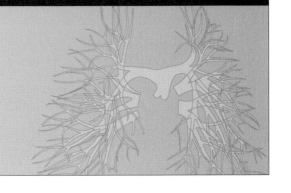

Associations have recently been noted between chronic obstructive pulmonary disease (COPD) and other systemic diseases including cardiovascular disease [1], diabetes mellitus [2], osteoporosis [3] and peptic ulcer disease [4]. These links persist even when common aetiologic factors such as cigarette smoking and steroid usage have been controlled for, raising the possibility of a common physiologic process.

The GOLD guidelines define chronic obstructive airways disease (COPD) as '. . . airflow limitation that is not fully reversible. This airflow limitation usually is both progressive and associated with an abnormal inflammatory response of the lungs to noxious particles or gases' [5].

The severity of this airflow obstruction, as assessed by the forced expiratory volume in 1 s (FEV_1), is a predictor of overall health status [6] and mortality from both respiratory disease [7] and all causes [8].

The inflammatory response to cigarette smoke is well known, yet it does not explain why only approximately 15% of smokers develop clinically important airflow obstruction. This suggests a genetic predisposition and elastase released from activated neutrophils has long been thought to be a significant mediator of the disease in this regard [9], especially in α_1-antitrypsin deficiency. The smoking mouse model has been used in recent studies to further elucidate the process and the mechanism appears to be driven by proinflammatory cytokines of which tumour necrosis factor α (TNF-α) seems key [10]. The role of these cytokines and the associated inflammation has been proposed to extend beyond the chest in COPD.

For reasons that are not clear, patients with COPD have higher baseline levels of several circulating inflammatory markers [11]. Whether the systemic inflammation is a primary or secondary phenomenon is also unknown at present. Specific subsets of patients with COPD have been identified and those with increased resting energy expenditure and decreased fat-free mass have more marked elevation of the acute phase C-reactive protein (CRP) and

lipopolysaccharide binding protein in the stable state [12]. Furthermore, patients with higher levels of systemic inflammation lack a response to nutritional supplementation [13].

It was initially thought that a low-grade systemic inflammation was produced by the 'overspill' of inflammatory mediators during the establishment of lung inflammation. However, the concentrations of soluble tumour necrosis factor receptor (sTNF-R) or interleukin 8 (IL-8) in sputum and plasma do not correlate, suggesting that a simple overspill explanation cannot be correct [14].

The central role of TNF-α in respect of this systemic inflammation is not only supported by animal models [10], but has also been implicated in the COPD phenotype with low body mass index [3]. Cytokine production by macrophages is increased by *in vitro* hypoxia [15] and systemic hypoxia may therefore explain the inverse correlation between arterial oxygen tension and circulating TNF-α and sTNF-R [15]. This would suggest that the systemic acute phase response is a secondary phenomenon.

Cardiovascular disease

The relative risk for future cardiovascular events has recently been shown to correlate to baseline CRP [16]. High levels of CRP and IL-6 have also been shown to significantly increase the risk of coronary heart disease in both men and women [17]. Individuals whose baseline value was greater than 3 mg/L had a relative risk of 1.79.

CRP is a type I acute phase protein and also part of the innate immune system. It is involved in the activation of the classic complement pathway by binding to bacteria. Complement binding can then occur, leading to bacterial phagocytosis or death. The protein has the ability to increase its concentration up to 1000-fold in the days following the start of an inflammatory process. It is known

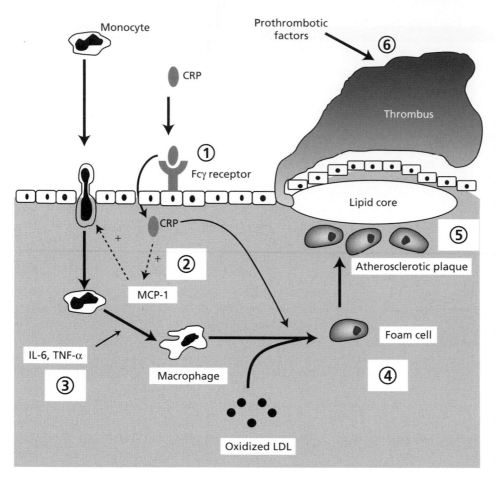

Figure 48.1 The inflammatory processes involved in atherosclerotic plaque formation. Endothelial cells bind CRP via the Fcγ receptor ①. It is then internalized and aids monocyte binding via the production of the chemokine MCP-1 ②. Activation continues leading to further cytokine release (including IL-6 and TNF-α) and differentiation of the monocytes into macrophages ③. CRP (in the presence of oxidized LDL) is also involved in the production of foam cells ④, which form the basis of an atherosclerotic plaque ⑤. Vascular occlusion can be amplified by increased thrombus formation ⑥. CRP, C-reactive protein; IL-6, interleukin 6; LDL, low density lipoprotein; MCP-1, monocyte chemotactic protein 1; TNF-α, tumour necrosis factor α.

to bind and cause lattice formation and precipitation leading to passive haemagglutination.

Macrophages have receptors for CRP, and CRP can increase cytokine production [18,19]. Recent work has pointed to the role of the Fcγ receptor in the actions of CRP [20], which may account for its effect on macrophages. During atherogenesis, CRP may deposit directly on to the arterial wall, assisting monocyte adherence through the production of the monocyte chemokine MCP-1. Production of other proinflammatory cytokines and differentiation of the monocytes into macrophages can occur with further activation. CRP can also facilitate foam cell production if oxidized low-density lipoproteins are present and foam cells are the building blocks of atherosclerotic plaques (Fig. 48.1).

Following a systemic respiratory tract infection, a well-recognized acute inflammatory response and increase in cytokine production occurs. The risk of having a myocardial infarction increases nearly fivefold and cerebrovascular event over threefold within the first 3 days of such an event [21]. Not only is the baseline CRP greater than 3 mg/L in almost half of COPD patients, but the rise during an acute exacerbation [22] is also associated with a rise in fibrinogen [23], which increases the prothrombotic risk.

These changes may explain the increased risk of vascular events and cardiovascular mortality in COPD, both in the stable state and particularly within a few months of hospital admission for an acute exacerbation [24]. These concepts have been related to those of the inflammatory mechanisms of insulin resistance [25].

Diabetes mellitus

Patients with COPD are nearly twice as likely to develop type 2 diabetes [26]. Indicators of inflammation in the absence of COPD can predict the development of diabetes and glucose disorders [2,27], and patients with type 2 diabetes mellitus are known to have increased circulating levels of TNF-α, IL-6 and CRP [28]. Because of these observations, the role of circulating cytokines in the pathogenesis of diabetes and insulin resistance has received increasing interest.

Numerous adipokines are secreted from adipose tissue, which markedly influence lipid and glucose/insulin metabolism. These include TNF-α and an adipose tissue-specific antagonist, the 'protective' adiponectin.

Nuclear factor-κB (NF-κB) is a transcription factor that is inactive when bound to its inhibitor but which can be activated by inflammatory cytokines including TNF-α [29]. Activation results in cytokine production, up-regulation of adhesion molecules and increased oxidative stress. These effects may provide a stimulating pathway that interferes with glucose metabolism and insulin sensitivity. Adiponectin antagonizes this pathway by reducing NF-κB activation [30].

Several clinical and experimental observations support the concept that inflammation, glucose intolerance and insulin resistance are intimately associated. This concept is summarized in Figure 48.2, which is derived from the proposal of Sonnenberg *et al.* [31]:

(a) In patients with weight gain and insulin resistance, TNF-α expression is increased [32]. This could represent a modulating effect because TNF-α stimulates lipolysis [33] but raised TNF-α levels are associated with hyperinsulinemia and insulin resistance [34].

(b) Obese patients have an increased acute phase response and associated insulin resistance [35].

(c) Reduced adiponectin levels, associated with insulin resistance and hyperinsulinemia [36] are seen in obese patients.

(d) In the obese insulin-resistant mouse, TNF-α inhibition improves insulin sensitivity [32].

Studies using thiazolidinediones have not only demonstrated decreased levels of inflammatory markers including TNF-α, soluble intercellular adhesion molecule 1 (ICAM-1), macrophage inflammatory protein 1 (MIP-1) and CRP, but also improved insulin action [37–39]. ICAM-1 is a member of the immunoglobulin superfamily and is involved in leukocyte recruitment and inflammation. MIP-1 is a proinflammatory cytokine of the CC subfamily and plays a key role in the induction and modulation of inflammatory responses. These results are consistent with a common inflammatory process or pathway linking COPD and type 2 diabetes [2] and are also in keeping with the theory that acute phase proteins have a predictive role in the development of type 2 diabetes.

Cachexia

Low body mass index (BMI), age and low arterial oxygen tension are known to be significant independent predictors of mortality in COPD [40]. Indeed, BMI is the first of the four variables used in the BODE index predicting the risk of death in COPD [41]. Loss of fat-free mass (FFM) is detrimental to respiratory and peripheral muscle function, exercise capacity and health status, and is an important supplementary prognostic parameter [42]. Both weight loss and loss of FFM are seen more commonly in emphysema and appear to be the result of a negative energy balance [43].

Patients can certainly become so breathless with severe COPD that maintaining an adequate oral intake becomes difficult. However, one physiologic response to starvation is a reduction in resting energy requirements [44]. In contrast, many COPD patients have been noted to have increased resting energy expenditure, associated with systemic inflammation [12,45]. In addition, cachectic patients exhibit preferential loss of FFM, enhanced protein degradation [46] and poor responsiveness to nutritional interventions [47,48]. Moreover, altered protein, lipid and carbohydrate metabolism is seen in cachexia and is thought to be related to systemic inflammation [48,49].

Muscle wasting in COPD therefore shows similarities to the cachexia seen in many other conditions including chronic heart failure, renal failure, cancer and acquired immunodeficiency syndrome. In these conditions, cachexia is not only associated with reduced survival [47,50–52], it is also related to poor functional status and health-related quality of life [53]. In all these conditions, circulating levels

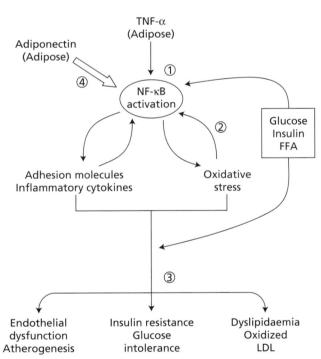

Figure 48.2 The roles of TNF-α, adiponectin and NF-κB in the metabolic syndrome. NF-κB activation is stimulated by TNF-α secreted from adipose tissue in conjunction with circulating glucose, FFA and insulin ①. The resulting increase in inflammatory cytokines, adhesion molecules and oxidative stress induce further activation of NF-κB ②. These pathways end with the clinical manifestations of the metabolic syndrome ③. Adiponectin directly antagonizes the effect on NF-κB ④. FFA, free fatty acid; LDL, low-density lipoprotein; NF-κB, nuclear factor κB; TNF-α, tumour necrosis factor α. Open arrows indicate inhibition; solid arrows stimulation.

of proinflammatory molecules including TNF-α, IL-1, IL-6, IL-8 and γ-interferon (INF-γ) are increased while levels of anabolic hormones including insulin-like growth factors and testosterone are decreased [53].

TNF-α has a key role in the muscle wasting and weight loss seen in COPD. It has several direct effects (anorexia, altered levels of circulating hormones and catabolic cytokines, and altered end organ sensitivities to them) that could promote muscle wasting [54]. These appear to be secondary to its main effect which is via the ubiquitin pathway.

This process is also mediated by NF-κB via the pathway previously described. In muscle cells, NF-κB can inhibit MyoD expression and thus interfere with skeletal muscle differentiation and repair. The MyoD gene plays a key role in the differentiation and determination of all skeletal muscle lineages. It can also increase ubiquitin/proteosome activity leading to increased protein loss (Fig. 48.3).

Reactive oxygen species (ROS) cause changes in TNF-α/NF-κB signalling, although their significance is not yet understood [55]. Inflammation and ROS do, however, appear to have a synergistic action on muscle breakdown [49] and because COPD is associated with increased oxidant stress [56] it is likely that this factor also has a role.

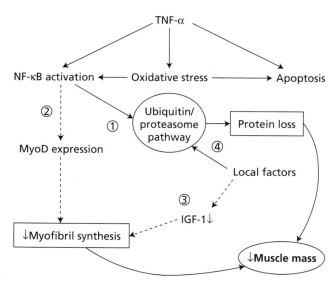

Figure 48.3 Pathogenic process implicated in muscle wasting in COPD. Circulating TNF-α binds to peripheral muscle cell receptors, thereby stimulating apoptosis and the production of ROS. The receptor binding also stimulates NF-κB activation, possibly enhanced by ROS. This results in protein loss, both directly through increased ubiquitin activity ①, or indirectly via decreased MyoD expression reducing myofibril synthesis ②. A decrease in muscle use will reduce IGF-1 production, decreasing myofibril synthesis ③, as well as increasing ubiquitin activity ④, amplifying protein loss. IGF, insulin-like growth factor; NF-κB, nuclear factor κB; ROS, reactive oxygen species; TNF-α, tumour necrosis factor α; TNFR, tumour necrosis factor receptor.

Smoking has been shown to have negative effects on markers of oxidative stress, as has COPD, particularly during exacerbations [57,58]. This increased oxidative stress may result in the inactivation of antiproteases, mucus hypersecretion, airspace epithelial damage, increased influx of neutrophils into lung tissue and the expression of pro-inflammatory mediators [59,60].

Inflammatory cell changes in peripheral blood have also been reported, including neutrophils and lymphocytes [61]. Patients with COPD have increased numbers of neutrophils in the lungs, increased activation of neutrophils in peripheral blood and an increase in circulating TNF-α and sTNF-R. It has been suggested that this indicates the importance of a TNF-α/neutrophil axis in maintaining the COPD phenotype [55,62].

Peptic ulcer disease

Patients with chronic bronchitis and emphysema are more likely to develop peptic ulceration [63]. Furthermore, studies in patients with gastric ulcers have found a decrease in FEV_1 and vital capacity in both smokers and non-smokers [4]. More recently, *Helicobacter* sero-positivity has been found to be increased in COPD patients (77.8 vs 54% in control subjects) [64]. In addition, genetic diversity between strains of *Helicobacter pylori* affects their virulence. Sero-positivity to the more proinflammatory phenotype expressing cytotoxin associated gene A (CagA) was present in almost twice as many patients as controls.

It has been hypothesized that the chronic activation of inflammatory mediators induced by *H. pylori* could amplify the development of COPD, although once again these associations may simply represent common factors such as smoking and socioeconomic status. The increased prevalence of the CagA-positive strain supports a common pathway hypothesis because this strain can stimulate the release of IL-1 and TNF-α [65], which may enhance the endothelial adhesion and migration of inflammatory cells into the lung. Whether such a process enhances the inflammatory response to cigarette smoke in the lungs is not known.

An alternative hypothesis is that overspill of *H. pylori* or its exotoxins may be inhaled into the lungs, leading to chronic airway inflammation and hence tissue damage. However, there is no direct evidence of this phenomenon in COPD.

Osteoporosis

Vertebral fractures are present in up to 50% of steroid naive males with COPD [66]. More recently, osteopaenia has been confirmed to be a feature of COPD and associated with an increase in circulating TNF-α [3]. Again, the association suggests a cause and effect.

High serum levels of IL-6 and TNF-α are related to postmenopausal osteoporosis [67]. Macrophages can differentiate into osteoclasts in the presence of marrow mesenchymal cells. Mesenchymal cells release the cytokine RANK ligand (RANKL), which is a member of the TNF-α superfamily. This process is enhanced by TNF-α and IL-1. TNF-α and IL-1 can also induce RANKL expression in marrow stromal cells and act synergistically with RANKL in osteoclastogenesis [68], although IL-6 can induce osteoclast formation independent of RANKL [69]. Other inflammatory conditions such as rheumatoid arthritis [70] and periodontal disease [71] produce RANKL via T-cell induction and it is therefore likely that a similar process occurs in COPD.

Proinflammatory cytokines may therefore have a central role in the osteoporosis associated with inflammatory disease. A close association between the proinflammatory processes and osteopaenia is supported by data confirming that that raloxifene was able to decrease TNF-α transcription and serum levels while increasing bone density [67].

Conclusions

In summary, several diseases are associated with similar inflammatory pathophysiology and coexist more commonly, suggesting that a common process is responsible for the clinical overlap. It is of course possible that the systemic inflammatory response to COPD precipitates disease processes at distant sites. Patients with COPD may present to other specialties because of the comorbidity and the diagnosis may be missed because of common symptoms in the overlapping conditions (e.g. dyspnoea as a result of cardiovascular disease or obesity). As effective anti-inflammatory therapy becomes available for COPD, it will be of importance not only to monitor the effect on the lungs but also any associated comorbidities. This may explain why inhaled corticosteroids in COPD are associated with decreased cardiovascular mortality [72] but clearly further studies are warranted to dissect this process in detail.

References

1 Sin DD, Man SF. Chronic obstructive pulmonary disease as a risk factor for cardiovascular morbidity and mortality. *Proc Am Thorac Soc* 2005;**2**:8–11.

2 Schmidt MI, Duncan BB, Sharrett AR *et al*. Markers of inflammation and prediction of diabetes mellitus in adults (Atherosclerosis Risk in Communities study): a cohort study. *Lancet* 1999;**353**:1649–52.

3 Bolton CE, Ionescu AA, Shiels KM *et al*. Associated loss of fat-free mass and bone mineral density in chronic obstructive pulmonary disease. *Am J Respir Crit Care Med* 2004;**170**:1286–93.

4 Kellow JE, Tao Z, Piper DW. Ventilatory function in chronic peptic ulcer: a controlled study of ventilatory function in patients with gastric and duodenal ulcer. *Gastroenterology* 1986;**91**:590–5.

5 Pauwels RA, Buist AS, Calverley PM, Jenkins CR, Hurd SS. Global strategy for the diagnosis, management, and prevention of chronic obstructive pulmonary disease. NHLBI/WHO Global Initiative for Chronic Obstructive Lung Disease (GOLD) Workshop summary. *Am J Respir Crit Care Med* 2001;**163**: 1256–76.

6 Ferrer M, Alonso J, Morera J *et al*. Chronic obstructive pulmonary disease stage and health-related quality of life. The Quality of Life of Chronic Obstructive Pulmonary Disease Study Group. *Ann Intern Med* 1997;**127**:1072–9.

7 Thomason MJ, Strachan DP. Which spirometric indices best predict subsequent death from chronic obstructive pulmonary disease? *Thorax* 2000;**55**:785–8.

8 Stavem K, Aaser E, Sandvik L *et al*. Lung function, smoking and mortality in a 26-year follow-up of healthy middle-aged males. *Eur Respir J* 2005;**25**:618–25.

9 Stockley RA. The neutrophil in acute and chronic lung disease. In: Bellingan G, Laurent G, eds. *Acute Lung Injury: From Inflammation to Repair*. Amsterdam: IOS Press, 2000: 69–84.

10 Churg A, Wang RD, Tai H *et al*. Tumor necrosis factor-alpha drives 70% of cigarette smoke-induced emphysema in the mouse. *Am J Respir Crit Care Med* 2004;**170**:492–8.

11 Gan WQ, Man SF, Senthilselvan A, Sin DD. Association between chronic obstructive pulmonary disease and systemic inflammation: a systematic review and a meta-analysis. *Thorax* 2004;**59**:574–80.

12 Schols AM, Buurman WA, Staal van den Brekel AJ, Dentener MA, Wouters EF. Evidence for a relation between metabolic derangements and increased levels of inflammatory mediators in a subgroup of patients with chronic obstructive pulmonary disease. *Thorax* 1996;**51**:819–24.

13 Creutzberg EC, Schols AM, Weling-Scheepers CA, Buurman WA, Wouters EF. Characterization of nonresponse to high caloric oral nutritional therapy in depleted patients with chronic obstructive pulmonary disease. *Am J Respir Crit Care Med* 2000;**161**(3 Pt 1):745–52.

14 Vernooy JH, Kucukaycan M, Jacobs JA *et al*. Local and systemic inflammation in patients with chronic obstructive pulmonary disease: soluble tumor necrosis factor receptors are increased in sputum. *Am J Respir Crit Care Med* 2002; **166**:1218–24.

15 Takabatake N, Nakamura H, Abe S *et al*. The relationship between chronic hypoxemia and activation of the tumor necrosis factor-alpha system in patients with chronic obstructive pulmonary disease. *Am J Respir Crit Care Med* 2000;**161** (4 Pt 1):1179–84.

16 Ridker PM, Rifai N, Rose L, Buring JE, Cook NR. Comparison of C-reactive protein and low-density lipoprotein cholesterol levels in the prediction of first cardiovascular events. *N Engl J Med* 2002;**347**:1557–65.

17 Pai JK, Pischon T, Ma J *et al*. Inflammatory markers and the risk of coronary heart disease in men and women. *N Engl J Med* 2004;**351**:2599–610.

18 Zahedi K, Tebo JM, Siripont J, Klimo GF, Mortensen RF.

Binding of human C-reactive protein to mouse macrophages is mediated by distinct receptors. *J Immunol* 1989;**142**:2384–92.

19 Ballou SP, Lozanski G. Induction of inflammatory cytokine release from cultured human monocytes by C-reactive protein. *Cytokine* 1992;**4**:361–8.

20 Devaraj S, Du Clos TW, Jialal I. Binding and internalization of C-reactive protein by Fcγ receptors on human aortic endothelial cells mediates biological effects. *Arterioscler Thromb Vasc Biol* 2005;**25**:1359–63.

21 Smeeth L, Thomas SL, Hall AJ *et al.* Risk of myocardial infarction and stroke after acute infection or vaccination. *N Engl J Med* 2004;**351**:2611–8.

22 Stockley RA, O'Brien C, Pye A, Hill SL. Relationship of sputum color to nature and outpatient management of acute exacerbations of COPD. *Chest* 2000;**117**:1638–45.

23 Wedzicha JA, Seemungal TA, MacCallum PK *et al.* Acute exacerbations of chronic obstructive pulmonary disease are accompanied by elevations of plasma fibrinogen and serum IL-6 levels. *Thromb Haemost* 2000;**84**:210–5.

24 Almagro P, Calbo E, Ochoa de Echaguen A *et al.* Mortality after hospitalization for COPD. *Chest* 2002;**121**:1441–8.

25 Fernandez-Real JM, Ricart W. Insulin resistance and chronic cardiovascular inflammatory syndrome. *Endocr Rev* 2003;**24**:278–301.

26 Rana JS, Mittleman MA, Sheikh J *et al.* Chronic obstructive pulmonary disease, asthma, and risk of type 2 diabetes in women. *Diabetes Care* 2004;**27**:2478–84.

27 Barzilay JI, Abraham L, Heckbert SR *et al.* The relation of markers of inflammation to the development of glucose disorders in the elderly: the Cardiovascular Health Study. *Diabetes* 2001;**50**:2384–9.

28 Pickup JC, Mattock MB, Chusney GD, Burt D. NIDDM as a disease of the innate immune system: association of acute-phase reactants and interleukin-6 with metabolic syndrome X. *Diabetologia* 1997;**40**:1286–92.

29 Reid MB, Li YP. Tumor necrosis factor-alpha and muscle wasting: a cellular perspective. *Respir Res* 2001;**2**:269–72.

30 Ouchi N, Kihara S, Arita Y *et al.* Adiponectin, an adipocyte-derived plasma protein, inhibits endothelial NF-κB signaling through a cAMP-dependent pathway. *Circulation* 2000;**102**:1296–301.

31 Sonnenberg GE, Krakower GR, Kissebah AH. A novel pathway to the manifestations of metabolic syndrome. *Obes Res* 2004;**12**:180–6.

32 Hotamisligil GS, Peraldi P, Budavari A *et al.* IRS-1-mediated inhibition of insulin receptor tyrosine kinase activity in TNF-alpha- and obesity-induced insulin resistance. *Science* 1996;**271**:665–8.

33 Porter MH, Cutchins A, Fine JB, Bai Y, DiGirolamo M. Effects of TNF-alpha on glucose metabolism and lipolysis in adipose tissue and isolated fat-cell preparations. *J Lab Clin Med* 2002;**139**:140–6.

34 Zinman B, Hanley AJ, Harris SB, Kwan J, Fantus IG. Circulating tumor necrosis factor-alpha concentrations in a native Canadian population with high rates of type 2 diabetes mellitus. *J Clin Endocrinol Metab* 1999;**84**:272–8.

35 Tamakoshi K, Yatsuya H, Kondo T *et al.* The metabolic syndrome is associated with elevated circulating C-reactive protein in healthy reference range, a systemic low-grade inflammatory state. *Int J Obes Relat Metab Disord* 2003;**27**:443–9.

36 Weyer C, Funahashi T, Tanaka S *et al.* Hypoadiponectinemia in obesity and type 2 diabetes: close association with insulin resistance and hyperinsulinemia. *J Clin Endocrinol Metab* 2001;**86**:1930–5.

37 Ghanim H, Garg R, Aljada A *et al.* Suppression of nuclear factor κB and stimulation of inhibitor κB by troglitazone: evidence for an anti-inflammatory effect and a potential antiatherosclerotic effect in the obese. *J Clin Endocrinol Metab* 2001;**86**:1306–12.

38 Haffner SM, Greenberg AS, Weston WM *et al.* Effect of rosiglitazone treatment on nontraditional markers of cardiovascular disease in patients with type 2 diabetes mellitus. *Circulation* 2002;**106**:679–84.

39 Ishibashi M, Egashira K, Hiasa K *et al.* Antiinflammatory and antiarteriosclerotic effects of pioglitazone. *Hypertension* 2002;**40**:687–93.

40 Schols AM, Slangen J, Volovics L, Wouters EF. Weight loss is a reversible factor in the prognosis of chronic obstructive pulmonary disease. *Am J Respir Crit Care Med* 1998;**157**(6 Pt 1):1791–7.

41 Celli BR, Cote CG, Marin JM *et al.* The body-mass index, airflow obstruction, dyspnea, and exercise capacity index in chronic obstructive pulmonary disease. *N Engl J Med* 2004;**350**:1005–12.

42 Dolan S, Varkey B. Prognostic factors in chronic obstructive pulmonary disease. *Curr Opin Pulm Med* 2005;**11**:149–52.

43 Engelen MP, Schols AM, Lamers RJ, Wouters EF. Different patterns of chronic tissue wasting among patients with chronic obstructive pulmonary disease. *Clin Nutr* 1999;**18**:275–80.

44 Schols AM. Nutritional and metabolic modulation in chronic obstructive pulmonary disease management. *Eur Respir J Suppl* 2003;**46**:81S–6S.

45 Baarends EM, Schols AM, Westerterp KR, Wouters EF. Total daily energy expenditure relative to resting energy expenditure in clinically stable patients with COPD. *Thorax* 1997;**52**:780–5.

46 Morrison WL, Gibson JN, Scrimgeour C, Rennie MJ. Muscle wasting in emphysema. *Clin Sci (Lond)* 1988;**75**:415–20.

47 Tisdale MJ. Biology of cachexia. *J Natl Cancer Inst* 1997;**89**:1763–73.

48 Schols AM, Soeters PB, Mostert R, Pluymers RJ, Wouters EF. Physiologic effects of nutritional support and anabolic steroids in patients with chronic obstructive pulmonary disease: a placebo-controlled randomized trial. *Am J Respir Crit Care Med* 1995;**152**(4 Pt 1):1268–74.

49 Debigare R, Cote CH, Maltais F. Peripheral muscle wasting in chronic obstructive pulmonary disease: clinical relevance and mechanisms. *Am J Respir Crit Care Med* 2001;**164**:1712–7.

50 Anker SD, Ponikowski P, Varney S *et al.* Wasting as independent risk factor for mortality in chronic heart failure. *Lancet* 1997;**349**:1050–3.

51 Kopple JD. Pathophysiology of protein-energy wasting in chronic renal failure. *J Nutr* 1999;**129**(1S Suppl):247S–51S.

52 Macallan DC. Wasting in HIV infection and AIDS. *J Nutr* 1999;**129**(1S Suppl):238S–42S.

53 Kotler DP. Cachexia. *Ann Intern Med* 2000;**133**:622–34.

54 Stewart CE, Newcomb PV, Holly JM. Multifaceted roles of TNF-alpha in myoblast destruction: a multitude of signal transduction pathways. *J Cell Physiol* 2004;**198**: 237–47.

55 Oudijk EJ, Lammers JW, Koenderman L. Systemic inflammation in chronic obstructive pulmonary disease. *Eur Respir J Suppl* 2003;**46**:5S–13S.

56 Barreiro E, de la Puente B, Minguella J *et al.* Oxidative stress and respiratory muscle dysfunction in severe chronic obstructive pulmonary disease. *Am J Respir Crit Care Med* 2005;**171**:1116–24.

57 Rahman I, Morrison D, Donaldson K, MacNee W. Systemic oxidative stress in asthma, COPD, and smokers. *Am J Respir Crit Care Med* 1996;**154**(4 Pt 1):1055–60.

58 Pratico D, Basili S, Vieri M *et al.* Chronic obstructive pulmonary disease is associated with an increase in urinary levels of isoprostane F2α-III, an index of oxidant stress. *Am J Respir Crit Care Med* 1998;**158**:1709–14.

59 Repine JE, Bast A, Lankhorst I. Oxidative stress in chronic obstructive pulmonary disease. Oxidative Stress Study Group. *Am J Respir Crit Care Med* 1997;**156**(2 Pt 1):341–57.

60 MacNee W, Rahman I. Is oxidative stress central to the pathogenesis of chronic obstructive pulmonary disease? *Trends Mol Med* 2001;**7**:55–62.

61 Sauleda J, Garcia-Palmer FJ, Gonzalez G, Palou A, Agusti AG. The activity of cytochrome oxidase is increased in circulating lymphocytes of patients with chronic obstructive pulmonary disease, asthma, and chronic arthritis. *Am J Respir Crit Care Med* 2000;**161**:32–5.

62 Lewis SA, Pavord ID, Stringer JR *et al.* The relation between peripheral blood leukocyte counts and respiratory symptoms, atopy, lung function, and airway responsiveness in adults. *Chest* 2001;**119**:105–14.

63 Arora OP, Kapoor CP, Sobti P. Study of gastroduodenal abnormalities in chronic bronchitis and emphysema. *Am J Gastroenterol* 1968;**50**:289–96.

64 Roussos A, Philippou N, Krietsepi V *et al.* Helicobacter pylori seroprevalence in patients with chronic obstructive pulmonary disease. *Respir Med* 2005;**99**:279–84.

65 Perri F, Clemente R, Festa V *et al.* Serum tumour necrosis factor-alpha is increased in patients with *Helicobacter pylori* infection and CagA antibodies. *Ital J Gastroenterol Hepatol* 1999;**31**:290–4.

66 McEvoy CE, Ensrud KE, Bender E *et al.* Association between corticosteroid use and vertebral fractures in older men with chronic obstructive pulmonary disease. *Am J Respir Crit Care Med* 1998;**157**(3 Pt 1):704–9.

67 Gianni W, Ricci A, Gazzaniga P *et al.* Raloxifene modulates interleukin-6 and tumor necrosis factor-alpha synthesis *in vivo*: results from a pilot clinical study. *J Clin Endocrinol Metab* 2004;**89**:6097–9.

68 Cenci S, Weitzmann MN, Roggia C *et al.* Estrogen deficiency induces bone loss by enhancing T-cell production of TNF-alpha. *J Clin Invest* 2000;**106**:1229–37.

69 Kudo O, Sabokbar A, Pocock A *et al.* Interleukin-6 and interleukin-11 support human osteoclast formation by a RANKL-independent mechanism. *Bone* 2003;**32**:1–7.

70 Kong YY, Feige U, Sarosi I *et al.* Activated T cells regulate bone loss and joint destruction in adjuvant arthritis through osteoprotegerin ligand. *Nature* 1999;**402**:304–9.

71 Teng YT, Nguyen H, Gao X *et al.* Functional human T-cell immunity and osteoprotegerin ligand control alveolar bone destruction in periodontal infection. *J Clin Invest* 2000;**106**: R59–67.

72 Sin DD, Man SF. Why are patients with chronic obstructive pulmonary disease at increased risk of cardiovascular diseases? The potential role of systemic inflammation in chronic obstructive pulmonary disease. *Circulation* 2003;**107**: 1514–9.

Current and future treatment

CHAPTER 49

Primary care

Daryl Freeman and David Price

Epidemiology

The facts and figures behind the disease processes collectively known as COPD are bleak. COPD is a progressive chronic condition and is already the third most common cause of death in the UK. By 2020 it is expected to be the third most common cause of death worldwide [1,2]. The most important cause of COPD in the developed world is cigarette smoking.

COPD is a major cause of morbidity and mortality. Approximately 6% of deaths in men and 4% in women are attributed to COPD [1]. There are approximately 30 000 deaths from COPD annually in the UK; approximately 5% of all deaths [3]. Of more concern, however, is the fact that COPD is the only common cause of death that is increasing [2].

Aetiology

COPD is an umbrella term encompassing chronic bronchitis and emphysema, and patients may have elements of both of these conditions. It is a chronic, slowly progressive disorder characterized predominantly by airways obstruction [4]. There is structural narrowing of the airways that is predominantly irreversible, with a combination of fibrosis, mucus hyperplasia and some alterations in vagal bronchomotor tone.

Agents (predominately cigarette smoke) causing COPD damage the airways and impair the defence and repair mechanisms within the respiratory system [5]. In addition, inflammation increases the thickness of the airway walls (an effect of smooth-muscle hyperplasia), which increases airways resistance throughout the lungs.

Diagnosis

Although a thorough history can give a reasonable indication of the diagnosis, spirometry is the gold standard [4,6].

A diagnosis of COPD is likely with a history of progressive symptoms: cough, dyspnoea, exacerbations and a smoking history of more than 20 pack-years in patients over the age of 40 years [4,6]. (One pack-year is the equivalent of smoking 20 cigarettes a day for 1 year.) The higher the number of pack-years, the greater the risk of COPD. The patients who are most likely to benefit from aggressive smoking cessation therapies are probably those with mild disease; however, these patients have relatively few symptoms at this stage and one of the challenges of caring for patients with COPD is identifying those with early disease. Many patients with COPD could be identified in primary care by targeting:

- smokers with symptoms (dyspnoea, cough, wheeze);
- patients on respiratory medication (particularly those with a positive smoking history); and
- patients who attend mainly in the winter months with symptoms or signs suggestive of a chest infection and a positive smoking history.

The late presentation of patients with COPD is a problem leading to underdiagnosis and under treatment [7]. A high index of suspicion is needed to identify patients earlier with COPD, and so management interventions, such as smoking cessation and drug therapies, can be instituted early. The presence of comorbid conditions is a frequent problem. In particular, other smoking-related illnesses such as heart failure and lung cancer, often coexist with COPD and often a generalist approach to 'the breathless patient' is needed at first.

Spirometry

A diagnosis of COPD depends on demonstrating an irreversible airway obstruction. Spirometry measures lung function and is the most reliable method for diagnosing COPD [8].

Spirometry measures the presence of airflow limitation. The two principal measurements are the forced expiratory volume in 1 s (FEV_1) and the forced vital capacity (FVC), which is the total volume of air that can be expelled from the lungs from maximum inhalation to maximum exhalation.

Table 49.1 Principles of interpreting spirometry.

1 Reduced $FEV_1 : FVC$ ratio (< 70%) demonstrates obstructive lung disease
2 Postbronchodilator FEV_1 < 80% predicted suggests COPD
3 A rise in FEV_1 of > 400 mL following an adequate dose of bronchodilator suggests a diagnosis of asthma
4 A normal $FEV_1 : FVC$ ratio with reduced FEV_1 indicates restriction and should prompt a referral to specialist care

FEV_1 forced expiratory volume in 1 s; FVC, forced vital capacity.

Airflow obstruction (and this may represent COPD or asthma) is suggested by a reduction in the $FEV_1 : FVC$ ratio to less than 70%; in addition, if the postbronchodilator FEV_1 is less than 80% predicted this signifies likely COPD.

Guidelines generally use FEV_1 as the method to assess severity. As far as assessing the severity of COPD is concerned, the NICE guidelines suggest that in addition to the lung function, other matters should be used to assess severity [9]. These include features such as breathlessness, body mass index (BMI), exacerbations, exercise limitation and presence/absence of cor pulmonale. Increasing severity of disease is associated with increasing morbidity and mortality (Table 49.1).

Smoking cessation

Smoking is the most preventable cause of premature death and disability in the developed world. One in four smokers will develop COPD, with the risk proportional to tobacco exposure [10]. Stopping smoking is the only intervention that has been shown to substantially slow the overall decline in lung function seen in COPD [11]. Brief smoking cessation advice given by GPs has been shown to be simple and effective [12]. The use of pharmacotherapy will further increase the cessation rates.

Nicotine replacement therapy

Nicotine replacement therapy (NRT) increases the chances of smoking cessation success [12] and over 80 research articles have shown a benefit. It gives smokers the opportunity to break their nicotine addiction by gradually reducing the amount of nicotine in the body. NRT is available as gum, patches, nasal sprays, inhalators and sublingual tablets.

Antidepressant therapy

Two drugs used to treat depression, bupropion SR (amfebuta-

mone) and nortriptyline have been used in smokers trying to quit. Bupropion SR is an antidepressant licenced in the USA, studies have shown that it may double cessation rates [13]. Side-effects include an increased risk of epileptiform seizure and the drug should be avoided in anyone at potential risk. Trials of nortriptyline also suggest that this can double cessation rates. Side-effects include nausea, sedation and urinary retention [14].

Treatment of stable COPD

The measurement of COPD severity is largely dependent on FEV_1 but a more holistic approach, including BMI, symptoms, exacerbations and exercise tolerance is more appropriate.

These same issues are important when assessing a response to a given treatment. As COPD is, by definition, a largely irreversible obstructive lung disease, it is unusual to see a significant spirometric response (and indeed an improvement of more than 400 mL with a trial of therapy would suggest a diagnosis of at least coexisting asthma). Other outcome measures are important in assessing response to treatment; these may include health status, symptoms, exacerbation rates and exercise tolerance (Table 49.2).

Drug therapy

Bronchodilators

Bronchodilators are the mainstay of pharmacological treatment for COPD. They are thought to reduce breathlessness by deflating the lung and reducing air trapping [16]. β_2-Agonists, anticholinergics and theophylline are effective bronchodilators; the choice of therapy depends on the individual's response to treatment.

Short-acting β_2-agonists (salbutamol, terbutaline)
Short-acting β_2-agonists (SABAs) help to relieve the symptoms of COPD. Studies have shown that SABAs can reduce dyspnoea, increase exercise capacity and improve health status [17].

Table 49.2 The Global COPD (GOLD) guidelines aims of treatment [15].

1 Prevention of disease progression
2 Relief of symptoms
3 Improved exercise tolerance
4 Improved health status
5 Prevention and treatment of complications
6 Prevention and treatment of exacerbations
7 Reduction of mortality from COPD
8 Prevention and reduction of side-effects of treatment

Long-acting β₂-agonists

The long-acting β_2-agonists (LABAs) formoterol and salmeterol work in a similar way to SABAs but have a longer duration of action, lasting up to 12 h. Studies have shown that in COPD, LABAs can increase FEV_1, increase exercise tolerance, improve health status, improve night-time symptoms and reduce exacerbation rates [3,18,19].

Short-acting anticholinergics (ipratropium bromide)

Ipratropium bromide is an effective bronchodilator, lasting approximately 4–6 h in patients with COPD; it may have additional beneficial effects such as drying of mucus. The drug is often used in combination with SABAs.

Long-acting anticholinergics (tiotropium)

Tiotropium is a once daily, anticholinergic bronchodilator. Early research suggests that it offers more sustained bronchodilatation, improves dyspnoea, health-related quality of life and exacerbations than four times daily treatment with ipratropium bromide [20,21].

Methylxanthines

Methylxanthines such as theophylline are usually reserved for more severe disease because of their narrow therapeutic range and the risk of side-effects. Multiple drug interactions (antibiotics, cigarette smoking), and the need for regular plasma drug levels, practically limit their use in everyday practice.

Inhaled corticosteroids (budesonide, fluticasone, beclometasone)

Inhaled corticosteroids (ICS) reduce exacerbations in COPD and may reduce decline in pulmonary function [22]. ICS should be used in patients with $FEV_1 \leq 50\%$ predicted who have frequent exacerbations (two or more in the preceding 12 months) [9].

Combination therapy for COPD

Combinations of drugs are now available: SABAs and anticholinergics, ICS and LABAs. Current guidelines support their use where the individual agents are recommended [23,24].

Mucolytics (carbocisteine, mecysteine hydrochloride)

Mucolytics may be considered in patients where production of sputum is a problem. The role of this class of therapy has recently been re-evaluated and recommended for consideration in patients with a chronic productive cough [9].

Antioxidants

N-acetylcysteine has been shown in recent studies to reduce exacerbations of COPD. However, its effectiveness has yet to be proven [25].

Oxygen therapy

As COPD progresses so does the likelihood of the patient developing pulmonary hypertension as a consequence of chronic hypoxaemia. Two studies have demonstrated the benefits of long-term oxygen therapy (LTOT) in this condition [26,27], and the last 20 years have seen a steady growth in the use of domiciliary LTOT.

There are clear criteria for referral for LTOT (see below) and assessment is usually carried out in secondary care.

Assessing the need for long-term oxygen therapy

LTOT assessment is indicated in patients who have a Pao$_2$ of less than 7.3 kPa when stable, or Pao$_2$ more than 7.3 kPa or less than 8.0 kPa when stable and one or more of the following: secondary polycythaemia, nocturnal hypoxaemia, oxygen saturation of less than 90% for more than 30% of the time, peripheral oedema, pulmonary hypertension.

Clearly, most primary care physicians do not have capillary gas analysers in their practice, so an empirical approach is required when deciding who may need referring for a LTOT assessment. The following are indications for referral for an LTOT assessment:

• Patients with oxygen saturation ≤ 92% on air
• Patients with signs of central cyanosis
• Patients with evidence of polycythaemia
• Patients with evidence of right heart failure (peripheral oedema, raised jugular venous pressure)
• Patients with severe COPD (FEV_1 less than 30% predicted)
• Some patients with moderate airflow obstruction may develop pulmonary hypertension, so assessment may be necessary in this group too.

LTOT is usually delivered via an oxygen concentrator backed up by a large cylinder and a smaller portable cylinder to maintain independence and mobility.

Exacerbations

COPD is not a stable disease and patients experience occasional worsening of symptoms or exacerbations. Most patients with an exacerbation can be managed at home by the primary health care team. Indications for consideration of admission include: ability to cope at home (requires assessment of support from carers), degree of breathlessness, presence of oedema and/or cyanosis, altered level of consciousness/increasing confusion or significant comorbidities (diabetes, heart failure, psychiatric problems).

Exacerbations also have an impact on health-care resources. For example, during the winter hospital admissions for COPD can increase the problem of bed shortages and lead to cancellation of surgical operations.

Treatment of exacerbations

Exacerbations are treated by increasing the dose of short-acting bronchodilator. This is usually a hand-held device, e.g. metered dose inhaler (MDI) + large volume spacer, but some patients may require a nebulizer (if the patient is hypercapnic this should be driven by air – not oxygen) [28]. In the absence of contraindications, a short course of oral steroids (prednisolone 30 mg/day for 10–14 days) should be used for patients with exacerbations – both at home and in those admitted to hospital [29]. The presence of green, purulent or excessive sputum suggests the presence of infection and so an antibiotic (choice of agent used should be based on advice from local prescribing/microbiology services) should be considered for 10–14 days.

Non-pharmacological treatments of COPD

Pulmonary rehabilitation

Pulmonary rehabilitation is a structured, individualized programme of exercise, physiotherapy and education for patients with COPD. It should be offered to all patients who are functionally disabled by their condition (in practice this means those with a Medical Research Council [MRC] score of 3 or above).

Pulmonary rehabilitation does not alter the course of the disease, or have any impact on mortality. However, it improves exercise capacity, physical functioning, quality of life and the patient's perception of control over their disease [30,31]. Pulmonary rehabilitation has been shown to reduce both symptoms and health-care utilization [32,33]. Indications for referral to pulmonary rehabilitation include:
• Confirmed diagnosis of COPD;
• MRC grade 3 or more (Table 49.3);
• Optimal medical treatment;
• No contraindications to exercise programme (e.g. unstable angina);

Table 49.3 The Medical Research Council (MRC) dyspnoea scale.

1 Not troubled by breathlessness unless on strenuous activity
2 Short of breath when hurrying or walking up a slight hill
3 Walks slower than contemporaries on the level because of breathlessness or has to stop for breath when walking at own pace
4 Stops to take a breath after approximately 100 m or a few minutes on the level
5 Too breathless to leave the house or breathless on dressing and undressing

• Able and willing to attend all the sessions;
• Neither use of LTOT nor being wheelchair bound due to COPD are contraindications and such patients should be encouraged to take part in rehabilitation programmes.

Anxiety and depression

Patients with COPD have many problems in addition to their medical condition; COPD strikes them at a time in their lives when they may have been looking forward to relative financial independence, retirement and more time to devote to their interests. It is not surprising therefore that studies of psychological factors in patients with COPD indicate that anxiety, depression and psychiatric symptoms are common [34].

Palliative care

Palliative care for patients with COPD is at best patchy. In the UK, 75% of people die from non-malignant causes and yet 95% of palliative care resources are used for malignant disease.

The care of the patient with terminal COPD is often up to the general practitioner or the patient's family or carers. Drugs used to treat breathlessness include benzodiazepines and opioids.

As with other aspects of managing the patients with COPD, a multidisciplinary approach to terminal care is vital and may involve the home nursing team, social services, charities such as the Marie Curie service and the primary health care team.

Structuring respiratory services in primary care

A regular structured review of asthma patients is shown to improve health outcomes regardless of whether the review is undertaken by a GP or a respiratory trained practice nurse [35].

Routine assessment

The most important part of assessing a patient with COPD is probably during the diagnosis, where the value of a thorough history followed by relevant examination and investigations cannot be overemphasized.

The routine follow-up of the patient with established COPD, however, takes a different course. Structured review is essential, and ideally will follow some form of protocol or computer template. Issues that should be covered during review appointments include those listed in Table 49.4. Clearly, not all these issues need reviewing at every

Table 49.4 Issues that could be covered during review appointments.

Routine review

Medication review
Understanding of drugs prescribed and when to take them
Inhaler technique assessment
Physician check for side-effects and possible interactions
    with other drugs or conditions (e.g. urinary retention
    with anticholinergics)
Use of rescue medications and use of self-management plans
    where used

Review of disease progression
Review of symptoms including objective score where
    possible (e.g. MRC dyspnoea score)
FEV_1 and *FVC* measurement
Review need for other investigations (e.g. CXR, FBC)
Review possibility of other diagnoses
Review need for referral for pulmonary rehabilitation
Review need for referral for long-term oxygen assessment
Exacerbations since last review

Immunization review
Has pneumococcal vaccination been given?
Does patient attend for annual influenza vaccination?

Smoking status
Encourage patient to give up smoking if still current smoker
Offer relevant smoking cessation therapies

Holistic review
Many patients become depressed as a consequence of
    the impact COPD has on their lives. Identification and
    treatment of depression should be part of the continuing
    review process
Many patients need encouragement to continue their
    everyday activities in spite of their breathlessness. Much of
    this is covered in a pulmonary rehabilitation programme,
    but advice about exercise, diet and walking should be part
    of the primary care structured review process
The patient's nutritional state should be reviewed at least
    annually. This should include recording their BMI and
    a review of their diet and appetite

BMI, body mass index; CXR, chest X-ray; FBC, full blood count; FEV_1, forced expiratory volume in 1 s; *FVC*, forced vital capacity; MRC, Medical Research Council.

appointment, but each clinic should have some form of formal annual review and a shorter intermediate review programme. Importantly, the patient, and not their disease, must remain at the centre of this process. It is often easier to discuss lung function and treatment options than to listen to the patient and try to understand their concerns, worries and expectations.

The future for the patient with COPD is looking brighter than it has for some time. There is increasing interest in the management of COPD, not only from the pharmaceutical industry, but governments are at last recognizing it as a priority area to target and treat (e.g. the British Department of Health has introduced a scheme whereby GPs are financially rewarded for diagnosing COPD). However, the management of patients with COPD remains a challenge and a responsibility for all in primary care.

Acknowledgements

The authors wish to acknowledge the administrative and secretarial support provided by Margaret Ross and Samantha Louw.

References

1 Crockett A. *Managing Chronic Obstructive Pulmonary Disease in Primary Care*. Oxford: Blackwell Science, 2000.
2 Barnes PJ. *Managing Chronic Obstructive Pulmonary Disease*. London: Science Press, 1999.
3 Halpin DMG. *COPD*. London: Harcourt Brace, 2001.
4 COPD Guidelines Group of the Standards of Care Committee of the BTS. BTS guidelines for the management of chronic obstructive pulmonary disease. *Thorax* 1997;**52**(Suppl 5): S1–28.
5 Turato G, Zuin R, Baroldo S *et al.* Lung pathology in chronic obstructive pulmonary disease. 2003. (Available at: http://www.copdprofessional.org/literature/big_articles/suetta.html. Accessed February, 2003.)
6 Godden DJ, Douglas A. *Clinicians Manual on Chronic Obstructive Pulmonary Disease*. London: Science Press, 2002.
7 Van Schayck CP, Chavannes NH. Detection of asthma and chronic obstructive pulmonary disease in primary care. *Eur Respir J* 2003;**21**(Suppl 39):16S–22S.
8 Celli BR. The importance of spirometry in COPD and asthma. *Chest* 2000;**117**:15S–19S.
9 National Institute for Clinical Excellence. *Chronic Obstructive Pulmonary Disease: Management of Chronic Obstructive Pulmonary Disease in Adults in Primary and Secondary Care*. NICE, February 2004.
10 Calverley PJ, Sondhi S. The burden of obstructive lung disease in the UK: COPD and asthma. *Thorax* 1998;**53**(Suppl 4):A83.
11 Fletcher C, Peto R. The natural history of chronic airflow obstruction. *BMJ* 1977;**1**:1645–8.
12 Silagy C, Stead LF. *Physician Advice for Smoking Cessation*. Oxford: Update Software, 2002.
13 Hughes JR, Stead LF, Lancaster T. *Antidepressants for Smoking Cessation* (Cochrane Review). Oxford: Update Software, 2002.
14 Wallstrom M, Nilsson F, Hirsch JM. A randomized, double-blind, placebo-controlled clinical evaluation of a nicotine sublingual tablet in smoking cessation. *Addiction* 2000;**95**: 1161–71.

15 Calverley PJ. *Chronic Obstructive Pulmonary Disease: The Key Facts*. London: British Lung Foundation, 1998.

16 Kanner RE. Early intervention in chronic obstructive pulmonary disease: a review of the Lung Health Study results. *Med Clin North Am* 1996;**80**:523–47.

17 Jones PW, Bosh TK. Quality of life changes in COPD patients treated with salmeterol. *Am J Crit Care Med* 2001;**163**:1087–92.

18 Appleton S, Smith B, Veale A, Bara A. Long-acting β_2-agonists for chronic obstructive pulmonary disease. *Cochrane Database Syst Rev* 2000;**3**:754–6.

19 Vincken W, van Noord JA, Bateman ED *et al.* Improved health outcomes in patients with COPD during 1 year's treatment with tiotropium. *Eur Respir J* 2002;**19**:209–16.

20 Casaburi R, Mahler DA, Jones PW *et al.* A long-term evaluation of once-daily inhaled tiotropioum in chronic obstructive pulmonary disease. *Eur Respir J* 2002;**19**:217–24.

21 Burge PS, Calverley PM, Jones PW *et al.* Randomised, double blind, placebo controlled study of fluticasone propionate in patients with moderate to severe chronic obstructive pulmonary disease: the Isolde trial. *BMJ* 2000;**320**:1279–303.

22 Szafranski W, Cukiev A, Ramirez A *et al.* Efficacy and safety of budesonide/formoterol in the management of chronic obstructive pulmonary disease. *Eur Respir J* 2003;**21**:74–81.

23 Calverley P, Pauwels R, Vestbo J *et al.* Trials of inhaled steroids and long-acting β_2-agonists group: combined salmeterol and fluticasone in the treatment of chronic obstructive pulmonary disease – a randomised controlled trial. *Lancet* 2003;**361**:449–56.

24 Gerrits CMJM, Herings RMC, Leufkens HGM, Lammers JJ. *N*-acetylcystein reduces the risk of re-hospitalisation among patients with chronic obstructive pulmonary disease. *Eur Respir J* 2003;**21**:795–8.

25 Medical Research Council Working Group. Long-term domiciliary oxygen therapy in chronic hypoxic cor pulmonale complicating chronic bronchitis emphysema. *Lancet* 1981;**1**:681–6.

26 Nocturnal Oxygen Therapy Trial Group. Continuous or nocturnal oxygen therapy in hypoxaemic chronic obstructive lung disease: a clinical trial. *Ann Intern Med* 1980;**93**:391–8.

27 Gravil JH, Al-Rawas OA, Cotton MM *et al.* Home treatment of exacerbations of chronic obstructive pulmonary disease by an acute respiratory assessment service. *Lancet* 1998; **351**:1853–5.

28 Thompson WH, Nielson CP, Carvalho EA. Controlled trials of oral prednisolone in outpatients with acute COPD exacerbation. *Am J Respir Crit Care Med* 1996;**1543**:407–12.

29 Folgering H, Dekhujzen R, Cox N, van Herwaarden C. The rationale of pulmonary rehabilitation. *Eur Respir Rev* 1991; **1**:490–7.

30 Hodgkin J, Conners G, Bell W. *Pulmonary Rehabilitation: Guidelines to Success*. Philadelphia: Lippincott, 1993.

31 Lacasse Y, Wong E, Guyatt GJ *et al.* Meta-analysis of respiratory rehabilitation in chronic obstructive pulmonary disease. *Lancet* 1996;**348**:1115–9.

32 Griffiths TL, Burr ML, Campbell IA *et al.* Results at 1 year of outpatient multidisciplinary pulmonary rehabilitation: a randomised controlled trial. *Lancet* 2000;**355**:362–8.

33 Karajgi BR, Rifkin A, Doddi S *et al.* The prevalence of anxiety disorders in patients with chronic obstructive pulmonary disease. *Am J Psychiatry* 1990;**147**:200–1.

34 Lindberg M, Ahlner J, Moller M *et al.* Asthma nurse practice: a resource-effective approach to asthma management. *Respir Med* 1999;**93**:584–8.

35 GOLD. Gold Initiative for Chronic Obstructive Lung Disease. 2005. (Available at: http://www.goldcopd.com/)

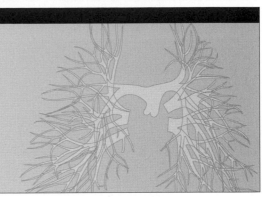

CHAPTER 50
Pulmonary rehabilitation

Richard ZuWallack

Definition and rationale

Individuals with chronic respiratory disease such as COPD often have distressing symptoms such as dyspnoea and fatigue, significant limitations in exercise capacity, limitations in activities of daily living and impaired quality of life. Pharmacological therapy, although a cornerstone in the symptomatic treatment of COPD [1], may fall short in the treatment in some or all of these important areas. Pulmonary rehabilitation complements this standard medical therapy.

Pulmonary rehabilitation was defined in the 1999 American Thoracic Society Statement on Pulmonary Rehabilitation as 'a multidisciplinary program of care for patients with chronic respiratory impairment that is individually tailored and designed to optimize physical and social performance and autonomy' [2]. It involves a spectrum of therapeutic strategies, including exercise training, self-management education, nutritional intervention, psychosocial support and promotion of long-term adherence, that are integrated into the lifelong management of the patient.

Pulmonary rehabilitation programmes involve patient assessment, exercise training, education, nutritional intervention and psychosocial support. In a broader sense, pulmonary rehabilitation includes a spectrum of intervention strategies integrated into the lifelong management of patients with chronic respiratory disease and involves a dynamic, active collaboration between the patient, family and health-care providers. These strategies address both the primary and the secondary impairments associated with respiratory disease.

This comprehensive interdisciplinary patient-centred intervention has virtually no effect on the lung function or respiratory physiological abnormalities of COPD, yet it frequently provides substantial and clinically meaningful benefits in important outcome areas such as dyspnoea, exercise performance, functional status and health-related quality of life. Pulmonary rehabilitation is effective because a considerable portion of the dyspnoea, fatigue, exercise limitation, and reductions in functional and health status is caused by the associated morbidity and comorbidity – which often responds to treatment. For example, while a patient with COPD has (by definition) some component of irreversible airflow limitation, he or she likely has deconditioning of the peripheral muscles resulting from inactivity [3], the use oral corticosteroids [4] or the presence of systemic inflammation associated with COPD [5]. These peripheral muscle effects contribute to the exertional dyspnoea and exercise limitation of COPD, and respond to exercise training. Table 50.1 lists some of the associated morbidities in COPD that potentially are responsive to comprehensive pulmonary rehabilitation.

Table 50.1 Some systemic effects of chronic respiratory disease that might be improved with pulmonary rehabilitation.

Nutritional depletion and body composition abnormalities, especially decreased muscle mass in the lower extremities [81,82]
Reduction in peripheral muscle oxidative enzymes [83]
Alterations in peripheral muscle fibre type [84]
Cardiovascular deconditioning
Poor pacing techniques
Maladaptive coping skills
Fear of dyspnoea-producing activities, depression
Adoption of a sedentary lifestyle with decreased participation in social events

Established positive outcomes from pulmonary rehabilitation

Pulmonary rehabilitation has proven to be a highly effective therapy that has positive outcomes in several areas

585

Table 50.2 The effectiveness of pulmonary rehabilitation in multiple outcome areas.

1 Reduced exertional dyspnoea and dyspnoea associated with daily activities [36,85,86–88]
2 Increased exercise endurance of the lower extremities [16,36,66,89]
3 Increased upper extremity endurance [22]
4 Increased peripheral muscle strength [29,30]
5 Increased strength and endurance of respiratory muscles [31,89]
6 Increased self-efficacy for walking [36]
7 Improved health status [9,22,66,88]
8 Reduced health-care utilization and increased cost effectiveness [66,90,91]

(Table 50.2). Note that this list of positive outcomes does not include improvement in pulmonary function or prolonged survival. Favourable changes in symptoms, exercise performance, activity levels and health-related quality of life occur despite this lack of change in pulmonary physiological measurements, such as the forced expiratory volume in 1 s (FEV_1). This reflects the effectiveness of pulmonary rehabilitation on the associated morbidity, such as peripheral muscle deconditioning. The lack of a demonstrated effect of pulmonary rehabilitation on survival probably reflects the limited number of controlled trials evaluating this variable (with relatively small numbers of randomized controlled trials), making them statistically underpowered to detect this change.

A brief history of pulmonary rehabilitation

Well before the advent of modern evidence-based medicine, clinicians had recognized that pulmonary rehabilitation or its components are effective in the treatment of chronic respiratory disease [6,7]. However, it has only been in the last decade or two that this intervention has become widely accepted as a state-of-the-art, scientifically proven therapy for chronic respiratory disease. This rise to prominence is underscored by the following:
1 Two major evidence-based reviews – by the combined efforts of the American College of Chest Physicians and the American Association of Cardiovascular and Pulmonary Rehabilitation [8], and a Cochrane meta-analysis [9] – that clearly demonstrate the effectiveness of pulmonary rehabilitation.
2 The National Emphysema Treatment Trial (NETT) [10], which considered pulmonary rehabilitation to be the gold standard of therapy with which lung volume reduction surgery was compared.

3 The endorsement of pulmonary rehabilitation by the Global Initiative for Obstructive Lung Disease (GOLD), by placing it in their treatment algorithm for individuals with moderate COPD [1].

A brief listing of several studies in the development of the science of pulmonary rehabilitation is given in Table 50.3. These studies, and others, have documented the effectiveness of pulmonary rehabilitation in multiple outcome areas. Current research has now shifted away from proving that pulmonary rehabilitation works, to determining ways to make it even more effective.

The process of pulmonary rehabilitation

Selection of candidates

Pulmonary rehabilitation is generally indicated for individuals with chronic respiratory disease who have persistent respiratory symptoms, decreased exercise capacity, a reduction in functional status (activity) or impairment in health-related quality of life despite standard medical therapy (Fig. 50.1), taken from the combined American Thoracic Society–European Respiratory Society statement, *Standards for the Diagnosis and Management of COPD* [11]. Note that a specific pulmonary physiological impairment, such a reduced FEV_1, is not in the above listing. Rather, the presence of distressing respiratory symptoms, activity limitation and reductions in participation dictate the need for pulmonary rehabilitation. Because the physiological measurements such as the FEV_1 correlate poorly with these important outcome areas [12], there are no specific pulmonary function inclusion criteria for pulmonary rehabilitation [13].

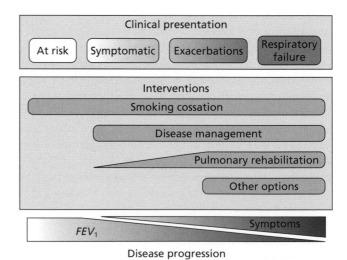

Figure 50.1 The combined American Thoracic Society–European Respiratory Society algorithm for management of stable COPD. FEV_1, forced expiratory volume in 1 s.

Table 50.3 Key studies in the development of the science of pulmonary rehabilitation.

Study	Design and findings
Casaburi et al. [16]	COPD patients randomized to exercise training involving higher work rates showed significantly more training effect than those with lower levels of exercise training. This was seen despite equalizing total amounts of work. This was the first randomized controlled study to show that physiological benefit from exercise training is possible in COPD patients and that this effect is dose-dependent
Reardon et al. [87]	COPD patients referred for pulmonary rehabilitation were randomized to either 6 weeks of pulmonary rehabilitation or standard therapy. Those who completed pulmonary rehabilitation had significant decreases in exertional dyspnoea and questionnaire-rated dyspnoea with activity. This is the first study to show that pulmonary rehabilitation improves dyspnoea. Subsequent studies by O'Donnell et al. [85] replicated these findings, and demonstrated that this improvement results from reduced ventilatory demand at iso-work levels
Goldstein et al. [88]	A randomized controlled trial demonstrating that pulmonary rehabilitation resulted in improvements in exercise performance and health-related quality of life
Ries et al. [36]	This was a large randomized trial comparing comprehensive pulmonary rehabilitation with education alone. It demonstrated the effectiveness of pulmonary rehabilitation in several areas, including exercise performance, dyspnoea, and self-efficacy for walking. It also showed that this improvement declined over time, reaching control group by 18–24 months
Maltais et al. [92]	This controlled study demonstrated the positive effect of exercise training on oxidative enzymes in peripheral muscles. This biochemical improvement correlated with reduced lactic acid production during exercise
Griffiths et al. [66]	This randomized trial of 200 Welsh patients with chronic respiratory disease compared outpatient pulmonary rehabilitation with standard medical therapy. In addition to showing an increase in exercise performance and health-related quality of life, pulmonary rehabilitation was shown for the first time in a prospective randomized trial to result in decreased health-care utilization: fewer days in the hospital and fewer primary care home visits. A subsequent study by this group demonstrated cost effectiveness of pulmonary rehabilitation [94]
Bourbeau et al. [91]	This large prospective randomized controlled trial compared a structured self-management programme with standard therapy for COPD. The intervention led to a reduction in health-care utilization and improved quality of life. This important study provides evidence that the self-management strategies employed in comprehensive pulmonary rehabilitation are effective, and provides support to the concept that pulmonary rehabilitation is more than just exercise training

Pulmonary rehabilitation should be considered as a potential intervention when standard (usually primarily pharmacological) therapy falls short in effectiveness. At present, patients with COPD comprise, by far, the largest group of respiratory disease referred for pulmonary rehabilitation. Patients referred to pulmonary rehabilitation often have one or more of the following symptoms, activity limitations or participation limitations [14]:

1 Severe dyspnoea and/or fatigue;

2 Decreased exercise capacity;

3 Limitations in functional status, especially higher order activities of daily living ;

4 Impaired health-related quality of life;

5 Interference with performance in employment;

6 Nutritional depletion and body composition abnormalities, such as COPD-associated cachexia;

7 Increased medical resource consumption resulting from chronic respiratory disease or its comorbidities.

Often, the referral to pulmonary rehabilitation had been reserved for advanced lung disease. While patients in this category will benefit from the intervention as long as they can participate in the programme [15], an earlier referral is preferable, because preventative strategies such as smoking cessation could be emphasized and different modes and higher intensities of exercise training could be utilized.

Exclusion criteria for pulmonary rehabilitation fall into two general areas:

1 An associated condition that might interfere with the rehabilitative process, such as disabling arthritis, or severe neurological, cognitive or psychiatric disease.

2 An associated condition that might place the participant at undue risk from exercise training, such as unstable angina. While a low level of motivation is a relative contraindication, it might improve with the intervention. Most – but by no means all – pulmonary rehabilitation programmes now allow active cigarette smokers to participate; in this circumstance the smoking cessation intervention becomes an important component of the process.

Components of a comprehensive pulmonary rehabilitation programme

Exercise training

Endurance and strength training of the upper and lower extremities is an essential component of comprehensive pulmonary rehabilitation [2]. Exercise performance in patients with COPD is frequently limited by peripheral muscle abnormalities and cardiovascular deconditioning, adding to the limitation imposed by airflow limitation, volume constraints related to hyperinflation and gas-exchange abnormalities. Thus, an early onset of anaerobic metabolism with lactic acidosis during low or moderate levels of exercise is observed [16]. The peripheral muscles in COPD are not frequently depleted [17], and also have alterations in fibre-type distribution and decreased metabolic capacity [18].

Exercise training for COPD is based on standard principles of intensity (higher levels of training produce more results), specificity (only those muscles trained show an effect) and reversibility (cessation of regular exercise training leads to loss of training effect) developed from studying normal individuals [19]. These principles have been applied to COPD patients, although there are relatively few studies that have evaluated exercise duration, exercise session duration or the number of sessions per week in this population. A dose-related increase in oxidative enzymes in the peripheral muscles accompanies the physiological adaptations to training [20], and this increase correlates with the concomitant reduction in lactic acid production [21]. A training effect is attainable in many patients with COPD, and higher levels of exercise results in a greater reduction in ventilation and lactate production at iso-work levels [16]. However, the greater increases in exercise performance from higher levels of training do not necessarily result in greater improvements in dyspnoea or health status [22].

Most pulmonary rehabilitation programmes emphasize endurance training of the lower extremities, often advocating sustained exercise for approximately 20–30 min, two to five times weekly. This type of training may utilize a stationary cycle ergometer, motorized treadmill, stair climbing or walking on a flat surface. Training is usually performed at levels at or greater than 50–60% of the estimated maximal workrate. For those unable to maintain this intensity for the recommended duration, interval training, consisting of 2–3 min of high intensity (60–80% maximal exercise capacity) training alternating with equal periods of rest, has similar results with less dyspnoea [23,24].

Few studies have evaluated the optimal duration of exercise training in pulmonary rehabilitation. One study showed that, on average, 7 weeks of pulmonary rehabilitation leads to a greater improvement in exercise performance than a 4-week intervention [25]. Recent COPD guidelines (GOLD) recommend (without providing much supportive evidence) at least 8 weeks of exercise training as part of a pulmonary rehabilitation programme. The total duration of exercise, although it is often standardized to the individual programme, should depend on the patient's underlying respiratory disease, the level of physical and cardiovascular conditioning, and continued demonstrated progress made during the exercise training sessions.

Although the strength of the upper extremity muscles is relatively preserved compared with that of the lower extremities in COPD [26,27], these muscles are very important in many activities of daily living and their use is associated with considerable dyspnoea. Both strength and endurance training of the upper extremities are probably important. Training is often through the use of arm ergometry, lifting free weights or dowels, or stretching elastic bands.

Because peripheral muscle weakness and/or depletion contribute to the exercise limitation in patients with COPD [28], strength training is a rational component of exercise training during pulmonary rehabilitation. Consequently, the current practice of pulmonary rehabilitation usually adds strength training to standard aerobic training. Weightlifting exercises training alone, involving the upper and lower extremities, increases muscle strength and endurance performance on a cycle ergometer [29]. This combination increases muscle strength and mass, but its additive effect on health status has not been proven [30].

Inspiratory muscle training increases strength and endurance of the inspiratory muscles in COPD [31,32]. However, the link between improvement in respiratory muscle strength or endurance and improvement in dyspnoea, exercise performance or health status is not firmly established [33]. Newer approaches that emphasize endurance training of the respiratory muscles at more precise percentages of maximal capacity are promising, although not yet proven.

Education and self-management strategies

Education is an integral component of virtually all comprehensive pulmonary rehabilitation programmes, providing information to the patient and the family on the respiratory disease and its treatment and helping to develop coping skills [34,35]. It encourages active participation in health care (collaborative self-management), thereby promoting adherence and self-management skills [36,37].

Education is usually provided both in both small group settings and on a one-to-one basis, tailored to the needs of the individual patient [38]. Advance directive discussions are an important component of pulmonary rehabilitation [39,40]. Generally, a number of standard topics are addressed in the educational sessions [41]; some of these are outlined in Table 50.4.

Table 50.4 Examples of educational topics in pulmonary rehabilitation [93].

Normal pulmonary anatomy and physiology of the lungs
Types of lung disease
Description and interpretation of medical tests
Breathing retraining techniques
Bronchial hygiene
Medications
Principles of exercise
Activities of daily living, energy conservation techniques
Nebulizers and supplemental oxygen
Symptom assessment and management
Proper nutrition
Psychosocial issues, dealing with fear of dyspnoea-producing
  activities
Ethical issues and advance directives
Recognizing and dealing with the acute exacerbation of
  COPD

Because education is integral to virtually all comprehensive pulmonary rehabilitation programmes, the effect of this specific component has not been adequately studied. However, a recent study evaluating self-management strategies (which are prominent in comprehensive pulmonary rehabilitation) applied to the home setting showed this form of therapy to be effective in improving health status and reducing utilization of medical resources.

Nutritional support

Decreased body weight and/or depletion in lean body mass are present in 20–35% of patients with stable COPD [42–44]. There are multiple causes of body composition abnormality in this disease, including increased energy expenditure [45,46] and systemic inflammation [5]. Nutritional depletion and body composition abnormalities are associated with decreased respiratory muscle strength [47,48], handgrip strength [49], exercise tolerance [47,50] and health related quality of life [51]. Additionally, depletion is a significant predictor of mortality in COPD, independent of FEV_1 [52]. Because of the associations with morbidity and mortality, nutritional intervention is a recommended component to comprehensive pulmonary rehabilitation.

Simple nutritional supplementation to underweight COPD patients has not met with much success, as evidenced by a recent meta-analysis that demonstrated only a 1.65-kg increase in weight following this type of intervention [53,54]. Because of these disappointing results with calorie supplementation alone, adjunctive treatment with anabolic steroids has been tried [54,55]. This has led to increases in weight, lean body mass, respiratory muscle strength, and arm and thigh muscle circumference [56]. To

date, however, improvements in these areas of impairment have not been convincingly demonstrated to be associated with improvements in exercise tolerance or functional status. Of considerably importance is a recent study that demonstrated that therapeutic increases in weight in COPD patients following therapy are related to increased long-term survival [57]. Further studies are needed to determine the optimal approach to treatment of nutritional depletion in chronic lung disease.

Psychosocial support

Psychosocial problems, including anxiety, depression, poor coping skills and decreased feelings of self-efficacy, contribute to the morbidity of COPD [58–60]. Intervention in these areas varies widely among pulmonary rehabilitation programmes, but often focuses on areas such as coping strategies [34,61] or stress management techniques such as muscle relaxation techniques, stress reduction and panic control. Improvement in anxiety may have the additional advantage of further decreasing dyspnoea [62]. Participation by family members or friends in pulmonary rehabilitation support groups is encouraged. Informal discussions of symptoms frequently present in chronic lung disease and common concerns may provide emotional support to patients and their families. Patients with substantial psychiatric disease as comorbidity should be referred for appropriate professional care outside of the programme.

There are only few studies evaluating the specific effect of pulmonary rehabilitation on psychological outcome [63], and none that evaluate this specific component of comprehensive rehabilitation on traditional outcomes. A randomized controlled trial of comprehensive pulmonary rehabilitation failed to demonstrate a significant effect on depression. However, in one non-controlled study of pulmonary rehabilitation, depression and anxiety levels decreased following 1 month of pulmonary rehabilitation. This programme included psychological counselling and stress management sessions twice weekly, in addition to standard exercise training and educational topics [64]. Of potential considerable importance, self-efficacy for walking increases with exercise training [36,65].

Promotion of long-term adherence

Pulmonary rehabilitation has impressive positive short-term effects in exercise capacity, dyspnoea relief and health-related quality of life. However, long-term effectiveness of this therapy tends to wane with time, with these outcomes often approaching those of the control group by 18–24 months [36,66–70]. Two factors are probably responsible for a substantial portion of this drop-off in effectiveness:
1 Exacerbations of underlying lung disease, leading to prolonged symptoms and a reassumption of a more sedentary lifestyle;

Table 50.5 Some examples of outcome assessment for pulmonary rehabilitation.

Exertional dyspnoea	Borg scale [94] or visual analogue scale [87] during exercise testing
Dyspnoea associated with daily activities	Modified Medical Research Council (MRC) questionnaire [95] Baseline and Transitional Dyspnoea Indexes (BDI/TDI) [96,97] San Diego Shortness of Breath Questionnaire [98]
Functional exercise capacity	Six-minute walk test, shuttle walk tests [99,100]
Laboratory measures of exercise performance	Cardiopulmonary exercise testing, treadmill endurance time [36,89]
Health-related quality of life	Chronic Respiratory Disease Questionnaire (CRQ) [101] St. George's Respiratory Questionnaire (SGRQ) [102] Medical Outcomes Study Short Form 36 (SF-36)
Functional performance	Pulmonary Functional Status Scale (PFSS) [103] Pulmonary Function Status and Dyspnoea Questionnaire (PFSDQ) [104]
Nutritional status/body composition	Body mass index, body composition using bioelectrical impedance or dual energy X-ray absorption (DEXA)
Psychological variables	Measurement of anxiety and depression using the Hospital Anxiety and Depression (HAD) questionnaire

2 A gradual decline in adherence with the post-rehabilitation exercise prescription [71].

Pulmonary rehabilitation programmes now routinely employ strategies to promote long-term adherence with post-rehabilitation instructions. One approach is to actively incorporate the principles of pulmonary rehabilitation such as regular exercise training into the home setting, with the hope that this would promote better long-term adherence with this intervention. This is supported indirectly by studies of home-based programmes, which suggest that gains achieved in this setting may be longer lasting than those of outpatient hospital-based programmes [72]. Additionally, giving a second course pulmonary rehabilitation following an exacerbation of COPD, emphasizing short periods of supervised exercise training to return the patient to baseline performance, might be a reasonable intervention in selected cases. Studies evaluating the potential effectiveness of these strategies or others are needed.

Outcome assessment

Outcome assessment is frequently performed in a pulmonary rehabilitation programme as part of a generalized audit of the effectiveness of the individual programme. Outcome areas often include dyspnoea, exercise performance and health-related quality of life. A listing of some commonly used outcome measures is listed in Table 50.5. Exercise tests such as the timed walk test, or the assessment of dyspnoea or health-related quality of life by a standardized questionnaire may also provide some information on the individual patient's response to therapy. Whether these outcome measures, which have been validated using groups of patients and are routinely used in overall pro-

gramme assessment, are useful in this individualized setting is not clear. Traditional one-on-one clinical assessment remains necessary for determining the effectiveness of pulmonary rehabilitation in the individual patient. Other outcome areas, such as health-care utilization or mortality, would require the collaboration of multiple pulmonary rehabilitation programmes to accrue the necessary number of patients for analysis.

Newer, adjunctive strategies in pulmonary rehabilitation

Non-invasive invasive positive pressure ventilation (NPPV), through its effect in helping unload the respiratory muscles, may improve breathlessness in COPD [73,74]. In one study of patients with more severe lung disease, this form of therapy allowed for exercise at a higher intensity, resulting in the achievement of a greater maximum exercise capacity [75]. Its role in pulmonary rehabilitation remains to be defined.

Some patients with very severe COPD, especially after a prolonged hospitalization for an exacerbation of the disease or those with substantial comorbidity, are unable to participate in exercise training effectively. One potential way around this is neuromuscular electrical stimulation using low-intensity electrical current to specific muscle groups, especially those of the lower limbs. To date, two trials have evaluated this modality of treatment [76,77]. In both studies, of respiratory patients with severe muscle weakness, transcutaneous neuromuscular electrical stimulation of lower limb muscles led to significant increases in skeletal muscle strength and exercise capacity.

Maximal bronchodilator therapy for COPD reduces the resistive work of breathing through increasing the calibre of airways and the elastic work of breathing through decreasing static and dynamic hyperinflation. These effects should allow for ventilatory-limited patients to exercise at higher training intensities. Because the training effect from exercise is dose-dependent, maximal bronchodilator therapy during pulmonary rehabilitation should improve outcome in this area. This was demonstrated in a recent study comparing exercise performance following pulmonary rehabilitation in a group of COPD patients who received the long-acting bronchodilator, tiotropium, with a group that received standard therapy with short-acting β-agonist bronchodilators. The group receiving the long-acting anticholingergic drug had a substantially greater improvement in treadmill endurance time.

Supplemental oxygen therapy reduces exertional dyspnoea in COPD, partly through reducing ventilatory drive [78,79]. A recent study demonstrated that supplemental oxygen therapy of non-hypoxaemic COPD patients allowed for exercise training at a higher intensity, resulting in greater gains from this therapy [80]. Whether this beneficial effect will continue when the patient finishes pulmonary rehabilitation and stops using supplemental oxygen remains to be determined.

References

1 Global Initiative for Chronic Obstructive Pulmonary Disease Workshop Report: www.goldcopd.com (accessed June 2005).

2 Pulmonary rehabilitation: Official statement of the American Thoracic Society. *Am J Respir Crit Care Med* 1999;**159**:1666–82.

3 Debigare R, Cote CH, Hould FS, LeBlanc P, Maltais F. *In vitro* and *in vivo* contractile properties of the vastus lateralis muscle in males with COPD. *Eur Respir J* 2003;**21**:273–8.

4 Decramer M, Lacquet LM, Fagard R, Rogiers P. Corticosteroids contribute to muscle weakness in chronic airflow obstruction. *Am J Respir Crit Care Med* 1994;**150**:11–6.

5 Schols AM, Buurman WA, Staal van den Brekel AJ, Dentener MA, Wouters EF. Evidence for a relation between metabolic derangements and increased levels of inflammatory mediators in a subgroup of patients with chronic obstructive pulmonary disease. *Thorax* 1996;**51**:819–24.

6 Barach AL. Breathing exercises in pulmonary emphysema and allied chronic respiratory disease. *Arch Phys Med Rehabil* 1955;**36**:379–90.

7 Haas A, Cardon H. Rehabilitation in chronic obstructive lung disease: a 5-year study of 252 male patients. *Med Clin North Am* 1969;**53**:593–606.

8 American College of Chest Physicians. American Association of Cardiovascular and Pulmonary Rehabilitation. Pulmonary rehabilitation: joint ACCP/AACVPR evidence-based guidelines. ACCP/AACVPR Pulmonary Rehabilitation Guidelines Panel. *Chest* 1997;**112**:1363–96.

9 Lacasse Y, Brosseau L, Milne S *et al.* Pulmonary rehabilitation for chronic obstructive pulmonary disease, *Cochrane Review*. The Cochrane Library, Issue 3, 2002. Oxford: Update Software.

10 National Emphysema Treatment Trial Research Group. A randomized trial comparing lung-volume-reduction surgery with medical therapy for severe emphysema. *N Engl J Med* 2003;**348**:2059–73.

11 http://www.thoracic.org/copd (Accessed 20 June 2005.)

12 Yusen RD. What outcomes should be measured in patients with COPD? *Chest* 2001;**119**:327–8.

13 AACVPR. *Guidelines for Pulmonary Rehabilitation Programs*, 3rd edn. Champaign, IL: Human Kinetics, 2004.

14 British Thoracic Society Standards of Care Subcommittee on Pulmonary Rehabilitation. BTS Statement. Pulmonary rehabilitation. *Thorax* 2001;**56**:827–34.

15 ZuWallack RL, PateK, Reardon JZ, Clark BA, Normandin EA. Predictors of improvement in the 12-minute walking distance following a six-week outpatient pulmonary rehabilitation program. *Chest* 1991;**99**:805–8.

16 Casaburi R, Patessio A, Ioli F *et al.* Reductions in exercise lactic acidosis and ventilation as a result of exercise training in patients with obstructive lung disease. *Am Rev Respir Dis* 1991;**143**:9–18.

17 Debigare R, Cote CH, Maltais F. Peripheral muscle wasting in chronic obstructive pulmonary disease: clinical relevance and mechanisms. *Am J Respir Crit Care Med* 2001;**64**:1712–7.

18 Maltais F, LeBlanc P, Whittom F *et al.* Oxidative enzyme activities of the vastus lateralis muscle and the functional status in patients with COPD. *Thorax* 2000;**55**:848–53.

19 American College of Sports Medicine. Position stand: the recommended quantity and quality of exercise for developing and maintaining cardiorespiratory and muscular fitness in healthy adults. *Med Sci Sports Exerc* 1990;**22**:265–74.

20 Maltais F, Leblanc P, Simard C *et al.* Skeletal muscle adaptation to endurance training in patients with chronic obstructive pulmonary disease. *Am J Respir Crit Care Med* 1996;**154**:442–7.

21 Sala E, Roca J, Marrades RM *et al.* Effects of endurance training on skeletal muscle bioenergetics in chronic obstructive pulmonary disease. *Am J Respir Crit Care Med* 1999;**159**: 1726–34.

22 Normandin EA, McCusker C, Connors ML *et al.* An evaluation of two approaches to exercise conditioning in pulmonary rehabilitation. *Chest* 2002;**121**:1085–91.

23 Coppoolse R, Schols AMWJ, Baarends EM *et al.* Interval versus continuous training in patients with severe COPD: a randomized clinical trial. *Eur Respir J* 1999;**14**:258–63.

24 Vogiatzis I, Nanas S, Roussos C. Interval training as an alternative modality to continuous exercise in patients with COPD. *Eur Respir J* 2002;**20**:12–19.

25 Green RH, Singh SJ, Williams J, Morgan MD. A randomised controlled trial of four weeks versus seven weeks of pulmonary rehabilitation in chronic obstructive pulmonary disease. *Thorax* 2001;**56**:143–5.

26 Bernard S, Leblanc P, Whittom F *et al.* Peripheral muscle weakness in patients with chronic obstructive pulmonary disease. *Am J Respir Crit Care Med* 1998;**158**:629–34.

27 Gosselink R, Troosters T, Decramer M. Peripheral muscle weakness contributes to exercise limitation in COPD. *Am J Respir Crit Care Med* 1996;**153**:976–80.

28 Hamilton N, Killian KJ, Summers E, Jones NL. Muscle strength, symptom intensity, and exercise capacity in patients with cardiorespiratory disorders. *Am J Respir Crit Care Med* 1995;**152**:2021–31.

29 Simpson K, Killian K, McCartney N, Stubbing DG, Jones NL. Randomised controlled trial of weightlifting exercise in patients with chronic airflow limitation. *Thorax* 1992;**47**:70–5.

30 Bernard S, Whittom F, LeBlanc P *et al.* Aerobic and strength training in patients with chronic obstructive pulmonary disease. *Am J Respir Crit Care Med* 1999;**159**:896–901.

31 Leith DE, Bradley M. Ventilatory muscle strength and endurance training. *J Appl Physiol* 1976;**41**:508–16.

32 Weiner P, Rasmi M, Berar-Yanay R *et al.* The cumulative effect of long-acting bronchodilators, exercise, and inspiratory muscle training in patients with advanced COPD. *Chest* 2000;**118**:672–8.

33 Lotters F, van Tol B, Kwakkel G, Gosselink R. Effects of controlled inspiratory muscle training in patients with COPD: a meta-analysis. *Eur Respir J* 2002;**20**:570–6.

34 Gilmartin ME. Patient and family education. *Clin Chest Med* 1986;**7**:619–27.

35 Neish CM, Hopp JW. The role of education in pulmonary rehabilitation. *J Cardiopulm Rehabil* 1988;**11**:439–41.

36 Ries AL, Kaplan RM, Limberg TM, Prewitt LM. Effects of pulmonary rehabilitation on physiologic and psychosocial outcomes in patients with chronic obstructive pulmonary disease. *Ann Intern Med* 1995;**122**:823–32.

37 Ries AL. Pulmonary rehabilitation. In: Tierney DF, ed. *Current Pulmonology*. St. Louis: Mosby, 1994: 441–67.

38 Hopp JW, Neish CM. Patient and family education. In: Hodgkin JE, Connors GL, Bell CW, eds. *Pulmonary Rehabilitation: Guidelines to Success*. Philadelphia: JB Lippincott, 1993: 72–85.

39 Heffner JE, Fahy B, Barbieri C. Advance directive education during pulmonary rehabilitation. *Chest* 1996;**109**:373–9.

40 Heffner JE, Fahy B, Hilling L, Barbieri C. Outcomes of advance directive education of pulmonary rehabilitation patients. *Am J Respir Crit Care Med* 1997;**155**:1055–9.

41 Patient Training. In: *AACVPR Guidelines for Pulmonary Rehabilitation Programs*. Champaign, IL: Human Kinetics, 1998.

42 Wilson DO, Rogers RM, Wright E, Anthonisen NR. Body weight in chronic obstructive pulmonary disease. *Am Rev Respir Dis* 1989;**139**:1435–8.

43 Gray-Donald K, Gibbons L, Shapiro SH, Macklem PT, Martin JG. Nutritional status and mortality in chronic obstructive pulmonary disease. *Am J Respir Crit Care Med* 1996;**153**: 961–6.

44 Wouters EFM, Schols AMWJ. Prevalence and pathophysiology of nutritional depletion in chronic obstructive pulmonary disease. *Respir Med* 1993;**87**(Suppl B):45–7.

45 Schols AM, Fredrix EW, Soeters PB, Westerterp KR, Wouters EF. Resting energy expenditure in patients with chronic obstructive pulmonary disease. *Am J Clin Nutr* 1991;**5**:983–7.

46 Goris AH, Vermeeren MA, Wouters EF, Schols AM, Westerterp KR. Energy balance in depleted ambulatory patients with chronic obstructive pulmonary disease: the effect of physical activity and oral nutritional supplementation. *Br J Nutr* 2003;**89**:725–31.

47 Schols AMWJ, Mostert R, Soeters PB, Wouters EFM. Body composition and exercise performance in patients with chronic obstructive pulmonary disease. *Thorax* 1991;**46**:695–9.

48 Nishimura Y, Tsutsumi M, Nakata H *et al.* Relationship between respiratory muscle strength and lean body mass in men with COPD. *Chest* 1995;**107**:1232–6.

49 Engelen MPKJ, Schols AMWJ, Baken WC, Wesseling GJ, Wouters EFM. Nutritional depletion in relation to respiratory and peripheral skeletal muscle function in out-patients with COPD. *Eur Respir J* 1994;**7**:1793–7.

50 Palange P, Forte S, Felli A *et al.* Nutritional status and exercise tolerance in patients with COPD. *Chest* 1995;**107**: 1206–12.

51 Shoup R, Dalsky G, Warner S *et al.* Body composition and health-related quality of life in patients with obstructive airways disease. *Eur Respir J* 1997;**10**:1576–80.

52 Marquis K, Debigare R, Lacasse Y *et al.* Midthigh muscle cross-sectional area is a better predictor of mortality than body mass index in patients with chronic obstructive pulmonary disease. *Am J Respir Crit Care Med* 2002;**166**:809–13.

53 Ferreira IM, Brooks D, Lacasse Y, Goldstein RS. Nutritional intervention in COPD: a systematic overview. *Chest* 2001; **119**:353–63.

54 Schols AM, Soeters PB, Mostert R, Pluymers RJ, Wouters EF. Physiologic effects of nutritional support and anabolic steroids in patients with chronic obstructive pulmonary disease: a placebo-controlled randomized trial. *Am J Respir Crit Care Med* 1995;**152**:1268–74.

55 Creutzberg EC, Wouters EF, Mostert R, Pluymers RJ, Schols AM. A role for anabolic steroids in the rehabilitation of patients with COPD? A double-blind, placebo-controlled, randomized trial. *Chest* 2003;**124**:1733–42.

56 Ferreira IM, Verreschi IT, Nery LE *et al.* The influence of 6 months of oral anabolic steroids on body mass and respiratory muscles in undernourished COPD patients. *Chest* 1998;**114**:19–28.

57 Schols AMWJ, Slangen J, Volovics L, Wouters EFM. Weight loss is a reversible factor in the prognosis of chronic obstructive pulmonary disease. *Am J Respir Crit Care Med* 1998; **157**:1791–7.

58 Agle DP, Baum GL. Psychosocial aspects of chronic obstructive pulmonary disease. *Med Clin North Am* 1977;**61**:749–58.

59 McSweeny AJ, Grant I, Heaton RK, Adams KM, Timms RM. Life quality of patients with chronic obstructive pulmonary disease. *Arch Intern Med* 1982;**142**:473–8.

60 Kaplan RM, Ries AL, Prewitt LM, Eakin E. Self-efficacy expectations predict survival for patients with chronic obstructive pulmonary disease. *Health Psychol* 1994;**13**: 366–8.

61 Neish CM, Hopp JW. The role of education in pulmonary rehabilitation. *J Cardiopulm Rehabil* 1988;**11**:439–41.

62 Renfroe KL. Effect of progressive relaxation on dyspnea and state anxiety in patients with chronic obstructive pulmonary disease. *Heart Lung* 1988;**17**:408–13.

63 Emery CF, Schein RL, Hauck ER, MacIntyre NR. Psychological and cognitive outcomes of a randomized trial of exercise among patients with chronic obstructive pulmonary disease. *Health Psychol* 1998;**17**:232–40.

64 Emery C, Leatherman NE, Burker EJ, MacIntyre NR. Psychological outcomes of a pulmonary rehabilitation program. *Chest* 1991;**100**:613–7.

65 Kaplan R, Atkins C. Specific efficacy expectations mediate exercise compliance in patients with COPD. *Health Psychol* 1984;**3**:223–42.

66 Griffiths TL, Burr ML, Campbell IA *et al*. Results at 1 year of outpatient multidisciplinary pulmonary rehabilitation: a randomised controlled trial. *Lancet* 2000;**355**:362–8.

67 Vale F, Reardon JZ, ZuWallack RL. The long-term benefits of outpatient pulmonary rehabilitation on exercise endurance and quality of life. *Chest* 1993;**103**:42–5.

68 Bestall JC, Paul EA, Garrod R *et al*. Longitudinal trends in exercise capacity and health status after pulmonary rehabilitation in patients with COPD. *Respir Med* 2003;**97**:173–80.

69 Guell R, Casan P, Belda J *et al*. Long-term effects of outpatient rehabilitation of COPD: a randomized trial. *Chest* 2000;**117**:976–83.

70 Troosters T, Gosselink R, Decramer M. Short- and long-term effects of outpatient rehabilitation in patients with chronic obstructive pulmonary disease: a randomized trial. *Am J Med* 2000;**109**:207–12.

71 Brooks D, Krip B, Mangovski-Alzamora S, Goldstein RS. The effect of postrehabilitation programmes among individuals with chronic obstructive pulmonary disease. *Eur Respir J* 2002;**20**:20–9.

72 Wijkstra PJ, Van der Mark TW, Kraan J *et al*. Long-term effects of home rehabilitation on physical performance in chronic obstructive pulmonary disease. *Am J Respir Crit Care Med* 1996;**153**:1234–41.

73 Keilty SEJ, Ponte J, Fleming TA, Moxham J. Effect of inspiratory pressure support on exercise tolerance and breathlessness in patients with severe stable chronic obstructive pulmonary disease. *Thorax* 1994;**49**:990–4.

74 Maltais F, Reissmann H, Gottfried SB. Pressure support reduces inspiratory effort and dyspnea during exercise in chronic airflow obstruction. *Am J Respir Crit Care Med* 1995;**151**:1027–33.

75 Hawkins P, Johnson LP, Nikoletou D *et al*. Proportional assist ventilation as an aid to exercise training in severe chronic obstructive pulmonary disease. *Thorax* 2002;**57**:853–9.

76 Zanotti E, Felicetti G, Maini M, Fracchia C. Peripheral muscle strength training in bed-bound patients with COPD receiving mechanical ventilation: effect of electrical stimulation. *Chest* 2003;**124**:292–6.

77 Bourjeily-Habr G, Rochester C, Palermo F, Snyder P, Mohsenin V. Randomised controlled trial of transcutaneous electrical muscle stimulation of the lower extremities in patients with chronic obstructive pulmonary disease. *Thorax* 2002;**57**:1045–9.

78 Garrod R, Paul EA, Wedzicha JA. Supplemental oxygen during pulmonary rehabilitation in patients with COPD with exercise hypoxaemia. *Thorax* 2000;**55**:539–43.

79 Somfay A, Porszasz J, Lee SM, Casaburi R. Dose–response effect of oxygen on hyperinflation and exercise endurance in non-hypoxaemic COPD patients. *Eur Respir J* 2001;**18**:77–84;169.

80 Emtner M, Porszasz J, Burns M, Somfay A, Casaburi R. Benefits of supplemental oxygen in exercise training in non-hypoxemic COPD patients. *Am J Respir Crit Care Med* 2003;**168**:1034–2.

81 Wouters EFM, Schols AMWJ. Prevalence and pathophysiology of nutritional depletion in chronic obstructive pulmonary disease. *Respir Med* 1993;**87**(Suppl B):45–7.

82 Schols AMWJ, Soeters PB, Dingemans MC *et al*. Prevalence and characteristics of nutritional depletion in patients with stable COPD eligible for pulmonary rehabilitation. *Am Rev Respir Dis* 1993;**147**:1151–6.

83 Maltais F, Simard AA, Simard C *et al*. Oxidative capacity of the skeletal muscle and lactic acid kinetics during exercise in normal subjects and in patients with COPD. *Am J Respir Crit Care Med* 1996;**153**:288–93.

84 Whittom F, Jobin J, Simard PM *et al*. Histochemical and morphological characteristics of the vastus lateralis muscle in COPD patients: comparison with normal subjects and effects of exercise training. *Med Sci Sports Exerc* 1998;**30**:1467–74.

85 O'Donnell DE, McGuire M, Samis L, Webb KA. The impact of exercise reconditioning on breathlessness in severe chronic airflow limitation. *Am J Respir Crit Care Med* 1995;**152**:2005–13.

86 Hernandez MTE, Rubio TM, Ruiz FO *et al*. Results of a home-based training program for patients with COPD. *Chest* 2000;**118**:106–14.

87 Reardon J, Awad E, Normandin E *et al*. The effect of comprehensive outpatient pulmonary rehabilitation on dyspnea. *Chest* 1994;**105**:1046–52.

88 Goldstein RS, Gort EH, Stubbing D, Avendano MA, Guyatt GH. Randomised controlled trial of respiratory rehabilitation. *Lancet* 1994;**344**:1394–7.

89 O'Donnell DE, McGuire M, Samis L, Webb KA. General exercise training improves ventilatory and peripheral muscle strength and endurance in chronic airflow limitation. *Am J Respir Crit Care Med* 1998;**157**:1489–97.

90 Griffiths TL, Phillips CJ, Davies S, Burr ML, Campbell IA. Cost effectiveness of an outpatient multidisciplinary pulmonary rehabilitation programme. *Thorax* 2001;**56**:779–84.

91 Bourbeau J, Julien M, Maltais F *et al*. Reduction in hospital utilization in patients with chronic obstructive pulmonary disease. *Arch Intern Med* 2003;**163**:585–91.

92 Maltais F, LeBlanc P, Simard C *et al*. Skeletal muscle adaptation to endurance training in patients with chronic obstructive pulmonary disease. *Am J Respir Crit Care Med* 1996;**154**:442–7.

93 American Association of Cardiovascular and Pulmonary Rehabilitation. *Guidelines for Pulmonary Rehabilitation Programs*, 2nd edn. Champaign, IL: Human Kinetics, 1998.

94 Borg GAV. Psychophysical bases of perceived exertion. *Med Sci Sports Exerc* 1982;**14**:377–81.

95 Bestall JC, Paul EA, Garrod R *et al*. Usefulness of the Medical

Research Council (MRC) dyspnoea scale as a measure of disability in patients with chronic obstructive pulmonary disease. *Thorax* 1999;**54**:581–6.

96 Mahler DA, Weinberg DH, Wells CK *et al*. The measurement of dyspnea: contents, interobserver agreement, and physiologic correlations of two new clinical indexes. *Chest* 1984;**85**:751–8.

97 Mahler DA, Tomlinson D, Olmstead EM, Tosteson ANA, O'Connor GT. Changes in dyspnea, health status, and lung function in chronic airway disease. *Am J Respir Crit Care Med* 1995;**151**:61–5.

98 Eakin EG, Resnikoff PM, Prewitt LM, Ries AL, Kaplan RM. Validation of a new dyspnea measure: the UCSD shortness of breath questionnaire. *Chest* 1998;**113**:619–24.

99 Singh SJ, Morgan MDL, Scott S, Walters D, Hardman AE. Development of a shuttle walking test of disability in patients with chronic airways obstruction. *Thorax* 1992;**47**:1019–24.

100 Revill SM, Morgan MDL, Singh SJ, Williams J, Hardman AE. The endurance shuttle walk: a new field test for the assessment of endurance capacity in chronic obstructive pulmonary disease. *Thorax* 1999;**54**:213–22.

101 Guyatt GH, Berman LB, Townsend M, Pugsley SO, Chambers LW. A measure of quality of life for clinical trials in chronic lung disease. *Thorax* 1987;**42**:773–8.

102 Jones PW, Quirk FH, Baveystock CM, Littlejohns P. A self-complete measure of health status for chronic airflow limitation. The St. George's Respiratory Questionnaire. *Am Rev Respir Dis* 1992;**145**:1321–7.

103 Weaver TE, Narsavage GL. Physiological and psychological variables related to functional status in chronic obstructive pulmonary disease. *Nurs Res* 1992;**41**:286–91.

105 Lareau SC, Meek PM, Roos PJ. Development and testing of the modified version of the Pulmonary Functional Status and Dyspnea Questionnaire (PFSDQ-M). *Heart Lung* 1998;**27**:159–68.

CHAPTER 51
Social support

Robin Stevenson

Many diseases have become prevalent because of society's failure to organize itself equitably. In the past, dysentery, cholera and tuberculosis were often related to overcrowding, poverty and poor sanitation. In the present time, the prevalence of COPD has a marked socioeconomic bias, greater than that described for ischaemic heart disease [1,2], and perhaps greater than for any other major disease [3]. The role of social support in COPD therefore merits close scrutiny.

By the 1950s, it was clear that there were marked social and occupational factors in the aetiology of COPD [1]. From 1930 until 1970, COPD mortality in men was consistently higher (approximately fourfold) in the UK than in the USA, whereas migrants from the UK to the USA had COPD mortality similar to the indigenous population [4]. From 1970 until the turn of the century, COPD mortality in UK men fell steadily, but a study using a general practice database showed that from the mid-1990s, prevalence rates for COPD in men appeared to plateau, whereas the prevalence in women rose and, by 1997, was similar in both men and women [5]. These epidemiological data indicate the importance of the socioeconomic component to COPD, which has been more obvious in the UK than in other Western countries and has resulted in COPD being described as the 'British Disease'. The precise nature of the environmental factors responsible for excess UK mortality has never been discovered. Current data since 1995 suggest that the UK is now behaving more like the USA [2].

Social bias in the prevalence of respiratory symptoms was described in 1979 [6]. Further studies from the 1970s onwards demonstrated a relationship between socioeconomic status and lung function impairment that was independent of smoking habits [7–12]. In a US study of male non-smokers, the difference in forced expiratory volume in 1 s (FEV_1) between the highest and lowest social classes was approximately 400 mL [13], and in the Copenhagen City Heart Study similar results were found after allowing for

smoking and were associated with a threefold increased risk of admission for COPD in the lowest socioeconomic group [14]. The risk factors related to social disadvantage include low birth weight, intrauterine effects of maternal smoking, frequency of childhood respiratory infections, poor housing conditions and atmospheric pollution [3,15]. Although these factors may contribute to the development of COPD, smoking is the main cause and the population-attributed risk of smoking for COPD in men is approximately 80%. In modern society, smoking is increasingly associated with low socioeconomic status. In the 1950s, cigarette smoking was common in all social strata, but since then it has become increasingly restricted to the lower end of the socioeconomic gradient. In 1998, 44% of men who lived in unskilled manual households smoked cigarettes, compared with 15% from professional households. Men from the unskilled manual group smoked on average 120 cigarettes per week whereas those from the professional group smoked an average of 91. In addition, men from manual socioeconomic groups were more likely to smoke high-tar cigarettes and to have started smoking at an earlier age [16]. Professional and managerial culture has become intolerant of smoking and this may account for the greater success of the higher social classes in quitting smoking [17].

If it is accepted that COPD increasingly occurs in the disadvantaged sections of society, then it would be expected that patients would be denied the benefits of the social support that is a feature of successful and prosperous population groups. There is evidence that social support is indeed less adequate in COPD than in other comparable diseases. A comparison between end-stage patients with cystic fibrosis and COPD who were awaiting lung transplantation showed that the cystic fibrosis patients had lower anxiety levels and better social support than the COPD patients [18]. In a series of health-related quality of life interviews of patients with COPD and non-small cell lung cancer, the latter group were less depressed and anxious and functioned better socially. Thirty per cent of the cancer patients had access to palliative care, whereas none of the COPD patients had similar support [19]. In a further comparative study of COPD and coronary artery disease, the COPD patients were less socially active, felt more disabled and had poorer health perception [20]. COPD patients on long-term oxygen therapy (LTOT) had poor quality of life which was partly attributed to social isolation [21], and hypoxaemic COPD patients showed impairment of quality of life associated with a reduction in social interaction and recreational pastimes [22]. In a study of patients with exacerbations of COPD, almost half lived alone and one-third still smoked [23]. In a small qualitative study, wives of patients with COPD complained of lack of support from friends, family and health-care providers [24].

There seems little doubt that patients and their carers feel that social support is lacking, but it is reasonable to ask if the provision of support is known to be beneficial and, not surprisingly, the evidence suggests that it is. A COPD questionnaire study found that high levels of social support correlated with reduced depression and anxiety [25] and quality of life has been shown to be related to family bonds, local neighbourliness and freedom from fear [26]. Patients with COPD who were dissatisfied with their level of social support or who felt isolated were less likely to adhere to a pulmonary rehabilitation programme [27]. From a literature search on rehabilitation between 1966 and 1996, an analysis of 22 randomized controlled trials (RCTs) showed that the inclusion of psychosocial support in the rehabilitation programme promoted compliance with the exercise regimen and improved quality of life [28]. A meta-analysis of 65 studies showed that rehabilitation plus a variety of psychosocial and behavioural interventions improved well-being, functional status and breathlessness [29]. In a population study, a correlation was found between social stress and COPD mortality [30], and early relapse after exacerbations of COPD has been shown to be more likely in widowed, separated or divorced patients [31].

The social environment is therefore not only instrumental in causing COPD, but also fails to provide support to the patients who contract the disease. If we accept the premise that society itself is largely responsible for creating the conditions under which COPD develops, then society should accept responsibility for the provision of appropriate support. Unfortunately, the criteria by which support can be considered appropriate are poorly defined. Cigarette smoking is the main risk factor for COPD and it would seem obvious that social support should be targeted primarily at smoking abstinence and cessation. Tobacco addicts have never received the degree of social support that has been available to alcohol or opiate addicts, perhaps because their addiction does not represent a threat to the civil order and does make a major contribution to government tax income.

There is little evidence that centrally funded social or behavioural interventions influence the use of addictive drugs such as tobacco, alcohol or opiates by socially deprived groups. Equally, the reduction in smoking in the more affluent classes probably owes more to peer pressure and the smoking behaviour of spouses and partners [17] than to health warnings on cigarette packets or to government-sponsored television campaigns. It may therefore be more profitable for society to support smoking cessation in individuals who are known to be at risk of COPD.

While it is true that quitting smoking benefits most smokers, the main effect on mortality relates to cardiovascular disease [32]. In patients with established COPD, mortality from respiratory disease may not be affected by smoking cessation and the benefit in terms of aborting the progress of COPD may be restricted to individuals with measurable impairment of lung function who are relatively asymptomatic [33]. There is good evidence that smoking cessation in patients with mild COPD reduces the rate of decline of FEV_1 to that of never-smokers [34], but the effect of quitting in patients with severe disease is not known.

Smokers with mild impairment of lung function will not easily be identified by GPs and many regions in the UK are now embarking on spirometry screening programmes organized by public health departments. Smoking cessation is more likely to be successful if an individual, recently apprised of his or her impaired spirometry, believes that he or she will benefit, rather than may benefit from smoking cessation. In the UK, nicotine replacement therapy and buproprion SR (amfebutamone) are now available on prescription but a community-based infrastructure is still needed to supply advice and support [35]. The continuation of spirometry screening will only be justified if at-risk people are recruited to a successful smoking cessation programme.

The priority for social support may be in relation to smoking cessation aimed at those with subclinical or mild disease, but it is clear that patients with established COPD not only lack support, but also would benefit if it were available. Low socioeconomic status is associated with weak family bonds, urban ghetto culture and juvenile street crime. Patients disabled by COPD are often afraid to leave their homes and become socially isolated. Some of these patients find support from the Internet. There are more than 6000 COPD support websites and almost 2000 COPD chat rooms in the UK. The British Lung Foundation created the Breathe Easy Club in 1991 and 120 Breathe Easy groups have been established in England, Scotland and Wales since 1992. Members of the club receive a quarterly magazine and are encouraged to meet together and to join the Penpals scheme. Breathe Easy also provides a banner under which patients with COPD can lobby for social support (Fig. 51.1).

COPD is a disease of inexorably worsening lung function

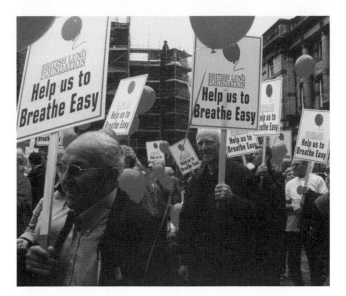

Figure 51.1 Breathe Easy Club members petitioning for liquid oxygen.

causing increasing disability. The majority of patients suffer from exacerbations which may occur as infrequently as once a year, but many will have three or more exacerbations annually. When assessed by the St. George's Respiratory Questionnaire, patients with frequent exacerbations have a poorer quality of life than those with less frequent exacerbations [36]. Exacerbations that require hospital admission may only affect a small proportion of the COPD population (less than 2% in one study) but the cost is disproportionate [37]. Hospital admissions are said to account for 35% of the annual health-care costs of COPD [38]. It is therefore understandable that many therapeutic interventions are designed to reduce exacerbation frequency or to minimize the length of hospital stay.

There have been various studies of domiciliary support by nurses and physiotherapists who have made regular home visits to stable COPD patients to provide support, education and monitoring of symptoms and treatment. Three RCTs have shown no benefit in exacerbation frequency or hospital admission [39–41]. However, three uncontrolled studies reported reductions in hospital admissions and emergency room attendance as a result of regular home visits by nurses or respiratory therapists [42–44]. In a Spanish RCT of COPD patients on LTOT, the intervention group had regular telephone calls and home visits with additional home or hospital visits on demand. The intervention group had fewer than one-third of the emergency department visits and slightly more than one-third of the hospital admissions of the control group in the follow-up period of 1 year, but did require many home and hospital visits [45]. This study may have shown a positive result because the patients were more severely ill than those in the other RCTs and therefore the effect of an intervention was more likely to be clinically evident. The authors felt that it was important that the same team was responsible for both hospital and home care.

The interventions above were described as hospital-based home care programmes, but similar initiatives are categorized as disease-specific self-management interventions. In a recent Canadian RCT of patients with advanced COPD who had at least one hospital admission for exacerbation in the previous year, the intervention group were assigned to a comprehensive education programme over a 2-month period with monthly telephone follow-up. Hospital admissions for COPD exacerbations were reduced by 40% in the intervention group compared with the usual care group and health status in the intervention group was also improved. Although admissions for exacerbations were reduced in the intervention group, the numbers of exacerbations in the two groups were not significantly different. The authors felt unable to separate the effect of education from the effect of direct support and counselling [46]. In other studies on less severely unwell patients, which have concentrated on self-management education without continuing support, inconclusive results on health-related quality of life have been observed [47].

The results of two studies from Spain and Canada [45,46] are important and need to be confirmed. However, they suggest that there are reasonable grounds for believing that continuing domiciliary support for patients with advanced stable COPD is cost-beneficial in reducing hospital admissions and may allow patients to cope with their disease more effectively.

In recent years, other interventions have received great attention because they are alleged to reduce exacerbation frequency. Several of the trials of inhaled steroids in stable COPD used exacerbation rate as a primary or secondary outcome measure. ISOLDE demonstrated a significant reduction of approximately 25% in exacerbation frequency [48]. The long-acting bronchodilator salmeterol reduced the time to first exacerbation [49] and two further large studies, comparing tiotropium with placebo [50] and ipratropium [51] have demonstrated a reduction in exacerbation rate. There are several observational studies that suggest that pulmonary rehabilitation reduces the frequency of COPD exacerbations [52–55]. An RCT showed that outpatient rehabilitation reduced the frequency of exacerbations but not the number of hospitalizations over a 2-year period [56].

Inhaled steroids, long-acting bronchodilators and pulmonary rehabilitation may therefore reduce exacerbation frequency, but domiciliary support may reduce hospitalization without necessarily affecting exacerbation frequency. These different forms of intervention may be complementary and domiciliary support may be just as important as, if

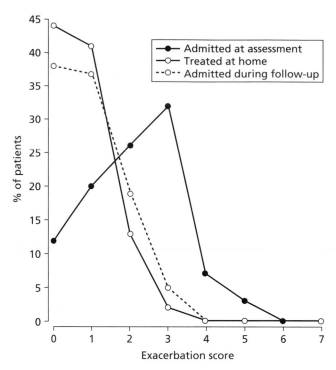

Figure 51.2 Exacerbation scores.

[59,63] and others identifying patients in emergency departments with the intention of preventing admission altogether [60,61]. Of the various approaches, the early supported discharge model is the simplest and most efficient. It targets patients who are using hospital resources and is economical of nurses' time because they do not need to be immediately available for prompt patient assessment in the emergency department. It also increases eligibility because improvement in FEV_1 is maximal in the first 24 h in hospital [65]. In a postal survey of UK hospitals in 2001, 28% of respondents offered a hospital at home service, most of which were run as early discharge schemes with only a minority relying solely on GP or emergency department referrals [66].

In conclusion, social support is relevant to all aspects of COPD. Its absence at the lower end of the socioeconomic gradient encourages the development of the disease and once established renders it more difficult to endure. When available, social support ameliorates the suffering caused by COPD, encourages smoking cessation and improves quality of life. It also reduces the cost and burden of hospital dependency and has earned its place in the front rank of COPD treatment modalities.

not more important than the more established treatment modalities.

Domiciliary support or 'hospital at home' has also been applied to the management of exacerbations of COPD. Many patients with exacerbations are suitable for home treatment with respiratory nurse supervision, because sophisticated monitoring is unnecessary, sudden deterioration is unlikely and once-daily observation is usually sufficient. Initial hospital assessment is important to confirm the diagnosis and exclude uncompensated respiratory acidosis. An uncontrolled study of home treatment by an acute respiratory assessment service (ARAS) showed that this development was safe, effective and popular with patients and GPs [57]. An exacerbation score derived from a European Respiratory Society consensus statement [58] was used to assess disease severity (Fig. 51.2).

Since the initial observational study, there have been six RCTs of hospital at home treatment carried out by specialist respiratory nurses [59–64]. All showed reduction in hospital admissions or bed utilization with no increase in morbidity, mortality or readmission rate. Of the larger studies, eligibility for home care averaged 35% and tended to correlate inversely with the FEV_1 at assessment. Direct GP referral achieves higher eligibility (approximately 70%) but it is not known how many of these patients would actually have been admitted to hospital [57]. The study design has varied, with some centres assessing patients on the day after admission with a view to early supported discharge

References

1 Goodman N, Lane RE, Rampling SB. Chronic bronchitis: an introductory examination of existing data. *BMJ* 1953;**2**: 237–43.

2 Pride NB, Soriano JB. Chronic obstructive pulmonary disease in the United Kingdom: trends in mortality, morbidity, and smoking. *Curr Opin Pulm Med* 2002;**8**:95–101.

3 Prescott E, Vestbo J. Socioeconomic status and chronic obstructive pulmonary disease. *Thorax* 1999;**54**:737–41.

4 Reid DD, Fletcher CM. International studies in chronic respiratory disease. *Br Med Bull* 1971;**27**:59–64.

5 Soriano JB, Maier WC, Egger P *et al.* Recent trends in physician diagnosed COPD in women and men in the UK. *Thorax* 2000;**55**:789–94.

6 Speizer FE, Tager IB. Epidemiology of chronic mucus hypersecretion and obstructive airways disease. *Epidemiol Rev* 1979;**1**:124–42.

7 Lebowitz MD. The relationship of socio-environmental factors to the prevalence of obstructive lung diseases and other chronic conditions. *J Chronic Dis* 1977;**30**:599–611.

8 Cohen BH, Ball WC Jr, Brashears S *et al.* Risk factors in chronic obstructive pulmonary disease (COPD). *Am J Epidemiol* 1977;**105**:223–32.

9 Higgins MW, Keller JB, Metzner HL. Smoking, socioeconomic status, and chronic respiratory disease. *Am Rev Respir Dis* 1977;**116**:403–10.

10 Marmot MG, Shipley MJ, Rose G. Inequalities in death: specific explanations of a general pattern? *Lancet* 1984;**1**: 1003–6.

11 Bakke PS, Hanoa R, Gulsvik A. Educational level and obstructive lung disease given smoking habits and occupational airborne exposure: a Norwegian community study. *Am J Epidemiol* 1995;**141**:1080–8.

12 Hole DJ, Watt GC, Davey-Smith G *et al*. Impaired lung function and mortality risk in men and women: findings from the Renfrew and Paisley prospective population study. *BMJ* 1996;**313**:711–5.

13 Stebbings JH Jr. Chronic respiratory disease among nonsmokers in Hagerstown, Maryland. IV. Effects of urban residence on pulmonary function values. *Environ Res* 1971;**4**:283–304.

14 Prescott E, Lange P, Vestbo J. Socioeconomic status, lung function and admission to hospital for COPD: results from the Copenhagen City Heart Study. *Eur Respir J* 1999;**13**:1109–14.

15 Marks GB, Burney PGJ. Diseases of the respiratory system. In: Charlton J, Murphy M, eds. *The Health of Adult Britain: 1841–1994*, vol. II. London: Stationary Office, 1997: 93–113.

16 Bridgwood A, Lilly R, Thomas M *et al*. Smoking. In: *Living in Britain: General Household Survey 1998*. London: Stationary Office, 2000: 115–43.

17 Osler M, Prescott E. Psychosocial, behavioural, and health determinants of successful smoking cessation: a longitudinal study of Danish adults. *Tob Control* 1998;**7**:262–7.

18 Burker EJ, Carels RA, Thompson LF, Rodgers L, Egan T. Quality of life in patients awaiting lung transplant: cystic fibrosis versus other end-stage lung diseases. *Pediatr Pulmonol* 2000;**30**:453–60.

19 Gore JM, Brophy CJ, Greenstone MA. How well do we care for patients with end-stage chronic obstructive pulmonary disease (COPD)? A comparison of palliative care and quality of life in COPD and lung cancer. *Thorax* 2000;**55**:1000–6.

20 Brown JS, Rawlinson ME, Hilles NC. Life satisfaction and chronic disease: exploration of theoretical model. *Med Care* 1981;**19**:1136–46.

21 Monso E, Fiz JM, Izquierdo J *et al*. Quality of life in severe chronic obstructive pulmonary disease: correlation with lung and muscle function. *Respir Med* 1998;**92**:221–7.

22 McSweeny AJ, Grant I, Heaton RK, Adams KM, Timms RM. Life quality of patients with chronic obstructive pulmonary disease. *Arch Intern Med* 1982;**142**:473–8.

23 Poole PJ, Bagg B, Brodie SM, Black PN. Characteristics of patients admitted to hospital with chronic obstructive pulmonary disease. *N Z Med J* 1997;**110**:272–5.

24 Bergs D. 'The Hidden Client': women caring for husbands with COPD – their experience of quality of life. *J Clin Nurs* 2002;**11**:613–21.

25 McCathie HC, Spence SH, Tate RL. Adjustment to chronic obstructive pulmonary disease: the importance of psychological factors. *Eur Respir J* 2002;**19**:47–53.

26 Guthrie SJ, Hill KM, Muers ME. Living with severe COPD: a qualitative exploration of the experience of patients in Leeds. *Respir Med* 2001;**95**:196–204.

27 Young P, Dewse M, Fergusson W, Kolbe J. Respiratory rehabilitation in chronic obstructive pulmonary disease: predictors of non-adherence. *Eur Respir J* 1999;**13**:855–9.

28 Lacasse Y, Guyatt GH, Goldstein RS. The components of a respiratory rehabilitation program: a systematic overview. *Chest* 1997;**111**:1077–88.

29 Devine EC, Pearcy J. Meta-analysis of the effects of psycho-educational care in adults with chronic obstructive pulmonary disease. *Patient Educ Couns* 1996;**29**:167–78.

30 Colby JP Jr, Linsky AS, Straus MA. Social stress and state-to-state differences in smoking and smoking related mortality in the United States. *Soc Sci Med* 1994;**38**:373–81.

31 Stehr DE, Klein BJ, Murata GH. Emergency department return visits in chronic obstructive pulmonary disease: the importance of psychosocial factors. *Ann Emerg Med* 1991;**20**:1113–6.

32 Pelkonen M, Tukiainen H, Tervahauta M *et al*. Pulmonary function, smoking cessation and 30 year mortality in middle aged Finnish men. *Thorax* 2000;**55**:746–50.

33 Anthonisen NR. Smoking, lung function, and mortality. *Thorax* 2000;**55**:729–30.

34 Anthonisen NR, Connett JE, Kiley JP *et al*. Effects of smoking intervention and the use of an inhaled anticholinergic bronchodilator on the rate of decline of FEV_1. The Lung Health Study. *JAMA* 1994;**272**:1497–505.

35 Richmond RL, Austin A, Webster IW. Three year evaluation of a programme by general practitioners to help patients to stop smoking. *BMJ* 1986;**292**:803–6.

36 Peach H, Pathy MS. Follow-up study of disability among elderly patients discharged from hospital with exacerbations of chronic bronchitis. *Thorax* 1981;**36**:585–9.

37 Guest JF. The annual cost of chronic obstructive pulmonary disease to the UK's National Health Service. *Dis Manag Health Outcomes* 1999;**5**:93–100.

38 Department of Health. *Hospital In-Patient Data Based on Hospital Episode Statistics 1992/93*. London: Stationary Office, 1993.

39 Cockcroft A, Bagnall P, Heslop A *et al*. Controlled trial of respiratory health worker visiting patients with chronic respiratory disability. *BMJ* 1987;**294**:225–8.

40 Hermiz O, Comino E, Marks G *et al*. Randomised controlled trial of home based care of patients with chronic obstructive pulmonary disease. *BMJ* 2002;**325**:938.

41 Littlejohns P, Baveystock CM, Parnell H, Jones PW. Randomised controlled trial of the effectiveness of a respiratory health worker in reducing impairment, disability, and handicap due to chronic airflow limitation. *Thorax* 1991;**46**:559–64.

42 Haggerty MC, Stockdale-Woolley R, Nair S. Respi-Care: an innovative home care program for the patient with chronic obstructive pulmonary disease. *Chest* 1991;**100**:607–12.

43 Roselle S, D'Amico FJ. The effect of home respiratory therapy on hospital readmission rates of patients with chronic obstructive pulmonary disease. *Respir Care* 1982;**27**:1194–9.

44 Clini E, Vitacca M, Foglio K, Simoni P, Ambrosino N. Long-term home care programmes may reduce hospital admissions in COPD with chronic hypercapnia. *Eur Respir J* 1996;**9**:1605–10.

45 Farrero E, Escarrabill J, Prats E, Maderal M, Manresa F. Impact of a hospital-based home-care program on the management of COPD patients receiving long-term oxygen therapy. *Chest* 2001;**119**:364–9.

46 Bourbeau JM, Julien MM, Maltais FM *et al*. Reduction of hospital utilization in patients with chronic obstructive pulmonary disease: a disease-specific self-management intervention. *Arch Intern Med* 2003;**163**:585–91.

47 Monninkhof E, van der Valk P, van der Palen J *et al*. Self-management education for patients with chronic obstructive pulmonary disease: a systematic review. *Thorax* 2003;**58**: 394–8.

48 Burge PS, Calverley PM, Jones PW *et al*. Randomised, double blind, placebo controlled study of fluticasone propionate in patients with moderate to severe chronic obstructive pulmonary disease: the ISOLDE trial. *BMJ* 2000;**320**:1297–303.

49 Mahler DA, Donohue JF, Barbee RA *et al*. Efficacy of salmeterol xinafoate in the treatment of COPD. *Chest* 1999; **115**:957–65.

50 Casaburi R, Mahler DA, Jones PW *et al*. A long-term evaluation of once-daily inhaled tiotropium in chronic obstructive pulmonary disease. *Eur Respir J* 2002;**19**:217–24.

51 Vincken W, van Noord JA, Greefhorst AP *et al*. Improved health outcomes in patients with COPD during 1 year's treatment with tiotropium. *Eur Respir J* 2002;**19**:209–16.

52 Foglio K, Bianchi L, Bruletti G *et al*. Long-term effectiveness of pulmonary rehabilitation in patients with chronic airway obstruction. *Eur Respir J* 1999;**13**:125–32.

53 Stewart DG, Drake DF, Robertson C *et al*. Benefits of an inpatient pulmonary rehabilitation program: a prospective analysis. *Arch Phys Med Rehabil* 2001;**82**:347–52.

54 Young P, Dewse M, Fergusson W, Kolbe J. Improvements in outcomes for chronic obstructive pulmonary disease (COPD) attributable to a hospital-based respiratory rehabilitation programme. *Aust N Z J Med* 1999;**29**:59–65.

55 Bowen JB, Thrall RS, ZuWallack RL, Votto JJ. Long-term benefits of short-stay inpatient pulmonary rehabilitation in severe chronic obstructive pulmonary disease. *Monaldi Arch Chest Dis* 1999;**54**:189–92.

56 Guell R, Casan P, Belda J *et al*. Long-term effects of outpatient rehabilitation of COPD: a randomized trial. *Chest* 2000;**117**: 976–83.

57 Gravil JH, Al Rawas OA, Cotton MM *et al*. Home treatment of exacerbations of chronic obstructive pulmonary disease by an acute respiratory assessment service. *Lancet* 1998;**351**: 1853–5.

58 Siafakas NM, Vermeire P, Pride NB *et al*. Optimal assessment and management of chronic obstructive pulmonary disease (COPD). The European Respiratory Society Task Force. *Eur Respir J* 1995;**8**:1398–420.

59 Cotton MM, Bucknall CE, Dagg KD *et al*. Early discharge for patients with exacerbations of chronic obstructive pulmonary disease: a randomized controlled trial. *Thorax* 2000;**55**:902–6.

60 Skwarska E, Cohen G, Skwarski KM *et al*. Randomized controlled trial of supported discharge in patients with exacerbations of chronic obstructive pulmonary disease. *Thorax* 2000;**55**:907–12.

61 Davies L, Wilkinson M, Bonner S, Calverley PM, Angus RM. 'Hospital at home' versus hospital care in patients with exacerbations of chronic obstructive pulmonary disease: prospective randomised controlled trial. *BMJ* 2000;**321**:1265–8.

62 Nicholson C, Bowler S, Jackson C *et al*. Cost comparison of hospital- and home-based treatment models for acute chronic obstructive pulmonary disease. *Aust Health Rev* 2001;**24**: 181–7.

63 Ojoo JC, Moon T, McGlone S *et al*. Patients' and carers' preferences in two models of care for acute exacerbations of COPD: results of a randomised controlled trial. *Thorax* 2002;**57**:167–9.

64 Hernandez C, Casas A, Escarrabill J *et al*. Home hospitalisation of exacerbated chronic obstructive pulmonary disease patients. *Eur Respir J* 2003;**21**:58–67.

65 Davies L, Angus RM, Calverley PM. Oral corticosteroids in patients admitted to hospital with exacerbations of chronic obstructive pulmonary disease: a prospective randomised controlled trial. *Lancet* 1999;**354**:456–60.

66 Johnson MK, Choo-Kang BSW, Sarvesvaran JS, Stevenson RD. Growth in hospital at home services for acute exacerbation of chronic obstructive pulmonary disease. *Thorax* 2001; **56**(Suppl 3):11 [Abstract].

CHAPTER 52
Long-term invasive mechanical ventilation

Gerard J. Criner

Patients receiving chronic invasive ventilation present an interesting set of problems because of the complex underlying medical or surgical disorders precipitating respiratory failure, coupled with the need for ventilation. As a result of devastating underlying medical or surgical illness, and a period of prolonged immobilization, and depending on whether the disorder requires treatment with high-dose systemic steroids or aminoglycosides, patients have substantial weakness of the extremities, as well as of respiratory and swallowing muscle groups. Therefore these patients pose unique and complex problems to the treatment team that mandates the use of a multidisciplinary approach to wean them successfully from mechanical ventilation, and to restore them to their prehospital functional status.

In this chapter, we detail our approach to the patient who requires chronic invasive ventilation. We emphasize the use of a multidisciplinary treatment plan.

Outcome of patients

Although several studies have reported on survival following long-term, chronic or prolonged mechanical ventilation, the studies vary significantly depending upon the definition of 'long-term' or 'chronic'. Some studies report chronic ventilation as being longer than 2 or 3 days, whereas others report as chronic those patients who have been ventilated for 30 days or longer. Regardless of the study definition of the period of ventilation, however, the mortality associated with prolonged ventilation is fairly high. Data previously published by the Health Care Financing Administration (HCFA) in the USA reported a mortality of 51% in Medicare beneficiaries who received mechanical ventilation for any length of time [1]. Previous studies reporting survival at hospital discharge in patients ventilated for 48 h or more, show mortalities that range anywhere from 36%

to 59%. Beside the duration of ventilation, patient age, the type of underlying medical or surgical illness precipitating respiratory failure and patient severity of illness are all-important factors that may affect outcome of patients receiving chronic ventilation. All of these factors vary substantially between studies.

Knaus [2] reported a hospital mortality rate of 59% in patients who were ventilated for at least 7 days with mean Acute Physiology and Chronic Health Evaluation II scores (APACHE II) of 11–15. Patients who were ventilated for comparable lengths of time but were more severely ill (APACHE II scores of 21–25) had significantly higher mortality (77%), in contrast with those with lower APACHE scores (APACHE II scores 1–15) who had decreased mortality rates (10%). These data suggest that the severity of illness is an important factor determining mortality in patients receiving prolonged ventilation.

Age has also been reported to be a significant factor affecting the outcome of patients receiving mechanical ventilation. Although some authors found a direct correlation between greater patient age and mortality [3], others have not observed such a relationship [4]. These studies commonly failed to control for other variables that may affect outcome, such as severity of illness or underlying disease-precipitating respiratory failure. As a result, the influence of age itself as an independent factor influencing mortality in patients receiving prolonged ventilation is not clear at the present time.

The disorder precipitating respiratory failure, however, seems to be important in affecting patient outcome. Patients with malignancy and respiratory failure who require mechanical ventilation have extremely limited survival of only several months, with mortality at 6 months approaching 100%. Several studies have shown improved survival and functional status in those patients receiving chronic ventilation for restrictive lung disorders, such as post-polio syndrome, muscular dystrophy and kyphoscoliosis. By

601

contrast, patients with obstructive disorders, such as chronic obstructive pulmonary disease (COPD) or bronchiectasis, have been reported to have a reduction in survival of the order of 50% compared with those with restrictive disorders [5]. In a study by Czorniak *et al.* [6], chronic ventilated COPD patients discharged home were less independent and more likely to require repeated hospitalization than patients discharged home with mechanical ventilation for neuromuscular chest wall disorders. In addition, COPD patients receiving home ventilation had a decrease in survival compared with those with neuromuscular diseases. Other reports have also confirmed the poor outcome of chronic ventilated patients with COPD [7].

The prehospital functional status may also be an important factor determining outcome in patients receiving prolonged ventilation. Carson *et al.* [8] reported the outcome in 133 consecutive patients who were admitted to a long-term acute care hospital where they received mechanical ventilation for 14 days or longer. Patients not functionally independent before admission had a much higher 1-year mortality compared with those who were functionally independent.

When reviewing data across studies, it appears that unselected patients receiving prolonged ventilation when not screened by the severity or nature of the underlying disease, evidence of multiple organ dysfunction, lack of rehabilitative potential and poor functional pre-admission status have much reduced survival and limited improvement in functional status and quality of life. Therefore, the outcome of prolonged mechanical ventilation, the treatment plan and the goals of patient care are heavily influenced by the patient population that is being described. With this in mind, the focus of this chapter is on those patients receiving chronic ventilation who are considered to have rehabilitative potential, lack multiorgan dysfunction and have a satisfactory pre-admission functional status.

Impact of multidisciplinary units on patient outcome

Several reports have shown that patients receiving prolonged ventilation are not relegated to a uniformly dismal outcome in terms of mortality and functional status, when patients are properly selected and receive aggressive rehabilitation. Data from two of the HCFA Chronic Ventilator Demonstration sites suggested that the survival of some patients requiring invasive long-term ventilation is better than previously reported. Gracey *et al.* [9] reported the outcomes in 206 consecutive patients admitted to the Mayo Clinic, Ventilator-Dependent Unit, during a 5-year study period. Two hundred and six patients who received mechanical ventilation for at least 6 h/day for 21 consecut-

ive days were admitted; 92% (190) survived to be discharged from the hospital, of whom 77% returned to their homes; 153 of the patients were weaned totally from mechanical ventilation, whereas 37 remained completely or partially ventilator dependent. Of the patients receiving mechanical ventilation at discharge, 73% received it only nocturnally. The 4-year survival of the patients was 53%. A significant percentage of the patients, however, suffered prolonged ventilation from postoperative conditions (60%), which may have been responsible for skewing the results to a more optimistic outcome than other reports covering a heavier concentration of medical patients.

The report from our HCFA Chronic Ventilator Demonstration Project clinical unit comprised 77 patients [10]. Of these, 74% had medical causes as the reason for ventilator dependence: neuromuscular disease (26%), advanced lung disease (29%), congestive heart failure (5%) and a variety of other medical disorders (40%). In spite of the differences between the two populations, our results were similar to those of Gracey *et al.* [9]. Ninety-three per cent of these HFCA patients were discharged alive, 82% were still alive at 6 months and 61% at 1-year follow-up. Eighty-six per cent of the patients were completely weaned from mechanical ventilation, whereas 11% required continuous ventilation and 10% had nocturnal ventilation at discharge. In patients discharged alive, there was a significant increase in functional status at 6 and 12 months' follow-up.

Overall, both of these studies suggest that when patients receiving chronic mechanical ventilation are properly selected, and following correction of the underlying process causing respiratory failure, they have an acceptable clinical outcome with a return to pre-admission functional status and successful home discharge.

Location of care

Generally, patients receive long-term ventilation benefit when that care is provided in a non-intensive care unit (non-ICU) location that is geared toward multidisciplinary rehabilitation. The advantages that a non-invasive

Table 52.1 Advantages of a non-invasive respiratory care unit over standard intensive care unit (ICU) care.

- Less expensive
- Unlocks ICU beds
- Transitions patients to home care
- Emphasis is on achieving maximal functional status despite the requirement for ventilator support
- Extend capabilities of medical/surgical programmes to treat patients with advanced lung disease

Table 52.2 Criteria for transfer of ventilator-dependent patients from intensive care unit (ICU) to ventilatory rehabilitation unit (VRU). (From Make *et al.* [11], with permission.)

	Respiratory stability	Non-respiratory medical stability
Airway	Tracheostomy for invasive ventilation, minimal aspiration	Sepsis controlled
Secretions	Manageable with infrequent suctioning	No uncontrolled haemorrhage
		No arrhythmias, CHF, unstable angina
Oxygen	Adequate oxygenation with $Fio_2 < 60\%$, $PEEP \leq 10$ cm H_2O ($SPo_2 \geq 90\%$)	
Ventilator settings	Stable, no sophisticated modes	No coma
Patient assessment	Comfortable, no increased WOB or dyspnoea	Secure IV access
Weaning technique	Tracheal collar	Secure alimentation route
NPPV	Tolerates breaks off, stable settings	

CHF, congestive heart failure; Fio_2, fractional inspired oxygen concentration; IV, intravenous; NPPV, non-invasive positive pressure ventilation; PEEP, positive end-expiratory pressure; SPo_2, saturation of oxygen by pulse oximetry; WOB, work of breathing.

respiratory care unit has over standard ICU care include a less expensive location and more effective transition for patients to eventual home care, or discharge to a non-acute care location (Table 52.1). The emphasis in those units is placed on achieving maximal functional status despite requirements for ventilatory support. Effective use of these units, moreover, extends the capabilities to treat patients having severe lung disease with advanced medical and surgical therapies in ICUs.

Before patients are transferred to a non-ICU location for ventilator care, they must meet certain requirements for respiratory and non-respiratory medical stability [11]. Criteria for respiratory–non-respiratory medical stability are shown in Table 52.2. In all cases, patients must have a stable airway place, as afforded by a tracheostomy; they must also have manageable secretions. They should not be on sophisticated modes of mechanical ventilation and have only modest requirements for supplemental oxygen or positive end-expiratory pressure (PEEP). In addition, patients should not have uncontrolled cardiac arrhythmia or ischaemia, unstable haematological or fluid and electrolyte disorders, and have secure routes for parenteral access for medications and also for alimentation.

At our facility, which was one of the four HCFA Chronic Ventilator Demonstration units, the complex problems of chronic ventilator patients are addressed by a team comprised of specialists including respiratory nurses, nutritionists, psychologists, respiratory physical speech therapists and social workers. The medical staff includes a rotating board certified pulmonary and critical care attending physician and a fellow in training. Weekly meetings are attended by all team members and are led by the medical director of

the unit. Patients who are admitted to this unit have been ventilated for at least 21 consecutive days, at least 6 h/day, and are required to have previously undergone at least two attempts at weaning from mechanical ventilation that failed. The emphasis in this unit is placed on rehabilitation and restoration of functional status, despite requirements for prolonged ventilation.

Special patient needs

Special needs of patients who require chronic invasive ventilation include evaluation of the optimum form of ventilator support. In addition, special attention must be paid to swallowing dysfunction, impaired communications skills, psychological dysfunction, optimization of nutrition, respiratory and whole body reconditioning and ever-changing medical conditions (Table 52.3).

Table 52.3 Special needs of chronically ventilated patients.

Need some form of mechanical ventilation or special respiratory treatment device
Patients requiring invasive ventilation require special attention to:
• Swallowing dysfunction
• Impaired communication skills
• Psychological dysfunction
Renutrition
Respiratory and whole body reconditioning
Close attention to new or changing medical conditions

Table 52.4 Psychological dysfunction in ventilator-dependent patients.

Intensive care unit (ICU) environmental factors
Monotonous, meaningless sensory input (e.g. alarms)
Sensory depravation
Sleep deprivation

Factors associated with mechanical ventilation
Hypoxaemia, illness, medication-induced short-term
  memory loss
Most report that inability to communicate is most important
  factor contributing to fear, or inability to rest or sleep
Lack of normal bodily function (e.g. eating, social
  interaction, ambulation)

In an effort to improve patient mobility and facilitate whole body rehabilitation, patients are transferred to a portable mechanical ventilator shortly after their admission to the unit. This enables patients not only to maximize their functional capabilities, but also to accustom those who require chronic intermittent or home mechanical ventilation to adjust their ventilator settings and receive instructions in its use if eventual home discharge with ventilation is required. In all cases, based on the underlying pathology causing respiratory failure, patients are evaluated for transition to nocturnal invasive ventilation or to the use of non-invasive ventilation.

Psychological dysfunction is an important issue in patients who receive chronic ventilation (Table 52.4). This is caused by a number of factors related to permanence in ICU, such as continuous input of monotonous sensory input from multiple audio alarms, sensory deprivation afforded by the sterile visual environment of an ICU and, finally, sleep deprivation – a significant and common finding in an ICU setting. Prior studies have shown that ICU patients are susceptible to sleep deprivation because of multiple factors, including the underlying disease, its severity, the administration of medications and the environment used to treat the disorder. Bentley *et al.* [12] demonstrated that the noise levels in the ICU compared negatively with that of a general medical floor. Furthermore, the noises are substantially greater and sustained throughout a 24-h period, a potentially important factor that could lead to a prolonged state of sleep deprivation while in the ICU. Other factors associated with the use of mechanical ventilation can also contribute to psychological dysfunction (see Table 52.4).

Most patients who survive an episode of respiratory failure requiring mechanical ventilation report that the inability to communicate is one of the single most important factors contributing to fear, or the inability to rest or sleep. Also, a lack of capability to perform normal bodily functions such as eating, talking or ambulation can also

contribute to a feeling of apathy, disorientation and social withdrawal.

In a study previously reported from our unit, Criner and Isaac [13] measured cognitive deficits in 28 consecutive ventilator-dependent patients. A significant number of them (40%) had problems with orientation, long- and short-term memory, language processing and reasoning. It was rare that a patient had no cognitive disorder, and more common that patients had multiple cognitive disorders.

Orientation techniques may be useful in helping to reverse the disorientation that accompanies the process of mechanical ventilation, as well as the environmental issues precipitated by the ICU environment. Visual orientation clues include large clocks, calendars and also a daily care plan, with personal effects such as pictures and other family items, and may orientate the patient back into the environment. Also, it has been shown that a nearby window open to the outside provides patients with visual clues such as the time of day and the season of the year, decreasing the incidence of delirium by two-thirds in ICU patients compared with those without visible windows to the outside [14].

Because speech is such an important issue in patients who have been chronically ventilated, attempts should be made to restore verbal communication in patients as soon as possible. At least, patients can communicate by verbal gestures such as mouthing, and if their hands are not impaired by disease, by writing. In a ventilated patient, however, a buccal resonator, electrolarynx or a one-way valve (Passy–Muir valve) worn over a deflated tracheostomy tube in line with the ventilator circuit, or while the patient is spontaneously breathing, can afford self-initiated speech. Patients who can communicate verbally are less likely to be anxious, and thus require less sedation, further fostering participation in rehabilitative efforts and hastening the weaning process.

Swallowing dysfunction is an important issue that faces patients who receive chronic invasive ventilation. We previously demonstrated that, in 35 consecutively ventilated patients receiving prolonged ventilation, swallowing dysfunction was common even in those not having an underlying neurological disease [15]. In that study, 34% of patients showed evidence of aspiration on bedside swallow evaluation, with 83% of them having abnormalities that would predispose them to aspiration of oropharyngeal contents on modified barium swallow using three different textures of barium (liquid, semi-solid and solid). The abnormalities in swallowing observed on bedside examination, or during the modified barium swallow, are shown in Tables 52.5 and 52.6.

In some patients who are unable to travel to a radiology suite to have a modified barium swallow, bedside fibreoptic endoscopic evaluation of swallowing (FEES) while patients are fed liquid, solid or semi-solid substances can provide

Table 52.5 Abnormalities found on bedside examination. (From Tolep *et al.* [15], with permission.)

	NMD (*n* = 5)	Non-NMD (*n* = 7)
Lingual control	3	2
Palatal elevation	1	0
Swallow reflex	4	0
Laryngeal elevation	2	4
Laryngeal control	2	1
Tainted secretions	1	5

NMD, neuromuscular disorder present; non-NMD, no neuromuscular disease present.

Table 52.6 Abnormal findings on modified barium swallow with visual fluoroscopy (*n* = 19). (From Tolep *et al.* [15], with permission.)

	NMD (*n* = 11)	Non-NMD (*n* = 8)
Lingual propulsion	6	8
Premature spillage	8	7
Swallow reflex	7	7
Aspiration	4	6
Vallecular stasis	8	5
Pyriform sinus stasis	8	5
Pharyngeal coating	7	6
Laryngeal elevation	6	3
Cricopharyngeal spasm	4	0

NMD, neuromuscular disorder present; non-NMD, no neuromuscular disease present.

useful information. After local anaesthesia of the nares, glottic examination using a laryngoscope or paediatric bronchoscope can determine whether there is decreased sensation of the oropharyngeal region, oedema of the arytenoids or larynx, pooling of secretions above the vocal cords, normal movement of the vocal cords, problems with premature spillage of oropharyngeal contents into the glottis or gross aspiration.

At our centre, patients who receive prolonged invasive ventilation are not allowed any oral intake until jointly evaluated by the speech therapist and pulmonologist at a bedside examination. Fibreoptic endoscopic evaluation of swallowing or modified barium swallow with videofluoroscope is used to evaluate swallowing function. The oropharyngeal and hypopharyngeal stages of swallowing with liquid, semi-solid and solid food textures are comprehensively evaluated, and rehabilitative techniques are developed as needed to minimize aspiration.

In some chronic ventilated patients, inspiratory muscle training may have a significant impact. At our institution, when patients are able to tolerate tracheal collar or T-piece weaning for at least 2 h/day, they begin inspiratory muscle training with an inspiratory muscle trainer; the load of which is placed at one-third of the maximum inspiratory pressure. The duration of breathing against the load is progressively increased to 15 min twice daily. The load and duration of inspiratory muscle training is then increased as the patient's tolerance increases. In a report by Aldrich *et al.* [16], inspiratory resistive training was used in 27 consecutive patients, ventilated for longer than 3 weeks. In the group as a whole, increases in maximum inspiratory pressure and vital capacity were observed. Patients who successfully underwent respiratory muscle training had a higher partial or total weaning rate than those who could not be trained. Inspiratory muscle training in chronically ventilated patients has not been studied in a prospective randomized controlled way. Most of the data suggest that patients with chronic respiratory failure suffer from respiratory muscle weakness rather than respiratory muscle fatigue, and that respiratory muscle training may have a reconditioning effort on restoring respiratory muscle strength and enhancing the patient's ability to wean from mechanical ventilation.

Besides inspiratory muscle training, focus is also placed on training the large groups of accessory inspiratory muscles of the chest wall, including the pectoralis, trapezius and serratus anterior muscles, which may act as accessory muscles of respiration. Several investigators [17–19], as shown in Table 52.7, have shown an increase in ventilatory muscle endurance, an increase in maximum inspiratory pressure and increased ability to cough after training the pectoralis muscles in normal individuals, cystic fibrosis patients or low tetraplegic patients. Although training the upper extremity muscles has not been validated in a perspective randomized controlled fashion, in chronic ventilator-dependent patients, it appears logical that strengthening and reconditioning skeletal muscles used as either primary or accessory muscles of ventilation may have a significant beneficial impact in those patients who suffer from chronic respiratory failure. As a result, patients admitted to our institution for chronic invasive ventilation have as part of their rehabilitative approach, upper extremity strengthening exercise performed to facilitate the inspiratory and expiratory actions of the pectoralis muscles, as well as improving the respiratory actions of other neck and chest wall muscle groups.

We believe that a multidisciplinary systematic approach to the global reconditioning of patients on prolonged mechanical ventilation will not only have a positive impact

Table 52.7 Effect of upper extremity training on ventilatory muscle strength and endurance.

Author/year [Ref.]	Subject	Results
Keens et al. 1977 [17]	Cystic fibrosis ($n = 7$)	57% increase in ventilatory muscle endurance
Clanton et al. 1987 [18]	Female swimmers ($n = 16$)	25% increase in MIP, 100% in ventilatory endurance
Estenne et al. 1989 [19]	C_1–C_8 quads ($n = 6$)	6 weeks of isometric pectoralis major training, increased ERV by 47%

ERV, expiratory reserve volume; MIP, maximum inspiratory pressure.

on improving function status and facilitate weaning from mechanical ventilation, but it also can have an important effect on the perception of patients and families about the care delivered while they receive chronic mechanical ventilation.

In one study, we measured the perception in patients and families about care delivered to the same group of patients cared for by the same team of pulmonary and critical care physicians in the ICU compared with the non-invasive respiratory care unit [20]. Interestingly, patients and families perceived the cognitive impairment (efforts to wean the patient) was less, and patient encouragement was greater in the Ventilator Rehabilitation Unit compared with the ICU. This had nothing to do with the change in the patient's severity of illness or change in the approach by the doctors, but was predominately related to the change in focus of care towards the patient as a whole, and that the environment of a non-invasive respiratory care unit was more conducive to rehabilitative efforts than the acutely intensive and chaotic environment of the ICU.

Data examining the outcome of patients who survive prolonged mechanical ventilation is limited, and there are many questions regarding the cost of care, their morbidity and mortality, and whether their quality of life is acceptable. We have recently reported on 25 consecutive patients who survived long-term invasive mechanical ventilation, and solicited information regarding their quality of life 18 months post-discharge from our non-invasive respiratory care unit [21]. Overall, we found that using Short Form 36 (SF-36) Sickness Impact Scores as a measure of quality of life, these patients were comparable to those patients suffering from hypothyroidism or rheumatoid arthritis, and substantially better than those who had chronic diseases such as COPD. Overall, the long-term survivors had satisfactory performance in the physical, psychological and social interaction domains of the SF-36 measures of quality of life. These data, although limited, suggest that patients who survive long-term invasive ventilation achieve a good quality of life that makes worthwhile the extraordinary efforts that they, their families and the staff made in their care during the period of prolonged mechanical ventilation.

Conclusions

Patients who require prolonged invasive mechanical ventilation pose a unique set of circumstances to the pulmonary and critical care practitioner. This requires a delineation of the primary cause for respiratory failure and, in most cases, a comprehensive multidisciplinary approach to the management of not only the primary disturbance causing respiratory failure, but the consequences that immobility, illness and prolonged ventilation have on swallowing and ambulatory function, psychosocial interaction and the ability to wean from mechanical ventilation.

The development of multidisciplinary rehabilitative units for patients requiring prolonged mechanical ventilation have showed not only a reduction in hospital costs and lengths of stay, but also an improvement in patient survival, functional status, reduction in ventilator days or need for mechanical ventilation at discharge and, overall, the achievement of a satisfactory quality of life.

References

1 Health Care Financing Administration. Ventilator-dependent demonstration. Presented at Technical Advisory Panel Meeting, Washington, DC, February 20, 1990.

2 Knaus WA. Prognosis with mechanical ventilation: the influence of disease, severity of disease, age and chronic health status on survival from an acute illness. *Am Rev Respir Dis* 1989;**140**(Suppl):S8–S13.

3 Kurek CJ, Cohen IL, Lambrinos J et al. Clinical and economic outcome of patients undergoing tracheostomy for prolonged mechanical ventilation in New York during 1993: analysis of 6353 cases under diagnosis related group 483. *Crit Care Med* 1997;**25**:983–8.

4 Meinders AJ, Van der Joeveen J, Weinders AE. The outcome of prolonged mechanical ventilation in elderly patients are: are the efforts worthwhile? *Age Ageing* 1996;**25**:353–6.

5 Robert D, Gerald M, Leger P. Domiciliary mechanical ventilation by tracheostomy for chronic respiratory failure. *Rev Fr Respir* 1983;**11**:923–36.

6 Czorniak MA, Gilmartin ME, Make BJ. Home mechanical ventilation: clinical course of patients with neuromuscular disease (NMD) and chronic obstructive pulmonary disease (COPD). *Am Rev Respir Dis* 1987;**15**:A194.

7 Votto J, Brancifort JM, Scalise PJ, Wollschlager CM, ZuWallack RL. COPD and other disease in chronically ventilated patients in a prolonged respiratory care unit: a retrospective 20-year survival study. *Chest* 1998;**113**:86–90.

8 Carson SS, Bach PB, Brzozowski L, Leff A. Outcomes after long-term acute care: an analysis of 133 mechanically ventilated patients. *Am J Respir Crit Care Med* 1999;**159**:1568–73.

9 Gracey DR, Hardy C, Naessens JM, Silverstein MC, Hubmayr RD. The Mayo Ventilator-Dependent Rehabilitation Unit: a 5-year experience. *Mayo Clin Proc* 1997;**72**:13–9.

10 Criner GJ, Kreimer DT, Pidlaoan L. Patient outcome following prolonged mechanical ventilation (MV) via tracheostomy. *Am Rev Respir Dis* 1993;**147**:A874.

11 Make BJ, Hill NS, Goldberg AI *et al*. Mechanical ventilation beyond the intensive care unit: report of a consensus conference of the American College of Chest Physicians. *Chest* 1998;**113**:289S.

12 Bentley S, Murphy F, Dudley H, Perceived noise in surgical wards and an intensive care area: an objective analysis. *BMJ* 1977;**2**:1503–6.

13 Criner GJ, Isaac L. Psychological problems in the ventilator-dependent patient. In: Tobin M, ed. *Principles and Practice of Mechanical Ventilation*. New York: McGraw-Hill; 1994: 1163–75.

14 Wilson M. Intensive care delirium. *Arch Intern Med* 1972; **130**:225–6.

15 Tolep K, Getch KL, Criner GJ. Swallowing dysfunction in patients requiring prolonged mechanical ventilation. *Chest* 1996;**109**:167–72.

16 Aldrich TK, Karpel JP, Uhrlass RM *et al*. Weaning from mechanical ventilation adjunctive use of inspiratory muscle resistive training. *Crit Care Med* 1989;**17**:143–7.

17 Keens TG, Krastens IRB, Wanamaker IM *et al*. Ventilatory muscle endurance training in normal subjects and patients with cystic fibrosis. *Am Rev Respir Dis* 1977;**116**:853–60.

18 Clanton T, Dixon G, Drake J, Gadek J. Effects of swim training on lung volumes and inspiratory muscle condition. *J Appl Physiol* 1987;**62**:39–46.

19 Estenne M, Kroop C, van Vaerehnbergh J, Heilporn A, De Troyer A. The effect of pectoralis muscle training in tetraplegia patients. *Am Rev Respir Dis* 1989;**139**:1218–22.

20 Isaac L, Criner GJ. Patient and family perceptions on weaning from mechanical ventilation in a specialized rehabilitation unit. *Am Rev Respir Dis* 1990;**141**:A411.

21 Chatila W, Kreimer DT, Criner GJ. Quality of life in survivors of prolonged mechanical ventilation. *Crit Care Med* 2001; **29**:737–42.

CHAPTER 53
Smoking cessation

Philip Tønnesen

Smoking cessation is a main intervention area in COPD in all stages. As stated in the GOLD guidelines: 'Smoking cessation is the single most effective – and cost-effective – intervention to reduce the risk of developing COPD and stop its progression (Evidence A)' [1].

However, for many years the intervention in this area had a low priority. This was likely because of clinicians' lack of knowledge that cigarette smoking results from an addiction to nicotine, combined with lack of skills in the area of smoking cessation. In addition, some clinicians adopted an unprofessional attitude towards smokers, blaming or scolding patients in the belief that quitting smoking was only a matter of willpower. Recently, increased attention has focused on both COPD per se and also on smoking cessation. In part, this may be because of the involvement of the pharmaceutical industry through the development of new therapeutic agents for these conditions. Also, several clinical guidelines about smoking cessation have helped focus attention in this area [2–4]. Despite this, relatively little research has focused on smoking cessation specifically in COPD. As a result, current approaches are generally similar to the approach in other smokers. Nevertheless, the major problem in smoking cessation for COPD patients is adequate implementation of current 'state of the art' care in daily clinical practice.

Nicotine receptors and the effect of nicotine

Tobacco dependence is a complex behaviour with both environmental and genetic influences. From twin studies, a substantial genetic component (approximately 50%) has been estimated [5]. The enzyme CYP 2A6 metabolizes nicotine to cotinine and smokers with a defective variant metabolize nicotine more slowly and exhibit reduced smoking.

Other candidate genes that affect smoking have been suggested, but inconsistent data exist regarding the effect of subgroups of dopamine receptors and function on the likelihood of initiation of smoking and nicotine dependence.

Nicotine acts on specific nicotine acetylcholine receptors, which consist of α- and β-subunits. In the brain, nicotine receptors are distributed in the mesolimbic system with particularly high density in the nucleus accumbens where nicotine augments the release of dopamine. Nicotine potentiation of neuronal dopamine release requires the β_2-subunit of the nicotine receptor. Mice lacking this subunit will not self-administer nicotine, supporting the concept of the increase in dopamine release associated with the acute rewarding effect of nicotine [6].

However, noradrenaline, acetylcholine, serotonin, glutamate, γ-aminobutyric acid and opioid peptide release are also affected by nicotine and these other mediators may also have a role in nicotine addiction [7]. Chronic smoking leads to an up-regulation of nicotine receptors which are also distributed in the prefrontal cortex and outside the central nervous system (CNS). Nicotine has peripheral actions, via nicotine receptors, that include release of adrenaline and stimulation of the carotid and aortic bodies with a slight increase in blood pressure and heart rate, tachypnoea and increased intestinal peristalsis. Nausea results from CNS stimulation. A lethal single dose of nicotine is approximately 60 mg and nicotine intoxication leads to central stimulation, respiratory paralysis and circulatory collapse.

Basic elements in smoking cessation

Cigarette smoking is a complex habit with nicotine dependence as the main component; however, psychological factors and habituation also have a role. Nicotine dependence is most often assessed by the use of a paper and pencil

Table 53.1 Fagerström Test for Nicotine Dependence (FTND) [8].

Item	Answers	Score
1 How soon after you wake up do you smoke your first cigarette?	Within 5 min	3
	6–30 min	2
	31–60 min	1
	61+	0
2 Do you find it difficult to refrain from smoking in places where it is forbidden (e.g. in church, at the library, in the cinema)?	Yes	1
	No	0
3 Which cigarette would you hate most to give up?	The first one in the morning	1
	All others	0
4 How many cigarettes per day do you smoke?	1–10	0
	11–20	1
	21–30	2
	31 or more	3
5 Do you smoke more frequently during the first hours after waking than during the rest of the day?	Yes	1
	No	0
6 Do you smoke if you are so ill that you are in bed most of the day (or absent from work)?	Yes	1
	No	0
	Total score	*0–10*

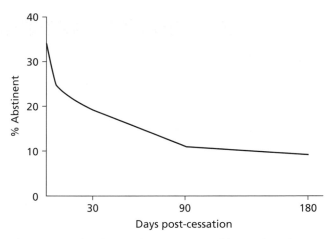

Figure 53.1 The classic relapse curve in addictive disorders such as cigarette smoking. (After Hughes [11].)

most often the case even in trials where the NRT is free of charge. Use of nicotine gum, inhaler or sublingual tablets on a fixed schedule (once or twice per hour) during the first 6–8 h of the day might increase nicotine substitution and enhance efficacy.

Support for smoking cessation should address the following elements: the use of pharmacological smoking cessation agents, handling of withdrawal symptoms, relapse prevention, weight gain and the benefits of quitting cigarettes. For many long-term COPD smokers, the first months after quitting is particularly hard and many miss the relaxing effect of smoking. The cigarette has been a friend for many years that the smoker will miss, and he or she will have to fight the withdrawal symptoms. In this situation, it is important for the clinician to have a supportive, positive and emphatic attitude to reinforce the quitter's motivation to stay abstinent.

The intensity of support provided to the smoker making a quit attempt will vary for many reasons. However, there is a dose–response effect of the time of each session and the number of sessions, and success rate increases with the intensity of intervention (Table 53.2) [2].

questionnaire (i.e. the Fagerström Test for Nicotine Dependence [FTND]) with a possible score from 0 to 10, where 6–10 reflects high nicotine dependence (Table 53.1) [8]. The most important of the seven questions seems to be 'Smoking within 30 minutes after awakening in the morning' corresponding to a low plasma nicotine concentration at that time.

Appoximately 4–8 h after quitting smoking, varying degrees of withdrawal symptoms appear including irritability, anxiety, restlessness, difficulty in concentration, depressed mood, increased appetite and craving for cigarettes. These peak in intensity after 1 week and then decline over several weeks to months [9,10].

The relapse rate for smokers following cessation is very similar to that for alcoholics and heroin users following abstinence. Relapse is highest during the first 3–6 weeks and then gradually declines (Fig. 53.1) [11]. This emphasizes the importance of support during the first few weeks after a quit day and that it is crucial the patient does not underdose nicotine replacement therapy (NRT) in the initial period after the quit date.

To accomplish this, a test period of NRT a few days before the quit day might help smokers become more familiar with how to use the NRT product. Underdosing of NRT is

Table 53.2 Intensity of intervention from Clinical Practice Guideline, *Treating Tobacco Use and Dependence* [2]. Based on meta-analysis (*n* = 45 studies).

Minimal (< 3 min) is effective (A)
[1-year quit rate: No contact: 11%; < 3 min: 13%]

Dose–response effect (person-to-person) (A)
[1-year quit rate: < 3 min: 13%; > 10 min: 22%]

Four or more sessions especially effective (A)
[1-year quit rate: 0–1 sessions: 12%; 4–8 sessions; 21%]

The treatment for smoking cessation consists of two elements: a pharmacological agent – NRT or bupropion SR (amfebutamone) – for 3 months which suppresses the withdrawal symptoms, thus allowing the subject to cope with the behavioural and psychological aspects of smoking; and a behavioural component consisting of advice, support and follow-up.

One of the most basic and important 'rules' is a complete abstinence from cigarettes from the quit day and avoidance of smoking even a single cigarette during the following 2 weeks. Consumption of only a few cigarettes in this period is predictive of relapse. In the CEASE study enrolling 3575 healthy smokers in 37 lung clinics in Europe, the 1-year success rate in subjects who smoked a few cigarettes during the first 2 weeks was 3% compared with 25% in subjects who were abstinent during the initial period [12].

Identification of the smoking COPD patient

To implement a smoking cessation programme in the individual chest unit it is important that the manager/chair of the department support the idea and allocate the necessary resources. Smoking cessation in the chest unit – inpatient or outpatient department – is best achieved with a team approach where all clinicians work together to potentiate the effect of intervention, as different types of clinician seem to be more efficacious in promoting smoking cessation than a single clinician type [2]. Another important element is the prescription of NRT or bupropion SR (Table 53.3).

Results from nine studies showed that the estimated intervention rate by clinicians with their patients who smoke increased from 39% to 66% with a screening system in place to identify smoking status [2]. Different systems have been used to increase identification rate. Stickers in nursing notes and/or in patient medical files can be useful.

Table 53.3 Smoking cessation in the chest unit for COPD patients.

Smoke-free units
Teamwork between different types of clinicians
Systematic identification of smokers
Strong advice to quit from physician
Smoking cessation counsellors
NRT and bupropion SR free of charge
Carbon monoxide assessments
Tobacco habits in medical file
Follow-up: clinic visits

NRT, nicotine replacement therapy.

Table 53.4 Example of medical file for smoking habits.

History	Action to be taken
Tobacco: never smoker	
Ex-smoker	Do not start (again)
Quit since: ___/___/___	Stop here
_____ cig./day	Advise to quit: yes/no
Pack-years: _____	NRT: dose/duration
Motivation to quit:	Bupropion SR:
no/maybe/yes	dose/duration
	Prescribe counselling
FTND-1: (0–3): ___	Brochure (diff. choices)
CO: ___ ppm (< 6–10)	Follow-up:
	visit/letter/phone/nurse/etc.

CO, carbon monoxide; FTND, Fagerström Test for Nicotine Dependence; NRT, nicotine replacement therapy.

Table 53.5 Proposal for accreditation standard for carbon monoxide assessment.

Standards	Specifications
Carbon monoxide air	1 app. per unit
Instruction for use	In national language
Training of staff	One responsible
Calibration	Every 3 months/log book
False-positive	Lactose malabsorption
False-negative	Too short breath
	holding/cut-off too high
A-puncture	Severe COPD/cut-off?
Cut-off for smokers	6–10 ppm

Routine inclusion of smoking habits in all patient medical files is another way of emphasizing the importance of this area (Table 53.4). It is important that one person have the responsibility for the smoking cessation programme when first implemented. Accreditation standards for smoking cessation programmes that include all elements required might facilitate programme implementation. An example of such an accreditation standard is the one proposed for the assessment of carbon monoxide (CO) in Table 53.5.

Verification of smoking status

The patient's report of smoking status combined with a biochemical verification of smoking status (CO and/or cotinine) is the usual way to confirm abstinence. A detailed history of smoking should be obtained: age when smoking started, number of cigarettes smoked per day, pack-years ([cigarettes per day × years, which may not be constant over the smoking history] : 20), prior quit attempts, prior use and effect of NRT and/or bupropion SR, motivation to quit, measure of nicotine dependency (question 1 in FTND: How soon after you wake do you smoke: within 5 min (3), within 6–30 min (2), within 31–60 min (1), later (0)) (Table 53.1). During examination of the patient, the smell of tobacco smoke in clothes, hair or skin, and yellow fingertips as well as a cigarette box is indicative of recent smoking.

CO is a product of combustion, and smokers have elevated levels of CO in both blood and expiratory air, while subjects using smokeless tobacco and/or NRT have levels indicative of non-smoking. The plasma half-life of CO is approximately 2 h during activity and 8 h during sleep. The CO level in expired air is 1–4 ppm in most non-smokers compared with 15–25 ppm in regular smokers, with a parallel increase in CO levels with increasing cigarette consumption. Through exposure to environmental tobacco smoke (ETS), non-smokers can attain expiratory CO levels of 6–9 ppm [13] and the cut-off between non-smokers and smokers is 8–10 ppm in most smoking cessation studies.

The correlation between arterial blood CO levels and expiratory air CO levels is high but in more severe COPD patients with decreased diffusion capacity, expiratory air CO might underestimate the blood levels and in light smokers, smoking 3–6 cigarettes daily, CO levels might be below 10 ppm.

The portable CO analyser is a relative simple, cheap and quick method to assess the CO level in expiratory air. It is important to hold the breath for 15–20 s to attain equilibrium between capillary and alveolar CO levels. The result is displayed immediately. False-positive values may be observed in subjects with lactose malabsorption and although an ethanol filter is present, high concentrations of ethanol in the breath may interfere with measurements. Drifting of the zero point may be observed if many smokers are tested consecutively. Calibration of the CO analyser is indicated every 3 months with a 50 ppm CO test gas. Without CO monitoring, approximately 10% of relapsers may state that they do not smoke.

Whenever an arterial blood sample is obtained in COPD patients on long-term oxygen therapy (LTOT), the CO level should also be analysed to identify smokers. Such individuals should be encouraged to stop smoking and should be specifically warned of the risk of fire.

The mean baseline expiratory air CO level in the CEASE study was 27 ppm (mean), (SD, 10 ppm) in 3575 smokers with a mean consumption of 27 cigarettes/day (SD, 10 ppm), all smokers consuming > 14 cigarettes/day [12]. In an Italian study of 550 consecutive patients with COPD and 100 patients on LTOT, arterial carboxyhaemoglobin was more than 2% (= 10 ppm) in 26% of the 550 COPD patients and in 21% of the patients on LTOT who smoked [14].

Plasma, saliva or urinary nicotine can be used to determine smoking status when taken in the afternoon; however, because of its short half-life of 2 h its not useful in assessing smoking more than 8–12 h previously. Cotinine, the major metabolite of nicotine with a half-life of 16–36 h, has a high specificity for tobacco use with a cut-off level indicating smoking of 15 ng/mL in saliva and plasma and 50 ng/mL in urine, if the patient does not use NRT.

Thiocyanate, with a half-life of 3–14 days, is a reasonable biomarker for heavy smoking, but is not good for detecting light smoking because of the contribution from dietary sources. The cut-off level of 78–88 µmol/L in plasma is commonly used [15].

Treatment

Figure 53.2 is a flow diagram for the management of the individual smoking COPD patient. All smoking COPD patients should be advised to quit smoking by the physician and the message should be repeated on subsequent visits and the advice to quit should be personalized and related to the individual patient (degree of reduced lung function, daily respiratory symptoms, other smoking-related risk factors). The advice to quit should be given independently of the smoker's motivation to quit.

If the smoker wants to quit, a target quit day should be set. If the patient is hospitalized – this should be regarded

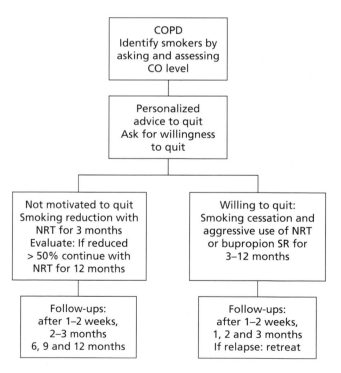

Figure 53.2 Handling of smoking in COPD patients. CO, carbon monoxide; NRT, nicotine replacement therapy.

as a window of opportunity – and a quit attempt should be started at once, irrespective of the patient's motivation to quit. Smoke-free units facilitate this process and should be implemented worldwide.

Nicotine replacement therapy

Nicotine is liberated from the acid cigarette smoke as a gas, inhaled to the lungs, transferred via the alveoli to the blood and is measurable in the brain in less than 8 s after inhalation. All the nicotine products that are used for the purpose of smoking cessation are absorbed through the skin or mucous membranes. The delivery of nicotine by these routes is much slower than by inhalation, and does not give the quick plasma concentration as does cigarette smoking. In addition, acidification of the mouth (e.g. by acidic food or beverages), by increasing the fraction of nicotine that is ionized, will further decrease absorption of oral formulations. Six hours after a 21-mg transdermal patch is applied, the blood level is approximately 10–17 ng/mL, in contrast to approximately 15–25 ng/mL within minutes after a cigarette [16].

The rapid absorption from cigarette smoke results in a transient high blood concentration. This has a greater psychoactive effect and likely biological effect that reinforces addiction, compared with the equivalent dose of nicotine delivered from gums or patches [17]. Compared with cigarette smoking, NRT produces lower plasma nicotine levels (i.e. one-third to half of the levels attained over several hours) and without the high peak levels. The slower absorption of nicotine from these products does not produce the same cardiovascular stimulation as does nicotine delivered by cigarette smoke [18].

The average 12-month success rate reported in most smoking cessation studies is approximately 15–25% [2].

The efficacy of NRT from a Cochrane meta-analysis reported an odds ratio for success of NRT compared with controls of 1.73 (95% CI, 1.62–1.85), with no statistical differences across the different formulations (Table 53.6) [19].

Nicotine transdermal patch

Absorption of nicotine from the transdermal nicotine patch is approximately 1 mg/h nicotine for 16 h (daytime patch) or for 24 h (24-h patch). Nicotine substitution is approximately 50% of the smoking level (21-mg patch/24 h and 15-mg patch/16 h) [16]. It is much easier to administer and use the patch than the gum. The recommended treatment duration is 8–12 weeks. Side-effects are mainly self-limited, mild, local skin irritation, occurring in 10–20% of users. A few per cent of subjects will terminate patch use because of more persistent and severe skin irritation in the nicotine

Table 53.6 Meta-analysis of controlled trials with nicotine replacement therapy from The Cochrane Register. Success rates sustained for 1 year [19,37].

NRT versus placebo	*1.73*
(108 studies)	(95% CI, 1.62–1.85)
Nicotine gum	1.66
Nicotine patch	1.76
Nicotine nasal spray	2.27
Nicotine inhaler	2.08
Nicotine sublingual tablet	1.73
Bupropion SR versus placebo	*1.97*
(16 studies)	(95% CI, 1.67–2.34)

CI, confidence interval; NRT, nicotine replacement therapy.

patch area [17]. Wearing the patch during waking hours (approximately 16 h/day) has been found to be as effective as wearing it for 24 h/day and there is no evidence that tapered therapy is better than abrupt withdrawal.

While the patch is a fixed delivery system, the delivered dose from the gum, inhaler, nasal spray and lozenge is dependent on the frequency of dosing. A basic advantage of these four products is the ability to self-titrate the dose as opposed to the patch, which delivers a fixed dose. Thus, it is possible to administer a dose whenever needed during the day; however, the principal disadvantage is potential underdosing. These products may also replace some of the habit patterns associated with smoking (e.g. handling reinforcement) along with providing nicotine replacement.

Nicotine chewing gum

With the use of nicotine gum throughout the day, blood levels of approximately one-third (for 2-mg gum) and two-thirds (for 4-mg gum) of the nicotine obtained through smoking are achieved.

In most studies the gum has been used for at least 6–12 weeks and, in some, up to 1 year, but individualization of treatment duration is recommended. As many as 10% of successful quitters still use the gum after 12 months [20–22]. While controversial, many believe that this long-term substitution of gum has fewer health risks than continued smoking.

Instruction in gum use is very important to increase effectiveness and adherence to therapy. Gum users should chew a piece of gum only 5–10 times until they can taste the nicotine. At that point, they should then let the gum rest in the cheek for a few minutes, while the nicotine is absorbed. This occurs through the buccal mucosa, and swallowing should be avoided. After this, they can chew again to expose a new surface of the gum, which will release more nicotine. Overexuberant chewing may release too much nicotine, which may be swallowed and may contribute to gastric side-effects. The gum can be chewed for approximately 20–30 min and, with proper use, approximately 0.8–1.0 mg nicotine is absorbed from a piece of 2-mg nicotine gum and 1.2–1.4 mg nicotine from a 4-mg piece. The principal disadvantage of gum use is potential underdosing, which might explain the lack of effect in several trials. Programmes with more intense counselling generally get better results with the gum, perhaps because these programmes include training in its use. The approximate dose equivalent with most nicotine patches is approximately 20 pieces of 2-mg gum, whereas the mean number of pieces of gum used daily is only around 5–6 in most studies, consistent with the general underdosing of the gum.

Side-effects of the gum consist mainly of mild, transient, local symptoms in the mouth, throat and stomach due to swallowed nicotine (e.g. nausea, vomiting, indigestion and hiccups). After adequate instruction most smokers can learn to use the gum properly but without instructions many will discontinue use or underdose themselves.

In the Lung Health Study, among 3094 smokers who were followed for 5 years, the use of the 2-mg gum appeared safe and did not produce cardiovascular problems or other adverse events even in subjects who continued to smoke and still used nicotine gum [23].

It is suggested that smokers be instructed to use the nicotine gum on a fixed schedule (e.g. every hour, from early morning, for at least 8–10 h) and use extra pieces of gum whenever needed.

Nicotine inhaler

An inhaler consists of a mouthpiece and a plastic tube with a porous plug impregnated with nicotine, which releases nicotine vapour when air is drawn through the plug. Most of the nicotine released by this device is absorbed through the mucosa of the mouth and throat. Very little of the nicotine is contained in particles of sufficient size to be inhaled into the lung. Each inhaler contains 10 mg nicotine and can release approximately 4–5 mg nicotine. In clinical use, each inhaler releases approximately 2–3 mg nicotine and the number of inhalers used daily averages 5–6. Thus, nicotine levels comparable with those found with use of the 2-mg nicotine gum are attainable (i.e. relatively low concentrations are achieved).

The inhaler may replace some of the habit patterns associated with smoking (e.g. oral and handling reinforcement) along with providing nicotine replacement. Current recommendations suggest at least four inhalers should be used per day, with the goal being 4–10 per day. The duration of use is generally 3 months with another 3 months of downtitration if needed. With rapid and frequent puffing it is possible to increase the delivered dose of nicotine. It has been suggested that the number of puffs on the inhaler should be around 10 times that of the usual puffing on a cigarette to get a similar amount of nicotine.

The efficacy of the inhaler in clinical trials is in the same range as the other NRT products [24–27].

Nicotine lozenge (sublingual tablet)

One to two sublingual tablets should be placed under the tongue where they will disintegrate within 20–30 min. The free nicotine released from the tablets will be absorbed through the oral mucous membrane. The dose delivered from the tablet is comparable with the 2-mg nicotine chewing gum. One tablet per hour is the recommended dosage, up to 20 per day (i.e. up to 2 tablets per hour). In highly dependent subjects, a maximum dose up to 40 tablets per day can be used. Swallowing results in delivery of nicotine to the stomach, which can cause side-effects but does not contribute to efficacy. Mild transient side-effects include hiccups, nausea and dyspepsia, and gingival bleeding. The tablets should be used for up to 3 months. The dosage is 8–20 (40) tablets per day or 1–2 tablets per hour, depending on withdrawal symptoms and craving [28].

Nicotine nasal spray

Nicotine nasal spray is an aqueous solution of nicotine (10 mg/mL) that delivers 0.5 mg nicotine per actuation [2]. When sprayed in the nose, nicotine is absorbed across the nasal mucosa, with peak blood levels being achieved in approximately 10 min. This delivery is much more rapid than that of other forms of NRT. In clinical trials, however, cessation rates are comparable with other NRT trials, with quit rates about double that of placebo. Side-effects include nasal irritation, which may be severe and is extremely common. The usual regimen is two actuations per dose (1 mg total) once or twice per hour, with a maximum total dosage of 40 mg/day.

Combination of NRT products and dose–response effects

There is conflicting evidence regarding the efficacy of the combination of two different nicotine products. In some studies the use of combinations has increased short-term cessation rates, but there is no consistent evidence of a long-term effect [19]. However, available data suggest that combinations can be used safely without symptoms of nicotine overdose such as weakness, nausea, sweating, palpitations and diarrhoea.

A small dose–response effect has been observed with the nicotine gum and patch. For highly nicotine-dependent

Table 53.7 Suggestions for use of four different nicotine replacement products.

	Patch	Gum	Inhaler	Lozenge
Absorption	Skin	Mouth	Mouth, throat	Mouth
Principle*	Fixed	Ad lib	Ad lib	Ad lib
Daily dose	1 patch 15–25 mg	1 piece/h 10–20 mg	6–10, 10–15 mg	8–20 tablets, 16–40 mg
Dose per piece	15 mg/16 h, 21 mg/24 h	2/4 mg	10 mg	1 mg/2 mg
Delivered dose	15 or 21 mg	0.8/1.4 mg	3–5 mg	0.8–1.0 mg
Duration of use	3 months	3 months (12 months)	3 months (6 months)	3 months (6 months)
Side-effects	Skin irritation	Hiccups, irritation in mouth, dyspepsia	Irritation in throat	Irritation in mouth, hiccups, dyspepsia
Precautions	Eczema	Dentures	Pharyngitis	Oral disease
Low dependency	+++	+++	+++	++
High dependency	+	+++	++	++

Combination treatment: patch plus either gum/inhaler or lozenge.

Long-term treatment or relapse situations: gum, inhaler or lozenge.

High-dependent subjects: patch 25 mg/16 h or 21 mg/24 h; 4 mg gum.

* Nicotine 'infusion' through the skin is constant with the patch.

smokers, 4-mg nicotine gum has been shown to result in a higher success rate than the 2-mg gum.

In subjects who relapse, repeated treatment should be undertaken at the earliest appropriate occasion. The success rate seems higher for subjects who had tried to quit previously without nicotine products, but most smokers achieve long-term abstinence only after several attempts.

In the Lung Health Study, where 3000 subjects were exposed to nicotine gum for up to 5 years, the concomitant use of cigarettes and NRT appeared to be safe and unrelated to any cardiovascular illness or other serious side-effects [23].

Thus, the current recommendation is to use one NRT product in most smokers. In the heavily dependent smoker, a combination of the patch with gum, inhaler or lozenge can be tried.

If the smoker has not tried NRT before, initial use of the patch is reasonable. First, it is easier for the patient and the physician. Secondly, self-selection of an NRT product does not increase success rate. If a patient has tried one of the NRT products earlier, a reasonable recommendation would be to try bupropion SR (see below) or another NRT product (Table 53.7). A test period with NRT for a few days before the target quit day to habituate the patient to the product might facilitate adequate initial dosing, which is important for success.

Effect of support

The effect of intensity of support is shown in Table 53.8. Three studies with a more intensive supportive programme

Table 53.8 Intensive group therapy or low intervention combined with nicotine replacement therapy or placebo. Continuous 12-month success rates. (Data from Hjalmarson *et al.* [25,29,30] and Tønnesen *et al.* [24,31,32].)

Intensive support (Hjalmarson)		Intensive support (Hjalmarson)	
Gum	29%	Placebo	16%
Nasal spray	27%	Placebo	15%
Inhaler	28%	Placebo	18%
Low support (Tønnesen)		Low support (Tønnesen)	
Inhaler	15%	Placebo	5%
Patch	17%	Placebo	4%
Bupropion SR	21%	Placebo	11%

with weekly group meetings showed high continuous success rates in both active NRT and placebo groups. In contrast, two other NRT studies with lower support but a very similar design reported much lower success rates, although the relative effect of NRT versus placebo was maintained [24,25,29–31]. The support in the bupropion SR study is moderate as are the success rates (Table 53.8) [32]. A meta-analysis evaluating behavioural interventions does not suggest that group therapy is more effective than individual counselling, but the total contact time per patient may be higher during group treatment [2].

Hypnosis and acupuncture have not proven to be of any effect in smoking cessation.

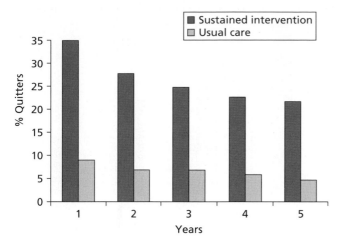

Figure 53.3 Lung Health Study: sustained abstinence ($n = 5587$.) (Data from Anthonisen *et al.* [33].)

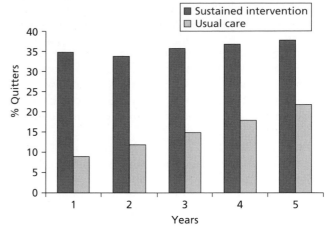

Figure 53.4 Lung Health Study: point prevalence ($n = 5587$) (Data from Anthonisen *et al.* [33].)

Lung Health Study I

The Lung Health Study I was a multicentre randomized study evaluating the rate of decline of lung function. It compared the effect of a smoking intervention versus usual care and also tested an inhaled anticholinergic bronchodilator or placebo. The study enrolled a total of 5887 subjects with mild COPD: a mean forced expiratory volume in 1 s (FEV_1) of 75% predicted (2.7 L [SD, 0.6 L]). They had a mean age of 48 years, with a smoking history of 40 pack-years [33]. During the first 3 months, an intensive 12-session smoking cessations programme took place, with the use of nicotine chewing gum plus adjunctive behavioural modification, with a relapse prevention programme every 4 months for 5 years. At entry, strong physician advice to quit was given, and a target-quit day was set. Two milligram nicotine gum was used aggressively.

The sustained quit rate was high in the intervention group and declined as usual over the years of the study. Continuous abstinence rates in the intervention group were 35% after 1 year, but had declined to 22% after 5 years. These compared with 10% after 1 year and 5% after 5 years in the control group (Fig. 53.3). However, the cross-sectional quit rate increased slightly during the 5 years of the study to 39% in the intervention group and 22% in the control group (Fig. 53.4). This supports the importance of subsequent quit attempts.

A major finding of the Lung Health Study I was that smoking cessation significantly reduced the age-related decline in FEV_1. The change in FEV_1 was −72 mL over 5 years for sustained quitters and −301 mL over 5 years for continuing smokers. Follow-up after 11 years showed that 22% (odds ratio [OR] = 4.45) of the subjects assigned to the inter-vention group maintained abstinence versus only 6% in the control group [34].

Overall, this large well-conducted study showed that aggressive and intensive smoking cessation programmes can produce high long-term quit rates in smokers with mild airway obstruction. Also, the improvement in the rate of the decline of FEV_1 supports the concept that smoking cessation is the first and most important intervention in smokers with mild COPD.

Bupropion SR

Bupropion SR (Zyban®, GlaxoWellcome) is an older antidepressant drug – an amino-ketone agent – with an inhibitory effect on noradrenaline and dopamine reuptake. In addition, it may also have direct effects on nicotine receptors. However, the exact mechanism by which bupropion SR aids in smoking cessation is not known.

Bupropion SR for 7–12 weeks is more effective than placebo. When combined with moderate behavioural support (weekly clinic visits during the first 7 weeks and follow-up), a 1-year sustained quit rate of 18–25% was observed for bupropion SR and 10% for placebo [35,36]. A meta-analysis of 16 studies found OR 1.97 (95% CI, 1.7–2.3) for 1-year success rate for active versus placebo therapy. This efficacy is in accordance with the success rates found in many studies with NRT that provided support in the same range. Thus, bupropion SR and NRT seem to be equally effective for smoking cessation (Table 53.6) [37]. Although when used for 1 year bupropion SR prolongs time to relapse, this difference in continuous abstinence rate was not significant from week 36 through to month 24 [38]. Thus, 7–12 weeks' treatment with bupropion

SR seems an adequate treatment duration for smoking cessation, although longer treatment prolongs time to relapse.

The recommended regimen for bupropion SR is 150 mg a.m. for 6 days prior to the quit date, in order to establish adequate brain levels. Therapy should then continue with 150 mg b.i.d. for 7–12 weeks. Success has been achieved in some individuals with a reduced dosage of 150 mg/day.

Although body-weight gain is significantly reduced during the drug treatment period with bupropion SR, this effect is lost after 1–2 years.

Recycling (i.e. repeated treatment with bupropion SR) in smokers treated previously with bupropion SR should be tried as this increased successful outcome in a randomized controlled trial of 450 smokers. In this study of relapsed smokers, a 6-month continuous success rate of 12% was observed for the bupropion SR group and 2% for the placebo group [39].

The most common adverse events from bupropion SR are insomnia (42%) and dry mouth (11%). In clinical trials, in approximately 10–12% of subjects, the treatment was stopped because of adverse events. The most serious adverse event was major motor seizures, which have been reported in 0.1% of patients treated with bupropion SR, and allergic reactions (1–2) with 0.1% of serious cases of hypersensitivity [40].

Bupropion SR is not indicated for individuals with an increased risk of seizures (e.g. epilepsy, history of head trauma, anorexia nervosa). Similarly, it is important not to increase the dose above 300 mg, and to administer the daily dose divided with an interval of at least 8 h. The last dose should not be taken later than 6 p.m. if insomnia is a problem.

In summary, bupropion SR is of similar efficacy to NRT and is generally well tolerated in smoking cessation. It is regarded a first-line medication in some guidelines [2]. As bupropion SR has a more severe side-effect profile, more contraindications and is only available on prescription, NRT is often regarded as first-line medication and bupropion SR as a second-line, although this is a matter of personal judgement. Some physicians who are comfortable with the medication will use bupropion SR as a first-line medication.

As another antidepressant, nortriptyline, has been shown to be effective in smoking cessation, it is not clear if the effect in smoking cessation of these two agents is drug-specific or a class effect. The dosage of nortriptyline in smoking cessation is 75–150 mg/day. However, several other antidepressants including selective serotonin reuptake inhibitors have not been found to be effective in smoking cessation (e.g. doxepin, fluoxetine, sertraline, moclobemide and venlafaxine) [37].

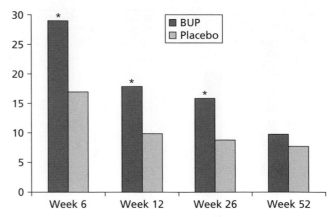

Figure 53.5 Continous quit rate in COPD patients with bupropion SR (BUP) versus placebo ($n = 404$). * = p-values of 0.002, 0.021, 0.04. (Data from Tashkin *et al.* [41] and Jarvis *et al.* [42].)

Bupropion SR COPD Study

One study has specifically evaluated bupropion SR in COPD patients. In this study, 404 COPD patients (15+ cigarettes per day) in 11 centres in the USA were allocated to bupropion SR for 3 months or placebo in a design that included moderately intensive behavioural support (i.e. 10 visits) with weekly individual sessions during the first 7 weeks (Fig. 53.5) [41]. Most patients had COPD with an $FEV_1 > 50\%$ although 15% had an $FEV_1 < 35$–49%. Cigarette consumption averaged 28 cigarettes per day and subjects had smoked an average of 52 pack-years. These subjects were relatively highly addicted with an average Fagerström score of 7 (maximal score 11). Abstinence rate was significantly higher at 6 months in the bupropion SR group versus placebo (16 vs 9%). After 1 year the significance was lost with a success rate of 10 vs 8%. These abstinence rates are much lower than those observed in similar studies with bupropion SR in healthy subjects [42], suggesting that COPD patients may be relatively 'hard core'. Nevertheless, the data support use of bupropion SR in this group.

Lung clinic interventions

Two large trials were conducted by the British Thoracic Society (BTS) in the UK in 1983 and 1990. One study comprised 1618 outpatients with respiratory disease attending a chest clinic [43]. Four methods were evaluated: physician advice, plus a booklet, plus placebo gum, and plus 2-mg nicotine chewing gum. The overall 1-year success rate for the entire population was 9.7% (95% CI, 8.3–11.3%) with no significant differences between the four groups.

The other study included two multicentre trials with outpatients attending hospital or chest clinics [44]. A total of 87% of the enrolled patients suffered from respiratory disease, mainly chronic bronchitis and emphysema.

In study A, the effect of physician advice to stop smoking was compared with the same advice plus a signed agreement to stop smoking by a target quit day plus two visits by a health visitor plus several letters. These two interventions were found to be equally effective. In study B, four groups were compared: physician advice versus advice plus a signed agreement versus advice plus letters versus advice plus letters plus a signed agreement. A signed agreement did not affect outcome but letters increased successful outcome from 5.1% to 8.7%. A secondary stratification and analysis of the two studies combined found that 5% stopped with advice alone; postal encouragement increased the success rate by more than half as much again; and outpatient visits seemed to increase the success rate. In conclusion, physician advice supported by encouraging letters and follow-up was found to be more effective than advice alone in a group of outpatients with respiratory disease.

In the lung clinic of the author, we have observed that minimal intervention (i.e. advice by nurses) increased 1-year quit rates from 3.6% to 8.7% [45] and that a nurse-directed smoking cessation programme which included nicotine patches increased quitting from 6% to 16% [46]. Similar programmes could easily be implemented as routine in most lung clinics.

Weight gain

Weight gain can be regarded as a withdrawal symptom. It occurs in part because of increased hunger and increased caloric intake, but metabolic effects may also have a role. As a result, a weight gain of 4–5 kg for abstainers after 1 year is found in most studies. About half of the participants in smoking cessation studies are specifically afraid of gaining weight, a problem that may be more prominent for females. Both NRT – especially nicotine gum – and bupropion SR can delay post-cessation weight gain. However, when NRT or bupropion SR are stopped, the ex-smoker will eventually end up with a similar weight gain as quitters who had not used medication [19,37].

In the Lung Health Study sustained quitters gained 5.2 kg (women) and 4.9 kg (men) in year 1 and experienced an additional gain of 3.4 kg (women) and 2.6 kg (men) in years 1–5. Over 5 years, 33% of the abstainers gained 10 kg in weight [47]. A weight gain after 3 months of 4.5 kg in men and 3.6 kg in women was found in the study with COPD patients and bupropion SR or placebo [41]. Weight gain prevention using caffeine plus ephedrine or a serotonergic anorexic drug – difenfluramine – did not increase the success rate for abstinence and, while weight gain was less in the prevention group during active treatment, there were no differences at 1 year [48]. In an open smoking cessation study with 287 females, nicotine gum combined with a behavioural weight control programme including a very low energy diet versus a control group without the diet resulted in an increase in success rate although there was no difference in weight gain after 1 year [49]. Thus, diet intervention and daily exercise might be a way to control excessive weight gain in the long term. For those COPD patients with low body mass index (BMI), this post-cessation weight increase might be an advantage together with increased appetite.

From the Lung Health Study it was reported that the weight gain in sustained quitters had a small negative effect on lung function; a reduction of forced vital capacity (*FVC*) of 17 mL/kg (men) and 11 mL/kg (women), and for FEV_1 of 11 mL/kg (men) and 6 mL/kg (women), respectively [50], but compared with the beneficial effect of smoking cessation this effect of weight gain is small.

Profile of COPD smokers

Why do COPD smokers achieve a lower success rate in smoking cessation? This might in part be because of selection, as the more motivated and less nicotine-dependent smokers with COPD probably successfully quit smoking when they suffered acute respiratory symptoms or were advised to stop smoking by their physician. In support of this, in a random population sample of smokers, subjects with COPD had a higher nicotine dependence and higher CO levels compared with smokers without COPD [51]. In addition, nearly half of all patients with COPD experience some depressive symptoms and 20% have had at least one major depressive episode. Depression is a predictor of relapse in smoking cessation, and the prevalence of this comorbidity may contribute to the refractoriness of smoking in COPD patients. Finally, there is an overrepresentation of the lower socio-economic classes among COPD patients, who also often have a poor social network and support system. Both lower social class and poor social support are predictors of failure in smoking cessation [52].

Approximately one-third of moderate to severe COPD patients evaluated in many clinical trials are still smoking. In a 1-year study of formoterol/budesonide with 812 COPD patients with a mean FEV_1 of 36% predicted normal, 34% were smokers [53]. In another 3-year study with fluticasone with 391 with mild COPD ($FEV_1 = 1.6$ L), 35% were smokers. Among 359 with severe COPD ($FEV_1 = 1.0$ L), 41% were smokers [54]. This group consists of more heavily dependent and persistent smokers and is representative of the group of COPD patients with frequent exacerbations and hospitalizations. Anticipated quit rates among these COPD patients would be lower than among healthy self-referred smokers enrolled in most smoking cessation studies.

There are limited data on the efficacy of smoking cessation interventions in COPD patients. Bupropion SR has efficacy in COPD patients compared with placebo, although quit rates are lower than in healthy subjects [41]. In two studies with patients with COPD and cardiovascular diseases, no effect of NRT was found, but NRT was used for an interval that was likely less than optimal (3 weeks and 4–6 weeks, respectively) [55,56].

A meta-analysis of 17 trials of smoking cessation interventions for hospitalized patients showed that 'intensive intervention' (inpatient contact plus follow-up for at least a month) was associated with higher quit rates than in controls (OR 1.82; 95% CI, 1.49–2.22, six trials). Results of NRT treatment in this group of patients were compatible with data from other trials, suggesting that NRT increases quit rates [57].

From a review of five smoking cessation studies with COPD patients, two of which were of high quality (see the discussion of the BTS studies above), it was concluded that a combination of psychosocial and pharmacological intervention was superior to no treatment or psychosocial therapy alone [58]. In a recent trial 370 COPD patients were enrolled in a smoking cessation study with low and high support and use of sublingual nicotine of placebo for 12 weeks [59]. They smoked a mean of 19.6 cigarettes/day with a mean of 42.7 pack-years and with a mean FEV_1 of 56% predicted. The 6 and 12 month point-prevalence abstinence rate for nicotine sublingual vs placebo was 23 vs 10% and 17 vs 10%, respectively. This success rate is in the same range as healthy smokers. Quality of life assessed by the *St. Georges's Respiratory Questionnaire* score improved significantly in abstainers vs non-abstainers; the changes in mean scores were −10.9 vs −2.9 for tatal score, and −28.6 vs 2.3 for symptom score, respectively. This is the first trial documenting that NRT is also effective in a COPD population.

Smoking reduction

The rationale for smoking reduction is as follows:
1 By using this approach it should be possible to recruit a new segment of smokers (i.e. smokers low in motivation to quit).
2 It should be possible to induce a permanent change in the smoking habit to maintain the reduced smoking level.
3 Compensatory smoking is not 100% so that reduction in smoking will result in reduced toxin exposure.
4 This concept will not interfere with smoking cessation.

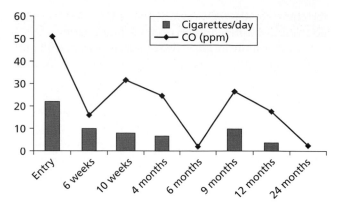

Figure 53.6 Smoking reduction (patient NN). CO, carbon monoxide.

Four randomized controlled trials used nicotine inhalers and nicotine gum and reported – surprisingly – a smoking cessation rate of approximately 10% after 2 years and a low reduction rate of 6% [60,61]. An example of a smoker who reduced and then quit is shown in Fig. 53.6. Regarding reduction, an analysis of 19 trials reported a reduction in cigarettes per day (CPD) of 25% (8 cigarettes) to 55% (23 cigarettes) in NRT groups compared with 13% (3 cigarettes) to 26% (8 cigarettes) in control groups [62].

However, there is no consistent evidence that smoking reduction per se will be followed by harm reduction. In a prospective population study, self-reported smoking reduction was not associated with lower risk of hospital admission for COPD, while quitting smoking was associated with a relative hazard of 0.57 for hospitalization [63]. In the same population, with a 16-year follow-up it was observed that smoking cessation reduces mortality and morbidity risk while smoking reduction did not [64].

An approach for COPD smokers not motivated to quit could be to prescribe NRT – nicotine gum or inhaler – for 2–3 months and recommended to reduce the number of cigarettes by at least 50% during the first 1–2 weeks and then to try to reduce further, although this concept has only been tested in healthy smokers. If the smoker has not reduced by more than 50% after 3 months NRT should be stopped. The goal is that smoking reduction will motivate this group of recalcitrant smokers to quit during this process.

Another way to attain smoking reduction and reduce the harm of smoking could be through tobacco product modification. The use of such products, however, raises a number of extremely controversial issues [65]. At the present time, there is no evidence supporting health benefits from their use. However, as it is likely that smoking will remain a highly prevalent condition, the development of a less hazardous cigarette might be an advantage. How such a product should be regulated and used will require careful scrutiny.

Research recommendations

There is a strong need to increase our knowledge of the efficacy of NRT and bupropion SR in COPD patients. Long-term treatment that includes combination pharmaco-therapy and group therapy might be of special value for the more severe COPD patient with a vulnerable social network. The influence of depression and psychiatric comorbidity on smoking cessation in COPD should be further explored. Correlation between nicotine dependence, motivation to quit and severity of COPD is another unexplored area.

The design of the Lung Health Study needs to be applied in studies enrolling severe COPD patients.

Pathophysiological studies need to be performed in smokers with mild to severe COPD before and after quitting, looking at lung function, inflammatory mediators and pulmonary imaging.

Studies of implementation of smoking cessation programmes in the chest clinic and quality control of this therapy could increase interest in this area. Standards for smoking cessation interventions and formal accreditation of this area might be a way to increase implementation of smoking cessation.

Several new agents for smoking cessation are being tested in clinical trials and these agents should also be tested in the COPD population. Although lower success rates may be observed among COPD patients compared with healthy smokers, knowledge of how these treatments work in special populations is crucial.

Conclusions

In summary, smoking cessation should be an integral part of the treatment of COPD patients. This is clearly stated in the recently published COPD guidelines: all COPD patients still smoking, regardless of age, should be encouraged to stop smoking and offered help with appropriate support to do so at every opportunity [65].

Every chest clinic should be smoke-free and have a teamwork-oriented organization for smoking cessation. As a result, every smoking COPD patient should be identified, advised to quit smoking and, if willing to quit, instructed in the use of NRT or bupropion SR and follow-up for the smoking cessation arranged. Every quit attempt should be given the maximal chance for success. Because both NRT and bupropion SR double long-term success in smoking cessation when used for 3 months, at least one should be used on every attempt.

The programme used in the Lung Health Study with an intensive initial smoking cessation programme with NRT, followed by boosters during subsequent visits, seems to be a design with a high sustained quit rate in COPD patients. Smoking should regarded as a chronic relapsing disorder, and it might be necessary to make several cessation attempts before permanent cessation is obtained. The COPD patient should be regarded as a hard-core smoker with the need for more aggressive therapy both with regard to NRT and behavioural support and might be a candidate for long-term NRT substitution.

References

1 NHLB/WHO Workshop. *Global Initiative for Chronic Obstructive Lung Disease*. US Department of Health and Human Services, National Institutes of Health, National Heart, Lung and Blood Institute, NIH Publ. No. 2701A, 2001.

2 Fiore MC, Bailey WC, Cohen SJ *et al*. *Treating Tobacco Use and Dependence*. Clinical Practice Guideline. Rockville, MD: US Department of Health and Human Services. Public Health Service, June 2000.

3 Raw M, McNeil A, West R. Smoking cessation guidelines and their cost effectiveness. *Thorax* 1998;**53**(Suppl 5):S1–37.

4 West R, McNeil A, Raw M. Smoking cessation guidelines for health professionals: an update. *Thorax* 2000;**55**:987–99.

5 Batra V, Patkar AA, Berrettini WH, Weinstein SP, Leone FT. The genetic determinants of smoking. *Chest* 2003;**123**: 1730–9.

6 Haustein KO. *Tobacco or Health? Physiological and Social Damages Caused by Tobacco Smoking*. Berlin: Springer, 2003: 59–77.

7 Watkins SS, Koob GF, Markou A. Neural mechanisms underlying nicotine addiction: acute positive reinforcement and withdrawal. *Nicotine Tob Res* 2000;**2**:19–37.

8 Fagerström KO, Heatherton TF, Kozlowski LT. Nicotine addiction and its assessment. *Ear Nose Throat J* 1991;**69**: 763–8.

9 Hughes JR, Gust SW, Skoog K, Keenan RM, Fenwick JW. Symptoms of tobacco withdrawal: a replication and extension. *Arch Gen Psychiatry* 1991;**48**:52–9.

10 American Psychiatric Association. *Diagnostic and Statistical Manual of Mental Disorders-IV*. Washington, DC: APA, 1994.

11 Hughes JR. Smoking cessation among self-quitters. *Health Psychol* 1992;**11**:331–4.

12 Tønnesen P, Paoletti P, Gustavsson G *et al*., members of the Steering Committee of CEASE on behalf of the European Respiratory Society. Higher dosage nicotine patches increase one-year smoking cessation rates: results from the European CEASE trial. *Eur Respir J* 1999;**13**:238–46.

13 Jarvis MJ, Russell MA, Saloojee Y. Expired air carbon monoxide: a simple breath test of tobacco smoke intake. *BMJ* 1980;**281**:484–5.

14 Rizzi M, Andreoli A, Greco M *et al*. Smoking habits in severe respiratory insufficiency, *Eur Respir J* 1995;214S.

15 SRNT Subcommittee on Biochemical Verification. Biochemical verification of tobacco use and cessation. *Nicotine Tob Res* 2002;**4**:149–59.

16 Fagerström KO, Säwe U, Tønnesen P. Therapeutic use of nicotine patches: efficacy and safety. *J Smoking Relat Dis* 1992;**3**:247–61.

17 Palme KJ, Brickley MM, Faulds D. Transdermal nicotine: a review of its pharmacodynamic and pharmacokinetic properties and therapeutic efficacy as an aid to smoking cessation. *Drugs* 1992;**44**:498–529.

18 Benowitz NL. Smoking-induced coronary vasoconstriction: implications for therapeutic use of nicotine. *J Am Coll Cardiol* 1993;**22**:648–9.

19 Silagy C, Lancaster T, Stead L, Mant D, Fowler G. Nicotine replacement therapy for smoking cessation. *Cochrane Database Syst Rev* 2004;**3**:CD000146.

20 Tønnesen P, Fryd V, Hansen M *et al*. Effect of nicotine chewing gum in combination with group counseling on the cessation of smoking. *N Engl J Med* 1988;**318**:15–8.

21 Puska P, Bjorkqvist S, Koskela K. Nicotine containing chewing gum in smoking cessation: a double-blind trial with half year follow-up. *Addict Behav* 1979;**4**:141–6.

22 Killen JD, Fortmann SP, Newman B, Varady A. Evaluation of a treatment approach combining nicotine gum with self-guided behavioral treatments for smoking relapse prevention. *J Consult Clin Psychol* 1990;**58**:85–92.

23 Murray RP, Bailey WC, Daniels K *et al*. Safety of nicotine polacrilex gum used by 3094 participants in the Lung Health Study. Lung Health Study Research Group. *Chest* 1996;**109**: 438–45.

24 Tønnesen P, Nørregaard J, Mikkelsen K, Jørgensen S, Nilsson F. A double-blind trial of a nicotine inhaler for smoking cessation. *JAMA* 1993;**269**:1268–71.

25 Hjalmarson A, Nilsson F, Sjöstrom L, Wiklund O. The nicotine inhaler in smoking cessation. *Arch Intern Med* 1997;**157**: 1721–8.

26 Leischow JJ, Nilsson F, Franzon M *et al*. Efficacy of the nicotine inhaler as an adjunct to smoking cessation. *Am J Health Behav* 1996;**20**:264–71.

27 Schneider NG, Olmstead R, Nilsson F *et al*. Efficacy of a nicotine inhaler in smoking cessation: a double-blind, placebo-controlled trial. *Addiction* 1996;**91**:1293–306.

28 Wallström M, Nilsson F, Hirch JM. A randomized, double-blind, placebo-controlled clinical evaluation of a nicotine sublingual tablet in smoking cessation. *Addiction* 2000;**95**:1161–71.

29 Hjalmarson AI. Effect of nicotine chewing gum in smoking cessation: a randomized, placebo-controlled, double-blind study. *JAMA* 1984;**252**:2835–8.

30 Hjalmarson A, Franzon M, Westin A, Wiklund O. Effect of nicotine nasal spray on smoking cessation: a randomized, placebo-controlled, double-blind study. *Arch Intern Med* 1994;**154**:2567–72.

31 Tønnesen P, Nørregaard J, Simonsen K, Säewe U. A double-blind trial of a 16-hour transdermal patch in smoking cessation. *N Engl J Med* 1991;**325**:311–5.

32 Tønnesen P, Tonstad S, Hjalmarson A *et al*. A multicentre, randomized, double-blind, placebo-controlled, 1-year study of bupropion SR for smoking cessation. *J Intern Med* 2003; **254**:184–92.

33 Anthonisen NR, Connett JE, Kiley JP *et al*. Effects of smoking intervention and the use of an inhaled anticholinergic bronchodilator on the rate of decline of FEV_1. The lung health study. *JAMA* 1994;**272**:1497–505.

34 Murray RP, Connett JE, Rand CS, Pan W, Anthonisen NR. Persistence of the effect of the Lung Health Study smoking intervention over 11 years. *Prev Med* 2002;**35**:314–9.

35 Hurt RD, Sachs DPL, Glover ED *et al*. A comparison of sustained release bupropion and placebo for smoking cessation. *N Engl J Med* 1997;**337**:1195–20.

36 Jorenby DE, Leischow SJ, Nides MA *et al*. A controlled trial of sustained-release bupropion, a nicotine patch, or both for smoking cessation. *N Engl J Med* 1999;**340**:685–91.

37 Hughes JR, Stead LF, Lancaster T. Antidepressants for smoking cessation. *Cochrane Database Syst Rev* 2004;**3**:CD000031.

38 Hays JT, Hurt RD, Rigotti NA *et al*. Sustained-release bupropion for pharmacologic relapse prevention after smoking cessation: a randomized, controlled trial. *Ann Intern Med* 2001;**18**:423–33.

39 Gonzales DH, Nides MA, Ferry LH *et al*. Bupropion SR as an aid to smoking cessation in smokers treated previously with bupropion: a randomized placebo-controlled study. *Clin Pharmacol Ther* 2001;**69**:438–44.

40 Kwan AL, Meiners AP, van Groorheest AC, Lekkerkerker JF. Risk of convulsions due to use of bupropion as an aid for smoking cessation. *Ned Tijdschr Geneeskd* 2001;**145**:277–8.

41 Tashkin DP, Kanner R, Bailey W *et al*. Smoking cessation in patients with chronic obstructive pulmonary disease: a double-blind, placebo-controlled, randomized trial. *Lancet* 2001;**357**:1571–75.

42 Jarvis MJ, Powell SR, Marsh HS. A meta-analysis of clinical studies confirms the effectiveness of bupropion SR in smoking cessation. Poster, 8th annual meeting Society for Research on Nicotine and Tobacco, Savannah (GA), 20–23th February 2002.

43 British Thoracic Society. Comparison of four methods of smoking withdrawal in patients with smoking related diseases. *BMJ* 1983;**286**:595–7.

44 Research Committee of the British Thoracic Society. Smoking cessation in patients: two further studies by the British Thoracic Society. *Thorax* 1990;**45**:835–40.

45 Tønnesen P, Mikkelsen K, Markholst C *et al*. Nurse-conducted smoking cessation in a lung clinic: a randomized controlled study. *Eur Respir J* 1996;**9**:2351–5.

46 Tønnesen P, Mikkelsen K. Smoking cessation with four nicotine replacement regimes in a lung clinic. *Eur Respir Dis* 2000;**16**:717–22.

47 O'Hara P, Connett JE, Lee WW *et al*. Early and late weight gain following smoking cessation in the lung health study. *Am J Epidemiol* 1998;**148**:821–30.

48 Nørregaard J, Jørgensen S, Mikkelsen KL *et al*. The effect of ephedrine plus caffeine on smoking cessation and post-cessation weight gain. *Clin Pharmacol Ther* 1996;**60**:679–86.

49 Danielsson T, Røssner S, Westin Å. Open randomized trial of intermittent very low energy diet together with nicotine gum for stopping smoking in women who gained weight in previous attempts to quit. *BMJ* 1999;**319**:490–4.

50 Wise RA, Enright PL, Connett JE *et al*. Effect of weight gain on pulmonary function after smoking cessation in the Lunge Health Study. *Am J Respir Crit Care Med* 1998;**157**:866–72.

51 Jimenez-Ruiz CA, Masa F, Miravitlles M *et al*. Smoking characteristics: differences in attitudes and dependence between healthy smokers and smokers with COPD. *Chest* 2001;**119**: 1365–70.

52 Wagena EJ, Zeegers MPA, van Schayck CP. Benefits and risks of pharmacological smoking cessation therapies in chronic obstructive pulmonary disease. *Drug Saf* 2003;**26**: 381–403.

53 Szafranski W, Cukier A, Ramirez A *et al*. Efficacy and safety of budesonide/formoterol in the management of chronic obstructive pulmonary disease. *Eur Respir Dis* 2002;**21**:74–81.

54 Jones PW, Willits LR, Burge PS, Calverley PMA. Disease severity and the effect of fluticasone propionate on chronic obstructive pulmonary disease exacerbations *Eur Respir J* 2003;**21**:68–73.

55 Campell IA, Prescott RJ, Tjeder-Burton SM. Smoking cessation in hospital patients given repeated advice plus nicotine or placebo chewing gum. *Respir Med* 1991;**85**:155–7.

56 Hand S, Edwards S, Campbell IA, Cannings R. Controlled trial of 3 weeks nicotine replacement treatment in hospital patients also given advice and support. *Thorax* 2002;**57**:715–8.

57 Rigotti NA, Munafo MR, Murphy MFG, Stead LF. Interventions for smoking cessation in hospitalized patients. *Cochrane Database Syst Rev* 2003;**1**:CD001837.

58 Wagena EJ, van der Meer RM, Ostelo RJ, Jacobs JE, van Schayck CP. The efficacy of smoking cessation strategies in people with chronic obstructive pulmonary disease: results from a systematic review. *Respir Med* 2004;**98**:805–15.

59 Tønnesen P, Mikkelsen K, Bremann L. Nurse-conducted smoking cessation in patients with COPD, using nicotine sublingual tablets and behavioral support. *Chest* 2006, in press.

60 Bolliger CT, Zellweger JP, Danielsson T *et al*. Smoking reduction with oral nicotine inhalers: double blind, randomised clinical trial of efficacy and safety. *BMJ* 2000;**321**:329–33.

61 Wennike P, Danielsson T, Landfeldt T, Westin Å, Tønnesen P. Smoking reduction promotes smoking cessation: results from a double blind, randomized, placebo-controlled trial of nicotine gum with 2-year follow-up. *Addiction* 2003;**98**:1395–402.

62 Hughes JR, Carpenter MJ. Can medications or behavioral treatment reduce smoking in smokers not trying to quit? A review. Proceedings of Society for research on nicotine and tobacco, 11th Annual Meeting, Prague, March, 2005 [Abstract].

63 Godtfredsen NS, Vestbo J, Osler M, Prescott E. Risk of hospital admission for COPD following smoking cessation and reduction: a Danish population study. *Thorax* 2002;**57**:967–72.

64 Godtfredsen NS, Holst C, Prescott E, Vestbo J, Osler M. Smoking reduction, smoking cessation and mortality: a 16-year follow-up of 19 732 men and women from the Copenhagen Centre for Prospective Population Studies. *Am J Epidemiol* 2002;**156**:994–1001.

65 Bates C, McNeill A, Jarvis M, Gray N. The future of tobacco product regulation and labelling in Europe: implications for the forthcoming European Union directive. *Tob Control* 1999;**8**:225–35.

66 NICE. Chronic obstructive pulmonary disease: national clinical guideline on management of chronic obstructive pulmonary disease in adults in primary and secondary care. *Thorax* 2004;**59**(Suppl 1):1–232. (www.nice.org.uk/CG012niceguideline.)

CHAPTER 54
Oxygen therapy in COPD

Brian Tiep and Rick Carter

Long-term oxygen therapy (LTOT) serves a critical role in the clinical management of patients with advanced lung disease. A map of the multiple considerations for LTOT is presented in Figure 54.1. Clinicians prescribe oxygen to protect the patient from the deleterious effects of tissue hypoxia. In addition, they prescribe it to improve survival, control dyspnoea, enhance exercise performance and maximize functional ability. The survival benefit of LTOT for severe hypoxaemia is well established [1,2]. There does not appear to be a survival benefit for patients with mild to moderate hypoxaemia [3]. However, there are other hypothesized benefits that await confirmation through well-designed clinical trials.

Oxygen for severely hypoxaemic patients appears to reduce hospitalization [4], improve pulmonary haemodynamics [5,6] and enhance psychomotor performance [7–10]. Nocturnal oxygen administration for patients who desaturate but who do not have obstructive sleep apnoea prevents nocturnal desaturations [11]; yet its impact on longevity remains unclear. Oxygen used during exercise prevents exercise-induced desaturation while improving exercise performance; however, its long-term benefits have not been fully defined. Providing oxygen during air travel in patients whose oxygen requirement on the ground is borderline, suggests good clinical judgement within the scope of our present state of knowledge, but its overall protective benefit is not yet known.

It is important to bear in mind that the introduction of oxygen into the lung is only the first of a series of steps that include oxygen transport, uptake and utilization at the cellular level. The movement of oxygen across the alveolar–capillary membrane, haemoglobin uptake and release, cardiovascular dynamics, cell membrane transport and mitochondrial utilization are essential processes of cellular respiration and life. These are also sites of potential barriers to oxygen transport. It is common for clinicians to focus attention on maintenance of arterial oxygen saturation because the data are easy to obtain, it is non-invasive and provides ongoing monitoring capabilities. However, that perspective should be widened to include haemoglobin and cardiovascular transport, while observing for adequate end-organ function. Therapeutically, aerobic exercise improves the totality of oxygen transport and thus becomes an essential intervention in maintaining cellular oxygenation while maximizing efficiency of the cardiopulmonary and bioenergetic systems.

Exercise imposes a higher metabolic demand, with a corresponding increase in oxygen uptake. In health, the lungs are quite capable of rapidly responding to the increase in metabolic demand and thereby do not impose a limitation to oxygen transport. In severe COPD, there is minimal lung function reserve as a result of the presence of airway obstruction with or without alveolar capillary block. An increase in ventilatory response often leads to progressive hyperinflation, contributes to ventilation–perfusion ($\dot{V}/\dot{Q}$) mismatching, higher V_D/V_T and a shortened red cell transit time – thereby widening the A–ā gradient. These adjustments undermine the competency of gas exchange. Hyperinflation places the respiratory muscles at a mechanical disadvantage, elevating the work of breathing and its associated metabolic needs. This effect, along with progressive muscle weakness – also a characteristic of this illness – creates a weaker and less effective ventilatory pump at a time of greater metabolic demand.

The collaborative benefits of oxygen therapy, exercise and an active lifestyle [12], while accommodating for an increase in metabolic requirement for oxygen, suggests that oxygen systems should adequately oxygenate patients during exertion and be very portable. The ideal portable system should be minimally intrusive and support an active lifestyle with moment-to-moment adjustments conforming to the physiological requirements.

Patients who require oxygen are frequently self-conscious and avoid social gatherings. To complicate the picture,

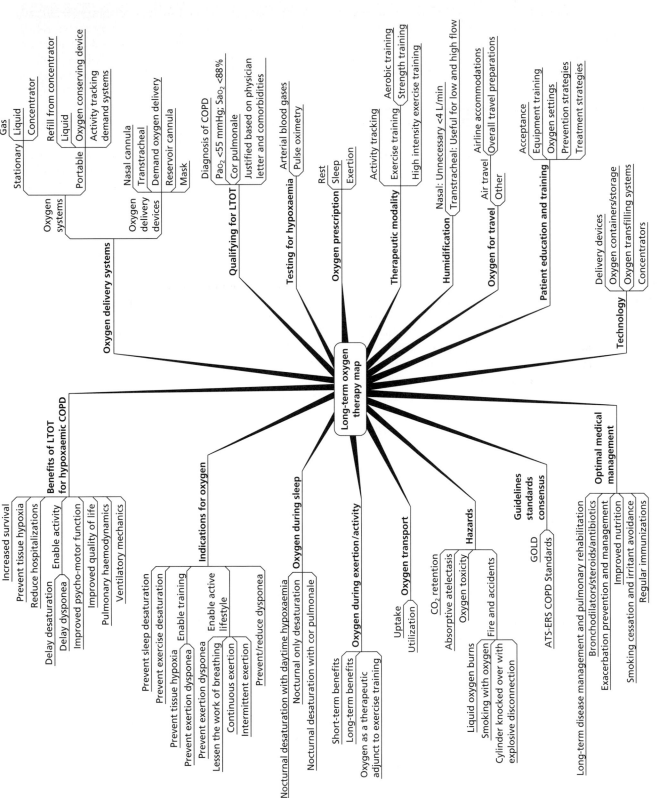

Figure 54.1 Map of considerations for long-term oxygen therapy (LTOT). ATS-ERS, American Thoracic Society and European Respiratory Society; CO_2, carbon dioxide; GOLD, Global Initiative on Obstructive Lung Disease; Pao_2, partial pressure of arterial oxygen (mmHg); Sao_2, arterial oxygen saturation (%).

patients often regard oxygen as a grim reminder that they have a relentlessly disabling illness. Consistent with the therapeutic goal, oxygen must be presented as being enabling. The patient must understand that oxygen serves a protective function and supports an active lifestyle. The patient should fully accept their oxygen and adhere to its prescription.

Physiological considerations

The cause of hypoxaemia bears on the clinical expectations from LTOT [13]. A low fraction of inspired oxygen (Fio_2), such as experienced at higher altitudes, is easily corrected by supplemental oxygen or return to sea level where the fractional content/driving pressure of oxygen in air is greater. Hypoventilation, which occurs during sleep apnoea, promotes a concomitant increase in $Paco_2$. Measures to improve ventilation are effective for improving oxygen transport and carbon dioxide (CO_2) removal. Diffusion impairment, which worsens during exercise – particularly in patients with pulmonary fibrosis – presents a major challenge to maintaining arterial oxygenation during exertion. Ventilation–perfusion mismatching is the usual reason why COPD patients become hypoxaemic and may also contribute to CO_2 retention, and usually responds to supplemental oxygen. Patients with a significant arterial–venous shunt defy correction of their hypoxaemia.

The consequences of hypoxaemia and tissue hypoxia are dependent on multiple factors. Severe acute hypoxia can cause rapid and irreversible tissue damage. Chronic hypoxia will variably impair cellular function and may progress to necrosis. This depends on the target tissue or cell line affected. Initially, the oxygen-deprived cell will resort to anaerobic glycolysis, with a resulting lactic acidosis. Cells can function temporarily within an anaerobic environment, but they do so inefficiently and uncomfortably. A rapid return to oxidative metabolism is necessary for re-establishment of a normal pH through removal of anaerobically generated lactic acid.

Recognition of signs of tissue hypoxia depends on the affected tissue [14]. Brain tissue hypoxia manifests as a loss of short-term memory, followed by euphoria, and impaired judgement. Severe cerebral hypoxia will trigger cerebral oedema, which is life-threatening. Cardiac muscle hypoxia is accompanied by tachycardia, a reduction in stroke volume, atrial and/or ventricular arrhythmia and congestive heart failure. Hypoxia in the lung causes pulmonary vasoconstriction that may lead to right heart failure, bronchospasm and weakened respiratory muscles. Lowering in gastric pH may be seen in conditions of tissue hypoxia and, although somewhat cumbersome, may be used to monitor the presence of tissue oxygenation.

The consequences of long-term hypoxaemia along with the impact of LTOT were addressed in two companion, landmark, randomly controlled clinical trials reported in early 1980s [1,2]. The British Medical Research Council (MRC) study randomly assigned hypoxaemic COPD patients to receive oxygen therapy 15 h/day (including the hours of sleep) versus no oxygen [1]. The survival benefit, which became apparent after 4 years, showed that 55% of the oxygen therapy group was alive versus 33% of the control group.

The National Institutes of Health Nocturnal Oxygen Therapy Trial (NOTT), performed at several centres in North America on a similar population of COPD patients, compared patients receiving oxygen 12 h/day (including the hours of sleep) versus 24 h/day [2]. Actually, the 24 h/day group used their oxygen an average of 19 h/day. Survival after 3 years was 70% for the continuous group versus 50% for the nocturnal oxygen therapy group. This survival difference became apparent after 12 months of oxygen use.

The results were more impressive when patients were stratified by the level of CO_2 retention [2]. A significant decrease in haematocrit and pulmonary vascular resistance was seen in the continuous oxygen group. However, these changes were not sufficient to explain the difference in survival. Autopsies on some of the NOTT patients failed to reveal a difference in pathology, which lends support to the conclusion that the observed survival difference may be related to the number of hours per day of oxygen therapy [15].

Because these two studies were performed on similar groups of patients with the common denominators being COPD and hypoxaemia, the results are often combined to present a unified message (Fig. 54.2): survival is positively

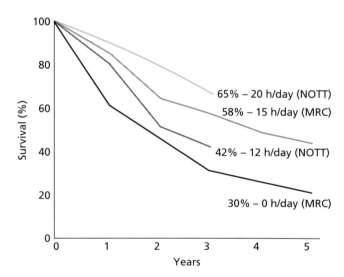

Figure 54.2 Combined results of the Medical Research Council (MRC) and National Institutes of Health Nocturnal Oxygen Therapy Trial (NOTT) studies. Survival is determined by the hours per day of oxygen therapy.

correlated with the number of hours per day of oxygen usage. However, several important areas were not specifically addressed. For example, we do not know if these patients benefited from oxygen during exertion or even if they used their oxygen during exertion. Also, even though implied by the MRC study, we do not know whether patients receiving oxygen during sleep improved their survival.

When LTOT was administered to a different group of patients with moderate hypoxaemia (partial pressure of arterial oxygen [Pao_2] 55–65 mmHg) no survival benefit could be demonstrated [3]. Younger age, better lung function as assessed using spirometry and higher body mass index (BMI) have been identified as positive predictors of survival. Certainly, survival is important but it does not relate to the many comorbidities encountered by the patients nor does it impact on the quality of life prior to mortality. Thus, we must also focus our attention toward other important and relevant endpoints. As will be shown in the sections that follow, oxygen has a positive effect on the ability to exert and exercise. Oxygen can improve the patient's ability to function, partly by reducing dyspnoea which discourages attempts to be active. Further, quality of life is improved, hospitalizations are decreased, enhanced neuropsychological performance is realized and there is the suggestion that oxygen may act as a reparative agent for the lung and other organs [16].

Hazards of oxygen therapy

Overall, oxygen therapy is safe. However, it is important to recognize conditions where oxygen, its associated equipment and patient misuse presents either clinical hazards, such as absorptive atelectasis, oxygen toxicity, CO_2 retention, or the risk of accidents relating to oxygen storage and handling.

Absorptive atelectasis

Oxygen administered in high concentrations may cause absorptive atelectasis and attenuation of hypoxic vasoconstriction [17]. Each of these responses may widen *V/Q* inequality. While some negative potential exists even at moderately low flows, the goal of LTOT is to prevent hypoxaemia. Thus, the benefits for correction of hypoxaemia support the administration of oxygen to a wide array of patients.

Oxygen toxicity

Patients experiencing prolonged exposure to oxygen, in high concentrations above 50%, may be subject to oxygen toxicity [18]. Oxygen toxicity is related to free radical load in the lung. The major end product of normal oxygen meta-

bolism is water. However, some oxygen molecules are not fully reduced and form reactive oxygen metabolites. These include superoxide anions, perhydroxy radicals, hydroxyl radicals and hydrogen peroxide. These free radicals are damaging to alveolar and tracheobronchial cells [19]. Normally, antioxidant enzymes, including metalloproteins (superoxide dismutase), catalase and glutathione peroxidase, protect cells by scavenging oxygen radicals. However, in the face of prolonged exposure to high concentrations of oxygen and/or chronic inflammation, the antioxidant system becomes overwhelmed, thereby permitting oxidative destruction of lung tissue.

Concern for oxygen toxicity generally begins at an Fio_2 of more than 50%. In the case of LTOT, pure oxygen is administered at a low flow that is rapidly diluted by a much higher flow of atmospheric air. This results in a Fio_2 that is much closer to atmospheric air than pure oxygen. For example, the most common oxygen setting is 2 L/min, which produces an Fio_2 of 27–28%. Even at 4 L/min the Fio_2 is usually less than 36%.

In considering the hazards of long-term exposure to low-flow LTOT, an uncontrolled autopsy study of COPD patients revealed exudative and proliferative changes consistent with oxygen toxicity [20]; however, there was no indication that these changes altered survival. Animal studies suggest that long-term exposure to 80% Fio_2 may stimulate greater levels of protective antioxidant enzymes. In general, the benefits of LTOT far outweigh the risks.

CO_2 retention

Concern that oxygen therapy will depress the respiratory drive and promote retention of CO_2 in COPD patients has led to inadequate oxygen prescriptions. Oxygen-induced hypercapnia does rarely occur, but it does not usually lead to respiratory acidosis. The cause of CO_2 retention in some patients has been the subject of debate. Originally, it was believed that patients with severe disease, particularly with CO_2 retention, possessed a defective CO_2 drive. Adaptively, they would then breathe from their hypoxaemia drive and administering oxygen would depress that drive. Aubier *et al.* [21] and Sassoon *et al.* [22] demonstrated an increase in V_D/V_T (V_D, physiological dead space; V_T, tidal volume) rather than a decrease in ventilation consistent with a widening of $\dot{V}a/\dot{Q}$ mismatch. Dunn *et al.* [23] found some evidence for depressed respiratory drive. Robinson *et al.* [24] found that a reduction in ventilation does occur in some patients during an exacerbation. Patients with lower room air oxygen saturation (%) (Sao_2) tended to be retainers and that providing high concentrations of oxygen had a specific effect on perfusion. In general, titrating oxygen flow so as to maintain Pao_2 between 60 and 65 mmHg can minimize the likelihood of hypercapnia and respiratory acidosis while providing adequate oxygenation. Initial oxygen delivery settings should be adjusted via arterial blood gas (ABG) rather than oximetry to assess Pa_{CO_2} and acid–base changes.

Many patients can tolerate chronic hypercapnia because of renal compensation that maintains their pH in the normal range. In fact, the ability of patients to tolerate hypercapnia may be an adaptive mechanism that minimizes their work of breathing. It is reasonable to accept chronic hypercapnia in this patient cohort. Thus, chronic hypercapnia may not always be a poor prognostic sign [25]. Adverse consequences of hypercapnia are related to acute acidaemia that can be detected by serial ABGs and the monitoring of mental status. In summary, correction of hypoxaemia takes precedence over concerns about CO_2 retention for patients with COPD.

Physical hazards

Oxygen therapy is safe and few accidents have been reported. Most major concerns relate to combustion. Some fires have been caused by patients lighting a cigarette as oxygen is flowing into their noses with destructive and sometimes fatal consequences [26]. The plastic cannula does not burn unless oxygen is flowing and a fire is lit. Hence, smoking in the presence of oxygen is to be strictly avoided.

Compressed gas oxygen is stored under pressure. It is possible, albeit rare, that an oxygen cylinder gets knocked over causing an explosive disconnection of the regulator, rendering the cylinder into a dangerous missile. Mishandling liquid oxygen systems can rarely lead to freeze burns during transfilling. Most accidents are completely avoidable by following manufacturers' directions and common sense.

LTOT and optimal medical management

Optimal medical management of a chronic illness with far-reaching systemic manifestations requires that the clinician maximize all aspects of care. COPD is chronic and progressive with episodes of acute exacerbations. However, all parts of the disease are treatable including most comorbidities. *V/Q* mismatching, a prevalent cause of hypoxaemia, is often worsened by bronchoconstriction, inflammation and hyperinflation, and *V/Q* mismatch tends to further widen during an exacerbation. Therefore, by addressing these components, the need for oxygen may be reduced. For the already hypoxaemic patient, oxygen appears to have a reparative effect over time – beyond simple therapeutic replacement. By reducing hypoxic vasoconstriction of the pulmonary arteries, *V/Q* matching is improved [16,27].

Hence, oxygen therapy performs a fundamental role in optimal medical management.

Again, the full route of oxygen transport requires regular clinical attention. Correction of anaemia, control of congestive heart failure and assuring adequate renal function are inherent components of medical management. An exercise programme delivered during the non-acute phase of the disease process will enhance oxygen transport and utilization and improve efficiency for many bodily functions.

Oxygen during sleep

A significant portion of the day is spent sleeping. Healthy persons commonly experience transient mild desaturations during sleep, particularly during rapid eye movement (REM) sleep. For the COPD patient, these desaturations are more common, more pronounced and tend to start from a lower baseline level. COPD patients with no sign of obstructive sleep apnoea (OSA) may undergo desaturations of 9–21% [28]. Thus, saturations dipping below 90% are frequent, with some patients spending more than 30% of the night below 90% [29].

The mechanisms vary but rapid shallow breathing with alveolar hypoventilation seem to be the major cause of sleep oxygen desaturation [11]. Nocturnal oxygen desaturation has also been attributed to suppression of the ventilatory drive that occurs largely during REM sleep, although it can occur in any stage including just after sleep onset. Other mechanisms include an increase in V_D/V_T and an increase in *V/Q* mismatch. Desaturation at night may not be totally predictable from daytime arterial blood gases, because sleep pattern abnormalities and their consequence on respiration may also contribute independent of the awake state [28].

Most COPD patients with well-corrected daytime saturation require an increase in oxygen flow during sleep in order to maintain an adequate saturation. This was recognized during the 1970s before the advent of modern oximeters. Patients in the NOTT study were prescribed an increase in flow of 1 L/min at night [2]. Patients with both hypercapnia and hypoxaemia are likely to desaturate at night [30]. Patients who desaturate at night have an increased risk of ventricular ectopy, higher pulmonary artery pressure and pulmonary vascular resistance and shortened survival [31]. In patients with nocturnal desaturation, adequate oxygenation during sleep may prevent or reverse those complications [32].

Nocturnal oxygen desaturation with adequate daytime saturations

Chaouat *et al.* [33] studied nocturnal desaturators with mild daytime hypoxaemia (Sao_2 greater than 88%) and compared them with non-desaturators for a total of 2 years [33]. The desaturators tended to be those with a slightly higher $Paco_2$ and pulmonary artery pressure (PAP), whereas the non-desaturators had no increase in their $Paco_2$ or PAP. This study concluded that nocturnal oxygen desaturation is specifically associated with CO_2 retention [33]. Other studies have concluded that disease severity, CO_2 retention and high BMI are predictive of nocturnal oxygen desaturation [34]. Fletcher *et al.* [35] found that COPD patients with severely impaired pulmonary mechanics along with CO_2 retention were more likely to desaturate during sleep.

Whether LTOT during sleep in this population improves survival or ameliorates the consequences of nocturnal desaturations warrants further study. The risks and concerns as previously described as well as from OSA research are substantial. A large multicentred trial studied patients with mild daytime hypoxaemia and noted that nocturnal oxygen therapy did not modify the evolution of pulmonary hypertension or delay the patient from meeting the criteria for LTOT. They did not detect a survival difference – albeit their population was small and the study did not last long enough to draw a definite conclusion [36]. On the other hand, Fletcher *et al.* [32], in a relatively small group of patients, found that oxygen therapy for nocturnal desaturation reduced pulmonary artery pressure with the suggestion of improved survival.

Overlap syndrome

Some patients have a coexistance of COPD and OSA – called overlap syndrome [37]. It is questionable whether the incidence of OSA is higher in COPD than the general population. Weitzenblum *et al.* [38] reported that 11% of their OSA patients had coexisting COPD. Patients with overlap syndrome may have an abnormally high rise in PAP during exercise [39]. The recommended approach for these patients is to perform a polysomnography and to address the OSA component [40] independent of the COPD.

Prescribing nocturnal oxygen

Patients who require LTOT because of daytime hypoxaemia will require nocturnal oxygen as well. If there are no symptoms of nocturnal desaturation, it is usually adequate to increase daytime setting by 1 L/m equivalent. Alternatively, a nocturnal saturation study can be utilized to establish the setting. In COPD patients with mild daytime hypoxaemia, who have cor pulmonale, right heart failure or erythrocytosis, nocturnal oxygen therapy may be warranted. Patients with mild daytime hypoxaemia in whom nocturnal desaturation has been documented can benefit from nocturnal oxygen therapy depending on the degree of

desaturation, percentage of the night below Sao_2 of 90% and tendency for hypercarbia. The supplementation of oxygen to patients with these characteristics remains a clinical judgement. Screening asymptomatic non-hypoxaemic patients for nocturnal oxygen desaturation is not warranted based on our present understanding.

Oxygen during exercise

Exercise hypoxaemia

Exercise training improves strength, endurance and confidence and lessens exertional dyspnoea – enabling an active lifestyle. In healthy individuals, the lungs easily meet oxygen uptake demands of exercising muscle by delivering adequate amounts of oxygen to the alveoli to participate in gas exchange thereby maintaining arterial oxygenation [41]. Red cell transit time can decrease from 0.75–1.0 s at rest to less than 0.5 s during exercise. D_L/Q as well as V/Q matching is maintained by recruiting previously non-communicating alveolar units to meet the oxygen delivery demands for cellular respiration/metabolism of active muscle tissues during exercise.

The pathophysiological progression of COPD eventually leads to hypoxaemia during exertion. During rest patients are generally not limited by lung diffusion or red cell transit time [42]. During exercise these factors come into play [43] along with a widening of the V/Q mismatch, progressive hyperinflation [44], an increase in oxygen cost and work of breathing [45], and suboptimal length–tension positioning of foreshortened ventilatory muscles. Otherwise stated, increasing oxygen uptake demands are met by inefficient lungs powered by a weakened ventilatory pump that drains a disproportionate share of the inspired oxygen.

Healthy individuals living at high altitude and exercising at low altitudes have improved performance and greater $\dot{V}O_{2max}$, whereas persons living at low altitude and exercising at high altitude had the opposite effect [46]. Thus, exercising in hypoxaemic conditions impairs performance and the resultant tissue hypoxia may be harmful. In COPD patients, exercise-induced hypoxaemia over the long term portends poor survival [47]. What remains to be determined is whether administering oxygen during exercise improves survival.

Short-term benefits of oxygen during exercise

Early studies demonstrated substantial short-term benefits of oxygen supplementation during exercise. Oxygen enables patients to exercise at higher workloads for longer periods, more intensely and with less dyspnoea [48–50]. There is less hyperinflation, which places the tidal loop in a more advantageous position along the flow–volume loop, decreasing the overall work of breathing thereby providing some relief to the compromised ventilatory muscles [44,51].

To some degree, higher exercise tolerance is made possible by depressing the carotid and aortic body chemosensors [52]. Oxygen can increase exercise tolerance by reducing minute ventilation at similar workloads [53]. A reduction in minute ventilation, which tolerates mild CO_2 retention, further eases the ventilatory burden. Oxygen administered during exercise may prevent transient increases in pulmonary artery pressure and pulmonary vascular resistance [54]. Oxygen therapy improves indices of oxidative metabolism in peripheral muscles. Some of the exercise metabolic indices remain abnormal, possibly indicating persistent cellular damage from chronic hypoxaemia [55]. Eaton et al. [56], in a randomized trial, showed that ambulatory oxygen can improve quality of life.

Oxygen to prevent exercise oxygen desaturation

McDonald et al. [57] compared delivery of oxygen versus compressed air using a portable cylinder with an oxygen-conserving device. They demonstrated immediate improvements in exercise performance, but failed to demonstrate longer term effects on exercise performance or quality of life. Survival benefits have not been demonstrated nor have functional improvements in rehabilitation performance over the long term [57–60]. Rooyackers et al. [59] compared training with oxygen versus room air. SaO_2 was never below 90%. Both groups improved exercise capacity and quality of life indices, but oxygen did not add to the benefits of training on room air [59]. Garrod et al. [60] showed a reduction of dyspnoea during exercise but no training effect from ambulatory oxygen therapy in a rehabilitation programme. Definitive studies combining pulmonary rehabilitation and disease management with oxygen therapy to prevent exercise desaturation are needed. Definitive research is required to fully understand the long-term benefits of preventing exercise desaturation. Clinical judgement suggests that exercise oxygen, delivered at the correct flow rate, is an important and essential component COPD disease management.

Oxygen to enhance exercise benefits

Exercise training in COPD patients is able to achieve a physiological training effect [61]. Previous investigations that studied the ability of hyperoxic mixtures to improve exercise and functional performance and boost $\dot{V}O_2$ to peripheral muscle have led to mixed results [52]. Early studies by Cotes and Gilson [48] in 1956 found progressive improvement in exercise performance up to FiO_2 of 0.5. Somfay et al.

[51] later demonstrated a dose-dependent reduction in hyperinflation and improvement in endurance with FiO_2 up to 0.5, with no further benefit at higher FiO_2. O'Donnell et al. [44] determined that exercise dyspnoea was ameliorated by lowering the ventilatory demand, reducing hyperinflation and decreasing lactate levels. Dean et al. [62] found a positive relationship between exercise performance and decreased dyspnoea, but minute ventilation, heart rate or right ventricular pressure remained unchanged. Mannix et al. [63] found that 30% oxygen lowered the oxygen cost of ventilation. Jolly et al. [49] observed no increase in exercise performance in non-destaturators in spite of the fact oxygen led to a substantial reduction in dyspnoea.

Muscle performance is improved with oxygen supplementation with no alteration in muscle kinetics [55,64]. The immediate effect of exercise oxygen is to reduce minute ventilation by slowing breath rate and reducing tidal volume. The net effect is to decrease the work of breathing by lowering minute ventilation at the cost of minimal CO_2 retention. The reduction in respiratory rate decreases hyperinflation, thereby alleviating dyspnoea [44]. The mechanism appears to be a blunting of the chemoreceptor response [55]. Maltais et al. [65], utilizing an FiO_2 of 0.75, demonstrated improvement in blood flow to the lower limb muscles.

Emtner et al. [66], in a randomized double-blinded trial, administered oxygen versus compressed room air to COPD patients ($FEV_1 = 36\%$ predicted), who were non-hypoxaemic at rest and did not desaturate below 89% during exercise. Patients participated in high-intensity training to 75% of maximum workload. Both groups benefited from exercise training, achieving greater endurance, higher exercise tolerance and lower respiratory rate, with the oxygen trained group performing significantly better. After training, the oxygen group performed better on constant work rate tests with lower breath rates, while breathing both room air and oxygen. Thus, oxygen is considered to be a therapeutic enabler for exercise training beyond simple protection against hypoxaemia.

Prescribing exercise oxygen

Patients should be evaluated using the same delivery devices they expect to use at home (e.g. nasal cannula or oxygen conserving device). Exercise testing is best carried out using muscle groups where dyspnoea is most pronounced (e.g. legs versus arms). The American Thoracic Society and European Respiratory Society (ATS-ERS) standards [67] recommend that exercise oxygen setting be titrated during a typical exercise such as a hallway walk. In daily life, most people tend to be inactive, interspersed with short bursts of activity approaching peak limits given the underlying impairment. In such circumstances, patients have little time to achieve a steady state. The resulting desaturation and ensuing dyspnoea discourages an active lifestyle. It is known that hypoxaemic COPD patients undergo many short periods of oxygen desaturation daily while complying with their oxygen prescription [68–71]. As such, a hallway walk at a steady pace may be inadequate to prevent these saturation dips. Also, many patients tend to forget to increase their oxygen setting during exertion – particularly for short intervals. Either the exercise setting must be increased or the setting adjustment needs to be automated. Recently, such a device has been announced, but studies in the home setting are recommended to determine its applicability.

Physiological qualification for LTOT

Guidelines for determining which patients will qualify for LTOT are based on the physiology and survival benefits as revealed in the MRC and NOTT studies [1,2]. Determination as to which patients will actually receive LTOT is heavily influenced by reimbursement, which varies by country. On the basis of both the MRC and NOTT studies, patients who meet the qualification criteria for home oxygen should use it continuously – at least 15 h/day [1,2].

Both ATS-ERS Standards and the Global initiative for Obstructive Lung Disease (GOLD) Guidelines qualify COPD patients for LTOT with Pao_2 less than 55 mmHg (7.3 kPa) or Sao_2 less than 88%. Patients may also qualify with Pao_2 between 55 and 60 mmHg (7.3–8.0 kPa) or Sao_2 of 89% with evidence of pulmonary hypertension, peripheral oedema indicating right heart failure, or polycythaemia [67,72].

Arterial blood gases

Initial qualification for LTOT should be based on arterial blood gases (ABG) measurement. It is more accurate than non-invasive oximetry and includes $Paco_2$, pH and Sao_2. GOLD recommends an ABG when the forced expiratory volume in 1 s (FEV_1) is less than 40% predicted or if there are signs of respiratory failure or right heart failure [72]. An early indicator of respiratory distress is dyspnoea; a late clinical sign of respiratory failure is cyanosis. Right heart failure is indicated by pedal oedema or an increase in jugular venous pressure. An added benefit is the ability to detect carboxyhaemoglobin in arterial blood through co-oximetry. This clinical knowledge may be used to reinforce smoking cessation or compliance.

Pulse oximetry

The Spo_2 represents the arterial oxygen saturation (Sao_2) measured by pulse oximetry. Oximetry Spo_2 closely tracks arterial Sao_2 under most conditions and is non-invasive.

With its continuous readout, oximetry has the advantage in being able to track changes over time. Spo_2 during exercise helps to determine the speed and extent of the desaturation response. Unfortunately, absolute values may not be accurate during exercise, particularly in patients with poor peripheral perfusion. Also, there is a time lag between desaturation and detection at the fingertip [73]. Verification of oximetry accuracy can be accomplished by obtaining ABG before and after exercise. A therapeutic use for pulse oximetry is as a biofeedback guide in conjunction with pursed lips breathing. The patient guided by the oximetry Spo_2 readout can learn to alter breathing patterns to increase Spo_2 and lessen dyspnoea [74].

Determining the LTOT prescription

An ABG drawn, while breathing room air, is used to determine whether the patient qualifies for LTOT. Concomitant oximetry provides a corresponding Spo_2 useful for flow adjustments. The ATS-ERS standards algorithm (Fig. 54.3) is a guide to adjusting oxygen settings. The resting flow rate can be adjusted via oximetry to Spo_2 of 92% or greater. Full equilibration may require 15 min or more. Concerns about hypercarbia may be addressed by drawing an ABG after the Spo_2 reaches 92%. If there is greater CO_2 retention, check the pH for acidosis. If the pH is balanced, that patient is chronically hypercapnic and no further adjustment is necessary.

COPD patients are encouraged live an active life and maintain an exercise programme. Accordingly, there should be a highly portable component to the oxygen system. The patient should be tested on the system being prescribed – particularly if an oxygen conserving device is included – during a typical or higher level of exertion than commonly experienced, such as walking with the oxygen flow setting titrated to achieve an Spo_2 of more than 92%. If dyspnoea is especially prevalent during arm exertion, the patient may also be tested while performing arm tasks. If an autoadjusting conserving device is prescribed, the setting should also be determined with the patient alternately sitting and walking.

Oxygen therapy during sleep is often set 1 L/min higher than daytime resting setting. If there are signs of cor pulmonale despite adequate daytime Spo_2, a sleep oximetry may be performed to establish fluctuations in Spo_2 and provide titration feedback to achieve an Spo_2 of more than 90%.

Oxygen systems

Oxygen is supplied and packaged as either compressed gas, liquid or oxygen concentrator. There are advantages and

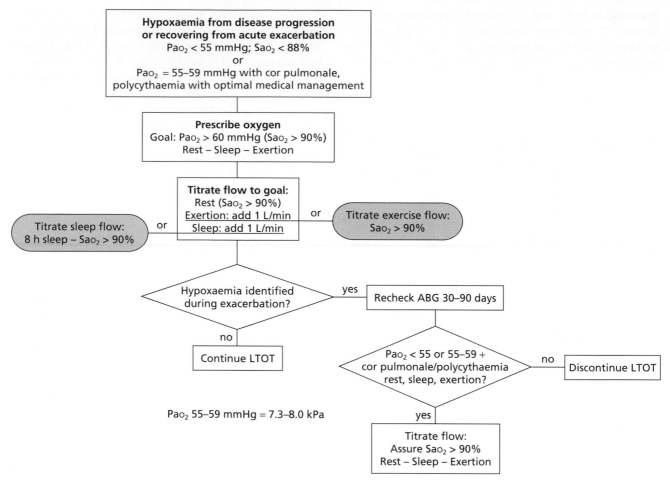

Figure 54.3 An algorithm for long-term oxygen therapy from the American Thoracic Society and European Respiratory Society (ATS-ERS) standards for the diagnosis and management of COPD. ABG, arterial blood gas; LTOT, long-term oxygen therapy; Pao_2, partial pressure arterial oxygen; Sao_2, arterial oxygen saturation.

disadvantages to each system depending on the needs of the individual patient, clinical application, and practical considerations such as availability, cost, ease of use, delivery to the home, and maintenance.

Compressed gas oxygen

Compressed gas oxygen is typically pressurized to 2200 psi and stored in steel or aluminum cylinders. The H cylinder is large, weighs over 200 lb (91 kg), stores 6900 L and lasts for 2.4 days set at 2 L/min. The E cylinder is a commonly used portable system; however, it is heavy and requires a cart. An aluminum E cylinder weighs 16–18 lb (7.3–8.2 kg) stores, 523 L, and lasts 5 h at 2 L/min. It must be wheeled on a cart that may add as much as 1 kg (2.2 lb) to the total weight. The M-6 aluminum cylinder weighs 4 lb (1.8 kg) and lasts about 1.2 h at 2 L/min. These cylinders are designed for use with an oxygen-conserving device that extends the cylinder life threefold or more. Transfillable

cylinders, which fill from an oxygen concentrator, enable patients to be free from home deliveries.

Oxygen concentrator

Oxygen concentrators extract oxygen directly from room air. Using a molecular sieve constructed of zeolite, oxygen is separated from nitrogen, which is returned to the room air. The purity at low flows is about 97% oxygen and drops to 94% at higher flows largely due to the presence of argon. Most oxygen concentrators are large consoles that operate on wall current. However, battery powered concentrators are now available – some weighing less than 10 lb with a battery that lasts approximately 50 min on a charge. The biggest advantages of standard concentrators are their low cost and high availability. Accordingly, concentrators are used as a stationary system in the home. Specialized concentrators are now available that refill small 4 lb portable cylinders that, combined with an oxygen conserving device, last up to 10 h at 2 L/min. Such systems are fully self-contained as they free the patient from home deliveries. These systems have demonstrated that they are easy for the patient to operate, are safe and reliable.

Liquid oxygen

Liquid oxygen is supercooled to convert it to its liquid state. It is stored in a special thermos called a Dewar flask. Because it is in its liquid state, a large volume of oxygen can be stored in a small, lightweight container. One liquid litre expands to nearly 1000 gaseous litres of oxygen. Liquid oxygen is easily transfilled by the patient from a larger stationary unit to a portable unit that patients can easily carry. Several manufactures now supply liquid portable oxygen systems with a built-in oxygen-conserving device. This further reduces the size and weight so that a unit that weighs 3.5 lb (1.6 kg) can provide up to 10 h of oxygen at a 2 L/min setting.

Oxygen delivery methods

Continuous-flow nasal cannulas

Continuous flow delivery via a standard dual prong nasal cannula provides a small flow of oxygen entrained in a much larger flow of inspired air. Each increase in litre flow of 1.0 L/min adds approximately 3–4% to the Fio_2 (Table 54.1). One model of delivery is based on a breath cycle of 3 s for a patient breathing 20 breaths/min [75]. COPD patients tend to have inspiratory–expiratory ratios of 1 : 2. This means that 1 s is devoted to inspiration and 2 s is devoted to exhalation. The last one-third of the inspiratory volume fills the dead space, which does not participate in gas exchange. Given that the breath slows at end-inspiration, approximately 0.5 s will be spent in filling the dead space. This leaves 0.5 s for early inhalation where filling of the alveolus and gas exchange takes place. That is the gas exchange window of opportunity [75].

Table 54.1 Approximate fraction of inspired oxygen (Fio_2) from continuous flow and reservoir cannula.

Oxygen setting	Fio_2 continuous flow (%)	Fio_2 reservoir cannula (%)
Room air	21	21
1 L/min	24	32
2 L/min	28	36
3 L/min	32	40
4 L/min	36	44
5 L/min	40	46

A patient delivered oxygen at 2 L/min using standard flow delivery will receive approximately 16.7 mL of oxygen in the first 0.5 s of inhalation. If mixed into the first 200 mL of inspired gas, this calculates to a Fio_2 of 27.6%. At 20 breaths/min the patient receives 333.3 mL (20×16.7 mL) of oxygen per minute. Thus, only 17% (333.3 mL/2000 mL) of the oxygen flow arrives during the gas exchange window of opportunity. The rest is largely wasted.

Reservoir cannulas

Reservoir cannulas function by storing oxygen during exhalation for delivery during the next inhalation [75]. A thin, compliant membrane creates the 20-mL chamber that expands and contracts in response to nasal airflow. Reservoir cannulas are supplied with continuous flow oxygen. The reservoir adds approximately 18 mL of oxygen to the inspiratory mixture, which is the equivalent of adding approximately 2 L/min to the Fio_2 (see Table 54.1).

Reservoir cannulas are available as an Oxymizer and Pendant [76,77]. In the Oxymizer, the reservoir is located immediately beneath the nose, whereas the Pendant stores oxygen in a chamber located at the anterior chest wall, as well as the tubing leading to the nasal prongs. Both the Oxymizer and the Pendant maintain the same efficacy. The Oxymizer is more noticeable but more comfortable than the Pendant. Reservoir cannulas are inexpensive and reliable, but do not support pursed lips breathing at low flows. Both reservoir cannulas have been utilized with success for high-flow oxygen delivery [78,79].

Transtracheal catheters

Transtracheal oxygen (TTO) is delivered through a small stoma placed surgically through the neck into the trachea. The objective is to deliver oxygen to the upper airway thereby reducing some dead space ventilation, improving *V/Q* and lessening the work of breathing [80]. This conserves oxygen and reduces inspired flow to achieve equivalent oxygenation to continuous flow nasal cannulas. The flow setting can be reduced by 50% at rest and 30% during exercise [81–84].

TTO has a cosmetic advantage because oxygen and its paraphernalia are removed from the face. Because oxygen flows directly into the trachea, TTO is able to reduce dyspnoea, minute ventilation, dead space and tension–time index of the diaphragm [84]. TTO candidates are usually active people who are both willing and able to follow a strict care protocol. A trained team of clinicians evaluates, educate and monitor patients [82,83]. TTO patients should not be heavy sputum producers nor experience frequent exacerbations. They should live within 2 h of the institution or have similar follow-up in their home community.

Demand delivery devices

Pulse demand oxygen delivery devices sense the beginning of inhalation – at which point they deliver a small oxygen pulse [85–89]. By delivering during the early part of inhalation, they conserve oxygen that would be otherwise wasted during late inhalation and exhalation. Demand pulsing devices vary in efficiency from 2 : 1 to 7 : 1 as compared with continuous flow. The more rapidly these devices respond while confining the pulse to the first 0.5 s of inhalation, the more efficacious the delivery [85].

Pulse demand oxygen delivery devices operate using several different technologies. The most efficient and effective devices sense the onset of inhalation electronically and deliver via a solenoid-controlled pulse. Pneumatic devices both sense and deliver pneumatically and thus do not require a battery. Newer devices now combine the low volume storage of liquid oxygen with oxygen conservation to create systems that are very small, portable and longlasting. An oxygen-conserving device that automatically tracks activity and adjusts for exertion is under evaluation. As such, oxygen becomes utilized as a therapeutic tool to assure better oxygenation during usual daily activities.

Many demand oxygen delivery devices are available. Some have undergone clinical studies but most have not. Some devices are relatively insensitive and slow to respond to the beginning of inhalation. Late delivery undoubtedly results in desaturation, particularly during exercise. Since patients vary in their breath pattern, pathology and how much airflow is parcelled to the nose versus mouth, Spo_2 testing using the device being contemplated during rest and exercise is essential to assure adequate oxygenation. It is important to select a device that is easy to use and has demonstrated reliability over the long haul because the typical patient breathes 16 breaths/min; 23 040 breaths/day; 8 409 600 breaths/year.

Humidification

There has been some concern that delivering oxygen will dry the nasal passages and the lungs. However, oxygen is provided at low flows relative to inhalation of atmospheric gas. As demonstrated in Table 54.1, oxygen represents a minor portion of inhalation. Moreover, oxygen flowing through the bubble humidifier is at room temperature; when it is raised to body temperature, the relative humidity falls. Finally, the nose is a very efficient and effective humidifier.

There is no evidence that humidification is necessary when oxygen is given by nasal cannula at flows less than 5 L/min [90]. There are no differences in subjective complaints or in severity of symptoms over time. This does not apply to patients receiving oxygen by tracheostomy or TTO therapy, in whom the upper airway has been bypassed by the catheter; for these patients, humidification of inspired gas is essential even at low flow rates (1 L/min). TTO patients at high risk for mucus ball formation, including those with oxygen flows more than 5 L/min, large amounts of mucus, or weak cough, may benefit from a servo-controlled heated humidifier because this device more efficiently humidifies inspired gas.

Patient education and training

Education and training is a continuous process that is central to oxygen supplementation, disease management and rehabilitation. One educational goal is help the patient understand their disease and how it impacts their life. Patients must be provided with an optimistic assessment of the enabling benefits of utilizing oxygen, as prescribed. They must be trained, and regularly evaluated, and reinforced with respect to the use of their equipment. The care and cleaning of equipment for proper functioning and prevention of infection is an essential component. It is especially important that patients and caregivers learn and develop the habits of appropriately adjusting oxygen delivery to rest, exertion and sleep. It is also imperative that patients and their caregivers received education regarding signs and symptoms of infection or other medical changes indicating worsening of their condition and to seek medical assistance at the first opportunity.

Conclusions

Human life depends on the adequate delivery of oxygen to the peripheral tissues. The process requires the efficient function of the respiratory pump, finely tuned matching of ventilation and circulation, and a fluid and efficient method of uptake, transport and delivery. The disruption of these steps with progressive COPD has dire consequences to the patient. The supplementation of oxygen is an important, essential and often misunderstood therapy in the management of hypoxaemic COPD patients. Oxygen is prescribed to prevent cellular hypoxia and end-organ destruction. It is a kind of replacement therapy – providing supplementation where the lungs have failed. Excellent studies have lent support to its life-saving benefits, as well as its ability to reduce mortality, improve psychomotor performance and prevent hospitalizations. A recent and exciting area of research is the use of oxygen as a tool to improve exercise performance and rehabilitation. Thus, oxygen also becomes a therapeutic tool. Technology has come through with the development of highly portable delivery devices, a portable oxygen concentrator, a concentrator that refills portable cylinders and an oxygen-conserving device that automatically adjusts to assure higher flows during usual exertion. For patients requiring oxygen supplementation, technological innovation, coupled with a better understanding of the patient, has provided realistic, reliable and cost-effective options for delivering oxygen and maintaining function.

References

1 Medical Research Council Working Party. Long-term domiciliary oxygen therapy in chronic hypoxic cor pulmonale complicating chronic bronchitis and emphysema. *Lancet* 1981;**1**:681–6.

2 Nocturnal Oxygen Therapy Trial Group. Continuous or nocturnal oxygen therapy in hypoxemic chronic obstructive lung disease. *Ann Intern Med* 1980;**93**:391–8.

3 Gorecka D, Gorzelak K, Sliwinski P *et al.* Effect of long-term oxygen therapy on survival in patients with chronic obstructive pulmonary disease with moderate hypoxaemia. *Thorax* 1997;**52**:674.

4 Ringbaek TJ, Viskum K, Lange P. Does long-term oxygen therapy reduce hospitalizations in hypoxemic chronic obstructive pulmonary disease? *Eur Respir J* 2002;**20**:30–42.

5 Alpert JS. Pulmonary hypertension and cardiac function in chronic obstructive pulmonary disease. *Chest* 1979;**75**:651–2.

6 Oswald-Mammosser ME, Weitzenblum E, Quoix E *et al.* Prognostic factors in COPD patients receiving long-term oxygen therapy: importance of pulmonary artery pressure. *Chest* 1995;**107**:1193–8.

7 Fix AJ, Daughton D, Kass I, Bell CW, Golden CJ. Cognitive functioning and survival among patients with chronic obstructive pulmonary disease. *Int J Neurosci* 1985;**27**:13–7.

8 Fix AJ, Golden CJ, Daughton D, Kass I, Bell CW. Neuropsychological deficits among patients with chronic obstructive pulmonary disease. *Int J Neurosci* 1982;**16**:99–105.

9 Heaton RK, Grant I, McSweeny AJ, Adams KM, Petty TL. Psychologic effects of continuous and nocturnal oxygen therapy in hypoxemic chronic obstructive pulmonary disease. *Arch Intern Med* 1983;**143**:1941–7.

10 Krop HD, Block AJ, Cohen E. Neuropsychologic effects of continuous oxygen therapy in chronic obstructive pulmonary disease. *Chest* 1973;**64**:317–22.

11 Caterall JR, Calverley PMA, McNee W *et al.* Mechanisms of transient nocturnal hypoxemia in hypoxic chronic bronchitis and emphysema. *J Appl Physiol* 1985;**159**:1689–703.

12 Tiep BL. Disease management of COPD with pulmonary rehabilitation. *Chest* 1997;**112**:1630–56.

13 West JB. Gas exchange. In: West JB, ed. *Pulmonary Physiology: The Essentials*. Baltimore, MD: Lippincott Williams and Wilkins, 2003: 17–28.

14 Leach RM, Treacher DF. ABC of oxygen: oxygen transport. 2. Tissue hypoxia. *BMJ* 1998;**317**:1370–3.

15 Jacques J, Cooney TP, Silvers GW *et al.* The lungs and causes of death in the nocturnal oxygen therapy trial. *Chest* 1984; **86**:230–3.

16 O'Donohue WJ. Effect of oxygen therapy on increasing arterial oxygen tension in hypoxemic patients with stable chronic obstructive pulmonary disease while breathing ambient air. *Chest* 1991;**100**:968–72.

17 Ploysongsang Y, Wiltse DW. Effects of breathing pattern and oxygen upon the alveolar arterial oxygen pressure difference in lung disease. *Respiration* 1985;**47**:39–47.

18 Jenkinson SG. Oxygen toxicity. *New Horiz* 1993;**1**:504–11.

19 Housset B, Hurbain I, Masliah J *et al.* Toxic effects of oxygen on cultured alveolar epithelial cells, lung fibroblasts and alveolar macrophages. *Eur Respir J* 1991;**4**:1066–75.

20 Petty TL, Stanford RE, Neff TA. Continuous oxygen therapy in chronic airway obstruction: observations on possible oxygen toxicity and survival. *Ann Intern Med* 1971;**75**:361–7.

21 Aubier M, Murciano D, Fournier M *et al.* Central respiratory drive in acute respiratory failure of patients with chronic obstructive pulmonary disease. *Am Rev Respir Dis* 1980;**122**: 191–9.

22 Sassoon CS, Hassell KT, Mahutte CK. Hyperoxic-induced hypercapnia in stable chronic obstructive pulmonary disease. *Am Rev Respir Dis* 1987;**135**:907–11.

23 Dunn WF, Nelson SB, Hubmayr RD. Oxygen-induced hypercarbia in obstructive pulmonary disease. *Am Rev Respir Dis* 1991;**144**:526–30.

24 Robinson TD, Freiberg DB, Regnis JA, Young IH. The role of hypoventilation and ventilation–perfusion redistribution in oxygen-induced hypercapnia during acute exacerbations of chronic obstructive pulmonary disease. *Am J Respir Crit Care Med* 2000;**161**:1524–9.

25 Aida A, Miyamoto K, Nishimura M *et al.* Prognostic value of hypercapnia in patients with chronic respiratory failure during long-term oxygen therapy. *Am J Respir Crit Care Med* 1998;**158**:188–93.

26 West GA, Primeau P. Non-medical hazards of long-term oxygen therapy. *Respir Care* 1983;**28**:906–12.

27 Weitzenblum E, Sautegeau A, Ehrhart M, Mammosser M, Pelletier A. Long-term oxygen therapy can reverse the progression of pulmonary hypertension in patients with chronic obstructive pulmonary disease. *Am Rev Respir Dis* 1985;**131**: 493–8.

28 Mohsenin V, Guffanti EE, Hilbert J, Ferranti R. Daytime oxygen saturation does not predict nocturnal oxygen desaturation in patients with chronic obstructive pulmonary disease. *Arch Phys Med Rehabil* 1994;**75**:285–9.

29 Weitzenblum E, Chaouat A, Charpentier C *et al.* Sleep-related hypoxaemia in chronic obstructive pulmonary disease: causes, consequences and treatment. *Respiration* 1997;**64**: 187–93.

30 Plywaczewski R, Sliwinski P, Nowinski A, Kaminksi D, Zielinski J. Incidence of nocturnal desaturation while breathing oxygen in COPD patients undergoing long-term oxygen therapy. *Chest* 2000;**117**:679–83.

31 Kimura H, Suda A, Sakuma T *et al.* Nocturnal oxyhemoglobin desaturation and prognosis in chronic obstructive pulmonary disease and late sequelae of pulmonary tuberculosis. *Intern Med* 1998;**37**:354–9.

32 Fletcher EC, Luckett RA, Goodnight-White S *et al.* A double-blind trial of nocturnal supplemental oxygen for sleep

desaturation in patients with chronic obstructive pulmonary disease and a daytime Pao_2 above 60 mmHg. *Am Rev Respir Dis* 1992;**145**:1070–6.

33 Chaouat A, Weitzenblum E, Kessler R *et al.* Outcome of COPD patients with mild daytime hypoxaemia with or without sleep-related oxygen desaturation. *Eur Respir J* 2001;**17**:848–55.

34 De Angelis G, Sposato B, Mazzei L *et al.* Predictive indexes of nocturnal desaturation in COPD patients not treated with long-term oxygen therapy. *Eur Rev Med Pharmacol Sci* 2001;**5**:173–9.

35 Fletcher EC, Scott D, Qian W *et al.* Evolution of nocturnal oxyhemoglobin desaturation in patients with chronic obstructive pulmonary disease and a daytime Pao_2 above 60 mmHg. *Am Rev Respir Dis* 1991;**145**:401–5.

36 Chaouat A, Weitzenblum E, Kessler R *et al.* A randomized trial of nocturnal oxygen therapy in chronic obstructive pulmonary disease patients. *Eur Respir J* 1999;**14**:997–9.

37 Flenley DC. Breathing during sleep. *Ann Acad Med Singapore* 1985;**14**:479–84.

38 Weitzenblum E, Krieger J, Oswald M *et al.* Chronic obstructive pulmonary disease and sleep apnea syndrome. *Sleep* 1992;**15**(Suppl):S33–5.

39 Hawrylkiewicz I, Palasiewicz G, Plywaczewski R, Sliwinski P, Zielinski J. Effects of nocturnal desaturation on pulmonary hemodynamics in patients with overlap syndrome (chronic obstructive pulmonary disease and obstructive sleep apnea). *Pneumonol Alergol Pol* 2000;**68**:28–36.

40 Nicholson D, Tiep B, Sadana G *et al.* Non-invasive positive pressure ventilation. *Curr Opin Pulm Med* 1999;**4**:66–75.

41 Hsia C. Recruitment of lung diffusing capacity: update of concept and application. *Chest* 2002;**122**:1774–83.

42 Hadeli KO, Siegel EM, Sherril DL, Beck KC, Enright PL. Predictors of oxygen desaturation during sub-maximal exercise in 8000 patients. *Chest* 2001;**120**:88–92.

43 Owens GR, Rogers RM, Pennock BE, Levin D. The diffusing capacity as a predictor of arterial oxygen desaturation during exercise in patients with COPD. *N Engl J Med* 1984;**310**:1218–21.

44 O'Donnell DE, D'Arsigny C, Fitzpatrick M, Webb KA. Exercise hypercapnia in chronic obstructive pulmonary disease: the role of lung hyperinflation. *Am J Respir Crit Care Med* 2002;**166**:663–8.

45 Alverti A, Macklem PT. How and why exercise is impaired in COPD. *Respiration* 2001;**68**:229–39.

46 Levine BD. Intermittent hypoxic training: fact and fancy. *High Alt Med Biol* 2002;**3**:177–93.

47 Fujii T, Kurihara N, Otsuka T *et al.* Relationship between exercise-induced hypoxemia and long-term survival in patients with chronic obstructive pulmonary disease. *Nihon Kyobu Shikkan Gakkai Zasshi* 1997;**35**:934–41.

48 Cotes JE, Gilson JC. Effect of oxygen on exercise ability in chronic respiratory insufficiency: use of portable apparatus. *Lancet* 1956;**1**:872–6.

49 Jolly EC, Di Boscio V, Aguirre L *et al.* Effects of supplemental oxygen during activity in patients with advanced COPD without severe resting hypoxemia. *Chest* 2001;**120**:437–43.

50 Lilker ES, Karnick A, Lerner L. Portable oxygen in chronic obstructive lung disease with hypoxemia and cor pulmonale. *Chest* 1975;**68**:236.

51 Somfay A, Porszasz J, Lee SM, Casaburi R. Dose–response effect of oxygen on hyperinflation and exercise endurance in non-hypoxemic COPD patients. *Eur Respir J* 2001;**18**:77–84.

52 Snider GL. Enhancement of exercise performance in COPD patients by hyperoxia: a call for research. *Chest* 2002;**122**:1830–6.

53 Carter R, Peavler M, Zinkgraf S, Williams J, Fields S. Predicting maximal exercise ventilation in patients with chronic obstructive pulmonary disease. *Chest* 1987;**92**:253–9.

54 Cotes JE, Pisa Z, Thomas AJ. Effects of breathing oxygen upon cardiac output, heart rate, ventilation, systemic and pulmonary blood pressure in patients with chronic lung disease. *Clin Sci* 1963;**25**:305–21.

55 Payen JF, Wuyam B, Levy P *et al.* Muscular metabolism during oxygen supplementation in patients with chronic hypoxemia. *Am Rev Respir Dis* 1993;**147**:592–8.

56 Eaton T, Garrett JE, Young P *et al.* Ambulatory oxygen improves quality of life of COPD patients: a randomised controlled study. *Eur Respir J* 2002;**20**:306–12.

57 McDonald CF, Blyth CM, Lazarus MD, Marschner I, Barter CE. Exertional oxygen of limited benefit in patients with chronic obstructive pulmonary disease and mild hypoxemia. *Am J Respir Crit Care Med* 1995;**152**:1616–9.

58 Ram FS, Wedzicha JA. 2002. Ambulatory oxygen for chronic obstructive pulmonary disease. *Cochrane Database Syst Rev* **2**:CD000238.

59 Rooyackers, JM, Dekhuijzen PN, Van Herwaarden CL, Folgering HT. Training with supplemental oxygen in patients with COPD and hypoxaemia at peak exercise. *Eur Respir J* 1997;**10**:1278–84.

60 Garrod R, Paul EA, Wedzicha JA. Supplemental oxygen during pulmonary rehabilitation in patients with COPD with exercise hypoxaemia. *Thorax* 2000;**55**:539–43.

61 Casaburi R, Porszasz J, Burns MR *et al.* Physiologic benefits of exercise training in rehabilitation of patients with severe chronic obstructive pulmonary disease. *Am J Respir Crit Care Med* 1997;**155**:1541–51.

62 Dean NC, Brown JK, Himelman RB *et al.* Oxygen may improve dyspnea and endurance in patients with chronic obstructive pulmonary disease and only mild hypoxemia. *Am Rev Respir Dis* 1992;**146**:941–5.

63 Mannix ET, Manfredi F, Palange P, Dowdeswell IRG, Farber MO. Oxygen may lower the O_2 cost of breathing in chronic obstructive lung disease. *Chest* 1992;**101**:910–5.

64 Somfay A, Pórszász J, Lee S, Casaburi R. Effect of hyperoxia on gas exchange and lactate kinetics following exercise onset in non-hypoxemic COPD patients. *Chest* 2002;**121**:393–400.

65 Maltais F, Simon M, Jobin J *et al.* Effects of oxygen on lower limb blood flow and O_2 uptake during exercise in COPD. *Med Sci Sports Exerc* 2001;**33**:916–22.

66 Emtner M, Porszasz J, Burns M, Somfay A, Casaburi R. Benefits of supplemental oxygen in exercise training in non-hypoxemic chronic obstructive pulmonary disease patients. *Am J Respir Crit Care Med* 2003;**168**:1034–42.

67 American Thoracic Society/European Respiratory Society Task Force. Standards for the Diagnosis and Management of Patients with COPD [Internet]. Version 1.2. New York: American Thoracic Society, 2004 [updated 2005 September 8]. (Available from: http://www.thoracic.org/copd)

68 Schenkel SN, Burdet L, de Muralt B *et al*. Oxygen saturation during daily activities in chronic obstructive pulmonary disease. *Eur Respir J* 1996;**9**:2584–9.

69 Sliwinski P, Lagosz M, Gorecka D *et al*. The adequacy of oxygenation in COPD patients undergoing long-term oxygen therapy assessed by pulse oximetry at home. *Eur Respir J* 1994;**7**:274–8.

70 Morrison D, Skwarski KM, MacNee W. The adequacy of oxygenation in patients with hypoxic chronic obstructive pulmonary disease treated with long-term domiciliary oxygen. *Respir Med* 1997;**91**:287–91.

71 Pilling J, Cutaia M. Ambulatory oximetry monitoring in patients with severe COPD: a preliminary study. *Chest* 1999;**116**:314–21.

72 Hurd S, Pauwels R. Global Initiative for Chronic Obstructive Lung Diseases (GOLD). *Pulm Pharmacol Ther* 2002;**15**:353–5.

73 Webb RK, Ralston C, Runciman WB. Potential errors in pulse oximetry. II. Effects of changes in saturation and signal quality. *Anesthesia* 1991;**46**:207–12.

74 Tiep BL, Burns M, Kao D, Madison R, Herrera J. Pursed lips breathing training using ear oximetry. *Chest* 1986;**90**:218–21.

75 Tiep BL. Continuous flow oxygen therapy and basis for improving the efficiency of oxygen delivery. In: Tiep BL, ed. *Portable Oxygen Therapy: Including Oxygen Conserving Methodology*. Mt Kisco, New York: Futura Publishing, 1991: 205–31.

76 Soffer M, Tashkin DP, Shapiro BJ *et al*. Conservation of oxygen supply using a reservoir nasal cannula in hypoxemic patients at rest and during exercise. *Chest* 1985;**89**:806–10.

77 Carter R, Williams JS, Berry J *et al*. Evaluation of the pendant oxygen-conserving nasal cannula during exercise. *Chest* 1986;**89**:806–10.

78 Sheehan JC, O'Donohue WJ. Use of a reservoir nasal cannula in hospitalized patients with refractory hypoxemia. *Chest* 1996;**110**:1S.

79 Dumont CP, Tiep BL. Using a reservoir nasal cannula in acute care. *Crit Care Nurse* 2002;**22**:41–6.

80 Heimlich HJ, Carr GC. The Micro-Trach: a seven-year experience with transtracheal oxygen therapy. *Chest* 1989;**95**: 1008–12.

81 Hoffman LA, Johnson JT, Wesmiller SW *et al*. Transtracheal delivery of oxygen: efficacy and safety for long-term continuous therapy. *Ann Otolol Rhinol Laryngol* 1991;**100**:108–15.

82 Christopher KL, Spofford BT, Petrun M *et al*. A program for transtracheal oxygen delivery: assessment of safety and efficacy. *Ann Intern Med* 1987;**107**:802–8.

83 Kampelmacher MJ, Deenstra M, Van Kesteren RG *et al*. Transtracheal oxygen therapy: an effective and safe alternative to nasal oxygen administration. *Eur Respir J* 1997;**10**:828–33.

84 Benditt JM, Pollock M, Roa J, Celli BR. Transtracheal delivery of gas decreases the oxygen cost of breathing. *Am Rev Respir Dis* 1993;**147**:1207–10.

85 Tiep BL, Christopher KL, Spofford BT *et al*. Pulsed nasal and transtracheal oxygen delivery. *Chest* 1990;**97**:364–8.

86 Bower JS, Brook CJ, Zimmer K, Davis D. Performance of a demand oxygen saver system during rest, exercise, and sleep in hypoxemic patients. *Chest* 1988;**94**:77.

87 Tiep BL, Nicotra MB, Carter R, Phillips R, Otsap B. Low-concentration oxygen therapy via a demand oxygen delivery system. *Chest* 1985;**87**:636–8.

88 Carter R, Tashkin D, Djahed B *et al*. Demand oxygen delivery for patients with restrictive lung disease. *Chest* 1989;**96**:1307.

89 Tiep BL, Barnett J, Schiffman G, Sanchez O, Carter R. Maintaining oxygenation via demand oxygen delivery during rest and exercise. *Respir Care* 2002;**47**:887–92.

90 Campbell EJ, Baker MD, Crites-Silver P. Subjective effects of humidification of oxygen for delivery by nasal cannula. *Chest* 1988;**93**:289–93.

CHAPTER 55
Surgical therapy for COPD

Fernando J. Martinez

COPD is a category of diseases with a varying pathophysiological basis but with a common picture of chronic airflow obstruction and hyperinflation [1]. Despite advances in medical therapy [2,3], many patients continue to experience incapacitating breathlessness and exercise limitation. Over the past several decades this has led to numerous surgical approaches to ameliorate symptoms in these patients.

History of surgical therapy for emphysema

Detailed discussions of the surgical history of emphysema management have been provided by several authors [4–6], with the surgical approaches reflecting the state of knowledge for their era. Early studies attempted to improve thoracic mobility, with procedures including costochondrectomy and transverse sternotomy [4,5], with unpredictable results. Later on, surgeons utilized techniques to decrease the size of the thoracic cage, including thoracoplasty and phrenicectomy, or to improve diaphragmatic architecture and function [4,5]. Although transient relief was noted, practical considerations limited widespread use [4,5]. Denervation was used to treat the chronic airflow obstruction, while various prosthetic devices supported the membranous trachea [5]. Significant morbidity and unpredictable results dampened the initial enthusiasm.

Brantigan *et al.* [7,8] hypothesized that by surgically removing lung volume one could restore radial traction on the terminal bronchioles, thereby improving airflow obstruction and improving diaphragmatic position and function. Although symptomatic improvement was reported in many patients, operative mortality was significant (18%) [7]. Widespread application of this technique never materialized. Over the subsequent 40 years various groups applied similar principles in small case series using various surgical techniques [9–14]. The current era of surgical lung volume reduc-

tion was ushered by Cooper *et al.* [15] who reported dramatic improvement with bilateral procedure performed via median sternotomy. Multiple investigators subsequently reported more limited improvements [16–19]. The results of the National Emphysema Treatment Trial (NETT) [21,22] have provided more definitive recommendations regarding the role of lung volume reduction surgery (LVRS) in patients with advanced emphysema.

Lung transplantation dates to the early 1960s, with 36 transplants performed between 1963 and 1974, 14 in patients with emphysema [22]. Uniformly poor results were described, with only three patients living more than 1 month. The major causes of death among the COPD patients were respiratory failure resulting from rejection, infection or bronchial disruption [23–25]. The first successful lung transplantation was performed as a heart–lung block for pulmonary vascular disease in 1981 [26]. The first successful single lung transplant (SLT) was reported in 1986 in patients with idiopathic pulmonary fibrosis. Because of differences in lung compliance, SLT was felt inappropriate for COPD patients [27,28]. Patterson *et al.* [29–31] reported successful double lung transplantation (DLT) in COPD patients, with Mal *et al.* [32] reporting successful SLT in COPD patients. SLT has become the predominant surgical therapy for advanced COPD [6,22].

Surgical techniques

An exhaustive description of the surgical techniques is outside the scope of this chapter. The important concepts are briefly reviewed here.

Bullectomy

Multiple techniques have been utilized to achieve resection of localized bullae, including standard lateral thoracotomy

636

[4], bilateral resection via median sternotomy (MS) [33], and video-assisted thoracoscopy (VATS) with stapling [34] or VATS with endoloop ligation [35].

LVRS without giant bullae

The approach to LVRS has included MS [36], standard thoracotomy and VATS [37]. Laser ablation has fallen out of favour as postoperative improvements were shown to be similar to stapled unilateral LVRS but with a higher complication rate [38]. Comparative studies have confirmed greater improvement with bilateral procedures [39,40], although not all investigators concur with this impression [41]. Results from the recently completed NETT study prospectively compared bilateral VATS with MS [21]. Similar morbidity and mortality were noted with both surgical techniques although the overall length of stay was longer for MS (10 days vs 9 days; $P = 0.01$). By 30 days after surgery, 70.5% of MS patients and 80.9% of VATS patients were living independently.

Lung transplantation

The current surgical approaches and principles of postoperative management are outside the scope of this chapter [22, 42–44]. Although controversy continues to revolve around the optimal transplant procedure in patients with COPD [45], increasing data have suggested improved long-term outcomes in COPD patients treated with DLT versus SLT [46–49]. These data are limited by the lack of prospective data collection and randomization to ensure comparable treatment groups. As such, clear recommendations require further data collection.

What are the results of surgery?

Short-term results

Bullectomy

Bullectomy appears to result in short-term benefit in highly selected patients [50–56]. Snider [57], in providing an elegant review of case series published from 1950 to the early 1990s, noted that none of the 22 studies included a control group and the majority were retrospective in nature, such that firm conclusions were difficult to reach. Nevertheless, improvement in hypoxaemia and hypercapnia were most frequently reported, with improvement in airflow being more heterogeneous. When measured, total lung capacity, residual volume and trapped gas generally decreased. In highly selected patients, cor pulmonale reversed if hypoxaemia and hypercapnia were present. Most authors described improvement in dyspnoea, with

several investigative groups reporting quantitative improvement in breathlessness. For example, the most recent series confirmed significant improvement in spirometry, residual volume (RV) and 6-minute walk distance [58].

LVRS without giant bullae

Since the early report of Cooper *et al.* in 1995 [15] numerous investigators have reported results of LVRS. Summaries of these studies have been reviewed by several authors [18,19]. Although several of these studies likely suffered from duplicate reporting of patient data, it is evident that major problems are consistently noted in the literature. These include:

1 Variable surgical techniques and selection criteria;

2 Short and often incomplete postoperative follow-up;

3 Retrospective data collection in most series; and

4 The absence of a control group in all but a few published reports.

Recently, however, results of several randomized controlled trials have clarified expectations [20,59–61].

Pulmonary function

Although Cooper *et al.* [15] initially documented an 82% improvement in forced expiratory volume in 1 s (FEV_1) after bilateral LVRS via MS, subsequent studies by this group and those of subsequent case series by others confirmed significant mean improvements in spirometry although to a lesser extent than initially suggested [18]. The NETT clearly demonstrated a modest improvement in FEV_1 for patients treated surgically compared with a modest decrement in medically treated patients (Fig. 55.1).

In general, bilateral surgical procedures have been associated with greater short-term improvement, although direct comparisons between unilateral and bilateral reduction are rare [39–41,62–66]. A multicentre prospective study comparing unilateral VATS LVRS ($n = 338$) with bilateral VATS LVRS ($n = 344$) noted greater pulmonary function improvement with the bilateral approach [66]. Unfortunately, no prospective randomized comparison exists although a strong suggestion is apparent of improved spirometric results in patients undergoing bilateral procedures. The results of laser procedures appear to be worse than those with stapling techniques. McKenna *et al.* [38] confirmed a greater short-term improvement in FEV_1 (32.9%) for those patients treated with staple resection than those undergoing laser reduction (13.4%). In addition, Keenan *et al.* [67] noted higher morbidity in a limited number of patients undergoing unilateral laser reduction ($n = 10$) compared with a group undergoing predominantly stapled resections ($n = 57$). As such, current laser technology has a limited role in LVRS.

Several investigators have compared the short-term physiological results of bilateral LVRS performed via VATS

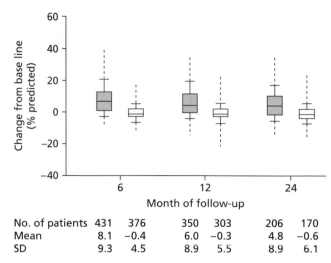

No. of patients	431	376	350	303	206	170
Mean	8.1	−0.4	6.0	−0.3	4.8	−0.6
SD	9.3	4.5	8.9	5.5	8.9	6.1

Figure 55.1 Box plots of changes from post-rehabilitation baseline in percentage of the predicted value for FEV_1 among National Emphysema Treatment Trial (NETT) patients who provided data after 6, 12 or 24 months of follow-up. High-risk patients were excluded. Solid boxes represent patients assigned to lung volume reduction surgery (LVRS); open boxes represent patients assigned to medical therapy. The line inside each box indicates the median value, the top and bottom of each box indicate the first and third quartiles, and the tails of the boxes extend to the most extreme values not considered to be outliers. Values outside the tails of the box plot are considered to be outliers. FEV_1, forced expiratory volume in 1 s; SD, standard deviation. (From the National Emphysema Treatment Trial Research Group [20], with permission.)

or MS. Kotloff *et al.* [63] noted no difference in short-term spirometric outcomes although the total in-hospital mortality was higher in the MS group (13.8 vs 2.5%). Wisser *et al.* [68] noted little difference in all outcomes between 15 patients treated with bilateral LVRS via MS compared with 15 undergoing bilateral thoracoscopic LVRS. These data corroborate the retrospective findings of other investigators [64,69]. In contrast, Ko and Waters [70] noted a higher total mortality (25%) in 19 patients undergoing bilateral LVRS via MS compared with 23 patients treated thoracoscopically (8%); the improvement in FEV_1 was higher in the VATS group (62 vs 28%). Data from the NETT have recently confirmed similar functional benefits between bilateral LVRS performed using MS or VATS [21].

The variance around the mean improvement in FEV_1 is demonstrated in remarkably few studies [63,71,72]. Figure 55.2 demonstrates the heterogeneity in spirometric response for the NETT. These data support the contention of others that 20–50% of patients show little short-term spirometric improvement after LVRS [73]. Interestingly, many patients who experience little spirometric improvement experience significant improvement in breathless-

ness, highlighting the limitation of FEV_1 as the sole measure of improvement [74].

Although published data are limited, lung volumes have generally decreased during short-term follow-up while the diffusing capacity of lung for carbon monoxide (DLCO) changes modestly [18]. Changes in resting arterial blood gases (ABGs) have also been heterogeneous [18]. For example, Albert *et al.* [75] noted minimal changes in ABGs for a group of patients as whole; some patients experienced significant improvement while others experienced worsening. In addition, no correlation was seen between ABG changes and the change in spirometry, lung volumes or DLCO.

Exercise capacity

The majority of investigators have confirmed improvements in simple measures of exercise capacity such as timed measures of walk distance [18]. Unfortunately, limited descriptions of the methodology utilized have been provided, which is particularly important for the 6-minute walk distance [76]. For example, NETT investigators have confirmed the effect of repeated testing and varying exercise format on outcomes in a large cohort of patients with severe emphysema [77]. Similarly, these investigators confirmed a modest improvement in 6-minute walk distance for the surgically treated patients compared with a consistent decrease in medically treated patients [20].

Similarly, numerous groups have reported results of cardiopulmonary exercise testing (CPET) [18], with consistent short-term increases in maximal work load, $\dot{V}O_2$ and $\dot{V}_E$ generally reported [71,74,78–82]. The improved maximal ventilation appears to be achieved through increased tidal volume, V_T, with little change in respiratory rate, f_b [71]; mean inspiratory and expiratory flows increased significantly while PaO_2 improved in 20 [71]. Benditt *et al.* [78] confirmed an improved exercise capacity after bilateral LVRS while noting decreased heart rate at similar work loads; the primary limitation to exercise was felt to be ventilatory. An improved V_T and physiological dead space at submaximal work loads during steady-state testing was associated with a decreased $PaCO_2$ during exercise in one series [80]. The NETT investigators confirmed an increase in maximal achieved wattage during oxygen supplemented cycle ergometry in surgical patients, while lesser improvement was noted in patients that continued aggressive medical management (Fig. 55.3) [20]. Additional results from another randomized trial have been recently published by Dolmage *et al.* [82]. These investigators documented an improved $\dot{V}O_{2\,peak}$ and power with a greater minute ventilation and tidal volume [82]. Importantly, an improvement in operational lung volumes was confirmed with LVRS. Importantly, the improvement in dyspnoea after surgery has been demonstrated to correlate best with decreased dynamic hyperinflation [74].

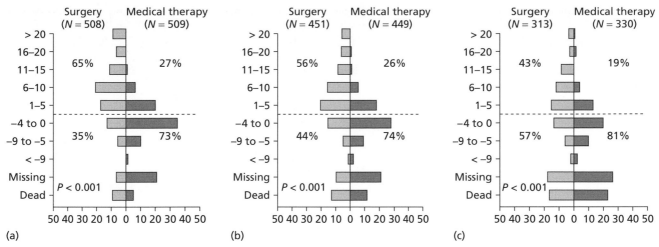

Figure 55.2 Histograms of changes from baseline in FEV_1 after 6, 12 and 24 months of follow-up. (a) Percentage of patients experiencing a change in FEV_1 per cent predicted 6 months after randomization to lung volume reduction surgery (LVRS) or medical therapy. (b) Percentage of patients experiencing a change in FEV_1 per cent predicted 12 months after randomization to LVRS or medical therapy. (c) Percentage of patients experiencing a change in FEV_1 per cent predicted 24 months after randomization to LVRS or medical therapy. Baseline measurements were performed after pulmonary rehabilitation. Patients previously identified as high risk were excluded. Patients who were too ill to complete the procedure or who declined to complete the procedure but did not explain why were included in the 'missing' category. P values were determined by the Wilcoxon rank-sum test. The degree to which the bars are shifted to the upper left of the chart indicates the degree of relative benefit of LVRS over medical treatment. The percentage shown in each quadrant is the percentage of patients in the specified treatment group with a change in the outcome falling into that quadrant. This was an intention-to-treat analysis. FEV_1, forced expiratory volume in 1 s. (From the National Emphysema Treatment Trial Research Group [20], with permission.)

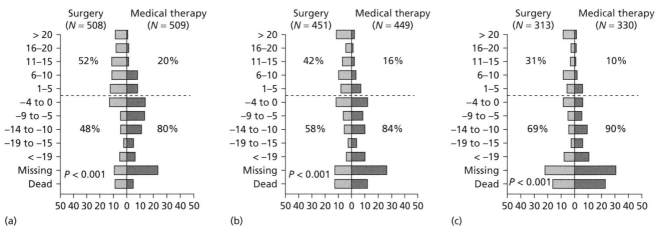

Figure 55.3 Histograms of changes from baseline in maximal achieved workload after 6, 12 and 24 months of follow-up. (a) Percentage of patients experiencing a change in maximal achieved work load predicted 6 months after randomization to lung volume reduction surgery (LVRS) or medical therapy. (b) Percentage of patients experiencing a change in maximum achieved work load 12 months after randomization to LVRS or medical therapy. (c) Percentage of patients experiencing a change in maximum achieved work load 24 months after randomization to LVRS or medical therapy. Baseline measurements were performed after pulmonary rehabilitation. Patients previously identified as high risk were excluded. Patients who were too ill to complete the procedure or who declined to complete the procedure but did not explain why were included in the 'missing' category. P values were determined by the Wilcoxon rank-sum test. The degree to which the bars are shifted to the upper left of the chart indicates the degree of relative benefit of LVRS over medical treatment. The percentage shown in each quadrant is the percentage of patients in the specified treatment group with a change in the outcome falling into that quadrant. This was an intention-to-treat analysis. (From the National Emphysema Treatment Trial Research Group [20], with permission.)

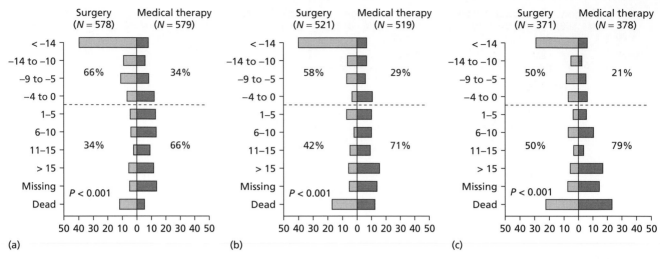

Figure 55.4 Histograms of changes from baseline in the University of California Shortness of Breath Questionnaire (UCSD SOBQ) after 6, 12 and 24 months of follow-up. (a) Percentage of patients experiencing a change in the UCSD SOBQ 6 months after randomization to lung volume reduction surgery (LVRS) or medical therapy. (b) Percentage of patients experiencing a change in the UCSD SOBQ 12 months after randomization to LVRS or medical therapy. (c) Percentage of patients experiencing a change in the UCSD SOBQ 24 months after randomization to LVRS or medical therapy. Baseline measurements were performed after pulmonary rehabilitation. Patients previously identified as high risk were excluded. Patients who were too ill to complete the procedure or who declined to complete the procedure but did not explain why were included in the 'missing' category. *P* values were determined by the Wilcoxon rank-sum test. The degree to which the bars are shifted to the upper left of the chart indicates the degree of relative benefit of LVRS over medical treatment. The percentage shown in each quadrant is the percentage of patients in the specified treatment group with a change in the outcome falling into that quadrant. This was an intention-to-treat analysis. (From the National Emphysema Treatment Trial Research Group [20], with permission.)

The short-term effects of LVRS on the pulmonary vascular response to exercise have been described by several investigative groups [83–85]. Most groups noted little change in pulmonary haemodynamics at rest or during exercise, although improvement in right heart function during exercise has been reported [86]. In contrast, Weg *et al.* [87] reported an elevation of resting pulmonary artery pressures 3 months after bilateral LVRS. Further prospective data are required to better define these changes and their clinical significance.

Medication and oxygen requirements
Several groups have described improvements in oxygen requirement after surgery [18,39,62,67,88–91]. For example, Cooper *et al.* [92] reported that of the 52% of patients using O_2 continuously before surgery, only 16% were using O_2 continuously 6 months after bilateral LVRS. Of the 92% who were using O_2 with exertion preoperatively, only 44% were doing so postoperatively. Similar data have been reported by others [38,68–70,91,93–95]. Several groups have noted discontinuation of oral steroid requirement after LVRS [15,62,69,88,89,92,96,97], although the majority of studies provided limited detail regarding specific steroid reduction protocols.

Health status
Several groups have demonstrated short-term improvement in the Medical Research Council (MRC) dyspnoea scoring system [15,38–40,62,92,98–102]. Others have confirmed similar improvement using the transitional dyspnoea index (TDI) of Mahler *et al.* [103]; the range of improvement has varied widely [15,67,71,74,88,90,92, 95,97,104–106]. The NETT investigators presented detailed assessment of breathlessness using the University of California Shortness of Breath Questionnaire (UCSD SOBQ), a symptom-based instrument validated in COPD [107]. Figure 55.4 demonstrates the heterogeneity of response noted, although a clear benefit is noted in the surgically treated group compared with medically managed patients. Some have suggested little difference in dyspnoea improvement between unilateral or bilateral LVRS [40], or between bilateral compared with unilateral LVRS [68], while others have reported better improvement with bilateral procedures [39].

The improvement in health status has been extensively reviewed [108]. Cooper *et al.* [15,92] confirmed short-term improvements using two generic instruments, the Medical Outcomes Survey-Short Form 36 (SF-36) and the Nottingham Health Profile (NHP), which have been

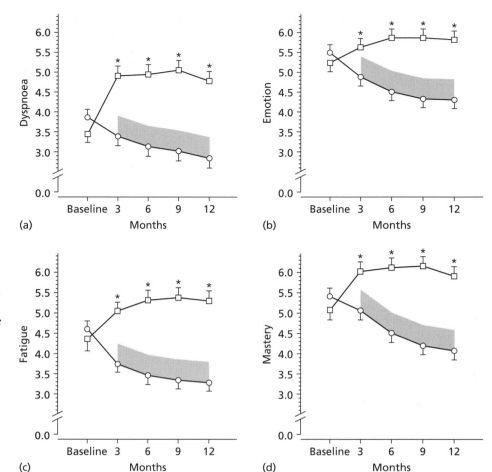

Figure 55.5 Panels (a–d) reflect the effect of surgery (□) and medical control treatment (○) on each of the four domains of the Chronic Respiratory Questionnaire (dyspnoea, emotional function, fatigue and mastery) at baseline and 3, 6, 9 and 12 months after randomization. Values at follow-up are adjusted least square mean (SE). The shaded area shows the minimum clinically important difference for each measure. (From Goldstein *et al.* [61], with permission.)

validated in COPD patients [109–111]. Similar results have been reported by other groups [69,80,112]. Several groups have described detailed analyses of health status as measured with the SF-36. Moy *et al.* [113] measured health-related quality of life (HRQL) with the SF-36 before and after comprehensive pulmonary rehabilitation and again after bilateral LVRS via VATS in 19 patients [114]. No significant change in any of the domains was noted after pulmonary rehabilitation although significant improvement was noted in vitality after LVRS. When compared with baseline, the combination of rehabilitation and bilateral LVRS resulted in significant improvement in four of the eight domains (physical functioning, role limitations because of physical problems, social functioning and vitality). Importantly, pulmonary rehabilitation accounted for most of the improvement in role limitations while LVRS accounted for most of the improvement in physical functioning, vitality and social functioning.

Change in health status measured with disease-specific instruments has been reported. Bagley *et al.* [91] described improvement in the Chronic Respiratory Questionnaire (CRQ) while Norman *et al.* [115] reported improvement

using the St. George's Respiratory Questionnaire (SGRQ). Canadian investigators noted clear improvement in the CRQ in patients treated surgically compared with a matched group randomized to medical therapy (Fig. 55.5) [61]. The NETT investigators noted significant improvement in the SGRQ of surgically treated patients compared with more modest effects [20]. Importantly, clinically significant improvement in SGRQ scores was seen in a minority of medically treated patients.

Lung transplantation

Pulmonary function

Spirometric improvement after both SLT and DLT has been consistently reported with lesser improvement generally reported in SLT recipients [46,94,116–125]. For example, Levine *et al.* [116] described functional results in 28 patients undergoing 29 SLT procedures; a rise in FEV_1 from a baseline of 16% predicted to 57% predicted at 3 months and 60% predicted at 6 months after SLT. Brunsting *et al.* [125] suggested that recipient chest wall factors determined postoperative pulmonary function, while Cheriyan *et al.* [126]

confirmed the importance of recipient factors by noting that pulmonary function after SLT reflected restriction of the transplanted lung and obstruction in the native lung with a decreased transpulmonary pressure. In an elegant study, Estenne *et al.* [127] confirmed hyperinflation of the native lung in all patients with a lower, yet stable, total lung capacity (TLC) in the allograft. The graft exhibited a normal functional residual capacity (FRC) suggesting the expansion of the rib cage allows preservation of the FRC in the transplanted lung. In contrast to SLT, DLT recipients experience a significantly higher FEV_1 with most series reporting values near normal [94,118,119].

Exercise capacity

Several early reports noted rising distance walked after SLT [117,121]. Early comparisons suggested a greater improvement in walk distance in emphysema patients undergoing SLT compared with DLT [46,118,124]. In contrast, others described similar 6-minute walk distance in patients after both types of transplantation for COPD [94,119].

Numerous investigators have confirmed persistent aerobic limitation after SLT or DLT with little evidence for ventilatory limitation [128,129]. In fact, short-term data reported by other investigators have been remarkably consistent [130–132]. Schwaiblmair *et al.* [133] demonstrated a severe aerobic limitation before transplantation which improved significantly after surgery. Importantly, no evidence of ventilatory limitation was noted after transplantation with a significant decrease in physiological dead space and $P(A–a)O_2$ at peak exercise.

Persistent aerobic limitation after transplantation has been consistently noted, with most reports supporting peripheral muscle dysfunction as the predominant cause of exercise limitation [134,135]. Pantoja *et al.* [136] examined nine lung transplant recipients (eight SLT, one DLT) 5–102 months after transplantation. In a subset, maximal voluntary contraction of the tibialis anterior muscle was decreased. Although maximal inspiratory pressures did not differ from control values, the maximal expiratory pressures were diminished by 30% relative to control ($P < 0.05$). The authors concluded that peripheral and expiratory muscle weakness, atrophy and reduction in muscular function with exercise was present in patients up to 3 years post-transplant [136]. Evans *et al.* [137] noted that quadriceps muscle intracellular pH was more acidic at rest and fell during exercise at a lower metabolic rate in transplant recipients versus healthy controls. In fact, the persistent decrease in $\dot{V}O_{2max}$ correlated closely with the metabolic rate at which muscle pH fell. Using non-invasive optical techniques, Tirdel *et al.* [138] reported that lung transplant recipients had a reduced maximum $\dot{V}O_2$ and an earlier onset of anaerobic threshold compared with matched healthy controls, suggesting an alteration in peripheral oxygen utilization by the myocyte. Wang *et al.* [139] extended these findings by analysing vastus lateralis muscle biopsies in lung transplant recipients following exercise. These biopsies demonstrated a lower mitochondrial adenosine triphosphate (ATP) production rate, lower activity of mitochondrial enzymes, a lower proportion of type 1 fibres and a higher lactate and inosine monophosphate content in the transplant recipients compared with controls. These findings were concordant with previous reports that reduced muscle calcium regulation and impaired potassium regulation after lung transplantation contributed to impaired muscle performance during exercise [140,141]. The cause of this peripheral muscle dysfunction post-transplantation remains unclear, although chronic disease, drug therapy, disuse and poor nutrition have all been suggested as contributing factors. For example, ciclosporin inhibits maximal coupled and uncoupled skeletal muscle mitochondrial respiration *in vitro* [142–144].

Health status

Gross *et al.* [145] administered to lung transplant candidates and recipients the Medical Outcome Study Health Survey (MOS 20), the Index of Well-Being, the Karnofsky Performance Status Index and questions assessing work history. Lung transplant candidates, most of who suffered from obstructive diseases, demonstrated significant impairment in health status. In those with sequential measurements, significant improvement was noted 6–12 months after transplantation. In a rare, prospective longitudinal study, TenVergert *et al.* [146] noted improvement in NHP 1 month after transplantation (13/24 patients with emphysema). Further improvement was noted during the first 4 postoperative months such that NHP scores were comparable to those of the general population. Cohen *et al.* [147] extended these findings by noting that pretransplant anxiety and psychopathology predicted post-transplant adjustment with greater anxiety predicting worse post-transplant quality of life.

Long-term results

Bullectomy

Fitzgerald *et al.* [51] reported results in 84 patients who underwent 95 surgical procedures performed over a greater than 20 year period. The mean follow-up was 7.3 years [51], with long-term follow-up available in 47 patients. Inconsistent maintenance of improvement was noted although some patients demonstrated improvement for 3–5 years. Pearson and Ogilvie [148] noted short-term improvement in 11 patients during a mean follow-up of 7.3 years, although a gradual decrement in physiological improvement was noted in most patients. During a mean follow-up of 4.5 years in 43 patients, Schipper *et al.* [58]

noted initial improvement in spirometry, residual volume and 6-minute walk distance, although a gradual worsening was noted over the years. Most authors have reported poorest long-term outcome in those individuals with greater degrees of emphysema in the remaining lung and greater underlying chronic bronchitis.

LVRS without giant bullae

Roue *et al.* [149] reported symptomatic improvement in 12/13 patients 6 months after LVRS (unilateral in 11). Although collection was incomplete, four of six patients with available data maintained a greater than 20% improvement in FEV_1 at 2 years, but neither of two patients maintained improvement at 4 years. Brenner *et al.* [150] noted a higher rate of drop in FEV_1 (0.255 ± 0.057 L/year) in those patients experiencing the greatest improvement in the initial 6 months after surgery (those treated with bilateral stapling). The lowest rate of drop was noted in those with the least initial improvement. Flaherty *et al.* [106] documented a gradual decrement in FEV_1 over the course of 3 years after bilateral LVRS, while the Washington University group has recently reported that the majority of 200 consecutive patients exhibited spirometric improvement 3 and 5 years after surgery [151].

Cordova *et al.* [152] noted a higher 6-minute walk distance in six patients 18 months after surgery compared with preoperative values; improvement in cardiopulmonary performance tended to be maintained 12 months after surgery. Flaherty *et al.* [106] also described maintenance of improvement in 6-minute walk distance despite spirometric decrement over 3 years after bilateral surgery. The NETT investigative group noted that surgical patients, in contrast to medically treated patients, were more likely to maintain improved maximal wattage during oxygen supplemented cardiopulmonary exercise testing up to 2 years after surgery [20].

Data regarding improved dyspnoea or health status have been limited. Appleton *et al.* [153] noted a sustained improvement in MRC scale and transitional dyspnoea scores during a mean of 51 months of follow-up. Cordova *et al.* [152] reported maintenance of improvement in sickness impact profile (SIP) in five of six patients with 18 months follow-up. Yusen *et al.* [151] reported improvement in MRC scores in 52% and 40% of patients 3 or 5 years after bilateral LVRS, respectively. Sixty nine per cent and 57% reported clinically significant improvement in the pulmonary function component and 65% and 54% in the dysponea component, 3 and 5 years after surgery, respectively. Similarly, the NETT investigators reported that surgical patients compared with medically treated patients were more likely to demonstrated clinically significant improvements in the SGRQ up to 2 years after surgery [20].

Lung transplantation

Clinical results

Data from the Registry of the International Society for Heart and Lung Transplantation suggests an approximately 80% 1 year, 50% 5 year and 35% 10 year survival for emphysema patients [48]. Long-term mortality seems positively related to increasing recipient age but appears less in patients with underlying emphysema [48]. The most frequent causes of late death include obliterative bronchiolitis, infection and malignancy [48,154].

Pulmonary function

Early reports noted that some patients demonstrated stability in FEV_1 improvement while others experienced a decline in pulmonary function after several months [116,121]. The importance of obliterative bronchiolitis on this loss of lung function has been reviewed recently [155,156]. Bjortuft *et al.* [123] compared pulmonary function in stable SLT recipients to recipients who developed histological obliterative bronchiolitis or obliterative bronchiolitis syndrome (BOS). Several groups have suggested that decrease in pulmonary function with BOS is particularly likely in SLT recipients [46,157]. Given the difficulty in histological confirmation of obliterative bronchiolitis, BOS has been defined physiologically as a persistent, greater than 20% drop in FEV_1 from the post-transplant baseline, in the absence of other acute conditions (airway complications, infection, congestive heart failure, reversible airway reactivity and systemic disease) [158]. Furthermore, BOS can be staged according to the drop in FEV_1 from the peak post-transplant value. Obliterative bronchiolitis is associated not only with a drop in pulmonary function but also by increased mortality [154,156].

Exercise capacity

Sundaresan *et al.* [46] noted persistent improvement in 6-minute walk distance after both SLT and DLT for COPD up to 4 years after transplantation. The same group has recently noted a mild decrease in 6-minute walk distance 5 years after transplantation [49]. Maximal achieved $\dot{V}o_2$ has been documented to change little in SLT or DLT recipients from 3 months to 1–2 years after transplantation [116,130]. As such, a significant limitation to exercise remains for patients after lung transplantation, although the effect of long-term aerobic training has not been described in this patient population.

Health status

Gross *et al.* [145] noted a similar result on the MOS 20 questionnaire in 17 recipients tested 19–36 months and 16 recipients tested greater than 36 months after transplantation when compared with responses 11 months after surgery. Importantly, recipients with BOS showed decrements in health status, particularly in the physical and social functioning and bodily pain. Similar results have been demonstrated by others [146,159,160].

Which patients should and which should not be considered for surgery?

Bullectomy

Most investigators have attempted to identify optimal surgical candidates using physiological tests and radiographical studies to identify compressed normal lung that is most likely to respond to bullectomy. These are summarized in Tables 55.1 and 55.2.

Clinical features

In general, optimal candidates suffer from persistent exertional limitation despite optimal medical therapy and pulmonary rehabilitation. A worse surgical result has been associated with older age in some series [51,52]. Some investigators have suggested a higher morbidity and worse long-term results in the presence of superimposed chronic bronchitis [51,52,56]. Although imperfect, a history of chronic sputum production and recurrent respiratory infections may provide a suggestion of such primary airway disease [1].

Physiological features

In general, ideal patients exhibit a 'restrictive' spirometric pattern with simultaneous elevation of the FRC and TLC

Table 55.1 Potential indications for classical bullectomy and lung volume reduction surgery (LVRS) in the absence of giant bullae. (Adapted from www.thoracic.org/copd/)

Parameter	Bullectomy	LVRS without giant bullae
Clinical	Young age (< 50 years)	Age < 75 years
		Clinical picture consistent with emphysema
	Rapid progressive dyspnoea despite maximal medical therapy	Dyspnoea despite maximal medical treatment pulmonary rehabilitation
	Ex smoker	Ex-smoker (> 6 months)
		Requiring < 20 mg prednisone/day
Physiological	Normal or slightly $\downarrow$ *FVC*	*FEV*$_1$ after bronchodilator < 45% prednisone
	FEV$_1$ > 40% prednisone	Hyperinflation:
	Little bronchoreversibility	TLC > 100% prednisone
	'High' trapped lung volume	RV > 150%
	Normal or near normal DLCO	Pao$_2$ > 45 mmHg
	Normal Pao$_2$ and Paco$_2$	Paco$_2$ < 60 mmHg
		Post-rehabilitation 6-min walk distance > 140 m
		Low post-rehabilitation maximal achieved cycle ergometry watts
Imaging	*CXR*	*CXR*
	Bulla > 1/3 hemithorax	Hyperinflation
	CT	*CT*
	Large and localized bulla with vascular crowding and normal, compressed pulmonary parenchyma around bulla	High-resolution CT confirming severe emphysema, ideally with upper lobe predominance
	Angiography	
	Vascular crowding with preserved distal vascular branching	
	Isotope scan	
	Well-localized matching defect with normal uptake and washout for underlying lung	

CT, computed tomography; CXR, chest X-ray; DLCO, diffusing capacity of lung for CO$_2$; *FEV*$_1$, forced expiratory volume in 1 s; *FVC*, forced vital capacity; Paco$_2$, arterial carbon dioxide tension; Pao$_2$, arterial oxygen tension.

Table 55.2 Potential contraindications for classical bullectomy and lung volume reduction surgery (LVRS) in the absence of giant bullae. (Adapted from www.thoracic.org/copd/)

Parameter	Bullectomy	LVRS without giant bullae

Clinical	Age > 50 years
	Comorbid illness
	Cardiac disease
	Pulmonary hypertension > 10% weight loss
	Frequent respiratory infections
	Chronic bronchitis
		Age > 75–80 years
		Comorbid illness that increases surgical mortality
		Clinically significant coronary artery disease
		Pulmonary hypertension (PA systolic > 45, PA mean > 35 mmHg)
		Surgical constraints:
		    Previous thoracic procedure
		    Pleuradesis
		    Chest wall deformity

Physiologic	$FEV_1 < 35\%$ prednisone 'Low' trapped gas volume Decreased DLCO	$FEV_1 \leq 20\%$ predicted and DLCO $\leq 20\%$ prednisone $\uparrow$ inspiratory resistance

Imaging	*CXR*
	Vanishing lung syndrome
	Poorly defined bullae
	
	CT
	Multiple ill-defined bullae in underlying lung
	
	Angiography
	Vague bullae; disrupted vasculature elsewhere
	
	Isotope scan
	Absence of target zones, poor washout in
	   remaining lung
		Homogeneous emphysema and $FEV_1 \leq 20\%$ predicted
		Non-upper lobe predominant emphysema and high
		   post-rehabilitation cycle ergometry maximal achieved wattage

CT, computed tomography; CXR, chest X-ray; DLCO, diffusing capacity of lung for carbon monoxide; FEV_1, forced expiratory volume in 1 s; PA, pulmonary artery.

[161]; severe obstruction, particularly when associated with smaller bullae, have been associated with poor long-term results [161]. One group noted the best improvement in patients with an FEV_1 of more than 40% predicted [162]. Significant bronchoreversibility has been proposed as an additional relative contraindication (see Table 55.2) [4,161]. Baseline elevation of the trapped gas volume has been noted in groups demonstrating better responses to classic bullectomy [51,161]. Some have utilized the DLCO as a marker of greater underlying emphysema; two groups have suggested a better response in those patients with higher DLCO and lack of exertional desaturation [50,162]. However, absolute thresholds are not available.

Imaging

Multiple groups have noted inferior surgical results in patients with bullae occupying less than one-third of the hemithorax, particularly for the long-term maintenance of functional improvement [51–53,163]. Angiography was a popular method used to identify crowded vasculature in compressed lung [161], although computed tomography (CT) has demonstrated a clear advantage. CT allows an assessment of the volume of air in bullae, the presence of compressed lung and an examination of the structure of the remaining lung tissue [53,161,164,165]. Some authors have advocated the use of radionuclide scans to assess the relative function of bullous and non-bullous areas, which may be particularly useful in identifying lung zones that appear normal or minimally involved on CT or chest radiograph [166].

Lung volume reduction without giant bullae

Clinical features

The clinical evaluation aims to identify patients with emphysema. As such, the presence of frequent respiratory infections and chronic copious sputum production may be useful in identifying patients with primary airway disease [167]. In addition, the clinical assessment should attempt to identify features predicting a higher mortality or likelihood of poor functional result (see Tables 55.1 and 55.2). Significant comorbidity, such as advanced cancer or multiorgan disease, is a reasonable contraindication (see Table 55.2). Coronary artery disease is frequently seen in this patient population [168], although it is not an absolute contraindication to surgery. Successful combined LVRS and cardiac surgery has been well documented [169,170]. Similarly, pulmonary hypertension has been described as a relative contraindication for LVRS [171], although prohibitive pulmonary hypertension is infrequent in this patient population [172–174]. The effect of milder pulmonary hypertension has not been prospectively studied [16]. Several groups have reported either no consistent change or a mild improvement in pulmonary artery pressure early after bilateral LVRS [84,85,175,176] or improved right ventricular function early after LVRS [83,86,177]. In contrast, some have reported worsening resting pulmonary hypertension after LVRS [87].

Less favourable outcomes have been reported in the presence of α_1-antitrypsin deficiency by some groups [36,178]. Cassina et al. [99] noted similar short-term clinical and physiological responses in 12 patients with α_1-antitrypsin deficiency compared with 18 patients with typical smoker's related emphysema; long-term response (12–24 months) was clearly poorer in those with α_1-antitrypsin deficiency [99]. Similarly, Gelb et al. [179] described only modest spirometric improvement after lower lobe LVRS via VATS in six patients with α_1-antitrypsin deficiency [179]. In contrast, one group has recently reported good long-term results in a group of emphysema patients with α_1-antitrypsin deficiency who were followed up to 5 years after thoracoscopic LVRS [180].

An impaired nutritional status, as measured by a lower body mass index or by decreased percentage of ideal body weight or fat-free mass index, has been associated with increased perioperative complications [181,182]. Importantly, clinical severity of disease has not proven a consistent contraindication [91,97,183,184].

Physiological features

Pulmonary function testing has proven instrumental in identifying optimal candidates for surgery (see Table 55.1). A lower limit of FEV_1 that identifies individuals at prohibitive risk has not been agreed upon, with some investigators reporting acceptable outcomes in patients with very severely decreased FEV_1 less than 500 mL [62,97,183,185]. As the mechanism of improvement in spirometry relates to improvement in elastic recoil [186], patients with airflow obstruction from structural emphysema appear to be the ones who benefit most from LVRS. Ingenito et al. [187] reported a relationship between low inspiratory resistance (as a measure of primarily airway disease) and short-term improvements in FEV_1. These same investigators have confirmed that measurement of inspiratory resistance provides additional information to emphysema distribution as defined by perfusion scintigraphy [188]. One group has recently confirmed that greater histopathological abnormalities of the smaller airways are associated with poorer short-term response to LVRS [189].

Although some have advocated LVRS only in those patients with a significant elevation of TLC [171], the RV and RV : TLC ratio may be better predictors of response [190]. Preliminary data have suggested that an elevated RV : TLC ratio may be the best physiological parameter to identify patients demonstrating improved quality of life, pulmonary function and exercise capacity after bilateral LVRS [191]. Importantly, the NETT did not identify lung volume as a predictor of mortality or functional improvement after bilateral LVRS [20].

Several investigators have suggested that a very low DLCO increases risk [67,90,192], but others have not confirmed these findings [185]. The NETT identified two subgroups of patients at particularly high risk of surgical mortality after bilateral LVRS [193]. One subgroup, composed of patients with a post-bronchodilator $FEV_1 \leq 20\%$ predicted and a DLCO $\leq 20\%$ predicted, experienced a much higher mortality with LVRS than with medical management (odds ratio [OR] 2.98; 95% confidence interval [CI], 1.3–7.7).

ABG abnormalities have been suggested to predict a bad outcome. Several investigators have suggested higher mortality in patients with hypercapnia [38,80,90,194], while others have not confirmed this finding [97,195–198]. The most definitive data come from the NETT where baseline $Paco_2$ was not associated with impaired outcome despite over 30% of randomized patients exhibiting baseline hypercapnia [20].

Preoperative exercise capacity has been documented to be a predictor of outcome by numerous investigators [90,183,194]. The most compelling data comes from the NETT, where one of the primary endpoints was maximal achieved work load achieved on a cycle ergometer while breathing supplemental oxygen [20]. A threshold of 40% of the baseline workload demonstrated a clear breakpoint in mortality for the overall study group; this corresponded to a work load of 25 watts (W) for females and 40 W for male patients [20]. These thresholds, in conjunction with computed tomography data, allowed a clear separation of non-high risk patients into four distinct categories (Fig. 55.6 and Table 55.3).

Imaging

Thoracic imaging is vital in the evaluation for LVRS [199], with most authorities considering topographical heterogeneity an important predictor of an optimal response from LVRS [16,18]. Some investigative groups have utilized chest radiographs to identify a favourable distribution of emphysema [200]. CT has proven particularly useful in this regard [201–203]. The severity of emphysema on CT may be associated with outcome after LVRS [204–206]. The

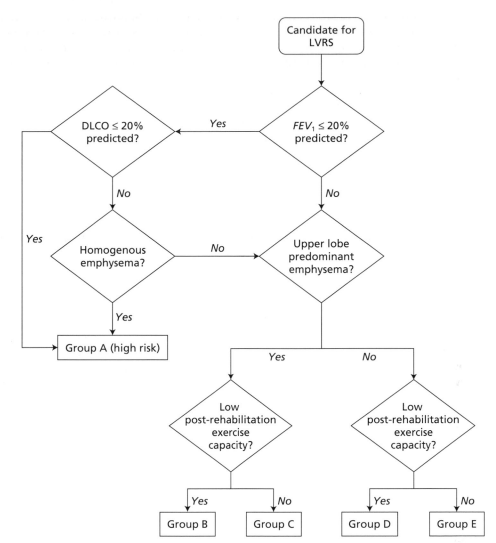

Figure 55.6 Diagnostic algorithm for patients being considered for lung volume reduction surgery (LVRS) based on data from the National Emphysema Treatment Trial (NETT) [20]. FEV_1, forced expiratory volume in 1 s; DLCO, diffusing capacity of lung for carbon monoxide. (From Martinez *et al.* [244], with permission.)

importance of emphysema heterogeneity has been consistently identified by many investigative groups [185,192, 206–212]. The most compelling data supporting the value of visual grading of emphysema distribution have been provided by NETT investigators [20]. Radiologists at 17 participating clinical centres classified HRCT scans as exhibiting predominantly upper lobe or non-upper lobe emphysema based on visual scoring of disproportionate disease between non-anatomical thirds divided equally from apex to base [213]. Using this method, in conjunction with the maximal achieved workload during oxygen supplemented maximal cycle ergometry, NETT investigators published two sentinel studies that clarified the role of CT imaging in the evaluation of patients for LVRS. An early manuscript identified an increased risk of surgical mortality in patients with severe obstruction ($FEV_1 \leq 20\%$ predicted) and either diffuse emphysema on HRCT or a DLCO $\leq 20\%$ predicted (relative risk [RR] 3.9; 95% CI, 1.9–9.0) [193]. Patients

with upper-lobe predominant emphysema and a low post-rehabilitation exercise tolerance exhibited a decreased risk of mortality (RR 0.47; $P = 0.005$) after LVRS compared with medical therapy [20]. Patients with non-upper lobe predominant emphysema and a high post-rehabilitation exercise capacity exhibited an increased risk of death during follow-up after LVRS (RR 2.06; $P = 0.02$) (see Table 55.3). Patients with upper lobe predominant emphysema and a high post-rehabilitation exercise capacity or patients with non-upper lobe predominant emphysema and a low post-rehabilitation exercise capacity did not have a survival advantage or disadvantage [20]. In addition, patients with upper lobe predominant emphysema treated surgically were more likely to improve their exercise capacity compared with medically treated patients (see Table 55.3). Figure 55.6 and Table 55.3 illustrate an approach to the evaluation of patients based on NETT data.

Unfortunately, the definition of emphysema heterogeneity

Table 55.3 Results of bilateral lung volume reduction surgery (LVRS) compared with medical therapy in patients with severe emphysema. Values in parentheses indicates percentage. Groups A–E refer to the patients as defined in Figure 55.6. (Adapted from National Emphysema Treatment Trial Research Group [20] and Martinez *et al.* [240], with permission.)

| Patients | 90-day mortality | | | Total mortality | | | |
	LVRS	Medical therapy	P value	LVRS	Medical therapy	Risk ratio*	P value
Group A	20/70 (28.6)	0/70 (0)	< 0.001	42/70	30/70	1.82	0.06
Group B	4/139 (2.9)	5/151 (3.3)	1.00	26/139	51/151	0.47	0.005
Group C	6/206 (2.9)	2/213 (0.9)	0.17	34/206	39/213	0.98	0.70
Group D	7/84 (8.3)	0/65 (0)	0.02	28/84	26/65	0.81	0.49
Group E	11/109 (10.1)	1/111 (0.9)	0.003	27/109	14/111	2.06	0.02

| Patients | Improvement in exercise capacity† | | | | Improvement in health-related quality of life‡ | | | |
	LVRS	Medical therapy	Odds ratio	P value	LVRS	Medical therapy	Odds ratio	P value
Group A	4/58 (7)	1/48 (2)	3.48	0.37	6/58 (10)	0/48 (0)	–	0.03
Group B	25/84 (30)	0/92 (0)	–	< 0.001	40/84 (48)	9/92 (10)	8.38	< 0.001
Group C	17/115 (15)	4/138 (3)	5.81	0.001	47/115 (41)	15/138 (11)	5.67	< 0.001
Group D	6/49 (12)	3/41 (7)	1.77	0.50	18/49 (37)	3/41 (7)	7.35	0.001
Group E	2/65 (3)	2/59 (3)	0.90	1.00	10/65 (15)	7/59 (12)	1.35	0.61

* Risk ratio for total mortality in surgically versus medically treated patients during a mean follow-up of 29.2 months.
† Increase in the maximal workload of more than 10 W from the patient's post-rehabilitation base-line value (24 months after randomization).
‡ Improvement in the health-related quality of life was defined as a decrease in the score on the St. George's Respiratory Questionnaire of more than 8 points (on a 100-point scale) from the patient's post-rehabilitation baseline score (24 months after randomization).

has varied widely [213]. As such, many investigators have utilized quantitative CT methodology to define disease heterogeneity. Several groups have confirmed moderately strong correlations between several quantitative CT values and outcome measures [106,214]. Nakano *et al.* [215] reported a positive correlation between the amount of amount of severe emphysema in the peripheral 50% of the lung and improvement in maximal achieved watts during cycle ergometry after LVRS [215]. This same group examined the relationship between the number and size of emphysematous lesions and the short-term response to LVRS [216]. The power law exponent (D) represents the slope of the relationship between the log of the cumulative number of emphysematous lesions and the log of the emphysema lesion size. As such, a steep slope and thus large D represents lungs with predominantly small lesions, while a shallow slope and small D suggests lungs with larger emphysematous lesions. A positive correlation was noted between the change in D and the change in maximal wattage achieved during cycle ergometry after surgery. As such, the authors suggested that patients with larger upper lobe lesions respond better to surgery than patients with small, uniformly distributed lesions [216].

Several groups have suggested that identifying heterogeneous perfusion during perfusion scanning may predict outcome after LVRS [217–219]. Thurnheer *et al.* [101] reported that functional improvement after surgery correlated better with physiological hyperinflation and emphysema heterogeneity as assessed by CT compared with perfusion heterogeneity assessed by scintigraphy. Hunsaker *et al.* [205] noted that patients with more heterogeneous emphysema, as determined by CT or *V/Q* imaging, tended to show a greater magnitude and likelihood for improved FEV_1. Cederlund *et al.* [220] noted little difference in emphysema heterogeneity classification based on CT or scintigraphy alone; the combination of the two was superior when contrasted with quantitative methodology as the 'gold standard'. It is likely that CT and scintigraphy demonstrate similar predictive ability in suggesting outcome after LVRS.

Lung transplantation

Given the significant morbidity and mortality associated with lung transplantation, careful patient selection is crucial. This is particularly relevant in COPD, as controversy

Table 55.4 General selection guidelines for candidate selection for lung transplantation in COPD patients. (Adapted from [225,227–229,241,242] and www.thoracic.org/copd/)

Relative contraindications
Age limits
    Heart-lung transplants ~ 55 years
    Double lung transplant ~ 60 years
    Single lung transplant ~ 65 years
Poorly or untreated, symptomatic osteoporosis
Oral corticosteroids > 20 mg/day prednisone
Ideal body weight < 70% or > 130%
Psychosocial problems
Requirement for invasive mechanical ventilation
Colonization with fungi or atypical mycobacteria

Absolute contraindications
Severe musculoskeletal disease affecting the thorax
Substance addiction within previous 6 months
Dysfunction of extrathoracic organ, particularly renal
    dysfunction
Human immunodeficiency virus infection
Active malignancy within 2 years except basal or squamous
    cell carcinoma of skin
Hepatitis B antigen positivity
Hepatitis C with biopsy-proven evidence of liver disease

Table 55.5 Disease-specific guidelines for candidate referral for lung transplantation in COPD patients. (Modified from [227,242,243].)

$FEV_1 < 20$–25% prednisone
$Pco_2 > 7.3$ kPa (55 mmHg)
Homogeneous emphysema distribution
Pulmonary hypertension

FEV_1, forced expiratory volume in 1 s; Pco_2, arterial carbon dioxide tension.

exists regarding whether a survival benefit is noted after lung transplantation in this condition [154,221–224]. A summary of potential selection criteria is contrasted with bullectomy and LVRS in Tables 55.4 and 55.5.

Clinical features

The initial evaluation should include an assessment of the general surgical risks associated with age, as older recipients have a significantly worse survival rate [48]. The Joint Statement of the American Society for Transplant Physicians, the American Thoracic Society, the European Respiratory Society and the International Society for Heart and Lung Transplantation suggests that potential age limits included approximately 55 years for HLT, 65 years for SLT and 60 years for DLT [225]. Several clinical characteristics are felt to represent absolute or relative contraindications as enumerated in Table 55.3 [22,225–230].

Physiological features

Physiological testing has been the most frequently used modality to assess prognosis in patients with COPD [231]. Numerous investigators have documented that the FEV_1 after bronchodilator administration is an important predictor of mortality in COPD [232–236]. An emphysema patient can be considered an appropriate candidate for transplantation when the FEV_1 is below 25% predicted

and/or the $Paco_2 \geq 55$ mmHg [225]. A recent study has suggested that a multidimensional index incorporating FEV_1, 6-minute walk distance, measurement of dyspnoea and body mass index predicts survival better in COPD than spirometry alone [237]. How this index will impact transplant listing decision making requires further investigation. Similarly, the presence of pulmonary hypertension with progressive deterioration should be considered an additional feature suggesting that transplantation should be considered an appropriate surgical intervention.

Imaging

Imaging techniques have a less defined role in the preoperative evaluation for lung transplantation. CT appears to alter the surgical approach to lung transplantation. Kazerooni *et al.* [238] noted a change in the determination of which lung was more severely diseased in 27/169 patients examined with preoperative chest radiography and CT. Of the 45 patients who subsequently underwent transplantation, CT prompted a change in the determination of which side to perform SLT in four. This same group has identified pulmonary nodules, suspicious for malignancy, in eight of 190 patients evaluated for lung transplantation [239]. As an active malignancy precludes transplantation, such a finding would clearly alter the candidacy of a patient for lung transplantation. Finally, the presence of unsuspected bronchiectasis could alter the decision to perform DLT in contrast to SLT.

Conclusions

Extensive literature has been published regarding surgical therapies for advanced COPD, with the most widely accepted directed at surgical relief of hyperinflation. Bullectomy and LVRS are established surgical techniques for a very limited number of patients. The patients with the poorest long-term outcomes appear to be those with the most abnormal respiratory function or greater extent of emphysema on imaging studies. Lung transplantation may serve as a viable therapeutic option for some of these COPD patients.

References

1 Martinez FJ. Diagnosing chronic obstructive pulmonary disease. The importance of differentiating asthma, emphysema and chronic bronchitis. *Postgrad Med* 1998;**103**:112–25.

2 Martinez FJ. Surgical therapy for chronic obstructive pulmonary disease: conventional bullectomy and lung volume reduction surgery in the absence of giant bullae. *Semin Respir Crit Care Med* 1999;**20**:351–64.

3 Sin DD, McAlister FA, Man SFP, Anthonisen NR. Contemporary management of chronic obstructive pulmonary disease: scientific review. *JAMA* 2003;**290**:2301–12.

4 Gaensler EA, Cugell DW, Knudson RJ, FitzGerald MX. Surgical management of emphysema. *Clin Chest Med* 1983;**4**:443–63.

5 Deslauriers J. History of surgery for emphysema. *Semin Thorac Cardiovasc Surg* 1996;**8**:43–51.

6 Meyers BF, Patterson GA. Chronic obstructive pulmonary disease. 10. Bullectomy, lung volume reduction surgery, and transplantation for patients with chronic obstructive pulmonary disease. *Thorax* 2003;**58**:634–8.

7 Brantigan O, Kress M, Mueller E. A surgical approach to pulmonary emphysema. *Am Rev Respir Dis* 1959;**39**:194–202.

8 Brantigan O, Mueller E. Surgical treatment of pulmonary emphysema. *Am Surg* 1957;**23**:789–804.

9 Delarue NC, Woolf CR, Sanders DE *et al*. Surgical treatment for pulmonary emphysema. *Can J Surg* 1977;**20**:222–31.

10 Even P, Sors H, Safran D *et al*. Hemodynamique des bulles d'emphyseme un nouveau syndrome: la tamponade cardiaque emphysemateuse. *Rev Fr Mal Respir* 1980;**8**:117–20.

11 Dahan M, Salerin F, Berjaud J *et al*. Interet de l'exploration hemodynamique dans les indications chirurgicales des emphysemes. *Ann Chir* 1989;**43**:669–72.

12 Crosa-Dorado VL, Pomi J, Perez-Penco EJ, Carriquiry G. Treatment of dyspnea in emphysema: pulmonary remodeling; hemo- and pneumostatic suturing of the emphysematous lung. *Res Surg* 1992;**4**:152–5.

13 Wakabayashi A. Thoracoscopic laser pneumoplasty in the treatment of diffuse bullous emphysema. *Ann Thorac Surg* 1995;**60**:936–42.

14 Wakabayashi A, Brenner M, Kayaleh RA *et al*. Thoracoscopic carbon dioxide laser treatment of bullous emphysema. *Lancet* 1991;**337**:881–3.

15 Cooper JD, Trulock EP, Triantafillou AN *et al*. Bilateral pneumectomy (volume reduction) for chronic obstructive pulmonary disease. *J Thorac Cardiovasc Surg* 1995;**109**:106–16; discussion 116–9.

16 Utz JP, Hubmayr RD, Deschamps C. Lung volume reduction surgery for emphysema: out on a limb without a NETT. *Mayo Clin Proc* 1998;**73**:552–6.

17 Benditt JO, Albert RK. Surgical options for patients with advanced emphysema. *Clin Chest Med* 1997;**18**:577–93.

18 Flaherty KR, Martinez FJ. Lung volume reduction surgery for emphysema. *Clin Chest Med* 2000;**21**:819–48.

19 Benditt JO. Surgical therapies for chronic obstructive pulmonary disease. *Respir Care* 2004;**49**:53–61.

20 National Emphysema Treatment Trial Research Group. A randomized trial comparing lung-volume-reduction surgery with medical therapy for severe emphysema. *N Engl J Med* 2003;**348**:2059–73.

21 National Emphysema Treatment Trial Research Group. Safety and efficacy of median sternotomy versus video assisted thoracic surgery for lung volume reduction surgery. *J Thorac Cardiovasc Surg* 2004;**127**:1350–60.

22 Dunitz JM, Hertz MI. Surgical therapy for COPD: lung transplantation. *Semin Respir Crit Care Med* 1999;**20**:365–73.

23 Wildevuur CRH, Benfield JR. A review of 23 human lung transplantation by 20 surgeons. *Ann Thorac Surg* 1970;**9**:489–515.

24 Veith FJ, Koerner SK. Problems in the management of lung transplant recipients. *Vasc Surg* 1974;**8**:273–82.

25 Veith FJ, Koerner SK, Siegelman SS *et al*. Single lung transplantation in experimental and human emphysema. *Ann Surg* 1973;**178**:463–76.

26 Reitz BA, Wallwork JL, Hunt SA *et al*. Heart-lung transplantation: successful therapy for patients with pulmonary vascular disease. *N Engl J Med* 1982;**306**:557–64.

27 Stevens PM, Johnson PC, Bell RL, Beall AC, Jenkins DE. Regional ventilation and perfusion after lung transplantation in patients with emphysema. *N Engl J Med* 1970;**282**:245–9.

28 Bates DV. The other lung. *N Engl J Med* 1970;**282**:277–9.

29 Patterson GA, Cooper JD, Dark JH, Jones MT. Experimental and clinical double lung transplantation. *J Thorac Cardiovasc Surg* 1988;**95**:70–4.

30 Patterson GA, Cooper JD, Goldman B *et al*. Technique of successful clinical double-lung transplantation. *Ann Thorac Surg* 1988;**45**:626–33.

31 Cooper JD, Patterson GA, Grossman R, Maurer J. Double-lung transplant for advanced chronic obstructive lung disease. *Am Rev Respir Dis* 1989;**139**:303–7.

32 Mal H, Andreassian B, Pamela F *et al*. Unilateral lung transplantation in end-stage pulmonary emphysema. *Am Rev Respir Dis* 1989;**140**:787–802.

33 Iwa T, Watanabe Y, Fukatani G. Simultaneous bilateral operations for bullous emphysema by median sternotomy. *J Thorac Cardiovasc Surg* 1981;**81**:732–7.

34 Dartevelle P, Macchiarini P, Chapelier A. Operative technique of bullectomy. *Chest Surg Clin North Am* 1995;**5**:735–49.

35 Liu HP, Chang CH, Lin PJ, Chu JJ, Hsieh MJ. An alternative technique in the management of bullous emphysema: thoracoscopic endoloop ligation of bullae. *Chest* 1997;**111**:489–93.

36 Cooper JD, Patterson GA. Lung volume reduction surgery for severe emphysema. *Semin Thorac Cardiovasc Surg* 1996;**8**:52–60.

37 Brenner M, Yusen R, McKenna R Jr *et al*. Lung volume reduction surgery for emphysema. *Chest* 1996;**110**:205–18.

38 McKenna RJ Jr, Brenner M, Gelb AF *et al*. A randomized, prospective trial of stapled lung reduction versus laser

bullectomy for diffuse emphysema. *J Thorac Cardiovasc Surg* 1996;**111**:317–22.

39 McKenna RJ Jr, Brenner M, Fischel RJ, Gelb AF. Should lung volume reduction for emphysema be unilateral or bilateral. *J Thorac Cardiovasc Surg* 1996;**112**:1331–8.

40 Argenziano M, Thorashow B, Jellen PA *et al.* Functional comparison of unilateral versus bilateral lung volume reduction surgery. *Ann Thorac Surg* 1997;**64**:321–7.

41 Oey IF, Waller DA, Bal S *et al.* Lung volume reduction surgery: a comparison of the long-term outcome of unilateral vs bilateral approaches. *Eur J Cardiothorac Surg* 2002;**22**:610–4.

42 Force SD, Choong C, Meyers BF. Lung transplantation for emphysema. *Chest Surg Clin North Am* 2003;**13**:651–67.

43 Trulock EP. Lung transplantation. *Am J Respir Crit Care Med* 1997;**152**:947–52.

44 Arcasoy SM, Kotloff RM. Lung transplantation. *N Engl J Med* 1999;**340**:1081–91.

45 Weill D, Keshavjee S. Lung transplantaion for emphysema: two lungs or one. *J Heart Lung Transplant* 2001;**20**:739–42.

46 Sundaresan RS, Shiraishi Y, Trulock EP *et al.* Single or bilateral lung transplantation for emphysema? *J Thorac Cardiovasc Surg* 1996;**112**:1485–95.

47 Meyer DM, Bennett LE, Novick RJ, Hosenpud JD. Transplantation for end-stage emphysema: influence of recipient age on survival and secondary end-points. *J Heart Lung Transplant* 2001;**20**:935–41.

48 Trulock EP, Edwards LB, Taylor DO *et al.* The Registry of the International Society for Heart and Lung Transplantation: Twentieth official adult lung and heart-lung transplant report – 2003. *J Heart Lung Transplant* 2003;**22**:625–35.

49 Cassivi SD, Meyers BF, Battafarano RJ *et al.* Thirteen-year experience in lung transplantation for emphysema. *Ann Thorac Surg* 2002;**74**:1663–9.

50 Hugh-Jones P, Whimster W. The etiology and management of disabling emphysema. *Am Rev Respir Dis* 1978;**117**:343–78.

51 Fitzgerald M, Keelan P, Angell D. Long-term results of surgery for bullous emphysema. *Surgery* 1974;**68**:566–82.

52 Laros C, Gellisen H, Bergstein PGM *et al.* Bullectomy for giant bullae in emphysema. *J Thorac Cardiovasc Surg* 1986;**91**:63–70.

53 Nickoladze GD. Functional results of surgery for bullous emphysema. *Chest* 1992;**101**:119–22.

54 Potgieter PD, Benatar SR, Hewitson RP, Ferguson AD. Surgical treatment of bullous lung disease. *Thorax* 1981;**36**:885–90.

55 Sung D, Payne W, Black L. Surgical management of giant bullae associated with obstructive airway disease. *Surg Clin North Am* 1973;**53**:913–20.

56 Petro W, Hubner Ch, Greschuchna D, MaaBen W, Konietzko N. Bullectomy. *Thorac Cardiovasc Surg* 1983;**31**:342–5.

57 Snider GL. Reduction pneumoplasty for giant bullous emphysema: implications for surgical treatment of non-bullous emphysema. *Chest* 1996;**109**:540–8.

58 Schipper PH, Meyers BF, Battafarano RJ *et al.* Outcomes after resection of giant emphysematous bullae. *Ann Thorac Surg* 2004;**78**:976–82.

59 Pompeo E, Marino M, Nofroni I, Matteucci G, Mineo TC, Pulmonary Emphysema Research Group. Reduction pneumoplasty versus respiratory rehabilitation in severe emphysema: a randomized study. *Ann Thorac Surg* 2000;**70**:948–54.

60 Geddes D, Davies M, Koyama H *et al.* Effect of lung-volume-reduction surgery in patients with severe emphysema. *N Engl J Med* 2000;**343**:239–45.

61 Goldstein RS, Todd TRJ, Guyatt GH *et al.* Influence of lung volume reduction surgery (LVRS) on health related quality of life in patients with chronic obstructive pulmonary disease. *Thorax* 2003;**58**:405–10.

62 Eugene J, Dajee A, Kayaleh R *et al.* Reduction pneumoplasty for patients with a forced expired volume in 1 second of 500 milliters or less. *Ann Thorac Surg* 1997;**63**:186–92.

63 Kotloff RM, Tino G, Bavaria JE *et al.* Bilateral lung volume reduction surgery for advanced emphysema: a comparison of median sternotomy and thoracoscopic approaches. *Chest* 1996;**110**:1399–406.

64 Yoshinaga Y, Iwasaki A, Kawahara K, Shirakusa T. Lung volume reduction surgery results in pulmonary emphysema: changes in pulmonary function. *Jpn J Thorac Cardiovasc Surg* 1999;**47**:445–51.

65 Nezu K, Kushibe K, Sawabata N *et al.* Thoracoscopic lung volume reduction surgery for emphysema: evaluation using ventilation–perfusion scintigraphy. *Jpn J Thorac Cardiovasc Surg* 1999;**47**:267–72.

66 Lowdermilk GA, Keenan RJ, Landreneau RJ *et al.* Comparison of clinical results for unilateral and bilateral thoracoscopic lung volume reduction. *Ann Thorac Surg* 2000;**69**:1670–4.

67 Keenan RJ, Landrenau RJ, Sciurba FC *et al.* Unilateral thoracoscopic surgical approach for diffuse emphysema. *J Thorac Cardiovasc Surg* 1996;**111**:308–16.

68 Wisser W, Tschernko E, Senbaklavaci O *et al.* Functional improvement after volume reduction: sternotomy versus videoendoscopic approach. *Ann Thorac Surg* 1997;**63**:822–8.

69 Hazelrigg SR, Boley TM, Magee MJ, Lawyer CH, Henkle JQ. Comparison of staged thoracoscopy and median sternotomy for lung volume reduction surgery. *Ann Thorac Surg* 1998;**66**:1134–9.

70 Ko CY, Waters PF. Lung volume reduction surgery: a cost and outcomes comparison of sternotomy versus thoracoscopy. *Am Surg* 1998;**64**:1010–3.

71 Keller CA, Ruppel G, Hibbett A, Osterloh J, Naunheim KS. Thoracoscopic lung volume reduction surgery reduces dyspnea and improves exercise capacity in patients with emphysema. *Am J Respir Crit Care Med* 1997;**156**:60–7.

72 Yusen RD, Trulock EP, Pohl MS, Biggar DG, Group The Washington University Emphysema Surgery: results of lung volume reduction surgery in patients with emphysema. *Semin Thorac Cardiovasc Surg* 1996;**8**:99–109.

73 Fessler HE, Wise RE. Lung volume reduction surgery: is less *really* more? *Am J Respir Crit Care Med* 1999;**159**:1031–5.

74 Martinez FJ, de Oca MM, Whyte RI *et al.* Lung-volume reduction improves dyspnea, dynamic hyperinflation, and respiratory muscle function. *Am J Respir Crit Care Med* 1997;**155**:1984–90.

75 Albert RK, Benditt JO, Hildebrandt J, Wood DE, Hlastala MP. Lung volume reduction surgery has variable effects on blood gases in patients with emphysema. *Am J Respir Crit Care Med* 1998;**158**:71–6.

76 Sciurba FC, Slivka WA. Six-minute walk testing. *Semin Respir Crit Care Med* 1998;**19**:383–92.

77 Sciurba F, Criner GJ, Lee SM *et al.* for the National Emphysema Treatment Trial Research Group. Six-minute walk distance in chronic obstructive pulmonary disease: reproducibility and effect of walking course layout and length. *Am J Respir Crit Care Med* 2003;**167**:1522–7.

78 Benditt JO, Lewis S, Wood DE, Klima L, Albert RK. Lung volume reduction surgery improves maximal O_2 consumption, maximal minute ventilation, O_2 pulse and dead space-to-tidal volume ration during leg cycle ergometry. *Am J Respir Crit Care Med* 1997;**156**:561–6.

79 Tschernko EM, Gruber EM, Jaksch P *et al.* Ventilatory mechanics and gas exchange during exercise before and after lung volume reduction surgery. *Am J Respir Crit Care Med* 1998;**158**:1424–31.

80 Ferguson GT, Fernandez E, Zamora MR *et al.* Improved exercise performance following lung volume reduction surgery for emphysema. *Am J Respir Crit Care Med* 1998; **157**:1195–203.

81 Criner GJ, Cordova FC, Furukawa S *et al.* Prospective randomized trial comparing bilateral lung volume reduction surgery to pulmonary rehabilitation in severe chronic obstructive pulmonary disease. *Am J Respir Crit Care Med* 1999;**160**:2018–27.

82 Dolmage TE, Waddell TK, Maltais F *et al.* The influence of lung volume reduction surgery on exercise in patients with COPD. *Eur Respir J* 2004;**23**:269–74.

83 Kubo K, Koizumi T, Fujimoto K *et al.* Effects of lung volume reduction surgery on exercise pulmonary hemodynamics in severe emphysema. *Chest* 1998;**114**:1575–82.

84 Oswald-Mammosser M, Kessler R, Massard G *et al.* Effect of lung volume reduction surgery on gas exchange and pulmonary hemodynamics at rest and during exercise. *Am J Respir Crit Care Med* 1999;**158**:1020–5.

85 Haniuda M, Kubo K, Fujimoto K *et al.* Different effects of lung volume reduction surgery and lobectomy on pulmonary circulation. *Ann Surg* 2000;**231**:119–25.

86 Mineo TC, Pompeo E, Rogliani P *et al.* for the Pulmonary Emphysema Research Group. Effect of lung volume reduction surgery for severe emphysema on right ventricular function. *Am J Respir Crit Care* 2002;**165**:480–94.

87 Weg IL, Rossoff L, McKeon K, Graver LM, Scharf SM. Development of pulmonary hypertension after lung volume reduction surgery. *Am J Respir Crit Care Med* 1999;**159**:552–6.

88 Naunheim KS, Keller CA, Krucylak PE *et al.* Unilateral video-assisted thoracic surgical lung reduction. *Ann Thorac Surg* 1996;**61**:1092–8.

89 Eugene J, Ott RA, Gogia HS *et al.* Video-thoracic surgery for treatment of end-stage bullous emphysema and chronic obstructive pulmonary disease. *Am Surg* 1995;**61**:934–6.

90 Hazelrigg S, Boley T, Henkle J *et al.* Thoracoscopic laser bullectomy: a prospective study with three-month results. *J Thorac Cardiovasc Surg* 1996;**112**:319–27.

91 Bagley PH, Davis SM, O'Shea M, Coleman AM. Lung volume reduction surgery at a community hospital: program development and outcomes. *Chest* 1997;**111**:1552–9.

92 Cooper JD, Patterson GA, Sundaresan RS *et al.* Results of 150 consecutive bilateral lung volume reduction procedures in patients with severe emphysema. *J Thorac Cardiovasc Surg* 1996;**112**:1319–30.

93 Daniel TM, Chan BBK, Bhaskar V *et al.* Lung volume reduction surgery: case selection, operative technique, and clinical results. *Ann Surg* 1996;**223**:526–33.

94 Gaissert HA, Trulock EP, Cooper JD, Sundaresan RS, Patterson GA. Comparison of early functional results after volume reduction or lung transplantation for chronic obstructive pulmonary disease. *J Thorac Cardiovasc Surg* 1996;**111**:296–307.

95 Bousamra M II, Haasler GB, Lipchik RJ *et al.* Functional and oximetric assessment of patients after lung reduction surgery. *J Thorac Cardiovasc Surg* 1997;**113**:675–82.

96 Miller JI, Lee RB, Mansour KA. Lung volume reduction surgery: lessons learned. *Ann Thorac Surg* 1996;**61**:1464–9.

97 Argenziano M, Moazami N, Thomashow B *et al.* Extended indications for lung volume reduction surgery in advanced emphysema. *Ann Thorac Surg* 1996;**62**:1588–97.

98 Bingisser R, Zollinger A, Hauser M *et al.* Bilateral volume reduction surgery for diffuse pulmonary emphysema by video-assisted thoracoscopy. *J Thorac Cardiovasc Surg* 1996; **112**:875–82.

99 Cassina PC, Teschler H, Konietzko N, Theegarten D, Stamatis G. Two-year results after lung volume reduction surgery in α_1-antitrypsin deficiency versus smoker's emphysema. *Eur Respir J* 1998;**12**:1028–32.

100 Stammberger U, Bloch KE, Thurnheer R *et al.* Exercise performance and gas exchange after bilateral video-assisted thoracoscopic lung volume reduction for severe emphysema. *Eur Respir J* 1998;**12**:785–92.

101 Thurnheer R, Engel H, Weder W *et al.* Role of lung perfusion scintigraphy in relation to chest computed tomography and pulmonary function in the evaluation of candidates for lung volume reduction surgery. *Am J Respir Crit Care Med* 1999;**159**:301–10.

102 Brenner M, McKenna RJ, Gelb AF *et al.* Dyspnea response following bilateral thoracoscopic staple lung volume reduction surgery. *Chest* 1997;**112**:916–23.

103 Mahler DA, Weinberg DH, Wells CK, Feinstein AR. The measurement of dyspnea: contents, interobserver agreement, and physiologic correlates of two new clinical indexes. *Chest* 1984;**85**:751–8.

104 Sciurba FC, Rogers RM, Keenan RJ *et al.* Improvement in pulmonary function and elastic recoil after lung-reduction surgery for diffuse emphysema. *N Engl J Med* 1996;**334**:1095–9.

105 Scharf SM, Rossoff L, McKeon K *et al.* Changes in pulmonary mechanics after lung volume reduction surgery. *Lung* 1998; **176**:191–204.

106 Flaherty KR, Kazerooni EA, Curtis JL *et al.* Short-term and long-term outcomes after bilateral lung volume reduction surgery: prediction by quantitative CT. *Chest* 2001;**119**: 1337–46.

107 Eakin EG, Resnikoff PM, Prewitt LM, Ries AL, Kaplan RM. Validation of a new dyspnea measure: the UCSD Shortness of Breath Questionnaire. University of California, San Diego. *Chest* 1998;**113**:619–24.

108 Yusen RD, Morrow LE, Brown KL. Health-related quality of life after lung volume reduction surgery. *Semin Thorac Cardiovasc Surg* 2002;**14**:403–12.

109 Mahler DA, Mackowiak JI. Evaluation of the short-form 36-item questionnaire to measure health-related quality of life in patients with COPD. *Chest* 1995;**6**:1585–9.

110 Nishimura K, Tsukino M, Hajiro T. Health-related quality of life in patients with chronic obstructive pulmonary disease. *Curr Opin Pulm Med* 1998;**4**:107–15.

111 Prieto L, Alonso J, Ferrer M, Anto JM, Group Quality of Life in COPD Study. Are results of the SF-36 Health Survey and the Nottingham Health Profile similar?: a comparison in COPD patients. *J Clin Epidemiol* 1997;**50**:463–73.

112 Anderson KL. Change in quality of life after lung volume reduction surgery. *Am J Crit Care* 1999;**8**:389–96.

113 Moy ML, Ingenito EP, Mentzer SJ, Evans RB, Reilly JJ Jr. Health-related quality of life improves following pulmonary rehabiliation and lung volume reduction surgery. *Chest* 1999;**115**:383–9.

114 Mineo TC, Ambrogi V, Pompeo E *et al*. Impact of lung volume reduction surgery versus rehabilitation on quality of life. *Eur Respir J* 2004;**23**:275–80.

115 Norman M, Hillerdal G, Orre L *et al*. Improved lung function and quality of life following increased elastic recoil after lung volume reduction surgery in emphysema. *Respir Med* 1998;**92**:653–8.

116 Levine SM, Anzueto A, Peters JI *et al*. Medium term functional results of single-lung transplantation for endstage obstructive lung disease. *Am J Respir Crit Care Med* 1994;**150**:398–402.

117 Kaiser LR, Cooper JD, Trulock EP, *et al*. The Washington University Lung Transplant Group. The evolution of single lung transplantation for emphysema. *J Thorac Cardiovasc Surg* 1991;**102**:333–41.

118 Patterson GA, Maurer JR, Williams TJ *et al*. Comparison of outcomes of double and single lung transplantation for obstructive lung disease. *J Thorac Cardiovasc Surg* 1991;**101**:623–32.

119 Low DE, Trulock EP, Kaiser LR *et al*. Morbidity, mortality, and early results of single versus bilateral lung transplantation for emphysema. *J Thorac Cardiovasc Surg* 1992;**103**:1119–26.

120 Cooper JD, Patterson GA, Trulock EP, Washington University Lung Transplant Group. Results of single and bilateral lung transplantaton in 131 consecutive recipients. *J Thorac Cardiovasc Surg* 1994;**107**:460–71.

121 Mal H, Sleiman C, Jebrak G *et al*. Functional results of single-lung transplantation for chronic obstructive lung disease. *Am J Respir Crit Care Med* 1994;**149**:1476–81.

122 Briffa NP, Dennis C, Higenbottam T *et al*. Single lung transplantation for end stage emphysema. *Thorax* 1995;**50**:562–4.

123 Bjortuft O, Geiran OR, Fjeld J *et al*. Single lung transplantation for chronic obstructive pulmonary disease: pulmonary function and impact of bronchiolitis obliterans syndrome. *Respir Med* 1996;**90**:553–9.

124 Bavaria JE, Kotloff R, Palevsky H *et al*. Bilateral versus single lung transplantation for chronic obstructive pulmonary disease. *J Thorac Cardiovasc Surg* 1997;**113**:520–8.

125 Brunsting LA, Lupinetti FM, Cascade PN *et al*. Pulmonary function in single lung transplantation for chronic obstructive pulmonary disease. *J Thorac Cardiovasc Surg* 1994;**107**:1337–45.

126 Cheriyan AF, Garrity ER, Pifarre R, Fahey PJ, Walsh JM. Reduced transplant lung volumes after single lung transplantation for chronic obstructive pulmonary disease. *Am J Respir Crit Care Med* 1995;**151**:851–3.

127 Estenne M, Cassart M, Poncelet P, Gevenois PA. Volume of graft and native lung after single-lung transplantation for emphysema. *Am J Respir Crit Care Med* 1999;**159**:641–5.

128 Miyoshi S, Trulock EP, Schaefers HJ *et al*. Cardiopulmonary exercise testing after single and double lung transplantation. *Chest* 1990;**97**:1130–6.

129 Gibbons WJ, Levine SM, Bryan CL *et al*. Cardiopulmonary exercise responses after single lung transplantation for severe obstructive lung disease. *Chest* 1991;**100**:106–11.

130 Williams TJ, Patterson GA, McClean PA, Zamel N, Maurer JR. Maximal exercise testing in single and double lung transplant recipients. *Am Rev Respir Dis* 1992;**145**:101–5.

131 Levy RD, Ernst P, Levine SM *et al*. Exercise performance after lung transplantation. *J Heart Lung Transplant* 1993;**12**:27–33.

132 Orens JB, Becker FS, Lynch JP III *et al*. Cardiopulmonary exercise testing following allogeneic lung transplantation for different underlying disease states. *Chest* 1995;**107**:144–9.

133 Schwaiblmair M, Reichenspurner H, Muller C *et al*. Munich Lung Transplant Group. Cardiopulmonary exercise testing before and after lung and heart-lung transplantation. *Am J Respir Crit Care Med* 1999;**159**:1277–83.

134 Williams TJ, Slater WR. Role of cardiopulmonary exercise testing in lung and heart-lung transplantation. In: Weisman I, Zeballos R, eds. *Clinical Exercise Testing*, vol. 32. Basel: Karger, 2002: 254–63.

135 Kerber AC, Szidon P, Kesten S. Skeletal muscle dysfunction in lung transplantation. *J Heart Lung Transplant* 2000;**19**:392–400.

136 Pantoja JG, Andrade FH, Stoki DS *et al*. Respiratory and limb muscle function in lung allograft recipients. *Am J Respir Crit Care Med* 1999;**160**:1205–11.

137 Evans AB, Al-Himyary AJ, Hrovat MI *et al*. Abnormal skeletal muscle oxidative capacity after lung transplantation by 31P-MRS. *Am J Respir Crit Care Med* 1997;**155**:615–21.

138 Tirdel GB, Girgis R, Fishman RS, Theodore J. Metabolic myopathy as a cause of the exercise limitation in lung transplant recipients. *J Heart Lung Transplant* 1998;**17**:1231–7.

139 Wang XN, Williams TJ, McKenna MJ *et al*. Skeletal muscle oxidative capacity, fiber type, and metabolites after lung transplantation. *Am J Respir Crit Care Med* 1999;**160**:57–63.

140 McKenna MJ, Fraser SF, Li JL *et al*. Impaired muscle Ca^{2+} and K^+ regulation contribute to poor exercise performance post-lung transplantation. *J Appl Physiol* 2003;**95**:1606–16.

141 Hall MJ, Snell GI, Side EA *et al.* Exercise, potassium, and muscle deconditioing post-thoracic organ transplantation. *J Appl Physiol* 1994;**77**:2784–90.

142 Hokanson JF, Mercier JG, Brooks GA. Cyclosporine A decreases rat skeletal muscle mitochondiral respiration *in vitro. Am J Respir Crit Care Med* 1995;**151**:1848–51.

143 Mercier JG, Hokanson JF, Brooks GA. Effects of cyclosporine A on skeletal muscle mitochondrial respiraton and endurance time in rats. *Am J Respir Crit Care Med* 1995;**151**:1532–6.

144 Biring MS, Fournier M, Ross DJ, Lewis MI. Cellular adaptations of skeletal muscles to cyclosporin. *J Appl Physiol* 1998;**84**:1967–75.

145 Gross CR, Savik K, Bolman RM III, Hertz MI. Long-term health status and quality of life outcomes of lung transplant recipients. *Chest* 1995;**108**:1587–93.

146 TenVergert EM, Essink-Bot ML, Geertsma A *et al.* The effect of lung transplantation on health-related quality of life: a longitudinal study. *Chest* 1998;**113**:358–64.

147 Cohen L, Littlefield C, Kelly P, Maurer J, Abbey S. Predictors of quality of life and adjustment after lung transplantation. *Chest* 1998;**113**:633–44.

148 Pearson MG, Ogilvie C. Surgical treatment of emphysematous bullae: late outcome. *Thorax* 1983;**38**:134–7.

149 Roue C, Mal H, Sleiman C *et al.* Lung volume reduction in patients with severe diffuse emphysema: a retrospective study. *Chest* 1996;**110**:28–34.

150 Brenner M, McKenna RJ Jr, Gelb AF, Fischel RJ, Wilson AF. Rate of FEV_1 change following lung volume reduction surgery. *Chest* 1998;**113**:652–9.

151 Yusen RD, Lefrak SS, Gierada DS *et al.* A prospective evaluation of lung volume reduction surgery in 200 consecutive patients. *Chest* 2003;**123**:1026–37.

152 Cordova F, O'Brien G, Furukawa S *et al.* Stability of improvement in exercise performance and quality of life following bilateral lung volume reduction surgery in severe COPD. *Chest* 1997;**112**:907–15.

153 Appleton S, Adams R, Porter S, Peacock M, Ruffin R. Sustained improvements in dyspnea and pulmonary function 3 to 5 years after lung volume reduction surgery. *Chest* 2003;**123**:1838–46.

154 Studer SM, Levy RD, McNeil K, Orens JB. Lung transplant outcomes; a review of survival, graft function, physiology, health-related quality of life and cost-effectiveness. *Eur Respir J* 2004;**24**:674–85.

155 Boehler A, Estenne M. Post-transplant bronchiolitis obliterans. *Eur Respir J* 2003;**22**:1007–18.

156 Chan A, Allen R. Bronchiolitis obliterans: an update. *Curr Opin Pulm Med* 2004;**10**:133–41.

157 Al-Kattan K, Tadjkarimi S, Cox A *et al.* Evaluation of the long-term results of single versus heart-lung transplantation for emphysema. *J Heart Lung Transplant* 1995;**14**:824–31.

158 Estenne M, Maure JR, Boehler A *et al.* Bronchiolitis obliterans syndrome 2001: an update of the diagnostic criteria. *J Heart Lung Transplant* 2002;**21**:297–310.

159 van Den Berg JW, Geertsma A, van der Bij W *et al.* Bronchiolitis obliterans syndrome after lung transplantation and health-related quality of life. *Am J Respir Crit Care Med* 2000;**161**:1937–41.

160 Anyanwu AC, McGuire A, Rogers CA, Murday AJ. Assessment of quality of life in lung transplantation using a simple generic tool. *Thorax* 2001;**56**:218–22.

161 Gaensler EA, Jederlinic PJ, FitzGerald MX. Patient work-up for bullectomy. *J Thorac Imaging* 1986;**1**:75–93.

162 Nakahara K, Nakaoka K, Ohno K *et al.* Functional indications for bullectomy of giant bulla. *Ann Thorac Surg* 1983; **35**:480–7.

163 Kinnear WJM, Tatterfield AE. Emphysematous bullae: surgery is best for large bullae and moderately impaired lung function. *BMJ* 1990;**300**:208–9.

164 Morgan MDL, Denison DM, Strickland B. Value of computed tomography for selecting patients with bullous lung disease for surgery. *Thorax* 1986;**41**:855–62.

165 Carr DH, Pride NB. Computed tomography in pre-operative assessment of bullous emphysema. *Clin Radiol* 1984;**35**:43–5.

166 Mehran RJ, Deslauriers J. Indications for surgery and patient work-up for bullectomy. *Chest Surg Clin North Am* 1995;**5**:717–34.

167 Flaherty KR, Kazerooni EA, Martinez FJ. Differential diagnosis of chronic airflow obstruction. *J Asthma* 2000;**37**: 201–23.

168 Thurnheer R, Muntwyler J, Stammberger U *et al.* Coronary artery disease in patients undergoing lung volume reduction surgery for emphysema. *Chest* 1997;**112**:122–8.

169 Whyte RI, Bria W, Martinez FJ, Lewis P, Bolling SF. Combined lung volume reduction surgery and mitral valve reconstruction. *Ann Thorac Surg* 1998;**66**:1414–6.

170 Schmid RA, Stammberger U, Hillinger S *et al.* Lung volume reduction surgery combined with cardiac interventions. *Eur J Cardiothorac Surg* 1999;**15**:585–91.

171 Lefrak SS, Yusen RD, Trulock EP *et al.* Recent advances in surgery for emphysema. *Ann Rev Med* 1997;**48**:387–98.

172 Bach DS, Curtis JL, Christensen PJ *et al.* Preoperative echocardiographic evaluation of patients referred for lung volume reduction surgery. *Chest* 1998;**114**:972–80.

173 Bossone E, Martinez FJ, Whyte RI *et al.* Dobutamine stress echocardiography for the preoperative evaluation of patients undergoing lung volume reduction surgery. *J Thorac Cardiovasc Surg* 1999;**118**:542–6.

174 Scharf SM, Iqbal M, Keller C *et al.* National Emphysema Treatment Trial (NETT) Research Group. Hemodynamic characterization of patients with severe emphysema. *Am J Respir Crit Care* 2002;**166**:314–22.

175 Thurnheer R, Bingisser R, Stammberger U *et al.* Effect of lung volume reduction surgery on pulmonary hemodynamics in severe pulmonary emphysema. *Eur J Cardiothorac Surg* 1998;**13**:253–8.

176 Haniuda M, Kubo K, Fujimoto K *et al.* Effects of pulmonary artery remodeling on pulmonary circulation after lung volume reduction surgery. *Thorac Cardiovasc Surg* 2003;**51**: 154–8.

177 Sciurba FC. Early and long-term functional outcomes following lung volume reduction surgery. *Clin Chest Med* 1997;**18**:259–76.

178 Teschler H, Thompson AB, Stamatis G. Short- and long-term functional results after lung volume reduction surgery for severe emphysema. *Eur Respir J* 1999;**13**:919–25.

179 Gelb AF, McKenna RJ, Brenner M, Fischel R, Zamel N. Lung function after bilateral lower lobe lung volume reduction surgery for α_1-antitrypsin emphysema. *Eur Respir J* 1999;**14**: 928–33.

180 Tutic M, Bloch KE, Lardinois D *et al*. Long-term results after lung volume reduction surgery in patients with α_1-antitrypsin deficiency. *J Thorac Cardiovasc Surg* 2004;**128**:408–13.

181 Mazolewski P, Turner JF, Baker M, Kurtz T, Little AG. The impact of nutritional status on the outcome of lung volume reduction surgery: a prospective study. *Chest* 1999;**116**: 693–6.

182 Nezu K, Yoshikawa M, Yoneda T *et al*. The effect of nutritional status on morbidity in COPD patients undergoing bilateral lung reduction surgery. *Thorac Cardiovasc Surg* 2001;**49**:216–20.

183 Naunheim KS, Hazelrigg SR, Kaiser LR *et al*. Risk analysis for thoracoscopic lung volume reduction: a multi-institutional experience. *Eur J Cardiothorac Surg* 2000;**17**:673–9.

184 Criner GJ, O'Brien G, Furukawa S *et al*. Lung volume reduction surgery in ventilator-dependent COPD patients. *Chest* 1996;**110**:877–84.

185 McKenna RJ Jr, Brenner M, Fischel RJ *et al*. Patient selection criteria for lung volume reduction surgery. *J Thorac Cardiovasc Surg* 1997;**114**:957–67.

186 Gelb AF, Brenner M, McKenna RJ Jr *et al*. Lung function 12 months following emphysema resection. *Chest* 1996;**110**: 1407–15.

187 Ingenito EP, Evans RB, Loring SH *et al*. Relation between preoperative inspiratory lung resistance and the outcome of lung-volume-reduction surgery for emphysema. *N Engl J Med* 1998;**338**:1181–5.

188 Ingenito EP, Loring SH, Moy ML *et al*. Comparison of physiological and radiological screening for lung volume reduction surgery. *Am J Respir Crit Care Med* 2001;**163**:1068–73.

189 Kim V, Criner GJ, Abdallah HY *et al*. Small airway morphometry and improvement in pulmonary function after lung volume reduction surgery. *Am J Respir Crit Care Med* 2005;**171**:40–7.

190 Fessler HE, Permutt S. Lung volume reduction surgery and airflow limitation. *Am J Respir Crit Care Med* 1998;**157**: 715–22.

191 Leyenson V, Furukawa S, Kuzma AM *et al*. Correlation of changes in quality of life after lung volume reduction surgery with changes in lung function, exercise, and gas exchange. *Chest* 2000;**118**:728–35.

192 Brenner M, Kayaleh RA, Milne EN *et al*. Thoracoscopic laser ablation of pulmonary bullae: radiographic selection and treatment response. *J Thorac Cardiovasc Surg* 1994;**107**: 883–90.

193 National Emphysema Treatment Trial Research Group. Patients at high risk of death after lung-volume-reduction surgery. *N Engl J Med* 2001;**345**:1075–83.

194 Szekely LA, Oelberg DA, Wright C *et al*. Preoperative predictors of operative morbidity and mortality in COPD patients undergoing bilateral lung volume reduction surgery. *Chest* 1997;**111**:550–8.

195 O'Brien GM, Furukawa S, Kuzma AM, Cordova F, Criner GJ. Improvements in lung function, exercise, and quality of life in hypercapnic COPD patients after lung volume reduction surgery. *Chest* 1999;**115**:75–84.

196 Shade D Jr, Cordova F, Lando Y *et al*. Relationship between resting hypercapnia and physiologic parameters before and after lung volume reduction surgery in severe chronic obstructive pulmonary disease. *Am J Respir Crit Care Med* 1999;**159**:1405–11.

197 Wisser W, Klepetko W, Senbaklavaci O *et al*. Chronic hypercapnia should not exclude patients from lung volume reduction surgery. *Eur J Cardiothorac Surg* 1998;**14**:107–12.

198 Mitsui K, Kurokawa Y, Kaiwa Y *et al*. Thoracoscopic lung volume reduction surgery for pulmonary emphysema patients with severe hypercapnia. *Jpn J Thorac Cardiovasc Surg* 2001;**49**:481–8.

199 Gierada DS. Radiologic assessment of emphysema for lung volume reduction surgery. *Semin Thorac Cardiovasc Surg* 2002;**14**:381–90.

200 Maki DD, Miller WT Jr, Aronchick JM *et al*. Advanced emphysema: preoperative chest radiographic findings as predictors of outcome following lung volume reduction surgery. *Radiology* 1999;**212**:49–55.

201 Kazerooni EA. Radiologic evaluation of emphysema for lung volume reduction surgery. *Clin Chest Med* 1999;**20**:845–61.

202 Goldin JG. Quantitative CT of the lung. *Radiol Clin North Am* 2002;**40**:45–58.

203 Madani A, Keyzer C, Gevenois PA. Quantitative computed tomography assessment of lung structure and function in pulmonary emphysema. *Eur Respir J* 2001;**18**:720–30.

204 Rogers RM, Coxson HO, Sciurba FC *et al*. Preoperative severity of emphysema predictive of improvement after lung volume reduction surgery: use of CT morphometry. *Chest* 2000;**118**:1240–7.

205 Hunsaker AR, Ingenito EP, Reilly JJ, Costello P. Lung volume reduction surgery for emphysema: correlation of CT and *V/Q* imaging with physiologic mechanisms of improvement in lung function. *Radiology* 2002;**222**:491–8.

206 Slone RM, Pilgram TK, Gierada DS *et al*. Lung volume reduction surgery: comparison of preoperative radiologic features and clinical outcome. *Radiology* 1997;**204**:685–93.

207 Weder W, Thurnheer R, Stammberger U *et al*. Radiologic emphysema morphology is associated with outcome after surgical lung volume reduction. *Ann Thorac Surg* 1997;**64**: 313–20.

208 Wisser W, Klepetko W, Kontrus M *et al*. Morphologic grading of the emphysematous lung and its relation to improvement after lung volume reduction surgery. *Ann Thorac Surg* 1998;**65**:793–9.

209 Hamacher J, Bloch KE, Stammberger U *et al*. Two years' outcome of lung volume reduction surgery in different morphologic emphysema types. *Ann Thorac Surg* 1999;**68**: 1792–8.

210 Wisser W, Senbaklavaci O, Ozpeker C *et al*. Is long-term functional outcome after lung volume reduction surgery predictable? *Eur J Cardiothorac Surg* 2000;**17**:666–72.

211 Pompeo E, Sergiacomi G, Nofroni I *et al*. Morphologic grading of emphysema is useful in the selection of candidates for unilateral or bilateral reduction pneumoplasty. *Eur J Cardiothorac Surg* 2000;**17**:680–6.

212 Bloch KE, Georgescu CL, Russi EW, Weder W. Gain and subsequent loss of lung function after lung volume reduction surgery in cases of severe emphysema with different morphologic patterns. *J Thor Cardiovas Surg* 2002;**123**:845–54.

213 Sciurba FC. Preoperative predictors of outcome following lung volume reduction surgery. *Thorax* 2002;**57**(Suppl 2): 47–52.

214 Gierada DS, Slone RM, Bae KT *et al*. Pulmonary emphysema: comparison of preoperative quantitative CT and physiologic index values with clinical outcome after lung-volume reduction surgery. *Radiology* 1997;**205**:235–42.

215 Nakano Y, Coxson HO, Bosan S *et al*. Core to rind distribution of severe emphysema predicts outcome of lung volume reduction surgery. *Am J Respir Crit Care Med* 2001;**164**: 2195–9.

216 Coxson HO, Whittall KP, Nakano Y *et al*. Selection of patients for lung volume reduction surgery using a power law analysis of the computed tomographic scan. *Thorax* 2003;**58**:510–4.

217 Jamadar DA, Kazerooni EA, Martinez FJ, Wahl RL. Semiquantitative ventilation–perfusion scintigraphy and single photon emission computed tomography for evaluation of lung volume reduction surgery candidates: description and prediction of clinical outcomes. *Eur J Nuclear Med* 1999; **26**:734–42.

218 Kotloff RM, Hansen-Flaschen J, Lipson DA *et al*. Apical perfusion fraction as a predictor of short-term functional outcomes following bilateral lung volume reduction surgery. *Chest* 2001;**120**:1609–15.

219 Wang SC, Fischer KC, Slone RM *et al*. Perfusion scintigraphy in the evaluation for lung volume reduction surgery: correlation with clinical outcome. *Radiology* 1997;**205**:243–8.

220 Cederlund K, Hogberg S, Jorfeldt L *et al*. Lung perfusion scintigraphy prior to lung volume reduction surgery. *Acta Radiologica* 2003;**44**:246–51.

221 DeMeester J, Smits JMA, Persijn GG, Haverich A. Lung transplant waiting list: differential outcome of type of end-stage lung disease, one year after registration. *J Heart Lung Transplant* 1999;**18**:563–71.

222 Demeester JD, Smits JMA, Persijn GG, Haverich A. Listing for lung transplantation: life expectancy and transplant effect, stratified by type of end-stage lung disease, the Eurotransplant Experience. *J Heart Lung Transplant* 2001;**20**:518–24.

223 Hosenpud JD, Bennett LE, Keck BM, Edwards EB, Novick RJ. Effect of diagnosis on survival benefit after lung transplantation for end-stage lung disease. *Lancet* 1998;**351**:24–7.

224 Charman SC, Sharples LD, McNeil KD, Wallwork J. Assessment of survival benefit after lung transplantation by patient diagnosis. *J Heart Lung Transplant* 2002;**21**:226–32.

225 Maurer JR, Frost AE, Estenne M, Higenbottam T, Glanville AR. International guidelines for the selection of lung transplant candidates. The International Society for Heart and Lung Transplantation, the American Thoracic Society, the American Society of Transplant Physicians, the European Respiratory Society. *Transplantation* 1998;**66**:951–6.

226 Lynch JP III, Martinez FJ. Lung transplantation: who's a candidate? *J Respir Dis* 1996;**17**:393–412.

227 Glanville AR, Estenne M. Indications, patient selection and timing of referral for lung transplantation. *Eur Respir J* 2003; **22**:845–52.

228 Di Boscio V, Sarli MA. Lung transplantation and osteoporosis: a review. *Clin Pulm Med* 1999;**6**:110–7.

229 Schafers HJ, Wagner TO, Demertzis S *et al*. Preoperative corticosteroids: a contraindication to lung transplantation? *Chest* 1992;**102**:1522–5.

230 Grady KL, Costanzo MR, Fisher S, Koch D. Preoperative obesity is associated with decreased survival after heart transplantation. *J Heart Lung Transplant* 1996;**15**:863–71.

231 Martinez FJ, Kotloff R. Prognostication in chronic obstructive pulmonary disease: implications for lung transplantation. *Semin Respir Crit Care Med* 2001;**22**:489–98.

232 Traver GA, Cline MG, Burrows B. Predictors of mortality in chronic obstructive pulmonary disease: a 15-year follow-up study. *Am Rev Respir Dis* 1979;**119**:895–902.

233 Anthonisen NR, Wright EC, Hodgkin JE, IPPB Trial Group. Prognosis in chronic obstructive pulmonary disease. *Am Rev Respir Dis* 1986;**133**:14–20.

234 Seersholm N, Dirksen A, Kok-Jensen A. Airway obstruction and two year survival in patients with severe α_1-antitrypsin deficiency. *Eur Respir J* 1994;**7**:1985–7.

235 Seersholm N, Kok-Jensen A. Survival in relation to lung function and smoking cessation in patients with severe hereditary α_1-antitrypsin deficiency. *Am J Respir Crit Care Med* 1995;**151**:369–73.

236 The Alpha-1 Antitrypsin Deficiency Registry Study Group. Survival and FEV_1 decline in individuals with severe deficiency of α_1-antitrypsin. *Am J Respir Crit Care Med* 1998; **158**:49–59.

237 Celli BR, Cote CG, Marin JM *et al*. The body-mass index, airflow obstruction, dyspnea, and exercise capacity index in chronic obstructive pulmonary disease. *N Engl J Med* 2004; **350**:1005–12.

238 Kazerooni EA, Chow LC, Whyte RI, Martinez FJ, Lynch JP III. Preoperative examination of lung transplant candidates: value of chest CT compared with chest radiography. *Am J Roentgenol* 1995;**165**:1343–8.

239 Kazerooni EA, Martinez FJ, Quint LE, Whyte RI. Quantitative helical CT indices of emphysema as predictors of outcome after lung volume reduction surgery. *Radiology* 1996;**201**(P):298.

240 Martinez FJ, Flaherty KR, Iannettoni M. Lung volume reduction surgery for emphysema. *Chest Surg Clin North Am* 2003;**13**:669–85.

241 Celli BR, MacNee W, ATS-ERS Task Force. Standards for the diagnosis and treatment of patients with COPD: a summary of the ATS-ERS position paper. *Eur Respir J* 2004;**23**:932–46.

242 American Thoracic Society. International guidelines for the selection of lung transplant candidates. *Am J Respir Crit Care Med* 1998;**158**:335–9.

243 Wouters EF. Management of severe COPD. *Lancet* 2004; **364**:883–95.

244 Martinez FJ, Flaherty KR, Iannettoni MD. Patient selection for lung volume reduction surgery. *Chest Surg Clin North Am* 2003;**13**:669–85.

CHAPTER 56
Anticholinergics in COPD

Theodore J. Witek, Jr

Bronchodilators are regarded as the mainstay of COPD pharmacotherapy [1–4] and the anticholinergic class of agents has proven over several decades to provide effective maintenance therapy [5]. This recognition of the value of anticholinergic therapy in COPD is anchored by the fascinating centuries of history of the medicinal properties of plants containing belladonna alkaloids and the present-day introduction of the new generation agent tiotropium. The recent introduction of tiotropium represents a significant advance in therapy, not only being the first inhaled once-daily agent, but also by its consistently better bronchodilatory effects relative to existing therapy as demonstrated in clinical trials [6–10].

This chapter briefly reviews the history and basic pharmacology of anticholinergics followed by a summary of the major clinical trials that have characterized the efficacy and safety of this class of agents in the treatment of COPD.

History

Uses of medicinal properties

The medicinal uses of inhaled antimuscarinics have been documented for centuries [11,12] and this history is made more fascinating by the fact that new generations of this class are being developed and introduced as innovative therapy at the present day.

In the time of Hippocrates, vapour inhalation was recorded and the use of the alkaloid in the treatment of asthma was cited in the 17th century. This practice was transferred from India to Great Britain where a more widespread use was observed in the 1800s. An interesting paper by Herxheimer in 1959 [13] described spirometric results following inhalation of asthma cigarettes containing atropine. Not only was his work among the first known to this author to evaluate spirometric therapeutic responses, it should not be overlooked that his insights to combine both

atropine and ephedrine was also novel in combination bronchodilator therapy.

Clearly, the ability of atropine as a bronchodilator was known, but its therapeutic utility was limited by systematic antimuscarinic side-effects. The first major advance was the discovery and development of ipratropium bromide, whose structure allowed preservation of bronchodilatation, but minimized absorption and side-effects [14,15]. Ipratropium bromide evolved to first-line maintenance treatment in COPD [16], and has been established as an effective and safe agent over decades of use. Its main disadvantage of four times daily dosing has recently been overcome with the latest generation compound tiotropium [17]. Tiotropium has significantly longer binding to muscarinic receptors than both atropine and ipratropium [18,19] with resultant functional consequences *in vitro* (Fig. 56.1) [20]. The clinical profile of these agents are detailed subsequently in this chapter.

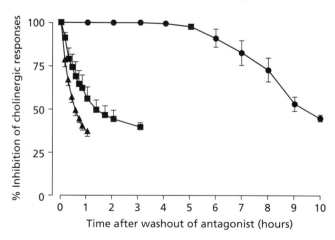

Figure 56.1 Time course of effects of BA679 BR (10^{-9} mol) (circles), ipratropium bromide (10^{-8} mol) (squares) and atropine (10^{-8} mol) (triangles) after washout of the test drugs in guinea pig trachea. Each value is the mean ± SEM of five animals. (From Takahashi *et al.* [20], with permission.)

Table 56.1 Muscarinic receptor subtypes nomenclature and characterization. (Derived from Roux *et al.* [101].)

Subtype	M_1	M_2	M_3
Selective antagonists (Range of affinity)	Pirenzepine $(M_1 > M_4 > M_3 \geq M_2)$ Telenzepine $(M_1 > M_4 > M_3 \geq M_2)$	Methoctramine $(M_2 \geq M_4 > M_1 \geq M_3)$ AF-DX 116 $(M_2 \geq M_4 > M_1 \geq M_3)$ Himbacine $(M_2 \geq M_4 > M_1 \geq M_3)$	4-DAMP $(M_3 \geq M_1 \geq M_4 > M_2)$ p-F-HHSiD $(M_3 \geq M_1 \geq M_4 > M_2)$
Genes	m_1	m_2	m_3
Localization in airway tissue	Parasympathetic ganglia Submucosal glands Alveolar walls	Postganglionic nerves Airway smooth muscle	Airway smooth muscle Submucosal glands Epithelial cells Endothelial cells

4-DAMP, 4-diphenylacetoxy-*N*-methylpiperidine.

Box 56.1 Excerpts from H. H. Dales' 1933 letter to American Physiologic Society on Anatomic Nervous System Nomenclature [22].

'Evidence has been rapidly accumulating in favour of the view that the effects of nervous impulses in the postganglionic fibres of the autonomic system are chemically transmitted, by substances liberated in relation to their endings, and directly acting on the effector cells'.

'My own earlier observations [1914] on acetylcholine had indicated a substance of this kind as a likely candidate for the function of transmitting the effects of impulses in peripheral parasympathetic fibres; and the evidence in recent years has all tended to increase the probability that this choline ester is the actual parasymphatetic transmitter'.

'Chemical transmission occurs at synapses in a symphathetic ganglion, and that the transmitter, even though the preganglionic fibres are anatomically sympathetic, is a substance indistinguishable from that which transmits the effects of postganglionic parasymphatetic impulses'.

'These observations bring into the physiological picture the other aspect of the action of acetylcholine, which I called "nicotine like". To avoid elaborate periphrasis, and to promote clear ideas, we seem to need words which will briefly indicate action by two kinds of chemical transmission, due in one case to some substance like adrenaline, in the other case to a substance like acetylcholine, so that we may distinguish between chemical function and anatomical origin. I suggest the words "adrenergic" and "cholinergic", respectively for use in this sense'.

Evolution of pharmacology

Muscarinic pharmacology had its modern foundation in 1914 when Sir Henry Dale [21] classified receptors for acetylcholine as nicotinic and muscarinic. Receptor subtyping was reported in 1980 and was rooted in the establishment of high (M_1) or low (M_2) affinity for the antagonist pirenzepine. This basis of using selective antagonists to classify subtypes was expanded with further division of the M_2 receptor into M_2, M_3 and M_4 (Table 56.1).

The description of the autonomic nervous system that has evolved over the past century encompasses many terms as one describes cholinergic nerves travelling down to the vagus nerve into parasympathetic ganglia within the airway. Its principal neurotransmitter, acetylcholine, is released at ganglionic synapses and postganglionic neuroeffector junctions. Acetylcholine acts at both nicotinic and muscarinic cholinergic receptors – the former located at parasympathetic ganglia and mediating ganglionic neurotransmission and the later located on postganglionic nerve fibres and on target cells such as epithelium, submucosal glands and airway smooth muscle. Nicotinic transmission at ganglia can be provoked by either acetylcholine or nicotine – transmission here can be interrupted by cholinergic blockers such as hexamenthonium or D-tubocurare. The acetylcholine released at postganglionic fibres has been termed muscarinic because transmission can be mimicked by muscarine. Effects resulting from muscarinic activity are blocked by antimuscarinics such as atropine; they are not blocked by curare. Thus, the evolution to the clinical referral of atropine and atropine-derived agents such as ipratropium and tiotropium as anticholinergics is correct; however, their description as antimuscarinics is more accurate. Box 56.1 lists excerpts from Dale's suggestions on such nomenclature in a 1933 note to the American Physiologic Society [22].

Basic pharmacology overview

Muscarinic receptors

The function of the various muscarinic receptor subtypes comes from observations in many species with the general understanding that M_1 receptors found in parasympathetic ganglia facilitate neurotransmission, M_2 receptors are localized to postganglionic cholinergic nerve terminals and provide a negative feedback modulation of acetylcholine release, and M_3 receptors are present on airway smooth muscle cells and mucosal glands with functional mediation of bronchoconstriction and glandular secretion (see Table 56.1). Several reviews describe investigations leading to this understanding [23–25].

Signal transduction

Ligand–receptor interaction of the muscarinic nature involves a biochemical pathway leading to an ultimate

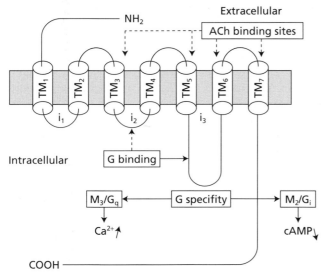

Figure 56.2 Guanosine triphosphate (GTP)-binding protein-coupled muscarinic cholinoceptor. This superfamily of receptors features seven transmembrane domains (TM_{1-7}). Acetylcholine binds to a cleft formed by the extracellular part of each of the seven TM domains and in particular to aminoacid residues located in the third, fifth, sixth and seventh TM regions. Among the three intracellular loops (i_1–i_3), i_2 and i_3 as well as the membrane proximal part of the intracellular tail of the receptor are implicated in G-protein coupling. Critical determinants for G-coupling selectivity are in i_3. M_2 cholinoceptors are coupled to G_i protein, leading to adenylyl cyclase inhibition and a decrease in cyclic adenosine monophosphate (cAMP). M_3 cholinoceptors are coupled to G_{q-11} protein, leading to phospholipase C activation and an increase in Ca^{2+}. (From Roux *et al*. [101], with permission from Elsevier.)

tissue response (e.g. contraction of airway smooth muscle; Fig. 56.2). While these events are complex, with several investigations advancing fundamental concepts, it is accepted that the neurotransmitter acetylcholine interacts with G proteins, stimulating phospholipose C (PLC) and the breakdown of membranes lipids (e.g. phosphatidylinositol polyphosphates → inositol phosphates [IP]) resulting in the release of intracellular calcium from the endoplasmic reticulum. These collective events lead to the end organ effect. Of most relevance in COPD are the airway smooth muscle contraction and possibly glandular secretion. Diacylglycerol is another second messenger which is associated with protein kinase C (PKC) activation. There have been some theories put forth that PKC could be involved in a slow, sustained contractile response where as IP may be more related to initiation of contraction [26–28].

The number, distribution and special function of these receptor subtypes in human lung tissue is not fully understood. In the human trachea, muscarinic receptors are likely of the M_2 and M_3 receptor subtype as they have low affinity for the M_1 specific antagonist pirenzepine [29]. Furthermore, mRNA for M_2 and M_3 receptors have been detected in human bronchi [30].

Potential cellular effects of relevance

While the focus of the role of bronchodilators in COPD has for decades been based on their ability to dilate airways via smooth muscle contraction, there has been a recent surge in interest in the role of inflammation in this disease, particularly in those with more severe illness and prone to frequent exacerbations. In fact, the consistent findings of reduced exacerbations evaluated as secondary endpoints in clinical trials of antimuscarinic bronchodilators have sparked interest. A potential effect can be both indirect and direct. First, prolonged maintenance of bronchial opening from the long-acting agent tiotropium may minimize physical forces that could lead to effects potentially associated with exacerbations [31]. Secondly, while acetylcholine has long been viewed solely as a neurotransmitter, it may have non-neuronal roles that may offer explanations for some of the favourable outcomes observed in clinical trials [32].

Disse [32] first raised the possible anti-inflammatory potential of antimuscarinics in this light, based on observations on the influence of acetylcholine on mast cells, epithial mediator release and alveolar macrophase chemotactic activity release. Additionally, recent evidence suggests a synergistic role of methylcholine with platelet-derived growth factor (PDGF) in potentiating mitogenesis in bovine tracheal smooth muscle cells [33].

While the clinical relevance of the role of antimuscarinics in the inflammatory arena is not clear, current observations prompt need for further characterization. For example, incubation of human lung tissue with acetylcholine (10^{-7} mol) showed increased histamine release with antigen exposure [34,35]. Furthermore, acetylcholine (10^{-7} to 10^{-4} mol) potentiated the release of 15-hydroxyeicosatetraenoic acid (15-HETE) and, to a lesser extent, prostaglandin E_2 (PGE_2), in the pressure of 10 μmol arachidonic acid [36]. Perhaps of more relevance to COPD is the cholinergic influence on the release of chemotactic activity by alveolar macrophages. Sato *et al.* [37] reported that chemotactic activity more than doubled in the presence of acetylcholine (10^{-7} to 10^{-5} mol). This stimulation of release was blunted by the M_3-selective antagonist 4-diphenylacetoxy-*N*-methylpiperidine (4-DAMP). As pointed out by Disse [32], acetylcholine concentrations in the range of 10^{-5} mol can be reached locally; therefore, a potential 'non-neuronal' therapeutic role of muscarinic blockage in the airways may be operating.

Clinical pharmacology overview

Pharmacodynamic effects in humans

The primary intended role of antimuscarinics in respiratory care is bronchodilatation. The basis for this effect rests on the role of the parasympathetic nervous system in regulating bronchomotor tone. In healthy individuals, indirect evidence for the presence of cholinergic airway tone can be seen in spirometric improvements following inhalation of atropine or ipratropium [38–40]. Dose-ordered reductions in airway resistance have also been observed in early human pharmacological studies with tiotropium [41]. The blunting of the response of the cholinergic agonist methacholine with tiotropium (Fig. 56.3) also provides a clinical demonstration of the pharmacological concept and agonist–antagonist interactions at the receptor level [42].

β-Adrenergic agonists dilate airways through functional antagonism (i.e. they functionally reverse or inhibit the action of another agonist). By way of this unspecific mechanism they can cover a broad range of bronchoconstrictive effects. In COPD, the agonist acetylcholine causes bronchoconstriction which can be functionally antagonized by giving an adrenergic agonist (Fig. 56.4). Competitive antagonism invokes competing of an agonist (e.g. acetylcholine) directly with an antagonist (e.g. tiotropium). The fact that anticholinergics provide equal or greater bronchodilatation than β-agonists is the basis for cholinergic tone being the major reversible component in COPD. Such is not the case in asthma.

The heightened cholinergic tone in COPD has been proposed based on greater bronchodilator responses in COPD versus healthy subjects, with the amount of bronchodilatation being directly proportional to severity of airflow limitation [38]. Other indirect support for a prominent role of the cholinergic system in COPD comes from the greater bronchodilatation most often observed with antimuscarinics versus β-adrenergic agonists [6,7,10].

Muscarinic receptors are located throughout the body and end-organ-driven pharmacodynamic effects can be anticipated based on concentrations at these sites which will be indirectly driven by the agent administered (e.g. potency) and the route of administration (e.g. inhalation). As there is not equal sensitivity to muscarinic receptor antagonists at the parasympathetic neuroeffector junctions in different end organs [43], dose–response effects can be observed clinically – as long described for atropine. The unintended pharmacodynamic effects that can be observed with inhaled therapeutic doses of ipratropium and tiotropium are minimized by their quaternary structure

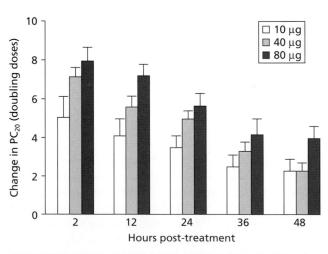

Figure 56.3 Change in PC_{20}, from placebo, for each dose of tiotropium at each time point after treatment, expressed in terms of doubling dose protection. (From O'Connor *et al.* [42], with permission.)

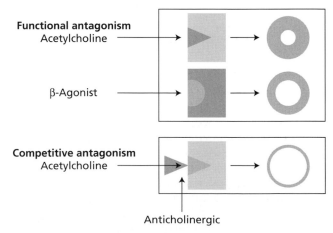

Figure 56.4 A schematic simplification of functional and competitive antagonism. The greater bronchodilatation with competitive antagonism of acetylcholine with anticholinergics versus that seen with functional antagonism via stimulation of β-receptors gives evidence that cholinergic tone is the major reversible competitor in COPD.

and less absorption, with the most commonly observed unintended pharmacodynamic effect being dry mouth [8]. The manifestation of dry mouth and the observation of reduced salivary secretion as the most sensitive antimuscarinic effect is supported by early clinical studies with tiotropium [41], where these effects were the first to manifest at high inhaled doses in the absence of heart rate or pupillary diameter changes.

The cholinergic system is involved in airway mucociliary system control [43], but a clear picture of clinical relevance does not emerge when considering endpoints such as sputum volume. For example, no reduction in sputum volume was observed after three times daily inhalation of 200 µg of either ipratropium [44] or oxitropium [45], while Ghafouri *et al.* [46] noted a significant reduction after 7 weeks of inhaled ipratropium (40 mg, q.i.d.). A reduction in sputum volume after 7 weeks' treatment with 200 µg oxitropium was also observed [47]. As the first two trials were of 4 weeks' duration, it may be that the duration of therapy is an important feature of any possible effect. Untoward effects of antimuscarinic therapy on mucociliary clearance have not been observed with quaternary agents such as ipratropium [45,48] and tiotropium [49].

The antimuscarinic effects of constipation (from decreased gastrointestinal tone and motility) and difficult urination (from decreased tone and contraction of urinary bladder) have been observed in small numbers in clinical trials with both ipratropium and tiotropium. Antimuscarinic action in the eye results in dilatation of pupils (mydriasis) and accommodation paralysis (cycloplegia). While these effects are uncommon in respiratory therapy, care should always be taken to avoid exposure of drug in the eye. Tachycardia and superventricular tachycardia have been observed in small numbers in controlled clinical trials.

Clinical observations

There are case reports and small-scale clinical trials on the response to atropine of healthy subjects and those with COPD [38,40,50]. These observations confirm the intended pharmacodynamic effect of bronchodilatation as measured by lung function tests as well as the fact that antimuscarinic side-effects manifest more commonly with the tertiary amine atropine. The clinical development programmes leading to regulatory reviews and approvals of ipratropium, alone and in combination with albuterol as well as tiotropium, have provided the largest body of evidence of the beneficial therapeutic window of this class of agents in COPD. Also, given the decades of experience with antimuscarinics such as ipratropium, observational studies and evaluation of patient databases have contributed further to our knowledge of the utility of these agents in COPD. While some observational and retrospective cohort analyses

have reported possible associations of antimuscarinics with increased risk of cardiovascular morbidity and mortality [51–53], no effects have been consistently shown [54], particularly after controlling for confounders such as disease severity [55,56].

Ipratropium

Among the early large-scale studies with ipratropium in COPD were the comparative studies with metaproterenol where its bronchodilator effect and safety were demonstrated [57,58] and the anticholinergic class of bronchodilators as foundation therapy was grounded. The largest controlled observation with ipratropium comes with the original Lung Health Study [59] where it was concluded that ipratropium bromide sustained its maintenance bronchodilatation over 5 years; however, there was no impact of ipratropium treatment on the longer term decline in forced expiratory volume in 1 s (FEV_1). A retrospective analysis of seven clinical trials comparing ipratropium with short-acting β-agonists in COPD found that baseline lung function improved with the anticholinergic over 90 days – an effect that was not seen with the β-agonist [60]. Additional present day studies with ipratropium come in the form of it being a gold standard comparator during the development of alternative delivery systems and long-acting β-agonists. For example, comparable efficacy and safety of chlorofluorocarbon (CFC) and hydrofluoroalkane (HFA) driven metered dose inhaler (MDI) ipratropium has been demonstrated [61,62]. The efficacy and safety of ipratropium have been confirmed in trials evaluating salmeterol [63,64] and formoterol [65]. In the salmeterol trials, the efficacy of ipratropium four times daily was reconfirmed and was similar to salmeterol twice daily. The effects of ipratropium on dyspnoea relief were more consistent than observed with salmeterol. In the formoterol trial [65], ipratropium (40 µg q.i.d.) significantly increased the area-under-the-curve over placebo for FEV_1; significantly greater responses were seen in the formoterol-treated patients, which can be caused, in part, by the fact that patients treated regularly with anticholinergic therapy were not allowed to participate in the study [66].

Short-acting anticholinergic–β-agonist combinations

Ipratropium was the first bronchodilator to focus its clinical development in COPD. Additionally, it was realized that with the polypharmacy common in COPD, many patients were co-prescribed a β-agonist with ipratropium. This was the basis for the development of the fixed combination of ipratropium bromide and albuterol, ultimately marketed as Combivent® [67]. The pharmacological basis for this therapy rested on the distinct mechanisms of action of

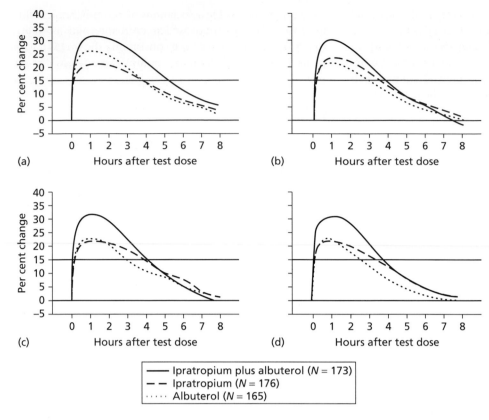

(a) Hours after test dose

(b) Hours after test dose

(c) Hours after test dose

(d) Hours after test dose

—— Ipratropium plus albuterol (N = 173)
– – Ipratropium (N = 176)
· · · · Albuterol (N = 165)

Figure 56.5 Percentage changes in mean forced expiratory volume in 1 s (FEV_1) from test day baselines. (a) Test day 1. (b) Test day 29. (c) Test day 57. (d) Test day 85. (From the Combivent Inhalation Study Group [70], with permission.)

antimuscarinics and sympathomimetics which supported the clinical research hypothesis that the combination would provide superior bronchodilatation than either agent administered alone. This was established in adequate and well-controlled clinical trials where the fixed combination provided significant increases in spirometric endpoints over the individual agents [68–70]. As illustrated in Figure 56.5, the additive benefit of the combination was consistent and maintained over the 3-month study period. In a retrospective analysis of these data, we also reported that more than 80% of patients receiving the combination of ipratropium bromide and albuterol had a 15% or greater increase in FEV_1, providing support for the concept of 'reversibility' in COPD [71].

Tiotropium

The functional and therapeutically relevant consequence of the prolonged receptor binding of tiotropium was first demonstrated in the form of sustained improvement in the FEV_1 of stable COPD patients, thus forming the basis for once daily therapy [72,73]. This effect observed from single-dose studies was confirmed in a 4-week dose–response trial [74] that set the stage for development of 18 μg tiotropium once daily for long-term maintenance therapy. One unique trial provided the first around-the-clock (every 3 h) assessment of spirometry in COPD [75]. This study pro-

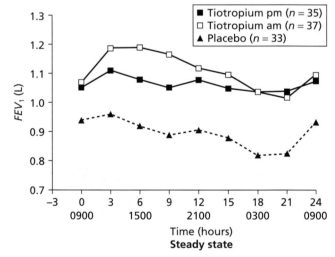

■ Tiotropium pm (n = 35)
□ Tiotropium am (n = 37)
▲ Placebo (n = 33)

Time (hours)
Steady state

Figure 56.6 Mean forced expiratory volume in 1 s (FEV_1) in litres over 24 h after 6 weeks (steady state) of tiotropium in the evening (p.m.), tiotropium in the morning (a.m.) or placebo. (From Calverley et al. [102], with permission.)

vided evidence for the effectiveness of tiotropium throughout its dosing interval as well as interesting insights into the circadian spirometric response in this patient group (Fig. 56.6).

The major development studies for tiotropium consisted of two replicate trials for each of the major comparators including usual care (placebo), ipratropium and salmeterol. In the individual and reported integrated analysis of these studies, tiotropium provided consistently better bronchodilatation than all comparators (Fig. 56.7) [7–9]. Spirometric responses were consistent in all trials, with the exception of one sister study versus salmeterol where the primary endpoint (trough FEV_1) was directionally, but not statistically significantly greater. Statistical significance favouring tiotropium over placebo and salmeterol was seen in all other spirometric endpoints (Fig. 56.8). The response

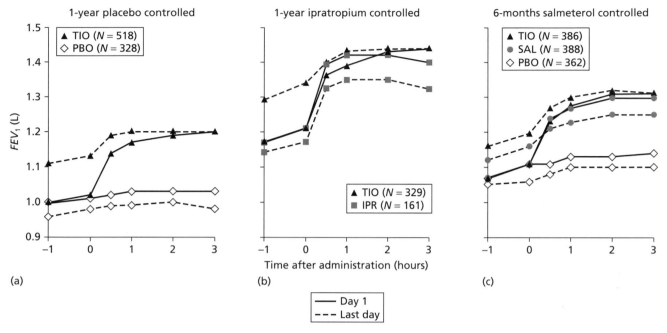

Figure 56.7 Spirometric response of tiotropium (TIO) compared with: (a) usual care (placebo [PBO]); (b) ipratropium (IPR); and (c) salmeterol (SAL). Figure derived from data in [7–9]. Data represents integrated data from two sister trials.

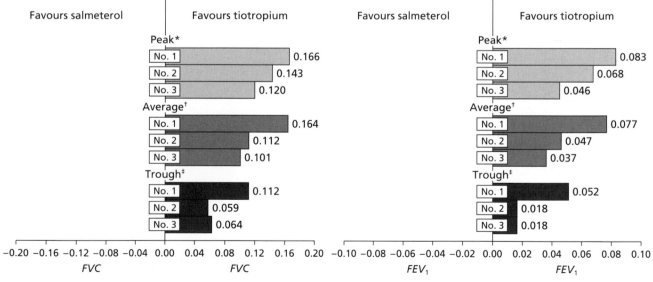

Figure 56.8 The spirometric results from three head-to-head trials of tiotropium versus salmeterol. * Peak represents maximum response over 3 h post-treatment administration; at 6 months for studies 1 and 2 and at 3 months for study 3. † Average is defined as normalized area-under-the-response curve post-treatment administration; for 12 h at 6 months for study 1, for 3 h at 6 months for study 2 and for 12 h at 3 months for study 3. ‡ Trough is the response value at the end of dosing interval – 12 h post-treatment for salmeterol and 24 h post-treatment for tiotropium; at 6 months for studies 1 and 2 and at 3 months for study 3. Further details provided in references [6,7,77]. * $P < 0.05$ tiotropium greater than salmeterol. Study 1 was a 6-month study with 12-h spirometry. Study 2 was a 6-month study with 3-h spirometry. Study 3 was a 3-month study with 12-h spirometry.

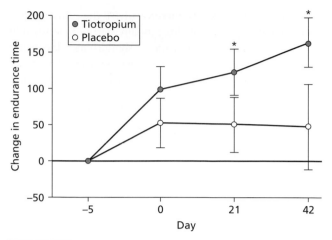

Figure 56.9 Changes in constant-load exercise endurance time are shown from baseline (day –5) for placebo and tiotropium. Data are presented as mean ± SEM. * $P < 0.05$ between groups. (From O'Donnell *et al.* [79] with permission.)

to tiotropium was maintained over 6 months, while the effects with salmeterol decreased over time [76]. A recent report from a completed third comparator trial once again showed significantly greater bronchodilatation of tiotropium over salmeterol, including the primary endpoint of the 12-h spirometric response [77].

In addition to the improved spirometry, tiotropium has been demonstrated to reduce hyperinflation as evidenced by a marked reduction in static lung volumes [78–80]. These mechanical changes are likely associated with the reduced dyspnoea observed in both the shorter term [79] and longer term trials [7–9], as measured by the validated Transition Dyspnea Index (TDI) [81–83]. Relief of hyperinflation at rest has also been accompanied by evidence from two independent clinical studies [79,84] that operating

lung volume is reduced and exercise tolerance, as assessed by endurance time, is improved (Fig. 56.9) [79,84]. Preliminary data have also revealed that tiotropium augments the effect of pulmonary rehabilitation [85]. The relationship between the mechanical and functional response has been advanced in the past decade by O'Donnell *et al.* [86], and the investigations with tiotropium now provide substantial evidence of the impact that sustained bronchodilatation can have.

Furthermore, the sustained bronchodilatation and its mechanical consequences are likely to be the basis for the observed improvements in health status. Here, tiotropium has been associated with improvements in all trials [6–8]. Understanding the improvements in health status with tiotropium, which is the ultimate goal of therapy, must consider both the mechanical benefits and the associated improvements in endpoints, reflecting the number and severity of exacerbations. Parameters associated with the worsening of disease have been evaluated as secondary endpoints in all of the major trials and consistent benefits have been observed (Table 56.2). Importantly, when exacerbations were evaluated as the primary endpoint in a cohort of US Veteran's Administration patients, tiotropium has shown to again be associated with a reduction [87]. Additionally, a report from over 1000 patients in France noted that tiotropium was significantly more effective than placebo in reducing the incidence, severity and duration of COPD exacerbations [88]. These effects can have their genesis in both the mechanical benefits (i.e. sustained 24-h bronchodilatation) as well as the potential anti-inflammatory effects that can accompany blockade of acetylcholine (see above). It is well known that exacerbations impact quality of life [89] and a retrospective analysis has shown that tiotropium blunts the impaired health status associated with frequent exacerbations [90].

Table 56.2 The balance of evidence in clinical endpoints associated with exacerbation of disease and the impact of tiotropium.

	Trial duration (weeks)			
Study/variable	49	52	26	26
Percentage of patients with at least one exacerbation	+ (0.03)	+ (0.01)	+ (0.064)	+ (0.0368)
Time to first exacerbation	+ (0.011)	+ (0.008)	+ (0.005)	+ (0.0337)
Number of exacerbations	+ (0.04)	+ (0.005)	+ (0.025)	+ (0.0028)
Percentage of patients with hospitalizations	+ (0.02)	+ (0.108)	+ (0.37)	+ (0.0557)
Time to first hospitalization	+ (0.007)	+ (0.048)	+ (0.137)	+ (0.0493)
Number of hospitalizations	+ (0.02)	+ (0.08)	+ (0.25)	+ (0.0131)

Numbers indicate the nominal P value associated with the comparison of tiotropium with the control (placebo or ipratropium). Plus (+) indicates that tiotropium was numerically superior to the control. Table based on trials reported in [7,9,10,87].

Long-acting anticholinergic–β-agonist combinations

Given the pharmacological premise that different modes of actions of anticholinergics and β-agonists on airway smooth muscle would result in additive bronchodilator response, there is no reason not to conclude that such effects would operate with agents with longer durations of effect. In a report describing the effects of ipratropium bromide administered concurrently with salmeterol, it was reported that significant increases in FEV_1 and reduced exacerbations only manifested with this combination and not with salmeterol alone [91]. A report evaluating the effects of tiotropium alone and in combination with formoterol [10] noted the greatest increase in FEV_1 with tiotropium and a significant added benefit when formoterol was added. Further studies characterizing this effect, along with expected growing clinical experience, will likely establish the roles of the bronchodilator combinations more firmly.

Therapeutic role in COPD

Inhaled anticholinergic therapy has gained wide acceptance as a foundation treatment in COPD, based in large part by the important role of the cholinergic nervous system in COPD. Treatment guidelines [92–95] and therapeutic reviews [13,96–100] published in the past decade have acknowledged this established role (Fig. 56.10). According to these reviews [1,2,4], bronchodilators are the primary intervention and mainstay of therapy, while other interventions such as inhaled steroids have restricted indication

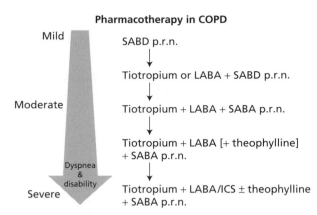

Figure 56.10 Pharmacological treatment of chronic obstructive pulmonary disease (COPD) based on increasing symptoms and disability. [+ theophylline] Add if tolerated: long-acting β$_2$-agonist (LABA) (i.e. formoterol or salmeterol); LABA combined with an inhaled corticosteroid in one preparation (LABA/ICS); short-acting β$_2$-agonist (SABA) (i.e. salbutamol); short-acting bronchodilator (SABD) (β$_2$-agonists or anticholinergics). p.r.n., as needed. (From O'Donnell *et al.* [95] with permission.)

(i.e. when additional treatment is required in severe disease). The recent introduction of tiotropium is an advance as its stable, long-lasting and sustained bronchodilatation achieved with a once daily regimen supports its role as foundation therapy and there is substantial and growing evidence of linked symptomatic and health status benefits (Fig. 56.11). Finally, its comparative efficacy versus salmeterol has been addressed in three trials (see Fig. 56.8) where tiotropium has provided consistently better bronchodilatation, with significantly greater spirometric responses during

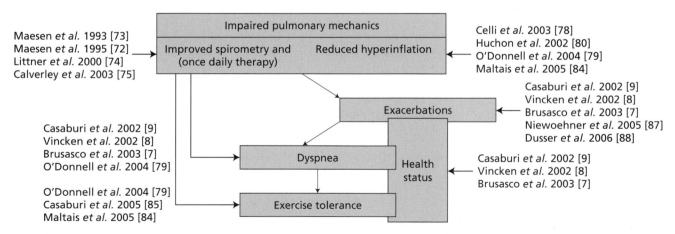

Figure 56.11 A simplified representation of the impairment, disability and involvement associated with COPD and the impact of tiotropium on relevant endpoints. The sustained bronchodilatation with tiotropium via inhibitor of cholinergic tone improves the altered pulmonary mechanisms as assessed by spirometry and static lung volume measures is supported by substantial and growing evidence. Reduced breathlessness and improved exercise tolerance as well as the reduction in the interrelation with improvements in health status are now established in the literature.

the day for peak and average, and significant or directional benefits in the trough value 24 h after tiotropium versus 12 h after salmeterol.

References

1 Barnes PJ. Chronic obstructive pulmonary disease. *N Engl J Med* 2000;**343**:269–80.

2 MacNee W, Calverley PMA. Chronic obstructive pulmonary disease. VII. Management of COPD. *Thorax* 2003;**58**:261–5.

3 Pauwels RA, Buist S, Calverley PMA *et al.* Global strategy for the diagnosis, management, and prevention of chronic obstructive pulmonary disease: NHLBI/WHO Global Initiative for Chronic Obstructive Pulmonary Disease (GOLD) Workshop summary. *Am J Respir Crit Care Med* 2001;**163**:1256–76.

4 Sutherland ER, Cherniack RM. Management of chronic obstructive pulmonary disease. *N Engl J Med* 2004;**350**: 2689–97.

5 Witek TJ. Anticholinergic bronchodilators. In: Rau JL, ed. *Respiratory Care Clinics of North America*. Philadelphia: W.B. Saunders, 1999: 521–36.

6 Donohue JF, van Noord JA, Bateman ED *et al.* A 6-month, placebo-controlled study comparing lung function and health status changes in COPD patients treated with tiotropium or salmeterol. *Chest* 2002;**122**:47–55.

7 Brusasco V, Hodder R, Miravitlles M *et al.* Health outcomes following treatment for six months with once daily tiotropium compared with twice daily salmeterol in patients with COPD. *Thorax* 2003;**58**:399–404.

8 Vincken W, Van Noord JA, Greefhorst APM *et al.* Improved health outcomes in patients with COPD during 1 year's treatment with tiotropium. *Eur Respir J* 2002;**19**:209–16.

9 Casaburi R, Mahler DA, Jones PW *et al.* A long-term evaluation of once-daily inhaled tiotropium in chronic obstructive pulmonary disease. *Eur Respir J* 2002;**19**:217–24.

10 van Noord JA, Aumann J-L, Janssens E *et al.* Comparison of tiotropium once daily, formoterol twice daily and both combined once daily in patients with COPD. *Eur Respir J* 2005; **26**:214–22.

11 Gandevia B. Historical review of the use of parasympatholytic agents in the treatment of respiratory disorders. *Postgrad Med J* 1995;**51**:13–20.

12 Chapman KR. History of anticholinergic treatment in airways disease. In: Gross NJ, ed. *Anticholinergic Therapy in Obstructive Airways Disease*. London: Franklin Scientific Publications, 1993: 9.

13 Herxheimer H. Atropine cigarettes in asthma emphysema. *BMJ* 1959;**2**:167.

14 Gross NJ. Ipratropium bromide. *N Engl J Med* 1988;**319**: 486–94.

15 Gross NJ. Safety and side effects of anticholinergic bronchodilators. In: Gross NJ, ed. *Anticholinergic Therapy in Obstructive Airway Disease*. London: Franklin Scientific Publications, 1993:116–27.

16 Ferguson GT, Cherniack RM. Management of chronic obstructive pulmonary disease. *N Engl J Med* 1993;**328**: 1017.

17 Witek TJ, Disse B. Inhaled antcholinergic therapy: applied pharmacology and interesting developments. *Curr Opin Investig Drugs* 2001;**2**:53–8.

18 Disse B, Reichl R, Speck G *et al.* BA 679 BR, a novel long-acting anticholinergic bronchodilator. *Life Sci* 1993;**52**: 537–44.

19 Haddad E, Mak JCW, Barnes PF. Characterization of [3H] BA 679, a slow-dissociating muscarinic receptor antagonist in human lung: radioligand binding and autoradiographic mapping. *Mol Pharmacol* 1994:**45**:899–907.

20 Takahashi T, Belvisi MG, Patel H *et al.* Effect of BA679 BR, a novel long-acting anticholinergic agent, on cholinergic neutrotransmission in guinea pig and human airways. *Am J Respir Crit Care Med* 1994;**150**:1640–5.

21 Dale HH. Action of certain esters and ethers of choline, and their relation to muscarine. *J Pharmacol Exp Ther* 1914;**6**: 147–90.

22 Dale HH. Nomenclature of fibres in autonomic system and their effects. *J Physiol* 1933;**80**:10P–11P.

23 Eglen RM, Hegde SS, Watson N. Muscarinic receptor subtypes and smooth muscle funtion. *Pharmacol Rev* 1996;**48**: 531–65.

24 Hall IP. Second messagers, ion channels, and pharmacology of airway smooth muscle. *Eur Respir J* 2000;**15**:1120–7.

25 Goyal RK. Muscarinic receptor subtypes: physiology and clinical implications. *N Engl J Med* 1989;**321**:1022.

26 Chilvers ER, Challiss J, Barnes PJ *et al.* Mass changes of inositol (1,4,5) triphosphate in trachealis muscle following agonist stimulation. *Eur J Pharmacol* 1989;**164**:587.

27 Nishizuka Y. Intracellular signaling by hydrolysis of phospholipids and activation of protein kinase C. *Science* 1992; **258**:607.

28 Tanaka C, Nishizuka Y. The protein kinase family for neuronal signaling. *Ann Rev Neurosci* 1994;**17**:551.

29 van Koppen CJ, Blanksteijn M, Klaassen BM *et al.* Autoradiographic visualization of muscarinic receptors in human bronchi. *J Pharmacol Exp Ther* 1988;**244**:760–4.

30 Mak JC, Baraniuk JN, Barnes PJ. Localization of muscarinic receptor subtypes in human and guinea-pig lung. *Am J Respir Dis* 1990;**141**:1559–68.

31 Tschumperlin DJ, Drazen JM. Mechanical stimuli to airway remodeling. *Am J Respir Crit Care Med* 2001;**164**:S90–4.

32 Disse B. Antimuscarinic treatment for lung diseases from research to clinical practice. *Life Sci* 2001;**68**:2557–64.

33 Gosens R, Nelemans SA, Grootte Bromhaar MM *et al.* Muscarinic M_3-receptors mediate cholinergic synergism of mitogenesis in airway smooth muscle. *Am J Respir Cell Mol Biol* 2003;**28**:257–62.

34 Kaliner M, Orange RP, Austen KF. Immunological release of histamine and slow reacting substance of anaphylaxis from human lung. IV. Enhancement by cholinergic and alpha adrenergic stimulation. *J Exp Med* 1972;**136**:556–67.

35 Morr H. Immunological release of histamine from human lung. II. Studies on acetylcholine. *Nature* 1978;**273**:473–4.

36 Salari H, Chang-Yeung M. Release of 15-hydroxyeicosatetraenoic acid (15-HETE) and prostaglandin E2 (PGE2) by cultured human bronchial epithelial cells. *Am J Respir Cell Mol Biol* 1989;**1**:245–50.

37 Sato E, Koyama S, Okubo Y, Kubo K, Sekiguchi M. Acetylcholine stimulates alveolar macrophages to release inflammatory cell chemotactic activity. *Am J Physiol* 1998; **274**:L970–9.

38 Gross NJ, Co E, Skorodin MS. Cholinergic bronchomotor tone in COPD: estimates of its amount in comparison with that in normal subjects. *Chest* 1989;**96**:984–7.

39 Taylor RG, McLagan J, Cook DG. Bronchodilator action of inhaled fenoterol and ipratropium in normal subjects: a teaching exercise for medical students. *Br J Clin Pharmac* 1989;**28**:709–13.

40 Gal TJ, Suratt PM. Atropine and glycopyrrolate effects on lung mechanics in normal man. *Anesth Analg* 1981;**60**:85–90.

41 Schilling JC, Witek TJ, Feifel U, Souhrada JF, Disse B. Safety and tolerability of supra-therapeutic doses of inhaled tiotropium (TIO). *Eur Respir J* 2000;**16**:361S.

42 O'Connor BJ, Towse LJ, Barnes PJ. Prolonged effect of tiotropium bromide on methacholine-induced bronchoconstriction in asthma. *Am J Respir Crit Care Med* 1996;**154**:876–80.

43 Brown HB, Taylor P. Muscarinic receptor agonists and antagonists. In: Hardman JG, Goodman Gilman A, Limbird LE, eds. *Goodman & Gilman's The Pharmacological Basis of Therapeutics*, 9th edn. Conshohocken: R.R. Donnelley and Sons, 1996: 141–60.

44 Taylor RG, Pavia D, Agnew JE *et al.* Effect of four weeks' high dose ipratropium bromide treatment on lung mucociliary clearance. *Thorax* 1986;**41**:295–300.

45 Pavia D, Lopez-Vidriero MT, Agnew JE *et al.* Effect of four-week treatment with oxitropium on lung mucociliary clearance in patients with chronic bronchitis or asthma. *Respiration* 1989;**55**:33.

46 Ghafouri MA, Patil KD, Kass I. Sputum changes associated with the use of ipratropium bromide. *Chest* 1984;**86**:387.

47 Tamaoki J, Chiyotani A, Tagaya B, Sakai N, Bomo K. Effect of long-term treatment with oxitropium bromide on airway secretion in chronic bronchitis and panbronchiolitis. *Thorax* 1994;**49**:545–8.

48 Pavia D, Batement JR, Sheahan NF *et al.* Clearance of lung secretions in patients with chronic bronchitis: effect of terbutaline and ipratropium bromide aerosols. *Eur Respir Dis* 1980;**61**:245.

49 Hasani A, Toms N, Agnew JE *et al.* The effect of inhaled tiotropium bromide on lung mucociliary clearance in patients with COPD. *Chest* 2004;**125**:1726–34.

50 Witek TJ, Dean NL, Schachter EN. Aerosolized atropine and relief of bronchospasm with cough: a case report. *Respir Care* 1980;**25**:570–2.

51 Anthonisen NR, Connett JE, Enright PL, Manfreda J, and the Lung Health Study Research Group. Hospitalizations and mortality in the Lung Health Study. *Am J Respir Crit Care Med* 2002;**166**:333–49.

52 Guite H, Dundas R, Burney PGB. Risk factors for death from asthma, chronic obstructive pulmonary disease, and cardiovascular disease after a hospital admission from asthma. *Thorax* 1999;**54**:301–7.

53 Ringbaek T, Viskum K. Is there an association between inhaled ipratropium and mortality in patients with COPD and asthma? *Respir Med* 2003;**97**:264–72.

54 Sin DD, Tu JV. Lack of association between ipratropium bromide and mortality in elderly patients with chronic obstructive airway disease. *Thorax* 2000;**55**:194–7.

55 Lanes S, Golisch W, Mikl J. Ipratropium and lung health study [Letter]. *Am J Respir Crit Care Med* 2003;**167**:2002.

56 Lanes SF, Garcia Rodriguez LA, Huerta C. Respiratory medications and risk of asthma death. *Thorax* 2002;**57**:683–6.

57 Braun SR, Levy SF. Comparison of ipratropium bromide and albuterol in chronic obstructive pulmonary disease: a three-center study. *Am J Med* 1991;**91**:28S–32S.

58 Taskhin DP, Ashutosh K, Bleecker ER *et al.* Comparison of the anticholinergic bronchodilator ipratropium bromide with metaproterenol in chronic obstructive pulmonary disease: a 90-day multi-center study. *Am J Med* 1986;**81**(Suppl FA): 81–9.

59 Anthonisen NR, Connett JE, Kiley JP *et al.* Effect of smoking intervention and the use of an inhaled anticholinergic bronchodilator on the rate of decline of FEV_1: The Lung Health Study. *JAMA* 1994;**272**:1497–505.

60 Rennard SI, Serby CW, Ghafouri MO, Johnson PA, Friedman M. Extended therapy with ipratropium is associated with improved lung function in patients with COPD. *Chest* 1996; **110**:62–70.

61 Taylor J, Kotch A, Rice K *et al.* and the Ipratropium Bromide HFA Study Group. Ipratropium bromide HFA inhalation aerosol is safe and effective in patients with chronic obstructive pulmonary disease (COPD). *Chest* 2001;**120**:1253–61.

62 Brazinsky SA, Lapidus RJ, Weiss LA *et al.* One-year evaluation of the safety and efficacy of ipratropium bromide HFA and CFC inhalation aerosols in patients with chronic obstructive pulmonary disease. *Clin Drug Invest* 2003;**23**:181–91.

63 Mahler DA, Donohue JF, Barbee RA *et al.* Efficacy of salmeterol xinafoate in the treatment of COPD. *Chest* 1999; **115**:957–65.

64 Rennard SI, Anderson W, ZuWallack R *et al.* Use of a long-acting inhaled β_2-adrenergic agonist, salmeterol xinafoate, in patients with chronic obstructive pulmonary disease. *Am J Respir Crit Care Med* 2001;**163**:1087–92.

65 Dahl R, Greefhorst LAPM, Nowak D *et al.* Inhaled formoterol dry powder versus ipratropium bromide in chronic obstructive pulmonary disease. *Am J Respir Crit Care Med* 2001;**164**:778–84.

66 Friedman M. Formoterol and ipratropium in COPD. *Am J Respir Crit Care Med* 2003;**167**:1579.

67 Wilson JD, Serby CW, Menjoge SS, Witek TJ. The efficacy and safety of combination bronchodilator therapy. *Eur Respir Rev* 1996;**6**:286–9.

68 Inhalation Aerosol Study Group. In chronic obstructive pulmonary disease, a combination of ipratropium and albuterol is more effective than either agent alone. *Chest* 1994;**105**: 1411–9.

69 Campbell S. For COPD, a combination of ipratropium bromide and albuterol sulfate is more effective than albuterol base. *Arch Intern Med* 1999;**159**:156–60.

70 The Combivent Inhalation Study Group. Routine nebulized ipratropium and albuterol together are better than either alone in COPD. *Chest* 1997;**112**:1514–21.

71 Dorinsky PM, Reisner C, Ferguson GT *et al.* The combination

of ipratropium and albuterol optimizes pulmonary function reversibility testing in patients with COPD. *Chest* 1999;**115**: 966–71.

72 Maesen FPV, Smeets JJ, Sldedsens TJH, Wald FDM, Cornelissen PJG. Tiotropium bromide, a new long-acting antimuscarinic bronchodilator: a pharmacodynamic study in patients with chronic obstructive pulmonary disease (COPD). *Eur Respir J* 1995;**8**:1506–13.

73 Maesen FPV, Smeets JJ, Costongs MAL, Wald FDM, Cornelissne PJG. BA 679 BR, a new long-acting anticumsarinic bronchodilator: a pilot dose-escalation study. *Eur Respir J* 1993;**6**:1031–6.

74 Littner MR, Ilowite JS, Tashkin DP *et al*. Long-acting bronchodilation with once daily dosing of tiotropium (SPIRIVA TM) in stable COPD. *Am J Respir Crit Care Med* 2000;**161**: 1136–42.

75 Calverley PMA, Lee A, Towse L *et al*. Effect of tiotropium bromide on circadian variation in airflow limitation in chronic obstructive pulmonary disease. *Thorax* 2003;**58**:855–60.

76 Donohue J, Menjoge S, Kesten S. Tolerance to the chronic bronchodilating effects of long-acting beta agonists in COPD. *Respir Med* 2003;**97**:1014–20.

77 Briggs DD Jr, Covelli H, Lapidus R *et al*. Improved daytime spirometric efficacy of tiotropium compared with salmeterol in patients with COPD. *Pulm Pharmacol Ther* 2005;**18**:397–404.

78 Celli B, ZuWallack R, Wang S, Kesten S. Improvement in resting inspiratory capacity and hyperinflation with tiotropium in COPD patients with increased static lung volumes. *Chest* 2003;**124**:1743–8.

79 O'Donnell DE, Fluege T, Gerken F *et al*. Effects of tiotropium in lung hyperinflation, dyspnoea and exercise tolerance in COPD. *Eur Respir J* 2004;**23**:832–40.

80 Huchon G, Verkindre C, Bart F *et al*. Improvements with tiotropium on endurance measured by the shuttle walking test (SWT) and on health related quality of life (HRQoL) in COPD patients. *Eur Respir J* 2002;**20**(Suppl 38):287S.

81 Mahler DA, Weinberg DH, Wells CK, Feinstein AR. The measurement of dyspnea: contents, interobserver agreement, and physiologic correlations of two new clinical indexes. *Chest* 1984;**85**:751–8.

82 Witek TJ, Mahler DA. Minimal important difference and patterns of response of the Transition Dyspnea Index. *J Clin Epidemiol* 2003;**56**:248–55.

83 Witek TJ, Mahler DA. Minimal important difference of the Transition Dyspnea Index in a multi-national clinical trial. *Eur Respir J* 2003;**21**:267–72.

84 Maltais F, Hamilton A, Marciniuk D *et al*. Improvements in symptom-limited exercise tolerance over eight hours with once daily tiotropium in patients with COPD. *Chest* 2005; **128**:1168–78.

85 Casaburi R, Kukafka D, Cooper CB, Witek TJ Jr, Kesten S. Improvement in exercise tolerance with the combination of tiotropium and pulmonary rehabilitation in patients with COPD. *Chest* 2005;**127**:809–17.

86 O'Donnell DE, Lam M, Webb KA. Measurement of symptoms, lung hyperinflation, and endurance during exercise in chronic obstructive pulmonary disease. *Am J Respir Crit Care Med* 1998;**158**:1557.

87 Niewoehner DE, Rice K, Cote C *et al*. Prevention of exacerbations of chronic obstructive pulmonary disease with tiotropium, a once-daily inhaled anticholinergic bronchodilator: a randomized trial. *Ann Intern Med* 2005;**143**: 317–26.

88 Dusser D, Bravo M-L, Iacono P, on behalf of the MISTRAL study group. The effect of tiotropium on exacerbations and airflow in patients with COPD. *Eur Respir J* 2006;**27**:1–9.

89 Seemungal T, Harper-Owen R, Bhowmik A *et al*. Respiratory viruses, symptoms, and inflammatory markers in acute exacerbations and stable chronic obstructive pulmonary disease. *Am J Respir Crit Care Med* 2001;**164**:1618–23.

90 Jones PW, Koch P, Menjoge SS, Witek TJ Jr. The impact of COPD exacerbations (EXAC) on health related quality of life (HRQL) is attenuated by tiotropium (TIO). *Am J Respir Crit Care Med* 2001;**163**:A771.

91 van Noord JA, de Munck DRAJ, Bantje TA *et al*. Long-term treatment of chronic obstructive pulmonary disease with salmeterol and the additive effect of ipratropium. *Eur Respir J* 2000;**15**:878–85.

92 ATS American Thoracic Society. Lung function testing: selection of reference values and interpretative strategies. *Am Rev Respir Dis* 1991;**144**:1202–18.

93 ERS Consensus Statement. Optimal assessment and management of chronic obstructive pulmonary disease (COPD). *Eur Respir J* 1995;**8**:1398.

94 Global Initiative for Chronic Obstructive Lung Disease. *Global Strategy for the Diagnosis, Management, and Prevention of Chronic Obstructive Pulmonary Disease NHLBI/WHO Workshop Report*. National Institutes of Health/National Heart, Lung and Blood Institute, April 2001.

95 O'Donnell DE, Hernandez P, Aaron S *et al*. Canadian Thoracic Society COPD Guidelines: Summary of highlights for family doctors. *Can Respir J* 2003;**10**:183–5.

96 Gross NJ. Outcome measurements in COPD: are we schizophrenic? *Chest* 2003;**123**:1325–7.

97 Tashkin DP, Cooper CB. The role of long-acting bronchodilators in the management of stable chronic obstructive pulmonary disease. *Chest* 2004;**125**:249–59.

98 Rees PJ. Tiotropium in the management of chronic obstructive pulmonary disease [Editorial]. *Eur Respir J* 2002;**19**:205–6.

99 Barr R, Bourbeau J, Camargo C, Ram F. Inhaled tiotropium for stable chronic obstructive pulmonary disease. *Cochrane Database Syst Rev* 2005 Apr 18;(2):CD002876.

100 Cooper CB, Tashkin DP. Recent developments in inhaled therapy in stable chronic obstructive pulmonary disease. *BMJ* 2005;**330**:640–4.

101 Roux E, Molimard M, Savineau J-P, Marthan R. Muscarinic stimulation of airway smooth muscle cells. *Gen Pharmacol* 1998;**31**:349–56.

102 Calverley PMA, Lee T, Towse L *et al*. Effect of tiotropium bromide on circadian variation in airflow limitation in chronic obstructive. *Thorax* 2003;**58**:855–60.

CHAPTER 57

β₂-Agonists

Malcolm Johnson

The pathophysiology of COPD may be considered as multi-component in nature [1]. It involves the large airways, small airways and lung parenchyma and comprises airway inflammation, structural changes, mucociliary dysfunction and a systemic component, all of which contribute to the airflow limitation characteristic of the disease.

Airway inflammation in stable COPD is characterized by increased numbers of inflammatory cells such as neutrophils, CD8⁺ T lymphocytes, monocytes–macrophages and mast cells, and elevated levels of inflammatory mediators such as interleukin 8 (IL-8), tumour necrosis factor α (TNF-α), leukotriene B_4 (LTB$_4$), RANTES, oxidants and proteases [1]. Exacerbations of COPD are associated with increased airway inflammation over stable disease and the increased presence of other cells such as eosinophils [2]. Inflammation in COPD is associated with many structural changes such as mural oedema, goblet cell hyperplasia and mucosal glandular hypertrophy in the large airways, fibrosis with collagen deposition and thickening of airway smooth muscle in the small airways and alveolar destruction in the parenchyma [3]. Airway inflammation is also associated with mucociliary dysfunction, including mucus hypersecretion, increased mucus viscosity and reduced mucociliary transport promoting bacterial colonization and mucosal damage [4]. COPD also has a number of systemic manifestations: weight loss, muscle weakness and reduced muscle mass [5] and a high incidence of disease co-morbidity [1].

Several pathophysiological mechanisms may therefore be responsible for airflow limitation in COPD. Because of this complexity of the disease, pharmacological agents that address more than one component of the underlying pathophysiology may have greater clinical efficacy.

Salbutamol, a short-acting β₂-agonist (SABA), has been used by patients with COPD over the past three decades to treat and prevent symptoms. It remains the standard bronchodilator for use in COPD-related acute bronchospasm and bronchitis. The major drawback with the first genera-tion of β₂-agonists is in their short duration of action (4–6 h). The need for a drug with more prolonged bronchodilator activity for use in COPD has been met with the development of the long-acting β₂-agonists (LABAs), salmeterol [6] and formoterol [7]. The aim of this chapter is to review the scientific and clinical evidence for the benefit of β₂-agonists in the treatment of COPD.

Mechanisms of action of β₂-agonists

β₂-Agonists exert their biological and therapeutic effects through β₂-adrenoceptors, members of the seven-transmembrane family of receptors, which are coupled to adenylate cyclase through a trimeric Gs-protein, consisting of α, β and γ subunits [8].

There is now good evidence that β₂-adrenoceptors exist in two forms, activated and inactivated, and that under resting conditions these two forms are in equilibrium [9]. The β₂-receptor is in the activated form when it is associated with the α-subunit of the G protein and guanosine triphosphate (GTP), and it is through this α-subunit that the receptor is coupled to adenylate cyclase (Fig. 57.1) to stimulate the conversion of adenosine triphosphate (ATP) to cyclic adenosine monophosphate (cAMP). It is probable that β₂-agonists have their effects by binding to and temporarily stabilizing receptors in their activated state [9]. cAMP catalyses the activation of protein kinase A (PKA), which in turn phosphorylates key regulatory proteins involved in the control of cell function [10]. cAMP also modulates intracellular calcium ion (Ca^{2+}) concentrations [11].

Salbutamol interacts directly with the active site of the β₂-adrenoceptor. Salmeterol, because of its lipophilic properties, partitions into the phospholipid membrane and diffuses laterally to approach the receptor through the cell membrane (see Fig. 57.1). The side-chain of salmeterol then binds to a discrete hydrophobic domain within the

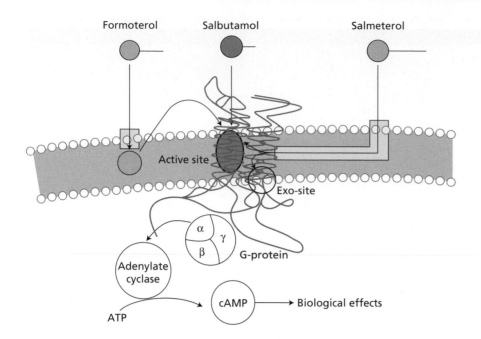

Figure 57.1 Interactions of salbutamol (short-acting β_2-agonist, SABA) and salmeterol and formoterol (long-acting β_2-agonists, LABAs) with the β_2-receptor. ATP, adenosine triphosphate; cAMP, cyclic adenosine monophosphate.

fourth transmembrane region of the β_2-adrenoceptor, called the exosite [12]. Binding to the exosite prevents the molecule from dissociating from the receptor and the saligenin head of salmeterol is then free to engage and disengage with the active site of the receptor, leading to a long concentration-independent duration of action [13]. Formoterol, which is moderately lipophilic, enters the membrane lipid bilayer and is retained as a depot (see Fig. 57.1). Subsequently, it gradually leaches out from the membrane to activate the receptor, imparting a prolonged concentration-dependent effect [14].

Effects of β_2-agonists on airway inflammation

Inflammatory cells

β_2-Receptors are present on a range of inflammatory cells that have been implicated in the pathophysiology of COPD (Table 57.1).

Table 57.1 Cellular β_2-receptor distribution.

Smooth muscle cells
Airway epithelial cells
Vascular endothelial cells
Inflammatory cells
Type II alveolar epithelial cells
Skeletal muscle cells
Fibroblasts

Anti-neutrophil effects of β_2-agonists

Neutrophils have relatively low β_2-receptor density [15]. Nevertheless, LABAs have been shown to reduce the number of neutrophils in the airway by inhibiting adhesion [16], accumulation [17], chemoattractant release [18] and by inducing apoptosis [19].

Adhesion of human neutrophils is attenuated by agents that elevate cAMP through inhibition of neutrophil Mac-1 cell surface expression. Salmeterol increased human neutrophil cAMP levels in a concentration-dependent manner [20]. Bloemen *et al.* [16] showed that salmeterol inhibited *N*-formyl-methionyl-leucyl-phenylalanine (fMLP) stimulated human neutrophil adhesion to human airway epithelial cells. The relevance of these findings to COPD patients is unclear.

In addition to their effects on adhesion, β_2-agonists also affect neutrophil accumulation [17]. In a clinical study of patients with mild asthma, salmeterol (50 μg b.i.d. for 6 weeks) treatment significantly reduced the number of neutrophils in bronchial biopsies [17]. The addition of salmeterol (50 μg b.i.d.) to low-dose inhaled corticosteroids (ICS) also reduced neutrophils in bronchoalveolar lavage (BAL; $P < 0.02$) from asthmatic patients with mild to moderate disease over 3 months [21]. Whether LABAs alone exhibit inhibitory effects on neutrophil accumulation in COPD has yet to be established.

IL-8 may be important in COPD pathophysiology because it is a chemoattractant and an activator for neutrophils. Three months' treatment with salmeterol (50 μg b.i.d.) reduced BAL IL-8 concentrations in asthmatics' ICS [21]. Compared with placebo, salmeterol also reduced the

Table 57.2 Effects of β$_2$-agonists on multicomponent pathophysiology of COPD.

Component	β$_2$-agonist effect	References
Mucociliary dysfunction		1
	Increased ciliary beating	32–35
	Increased mucociliary transport	37–41
	Decreased mucosal damage	54, 55
	Increased mucus hydration	45
Airway inflammation		1
	Anti-neutrophil activity	16–24
	Inhibition of monocytes/macrophages	26–29
	Reduction in IL-8, oxidant and PAF release	21–24
	Attenuation of mucosal oedema	31, 50, 51
	Increased surfactant secretion	49
Structural changes		1
	Inhibition of smooth muscle cell and fibroblast proliferation	61
	Inhibition of fibroblast contraction and differentiation	62, 63
Systemic component		1
	Increased respiratory muscle contractility	65–67

IL-8, interleukin 8; PAF, platelet-activating factor.

concentrations of myeloperoxidase and lipocalin (indicators of neutrophil activation) in bronchoalveolar lavage fluid (BALF) [17]. Formoterol and salmeterol [20,22,23] caused down-regulation of neutrophil respiratory burst (oxygen production) in response to fMLP, while salbutamol was without effect. Salmeterol also inhibited fMLP-induced intracellular calcium flux, phospholipase A$_2$ activity and synthesis of platelet-activating factor (PAF) [24]. This may be relevant because PAF has been associated with ciliary dysfunction, cytotoxicity and impaired mucociliary clearance [25]. Therefore, LABAs have the potential to decrease neutrophil activation in patients with COPD and may be useful in reducing the cytotoxic effects of neutrophil-derived oxidants at sites of inflammation within the airways (Table 57.2).

When neutrophils fail to undergo apoptosis, or programmed cell death, they die by lysis releasing their cellular components into the airways. In contrast to corticosteroids, LABAs can induce apoptosis in human neutrophils [19]. Salmeterol has been shown to increase apoptosis in human neutrophils via activation of the β$_2$-adrenoceptor and elevation of intracellular cAMP [19]. Although at present there are no published studies investigating the effect of formoterol on neutrophil apoptosis, it is likely to have similar activity to salmeterol.

A possible reduction by LABAs in the number of neutrophils in airway tissue and in the airway lumen may contribute to clinical efficacy in COPD.

Effects of β$_2$-agonists on monocytes–macrophages

Peripheral blood monocytes express high numbers of β$_2$-receptors, and there have been a number of reports of β$_2$-agonist inhibition of cytokine release from human monocytes *in vitro* [26]. For example, LABAs have been shown to inhibit TNF-α and IL-8 release from monocytes predominantly via the β$_2$-receptor through the generation of cAMP and activation of PKA. Maximum inhibition occurred at 10^{-8} mol/L [27]. Both salmeterol and formoterol also inhibited LTB$_4$ and IL-1β secretion from human blood monocytes by a β$_2$-receptor-independent mechanism, but only salmeterol lowered the secretion of prostaglandin E$_2$ (PGE$_2$) [28]. In contrast, the differentiated macrophage, with lower β$_2$-receptor density, exhibits reduced sensitivity to β$_2$-agonists. Concentrations of formoterol and salmeterol in excess of 10^{-6} mol/L were required to inhibit superoxide, protease and thromboxane B$_2$ release from alveolar macrophages *in vitro* [29].

Mucosal oedema

Many of the mediators released by inflammatory cells have the potential to induce tissue oedema, which is initiated by increased microvascular permeability to plasma proteins in the airway. Hill *et al.* [30] showed an inverse relationship between protein concentrations in BALF from COPD patients and lung function. A recent study has suggested that β$_2$-agonists may have a beneficial effect on pulmonary oedema [31]. Inhaled salmeterol (100 μg) decreased the incidence of high-altitude pulmonary oedema (assessed radiologically) by more than 50% compared with placebo, at the same time as arterial O_2 saturation increased. The relevance of this observation to mural oedema in COPD remains to be established.

Effects of β₂-agonists on the airway epithelium

Airway inflammation in COPD is associated with both epithelial and mucociliary dysfunction [1].

Mucociliary dysfunction

During exacerbations of COPD, the airways can be obstructed by mucus as a result of increased production, altered rheology, as well as by defective mucociliary clearance.

Mucociliary clearance

Stimulation of epithelial β₂-receptors by β₂-agonists increases ciliary beat frequency (CBF) and mucociliary transport (MCT). Salbutamol and salmeterol increased CBF in human nasal epithelial cells, with salmeterol being active at 100-fold lower concentrations than salbutamol [32]. A similar study with human bronchial epithelium revealed that, while salbutamol induced a transient increase in CBF, salmeterol caused a significant increase for 24 h [33]. Salmeterol (10^{-7} M) increased CBF from 8.6 Hz to 10.0 Hz in epithelial cells taken from COPD patients [34]. At lower concentrations, salmeterol, while having no effect itself, inhibited *Pseudomonas aeruginosa* (PA) pyocyanin-induced reduction in CBF [35]. At present, there are no published accounts on the effect of formoterol on CBF.

Short-acting β₂-agonists such as salbutamol and terbutaline have been reported to increase MCT *in vivo* [36]. This has also been shown with salmeterol and formoterol. Studies in healthy subjects showed that salmeterol (50 μg) significantly increased mucociliary transport compared with placebo [37,38]. A clinical study with salmeterol in asthmatic patients indicated a modest enhancement of mucociliary function [39]. Formoterol (24 μg b.i.d. for 7 days) has also been shown to significantly increase mucociliary clearance in bronchitic patients [40]. In contrast, the long-acting anticholinergic, tiotropium, had no significant effect on mucociliary clearance in COPD [41].

Airway secretions

The efficiency of mucociliary clearance is also affected by the amount and physical properties of airway secretions. Both α-adrenergic and β₂-receptors are present on submucosal gland mucous cells [42], but earlier studies did not report consistent effects of β₂-agonists on mucus viscosity and glycoprotein secretion [43]. However, a recent study [44] has shown that the LABA, salmeterol, but not the SABA, salbutamol, potentiates the inhibitory effect of corticosteroids on mucin secretion by airway epithelial cells. This effect of salmeterol was synergistic in nature, decreasing the IC_{50} for fluticasone propionate (FP) from 1.8 nM to 0.3 nM [44]. There is a growing body of literature [45] that supports the role of β₂-agonists in increasing mucus hydration, thereby possibly reducing viscosity and thus aiding effective mucociliary transport.

Cigarette smoke is known to adversely affect surfactant [46] and Anzueto *et al.* [47] showed that aerosolized surfactant resulted in an improvement in mucociliary transport in patients with stable chronic bronchitis. Surfactant may also modulate the function of respiratory inflammatory cells [48]. β₂-Agonists enhance secretion of surfactant (phosphatidylcholine, PC) by type II epithelial cells. Salmeterol stimulated PC secretion by up to 60% with a duration of action of more than 6 h [49]. More investigations evaluating the potential benefits of β₂-agonists in modulating surfactant secretion are needed.

Finally, β₂-agonists increase fluid clearance (reabsorption) by stimulating apical sodium uptake and sodium/potassium-adenosine triphosphatase activity in type II cells [50]. Terbutaline stimulated clearance of alveolar fluid through amiloride-sensitive and amiloride-insensitive pathways [51] and salmeterol increased alveolar fluid clearance in human lung explants instilled with iso-osmolar albumin solution [52]. Augmented fluid clearance with LABAs could contribute to a reduction in exacerbations of COPD.

Mucosal damage

Recurrent bacterial infection is a hallmark of COPD. With increased mucus accumulation in the airways and compromised mucociliary clearance, patients with stable COPD are frequently colonized by bacteria such as unencapsulated *Haemophilus influenzae* (HI), *Streptococcus pneumoniae* (SP) and *Moraxella catarrhalis* [52]. Bacteria damage the respiratory epithelium by releasing toxins, proteases, oxidants and other mediators, and by stimulating recruitment of inflammatory cells, which release pro-inflammatory mediators.

LABAs have a cytoprotective effect on the respiratory epithelium against microorganisms [54,55]. Salmeterol inhibited the invasiveness of SP and HI into airway epithelial cells, partly due to decreased expression of PAF receptors on the cell surface [53]. Salmeterol protected the respiratory epithelium against ultrastructural damage (cytoplasmic blebbing, mitochondrial damage) induced by the PA-derived toxin, pyocyanin and elastase [54]. This effect, which was mediated via β₂-receptors, was not apparent with SABAs or the anticholinergic, ipratropium bromide [54]. Salmeterol also protected the respiratory epithelium against HI-induced damage [55], with preservation of the number of both ciliated and unciliated cells and a concomitant reduction in epithelial stripping, as well as inhibition of the number of bacteria adhering to the respiratory mucosa [55]. A cytoprotective effect of formoterol has not been reported but, if used in sufficient concentrations to increase cAMP over time, is likely to have the same activity. It is encouraging that the concentration range of salmeterol for epithelial cytoprotective activity is similar to that observed in human peripheral lung tissue *in vivo*, following an inhaled dose of 50 μg [56].

De Bentzmann *et al.* [57] showed that salmeterol significantly reduced transepithelial permeability, as assessed by transepithelial resistance, mannitol flux and diffusion of a low molecular weight tracer, and prevented degradation of epithelial cell tight junctional proteins such as ZO1 and vinculin. Maintenance of tight junction integrity by salmeterol may be caused by prevention of bacterial-induced reductions in intracellular cAMP or, more importantly, by up-regulation of junctional protein expression [55]. Preservation of the number of ciliated cells and stimulation of ciliary beating by salmeterol may protect the respiratory epithelium against bacterial-induced damage by preventing bacterial adherence and by reducing the concentration of bacterial toxins in the microenvironment of the mucosal surface.

A reduction by LABA in the number of bacteria adhering to the epithelium may render patients less prone to acute bacterial infections. The incidence of respiratory infections in a 16-week study [58] in COPD patients was 15% with placebo, compared with 8% with salmeterol ($P < 0.005$). This was confirmed in a second study of salmeterol in COPD [59], where the incidence of bronchitis was 1%, compared with 8% in the placebo group ($P < 0.001$). Thus, it appears that salmeterol offers some protection against respiratory infections, perhaps by having a cytoprotective effect on the airway epithelium [60].

Potential effects of β₂-agonists on structural changes in COPD

The clinical relevance of airway smooth-muscle and fibroblast proliferation in patients with COPD remains to be determined. Salbutamol and salmeterol-inhibited human airway smooth-muscle cell proliferation *in vitro* induced by mitogens, such as thrombin, an effect that was mediated by an increase in cAMP and an action on cyclin D_1 [61]. Similarly, β₂-agonists also attenuated fibroblast contraction *in vitro* [62] and the differentiation of fibroblasts to myofibroblasts [63], suggesting a potential antifibrotic activity (see Table 57.2). Again, it is encouraging that human peripheral lung tissue concentrations of salmeterol [56] exceed that shown to have antiproliferative activity *in vitro* [61]. Furthermore, although carried out in asthmatic patients, a recent study has shown that salmeterol, when added to ICS, reduces the degree of ongoing angiogenesis [64], a recognized component of airway remodelling.

Effects of β₂-agonists on the systemic component of COPD

Recent evidence suggests that β₂-agonists may have beneficial effects on respiratory muscle contractility and therefore improve the mechanics of breathing in COPD [65,66]. In healthy subjects, salbutamol (10–20 μg i.v.) was shown to increase minute ventilation, tidal volume and respiratory flow, both at rest and under conditions of CO_2 stimulation [65]. This was associated with enhanced contractility of parasternal muscles, a surrogate for the diaphragm. Importantly, this effect was also observed with inhaled salmeterol (50 and 100 μg) where increases in minute ventilation were paralleled by enhanced parasternal contractility, independent of changes in pulmonary mechanics and heart rate [66].

The clinical relevance of these findings has now been investigated in COPD patients. Salmeterol/FP combination produced a significant increase in both ventilation and parasternal muscle contractility in severe COPD patients who were bronchodilator unresponsive and had minimal improvement in gas trapping [67]. It is an interesting possibility that the action of salmeterol may be similar to the recognized 'theophylline effect' on the diaphragm and other respiratory muscles [68], and may be particularly crucial at later stages of the disease.

Clinical efficacy of β₂-agonists in patients with COPD

β₂-Agonists are recommended in treatment guidelines for COPD [66] as they improve lung function, reduce symptoms and protect against exercise-induced dyspnoea. Several clinical studies have investigated the effect of LABAs in COPD and have shown them to provide important benefits in symptomatic patients (Table 57.3). Both salmeterol [70] and formoterol [71] significantly improve lung function (forced expiratory volume in 1 s [FEV_1], forced vital capacity [FVC] and peak expiratory flow rate [$PEFR$]) and appear to be more effective than SABAs. Other improvements include a reduction in breathlessness, hyperinflation, nighttime awakenings, rescue medication usage and respiratory tract infections, an increase in health status and a decrease in exacerbations and hospitalizations [72–74].

LABAs versus placebo

A 12-week study examined the onset and duration of action of salmeterol in COPD [75]. Clinically significant bronchodilator activity (≥ 0.1 L increase in FEV_1) occurred

Table 57.3 Clinical efficacy and safety of long-acting β₂-agonists (LABAs) in COPD.

	References
Efficacy	
Increased lung function:	
FEV_1	59, 70–72, 75–86, 90–94, 126
FVC	72, 76, 80–85, 91, 126
PEFR	78, 79, 85, 92
Inspiratory capacity	90
Decreased lung hyperinflation	72, 90
Decreased dyspnoea	59, 72, 85, 88, 90, 91
Increased health status	59, 71, 73, 85, 86, 93, 94
Decreased rescue medication use	85, 86, 93, 94
Decreased night-time awakenings	85, 93
Decreased respiratory tract infections	58, 59
Decreased hospitalizations	74
Decreased exacerbations	78
Increased survival	122
Safety	
No effect oxygen saturation at rest or during exercise	139
No clinically significant effect on heart rate, ECG, QTC interval or blood pressure	139, 140

ECG, electrocardiogram; FEV_1, forced expiratory volume in 1 s; *FVC*, forced vital capacity; PEFR, peak expiratory flow rate.

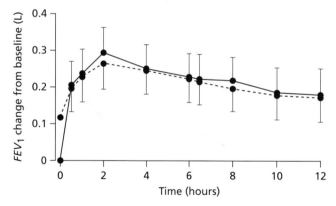

Figure 57.2 Effects of salmeterol (50 µg b.i.d. for 12 weeks) on forced expiratory volume in 1 s (FEV_1) in patients with COPD. FEV_1 (L) as change from baseline following a dose of salmeterol (50 µg) was measured over 12 h at week 0 (solid line) and week 12 (dashed line) of treatment. (From Rennard *et al.* [85] with permission.)

on day 1 after 24 min. This was maintained throughout the study. The duration of action was 10.9 and 11.7 h on day 1 and day 84, respectively. The bronchodilator response to LABAs in COPD therefore shows no evidence of tolerance (Fig. 57.2).

The efficacy and safety of 50 and 100 µg salmeterol b.i.d. was studied in COPD patients over 16 weeks [70]. FEV_1

improved significantly in the salmeterol group compared with placebo ($P < 0.001$), and significant reversibility to salmeterol was present in patients classified as not reversible to salbutamol at baseline. Maesen *et al.* [76] also demonstrated that inhaled formoterol caused long-lasting dose-dependent lung function improvement in COPD patients poorly reversible to terbutaline.

Treatment with LABAs significantly decreased daytime and night-time symptom scores, improved dyspnoea and reduced hyperinflation. In a randomised, double-blind crossover study over 2 weeks, salmeterol (50 µg b.i.d.) increased inspiratory capacity, tidal volume, mean inspiratory and expiratory flow, ventilation, oxygen uptake and carbon dioxide output [77]. These improvements were accompanied by increased peak exercise endurance [77]. These effects were associated with a clinically significant improvement in health status (quality of life) with salmeterol and formoterol, which correlated with patient and physician assessments of treatment efficacy [73].

In a 12-month randomized double-blind parallel group, placebo-controlled study in COPD [78], end-of-treatment predose FEV_1 was 1323 mL following salmeterol (50 µg b.i.d.) compared with 1264 mL with placebo ($P < 0.0001$). The rate of exacerbations was 1.04 and 1.30/year in the salmeterol and placebo groups, respectively; a reduction of 20% ($P = 0.003$). Exacerbations that required oral corticosteroids were also reduced by 29% in the salmeterol group [78].

A similar 12-month study [79] in a more severe COPD population (FEV_1 of less than 50%) showed an improvement in post-dose FEV_1 with formoterol (4.5 µg b.i.d.) of 140 mL (14%) compared with placebo. Reductions in severe exacerbations were, however, only 2% and the decrease in oral steroid use was 3% [79].

Salmeterol versus formoterol

Salmeterol and formoterol are both effective in improving airflow limitation in patients with COPD. Cazzola et al. [80] showed that salmeterol (50 µg) induced a dose-independent bronchodilator response, which lasted longer than formoterol (12 or 24 µg). However, in another study [81], there was no significant difference in the duration of action of salmeterol and formoterol (both less than 12 h). Disparity in these results may be explained by differences in the severity of disease. In a later dose-ranging study, Cazzola et al. [82] showed that both salmeterol (25, 50 and 75 µg) and formoterol (12, 24 and 36 µg) induced an increase in FVC and FEV_1 over 12 h in patients with partially reversible but severe COPD.

In some studies [83], formoterol has been shown to induce bronchodilatation more rapidly than salmeterol. Celik et al. [83] showed formoterol and salmeterol induced a clinically and statistically significant improvement in FEV_1 compared with placebo, after 10 and 20 min, respectively. This difference between salmeterol and formoterol is, however, lost on chronic dosing because bronchodilatation is still evident 12 h after the last dose [80,82].

LABAs: comparison with other therapies

In patients with stable COPD, LABAs have been shown to be more effective than short-acting anticholinergic agents or theophylline.

LABAs versus anticholinergics

Several studies have compared salmeterol with ipratropium bromide in terms of safety and efficacy in COPD patients [59,84,85]. Salmeterol showed a greater improvement in FEV_1 compared with ipratropium bromide or placebo [59]. Patients treated with ipratropium bromide experienced a trough in FEV_1 after 6 h because of its shorter duration of action, whereas those receiving salmeterol had a sustained improvement in FEV_1 over 12 h. Salmeterol also improved morning peak expiratory flow (PEF), evening PEF and night-time shortness of breath ($P = 0.04$) compared with ipratropium bromide. These beneficial effects were apparent in those patients who were responsive as well as those unresponsive to salbutamol at baseline. Patients with partially reversible COPD, pretreated with salmeterol, responded normally to salbutamol when required for rescue therapy [84].

While one study demonstrated that salmeterol extended the time to first exacerbation [59], this was not confirmed in a second study [85], where the percentage of patients experiencing one or more COPD exacerbations over the 12-week treatment period were 30.4, 28.8 and 26.8% for the placebo, salmeterol and ipratropium groups, respectively. However, 20 patients (14.8%) in the placebo group experienced their first exacerbation during week 1, compared with six patients (4.6%) in the salmeterol group. Interestingly, the trend for salmeterol to reduce exacerbations does not appear to be an effect associated with SABA.

A number of studies have also compared formoterol with ipratropium bromide. Dahl et al. [86] studied the efficacy and safety of 12 weeks of treatment with formoterol (12 and 24 µg b.i.d.) or ipratropium bromide (40 µg q.i.d.) in patients with COPD. In terms of improving FEV_1, both doses of formoterol were significantly superior to ipratropium bromide. In addition, the onset of action of formoterol (less than 5 min), was faster than that of ipratropium bromide, and the duration of action was at least 12 h [86]. Formoterol also significantly improved quality of life and reduced the number of 'bad' days (more than 20% reduction in PEF and/or at least double symptom score) compared with ipratropium bromide [86].

Inhaled SABAs have been shown to reduce dynamic hyperinflation during exercise, thus improving breathlessness on exertion [87,88]. This may be an effect of β_2-agonists in improving lung emptying, resulting in reduced lung volumes. In this context, reduction in end-expiratory lung volume following β-agonist bronchodilators is better correlated with improved dyspnoea than FEV_1 [84]. In a recent study [89], the effect of 1 week of treatment with 4.5, 9.0 or 18.0 µg formoterol b.i.d. on exercise capacity was compared with that of 80 µg ipratropium bromide t.i.d. or placebo, using a bicycle ergometer test. All three doses of formoterol significantly prolonged the time to exhaustion, which was comparable to the effect of 80 µg ipratropium t.i.d. The maximum Borg dyspnoea scale was unaffected. Similar data were reported by Ayers et al. [90] and Patakas et al. [91], who evaluated the effect of salmeterol in an ergometry and a treadmill exercise test, respectively. The mean distance walked did not increase by more than 9.1 m (10 yards) during the 12-week treatment period [91]. However, salmeterol significantly reduced the prewalk dyspnoea score, but there were no significant differences in postwalk Borg scores at the end of the study period.

A 6-month study has compared the effects of salmeterol (50 µg b.i.d.) with tiotropium (18 µg o.d.) in COPD [92]. In terms of lung function, mean trough FEV_1 responses were approximately 50 mL higher with tiotropium than salmeterol, increases in morning PEFR were 11% and 9% in the tiotropium and salmeterol groups, respectively, and there were equal reductions in lung hyperinflation [92]. Both groups reduced the need for rescue medication to the same extent, and there were fewer exacerbations (36.8%, tiotropium; 38.5%, salmeterol) compared with placebo (45.8%).

LABAs versus theophylline

In the long-term treatment of patients with COPD, LABAs were shown to be more effective than oral (dose-titrated) theophylline. Salmeterol (50 µg b.i.d.) was statistically more effective than theophylline in improving FEV_1 and morning PEF, and in increasing the percentage of days and nights without symptoms [93]. Salmeterol was also significantly superior to theophylline in reducing the need for additional salbutamol during the day and night and increasing patient quality of life [93]. Similar findings have been reported for formoterol over 12 months [94]. Treatment-related adverse events were more frequent among patients receiving theophylline.

Combination therapy with LABAs and corticosteroids

Interactions between $β_2$-agonists and corticosteroids

A complementary effect occurs when the response of two or more drugs combined produces a greater effect than either drug alone. An additive effect is where the combined response of two or more drugs equals the sum of the response of the individual drugs. A synergistic effect occurs when the combined response of two or more drugs is greater than the sum of the response of the individual drugs.

Complementary interactions at the molecular and receptor levels

Corticosteroids (CS) increase the synthesis of $β_2$-receptors and reduce receptor desensitization [95]. $β_2$-Agonists, particularly LABAs, modulate glucocorticoid receptors (GRs) by priming the GR for subsequent corticosteroid binding and by increasing the translocation of the GR from the cell cytosol to the nucleus [96,97]. GRs are modulated by phosphorylation which leads to activation, and dephosphorylation which leads to inactivation [98]. LABA-induced GR priming is achieved by mitogen-activated protein kinase (MAPK) dependent phosphorylation [99]. When salmeterol or formoterol stimulate the $β_2$-receptor, the G-αs subunit disassociates and the residual βγ-subunit of the G-protein initiates an intracellular signalling cascade, culminating in the activation of MAPK [100]. This has been demonstrated with salmeterol in cells transfected with a MAPK-luciferin/luciferase reporter construct and directly, by isolation of phospho-MAPK [101].

Activation of the MAPK pathway by the LABA requires that the $β_2$-receptor is phosphorylated, probably by PKA. MAPK then phosphorylates the GR at a number of proline-directed serine residues in the N-terminus region of the receptor [102]. Phosphorylated GR has been detected in cells, containing both $β_2$-receptors and GRs, when stimulated with salmeterol in the presence of radiolabelled phosphate [103]. An increase in negative charge at the N-terminal domain of the receptor resulting from phosphorylation may lead to a conformational change in the GR protein, leading to the 'priming' event and rendering the receptor more sensitive to steroid-dependent activation.

Translocation of the GR from the cell cytosol to the nucleus is a fundamental step in the anti-inflammatory activity of ICS. GR translocation has been shown to be increased by the addition of a LABA in vitro [96,97] and in some cases in vivo [104]. The mechanism of this effect has been further investigated. Salmeterol and formoterol have been shown to activate a CCAAT enhancer binding protein (C/EBP-α) in airway smooth muscle cells [105] and in epithelial cells). The synchronous activation of GR by CS and of C/EBP-α by LABA allows a heterodimer between GR and C/EBP-α to form, increasing the activation of the receptor and nuclear translocation [105]. Haque et al. [106] showed that the combined inhalation of salmeterol (50 µg) and FP (100 µg) by COPD patients increased the nuclear translocation of GR in sputum macrophages significantly more than the same dose of FP alone and equivalent to a fivefold higher dose of steroid [106]. Whereas budesonide (BUD) (800 µg) also significantly increased the translocation of the GR from the cytosol into the nuclei of peripheral blood leucocytes, the combination with formoterol (24 µg) did not enhance this effect versus BUD alone.

Complementary anti-inflammatory effects of LABAs and corticosteroids

Complementary cellular effects of LABAs and CS that may be of relevance in COPD have been demonstrated in vitro in terms of inhibition of inflammatory mediator release [107–109], protection of the respiratory mucosa against bacterial-induced damage [110], inhibition of neutrophil chemoattractant release [107–109], eosinophilic oxidative burst [111] and myofibroblast differentiation [63], and stimulation of T-lymphocyte apoptosis [112].

Dowling et al. [110] reported that incubation of human respiratory mucosa with either salmeterol or FP alone, significantly inhibited PA-induced epithelial damage and loss of ciliated cells in a concentration-dependent manner. However, when a combination of salmeterol and FP was used, the loss of cilia from the epithelial surface was synergistically reduced [110].

IL-8 is a major neutrophil chemoattractant involved in the pathogenesis of COPD. Pang and Knox [107] showed that TNF-α-induced IL-8 release from human airway smooth-muscle cells was markedly inhibited by FP, but unaffected by salmeterol. However, a combination of salmeterol with FP synergistically enhanced the inhibition induced by the CS. Cigarette smoke-induced release of IL-8 from human monocyte-derived macrophages was synergistically inhibited by a combination of FP and salmeterol. Similar results were reported in human alveolar macrophages isolated from the BALF of COPD patients. FP (10^{-8}–10^{-12} mol/L) inhibited IL-8 and TNF-α production in a dose-dependent manner, while salmeterol was without effect [108]. Combining both drugs resulted in a greater inhibition of cytokine production than FP alone [108]. Combination therapy with FP (10^{-9} or 10^{-10} mol/L) and salmeterol (10^{-9} mol/L) also synergistically inhibited rhinovirus-induced IL-8 and RANTES release from bronchial epithelial cells [109].

Inhibition of cytokine release by CS is thought to be caused by reduced activation of transcription factors such as GATA-3 and nuclear factor κB (NF-κB) (via IKKβ), Maneechotesuwan et al. [113] showed that GATA-3 nuclear localization in peripheral blood mononuclear cells was decreased by inhaled FP (both 100 and 500 μg) but unaffected by salmeterol (50 μg). However, a combination of salmeterol (50 μg) with the lower dose of FP (100 μg) synergistically reduced GATA-3 nuclear expression [113]. Similarly, in human bronchial epithelial cells FP caused a dose-dependent inhibition of IKKβ phosphorylation [114]. The combination of FP and salmeterol caused an inhibition of IKKβ phosphorylation which was significantly greater than FP alone (0.01 μmol/L) and similar to that achieved by a higher concentration of FP (0.1 μmol/L). A number of studies have now investigated the anti-inflammatory effects of LABA/ICS combinations.

In COPD patients, the combination of salmeterol and FP at a dose of 50/500 μg b.i.d. significantly ($P < 0.04$) reduced neutrophils in induced sputum over 13 weeks [115]. Similarly, whereas FP (500 μg b.i.d.) alone increased neutrophil numbers in airway tissue from COPD patients, this was not observed [116] when salmeterol was added to the inhaled corticosteroid.

In a study in COPD, the salmeterol/FP combination (50/500 μg b.i.d.), but not FP alone, reduced macrophages ($CD68^+$ cells) in airway tissue over 3 months of treatment [116]. However, a second study [115] failed to show an effect compared with placebo.

There is evidence for a key role for the $CD8^+$ T-lymphocyte in the pathophysiology of COPD and an elevated CD8/CD4 ratio has been reported [2]. Three studies [115–117] have investigated the effect of salmeterol/FP combination therapy on airway T-lymphocyte populations in COPD patients. Both $CD8^+$ and $CD4^+$ cells were significantly reduced over 3 months [115–117] and this

effect was greater than that observed with FP alone [116,117]. In addition, cells staining positive for mRNA for TNF-α and IFN-γ were also suppressed [115]. These broad spectrum anti-inflammatory effects observed when a LABA is added to an ICS may have relevance to the enhanced clinical benefit in COPD.

Elevated numbers of eosinophils have been found in the induced sputum, bronchial biopsies and lamina propria of COPD patients, particularly during an exacerbation [2]. Both formoterol (1–10 nmol/L) and BUD (1–100 nmol/L) when administered separately inhibit superoxide generation from peripheral blood eosinophils. Combination of a low concentration of BUD (0.1 nmol/L) with formoterol (1 nmol/L) inhibited eosinophilic oxidative burst with an effect that was more than additive [111]. Another key element in the anti-inflammatory effects of ICS is their ability to shorten the survival of inflammatory cells in airway tissue. In T lymphocytes, apoptosis in response to FP, at both low and higher concentrations, was enhanced by the addition of salmeterol [112].

Airway remodelling occurs in both asthma and COPD [1,2] and has been shown to be associated with increased numbers of activated fibroblasts, many of which have the phenotypic characteristics of myofibroblasts (i.e. express α-smooth muscle actin [SMA]). Giuliani et al. [63] showed that transforming growth factor β₁ (TGF-β₁), a cytokine present in increased quantities in COPD, induced a dose-dependent increase in the number of SMA-positive cells in primary human airway fibroblast culture. This TGF-β₁-induced myofibroblast differentiation was effectively down-regulated by salmeterol and FP. Both agents administered together produced a synergistic inhibitory effect [63].

Clinical efficacy of LABA/ICS combination therapy

What is the clinical rationale for combining LABAs with ICS in the treatment of COPD? First, LABAs are potent bronchodilators and have non-bronchodilator activity [18], which may be relevant to their efficacy in COPD. Secondly, LABAs and ICS influence different aspects of COPD pathophysiology, so together they may provide an additive therapeutic effect. Finally, there is some evidence of synergy between LABAs and ICS in COPD which may be important in improving the overall clinical efficacy of the combination.

The efficacy of inhaled salmeterol/fluticasone propionate 50/250 or 50/500 μg b.i.d. compared with its components or placebo in the treatment of patients with COPD was initially evaluated in three randomized double-blind placebo-controlled 24-week multicentre trials [118–120].

In the first study [118], a significantly greater increase in predose FEV_1 at endpoint was observed after combination therapy (15%) compared with salmeterol (10%; $P = 0.012$)

and placebo (2%; $P < 0.0001$). An increase in 2-h postdose FEV_1 was also observed after treatment with the combination (261 mL) compared with FP (138 mL; $P < 0.001$) and placebo (28 mL; $P < 0.001$). There were greater improvements in the Transitional Dyspnoea Index (TDI) with salmeterol/FP (2.1) compared with FP (1.3; $P = 0.033$), salmeterol (0.9; $P < 0.001$), and placebo (0.4; $P < 0.0001$). There was an associated reduction in the need for rescue salbutamol use (1.2 puffs/day) and an increase of 16.3% in rescue-free days compared with placebo [118]. Health status (Chronic Respiratory Disease Questionnaire, CRDQ) also improved significantly (score 10.0).

Similar findings were obtained in a second study [119], where PEFR increased by 30.7 L/min over baseline, compared with 0.8, 14.4 and 11.3 L/min for placebo, salmeterol and FP, respectively. This was associated with a change in TDI of 1.7 [119].

The trial of inhaled steroids and long-acting β_2-agonists (TRISTAN) [78] was the first long-term study to investigate the efficacy and safety of LABA/ICS combination therapy for the treatment of COPD patients. COPD patients were randomized to treatment with either salmeterol (50 µg b.i.d.), FP (500 µg b.i.d.), salmeterol/FP (50/500 µg b.i.d.) or placebo for 12 months in a double-blind parallel-group placebo-controlled design.

There was good evidence of the beneficial effects of combining a LABA with an ICS in this COPD patient population. Combination therapy improved pretreatment FEV_1 significantly ($P < 0.001$) more than placebo (treatment difference 133 mL), salmeterol (73 mL) or FP (95 mL) alone [78]. This was also seen with FVC and PEF. The improvement in PEF was evident within 1 week of treatment and was sustained throughout the year. The improvement in FVC observed for combination therapy may be indicative of improved exercise performance. Combination treatment was also the only treatment to produce a clinically significant improvement in health status (St. George's Respiratory Questionnaire, SGRQ), and produced the greatest reduction in daily symptoms, particularly breathlessness, and this was evident within 1 week of treatment. The exacerbation rate significantly fell by 25% ($P < 0.001$) in the combination group and by 20% and 19% in the salmeterol and FP group, respectively, compared with placebo (Fig. 57.3). The treatment effect was more pronounced in the more severe patients (baseline FEV_1 less than 50% predicted), where exacerbations requiring oral corticosteroids were reduced by 39% ($P < 0.001$) in the combination group [78]. The absence of a statistical, significant gender interaction in this study indicates that the salmeterol/fluticasone combination therapy was equally effective in both women and men with COPD [121].

Possible evidence of clinical synergy was obtained from predose FEV_1 and rescue medication use in the more severe patient subgroup [78]. By week 52, predose FEV_1 in the

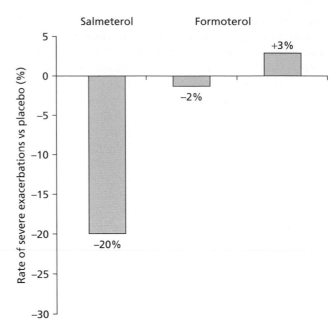

Figure 57.3 Effect of long-acting β_2-agonists (LABAs) on exacerbations in COPD. COPD patients were treated for 1 year with: (a) salmeterol (50 µg b.i.d.) or placebo; or (b) formoterol (4.5 µg b.i.d.) or placebo. The rate of severe exacerbations (requiring use of oral steroids and/or antibiotics and/or hospitalizations resulting from respiratory symptoms) was calculated as differences (%) from placebo. (Data from Calverley *et al.* [78] and Szafranski *et al.* [79].)

combination group had increased by 10% ($P < 0.001$) compared with 2% in both the salmeterol and FP groups, and had decreased by 3% in the placebo group [78]. Similarly, median percentage of days without reliever medication were 0% for placebo, 3% for salmeterol, 2% for FP and 14% for combination therapy ($P < 0.004$).

The efficacy and safety of BUD/formoterol in a single inhaler compared with either agent alone has also recently been evaluated in patients with moderate to severe COPD [79]. COPD patients were randomized to treatment with either formoterol (4.5 µg b.i.d.), BUD (400 µg b.i.d.), formoterol/BUD (4.5/400 µg b.i.d.) or placebo for 12 months in a double-blind parallel-group placebo-controlled study. The results of this study showed BUD/formoterol improved FEV_1 versus placebo (15%) and versus ICS (9%), but not compared with formoterol, and reduced symptom scores and use of relief medication versus BUD alone [79]. Improvements in morning and evening PEF were maintained over the 12 months of the study. The mean number of severe exacerbations (see Fig. 57.3) was equally reduced by BUD (23%) and BUD/formoterol (24%), but unchanged by formoterol alone (2%). Mild exacerbations were reduced by 62% with combination therapy compared with 55% for formoterol and 41% for budesonide [79].

These findings suggest that treatment of the underlying

multicomponent pathophysiology of COPD with both LABAs and ICS is necessary for improved control of the disease in many patients. Support for this approach was provided by a retrospective cohort study of COPD patients [122], which revealed that regular use of salmeterol/FP combination therapy was associated with significantly greater 3-year survival than those patients taking short-acting bronchodilators. A Landmark study, Towards a revolution in COPD Health (TORCH) is underway to assess the impact of salmeterol/FP combination therapy on all-cause mortality over 3 years in COPD [123].

Combination of β$_2$-agonists and anticholinergics

Beneficial effects have been reported previously when salbutamol is added to anticholinergic therapy in COPD [124]. Van Noord *et al.* [125] more recently examined the effect of the combination of 50 μg salmeterol b.i.d. and 40 μg ipratropium bromide q.i.d. They showed that ipratropium bromide and salmeterol improved FEV_1 to a significantly greater extent than salmeterol alone. This has been confirmed in another study over 24 weeks [126]. However, patients did not experience any additional benefit in symptom control when salmeterol and ipratropium bromide were administered together [126]. The combination of 12 μg formoterol b.i.d. and 40 μg ipratropium bromide q.i.d. has also been shown to be superior to formoterol alone in improving morning PEF and FEV_1 in patients with COPD [127]. A second study showed that the effects of formoterol/ipratropium over 3 weeks were significantly superior to salbutamol/ipratropium [128]. The effect of tiotropium in combination with LABAs has also been evaluated. The acute effects of adding salmeterol (50 μg) and tiotropium (18 μg) has been studied in patients with stable COPD [129,130]. At 12 h, the mean increase in FEV_1 for the salmeterol/tiotropium combination was significantly ($P = 0.009$) greater than for salmeterol alone [129]. Salmeterol and tiotropium produced a further increase in FEV_1 and FVC over that observed with either alone [130]. Combination therapy of salmeterol and tiotropium also resulted in the greatest reduction in dynamic hyper-inflation compared with single agent therapy [131]. Finally, one study has shown that the triple combination of salmeterol/FP/tiotropium was superior to the dual combinations in improving lung function in COPD patients [132].

Combination of β$_2$-agonists and theophylline

Both SABAs [133] and LABAs [134,135] have been studied in combination with theophylline. The beneficial effects of the combination of 50 μg salmeterol b.i.d. and theophylline (titrated to 10–20 μg/mL) over 12 weeks of treatment has recently been shown in two large multicentre studies [134,135]. By week 4, the combination of salmeterol and theophylline was significantly superior in improving FEV_1 than either salmeterol or theophylline alone, and this benefit was maintained over the 12 weeks. In addition, significantly fewer patients in the combination group had exacerbations, and the TDI was also significantly improved [134]. At each 4-week period, salbutamol use was significantly decreased in both the combination and salmeterol-alone groups. Although no studies examining the combination of formoterol and theophylline have been published, it is likely that formoterol would have similar activity to salmeterol. One study has evaluated salbutamol and theophylline in combination with ipratropium bromide or placebo and has demonstrated benefit of the triple combination in some patients [136].

Safety of β$_2$-agonists in COPD

Patients with COPD are known to be at increased risk of cardiovascular disease [137]. Pharmacologically predictable cardiovascular adverse effects of β$_2$-agonists include tachycardia, hypokalaemia and worsening ventilation–perfusion (V/Q) matching [138].

The systemic effects of a single dose of salmeterol (50 μg) and formoterol (12–24 μg) have been studied in patients with a history of 'mild to moderate' cardiac arrhythmias and hypoxaemia (Pao$_2$ < 60 mmHg). Mean maximum heart rate increased by approximately 6 beats/min and mean plasma potassium concentrations decreased by 0.45 mmol/L after inhalation of salmeterol [139]. The effects of formoterol (12 μg) on these parameters were generally similar to those of salmeterol; however, the effects of a higher dose of formoterol (24 μg) were more marked. The number of patients experiencing supraventricular premature beats or isolated ventricular premature beats (VPB) was similar after inhalation of placebo or salmeterol. Complex ventricular arrhythmias (multiform or paired VPBs) were reported only after inhalation of formoterol. The authors concluded that 50 μg salmeterol and 12 μg formoterol had a higher 'safety margin' than 24 μg formoterol in COPD patients with pre-existing cardiac arrhythmias and hypoxaemia [139]. A pooled analysis of salmeterol treatment in COPD for 12 weeks to 1 year showed no clinically significant differences from placebo in electrocardiogram (ECG), QTC interval or 24-h heart rate [140].

The concern that LABA bronchodilators may induce a mismatch between ventilation and perfusion, resulting in a degree of oxygen desaturation was examined in a three-way cross-over study [141], which showed that salmeterol, ipratropium bromide and salbutamol all induced an equally small and transient fall in Pao_2. The nadir in Pao_2 was greatest (3.5 mmHg; $P < 0.05$ vs baseline) after inhalation of salbutamol (200 µg), lowest after ipratropium bromide (1.4 mmHg) and intermediate (2.8 mmHg; $P < 0.05$ vs baseline) after salmeterol (50 µg). Compared with baseline, $Paco_2$ and arterial pH values did not change significantly [141]. The observed effects of salmeterol and salbutamol on Pao_2 are therefore unlikely to be of clinical significance. Similarly, there was no evidence that LABAs used in combination therapy increased the risk of hypokalaemia in COPD patients [78].

Conclusions

The pathophysiology of COPD is complex and multicomponent in nature. Pharmacological intervention, which addresses a number of elements of the underlying processes, may have greater clinical impact on the disease. β_2-Agonists, particularly LABAs, have both bronchodilator and non-bronchodilator activity (see Table 57.2) that may be relevant to their efficacy in COPD (see Table 57.3). They have been shown to increase lung function, decrease symptoms, reduce exacerbations, increase health status, decrease hospitalizations and prolong survival. Combinations of LABAs and ICS have superior efficacy than either LABAs alone or other LABA combined therapies, and this may be the result of their effects being additive or, in some cases, synergistic in nature.

Acknowledgement

The author would like to thank Cathy Henderson for her assistance in preparing this manuscript.

References

1 Agusti AGN. COPD, a multicomponent disease: implications for management. *Resp Med* 2005;**99**:670–82.

2 Jeffery PK. Differences and similarities between chronic obstructive pulmonary disease and asthma. *Clin Exp Allergy* 1999;**29**:14–26.

3 Jeffery P. Morphology of the airway wall in asthma and in chronic obstructive pulmonary disease. *Am Rev Respir Dis* 1991;**143**:1152–8.

4 Sethi S. Bacterial infection and the pathogenesis of COPD. *Chest* 2000;**117**:286S–91S.

5 Wouters EFM. Muscle weakness in chronic obstructive pulmonary disease. *Eur Respir Rev* 2000;**10**:349–53.

6 Brittain RT. Approaches to a long-acting selective β_2-adrenoceptor stimulant. *Lung* 1990;**168**:111–4.

7 Pauwels R. Rate of onset and duration of action of beta-2-agonists: comparison of inhaled formoterol with salbuta-

mol. In: Barnes PJ, Matthys H, eds. *Formoterol, A New Generation Beta-2-Agonist*. Toronto: Hogrefe & Huber, 1990: 35–9.

8 Robison GA, Butcher RW, Sutherland EW. Adenyl cyclase as an adrenergic receptor. *Ann N Y Acad Sci* 1967;**319**: 703–23.

9 Onaran HO, Costa T, Rodbard D. Subunits of guanine nucleotide-binding proteins and regulation of spontaneous receptor activity: thermodynamic model for the interaction between receptors and guanine nucleotide-binding protein subunits. *Mol Pharmacol* 1993;**43**:245–56.

10 Johnson M. The β-adrenoceptor. *Am J Respir Crit Care Med* 1998;**158**:S146–53.

11 Johnson M, Coleman RA. *Mechanisms of Action of β_2-Adrenoceptor Agonists*. Cambridge: Blackwell, 1995: 1278–95.

12 Green SA, Spasoff AP, Coleman RA, Johnson M, Liggett SB. Sustained activation of a G-protein-coupled receptor via anchored agonist binding. *J Biol Chem* 1996;**271**:24029–35.

13 Johnson M, Butchers PR, Coleman RA *et al.* The pharmacology of salmeterol. *Life Sci* 1993;**52**:2131–47.

14 Anderson GP. Formoterol: pharmacology, molecular basis of agonism and mechanism of long duration of a highly potent and selective β_2-adrenoceptor agonist bronchodilator. *Life Sci* 1993;**52**:2145–60.

15 Johnson M. Effects of β_2-agonists on resident and infiltrating inflammatory cells. *J Allergy Clin Immunol* 2002;**110**: S282–90.

16 Bloemen P, van den Tweel M, Henricks P *et al.* Increased cAMP levels in stimulated neutrophils inhibit their adhesion to human bronchial epithelial cells. *Am J Physiol* 1997;**272**: L580–7.

17 Jeffery P, Venge P, Gizycki M *et al.* Effects of salmeterol on mucosal inflammation in asthma: a placebo-controlled study. *Eur Respir J* 2002;**20**:1378–85.

18 Johnson M, Rennard S. Alternative mechanisms for long-acting beta$_2$-adrenergic agonists in COPD. *Chest* 2001;**120**: 258–70.

19 Lee E, Smith J, Robertson T *et al.* Salmeterol and inhibitors of phosphodiesterase 4 (PDE-4) induce apoptosis in neutrophils from asthmatics: β-adrenergic receptor-mediated salmeterol activity and additive effects with PDE4 inhibitors. *Am J Respir Cell Mol Biol* 1999;**159**:A329.

20 Ottonello L, Morone P, Dapino P *et al.* Inhibitory effect of salmeterol on the respiratory burst of adherent human neutrophils. *Clin Exp Immunol* 1996;**106**:97–102.

21 Ward C, Li X, Wang N *et al.* Salmeterol reduces BAL IL-8 levels in asthmatics on low dose inhaled corticosteroids. *Eur Respir J* 1998;**28**:380S.

22 Anderson R, Feldman C, Theron A *et al.* Anti-inflammatory, membrane-stabilizing interactions of salmeterol with human neutrophils *in vitro. Br J Pharmacol* 1996;**117**:1387–94.

23 Nials AT, Coleman RA, Johnson M *et al.* The duration of action of non-β_2-adrenoceptor mediated responses to salmeterol. *Br J Pharmacol* 1997;**120**:961–7.

24 Banner K, Moriggi E, Da Ros B *et al.* The effect of selective phosphodiesterase 3 and 4 isoenzyme inhibitors and established anti-asthma drugs on inflammatory cell activation. *Br J Pharmacol* 1996;**119**:1255–61.

25 Klettke U, Luck W, Wahn U et al. Platelet-activating factor inhibits ciliary beat frequency of human bronchial epithelial cells. *Allergy Asthma Proc* 1990;**20**:115–8.

26 Pennings HJ, Dentener MA, Buurman WA, Wouters EFM. Salbutamol and salmeterol modulate cytokine production by peripheral blood monocytes. *Eur Respir J* 1995;**8**(Suppl 19):1871.

27 Pantelidis P, Hayes KL, Vardey C, Du Bois RM. Modulation of monocyte cytokine secretion by β$_2$-agonists: a comparison of salbutamol and salmeterol. *Eur Respir J* 1995;**8**(Suppl 19):2692.

28 Linden M. The effects of β$_2$-adrenoceptor agonists and a corticosteroid, budesonide, on the secretion of inflammatory mediators from monocytes. *Br J Pharmacol* 1992;**107**:156–60.

29 Baker A, Palmer J, Johnson M, Fuller R. Inhibitory actions of salmeterol on human airway macrophages and blood monocytes. *Eur J Pharmacol* 1994;**264**:301–6.

30 Hill A, Bayley D, Campbell E, Hill S, Stockley R. Airways inflammation in chronic bronchitis: the effects of smoking and α$_1$-antitrypsin deficiency. *Eur Respir J* 2000;**15**: 886–90.

31 Sartori C, Allemann Y, Duplain H et al. Salmeterol for the prevention of high-altitude pulmonary edema. *N Engl J Med* 2002;**346**:1631–6.

32 Rusznak C, Sapsford RJ, Devalia JL et al. Influence of albuterol and salmeterol on ciliary beat frequency of cultured human bronchial epithelial cells. *Thorax* 1991;**46**:782P.

33 Devalia J, Sapsford R, Rusznak C, Toumbis M, Davies R. The effects of salmeterol and salbutamol on ciliary beat frequency of cultured human bronchial epithelial cells, *in vitro*. *Pulm Pharmacol* 1992;**5**:257–63.

34 Piatti G, Ambrosetti U, Dal Sasso M et al. Effects of salmeterol on ciliary beat and mucus rheology in COPD patients. *Eur Resp J* 2003;**22**:78S.

35 Kanthakumar K, Cundell DR, Johnson M et al. Effect of salmeterol on human nasal epithelial cell ciliary beating: inhibition of the ciliotoxin, pyocyanin. *Br J Pharmacol* 1994; **112**:493–8.

36 Foster WM, Bergofsky EH, Bohning DE, Lippman M, Albert RE. Effect of adrenergic agents and their mode of action on mucociliary clearance in man. *J Apply Physiol* 1976;**41**: 146–52.

37 Chambers CB, Corrigan BW, Newhouse MT. Salmeterol (S) speeds mucociliary transport (MCT) in healthy subjects. *Am J Respir Cell Mol Biol* 1999;**159**:A636.

38 Tay HL, Armogum N, Tan LK. Nasal mucociliary clearance and salmeterol. *Clin Otolaryngol Allied Sci* 1997;**22**:68–70.

39 Hasani A, Toms N, O'Connor J et al. The effect of salmeterol xinafoate on lung mucociliary clearance in patients with stable asthma. *Eur Respir J* 1998;**12**(Suppl 28):180S.

40 Melloni B, Germouty J. The influence of a new beta agonist: formoterol on mucociliary function. *Rev Mal Respir* 1992; **9**:503–7.

41 Hasani A, Toms N, Creer DD et al. Effect of inhaled tiotropium on tracheobronchial clearance in patients with COPD. *Eur Respir J* 2001;**18**:245S.

42 Pack RJ, Richardson PS, Smith IC et al. The functional significance of the sympathetic innervation of mucous glands in the bronchi of man. *J Physiol* 1988;**403**:211–9.

43 Phipps RJ, Williams IP, Richardson PS et al. Sympathomimetic drugs stimulate the output of secretory glycoproteins from human bronchi *in vitro*. *Clin Sci* 1982;**63**:23–8.

44 Reddy S, Johnson M, Barnes PJ, Rogers DF. The long-acting β$_2$-agonist salmeterol, but not the short-acting β$_2$-agonist salbutamol, potentiates the inhibitory effect of fluticasone propionate on mucin secretion by BEAS-2B cells. *Proc Am Thor Soc* 2006;**3**:A689.

45 Wanner A, Salathe M, O'Riordan TG. Mucociliary clearance in the airways. *Am J Respir Crit Care Med* 1996;**154**:1868–902.

46 Lusuardi M, Capelli A, Carli S et al. Role of surfactant in chronic obstructive pulmonary disease: therapeutic implications. *Respiration* 1992;**59**(Suppl 1):28–32.

47 Anzueto A, Jubran A, Ohar JA et al. Effects of aerosolized surfactant in patients with stable chronic bronchitis: a prospective randomized controlled trial. *JAMA* 1997;**278**: 1426–31.

48 Pikaar JC, Voorhout WF, van Golde LM et al. Opsonic activities of surfactant proteins A and D in phagocytosis of Gram-negative bacteria by alveolar macrophages. *J Infect Dis* 1995;**172**:481–9.

49 Kumar V, Kresch M. Effects of salmeterol (S) on phosphatidylcholine (PC) secretion by type II cells. *Pediatr Res* 1996;**39**:337A.

50 Sakuma T, Okaniwa G, Nakada T et al. Alveolar fluid clearance in the resected human lung. *Am J Respir Crit Care Med* 1994;**150**:305–10.

51 Sakuma T, Folkesson H, Suzuki S et al. Salmeterol increases alveolar epithelial fluid clearance in both *in vitro* and *ex vivo* rat lungs, as well as in *ex vivo* human lungs. *Am J Respir Cell Mol Biol* 1996;**153**:A195.

52 Murphy TF, Sethi S. Bacterial infection in chronic obstructive pulmonary disease. *Am Rev Respir Dis* 1992;**146**:1067–83.

53 Barbier M, Franco-Capo M, Agusti A, Alberti S. Effects of salmeterol and fluticasone on the expression of the PAFr and the invasiveness of *Streptococcus pneumoniae* and *Haemophilus influenzae* into airway epithelial cells. *J Chemo Infect* 2005;**19**:22.

54 Dowling RB, Rayner CF, Rutman A et al. Effect of salmeterol on *Pseudomonas aeruginosa* infection of respiratory mucosa. *Am J Respir Crit Care Med* 1997;**155**:327–36.

55 Dowling RB, Johnson M, Cole PJ et al. Effect of salmeterol on *Haemophilus influenzae* infection of respiratory mucosa *in vitro*. *Eur Respir J* 1998;**11**:86–90.

56 Johnson M. Mechanisms of action of β$_2$-adrenoceptor agonists. In: Busse WW, Holgate St, eds. *Asthma and Rhinitis*. Oxford, UK: Blackwell, 2000: 1541–57.

57 de Bentzmann S, Kiletzky C, Hinnrasky J, Zahm J, Puchelle E. Salmeterol protects airway epithelium from bacterial injury by preventing tight junction degradation. *Am J Respir Crit Care Med* 2002;**165**:A652.

58 Boyd G, Morice AH, Pounsford JC et al. An evaluation of salmeterol in the treatment of chronic obstructive pulmonary disease (COPD). *Eur Respir J* 1997;**10**:815–21.

59 Mahler DA, Donohue JF, Barbee RA et al. Efficacy of salmeterol xinafoate in the treatment of COPD. *Chest* 1999;**115**: 957–65.

60 James MH, Johnson M. Effect of salmeterol on respiratory tract infections. *Eur Respir J* 1996;**23**:264S.

61 Harris T, Koutsoubos V, Guida E *et al.* Salmeterol modulates cell proliferation and cyclin D1 protein levels in thrombin-stimulated human cultured airway smooth muscle via an action independent of the β_2-adrenoceptor. *Am J Respir Crit Care Med* 1999;**159**:A530.

62 Mio T, Adachi Y, Carnevali S *et al.* Beta-adrenergic agonists attenuate fibroblast-mediated contraction of released collagen gels. *Am J Physiol* 1996;**70**:L829–35.

63 Giuliani M, Serpero L, Petecchia L *et al.* Inhibitory activity of fluticasone propionate and salmeterol on TGF- β-induced expression of alpha-smooth muscle actin (alpha-SMA) by human primary airway fibroblasts. *Am J Respir Crit Care Med* 2003;**167**:A206.

64 Orsida B, Ward C, Li X *et al.* Effect of a long-acting β_2-agonist over 3 months on airway wall remodelling in asthma. *Am J Respir Crit Care Med* 2001;**164**:117–21.

65 Easton P, Yokoba M, Hawes H *et al.* Salbutamol effects on parasternal muscle activity and ventilation in humans. *Am J Respir Crit Care Med* 2000;**161**:A117.

66 Hawes HG, Yokoba M, Katagiri M *et al.* Inhaled salmeterol increases parasternal EMG activity. *Am J Respir Crit Care Med* 2003;**167**:A413.

67 Easton PA, Wilde FR, Yokoba M *et al.* Effect of inhaled salmeterol/fluticasone on ventilation and parasternal EMG activity in severe COPD. *Proc Am Thor Soc* 2006;**3**:A112.

68 Jenne JW, Siever JR, Druz WS *et al.* The effect of maintenance theophylline therapy on lung work in severe chronic obstructive pulmonary disease while standing and walking. *Am Rev Respir Dis* 1984;**130**:600–5.

69 Pauwels R, Buist A, Calverley P, Jenkins C, Hurd S. Global strategy for the diagnosis, management and prevention of chronic obstructive pulmonary disease. NHLBI/WHO Global Initiative for Chronic Obstructive Lung Disease (GOLD) workshop summary. *Am J Respir Crit Care Med* 2001;**163**:1256–76.

70 Ulrik C. Efficacy of inhaled salmeterol in the management of smokers with chronic obstructive pulmonary disease: a single centre randomised, double blind, placebo controlled, crossover study. *Thorax* 1995;**50**:750–4.

71 Aalbers R, Ayres J, Backer V *et al.* Formoterol in patients with chronic obstructive pulmonary disease: a randomized, controlled, 3-month trial. *Eur Respir J* 2002;**19**:936–43.

72 Ramirez-Venegas A, Ward J, Lentine T *et al.* Salmeterol reduces dyspnoea and improves lung function in patients with COPD. *Chest* 1997;**112**:336–40.

73 Jones PW, Bosh TK. Quality of life changes in COPD patients treated with salmeterol. *Am J Respir Crit Care Med* 1997;**155**:1283–9.

74 Kiri VA, Soriano JB, Viegi G, Testi R. Inhaled corticosteroids (ICS) are more effective in reducing the risk of re-hospitalisation or death in severe COPD patients when used with long-acting beta-agonists (LABA) than with short-acting beta-agonists (SABA). *Am J Respir Crit Care Med* 2003;**167**:A317.

75 Watkins M, Wire P, Yates J *et al.* Sustained FEV_1 increases in COPD patients induced by salmeterol 50 μg twice daily via the Diskus inhaler. *Am J Respir Crit Care Med* 2002;**165**:A228.

76 Maesen BLP, Westermann CJJ, Duurkens VAM *et al.* Effects of formoterol in apparently poorly reversible chronic obstructive pulmonary disease. *Eur Respir J* 1999;**13**:1103–8.

77 O'Donnell DE, Voduc N, Fitzpatrick M, Webb KA. Effect of salmeterol on the ventilatory response to exercise in chronic obstructive pulmonary disease. *Eur Respir J* 2004;**24**:86–94.

78 Calverley P, Paulwels R, Vestbo J *et al.* Combined salmeterol and fluticasone in the treatment of chronic obstructive pulmonary disease: a randomised controlled trial. *Lancet* 2003;**361**:449–56.

79 Szafranski W, Cukler A, Ramirez A *et al.* Efficacy and safety of budesonide/formoterol in the management of chronic obstructive pulmonary disease. *Eur Respir J* 2003;**21**:74–81.

80 Cazzola M, Santangelo G, Piccolo A *et al.* Effect of salmeterol and formoterol in patients with chronic obstructive pulmonary disease. *Pulm Pharmacol* 1994;**7**:103–7.

81 Cazzola M, Di Perna F, Califano C *et al.* Formoterol Turbuhaler (F) vs salmeterol Diskus (S) in patients with partially reversible stable COPD. *Am J Respir Crit Care Med* 1999;**159**:A798.

82 Cazzola M, Matera M, Santangelo G *et al.* Salmeterol and formoterol in partially reversible severe chronic obstructive pulmonary disease: a dose–response study. *Respir Med* 1995;**89**:357–62.

83 Celik G, Kayacan O, Beder S *et al.* Formoterol and salmeterol in partially reversible chronic obstructive pulmonary disease: a crossover, placebo-controlled comparison of onset and duration of action. *Respiration* 1999;**66**:434–9.

84 Matera M, Cazzola M, Vinciguerra A *et al.* A comparison of the bronchodilating effects of salmeterol, salbutamol and ipratropium bromide in patients with chronic obstructive pulmonary disease. *Pulm Pharmacol* 1995;**8**:267–71.

85 Rennard S, Anderson W, ZuWallack K *et al.* Use of a long-acting inhaled beta$_2$-adrenergic agonist, salmeterol xinafoate, in patients with chronic obstructive pulmonary disease. *Am J Respir Crit Care Med* 2001;**163**:1087–92.

86 Dahl R, Greefhorst L, Nowark D *et al.* Inhaled formoterol dry powder versus ipratropium bromide in chronic obstructive pulmonary disease. *Am J Respir Crit Care Med* 2001;**164**:778–84.

87 Mahler DA. The effect of inhaled β_2-agonists on clinical outcomes in chronic obstructive pulmonary disease. *J Allergy Clin Immunol* 2002;**110**:S298–303.

88 Belman MJ, Botnick WC, Shin JW. Inhaled bronchodilators reduce dynamic hyperinflation during exercise in patients with chronic obstructive pulmonary disease. *Am J Respir Crit Care Med* 1996;**153**:967–75.

89 Weiner P, Magadle R, Berar-Yanay N *et al.* The cumulative effect of long-acting bronchodilators, exercise and inspiratory muscle training on the perception of dyspnea in patients with advanced COPD. *Chest* 2000;**118**:672–8.

90 Ayers RA, Meija J, Ward T *et al.* Comparison of sameterol (42 μg) and ipratropium bromide (72 μg) on dynamic hyperinflation and dyspnea during exercise in patients with COPD. *Am J Respir Crit Care Med* 2000;**161**:A749.

91 Patakas D Andreadis D, Mavrofridas E *et al.* Comparison of the effects of salmeterol and ipratropium bromide on exercise performance and breathlessness in patients with stable chronic obstructive pulmonary disease. *Respir Med* 1998;**92**:1116–21.

92 Donohue J, van Noord, Bateman E *et al*. A 6-month placebo-controlled study comprising lung function and health status in COPD patients treated with tiotropium or salmeterol. *Chest* 2002;**122**:47–55.

93 Taccola M, Bancalari L, Ghignono G *et al*. Salmeterol versus slow-release theophylline in patients with reversible obstructive pulmonary disease. *Monaldi Arch Chest Dis* 1999;**54**:302–6.

94 Rossi A, Kristufek P, Levine BE *et al*. Comparison of the efficacy, tolerability and safety of formoterol dry powder and oral, slow-release theophylline in the treatment of COPD. *Chest* 2002;**121**:1058–69.

95 Baraniuk J, Ali M, Brody D *et al*. Glucocorticoids induce beta$_2$-adrenergic receptor function in human nasal mucosa. *Am J Respir Crit Care Med* 1997;**155**:704–10.

96 Eickelberg O, Roth M, Lorx R *et al*. Ligand-independent activation of the glucocorticoid receptor by beta 2-adrenergic receptor agonists in primary human lung fibroblasts and vascular smooth muscle cells. *J Biol Chem* 1999;**274**:1005–10.

97 Haque RA, Johnson M, Adcock IM, Barnes PJ. Addition of salmeterol to fluticasone prolongs the retention of glucocorticoid receptors within the nucleus of BEAS-2B cells and enhances downstream glucocorticoid effects. *Proc Am Thor Soc* 2006;**3**:A78.

98 Adcock IM, Maneechotesuwan K, Usmani O. Molecular interactions between glucocorticoids and long-acting β$_2$-agonists. *J Allergy Clin Immunol* 2002;**110**:S261–8.

99 Johnson M. Combination therapy for asthma: complementary effects of long-acting β$_2$-agonists and corticosteroids. *Curr Allergy Clin Immunol* 2002;**15**:16–22.

100 Daaka Y, Luttrell L, Lefkowitz R. Switching off the coupling of the beta-2-adrenergic receptor to different G-proteins by protein kinase A. *Nature* 1997;**390**:88–91.

101 Latif M, Hill S. Salmeterol induction of mitogen-activated protein kinase (MAPK) in transfected HEK cells. *Br J Pharmacology* 2001;**32**:159.

102 Bodwell JE, Hu J-M, Orti E, Munck A. Hormone-induced hyperphosphorylation of specific phosphorylated sites in the mouse glucocorticoid receptor. *J Steroid Biochem Mol Biol* 1995;**52**:135–40.

103 Evans M, Bloom J. Salmeterol increases fluticasone propionate-induced suppression of NFκB-mediated gene transcription in human bronchial epithelial cells. *Am J Respir Cell Mol Biol* 2001;**15**:18–27.

104 Usmani O, Maneechotesuwan K, Adcock I, Barnes P. Glucocorticoid receptor activation following inhaled fluticasone and salmeterol. *Am J Respir Crit Care Med* 2005;**172**: 704–12.

105 Roth M, Johnson PR, Rudiger JJ *et al*. Interaction between glucocorticoids and β$_2$-agonists on bronchial airway smooth muscle cells through synchronized cellular signalling. *Lancet* 2002;**360**:1293–9.

106 Haque RA, Torrego A, Essilfie-Quaye S *et al*. Effect of salmeterol and fluticasone on glucocorticoid receptor translocation in sputum macrophages and peripheral blood mononuclear cells from patients with chronic obstructive pulmonary disease. *Proc Am Thor Soc* 2006;**3**:A848.

107 Pang L, Knox AJ. Synergistic inhibition by the β$_2$-aonists and corticosteroids on tumor necrosis factor alpha-induced interleukin-8 release from cultured human airway smooth muscle cells. *Am J Respir Cell Mol Biol* 2000;**22**:1–7.

108 Seeto L, Johnson M, Hendel N, Lim S. Effect of dexamethasone and salmeterol on alveolar macrophage cytokine production in patients with chronic obstructive pulmonary disease (COPD). *Am J Respir Crit Care Med* 2002;**165**:A597.

109 Edwards MR, Johnson M, Johnston SL. Combination therapy: synergistic suppression of virus-induced chemokines in airway epithelial cells. *Am J Respir Cell Mol Biol* 2006;**34**: 616–24.

110 Dowling R, Johnson M, Cole P, Wilson R. Effect of fluticasone propionate and salmeterol on *Pseudomonas aeruginosa* infection of the respiratory mucosa *in vitro*. *Eur Respir J* 1999;**14**:363–9.

111 Miller-Larsson A, Persdotter S, Lexmuller K, Lindahl M, Brattsand R. Synergistic inhibition of oxidative burst in human eosinophils by combination treatment with formoterol and budesonide. *Eur Respir J* 2001;**18**:48S.

112 Chiappara G, Merendino A, Bruno A *et al*. Evaluation of apoptosis in T-lymphocytes and neutrophils in steroid-dependent asthma. *Am J Respir Crit Care Med* 2001;**163**:A188.

113 Maneechotesuwan K, Usmani OS, Adcock IM, Barnes PJ. The modulation of GATA-nuclear localization by fluticasone and salmeterol. *Am J Respir Crit Care Med* 2002;**165**: A620.

114 Gagliardo R, Merendino A, Pompeo F *et al*. IKKβ phosphorylation is modulated by the combination of glucocorticosteroids and long-acting β$_2$-agonists in human bronchial epithelial cells. *Am J Respir Crit Care Med* 2003;**167**:A653.

115 Barnes NC, Qiu YQ, Pavord ID *et al*. Anti-inflammatory effects of salmeterol/fluticasone propionate in chronic obstructive pulmonary disease. *Am J Respir Crit Care Med* 2006;**173**(7):736–43.

116 Yamauchi Y, Christodoulopoulos P, Maltais F, Bourbeau J, Hamid Q. The effect of salmeterol/fluticasone combination on airway inflammation in COPD compared to fluticasone. *Proc Am Thor Soc* 2006;**3**:A113.

117 Gosman MME, Lapperre TS, Snoeck-Stroband JB *et al*. Effect of 6 months therapy with inhaled fluticasone propionate (FP) with or without salmeterol (S) on bronchial inflammation in COPD. *Proc Am Thor Soc* 2006;**3**:A111.

118 Mahler DA, Wire P, Horstman D *et al*. Effectiveness of fluticasone propionate and salmeterol combination delivered via the Diskus device in the treatment of chronic obstructive pulmonary disease. *Am J Respir Crit CCare Med* 2002;**166**: 1084–91.

119 Mahler DA, Wong E, Giessel G *et al*. Improvements in *FEV$_1$* and symptoms in COPD patients following 24 weeks of twice daily treatment with salmeterol 50/fluticasone propionate 500 combination. *Am J Respir Crit Care Med* 2001;**163**:A279.

120 Hanania NA, Ramsdell J, Payne K *et al*. Improvements in airflow and dyspnea in COPD patients following 24 weeks treatment with salmeterol 50 μg and fluticasone propionate 250 μg alone or in combination via the Diskus. *Am J Respir Crit Care Med* 2001;**163**:A279.

121 Vestbo J, Calverley P, Pauwels R *et al*. Absence of gender susceptibility to the combination of salmeterol and

fluticasone in the treatment of chronic obstructive pulmonary disease. *Eur Respir J* 2002;**20**:241S.

122 Soriano J, Vestbo J, Pride N *et al*. Survival in COPD patients after regular use of fluticasone propionate and salmeterol in general practice. *Eur Respir J* 2002;**20**:819–25.

123 The TORCH Study Group. The TORCH (Towards a Revolution in COPD Health) Survival Study protocol. *Eur Respir J* 2004;**24**:206–10.

124 CIAS Group. In chronic obstructive pulmonary disease, a combination of ipratropium and albuterol is more effective than either agent alone. *Chest* 1994;**105**:1411–9.

125 Van Noord J, De Munck D, Bantje T *et al*. Efficacy and safety of salmeterol and ipratropium bromide in patients with chronic obstructive pulmonary disease. *Am J Respir Crit Care Med* 1998;**157**:A799.

126 Van Noord JA, Bantje TA, Eland ME, Korducki L, Cornelissen PJ. Long-term treatment of chronic obstructive pulmonary disease with salmeterol and the additive effect of ipratropium. *Eur Respir J* 2000;**15**:878–85.

127 Sichletidis L, Kottakis J, Marcou S *et al*. Bronchodilatory responses to formoterol, ipratropium, and their combination in patients with stable COPD. *Int J Clin Pract* 1999;**53**: 185–8.

128 D'Urzo AD, De Salvo MC, Ramirez-Rivera A *et al*. FOR-INT-03 Study Group. In patients with COPD, treatment with a combination of formoterol and ipratropium is more effective than a combination of salbutamol and ipratropium: a 3-week, randomized, double-blind, within-patient, multi-centre study. *Chest* 2001;**119**:1347–56.

129 Cazzola M, Centanni S, Santus P *et al*. The functional impact of adding salmeterol and tiotropium in patients with stable COPD. *Resp Med* 2004;**98**:1214–21.

130 Van Noord JA, Aumann J, Janssens E, Mueller A, Cornelissen PJG. A comparison of the 24-hour broncho-dilator effect of tiotropium (QD TIO), salmeterol BID (SALM) or their combination in COPD. *Proc Am Thor Soc* 2005;**2**:A542.

131 Van Noord JA, Smeets JJ, Otte A *et al*. The effect of tiotropium, salmeterol and its combination on dynamic hyperinflation in COPD. *Proc Am Thor Soc* 2005;**2**:A542.

132 Villar AB, Pombo CV. Bronchodilator efficacy of combined salmeterol and tiotropium in patients with chronic obstructive pulmonary disease. *Archivos de Bronconeumolgia* 2005; **41**(3):130–4.

133 Taylor DR, Buick B, Kinney C *et al*. The efficacy of orally administered theophylline, inhaled salbutamol, and a combination of the two as chronic therapy in the management of chronic bronchitis with reversible air-flow obstruction. *Am Rev Respir Dis* 1985;**131**:747–51.

134 Knobil K, Emmett A, Reilly D *et al*. Combination therapy with salmeterol and theophylline for COPD. *Am J Respir Crit Care Med* 2000;**161**:A804.

135 ZuWallack RL, Mahler DA, Reilly D *et al*. Salmeterol plus theophylline combination therapy in the treatment of COPD. *Chest* 2001;**119**:1661–70.

136 Nishimura K, Koyama H, Ikeda A *et al*. The additive effect of theophylline on a high-dose combination of inhaled salbutamol and ipratropium bromide in stable COPD. *Chest* 1995;**107**:718–23.

137 Lamb D. Pathology of COPD. In: Brewis RAL, Gibson GJ, Geddes DM, eds. *Respiratory Medicine*. London: Bailliere-Tindall, 1990: 497–507.

138 Bennett J, Smyth E, Pavord I *et al*. Systemic effects of albuterol and salmeterol in patients with asthma. *Thorax* 1994;**49**:771–4.

139 Cazzola M, Imperatore F, Salzillo A *et al*. Cardiac effects of formoterol and salmeterol in patients suffering from COPD with pre-existing cardiac arrythmias and hypoxemia. *Chest* 1998;**114**:411–5.

140 Reisner, C, Funck-Brentano C, Fischer T, Darken P, Rickard K. Cardiovascular safety of salmeterol in patients with COPD. *Chest* 2003;**123**:1817–24.

141 Gross NJ, Bankwala Z. Effects of an anticholinergic bron-chodilator on arterial blood gases of hypoxemic patients with chronic obstructive pulmonary disease: comparison with a beta-adrenergic agent. *Am Rev Respir Dis* 1987;**136**:1091–4.

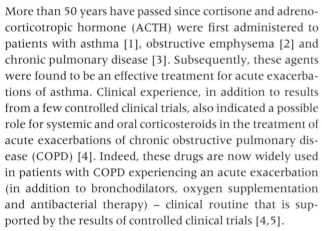

CHAPTER 58
Corticosteroids

Olof Selroos

More than 50 years have passed since cortisone and adreno-corticotropic hormone (ACTH) were first administered to patients with asthma [1], obstructive emphysema [2] and chronic pulmonary disease [3]. Subsequently, these agents were found to be an effective treatment for acute exacerbations of asthma. Clinical experience, in addition to results from a few controlled clinical trials, also indicated a possible role for systemic and oral corticosteroids in the treatment of acute exacerbations of chronic obstructive pulmonary disease (COPD) [4]. Indeed, these drugs are now widely used in patients with COPD experiencing an acute exacerbation (in addition to bronchodilators, oxygen supplementation and antibacterial therapy) – clinical routine that is supported by the results of controlled clinical trials [4,5].

The role of inhaled corticosteroids in COPD has for some time been unclear. Debates have taken place [6,7] but no consensus agreement has yet been reached [8]. New studies evaluating the efficacy of the combination of inhaled corticosteroids and long-acting inhaled β_2-agonists in patients with COPD (GOLD stage III–IV) are of great interest as they show significant effects not only on airway function variables, but also on important outcome measures such as prevention of COPD exacerbations and health-related quality of life [9–11].

This chapter reviews some of the established studies in this field, with a particular focus on more recent clinical trials of inhaled corticosteroids and their combinations with long-acting inhaled β_2-agonists in the treatment of COPD.

Acute exacerbations of COPD

Systemic corticosteroids

The first double-blind placebo-controlled clinical study evaluated the efficacy of methylprednisolone in 44 consecutive hospitalized patients with chronic bronchitis and acute respiratory insufficiency defined as an arterial Po_2 ≤ 60 mmHg [12]. Treatment consisted of either 0.5 mg/kg body weight intravenous methylprednisolone ($n = 22$) or placebo ($n = 22$) every 6 h for 72 h, in addition to ampicillin, oxygen, intravenous aminophylline and inhaled isoprenaline. Pre- and postbronchodilator forced expiratory volume in 1 s (FEV_1) were measured three times daily. Methylprednisolone improved airflow more than placebo; the improvements in both pre- and postbronchodilator FEV_1 were greater in the corticosteroid-treated group ($P < 0.001$ for both). Twelve patients in the corticosteroid group had improvements in FEV_1 ≥ 40% by 72 h compared with three patients in the placebo group ($P < 0.01$).

Thompson *et al.* [13] performed a 10-day double-blind placebo-controlled study in 27 outpatients with an acute exacerbation of COPD. An exacerbation was defined as subjective worsening of chronic baseline dyspnoea or cough for more than 24 h and necessitating a hospital visit. An at least 25% increase in inhaled β_2-agonist use for more than 24 h was also required, or an increase in sputum production and/or purulence. Postbronchodilator FEV_1 should be less than 60% of predicted normal. Treatment consisted of a 9-day course of prednisone – 60, 40 and 20 mg/day for 3 days each – or placebo, in addition to the patient's previous medication and increased doses of inhaled β_2-agonists. Assessments of treatment were made at baseline and on days 3 and 10. The primary endpoint was a treatment failure defined as hospitalization or prescription of oral corticosteroids because of dyspnoea. The failure rate was 0/13 in the prednisone group and 8/14 in the placebo group ($P = 0.002$). Treatment with prednisone also resulted in a more rapid improvement in arterial Po_2 ($P = 0.002$), alveolar–arterial oxygen gradient ($P = 0.04$), FEV_1 ($P = 0.006$) and peak expiratory flow (PEF) ($P = 0.009$) and in a trend towards more rapid improvement in dyspnoea scale scores.

A large double-blind randomized study evaluated the efficacy of intravenous hydrocortisone versus placebo in 113 patients attending the emergency room because of an acute COPD exacerbation [14]. FEV_1 and $FEV_1 : FVC$ (forced vital capacity) ratio should be less than 60% of predicted normal. In addition to identical high-dose bronchodilator therapy, the patients received 100 mg hydrocortisone every 4 h for 4 days, or placebo. Of those patients receiving steroids, 22 achieved a more than 40% improvement in PEF by 6 h and 17 achieved similar results in FEV_1. In the placebo-treated group the corresponding figures were 13 and 8, respectively. More patients in the hydrocortisone group could be discharged within 24 h (16 vs 10) and fewer patients relapsed within 2 weeks requiring hospitalization (0 vs 3).

Davies et al. [5] recruited patients with non-acidotic exacerbations of COPD to a double-blind placebo-controlled study. Patients were randomized to treatment with 30 mg oral prednisolone once daily ($n = 29$) or placebo ($n = 27$) for 14 days in addition to standard treatment with nebulized bronchodilators, antibiotics and oxygen. Daily assessments of lung function and symptoms were performed and patients were recalled at 6 weeks for a follow-up examination. Postbronchodilator FEV_1 increased more rapidly and to a greater extent in the steroid-treated group (Fig. 58.1), with percentage predicted FEV_1 rising from 26% to 32% in the placebo group, and from 28% to 42% in the prednisolone

group ($P < 0.0001$). Up to day 5 of hospital stay, postbronchodilator FEV_1 increased by 90 mL/day in the prednisolone group compared with 30 mL/day in the placebo group. Hospital stays were shorter in the steroid-treated group (9 days vs 7 days; $P = 0.027$). Groups did not differ at 6-week follow-up.

The largest study has been reported by Niewoehner et al. [15]. This double-blind 6-month multicentre study conducted at 25 Veterans Affairs medical centres in the USA included 271 eligible patients of 1840 potential study candidates. The main inclusion criteria were age over 50 years, a smoking history of $\geq$ 30 pack-years, a history of COPD exacerbations and an $FEV_1 \leq 1.5$ L or inability to perform spirometry because of dyspnoea. The main exclusion criterion was use of systemic steroids in the previous 30 days. Patients were randomized to treatment with 125 mg intravenous methylprednisolone every 6 h for 3 days followed by oral prednisone in decreasing doses (60 to 20 mg) for 2 weeks ($n = 80$) or 8 weeks ($n = 80$), or to placebo ($n = 111$). The primary variable of efficacy was the rate of treatment failures, which was significantly higher in the placebo group than in the combined steroid group (at 30 days 33% vs 23%; $P = 0.04$: at 90 days 48% vs 37%; $P = 0.04$). Steroid treatment was also associated with a shorter stay in hospital (8.5 days vs 9.7 days for placebo; $P = 0.03$) and with a greater improvement in FEV_1 of approximately 100 mL by the first day after enrolment. No differences were found between the two steroid treatments for any of the variables. Significant treatment effects were not seen at 6 months' follow-up. Patients receiving steroid treatment were more likely to have hyperglycaemia than placebo-treated patients (15% vs 4%; $P = 0.002$).

Sayiner et al. [16] performed a single-blind randomized study in 36 patients with severe COPD exacerbations. Their mean FEV_1 was 0.6 L and Pao_2 46 mmHg. They were randomized to treatment with 0.5 mg/kg body weight intravenous methylprednisolone every 6 h for 3 days followed by 0.5 mg/kg every 12 h for 3 days and 0.5 mg/kg once daily for 4 days, or to the same treatment for the first 3 days and thereafter placebo (saline) injections. Both groups showed improvements in Pao_2 and FEV_1 levels, but these were significantly better in the 10-day active treatment group ($P = 0.012$ and 0.019, respectively). Dyspnoea also improved more in the 10-day treatment group. No difference in exacerbation rate was observed during a 6-month follow-up period. The authors conclude that a 10-day course of steroid treatment is more effective than a 3-day course.

A recent meta-analysis on eight studies fulfilling defined criteria found that in five studies significant improvement in FEV_1 (more than 20%) was associated with administration of corticosteroids [17]. The authors concluded that short courses of systemic corticosteroids in acute exacerbations of

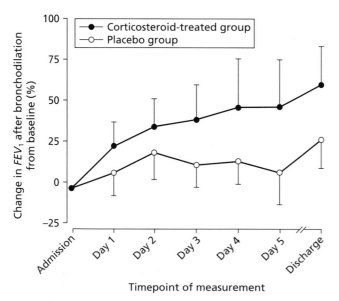

Figure 58.1 Change in absolute postbronchodilator forced expiratory volume in 1 s (FEV_1) from admission by day of study in active and placebo groups. Means (95% confidence interval) are shown. (From Davies et al. [15] with permission.)

COPD have been shown to improve spirometric and clinical outcomes (good quality evidence for both).

Conclusions

Controlled clinical studies and a meta-analysis show that systemic corticosteroids are beneficial for the treatment of acute exacerbations of COPD in patients not recently treated with corticosteroids. Compared with placebo, systemic corticosteroids improve short-term FEV_1 by approximately 100 mL during acute exacerbations [4]. They can reduce the length of stay in hospitalized patients by 1–2 days and reduce the absolute number of treatment failures by approximately 10% [4]. The importance of treatment duration has been investigated in a few studies which suggest that a 10–14-day course of corticosteroids is most beneficial. A 3-day course was less effective than a 10-day course [16] and no advantage was seen with an 8-week course compared with a 2-week course [15]. Hyperglycaemia has been the most frequently reported adverse event.

Nebulized corticosteroids

The benefits of systemic corticosteroid therapy as described above may be limited by the risk of adverse effects. In addition to hyperglycaemia, adrenal suppression has been reported after short-term use of high doses of systemic corticosteroids [18]. Nebulized therapy has therefore attracted attention. A double-blind randomized placebo-controlled multicentre study investigated the use of a nebulized corticosteroid, budesonide, compared with prednisolone for the treatment of acute exacerbations of COPD [19]. A total of 199 patients were included. They received 2 mg nebulized budesonide every 6 h for 72 h, 30 mg oral prednisolone every 12 h, or placebo in addition to standard treatment with nebulized β_2-agonists, ipratropium, antibiotics and oxygen. Both active treatments resulted in significant improvements in postbronchodilator FEV_1 compared with placebo and without a significant difference in the change in FEV_1 between the two. However, prednisolone was associated with a higher incidence of hyperglycaemia than budesonide treatment.

In a double-blind study, 40 patients with moderate to severe acute exacerbations of COPD were randomized to treatment with 8 mg/day nebulized budesonide or 40 mg/day intravenous prednisolone for 10 days [20]. Similar improvements were seen in both groups for airway function (PEF), Sao_2 and Pao_2 ($P < 0.001$) and without statistically significant differences between the groups. No adverse events were recorded.

Based on these two studies, it appears that nebulized budesonide may represent an alternative to systemic corticosteroids for the treatment of acute exacerbations of COPD.

Stable COPD

Oral corticosteroids

Short-term studies

A large number of short-term studies (duration of treatment ≤ 3 months) have evaluated the efficacy of oral prednisone or prednisolone in patients with stable COPD. The results have varied greatly as inclusion criteria have differed, the number of patients has usually been small and it has been difficult to determine how well patients with asthma have been excluded. Nevertheless, the results of these early studies suggest that some COPD patients benefit from treatment with corticosteroids. Eosinophilia of blood [21], sputum [22], variability of FEV_1 [21] and response to inhaled β_2-agonists [22] were cited as criteria for differentiating steroid responders from non-responders.

Callahan *et al.* [23] performed a meta-analysis by selecting 33 studies published since 1951. The quality of the studies was assessed by three investigators using nine selected criteria. Ten studies met all nine criteria. Response to treatment was defined as a 20% or greater increase in FEV_1 from baseline. A calculated mean effect size in the studies was 10% (95% confidence interval [CI], 2–18%) and varied from 0% to 56%. This result suggests that patients treated with oral steroids approximately 10% more often than placebo-treated patients will improve FEV_1 by 20% or more.

Responders and non-responders

Nisar *et al.* [24] showed that approximately 40% of patients with stable, moderate to severe COPD demonstrated a significant increase in FEV_1 when receiving a 2-week course of oral corticosteroids. However, it was not possible to separate responders from non-responders based on baseline characteristics as no clinical differences were found between the groups. A reversibility test with a bronchodilator is neither very sensitive in identifying patients who may respond with a significant change in FEV_1 with a corticosteroid [25].

A further attempt to identify steroid responders was undertaken by Pizzichini *et al.* [26]. In a single-blind cross-over study in 18 patients, they investigated whether an increased proportion of sputum eosinophils (≥ 3%) predicts an effect in smokers with severe COPD. The included patients had a mean FEV_1 of less than 30% predicted normal. Treatment consisted of 30 mg/day prednisone for 2 weeks, or placebo. In patients with sputum eosinophilia ($n = 8$), prednisone, as compared with placebo, produced a statistically significant and clinically important mean effect on effort dyspnoea ($P = 0.008$) and health-related quality of life ($P = 0.01$). A mean increase in FEV_1 of 0.11 L was found ($P = 0.05$).

Long-term studies

COPD guidelines published in the 1990s recommended long-term use of oral corticosteroids in patients with COPD who had demonstrated a response in a 2-week test with prednisolone [27–29]. However, there is little scientific support for such a statement. On the contrary, the more recent GOLD and ATS/ERS guidelines clearly state that 'long-term treatment with oral glucocorticosteroids is not recommended in COPD' [30,31], mainly because of lack of demonstrated efficacy in prospective controlled clinical trials and the risk of systemic glucocorticoid side-effects.

The available information on long-term therapy with oral corticosteroids comes from retrospective studies. Postma *et al.* [32] reported 14–18 years' data from a series of 79 patients with severe COPD (FEV_1 less than 1 L). These patients had used 10–15 mg/day prednisolone in the beginning, and later lower doses, if possible. The investigators noticed three patterns of response: no change; initial increase in FEV_1 followed by a decrease; and a linear progression. At an oral dose of 7.5 mg/day or less, FEV_1 decreased, but often after a considerable time-lag (6–32 months). The results indicated that, in doses above 7.5 mg/day, prednisolone may slow down the progression of COPD. However, the treatment was associated with a considerable number of severe side-effects. In a later study, the same authors reported long-term findings in 139 non-allergic patients with less severe disease (FEV_1 more than 1.2 L; FEV_1/VC (vital capacity) 40–55%) [33]. Again they noticed the same three patterns of response as mentioned above, and a further group of patients with an initial decline in FEV_1 followed by an increase. The conclusion was similar: in a dose above 7.5 mg/day, prednisolone may slow down the progression of COPD.

The value of long-term treatment with oral corticosteroids was more recently evaluated in a double-blind prednisolone withdrawal study [34]. A total of 42 steroid-dependent patients out of 164 candidates, who had used prednisolone at least for the last 6 months, agreed to participate in the study. Patients were randomized to continuous treatment with prednisolone ($n = 20$) or to a regimen where the prednisolone dose was reduced by 5 mg/week. Patients were stratified according to baseline prednisolone doses: 5–10 mg/day prednisolone or more than 10 mg. Both groups could receive open label 40 mg/day prednisolone for 10 days for treatment of exacerbations. A total of 33 patients (87%) used an inhaled corticosteroid at baseline and all patients continued treatment with 1600 g/day triamcinolone acetonide throughout the study. No statistically significant differences were found between the groups in number of acute exacerbations, spirometric values, dyspnoea or health-related quality of life. At the end of the study the average daily prednisolone doses (mean ± standard deviation [SD]) were 10.7 ± 5.2 mg in the continuous group and 6.3 ± 6.4 mg in the 'on demand' group ($P = 0.003$), which also had lost 4.6 ± 2.0 kg (mean ± SD) of body weight compared with an increase of 0.5 ± 3.5 kg ($P = 0.007$) in the continuous prednisolone group. The results of this study, although in a small number of patients, show that continuous treatment with oral corticosteroids is of minor benefit in patients with COPD, but causes systemic glucocorticoid side-effects.

Conclusions

Few prospective controlled studies have been performed with oral corticosteroids in patients with stable COPD. The effect size has been small. Long-term treatment is not recommended because of the risk of systemic side-effects.

Inhaled corticosteroids

For some time it has been unclear whether inhaled corticosteroids have a role in the treatment of patients with COPD.

Short-term studies

It has been a common understanding that inhaled corticosteroids do not affect the type of inflammation present in patients with COPD [7]. The benefit of systemic corticosteroids in patients with acute exacerbations of COPD has been explained as a consequence of existing eosinophilia in that condition [35].

There are, however, observations that inhaled corticosteroids do affect the cellular findings in bronchial biopsies and in sputum in patients with stable COPD, too. Hattotuwa *et al.* [36] studied the effect of FP 500 μg b.i.d. over a 3-month period in a randomized, double-blind, placebo-controlled study in 30 patients. The significant finding was a reduction in the CD8 : CD4 ratio in the epithelium and of the numbers of subepithelial mast cells in the FP group.

Gan *et al.* [37] performed a meta-analysis on six inhaled corticosteroid studies with a duration of 2–12 weeks in which sputum analyses had been performed. There were two studies with budesonide, BDP and FP each and with a total of 162 patients. In three studies with a cumulative dose ≥ 60 mg or longer duration (≥ 6 weeks), inhaled corticosteroids were uniformly effective in reducing the total cell, neutrophil, and lymphocyte counts. In contrast, the three studies with lower cumulative doses and of shorter duration of therapy did not demonstrate a favourable effect.

It therefore appears that inhaled corticosteroids may affect cellular components in COPD which are of importance for the pathogenesis and progression of the disease.

In 1998, Barnes *et al.* [38] reviewed the literature on inhaled corticosteroids and COPD and identified more than 100 trials, but only 12 randomized placebo-controlled studies. Most of the studies were short term, varying in duration from 10 days to 12 weeks. None of the studies measuring bronchial hyperresponsiveness were able to document a change in the provocative concentration of histamine or methacholine causing a 20% decrease in FEV_1 (PC_{20}). All but one failed to show significant improvements in FEV_1. The exception was a double-blind randomized study with 250 µg beclomethasone dipropionate (BDP) q.i.d. ($n = 20$), or placebo ($n = 10$) for 6 weeks [39]. Bronchoalveolar lavage was performed before and after treatment and showed improvement in epithelial permeability (statistically significant changes in epithelial lining fluid albumin, lactoferrin and lysozyme) and a reduction in sample cell count ($P = 0.048$). A bronchitis index was calculated based on visual inspection during bronchoscopy and this index improved during treatment ($P = 0.02$). Also, the spirometric indices (FEV_1, FVC and forced expiratory flow during 25 to 75% of VC ($FEF_{25-75\%}$)) improved significantly compared with placebo. A more recent double-blind cross-over study compared the efficacy of 440 µg fluticasone propionate (FP) b.i.d. (delivered dose, corresponding to 500 µg b.i.d. of metered dose) with placebo for 3 months each in 36 patients with COPD (median age 69 years; mean $FEV_1 \pm$ SD, 1.10 ± 0.43 L; median pack-years 50) [40]. A total of 52 patients had been included but 16 (12 on placebo) were withdrawn for various reasons. Six (five on placebo) were withdrawn because of acute COPD worsening. FP treatment resulted in higher prebronchodilator FEV_1 (1.17 vs 1.07 L; $P = 0.001$), higher Pao_2 (67 vs 64 mmHg; $P = 0.002$) and better dyspnoea score on the chronic respiratory questionnaire (3.70 vs 3.47; $P = 0.03$). A trend towards fewer exacerbations during FP treatment compared with placebo did not reach a level of statistical significance.

Short-term studies comparing inhaled corticosteroids with oral corticosteroids have usually found the latter to be slightly more effective, although differences have not been statistically significant [38].

Conclusions

Most short-term studies with inhaled corticosteroids in patients with COPD have not shown efficacy compared with placebo. Individual patients have responded to treatment with improved airway function, but as a general rule these patients have exhibited signs of an asthmatic bronchitis (e.g. eosinophilia in blood or sputum, atopy or an increased bronchial hyperresponsiveness).

Medium-term studies

Medium-term studies are defined as clinical trials with a duration of 6–30 months. Eight randomized trials were identified in the literature [41–48]. Of these, three studies [42–44] have been included in a meta-analysis [49]. Baseline characteristics of patients with COPD included in the studies and the main findings are summarized in Table 58.1.

Dompeling *et al.* [41] studied the effect of BDP in a group of 28 COPD (and 28 asthma) patients with a rapid decline in FEV_1, selected from a previous bronchodilator study [50]. Smoking history and FEV_1 levels had been similar in the two groups and overlaps had probably existed. Both groups showed a mean fall in FEV_1 during the first 2 years of approximately 160 mL/year. After starting treatment with BDP, the patients showed significant improvements in prebronchodilator FEV_1 in the first 6 months, and thereafter the fall in FEV_1 continued over the next 6 months. Treatment with BDP was then extended for a second year [51]. At that time 22 COPD patients had been followed for 4 years. Postbronchodilator FEV_1 was not affected by treatment with BDP (see Table 58.1). Early improvements in symptoms (months 7–12) was not observed later. Some patients discontinued their treatment with BDP and this did not affect the subsequent decline in FEV_1 [52].

The Dutch Chronic Non-Specific Lung Disease Study Group [42] reported the results of a 2.5-year study in which patients with asthma or COPD were included based on degree of airway obstruction and bronchial hyperresponsiveness. Patients were randomized to regular treatment with 0.5 mg terbutaline q.i.d. with the addition of 40 µg ipratropium q.i.d., 200 µg BDP q.i.d. via pressurized metered dose inhaler (pMDI), or placebo. There were equal numbers of smokers, ex-smokers and non-smokers. Approximately half of the patients were skin test positive with common allergens, or had increased levels of immunoglobulin E (IgE). The same proportion had previously been treated with an inhaled corticosteroid. Based on symptoms, the series could be divided into subgroups of 99 patients with asthma, 88 with asthmatic bronchitis, 51 with COPD and 36 with an undefined diagnosis of airway obstruction. The primary variable of efficacy was the withdrawal rate, mainly because of exacerbations, which was significantly lower in the BDP group (see Table 58.1) than in the placebo group. The patients who were withdrawn had a lower mean FEV_1 (61% vs 65% predicted normal) and lower geometric mean PC_{20} (0.19 vs 0.31 mg/mL) than the rest of the patients.

Derenne [43] randomized 194 patients with COPD (mean reversibility with 400 µg salbutamol 3.3% predicted) to treatment for 2 years with BDP or placebo. An intention-to-treat analysis in 170 patients showed a decrease in FEV_1 in the placebo group and an increase in the BDP group (see Table 58.1). The result thus indicated that treatment with BDP could maintain the FEV_1 on a pretreatment level for 2 years.

Renkema *et al.* [44] followed 58 non-allergic patients with COPD and moderate airflow limitation for 2 years in a double-blind randomized study. The patients were treated with budesonide alone, budesonide plus oral prednisolone, or placebo (see Table 58.1). Assessments were performed

Table 58.1 Double-blind randomized 6–24 month studies with inhaled corticosteroids in patients with COPD.

Author [Ref.]	COPD study population Study duration	No. of patients, R/C Mean age Inhaled corticosteroid, daily dose	Per cent smokers Smoking history	Mean FEV_1 (mean ± SD) and FEV_1 % predicted	Decline in FEV_1 (mL/time)	Exacerbations Symptoms
Dompeling et al. [41]	Selected as a group of rapid decliners (≥ 80 mL/year) from a previous bronchodilator study	28 54 years BDP 800 µg vs placebo	65% 23 pack-years	70 ± 16% predicted	0–6 months: BDP −10 mL/year, NS from earlier annual decline of −77 mL/year 7–12 months: BDP −75 mL/year (NS) (postbronchodilator)	7–12 months: sign reduction in symptoms, no reduction in exacerbation rate
Kerstjens et al. [42]	Age 18–60 years Symptom-based diagnosis of COPD PC_{20} histamine < 8 mg/mL Dutch multicentre 30 months	274* 39.6 years BDP 800 µg vs placebo	36% Pack-years not reported	2.33 L 64% (29–115%)	COPD subgroup: 'initial treatment effect maintained', figures not given Median slopes 3–30 months: BDP −33 mL/year, P −64 mL/year (NS) (prebronchodilator)	Sign fewer withdrawals in the BDP group, 0.25/year vs 0.72/year in P group mainly due to exacerbations ($P < 0.001$) 0–3 months: Increase in FEV_1 by 10.3% points in the BDP group vs 1.0% decrease in P ($P < 0.001$) 3–30 months: no difference in FEV_1 slopes
Derenne [43]	Age ≤ 75 years Prednisone non-responders French multicentre 24 months	194/170 63 years BDP 1500 µg vs placebo	90% Pack-years > 0	1.3 L	BDP +1.44% P −0.62% ($P = 0.05$) over a 2-year period (?)	Not reported
Renkema et al. [44]	Age < 70 years Male outpatients in the Netherlands 24 months	58 56 years BUD 1600 µg vs BUD 1600 µg plus 5 mg prednisolone and placebo	45% Pack-years not reported	1.98 ± 0.61 L	BUD −30 BUD plus prednisolone −40 P −60 mL/year (NS)	Sign reduction in symptom scores after 12 and 24 months in both BUD groups vs P

Study	Population/setting	n/Age/Treatment	Smoking	FEV_1	Treatment effect	Outcome
Paggiaro et al. [45]	Age 50–70 years 13 centres in Europe 6 months	281/235 63 years FP 1000 μg vs placebo	49% Pack-years not reported	1.57 ± 0.60 L 55(17)–59(18)%	FP + 110, P −40 mL 0–6 months ($P < 0.001$)	Fewer exacerbations in FP group (NS) but sign less severe. Sign difference in improvement in 6-min walking test and reduction in cough score and sputum volume. No difference in dyspnoea score
Bourbeau et al. [46]	Age > 40 years Prednisone non-responders Outpatients at a university affiliated hospital 6 months	79/20 66 years BUD 1600 μg vs placebo	39% 51 pack-years	0.93 ± 0.32 L 36(12)–37(10)%	No treatment difference between the groups at 3 or 6 months; −12 mL (−88 to 63) and −4 mL (−95 to 87) (prebronchodilator)	No difference between the groups in 6-min walking test or QoL
Weir et al. [47]	Not specified Two centres in the UK 24 months	98/59 66 years BDP 1500 or 2000 μg vs placebo	39% 55 pack-years	1.21 ± 0.06 L (completers) 0.93 ± 0.07 (withdrawn patients) (mean ± SEM) 40%	BDP −21, P −57 95% CI −80 to +8 mL/year (postbronchodilator)	BDP 0.36, P 0.57 exacerbations/year (NS). More exacerbations in patients with more severe disease (NS) No difference in dyspnoea index, QoL or PC_{20} histamine
Senderovitz et al. [48]	Age 18–75 years Outpatients bronchodilator no-responders, five centres in Denmark 6 months	40/26 54 years BUD 800 μg vs placebo	Not reported	1.49 L (median) range 0.8–2.45 L	BUD −0.02 L P −0.125 L ($P = 0.106$) (postbronchodilator)	No difference in number of exacerbations or symptom scores

BDP, beclomethasone dipropionate; BUD, budesonide; CI, confidence interval; FEV_1, forced expiratory volume in 1 s; FP, fluticasone propionate; NS, not statistically significant; P, placebo; PC_{20}, provocative concentration causing a 20% decrease in FEV_1; QoL, quality of life; R/C, randomized/completed; SD, standard deviation.

* Asthma, $n = 99$; COPD, $n = 51$; 'asthmatic bronchitis,' $n = 88$; not classified, $n = 36$.

every second month. Eleven patients discontinued the study – seven because of COPD deterioration (five in the placebo group and two in the combined treatment group). The median prebronchodilator decline in FEV_1 in the three groups is shown in Table 58.1, with the lowest mean decline in the budesonide group. However, the variations were large and the differences between the groups were not statistically significant. Symptoms scores calculated at baseline and after treatment for 1 and 2 years decreased significantly in the active treatment groups compared with placebo.

Paggiaro *et al.* [45] conducted a study comparing FP with placebo in patients with moderate COPD (mean bronchodilator reversibility 0.8–1.7% of predicted FEV_1; see Table 58.1). Treatment with FP significantly improved FEV_1, FVC, morning PEF, symptom scores for median cough and sputum volume, prolonged the 6-min walking distance, and reduced the severity of exacerbations but not the exacerbation rate.

Bourbeau *et al.* [46] included patients with moderate to severe COPD, not responding to 40 mg oral prednisolone, into a study comparing the efficacy of budesonide with placebo (see Table 58.1). Only 11 patients in the budesonide group and nine in the placebo group were able to complete the study. No statistically significant difference in the change in FEV_1 over time was seen between the groups up to 6 months. At 12 months there were too few patients left for an evaluation. No changes in the 6-min walking test or in quality of life assessed by the Chronic Respiratory Disease Questionnaire were found.

Weir *et al.* [47] randomized 98 COPD patients into a study where they received BDP 1500 or 2000 µg/day depending on body weight, or placebo. A total of 59 patients completed the study. The annual decline in FEV_1 was slower in patients treated with BDP but the difference compared with placebo was not significant (see Table 58.1). The exacerbation rate was also lower in the BDP group but again the difference versus placebo was not significant. No difference in dyspnoea scores was found.

Senderovitz *et al.* [48] performed a 6-month study in 40 patients with a mean FEV_1 of 1.49 L and not responding to inhaled β_2-agonists with a FEV_1 increase of 15%. A total of 26 patients completed the study. Patients were randomized to treatment with budesonide ($n = 14$) or placebo. At the end of the study the median decrease in postbronchodilator FEV_1 was smaller in the budesonide group than in the placebo group (see Table 58.1). There was no difference between the groups in the number of exacerbations or symptoms.

A meta-analysis [49] included data from two studies [42,44], and the otherwise unpublished study by Derenne [43]. The main question of the analysis was whether inhaled corticosteroids were able to slow down the decline in FEV_1 in patients with COPD. Patients with asthmatic features ($n = 101$) were excluded from the analysis, which was then based on 95 of the initially 140 steroid-treated and on 88 of the placebo-treated patients. The patients in the steroid group had mainly been treated with 1500 µg/day BDP, and a few with 1600 µg/day budesonide or 800 µg/day BDP. The mean age of the patients was 61 years and their mean FEV_1 45% of predicted normal. The estimated 2-year difference in prebronchodilator FEV_1 was 34 mL/year (95% CI, 5–63 mL/year). The postbronchodilator FEV_1 showed a difference of 39 mL/year (95% CI, −6 to 84 mL/year). The number of exacerbations did not differ between the groups.

The effect of FP was furthermore investigated in a placebo-controlled study in 23 COPD patients with increased bronchial hyperresponsiveness [53]. These patients received 500 µg FP b.i.d. or placebo for 6 months. Treatment with FP did not affect the degree of hyperresponsiveness but resulted in an unchanged level of airway function, whereas a decline in FEV_1 was seen in the placebo group. FP treatment resulted in small changes in biopsy indeces of airway inflammation.

Conclusions

The individual medium-term studies did not show an effect on the annual decline in FEV_1 with the exception of one study [43], which has been reported only as an abstract. In a meta-analysis of three studies carefully excluding patients with asthma, a statistically significant effect in prebronchodilator FEV_1 was seen between treated and untreated patients, but not in postbronchodilator FEV_1 [49]. Bronchial hyperresponsiveness remained unaffected in a small group of patients [53]. Severity of exacerbations was influenced in one study together with improvements in a number of clinical variables [45].

Long-term studies

Four 3-year studies have been performed in patients with different degrees of COPD severity, with the aim of evaluating the effect of an inhaled corticosteroid on the decline in FEV_1 [54–57]. These studies are summarized in Table 58.2.

The Copenhagen City Heart Study (CCHS) started in the mid-1970s with a random age-starfified sample of 19 327 individuals [54]. Between 1992 and 1994, 10 127 individuals were questioned about their respiratory symptoms and spirometry was performed. Subjects with an FEV_1 : VC ratio of ≤ 70% and no self-reported asthma were referred to the study for further examination. Reversibility tests with a β_2-agonist and with oral prednisolone were conducted, and individuals with a reversibility more than 15% in one or both of the tests were excluded from the study. A total of 290 patients (40% being symptom-free) were finally randomized to treatment with budesonide or placebo (see Table 58.2). The mean age of the patients was 59 years,

Table 58.2 Summary of placebo-controlled, parallel-group, 3-year studies with inhaled corticosteroids in patients with COPD.

Author [Ref.]	Study population	No. of patients Mean age Inhaled corticosteroid, daily dose	Per cent smokers Smoking history	Mean FEV_1 (mean ± SD) and FEV_1% predicted	Decline in postbronchodilator FEV_1, mL/year	Other effects
Vestbo et al. [54]	Age 30–70 years, single centre, community survey programme	290 59 years BUD Turbuhaler 600 µg b.i.d. for 6 months, then 400 µg b.i.d. for 2.5 years	77% Pack-years not reported	2.37 ± 0.82 L (postbronchodilator) 86 ± 21%	BUD −49, P −46 ($P = 0.7$)	No significant effects on symptoms and exacerbations
Pauwels et al. [55]	Age 30–75 years, population-based, nine European countries	1277 52 years BUD Turbuhaler 400 µg b.i.d.	100% 39 pack-years	2.54 ± 0.64 L (prebronchodilator) 76.8 ± 12.4%	First 6 months: BUD +17, P −81 ($P < 0.001$) 9–36 months: BUD −57, P −69 ($P = 0.39$)	More beneficial effects in subjects who had smoked less
Burge et al. [56]	Age 40–75, outpatients, 18 centres in the UK	751 64 years FP pMDI 500 µg b.i.d.	38% 44 pack-years	1.24 ± 0.45 L (prebronchodilator) 50.1 ± 14.9%	FP −50, P −59 ($P = 0.16$)	Significant reduction in exacerbation rate, less withdrawals due to respiratory disease and improved QoL
Lung Health Study Research Group [57]	Age 40–75 years, screened for lung health smoking cessation study, 10 centres in USA and Canada	1116 56 years TA pMDI 600 µg b.i.d.	90% Current smoking 23.5 ± 12.7 cigarettes/day	2.13 ± 0.63 L 64.1 ± 13.3 (prebronchodilator)	TA −44, P −47 ($P = 0.50$)	Fewer respiratory symptoms, fewer physician visits, improved BHR in TA group

BHR, bronchial hyperresponsiveness; b.i.d., twice daily; BUD, budesonide; FEV_1, forced expiratory volume in 1 s; FP, fluticasone propionate; P, placebo; pMDI, pressurized metered dose inhaler; QoL, quality of life; SD, standard deviation; TA, triamcinolone acetonide.

40% were women and 77% were current smokers. Overall, patients had very mild COPD (mean FEV_1 86% of predicted normal). There was no difference between groups for the decline in FEV_1, exacerbation rates or presence of respiratory symptoms.

The EUROSCOP (European Respiratory Study on Chronic Obstructive Pulmonary Disease) was a double-blind placebo-controlled trial evaluating the effect of budesonide compared with placebo [55]. After a smoking cessation period, subjects who were unable to stop smoking ($n = 1277$) were included and 912 of those (71%) completed the study. The reasons for withdrawal – non-compliance, adverse events and loss of follow-up – were similar in both groups. The patients' mean age was 52 years, 27% were women and mean FEV_1 was 77% of predicted normal. During the first 6 months of the study, FEV_1 improved at a rate of 17 mL/year in the budesonide group compared with a decline of 81 mL/year in the placebo group ($P < 0.001$). Subsequently, the annual decline in postbronchodilator FEV_1 was not statistically significantly different between

the groups (see Table 58.2). However, during this period more patients in the placebo group showed a rapid decline in FEV_1 (more than 60 mL/year): 55% of patients in the placebo group compared with 49% in the budesonide group ($P = 0.06$). Of the 912 subjects completing the study, the median decline in FEV_1 over the 3-year period was 140 mL with budesonide and 180 mL with placebo ($P = 0.05$). Subjects with a smoking history of less than 36 pack-years at enrolment had a reduction of 190 mL with placebo and 120 mL with budesonide ($P < 0.001$) (Fig. 58.2). There was no difference in decline in FEV_1 in subjects with a smoking history of more than 36 pack-years ($P = 0.57$). The incidence of exacerbations was not evaluated. A *post hoc* analysis revealed that treatment with budesonide had significantly reduced the incidence of cardio-vascular events [58]. A frequency of 6% was seen in the placebo group compared with 3% in the budesonide group ($P < 0.05$). This may indicate that treatment with inhaled corticosteroids can also influence systemic components of COPD.

The ISOLDE (Inhaled Steroids in Obstructive Lung

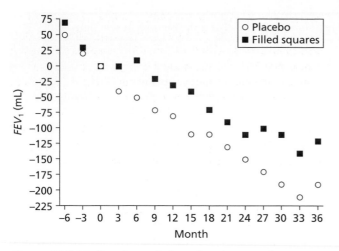

Figure 58.2 Median change in forced expiratory volume in 1 s (*FEV*₁) as compared with the value at randomization (month 0) in the placebo and budesonide groups in patients with ≤ 36 pack-year smoking history. (From Pauwels *et al.* [55] with permission.)

Disease in Europe) study included symptomatic patients with COPD (i.e. with more severe illness than those in the two studies cited above) [56]. A total of 751 patients with a mean baseline postbronchodilator *FEV*₁ of 1.4 L (50% of predicted normal) were included. Patients with a bronchodilator reversibility to 400 μg salbutamol of more than 10% predicted normal were excluded from the study. Patients were treated for 3 years with 1000 μg/day FP or placebo (see Table 58.2). No difference in the annual decline of *FEV*₁ was observed between the groups (see Table 58.2). However, the predicted mean *FEV*₁ in the FP group at 3 and 36 months was 76 and 100 mL higher, respectively, compared with placebo (mixed effects model; *P* < 0.001). There was no significant correlation between the *FEV*₁ response to oral corticosteroids or FP (*P* = 0.056). The rate of exacerbations (defined as a worsening of respiratory symptoms requiring treatment with oral corticosteroids and/or antibiotics) was lower in the FP group (0.99 per year compared with 1.32 per year in the placebo group) as were the withdrawals because of respiratory symptoms (19% compared with 25% in the placebo group; *P* = 0.034). The rate of decline in respiratory health status was significantly lower in the FP group compared with placebo (total respiratory questionnaire score: 3.2 vs 2.0 units/year, respectively; *P* = 0.004). This difference was interpreted as a delay in average time for clinically important reduction in health status from 15 to 24 months.

The Lung Health Study II was a randomized placebo-controlled trial in the USA [57]. Smokers and ex-smokers who had participated in the previous Lung Health Study I [59] and who had a baseline *FEV*₁ of 30–90% of predicted normal and a *FEV*₁ : *FVC* ratio of less than 70% were

recruited. Of these, 1116 patients were randomized to treatment with triamcinolone or placebo (see Table 58.2). The patients' mean age was 56 years and mean postbronchodilator *FEV*₁ was 68% of predicted normal. The mean duration of follow-up was 40 months. During the study, the rate of decline of postbronchodilator *FEV*₁ was not statistically significantly different between the groups (see Table 58.2). However, the steroid-treated patients experienced fewer respiratory symptoms (*P* = 0.005) and had fewer visits to a physician because of respiratory problems (*P* = 0.03) compared with those receiving placebo. Furthermore, patients receiving triamcinolone showed lower airway reactivity in response to methacholine challenge at 9 and 33 months (both *P* = 0.02).

Meta-analyses of the long-term studies

Two recent meta-analyses evaluated the effect of inhaled corticosteroids on the decline in *FEV*₁. Highland *et al.* [60] included six studies with 3571 patients in their review [44,47,54–57] and reported that the summary estimate for the difference in *FEV*₁ decline between placebo and active treatment was –5.0 ± 3.2 mL/year (95% CI, –11.2–1.2 mL/year; *P* = 0.11). The authors concluded that inhaled corticosteroids use was not associated with the annual rate of *FEV*₁ decline. Using data from the same plus two additional studies [42,43], Sutherland *et al.* [61] included 3715 patients in their analysis. In this meta-analysis, treatment with inhaled corticosteroids was shown to reduce the rate of *FEV*₁ decline by 7.7 mL/year (95% CI, 1.3–14.2 mL/year; *P* = 0.02). A meta-analysis of high-dose regimens revealed an even greater effect of 9.9 mL/year (95% CI, 2.3–17.5 mL/year; *P* = 0.01) compared with the meta-analysis of all studies. The authors concluded that inhaled corticosteroid treatment for ≥ 2 years slows the rate of decline in lung function in patients with COPD.

How is it possible that two meta-analyses performed at the same time and using similar datasets can reach different conclusions? The similarities and differences between the two analyses were reviewed by Burge and Lewis [62]. The difference appears to partly depend the results of a study in patients with early COPD [54]. The benefits of inhaled corticosteroids in this largely asymptomatic patient group is limited. In their analyses, Highland *et al.* presumed a 3.1 mL/year greater rate of *FEV*₁ decline in the budesonide group, while Sutherland *et al.* correctly interpreted the data as showing a 3.1 mL/year improvement in *FEV*₁ in patients receiving an inhaled corticosteroid. Furthermore, differences in the interpretation of standard errors (*P* values) and choice of patient groups (in studies involving subgroups of patients) are further confounding factors. In other words, these vastly different conclusions stemmed directly from differences in the interpretation of almost identical datasets [62]. However, based on detailed reviews of these recent meta-analyses and the results of long-term clinical studies, it can be concluded that treatment with inhaled corticosteroids do modify disease progression and slow the decline in FEV_1 in patients with COPD.

Conclusions

The four long-term studies of inhaled corticosteroids in patients with mild to moderate COPD did not show a significant effect on the decline in postbronchodilator FEV_1 compared with placebo. A recent meta-analysis, however, demonstrated a significant effect on the rate of decline of FEV_1, which was even greater in patients on a high-dose inhaled corticosteroid regimen. In addition, an increase in FEV_1 has been observed during the first 3–6 months of treatment and a lower reactivity in response to methacholine was seen in one study, where it was investigated. Improvements in respiratory symptoms and health-related quality of life have also been reported. A reduction in exacerbation rate was found in the two studies that included patients with more severe COPD.

Responders and non-responders

Several studies have investigated whether the response to a 2-week course of oral corticosteroids can predict the subsequent benefit of treatment with an inhaled corticosteroid. Selroos [63] investigated whether a 10-day course of oral prednisolone (30–40 mg/day) could predict the future response to an inhaled corticosteroid. A group of 52 patients with stable COPD and no significant response to an inhaled β_2-agonist were included. Their mean $FEV_1 \pm SD$ was 1.7 ± 0.4 L. Of these, 12 steroid responders were identified (increase in $FEV_1 \geq 15\%$). Subsequently all 52 patients received 1600 µg/day budesonide for 6 months. During this phase, nine of the prednisolone responders maintained their improved airway function. Moreover, eight of the initial 40 non-responders to prednisolone demonstrated a significant improvement with budesonide. Thus, responders could not be identified and the benefit of long-term treatment with budesonide could not be predicted based on the short course of oral prednisolone.

Boothman-Burrell *et al.* [64] performed a double-blind placebo-controlled cross-over study in 18 patients with COPD. Treatment consisted of 1000 µg BDP or placebo twice daily for 3 months. At the end of each treatment period patients received 30 mg prednisone for 10 days. The two treatment phases were separated by a 1-month wash-out period. The predictive value of the prednisone response was 0% and 81% for a positive and negative outcome, respectively.

Davies *et al.* [65] performed a study in 127 patients with stable COPD (mean FEV_1 of less than 40% of predicted normal). Initial spirometry was performed after treatment with 5 mg nebulized salbutamol, and after a 2-week course of oral prednisolone. Thereafter, patients were treated by two physicians with different treatment policies. One prescribed inhaled BDP (800 µg/day) to all patients, whereas the other gave BDP only to those with a positive prednisolone test. Results of 104 patients were evaluated after treatment for 1 year. Of these, 31% were unresponsible to salbutamol and prednisolone at baseline, 46% were responsive to salbutamol but not to prednisolone, and 23% responded to both. The results showed that after treatment for 1 year the prednisolone responders had higher FEV_1 values and less symptoms ($P < 0.02$ for both) than the steroid non-responders, indicating a value of the prednisolone test on a group level. However, there were more ex-smokers and more patients with blood eosinophilia among the responders.

Reversibility tests from 1048 patients with airway obstruction and with a FEV_1 of less than 60% of predicted normal and a $FEV_1 : FVC$ ratio less than 60% were analysed in another study before and after a 7-day course of 30 mg prednisone [66]. Spirometry was performed before and 30 min after inhalation of 300 µg salbutamol and 60 µg ipratropium bromide. The frequency distribution of the bronchodilator and steroid responses (in addition to the combinations of responses) were all unimodal, making any distinction between nosological subgroups arbitrary. Similarly, in another Danish study [54], the predictive value of a 2-week course of 37.5 mg prednisolone on the effects of 6 months' treatment with budesonide or placebo was evaluated in 37 patients with stable COPD. No significant differences in spirometry values, symptoms or number of exacerbations were found between the budesonide and placebo groups. The authors concluded that a 2-week course of prednisolone was of no value in choosing subsequent long-term therapy.

Before the double-blind phase of the 3-year ISOLDE study (FP vs placebo), patients received a 2-week course of 0.6 mg/kg/day oral prednisolone during which the response in terms of FEV_1 improvement was registered. A reversibility test with salbutamol was also conducted. Neither the short-term response to bronchodilator treatment nor the response to prednisolone could predict the long-term response [67,68].

Conclusion

A 2-week course with oral prednisolone is unnecessary to perform as it has no predctive value for the subsequent response to an inhaled corticosteroid.

Withdrawal of inhaled corticosteroids

In patients with COPD, it is often easier to detect a change in response when treatment is stopped.

Run-in phase data from a total of 272 patients recruited for the ISOLDE study [56] were analysed in an observational study [69]. Of the patients entering the 8-week run-in phase, 160 had been treated with an inhaled corticosteroid prior to study entry, whereas 112 had not. All patients were clinically stable for at least 6 weeks; there were no differences in baseline lung function, bronchodilator reversibility or smoking history between patients previously receiving an inhaled corticosteroid, compared with those who had not. Inhaled corticosteroid treatment was discontinued during the first week of the 8-week run-in period before randomization. During the remaining 7 weeks, 38% of patients previously treated with inhaled steroids experienced an acute exacerbation of COPD compared with 6% of those patients not receiving prior inhaled corticosteroid treatment. The daily dose of inhaled steroids in the year preceding the study was slightly higher in patients who experienced an exacerbation, compared with those who did not have an acute worsening; however, this difference was not statistically significant. There was no correlation between the total dose of inhaled or oral corticosteroids used in the year before the study and the time to first exacerbation.

O'Brian *et al.* [70] investigated what happened when inhaled corticosteroid treatment was stopped in a group of 24 men with moderate to severe COPD (mean age 67 years; mean FEV_1 1.6 L = 47% of predicted normal). This was a double-blind randomized placebo-controlled cross-over study. Patients entering the study received 100 µg BDP q.i.d. or placebo for 3 weeks and had a 3-week wash-out period before receiving the alternate treatment. They underwent lung function tests (spirometry, diffusion capacity), had health-related quality of life (HRQL) testing, sputum examination for inflammatory markers, and performed a 6-min walking test before randomization and 3 weeks after each treatment period. Fifteen patients completed the study. Even if the BDP dose was relatively low, the results showed that withdrawal of treatment resulted in a statistically significant deterioration in lung function and increase in exercise-induced dyspnoea.

The COPE study was a 6-month single-centre parallel-group double-blind study evaluating the effect of withdrawal of inhaled FP after 4 months' treatment in a group of patients with COPD [71]. Overall, 509 of the 615 patients recruited to the study were eligible for inclusion. A total of 263 patients started an open-label 4-month treatment phase with 500 µg FP b.i.d. and 40 µg ipratropium q.i.d. to optimize their clinical status. Their mean age was 64 years, 84% were men, and baseline postbronchodilator FEV_1 was 54% of predicted normal. More than 80% of the patients had previously used an inhaled corticosteroid. After the open-label phase, patients were randomized to continuous treatment with FP ($n = 123$) or placebo ($n = 121$) for 6 months and contacted the study centre as soon as there was a change in their well-being. Exacerbations (defined as a worsening of respiratory symptoms requiring treatment

with oral corticosteroids or antibiotics) occurred in 47% of the patients receiving FP compared with 57% in the placebo group. The hazard ratio for the first exacerbation was 1.5 (95% CI, 1.1–2.1) with placebo compared with FP. A total of 26 patients (22%) in the placebo group had a recurrent rapid exacerbation and were changed to open-label FP treatment, compared with six patients (5%) receiving FP. The relative risk for this was 4.4 (95% CI, 1.9–10.3). Statistically significant differences in health status (St. George's Respiratory Questionaire [SGRQ]) total scores, activity and symptom domain scores were observed between the groups. There were no differences in postbronchodilator FEV_1, excertion dyspnoea (Borg scale), or in distance walked during 6 min with active treatment or placebo.

Conclusions

Withdrawal of inhaled corticosteroids in patients with moderate to severe COPD has resulted in an increased incidence of exacerbations compared with continuous treatment, and in deterioration of health-related quality of life. The results indicate that inhaled corticosteroids should be withdrawn with caution in patients with COPD. Indeed, patients should be monitored carefully as the effect of inhaled corticosteroids may be more apparent after treatment has been withdrawn.

Effect of inhaled corticosteroids on acute exacerbations

COPD exacerbations are serious events which may be life-threatening [72]. Frequent exacerbations impair health-related quality of life [73] and lung function decline is faster in patients with frequent exacerbations compared with patients having no or only a few exacerbations [74]. To date, there is no universal definition of a COPD exacerbation, which makes comparison of the preventive effects of treatment on exacerbations difficult [75]. However, action-driven definitions of exacerbations (episodes requiring medical intervention with oral corticosteroids and/ or antibiotics and/or hospitalization) are considered more objective than symptom-based definitions to compare therapeutic interventions in a clinical trial setting [76].

In the ISOLDE study, exacerbations were defined as events requiring treatment with oral corticosteroids or antibiotics. The study showed a 25% reduction in the yearly rate of exacerbations in patients treated with FP compared with placebo ($P = 0.026$) [56], but did not indicate which patients showed greatest benefit. Jones *et al.* [77] performed a *post hoc* analysis of these data and divided the study population into those with mild ($FEV_1 \geq 50\%$ predicted normal) and moderate to severe (FEV_1 of less than 50% predicted normal) disease. There were 391 patients with mild COPD (195 FP-treated) and 359 with moderate

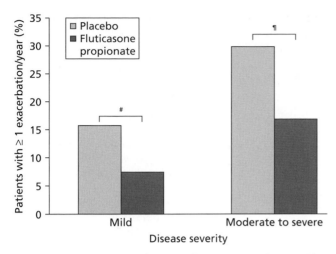

Figure 58.3 Percentage of patients having ≥ 1 corticosteroid-treated exacerbation per year in placebo and fluticasone propionate treated groups split by disease severity. #, *P* = 0.02; ¶, *P* = 0.01. (From Jones *et al.* [77] with permission.)

to severe disease (180 FP-treated). Over the 3-year study period, 29% of patients with mild disease and 16% of patients with moderate to severe disease had no exacerbations; the median exacerbation rate was significantly lower in the mild disease group (*P* < 0.0001). There were significantly fewer exacerbations in the FP group (0.99 exacerbations per year) compared with placebo (1.32 exacerbations per year; *P* = 0.026). This significant effect was largely confined to the moderate to severe group: median number of exacerbations per year was 1.47 and 1.75 in the FP and placebo groups, respectively (*P* < 0.022). In patients with moderate to severe disease, 52% had a corticosteroid-treated exacerbation compared with 30% of those in the mild group (*P* < 0.0001). The rate of these exacerbations was significantly lower in FP-treated patients compared with placebo (*P* < 0.001). FP reduced the number of patients experiencing one or more exacerbations per year by half in both patient groups (Fig. 58.3). Reversibility to bronchodilator or prednisolone did not identify patients in whom FP had an effect on exacerbations.

In a 6-month study comparing FP with placebo, active treatment reduced the incidence of severe exacerbations (defined as a need for hospitalization) [45]. Thus, an effect on the severity of exacerbations was demonstrated. In this shorter term study, however, no effect on the time to the first exacerbation was found. A meta-analysis based on nine studies with 3976 patients [44–48,54–57], including four with a systemic steroid run-in phase, reported a 30% reduction in COPD exacerbations (risk ratio 0.70; 95% CI, 0.58–0.84) with inhaled corticosteroid treatment [8].

Three placebo-controlled 12-month studies have compared the efficacy of combinations of an inhaled corticosteroid and an inhaled long-acting β$_2$-agonist (fluticasone/

salmeterol and budesonide/formoterol) with the individual monocomponents in patients with moderate to severe COPD [9–11]. Exacerbations were an important endpoint in these studies, and further information has been obtained that relates to the efficacy of inhaled corticosteroids alone on the incidence and rate of exacerbations. These studies are discussed later in this chapter.

Conclusions
The effect of inhaled corticosteroids on COPD exacerbations defined as action-driven events (a course of oral corticosteroids and/or antibiotics and/or hospitalization) appears to be confined to patients with moderate to severe disease. Reversibility to treatment with a β$_2$-agonist or oral prednisolone does not predict the efficacy. Treatment with inhaled corticosteroids has been shown to reduce both the severity of exacerbations and the number and rate of severe exacerbations.

Inhaled corticosteroids and survival/mortality

Frequent exacerbations are associated with increased mortality in COPD [78,79]. Deterioration in health-related quality of life appears to be the best predictor of rehospitalization and mortality in COPD [80]. Several studies have also shown that exacerbations necessitating hospitalization increase the mortality in COPD [81–83]. To date, no prospective studies to evaluate the effect of treatment with inhaled corticosteroids on mortality have been reported. In the meta-analysis by Alsaeedi *et al.* [8], which included five randomized placebo-controlled trials measuring this endpoint, a 16% reduction in mortality compared with non-inhaled corticosteroid treatment was observed. However, this reduction was not statistically significant.

Sin and Tu [84] conducted a population-based cohort study using databases in Ontario, Canada (*n* = 22 620) to determine the association between inhaled corticosteroid therapy and the combined risk of repeat hospitalization and all-cause mortality in elderly patients (mean age 75 years) with COPD. Patients who received inhaled corticosteroid therapy within 90 days after discharge from hospital had 24% fewer repeat hospitalizations for COPD (95% CI, 20–29%) and were 29% less likely to die during 1 year of follow-up after adjustment for a number of confounding factors (95% CI, 22–35%). Very similar results were reported by Soriano *et al.* [85] who used an UK General Practice Research Database (*n* = 4665) and demonstrated that regular use of inhaled corticosteroids was associated with increased survival of COPD patients managed in primary care compared with patients receiving bronchodilators other than long-acting inhaled β$_2$-agonists and no inhaled corticosteroids. They also compared rehospitalization in a retrospective cohort of 3636 patients with COPD and found the use of inhaled corticosteroid (with or

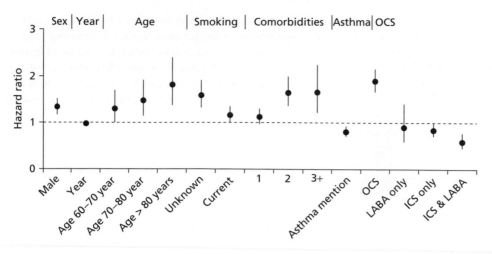

Figure 58.4 Multivariate analysis of time to rehospitalization or death in patients with COPD using inhaled corticosteroids (ICS) and long-acting β-agonists (LABAs). OCS, oral corticosteroids. (From Soriano *et al.* [86] with permission.)

without a long-acting β₂-agonist) was associated with a reduction of rehospitalization or death (Fig. 58.4) [86]. The use of inhaled corticosteroids in this database cohort was shown to be associated with markers of increased disease severity, but not with a number of other potential confounding factors that could explain the benefits observed in mortality or risk of hospitalization [87].

In another study, Sin and Man [88] used hospital discharge data from Alberta, Canada (*n* = 6740) for COPD patients ≥ 65 years and reported a 25% relative reduction in risk for all-cause mortality in patients on inhaled corticosteroids. Furthermore, patients receiving medium or high-dose therapy showed lower risks than patients receiving low doses of inhaled corticosteroids.

Reductions in mortality of 40–42% in COPD patients using inhaled corticosteroids have been reported in other studies. Mapel *et al.* conducted a cohort study to examine the relationship between survival and use of inhaled corticosteroids and/or long-acting inhaled β₂-agonists in COPD (*n* = 1288) and compared the results with those of a control group (*n* = 397) [89]. They found that COPD patients who used an inhaled corticosteroid alone or in combination with a long-acting β₂-agonist had substantially improved survival even after adjustment for asthma and other confounding factors. However, a time-dependent analysis based on seven Veterans Administration clinics in the USA (inhaled corticosteroids *n* = 2654; no inhaled corticosteroids *n* = 5398) demonstrated no reduction in mortality in the corticosteroidtreated population compared with the control group [90].

It has been argued that the effects of inhaled corticosteroids on survival and mortality in these non-randomized cohort studies may be confounded by a number of factors [91], most notably 'the immortal time bias'. This type of survival bias occurs when assessing exposure to inhaled corticosteroids after some patients have died, meaning that those who survive have a theoretically greater amount of time to receive therapy with an inhaled corticosteroid.

However, even after adjusting for this effect and reanalysis of the data, Sin *et al.* [92] reported that inhaled corticosteroid treatment was still associated with a 21% reduction in hospitalization and mortality rate. Furthermore, at least one of the cohort studies [89] appears to be free from such bias, suggesting that this effect is real. An additional analysis showed that in patients with COPD, the use of inhaled corticosteroids for 3 years in those with moderate to severe disease improved quality-adjusted life expectancy at a cost that was similar to that of other therapies commonly used in clinical practice [93].

Finally, Sin *et al.* [94] conducted a pooled analysis, based on intention to treat, of individual patient data from seven randomised studies (*n* = 5085) [9–11,54–57]. The effects of inhaled corticosteroids and placebo were compared over at least 12 months in patients with stable COPD. Inhaled corticosteroids reduced all-cause mortality by about 25%. The beneficial effect appeared to be especially noticeable in women and former smokers. Also patients with COPD and respiratory insufficiency requiring domiciliary oxygen treatment with inhaled corticosteroids have improved survival [95].

Conclusions

Some retrospective cohort studies, but not all, have indicated a reduced risk for rehospitalization and mortality in COPD patients using inhaled corticosteroids after treatment in hospital for an acute exacerbation of COPD compared with patients not using inhaled corticosteroids. The improved quality-adjusted life expectancy has been achieved without an increase in costs. Results of prospective studies are warranted.

Inhaled corticosteroids and long-acting inhaled β₂-agonists

Six placebo-controlled studies have been published evaluating the efficacy of an inhaled corticosteroid and a long-acting inhaled β₂-agonist (fluticasone/salmeterol and budesonide/formoterol) in the same inhaler [9–11,96–99] in comparison with the monocomponents (i.e. inhaled corticosteroid alone and a long-acting inhaled β_2-agonist alone) and placebo. These studies are summarized in Table 58.3. Three 12-month studies were designed specifically to evaluate the effect of combination therapies on exacerbations in patients with COPD [9–11].

In a 12-month parallel-group study with four treatment arms, 500 µg FP, 50 µg salmeterol and 500 µg FP/50 µg salmeterol b.i.d. were compared with placebo in 1465 patients with COPD (GOLD stage II–IV) [10]. Combination treatment with FP/salmeterol significantly improved FEV_1 compared with placebo (treatment difference 133 mL; $P < 0.0001$); a significant difference was also observed with FP alone (95 mL; $P < 0.0001$). The mean exacerbation rate (defined as a worsening of COPD symptoms requiring antibiotics, oral corticosteroids, or both) per patient per year was also reduced by 25% ($P < 0.0001$) with FP/salmeterol, and by 20% ($P = 0.0027$) and 19% ($P = 0.0033$) with salmeterol and FP, respectively, compared with placebo. There were no significant differences between active treatment groups with regard to reduction in exacerbation frequency or time to first exacerbation. A statistically significant improvement in health status (as measured by SGRQ total score) was observed at 12 months in the FP/salmeterol treatment group compared with placebo (treatment difference –2.2 [$P = 0.0003$]) and FP (treatment difference –1.4 [$P = 0.021$]).

Szafranski et al. [9] enrolled 812 patients with COPD (GOLD stages III–IV) into a 12-month placebo-controlled study. Patients were randomized to treatment with either 400 µg budesonide b.i.d., 9 µg formoterol b.i.d., 400 µg budesonide/9 µg formoterol b.i.d. (Symbicort 160/4.5 µg labelled as delivered doses), or placebo. During the 12-month study period, all active treatments increased FEV_1 compared with placebo (budesonide/formoterol, 15% [$P < 0.001$], formoterol, 14% [$P < 0.001$] and budesonide, 9% [$P < 0.001$]). Budesonide/formoterol was more effective than budesonide alone at improving lung function ($P < 0.001$). In addition, budesonide/formoterol sustained improvements in FEV_1 throughout the study period, compared with both budesonide and placebo.

Patients treated with budesonide/formoterol and budesonide alone had fewer exacerbations requiring the use of oral corticosteroids and/or antibiotics and/or hospitalization (1.4 and 1.6 per patient per year, respectively) compared with 1.8 for formoterol and 1.9 for placebo ($P < 0.05$ budesonide/formoterol vs placebo and formoterol). The lowest number of oral corticosteroid courses per patient per year was observed with budesonide/formoterol (0.74) and budesonide (0.76) treatment compared with formoterol (1.04) and placebo (1.07). Both budesonide/formoterol and budesonide treatment reduced the number of oral corticosteroid courses required to treat an exacerbation (31%

[$P = 0.027$] and 29% [$P = 0.045$], respectively). Furthermore, budesonide/formoterol, but not budesonide alone, significantly improved SGRQ total score compared with placebo ($P < 0.01$) during the study. The mean change in SGRQ total score with budesonide/formoterol compared with placebo (–3.9) approached clinical relevance (where a change of 4 points represents a clinically important difference relevant to the patient).

Calverley et al. [11] recruited 1022 COPD patients of a similar type to those recruited by Szafranski et al. [9] in another 12-month placebo-controlled study. In this study, treatment was intensified with 30 mg oral prednisolone once daily and 9 µg formoterol b.i.d. during a 2-week run-in period to optimize patients' level of disease control. This type of design was used to test a clinically relevant situation (i.e. whether short-term improvements achieved after treatment intensification could be maintained with inhaled therapy). Patients were randomized to treatment as outlined in the Szafranski et al. study [9]. Budesonide/formoterol maintained improvements in FEV_1 achieved with treatment intensification. In contrast, FEV_1 declined rapidly in the other active treatment groups and placebo. This difference was significant with budesonide//formoterol compared with placebo (14%; $P = 0.001$), budesonide (11%; $P < 0.001$) and formoterol (5%; $P = 0.002$), but not with budesonide versus placebo (2%). The median time to first exacerbation requiring medical intervention (oral antibiotics and/or corticosteroids or hospitalization) with budesonide/formoterol in combination and budesonide alone was 254 days and 178 days, respectively, compared with 154 days with formoterol (a long-acting bronchodilator – the current standard of care) and 96 days in the placebo group. In this study, the statistical power was in the hazard rate or time to first exacerbation analysis: –28.5% for budesonide/formoterol versus placebo ($P < 0.01$), –30% versus formoterol ($P = 0.003$) and –21% versus budesonide ($P = 0.033$). Combination therapy and budesonide alone was also associated with a lower mean exacerbation rate (1.4 and 1.6 exacerbations per patient per year, respectively) compared with placebo (1.8) and formoterol (1.9). Importantly, budesonide/formoterol also prolonged the time to first oral corticosteroid course compared with placebo (–42% versus placebo; $P < 0.001$) as did budesonide (–14% vs placebo; $P = 0.009$). The effect of budesonide/formoterol was greater than the sum of its constituent components. With regard to improvements in exacerbation status, budesonide/formoterol significantly improved SGRQ total score compared with other active treatments and placebo. All active treatment groups improved the total score versus placebo, but the greatest difference and clinically significant difference (–7.5) was observed with budesonide/formoterol. Inhaled corticosteroid and long-acting inhaled β_2-agonist combination therapy improved symptoms and use of reliever medication in all three 12-month studies.

Table 58.3 Summary of placebo-controlled COPD studies investigating the efficacy of combinations of an inhaled corticosteroid and an inhaled long-acting β_2-agonist compared with the inhaled steroid and the inhaled β_2-agonist alone.

Author [Ref.]	Inhaled steroid Daily dose	Inhaled β_2-agonists Daily dose	Study duration (weeks)	No. of randomized patients	Mean age (years)	Mean no. of pack years	Baseline FEV_1 (L)	FEV_1 PN (%)	Bronchodilator reversibility	% Patients using inhaled steroids	Results FEV_1	Rate of severe exacerbations	HRQL
Szafranski et al. [9]	BUD 400 μg b.i.d.	F 9 μg b.i.d.	52	812	64	44	0.99	36	6.0% of PN	26	Postdose +15% vs P, 9% vs BUD	24% reduction vs P, 23% vs F	SGRQ Compared with P statistically significant effect on total score and symptom and impact domains
Calverley et al. [10]	FP 500 μg b.i.d.	SM 50 μg b.i.d.	52	1465	63	42–44	1.2–1.3	44–45	3.7–4.0% of PN	49–54	Predose +133 mL vs P	25% reduction vs P, no difference vs FP or SM	SGRQ Statistically significant change compared with P and FP
Calverley et al. [11]	BUD 400 μg b.i.d.	F 9 μg b.i.d.	52	1022	64	39	0.99	36	6.0% of PN	48	Postdose +14% vs P, 11% vs BUD, 5% vs F	24% reduction vs P, 26% vs F	SGRQ Compared with P, statistically significant effect on total score and on symptom, activity and impact domains
Mahler et al. [96]	FP 500 μg b.i.d.	SM 50 μg b.i.d.	24	691	62–64	53–60	1.2–1.3	40–41	19–21%	33–49	Predose +14.5% vs P	Not reported	CRDQ Clinically important increase from baseline. Statistically significant vs P and FP
Dal Negro et al. [97]	FP 250 μg b.i.d.	SM 50 μg b.i.d.	52	18 (6 each of FP/SM, SM and P)	50–78	40–43	1.4–1.5	48–50	3.0–3.5%	Not reported	+7.3% over baseline	7 in 6 patients, 25 in 6 patients on P	Not reported
Hanania et al. [98]	FP 250 μg b.i.d.	SM 50 μg b.i.d.	24	723	63–65	53–60	1.2–1.3	41–42	20–21%	35–55	Predose +161 mL vs P	Not reported	SGRQ Compared with P statistically significant effect on total score

b.i.d., twice daily; BUD, budesonide; CRDQ, Chronic Respiratory Disease Questionnaire; F, formoterol; FEV_1, forced expiratory volume in 1 s; FP, fluticasone propionate; HRQL, health-related quality of life; P, placebo; PN, predicted normal; SGRQ, St. Georges's Respiratory Questionnaire; SM, salmeterol.

Using the UK General Practice Research Database Kiri et al. [99] obtained 437 pairs of patients with moderate-to-severe COPD who either used an inhaled corticosteroid together with a long-acting or a short-acting inhaled β_2-agonist. In a multivariate analysis they found a 38% risk reduction ($P < 0.007$) among patients given the inhaled steroid with the long-acting relative to those using the short-acting bronchodilator.

Numbers needed to treat
The 'number needed to treat' (NNT) was developed to provide a simple, clinically relevant measure of treatment effects [100]. In COPD the NNT values, defined as the number of patients who need to be treated with the combination inhaler for 1 year to avoid one severe exacerbation compared with the long-acting bronchodilator alone, has been calculated. For budesonide/formoterol the NNT values in the studies by Szafranski *et al.* [9] and Calverley *et al.* [11] were 2.1 and 2.4 [101]. The corresponding value in the study by Calverley *et al.* [10] for salmeterol/fluticasone have been 14 [102]. This figure has to be interpreted with caution as no statistically significant difference in exacerbation rates was seen in the study between salmeterol and the combination product, which is necessary for a proper calculation of NNT values.

Conclusions
In patients with moderate to severe COPD (*FEV*$_1$ less than 50% of predicted normal) combination treatment with an inhaled corticosteroid and a long-acting β_2-agonist in the same inhaler has provided clinically important and statistically significant effects. A clear reduction in exacerbations rates, time to first severe exacerbation and in symptoms, together with great improvements in health-related quality of life, have been observed.

Tolerability and safety of corticosteroids in COPD

The safety and tolerability of inhaled corticosteroids in patients with asthma have been well documented in several papers (e.g. Barnes *et al.* [38]). However, patients with COPD differ from those with asthma and results obtained in studies of healthy subjects or patients with asthma may not be applicable to those with COPD, who are often older and have a significant smoking history with other concomitant smoking-related diseases. In addition, patients are often physically inactive because of respiratory problems such as dyspnoea. It may be difficult therefore to distinguish between treatment-induced adverse effects and the symptoms and signs caused by tobacco smoking and comorbidities.

Many studies in patients with asthma have reported changes in markers of hypothalamic–pituitary–adrenal (HPA) function and bone formation; however, clinical risks

in terms of adrenal crisis or bone fractures are rare. The adverse effects and the benefit–risk ratio of inhaled corticosteroids in the treatment of patients with COPD have recently been reviewed [103,104].

This review focuses on the pharmacokinetics of inhaled corticosteroids in patients with COPD and adverse effects reported in the long-term placebo-controlled studies.

Pharmacokinetics
Few controlled studies have evaluated the pulmonary pharmacokinetics of inhaled corticosteroids in patients with COPD. Providing the patient's inhalation effort is acceptable, studies with budesonide have shown no difference in kinetics between patients with COPD and healthy subjects, but a higher systemic availability for FP than for budesonide [105]. For FP, significant differences have been observed between healthy control subjects and patients with asthma [106,107] and COPD [108], with systemic effects in healthy subjects being greater than in patients with airway obstruction. For FP a linear relation has been found between the degree of airway obstruction and the systemic activity of FP [109]. A plausible explanation for the difference in systemic activity between budesonide and FP may be the difference in water–lipid solubility between the substances. FP is significantly less water soluble, has a much higher volume of distribution with a corresponding significantly longer elimination half-life, and is therefore retained for a longer time in the tissues.

The results of FP studies demonstrating a difference between patients and healthy subjects may be caused by a more central drug deposition in patients. A centrally deposited lipophilic substance may be more easily transported away from the airways by the mucociliary clearance than a more peripherally deposited one, thus resulting in less systemic activity.

Topical adverse effects
Adverse effects associated with inhaled corticosteroid treatment include voice problems (hoarseness, dysphonia), sore throat and oropharyngeal candidiasis. They are generally caused by the deposition of corticosteroids in the oropharynx and on the vocal cords, but are more frequent in people misusing their voice (e.g. teachers, switch board operators, sport coaches). They also depend on dosing frequency and the total daily dose, but not on duration of treatment [110]. The choice of delivery device also influences the incidence of local side-effects [110]. Inhalation through devices with an inherent resistance (e.g. Turbuhaler) opens up the vocal cords and thereby minimize deposition on the vocal cords. A significant reduction in the frequency of local side-effects was observed in a 4-year study in 154 patients with obstructive airway diseases (29 with COPD) treated with an inhaled corticosteroid (BDP or budesonide pMDI attached

to a large volume spacer) for 2 years, when they changed treatment to budesonide delivered via Turbuhaler for the next 2 years [111].

In the EUROSCOP study, 5% of budesonide and 2% of placebo-treated patients had oropharyngeal candidiasis ($P < 0.001$) and 7% and 5% of patients, respectively, reported hoarseness or sore throat [55]. In the ISOLDE trial, 21% of the patients in the FP group had dysphonia or sore throat compared with 12% in the placebo group [56]. *Candida* infections were found in 11% and 7%, respectively.

In the corticosteroid/long-acting β_2-agonist combination studies, more topical adverse events were reported in the groups receiving treatment with the inhaled corticosteroid than in the placebo and long-acting β_2-agonist groups. In the 6-month study by Mahler *et al.* [96] candidiasis was found in less than 1% in the placebo and salmeterol groups but in 10% in the FP and 7% in the combined FP/salmeterol groups. In the 12-month study with the same treatments [10], the frequency of oropharyngeal candidiasis was 1% during treatment with placebo and salmeterol, and 6% during the treatments including FP.

Systemic adverse effects

Hypothalamic–pituitary–adrenal axis

Treatment with oral corticosteroids in daily doses of more than 7.5 mg usually causes signs of suppression of the HPA axis and patients may develop moon face, acne, arterial hypertension, osteoporosis with bone fractures, disturbed carbohydrate metabolism, mental and behavioural disturbances, and other signs and symptoms. Few systemic side-effects have been reported with inhaled corticosteroid treatment, but it should be remembered that individual susceptibility – in addition to dose–response for systemic effects – does exist.

In the 6-month study in which patients received 1000 μg/day FP or placebo, the mean serum cortisol level was significantly lower with FP at 6 months (345 nmol/L) compared with placebo (385 nmol/L; $P = 0.02$), but no obvious clinical signs of adverse effects were seen [45]. A total of 19 patients (14% of 134 patients) in the FP group and 13 patients (11% of 116 patients) in the placebo group had cortisol values below the reference range.

In the ISOLDE study, morning serum cortisol was measured at baseline and every 6 months during treatment in 372 FP-treated and 370 placebo-treated patients [56]. A small – but statistically significant – decrease in mean values was observed in the FP group ($P = 0.03$). Overall, 5% of the FP-treated patients had values below the normal range.

Osteoporosis and fractures

Long-term oral corticosteroid treatment is associated with osteoporosis and an increased risk of fractures. In a study in 117 patients with chronic lung diseases, the cumulative

prednisolone dose was strongly related to fracture risk, and this effect was found to be independent of its more modest impact on bone mineral density [112].

Several studies in patients with asthma have failed to identify an increased frequency of bone fractures or lower bone density in patients receiving long-term inhaled corticosteroid therapy [38]. However, a population-based case–control study in the UK suggested that there is a dose–response relationship between inhaled corticosteroid use and hip fractures, even after adjusting for the annual number of courses of oral corticosteroids [113]. In older subjects, the recent use of inhaled corticosteroids was associated with a dose-related increase in hip fractures.

In the placebo-controlled EUROSCOP study, patients with mild COPD received 800 μg/day budesonide [55]. Bone mineral density (BMD) was measured at the L2–L4 vertebrae and femoral neck, trochanter and Ward triangle by dual-energy X-ray absorptiometry at baseline and after 6, 12, 24 and 36 months in 82 budesonide and 79 placebo-treated patients. No detrimental effect of budesonide treatment was observed [114]. Radiographs of the thoracic and lumbar spine (before and after 3 years' study treatment) were also obtained in 322 budesonide and 331 placebo-treated patients. At randomization, 43 patients (13%) in the budesonide group and 38 (12%) in the placebo group had at least one vertebral fracture. At the end of the study, five new fractures occurred in the budesonide group and three in the placebo group. This difference was not statistically significant.

In the ISOLDE study, 751 patients were followed for 3 years during treatment with 1000 g/day FP [56]. The incidence of bone fractures was low in both treatment groups (FP 2%; placebo 4.5%).

In the Lung Health Study, 559 patients were treated with 1200 μg/day triamcinolone for 3 years [57]. Bone density values for the lumbar spine were available at baseline and after treatment for 1 and 3 years in 328 patients, and for the femoral neck in 359 patients. For femoral neck, the percentage of change (mean ± SE) from baseline to 3 years was $-2.00 \pm 0.35\%$ in the inhaled corticosteroid group and $-0.22 \pm 0.32\%$ with placebo ($P < 0.001$). For lumbar spine, the percentage of change was $-0.35 \pm 0.33\%$ in the steroid-treated group and $+0.98 \pm 0.36\%$ in the placebo group ($P = 0.007$). Fractures were not reported.

Postcapsular cataracts

The incidence of cataracts in the EUROSCOP study was less than 5% and was equally distributed between budesonide and placebo-treated patients [55]. In the ISOLDE study, the incidence of cataracts was 1.3% in the FP group and 1.9% in the placebo group [56]. The Lung Health Study group reported a much higher incidence of cataracts, but this was equally distributed between triamcinolone and placebo treatments (22% vs 20%) [57].

Skin bruises

Oral and high-dose inhaled corticosteroid treatments are associated with an increased incidence of purpura and dermal thinning compared with low-dose inhaled corticosteroid and placebo treatments [115]. The tendency to bruise easily is a well-known adverse effect of inhaled corticosteroid treatment. A study of patients with asthma showed that the prevalence of bruising increased with age, dose of inhaled corticosteroids and duration of treatment [116].

In the EUROSCOP study, bruising on a defined area of the forearm was recorded on a regular basis [55]. At clinic visits, bruising was found in 10% of patients taking budesonide compared with 4% in the placebo group ($P < 0.001$). In the ISOLDE study, which included spontaneous reporting of adverse events, 7% of FP-treated and 4% of placebo-treated patients reported bruising [56]. In the Lung Health Study, in which younger patients were enrolled, the annual incidence of bruising was 0.8% in the triamcinolone group compared with 0.4% in the placebo group (based on patient questioning every 3 months) [57].

It should be noted that, as there are methodological differences between the various studies, the incidence of adverse events reported may differ. In general terms, however, an inhaled corticosteroid with a high systemic bioavailability results in a higher systemic activity than a compound with a low systemic availability when administered at equally effective clinical doses. Data of comparative studies in patients with COPD are lacking.

Other adverse effects

The EUROSCOP study reported similar incidences of diabetes, myopathy, and cardiovascular and gastrointestinal disorders in both the budesonide and placebo groups [55]. The ISOLDE study [56] and the Lung Health Study [57] did not mention these adverse effects. None of the four recent long-term studies reported an increased risk of respiratory or systemic infections in the groups of patients using inhaled corticosteroids [54–57].

Conclusions

Corticosteroids have an important place in the treatment of patients with COPD. Systemic corticosteroids are beneficial for the treatment of acute exacerbations, but should not be used for maintenance treatment because of the associated risk of side-effects.

The role of inhaled corticosteroids in COPD management has been debated for some time. Short- and medium-term studies of inhaled corticosteroids have generally documented small effects of treatment, mostly in patients or subgroups with features of asthma, although an overall improvement in FEV_1 and an effect on decline in FEV_1 have

been reported. The four long-term placebo-controlled studies that have more rigorously excluded patients with asthma and have evaluated the effects of inhaled corticosteroids on FEV_1 decline were all negative; there was no significant difference between active treatment and placebo. Thus, no disease-modifying effect could be demonstrated. However, compared with placebo, an initial improvement over the first 3–6 months was demonstrated with inhaled corticosteroid treatment and one study showed an effect on bronchial hyperresponsiveness. Nevertheless, a meta-analysis of the four studies demonstrated a statistically significant effect on the FEV_1 decline in the order of 7–10 mL/year, which may represent a clinically meaningful improvement for the patient.

Inhaled corticosteroid treatment modifies the severity of acute exacerbations, reduces the risk of severe exacerbations, reduces symptoms associated with COPD, and improves health status and exercise tolerance. Patients with more severe disease (FEV_1 of less than 50% of predicted normal, rapid decline in FEV_1), a short smoking history and asthma-like features respond better than the rest of the patient population. Inhaled corticosteroid treatment may also reduce the number of rehospitalizations and deaths from a worsening of COPD. Importantly, discontinuing treatment with inhaled corticosteroids in patients with COPD has been shown to increase the risk of experiencing an exacerbation. Reversibility testing with bronchodilators or oral corticosteroids is not indicative of a treatment effect, as they do not predict the response to subsequent long-term treatment with inhaled corticosteroids. To date, no dose–response studies have been reported; however, the daily doses used are those believed to be safe in the long term.

Dysphonia and oropharyngeal candidiasis are the most frequently reported local adverse effects when using inhaled corticosteroids. Systemic side-effects are dose-dependent but are rare with clinically approved doses. Indeed, less lipophilic inhaled corticosteroids (e.g. budesonide with a high first-pass metabolism in the liver) are associated with an improved adverse event profile, compared with older agents such as BDP and triamcinolone, and more lipophilic compounds such as FP. It may be difficult to distinguish between COPD- and smoking-related adverse events, and those caused by treatment with inhaled corticosteroids. Nevertheless, the benefit–risk ratio for inhaled corticosteroids is clearly positive in the subgroups of patients with COPD mentioned previously. Whether inhaled corticosteroid treatment in patients with COPD is also cost-effective depends on the frequency of exacerbations – which can now be prevented. Further prospective controlled studies evaluating the effect of inhaled corticosteroids on long-term mortality are warranted.

At this stage, it seems appropriate to recommend treatment with inhaled corticosteroids for all patients with frequent exacerbations and for those with poor airway function and HRQL. To date, patients with mild COPD as a group have not been shown to benefit from treatment with inhaled corticosteroids or inhaled corticosteroid/long-acting inhaled β_2-agonist combinations in clinical trials. However, the recent meta-analysis by Sutherland et al. [61] reported positive treatment benefits in patients with COPD, including those with mild disease. The recent results with combination therapy are clinically important as they demonstrate improved treatment benefits compared with inhaled corticosteroids alone in patients at risk of COPD exacerbations.

References

1 Carryer HM, Prickman LE, Maytum CK. Effects of cortisone on bronchial asthma and hayfever occurring in subjects sensitive to ragweed pollen. *Proc Mayo Clin* 1950;**25**:282–7.

2 Lukas D. Some effects of adrenocorticotropic hormone and cortisone on pulmonary function of patients with obstructive emphysema. *Am Rev Tuberc* 1951;**64**:279–94.

3 Gladstone M, Weisenfeld S, Benjamin B, Rosenbluth MB. Effect of ACTH in chronic lung disease. *Am J Med* 1951;**10**: 166–81.

4 Niewoehner DE. The role of systemic corticosteroids in acute exacerbations of chronic obstructive pulmonary disease. *Am J Respir Med* 2002;**1**:243–8.

5 Davies L, Angus RM, Calverley PMA. Oral prednisolone in patients admitted to hospital with exacerbations of chronic obstructive pulmonary disease: a prospective randomised controlled trial. *Lancet* 1999;**354**:456–60.

6 Calverley PMA. Inhaled corticosteroid are beneficial in chronic obstructive pulmonary disease. *Am J Respir Crit Care Med* 2000;**161**:341–2; discussion 344.

7 Barnes PJ. Inhaled corticosteroid are not beneficial in chronic obstructive pulmonary disease. *Am J Respir Crit Care Med* 2000;**161**:342–4; discussion 344.

8 Alsaeedi A, Sin DD, McAlister FA. The effects of inhaled corticosteroids in chronic obstructive pulmonary disease: a systematic review of randomized placebo-controlled trials. *Am J Med* 2002;**113**:59–65.

9 Szafranski W, Cukier A, Ramirez A et al. Efficacy and safety of budesonide/formoterol in the management of chronic obstructive pulmonary disease. *Eur Respir J* 2003;**21**:74–81.

10 Calverley P, Pauwels R, Vestbo J et al. Combined salmeterol and fluticasone in the treatment of chronic obstructive pulmonary disease: a randomised controlled trial. *Lancet* 2003; **361**:449–56.

11 Calverley PM, Boonsawat W, Cseke Z et al. Maintenance therapy with budesonide and formoterol in chronic obstructive pulmonary disease. *Eur Respir J* 2003;**22**:912–9.

12 Albert RK, Martin TR, Lewis SW. Controlled clinical trial of methylprednisolone in patients with chronic bronchitis and acute respiratory insufficiency. *Ann Intern Med* 1980;**92**: 753–8.

13 Thompson WH, Nielson CR, Carvalho P, Charan NB,

Crowley JJ. Controlled trial of oral prednisone in outpatients with acute COPD exacerbation. *Am J Respir Crit Care Med* 1996;**154**:407–12.

14 Bullard MJ, Liaw S-J, Tsai Y-H, Min HP. Early corticosteroid use in acute exacerbations of chronic airflow obstruction. *Am J Emerg Med* 1996;**14**:139–43.

15 Niewoehner DE, Erbland ML, Deupree RH et al. Effect of systemic glucocorticoids on exacerbations of chronic obstructive pulmonary disease. *N Engl J Med* 1999;**340**:1941–7.

16 Sayiner A, Aytemur ZA, Cirit M, Ünsal I. Systemic glucocorticoids in severe exacerbations of COPD. *Chest* 2001;**119**: 726–30.

17 Singh JM, Palda VA, Stanbrooth MB, Chapman KR. Corticosteroid therapy for patients with acute exacerbations of chronic obstructive pulmonary disease: a systematic review. *Arch Intern Med* 2002;**162**:2527–36.

18 Henzen C, Suter A, Lerch E et al. Suppression and recovery of adrenal response after short-term, high-dose glucocorticoid treatment. *Lancet* 2000;**355**:542–5.

19 Maltais F, Ostinelli J, Bourbeau J et al. Comparison of nebulized budesonide and oral prednisolone with placebo in the treatment of acute exacerbations of chronic obstructive pulmonary disease: a randomized controlled trial. *Am J Respir Crit Care Med* 2002;**165**:698–703.

20 Mirici A, Meral M, Akgun M. Comparison of the efficacy of nebulised budesonide with parenteral corticosteroids in the treatment of acute exacerbations of chronic obstructive pulmonary disease. *Clin Drug Invest* 2003;**23**:55–62.

21 Harding SM, Freedman S. A comparison of oral and inhaled steroids in patients with chronic airways obstruction: features determining response. *Thorax* 1978;**33**:214–8.

22 Shim C, Stover DE, Williams MH Jr. Response to corticosteroids in chronic bronchitis. *J Allergy Clin Immunol* 1978;**62**: 363–7.

23 Callahan CM, Dittus RS, Katz BP. Oral corticosteroid therapy for patients with stable chronic obstructive pulmonary disease: a meta-analysis. *Ann Intern Med* 1991;**114**: 216–23.

24 Nisar M, Walshaw M, Earis JE, Pearson MG, Calverley PMA. Assessment of reversibility of airway obstruction in patients with chronic obstructive airways disease. *Thorax* 1990;**45**: 190–4.

25 Weir DC, Burge PS. Effects of high dose inhaled beclomethasone dipropionate, 750 µg and 1500 µg twice daily and 40 mg per day oral prednisolone on lung function, symptoms and bronchial hyper-reactivity in patients with non-asthmatic chronic airway obstruction. *Thorax* 1993;**48**: 309–16.

26 Pizzichini E, Pizzichini MMM, Gibson P et al. Sputum eosinophilia predicts benefit from prednisone in smokers with chronic obstructive bronchitis. *Am J Respir Crit Care Med* 1998;**158**:1511–7.

27 American Thoracic Society. Standards for the diagnosis and care of patients with chronic obstructive pulmonary disease (COPD). *Am J Respir Crit Care Med* 1995;**152**:S77–120.

28 Siafakas NM, Vermeire P, Pride NB et al. Optimal assessment and management of chronic obstructive pulmonary disease (COPD). *Eur Respir J* 1995;**8**:1398–420.

29 British Thoracic Society. Guidelines for the management of chronic obstructive pulmonary disease. *Thorax* 1997;**52** (Suppl 5):S1–28.

30 Global Initiative for Chronic Obstructive Lung Disease (GOLD). (2002) Global Strategy for the Diagnosis, Management, and Prevention of Chronic Obstructive Pulmonary Disease NHLBI/WHO Workshop Report. http://www. goldcopd.com

31 Celli BR, MacNee W for the ATS/ERS task force. Standards for the diagnosis and treatment of patients with COPD: a summary of the ATS/ERS position paper. *Eur Respir J* 2004; **23**:932–46.

32 Postma DS, Steenhuis EJ, van der Weele LT, Sluiter HJ. Severe chronic airflow obstruction: can corticosteroids slow down progression? *Eur J Respir Dis* 1985;**67**:56–64.

33 Postma DS, Peters I, Steenhuis EJ, Sluiter HJ. Moderately severe chronic airflow obstruction: can corticosteroids slow down obstruction? *Eur Respir J* 1988;**1**:22–6.

34 Rice KL, Rubins JB, Lebahn F *et al.* Withdrawal of chronic systemic corticosteroids in patients with COPD. *Am J Respir Crit Care Med* 2000;**162**:174–8.

35 Saetta M, Di Stefano A, Maestrelli T *et al.* Airway eosinophilia in chronic bronchitis during exacerbations. *Am J Respir Crit Care Med* 1994;**150**:1646–52.

36 Hattotuwa KL, Gizycki MJ, Ansari TW, Jeffery PK, Barnes NC. The effects of inhaled fluticasone on airway inflammation in chronic obstructive pulmonary disease. A double-blind, placebo-controlled biopsy study. *Am J Respir Crit Care Med* 2002;**165**:1592–6.

37 Gan WQ, Man SFP, Sin DD. Effects of inhaled corticosteroids on sputum cell counts in stable chronic obstructive pulmonary disease: a systematic review and a meta-analysis. *BMC Pulm Med* 2005;**5**:3.

38 Barnes PJ, Pedersen S, Busse WW. Efficacy and safety of inhaled corticosteroids: new developments. *Am J Respir Crit Care Med* 1998;**157**:S1–53.

39 Thompson AB, Mueller MB, Heires AJ *et al.* Aerosolized beclomethasone in chronic bronchitis: improved pulmonary function and diminished airway inflammation. *Am Rev Respir Dis* 1992;**146**:389–95.

40 Thompson WH, Carvalho P, Souza JP, Charan NB. Controlled trial of inhaled fluticasone propionate in moderate to severe COPD. *Lung* 2002;**180**:191–201.

41 Dompeling E, van Schayck CP, Molema J *et al.* Inhaled beclomethasone improves the course of asthma and COPD. *Eur Respir J* 1992;**5**:945–52.

42 Kerstjens HAM, Brand PLP, Hughes MD *et al.* A comparison of bronchodilator therapy with and without inhaled corticosteroid therapy for obstructive airway disease: Dutch Chronic Non-Specific Lung Disease Study Group. *N Engl J Med* 1992;**327**:1413–9.

43 Derenne JP. Effects of high-dose inhaled beclomethasone on the rate of decline in FEV_1 in patients with chronic obstructive pulmonary disease: results of a 2 year prospective multicentre study. *Am J Respir Crit Care Med* 1995;**151**:A463.

44 Renkema TEJ, Schouten JP, Koeter GH, Postma DS. Effects of long-term treatment with corticosteroids in COPD. *Chest* 1996;**109**:1156–62.

45 Paggiaro PL, Dahle R, Bakran I *et al.* Multicentre randomised placebo-controlled trial of inhaled fluticasone propionate in patients with chronic obstructive pulmonary disease. *Lancet* 1998;**351**:773–80.

46 Bourbeau J, Rouleau MY, Boucher S. Randomised controlled trial of inhaled corticosteroids in patients with chronic obstructive pulmonary disease. *Thorax* 1998;**53**: 477–82.

47 Weir DC, Bale GA, Bright P, Sherwood Burge P. A double-blind placebo-controlled study of the effect of inhaled beclomethasone dipropionate for 2 years in patients with non-asthmatic chronic obstructive pulmonary disease. *Clin Exp Allergy* 1999;**29**(Suppl 2):125–8.

48 Senderovitz T, Vestbo J, Frandsen J *et al.* Steroid reversibility test followed by inhaled budesonide or placebo in outpatients with stable chronic obstructive pulmonary disease. *Respir Med* 1999;**93**:715–8.

49 van Grunsven PM, van Schayck CP, Derenne JP *et al.* Long term effects of inhaled corticosteroids in chronic obstructive pulmonary disease: a meta-analysis. *Thorax* 1999;**54**:7–14.

50 van Schayck CP, Dompeling E, van Heerwaarden CLA *et al.* Bronchodilator treatment in moderate asthma and chronic bronchitis: continuous or on demand? A randomised controlled study. *BMJ* 1991;**303**:1426–31.

51 Dompeling E, van Schayck CP, van Grunsven PM *et al.* Slowing the deterioration of asthma and chronic obstructive pulmonary disease observed during bronchodilator therapy by adding inhaled corticosteroids: a 4-year prospective study. *Ann Intern Med* 1993;**118**:770–8.

52 van Schayck CP, van den Broek PJJA, den Otter JJ *et al.* Periodic treatment regimens with inhaled steroids in asthma and chronic obstructive pulmonary disease. Is it possible? *JAMA* 1995;**274**:161–4.

53 Verhoeven GT, Hegmans JPJJ, Mulder PGH *et al.* Effects of fluticasone propionate in COPD patients with bronchial hyperresponsiveness. *Thorax* 2002;**57**:694–700.

54 Vestbo J, Sørensen T, Lange P, Brix A, Viskum K. Long-term effect of inhaled budesonide in mild and moderate chronic obstructive pulmonary disease: a randomised controlled study. *Lancet* 1999;**353**:1819–23.

55 Pauwels RA, Löfdahl C-G, Laitinen LA *et al.* Long-term treatment with inhaled budesonide in persons with mild chronic obstructive pulmonary disease who continue smoking. *N Engl J Med* 1999;**340**:1948–53.

56 Burge PS, Calverley PMA, Jones PW *et al.* Randomised, double blind, placebo controlled study of fluticasone propionate in patients with moderate to severe chronic obstructive pulmonary disease: the ISOLDE study. *BMJ* 2000;**320**: 1297–303.

57 The Lung Health Study Research Group. Effect of inhaled triamcinolone on the decline in pulmonary function in chronic obstructive pulmonary disease. *N Engl J Med* 2000; **343**:1902–9.

58 Löfdahl C-G, Postma D, Pride N, Boe J, Thorén A. Does inhaled budesonide protect against cardio-ischemic events in mild-moderate COPD. A post-hoc evaluation of the EUROSCOP study. *Eur Respir J* 2005;**26**(Suppl 49):360s.

59 Anthonisen NR, Connett JE, Kiley JP *et al.* Effects of smoking

intervention and the use of an inhaled anticholinergic bronchodilator on the rate of decline of FEV_1. *JAMA* 1994; **272**:1497–505.

60 Highland KB, Strange C, Heffner JE. Long-term effects of inhaled corticosteroids on FEV_1 in patients with chronic obstructive pulmonary disease: a meta-analysis. *Ann Intern Med* 2003;**138**:969–73.

61 Sutherland ER, Allmers H, Ayas NT, Venn AJ, Martin RJ. Inhaled corticosteroids reduce the progression of airflow limitation in chronic obstructive pulmonary disease: a meta-analysis. *Thorax* 2003;**58**:937–41.

62 Burge PS, Lewis SA. So inhaled steroids slow the rate of decline of FEV_1 in patients with COPD after all? *Thorax* 2003;**58**:911–3.

63 Selroos O. The effects of inhaled corticosteroids on the natural history of obstructive lung diseases. *Eur Respir Rev* 1991;**1**:369–78.

64 Boothman-Burrell D, Delany SG, Flannery EM, Hancox RJ, Taylor DR. The efficacy of inhaled corticosteroids in the management of non-asthmatic chronic airflow obstruction. *N Z Med J* 1997;**110**:370–3.

65 Davies L, Nisar M, Pearson MG *et al.* Oral corticosteroid trials in the management of stable chronic obstructive pulmonary disease. *Q J Med* 1999;**92**:395–400.

66 Dirksen A, Christensen H, Evald T *et al.* Bronchodilator and corticosteroid reversibility in ambulatory patients with airways obstruction. *Dan Med Bull* 1991;**38**:486–9.

67 Burge PS, Calverley PMA, Jones PW, Spencer S, Anderson JA. Prednisolone response in patients with chronic obstructive pulmonary disease: results from the ISOLDE study. *Thorax* 2003;**58**:654–8.

68 Calverley PMA, Burge PS, Spencer S, Anderson JA, Jones PW. Bronchodilator reversibility testing in chronic obstructive pulmonary disease. *Thorax* 2003;**58**:659–64.

69 Jarad NA, Wedzicha JA, Burge PS, Calverley PMA. An observational study of inhaled corticosteroid withdrawal in stable chronic obstructive pulmonary disease. *Respir Med* 1999;**93**:161–6.

70 O'Brian A, Russo-Magno P, Karki A *et al.* Effects of withdrawal of inhaled steroids in men with severe irreversible airflow obstruction. *Am J Respir Crit Care Med* 2001;**164**:365–71.

71 van der Valk P, Monninkhof E, van der Palen J, Zielhuis G, Herwaarden C. Effect of discontinuation of inhaled corticosteroids in patients with chronic obstructive pulmonary disease: the COPE study. *Am J Respir Crit Care Med* 2002; **166**:1358–63.

72 Spencer S, Calverley PM, Burge PS, Jones PW. Impact of preventing exacerbations on deterioration of health status in COPD. *Eur Respir J* 2004;**23**:698–702.

73 Seemungal TA, Donaldson GC, Paul EA *et al.* Effect of exacerbation on quality of life in patients with chronic obstructive pulmonary disease. *Am J Respir Crit Care Med* 1998; **57**:1418–22.

74 Donaldson GC, Seemungal TA, Bhowmik A, Wedzicha JA. Relationship between exacerbation frequency and lung function decline in chronic obstructive pulmonary disease. *Thorax* 2002;**57**:847–52.

75 Burge S, Wedzicha JA. COPD exacerbations: definitions and classifications. *Eur Respir J* 2003;**21**(Suppl 41):46S–53S.

76 Vestbo J. What is an exacerbation of COPD? *Eur Respir Rev* 2004;**13**:6–13.

77 Jones PW, Willits LR, Burge PS, Calverley PMA. Disease severity and the effect of fluticasone propionate on chronic obstructive pulmonary disease exacerbations. *Eur Respir J* 2003;**21**:68–73.

78 Garcia-Aymerich J, Monsó E, Marrades RM *et al.* Risk factors for hospitalization for chronic obstructive pulmonary disease exacerbation. EFRAM study. *Am J Respir Crit Care Med* 2001;**164**:1002–7.

79 Soler-Cataluña JJ, Martínez-Garcia MÁ, Román Sánchez P *et al.* Severe acute exacerbations and mortality in patients with chronic obstructive pulmonary disease. *Thorax* 2005; **60**:925–31.

80 Osman LM, Godden DJ, Friend JAR, Legge JS, Douglas JG. Quality of life and hospital-readmission in patients with chronic obstructive pulmonary disease. *Thorax* 1997;**52**:67–71.

81 Almagro P, Calbo E, Ochoa de Echagüen A *et al.* Mortality after hospitalization for COPD. *Chest* 2002;**121**:1441–8.

82 Eriksen N, Hansen EF, Munch EP, Rasmussen FV, Vestbo J. Chronic obstructive pulmonary disease. Admission, course and prognosis (in Danish). *Ugeskr Laeger* 2003;**165**:3499–502.

83 Groenewegen KH, Schols AMWJ, Wouters EFM. Mortality and mortality-related factors after hospitalization for acute exacerbation of COPD. *Chest* 2003;**124**:459–67.

84 Sin DD, Tu JV. Inhaled corticosteroids and the risk of mortality and readmission in elderly patients with chronic obstructive pulmonary disease. *Am J Respir Crit Care Med* 2001;**164**:580–4.

85 Soriano JB, Vetsbo J, Pride NB *et al.* Survival in COPD patients after regular use of fluticasone propionate and salmeterol in general practice. *Eur Respir J* 2002;**20**:819–25.

86 Soriano JB, Kiri VA, Pride NB, Vestbo J. Inhaled corticosteoids with/without long-acting β-agonists reduce the risk of rehospitalization and death in COPD patients. *Am J Respir Med* 2003;**2**:67–74.

87 Spencer MD, Vestbo J, Soriano JB. The beneficial effects of inhaled corticosteroid use in observational studies of COPD are unlikely to be explained by unmeasured confounders. *Am J Respir Crit Care Med* 2003;**167**:A90.

88 Sin DD, Man SFP. Inhaled corticosteroids and survival in chronic obstructive pulmonary disease: does the dose matter? *Eur Respir J* 2003;**21**:260–6.

89 Mapel DW, Hurley JS, Roblin D *et al.* Survival of COPD patients using inhaled corticosteroids and long-acting beta agonists. *Respir Med* 2006;**100**:595–609.

90 Fan SF, Bryson CL, Curtis JR *et al.* Inhaled corticosteroids in chronic obstructive pulmonary disease and risk of death and hospitalization. Time-dependent analysis. *Am J Respir Crit Care Med* 2003;**168**:1488–94.

91 Suissa S. Effectiveness of inhaled corticosteroids in chronic obstructive pulmonary disease: immortal time bias in observational studies. *Am J Respir Crit Care Med* 2003;**168**:49–53.

92 Sin DD, Man SF, Tu JV. Inhaled glucocorticoids in COPD: immortal time bias. *Am J Respir Crit Care Med* 2003;**168**:126–7.

93 Sin DD, Golmohammadi K, Jacobs P. Cost-effectiveness of inhaled corticosteroids for chronic obstructive pulmonary disease according to disease severity. *Am J Med* 2004;**116**: 325–31.

94 Sin DD, Anderson JA, Anthonisen NR *et al.* Inhaled corticosteroids and mortality in chronic obstructive pulmonary disease. *Thorax* 2005;**60**:992–7.

95 Tkacova R, Toth S, Sin DD. Inhaled corticosteroids and survival in COPD patients receiving long-term home oxygen therapy. *Respir Med* 2006;**100**:385–92.

96 Mahler DA, Wire P, Horstman D *et al.* Effectiveness of fluticasone propionate and salmeterol combination delivered via the Diskus device in the treatment of chronic obstructive pulminary disease. *Am J Respir Crit Care Med* 2002;**166**: 1084–91.

97 Dal Negro RW, Pomari C, Tognella S, Micheletto C. Salmeterol and fluticasone 50 μg/250 μg b.i.d. in combination provides a better long-term control than salmeterol 50 μg b.i.d. alone and placebo in COPD patients already treated with theophylline. *Pulm Pharmacol Ther* 2003;**16**:241–6.

98 Hanania NA, Darken P, Horstman D *et al.* The efficacy and safety of fluticasone propionate (250 μg)/salmeterol (50 μg) combined in the Diskus inhaler for the treatment of COPD. *Chest* 2003;**124**:834–43.

99 Kiri VA, Bettoncelli G, Testi R, Viegi G. Inhaled corticosteroids are more effectrive in COPD patients when used with LABA than with SABA. *Respir Med* 2005;**99**:1115–24.

100 Laupacis A, Sackett DL, Roberts RS. As assessment of clinically useful measures of the consequenses of treatment. *N Engl J Med* 1988;**318**:1728–33.

101 Halpin DMG. Evaluating the effectiveness of combination therapy to prevent COPD exacerbations: the value of NNT analysis. *Int J Clin Pract* 2005;**59**:1187–94.

102 Cazzola M. Application of number needed to treat (NNT) as a measure of treatment effect in respiratory medicine. *Treat Respir Med* 2006;**5**:79–84.

103 McEvoy CE, Niewoehner DE. Adverse effects of corticosteroid therapy for COPD: a critical review. *Chest* 1997;**111**: 732–43.

104 Bonay M, Bancal C, Crestani B. Benefits and risks of inhaled corticosteroids in chronic obstructive pulmonary disease. *Drug Saf* 2002;**25**:57–71.

105 Thorsson L, Edsbäcker S, Källén A, Löfdahl C-G. Pharmacokinetics and systemic activity of fluticasone via Diskus and pMDI and of budesonide via Turbuhaler. *Br J Clin Pharmacol* 2001;**52**:529–38.

106 Harrison TW, Wiseiewski A, Honour J, Tattersfield AE. Comparison of the systemic effects of fluticasone propionate and budesonide given by dry powder inhaler in healthy and asthmatic subjects. *Thorax* 2001;**56**:186–91.

107 Harrison TW, Tattersfield AE. Plasma concentrations of fluticasone propionate and budesonide following inhalation from dry powder inhalers by healthy and asthmatic subjects. *Thorax* 2003;**58**:258–60.

108 Singh SD, Whale C, Houghton N *et al.* Pharmacokinetics and systemic effects of inhaled fluticasone propionate in chronic obstructive pulmonary disease. *Br J Clin Pharmacol* 2003;**55**:375–81.

109 Weiner P, Berar-Yanay N, Davidovich A, Magadle R. Nocturnal cortisol secretion in asthmatic patients after inhalation of fluticasone propionate. *Chest* 1999;**116**:931–4.

110 Toogood JH, Jennings B, Baskerville J, Anderson J, Johansson SA. Dosing regimen of budesonide and occurrence of oropharyngeal complications. *Eur J Respir Dis* 1984; **65**:35–44.

111 Selroos O, Backman R, Forsén K-O *et al.* Local side-effects during 4-year treatment with inhaled corticosteroids: a comparison between pressurized metered-dose inhalers and Turbuhaler. *Allergy* 1994;**49**:888–90.

112 Walsh LJ, Lewis SA, Wong CA *et al.* The impact of oral corticosteroid use on bone mineral density and vertebral fracture. *Am J Respir Crit Care Med* 2002;**166**:691–5.

113 Hubbard RB, Smith CJP, Smeeth L, Harrison TW, Tattersfield AE. Inhaled corticosteroids and hip fractures: a population-based case–control study. *Am J Respir Crit Care Med* 2002;**166**:1563–6.

114 Johnell O, Pauwels R, Löfdahl C-G *et al.* Bone mineral density in patients with chronic obstructive pulmonary disease treated with budesonide Turbuhaler. *Eur Respir J* 2002;**19**:1058–63.

115 Capewell S, Reynolds S, Shuttleworth D, Edwards C, Finlay AY. Purpura and dermal thinning associated with high dose inhaled corticosteroids. *BMJ* 1990;**300**:1548–51.

116 Mak VHF, Melchor R, Spiro SG. Easy bruising as a side-effect of inhaled corticosteroids. *Eur Respir J* 1992;**5**:1068–74.

CHAPTER 59

Phosphodiesterase 4 inhibitors in the treatment of COPD

Hermann Tenor, Daniela S. Bundschuh, Christian Schudt, Dirk Bredenbröker and Armin Hatzelmann

Characterization and understanding of the molecular mechanisms underlying the control of airway integrity have led to the identification of new targets for drug development. The mechanism of 3′,5′-cyclic adenosine monophosphate (cAMP)-mediated modulation of inflammation and bronchiolar tone is illustrated in Figure 59.1 [1,2]. In this context, inhibitors selective for cAMP-hydrolysing phosphodiesterase 4 (PDE4) represent a new class of agents with anti-inflammatory activities that appear to confer significant benefits in animal models of airway disease and

therapeutic efficacy in patients with chronic obstructive pulmonary disease (COPD). Indeed, many of the immune effector cells implicated in the pathogenesis of COPD – neutrophils, macrophages and CD8[+] T cells – express PDE4. Hence, targeting PDE4 provides an opportunity for the design of new drugs. The anti-inflammatory activity of PDE4 inhibitors may improve clinical symptoms and potentially alter or modify disease progression. Thus, PDE4 inhibitors could represent novel drugs that may overcome limitations of existing therapies.

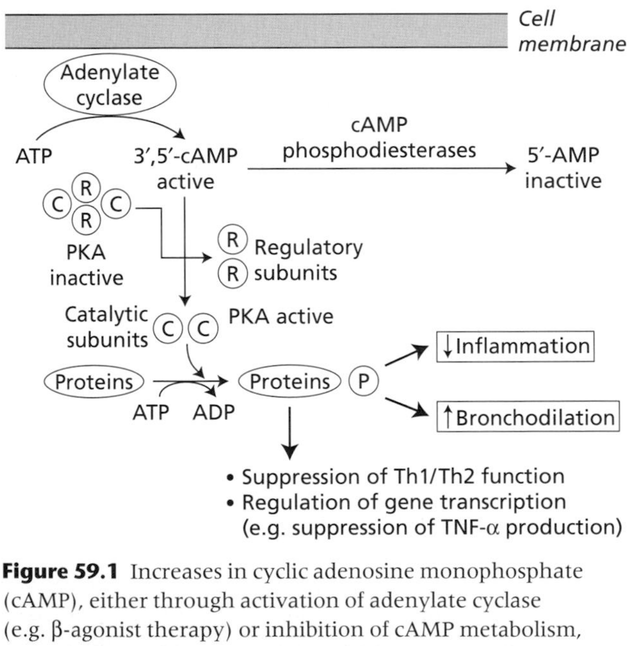

This chapter provides a state-of-the-art review and update on PDE4 inhibitors in COPD, including a review of the rationale, known mechanisms of action, clinical profile and development status of the leading agents. The chapter concludes with an outlook on future perspectives for PDE4 inhibitors in the treatment of COPD.

Figure 59.1 Increases in cyclic adenosine monophosphate (cAMP), either through activation of adenylate cyclase (e.g. β-agonist therapy) or inhibition of cAMP metabolism, activate protein kinase A (PKA), which in turn catalyses the phosphorylation of proteins that result in anti-inflammatory effects or bronchorelaxation [1]. ADP, adenosine diphosphate; ATP, adenosine triphosphate; P, phosphate; Th, T-helper cell; TNF-α, tumor necrosis factor α. (Adapted with permission from ALTANA Pharma AG [2].)

Phosphodiesterases

Cellular levels of cyclic nucleotides are regulated through activation of adenylate and guanylate cyclase and rapid inactivation by PDEs. With respect to the latter, at least 11 families have been characterized based on substrate specificity and sensitivity to PDE inhibitors [3]. These isozymes catalyse the hydrolysis of cyclic nucleotides cAMP and cyclic guanosine monophosphate (cGMP) to 5′-AMP and 5′-GMP, respectively, in a highly regulated manner. More than 50 isoforms or splice variants of PDEs have been identified. Of the human PDE isozymes described, PDE4, 7 and 8, are specific for cAMP; PDE1A, 5, 6 and 9 are selective for cGMP; and PDE1B, 1C, 2, 3, 10 and 11 have dual specificity for cAMP and cGMP. In turn, many of these PDE isozymes have been found in human lung tissue (e.g. PDE1, 3, 4 and 7).

The relative success of theophylline – considered a non-selective inhibitor of PDEs among other mechanisms of action such as adenosine receptor antagonism – in the treatment of airway disease has provided a rationale for pursuing PDE inhibitors. However, the non-selective activity of theophylline has generally been associated with substantial adverse effects (e.g. intractable seizures, persistent vomiting and cardiac arrhythmias), which, in turn, have limited the use of this non-selective agent in COPD. Of particular importance is that many of the PDE isozymes, particularly the PDE4 isozyme, have been localized to inflammatory and immunocompetent cells, including neutrophils, CD8[+] T cells and macrophages, among others [4,5]. These findings provided the impetus for development and clinical testing of PDE inhibitors with greater selectivity for particular isozymes.

Of the 11 PDE families, the PDE4 family has been of most interest to investigators for the treatment of inflammatory diseases of the airways because of the localization of these enzymes in lung structures and broad distribution in pro-inflammatory and immunocompetent cells.

Phosphodiesterase 4

There are four PDE4 subtypes (PDE4A, B, C and D); each is the product of a separate gene, the expression of which results in a myriad of gene splice variants [6]. All of the PDE4 variants have complete specificity for cAMP [3]; however, inhibitors may display some preferences for a particular subtype. Likewise, different effector cells exhibit differing sensitivities to PDE4 inhibitors [7]. Investigations are ongoing to further elucidate the role of PDE4 splice variant diversity and cellular and subcellular localization of these proteins.

Isoforms from all four PDE4 gene variants are found in the human lung [6,8–10]. PDE4 is a major regulator of cAMP metabolism in a variety of pro-inflammatory and immune cells associated with COPD [11–13], including neutrophils [5], macrophages, CD8[+] T cells [4] and eosinophils [5]. In animal and human tissue studies, PDE4 has also been localized to epithelial cells, endothelial cells, fibroblasts and smooth muscle cells [14–18].

Tissue-specific expression of various splice variants should be considered in understanding how these gene products contribute to cellular responses to cAMP. This may, in part, account for the differential sensitivities of the various effector cells to inhibition via PDE4 inhibitors.

PDE4 inhibitors – anti-inflammatory activity

Biological activity of PDE4 inhibitors can be broadly categorized into effects on pro-inflammatory effector cells or pathways [4,14,16,19–32]. The majority of studies have been performed in *in vitro* systems, many of which involved human cells or tissues, and in animal models of inflammation.

The bronchodilatory activities of non-selective PDE4 inhibitors such as theophylline are generally well recognized. Briefly, PDE4 inhibitor-induced bronchodilatation is mediated through increases in intracellular cAMP and subsequent relaxation of bronchiolar smooth muscle (see Fig. 59.1) [1,2]. On the other hand, controversy remains on the effects of PDE4 inhibitors on their own in human bronchial smooth muscle contractility. In fact, acute bronchodilatory activity in patients with COPD has not been observed with selective PDE4 inhibitors; therefore, these newer agents are not considered bronchodilators [33].

Of greater interest with respect to modulating the natural history of COPD are the potential anti-inflammatory effects of PDE4 inhibitors. The *in vitro* and preclinical anti-inflammatory activities have been of considerable interest, and potential anti-inflammatory effects of PDE4 inhibitors are illustrated in Figure 59.2 [2].

The best-characterized cellular component implicated in the pathophysiology of COPD is the neutrophil. COPD is associated with a marked increase in the number and activation level of neutrophils [19–21]. Additionally, neutrophils from patients with COPD produce more reactive oxygen species (ROS), which may support pulmonary inflammation [22]. Inhibitors of PDE4 also suppress neutrophil ROS and leukotriene B_4 (LTB_4) generation, degranulation, CD11b presentation and chemotaxis. Additionally, the PDE4 inhibitor BAY 19-8004 inhibited lipopolysaccharide (LPS)-induced neutrophil influx in a rat model of neutrophilic lung inflammation [24].

Another inflammatory cell implicated in the pathogenesis of airway disease is the CD8[+] T lymphocyte. Indeed, smokers with symptoms of chronic bronchitis and chronic airflow limitation demonstrate an increased proportion of CD8[+] T lymphocytes infiltrating the peripheral airway walls [19]. PDE4 isozymes regulate the levels of cAMP in these cells and, as a result, suppress proliferation. Indeed, in CD8[+] human peripheral blood T lymphocytes, treatment with rolipram significantly ($P < 0.05$) reduced mitogen-evoked production of interleukin-2 (IL-2) and γ-interferon (IFN-γ) [4]. Translating this into the clinic, in a trial comparing cilomilast with placebo, Gamble *et al.* [26] reported a significant ($P < 0.01$) reduction in CD8[+] T cells in bronchial biopsies from cilomilast-treated COPD patients. This was the first report of PDE4-mediated reduction in CD8[+] T cells over the clinical dosing range.

Macrophages represent a major source of TNF-α, and overproduction of TNF-α is believed to have a pathogenic role in COPD. Macrophages are increased in the sputum of smokers with chronic bronchitis [19]. The potential role of cAMP and PDE4 in mediating LPS-activated TNF-α responses was investigated in mice deficient in PDE4B and PDE4D [25]. In that study, LPS induction of TNF-α was decreased by approximately 90% in mice deficient in

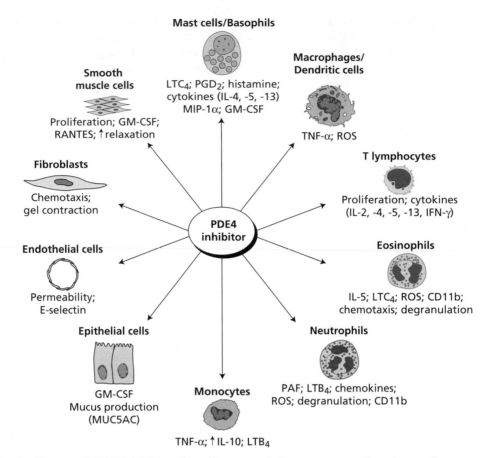

Figure 59.2 Phosphodiesterase 4 (PDE4) inhibitors broadly target cellular components of respiratory diseases, e.g. COPD. In animal models and *in vitro* experiments, PDE inhibitors may reduce proliferation and infiltration of inflammatory cells and decrease the release of inflammatory and cytotoxic mediators (e.g. pro-inflammatory cytokines). GM-CSF, granulocyte–macrophage colony-stimulating factor; IFN-γ, γ-interferon; IL, interleukin; LTB$_4$, leukotriene B$_4$; LTC$_4$, leukotriene C$_4$; MIP-1α, macrophage inflammatory protein 1α; PAF, platelet activating factor; PGD$_2$, prostaglandin D$_2$; RANTES, regulated on activation, normal T cell expressed and secreted; ROS, reactive oxygen species; TNF-α, tumour necrosis factor α. (Adapted with permission from ALTANA Pharma AG [2].)

PDE4B, suggesting a possible role for PDE4 inhibitors in controlling this response [25].

Additionally, therapies that mitigate the fibrotic process (i.e. fibrotic scar) caused by repeated repair processes may be able to slow progressive loss of function in many lung diseases. For example, fibroblast accumulation in and subsequent contraction of the surrounding matrix of small airways is associated with airway lumen narrowing. This can potentially lead to progressive loss of lung function in patients with COPD [16]. cAMP has been shown to regulate fibroblast chemotaxis and contraction. Kohyama *et al.* [16] showed that the PDE4 inhibitors rolipram and cilomilast suppressed fibroblast chemotaxis and fibroblast-mediated collagen gel contraction, at least suggesting that these agents have the potential to suppress fibroblast activity and block the development of progressive fibrosis.

Because epithelial cells have a critical role in airway inflammation, agents that inhibit pro-inflammatory medi-

ator release may help control COPD. PDE4 is a predominant PDE isozyme expressed in airway epithelial cells [14,29]. One report [30] demonstrated that the selective PDE4 inhibitor rolipram concentration-dependently inhibited IL-1β-induced release of granulocyte–macrophage colony-stimulating factor (GM-CSF) from BEAS2B human bronchial epithelial cells with IC50 of about 1 μM and a maximum inhibition of 80% at 10 μM. Human bronchial epithelial cells orchestrate mucociliary clearance, an important airway defense mechanism. Mucus overproduction may contribute to peripheral airway obstruction in COPD. PDE4 inhibitors were shown to reduce MUC5AC from human lung epithelial cells [34]. Cl-secretion over the CFTR channel that is activated by cAMP contributes to maintain the critical height of periciliary liquid required for ciliary mucus transportation supporting pathogen clearance. Cigarette smoke decreased CFTR expression and function *in vitro* and an acquired CFTR deficiency was reported in the nasal respiratory epithelium of cigarette smokers [35]. Selective inhibition of PDE4 was shown to support CFTR activity in Calu-3 airway epithelial cells [36]. In a rat model of neutrophilic lung inflammation, the selective PDE4 inhibitor BAY 19-8004 reduced mucus hypersecretion, as indicated by a decrease in MUC5 mRNA expression *in vivo* [24].

Taken together, the results of these studies suggest that PDE4 inhibition has potentially far-reaching effects on inflammatory cells and pathways involved in the pathogenesis of COPD. Potential anti-inflammatory effects of PDE4 inhibition are likely to account, at least in part, for the clinical efficacy and therapeutic benefits increasingly reported in clinical trials of PDE4 inhibitor therapy in patients with COPD and other inflammatory diseases of the airways.

Non-selective PDE inhibitors

Theophylline

The methylxanthine theophylline (3,7-dihydro-1,3-dimethyl-1H-purine-2,6-dione), has been used as a bronchodilator in patients with COPD for decades (Fig. 59.3a) [37–44]. Theophylline acts non-selectively through inhibition of all major PDE isozymes and adenosine receptor antagonism, and has broad activity in animal models and in patients with COPD [45]. Theophylline exhibits a narrow therapeutic index, with a concentration of more than 50 μM

required to inhibit PDEs in airway smooth muscles (bronchodilatation) [45,46], and therefore has modest activity as a primary bronchodilator. In addition, theophylline inhibits the activation of some key inflammatory cells *in vitro*; however, concentrations required are greater than those that could likely be achieved therapeutically in patients [47]. Thus, the contribution of these latter effects to the clinical efficacy of theophylline is still under debate.

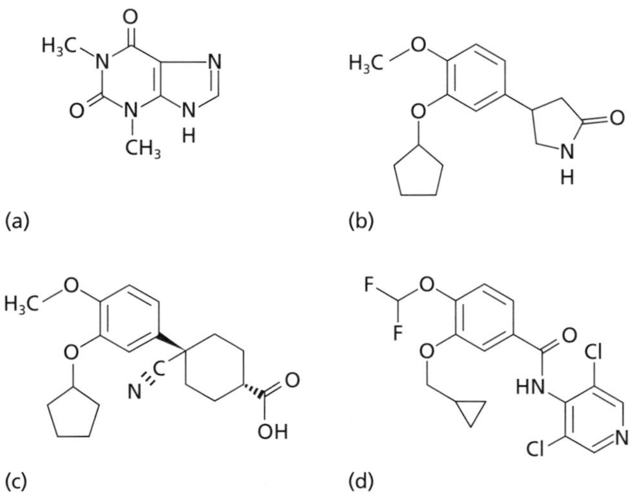

Theophylline at concentrations as low as 1 μM, i.e. well within the therapeutic range have recently been reported to restore the reduced HDAC activity and responsiveness to glucocorticoids that is observed in macrophages from smokers with COPD [48]. Theophylline exhibits variable interpatient pharmacokinetics and, consequently, drug levels are difficult to predict and drug blood level monitoring is required. Oral formulations exhibit a slow onset of action and sustained-release formulations are preferred because they provide more predictable pharmacokinetics [49]. Theophylline also exhibits a variety of drug interactions, limiting its usefulness in a patient population with a variety of comorbidities.

Although variable effects on exercise tolerance and clinical symptoms (e.g. dyspnoea) have been reported [40,43], theophylline is only recommended as third-line therapy in the treatment of COPD. However, a meta-analysis did not recommend theophylline in the treatment of COPD exacerbations [50]. Further, because of its non-selective inhibition of PDEs, adenosine receptor antagonism, stimulation of calcium mobilization, and inhibition of phosphoinositide 3-kinase, theophylline is associated with a high incidence of side-effects within its therapeutic range. For example, serious side-effects such as cardiac arrhythmias and seizures have been associated with non-selective adenosine receptor antagonism [38,51]. Because of the limited value of theophylline formulations in patients with COPD, researchers have focused on PDE4 inhibitors with improved therapeutic ratios and safety profiles.

(a)   (b)

(c)   (d)

Figure 59.3 Chemical structures of: (a) the non-selective inhibitor theophylline; (b) the first-generation phosphodiesterase 4 (PDE4) inhibitor rolipram, and the selective PDE4 inhibitors; (c) cilomilast; and (d) roflumilast (b–d). (Adapted from PharmaPress Ltd and Martin [37] with permission.)

Selective PDE4 inhibitors

Rolipram

Rolipram (4-[3-cyclopentyloxy-4-methoxyphenyl]-2-pyrrolidinone) is an archetypal PDE4 inhibitor that exhibits a multitude of biological effects, including anti-inflammatory activities (see Fig. 59.3b) [37,52,53]. Because of its ability to cross the blood–brain barrier, this agent was initially investigated in the treatment of depression [53–55]. Rolipram is selective for PDE4 and does not appreciably inhibit PDE 1, 2, 3 or 5 [7]. The PDE4 enzyme exists in at least two conformations, with rolipram selectivity for these two conformations differing by more than 100-fold

[56]. To distinguish these two types of rolipram selectivity, investigators have identified these two conformations as either the high-affinity rolipram binding site (HARBS) or the low-affinity rolipram binding site (LARBS) [57]. The high-affinity interaction with rolipram and PDE4 is thought to be related to the presence of metal cofactors (e.g. Mg^{2+}) located in the active site of PDE4 [58,59]. Preferential binding to the HARBS has been suspected to be responsible for central nervous system (e.g. nausea and emesis) and cardiovascular effects.

Because of its ability to inhibit pulmonary eosinophilia, airway inflammation, oedema and airway hyperreactivity *in vitro* and in animal models [18,60–65], rolipram was investigated as a potential treatment for asthma. However, it exhibited a low therapeutic ratio and unfavourable side-effect profile, including nausea and emesis thought to be linked to its high affinity binding to the HARBS conformation, thereby restricting its therapeutic utility [66,67]. Therefore, safety issues, including dose-limiting gastro-intestinal adverse events, stopped clinical development of rolipram. Despite its failure as a clinically useful agent in the treatment of inflammatory airway diseases, rolipram is currently valued as a standard or control agent for *in vitro* and preclinical studies with newer, more selective PDE4 inhibitors. The remainder of the chapter focuses on the only two PDE4 inhibitors in late-stage clinical development in the treatment of COPD: cilomilast and roflumilast.

Cilomilast

Cilomilast (SB 207499; *cis*-4-cyano-4-[3-(cyclopentyloxy)-4-methoxy-phenyl]cyclohexanecarboxylic acid) is a PDE4 inhibitor that was originally under clinical investigation in the treatment of asthma, but development for this indication was discontinued because of poor efficacy (see Fig. 59.3c) [37]. Cilomilast is selective for PDE4 and does not appreciably inhibit PDE1, 2, 3 or 5 at concentrations ≤ 10 μM [68]. Of the four isoforms in the PDE4 family, cilomilast is approximately 10-fold more selective for PDE4D than the other three isoforms (PDE4A, B and C) [69]. For example, the IC_{50} of cilomilast is 13 nM for PDE4D, compared with the next highest selectivity of 120 nM for PDE4B [69]. In addition, cilomilast has approximately equal affinity for the two conformations of PDE4, LARBS and HARBS, whereas rolipram has a 60-fold greater affinity (i.e. lower IC_{50}) for the HARBS conformation (Table 59.1) [68]. This results in a higher cilomilast selectivity for the preferred PDE4 conformation, LARBS, and has translated into an improved therapeutic ratio compared with rolipram.

Preclinical and human *ex vivo* data

Several studies in animal models and human samples have

Table 59.1 Phosphodiesterase 4 inhibitor affinity for phosphodiesterase 4 conformations. (Data from Christensen *et al.* [68].)

Agent	IC_{50}, nM		LARBS/HARBS ratio
	LARBS	**HARBS**	
Rolipram	300	5	60
Cilomilast	95	120	0.8

HARBS, high-affinity rolipram binding site; IC_{50}, 50% inhibitory concentration; LARBS, low-affinity rolipram binding site.

investigated the anti-inflammatory potential of cilomilast in the treatment of COPD. Dose-dependent inhibition of LPS-induced pulmonary inflammation has been reported in a rat model of pulmonary neutrophilia, and attenuation of pulmonary neutrophilia and oedema has been observed in a guinea pig model of pulmonary neutrophilia [70,71]. In a human monocyte adoptive transfer model, 50 mg/kg oral cilomilast inhibited LPS-stimulated TNF-α production by 79% compared with vehicle [72]. This was similar to the level of inhibition by rolipram and has been confirmed in other studies [73].

Studies have also indicated that cilomilast was comparably potent with rolipram to inhibit fMLP-induced neutrophil degranulation, however maximum inhibition was modest with approximately 30% [73,74]. Further, bronchial epithelial and sputum cells were obtained from patients with moderate COPD or from normal controls and were cultured for 24 h in the presence or absence of 1 μM cilomilast (final concentration determined by a series of dose–response curves) [75]. Cilomilast reduced TNF-α release in both bronchial epithelial and sputum cells ($P = 0.005$), suppressed GM-CSF release in sputum cells ($P = 0.003$), but did not significantly inhibit IL-8 secretion.

Fibroblast accumulation is thought to have a role in the fibrosis of small airways, and has been associated with airway lumen narrowing. The activity of cilomilast was tested in two *in vitro* models of tissue remodelling: a model of recruitment of fibroblasts to sites of ongoing fibrosis and a model of the wound repair process that in the airway directly leads to airway narrowing [16]. Cilomilast 10 μM inhibited human fetal lung fibroblast chemotaxis toward the chemoattractant fibronectin to 40.5 ± 7.3% ($P < 0.05$) of control. The PDE4 inhibitor also significantly inhibited fibroblast-mediated type I collagen gel contraction reflected by an approximately 1.7-fold increase in collagen gel size with 10 μM cilomilast compared to control.

In another study, which used the three-dimensional type I collagen gel culture system with human fetal lung fibroblasts incubated with TNF-α (to induce matrix metalloproteinases [MMPs]) and neutrophil elastase (to activate MMPs), cilomilast inhibited the degradation of the collagen matrix secondary to suppressing MMP-1 and MMP-9 release and MMP-1 activation [76]. In view of recent evidence that neutrophil elastase (NE) triggers oxidant stress (77) and activates EGFR and downstream signalling [78] in lung fibroblasts that by inference are linked through MMP activation as this cascade is well-described in airway epithelial cells one may postulate that the PDE4 inhibitor restricts MMP activation by reducing NE-induced oxygen radical formation.

In addition to animal and *in vitro* models, patients have been tested for the ability of cilomilast to mitigate inflammatory pathways in the lung. In a 12-week study designed to measure the anti-inflammatory effects of cilomilast, patients ($n = 59$) with moderate COPD were randomized to receive 15 mg cilomilast twice daily (b.i.d.) or placebo [26]. Induced sputum differential cell counts were obtained at baseline; weeks 1, 2, 4, 8, 10 and 12; and 7–10 days after study completion; and bronchial biopsies were obtained at baseline and week 10. Cilomilast did not alter neutrophil elastase and IL-8 concentrations or result in significant changes from baseline in percentage of sputum neutrophils during treatment. However, Poisson regression analysis showed a significant ($P < 0.01$) reduction of 48% for $CD8^+$ T-lymphocyte subsets and a significant ($P = 0.001$) reduction of 47% for $CD68^+$ macrophages compared with placebo. Although not powered to show changes in pulmonary function, there was no cilomilast treatment-related effect on forced expiratory volume in 1 s (FEV_1). Overall, these data suggest that cilomilast has the potential to exert anti-inflammatory effects *in vivo*.

Pharmacokinetics

The pharmacokinetics of intravenous and oral administration of cilomilast has been evaluated in 16 healthy men [79]. Two separate experiments were performed in volunteers receiving 4 mg cilomilast by intravenous administration over 1 h or a single 15-mg oral dose (Table 59.2) [79]. Similar pharmacokinetic profiles were observed with the two modes of administration, with dose-dependent pharmacokinetics and a low cilomilast clearance rate. A half-life of approximately 8 h suggested that cilomilast b.i.d. dosing would be an appropriate regimen for further clinical studies. Cilomilast also had a high oral bioavailability, with a mean absolute bioavailability of 103% (95% confidence interval [CI], 98–109%) for a 15-mg tablet. The dose linearity of oral cilomilast up to 15 mg b.i.d. has also been confirmed in a randomized placebo-controlled dose-ranging study [80]. Because pharmacokinetics and oral bioavailability can be affected by time of administration and coadministration with other medications, several studies were conducted to determine potential pharmacokinetic alterations for cilomilast and other medications.

The effect of food absorption on cilomilast bioavailability was evaluated in 28 healthy volunteers who were administered two single 15-mg oral doses of cilomilast: 1 dose after a 10-h overnight fast and 1 dose 5 min after a high-fat breakfast (see Table 59.2) [79]. Overall, data suggested that coadministration with food did not affect cilomilast bioavailability. In addition, neither coadministration of an antacid [79] nor timing (morning or evening) of drug administration (see Table 59.2) [79] appreciably affected the pharmacokinetics of cilomilast.

Pharmacodynamic studies in healthy volunteers indicated no significant drug interactions between cilomilast and digoxin, erythromycin, salbutamol, theophylline or warfarin [81–85]. In renally impaired patients, the half-life and unbound cilomilast area under the curve (AUC) increased progressively with increasing renal impairment because of decreases in unbound cilomilast clearance and plasma protein binding [86]. In addition, renal clearance of the active metabolite of cilomilast decreased with increasing renal impairment, with the unbound AUC ratio of the metabolite to cilomilast in severe renal impairment (creatinine clearance less than 30 mL/min) twice that observed in healthy volunteers. The investigators recommended that cilomilast not be administered to patients with severe renal impairment.

Efficacy in COPD

The efficacy of cilomilast has been investigated in a number of clinical studies. A 6-week placebo-controlled dose-ranging trial was conducted to determine the efficacy, safety and dose–response of cilomilast in patients with COPD [87]. Patients ($n = 424$) were randomized to receive 5, 10 or 15 mg cilomilast b.i.d. or matching placebo for 6 weeks. A total of 355 patients completed the study. Only patients treated at the highest dose level experienced consistent improvements in both prebronchodilator and postbronchodilator pulmonary function tests. Patients treated with 15 mg cilomilast b.i.d. had a significantly greater increase in mean trough prebronchodilator FEV_1 compared with placebo at week 6 ($P < 0.0001$) [87]. At week 6, there were also significant improvements in mean postbronchodilator FEV_1 ($P < 0.0096$), prebronchodilator forced vital capacity (FVC; $P = 0.001$) and peak expiratory flow rate ($P < 0.0001$) compared with placebo. However, there were no significant differences between placebo and the three dose levels of cilomilast in quality of life measures from the St. George's Respiratory Questionnaire (SGRQ).

Four pivotal, randomized double-blind placebo-controlled parallel-group phase III studies ($n = 647–825$ per study) were conducted to determine the efficacy of cilomilast in patients with COPD that was poorly reversible ($\leq 15\%$ or

Table 59.2 Mean pharmacokinetic parameters for cilomilast. (Adapted from Zussman *et al.* [79] with permission.)

Parameter	Route* IV (*n* = 16)	Route* Oral (*n* = 15)	Food status† Fasted (*n* = 28)	Food status† Fed (*n* = 28)	Food status† Point estimate (90% CI)	Time of administration‡ Morning (*n* = 24)	Time of administration‡ Evening (*n* = 24)	Time of administration‡ Point estimate (95% CI)
C_{max}, µg/L (SD)	385 (88)	1113 (229)	1510 (259)	930 (220)	0.61§ (0.55–0.67)	881 (262)	849 (249)	0.97 (0.84–1.11)
T_{max}, h (range)	NR	1.50¶ (1.00–4.02)	1.76# (0.5–3.03)	4.00# (1.00–11.07)	2.13# (1.48–3.00)	3.66¶ (0.50–8.03)	3.50¶ (1.02–8.00)	0** (−1.01–1.00)
$AUC_{0-\infty}$, µg/h/L (SD)	2236 (551)††	8644 (2103)	11 274 (2579)	10 813 (2789)	0.95§ (0.91–0.99)	9385 (2496)	8299 (1986)	0.89 (0.84–0.94)
$t_{1/2}$, h (SD)	7.95 (1.94)	8.14 (1.63)	7.17 (1.64)	7.24 (1.29)	NR	7.54 (1.35)	6.73 (1.11)	−0.81‡‡ (−1.13–0.49)
CL, L/h (SD)	1.94 (0.49)	NR	NR	NR	NR	NR	NR	NR
V_{ss}, L (SD)	16.5 (3.3)	NR	NR	NR	NR	NR	NR	NR

* Cilomilast 4 mg intravenous dose infused over 1 h or cilomilast 15 mg oral dose administered while fasting.

† Two single 15-mg oral doses of cilomilast; one dose administered after a 10-h overnight fast and one dose administered 5 min after a high-fat breakfast.

‡ Two single 15-mg oral doses of cilomilast; one dose administered at approximately 8:30 a.m., 10 min after a meal, and one dose administered at approximately 8:30 p.m., 10 min after a meal.

§ Geometric mean ratio (fed/fasted).

¦ Geometric mean ratio (evening/morning).

¶ Data are median (range).

Data are median (range), median difference (fed–fasted) and 95% CI.

** Median difference (evening–morning).

†† *n* = 15.

‡‡ Mean difference (evening–morning).

$AUC_{0-\infty}$, area under the concentration–time curve from 0 to infinity; C_{max}, maximum (plasma) concentration; CI, confidence interval; CL, total (plasma) clearance; IV, intravenous; NR, not reported; SD, standard deviation; T_{max}, time to C_{max}; $t_{1/2}$, half-life; V_{ss}, volume of distribution at steady state.

≤ 200 mL) by albuterol [88,89]. Patients were treated with 15 mg cilomilast b.i.d. or placebo b.i.d. for 24 weeks after a 4-week single-blind run-in period. A primary endpoint in these studies was the change from baseline in trough FEV_1.

Only two of the four studies demonstrated a significant change from baseline in trough FEV_1 at study endpoint versus placebo (Fig. 59.4) [88,89]. Three of the four studies showed only a 30–40 mL improvement (i.e. mean change from baseline) in FEV_1 for patients treated with cilomilast. In addition, there was a decline in placebo trough FEV_1 for three of the four trials, particularly during the first few weeks of the study, which could not be adequately explained by investigators. Based on the data, cilomilast did not substantially improve lung function but appeared to delay a decline in (i.e. maintained) lung function (see Fig. 59.4) [88]. However on 5 September 2003, the Pulmonary-Allergy Drugs Advisory Committee of the US Food and Drug Administration stated that one could not draw this conclusion based on the short duration (6 months) of the study. Therefore, this committee did not recommend

approval of cilomilast for the maintenance of lung function (FEV_1) and recommended that longer term studies (e.g. 1 year) be conducted.

Reports from one of the pivotal phase III studies noted significant improvements in several lung function parameters, such as FVC ($P = 0.001$) and trough 25–75% forced expiratory flow ($P = 0.003$) in patients treated with cilomilast compared with placebo [90,91]. In addition to improvement in lung function, the risk of a patient experiencing ≥ 1 COPD exacerbation (i.e. self-treated, physician intervention or hospitalization) was reduced by 44% ($P = 0.0001$) [92]. For any exacerbation, 74% of patients treated with cilomilast were exacerbation-free compared with 62% of patients treated with placebo ($P = 0.0077$).

For the four pivotal phase III studies, the change from baseline in total score of the SGRQ was a primary efficacy variable in addition to the change from baseline in trough FEV_1. However, only one (Study 039) of the four studies demonstrated a statistically significant and minimal clinically meaningful (more than 4-point change) improvement

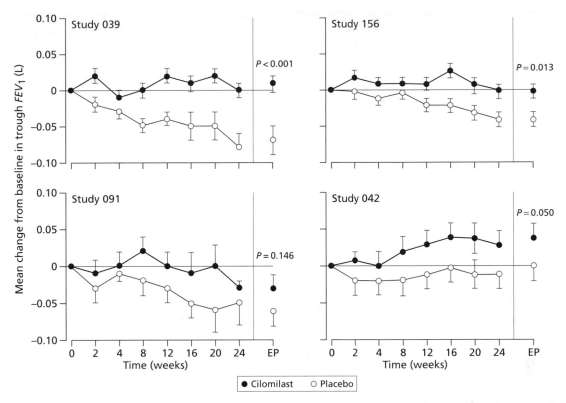

Figure 59.4 Mean change from baseline in trough forced expiratory volume in 1 s (FEV_1) with 15 mg cilomilast twice daily (b.i.d.) versus placebo for four pivotal randomized double-blind phase III trials. EP, endpoint. (Adapted from US Food and Drug Administration [88].)

in SGRQ total score [89]. In addition, this study noted significant improvements at the study endpoint for Short Form-36 scores for physical function ($P = 0.017$) and general health perceptions ($P = 0.02$) compared with placebo treatment [90].

A prospective analysis was also conducted to determine health-care utilization in patients treated with 15 mg cilomilast b.i.d. ($n = 431$) versus placebo ($n = 216$) during one of the pivotal 6-month double-blind trials [93]. Cilomilast was associated with significantly ($P = 0.004$) less cumulative health-care resource utilization (11.0% versus 21.1% for placebo), including physician visits ($P = 0.002$), emergency room visits ($P = 0.004$) and hospitalizations ($P = 0.021$).

Safety in COPD

Cilomilast was generally well tolerated in a series of phase II and III studies. In a dose-ranging study, the most common drug-related adverse event was nausea, reported in 1%, 1%, 12% and 11% of patients in the placebo, 5, 10 and 15 mg dose groups, respectively [87]. The most common serious adverse event was COPD exacerbation. In addition, the most common reason for withdrawal from the study was respiratory disorder, which occurred more often in the placebo ($n = 6$) and 5 mg cilomilast ($n = 6$) dose groups. Overall, there was no cilomilast dose-related trend or signi-

ficant difference in incidence versus placebo for any serious adverse event.

A pooled analysis of 6-month phase III studies indicated that, collectively, gastrointestinal adverse events were the most common complication, reported more often in patients treated with cilomilast compared with placebo (Table 59.3) [94]. For example, nausea was reported in 12% of 1374 patients treated with cilomilast compared with 4% of 684 patients treated with placebo. In addition, diarrhoea, abdominal pain, dyspepsia and vomiting were also reported more frequently in patients treated with cilomilast compared with placebo (see Table 59.3) [94]. Gastrointestinal adverse events were generally self-limited and were mild to moderate in intensity. However, gastrointestinal adverse events were the most frequent reason for discontinuations because of adverse events [89]. Cilomilast preferentially binds PDE4D, and animal studies have suggested that preferential inhibition of PDE4D may account for side-effects such as vomiting [95].

Roflumilast

Roflumilast (3-cyclopropylmethoxy-4-difluoromethoxy-N-[3,5-dichloropyridyl-4-yl]-benzamide) [96] is a PDE4 inhibitor currently in phase III clinical development for

Table 59.3 Cilomilast: most frequently reported adverse events. (Adapted from Compton *et al.* [94] with permission.)

Adverse event	Patients, n (%)	
	Cilomilast ($n = 1374$)	Placebo ($n = 684$)
COPD exacerbation	422 (30.7)	266 (38.9)
Diarrhoea	175 (12.7)	41 (6.0)
Nausea	172 (12.5)	28 (4.1)
Abdominal pain	157 (11.4)	39 (5.7)
Upper respiratory tract infection	111 (8.1)	51 (7.5)
Headache	101 (7.4)	43 (6.3)
Dyspepsia	83 (6.0)	17 (2.5)
Vomiting	76 (5.5)	7 (1.0)

COPD, Chronic obstructive pulmonary disease.

the treatment of COPD and asthma (see Fig. 59.3d) [37]. Compared with cilomilast and rolipram, roflumilast has more than 100-fold higher potency in inhibiting PDE4, as reflected by IC_{50} values of 0.8 nM for roflumilast versus 120 nM for cilomilast and 210 nM for rolipram [7]. *In vivo*, roflumilast is metabolized to roflumilast N-oxide. Both the potent PDE4 inhibition ($IC_{50} = 2$ nM) and selectivity of roflumilast are preserved by roflumilast N-oxide. Because of its long half-life, the active metabolite substantially contributes to the overall clinical efficacy of roflumilast.

Preclinical and *in vitro* data

Evidence from *in vitro* and *in vivo* studies supports the broad anti-inflammatory activity of roflumilast because its target, PDE4, is widely expressed in cells involved in inflammation. The potency of roflumilast and its active metabolite, roflumilast N-oxide, has been demonstrated in many *in vitro* cell models. Half-maximum inhibition values in the lower nanomolar range suppressed human cell functions (Table 59.4) [7] and corresponded well to inhibition of PDE4 activity in a cell-free system. The maximum efficacy attained with a PDE4 inhibitor in functional cell-based assays *in vitro* is dictated by the additional expression of PDE families other than PDE4. In addition, a threshold cAMP concentration is a prerequisite for the activity of a PDE4 inhibitor. Neutrophils, eosinophils and monocytes isolated from human peripheral blood almost exclusively express PDE4. As a consequence, maximum inhibition (efficacy) by roflumilast or roflumilast N-oxide of LPS-induced TNF-α synthesis in monocytes is approximately 80%, and complete inhibition of fMLP-stimulated LTB_4 synthesis from neutrophils is observed.

Macrophages for preclinical studies are obtained by *in vitro* differentiation of monocytes incubated in human AB serum for several days. This transition to monocyte-derived macrophages is associated with up-regulation of genes for PDE3 and PDE1 and reduced expression of PDE4 [32]. Macrophages differentiated from monocytes in human AB serum are considered to be similar to human alveolar macrophages and, importantly, have a comparable PDE expression profile [97]. In contrast to monocytes, a PDE4 inhibitor alone has virtually no effect on LPS-induced TNF-α generation in monocyte-derived macrophages. Even at a concentration of 10 nM prostaglandin E_2 (PGE_2) to stimulate cAMP formation, the maximum inhibition attained with PDE4 inhibitors was only 20%. In addition,

Table 59.4 Inhibition of inflammatory activities by phosphodiesterase 4 inhibitors. (Adapted with permission from Hatzelmann *et al.* [7].)

Cell type	Measured parameter	IC value, nM	Roflumilast	Roflumilast N-oxide	Cilomilast	Rolipram
Neutrophil	ROS	IC_{35}	4	8	60	20
	LTB_4	IC_{50}	2	5	40	11
Monocyte	TNF-α	IC_{40}	21	17	1300	330
Macrophage	TNF-α	IC_{35}	13	12	130	10
DC	TNF-α	IC_{20}	5	4	200	40
$CD4^+$ T cell	Proliferation	IC_{30}	7	10	900	330
	IL-2	IC_{20}	1	1	400	200
	IL-4	IC_{30}	7	3	1300	600
	IL-5	IC_{25}	13	6	3000	500
	IFN-γ	IC_{35}	8	3	700	130

Values indicate the concentrations at which half-maximum concentrations were achieved.

DC, dendritic cell; IC, inhibitory concentration; IL, interleukin; IFN-γ, γ-interferon; LTB_4, leukotriene B_4; ROS, reactive oxygen species; TNF-α, tumour necrosis factor α.

concomitant inhibition of PDE3 did not augment the efficacy of PDE4 inhibitors. However, in the presence of both 1 μM motapizone to inhibit PDE3 and 10 nM PGE_2 to stimulate cAMP formation, roflumilast concentration-dependently suppressed LPS-induced TNF-α formation to a maximum of approximately 70%. These results reflect additional PDE3 expression and subthreshold baseline cAMP synthesis in macrophages. Under these experimental conditions, the administration of a PDE3 inhibitor in the presence of a cAMP-generating system enables the PDE4 inhibitor to suppress LPS-induced TNF-α synthesis [32,97].

How might these findings translate to the clinical situation in COPD? Activated macrophages in distal airways produce mediators such as TNF-α, MMP-12, ROS and LTB_4 that may orchestrate inflammation and remodelling in COPD. For example, mice deficient in macrophage elastase (MMP-12) were not susceptible to cigarette smoke-induced emphysema [98]. Importantly, transgenic pulmonary expression of constitutive or inducible TNF-α was associated with characteristics of emphysema (e.g. alveolar airspace enlargement) [99,100]. In inducible TNF-α transgenic mice, macrophage metalloelastase (MMP-12) mRNA was enhanced, and increased numbers of $CD8^+$ T cells were observed in the lung parenchyma [100]. Conversely, TNF-α receptor deficient mice did not exhibit an acute cigarette smoke-induced increase in neutrophils and macrophages (obtained by bronchoalveolar lavage) or markers of connective tissue breakdown, such as desmosine or hydroxyproline [101]. Data from a recent study [102] indicated that TNF-α levels might determine the extent of neutrophilic airway infiltration via up-regulation of E-selectin in endothelial cells. In addition, alveolar macrophages exposed to cigarette smoke *in vitro* produced substantial amounts of TNF-α [102]. Cigarette smoke also contains bioactive amounts of LPS that may further contribute to macrophage TNF-α formation [103].

Overall, these data strongly support a pre-eminent role for macrophage-produced TNF-α in the different manifestations of COPD. Although ineffective by itself, a PDE4 inhibitor such as roflumilast strongly suppresses LPS-induced TNF-α generation in the presence of PGE_2 if PDE3 activity is blocked. In COPD patients, an increase in exhaled PGE_2 levels was shown [104] and probably reflects elevated prostaglandin generation in airway cells. In fact, there are many cellular sources of up-regulated PGE_2 associated with lung inflammation [105], including fibroblasts [106], smooth muscle cells [107] and alveolar macrophages [108].

Expression of inducible nitric oxide synthase (iNOS) was increased in cells such as neutrophils or macrophages recovered from induced sputum of patients with COPD [109]. Human macrophages express NO-sensitive guanylyl cyclase [110], and up-regulated NO generation in COPD may increase cGMP levels in pulmonary macrophages. cGMP is a strong inhibitor of PDE3 activity and, therefore,

iNOS-derived NO might translate into PDE3 inhibition in endogenous macrophages. Taken together, it may be hypothesized that excessive cellular activation and infiltration within the small airways of patients with COPD create clinically relevant PGE_2 concentrations and PDE3 inhibition, thus allowing potent suppression of human lung macrophage TNF-α generation by roflumilast. The presence of PGE_2 or other mediators in COPD may further up-regulate PDE4 activity in the lung macrophages. In fact, it is well known that PDE4 is subject to extensive regulation on both the transcriptional and post-transcriptional levels [111]. For example, in human monocytes LPS enhances PDE4B2 expression [112]. Such increased levels of PDE4 may then further accentuate the efficacy of a PDE4 inhibitor.

Contrary to the situation in the small airways in patients with COPD, roflumilast may have little effect on macrophages in larger airways, and this may be advantageous given the role of macrophages in host defence. In addition, at least in asthma, the relative resistance of macrophages toward PDE4 inhibitors might be considered favourable because a subpopulation of immunosuppressive alveolar macrophages has been shown to inhibit bronchial T-cell reactivity [113].

The ability of roflumilast to interfere with $CD4^+$ T-cell proliferation and cytokine generation has been investigated [7]. $CD4^+$ T cells were purified from human peripheral blood using an immunomagnetic procedure. Cells were then preincubated with various PDE4 inhibitors and co-stimulated with anti-CD3 (0.3 μg/well) and anti-CD28 (3 μg/mL) for 72 h. As a surrogate of proliferation, incorporation of [^{3}H]-thymidine was assessed during the final 18 h of incubation. Cytokine levels from culture supernatants were also measured after the incubation period. Roflumilast and roflumilast N-oxide suppressed [^{3}H]-thymidine incorporation and inhibited production of IL-2, IL-4 and IFN-γ, with half-maximum efficacy values between 1 and 8 nmol. Maximum inhibition (efficacy) by roflumilast ranged from 40% for IL-2 synthesis to 70% for IFN-γ formation.

Previous studies have shown that the PDE4 inhibitor rolipram reduced anti-CD3/anti-CD28-induced IL-13 formation by human T cells by up to 40% [114]. Resting $CD4^+$ T cells primarily express PDE4 and PDE3, but also express PDE7 [4,97]. Co-stimulation with anti-CD3/anti-CD28 induced novel expression of PDE1B protein [114]. In the presence of a PDE3 inhibitor, which by itself has little effect, the efficacy of a PDE4 inhibitor in suppressing T-cell functions was increased, reflecting the functional role of the additionally expressed PDE3 [4,115]. Thus, the incomplete inhibition of $CD4^+$ T-cell functions by PDE4 inhibitors indicates that other PDE isozymes may also contribute to cAMP regulation in relevant subcellular compartments of T lymphocytes. The T cells that were co-stimulated with anti-CD3/anti-CD28 responded with a rapid and transient increase in PDE4 activity [114] that was insensitive to cycloheximide or actinomycin D. The increased PDE4 activity may originate in a recruitment of PDE4B2 to the CD3–T-cell receptor (TCR) complex after CD3 ligation that is associated with tyrosine phosphorylation of this PDE4 splicing variant [116]. Stimulation of human T cells stably transfected with a tetracycline-sensitive PDE4B2 construct by activated antigen-presenting cells rapidly up-regulated tetracycline-triggered PDE4 activity. This was associated with recruitment to the lipid raft membrane microdomains close to the immunological synapse. These PDE4B2-transfected cells generated greater amounts of IL-2 after specific antigen stimulation compared with wild type lymphocytes [117], supporting findings that PDE4 inhibitors such as roflumilast reduce IL-2 synthesis.

These data provide conclusive evidence that recruitment of PDE4B2 to the TCR complex – and its subsequent activation – alleviates T-cell activation induced by specific antigen presentation. This is probably based on down-regulation of cAMP within the lipid raft subcellular signalling complex. It may be inferred that PDE4 inhibitors, by targeting the enzyme in its strategic position near the TCR, increase cAMP levels in the lipid raft signalling complex and result in efficient reduction of T-cell activation. Long-term transcriptional regulation of PDE4 by cAMP-generating systems has been described in human T cells. Incubation with fenoterol or 8-bromo-cAMP for several hours resulted in enhanced PDE4 activity, particularly PDE4D2 [118].

Up-regulation of cAMP-dependent PDE4 has been discussed as an important mechanism of heterologous desensitization to β_2-agonists. In fact, use of PDE4 inhibitors has been suggested to delay tolerance to therapeutic β_2-agonists and endogenous catecholamines or PGE$_2$ [119].

In COPD, the role of CD8$^+$ T cells has been a key focus because these cells appear to be increased both in the airway mucosa and regional lymph nodes [120]. Comparable to CD4$^+$ T cells, PDE3, PDE4 and PDE7 activities were detected in unstimulated CD8$^+$ T cells [4,97]. Roflumilast and roflumilast-N-oxide potently reduced antiCD3/antiCD28-induced granzyme B and IL-2 release from [3H] thymidine incorporation in purified human peripheral blood CD8+ T-cells with IC50 from 1–10 nM and in presence of 10 µM motapizone to block PDE3 [121].

Comparison of potencies of the PDE4 inhibitors roflumilast, roflumilast N-oxide, rolipram and cilomilast for their inhibition of monocyte and macrophage TNF-α synthesis and CD4$^+$ T-cell functions (e.g. proliferation, cytokine generation), versus inhibition of neutrophil LTB$_4$ and ROS release revealed that rolipram and cilomilast were substantially less potent inhibitors of monocytes and T lymphocytes than of neutrophils [7]. Conversely, the potencies of roflumilast and roflumilast N-oxide in suppressing monocyte, T cell, macrophage and neutrophil functions were comparable (see Table 59.4) [7]. The ability of rolipram to reduce neutrophil (IC$_{50}$ = 11 nM for LTB$_4$ and 20 nmol for ROS) and macrophage (IC$_{50}$ = 10 nM for TNF-α formation) functions was greater than for inhibition of PDE4 activity (IC$_{50}$ = 210 nM) [7]. This was not the case with roflumilast and roflumilast N-oxide, in which potency levels for inhibition of neutrophil and macrophage functions were slightly lower compared with PDE4 inhibition. Monocyte and T-cell functions, however, were attenuated with a potency corresponding to levels of inhibition of PDE4 activity by all of the PDE4 inhibitors tested.

PDE4 proteins assume at least two interconvertible conformational states, which may be distinguished by their binding of rolipram with different affinities. Association of PDE4 inhibitors with the LARBS conformation is reflected by inhibition of catalytic activity. Binding of PDE4 inhibitors to the HARBS conformation is assessed by competition assays with [^{3}H]-rolipram. For rolipram, binding to the HARBS was observed at an IC$_{50}$ of approximately 5 nM whereas inhibition of catalytic activity corresponding to the LARBS was observed at an IC$_{50}$ of approximately 120 nM [74]. Studies with various PDE4 inhibitors demonstrated that reduction of neutrophil functions correlated with the HARBS (i.e. inhibition of [^{3}H]-rolipram binding), whereas suppression of monocytes was correlated with the LARBS (i.e. inhibition of PDE4 catalysis) [74]. In addition, evidence published during the past decade indicates that interaction of compounds with the HARBS correlates with emesis and other central nervous system-related effects [122–124]. For rolipram, preferential binding to the HARBS versus the LARBS explains its more potent inhibition of neutrophil LTB$_4$ and ROS generation versus monocyte TNF-α synthesis and PDE4 catalytic activity and the early occurence of emesis. Roflumilast attenuates the above-mentioned neutrophil and monocyte functions with comparable potency. Indeed, roflumilast was shown to bind HARBS and LARBS with comparable affinity (Ki = 1.5–3 nM) [125] and this may finally allow that improvement of lung function in COPD associated with low emetic risk as observed in clinical studies with roflumilast.

The binding of cilomilast to HARBS and LARBS has been reported as approximately equal [71]. However, in our laboratory cilomilast was about 25-fold more potent in inhibiting neutrophil LTB$_4$ or ROS generation than monocyte TNF-α synthesis [7]. The preferential inhibition of PDE4D (IC50 = 4 nM) over PDE4B (IC50 = 99 nM) [126] by cilomilast might explain this finding. In contrast, roflumilast and roflumilast N-oxide inhibited PDE4A, B and D equipotently [127]. Generation of LPS-induced TNF-α appears to be governed by PDE4B, as lipopolysaccharide-induced TNF-α formation was nearly eliminated in PDE4B –/– mice [25].

Whether neutrophil ROS and LTB4 formation is primarily regulated by PDE4D over PDE4B remains to be explored.

It was shown that neutrophils exhibit PDE4D > PDE4B however, both subtypes are equally involved in neutrophil chemotaxis [128]. In summary, *in vitro* assays with inflammatory cells PDE4 reflected the higher potency of roflumilast over cilomilast to inhibit PDE4 and this was particularly marked in monocytes and T lymphocytes. In parallel, roflumilast was more potent than cilomilast to reduce LPS-induced plasma TNF-α *in vivo* (EC50 of 0.2 vs. 93 μmol/kg, respectively) [96].

Recently, the potency and efficacy of roflumilast and its active metabolite were explored in other *in vitro* and *in vivo* systems of relevance in COPD. Neutrophil studies were complemented by findings that roflumilast and roflumilast N-oxide reduced fMLP-induced degranulation (i.e. release of neutrophil elastase, MPO and MMP-9) with IC50 = 1–2 nM [129] and also CD11b presentation [130]. Considering airway epithelial cells roflumilast strongly suppressed MUC5AC mRNA and protein in cultured human bronchial slices and in A549 cells, roflumilast was more potent than cilomilast or rolipram in this respect. [34]. These data indicate that roflumilast may assist to reduce mucus overproduction in peripheral airways in COPD. Roflumilast or roflumilast N-oxide suppressed an array of functions in cell types involved in pulmonary remodelling in COPD. In human lung fibroblasts roflumilast N-oxide inhibited TNF-α induced up-regulation of ICAM-1 cell adhesion molecule and Eotaxin release with IC50 around 1–3 nM. In addition, TGFβ1 induced expression of α-smooth muscle actin, a surrogate of myofibroblast transition was reduced by roflumilast N-oxide [131]. Further, roflumilast (1 μM) reduced TGFβ1 induced chemotaxis and collagen gel contraction [132]. In human pulmonary artery smooth muscle cells roflumilast decreased [3H]thymidine incorporation triggered by PDGF with IC50 = 4.4 nM in presence of 3 nM cicaprost [133]. Human airway smooth muscle cells produce extracellular matrix proteins and roflumilast (1 μM) suppressed TGFβ-induced CTGF, collagen I and fibronectin in bronchial rings and deposition of fibronectin from bronchial smooth muscle cells [134]. Roflumilast and its N-oxide potently reduced serum-induced [3H]thymidine incorporation in these cells with IC50 = 1–3 nM [135]. *In vivo*, roflumilast at 0.1–10 μmol/kg p.o. dose-dependently inhibited leucocyte-endothelial interaction triggered by LPS as assessed by intravital microscopy in rats [130]. Importantly, roflumilast (5 mg/kg/d p.o.) prevented cigarettesmoke induced emphysema in mice in a chronic study over 7 months [136]. From these results one may hypothesize that roflumilast alleviates airway and pulmonary vascular remodelling in COPD. In summary, preclinical data suggest a therapeutic benefit of roflumilast in COPD.

Pharmacokinetics

The pharmacokinetics of intravenous and oral administration of roflumilast has been evaluated in a randomized, two-period cross-over study [137]. Twelve healthy male volunteers received a single oral dose of 500 μg and an intravenous 150 μg dose infused over a 15-min period. After infusion, the plasma concentration of roflumilast showed a rapid distribution and long apparent terminal plasma disposition half time of about 15 h. The active metabolite roflumilast N-oxide achieved a plateau-like concentration about 4 h after infusion (C_{max} at about 8 h). This concentration was maintained for several hours and declined slowly with an apparent terminal fall time of 23 h. Roflumilast N-oxide accounts for about 87% of PDE4 inhibitor exposition. Absolute bioavailability of oral 500 μg roflumilast (relative to the short-term i.v. infusion) was high with 79% [137].

A double-blind parallel-group dose-ranging study was conducted in 18 healthy volunteers to determine the pharmacokinetics of roflumilast and roflumilast N-oxide, the active metabolite of roflumilast [138]. Volunteers received 500 μg roflumilast once daily during days 1–7, 750 μg once daily during days 8–14 and 1000 μg once daily during days 15–21. Pharmacokinetic parameters for days 7, 14 and 21 are shown in Table 59.5. Roflumilast exhibited linear pharmacokinetics in the dose range of 500–1000 μg. Roflumilast and roflumilast N-oxide exhibited a prolonged half-life of approximately 15 and 20 h, respectively, providing a rationale for a once-daily dosing regimen. Roflumilast was well tolerated at all dose levels tested. From the AUC values obtained after repeated dosing over 7 days it is obvious that roflumilast N-oxide accounted for > 90% of PDE4 inhibitor exposition. Considering binding to human plasma proteins for roflumilast and roflumilast-N-oxide being 98.9% and 96.6%, respectively, the pharmacokinetic profile at day 7 following repeated dosing with 500 μg once daily roflumilast as currently used in clinical trials reveals plasma concentrations of 1–2 nM unbound roflumilast-N-oxide within the dosing periods. At these concentrations PDE4 activity and numerous cellular functions are inhibited by approximately 50%.

Concomitant drug administration and time of administration were investigated to determine potential pharmacokinetic alterations for roflumilast and other medications. The effect of food intake on the pharmacokinetics of roflumilast and roflumilast N-oxide was evaluated in a two-period cross-over study [139]. Twelve healthy volunteers received a single 500-μg oral dose of roflumilast in a fasted state and after a high-fat breakfast [139]. Similar to findings with cilomilast [79], point estimates (test/reference ratios for maximum concentration [C_{max}]) indicated that a high-fat meal reduced the absorption. The point estimate for C_{max} for roflumilast was 0.59 (90% CI, 0.49–0.70) and was 0.95 (90% CI, 0.90–1.01) for roflumilast N-oxide. This indicated that C_{max} was reduced for roflumilast but not for the active

Table 59.5 Geometric mean pharmacokinetic parameters for roflumilast. (Data from Bethke *et al.* [138].)

Parameter	Oral multiple dose* Roflumilast			Roflumilast N-oxide		
	500 µg (*n* = 18)	750 µg (*n* = 18)	1000 µg (*n* = 18)	500 µg (*n* = 18)	750 µg (*n* = 18)	1000 µg (*n* = 18)
C_{max}, µg/L (68% range)	4.7 (3.7–6.1)	8.2 (6.0–11.0)	11.1 (8.3–15.0)	20.7 (17.2–24.8)	33.7 (27.3–41.7)	50.6 (43.7–58.5)
$AUC_{0-\infty}$, µg/h/L (68% range)	32.6 (24.0–44.4)	50.8 (36.9–70.0)	65.9 (49.5–87.8)	347.2 (284.7–423.3)	587.3 (462.3–746.2)	799.9 (638.5–1002.1)
$t_{1/2}$, h (68% range)	14.3 (10.05–21.75)	13.7 (12.38–19.90)	14.7 (9.0–22.8)	NR (8.7–21.7)	NR (10.4–20.7)	19.6 (15.1–25.6)

* Dose-escalation study of 7-day dose regimen for each dose with pharmacokinetic parameter measurements on day 7 for each dose.
$AUC_{0-\infty}$, area under the concentration–time curve from 0 to infinity; C_{max}, maximum plasma concentration; IV, intravenous; NR, not reported; $t_{1/2}$, half-life.

metabolite. The point estimate for AUC for roflumilast was 1.12 (90% CI, 1.00–1.25) and was 0.91 (90% CI, 0.79–1.04) for roflumilast N-oxide, indicating that AUC values for roflumilast and the active metabolite were not affected by food intake. Therefore, administration of roflumilast with or without food did not affect the bioavailability of roflumilast or roflumilast N-oxide.

Potential influences of time of administration on pharmacokinetic parameters were evaluated in a two-period cross-over study conducted in 16 healthy volunteers who received a single oral dose of 500 µg roflumilast in the morning or in the evening [140]. During the first 12-h time period after drug administration, the pharmacokinetics of roflumilast varied between morning and evening administration with regard to C_{max} (marginally lower with evening dosing) and time to C_{max} (slightly longer with evening dosing). In contrast, AUC did not differ between the times of administration, suggesting that exposure to roflumilast and roflumilast N-oxide was unaffected. Overall, the time of roflumilast administration (morning or evening) did not significantly influence the pharmacokinetics of roflumilast or roflumilast N-oxide.

Pharmacodynamic studies in healthy volunteers have also indicated no effect of smoking status on the pharmacokinetics of roflumilast and roflumilast N-oxide [141]. Furthermore, no relevant drug interactions between roflumilast and budesonide, salbutamol or warfarin have been observed [141–144]. A study of 12 patients with severe renal impairment (creatinine clearance ≥ 10 and ≤ 30 mL/min) and 12 healthy control-matched volunteers found no statistically significant difference in pharmacokinetic characteristics between the two groups [145]. In contrast to cilomilast, no dose adjustment for roflumilast is expected to be required in patients with severe renal impairment.

Efficacy and safety of COPD

Preliminary clinical phase II data suggested that roflumilast could improve lung function in patients with COPD while being well tolerated [146,147].

The efficacy and safety of roflumilast have been further investigated in a large phase III double-blind dose-ranging parallel-group study [148]. Patients with moderate to severe COPD were randomized to receive placebo (*n* = 280), oral roflumilast 250 µg (*n* = 576) or 500 µg (*n* = 555) once daily for 24 weeks after an initial 4-week run-in period. Treatment with both roflumilast doses resulted in statistically significant improvements in pre- and post-bronchodilator FEV_1 (Fig. 59.5) versus placebo, with differences of 88 mL (pre-bronchodilator FEV_1) and 97 mL (post-bronchodilator FEV_1) with 500 µg roflumilast [148]. Significant improvements with roflumilast versus placebo were also seen for further lung function variables (*FVC*, FEV_6 and FEF_{25-75}, all post-bronchodilator [148]).

Roflumilast was well tolerated at both dose levels tested (Table 59.6) [148]. The incidence of adverse events was comparable between placebo (62%) and the two treatment groups (66–67%) [148]. In the 500 µg dose group, the most commonly reported gastrointestinal events were nausea and diarrhoea, occurring in 9% and 5% of patients, respectively. These adverse events were generally mild to moderate in intensity. Vomiting was rare (≤ 1%) in both dose groups and was similar to the incidence reported in patients treated with placebo. Importantly, roflumilast displayed an improved gastrointestinal side-effect profile compared with cilomilast (see Table 59.3) [94], which caused a higher incidence of gastrointestinal adverse events (e.g. 12.5% for nausea). Roflumilast and its N-oxide show no preference for the PDE4 D-subtype and no preference for the HARBS [125] which may explain why roflumilast

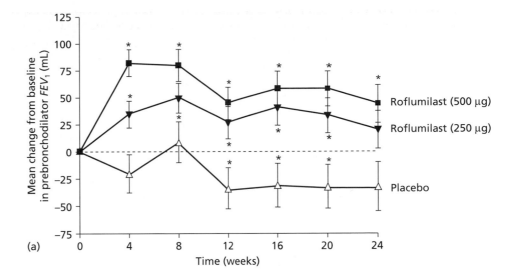

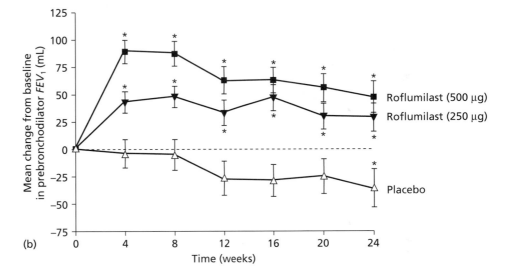

Figure 59.5 Mean change from baseline in pre-bronchodilator (a) and post-bronchodilator (b) forced expiratory volume in 1 s (FEV_1) with roflumilast 250 or 500 µg once daily. Data are least square means ± standard errors. * $p < 0.05$ versus baseline. (Adapted from Rabe *et al.* [148].)

shows a more favourable gastrointestinal safety profile compared with cilomilast.

Further data that support the promising role of roflumilast in the treatment of COPD come from a recently completed study which involved more than 1500 patients with severe to very severe COPD. In this study 500 µg oral roflumilast once daily administered for 12 months led to a significant improvement in pre- and post-bronchodilator FEV_1 [149] and resulted in fewer exacerbations in patients with very severe COPD [150] who are likely to exacerbate more frequently. Due to these promising treatment outcomes with 500 µg oral roflumilast once daily, further trials are currently underway.

Future role of PDE4 inhibitors

Currently, there is no disease-modifying (i.e. controller)

therapy available that effectively addresses the underlying pathology of COPD. In present-day practice, medications (e.g. anticholinergics and long-acting β-agonists) are administered to treat or control the symptoms of the disease. However, the anti-inflammatory activities (e.g. neutrophil, macrophage or CD8+ cell-targeted) associated with improved PDE4 inhibitors may provide an opportunity to interfere with the pathophysiology of COPD and positively influence the disease rather than solely treat the symptoms. Significant improvements in lung function, reduction in exacerbation rates and improvement in quality of life have already been demonstrated in clinical trials. In this context, selective PDE4 inhibitors will likely have an important value as first-line therapy in the treatment and management of COPD. Further studies are needed to elucidate the long-term effects of PDE4 inhibitors on the cause and progression of COPD. Future studies may also identify additional health-related benefits with the administration of PDE4

Table 59.6 Roflumilast: most frequently reported adverse events. (Adapted from Rabe *et al.* [148])

| | Patients (%) | | |
| | | Roflumilast | |
Adverse event	Placebo *n* = 280	250 µg *n* = 576	500 µg *n* = 555
COPD exacerbation*	65 (23)	135 (23)	113 (20)
Nasopharyngitis	19 (7)	42 (7)	46 (8)
Diarrhoea NOS	6 (2)	28 (5)	50 (9)
Upper respiratory tract infection	14 (5)	27 (5)	23 (4)
Nausea	2 (1)	16 (3)	27 (5)

* Only moderate and severe exacerbations were reported as adverse events.
COPD, chronic obstructive pulmonary disease; NOS, not otherwise specified.

inhibitors, particularly in combination with other once-daily maintenance therapies, such as inhaled anticholinergic drugs (e.g. tiotropium) and long-acting β-agonists.

Because the pathogenesis and clinical manifestations of COPD are not restricted to pulmonary inflammation and structural airway remodelling, the role of PDE4 inhibitors in modifying the systemic manifestations (e.g. skeletal muscle atrophy) of COPD will be of significant interest. For example, systemic oxidative stress, modifications in circulating inflammatory cells (e.g. neutrophils) and increased levels of proinflammatory cytokines (e.g. TNF-α) in the peripheral circulation have all been observed in patients with COPD [151–153]. In addition, skeletal muscle apoptosis (i.e. wasting) is also a frequently observed complication of COPD. Studies have suggested that inflammatory cytokines (e.g. TNF-α) may contribute to muscle wasting and protein loss via a nuclear factor κB-dependent pathway [153]. Further, this signalling pathway is regulated by endogenous ROS [153]. Additional studies have shown that systemic inflammation can produce iNOS in skeletal muscle, stimulating NO production [154]. These data have been supported by clinical studies [155]. Although data are lacking that explore the effects of PDE4 inhibitors on systemic inflammation and iNOS expression in skeletal muscle, *in vitro* data have shown that PDE4 inhibitors are beneficial in down-regulating cytokine-induced iNOS expression and NO production in human chondrocytes [156]. Therefore, future studies with PDE4 inhibitors may identify systemic benefits for patients with COPD. The anti-inflammatory activities and potential systemic effects of PDE4 inhibitors in patients with COPD represent a challenging area for further research.

Conclusions

PDE4 has a critical role in the disease pathophysiology of COPD, including key activities in inflammatory cells (e.g. neutrophils) and inflammatory cytokine profiles. With the current lack of disease-modifying agents available in the COPD armamentarium, PDE4 inhibitors provide a novel opportunity to shift or change the treatment paradigm for COPD. Comprehensive preclinical data support the potent anti-inflammatory properties of selective PDE4 inhibitors. The more favourable safety profiles (e.g. gastrointestinal adverse events) observed with newer generation PDE4 inhibitors (e.g. roflumilast) are encouraging. Furthermore, data with selective PDE4 inhibitors support sustained lung function improvements, reduction in COPD exacerbations and improved health-related quality of life benefits with long-term therapy.

The PDE4 inhibitors cilomilast and roflumilast share some important characteristics (e.g. high bioavailability, oral dosing capabilities, low risk of drug–drug interactions). However, with regard to efficacy and safety, key differences between cilomilast and roflumilast have shown that roflumilast may provide a higher therapeutic index for patients with COPD. For example, roflumilast has an improved therapeutic ratio and is more potent than cilomilast in inhibiting PDE4 activity. The pharmacokinetics of roflumilast and its active metabolite, roflumilast N-oxide, allow once daily dosing versus twice daily dosing for cilomilast. Roflumilast shows efficacy in both COPD and asthma and is in late-stage clinical development for both indications, whereas clinical development of cilomilast was discontinued in asthma because of poor efficacy.

The next decade promises exciting new opportunities in the management of COPD – targeting the disease pathophysiology (i.e. disease modifying) rather than just the clinical symptoms. Importantly, long-term studies on morbidity and mortality in patients treated with selective PDE4 inhibitors are anticipated and may further validate PDE4 inhibitors for effective treatment of COPD.

References

1 Giembycz MA, Raeburn D. Putative substrates for cyclic nucleotide-dependent protein kinases and the control of airway smooth muscle tone. *J Auton Pharmacol* 1991;**11**:365–98.

2 Data on file. Konstanz, Germany; Altana Pharma AG. 2003.

3 Houslay MD, Sullivan M, Bolger GB. The multienzyme PDE4 cyclic adenosine monophosphate-specific phosphodiesterase family: intracellular targeting, regulation, and selective inhibition by compounds exerting anti-inflammatory and antidepressant actions. *Adv Pharmacol* 1998;**44**:225–342.

4 Giembycz MA, Corrigan CJ, Seybold J, Newton R, Barnes

PJ. Identification of cyclic AMP phosphodiesterases 3, 4 and 7 in human CD4+ and CD8+ T-lymphocytes: role in regulating proliferation and the biosynthesis of interleukin-2. *Br J Pharmacol* 1996;**118**:1945–58.

5 Pryzwansky KB, Madden VJ. Type 4A cAMP-specific phosphodiesterase is stored in granules of human neutrophils and eosinophils. *Cell Tissue Res* 2003;**312**:301–11.

6 Obernolte R, Ratzliff J, Baecker PA *et al.* Multiple splice variants of phosphodiesterase PDE4C cloned from human lung and testis. *Biochim Biophys Acta* 1997;**1353**:287–97.

7 Hatzelmann A, Schudt C. Anti-inflammatory and immunomodulatory potential of the novel PDE4 inhibitor roflumilast *in vitro*. *J Pharmacol Exp Ther* 2001;**297**:267–79.

8 Rena G, Begg F, Ross A *et al.* Molecular cloning, genomic positioning, promoter identification, and characterization of the novel cyclic AMP-specific phosphodiesterase PDE4A10. *Mol Pharmacol* 2001;**59**:996–1011.

9 Huston E, Lumb S, Russell A *et al.* Molecular cloning and transient expression in COS7 cells of a novel human PDE4B cAMP-specific phosphodiesterase, HSPDE4B3. *Biochem J* 1997;**328**:549–58.

10 Bolger GB, Erdogan S, Jones RE *et al.* Characterization of five different proteins produced by alternatively spliced mRNAs from the human cAMP-specific phosphodiesterase PDE4D gene. *Biochem J* 1997;**328**:539–48.

11 Dent G, Giembycz MA, Evans PM, Rabe KF, Barnes PJ. Suppression of human eosinophil respiratory burst and cyclic AMP hydrolysis by inhibitors of type IV phosphodiesterase: interaction with the beta adrenoceptor agonist albuterol. *J Pharmacol Exp Ther* 1994;**271**:1167–74.

12 Giembycz MA. Could isoenzyme-selective phosphodiesterase inhibitors render bronchodilator therapy redundant in the treatment of bronchial asthma? *Biochem Pharmacol* 1992;**43**:2041–51.

13 Torphy TJ, Undem BJ. Phosphodiesterase inhibitors: new opportunities for the treatment of asthma. *Thorax* 1991;**46**:512–23.

14 Dent G, White SR, Tenor H *et al.* Cyclic nucleotide phosphodiesterase in human bronchial epithelial cells: characterization of isoenzymes and functional effects of PDE inhibitors. *Pulm Pharmacol Ther* 1998;**11**:47–56.

15 Le Jeune IR, Shepherd M, Van Heeke G, Houslay MD, Hall IP. Cyclic AMP-dependent transcriptional up-regulation of phosphodiesterase 4D5 in human airway smooth muscle cells: identification and characterization of a novel PDE4D5 promoter. *J Biol Chem* 2002;**277**:35980–9.

16 Kohyama T, Liu X, Wen FQ *et al.* PDE4 inhibitors attenuate fibroblast chemotaxis and contraction of native collagen gels. *Am J Respir Cell Mol Biol* 2002;**26**:694–701.

17 Campos-Toimil M, Lugnier C, Droy-Lefaix MT, Takeda K. Inhibition of type 4 phosphodiesterase by rolipram and *Ginkgo biloba* extract (EGb 761) decreases agonist-induced rises in internal calcium in human endothelial cells. *Arterioscler Thromb Vasc Biol* 2000;**20**:E34–40.

18 Thompson WJ, Ashikaga T, Kelly JJ *et al.* Regulation of cyclic AMP in rat pulmonary microvascular endothelial cells by rolipram-sensitive cyclic AMP phosphodiesterase (PDE4). *Biochem Pharmacol* 2002;**63**:797–807.

19 Saetta M, DiStefano A, Turato G *et al.* CD8+ T-lymphocytes in peripheral airways of smokers with chronic obstructive pulmonary disease. *Am J Respir Crit Care Med* 1998;**157**:822–6.

20 Noguera A, Batle S, Miralles C *et al.* Enhanced neutrophil response in chronic obstructive pulmonary disease. *Thorax* 2001;**56**:432–7.

21 Burnett D, Chamba A, Hill SL, Stockley RA. Neutrophils from subjects with chronic obstructive lung disease show enhanced chemotaxis and extracellular proteolysis. *Lancet* 1987;**2**:1043–6.

22 Langen RC, Korn SH, Wouters EF. ROS in the local and systemic pathogenesis of COPD. *Free Radic Biol Med* 2003;**35**:226–35.

23 Blease K, Burke-Gaffney A, Hellewell PG. Modulation of cell adhesion molecule expression and function on human lung microvascular endothelial cells by inhibition of phosphodiesterases 3 and 4. *Br J Pharmacol* 1998;**124**:229–37.

24 Fitzgerald MF, Spicer J, Clark E, Bowyer N. Efficacy of the selective phosphodiesterase (PDE) 4 inhibitor, BAY 19-8004, in a rat model of neutrophilic lung inflammation [poster abstract online] Available at: https://www.ersnetsecure.org/public/prg_congres.abstract?ww_i_presentation=775. Accessed 14 October 2003.

25 Jin SLC, Conti M. Induction of the cyclic nucleotide phosphodiesterase PDE4B is essential for LPS-activated TNF-α responses. *Proc Natl Acad Sci USA* 2002;**99**:7628–33.

26 Gamble E, Grootendorst DC, Brightling CE *et al.* Anti-inflammatory effects of the phosphodiesterase-4 inhibitor cilomilast (Ariflo) in chronic obstructive pulmonary disease. *Am J Respir Crit Care Med* 2003;**168**:976–82.

27 Trifilieff A, Wyss D, Walker C, Mazzoni L, Hersperger R. Pharmacological profile of a novel phosphodiesterase 4 inhibitor, 4-(8-benzo[1,2,5]oxadiazol-5-yl-[1,7]naphthyridin-6-yl)-benzoic acid (NVP-ABE171), a 1,7-naphthyridine derivative, with anti-inflammatory activities. *J Pharmacol Exp Ther* 2002;**301**:241–8.

28 Santamaria LF, Palacios JM, Beleta J. Inhibition of eotaxin-mediated human eosinophil activation and migration by the selective cyclic nucleotide phosphodiesterase type 4 inhibitor rolipram. *Br J Pharmacol* 1997;**121**:1150–4.

29 Fuhrmann M, Jahn HU, Seybold J *et al.* Identification and function of cyclic nucleotide phosphodiesterase isoenzymes in airway epithelial cells. *Am J Respir Cell Mol Biol* 1999;**20**:292–302.

30 Meja KM, Catley MC, Cambridge LM *et al.* Adenovirus-mediated delivery and expression of a cAMP-dependent protein kinase inhibitor gene to BEAS-2B epithelial cells abolishes the anti-inflammatory effects of rolipram, salbutamol, and prostaglandin E2: A comparison with H-89. *J Pharmacol Exp Ther* 2004;**309**:833–44.

31 Brideau C, Van Staden C, Styhler A, Rodger IW, Chan CC. The effects of phosphodiesterase type 4 inhibitors on tumour necrosis factor-alpha and leukotriene B₄ in a novel human whole blood assay. *Br J Pharmacol* 1999;**126**:979–88.

32 Gantner F, Kupferschmidt R, Schudt C, Wendel A, Hatzelmann A. *In vitro* differentiation of human monocytes to macrophages: change of PDE profile and its relationship

to suppression of tumour necrosis factor-α release by PDE inhibitors. *Br J Pharmacol* 1997;**121**:221–31.

33 Grootendorst DC, Gauw SA, Baan R *et al*. Does a single dose of the phosphodiesterase 4 inhibitor, cilomilast (15 mg), induce bronchodilation in patients with chronic obstructive pulmonary disease? *Pulm Pharmacol Ther* 2003;**16**:115–20.

34 Mata M, Sarria B, Buenestado A, *et al*. Phosphodiesterase 4 inhibition decreases MUC5AC expression induced by epidermal growth factor in human airway epithelial cells. *Thorax*. 2005;**60**:144–52.

35 Cantin AM, Hanrahan JW, Bilodeau G, *et al*. Cystic fibrosis transmembrane conductance regulator function is suppressed in cigarette smokers. *Am J Respir Crit Care Med*. 2006;**173**:1139–44.

36 Barnes AP, Livera G, Huang P *et al*. Phosphodiesterase 4D forms a cAMP diffusion barrier at the apical membrane of the airway epithelium. *J Biol Chem* 2005;**280**:7997–8003.

37 Martin TJ. PDE4 inhibitors: a review of the recent patent literature. *IDrugs* 2001;**4**:312–38.

38 Uniphyl® Tablets [package insert]. Stamford, CT: Purdue Fredrick Company; 2002.

39 Murciano D, Auclair MH, Pariente R, Aubier M. A randomized, controlled trial of theophylline in patients with severe chronic obstructive pulmonary disease. *N Engl J Med* 1989;**320**:1521–5.

40 Ram FS, Jones PW, Castro AA *et al*. Oral theophylline for chronic obstructive pulmonary disease. *Cochrane Database Syst Rev* 2002:CD003902.

41 Tsukagoshi H, Shimizu Y, Iwamae S *et al*. Evidence of oxidative stress in asthma and COPD: potential inhibitory effect of theophylline. *Respir Med* 2000;**94**:584–8.

42 Culpitt SV, de Matos C, Russell RE *et al*. Effect of theophylline on induced sputum inflammatory indices and neutrophil chemotaxis in chronic obstructive pulmonary disease. *Am J Respir Crit Care Med* 2002;**165**:1371–6.

43 Mahler DA. The role of theophylline in the treatment of dyspnea in COPD. *Chest* 1987;**92**:2S–6.

44 Barnes PJ. Theophylline: new perspectives for an old drug. *Am J Respir Crit Care Med* 2003;**167**:813–8.

45 Rabe KF, Magnussen H, Dent G. Theophylline and selective PDE inhibitors as bronchodilators and smooth muscle relaxants. *Eur Respir J* 1995;**8**:637–42.

46 Ito K, Lim S, Caramori G *et al*. A molecular mechanism of action of theophylline: induction of histone deacetylase activity to decrease inflammatory gene expression. *Proc Natl Acad Sci USA* 2002;**99**:8921–6.

47 Torphy TJ. Phosphodiesterase isozymes: molecular targets for novel antiasthma agents. *Am J Respir Crit Care Med* 1998;**157**:351–70.

48 Cosio BG, Tsaprouni L, Ito K, Jazrawi E, Adcock IM, Barnes PJ. Theophylline restores histone deacetylase activity and steroid response in COPD macrophages. *J Exp Med* 2004;**200**:689–95.

49 BTS guidelines for the management of chronic obstructive pulmonary disease. The COPD Guidelines Group of the Standards of Care Committee of the BTS. *Thorax* 1997;**52**(Suppl 5):S1–28.

50 Barr RG, Rowe BH, Camargo CA. Methylxanthines for exacerbations of chronic obstructive pulmonary disease. *Cochrane Database Syst Rev* 2003:CD002168.

51 Tsiu SJ, Self TH, Burns R. Theophylline toxicity: update. *Ann Allergy* 1990;**64**:241–57.

52 Sekut L, Yarnall D, Stimpson SA *et al*. Anti-inflammatory activity of phosphodiesterase (PDE)-IV inhibitors in acute and chronic models of inflammation. *Clin Exp Immunol* 1995;**100**:126–32.

53 Zhu J, Mix E, Winblad B. The antidepressant and anti-inflammatory effects of rolipram in the central nervous system. *CNS Drug Rev* 2001;**7**:387–98.

54 Nibuya M, Nestler EJ, Duman RS. Chronic antidepressant administration increases the expression of cAMP response element binding protein (CREB) in rat hippocampus. *J Neurosci* 1996;**16**:2365–72.

55 Sommer N, Loschmann PA, Northoff GH *et al*. The antidepressant rolipram suppresses cytokine production and prevents autoimmune encephalomyelitis. *Nat Med* 1995;**1**: 244–8.

56 Souness JE, Rao S. Proposal for pharmacologically distinct conformers of PDE4 cyclic AMP phosphodiesterases. *Cell Signal* 1997;**9**:227–36.

57 Schneider HH, Schmiechen R, Brezinski M, Seidler J. Stereospecific binding of the antidepressant rolipram to brain protein structures. *Eur J Pharmacol* 1986;**127**:105–15.

58 Liu S, Laliberte F, Bobechko B *et al*. Dissecting the cofactor-dependent and independent bindings of PDE4 inhibitors. *Biochemistry (Mosc)* 2001;**40**:10179–86.

59 Laliberte F, Han Y, Govindarajan A *et al*. Conformational difference between PDE4 apoenzyme and holoenzyme. *Biochemistry (Mosc)* 2000;**39**:6449–58.

60 Lagente V, Moodley I, Perrin S, Mottin G, Junien JL. Effects of isozyme-selective phosphodiesterase inhibitors on eosinophil infiltration in the guinea-pig lung. *Eur J Pharmacol* 1994;**255**:253–6.

61 Howell RE, Jenkins LP, Fielding LE, Grimes D. Inhibition of antigen-induced pulmonary eosinophilia and neutrophilia by selective inhibitors of phosphodiesterase types 3 or 4 in Brown Norway rats. *Pulm Pharmacol* 1995;**8**:83–9.

62 Toward TJ, Broadley KJ. Airway function, oedema, cell infiltration and nitric oxide generation in conscious ozone-exposed guinea-pigs: effects of dexamethasone and rolipram. *Br J Pharmacol* 2002;**136**:735–45.

63 Rabinovici R, Feuerstein G, Abdullah F *et al*. Locally produced tumor necrosis factor-alpha mediates interleukin-2-induced lung injury. *Circ Res* 1996;**78**:329–36.

64 Santing RE, Olymulder CG, Van der Molen K, Meurs H, Zaagsma J. Phosphodiesterase inhibitors reduce bronchial hyperreactivity and airway inflammation in unrestrained guinea pigs. *Eur J Pharmacol* 1995;**275**:75–82.

65 Underwood DC, Osborn RR, Novak LB *et al*. Inhibition of antigen-induced bronchoconstriction and eosinophil infiltration in the guinea pig by the cyclic AMP-specific phosphodiesterase inhibitor, rolipram. *J Pharmacol Exp Ther* 1993;**266**:306–13.

66 Bobon D, Breulet M, Gerard-Vandenhove MA *et al*. Is phosphodiesterase inhibition a new mechanism of antidepressant action? A double blind double-dummy study between rolipram and desipramine in hospitalized major

and/or endogenous depressives. *Eur Arch Psychiatry Neurol Sci* 1988;**238**:2–6.

67 Hebenstreit GF, Fellerer K, Fichte K *et al*. Rolipram in major depressive disorder: results of a double-blind comparative study with imipramine. *Pharmacopsychiatry* 1989;**22**:156–60.

68 Christensen SB, Guider A, Forster CJ *et al*. 1,4-Cyclohexane-carboxylates: potent and selective inhibitors of phosphodiesterase 4 for the treatment of asthma. *J Med Chem* 1998;**41**:821–35.

69 Giembycz MA. Development status of second generation PDE4 inhibitors for asthma and COPD: the story so far. *Monaldi Arch Chest Dis* 2002;**57**:48–64.

70 Spond J, Chapman R, Fine J *et al*. Comparison of PDE 4 inhibitors, rolipram and SB 207499 (Ariflo), in a rat model of pulmonary neutrophilia. *Pulm Pharmacol Ther* 2001;**14**:157–64.

71 Torphy TJ, Barnette MS, Underwood DC *et al*. Ariflo (SB 207499), a second generation phosphodiesterase 4 inhibitor for the treatment of asthma and COPD: from concept to clinic. *Pulm Pharmacol Ther* 1999;**12**:131–5.

72 Griswold DE, Webb EF, Badger AM *et al*. SB 207499 (Ariflo), a second generation phosphodiesterase 4 inhibitor, reduces tumor necrosis factor α and interleukin-4 production in vivo. *J Pharmacol Exp Ther* 1998;**287**:705–11.

73 Barnette MS, Christensen SB, Essayan DM *et al*. SB 207499 (Ariflo), a potent and selective second-generation phosphodiesterase 4 inhibitor: *in vitro* anti-inflammatory actions. *J Pharmacol Exp Ther* 1998;**284**:420–6.

74 Barnette MS, Bartus JO, Burman M *et al*. Association of the anti-inflammatory activity of phosphodiesterase 4 (PDE4) inhibitors with either inhibition of PDE4 catalytic activity or competition for [3H]rolipram binding. *Biochem Pharmacol* 1996;**51**:949–56.

75 Profita M, Chiappara G, Mirabella F *et al*. Effect of cilomilast (Ariflo) on TNF-α, IL-8, and GM-CSF release by airway cells of patients with COPD. *Thorax* 2003;**58**:573–9.

76 Kohyama T, Liu X, Zhu YK *et al*. Phosphodiesterase 4 inhibitor cilomilast inhibits fibroblast-mediated collagen gel degradation induced by tumor necrosis factor-α and neutrophil elastase. *Am J Respir Cell Mol Biol* 2002;**27**:487–94.

77 Aoshiba K, Yasuda K, Yasui S *et al*. Serine proteases increase oxidative stress in lung cells. *Am J Physiol* 2001;**281**:L556–64.

78 Di Camillo S, Carreras I, Panchenko MV *et al*. Elastase-released epidermal growth factor recruits epidermal growth factor receptor and extracellular signal-regulated kinases to down-regulate tropoelastin mRNA in lung fibroblasts. *J Biol Chem* 2002;**277**:18938–46.

79 Zussman BD, Davie CC, Kelly J *et al*. Bioavailability of the oral selective phosphodiesterase 4 inhibitor cilomilast. *Pharmacotherapy* 2001;**21**:653–60.

80 Murdoch RD, Cowley H, Upward J *et al*. The safety and tolerability of Ariflo™ (SB 207499), a novel and selective phosphodiesterase 4 inhibitor, in healthy male volunteers [Abstract]. *Am J Respir Crit Care Med* 1998;**157**(Suppl):A409.

81 Kelly J, Murdoch RD, Clark DJ, Webber DM, Fuder H. Warfarin pharmacodynamics unaffected by cilomilast. *Ann Pharmacother* 2001;**35**:1535–9.

82 Murdoch RD, Cowley H, Kelly J, Higgins R, Webber D. Cilomilast (Ariflo) does not potentiate the cardiovascular effects of inhaled salbutamol. *Pulm Pharmacol Ther* 2002;**15**:521–7.

83 Zussman BD, Kelly J, Murdoch RD *et al*. Cilomilast: pharmacokinetic and pharmacodynamic interactions with digoxin. *Clin Ther* 2001;**23**:921–31.

84 Kelly J, Walls C, Murdoch R *et al*. No interaction when erythromycin is co-administered with cilomilast at steady state [Abstract]. *Am J Respir Crit Care Med* 2002;**165**(Suppl):A536.

85 Kelly J, Murdoch RD, Schofield JP, Webber D, Zussman B. The safety of cilomilast (Ariflo) co-administration with oral theophylline: cardiovascular profile [Abstract]. *Am J Respir Crit Care Med* 2001;**163**(Suppl):A79.

86 Zussman B, Kelly J, Rost K *et al*. The effect of renal impairment on the disposition of cilomilast, a novel and selective oral PDE4 inhibitor [Abstract]. *Am J Respir Crit Care Med* 2002;**165**(Suppl):A596.

87 Compton CH, Gubb J, Nieman R *et al*. Cilomilast, a selective phosphodiesterase-4 inhibitor for treatment of patients with chronic obstructive pulmonary disease: a randomised, dose-ranging study. *Lancet* 2001;**358**:265–70.

88 US Food and Drug Administration. NDA 21-573, Ariflo™ tablets 15 mg, by GlaxoSmithKline, for use in chronic obstructive pulmonary disease (COPD). Available at: http://www.fda.gov/ohrms/dockets/ac/03/slides/3976s1.htm. Accessed 15 October 2003.

89 US Food and Drug Administration. Ariflo™ [PADAC briefing document]. Available at: http://www.fda.gov/ohrms/dockets/ac/03/briefing/3976b1.htm. Accessed 14 October 2003.

90 Edelson JD, Compton C, Nieman R *et al*. Cilomilast (Ariflo®) improves health status in patients with COPD: results of a 6-month trial [Abstract]. *Am J Respir Crit Care Med* 2001;**163**(Suppl):A277.

91 Edelson JD, Compton C, Nieman R *et al*. Cilomilast (Ariflo®), a potent, selective inhibitor of phosphodiesterase 4, improves lung function in COPD patients: results of a 6-month trial [Abstract]. *Am J Respir Crit Care Med* 2001;**163**(Suppl):A277.

92 Kelsen SG, Rennard SI, Chodosh S *et al*. COPD exacerbation in a 6-month trial of cilomilast (Ariflo®), a potent, selective phosphodiesterase 4 inhibitor [Abstract]. *Am J Respir Crit Care Med* 2002;**165**(Suppl):A271.

93 Bagchi I, Bakst AW, Edelson JE, Amit O. Cilomilast reduces healthcare resource utilization of chronic obstructive pulmonary disease patients [Abstract]. *Am J Respir Crit Care Med* 2001;**163**(Suppl):A507.

94 Compton CH, Edelson JD, Cedar E *et al*. Cilomilast (Ariflo®) 15 mg BID safety in a 6-month clinical trial program [Abstract]. *Am J Respir Crit Care Med* 2001;**163**(Suppl):A909.

95 Robichaud A, Stamatiou PB, Jin SLC *et al*. Deletion of phosphodiesterase 4D in mice shortens α_2-adrenoceptor-mediated anesthesia, a behavioral correlate of emesis. *J Clin Invest* 2002;**110**:1045–52.

96 Bundschuh DS, Eltze M, Barsig J *et al*. *In vivo* efficacy in airway disease models of roflumilast, a novel orally active PDE4 inhibitor. *J Pharmacol Exp Ther* 2001;**297**:280–90.

97 Tenor H, Staniciu L, Schudt C *et al*. Cyclic nucleotide phosphodiesterases from purified human CD4+ and CD8+ T lymphocytes. *Clin Exp Allergy* 1995;**25**:616–24.

98 Hautamaki RD, Kobayashi DK, Senior RM, Shapiro SD. Requirement for macrophage elastase for cigarette smoke-induced emphysema in mice. *Science* 1997;**277**:2002–4.

99 Fujita M, Shannon JM, Irvin CG *et al*. Overexpression of tumor necrosis factor-alpha produces an increase in lung volumes and pulmonary hypertension. *Am J Physiol Lung Cell Mol Physiol* 2001;**280**:L39–49.

100 Vuillemenot BR, Rodriguez JF, Hoyle GW. Lymphoid tissue and emphysema in the lungs of transgenic mice inducibly expressing TNF-α. *Am J Respir Cell Mol Biol* 2004;**30**:438–48.

101 Churg A, Dai J, Tai H, Xie C, Wright JL. Tumor necrosis factor-alpha is central to acute cigarette smoke-induced inflammation and connective tissue breakdown. *Am J Respir Crit Care Med* 2002;**166**:849–54.

102 Churg A, Wang RD, Tai H *et al*. Macrophage metalloelastase mediates acute cigarette smoke-induced inflammation via tumor necrosis factor-alpha release. *Am J Respir Crit Care Med* 2003;**167**:1083–9.

103 Hasday JD, Bascom R, Costa JJ, Fitzgerald T, Dubin W. Bacterial endotoxin is an active component of cigarette smoke. *Chest* 1999;**115**:829–35.

104 Montuschi P, Kharitonov SA, Ciabattoni G, Barnes PJ. Exhaled leukotrienes and prostaglandins in COPD. *Thorax* 2003;**58**:585–8.

105 Vancheri C, Mastruzzo C, Sortino MA, Crimi N. The lung as a privileged site for the beneficial actions of PGE$_2$. *Trends Immunol* 2004;**25**:40–6.

106 Keerthisingam CB, Jenkins RG, Harrison NK *et al*. Cyclooxygenase-2 deficiency results in a loss of the antiproliferative response to transforming growth factor-beta in human fibrotic lung fibroblasts and promotes bleomycin-induced pulmonary fibrosis in mice. *Am J Pathol* 2001; **158**:1411–22.

107 Belvisi MG, Saunders M, Yacoub M, Mitchell JA. Expression of cyclo-oxygenase-2 in human airway smooth muscle is associated with profound reductions in cell growth. *Br J Pharmacol* 1998;**125**:1102–8.

108 Monick MM, Robeff PK, Butler NS *et al*. Phosphatidylinositol 3-kinase activity negatively regulates stability of cyclooxygenase 2 mRNA. *J Biol Chem* 2002;**277**:32992–3000.

109 Ichinose M, Sugiura H, Yamagata S, Koarai A, Shirato K. Increase in reactive nitrogen species production in chronic obstructive pulmonary disease airways. *Am J Respir Crit Care Med* 2000;**162**:701–6.

110 Heinloth A, Brune B, Fischer B, Galle J. Nitric oxide prevents oxidised LDL-induced p53 accumulation, cytochrome C translocation, and apoptosis in macrophages via guanylate cyclase stimulation. *Atherosclerosis* 2002;**162**:93–101.

111 Conti M, Richter W, Mehats C *et al*. Cyclic AMP-specific PDE4 phosphodiesterases as critical components of cyclic AMP signaling. *J Biol Chem* 2003;**278**:5493–6.

112 Wang P, Wu P, Ohleth KM, Egan RW, Billah MM. Phosphodiesterase 4B2 is the predominant phosphodiesterase species and undergoes differential regulation of gene expression in human monocytes and neutrophils. *Mol Pharmacol* 1999;**56**:170–4.

113 Poulter LW, Janossy G, Power C, Sreenan S, Burke C. Immunological/physiological relationships in asthma: potential regulation by lung macrophages. *Immunol Today* 1994;**15**:258–61.

114 Kanda N, Watanabe S. Regulatory roles of adenylate cyclase and cyclic nucleotide phosphodiesterases 1 and 4 in interleukin-13 production by activated human T cells. *Biochem Pharmacol* 2001;**62**:495–507.

115 Schudt C, Tenor H, Hatzelmann A. PDE isoenzymes as targets for anti-asthma drugs. *Eur Respir J* 1995;**8**:1179–83.

116 Baroja ML, Cieslinski LB, Torphy TJ, Wange RL, Madrenas J. Specific CD3 epsilon association of a phosphodiesterase 4B isoform determines its selective tyrosine phosphorylation after CD3 ligation. *J Immunol* 1999;**162**:2016–23.

117 Arp J, Kirchhof MG, Baroja ML *et al*. Regulation of T-cell activation by phosphodiesterase 4B2 requires its dynamic redistribution during immunological synapse formation. *Mol Cell Biol* 2003;**23**:8042–57.

118 Seybold J, Newton R, Wright L *et al*. Induction of phosphodiesterases 3B, 4A4, 4D1, 4D2, and 4D3 in Jurkat T-cells and in human peripheral blood T-lymphocytes by 8-bromo-cAMP and Gs-coupled receptor agonists: potential role in β$_2$-adrenoreceptor desensitization. *J Biol Chem* 1998;**273**: 20575–88.

119 Giembycz MA. Phosphodiesterase 4 and tolerance to beta 2-adrenoceptor agonists in asthma. *Trends Pharmacol Sci* 1996;**17**:331–6.

120 Saetta M, Baraldo S, Turato G *et al*. Increased proportion of CD8+ T-lymphocytes in the paratracheal lymph nodes of smokers with mild COPD. *Sarcoidosis Vasc Diffuse Lung Dis* 2003;**20**:28–32.

121 Tenor H, Burgbacher B, Schudt C *et al*. Effects of roflumilast and other PDE4 inhibitors on human CD8+ T-cell functions. *Eur Respir J* 2005;**26**:Suppl. 49, 716s.

122 Barnette MS. Challenges for drug discovery [Abstract]. Presented at: New drugs for asthma III. July 1994; Montebello, Quebec.

123 Duplantier AJ, Biggers MS, Chambers RJ *et al*. Biarylcarboxylic acids and -amides: inhibition of phosphodiesterase type IV versus [3H] rolipram binding activity and their relationship to emetic behavior in the ferret. *J Med Chem* 1996;**39**:120–5.

124 Schmiechen R, Schneider HH, Wachtel H. Close correlation between behavioural response and binding *in vivo* for inhibitors of the rolipram-sensitive phosphodiesterase. *Psychopharmacology (Berl)* 1990;**102**:17–20.

125 Zhao Y, Zhang HT, O'Donnell JM. Inhibitor binding to type 4 phosphodiesterase (PDE4) assessed using [3H]piclamilast and [3H]rolipram. *J Pharmacol Exp Ther* 2003;**305**(2):565–72.

126 Torphy TJ, Christensen SB, Barnette MS *et al*. Molecular basis for an improved therapeutic index of SB207499, a second generation phosphodiesterase 4 inhibitor [Abstract]. *Eur Respir J* 1997;**10**:313S.

127 Claveau D, Chen SL, O'Keefe S *et al*. Preferential inhibition of T helper 1, but not T helper 2 cytokines *in vitro* by L-826, 141[4-{2-(3,4-Bis-difluoromethoxyphenyl)-2-{4-(1,1,1,3,3, 3-hexafluoro-2-hydroxypropan-2-yl)-phenyl)-ethyl}-3-methylpyridine-1-oxide], a potent and selective phosphodiesterase 4 inhibitor. *J Pharmacol Exp Ther* 2004;**310**:752–60.

128 Ariga M, Neitzert B, Nakae S *et al*. Nonredundant function of phosphodiesterases 4D and 4B in neutrophil recruitment to the site of inflammation. *J Immunol* 2004;**173**:7531–38.

129 Jones NA, Boswell-Smith V, Lever R, Page CP. The effect of selective phosphodiesterase isoenzyme inhibition on neutrophil function *in vitro*. *Pulm Pharmacol Ther* 2005;**18**: 93–101.

130 Sanz MJ, Abu-Taha M, Naim-Abu-Nabah Y, Cortijo J, Morcillo EJ. Roflumilast inhibits leucocyte endothelial cell interactions *in vivo*. *Eur Respir J* 2006;**28**:Suppl. 224s.

131 Boero S, Silvestri M, Sabatini F, Nachira A, Rossi GA. Inhibition of human lung fibroblast functions by roflumilast N-oxide. *Eur J Respir* 2006;**28**:Suppl, 662s.

132 Togo S, Liu X, Kobayashi T *et al*. The PDE4 inhibitors roflumilast and rolipram modulate fibroblast collagen gel contraction and chemotaxis mediated by autocrine PGE2 synthesis induced by transforming growth factor β1. *Proc Am Thorac Soc* 2006;**3**:547–8.

133 Growcott EJ, Spink KG, Ren X *et al*. Phosphodiesterase 4 expression and anti-proliferative effects in human pulmonary artery smooth muscle cells. *Respir Res* 2006;**7**:9.

134 Burgess JK, Oliver BGG, Poniris MH *et al*. A phosphodiesterase 4 inhibitor inhibits matrix protein deposition in airways *in vitro*. *J Allergy Clin Immunol* 2006;**118**:649–57.

135 Tenor H, Schatton E, Schudt C, Hatzelmann A. Effects of roflumilast and other PDE4 inhibitors on [3H]thymidine incorporation in human bronchial smooth muscle cells. *Eur Respir J* 2005;**26**:Suppl. 49, 717s.

136 Martorana PA , Beume R, Lucatelli M, Wollin L, Lungarella G. Roflumilast fully prevents emphysema in mice chroncially exposed to cigarette smoke. *Am J Respir Crit Care Med* 2005;**172**:848–853.

137 Zech K, David M, Seiberling M *et al*. High oral absolute bioavailability of roflumilast, a new, orally active, once daily PDE4 inhibitor [Abstract]. *Eur Respir J* 2001;**18**(Suppl 33):20S.

138 Bethke T, Hauns B, Zech K, David M, Wurst W. Dose linearity of roflumilast, a new selective PDE4 inhibitor. *AJRCCM* 2002;**165**:A595.

139 Hauns B, Hermann R, Huennemeyer A, Herzog R, Hauschke D, Zech K, Bethke TD. Investigation of a potential food effect on the pharmacokinetics of roflumilast, an oral, once-daily phosphodiesterase 4 inhibitor in healthy subjects. *J Clin Pharmacol* 2006, in press.

140 Hauns B, Huennemeyer A, Seiberling M *et al*. Investigation of pharmacokinetics of roflumilast and roflumilast N-oxide after single morning or evening oral administration of 500 μg roflumilast in healthy subjects: an open, randomized, two-period crossover study [Abstract]. *Am J Respir Crit Care Med* 2003;**167**(Suppl):A92.

141 Hünnemeyer A, Hauns B, Drollmann A *et al*. Pharmacokinetics of roflumilast and its active metabolite, roflumilast-N-oxide, is not influenced by smoking [Abstract]. *Am J Respir Crit Care Med* 2002;**165**(Suppl):A594.

142 Hünnemeyer A, Bethke T, David M *et al*. No interaction of roflumilast and its active metabolite, roflumilast-N-oxide, with inhaled budesonide [Abstract]. *Am J Respir Crit Care Med* 2002;**165**(Suppl):A595.

143 Bethke TD, Giessmann T, Westphal K, Weinbrenner A, Hauns B, Hauschke D, David M, Lahu G, Zech K, Hermann R, Siegmund W. Roflumilast, a once-daily oral phophodiesterase 4 inhibitor, lacks relevant pharmacokinetic interaction with inhaled salbutamol when co-administered in healthy subjects. *Int. J Clin Pharmacol Therapeut.* 2006; in press.

144 Hauns B, Huennemeyer A, Duursema L *et al*. Roflumilast and its active metabolite roflumilast N-oxide do not interact with R- and S-warfarin [Abstract]. *Eur Respir J* 2003;**22** (Suppl 45):103S.

145 Bethke T, Hartmann M, Zech K *et al*. No dose adjustment of roflumilast in patients with severe renal impairment [Abstract]. *Am J Respir Crit Care Med* 2002;**165**(Suppl): A594.

146 Leichtl S, Syed J, Bredenbröker D, Rathgeb F, Wurst W. Efficacy of once-daily roflumilast, a new, orally active, selective phosphodiesterase 4 inhibitor, in chronic obstructive pulmonary disease [abstract]. *Am J Respir Crit Care Med* 2002;**165**(Suppl):A229.

147 Bredenbröker D, Syed J, Leichtl S, Rathgeb F, Wurst W. Safety of once-daily roflumilast, a new, orally active, selective phosphodiesterase 4 inhibitor, in patients with COPD [Abstract]. *Am J Respir Crit Care Med* 2002;**165**(Suppl): A595.

148 Rabe KF, Bateman ED, O'Donnell D, Witte S, Bredenbroker D, Bethke TD. Roflumilast – an oral anti-inflammatory treatment for chronic obstructive pulmonary disease: a randomised controlled trial. *Lancet* 2005;**366**(9485):563–571.

149 Calverley PM, Sanchez-Toril F, McIvor RA, Teichmann P, Bredenbroker D, Fabbri LM. Effect of roflumilast on lung function: a 1-year study in patients with severe to very severe COPD. *Proc Am Thorac Soc* 2006;**3**:A725.

150 Fabbri LM, Sanchez-Toril F, McIvor RA, Teichmann P, Bredenbroker D, Calverley PM. Effect of roflumilast on exacerbations: a 1-year study in patients with severe to very severe COPD. *Proc Am Thorac Soc* 2006;**3**:A841.

151 Wouters EFM, Creutzberg EC, Schols AMWJ. Systemic effects in COPD. *Chest* 2002;**121**(Suppl):127S–30S.

152 Agusti AGN, Noguera A, Sauleda J *et al*. Systemic effects of chronic obstructive pulmonary disease. *Eur Respir J* 2003; **21**:347–60.

153 Li YP, Schwartz RJ, Waddell ID, Holloway BR, Reid MB. Skeletal muscle myocytes undergo protein loss and reactive oxygen-mediated NF-κB activation in response to tumor necrosis factor α. *FASEB J* 1998;**12**:871–80.

154 Williams G, Brown T, Becker L, Prager M, Giroir BP. Cytokine-induced expression of nitric oxide synthase in C2C12 skeletal muscle myocytes. *Am J Physiol* 1994;**267**: R1020–5.

155 Agusti A, Morla M, Sauleda J *et al*. NF-kappaB activation and iNOS upregulation in skeletal muscle of patients with COPD and low body weight. *Thorax* 2004;**59**:483–7.

156 Tenor H, Hedbom E, Hauselmann HJ, Schudt C, Hatzelmann A. Phosphodiesterase isoenzyme families in human osteoarthritis chondrocytes: functional importance of phosphodiesterase 4. *Br J Pharmacol* 2002;**135**:609–18.

CHAPTER 60
Antibiotic therapy in patients with COPD

Michael S. Niederman

Patients with chronic bronchitis commonly have disease exacerbations, and antibiotics are commonly used as part of the therapy for this condition, even though bacterial infection is present in no more than 50% of excacerbations. Although a recent meta-analysis has concluded that antibiotics are of benefit, compared to placebo, for acute exacerbations of chronic bronchitis (AECB), not all patients require such therapy [1]. One way to decide who should be treated is to count the number of 'cardinal symptoms' of exacerbation: increased dyspnoea, increased sputum volume and increased sputum purulence. In one study, Anthonisen *et al.* [2] graded exacerbations as type I if all three symptoms were present; type II if only two symptoms were present; and type III if only one symptom was present, and found a benefit for antibiotic therapy in the 80% of patients with either type I or II exacerbations. Even if antibiotics are used, some experts believe that the choice of a specific agent is not important with regard to patient outcome [3]. In fact, a recent consensus statement of the Amercian College of Physicans and the American College of Chest Physicians, as well as the GOLD guidelines for COPD support this concept [4]. In spite of this view, guidelines for the therapy of AECB have been published, and they take the approach that there are differences in the bacteriology of exacerbations in different patient populations, necessitating that therapy be given in different ways for different subsets of patients [5]. Implicit in these guidelines is the belief that the benefits of antibiotics may be more dramatic for patients with more severe illness, where the impact of no therapy, or failed therapy, may be catastrophic leading to hospitalization and even mechanical ventilation.

This discussion explores the use of antibiotics in COPD patients, focusing primarily on their role in acute exacerbations, but also considering the issue of pneumonia in the COPD patient. The rationale for the use of antibiotics in exacerbations, as well as the target organisms and principles of antibiotic usage are examined. Finally, the concept that specific antibiotics should be used in specific patients is discussed.

Why should antibiotics be used in AECB?

Patients usually have exacerbations of COPD each year, with only one-third of all patients having less than three episodes, one-third having three episodes and one-third having four or more episodes [6]. One recent study examined the cost of treating AECB in the USA, although the estimates related to total outpatient cost were limited by the available data, and thus the study probably underestimated the number of outpatients treated annually [7]. Using 1994 data, the authors estimated that there were 280 000 admissions for AECB and over 10 million outpatient visits for this illness, a ratio of 30 : 1 for outpatient management versus inpatient care. For the admitted patients, the mean length of stay for those 65 years and older was 6.3 days at a total cost of 1.1 billion dollars, while younger patients had a mean length of stay of 5.8 days at a total cost of 419 million dollars. For the outpatients, 5.8 million episodes are in those aged 65 or older, while 4.2 million episodes were in the younger population. When care was given out of the hospital, for those treated in an office, emergency room or hospital clinic, the cost of an exacerbation was $74, $76 and $159, respectively [7]. In contrast, for an inpatient, the average cost was $5516 per episode. In both the outpatient and inpatient setting, antibiotics made up a small amount of total cost, accounting for 15% and 11%, respectively, of all costs. The data in this study make it very clear that if an antibiotic is used during exacerbation, and it can prevent hospitalization, it will be a highly cost-effective therapy, given the large difference in the cost of care in these two settings.

The arguments in favour of using antibiotics in many patients with exacerbations come from several areas (Table 60.1):

Table 60.1 Why antibiotics should be used in acute exacerbations of chronic bronchitis.

Bacteriological data show a role for bacteria in exacerbations
- Quantitative cultures
- Strain-specific data

Serological data show a role for bacteria in exacerbations
- Strain-specific antibody responses for *Haemophilus influenzae*

Inflammatory events in the airway are linked to bacteria
- Antibiotics might prevent progressive airways damage by breaking the vicious cycle of infection and airway injury

Antibiotics lead to a reduced duration of symptoms and more patients with a clinical cure and fewer with a clinical deterioration than placebo
- May help avoid hospitalization
- May help return to work sooner
- Certain agents may prolong time between exacerbations

May prevent some severe airway infections from progressing to pneumonia

1 Bacteriological and serological data show a role for bacterial infection in acute exacerbations.
2 Inflammatory events in the airway can be linked to the presence of bacteria, and the elimination of bacteria is associated with reduced signs of inflammation.
3 Prospective randomized placebo-controlled trials show a benefit for antibiotics, especially in more severe exacerbations.
4 Antibiotics may prevent some patients with severe exacerbations from progressing to pneumonia.

Bacteriological and serological data showing a role of bacteria in exacerbations

When sputum is cultured from a patient with chronic bronchitis, bacteria are often present, with non-typable *Haemophilus influenzae*, pneumococcus and *Moraxella catarrhalis* being the most commonly recovered pathogens. The uncertainty about the role of bacteria in AECB results from the observation that the same organisms may be present when the patient is clinically stable or when the patient is having an acute exacerbation, reflecting the fact that these patients have chronic tracheobronchial colonization. While most bacteriological data are qualitative, a number of studies have examined quantitative cultures of lower respiratory tract secretions using a bronchoscopic protected specimen brush in this population, and demonstrated that many patients with exacerbations have large numbers of bacteria, often more than are present in the absence of exacerbation symptoms [8–11]. To date, at least four

studies have used quantitative cultures and found that at least 50% of patients with exacerbations (as opposed to fewer who are stable) have concentrations of bacteria in their lower airways that are comparable to the concentrations that are present in patients with pneumonia (more than 1000 colony-forming units [CFU]/mL) [8–11]. Thus, exacerbations can be accompanied by as many organisms as are present during invasive infection. In one outpatient study of 40 stable patients, only 25% had organisms present at more than 1000 CFU/mL, while 52% of 29 patients with exacerbations had concentrations of bacteria at this level [9]. In fact, if a concentration of more than 10 000 CFU/mL was used, then only 5% of the stable patients had these many bacteria, compared with 24% of the patients with exacerbation.

Still, the question remains, how is it possible for bacteria to cause exacerbations if the same organisms are present when a patient is stable or when the patient is ill. This issue was recently evaluated by Sethi *et al.* [12] who studied the bacteriology of respiratory secretions in a longitudinal study of outpatients with chronic bronchitis. Using molecular typing, they found that even when patients had the same organism in the airway over time, the specific surface-exposed epitopes changed, because patients were acquiring new 'strains' of the same organism. They found that when a new strain was acquired of either pneumococcus, *H. influenzae* or *M. catarrhalis*, the likelihood of exacerbation was increased more than twofold. In fact, the authors found that 33% of clinic visits associated with acquisition of a new bacterial strain were accompanied by an exacerbation, compared with 15.4% of visits without the acquisition of a new bacterial strain [12]. These findings answer the question as to how it is possible for bacteria to cause exacerbations, while having the same organism present persistently. In addition, they provide a mechanism for bacteria to be pathogenic; the organisms lead to exacerbation once they are of a new strain type, and are able to evade host defences.

More recently, the same authors have found that the acquisition of a new strain is associated with a strain-specific antibody response, at least for new strains of *H. influenzae*, but this phenomenon still needs to be studied for other organisms. They found that if patients acquired a new strain at the time of an exacerbation, a specific antibody response to this strain (by ELISA assay) was present 58.3% of the time, while only 15.2% of exacerbations characterized by the presence of a persistent strain were accompanied by an antibody response [13]. Similar findings were seen when bactericidal antibodies were measured. The specificity of the bactericidal antibody response was demonstrated because only 12% of heterologous strains of *H. influenzae* were killed by new bactericidal antibodies that developed after an exacerbation. These findings are consistent with previous serological studies that did not demonstrate an antibody response to laboratory strains of *H. influenzae* following an exacerbation because these strains can be viewed as heterologous, and not homologous. In the instance of persistence of a pre-existing strain at the time of exacerbation, the absence of an antibody response implies that another bacteria (to which antibodies were not measured), or a virus, could have caused the exacerbation.

Inflammation and the vicious cycle hypothesis

The presence of bacteria in the airway of the COPD patient is met by an inflammatory response that arises from the bacteria themselves (through the production of exoproducts) and the patient's response to bacteria (primarily through neutrophilic by-products). The presence of bacteria in the airway is associated with a variety of inflammatory cytokines, and the levels of these products are increased when bacteria are present, compared with when they are absent, and when the sputum appears purulent [14,15]. The vicious cycle hypothesis states that the presence of bacteria in the airways initiates inflammation, which in turn injures the lung and the injury propagates favourable growth conditions for the bacteria to persist [16,17]. One by-product of inflammation is neutrophilic elastase, an enzyme that could lead to lung tissue destruction. Thus, the presence of bacteria in the airway could lead to inflammation, which in turn leads to more favourable growth conditions for bacteria, more inflammation and more growth and, as this cycle continues, inflammatory enzymes accelerate the loss of lung function.

In spite of this idea, only one of four prospective studies have shown that a more rapid decline in lung function occurs in patients with more frequent exacerbations (16). More recently, a 4-year study of 109 patients categorized individuals into high and low frequency of exacerbations, and found that those with frequent exacerbations had a faster decline in forced expiratory volume in 1 s (FEV_1) than those with infrequent exacerbations [18]. Although the vicious cycle concept is still unproven in COPD, it is a more clearly established mechanism in patients with another closely related obstructive lung disease, bronchiectasis.

Secondary bacterial infection can follow viral bronchitis

Many patients with AECB have preceding viral infections, which could serve either as the cause of exacerbation, or could create conditions in the airway that predispose to secondary bacterial infection [19]. In a study of 83 patients with COPD, 64% of exacerbations were preceded by cold symptoms within the previous 18 days. In the group as a whole, 39% of exacerbations had a virus detected during the period of symptoms, and the presence of virus was associated with symptoms of sore throat, but not with any of the symptoms of purulent sputum, increased sputum volume or increased dyspnoea [20]. Of the viruses found, rhinovirus was present in 58% of exacerbations, and the next most common agents were respiratory syncytial virus and coronavirus. Another study used case–control methodology to evaluate 85 patients with AECB and 42 patients with stable COPD [21]. Respiratory viruses were present in the sputum and nasal lavage in 56% of exacerbations and in 19% without exacerbation. The most common viruses were picornavirus, influenza A and respiratory syncytial virus. More recently, Tan *et al.* [22] examined respiratory secretions from 14 patients hospitalized with COPD and used the polymerase chain reaction to detect six common respiratory viruses. Overall, 64% had a virus present, with influenza, picornavirus and adenovirus predominating [22].

If antibiotics are used empirically for AECB, and many patients have documented viral infection, does this mean antibiotics are not of value? This remains uncertain, because antibiotics could prevent secondary bacterial infections that result from the airway changes induced by viral infection. Smith *et al.* [23] observed an increased rate of culturing *H. influenzae* from the respiratory secretions of patients with documented influenza infection. Colonization rates first increased 7 days after influenza infection, and persisted at increased levels for at least 30 days. The authors also observed a similar trend after herpesvirus and rhinovirus infection, but this trend was not as significant as after influenza. In addition, herpesvirus infection was associated with an increased likelihood of bronchial secretions being colonized by *Streptococcus pneumoniae*. More data are needed to determine whether antibiotics can prevent secondary colonization and if so, whether this therapy is associated with less frequent bacterial exacerbations and with clinical benefit.

Outcomes of antibiotic therapy trials in AECB

There are data from a variety of sources that show a benefit for antibiotics in patients with AECB. A number of prospective, randomized, placebo-controlled trials of antibiotics in chronic bronchitis have shown some benefit during acute exacerbations, but no benefit if used to prevent exacerbations [1,2,17]. One recent meta-analysis evaluated nine randomized and placebo-controlled trials of antibiotic therapy in AECB, conducted between 1957 and 1992 [1], and showed a small beneficial effect of antibiotic therapy when the endpoints were overall benefit and change in peak flow rate. Another analysis of placebo-controlled trials for AECB, conducted by Ball [24], reached similar conclusions. A consensus statement of the American College of Physicians and American College of Chest Physicians evaluated 11 randomized placebo-controlled studies of antibiotics and concluded that this therapy had benefit, but primarily in patients with more severe and symptomatic exacerbations [4,25]. This analysis did recognize that most of the trials were performed in an era before antibiotic resistance was common, and the benefit of new, more broad-spectrum antibiotics could not be directly defined [4,25]. Two other studies of relevance to this issue were not included in any of the large analyses. One was an Italian study comparing amoxicillin/clavulanate to placebo, which showed a benefit for antibiotics, especially for patients with severe lung dysfunction, defined as an FEV_1 of less than 33% of predicted [26]. The other study was a retrospective evaluation of patients discharged from a US emergency department with and without antibiotics, following an acute exacerbation of COPD [27]. In that study, 362 emergency visits were evaluated, and 92 patients did not receive antibiotics, while 270 did. The relapse rate was significantly lower for antibiotic-treated patients compared with those without therapy (19% vs 32%). In addition, there was a trend to fewer hospitalizations for the antibiotic-treated patients. Interestingly, although the failure to use antibiotics led to a higher relapse rate than antibiotic therapy, the use of amoxicillin led to the highest relapse rate of all, implying that an ineffective therapy (which amoxicillin could be, for a variety of reasons) was worse than no therapy. A multivariate analysis supported the finding of reduced relapse risk with antibiotics, implying that even after correcting for confounding factors, antibiotic therapy had benefit.

Probably the best single study of AECB was that of Anthonisen *et al.* [2], reported in 1987 from Canada. A total of 362 exacerbations in 173 patients were evaluated in a placebo-controlled, randomized, double-blinded study design. When patients were treated with an antibiotic, therapy was continued for 10 days, and the antibiotics used were either co-trimoxazole, amoxicillin or doxycycline. The authors used these antibiotics interchangeably, believing that any antibiotic was equally effective, an assumption that may not be correct, because of our current understanding of differences among patients and because of an increased frequency of antibiotic resistance, compared with the early 1980s. In the study, each exacerbation was graded as type I, II or III, according to the number of cardinal symptoms present. Approximately 40% of all exacerbations were the most severe, type I, with all three cardinal symptoms present; 40% were type II with two symptoms present; and 20% were type III, having only one symptom present. Antibiotic-treated patients did significantly better than placebo-treated patients, showing a more rapid return of peak flow, a greater percentage of patients showing clinical success and a smaller percentage showing clinical failure. The benefits of antibiotic therapy were most clearly evident in patients with at least two cardinal symptoms present: the 80% of individuals with type I or II exacerbations. Patients with type III exacerbations had a high spontaneous resolution rate, and antibiotics were no better than placebo.

The data from Anthonisen *et al.*'s [2] study suggest that antibiotics should be given to patients who have at least two of the three cardinal symptoms present. This is a clinical approach, which is more likely to be useful than simply reserving antibiotics for episodes that are suspected to be bacterial and not viral in origin. Even though as many as half of all episodes are non-bacterial, there are data suggesting that clinical features cannot reliably distinguish these episodes from bacterial exacerbations, although sputum purulence may help [15]. In one study of 54 patients with severe (requiring mechanical ventilation) episodes of bronchial infection complicating COPD, 27 patients had bacteria recovered from the airway, using a bronchoscopic protected specimen brush sampling technique [8]. When patients with secretions containing bacteria were compared with those with sterile secretions, there were no differences with regard to duration of symptoms, fever, white blood cell count or degree of hypoxaemia.

Antibiotics could reduce the burden of bacteria in the airway and prevent pneumonia

Often, a stable bronchitic patient has chronic tracheobronchial colonization, but with fewer bacteria than are present during an exacerbation. If a sputum Gram's stain is performed, patients have fewer than two organisms per oil immersion field when stable, but more than 8–18 per field at the time of an exacerbation [28]. Several bronchoscopy studies have examined the concentration of bacteria in the airway of chronic bronchitis patients studied when stable, and during an exacerbation. Monso *et al.* [9] performed protected specimen brush (PSB) sampling in 40 stable outpatients with COPD and 29 outpatients with acute exacerbations. In that study, 25% of the stable patients and 52% of the exacerbation patients had positive respiratory secretion cultures. Quantitatively, patients with an exacerbation had more bacteria, with 24% having more than 10^4 organisms/mL, compared with only 5% of the stable patients having this finding. Similar findings have been made in patients with more severe illness, but the specific bacteria that are present may differ. In one study of 50 mechanically ventilated patients with COPD, 72% had potentially pathogenic organisms present, including *Pseudomonas aeruginosa* or other enteric Gram-negative bacteria in 28% of patients [10]. In another similar study of 54 patients with severe exacerbations, requiring mechanical ventilation, Fagon *et al.* [8] found that nearly half of the patients had more than 10^3 organisms/mL on a PSB sample.

Because PSB has been used to define the presence or absence of pneumonia in hospitalized patients with lung infiltrates, and because a concentration of more than 10^3 organisms/mL is thought to indicate the presence of pneumonia, it is clear that many patients with AECB have as many bacteria in their airway as if they had pneumonia. These observations suggest that for a more severe exacerbation, associated with a high concentration of bacteria, antibiotics could theoretically reduce this bacterial burden, and possibly prevent some patients from progressing to parenchymal lung infection (such as pneumonia). In support of this possibility is one study of 93 patients with severe exacerbations who were randomized to an antibiotic (ofloxacin) or placebo while managed in the hospital with mechanical ventilation. The antibiotic-treated patients had a significantly lower in-hospital and intensive care unit (ICU) mortality, primarily related to the avoidance of pneumonia [29]. In fact, significantly fewer antibiotic-treated patients developed pneumonia, compared with placebo-treated patients, and the need for additional antibiotics was lower for the antibiotic-treated patients. Thus, for severe exacerbations, antibiotics are clearly beneficial, primarily by reducing bacterial burden and preventing pneumonia.

The relationship of pneumonia to AECB

While some patients with AECB may progress to pneumonia, and antibiotics are potentially useful to avoid this complication, the distinction between airway and parenchymal infection in COPD patients is sometimes unclear. In 1996, Torres *et al.* [30] documented that pneumonia is common in certain COPD patients. Among 124 COPD patients with community-acquired pneumonia, the mean age was 56 years, 19% had chronic respiratory failure (hypoxaemia or hypercarbia), 25% had a previous episode of pneumonia, and the mean FEV_1 was 40% of predicted normal. Almost all patients had symptoms of fever (83%), increased dyspnoea (93%) and cough (85%). The predominant pathogen was pneumococcus (in 43% of those with an aetiological diagnosis), followed by *Chlamydia pneumoniae* (12%), *Haemophilus influenzae* (9%) and *Legionella pneumophila* (9%).

Lieberman *et al.* [31] have recently reported their experience with 219 patients with symptomatic exacerbations of COPD and compared the clinical risks and presenting features of those with pneumonia during an exacerbation and those with no lung infiltrate. The population had at least one of the three cardinal symptoms of exacerbation, but there was no significant difference in the number of symptoms present when the patients had pneumonia, compared with when they did not. Overall, 26% of the pneumonia patients and 22% of the non-pneumonic patients had a type III exacerbation, with only one of the three cardinal

symptoms present. Thus, if antibiotics were withheld in all COPD patients with only one such symptom, some with pneumonia would not have been treated. Thus, to identify this population, a chest radiograph is needed. The patients who did have pneumonia had an abrupt onset of symptoms, fever, focal crepitations on examination and severe hypoxaemia more often than those without pneumonia. Those with pneumonia had a higher mortality rate, a greater need for mechanical ventilation and a longer duration of hospitalization. Based on these findings, it may be important to realize that the distinction between pneumonia and acute airway infection is often difficult to make clinically but, because the outcomes are so different, a chest radiograph may be valuable to identify rapidly those with parenchymal lung infection. Given the difficulty of clinically separating pneumonia from bronchitis in the COPD patient and the ability of antibiotics to prevent some patients from developing pneumonia, the value of antibiotics for those with severe exacerbations seems clear.

Likely bacteria in AECB and the frequency of antibiotic resistance

Spectrum of pathogens and the frequency of antibiotic resistance

The exact frequency of bacterial infection in AECB is debated, and the role of viruses, allergens and airway irritants in exacerbations is difficult to estimate. However, as many as half of all exacerbations may be associated with bacteria and the three most common organisms present during AECB are *H. influenzae*, pneumococcus and *M. catarrhalis*, with the frequency of these organisms, and the likelihood that they are antibiotic resistant, varying with the country, specific patient features and the severity of exacerbation. In outpatients with exacerbations of mild severity, *H. influenzae* predominates, followed by the other organisms (pneumococcus and *M. catarrhalis*), but Gram-negative infection is relatively uncommon [9]. In patients with severe exacerbation, *H. influenzae* is less common, with *H. parainfluenzae* being the most common organism isolated from bronchoscopy samples, and Gram-negative bacteria are also frequently isolated [8].

Haemophilus influenzae is generally the most common isolate in patients with AECB, but is usually non-encapsulated and thus non-typable. In recent years, these organisms have developed a high frequency of beta-lactamase production, with as many as 40% having these enzymes present, a finding which makes traditional beta-lactam antibiotics (such as ampicillin or amoxicillin) potentially ineffective. While as many as 40% of *H. influenzae* produce this enzyme, some organisms produce so much of this product that they can even be resistant to amoxicillin/clavulanate [32]. In addition, in one study, 2.5% of these organisms were ampicillin resistant through another mechanism, alteration of penicillin-binding proteins [32]. Beta-lactamase production is even more common with *M. catarrhalis*, and one study found these enzymes in 95% of 723 isolates [33]. If infection with this Gram-negative coccus is likely, then beta-lactam resistance should be assumed to be present.

Pneumococcal resistance to common antibiotics is increasingly frequent, being present in as many as 40% of all isolates, although much of this resistance is intermediate and not high-level resistance, and thus the implications of resistance to antibiotic therapy are uncertain [34,35]. Resistance is more likely if patients have identified risk factors, including: age over 65 years, alcoholism, beta-lactam therapy within the past 3 months, multiple medical comorbidities and immunosuppressive illness [35,36]. In addition, resistance can occur to multiple other antibiotic classes, including macrolides and quinolones. Throughout the 1990s, the frequency of macrolide-resistant pneumococcus rose to over 30%, but in the USA, much of this was caused by an efflux-mediated mechanism (*mef* gene) allowing the bacteria to remove the antibiotic from the cytoplasm, rather than altered binding of the macrolide to the bacterial ribosome (*erm* gene) [37]. The magnitude of resistance associated with the *mef* mechanism is much lower than the magnitude of resistance due to the *erm* mechanism, and this may explain why macrolides have generally continued to be successful for the therapy of AECB and community-acquired pneumonia (CAP) [38]. Efflux resistance may not be clinically relevant because it is a relatively low level of resistance, but also because it may be overcome by adequate dosing of macrolides, combined with good penetration at the site of infection.

In recent years, the use of quinolones has exploded, often in situations where they are not indicated [39], and consequently pneumococcal resistance to these agents has begun to emerge. Among the commonly used quinolones for AECB, the relative activity against pneumococci, from most to least active is: gemifloxacin, moxifloxacin, gatifloxacin, levofloxacin and ciprofloxacin [40,41]. Pneumococcal resistance has occurred most commonly to the least active pneumococcal agents, but appears to be a particular problem for the COPD patient. In adults, the airway of the COPD patient has been the breeding ground for pneumococcal resistance to a variety of agents, including the new quinolones [42]. This can be explained because these patients are chronically colonized, frequently immunosuppressed (with corticosteroids), elderly and exposed to repeated courses of antibiotics, and all of these factors are known to promote the emergence of antibiotic resistance [36]. One concern has been that repeated exposures to less active agents can promote resistance to the entire class of

quinolones [43], and thus there may be some advantage to selecting the most active anti-pneumococcal agent in the class in an effort to assure efficacy and minimize the subsequent emergence of resistance.

In a large number of studies, investigators have found that recent exposure to any antibiotic predicts subsequent pneumococcal resistance to that same class of antibiotics. This finding has been shown for beta-lactams, if used within the last 3 months [36]; macrolides (although only for the *mef* mechanism of resistance) [37]; and quinolones, if used in the last 12 months [42]. One recent study has found that use of macrolides or beta-lactams within the past 6 months predisposes patients with bacteraemic pneumococcal pneumonia to a high rate of infection with penicillin non-susceptible organisms [44]. Interestingly, this finding did not apply to recent quinolone use, but even if quinolones do not promote penicillin-resistant pneumococci, repeated use can predispose to quinolone-resistant pneumococci [45]. In view of these data, one strategy for minimizing future resistance in pneumococci for the AECB patient is 'patient-specific antibiotic rotation', a strategy that requires the patient to be treated for subsequent exacerbations with a different class of antibiotic than was used in previous exacerbations. The value of this approach still needs confirmation but, in the past, many patients with AECB received the same antibiotic repeatedly, for multiple exacerbations, and this approach may have been driving antibiotic resistance to a high frequency in this population.

The role of atypical pathogens in AECB is uncertain, but some studies have found a high frequency of infection with *Mycoplasma pneumoniae* and *Chlamydia pneumoniae* in exacerbation patients, and these pathogens may coexist with bacterial pathogens [46]. In one study, patients with positive serology for *C. pneumoniae* at the time of exacerbation had the same frequency of cough, dyspnoea, fever, sputum production, tachypnoea and tachycardia as patients with negative serology [46]. These findings do not definitively establish an aetiological role for these organisms, and many therapy trials have not shown superiority when an antibiotic regimen is used that covers atypical organisms, compared with one that does not.

Enteric Gram-negative bacteria, including *Pseudomonas aeruginosa*, have also been isolated from some patients with AECB [47,48]. Although the frequency of these pathogens is not high in all patients, they are much more common in those who are admitted to hospital, especially in patients with severe airflow obstruction and in those with respiratory failure requiring mechanical ventilation [47,48]. In fact, when patients had an $FEV_1 \leq 35\%$ of predicted, more than half of the pathogens isolated from patients admitted with an exacerbation in one study had Gram-negative organisms present, including *P. aeruginosa* [47]. Although not all investigators have confirmed this finding, these organisms have also been reported to be more common in patients with an *FEV*$_1$ of less than 50% than in patients with better lung function [48], and these organisms were present in nearly 30% of patients with severe exacerbations requiring mechanical ventilation [10].

Relationship of bacteriology to specific patient features

The identity of the likely bacterium present during an acute exacerbation is variable and related to a number of patient features including: severity of exacerbation, age (≥ 65 years), frequency of exacerbations, presence of comorbid cardiopulmonary disease, frequency of antibiotic therapy, use of corticosteroids and the severity of obstructive airways disease (*FEV*$_1$ as a percentage of predicted) [5,6,47,48].

Bronchoscopic studies have shown that as the severity of exacerbation increases, the bacteriology of the exacerbation becomes more complex, involving more Gram-negatives, and more antibiotic-resistant pathogens. For stable outpatients with AECB, the three common 'core organisms' (*H. influenzae*, pneumococcus and *M. catarrhalis*) predominate. However, in patients requiring mechanical ventilation for AECB, Gram-negative organisms are seen with increasing frequency [8,10]. In addition, these organisms are also more common in patients with severe airflow obstruction, defined in different studies as an *FEV*$_1$ (as % predicted) below 50% or 35% [47,48].

Other studies have identified the frequency of exacerbations and the presence of comorbid cardiopulmonary disease as factors to be considered in defining patients who are infected with pathogens that are difficult to treat with standard antibiotic therapy. In one study of 471 outpatients with AECB, the likelihood of a patient having a recurrence after therapy for exacerbation was related to the presence of underlying cardiopulmonary disease, and the history of how many exacerbations were present in the preceding year [6]. If patients had less than three exacerbations per year, then the recurrence rate was 9.1%, compared with a 13.1% rate in those with 3–4 exacerbations per year and 18.4% in those with more than four exacerbations per year. A factor such as age is also important in predicting bacteriology, because age over 65 years has been identified as a risk factor for airway colonization by Gram-negative organisms, and for antibiotic resistance if pneumococcus is present [35,36,49].

In one recently published guideline for antibiotic therapy of AECB, many of these patient features were used to predict the likely pathogens causing exacerbation [5]. Such stratification serves two purposes: first, to predict the likely pathogens and the likelihood of antibiotic resistance and, secondly, to identify patients who may do poorly with an exacerbation if not given a rapidly effective therapy. For stratification purposes, complicated AECB patients, at risk for beta-lactam resistance and Gram-negative infection, are those with *FEV*$_1$ of less than 50% predicted, more than four exacerbations per year, cardiac disease, use of home oxygen, chronic oral steroid therapy and use of antibiotics in the past 3 months. Patient features that make *Pseudomonas* and multidrug-resistant Gram-negative organisms more likely are the presence of an *FEV*$_1$ of less than 35% predicted or the presence of more than one of the risk factors listed above.

Principles of antibiotic use

Mechanisms of bacterial killing

Antibiotics disrupt bacterial growth by preventing the formation of an intact cell wall, by interfering with protein synthesis or by inhibiting common metabolic pathways [50,51]. Agents that interfere with cell wall synthesis or with other key metabolic functions of the organism can kill bacteria and are termed 'bactericidal'. These agents include penicillins, cephalosporins, aminoglycosides, fluoroquinolones, vancomycin, rifampin and metronidazole. Agents that inhibit the growth of bacteria and rely on host defences to eliminate the organisms are termed 'bacteriostatic' and these agents include the macrolides, tetracyclines, sulfa drugs, chloramphenicol and clindamycin. The distinction between bacteriostatic and bacteriocidal agents may be most relevant in patients with impaired neutrophil function (neutropenia) or in those with deep-seated infections such as endocarditis or meningitis. However, in the therapy of AECB, these distinctions may not be clinically relevant, and the value of an agent is probably best predicted by its activity against the aetiological pathogen. In fact, in one analysis, there was a strong correlation ($r = 0.9$) between the ability of an antibiotic to eradicate an organism from the sputum with the clinical response rate, regardless of the mechanism of bacterial killing [52]. These findings suggest that the activity of an antibiotic, relative to the susceptibility of the aetiological pathogen, is the most important determinant of clinical outcome.

The activity of an antimicrobial agent can be defined by the minimum inhibitory concentration (MIC) required to inhibit *in vitro* the growth of 90% of a standard sized inoculum in broth culture. The lower the MIC number is, the more active an agent is against its target pathogen. However, the use of MIC values to predict antimicrobial effect only takes into account whether an agent can achieve adequate levels in serum. When an infection is in the airways, as in patients with AECB, then the MIC value may not adequately predict killing in the lung. Thus, if an agent penetrates well into respiratory secretions (such as a quinolone) and its concentrations in the airway exceed serum levels, the MIC values may underestimate the antibacterial effect [53]. Conversely a poorly penetrating agent (such as an aminoglycoside) may be less effective clinically at certain sites of respiratory infection than expected on the basis of *in vitro* MIC values.

Even if an antibiotic reaches the site of airway infection, not all bactericidal agents kill bacteria in the same fashion, and this information should be used to optimize dosing regimens [54]. Certain agents, especially the quinolones and aminoglycosides, kill bacteria in what has been described as a 'concentration dependent fashion', meaning that the higher the serum level relative to the MIC and the higher the area under the concentration–time curve (AUC) relative to the MIC, the more effective the agent. Optimization of the peak/MIC ratio or the AUC/MIC (defined as the area under the inhibition curve, or AUIC), can lead to more rapid killing of bacteria and less chance of selecting for resistance [53–55]. In theory, the optimal way to administer these agents would be to take a 24-h dose and administer it once a day to achieve high peak concentrations. In addition, increasing the dosage to the highest level tolerated can also optimize these pharamcokinetic parameters. In the case of quinolone therapy of pneumonia, increasing the dosage of ciprofloxacin or levofloxacin to 400 mg every 8 h or 750 mg/day, respectively, has led to more rapid resolution of symptoms and the ability to eradicate organisms that would be unable to be eradicated at lower doses [56,57]. However, there are agents that do not achieve a greater effect with higher concentrations, but rather kill in relation to how long they exceed the MIC of the target organism, and the activity of these agents can be enhanced by maximizing time above the MIC of the target organism. For these drugs, optimal effect could be achieved by prolonged serum concentrations that are above the MIC, but it is not necessary to have these concentrations exceed the MIC value by more than a factor of 4, or to exceed the MIC of the target organism for more than 40% of the dosing interval [54]. Optimal dosing of these agents could be achieved with prolonged release preparations (such as the new formulation of amoxicillin/clavulanate), or by continuous intravenous infusion.

Craig [54] has recently reviewed and clarified some of these concepts related to bactericidal killing mechanisms. Agents that kill in a concentration-dependent fashion include the aminoglycosides, the fluoroquinolones and metronidazole (Table 60.2). Studies with quinolones have shown that in the therapy of pneumococcus with levofloxacin, both clinical and microbiological success were more likely if the peak/MIC ratio exceeded 12 [55]. In addition, it is necessary to maintain a peak/MIC ratio of at least 8–10 to prevent the emergence of resistance during therapy [53–55]. In studies of critically ill patients with

Table 60.2 Pharmacokinetics of common antibiotics.

Bactericidal in a concentration-dependent fashion
(Optimize peak/MIC ratio or AUC/MIC ratio)
Aminoglycosides*
Fluoroquinolones*
Metronidazole

Bactericidal in a time-dependent fashion
(Once concentration is 4–5 times MIC, optimize time above MIC to at least 40% of the dosing interval)
Beta-lactams†
Vancomycin
Clindamycin
Macrolides

AUC, area under the curve; MIC, minimum inhibitory concentration.
* Prolonged postantibiotic effect against Gram-negative bacteria.
† Little or no postantibiotic effect against Gram-negative bacteria.

ciprofloxacin, the best predictor of clinical and microbiological efficacy against *P. aeruginosa* was an AUC/MIC ratio of at least 125 [58]. The efficacy of aminoglycosides has also been related to both the AUC/MIC and peak/MIC ratios [54]. Agents that kill in a time-dependent fashion have a saturation of killing effect once the concentrations exceed 4–5 times the MIC, and time of exposure above MIC is the key to their effect. In this group of antimicrobials are beta-lactam antibiotics, vancomycin, clindamycin and the macrolides. In designing dosing regimens, it is important to realize that it may not be necessary to keep the concentration of antibiotics above the MIC for the entire dosing interval. Craig [54] has shown in animal models that with penicillins and cephalosporins, bacteriological cure will occur 85–100% of the time if the concentration of these agents exceed the MIC for at least 40% of the dosing interval. Maximal killing occurs once concentrations exceed the MIC for 60–70% of the dosing interval.

Another killing mechanism that may have relevance for some antibiotics is the postantibiotic effect (PAE), which refers to the continued suppression of bacterial growth after the concentration of the antibiotic falls below the MIC of the target organism [54]. While most antibiotics have a PAE against Gram-positive organisms, prolonged PAEs against Gram-negative organisms occur with the aminoglycosides, quinolones, tetracyclines and macrolides. Little or no PAE against Gram-negative organisms occurs with beta-lactam agents with the exception of the carbapenems (imipenem and meropenem). Fortunately, the agents with a prolonged PAE tend to be the same agents that kill in a concentration-dependent fashion, and this is why once daily dosing of agents such as the aminoglycosides has been successful [59]. With once daily dosing, high peaks are achieved, thus maximizing concentration-dependent killing; low troughs result, thus minimizing nephrotoxicity; and the prolonged PAE is relied upon to keep killing bacteria at the times when low trough concentrations occur. A recent meta-analysis has shown the efficacy and safety of once daily aminogylcoside dosing, although this type of regimen is not substantially safer or more effective than traditional regimens [59]. In the therapy of complicated AECB, aminoglycosides are sometimes required, but aerosol therapy is now an option, and this approach may overcome some of the concerns with the dosing and toxicity of systemic aminoglycosides.

Table 60.3 Penetration of common antibiotics into respiratory secretions.

Good penetration (generally lipid soluble and inflammation independent)
Fluoroquinolones
Macrolides: including azithromycin and clarithromycin
Tetracyclines
Co-trimoxazole

Poor penetration (generally lipid insoluble and inflammation dependent)
Aminoglycosides
Beta-lactams: penicillins, cephalosporins

Penetration to site of infection and route of administration

In the therapy of AECB, the antibiotic must reach the bronchial mucosa, the primary site of infection, in order to be effective. Antibiotics can concentrate in a variety of sites in the lung, including the sputum, the bronchial epithelium, the lung parenchyma, the epithelial lining fluid and phagocytic cells [60]. Although it is unclear which site is most relevant in the therapy of AECB, concentrations in the mucosa and sputum are probably the most important. Some drugs reach lung tissue only when inflammation is present, while others, primarily lipid-soluble agents, are inflammation independent and can penetrate in the absence of increased capillary permeability. These lipid-soluble agents include the macrolides, tetracyclines, quinolones and co-trimoxazole, and all of these agents can achieve good penetration into the sputum or the bronchial mucosa. Penetration of the antibiotic is reflected by how high the sputum level is, relative to the MIC of the target organism. For a quinolone such as ciprofloxacin, the sputum/MIC ratio for *H. influenzae* and *M. catarrhalis* exceeds a value of 60. The macrolide azithromycin has a sputum/MIC ratio for *H. influenzae* and pneumococcus that also exceeds 60. Although the ratio for clarithromycin against *H. influenzae* is considerably lower, the ratio for the agent against pneumococcus exceeds a value of 250 [61]. In addition, agents such as the macrolides, quinolones and clindamycin are actively transported into phagocytic cells and achieve very high levels at this site. The clinical relevance of these findings remains uncertain, but may explain why some agents remain clinically effective when good bronchial penetration occurs even when serum levels are not high, relative to the MIC of the target organism. The agents that are relatively lipid insoluble, and thus penetrate poorly and are inflammation dependent include the aminoglycosides, the penicillins and the cephalosporins (Table 60.3).

The route of administration may also impact on pharmacokinetics and respiratory concentrations. If an agent is given intravenously, the serum levels peak rapidly, while oral administration generally leads to a lower peak level, but antibiotics can be formulated for slow release after oral administration, and allow for prolonged concentration in the serum (as with extended-release preparations of amoxicillin/clavulanate and clarithromycin). One way to avoid concerns about antibiotic penetration is to deliver the antibiotic via the aerosol route. There are no good studies of this approach in AECB, but aerosolized aminoglycosides have been used as adjunctive therapy for pneumonia and nosocomial tracheobronchitis, as well as for exacerbations of airway diseases such as bronchiectasis and cystic fibrosis [62]. In one placebo-controlled trial, inhaled tobramycin was used twice daily for 4 weeks in bronchiectasis patients who were colonized with *P. aeruginosa*, and the treatment led to a reduction in bacterial count but no change in the frequency of exacerbation or antibiotic use; however, the number of patients studied was small [62].

Ease of use of common antibiotics and frequency of administration

As with any therapy, the patient must complete a full course of therapy with an antibiotic to assure maximal efficacy. Previous studies have shown that compliance with short-term antibiotic regimens ranges from 56% to 89% [63]. Patients are less likely to comply with a prescribed regimen if they are already taking multiple medications, if side-effects occur, if dosing is more than twice a day, if use conflicts with their lifestyle and if the consequences of non-compliance seem minimal. In a Gallup survey, 54% of all Americans reported that they did not finish a course of antibiotics as prescribed. In fact, 54% stopped antibiotics once they felt better, even if they had not finished a full course of therapy [64]. In addition, many reported missing a scheduled dose. When questioned, 82% of the respondents prefered an antibiotic that can be given once or twice a day, and only 5% were willing to be treated for a 14-day course [64].

These findings should be considered when prescribing an antibiotic for AECB. Fortunately, a number of appropriate antibiotics can be given once or twice daily. Once daily dosing is available with azithromycin and extended-release clarithromycin, telithromycin and the new quinolones (gatifloxacin, levofloxacin and moxifloxacin). Other oral antibiotics are also available for once daily dosing, but do not represent ideal drugs from an antimicriobial spectrum and these include cefixime, ceftibutin and dirithromycin. Twice daily dosing is available with amoxicillin/clavulanate, cefpodoxime, cefprozil, ceftibutin, cefuroxime, ciprofloxacin, clarithromycin, doxycline, ofloxacin and co-trimoxazole. In general, patients with AECB should receive one of these agents because it is unlikely that an agent given more often will be taken as prescribed.

Duration of therapy

Most clinical trials in AECB have used durations of therapy of 7–10 days. However, a number of recent trials have successfully used shorter durations of therapy, especially with agents that are active against drug-resistant pathogens. Thus, 5 days of therapy has been adequate for the new quinolones, the ketolide telithromycin, and 3-day therapy has been effective for azithromycin and quinolones, in selected populations [65–72].

Desired features of an ideal antibiotic for AECB

Although a current evidence-based consensus statement concluded that all antibiotics are equivalent in AECB, there may be some advantages to specific agents, particularly in certain patient populations [5]. However, this is difficult to prove, because most studies of AECB therapy have been conducted for the purposes of licensing a new antimicrobial and have been designed to include just enough patients to show equivalence between the tested agents. In addition, these antibiotic trials have rarely defined different therapies for different types of patients, lumping patients of all disease severity together in one clinical trial. Several newer trials, described below, have suggested that certain agents may have value over other agents for specific patient populations [67,73,74]. Ideally, an antibiotic that is used for AECB should have several features (Table 60.4):

1 Activity against the most common and most likely (for each patient type) aetiological pathogens, but certainly with activity against *H. influenzae*, pneumococcus and *M. catarrhalis*;

2 resistance to destruction by bacterial beta-lactamases;

3 good penetration into the sputum and bronchial mucosa;

4 easy to take (no more than twice daily), with few side-effects; and

Table 60.4 Characteristics of the ideal antibiotic for acute exacerbations of chronic bronchitis.

Active against the likely pathogens for each patient type:
• Always active against pneumococcus, *Haemophilus influenzae*, and possibly atypical pathogens
• In selected patients, active against resistant organisms and enteric Gram-negative bacteria

Resistant to destruction by bacterial beta-lactamases (*H. influenzae* and *Moraxella catarrhalis*)

Good penetration into sputum and bronchial tissue
• High sputum/MIC ratio against target organisms

Likelihood of compliance with the prescribed regimen is high: once or twice daily dosing, few side-effects

Cost effective
• Prevention of hospitalization, prolonged time between exacerbations

MIC, minimum inhibitory concentration.

5 cost effective, considering factors such as prevention of hospitalization and prolongation of time between exacerbations.

Properties of specific antimicrobial agents

A number of agents are commonly used to treat patients with AECB. They generally fall into the following drug classes: macrolides and azalides (erythromycin, clarithromycin and azithromycin), tetracyclines, ketolides, co-trimoxazole, beta-lactams (penicillins and cephalosporins) and fluoroquinolones.

Macrolides

Macrolides are bacteriostatic agents that bind to the 50S ribosomal subunit of the target bacteria and inhibit RNA-dependent protein synthesis. The macrolides have good activity against pneumococci, as well as atypical pathogens (*C. pneumoniae*, *M. pneumoniae*, *Legionella*), but the older erythromycin-type drugs are not active against *H. influenzae*, can interact with theophylline to increase levels and have poor intestinal tolerance, making it difficult to use these agents in patients with AECB. The newer macrolide agents include azithromycin (also referred to as an azalide) and clarithromycin. These agents have enhanced activity against *H. influenzae* (including beta-lactamase producing strains) although, on an MIC basis, azithromycin is more active [50,51]. The macrolides are also active against *M. catarrhalis*, although the newer agents have enhanced activity against this pathogen compared with the older agents. Among the newer macrolides, azithromycin is more active than erythromycin against not only *H. influenzae* and *M. catarrhalis*, but also *M. pneumoniae*. However, clarithromycin is more active against *S. pneumoniae*, *Legionella* and *C. pneumoniae* [50,51]. Azithromycin has no theophylline interaction, while clarithromycin has the same potential for interaction as erythromycin.

Both of the newer agents have better intestinal tolerance than erythromycin and penetrate well into sputum, lung tissue and phagocytes. Clarithromycin, which has an active 14-hydroxy metabolite that is antibacterial, is administered twice a day orally at a dose of 500-mg for 7–10 days in the treatment of AECB. A new preparation of extended-release clarithromycin is administered as a 1000-mg dose once daily and has been effective with a 7-day course of therapy [75]. Azithromycin has a longer half-life than clarithromycin, and concentrates in tissues, achieving very low serum levels when administered orally. The dose for oral therapy of AECB is 500 mg on day 1, followed by 250 mg/day on days 2–5. Alternatively, this drug can be administered for AECB in a dosage of 500 mg/day for 3 days, and this regimen has efficacy comparable to other agents administered for a longer duration [69,70]. For the hospitalized patient, an intravenous preparation of azithromycin is available and is administered at 500 mg/day, with the duration defined by the clinical course of the patient

Although macrolides remain an important therapeutic option for AECB, pneumococcal resistance is becoming increasingly common, being present in as many as 35–40% of all pneumococci [37]. In addition, macrolide resistance can also coexist with penicillin resistance, and as many as 30–40% of penicillin-resistant pneumococci are also erythromycin resistant [36,37]. The clinical relevance of these *in vitro* findings remains to be defined. However, there are two forms of macrolide resistance: one involving efflux of the antibiotic from the bacterial cell, and the other involving altered ribosomal binding of the antibiotic. The former mechanism is associated with much lower levels of resistance than the latter, and is present in two-thirds of the macrolide-resistant pneumococci in the USA. The latter form of resistance is fortunately less common because, if present, it is unlikely that macrolide therapy for pneumococcal infection would be effective.

Clinical trials of macrolides in AECB have documented efficacy for clarithromycin (including the extended-release preparation) and azithromycin [69,70,75,76]. In general, these agents have been equivalent to other classes of antibiotics, including quinolones (azithromycin versus levofloxacin and moxifloxacin, clarithromycin versus gatifloxacin), and beta-lactams (clarithromycin and azithromycin equivalent to amoxicillin/clavulanate) [65,70,76–79]. In spite of general equivalence to other, newer agents, in one retrospective analysis, azithromycin was among a group of antibiotics that led to less relapses and a prolonged duration of time from one exacerbation to the next compared with older agents, in patients with recurrent exacerbations [73]. However, in a comparative study with a quinolone (gemifloxacin), clarithromycin was less effective in preventing relapses, particularly if the pathogen was *H. influenzae* [67].

Macrolides have other effects beyond their antibacterial action, and may be anti-inflammatory, reducing the amount of sputum production in chronic bronchitis patients [80]. The role of macrolides in preventing exacerbations of COPD through their anti-inflammatory actions is unknown, but chronic macrolide therapy has been shown to reduce the frequency of exacerbations in patients with cystic fibrosis [81].

Tetracyclines

The tetracyclines, like the macrolides, are also bacteriostatic agents, which act by binding the 30S ribosomal subunit and interfering with protein synthesis. These agents can be used in AECB because they are active against *H. influenzae* and atypical pathogens, but there are reports of increasing resistance among pneumococci [50,51]. In the USA, pneumococcal resistance to tetracyclines may be approaching 20%, and may exceed 50% among organisms with high-level penicillin resistance [5]. Photosensitivity is the major side-effect, limiting the use of these agents in sun-exposed patients.

Ketolides

This new class of antibiotics is a semi-synthetic derivative of the macrolides, with a 14-member ring structure, and substitution of a keto group at the C3 site. These agents act to inhibit ribosomal protein synthesis in bacteria, by binding to two different sites on the 50S ribosomal subunit and, because of enhanced binding affinity and the binding to multiples sites, are able to avoid some of the resistance problems associated with the macrolides [82]. In addition, this class of antibiotics has a poor affinity for the pneumococcal efflux pump. Because of these characteristics, ketolides are active against pneumococci that are macrolide resistant by either the *erm* or *mef* mechanism. Ketolides are also active against *H. influenzae*, but *in vitro* activity is not quite as high as with azithromycin. In clinical trials, the eradication rate of *H. influenzae* by telithromycin has been 84% [82]. In addition, these agents have activity against the atypical pathogens. Ketolides concentrate well in the respiratory tract and in white blood cells, and kill bacteria in a concentration-dependent fashion, unlike the macrolides which kill in a time-dependent manner. In clinical trials, a ketolide, telithromycin, has been evaluated and has been administered at 800 mg/day for 5 days. This regimen has been compared with a 10-day course of amoxicillin/

clavulanic acid (500 mg t.i.d.) or cefuroxime (500 mg b.i.d.) and found to be equivalent [66,82]. Telithromycin was as active as comparators in patients above the age of 65 years, in those with worse lung function and in those with multiple comorbid illnesses. Bacteriological success was equivalent to comparators when the infecting pathogen was either pneumococcus or *H. influenzae* [82]. Side-effects are primarily intestinal with nausea and diarrhoea occurring in some patients, but liver function abnormalities and cardiac QT prolongation have been reported, but are uncommon. There does not appear to be an interaction with theophylline.

Co-trimoxazole

This combination antibiotic has been used as a mainstay for the therapy of AECB because of its antimicrobial spectrum, ease of use and low cost [83]. It has bactericidal activity against pneumococcus, *H. influenzae* and *M. catarrhalis*, but not against atypical pathogens. Recently, it has become less popular because of the emergence of pneumococcal resistance at rates of at least 30%, because 80–90% of organisms that are penicillin-resistant are also resistant to co-trimoxazole [36]. The sulfa component of the drug inhibits the bacterial enzyme responsible for forming the immediate precursor of folic acid, dihydropteroic acid. Trimethoprim is synergistic with the sulfa component because it inhibits the activity of bacterial dihydrofolate reductase. Co-trimoxazole is available in a fixed combination of 1 : 5 (trimethoprim : sulfamethoxazole), and is given as either 80/400 or 160/800 mg orally twice a day for 10 days, but the dosage should be adjusted in renal failure. An intravenous preparation is also available. Side-effects generally result from the sulfa component and include rash, gastrointestinal upset and occasional renal failure (especially in elderly patients).

Beta-lactam antibiotics

These bactericidal antibiotics, which include the penicillins, cephalosporins and other agents, have in common the presence of a beta-lactam ring, which is bound to a five-membered thiazolidine ring in the case of the penicillins and to a six-membered dihydrothiazine ring in the case of the cephalosporins [50,51]. Modifications in the thiazolidine ring can lead to agents such as the penems (imipenem and meropenem), while absence of the second ring structure characterizes the monobactams (aztreonam). These agents can also be combined with beta-lactamase inhibitors such as sulbactam, tazobactam or clavulanic acid to create the beta-lactam/beta-lactamase inhibitor drugs. These combination agents extend the antimicrobial spectrum of the beta-lactams by providing a substrate (sulbactam, clavulanic acid, tazobactam) for the bacterial beta-lactamases, thereby preserving the antibacterial activity of the parent compound. Beta-lactam antibiotics work by interfering with the synthesis of bacterial cell wall peptidogylcans by binding to bacterial penicillin-binding proteins.

The penicillins used for AECB include the aminopenicillins (ampicillin, amoxicillin) and the beta-lactam/beta-lactamase inhibitor combinations. The anti-pseudomonal penicillins (piperacillin, ticarcillin) are available only intravenously, and as a beta-lactamase inhibitor combination (piperacillin/tazobacteam, ticarcillin/clavulanate) and are not commonly used for AECB. The beta-lactamase inhibitor combination most commonly used for oral therapy of AECB is amoxicillin/clavulanate. The addition of clavulanic acid makes this agent resistant to bacterial beta-lactamases, an important concern in patients with AECB, but some *H. influenzae* organisms can hyperproduce these enzymes and even be resistant to amoxicillin/clavulanate [33].

Amoxicillin/clavulanate had been given as 500/125 mg t.i.d or 875/125 mg b.i.d. for 10 days, and has been effective therapy for AECB. Clinical trials have shown equivalence to azithromycin and to moxifloxacin, when given for 7–10 days [26,83–85]. It may offer an advantage over amoxicillin alone, because this agent is susceptible to destruction by bacterial beta-lactamases, a feature that may explain the observation of high failures rates with amoxicillin (54%) but not with amoxicillin/clavulanate (9%) in patients presenting to an emergency department with AECB [27]. Recently, with concerns about pneumococcal resistance, a new preparation of amoxicillin/clavulanate has been developed with a slow release formulation and with more amoxicillin relative to clavulanate, and the dosage is 2000/125 mg b.i.d. This new preparation would be active against resistant pneumococci with MIC values of at least 2 mg/L. Although this high-dose preparation is not approved in the USA for AECB therapy, clinical trials have shown efficacy similar to levofloxacin and clarithromycin [78].

The cephalosporins span from first to fourth generation, but the fourth-generation agents are not available for oral therapy of AECB [83,86]. The earlier agents were generally active against Gram-positive organisms, but did not have extended activity for the more complex Gram-negative organisms, or anaerobes, and were susceptible to destruction by bacterial beta-lactamases. The newer generation agents are generally more specialized, with broad-spectrum activity and with more mechanisms to resist breakdown by bacterial enzymes. The second-generation and newer agents are resistant to bacterial beta-lactamases, and the oral agents that are active against resistant pneumococci include cefuroxime, cefprozil and cefpodoxime [86]. The intravenous third- and fourth-generation agents active against penicillin-resistant pneumococci include ceftriaxone, cefotaxime and cefepime, while ceftazidime is less reliable against this organism. Intravenous agents are occasionally used in hospitalized patients, and cefepime and ceftazidime have activity against *P. aeruginosa*. Although cephalosporins have been used successfully to treat AECB, they have not always been as successful as quinolones, amoxicillin/clavulanate and the macrolides in patients with recurrent infections [73], but have been effective at preventing relapses in AECB among patients seen in an emergency room setting [27].

Fluoroquinolones

These bactericidal agents act by inhibiting bacterial DNA gyrase and thus interfere with DNA replication, repair, transcription and other cellular processes [40,53]. DNA gyrase is only one form of a bacterial topoisomerase enzyme that is inhibited by quinolones, and activity against other such enzymes is part of the effect of a variety of quinolones [40,83]. The earlier quinolones (such as ciprofloxacin and ofloxacin) are active primarily against DNA gyrase, which accounts for their good activity against Gram-negative organisms. The newer agents (gatifloxacin, gemifloxacin, levofloxacin and moxifloxacin) bind both DNA gyrase and topoisomerase IV, and have extended their activity to Gram-positive organisms, including drug-resistant *Streptococcus pneumoniae* (DRSP). Resistance to quinolones can occur through mutations in the topoisomerase enzymes, by altered permeability of the bacterial cell wall or by efflux. The quinolones kill in a concentration-dependent fashion, and thus optimal antibacterial activity can be achieved with infrequent dosing, and with high peak concentrations and high AUCs. In addition, because quinolones have a PAE against both Gram-positive and Gram-negative organisms, they can continue to kill even after local concentrations fall below the MIC of the target organism [53]. These properties make the quinolones well-suited to infrequent dosing, with the ideal being once daily dosing, particularly given the relatively long half-life of the newer compounds. The only factor limiting a switch to once daily dosing for all quinolones is the toxicity associated with high doses of some agents (such as ciprofloxacin), particularly concerns related to neurotoxicity and possible seizures.

There are two features of quinolones that make them well-suited to respiratory infections. First, they penetrate well into respiratory secretions and inflammatory cells, achieving concentrations that usually exceed serum levels, and thus these agents may be clinically more effective than predicted by MIC values. This may explain the observation that quinolones are often better than other agents in prolonging the 'disease-free' interval between exacerbations [87]. Secondly, these agents are highly bioavailable with oral administration and thus similar levels can be reached if administered orally or intravenously. This has allowed some patients to remain on oral therapy out of the hospital and still receive a highly active antimicrobial regimen.

The fluoroquinolones have excellent antimicrobial activity against beta-lactamase producing *H. influenzae*

and *M. catarrhalis*, making them very useful for patients with AECB. However, the newer agents (gatifloxacin, gemifloxacin, levofloxacin and moxifloxacin) extend the activity of the quinolones by Gram-positive activity, as well as by being more active against *C. pneumoniae* and *M. pneumoniae* than the older agents [53]. The new agents are also highly effective against *L. pneumophila*. However, if *P. aeruginosa* is the target organism, then only ciprofloxacin (750 mg b.i.d. orally or 400 mg 8-hourly intravenously) or levofloxacin (750 mg/day) are active enough for clinical use. Because the older agents, ciprofloxacin and ofloxacin, have borderline activity against pneumococcus, if they are used for AECB, the dose must be increased, and in one study, ciprofloxacin was administered at 750 mg b.i.d., and led to efficacy in the therapy of complex patients with AECB [88].

Among the newer agents, their *in vitro* activity against pneumococcus is variable, with the agents listed in the order of most to least active (on an MIC basis) as: gemifloxacin, moxifloxacin, gatifloxacin and levofloxacin (Table 60.5) [40,41,53]. All of these agents also have long half-lives, generally allowing for once daily dosing, although the half-lives of these drugs vary from 6 h for levofloxacin to more than 15 h for moxifloxacin and gemifloxacin. The agents also differ in the degree of protein binding, with agents that have a low degree of binding having higher free concentrations in the serum. The relevance of this feature to clinical outcome is uncertain, but agents such as levofloxacin and moxifloxacin are not highly protein bound. Although the new agents are highly active against pneumococci, both penicillin sensitive and resistant organisms, there is some concern that with widespread use, pneumococcal resistance to these agents will increase [40,41,43]. In addition, one recent study has shown that as organisms become penicillin resistant, they are also more likely to be quinolone resistant [41]. With this in mind, pneumococci are more likely to be resistant to the agents with the lowest pneumococcal activity (as listed above). Although

Table 60.5 Activity of fluoroquinolones against pneumococcus.

Agent	MIC 90 (mg/L)	C_{max} (mg/L)
Ciprofloxacin (500 mg)	2.0	3.0
Gatifloxacin (400 mg)	0.5	4.2
Gemifloxacin (320 mg)	0.125	1.5
Levofloxacin (500 mg)	1.0	5.7
Moxifloxacin (400 mg)	0.25	4.5

C_{max}, maximum plasma concentration; MIC, minimum inhibitory concentration.

resistance of pneumococci to quinolones is still not common, it has developed in Asia, particularly to levofloxacin, in COPD patients who have been given repeated courses of therapy [89]. Other risk factors for quinolone resistance among pneumococci are recent hospitalization and residence in a nursing home. One concern for the future efficacy of the quinolones in AECB patients has been their widespread use in outpatients with a variety of illnesses, who may be better treated with another antibiotic or who may not even need antibiotic therapy [39].

One major distinction among these new quinolones is their profile of toxic side-effects. A number of agents have been removed from clinical use because of toxicities such as QT prolongation (grepafloxacin), phototoxicity (sparfloxacin) and liver necrosis (trovafloxacin). Recently, gatifloxacin use has been curtailed because of drug-induced glucose abnormalities (hypo- and hyperglycaemia), especially in diabetics. The side-effects of the other new agents have generally been minimal but, as with any therapy, the risks of use should be weighed against the benefits.

In clinical trials, all of the newer agents have been effective with 5 days of therapy. The dosing of gatifloxacin is 400 mg/day, gemifloxacin 320 mg/day, levofloxacin 500 mg/day and moxifloxacin 400 mg/day. In many situations, the newer agents are considered to be therapeutically equivalent, but some investigators have considered that the risk of promoting pneumococcal quinolone resistance may be higher with agents that have higher MIC values, and thus have recommended using the most active agents preferentially [40]. When compared with other classes of antibiotics, the quinolones have the ability to prolong the disease-free interval, a feature that was first described with ciprofloxacin [67,74,87].

While most studies have not shown quinolones to be more effective than other antibiotics used to treat AECB, two recent studies have reported improved outcomes with the newer agents [67,74]. In one study, 320 mg/day gemifloxacin for 5 days was compared with 500 mg clarithromycin b.i.d. for 7 days and, although both agents showed similar clinical success rates initially, gemifloxacin led to a higher bacteriological success rates, especially for *H. influenzae* [67]. In addition, gemifloxacin-treated patients had fewer recurrences after 26 weeks, and fewer hospitalizations. In another study, 5 days of moxifloxacin was compared with therapy with one of three standard agents given for 7 days (amoxicillin, cefuroxime or clarithromycin) [74]. Patients in this study had established chronic bronchitis with at least two exacerbations in the preceding year, and those given moxifloxacin had less need for additional antibiotics and a longer disease-free interval than those given the comparator. These two studies are interesting because they focused on long-term endpoints, and documented a potential advantage of the new quinolones compared with other accepted therapies of AECB. The fact that differences only became evident when outcomes other than short-term results were evaluated may explain why many prior studies concluded that all antibiotics used for AECB are equivalent.

Cost effectiveness of antibiotic therapy in AECB

Although it is difficult to determine how to best define the cost effectiveness of antibiotic therapy, it is quite clear that multiple factors, in addition to acquisition cost, should be considered. For example, an agent that costs little to buy, but has limited efficacy, might cause a patient to miss several days of work, and thus be less cost effective than a more expensive agent that was able to cure the patient rapidly. Other economic endpoints that should be considered in defining a cost-effective antibiotic for AECB include the prevention of hospitalization, the duration of disease-free interval, the need for other medications and the development of antimicrobial resistance [90,91].

One study looking at this issue was a prospective randomized trial of quinolone therapy (with ciprofloxacin) versus usual care, involving 240 patients with AECB managed by their family physicians [90]. For the group as a whole, quinolone therapy was not substantially better than usual care, but for certain patient subsets it appeared to have some advantage. Ciprofloxacin was associated with a better clinical outcome and lower cost for patients who had moderate or severe bronchitis (severity of the acute episode), at least four episodes of AECB in the preceding year, more than 10 years illness, age of at least 56 years and at least three comorbities, once again confirming the concept that empirical therapy should be modified for different patient groups. All of these findings suggest that if patient profiling is used to prescribe antibiotics, then the benefits of therapy with specific agents for specific patients will be enhanced. Similarly, the study of gemifloxacin versus clarithromycin documented cost efficacy for the quinolone, primarily by the avoidance of hospitalization, physician visits and lost work productivity [92].

Therapy for AECB using patient subsets: should different patients be treated with different therapies?

The bacteriology of exacerbations may vary with specific patient features, and in certain populations, specific therapies may have more value than others. In addition, as patients become increasingly ill, both acutely and chronically, the consequences of ineffective antibiotic therapy of AECB may become more important. Therefore, a number of guidelines have been developed that suggest patient stratification approaches and suggested therapies for each subset. Most of the guidelines about exacerbations of COPD either do not recommend specific antibiotics or recommend that any antibiotic can be used in any patient population. For example, the statement of the American College of Physicians and the American Society of Internal Medicine, published jointly with the American College of Chest Physicians states 'to date, no randomized, placebo-controlled trials have proved the superiority of the newer broad-spectrum antibiotics' in patients who are likely to have resistant organisms present [4]. Recently, a Candian guideline was published that made recommendations for specific antibiotic choices for different populations, defined on the basis of the presence of risk factors for treatment failure [5].

In the Canadian guideline, the risk factors for treatment failure in AECB included: frequent exacerbations (odds ratio of 2.11 for those with more than four exacerbations per year), more severe lung dysfunction, ischaemic heart disease or congestive heart failure, increasing age, use of maintenance steroids, use of home oxygen and chronic mucus hypersecretion [5]. Many of these factors also increase risk for hospitalization including cardiopulmonary disease (odds ratio of 8.9), patients with disease of long duration and in those with severe lung dysfunction. Based on these features, the authors identified three groups of patients with AECB: the simple bronchitic, the complicated bronchitic and the patient with chronic suppurative bronchitis (Table 60.6) [5].

Therapy for all patients should target the group of 'core organisms' that are possible for any patient with exacerbation, and these include *H. influenzae* (usually non-typable), *M. catarrhalis*, *S. pneumoniae* and *H. parainfluenzae*. The patient who is at risk for only these organisms is the 'simple bronchitic', defined as a patient with at least two of the three cardinal symptoms of exacerbation, but with no risk factors for treatment failure or hospitalization. This population has an FEV_1 of more than 50% predicted, less than four exacerbations per year and no underlying cardiac disease. These patients are less likely to have resistant pathogens, and could even tolerate treatment failure (although not highly likely) without requiring hospitalization. Therapy for this population was recommended to be a newer macrolide (azithromycin or clarithomycin), a cephalosporin, amoxicillin, co-trimoxazole, or tetracycline (doxycycline); but, in the case of a treatment failure, a fluroquinolone or beta-lactam/beta-lactamase inhibitor combination could be used as alternative therapies. It is still uncertain, if the patient resides in an area with high rates of antibiotic resistance, whether agents such as amoxicillin and co-trimoxazole will remain as reliable choices.

The complicated patient is more likely to have a resistant pathogen, and is also defined as having at least one adverse outcome risk factor such as: FEV_1 of less than 50% pre-

Table 60.6 Patient stratification and suggested therapy for acute exacerbations of chronic bronchitis. (Only treat those with at least two of the cardinal symptoms of exacerbation.)

Simple bronchitic
$FEV_1 > 50\%$ predicted, < 4 exacerbations/year, and no underlying cardiac disease
- Newer macrolide, cephalsosporin, doxycycline
- Amoxicillin, co-trimoxazole (may be a concern in areas with high rates of antibiotic resistance)
- For non-responders: fluroquinolone, beta-lactam/beta-lactamase inhibitor combination

Complicated bronchitic
At least one of: $FEV_1 < 50\%$ predicted, > 4 exacerbations/year, cardiac disease, need for home oxygen, use of chronic oral corticosteroids, antibiotic use in the past 3 months
- Fluoroquinolone, beta-lactam/beta-lactamase inhibitor
- Consider azithromycin if only one risk factor

Chronic suppurative bronchitis
Constant purulent sputum, and at least one of: bronchiectasis, $FEV_1 < 35\%$ predicted, multiple exacerbations
- Sputum culture may be useful in this group
- Ciprofloxacin orally
- Maybe a role for inhaled aminoglycosides
- Parenteral therapy if admitted

FEV_1, forced expiratory volume in 1 s.

dicted, more than four exacerbations per year, cardiac disease, use of home oxygen, chronic oral steroid use or antibiotic use in the last 3 months. For this population, the recommended therapies were a fluroquinolone, or a beta-lactam/beta-lactamase inhibitor combination, but other groups have considered azithromycin to be an acceptable alternative for patients with only one adverse outcome risk factor [77].

The chronic suppurative bronchitic patient is defined as having constant purulent sputum, usually with bronchiectasis or an FEV_1 of less than 35% predicted, or with multiple risk factors such as frequent exacerbations. These patients can be infected with resistant Gram-negative organisms, and thus therapy should be tailored to culture data from sputum samples, but empirical therapy should be directed against *P. aeruginosa*, with ciprofloxacin in outpatients and generally parenteral therapy in hospitalized patients [5].

This stratification scheme must be viewed as a hypothesis that requires prospective verification. Future studies are needed to document that, if patients are managed with this approach to therapy, outcomes are improved. However, retrospective data do support this general approach. In one study, the value of using newer, and more expensive antibiotics was documented as being both beneficial and cost effective in a population of patients that could be described as mildly complicated. In this study, a group of 60 patients had, on average, more than three exacerbations (a total of 224 exacerbations) and therapy was categorized by the authors as being with first-line (amoxicillin, tetracycline, erythromycin, co-trimoxazole), second-line (cephalosporins) or third-line (amoxicillin/clavulanate, azithromycin, ciprofloxacin) agents [73]. Patients who received third-line agents failed less often than those who received first-line agents (7% vs 19%; $P < 0.05$) [73]. In addition, those given third-line agents were hospitalized less often, and their time between exacerbations was significantly longer than for those given first-line agents. Another study, using a pharmacoeconomic model to evaluate 1102 patients with AECB in previously reported randomized trials, concluded that macrolide therapy and therapy with amoxicillin/clavulanate was more cost effective than therapy with ampicillin and older cephalosporins [91].

In the future, the value of new agents will need to be studied using both traditional and novel endpoints. Thus, in addition to clinical and microbiological success, future studies will need to examine time to clinical resolution, time to return to work or other productive activity, disease-free interval, and the ability of a selected therapy to minimze the future potential for antibiotic resistance.

References

1 Saint S, Bent S, Vittinghoff E, Grady D. Antibiotics in chronic obstructive pulmonary disease exacerbations: a meta-analysis. *JAMA* 1995;**273**:957–60.

2 Anthonisen NR, Manfreda J, Warren CPW *et al.* Antibiotic therapy in exacerbations of chronic obstructive pulmonary disease. *Ann Intern Med* 1987;**106**:196–204.

3 American Thoracic Society. Standards for the diagnosis and care of patients with chronic obstructive pulmonary disease. *Am J Respir Crit Care Med* 1995;**152**:S77–120.

4 Snow V, Lascher S, Mottur-Pilson C *et al.* Evidence base for management of acute exacerbations of chronic obstructive pulmonary disease. *Ann Intern Med* 2001;**134**: 595–9.

5 Balter MS, LaForge J, Low DE, Mandell L, Grossman RF, and the Chronic Bronchitis Working Group. Canadian guidelines for the management of acute exacerbations of chronic bronchitis. *Can Respir J* 2003;**10**(Suppl B):3B–32B.

6 Ball P, Harris JM, Lowson D *et al.* Acute infective exacerbations of chronic bronchitis. *Q J Med* 1995;**88**:61–8.

7 Niederman MS, McCombs JS, Unger AN, Kumar A, Popovian R. Treatment cost of acute exacerbations of chronic bronchitis. *Clin Ther* 1999;**21**:576–91.

8 Fagon JY, Chastre J, Trouillet JL *et al.* Characterization of distal bronchial microflora during acute exacerbation of chronic bronchitis: use of the protected specimen brush technique in 54 mechanically ventilated patients. *Am Rev Respir Dis* 1990;**142**:1004–8.

9 Monso E, Ruiz J, Rosell A *et al.* Bacterial infection in chronic obstructive pulmonary disease: a study of stable and exacerbated outpatients using the protected specimen brush. *Am J Respir Crit Care Med* 1995;**152**:1316–20.

10 Soler N, Torres A, Ewig S *et al.* Bronchial microbial patterns in severe exacerbations of chronic obstructive pulmonary disease (COPD) requiring mechanical ventilation. *Am J Respir Crit Care Med* 1998;**157**:1498–505.

11 Zalacain R, Sobradillo V, Amilibia J *et al.* Predisposing factors to bacterial colonization in chronic obstructive pulmonary disease. *Eur Respir J* 1999;**13**:343–8.

12 Sethi S, Evans N, Grant BJB, Murphy TF. New strains of bacteria and exacerbations of chronic obstructive pulmonary disease. *N Engl J Med* 2002;**347**:465–71.

13 Sethi S, Wrona C, Grant BJB, Murphy TF. Strain specific immune response to *Haemophilus influenzae* in chronic obstructive pulmonary disease. *Am J Respir Crit Care Med* 2004;**169**:448–53.

14 Sethi S, Muscarella K, Evans N *et al.* Airway inflammation and etiology of acute exacerbations of chronic bronchitis. *Chest* 2000;**118**:1557–65.

15 Stockley RA, O'Brien C, Pye A, Hill SL. Relationship of sputum color to nature and outpatient management of acute exacerbations of COPD. *Chest* 2000;**117**:1638–45.

16 Murphy TF, Sethi S. Bacterial infection in chronic obstructive pulmonary disease. *Am Rev Respir Dis* 1992;**146**:1067–83.

17 Murphy T, Sethi S, Niederman M. The role of bacteria in exacerbations of COPD: a constructive view. *Chest* 2000;**118**: 204–9.

18 Donaldson GC, Seemungal TAR, Bhowmik A, Wedzicha JA. Relationship between exacerbation frequency and lung function decline in chronic obstructive pulmonary disease. *Thorax* 2002;**57**:847–52.

19 Hogg JC. Chronic bronchitis: the role of viruses. *Semin Respir Infect* 2000;**15**:32–40.

20 Seemungal T, Harper-Owen R, Bhowmik A *et al.* Respiratory viruses, symptoms, and inflammatory markers in acute exacerbations and stable chronic obstructive pulmonary disease. *Am J Respir Crit Care Med* 2001;**164**:1618–23.

21 Rhode G, Wiethege A, Borg I *et al.* Respiratory viruses in exacerbations of chronic obstructive pulmonary disease requiring hospitalization: a case–control study. *Thorax* 2003; **58**:37–42.

22 Tan WC, Xiang X, Qui D *et al.* Epidemiology of respiratory viruses in patients hospitalized with near-fatal asthma, acute exacerbations of asthma, or chronic obstructive pulmonary disease. *Am J Med* 2003;**115**:272–7.

23 Smith CB, Golden C, Klauber MR *et al.* Interaction between viruses and bacteria in patients with chronic bronchitis. *J Infect Dis* 1976;**134**:552–61.

24 Ball P. Epidemiology and treatment of chronic bronchitis and its exacerbations. *Chest* 1995;**108**:43S–52S.

25 Bach PB, Brown C, Gelfand SE, McCrory DC. Management of acute exacerbations of chronic obstructive pulmonary disease: a summary and appraisal of published evidence. *Ann Intern Med* 2001;**143**:600–20.

26 Allegra L, Blasi F, deBernardi B *et al*. Antibiotic treatment and baseline severity of disease in acute exacerbations of chronic bronchitis: a re-evaluation of previously published data of a placebo controlled randomized study. *Pulm Pharmacol Ther* 2001;**14**:149–55.

27 Adams S, Melo J, Luther M, Anzueto A. Antibiotics are associated with lower relapse rates in outpatients with acute exacerbations of COPD. *Chest* 2000;**117**:1345–52.

28 Baigelman W, Chodosh S, Pizzuto D *et al*. Quantitative sputum Gram stains in chronic bronchial disease. *Lung* 1979; **156**:265–70.

29 Nouira S, Marghli S, Belghith M *et al*. Once daily oral ofloxacin in chronic obstructive pulmonary disease exacerbation requiring mechanical ventilation: a randomized placebo-controlled trial. *Lancet* 2001;**358**:2020–5.

30 Torres A, Dorca J, Zalacain R *et al*. Community-acquired pneumonia in chronic obstructive pulmonary disease: a Spanish multicenter study. *Am J Respir Crit Care Med* 1996; **154**:1456–61.

31 Lieberman D, Lieberman D, Glefer Y *et al*. Pneumonia vs. non-pneumonic acute exacerbations of COPD. *Chest* 2002;**122**:1264–70.

32 Doern GV, Brueggemann AB, Pierce G, Holley HP Jr, Rauch A. Antibiotic resistance among clinical isolates of *Haemophilus influenzae* in the United States in 1994 and 1995 and detection of beta-lactamase-positive strains resistant to amoxicillin-clavulanate: results of a national multicenter surveillance study. *Antimicrob Agents Chemother* 1997;**41**:292–7.

33 Doern GV, Brueggemann AB, Pierce G *et al*. Prevalence of antimicrobial resistance among 723 outpatient clinical isolates of *Moraxella catarrhalis* in the United States in 1994 and 1995: results of a 30-center national surveillance study. *Antimicrob Agents Chemother* 1997;**40**:2884–6.

34 Doern G, Pfaller M, Kugler K *et al*. Prevalence of antimicrobial resistance among respiratory tract isolates of *Streptococcus pneumoniae* in North America: 1997 results form the SENTRY antimicrobial surveillance program [see comments]. *Clin Infect Dis* 1998;**27**:764–70.

35 Ewig S, Ruiz M, Torres A *et al*. Pneumonia acquired in the community through drug-resistant *Streptococcus pneumoniae*. *Am J Respir Crit Care Med* 1999;**159**:1835–42.

36 Clavo-Sánchez AJ, Girón-González JA, López-Prieto D *et al*. Multivariate analysis of risk factors for infection due to penicillin-resistant and multidrug-resistant *Streptococcus pneumoniae*: a multicenter study. *Clin Infect Dis* 1997;**24**:1052–9.

37 Hyde TB, Gay K, Stephens DS *et al*. Macrolide resistance among invasive *Streptococcus pneumoniae* isolates. *JAMA* 2001;**286**:1857–62.

38 Lonks JR, Garau J, Gomez L *et al*. Failure of macrolide antibiotic treatment in patients with bacteremia due to erythromycin-resistant *Streptococcus pneumoniae*. *Clin Infect Dis* 2002;**35**:556–64.

39 Lautenbach E, Larosa LA, Kasbelar N *et al*. Fluoroquinolone utilization in the emergency departments of academic medical centers: prevalence of, and risk factors for, inappropriate use. *Arch Intern Med* 2003;**163**:601–5.

40 Scheld WM. Maintaining fluroroquinolone class efficacy: review of influencing factors. *Emerg Infect Dis* 2003;**9**:1–9.

41 Chen DK, McGeer A, De Azavedo JC *et al*. Decreased susceptibility of *Streptococcus pneumoniae* to fluoroquinolones in Canada. *N Engl J Med* 1999;**341**:233–9.

42 Ho PL, Tse WS, Tsang KW *et al*. Risk factors for acquisition of levofloxacin-resistant *Streptococcus pneumoniae*: a case–control study. *Clin Infect Dis* 2001;**32**:701–7.

43 Urban C, Rahman N, Zhao X *et al*. Fluoroquinolone-resistant *Streptococcus pneumoniae* associated with levofloxacin therapy. *J Infect Dis* 2001;**184**:794–8.

44 Ruhe JJ, Hasbu R. *Streptococcus pneumoniae* bacteremia: duration of previous antibiotic use and association with penicillin resistance. *Clin Infect Dis* 2003;**36**:1132–8.

45 Anderson KB, Tan JS, File TM *et al*. Emergence of levofloxacin-resistant pneumococci in immunocompromised adults after therapy for community-acquired pneumonia. *Clin Infect Dis* 2003;**37**:376–81.

46 Mogulkoc N, Karakurt S, Isalska B *et al*. Acute purulent exacerbation of chronic obstructive pulmonary disease and *Chlamydia pneumoniae* infection. *Am J Respir Crit Care Med* 1999;**160**:349–53.

47 Eller J, Ede A, Schaberg T *et al*. Infective exacerbations of chronic bronchitis: relation between bacteriologic etiology and lung function. *Chest* 1998;**113**:1542–8.

48 Miravitlles M, Espinosa C, Fernandez-Laso E *et al*. Relationship between bacterial flora in sputum and functional impairment in patients with acute exacerbations of COPD. Study Group of Bacterial Infection in COPD. *Chest* 1999;**16**:40–6.

49 Niederman MS. Pathogenesis of airway colonization: lessons learned from studies of bacterial adherence. *Eur Respir J* 1994;**7**:1737–40.

50 Mandell LA. Antibiotics for pneumonia therapy. *Med Clin North Am* 1994;**78**:997–1014.

51 Niederman MS. The principles of antibiotic use and the selection of empiric therapy for pneumonia. In: Fishman A, ed. *Pulmonary Diseases and Disorders*, 3rd edn. New York: McGraw-Hill, 1997; 1939–49.

52 Pechere JC, Lacey L. Optimizing economic outcomes in antibiotic therapy of patients with acute bacterial exacerbations of chronic bronchitis. *J Antimicrob Chemother* 2000;**45**: 19–24.

53 Niederman MS. Treatment of respiratory infections with quinolones. In: Andriole V, ed. Th*e Quinolones*, 2nd edn. San Diego, CA: McGraw-Hill, 1998; 229–50.

54 Craig WA. Pharmacokinetic/pharmacodynamic parameters: rationale for antimicrobial dosing of mice and men. *Clin Infect Dis* 1998;**26**:1–12.

55 Preston SL, Drusano GL, Berman AL *et al*. Pharmaco-dynamcis of levofloxacin: a new paradigm for early clinical trials. *JAMA* 1998;**279**:125–9.

56 Fink MP, Snydman DR, Niederman MS *et al*. Treatment of severe pneumonia in hospitalized patients: results of a multicenter, randomized, double-blind trial comparing intra-venous ciprofloxacin with imipenem-cilastatin. *Antimicrob Agents Chemother* 1994;**38**:547–57.

57 Dunbar LM, Wunderink RG, Habib MP *et al*. High-dose, short-course levofloxacin for community-acquired pneumonia: a new treatment paradigm. *Clin Infect Dis* 2003;**37**:752–60.

58 Forest A, Nix DE, Ballow CH *et al*. Pharmacodynamics of intravenous ciprofloxacin in seriously ill patients. *Antimicrob Agents Chemother* 1993;**37**:1073–81.

59 Hatala R, Dinh T, Cook DJ. Once-daily aminoglycoside dosing in immunocompetent adults: a meta-analysis. *Ann Intern Med* 1996;**124**:717–25.

60 Honeybourne D. Antibiotic penetration into lung tissues. *Thorax* 1994;**49**:104–6.

61 Sonnesyn SW, Gerding DN. Antimicrobials for the treatment of respiratory infection. In: Niederman MS, Sarosi GA, Glassroth J, eds. *Respiratory Infections: A Scientific Basis for Management*. Philadelphia: W.B. Saunders, 1994: 511–37.

62 Barker AF, Couch L, Fiel SB *et al*. Tobramycin solution for inhalation reduces sputum *Pseudomonas aeruginosa* density in bronchiectasis. *Am J Respir Crit Care Med* 2000;**162**:481–5.

63 Gantz N. Patient compliance in the management of adult respiratory infections. *Internal Medicine for the Specialist* 1990; **10**:1–3.

64 Gallup Organization. *Consumer Attitudes Toward Antibiotic Use*. American Lung Association Publication, 1995.

65 Gotfried MH, DeAbate CA, Fogarty C, Mathew CP, Sokol WN. Comparison of 5-day, short-course gatifloxacin therapy with 7-day gatifloxacin therapy and 10-day clarithromycin therapy for acute exacerbation of chronic bronchitis. *Clin Ther* 2001;**23**:97–107.

66 Zervos MJ, Heyder AM, Leroy B. Oral telithromycin 800 mg once daily for 5 days versus cefuroxime axetil 500 mg twice daily for 10 days in adults with acute exacerbations of chronic bronchitis. *J Int Med Res* 2003;**31**:157–69.

67 Wilson R, Schentag JJ, Ball P *et al*. A comparison of gemifloxacin and clarithromycin in acute exacerbations of chronic bronchitis and long-term clinical outcomes. *Clin Ther* 2002;**24**:639–52.

68 Guay D. Short-course antimicrobial therapy of respiratory tract infections. *Drugs* 2003;**63**:2169–84.

69 Cazzola M, Vinciguerra A, Di Perna F *et al*. Comparative study of dirithromycin and azithromycin in the treatment of acute bacterial exacerbations of chronic bronchitis. *J Chemother* 1999;**11**:119–25.

70 Gris P. Once-daily, 3-day azithromycin versus a three-times-daily, 10-day course of co-amoxiclav in the treatment of adults with lower respiratory tract infections: results of a randomized, double-blind comparative study. *J Antimicrob Chemother* 1996;**37**(Suppl C):93–101.

71 Saravolatz LD, Leggett J. Gatifloxacin, gemifloxacin, and moxifloxacin: the role of three newer fluoroquinolones. *Clin Infect Dis* 2003;**37**:1210–5.

72 Grassi C, Casali L, Curti E *et al*. SMART Study Group. Studio Multicentrico con Moxifloxacina nel Trattamento delle Riacutizzazioni de Bronchite Cronica. Efficacy and safety of short course (5-day) moxifloxacin vs 7-day ceftriaxone in the treatment of acute exacerbations of chronic bronchitis (AECB). *J Chemother* 2002;**14**:597–608.

73 Destache CJ, Dewan N, O'Donahue WJ, Campbell JC, Angelillo VA. Clinical and economic considerations in the treatment of acute exacerbations of chronic bronchitis. *J Antimicrob Chemother* 1999;**43**(Suppl A):107–13.

74 Wilson, R, Allegra L, Hudson G *et al*. Short-term and long-term outcomes of moxifloxacin compared to standard antibiotic treatment of chronic bronchitis. *Chest* 2004;**125**:953–64.

75 Weiss K, Vanjaka A, and the Canadian Clarithromycin Study Group on Bronchitis. An open-label, randomized, multi-center, comparative study of the efficacy and safety of 7 days of treatment with clarithromycin extended-release tablets versus clarithromycin immediate-release tablets for the treatment of patients with acute bacterial exacerbation of chronic bronchitis. *Clin Ther* 2002;**24**:2105–22.

76 Amsden GW, Baird IM, Simon S, Treadway G. Efficacy and safety of azithromycin vs. levofloxacin in the outpatient treatment of acute bacterial exacerbations of chronic bronchitis. *Chest* 2003;**123**:772–77.

77 DeAbate CA, Mathew CP, Warner JH, Heyd A, Church D. The safety and efficacy of short course (5-day) moxifloxacin vs. azithromycin in the treatment of patients with acute exacerbation of chronic bronchitis. *Respir Med* 2000;**94**:1029–37.

78 File TM, Jacobs MR, Poole MD *et al*. Outcome of treatment of respiratory tract infections due to *Streptococcus pneumoniae*, including drug-resistant strains, with pharmacokinetically enhanced amoxycillin/clavulanate. *Int J Antimicrob Agents* 2002;**20**:235–47.

79 Anzueto A, Fisher CL Jr, Busman T, Olson CA. Comparison of the efficacy of extended-release clarithomycin tablets and amoxicillin/clavulanate tablets in the treatment of acute exacerbation of chronic bronchitis. *Clin Ther* 2001;**23**:72–86.

80 Tagaya E, Tamaoki J, Kondo M, Nagai A. Effect of a short course of clarithromycin therapy on sputum production in patients with chronic airway hypersecretion. *Chest* 2002;**122**: 213–8.

81 Saiman L, Marshall BC, Mayer-Hamblett N *et al*. Macrolide Study Group. Azithromycin in patients with cystic fibrosis chronically infected with *Pseudomonas aeruginosa*: a randomized controlled trial. *JAMA* 2003;**290**:1749–56.

82 Low DE, Brown S, Felmingham D. Clinical and bacteriological efficacy of the ketolide telithromycin against isolates of key respiratory pathogens: a pooled analysis of phase III studies. *Clin Microbiol Infect* 2004;**10**:27–36.

83 Anzueto A. Acute exacerbations of chronic bronchitis. *Curr Treat Options Infect Dis* 2002;**4**:129–40.

84 Beghi G, Berni F, Carratu L *et al*. Efficacy and tolerability of azithromycin versus amoxicillin/clavulanic acid in acute purulent exacerbation of chronic bronchitis. *J Chemother* 1995;**7**:146–52.

85 Schaberg T, Ballin I, Huchon G *et al*. AECB Study Group. A multinational, multicentre, non-blinded, randomized study of moxifloxacin oral tablets compared with co-amoxiclav oral tablets in the treatment of acute exacerbation of chronic bronchitis. *J Int Med Res* 2001;**29**:314–28.

86 Chodosh S, McCarty J, Farkas S *et al*. Randomized, double-blind study of ciprofloxacin and cefuroxime axetil for treatment of acute bacterial exacerbations of chronic bronchitis. The Bronchitis Study Group. *Clin Infect Dis* 1998;**27**:722–9.

87 Chodosh S. Treatment of chronic bronchitis: state of the art. *Am J Med* 1991;**91**(6A):87S–92S.

88 Anzueto A, Niederman MS, Tillotson GS, and the Bronchitis Study Group. Etiology, susceptibility, and treatment of acute bacterial exacerbations of complicated chronic bronchitis

in the primary care setting: ciprofloxacin 750 mg BID vs clarithromycin 500 mg BID. *Clin Ther* 1998;**20**:885–900.

89 Ho PL, Tse WS, Tsang KW *et al.* Risk factors for acquisition of levofloxacin-resistant *Streptococcus pneumoniae*: a case–control study. *Clin Infect Dis* 2001;**32**:701–7.

90 Grossman R, Mukherjee M, Vaughan D *et al.* A 1-year community-based health economic study of ciprofloxacin vs. usual antibiotic treatment in acute exacerbations of chronic bronchitis: the Canadian ciprofloxacin health economic study group. *Chest* 1998;**113**:131–41.

91 Quenzer RW, Pettit KG, Arnold RJ, Kaniecki DJ. Pharmacoeconomic analysis of selected antibiotics in lower respiratory tract infection. *Am J Manag Care* 1997;**3**:1027–36.

92 Halpern MT, Palmer CS, Zodet M, Kirsch J. Cost-effectiveness of gemifloxacin: results from the GLOBE study. *Am J Health Syst Pharm* 2002;**59**:1357–65.

CHAPTER 61
Antioxidants

Claudio F. Donner

In the normal lung, the balance between antioxidants and oxidants is sufficient to keep the airway lining fluids and extracellular spaces in a highly reduced state and enable normal physiological functions. Any increase in oxidants or decrease in antioxidants can disrupt this balance. The state of imbalance is collectively referred to as oxidative stress and is associated with diverse airway pathologies including asthma, COPD and interstitial lung disease [1,2].

In the last few years, the possible association between free radical-induced oxidative damage in the lung and the development of cigarette smoke-related pathologies (e.g. COPD, lung cancer) has received considerable attention. There is growing evidence of the role of oxidative stress in

COPD [3–5]. Oxygen radicals from endogenous (priming of inflammatory cells) and exogenous sources (cigarette smoke) induce parenchyma and airways wall damage in the lung, as well as interferring in the inflammation process by activation of transcription factors (Fig. 61.1).

Extracellular superoxide dismutase (ECSOD) is the primary extracellular antioxidant enzyme in the lung and is most highly expressed in airway and vascular walls (Fig. 61.2) [2]. The antioxidant defence of the lung seems incapable of controlling the process, as results from measurement of markers of oxidative stress in COPD patients [5,6]. Enhancing the antioxidant defence could be an attractive strategy for the treatment of COPD. An ideal antioxidant would be very specific and not interfere with the normal oxidative function essential for the inflammatory response for several metabolic reactions. A number of metal complexes have been described as superoxide dismutase (SOD) mimetics. AEOL 10113 and AEOL 10150 are positively charged, and the positive charges on the four pyridyl or

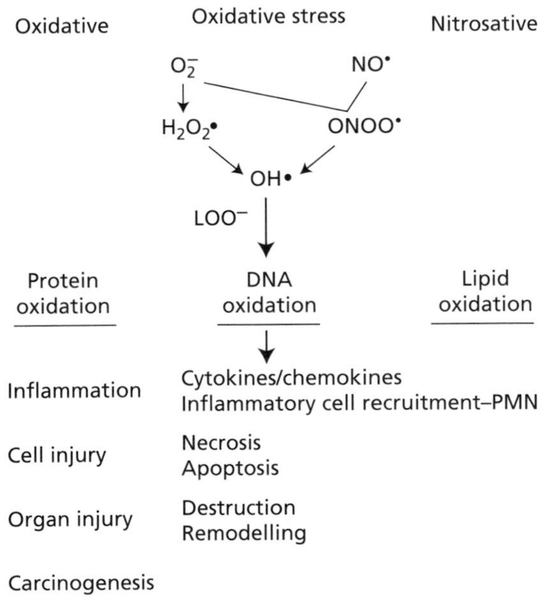

Oxidative   Oxidative stress   **Nitrosative**

$$O_2^-\quad\quad NO^{\bullet}$$
$$H_2O_2^{\bullet}\quad\quad ONOO^{\bullet}$$
$$OH^{\bullet}$$
$$LOO^-$$

Protein oxidation	DNA oxidation	Lipid oxidation

Inflammation   Cytokines/chemokines
Inflammatory cell recruitment–PMN

Cell injury   Necrosis
Apoptosis

Organ injury   Destruction
Remodelling

Carcinogenesis

Figure 61.1 Comparative levels of extracellular superoxide dismutase (ECSOD) in various tissues, showing the unique expression in the lung. (From First ERS Lung Science Conference, Taormina, 2003. Copyright J. Crapo.)

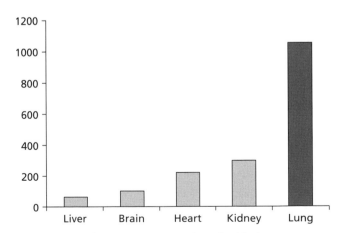

Figure 61.2 Schematic representation of oxidative stress. (From First ERS Lung Science Conference, Taormina, 2003. Copyright J. Crapo.)

imidizol groups in these compounds give them distribution and function profiles that mimic ECSOD. Thus, AEOL 10113 and AEOL 10150 possess a broad range of antioxidant activities including mimicking SOD and catalase, and scavenging both lipid peroxides and peroxynitrite [7–9]. Natural antioxidants, such as vitamins, and synthetic ones, such as *N*-acetylcysteine, have been investigated in the clinical setting. However, few compounds have been studied in randomized controlled trials.

In this chapter, antioxidants used in the clinical setting are discussed.

Oxidants and antioxidants

Reactive oxygen species (ROS, or oxidants) and antioxidants have an essential role in aerobic life. Most of the oxygen taken into the body is expelled as CO_2; however, some molecular oxygen (O_2) is converted to water. For this reaction four electrons must be added to the oxygen molecule. Conversion of oxygen to water can result in the formation of several oxygen free radicals (O_2, H_2O_2, OH).

ROS and free radicals are molecules with an impaired number of electrons in the external orbit. Because of the instability in the molecular structure, these compounds are very reactive and interact with fat and proteins, altering cellular structure. Activated phagocytic cells (e.g. neutrophils, macrophages) generate ROS [10]. ROS are present in all cellular compartments: lysosomes, peroxisome, endoplasmatic reticulum, mitochondria, cell membranes and cytoplasm. The oxidants formed by the activated cells are not only present intracellularly but also reach the extracellular environment, reacting with proteins and fat molecules causing cellular or tissue damage, which can result in chronic inflammation [11].

Cigarette smoke is a potent source of inhaled oxidants and free radicals present in both gas and tar phase [12]. Cigarette smoke contains approximately 10–15 oxidant molecules per puff and in aqueous solution it can generate hydrogen peroxide and superoxide radicals [13,14].

The organism is protected from oxidative damage by a wide screen of antioxidants. Natural antioxidants can be divided into enzymatic (superoxide dismutase, glutathione, catalase), non-enzymatic synthesized (uric acid, glutathione) and dietary vitamins (vitamins E and C, beta-carotene).

When the amount of oxidants exceeds the available antioxidant defence, oxidative stress ensues. Oxidative stress has been implicated in the pathology of numerous diseases such as atherosclerosis, diabetes, ischaemia–reperfusion injury and cancer. The lung, widely exposed to oxidative injury, is highly dependent on its antioxidant screen. Several chronic (COPD, idiopathic pulmonary fibrosis [IPF], asthma) and non-chronic (adult respiratory distress syndrome [ARDS], cancer) lung deseases have been related to oxidative stress [11].

Oxidative stress and COPD

Oxidants

An increased number of ROS from exogenous and endogenous sources are present in the lung of COPD patients (Fig. 61.3). Cigarette smoke is irreversibly linked to COPD. Inhaled ROS are derived from tobacco smoke and air pollution. In addition, cigarette smoke induces iron release from ferritin, essential for oxidative processes (Fig. 61.4).

Endogenously ROS are generated by phagocytic cells (neutrophils and macrophages) [10,15]. Activated macrophages and polymorphonuclear neutrophils (PMNs) from smokers release more ROS than cells derived from non-smokers [3,10]. There is evidence that cigarette smoke exposure provokes an accumulation of macrophages and neutrophils [16] in respiratory bronchiole and alveolar septum. Di Stefano *et al.* [17] described an increase of macrophages in bronchial mucosa of patients with chronic bronchitis. This situation escalates during exacerbations when neutrophils and eosinophils increase even further, compared with stable patients [18]. In conclusion, the

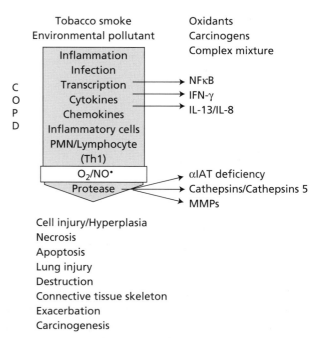

Figure 61.3 Schematic representation of oxidative stress in COPD. IFN-γ, γ-interferon; IL, interleukin; MMP, matrix metalloproteinase; NFκB, nuclear factor κB. (From First ERS Lung Science Conference, Taormina, 2003. Copyright J. Crapo.)

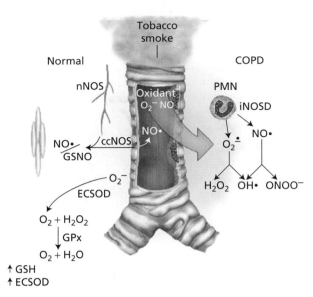

Figure 61.4 Oxidative stress resulting from tobacco smoke in normal subjects and in COPD. ccNOS, constitutive calcium/calmodulin regulated nitric oxide synthase; ECSOD, extracellular superoxide dismutase; GPx, glutathione peroxidase; GSH, glutathione; GSNO, NO-donor S-nitrosoglutathione; iNOSD, inducible nitric oxide synthase; nNOS, neuronal nitric oxide synthase; NO, nitric oxide; ONOO−, peroxynitrite; PMN, polymorphonuclear neutrophil. (From First ERS Lung Science Conference, Taormina, 2003. Copyright J. Crapo.)

number of inflammatory cells is higher in COPD and therefore their potential production of ROS is greater.

Jorres and Magnussen [13] suggested that the cellular activation and tissue damage in COPD patients should be associated with uncontrolled and not site-specific production of ROS, which can generate a chain reaction perpetuating these alterations.

Antioxidants

Pulmonary antioxidants are widely distributed and include both enzymatic and non-enzymatic systems. The intracellular antioxidant system comprises vitamins E and C, beta-carotene and glutathione (GSH). Extracellular fluid contains high levels of antioxidants but is relatively poor in enzymes. GSH in particular is critical in antioxidant pulmonary defence [11].

GSH, a low molecular tripeptide (L-gamma-glutamyl-L-cysteinylglycine) is an important intracellular water-soluble antioxidant. It is present in airways epithelial cells and in pulmonary endothelial cells. In the lung, GSH is also present extracellularly and it reaches high concentrations in the lung epithelial lining fluid (ELF). The concentration of GSH in ELF is approximately 100-fold higher than in plasma. The GSH redox cycle is considered the most

important mechanism for reduction of intracellular hydroperoxides [15]. The antioxidant action of GSH will lead to formation of a non-radical end product: GSSG, oxidized glutathione. Conversely, GSSG can be reduced again to GSH by the enzyme glutathione reductase, enabling the cell to keep a ratio of GSH/GSSG.

Besides its function in maintaining a reducing environment, GSH is also a cofactor for various protective enzymes against oxidative stress. Furthermore, GSH has been implicated in immunomodulation and the inflammatory response [19].

Several animal and human studies [19] show that cigarette smoke alters GSH levels in the lung. An acute fall, as a direct consequence of smoking, is followed by a persistent increase. Smokers have an elevated GSH and GSH peroxidase activity in ELF [20]. Animal and human studies demonstrated that increased GSH levels increase lung permeability [21,22], suggesting a critical role for GSH in maintaining epithelial barrier function. Linden et al. [23] found an increased concentration of total GSH in bronchoalveolar lavage (BAL) fluid of chronic bronchitis patients. The GSH concentration was inversely correlated with the forced expiratory volume in 1 s (FEV_1) of these patients.

Rahman and MacNee [11] suggest that the intracellular redox state of the cell has a key role in the regulation and potentiation of the inflammatory response in the cell. Oxidants are implicated in the inflammatory response of the cell via activation of redox-sensitive transcription factors such as nuclear factor κB (NF-κB) and activatory protein-1 (AP-1). Depletion of GSH or alteration in the balance of GSH/GSSG in favour of the oxidized form causes degradation of the inhibitor form of NF-κB and consequently its activation. NF-κB is involved in gene regulation of pro-inflammatory cytokines (e.g. tumour necrosis factor α [TNF-α], interleukin 6 [IL-6], IL-8, vascular cell adhesion molecule 1 [VCAM-1] and intercellular adhesion molecule 1 [ICAM-1]). The activation of the cytokines, caused by oxidative stress, will amplify the inflammatory response, creating a chain reaction.

The same authors show that GSH regulation is one of the factors involved in genetic susceptibility to oxidant-mediated lung damage. Furthermore, GSH redox state and oxidative stress are involved in the expression of pro-inflammatory and antioxidant genes.

Alteration in GSH concentration in BAL and ELF has also been described in several inflammatory pathologies: ARDS [24], IPF [25], cystic fibrosis and asthma [26].

Evidence of oxidative stress in COPD

The short half-life of oxidants makes their direct measurement *in vivo* difficult. In the last few years, several techniques have been developed that permit the measurement of markers of oxidative stress in COPD patients, using less invasive methods. Increased evidence of oxidative stress in the lung was presented by Maier et al. [27], who showed elevated levels of oxidized methionine residues of α_1-proteinase inhibitor in BAL of smokers with chronic bronchitis. Dekhuijzen et al. [6] found increased levels of hydrogen peroxide (H_2O_2) in exhaled breath of COPD patients. Higher levels were found during exacerbations. More recently, Montuschi et al. [28] demonstrated increased levels of 8-isoprostane in exhaled air, a marker of lipid peroxidation, confirming the previous data of Pratico et al. [29] for the same marker in urine. Elevated plasma levels of thiobarbituric acid-reactive substances (TBARS), another marker of lipid peroxidation, were found in stable and exacerbated COPD patients [30]. Finally, decreased antioxidant capacity in plasma (TEAC) was described by Rahman et al. [12] in smokers and in patients with acute exacerbations of COPD. These data confirm the presence of an imbalance between oxidants and antioxidants in COPD and support the use of antioxidants in this pathology.

Pharmacological intervention

The use of antioxidants may be an interesting strategy in the prevention of radical-induced damage. The lung protects itself through several antioxidant systems, including thiol compounds, vitamins and enzymes. Enzymes such as SOD and catalase are large mass polymers, which prevents their intracellular transport and their use by the oral route; therefore their use has been limited to experimental studies. Only thiols and vitamins have been studied in the clinical setting.

Thiols

GSH and cysteine are the most important antioxidant thiols in the lung. Intracellular synthesis of GSH depends on the availability of its natural precursor, L-cysteine [31]. Cysteine has a poor resorption, it is rapidly oxidized and is toxic. These disadvantages are prevented by acetylation of the molecule.

Exogenous GSH must be broken down to the constituent aminoacids. A GSH preparation is available for intravenous use but has never been tested in chronic pulmonary diseases.

N-acetylcysteine

N-acetylcysteine (NAC) is a sulphydryl group (SH) containing aminoacid residue with an acetyl group on the nitrogen. The thiol group is crucial for its therapeutic effect. NAC has been used in Europe as a mucolytic agent. The mucolytic action, a result of cleavage of disulphide bonds between mucines and consequent decrease of the viscosity of the mucus, was described by Sheffner et al. [32] in the 1970s. More recently, the therapeutic effect of NAC has been primarily ascribed to its antioxidant properties.

NAC is biotransformed very effectively, which explains its low bioavailability. After oral administration, NAC is deacetylated to L-cysteine. Cysteine has a central role in the endogenous thiol metabolism and may be transformed into a large number of molecules, including GSH.

In analogy with the well-established mechanism of action of NAC against liver toxicity resulting from paracetamol (acetaminophen) intoxication [33], GSH has been seen as a link between NAC and therapeutic effects in chronic bronchitis.

Pharmacokinetics

After oral intake of 600 mg/day, the intestinal absorption of NAC is rapid; it can be measured in the plasma after 60 min [34]. NAC is partially deacetylated at intestinal mucosa level and undergoes an intense metabolism after the first hepatic passage. As a consequence, the bioavailability of the unchanged molecule is apparently low (10%). At this dose, NAC could not be detected in BAL fluid [35]. It is important to bear in mind, however, that it is at the hepatic level that its principal conversion into GSH takes place. An increase in bioavalability has been reported after higher doses.

After administration of NAC, plasma level increases in cysteine, GSH and thiolic groups have been measured [35,36]. Also, increased levels of GSH in the lung were measured [36]. However, in COPD patients, after an oral dose of 600 mg NAC, the plasma concentrations of GSH were unchanged, whereas 600 mg NAC three times daily increased GSH plasma concentrations [37]. These data were confirmed by Behr et al. [38] in patients with IPF, who also demonstrated a significant increase in total concentration of GSH both in ELF and in the cells after oral administration of 1800 mg/day NAC.

Pendyala and Creaven [39] found a significant increase in GSH in the circulating lymphocytes in healthy volunteers after a single administration of 800 mg/m². Repeated administrations caused an increase in GSH concentration of approximately 20% over baseline.

To understand the effect of NAC on cysteine and GSH levels it is important to note that plasma levels are often non-representative of the situation in the lung because of compartmentalization of GSH need and availability. Furthermore, studies performed after coadministration of NAC (2 g) and paracetamol (2 g) to healthy volunteers showed an increase in cysteine and GSH levels in plasma, when a single administration of NAC was without effect [27,40]. This result suggests that the incorporation of NAC into GSH is dependent on the increased demand, as during oxidative stress.

Rationale for the use of NAC in COPD

NAC can interfere in the pathophysiology of COPD in different ways. Thiol groups are rich in electrons and can act as scavengers, reductans and antioxidants. NAC exerts a direct antioxidant effect through its free thiol group interacting with electrophilic groups of ROS [41]. Aruoma *et al.* [42] investigated the antioxidant action of NAC against hydrogen peroxide, hydroxyl radical, superoxide and hypochlorous acid. NAC is a powerful scavenger of hypochlorous acid and hydroxyl radical, while the reaction with hydrogen peroxide was noted to be slow. NAC's effect in reducing elastase activity was ascribed to the property of scavenging hypochlorous acid.

Besides this direct scavenger effect, NAC's working mechanism has to be related to its function as a GSH precursor. Maintaining adequate intracellular levels of GSH is essential for overcoming the effects of toxic agents such as cigarette smoke. Moldeus *et al.* [41] showed that NAC prevents the decrease of pulmonary GSH in a rat cigarette smoke exposure model and protects the lung against the effects of cigarette smoke. The studies of NAC as a precursor of GSH in humans have been discussed above (see p. 749).

Jeffery *et al.* [43] proved that NAC inhibits mucous cell hyperplasia in rats exposed to cigarette smoke, with the greatest effect in peripheral small airways. Furthermore, NAC tended to reduce the magnitude of permeability changes of the airways mucosa.

Several studies have studied the effect of NAC on inflammatory cells. Kharazmi *et al.* [44] studied the effect of NAC on neutrophils and monocytes *in vitro* and *in vivo*. *In vitro*, NAC was shown to inhibit the chemotaxis and oxidative-burst response of neutrophils and monocytes at approximately millimolar concentration. In a study of healthy volunteers, a single dose (400 mg) of NAC provoked a significant reduction of neutrophil chemoluminescence response following zymosan activation. The author concluded that the inhibition of migration and generation of ROS by phagocytic cells could be of major importance in preventing tissue damage in patients with chronic inflammatory disorders [45]. Three studies were performed to study the effect of NAC on inflammatory cells and mediators in BAL fluid in smokers [46–48]. The results can be summarized as a tendency towards normalization of cell composition with an increase in the proportion of lymphocytes. Activation was reduced as well as lactoferrin. The activity of alveolar macrophages was also measured; an increase in leukotriene B_4 production, a reduction of the production of ROS and an increase in the phagocytic activity of the cells was found.

Marui *et al.* [49] showed the ability of NAC to inhibit the expression of VCAM-1 in human endothelial cells. De Backer *et al.* [50] found a decrease of sputum eosinophil cationic protein (ECP) levels and reduction of PMN adhesion with a dose of 600 mg/day NAC to COPD patients.

Effect on bacterial colonization

Riise *et al.* [51] described for the first time an effect of NAC on bacterial colonization in a population of smokers with or without chronic obstruction. Patients with chronic obstruction presented the highest number of bacterial colonies. The intrabronchial bacterial colonization was significantly lower ($P < 0.05$) in patients treated with NAC (600 mg/day for several months).

It has already been demonstrated that NAC inhibits bacterial adhesion to epithelial cells [52,53] and that it stimulates the phagocytic activity of macrophages in smokers. More recently, Oddera *et al.* [54] demonstrated *in vitro* that NAC stimulates the intracellular killing of *Staphylococcus aureus* by alveolar macrophages and polymorphonuclear leucocytes of peripheral blood. Riise *et al.* [55] demonstrated that NAC reduces the ability of bacteria (*Streptococcus pneumonia* and *Haemophilus influenza*) to adhere to human oropharyngeal epithelial cells. Very recently, an Italian group (Schito University of Genoa) investigated the effect of NAC (in concentration from 0.07–8.0 mg/mL) to inhibit the formation of biofilms in *S. aureus* cultures. NAC was found to inhibit the formation of biofilms in all cultures [56].

A significant number of COPD exacerbations are associated with respiratory viral infection. The role of oxidative stress in relation to viral infections (influenza, rhinovirus) has been recently evaluated. Viral induction of oxidative stress in respiratory cells has been described by Biagioli *et al.* [57]. Rhinovirus induces the production of ROS and consequently stimulates the activation of NF-κB, a key step in the signal transduction pathway leading to IL-8 production. The same authors demonstrated that NAC blocked IL-8 production in a dose-dependent way by down-regulation of the NF-κB activation, as also observed by Knobil *et al.* [58]. Pretreatment with NAC attenuated the virus-induced NF-κB activation and IL-8 release caused by influenza virus in epithelial cells. Further evidence was offered by the work of Ungheri *et al.* [59]. Mice infected intranasally by influenza virus APR/8 showed high BAL levels of xantineoxidase, TNF and IL-6. Oral administration of NAC (1 g/kg/day) significantly reduced the mortality rate of the infected mice.

Systemic effect

In recent years there has been a growing tendency to consider COPD as a systemic disease. Thiols are implicated in several enzymatic reactions in the organism and therefore have an important metabolic role not only in the lung, but also in other systems such as the muscles.

An interesting study was performed by Santini *et al.* [60], who demonstrated that in COPD patients, red blood cells (RBC) have a low thiol concentration and are morphologically damaged, with possible consequences for oxygen exchange. NAC (1.2 or 1.8 g/day for 2 months) was able to improve the shape of the RBC and elevate the thiol concentration [61]. Quing Lu *et al.* [62] found that treatment with NAC (600 mg/day for 2 weeks) has a positive impact on the smoking-induced negative effects on microcirculatory flow. This effect was enhanced in habitual smokers, suggesting that NAC could improve tissue oxygenation.

Clinical efficacy

In several controlled trials conducted in a large number of chronic bronchitis patients, NAC proved evidence for reduction in symptoms, incidence and duration of exacerbations [63,64] and number of sick days [65]. These results were not reproducible in all the studies [66] and the group of patients studied was not very homogeneous.

To check the efficacy of NAC, Grandjean *et al.* [67] and Stey *et al.* [68] performed a meta-analysis on the results of double-blind placebo controlled clinical trials with common endpoint exacerbations rate, duration of 12–24 weeks, dosage 400–600 mg and similar definition of exacerbations. The Grandjean meta-analysis resulted in a 23% reduction of exacerbations in favour of NAC. The systematic review by Stey *et al.* [68] considered 11 trials with 2001 analysed patients selected following preset criteria. Nine of the eleven trials reported prevention of any exacerbation as the outcome in 1456 patients. With NAC, 48.5% of patients were free of any exacerbation compared with 31.2% in the placebo group. This result was statistical significant; relative benefit = 1.56 (95% confidence interval [CI], 1.37–1.77), with a number needed to treat of 5.8 (95% CI, 4.5–8.1). Only one trial reported the number of patients having exacerbations requiring hospitalization [69]. With NAC, 1.6% of patients were hospitalized within the 24-week study period against 3.4% in the placebo group. The difference was not statistically significant. Stey *et al.* [68] also reported a significant improvement in symptoms: 61.4% in the NAC patients against 34.6% in the placebo group. The tolerability of NAC was very good and comparable to placebo. Comparable results were obtained in a meta-analysis performed by the Cochrane group [70] on mucolytic agents including NAC.

These data seem to suggest that NAC has an effect in reducing the exacerbation rate in the same order of magnitude as other compounds (e.g. inhaled corticosteroids [ICS]), but in a mild disease population. A large number of national and international (Global Initiative for Chronic Obstructive Lung Disease [GOLD], Swiss, Dutch, Spanish, German) guidelines classify NAC as an antioxidant and claim that NAC could have a role in the treatment of patients with recurrent exacerbations [71].

There are few reports on the effect of NAC on other parameters of COPD: FEV_1 decline and quality of life (QoL). Hansen *et al.* [72] studied the effect of 600 mg NAC twice daily on the well-being status of 165 patients with mild to moderate obstruction (FEV_1 of less than 50%), using the General Health Questionnaire (GHQ). NAC was significantly superior to placebo in terms of favourable effect on GHQ score.

Data on the monitoring of lung function were collected in an open, randomized and stratified trial [73] in 113 COPD patients identified in a large population participating in an epidemiological surrey (Olin study) in northern Sweden. After 2 years, a significant reduction in FEV_1 decline ($P < 0.03$) in the NAC group was reported. A beneficial effect of NAC was still present after 5 years.

Some interesting data appear on the effect of NAC on markers of oxidative stress. Kasielski and Nowak [74] described a reduction of H_2O_2 in exhaled breath concentrate (EBC) in stable COPD patients treated for 12 months with 600 mg NAC versus placebo. This effect has been confirmed by De Benedetto *et al.* [75] using 1.2 g NAC.

To assess the effect of NAC on the most significant parameters in COPD (exacerbations, FEV_1 decline and QoL) and to justify its long-term use, two phase 3, randomized, placebo-controlled multicentre studies were started. The BRONCUS (Bronchitis Randomised On NAC and Cost-Utility Study) [76] began in June 1997. Patients are treated for 3 years with 600 mg/day NAC on top of standard treatment (including ICS). The main goals of the study are: reduction of exacerbation rate, decline of FEV_1, QoL assessment and pharmacoeconomic analysis. A total of 523 patients with mild to moderate disease have been recruited. In a group of COPD patients with milder disease, recruited from general practice, the effect of NAC (600 mg/day for 3 years) on exacerbation rate and cost effectiveness has been compared with fluticasone and placebo. The BRONCUS study has demonstrated that 600 mg/day NAC in COPD patients had effects on pulmonary function and exacerbation rate. It improved FEV_1 and vital capacity (VC) initially in patients with FEV_1 of less than 50% of predicted but did not affect the annual decline in these variables. It reduced hyperinflations. It reduce yearly exacerbation rates, with 22% of the patients not taking inhaled corticosteroids [77].

Vitamins

There is clear epidemiological evidence that dietary intake of antioxidant vitamins (vitamins E and C and α-tocopherol) is positively associated with lung function and respiratory symptoms. Large epidemiological studies such as NHANES 1–3 [78–80] demonstrated that higher levels of antioxidant nutrients are associated with better lung function. Vitamin E in particular could be important in protecting surfactant lipids against oxidation and subsequent lung injury. A temporary vitamin E deficiency induces a reversible change of the expression of pro- and anti-inflammatory markers and of markers defining apoptosis, and reduces surfactant lipid synthesis in alveolar type II cells [81]. The question is whether supplementation of vitamins, outside the dietary intake, can provide benefit to patients. Fairfield and Fleicher [81], in a recent review, found little convincing evidence in favour of supplementation for chronic disease prevention; fruit and vegetables contain a variety of other compounds that may be protective [82]. Bender, in an editorial in the *British Medical Journal* [83], concluded that supplementation will be of little benefit unless intake is inadequate as a result of poor diet.

Conclusions

Smoking, acute exacerbation of COPD and asthma are all associated with a marked oxidant–antioxidant imbalance and with signs of oxidative stress. COPD and asthma are growing worldwide, and represent an ever-increasing burden on national health costs. However, it is not easy to obtain definitive proof that oxidants have a decisive role in the pathogenesis and evolution of these diseases. Because asthma and COPD are chronic progressive diseases, long-term studies in large case series are required. One of the most significant aspects is that the lung oxidant–antioxidant balance is abnormal in cigarette smokers; however, it remains unclear why only certain cigarette smokers develop COPD while others do not. The answer to this question is related to an improved understanding of the nature of the oxidant–antioxidant balance, as well as of the genetic factors and other intrinsic factors, including dietary, that control this balance. In view of these uncertainties, it is not possible to date to specifically document the benefit of antioxidant therapy. Nevertheless, there are some antioxidants that have been sufficiently well investigated and appear very close to giving a definitive positive response concerning their efficacy in the treatment of COPD. In this context, *in vitro* and *in vivo* data show that NAC protects the lungs against toxic agents by increasing pulmonary defence mechanisms through its direct antioxidant role in the rate and severity of exacerbations, and its indirect role as a precursor of GSH synthesis. The long-term use of the drug in COPD patients results in an improvement in respiratory symptoms and in a decrease in the exacerbation rate.

It should be emphasized that there are numerous and important studies in progress, unfortunately often limited to the experimental setting, on new substances that will have an important role in antioxidant therapy in the future.

References

1 Bowler RP, Crapo JD. Oxidative stress in allergic respiratory diseases. *J Allergy Clin Immunol* 2002;**110**:349–56.

2 Kinnula VL, Crapo JD. Superoxide dismutases in the lung and human lung diseases. *Am J Respir Crit Care Med* 2003;**167**:1600–19.

3 Repine JE, Lankhorst ILM, Debacker WA *et al.* Oxidative stress in chronic obstructive pulmonary disease. *Am J Respir Crit Care Med* 1997;**156**:341–57.

4 Rahman I, MacNee W. Lung glutathione and oxidative stress: implications in cigarette smoke-induced airway disease. *Am J Physiol* 1999;**277**:L1067–88.

5 Barnes PJ. Chronic obstructive pulmonary disease. *N Engl J Med* 2000;**343**:269–80.

6 Dekhuijzen PNR, Aben KKH, Dekker I *et al.* Increased exhalation of hydrogen peroxide in patients with stable and unstable COPD. *Am J Respir Crit Care Med* 1996;**154**:813–6.

7 Smith KR, Uyeminami DL, Kodavanti UP *et al.* Inhibition of tobacco smoke-induced lung inflammation by a catalytic antioxidant. *Free Radic Biol Med* 2002;**33**:1106–14.

8 Chang L-Y, Crapo JD. Inhibition of airway inflammation and hyperreactivity by an antioxidant memetic. *Free Radic Biol Med* 2002;**33**:379–86.

9 Ross AD, Sheng H, Warner DS *et al.* Hemodynamic effects of metalloporphyrin catalytic antioxidants: structure–activity relationships and species-specificity. *Free Radic Biol Med* 2002;**33**:1657–69.

10 Hoidal JR, Fox RB, LeMarbe PA *et al.* Altered oxidative metabolic responses *in vitro* of alveolar macrophages from asymptomatic cigarette smokers. *Am Rev Respir Dis* 1981;**123**:85–9.

11 Rahman I, MacNee W. Oxidative stress and regulation of glutathione in lung inflammation. *Eur Respir J* 2000;**16**:534–54.

12 Rahman I, MacNee W. Oxidant–antioxidant imbalance in smokers and chronic obstructive pulmonary disease. *Thorax* 1996;**51**:348–50.

13 Jorres RA, Magnussen H. Oxidative stress in COPD. *Eur Respir Rev* 1997;**43**:131–5.

14 Heffner JB, Repine JE. Pulmonary strategies of anitoxidant defense. *Am Rev Respir Dis* 1989;**140**:531–54.

15 Rahman I, MacNee W. Role of oxidants–antioxidants in smoking-induced lung diseases. *Free Radic Biol Med* 1996;**21**:669–81.

16 Ludwig PW, Schwartz BA, Hoidal JR, Niewoehner D. Cigarette smoking causes accumulation of polymorphonuclear leukocytes in alveolar septum. *Am Rev Respir Dis* 1985;**131**:828–30.

17 Di Stefano A, Caramori G, Oates T *et al.* Morphological and cellular basis for airflow limitation in smokers. *Eur Respir J* 2002;**20**:556–63.

18 Saetta M, Di Stefano A, Maestrelli P *et al.* Airway eosinophilia in chronic bronchitis during exacerbations. *Am J Respir Crit Care Med* 1994;**150**:1646–52.

19 Rahman ID, Morrison K, Donaldson, MacNee W. Systemic oxidative stress in asthma, COPD, and smokers. *Am J Respir Crit Care Med* 1996;**154**:1055–60.

20 Cantin AMS, North L, Hubbard R, Crystal RG. Normal alveolar epithelial lining fluid contains high levels of glutathione. *J Appl Physiol* 1987;**63**:152–7.

21 Linden M, Hakansson L, Olsson K, *et al*. Glutathione in bronchoalveolar lavage fluid from smokers is related to humoral markers of inflammatory cell activity. *Inflammation* 1989;**13**:651–8.

22 Li XY, Donaldson K, Rahman I, MacNee W. An investigation of the role of glutathione in the increased permeability induced by cigarette smoke *in vivo* and *in vitro*. *Am J Respir Crit Care Med* 1994;**149**:1518–25.

23 Linden M, Rasmussen JB, Pitulainen E *et al*. Airway inflammation in smokers with non-obstructive and obstructive chronic bronchitis. *Am Rev Respir Dis* 1993;**148**:1226–32.

24 Pacht ER, Timerman AP, Lykens MG, Merola AJ. Deficiency of alveolar fluid glutathione in patients with sepsis and the adult respiratory distress syndrome. *Chest* 1991;**100**:1397–403.

25 Cantin AM, Hubbard RC, Crystal RG. Glutathione deficiency in the epithelial lining fluid of the lower respiratory tract in idiopathic pulmonary fibrosis. *Am Rev Respir Dis* 1989;**139**:370–2.

26 Smith LJ, Houston M, Andarson J. Increased levels of glutathione in bronchoalveolar lavage fluid from patients with asthma. *Am Rev Respir Dis* 1993;**147**:1461–4.

27 Maier KL, Leuschel L, Costabel U. Increased oxidized methionine residues in BAL fluid proteins in acute or chronic bronchitis. *Eur Respir J* 1992;**5**:651–8.

28 Montuschi P, Corradi M, Ciabattoni G *et al*. Breath condensate analysis of 8-isoprostane: a new approach for assessment of oxidative stress in patients with chronic obstructive pulmonary disease [Abstract]. *Am J Respir Crit Care Med* 1999;**159**(Suppl):A798.

29 Pratico D, Basili S, Vieri M *et al*. Chronic obstructive pulmonary disease is associated with an increase in urinary levels of isoprostane $F_2\alpha$-III, an index of oxidative stress. *Am J Respir Crit Care Med* 1998;**158**:1709–14.

30 Petruzzelli S, Hietanen E, Bartsch H *et al*. Pulmonary lipid peroxidation in cigarette smokers and lung patients. *Chest* 1990;**98**:930–5.

31 Meister A, Anderson ME. Glutathione. *Ann Rev Biochem* 1983;**52**:711–60.

32 Sheffner A, Medler EM, Jacobs LW, Sarett HP. The *in vitro* reduction in viscosity of human tracheobronchial secretions by acetylcysteine. *Am Rev Respir Dis* 1964;**90**:721–9.

33 Prescott LF. Treatment of severe acetaminophen poisoning with intravenous acetylcysteine. *Arch Intern Med* 1981;**141**:358–9.

34 Maddock J. Biological properties of acetylcysteine: assay development and pharmacokinetic studies. *Eur J Respir Dis* 1980;**61**(Suppl 111):52–8.

35 Cotgreave IA, Eklund A, Larsson K, Moldeus P. No penetration of orally administered *N*-acetylcysteine into bronchoalveolar lavage fluid. *Eur J Respir Dis* 1987;**70**:73–7.

36 Bridgeman MM, Marsden M, MacNee W, Flenley DC, Ryle AP. Cysteine and glutathione concentrations in plasma and bronchoalveolar lavage fluid after treatment with *N*-acetylcysteine. *Thorax* 1991;**46**:39–42.

37 Bridgeman MM, Marsden M, Selby C, Morrison D, MacNee W. Effect of *N*-acetylcysteine on the concentrations of thiols in plasma, bronchoalveolar lavage fluid, and lung tissue. *Thorax* 1994;**49**:670–5.

38 Behr J, Maier K, Degenkolb B *et al*. Antioxidative and clinical effects of high-dose *N*-acetylcysteine in fibrosing alveolitis. *Am J Respir Crit Care Med* 1997;**158**:1897–901.

39 Pendyala L, Creaven PJ. Pharmacokinetic amd pharmacodynamic studies of *N*-acetylcysteine, a potential chemopreventive agent during a phase I trial. *Cancer Epidemiol Biomarks Prev* 1995;**4**:245–51.

40 Burgunder JM, Varriale A, Lauterburg BH. Effect of *N*-acetylcysteine on plasma cysteine and glutathione following pacaetamol administration. *Eur J Clin Pharmacol* 1989;**36**:127–31.

41 Moldeus P, Cotgreave IA, Berggren M. Lung protection by a thiol-containing antioxidant: *N*-acetylcysteine. *Respiration* 1986;**50**:31–42.

42 Aruoma OI, Halliwell B, Hoey BM, Butler J. The antioxidant action of *N*-acetylcysteine: its reaction with hydrogen peroxide, hydroxyl radical, superoxide, and hypochlorous acid. *Free Radic Biol Med* 1989;**6**:593–7.

43 Jeffery PK, Rogers DF, Ayers MM. Effect of oral acetylcysteine on tobacco smoke-induced secretory cell hyperplasia. *Eur J Respir Dis* 1985;**66**(Suppl 139):117–22.

44 Kharazmi A, Nielson H, Schiotz PO. *N*-acetylcysteine inhibits human neutrophil and monocyte chemotaxis and oxidative metabolism. *Int J Immunopharmacol* 1988;**10**:39–46.

45 Kharazmi A. The anti-inflammatory properties of *N*-acetylcysteine. *Eur Respir Rev* 1992;**2**:32–4.

46 Linden M, Wieslander E, Eklund A, Larsson K, Brattsand R. Effects of oral *N*-acetylcysteine on cell content and macrophage function in bronchoalveolar lavage from healthy smokers. *Eur Respir J* 1988;**1**:645–50.

47 Bergstrand H, Björnson A, Eklund A *et al*. Stimuli-induced superoxide radical generation *in vitro* by human alveolar macrophages from smokers: modulation by *N*-acetylcysteine treatment *in vivo*. *J Free Radic Biol Med* 1986;**2**:119–27.

48 Eklund A, Eriksson O, Hakansson L *et al*. Oral *N*-acetylcysteine reduces selected humoral markers of inflammatory cell activity in BAL fluid from healthy smokers: correlation to effects on cellular variables. *Eur Respir J* 1988;**1**:832–8.

49 Marui N, Offermann MK, Swerlick R *et al*. Vascular cell adhesion molecule-1 (VCAM-1) gene transcription and expression are regulated through an antioxidant-sensitive mechanism in human vascular endothelial cells. *J Clin Invest* 1993;**92**:1866–74.

50 De Backer W, van Overveld F, Vandekerckhove K. Sputum ECP levels in COPD patients decrease after treatment with *N*-acetylcysteine (NAC). *Eur Respir J* 1997;**12**:225S.

51 Riise GC, Larsson S, Larsson P, Jeansson S, Andersson BA. The intrabronchial microbial flora in chronic bronchitis patients: a target for *N*-acetylcysteine therapy? *Eur Respir J* 1994;**7**:94–101.

52 Niederman MS, Rafferty TD, Sasaki CT *et al*. Comparison of bacterial adherence to ciliated and squamous epithelial cells obtained from the human respiratory tract. *Am Rev Respir Dis* 1983;**127**:85–90.

53 Andersson B, Larsson S, Riise G. Inhibition of adherence of *Streptococcus pneumoniae* and *Haemophilus influenzae in vitro* by therapeutic compounds. *Am Rev Respir Dis* 1991;**143**:A289.

54 Oddera S, Silvestri M, Sacco O *et al*. *N*-acetylcysteine enhances *in vitro* the intracellular killing of *Staphylococcus aureus* by human alveolar macrophages and blood polymorphonuclear leukocytes partially protects phagocytes from self-killing. *J Lab Clin Med* 1994;**124**:293–301.

55 Riise GC, Qvarfordt I, Larsson S, Eliasson V, Andersson BA. Inhibitory effect of *N*-acetylcysteine on adherence of *Streptococcus pneumoniae* and *Haemophilus influenzae* to human oropharyngeal epithelial cells *in vitro*. *Respiration* 2000;**67**: 552–8.

56 Bozzolasco M, Debbia EA, Schito GC. Rilevanza dei biofilm batterici nelle infezioni respiratorie: problematiche terapeutiche e possibili soluzioni. *GIMMOC* 2002;**6**:203–15.

57 Biagioli MC, Kaul P, Singh I, Turner RB. The role of oxidative stress in rhinovirus induced elaboration of IL-8 by respiratory epithelial cells. *J Free Radic Biol Med* 1999;**26**:454–62.

58 Knobil K, Choi AM, Weigand GW, Jacoby DB. Role of oxidants in influenza virus-induced gene expression. *Am J Physiol* 1998;**274**:L134–42.

59 Ungheri D, *et al*. Protective effect of *N*-acetylcysteine in a model of influenza infection in mice. *Int J Immunopathol Pharmacol* 2000;**13**:123–8.

60 Santini MT, Straface E, Cipri A *et al*. Structural alterations in erythrocytes from patients with chronic obstructive pulmonary disease. *Haemostasis* 1997;**27**:201–10.

61 Schmid G, Li Bianchi E, Straface E *et al*. *N*-acetylcysteine (NAC) counteracts erythrocyte damages and is useful in the management of COPD. *Am J Respir Crit Care Med* 2002;**165**: A227.

62 Quing Lu, Bjorkhem I, Xiu RJ, Henriksson P, Freyschuss A. *N*-acetylcysteine improves microcirculatory flow during smoking: new effects of an old drug with possible benefits for smokers. *Clin Cardiol* 2001;**24**:511–5.

63 Boman G, Backer U, Larsson S, Melander B, Wahlander L. Oral acetylcysteine reduces exacerbation rate in chronic bronchitis: report of a trial organized by the Swedish Society for Pulmonary Diseases. *Eur J Respir Dis* 1983;**64**:405–15.

64 Multicenter Study Group. Long-term oral acetylcysteine in chronic bronchitis: a double-blind controlled study. *Eur J Respir Dis* 1980;**61**(Suppl 111):93–108.

65 Rasmussen JB, Glennon C. Reduction in days of illness after long-term treatment with *N*-acetylcysteine controlled-release tablets in patients with chronic bronchitis. *Eur Respir J* 1988;**1**:351–5.

66 British Thoracic Society Research Committee. Oral *N*-acetylcysteine and exacerbation rates in patients with chronic bronchitis and severe airways obstruction. *Thorax* 1985;**40**:832–5.

67 Grandjean EM, Berthet P, Ruffmann R, Leuenberger P. Efficacy of oral long-term *N*-acetylcysteine in chronic bronchopulmonary disease: a meta-analysis of published double-blind, placebo-controlled clinical trials. *Clin Ther* 2000;**22**:209–21.

68 Stey C, Steurer J, Bachmann S, Medici TC, Tramer MR. The effect of oral *N*-acetylcysteine in chronic bronchitis: a quantitative systematic review. *Eur Respir J* 2000;**16**:253–62.

69 Parr GD, Huitson A. Oral Fabrol (oral *N*-acetyl-cysteine) in chronic bronchitis. *Br J Dis Chest* 1987;**81**:341–8.

70 Poole PJ, Black PN. Oral mucolytic drugs for exacerbations of chronic obstructive pulmonary disease: systematic review. *BMJ* 2001;**322**:1271–4.

71 Pauwels RA, Buist AS, Calverley PMA, Jenkins CR, Hurd SS, and on behalf of the GOLD Scientific Committee. Global strategy for the diagnosis, management, and prevention of chronic obstructive pulmonary disease: NHLBI Global Initiative for Chronic Obstructive Lung Disease (GOLD) Workshop Summary. *Am J Respir Crit Care Med* 2001;**163**: 1256–76.

72 Hansen NCG, Skriver A, Brorsen-Riis L *et al*. Orally administered *N*-acetylcysteine may improve general well-being in patients with mild chronic bronchitis. *Respir Med* 1994;**88**: 531–5.

73 Lundbäck B, Lindström M, Andersson S *et al*. Possible effect of acetylcystein on lung function. *Eur Respir J* 1992;**5**(Suppl 15): 289S.

74 Kasielski M, Nowak D. Long-term administration of *N*-acetylcysteine decreases hydrogen peroxide exhalation in subjects with chronic obstructive pulmonary disease. *Respir Med* 2001;**95**:448–56.

75 De Benedetto F, Aceto A, Formisano S *et al*. Long-term treatment with *N*-acetylcysteine (NAC) decreases hydrogen peroxide level in exhaled air of patients with moderate COPD. *Am J Respir Crit Care Med* 2001;**163**:A725.

76 Decramer M, Dekhuijzen PNR, Troosters T *et al*. The Bronchitis Randomized On NAC Cost Utility Study (BRONCUS): hypothesis and design. BRONCUS Trial Committee. *Eur Respir J* 2001;**17**:329–36.

77 Decramer M, Rutten-van Molken M, Dekhuijzen PN *et al*. Effects of *N*-acetylcysteine on outcomes in chronic obstructive pulmonary disease (Bronchitis Randomized on NAC Cost-Utility Study, BRONCUS): a randomised placebo-controlled trial. *Lancet* 2005;**365**(9470):1552–60.

78 Mannino DM, Homa DM, Akinbami LJ, Ford ES, Redd SC. Chronic obstructive pulmonary disease surveillance: United States, 1971–2000. *MMWR Surveill Summ* 2002;**51**:1–16.

79 Hu G, Cassano PA. Antioxidants, nutrients and pulmonary function: the Third National Health and Nutrition Examination Survey (NHANES III). *Am J Epidemiol* 2000;**151**:975–81.

80 Schwartz J, Weiss ST. Relationship between dietary vitamin C intake and pulmonary function in the First National Health and Nutrition Examination Survey (NHANES I). *Am J Clin Nutr* 1994;**59**:110–4.

81 Fairfield KM, Fleicher RH. Vitamins for chronic disease prevention in adults: scientific review. *JAMA* 2002;**287**:5116–26.

82 Kolleck I, Sinha P, Ruestow B. Vitamin E as an antioxidant of the lung: mechanisms of vitamin E delivery to alveolar type II cells. *Am J Respir Crit Care Med* 2002;**166**:S62–6.

83 Bender D. Daily doses of multivitamin tablets. *BMJ* 2002;**325**: 173–4.

CHAPTER 62
Mucolytics for COPD

Duncan F. Rogers and Bruce K. Rubin

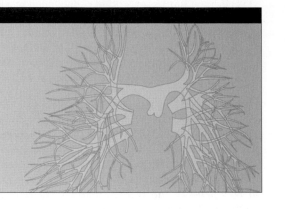

The role of airway mucus hypersecretion in the patho-physiology of chronic obstructive pulmonary disease (COPD) is debated. Similarly, the use of mucolytic medications in the clinical management of COPD is controversial. Mucus hypersecretion, implicit in the clinical term chronic bronchitis, is one of three pathophysiological entities comprising COPD. The other two components are chronic bronchiolitis (small airways disease) and emphysema (alveolar destruction) [1]. The relative contribution of each component to pathophysiology varies between patients, with the impact of mucus hypersecretion on morbidity and mortality varying accordingly. Thus, although previously included in definitions of COPD [2], the term 'mucus hypersecretion' is omitted from current definitions [3]. Nevertheless, there are many patients in whom airway hypersecretion has clinical significance; for example, patients prone to chest infections [4]. Consequently, development of pharma-cotherapeutic compounds to inhibit mucus hypersecretion in these patients is warranted. This chapter:

1 assesses the contribution of airway mucus hypersecretion to the pathophysiology of the 'bronchitic' component of COPD;

2 considers the clinical impact of mucus hypersecretion in COPD; and

3 discusses use of mucolytic and related drugs in the treatment of COPD.

The chapter begins with an overview of airway mucus, mucins and sputum.

Airway mucus and mucins

In health, a thin film of slimy liquid protects the airway surface [5]. The liquid is often referred to as 'mucus' and is a non-homogeneous 1–2% aqueous solution of electrolytes, enzymes and antienzymes, oxidants and antioxidants, bacterial products, antibacterial agents, cell-derived mediators and proteins, plasma-derived mediators and proteins, and cell debris such as DNA. The mucus forms a bilayer, comprising an upper mucous gel layer and a lower sol layer, with a thin layer of surfactant separating the two [6,7]. Cilia beat in the sol layer, often termed periciliary fluid. Inhaled particles are trapped in the gel layer and, by transportation on the tips of beating cilia, are removed from the airways, a process termed mucociliary clearance. The mucus gel requires an optimal combination of relatively low viscosity and preserved elasticity for efficient ciliary interaction [8]. Viscoelasticity is conferred primarily by high molecular weight mucous glycoproteins, termed mucins, which comprise up to 2% by weight of the mucus [9]. Respiratory tract mucins are produced by epithelial goblet cells [10] and sub-mucosal glands [11], and are long, thread-like molecules composed of monomers joined end-to-end by disulphide bridges. The monomers comprise a highly glycosylated (70–80%) linear peptide sequence, termed apomucin, that is encoded by specific mucin (*MUC*) genes. Eighteen human mucin genes, to date, have been cloned and over 20 identified [12; see also 9, 13–15]. At least 12 are expressed as mRNA in the lower respiratory tract [12]. In the normal, healthy lung, *MUC1*, *MUC4* are expressed at the apical surface of the respiratory epithelium; *MUC2*, *MUC5AC* are generally expressed in goblet cells of the superficial airway epithelium; *MUC5B*, *MUC8*, *MUC19* are expressed in mucosal cells of submucosal glands; *MUC7* is not well-expressed normally and when expressed is localized to the serosal cells of submucosal glands; *MUC11*, *MUC13*, *MUC15*, *MUC20* are also known to be expressed as mRNA in lung tissue [12].

Mucus properties

Before consideration of medications that may affect mucus properties and, hence, mucus clearance, it is essential to understand and define these properties. Often, mucoactive medications are defined by their presumed action on the mucus gel.

Periciliary fluid viscosity and depth affect mucociliary clearance. If this fluid is too viscous the cilia will not be able to beat effectively, and the decreased ciliary velocity will decrease mucociliary clearance. This principle is well established for water-propelling cilia, but for the periciliary fluid in the two-layer airway mucociliary system, periciliary fluid viscosity is unknown. Active ion transport and associated transepithelial water flux are probably important in modulating periciliary fluid viscosity [16]. Transepithelial protein fluxes may also contribute to periciliary fluid viscosity [17]. The efficient transfer of momentum between the cilia and the mucus layer requires the cilia to be firmly in contact with the mucus during their forward stroke, while minimally interacting with it during the return stroke. Thus, mucociliary clearance will also decrease if the periciliary fluid is either too deep or too shallow. The characteristics of mucus that affect mucociliary clearance are depth and viscoelasticity [18]. Although mucus that is too deep hinders clearance by cilia, it may be better suited to clearance by cough [19].

Rheology is the study of the deformation (strain) of matter with applied stress. Viscosity (energy loss or G′) is a property of liquids and an ideal or Newtonian liquid can be described strictly in terms of viscosity. An ideal or Hookian solid is described entirely by elasticity or energy storage (G″) with an applied stress. A non-Newtonian gel such as mucus has both viscous and elastic properties. Both viscosity and elasticity are needed for airway secretion clearance. The elastic component is essential for beating cilia to transmit kinetic energy to the mucus. Viscosity is also essential for effective clearance. Patients who have liquid-like mucus, often termed 'bronchorrhoea', are unable to clear secretions effectively. Mucociliary clearance is much more sensitive to high levels of viscosity, although high levels of elasticity may also impede ciliary transport [20]. A balance between these factors must be maintained for optimal efficiency of mucociliary clearance [21].

Sputum

Expectoration of sputum is a sign of respiratory disease and indicates excessive production (hypersecretion) and retention (impaired clearance) of mucus, as occurs in patients with COPD, respiratory infection, asthma, bronchiectasis and cystic fibrosis (CF). When excessive secretions are expectorated, this substance is called sputum.

The characteristics of mucus change with infection and inflammation. Inflammation leads to mucus hypersecretion, ciliary dysfunction and changes in the composition and property of airway secretions. Inflammatory cells, particularly neutrophils, which are recruited to the airway to combat infection, disappear from the airway either through programmed cell death (apoptosis) or by necrosis. Necrotic neutrophils release pro-inflammatory mediators that damage the epithelium and recruit more inflammatory cells. They also release DNA and filamentous actin (F-actin) from the cytoskeleton. DNA and F-actin copolymerize to form a second rigid network within airway secretions [22]. Neutrophil-derived myeloperoxidase imparts a characteristic green colour to inflamed airway secretions, and thickened and green secretions are usually described as purulent.

Pathophysiology of mucus hypersecretion in COPD

Mucus hypersecretion in COPD has characteristic features. It was thought that COPD mucus hypersection was similar to hypersection in asthma and CF. However, it is clear now that there is almost no mucin in the CF airway and with chronic CF or bronchiectasis, the airways fill with similar to pus rather than mucin [23]. Differences in mucus pathophysiology between COPD and asthma have been considered previously [24], and are summarized in Figure 62.1. Mucociliary clearance is also impaired in COPD and is discussed in detail elsewhere in the present volume. In addition, the pulmonary inflammation of COPD (essentially a macrophage-driven neutrophilia) that induces the hypersecretory phenotype of COPD is different from asthma [1].

Sputum production can be up to 100 mL/day in some patients and is associated with excessive airway mucus [25–27]. The increased mucus is associated with goblet cell hyperplasia [25,28] and submucosal gland hypertrophy [25,26,29,30]. Of note is that gland mucous cells are markedly increased relative to serous cells [29]. This is in contrast to asthma where the glands are hypertrophied but otherwise morphologically normal. Gland size correlates with amount of luminal mucus and daily sputum volume [29].

Not all COPD patients exhibit all of the above features of hypersecretion. Not all patients expectorate, not all patients have goblet cell hyperplasia [26,31], and there is overlap in gland size with healthy non-smokers, and between sputum producers and non-producers [28,30,32–34]. Thus, although considered a general feature of COPD, mucus hypersecretion is not always diagnostic.

The mucin composition of airway mucus in patients with COPD may be abnormal. For example, most chronic smokers produce a relatively rigid mucus with more sialic acid and fewer fucose residues [35]. Mucins in sputum from patients with COPD are less acidic than in sputum from control subjects [36], which may relate to altered glycosylation. *MUC5AC* and a low charge glycoform of *MUC5B* are the major mucin species in patients with COPD [37–40], with the low charge glycoform increased above normal levels [41]. Although COPD patients often have airway

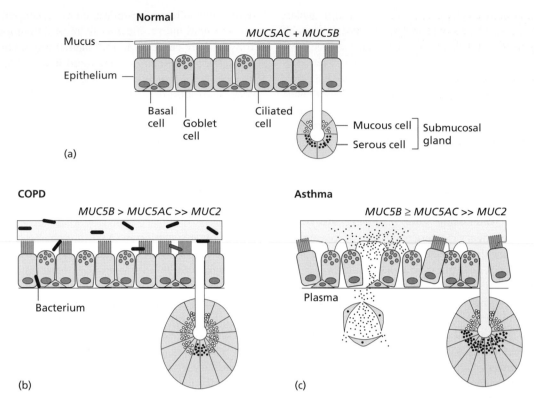

Figure 62.1 Schematic diagram of differences in airway mucus pathophysiology between COPD and asthma. Compared with normal (a), in COPD (b) there is increased luminal mucus, goblet cell hyperplasia, submucosal gland hypertrophy (with an increased proportion of mucous to serous cells), an increased ratio of mucin (*MUC*) *5B* (low charge glycoform) to *MUC5AC* and respiratory infection. In asthma (c) there is increased luminal mucus, marked goblet cell hyperplasia, submucosal gland hypertrophy (although without a marked increase in mucous/serous cell ratio), 'tethering' of mucus to goblet cells, and plasma exudation. Many of these differences require confirmation from greater numbers of subjects.

infection it is not clear how this may be related to the change in *MUC5B* glycoforms [3].

In contrast to normal airways, airway goblet cells in COPD patients contain not only *MUC5AC* but also *MUC5B* [39,42] and *MUC2* [9]. This distribution is different to that in patients with asthma or CF, where *MUC5AC* and *MUC5B* show a similar distribution to normal controls [43,44]. Although found inconsistently [27,38], *MUC2* may be increased in inflamed airways, including in CF or COPD [9,41,45].

Epidemiology of mucus hypersecretion in COPD

The contribution of mucus to pathophysiology and clinical symptoms in COPD is controversial [24]. Epidemiological studies sampling hundreds to thousands of subjects in the late 1970s and 1980s found scant evidence for the involvement of mucus in either the mortality or accelerated agerelated decline in lung function associated with COPD [46–50]. In all studies, expectorated sputum volume

(sometimes called sputum production) was used as an index of mucus hypersecretion. The relationship between sputum volume and mucus hypersecretion is unclear, particularly in the small airways, the main site of airflow obstruction. The consensus of the studies was that airflow obstruction and mucus hypersecretion were largely independent disease processes.

In contrast, a number of studies in the late 1980s and 1990s found positive associations between sputum production and decline in lung function, hospitalization and death [51–55]. Some of these reports were re-examinations of the same patients, now older, reported previously. The increased risk of death in patients with excessive sputum appears to be brought about by the severity and chronicity of disease and the frequency of infectious exacerbations [4]. Thus, although not associated with disease progression in all cases, mucus hypersecretion contributes to morbidity and mortality in certain groups of patients with COPD, particularly those prone to infection, and possibly as patients age. This highlights the potential importance of developing drugs that inhibit mucus hypersecretion in these patients.

Preliminary considerations for mucolytic therapy of COPD

From the above it may be seen that there is some debate concerning both the pathophysiological and clinical significance of mucus hypersecretion in COPD and, therefore, the therapeutic value of drugs affecting mucus properties. This is evident in the observation that mucolytic agents are not recommended in current guidelines for management of stable COPD [3]. Nevertheless, the clinical symptoms of cough and sputum production, coupled with a perception of the importance of mucus hypersecretion in the pathophysiology of COPD, has prompted renewed interest in research into airway hypersecretion and, in concert, in development of drugs targeting mucus. Because COPD has specific trigger factors and mucus hypersecretory phenotype (see Fig. 62.1), COPD-specific drugs may be required to fulfil the theoretical requirements for treatment of hypersecretion (Table 62.1). There are many medications available that purport to alleviate airway mucus hypersecretion. The mechanism of action of these compounds is mostly unknown or incompletely characterized. For example, *N*-acetylcysteine (NAC) is considered a mucolytic drug, although this activity is not well documented [56], and it is not found in airway secretions after oral dosing [57]. NAC has antioxidant properties [58], and may also have antibacterial activity [59,60]. Ambroxol is another drug with possible multiple mechanisms of action, including antioxidant activity [61] and enhancement of surfactant secretion [62]. Thus, any beneficial clinical effects of mucolytic treatment are not necessarily a result of decreasing mucus viscosity – the definition of a mucolytic.

In the following discussion, compounds will be classified as mucolytics, mucoregulators, expectorants or abhesives according to the following characteristics. Respiratory mucins, in common with other mucins, contain disulphide bonds that contribute to mucus viscosity and gel formation [63,64]. Herein, the term mucolytic refers to compounds with free sulphydryl groups that hydrolyse disulphide bonds and reduce mucus viscosity. Other compounds such as proteolytic enzymes and DNase also break up mucus, but do so via mechanisms other than dissociating disulphide bonds in mucin molecules and, as such, are not classic mucolytics and are often termed peptide mucolytics. Other drugs do not have free sulphydryl groups, or otherwise break up mucus. Nevertheless, in experimental studies they have beneficial actions on various aspects of mucus properties. These compounds are termed non-thiol mucolytics herein. Expectorants probably increase secretion to a point where sufficient mucus is produced to enable it to be coughed up. Expectorants may also hydrate mucus and, thereby, enhance mucociliary clearance. These drugs may also be irritants and facilitate cough to dislodge mucus. Oral expectorants are considered to increase secretion by triggering a vagal reflex via nerve endings in the gastric mucosa. Abhesives reduce mucus adhesiveness, thereby enhancing mucociliary clearance by increasing the efficiency of energy transfer from the cilia. The effectiveness of cough in dislodging secretions will also be enhanced because sputum tenacity, the product of adhesivity and cohesivity (Fig. 62.2), has a marked influence on cough clearance [65].

Mucolytics

N-acetylcysteine

N-acetylcysteine (NAC) is a commonly prescribed mucolytic compound [66] that decreases mucus viscosity *in vitro* [67,68]. In a rat model of chronic bronchitis, oral NAC inhibited cigarette smoke-induced goblet cell hyperplasia [69] and associated mucus hypersecretion [70], when given concurrently with the smoke. More importantly from a clinical and therapeutic standpoint, NAC reduced the time taken for goblet cell numbers to return to normal after cessation of smoke exposure [71]. This may have relevance to treatment of patients with COPD who quit smoking.

Table 62.1 Theoretical requirements for treatment of mucus pathophysiology in COPD.

Overall effect	Component effects
Facilitate mucus clearance (short-term relief of symptoms)	Reduce mucus viscosity (?increase elasticity)
	Increase ciliary function
	Induce cough
Reverse hypersecretory phenotype (long-term benefit)	Reduce submucosal gland size
	Correct increased gland mucous/serous cell ratio
	Reduce goblet cell number
	Reverse increased LCGF-*MUC5B/MUC5AC* ratio
LCGF, low charge glycoform; MUC, mucin gene product.	

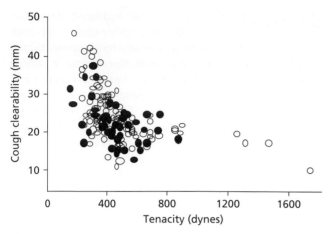

Figure 62.2 Tenacity (dynes) is the product of cohesivity and work of adhesion. Sputum tenacity and air flow are the two strongest predictors of cough clearability.

The pharmacokinetics of NAC depend upon the route of administration. Aerosolized inhaled NAC directly reduces mucus viscosity whereas oral NAC has low bioavailability [72], although it is deacetylated to cysteine whose thiol group possesses reducing and antioxidant properties [73]. NAC cannot be detected in plasma or bronchoalveolar lavage fluid following oral dosing for up to 2 weeks [57,74], although increases in plasma cysteine concentrations were reported [57], with associated increased levels of glutathione (GSH) in both plasma [57,74] and lung [57]. However, in patients with COPD, high doses of NAC (600 mg three times daily) are required to elevate plasma GSH levels [75].

Clinical trial data on NAC are variable, and may be related to route of administration. For example, inhaled NAC in patients with chronic bronchitis did not improve dyspnoea, cough, sputum production, lung function or feelings of well-being after treatment for 16 weeks [76]. In contrast, oral NAC increased sputum volume, decreased sputum thickness and improved scores for dyspnoea and ease of expectoration in chronic bronchitis patients [77]. The study also reported improvements in lung function compared with the placebo group, although this should be treated with caution because of differences in lung function between the two groups at baseline. A large placebo-controlled trial in patients with chronic bronchitis found that oral NAC treatment (200 mg twice daily) decreased symptom scores for sputum volume, degree of purulence, 'thickness' of sputum and difficulty in expectoration and severity of cough [78].

A common theme of clinical trials with NAC is reductions in exacerbations [78–80], although this is not always the case [81]. The latter study differed from the former two studies in that patients not only had chronic bronchitis but also severe airways obstruction. Oral NAC (300 mg twice daily as slow-release tablets) also reduces days off work because of illness in patients with chronic bronchitis [82], while 600 mg twice daily sustained-release NAC improves 'general well-being' [83]. This result should be interpreted with caution because there was an imbalance between groups in 'well-being' scores at the start of the trial.

In the largest and most complete randomized, placebo-controlled, and well-powered study of NAC in COPD to date, 523 patients from 50 European centres were assigned to 600 mg daily NAC or placebo. After 3 years, neither the annual number of exacerbations nor the yearly rate of decline in FEV_1 differed between treatment and control groups. From these data it appears that NAC is ineffective at preventing deterioration in lung function or preventing exacerbations in patients with COPD [84]

Nacystelyn

Nacystelyn is a lysine salt of NAC that has mucolytic and antioxidant properties, and a neutral pH which, when compared with the more acidic NAC (pH 2.2), reduces unwanted side-effects when aerosolized into the lung [85,86]. *In vivo*, nacystelyn has greater mucolytic activity than NAC [87], and *in vitro* has greater antioxidant activity in inhibiting the oxidative burst of human peripheral blood neutrophils [88]. Inhaled nacystelyn has been given to CF patients but, to date, there are no data available regarding its use in COPD.

Methylcysteine hydrochloride

Methylcysteine hydrochloride (mecysteine) is a mucolytic indicated for reduction of sputum viscosity [89]. In a double-blind placebo-controlled trial in chronic bronchitis patients with uncontrolled productive cough, oral methylcysteine markedly decreased sputum viscosity at all time points assessed, increased sputum volume, albeit at one time point only, and improved the subjective assessment of both ease of expectoration and severity and frequency of cough [90]. No side-effects of clinical significance were reported. Further clinical trials of the use of this drug in COPD are warranted.

2-Mercaptoethane sulphonate sodium

2-Mercaptoethane sulphonate sodium (MESNA) is a mucolytic agent that reduces the viscosity of aspirated mucus from patients following surgery [91]. In rabbits, MESNA was the least irritating to the tracheal epithelium of three mucolytic agents examined [92]. In surgical cases requiring mucolytic therapy for mucus retention in the lung, MESNA instillation liquefied the secretions and facilitated aspiration [91]. There were no side-effects. Specific studies in COPD are required.

Non-thiol mucolytics

Carbocysteine

Carbocysteine (S-carboxymethylcysteine) is a cysteine derivative with a blocked sulphydryl group, and so does not directly break disulphide bonds [93]. Consequently, carbocysteine does not reduce the viscosity of canine tracheal mucus *in vitro* [94] or human nasal mucus [95], but did reduce sputum viscosity in patients with chronic bronchitis who produced viscous secretions [96]. The therapeutic effect of carbocysteine may be via stimulation of intracellular sialyl transferase activity [97]. As a result, newly synthesized mucus would have an increased content of sialomucins and a decreased content of fucomucins. In a rat model of chronic bronchitis, carbocysteine inhibited tracheal mucus hypersecretion [70].

Carbocysteine has been reported to have variable effects in clinical trials. For example, in one study, carbocysteine had no effect on lung clearance, cough, weight of sputum expectorated, lung function or subjective improvement in patients with chronic bronchitis [98]. In contrast, in a 3-month double-blind controlled study of 82 patients with chronic bronchitis, carbocysteine reduced sputum viscosity, increased sputum volume and ease of expectoration, reduced cough frequency, improved lung function and reduced dyspnoea [99]. Similarly, in another double-blind placebo-controlled study in 20 male patients, 2 weeks of oral carbocysteine enhanced the viscoelastic properties of the bronchial secretions, improved clinical parameters, although with no change in lung function [100]. Carbo-cysteine also increased penetration of amoxicillin into bronchial secretions in patients with chronic bronchitis [101], an effect that may be beneficial during infective exacerbations.

Carbocysteine-lys

Carbocysteine-lys is a lysine salt of carbocysteine that diffuses into bronchial mucus [102] and has modest mucolytic activity [103]. Four days' treatment of patients with chronic bronchitis with carbocysteine-lys decreased sputum viscosity and increased mucociliary transport for up to 8 days after cessation of treatment [104]. In a 6-month multicentre double-blind placebo-controlled trial in 622 COPD patients, carbocysteine-lys reduced exacerbations and antibiotic use compared with placebo controls [105]. However, intermittent carbocysteine-lys therapy (1-week courses alternating with 1 week of placebo) was not effective. No serious adverse effects were reported.

Erdosteine

Erdosteine (N-(carboxymethylthioacetyl)-homocysteine thiolactone) is a synthetic derivative of the naturally occurring amino acid methionine that was developed as a mucolytic for use in COPD patients [106]. Erdosteine contains two blocked sulphydryl groups that are 'exposed' after hepatic metabolism of the drug. The freed sulphydryl groups break down disulphide bonds in mucins [106], and also confer free radical scavenging and antioxidant properties. Erdosteine 300 mg three times daily significantly reduced the viscosity of sputum in 20 male patients with COPD without altering elasticity [107]. These changes were accompanied by reductions in mucin concentration and dry weight. The same dose of drug improved mucociliary transport in 16 former smokers with chronic bronchitis [108].

Erdosteine also appears to have antioxidant activity, leading to significant increases in levels of functional α_1-antitrypsin (an endogenous antielastase) in healthy smokers [109]. In addition, erdosteine enhances antibiotic penetration into sputum. Twenty four patients with an infective exacerbation of chronic bronchitis were treated with amoxicillin (500 mg three times daily) plus either erdosteine or placebo in a double-blind trial [110]. There was a significantly higher concentration of amoxicillin in the sputum of the erdosteine group, with more rapid sterilization of the sputum. Erdosteine was evaluated in 237 patients with exacerbations of COPD, comparing treatment with amoxicillin (500 mg three times daily) plus erdosteine (300 mg twice daily) with amoxicillin plus placebo [111]. Sputum viscosity and clinical assessment improved with combined therapy, but without changes in sputum volume, body temperature or lung function.

Stepronin

Stepronin (2-(α-theoylthio)propionylglycine lysine salt), like erdosteine, is not itself mucolytic but is metabolised in the intestine to remove a thenoyl moiety and release thiopropionylglycine, which has a free sulphydryl group that breaks disulphide bonds [112]. It also reduces secretion in cat isolated tracheal submucosal glands [113]. Launched in Italy in 1981 [114], stepronin was developed to treat chronic bronchitis associated with mucus hypersecretion. Side-effects are rare, although cell-mediated hypersensitivity to stepronin has been reported [115].

Expectorants

Bromhexine

Bromhexine (N-methyl-N-cyclohexane-3,5-dibromo-2-aminobenzylamine hydrochloride) is derived from the alkaloid vasicine (*Adhatoda vasica nees*). Bromhexine reduces the elasticity and viscosity of mini-pigis tracheal mucus after oral dosing [116] and stimulates mucus secretion by canine tracheal submucosal glands, but not goblet cells [117]. In a multicentre placebo-controlled trial of 237 patients with COPD, oral bromhexine (30 mg twice daily) significantly decreased sputum volume and improved sputum 'quality' and ease of expectoration, cough, dyspnoea, lung function a nd the physician's overall assessment [118]. Similar to erdosteine and ambroxol (see above), bromhexine increases penetration of antibiotics, amoxicillin and erythromycin, into sputum [119,120].

Ambroxol

Ambroxol is a metabolite of bromhexine (see above) and is probably an expectorant because it stimulates mucus secretion [121]. It does not exhibit anti-inflammatory activity in patients with chronic bronchitis [122]. The effect of ambroxol on mucociliary clearance is variable. For example, ambroxol significantly increased mucociliary transport in one double-blind cross-over study in 12 heavy smokers with chronic bronchitis [123]. In contrast, in another double-blind placebo-controlled trial in 30 patients with COPD and asthma, ambroxol increased mucociliary clearance in only one out of five regions of the lung, compared with an increase in four out of five regions following a β_2-adrenoceptor agonist [124]. Similar results were found in 14 patients with simple chronic bronchitis [125].

The clinical efficacy of ambroxol is also equivocal. For example, in a controlled study in 60 patients with 'bronchial stasis', 120 mg/day ambroxol increased ease of expectoration and sputum volume, and reduced cough severity and sputum viscosity [126]. In another controlled study, ambroxol improved subjective symptoms and phlegm loosening in 92 patients with chronic bronchitis, but did not improve lung function or diary card entries [127]. In contrast, in a similarly designed study in 90 patients with stable chronic bronchitis who had difficulty clearing secretions, there was no clinical advantage in taking ambroxol [128]. In a 6-month multicentre double-blind controlled trial, ambroxol significantly reduced the frequency of exacerbations in 104 patients with chronic bronchitis compared with 104 patients taking placebo [129]. A similar reduction in frequency of exacerbations was seen in a larger trial of 5635 patients, although the results should be interpreted with caution as the trial was open, prospective and had no control group [130]. In a study in 24 patients with infectious exacerbations of COPD, ambroxol increased the concentration of the antibiotic ofloxacin in lung lavage alveolar cells, although there were no increases in concentration in plasma or bronchial biopsy specimens [131]. Ambroxol was well tolerated in all studies.

Iodides

Although iodides, in particular saturated solutions of potassium iodide (SSKI), have long been used as expectorants, clinical efficacy has not been demonstrated and their use is not recommended because they may induce thyroid disease [132]. A potentially less toxic product is 'iodinated' glycerol (iodopropylidene glycerol), which has been shown to be an effective expectorant in patients with excessive sputum production [133]. However, clinical data are equivocal. For example, in a randomized double-blind placebo-controlled study in 361 patients with chronic bronchitis, 2 months' treatment with iodinated glycerol tablets reduced chest discomfort and frequency and severity of cough, increased ease of expectoration and improved patients' subjective assessment of well-being [134]. However, the physician's evaluation of patients showed no significant difference between treatment and placebo groups, and the study lacked objective measurements of pulmonary function or sputum clearance. Similarly, another placebo-controlled trial found no significant changes in pulmonary function, clinical scores or sputum properties following 16 weeks' treatment with iodinated glycerol [135]. Although considered safe in clinical trials [134,135], iodinated glycerol is associated with adverse side-effects, including hypothyroidism, hyperthyroidism and goitre [136–140]. Chronic iodine poisoning has been reported with long-term use [141].

Domiodol (iodoethylene glycerol) is another iodinated organic compound [142]. In a placebo-controlled cross-over study, domiodol significantly increased volume of secretions and aided ease of expectoration in chronic bronchitis patients [143]. However, the lack of convincing clinical evidence coupled with concerns regarding safety suggests that iodine and iodinated compounds should not be used as mucoregulatory drugs in COPD.

Adhesives

Surfactant can reduce sputum adhesiveness and enhance mucus clearance, thereby improving lung function (Fig. 62.3). Patients with chronic bronchitis have a reduced amount of bronchial surfactant [144], and also have abnormal sputum phospholipid composition [145,146], factors that would tend to decrease clearance. Consequently, decreasing tenacity with surfactant enhances the effectiveness of cough [147]. Fourteen days of aerosolized surfactant (607.5 mg dipalymotyl phosphotidal choline/day) increased *in vitro* sputum transportability, improved forced expiratory volume in 1 s (FEV_1) and forced vital capacity (FVC) by more than 10%, and decreased trapped thoracic gas (residual volume/total lung capacity [RV/TLC] ratio) by more than 6% in patients with stable chronic bronchitis [148]. This effect persisted for

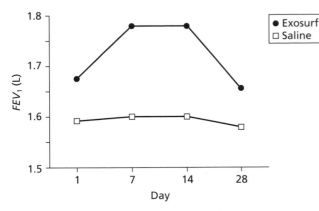

Figure 62.3 Surfactant therapy in cystic fibrosis. Fourteen days of aerosolized surfactant (Exosurf at 607.5 mg dipalymotyl phosphotidal choline/day) increased *in vitro* sputum cough transportability and improved forced expiratory volume in 1 s (*FEV*$_1$) by more than 10% in patients with stable cystic fibrosis. Pulmonary function returned to baseline within 2 weeks of stopping therapy. (From B.K. Rubin, unpublished data.)

at least a week after treatment was completed. Interestingly, ambroxol is thought to stimulate surfactant secretion.

Some of the expectorant activity of mucolytic and related compounds may be attributed to abhesive action. Decreasing the viscosity of a mucous plug might, theoretically, reduce cough clearance by decreasing the height of the mucus layer. However, if a mucolytic decreased mucus mechanical impedance at the epithelial surface (i.e. frictional adhesive forces), it might 'unstick' secretions from the underlying ciliated epithelium, thereby making airflow-dependent clearance more efficient.

Peptide mucolytics

Recombinant human DNase (dornase alfa)

DNA, released in large amounts from necrosed neutrophils, increases mucus viscosity in purulent lung secretions. Recombinant human DNase I (dornase alfa) has been developed for treatment of mucus hypersecretion in CF [149,150]. Dornase alfa reduces the viscosity of purulent sputum from CF patients (see Plate 62.1; colour plate section falls between pp. 354 and 355) and, in a clinical trial, dornase alfa inhalation decreased the surface adhesivity (and thus the tenacity) of CF sputum, with an associated improvement in lung function [151]. In contrast, in patients with bronchiectasis not caused by CF, dornase alfa did not alter sputum transportability, lung function, dyspnoea or quality of life [152].

Dornase alfa also reduces the viscosity and favourably

alters the surface properties of purulent sputum *in vitro* from patients with chronic bronchitis [153]. Phase II and III clinical trials of the effects of dornase alfa in COPD are, to date, reported only in abstract form, with limited data on patient characteristics, disease severity and concomitant treatment [154–156]. The results of these studies are equivocal. Consequently, at present, dornase alfa is recommended only for use in patients with CF [157].

Gelsolin

Actin is the most prevalent cellular protein in the body, having a vital role in maintaining the structural integrity of cells. In addition to DNA (see above), necrozing cells also release significant quantities of actin. The actin in turn interacts with mucus to increase its viscosity. Gelsolin is the recombinant form of the natural actin-severing agent and reduces sputum viscosity in patients with CF [158]. Clinical trials of gelsolin in patients with respiratory diseases, including chronic bronchitis, have not been reported.

Conclusions

Current guidelines do not recommend mucolytics in the management of COPD [3]. Despite this, numerous mucolytic and related drugs are available worldwide, with *N*-acetylcysteine, bromhexine and carbocysteine listed extensively in international pharmacopoeiae [66]. The discrepancy between drug listing and recommended treatment is related to the inconsistency in data from clinical trials of mucolytic drugs [159]. Many mucoactive compounds have an impressive preclinical profile but subsequently are entered into imprecise clinical trials of a design leading to ambiguity in interpretation. Two meta-analyses of clinical trials in COPD, one on mucolytics [160], the other on *N*-acetylcysteine [161], excluded 70–80% of the reported trials because they did not conform to standard criteria including being double blind and placebo controlled, of sufficient duration and of sufficient power, and with well-defined primary endpoints or outcome measures. Better clinical studies are required and should conform to current guidelines for clinical trials of mucolytics [162,163]. Data on rate of hospital admissions in response to mucolytic treatment would be useful because this outcome measure contributes greatly to the costs of treating severe COPD. Two systematic reviews analysed clinical trials in COPD, one for mucolytics and exacerbations [80], the other for *N*-acetylcysteine [161], and concluded that treatment for 2–6 months with oral mucolytic drugs was associated with a 23–29% reduction in exacerbation rate.

The conclusion from the present chapter and the meta-analyses [80,160] is that maintenance treatment with mucolytic or related drugs is not associated with significant improvements in lung function in patients with COPD. However, treatment with certain mucolytic drugs is associated with a reduction in exacerbations and days of illness [80,161]. The cost effectiveness of treatment of this patient group for up to 6 months a year is debatable [164]. However, the analysis of Poole and Black [80] indicates that patients with more severe COPD benefit more from treatment with mucolytics. Consequently, maintenance mucolytic treatment of patients with severe COPD should be cost effective, and future clinical trials should examine the value of mucolytic drugs in this difficult patient group.

References

1 Barnes PJ. New concepts in chronic obstructive pulmonary disease. *Annu Rev Med* 2003;**54**:113–29.

2 Fletcher CM, Pride NB. Definitions of emphysema, chronic bronchitis, asthma, and airflow obstruction: 25 years on from the Ciba symposium. *Thorax* 1984;**39**:81–5.

3 National Heart Lung and Blood Institute, World Health Organisation. Global initiative for chronic obstructive lung disease. Publication no. 2701. National Institutes of Health, 2001.

4 Prescott E, Lange P, Vestbo J. Chronic mucus hypersecretion in COPD and death from pulmonary infection. *Eur Respir J* 1995;**8**:1333–8.

5 Knowles MR, Boucher RC. Mucus clearance as a primary innate defense mechanism for mammalian airways. *J Clin Invest* 2002;**109**:571–7.

6 Morgenroth K, Bolz J. Morphological features of the interaction between mucus and surfactant on the bronchial mucosa. *Respiration* 1985;**47**:225–31.

7 Schurch S, Gehr P, Im H, V, Geiser M, Green F. Surfactant displaces particles toward the epithelium in airways and alveoli. *Respir Physiol* 1990;**80**:17–32.

8 Davis B, Roberts AM, Coleridge HM, Coleridge JC. Reflex tracheal gland secretion evoked by stimulation of bronchial C-fibers in dogs. *J Appl Physiol* 1982;**53**:985–91.

9 Davies JR, Herrmann A, Russell W *et al.* Respiratory tract mucins: structure and expression patterns. In: Chadwick DJ, Goode JA, eds. *Mucus Hypersecretion in Respiratory Disease*. Chichester: John Wiley & Sons, 2002: 76–88.

10 Rogers DF. The airway goblet cell. *Int J Biochem Cell Biol* 2003;**35**:1–6.

11 Finkbeiner WE. Physiology and pathology of tracheobronchial glands. *Respir Physiol* 1999;**118**:77–83.

12 Rose MC, Voynow JA. Respiratory tract mucin genes and mucin glycoproteins in health and disease. *Physiol Rev* 2006;**86**:245–78.

13 Dekker J, Rossen JW, Buller HA, Einerhand AW. The MUC family: an obituary. *Trends Biochem Sci* 2002;**27**:126–31.

14 Gum JR Jr, Crawley SC, Hicks JW, Szymkowski DE, Kim YS. MUC17, a novel membrane-tethered mucin. *Biochem Biophys Res Commun* 2002;**291**:466–75.

15 Wu GJ, Wu MW, Wang SW *et al.* Isolation and characterization of the major form of human MUC18 cDNA gene and correlation of MUC18 over-expression in prostate cancer cell lines and tissues with malignant progression. *Gene* 2001;**279**:17–31.

16 Boucher RC. Human airway ion transport. Part 1. *Am J Respir Crit Care Med* 1994;**150**:271–81.

17 Govindaraju K, Cowley EA, Eidelman DH, Lloyd DK. Analysis of proteins in microsamples of rat airway surface fluid by capillary electrophoresis. *J Chromatogr B Biomed Sci Appl* 1998;**705**:223–30.

18 King M, Rubin B. Mucus physiology and pathophysiology: therapeutic aspects. In: Derenne JP, Similowski T, Whitelaw WA, eds. *Chronic Obstructive Lung Disease*. New York: Marcel Dekker, 1996: 391–411.

19 Bennett WD, Foster WM, Chapman WF. Cough-enhanced mucus clearance in the normal lung. *J Appl Physiol* 1990;**69**:1670–5.

20 King M. Rheological requirements for optimal clearance of secretions: ciliary transport versus cough. *Eur J Respir Dis Suppl* 1980;**110**:39–45.

21 Puchelle E, Zahm JM, Girard F *et al.* Mucociliary transport *in vivo* and *in vitro*: relations to sputum properties in chronic bronchitis. *Eur J Respir Dis* 1980;**61**:254–64.

22 Tomkiewicz RP, Kishioka C, Freeman J, Rubin BK. DNA and actin filament ultrastructure in cystic fibrosis sputum. In: Baum G, ed. *Cilia, Mucus and Mucociliary Interactions*. New York: Marcel Dekker, 1998: 333–41.

23 Henke MO, Renner A, Huber RM, Seeds MC, Rubin BK. MUC5AC and MUC5B mucins are decreased in cystic fibrosis airways secretions. *Am J Respir Cell Mol Biol* 2004;**31**:86–91.

24 Rogers DF. Mucus pathophysiology in COPD: differences to asthma, and pharmacotherapy. *Monaldi Arch Chest Dis* 2000;**55**:324–32.

25 Reid L. Pathology of chronic bronchitis. *Lancet* 1954;**i**:275–8.

26 Aikawa T, Shimura S, Sasaki H *et al.* Morphometric analysis of intraluminal mucus in airways in chronic obstructive pulmonary disease. *Am Rev Respir Dis* 1989;**140**:477–82.

27 Steiger D, Fahy J, Boushey H, Finkbeiner WE, Basbaum C. Use of mucin antibodies and cDNA probes to quantify hypersecretion *in vivo* in human airways. *Am J Respir Cell Mol Biol* 1994;**10**:538–45.

28 Mullen JB, Wright JL, Wiggs BR, Pare PD, Hogg JC. Structure of central airways in current smokers and ex-smokers with and without mucus hypersecretion: relationship to lung function. *Thorax* 1987;**42**:843–8.

29 Reid L. Measurement of the bronchial mucous gland layer: a diagnostic yardstick in chronic bronchitis. *Thorax* 1960;**15**:132–41.

30 Restrepo G, Heard BE. The size of the bronchial glands in chronic bronchitis. *J Pathol Bacteriol* 1963;**85**:305–10.

31 Glynn AA, Michaels L. Bronchial biopsy in chronic bronchitis and asthma. *Thorax* 1960;**15**:142–53.

32 Hayes JA. Distribution of bronchial gland measurement in a Jamaican population. *Thorax* 1960;**24**:619–22.

33 Thurlbeck WM, Angus CW, Paré JAP. Mucous gland hypertrophy in chronic bronchitis, and its occurrence in smokers. *Br J Dis Chest* 1963;**57**:73–8.

34 Thurlbeck WM, Angus GE. A distribution curve for chronic bronchitis. *Thorax* 1964;**19**:436–42.

35 Lopez-Vidriero MT. Airway mucus: production and composition. *Chest* 1981;**80**(Suppl):799–804.

36 Davies JR, Hovenberg HW, Linden CJ *et al.* Mucins in airway secretions from healthy and chronic bronchitic subjects. *Biochem J* 1996;**313**:431–9.

37 Thornton DJ, Carlstedt I, Howard M *et al.* Respiratory mucins: identification of core proteins and glycoforms. *Biochem J* 1996;**316**:967–75.

38 Hovenberg HW, Davies JR, Herrmann A, Linden CJ, Carlstedt I. MUC5AC, but not MUC2, is a prominent mucin in respiratory secretions. *Glycoconj J* 1996;**13**:839–47.

39 Wickstrom C, Davies JR, Eriksen GV, Veerman EC, Carlstedt I. MUC5B is a major gel-forming, oligomeric mucin from human salivary gland, respiratory tract and endocervix: identification of glycoforms and C-terminal cleavage. *Biochem J* 1998;**334**:685–93.

40 Sheehan JK, Howard M, Richardson PS, Longwill T, Thornton DJ. Physical characterization of a low-charge glycoform of the MUC5B mucin comprising the gel-phase of an asthmatic respiratory mucous plug. *Biochem J* 1999;**338**:507–13.

41 Kirkham S, Sheehan JK, Knight D, Richardson PS, Thornton DJ. Heterogeneity of airways mucus: variations in the amounts and glycoforms of the major oligomeric mucins MUC5AC and MUC5B. *Biochem J* 2002;**361**:537–46.

42 Chen Y, Zhao YH, Di YP, Wu R. Characterization of human mucin 5B gene expression in airway epithelium and the genomic clone of the amino-terminal and 5′-flanking region. *Am J Respir Cell Mol Biol* 2001;**25**:542–53.

43 Groneberg DA, Eynott PR, Lim S *et al.* Expression of respiratory mucins in fatal status asthmaticus and mild asthma. *Histopathology* 2002;**40**:367–73.

44 Groneberg DA, Eynott PR, Oates T *et al.* Expression of MUC5AC and MUC5B mucins in normal and cystic fibrosis lung. *Respir Med* 2002;**96**:81–6.

45 Davies JR, Svitacheva N, Lannefors L, Kornfalt R, Carlstedt I. Identification of MUC5B, MUC5AC and small amounts of MUC2 mucins in cystic fibrosis airway secretions. *Biochem J* 1999;**344**:321–30.

46 Fletcher C, Peto R. The natural history of chronic airflow obstruction. *BMJ* 1977;**1**:1645–8.

47 Kauffmann F, Drouet D, Lellouch J, Brille D. Twelve years spirometric changes among Paris area workers. *Int J Epidemiol* 1979;**8**:201–12.

48 Higgins MW, Keller JB, Becker M *et al.* An index of risk for obstructive airways disease. *Am Rev Respir Dis* 1982;**125**:144–51.

49 Peto R, Speizer FE, Cochrane AL *et al.* The relevance in adults of air-flow obstruction, but not of mucus hypersecretion, to mortality from chronic lung disease: results from 20 years of prospective observation. *Am Rev Respir Dis* 1983;**128**:491–500.

50 Ebi-Kryston KL. Respiratory symptoms and pulmonary function as predictors of 10-year mortality from respiratory disease, cardiovascular disease, and all causes in the Whitehall Study. *J Clin Epidemiol* 1988;**41**:251–60.

51 Annesi I, Kauffmann F. Is respiratory mucus hypersecretion really an innocent disorder? A 22-year mortality survey of 1061 working men. *Am Rev Respir Dis* 1986;**134**:688–93.

52 Vestbo J, Prescott E, Lange P. Association of chronic mucus hypersecretion with FEV_1 decline and chronic obstructive pulmonary disease morbidity. Copenhagen City Heart Study Group. *Am J Respir Crit Care Med* 1996;**153**:1530–5.

53 Lange P, Nyboe J, Appleyard M, Jensen G, Schnohr P. Relation of ventilatory impairment and of chronic mucus hypersecretion to mortality from obstructive lung disease and from all causes. *Thorax* 1990;**45**:579–85.

54 Speizer FE, Fay ME, Dockery DW, Ferris BG Jr. Chronic obstructive pulmonary disease mortality in six US cities. *Am Rev Respir Dis* 1989;**140**:S49–55.

55 Sherman CB, Xu X, Speizer FE *et al.* Longitudinal lung function decline in subjects with respiratory symptoms. *Am Rev Respir Dis* 1992;**146**:855–9.

56 Houtmeyers E, Gosselink R, Gayan-Ramirez G, Decramer M. Effects of drugs on mucus clearance. *Eur Respir J* 1999;**14**:452–67.

57 Bridgeman MM, Marsden M, MacNee W, Flenley DC, Ryle AP. Cysteine and glutathione concentrations in plasma and bronchoalveolar lavage fluid after treatment with *N*-acetylcysteine. *Thorax* 1991;**46**:39–42.

58 Kiefer P, Vogt J, Radermacher P. From mucolytic to anti-oxidant and liver protection: new aspects in the intensive care unit career of *N*-acetylcysteine. *Crit Care Med* 2000;**28**:3935–6.

59 Riise GC, Larsson S, Larsson P, Jeansson S, Andersson BA. The intrabronchial microbial flora in chronic bronchitis patients: a target for *N*-acetylcysteine therapy? *Eur Respir J* 1994;**7**:94–101.

60 Riise GC, Qvarfordt I, Larsson S, Eliasson V, Andersson BA. Inhibitory effect of *N*-acetylcysteine on adherence of *Streptococcus pneumoniae* and *Haemophilus influenzae* to human oropharyngeal epithelial cells *in vitro*. *Respiration* 2000;**67**:552–8.

61 Nowak D, Antczak A, Krol M, Bialasiewicz P, Pietras T. Antioxidant properties of Ambroxol. *Free Radic Biol Med* 1994;**16**:517–22.

62 Wang Y, Griffiths WJ, Curstedt T, Johansson J. Porcine pulmonary surfactant preparations contain the antibacterial peptide prophenin and a C-terminal 18-residue fragment thereof. *FEBS Lett* 1999;**460**:257–62.

63 Thornton DJ, Davies JR, Carlstedt I, Sheehan JK. Structure and biochemistry of human respiratory mucins. In: Rogers DF, Lethem MI, eds. *Airway Mucus: Basic Mechanisms and Clinical Perspectives*. Basel: Birkhäuser Verlag, 1997: 19–39.

64 Davies JR, Carlstedt I. Respiratory tract mucins. In: Salthe M, ed. *Cilia and Mucus: from Development to Respiratory Defense*. New York: Marcel Dekker, 2001: 167–78.

65 Albers GM, Tomkiewicz RP, May MK, Ramirez OE, Rubin BK. Ring distraction technique for measuring surface tension of sputum: relationship to sputum clearability. *J Appl Physiol* 1996;**81**:2690–5.

66 Rogers DF. Mucoactive drugs for asthma and COPD: any place in therapy? *Expert Opin Investig Drugs* 2002;**11**:15–35.

67 Sheffner AL, Medler EM, Jacobs LW, Sarett HP. The *in vitro* reduction in viscosity of human tracheobronchial secretions by acetylcysteine. *Am Rev Respir Dis* 1964;**90**:721–9.

68 Rhee CS, Majima Y, Cho JS *et al.* Effects of mucokinetic drugs on rheological properties of reconstituted human nasal mucus. *Arch Otolaryngol Head Neck Surg* 1999;**125**: 101–5.

69 Rogers DF, Jeffery PK. Inhibition by oral *N*-acetylcysteine of cigarette smoke-induced 'bronchitis' in the rat. *Exp Lung Res* 1986;**10**:267–83.

70 Rogers DF, Turner NC, Marriott C, Jeffery PK. Oral *N*-acetylcysteine or *S*-carboxymethylcysteine inhibit cigarette smoke-induced hypersecretion of mucus in rat larynx and trachea *in situ. Eur Respir J* 1989;**2**:955–60.

71 Rogers DF, Godfrey RW, Majumdar S, Jeffery PK. Oral *N*-acetylcysteine speeds reversal of cigarette smoke-induced mucous cell hyperplasia in the rat. *Exp Lung Res* 1988;**14**: 19–35.

72 Borgstrom L, Kagedal B, Paulsen O. Pharmacokinetics of *N*-acetylcysteine in man. *Eur J Clin Pharmacol* 1986;**31**:217–22.

73 Bonanomi L, Gazzaniga A. Toxicological, pharmacokinetic and metabolic studies on acetylcysteine. *Eur J Respir Dis Suppl* 1980;**111**:45–51.

74 Cotgreave IA, Eklund A, Larsson K, Moldeus PW. No penetration of orally administered *N*-acetylcysteine into bronchoalveolar lavage fluid. *Eur J Respir Dis* 1987;**70**:73–7.

75 Bridgeman MM, Marsden M, Selby C, Morrison D, MacNee W. Effect of *N*-acetyl cysteine on the concentrations of thiols in plasma, bronchoalveolar lavage fluid, and lung tissue. *Thorax* 1994;**49**:670–5.

76 Dueholm M, Nielsen C, Thorshauge H *et al. N*-acetylcysteine by metered dose inhaler in the treatment of chronic bronchitis: a multi-centre study. *Respir Med* 1992;**86**:89–92.

77 Aylward M, Maddock J, Dewland P. Clinical evaluation of acetylcysteine in the treatment of patients with chronic obstructive bronchitis: a balanced double-blind trial with placebo control. *Eur J Respir Dis Suppl* 1980;**111**:81–9.

78 Multicentre Study Group. Long-term oral acetylcysteine in chronic bronchitis: a double-blind controlled study. *Eur J Respir Dis* 1980;**61**(Suppl):93–108.

79 Boman G, Backer U, Larsson S, Melander B, Wahlander L. Oral acetylcysteine reduces exacerbation rate in chronic bronchitis: report of a trial organized by the Swedish Society for Pulmonary Diseases. *Eur J Respir Dis* 1983;**64**:405–15.

80 Poole PJ, Black PN. Oral mucolytic drugs for exacerbations of chronic obstructive pulmonary disease: systematic review. *BMJ* 2001;**322**:1271–4.

81 British Thoracic Society Research Committee. Oral *N*-acetylcysteine and exacerbation rates in patients with chronic bronchitis and severe airways obstruction. *Thorax* 1985;**40**:832–5.

82 Rasmussen JB, Glennow C. Reduction in days of illness after long-term treatment with *N*-acetylcysteine controlled-release tablets in patients with chronic bronchitis. *Eur Respir J* 1988;**1**:351–5.

83 Hansen NC, Skriver A, Brorsen-Riis L *et al.* Orally administered *N*-acetylcysteine may improve general well-being in patients with mild chronic bronchitis. *Respir Med* 1994;**88**:531–5.

84 Decramer M, Rutten-van Molken M, Dekhuijzen PN *et al.* Effects of *N*-acetylcysteine on outcomes in chronic obstructive pulmonary disease (bronchitis randomized on NAC cost-utility study, BRONCUS): a randomised placebo-controlled trial. *Lancet* 2005;**365**(9470):1552–60.

85 Marriott C, Ingham S, Coffiner M, Fossion J, Maes P. Determination of the mode of action of a novel mucolytic agent, nacystelyn. *Eur Respir J* 1993;**6**(Suppl):438S.

86 Gillissen A, Jaworska M, Orth M *et al.* Nacystelyn, a novel lysine salt of *N*-acetylcysteine, to augment cellular antioxidant defence *in vitro. Respir Med* 1997;**91**:159–68.

87 Tomkiewicz RP, App EM, De Sanctis GT *et al.* A comparison of a new mucolytic *N*-acetylcysteine L-lysinate with *N*-acetylcysteine: airway epithelial function and mucus changes in dog. *Pulm Pharmacol* 1995;**8**:259–65.

88 Nagy AM, Vanderbist F, Parij N *et al.* Effect of the muco-active drug nacystelyn on the respiratory burst of human blood polymorphonuclear neutrophils. *Pulm Pharmacol Ther* 1997;**10**:287–92.

89 British Medical Association and the Royal Pharmaceutical Society of Great Britain. *British National Formulary.* London: British Medical Association and the Royal Pharmaceutical Society of Great Britain, 2001.

90 Aylward M, Bater PA, Davies DE *et al.* Clinical therapeutic evaluation of methylcysteine hydrochloride in patients with chronic obstructive bronchitis: a balanced double-blind trial with placebo control. *Curr Med Res Opin* 1978;**5**:461–71.

91 Tekeres M, Horvath A, Bardosi L, Kenyeres P. Clinical studies on the mucolytic effect of MESNA. *Clin Ther* 1981; **4**:56–60.

92 Konradova V, Vavrova V, Sulova J. Comparison of the effect of three oral mucolytics on the ultrastructure of the tracheal epithelium in rabbits. *Respiration* 1985;**48**:50–7.

93 Brown DT. Carbocysteine. *Drug Intell Clin Pharm* 1988;**22**: 603–8.

94 Martin R, Litt M, Marriott C. The effect of mucolytic agents on the rheologic and transport properties of canine tracheal mucus. *Am Rev Respir Dis* 1980;**121**:495–500.

95 Majima Y, Hirata K, Takeuchi K, Hattori M, Sakakura Y. Effects of orally administered drugs on dynamic viscoelasticity of human nasal mucus. *Am Rev Respir Dis* 1990;**141**:79–83.

96 Braga PC, Allegra L, Bossi R *et al.* Identification of subpopulations of bronchitic patients for suitable therapy by a dynamic rheological test. *Int J Clin Pharmacol Res* 1989;**9**: 175–82.

97 Havez R, Degand P, Roussel P, Randoux A. Mode d'action biochimique des derives de la cysteine sur le mucus bronchique. *Poumon Coeur* 1970;**26**:81–90.

98 Thomson ML, Pavia D, Jones CJ, McQuiston TA. No demonstrable effect of *S*-carboxymethylcysteine on clearance of secretions from the human lung. *Thorax* 1975;**30**:669–73.

99 Edwards GF, Steel AE, Scott JK, Jordan JW. *S*-carboxymethylcysteine in the fluidification of sputum and treatment of chronic airway obstruction. *Chest* 1976;**70**: 506–13.

100 Puchelle E, Aug F, Polu JM. Effect of the mucoregulator *S*-carboxy-methyl-cysteine in patients with chronic bronchitis. *Eur J Clin Pharmacol* 1978;**14**:177–84.

101 Braga PC, Scaglione F, Scarpazza G *et al*. Comparison between penetration of amoxicillin combined with carbocysteine and amoxicillin alone in pathological bronchial secretions and pulmonary tissue. *Int J Clin Pharmacol Res* 1985;**5**:331–40.

102 Braga PC, Borsa M, De Angelis L *et al*. Pharmacokinetic behavior of *S*-carboxymethylcysteine-Lys in patients with chronic bronchitis. *Clin Ther* 1982;**4**:480–8.

103 Braga PC, Bossi R, Allegra L. Evaluation of the elastic and viscous components of bronchial mucus before and after *S*-carboxymethylcysteine-Lys treatment. *Int J Clin Pharmacol Res* 1984;**4**:121–7.

104 Braga PC, Allegra L, Rampoldi C, Ornaghi A, Beghi G. Long-lasting effects on rheology and clearance of bronchial mucus after short-term administration of high doses of carbocysteine-lysine to patients with chronic bronchitis. *Respiration* 1990;**57**:353–8.

105 Allegra L, Cordaro CI, Grassi C. Prevention of acute exacerbations of chronic obstructive bronchitis with carbocysteine lysine salt monohydrate: a multicenter, double-blind, placebo-controlled trial. *Respiration* 1996;**63**:174–80.

106 Dechant KL, Noble S. Erdosteine. *Drugs* 1996;**52**:875–81.

107 Marchioni CF, Moretti M, Muratori M *et al*. Effects of erdosteine on sputum biochemical and rheologic properties: pharmacokinetics in chronic obstructive lung disease. *Lung* 1990;**168**:285–93.

108 Olivieri D, Del Donno M, Casalini A, D'Ippolito R, Fregnan GB. Activity of erdosteine on mucociliary transport in patients affected by chronic bronchitis. *Respiration* 1991;**58**:91–4.

109 Vagliasindi M, Fregnan GB. Erdosteine protection against cigarette smoking-induced functional antiprotease deficiency in human bronchiolo-alveolar structures. *Int J Clin Pharmacol Ther Toxicol* 1989;**27**:238–41.

110 Ricevuti G, Mazzone A, Uccelli E, Gazzani G, Fregnan GB. Influence of erdosteine, a mucolytic agent, on amoxycillin penetration into sputum in patients with an infective exacerbation of chronic bronchitis. *Thorax* 1988;**43**:585–90.

111 Marchioni CF, Polu JM, Taytard A *et al*. Evaluation of efficacy and safety of erdosteine in patients affected by chronic bronchitis during an infective exacerbation phase and receiving amoxycillin as basic treatment (ECOBES, European Chronic Obstructive Bronchitis Erdosteine Study). *Int J Clin Pharmacol Ther* 1995;**33**:612–8.

112 Braga PC, Bossi R, Allegra L. Rheological modifications of mucus in chronic bronchitic patients after treatment with stepronine-lysine salt. *Drugs Exp Clin Res* 1987;**13**:707–10.

113 Yamada K, Satoh M, Shimura S *et al*. An expectorant, stepronin, reduces airway secretion *in vitro*. *Respiration* 1994;**61**:42–7.

114 Davis SS, Cox A, Marriott C, Readman AS, Barrett-Bee K. A new mucotropic agent: *in vitro* and *in vivo* evaluation of 2-alpha-thenoylthiopropionylglycine (bronchoplus). *Eur J Respir Dis* 1985;**67**:94–102.

115 Romano A, Di Fonso M, Mormile F *et al*. Accelerated cell-mediated broncho-obstructive reaction to inhaled stepronin: a case report. *Allergy* 1996;**51**:269–71.

116 Martin GP, Loveday BE, Marriott C. The effect of bromhexine hydrochloride on the viscoelastic properties of mucus from the mini-pig. *Eur Respir J* 1990;**3**:392–6.

117 Yanaura S, Takeda H, Nishimura T, Misawa M. [Histological and histochemical changes of tracheal secretory cells following bromhexine treatment (author's translation)]. *Nippon Yakurigaku Zasshi* 1981;**77**:559–68.

118 Valenti S, Marenco G. Italian multicenter study on the treatment of chronic obstructive lung disease with bromhexine: a double-blind placebo-controlled trial. *Respiration* 1989; **56**:11–5.

119 Taskar VS, Sharma RR, Goswami R, John PJ, Mahashur AA. Effect of bromhexeine on sputum amoxycillin levels in lower respiratory infections. *Respir Med* 1992;**86**:157–60.

120 Bergogne-Berezin E, Berthelot G, Kafe HP, Dournovo P. Influence of a fluidifying agent (bromhexine) on the penetration of antibiotics into respiratory secretions. *Int J Clin Pharmacol Res* 1985;**5**:341–4.

121 Disse BG. The pharmacology of ambroxol: review and new results. *Eur J Respir Dis Suppl* 1987;**153**:255–62.

122 Lusuardi M, Capelli A, Salmona M *et al*. Intraluminal inflammation in the airways of patients with chronic bronchitis after treatment with Ambroxol. *Monaldi Arch Chest Dis* 1995;**50**:346–51.

123 Olivieri D, Marsico SA, Del Donno M. Improvement of mucociliary transport in smokers by mucolytics. *Eur J Respir Dis Suppl* 1985;**139**:142–5.

124 Weiss T, Dorow P, Felix R. Effects of a beta adrenergic drug and a secretolytic agent on regional mucociliary clearance in patients with COLD. *Chest* 1981;**80**(Suppl):881–5.

125 Ericsson CH, Juhasz J, Mossberg B *et al*. Influence of ambroxol on tracheobronchial clearance in simple chronic bronchitis. *Eur J Respir Dis* 1987;**70**:163–70.

126 Germouty J, Jirou-Najou JL. Clinical efficacy of ambroxol in the treatment of bronchial stasis: clinical trial in 120 patients at two different doses. *Respiration* 1987;**51**(Suppl 1):37–41.

127 Ericsson CH, Juhasz J, Jonsson E, Mossberg B. Ambroxol and simple chronic bronchitis: effects on subjective symptoms and ventilatory function. *Respiration* 1987;**51**(Suppl 1): 33–6.

128 Guyatt GH, Townsend M, Kazim F, Newhouse MT. A controlled trial of ambroxol in chronic bronchitis. *Chest* 1987;**92**:618–20.

129 Olivieri D, Zavattini G, Tomasini G *et al*. Ambroxol for the prevention of chronic bronchitis exacerbations: long-term multicenter trial. Protective effect of ambroxol against winter semester exacerbations: a double-blind study versus placebo. *Respiration* 1987;**51**(Suppl 1):42–51.

130 Anon. Prevention of chronic bronchitis exacerbations with ambroxol (mucosolvan retard): an open, long-term, multicenter study in 5635 patients. *Respiration* 1989;**55**(Suppl 1): 84–96.

131 Paganin F, Bouvet O, Chanez P *et al*. Evaluation of the effects of ambroxol on the ofloxacin concentrations in bronchial tissues in COPD patients with infectious exacerbation. *Biopharm Drug Dispos* 1995;**16**:393–401.

132 Ziment I. History of the treatment of chronic bronchitis. *Respiration* 1991;**58**(Suppl 1):37–42.

133 Pavia D, Agnew JE, Glassman JM *et al*. Effects of iodopropylidene glycerol on tracheobronchial clearance in stable, chronic bronchitic patients. *Eur J Respir Dis* 1985;**67**:177–84.

134 Petty TL. The National Mucolytic Study. Results of a randomized, double-blind, placebo-controlled study of iodinated glycerol in chronic obstructive bronchitis. *Chest* 1990;**97**:75–83.

135 Rubin BK, Ramirez O, Ohar JA. Iodinated glycerol has no effect on pulmonary function, symptom score, or sputum properties in patients with stable chronic bronchitis. *Chest* 1996;**109**:348–52.

136 Gomolin IH. More on the toxicity of iodinated glycerol. *J Am Geriatr Soc* 1989;**37**:486–7.

137 Drinka PJ, Nolten WE. Effects of iodinated glycerol on thyroid function studies in elderly nursing home residents. *J Am Geriatr Soc* 1988;**36**:911–3.

138 Gomolin IH. Iodinated glycerol-induced hypothyroidism. *Drug Intell Clin Pharm* 1987;**21**:726–7.

139 Huseby JS, Bennett SW, Hagensee ME. Hyperthyroidism induced by iodinated glycerol. *Am Rev Respir Dis* 1991;**144**: 1403.

140 Block SH. Goiter complicating therapy with iodinated glycerol (Organidin). *J Pediatr* 1973;**83**:84–6.

141 Geurian K, Branam C. Iodine poisoning secondary to long-term iodinated glycerol therapy. *Arch Intern Med* 1994;**154**: 1153–6.

142 De Rosa G, Donati C, Hodel CM. Domiodol. In: Braga PC, Allegra L, eds. *Drugs in Bronchial Mucology*. New York: Raven Press, 1989: 239–49.

143 Ferrari S, Donati C, Legnani W. Studio clinico controllato dell'attivata terapeutica del domiodolo. *Riv Patol Clin* 1981; **36**:139–54.

144 Finley TN, Ladman AJ. Low yield of pulmonary surfactant in cigarette smokers. *N Engl J Med* 1972;**286**:223–7.

145 Higenbottam T. Pulmonary surfactant and chronic lung disease. *Eur J Respir Dis Suppl* 1987;**153**:222–8.

146 Girod S, Galabert C, Lecuire A, Zahm JM, Puchelle E. Phospholipid composition and surface-active properties of tracheobronchial secretions from patients with cystic fibrosis and chronic obstructive pulmonary diseases. *Pediatr Pulmonol* 1992;**13**:22–7.

147 Rubin BK. Therapeutic aerosols and airway secretions. *J Aerosol Med* 1996;**9**:123–30.

148 Anzueto A, Jubran A, Ohar JA et al. Effects of aerosolized surfactant in patients with stable chronic bronchitis: a prospective randomized controlled trial. *JAMA* 1997;**278**: 1426–31.

149 Shak S, Capon DJ, Hellmiss R, Marsters SA, Baker CL. Recombinant human DNase I reduces the viscosity of cystic fibrosis sputum. *Proc Natl Acad Sci USA* 1990;**87**:9188–92.

150 Shak S. Aerosolized recombinant human DNase I for the treatment of cystic fibrosis. *Chest* 1995;**107**(Suppl):65S–70S.

151 Shah PL, Scott SF, Knight RA et al. In vivo effects of recombinant human DNase I on sputum in patients with cystic fibrosis. *Thorax* 1996;**51**:119–25.

152 Wills PJ, Wodehouse T, Corkery K et al. Short-term recombinant human DNase in bronchiectasis: effect on clinical state and in vitro sputum transportability. *Am J Respir Crit Care Med* 1996;**154**:413–7.

153 Puchelle E, Zahm JM, de Bentzmann S et al. Effects of rhDNase on purulent airway secretions in chronic bronchitis. *Eur Respir J* 1996;**9**:765–9.

154 Thompson AB, Fuchs H, Corkery K, Pun E, Fick RB. Phase II trial of recombinant human DNase for the therapy of chronic bronchitis. *Am Rev Respir Dis* 1993;**147**(Suppl):A318.

155 Fick RB, Anzeuto A, Mahutte KMott-CSG. Recombinant DNase mortality reduction in acute exacerbations of chronic bronchitis. *Clin Res* 1994;**42**:294A.

156 Bone RC, Fuchs H, Fox NL et al. The chronic obstructive pulmonary disease mortality endpoint trial. *Chest* 1995;**108** (Suppl):R.

157 Hudson TJ. Dornase in treatment of chronic bronchitis. *Ann Pharmacother* 1996;**30**:674–5.

158 Vasconcellos CA, Allen PG, Wohl ME et al. Reduction in viscosity of cystic fibrosis sputum in vitro by gelsolin. *Science* 1994;**263**:969–71.

159 Fuloria M, Rubin BK. Evaluating the efficacy of mucoactive aerosol therapy. *Respir Care* 2000;**45**:868–73.

160 Poole PJ, Black PN. Mucolytic agents for chronic bronchitis or chronic obstructive pulmonary disease. *Cochrane Database Syst Rev* 2000;**2**:CD001287.

161 Grandjean EM, Berthet P, Ruffmann R, Leuenberger P. Efficacy of oral long-term *N*-acetylcysteine in chronic broncho-pulmonary disease: a meta-analysis of published double-blind, placebo-controlled clinical trials. *Clin Ther* 2000;**22**:209–21.

162 Task Group on Mucoactive Drugs. Recommendations for guidelines on clinical trials of mucoactive drugs in chronic bronchitis and chronic obstructive pulmonary disease. *Chest* 1994;**106**:1532–7.

163 Del Donno M, Olivieri D. Mucoactive drugs in the management of chronic obstructive pulmonary disease. *Monaldi Arch Chest Dis* 1998;**53**:714–9.

164 Grandjean EM, Berthet PH, Ruffmann R, Leuenberger P. Cost-effectiveness analysis of oral *N*-acetylcysteine as a preventive treatment in chronic bronchitis. *Pharmacol Res* 2000;**42**:39–50.

CHAPTER 63

End-of-life and palliative care for patients with COPD

John E. Heffner and Ann L. Heffner

Patients with moderate to severe chronic obstructive pulmonary disease (COPD) experience a progressive disorder characterized by breathlessness, decreased exercise tolerance and episodes of acute exacerbations of airway obstruction. Each exacerbation presents a risk of respiratory failure that may require intubation and ventilatory support. Although most hospitalized patients with COPD managed by mechanical ventilation survive to hospital discharge, a subset of patients with far advanced disease and poor baseline quality of life have a low probability of weaning from mechanical ventilation and regaining their prehospitalization functional capacity. Such patients face either a prolonged period of ventilatory support at the end of life or considerations of withdrawal of life support after a trial of aggressive restorative care. Other patients with end-stage COPD may elect to avoid hospitalization during the final stages of their disease if the burden of life-supportive care exceeds its anticipated benefit.

Meeting the needs of patients with moderate to severe COPD at the end of life requires advance care planning and appropriate palliative services directed by skilled caregivers [1,2]. Unfortunately, most observers note extensive deficiencies in the USA with the provision of care to patients with terminal medical conditions [3]. Recently, even greater deficiencies in end-of-life and palliative care have been noted to exist for patients with COPD as compared with other terminal conditions, such as lung cancer [4,5], even though patients with chronic lung disease have similar physical and psychosocial needs [6].

Although the reasons for these deficiencies are uncertain, lack of patient desire for comprehensive end-of-life care does not appear to contribute. Patients with advanced symptomatic COPD desire information about life-supportive care and advance care planning [7] but voice disappointment with the amount of educational information typically provided by their physicians [8].

This chapter focuses on the nature of the ethical decisions faced by patients with advanced COPD and describes general approaches to advance care planning and palliative care. Expert clinicians who have pioneered the modern management of COPD have deep roots in offering a message of hope, aspirations for a high quality of life, and comprehensive supportive care to promote an active and functional lifestyle for patients [9,10]. We believe end-of-life care and advance care planning fits well into this rich medical tradition.

Outcome predictions and advance care planning

Patients hospitalized for an acute exacerbation of their airway disease represent a subgroup of patients with COPD who have a guarded prognosis. Although 89% of patients survive the initial hospitalization [3], hospital survival decreases to 76% if intubation and mechanical ventilation are required [4]. Survival measured at 1 year after hospitalization decreases to 59%, which is a marker for the underlying severity of COPD among patients who require hospitalization for exacerbations [11]. Those patients who survive hospitalization frequently experience a poor quality of life after discharge because of unremitting respiratory symptoms [11].

Clinicians faced with assisting patients with advance care planning would benefit from accurate prognostic information that could guide an individual patient toward understanding his or her likely clinical course. Such information would enable the patient and their family to weigh the relative benefits and burdens of life-supportive care as they consider their wishes regarding the desired level of medical care. Unfortunately, the ability to predict clinical outcome of hospitalized patients with COPD is marginal at best. No clinical characteristics available at the time of hospital admission identify with sufficient accuracy which patients will follow an unfavourable clinical course [12–14]. Available systems utilize a complex combination of clinical factors to estimate the probability of a specific outcome for populations of patients and lose validity when applied to individual patients with COPD. Moreover, most prediction models presented in the literature have not been validated in independent cohorts. Also, the Study to Understand Prognoses and Preferences for Outcome and Risks of Treatment (SUPPORT) demonstrated that physicians have limited ability to incorporate prognosticating information into their clinical practices [3].

The ability to predict the mortality of ambulatory patients is even more challenging. Single variables, such as forced expiratory volume in 1 s (FEV_1), have limited predictive accuracy for individual patients [15]. Multidimensional disease staging systems that consider variables such as dyspnoea, health status and exercise capacity are only now being developed [16]. Fan *et al.* [17] recently demonstrated that quality of life, as assessed by a condition-specific measure (Seattle Obstructive Lung Disease Questionnaire), was a strong predictor of hospitalization and all-cause mortality. The application of these measures to specific patients to assist advance care planning awaits further investigation.

Without accurate predictors of clinical outcomes for individual patients, caregivers must recognize the ethical dilemmas that arise in caring for patients with advanced COPD, assist patients with the uncertainties of advance care planning and understand the perspectives of patients with advanced lung disease who may face end-of-life decisions. Autonomy is the predominant ethical principle that drives end-of-life decision-making in the USA [18]. Most patients with advanced COPD wish to make their own decisions regarding life-supportive care even after they lose decision-making capacity. More than 80% of patients with advanced COPD enrolled in pulmonary rehabilitation programmes would choose to direct decisions regarding intubation and mechanical ventilation by either communicating with their physicians directly or through an appointed surrogate or instrument of advance care planning [7].

To make informed decisions, patients need knowledge of the nature of alternative therapeutic decisions (e.g. intubation, mechanical ventilation, tracheotomy) and their probable outcomes. The complexity of advanced life-supportive care requires physicians to discuss these interventions with patients in advance of their need. Unfortunately, only 19% of patients with advanced lung disease enrolled in pulmonary rehabilitation programmes have discussed with their physicians the appropriateness of life-supportive care relative to their lung condition and 15% have discussed the nature of intubation and mechanical ventilation [7]. Consequently, less than 15% of patients with advanced lung disease have confidence that their physicians understand their end-of-life wishes, even though most of these patients have strong opinions regarding end-of-life care [7]. A clear understanding of the potential value of life-supportive care is important because patients with terminal conditions, such as lung cancer, usually retain a more optimistic and less accurate estimate of their survival compared to their physicians [19]. Patients with severe lung disease alter their willingness to accept life-supportive care once informed of a low likelihood of survival or recovery to an acceptable functional status [7,20].

Multiple studies confirm that patients with a broad category of conditions and their physicians agree that physicians should initiate discussions about end-of-life care [7,21,22]. Many barriers exist, however, to the completion of these discussions. Most studies that examine these barriers demonstrate that physicians identify more barriers than patients [23]. The majority of these barriers pertain to concern that patients will not be receptive to these discussions or that the patient's condition has not yet advanced enough to warrant these discussions [23–25].

Multiple interventions to promote more patient–physician discussions related to advance care planning have been examined. Unfortunately, policy interventions, case manager facilitators in inpatient settings, computer prompts to electronic medical records and physician education have provided only marginal effects [3,26–28]. Greater research is needed to understand the barriers that limit the occurrence of these discussions [24]. The variability of the barriers to these communications suggests that multiple interventions, both educational and health system related, are required [23,29].

In face of these barriers, physicians should develop their own strategies for inviting their patients with COPD to discuss advance care planning. An increasing body of knowledge has developed to assist physicians in initiating end-of-life discussions with their patients [30–34]. These strategies recommend that physicians introduce these discussions in a manner that does not trigger understandable patient reactions that their physicians have new concerns about their imminent death, a sense of hopelessness or futility, a negative view of their disease status, or an interest in abandoning restorative care. Introducing these discussions during intervals of stable or good health defuse some of these concerns. Also, specific measures have been recommended to assist patients' acceptance of these discussions. These measures include neutral topic introductions, certain prompting cues and phrasing, focused listening, efforts to gain patient goals and values, clarifying strategies, avoiding too much discussion about specific treatment details, and a series of open-ended questions (Table 63.1) [30–39].

Although most patients with advanced lung disease desire advance care planning discussions with their physicians, a small minority (less than 5%) do not because of concerns that these discussions may provoke anxiety [7].

Table 63.1 Open-ended questions to promote end-of-life discussions with patients. (Adapted from Lo *et al.* [35].)

General

What are your greatest concerns about your illness?

What are your and your family's thoughts about your care?

What are your greatest hopes and fears related to your illness?

Tell me about the most difficult part of this illness?

What would you hope for the future?

When you think about your future, what is most important to you?

Questions to determine patient interest in spiritual and existential matters

In thinking about this illness, is faith (religion, spirituality) important to you?

In earlier times before your illness, has faith (religion, spirituality) been important to you?

Are you able to talk with someone about religious matters?

Would you wish to talk about religious matters with someone?

Questions for patients who wish to pursue spiritual and existential matters

What would you like to accomplish during the rest of your life?

Do you have thoughts as to why you became ill?

If you were to die today, what would be left undone?

What do you think happens after you die?

What legacy do you want to leave your family were you to die today?

After your death, what do you want your family to remember about you?

Most patients with chronic health conditions, however, do not find these discussions anxiety provoking, and some studies note more end-of-life information from physicians decrease depression scores [7,30,40–43]. Patients who initially refuse these discussions may become more receptive after they receive general information regarding the nature of their disease and the progressive course of COPD [44]. Patients may benefit from reading materials on advance care planning in preparation for physician discussions.

Even when patient–physician discussions about end-of-life care occur, they frequently do not achieve the patient's goals. Patients with COPD and other terminal conditions prefer to receive straightforward, honest and relevant information about their specific prognosis and circumstances [8,45,46]. Unfortunately, physicians often deliberately soften their discussion of prognosis when they sense patients harbour more optimistic prognostic outlooks in an effort to avoid extinguishing hope [47]. Also, physicians spend 75% of such conversations talking and allow little time for patients to state their wishes for therapy and personal values

[48–50]. Few data exist regarding interventions to enhance these discussions. Randomized trials demonstrate that an intensive communication skills workshop over several days can improve physician communication skills [37].

Timing and setting for advance care planning

Most patients with advanced lung disease prefer discussions about advance care planning to occur in outpatient settings during periods of stable health [7]. Physicians usually defer these discussions until patients have far advanced disease. McNeely *et al.* [25] observed that pulmonary physicians delayed discussions with their patients about end-of-life care until their patients experienced recent hospitalizations and marked decreases in FEV_1. Sullivan *et al.* [24] noted that physicians used clinical metrics, such as poor nutritional status or low FEV_1, to trigger end-of-life discussions. In contrast, patients with COPD demonstrate an interest in receiving this information regardless of the severity of their disease. Heffner *et al.* [7] demonstrated that no measure of lung disease severity was associated with desire among pulmonary rehabilitation patients to discuss end-of-life issues with their physicians. Pfeifer *et al.* [51] reported that the desire for an end-of-life discussion with their physicians expressed by 100 patients with COPD presenting for pulmonary function testing was not associated with FEV_1, oral corticosteroid use, functional status score, hospitalizations in the past year or previous mechanical ventilation.

Ideally, these discussions should occur with the first diagnosis of COPD as soon as a primary care provider establishes a therapeutic relationship. Generally, the caregiver most closely involved with the patient's care should initiate these discussions, which has been termed 'captaincy' [52]. In the absence of physician initiative, however, other caregivers can promote the completion of these discussions by educating patients to expect that these discussions should occur.

One study heightened these patient expectations through an educational programme on advance care planning in a pulmonary rehabilitation programme [7]. Patients enrolled in pulmonary rehabilitation consider their non-physician rehabilitation programme educators as acceptable sources of information on life-supportive care [7]. A before–after study demonstrated that end-of-life education in pulmonary rehabilitation increases the adoption rate for instruments of advance care planning and completion of patient–physician discussions about end-of-life care [20]. Although 70% of pulmonary rehabilitation programme directors consider end-of-life education as an appropriate component of their curriculum, fewer than 10% of programmes in the USA provide their enrolled patients these educational opportunities [53].

Nature of advance care planning

Advance care planning has traditionally focused on methods to address plans for the use of life-sustaining treatments. Methods have included written advance directives, surrogate decisions by families, friends or physicians, and discussions between patients and their physicians.

Advance care planning with the completion of formal written instruments, such as living wills and durable powers of attorney for health care, were met with optimism when introduced into health care that would allow the patient to direct their own end-of-life care or identify a proxy who could convey the patient's wishes after the patient lost decision-making capacity. These documents, however, face major barriers in implementation and have not achieved their goals of promoting patient autonomy [54,55]. Only 10–20% of patients complete advance directives and these instruments, when present, have limited impact on future care [56–60]. Also, the decisions of surrogates correspond poorly with the wishes and desires of the patient for whom decisions are being made [56]. Uncertainty in the minds of surrogates regarding the appropriateness of their decisions often lead them to favour more intense life-supportive interventions that warranted by the patient's previously expressed wishes or the likelihood of a favourable clinical outcome [56,59,61–63].

The utility of advance directives may be improved if they are tailored to a specific patient's underlying condition and clinical events that they will most likely experience [64,65]. However, because most patients request that physicians and surrogates overrule their wishes contained within advance directives if unique clinical circumstances occur [66,67], written advance directives should be considered for most patients as general statements regarding treatment preferences rather than specific directives that cannot be altered. This indicates that both medical and ethical decision making at the end of life is a shared process and the principle of beneficence on the part of both the physician and the family may at times equal or override patient autonomy [68,69].

Limitations of written advance directives and surrogate decision making prompt medical professionals to adopt a broader approach to advance care planning that incorporates the patient's perspective [70]. Most physicians consider advance directives to be operational tools to determine which life-sustaining interventions should be applied in various clinical circumstances. In contrast, patients have more comprehensive goals that centre on preparing for death, achieving a sense of control over their lives, and fortifying personal relationships with friends and families. Patient goals, therefore, are less operational and more orientated toward their psychological, emotional and spiritual needs.

Consequently, the emphasis of discussions on end-of-life care may shift from patient–physician discussions on the use of life-supportive interventions to patient–family–friend communication. This communication has a purpose of strengthening relationships and sharing decisions regarding life-supportive care through mutual support. Physicians, with their patient's permission, can promote this dialogue by involving families in advance care planning and encouraging discussions within families regarding the end-of-life decisions that patients may eventually face [18]. Caregivers can enrich these discussions by providing the patient with educational materials and resources that enhance informed decisions. In this model, emphasis shifts from the completion of written advance directives to an ongoing dialogue between patients, caregivers and families regarding the prognosis of the patient's condition, likely outcomes of various treatment interventions, and the values and goals that the patient would wish to have fulfilled [70].

Physicians frequently overlook the spiritual context of these discussions. Most patients with pulmonary or other medical conditions wish to discuss spiritual and religious topics with their physicians [19,46,71]. Physicians, however, either omit or perform poorly in conversations about the spiritual needs of their patients, despite guidance in the literature for approaching these discussions [35,72]. Physicians in this setting are challenged to balance the need to maintain their professional boundaries yet recognize their patient's spiritual concerns in the clinical environment [73].

Withdrawal of life-supportive care

Comprehensive advance care planning for patients with COPD assists in the identification of patients with far advanced symptomatic disease who wish to withhold ventilatory support at the end of life. Other patients with end-stage disease who fail a trial of aggressive restorative care benefit from a humane withdrawal of life support after it is initiated. Extensive legal, ethical and moral justification exists for the withdrawal of life-supportive care at the end of life when it is no longer desired or no longer provides comfort to the patient [74]. Less consensus exists regarding the specific practical steps for withdrawing life-supportive care. Observational studies demonstrate extensive practice variation both within and between institutions in the timing and methods of life-support withdrawal [75–78].

For patients with COPD receiving ventilatory support, practical steps begin with a validation of the decision to withdraw life support with the patient (when possible), family and all team members who participate in patient care. This process 'shares the burden of decision making'

[79]. Informed consent is then obtained. Although the sequencing and manner for withdrawal of life support is complex and varies on the basis of patient, family and institutional needs, an explicit and organized approach improves patient care [80]. Preprinted order sheets and established policies and procedures enhance amelioration of patient and family discomfort and promote the acceptance of the process by bedside caregivers [81].

Essential elements of an organized approach include adequate treatment of the patient's pain, anxiety and suffering that is present or anticipated to occur after withdrawal of ventilatory support. Patient surrogates and family members of patients dying in the intensive care unit (ICU) rank pain control, availability of family at the bedside, and efforts to address dyspnoea as the most important factors that promote a peaceful and satisfying death experience [82]. Aggressive symptom control with opioids and sedatives, even if such treatment accelerates death, has received endorsement under the 'principle of double effect', which allows such treatment if the *intent* is not to hasten death [83]. In actual practice, the amount of morphine used during withdrawal of life support does not correlate with the duration of survival, which is a function of ventilatory status at the time support is withdrawn [81]. Careful planning is required to manage the patient who has received neuromuscular paralytic agents before the decision to withdraw support [84]. Several reviews provide extensive discussions of the practical aspects of the withdrawal of life-supportive care [79,80,84].

Palliative care

Hospitalized patients with acute exacerbations of COPD who choose to have life-supportive care withheld or withdrawn require expert care to relieve their pain and suffering and manage their end-of-life care [85]. Special considerations are required for terminal patients with COPD who choose to avoid hospitalization and die at home. Both groups of patients may experience distressing physiological symptoms of pain, cough, dyspnoea, anxiety, agitation, confusion, fatigue and depression [86,87]. Patients may also experience discomfort related to their sense of completion with their life affairs, meaning to their life, and relationships with their family and friends. Unresolved issues in these areas can cause 'existential suffering' at the end of life, which often surpasses physiological symptoms as a source of distress for dying patients [88,89]. Caregivers versed in palliative care can address these symptoms and experiences to improve the quality of life in the last days of patients' lives.

The goals of palliative care encompass the comprehensive management of physical, psychological, social and spiritual needs of patients [90]. It attempts to improve the life of not only ill patients, but also for family members through the interaction of an interdisciplinary team of physicians, nurses, social workers, home health agencies, pharmacists, chaplains, and physical and occupational therapists. Although death is nearly always hard, palliative care services work to ensure that death is not horrible. Palliative principles of managing symptoms at the end of life derive from hospice care and focus on both pharmacological and non-pharmacological interventions (Tables 63.2 and 63.3) [83,87,91–94].

Patients hospitalized with endstage COPD in an acute care setting benefit from the coordinated services provided by a hospital-based multidisciplinary palliative care team [95]. These teams provide the necessary skills to control physical and psychological symptoms and assist patients to die with as much comfort as possible. In the absence of a coordinated team approach to palliative care in the inpatient setting, families of dying patients report that as many as 50% of patients experience moderate to severe pain during the last days of their lives [96].

Palliative care for the hospitalized patient with COPD begins with goal setting. Efforts to set goals for individual patients should be proactive and deliberate, with attention to the needs of the individual patient. Initial questions that assist goal setting include: 'What is best for this patient and the patient's family?', 'What can we achieve?' and 'How can we go about achieving it?' [97]. The role of the critical care or ward nurse in identifying when treatment goals require revision to emphasize palliative over restorative care is critical because of the extensive opportunities nurses have to interact with patients and families. The palliative care team considers the family in setting goals to support family members in their roles as surrogate decision-makers and to address their needs for care themselves. Addressing family needs requires a shift toward 'family-focused care', which requires hospital administrative and services changes akin to the dramatic shift in inpatient obstetric services that included the family in labour and delivery [98]. Shannon [98] reviews the elements of 'family-focused care' and practical measures to address family needs during the death of a hospitalized patient.

After goal setting, symptom assessment assists the selection of palliative care interventions and the monitoring of their effect [95]. Objective assessment tools for pain allow implementation of treatment algorithms that provide rapid dosage escalations or drug changes to control symptoms quickly [99–102]. Assessment techniques for the hospitalized patient with pain utilize verbal and non-verbal methods that incorporate physiological measures of pain [96,103,104]. Puntillo [97] has reviewed available assessment tools for the inpatient setting.

In managing dyspnoea at the end of life, objective

Table 63.2 Pharmacological interventions to improve symptoms for patients with COPD at the end of life.

Indication	Drug	Commonly used doses
Dyspnoea	Morphine	
	Oral	5–10 mg every 4 h
	Rectal	5–10 mg every 4 h
	IV, SC	Titrate to relieve dyspnoea
	Nebulized	5 mg in 2 mL normal saline every 4 h with hand-held nebulizer. Benefit from this route of administration remains controversial
	Benzodiazepines	
	Lorazepam oral, sublingual, IV	1–2 mg every 1–4 h
	Diazepam oral, IV (IV risks phlebitis)	2.5–25 mg/day
	Midazolam SC, IV, sublingual	5–10 mg SC then 10–30 mg continuous subcutaneous infusion/24 h
Cough	Opioids	
	Codeine linctus oral	30–60 mg every 4 h
	Morphine linctus oral	2.5–5 mg every 4 h
	Methadone linctus oral	2 mg every 4 h
	Inhaled anaesthetics	
	Bupivacaine 0.25%	5 mg every 4–6 h
Retained secretions	Anticholinergic agents	
	Scopolamine hydrobromide SC	0.4–0.6 mg every 4–6 h then 1.2–1.6 mg/24 h continuous SC infusion
	Transdermal patch	Every 72 h
	Hyoscyamine SC	0.25–0.5 mg every 4–6 h
	Mucokinetic agents	
	Carbocysteine oral	750 mg t.i.d.

IV, intravenous; SC, subcutaneous; t.i.d., three times daily.

Table 63.3 Non-pharmacological interventions to relieve intractable dyspnoea at the end of life.

Non-invasive positive pressure ventilation – Face mask ventilation has been used for patients who refuse intubation and mechanical ventilation to relieve intractable suffering and maintain cognition at the end of life [117]
Patient positioning
Relaxation techniques
Guided imagery
Fans with directed cool air
Pursed-lip breathing
Diaphragmatic training
Energy conservation techniques

measures of dyspnoea can guide therapy but are rarely used [94], in contrast to the frequent use of pain scales for guiding analgesia therapy. Absence of objective measures promote under-recognition of the need to treat severe dyspnoea, which is experienced by 56% of COPD patients during their terminal hospitalization [4]. Uncontrolled dyspnoea produces anxiety, fear and dread, and warrants aggressive management. Unfortunately, specific interventions to relieve dyspnoea do not exist, which requires physicians to use opioids and sedatives that partially relieve dyspnoea and also manage the associated distress of anxiety, discomfort and fear (see Tables 63.2 and 63.3). Recent systematic reviews of sedative therapy for symptom relief in the terminally ill recognize that sedatives 'relieve intolerable and refractory distress by the reduction in patient consciousness' [105]. Although depression of consciousness is not the primary goal of palliative sedation therapy for dyspnoeic patients, it becomes a necessary by-product of palliative care.

Use of sedatives for the non-intubated patient with disabling dyspnoea at the end of life commonly engenders physicians' concern that they will be participating in a form of euthanasia or will become subject to legal action [106]. Forty percent of surveyed neurologists in one study, for instance, believed that administering intravenous morphine to severely dyspnoeic patients with amyotrophic lateral sclerosis would be considered euthanasia [107]. Caregivers can gain confidence in aggressively using sedatives to relieve severe dyspnoea if they direct therapy with pre-established treatment algorithms and guidelines to direct therapy. These guidelines explicitly express the purpose of sedative and opioid therapy, which is to relieve symptoms and distress rather than to accelerate death. Clear indications for advancing therapy document the purpose of dosing schedules and prevent misinterpretations of intent. Family requests to advance therapy to bring death and end patient suffering more quickly signal the need for family support rather than an acceleration of therapy.

Recent data further support the conclusion that symptom relief for dying patients represents aggressive palliative care rather than euthanasia. Sykes *et al.* [108] reported that adequate sedative therapy to relieve symptoms rarely accelerates death or invokes the principle of double effect. Similarly, Wilson *et al.* [101] demonstrated that patients who receive morphine after withdrawal of ventilatory support have a longer survival time than patients who do not, which suggests a protective effect from physiological stress-related consequences of severe dyspnoea. Daly *et al.* [81] did not observe a correlation between sedative and opioid use after withdrawal of mechanical ventilation and survival time. Ongoing dialogues regarding end-of-life care within hospitals and other clinical units draw on available resources that separate myths from realities of sedative palliative care to promote quality patient care [109,110].

Hospice services provide opportunities for respite care, assisted living and end-of-life care [11,112], which unfortunately is frequently neglected for terminal patients with COPD [113,114]. Spouses of patients with advanced COPD often endure negative impacts on the quality of their own lives [115]. Neglect in offering patients and their families appropriate resources for supportive end-of-life care results in unnecessary admissions to acute care hospitals for worsening respiratory symptoms. Many episodes of worsening dyspnoea in patients coming to the end of life can be avoided in a reliable care system with effective treatment of dyspnoea (with assurance of terminal sedation if warranted) and with comprehensive advance care planning. Most patients eventually choose not to use ventilator support, or to use it only for a time-limited span, if they can be sure of competent relief of terrifying dyspnoea [116].

Conclusions

Patients with moderate to severe COPD as defined by FEV_1 face a high likelihood that their disease adversely affects the quality of their lives. The progressive course of COPD punctuated by episodes of acute respiratory failure necessitates decisions about the relative benefit and burdens of life-supportive care. In facing these decisions, patients and families benefit from advance care planning initiated by physicians during intervals of stable health. Physicians should not reserve these discussions for patients with endstage disease considering that severity of COPD is not associated with patient interest in and receptiveness for these discussions. Once the burden outstrips the benefits of aggressive life restorative care, pulmonary and critical care physicians must skillfully engage the patient in discussions that promote 'shared decision making' about end-of-life care. These decisions allow the introduction of palliative services to control symptoms and the initiation of an appropriate treatment plan that meets the patient's life values and goals during the terminal stages of COPD. Caregivers' skilled understanding of ethical issues related to end-of-life and palliative care prevent the dying patient with COPD and his or her family from experiencing death as a horrible event.

References

1 Field MJ, Cassel CK. *Approaching Death: Improving Care at the End of Life*. Washington DC: National Academy Press, 1997.

2 Council on Scientific Affairs, American Medical Association. Good care of the dying patient. *JAMA* 1996;**275**:474–8.

3 The SUPPORT Principal Investigators. A controlled trial to improve care for seriously ill hospitalized patients: the study to understand prognoses and preferences for outcomes and risks of treatments (SUPPORT). *JAMA* 1995;**274**:1591–8.

4 Claessens MT, Lynn J, Zhong Z *et al.* Dying with lung cancer or chronic obstructive pulmonary disease: insights from SUPPORT: Study to Understand Prognoses and Preferences for Outcomes and Risks of Treatments. *J Am Geriatr Soc* 2000;**48**(Suppl):S146–53.

5 Gore JM, Brophy CJ, Greenstone MA. How well do we care for patients with end stage chronic obstructive pulmonary disease (COPD)? A comparison of palliative care and quality of life in COPD and lung cancer. *Thorax* 2000;**55**:1000–6.

6 Edmonds P, Karlsen S, Khan S, Addington-Hall J. A comparison of the palliative care needs of patients dying from chronic respiratory diseases and lung cancer. *Palliat Med* 2001;**15**:287–95.

7 Heffner JE, Fahy B, Hilling L, Barbieri C. Attitudes regarding advance directives among patients in pulmonary rehabilitation. *Am J Respir Crit Care Med* 1996;**154**:1735–40.

8 Curtis JR, Wenrich MD, Carline JD *et al.* Patients' perspectives on physician skill in end-of-life care: differences between patients with COPD, cancer, and AIDS. *Chest* 2002;**122**:356–62.

9 Hodgkin JE, Balchum OJ, Kass I *et al.* Chronic obstructive airway diseases: current concepts in diagnosis and comprehensive care. *JAMA* 1975;**232**:1243–60.

10 Petty TL. Supportive therapy in COPD. *Chest* 1998;**113** (Suppl):256S–62S.

11 Lynn J, Ely EW, Zhong Z *et al*. Living and dying with chronic obstructive pulmonary disease. *J Am Geriatr Soc* 2000;**48** (Suppl):S91–100.

12 Almagro P, Calbo E, Ochoa de Echaguen A *et al*. Mortality after hospitalization for COPD. *Chest* 2002;**121**:1441–8.

13 Nevins ML, Epstein SK. Predictors of outcome for patients with COPD requiring invasive mechanical ventilation. *Chest* 2001;**119**:1840–9.

14 Fox E, Landrum-McNiff K, Zhong Z *et al*. Evaluation of prognostic criteria for determining hospice eligibility in patients with advanced lung, heart, or liver disease. SUPPORT Investigators: Study to Understand Prognoses and Preferences for Outcomes and Risks of Treatments [see comments]. *JAMA* 1999;**282**:1638–45.

15 Nishimura K, Izumi T, Tsukino M, Oga T. Dyspnea is a better predictor of 5-year survival than airway obstruction in patients with COPD. *Chest* 2002;**121**:1434–40.

16 Oga T, Nishimura K, Tsukino M, Sato S, Hajiro T. Analysis of the factors related to mortality in chronic obstructive pulmonary disease: role of exercise capacity and health status. *Am J Respir Crit Care Med* 2003;**167**:544–9.

17 Fan VS, Curtis JR, Tu SP, McDonell MB, Fihn SD. Using quality of life to predict hospitalization and mortality in patients with obstructive lung diseases. *Chest* 2002;**122**: 429–36.

18 Jennings B, Callahan D, Caplan AL. Ethical challenges of chronic illness. *Hastings Cent Rep* 1988;**18**(Suppl):1–16.

19 Weeks JC, Cook EF, O'Day SJ *et al*. Relationship between cancer patients' predictions of prognosis and their treatment preferences. *JAMA* 1998;**279**:1709–14.

20 Heffner JE, Fahy B, Hilling L, Barbieri C. Outcomes of advance directive education of pulmonary rehabilitation patients. *Am J Respir Crit Care Med* 1997;**155**:1055–9.

21 Layson RT, Adelman HM, Wallach PM *et al*. Discussions about the use of life-sustaining treatments: a literature review of physicians' and patients' attitudes and practices. End of Life Study Group. *J Clin Ethics* 1994;**5**:195–203.

22 Johnston SC, Pfeifer MP, McNutt R. The discussion about advance directives: patient and physician opinions regarding when and how it should be conducted. *Arch Intern Med* 1995;**155**:1025–30.

23 Curtis JR, Patrick DL, Caldwell ES, Collier AC. Why don't patients and physicians talk about end-of-life care? Barriers to communication for patients with acquired immunodeficiency syndrome and their primary care clinicians [see comments]. *Arch Intern Med* 2000;**160**:1690–6.

24 Sullivan KE, Hébert PC, Logan J, O'Connor AM, McNeely PD. What do physicians tell patients with end-stage COPD about intubation and mechanical ventilation? *Chest* 1996; **109**:258–64.

25 McNeely PD, Hebert PC, Dales RE *et al*. Deciding about mechanical ventilation in end-stage chronic obstructive pulmonary disease: how respirologists perceive their role. *CMAJ* 1997;**156**:177–83.

26 Reilly BM, Wagner M, Magnussen R *et al*. Promoting inpatient directives about life-sustaining treatments in a community hospital: results of a 3-year time-series intervention trial. *Arch Intern Med* 1995;**155**:2317–23.

27 Landry FJ, Kroenke K, Lucas C, Reeder J. Increasing the use of advance directives in medical outpatients. *J Gen Intern Med* 1997;**12**:412–5.

28 Sulmasy DP, Marx ES. A computerized system for entering orders to limit treatment: implementation and evaluation. *J Clin Ethics* 1997;**8**:258–63.

29 Curtis JR, Patrick DL, Shannon SE *et al*. The family conference as a focus to improve communication about end-of-life care in the intensive care unit: opportunities for improvement. *Crit Care Med* 2001;**29**(Suppl):N26–33.

30 Pfeifer MP, Sidorov JE, Smith AC *et al*. Discussion of end of life medical care by primary care physicians and patients: a multicenter study using qualitative interviews. *J Gen Intern Med* 1994;**9**:82–8.

31 Balaban RB. A physician's guide to talking about end-of-life care. *J Gen Intern Med* 2000;**15**:195–200.

32 Carrese J. Out of darkness: shedding light on end-of-life care. *J Gen Intern Med* 2001;**16**:68–9.

33 Roter DL, Larson S, Fischer GS, Arnold RM, Tulsky JA. Experts practice what they preach: a descriptive study of best and normative practices in end-of-life discussions. *Arch Intern Med* 2000;**160**:3477–85.

34 Quill TE. Perspectives on care at the close of life. Initiating end-of-life discussions with seriously ill patients: addressing the 'elephant in the room'. *JAMA* 2000;**284**:2502–7.

35 Lo B, Quill T, Tulsky J. Discussing palliative care with patients. ACP-ASIM End-of-Life Care Consensus Panel. American College of Physicians/American Society of Internal Medicine. *Ann Intern Med* 1999;**130**:744–9.

36 Buckman R. Breaking bad news: why is it still so difficult? *BMJ* 1984;**288**:1597–9.

37 Fallowfield L, Jenkins V, Farewell V *et al*. Efficacy of a Cancer Research UK communication skills training model for oncologists: a randomised controlled trial. *Lancet* 2002;**359**: 650–6.

38 Ptacek JT, Eberhardt TL. Breaking bad news: a review of the literature. *JAMA* 1996;**276**:496–502.

39 Quill TE, Townsend P. Bad news: delivery, dialogue, and dilemmas. *Arch Intern Med* 1991;**151**:463–8.

40 Reilly BM, Magnussen CR, Ross J *et al*. Can we talk? Inpatient discussions about advance directives in a community hospital. *Arch Intern Med* 1994;**154**:2299–308.

41 Bedell SE, Delbanco TL. Choices about cardiopulmonary resuscitation in the hospital: when do physicians talk with patients? *N Engl J Med* 1984;**310**:1089–93.

42 Stolman CJ, Gregory JJ, Dunn D, Ripley B. Evaluation of the do not resuscitate orders at a community hospital. *Arch Intern Med* 1989;**149**:1851–6.

43 Kellogg FR, Crain M, Corwin J, Brickner PW. Life-sustaining interventions in frail elderly persons: talking about choices. *Arch Intern Med* 1992;**152**:2317–20.

44 Steinbrook R, Lo B, Moulton J *et al*. Preferences of homosexual men with AIDS for life-sustaining treatment. *N Engl J Med* 1986;**314**:457–60.

45 Wenrich MD, Curtis JR, Shannon SE *et al*. Communicating with dying patients within the spectrum of medical care from terminal diagnosis to death. *Arch Intern Med* 2001;**161**: 868–74.

46 Jenkins V, Fallowfield L, Saul J. Information needs of patients with cancer: results from a large study in UK cancer centres. *Br J Cancer* 2001;**84**:48–51.

47 The AM, Hak T, Koeter G, van Der Wal G. Collusion in doctor–patient communication about imminent death: an ethnographic study. *BMJ* 2000;**321**:1376–81.

48 Tulsky JA, Chesney MA, Lo B. How do medical residents discuss resuscitation with patients? *J Gen Intern Med* 1995;**10**:436–42.

49 Tulsky JA, Fischer GS, Rose MR, Arnold RM. Opening the black box: how do physicians communicate about advance directives? *Ann Intern Med* 1998;**129**:441–9.

50 Fischer GS, Tulsky JA, Rose MR, Siminoff LA, Arnold RM. Patient knowledge and physician predictions of treatment preferences after discussion of advance directives. *J Gen Intern Med* 1998;**13**:447–54.

51 Pfeifer MP, Mitchell CK, Chamberlain L. The value of disease severity in predicting patient readiness to address end-of-life issues. *Arch Intern Med* 2003;**163**:609–12.

52 Pellegrino ED. Emerging ethical issues in palliative care. *JAMA* 1988;**279**:1521–2.

53 Heffner JE, Fahy B, Barbieri C. Advance directive education during pulmonary rehabilitation. *Chest* 1996;**109**:373–9.

54 Miles SH, Koepp R, Weber EP. Advance end-of-life treatment planning: a research review. *Arch Intern Med* 1996;**156**:1062–8.

55 Tonelli MR. Pulling the plug on living wills: a critical analysis of advance directives. *Chest* 1996;**110**:816–22.

56 Ditto PH, Danks JH, Smucker WD *et al.* Advance directives as acts of communication: a randomized controlled trial. *Arch Intern Med* 2001;**161**:421–30.

57 Teno J, Lynn J, Phillips RS *et al.* Do formal advance directives affect resuscitation decisions and the use of resources for seriously ill patients? *J Clin Ethics* 1994;**51**:23–30.

58 Teno J, Lynn J, Wenger N *et al.* Advance directives for seriously ill hospitalized patients: effectiveness with the Patient Self-Determination Act and the SUPPORT intervention. *J Am Geriatr Soc* 1997;**45**:500–7.

59 Covinsky KE, Fuller JD, Yaffe K *et al.* Communication and decision-making in seriously ill patients: findings of the SUPPORT project. The Study to Understand Prognoses and Preferences for Outcomes and Risks of Treatments. *J Am Geriatr Soc* 2000;**48**(Suppl):S187–93.

60 Teno JM, Stevens M, Spernak S, Lynn J. Role of written advance directives in decision making: insights from qualitative and quantitative data. *J Gen Intern Med* 1998;**13**:439–46.

61 Emanuel EJ, Emanueal LL. Proxy decision-making for incompetent patients: an ethical and empirical analysis. *JAMA* 1992;**267**:2067–71.

62 Suhl J, Simons P, Reedy T, Garrick T. Myth of substituted judgement: surrogate decision making regarding life support is unreliable. *Arch Intern Med* 1994;**154**:90–6.

63 Hare J, Pratt C, Nelson C. Agreement between patients and their self-selected surrogates on difficult medical decisions. *Arch Intern Med* 1992;**152**:1049–54.

64 Heffner JE. End-of-life ethical decisions. *Semin Respir Crit Care Med* 1998;**19**:271–82.

65 Lanken PN, Ahlheit BD, Crawford S *et al.* Withholding and withdrawing life-sustaining therapy. *Am Rev Respir Dis* 1991;**144**:726–31.

66 Mazur DJ, Hickman DH. Patients' preferences for risk disclosure and role in decision making for invasive medical procedures. *J Gen Intern Med* 1997;**12**:114–7.

67 Seghal A, Galbraith A, Chesney M *et al.* How strictly do dialysis patients want their advance directives followed? *JAMA* 1992;**267**:59–63.

68 Cassell EJ. The principles of the Belmont report revisited: how have respect for persons, beneficence, and justice been applied to clinical medicine? *Hastings Cent Rep* 2000;**30**:12–21.

69 Teno JM, Nelson HL, Lynn J. Advance care planning: priorities for ethical and empirical research. *Hastings Cent Rep* 1994;**24**:S32–6.

70 Martin DK, Thiel EC, Singer PA. A new model of advance care planning. *Arch Intern Med* 1999;**159**:86–92.

71 Ehman JW, Ott BB, Short TH, Ciampa RC, Hansen-Flaschen J. Do patients want physicians to inquire about their spiritual or religious beliefs if they become gravely ill? *Arch Intern Med* 1999;**159**:1803–6.

72 Lo B, Ruston D, Kates LW *et al.* Discussing religious and spiritual issues at the end of life: a practical guide for physicians. *JAMA* 2002;**287**:749–54.

73 Post SG, Puchalski CM, Larson DB. Physicians and patient spirituality: professional boundaries, competency, and ethics. *Ann Intern Med* 2000;**132**:578–83.

74 Luce JM. Withholding and withdrawal of life support: ethical, legal, and clinical aspects. *New Horiz* 1997;**5**:30–7.

75 Kollef MH. Private attending physician status and the withdrawal of life-sustaining interventions in a medical intensive care unit population. *Crit Care Med* 1996;**24**:968–75.

76 Faber-Langendoen K, Bartels DM. Process of forgoing life-sustaining treatment in a university hospital: an empirical study. *Crit Care Med* 1992;**20**:570–7.

77 Asch DA, Faber-Langendoen K, Shea JA, Christakis NA. The sequence of withdrawing life-sustaining treatment from patients. *Am J Med* 1999;**107**:153–6.

78 Keenan SP, Busche KD, Chen LM *et al.* A retrospective review of a large cohort of patients undergoing the process of withholding or withdrawal of life support. *Crit Care Med* 1997;**25**:1324–31.

79 Prendergast TJ, Puntillo KA. Withdrawal of life support: intensive caring at the end of life. *JAMA* 2002;**288**:2732–40.

80 Rubenfeld GD, Crawford SW. Principles and practice of withdrawing life-sustaining treatment in the ICU. In: Curtis JR, Rubenfeld GD, eds. *Managing Death in the Intensive Care Unit: The Transition from Cure to Comfort*. Oxford: Oxford University Press, 2001: 127–47.

81 Daly BJ, Thomas D, Dyer MA. Procedures used in withdrawal of mechanical ventilation. *Am J Crit Care* 1996;**5**:331–8.

82 Loss CR, Ely EW, Bowman C *et al.* Quality of death in the ICU: comparing the perceptions of family with multiple professional care providers. *Am J Respir Crit Care Med* 2001;**163**:A896.

83 Sulmasy DP, Pellegrino ED. The rule of double effect: clearing up the double talk. *Arch Intern Med* 1999;**159**:545–50.

84 Truog RD, Burns JP, Mitchell C, Johnson J, Robinson W. Pharmacologic paralysis and withdrawal of mechanical ventilation at the end of life. *N Engl J Med* 2000;**342**:508–11.

85 Youngner SJ, Lewandowsky W, McClish DK *et al*. 'Do not resuscitate' orders: incidence and implications in a medical intensive care unit. *JAMA* 1985;**253**:54–7.

86 Lynn J, Teno JM, Phillips RS *et al*. Perceptions by family members of the dying experience of older and serioulsy ill patients. *Ann Intern Med* 1997;**126**:97–106.

87 Rousseau P. Non-pain symptom management in terminal care. *Clin Geriatric Med* 1996;**12**:313–27.

88 Rousseau P. Existential suffering and palliative sedation: a brief commentary with a proposal for clinical guidelines. *Am J Hosp Palliat Care* 2001;**18**:151–3.

89 Walton O, Weinstein SM. Sedation for comfort at end of life. *Curr Pain Headache Rep* 2002;**6**:197–201.

90 Task Force on Palliative Care. Precepts of palliative care. *J Palliat Care* 1998;**1**:109–12.

91 Papa-Kanaan JM, Sicilian L. Ethical issues in the chronically critically ill patient. *Clin Chest Med* 2001;**22**:209–17.

92 Hansen-Flaschen J. Advanced lung disease: palliation and terminal care. *Clin Chest Med* 1997;**18**:645–55.

93 Janssens JP, de Muralt B, Titelion V. Management of dyspnea in severe chronic obstructive pulmonary disease. *J Pain Symptom Manage* 2000;**19**:378–92.

94 Webb M, Moody LE, Mason LA. Dyspnea assessment and management in hospice patients with pulmonary disorders. *Am J Hosp Palliat Care* 2000;**17**:259–64.

95 Foley KM. Pain and symptom control in the dying ICU patient. In: Curtis JR, Rubenfeld GD, eds. *Managing Death in the Intensive Care Unit*. Oxford: Oxford University Press, 2001: 103–25.

96 Desbiens NA, Mueller-Rizner N, Connors AF Jr, Wenger NS, Lynn J. The symptom burden of seriously ill hospitalized patients. SUPPORT Investigators: Study to Understand Prognoses and Preferences for Outcome and Risks of Treatment. *J Pain Symptom Manage* 1999;**17**:248–55.

97 Puntillo KA. The role of critical care nurses in providing and managing end-of-life care. In: Curtis JR, Rubenfeld GD, eds. *Managing Death in the Intensive Care Unit*. Oxford: Oxford University Press, 2001: 149–64.

98 Shannon SE. Helping families prepare for and cope with a death in the ICU. In: Curtis JR, Rubenfeld GD, eds. *Managing Death in the Intensive Care Unit*. Oxford: Oxford University Press, 2001: 165–91.

99 Bookbinder M, Coyle N, Kiss M *et al*. Implementing national standards for cancer pain management: program model and evaluation. *J Pain Symptom Manage* 1996;**12**:334–47; discussion 331–3.

100 Ingham JM, Portenoy RK. Symptom assessment. *Hematol Oncol Clin North Am* 1996;**10**:21–39.

101 Wilson WC, Smedira NG, Fink C, McDowell JA, Luce JM. Ordering and administration of sedatives and analgesics during the withholding and withdrawal of life support from critically ill patients. *JAMA* 1992;**267**:949–53.

102 Tittle M, McMillan SC. Pain and pain-related side effects in an ICU and on a surgical unit: nurses' management. *Am J Crit Care* 1994;**3**:25–30.

103 Caswell DR, Williams JP, Vallejo M *et al*. Improving pain management in critical care. *Jt Comm J Qual Improv* 1996; **22**:702–12.

104 Puntillo KA, Miaskowski C, Kehrle K *et al*. Relationship between behavioral and physiological indicators of pain, critical care patients' self-reports of pain, and opioid administration. *Crit Care Med* 1997;**25**:1159–66.

105 Morita T, Tsuneto S, Shima Y. Definition of sedation for symptom relief: a systematic literature review and a proposal of operational criteria. *J Pain Symptom Manage* 2002;**24**:447–53.

106 Solomon MZ, O'Donnell L, Jennings B *et al*. Decisions near the end of life: professional views on life-sustaining treatments. *Am J Public Health* 1993;**83**:14–23.

107 Carver AC, Vickrey BG, Bernat JL *et al*. End-of-life care: a survey of US neurologists' attitudes, behavior, and knowledge. *Neurology* 1999;**53**:284–93.

108 Sykes N, Thorns A. Sedative use in the last week of life and the implications for end-of-life decision making. *Arch Intern Med* 2003;**163**:341–4.

109 Mount B. Morphine drips, terminal sedation, and slow euthanasia: definitions and facts, not anecdotes. *J Palliat Care* 1996;**12**:31–7.

110 Portenoy RK. Morphine infusions at the end of life: the pitfalls in reasoning from anecdote. *J Palliat Care* 1996;**12**:44–6.

111 Stuart B, Alexander C, Arenella C *et al*. *Medical Guidelines for Determining Prognosis in Selected Non-Cancer Diseases*, 2nd edn. Arlington, VA: National Hospice Organization, 1996.

112 Abrahm JL, Hansen-Flaschen J. Hospice care for patients with advanced lung disease. *Chest* 2002;**121**:220–9.

113 Emanuel EJ, Fairclough DL, Slutsman J *et al*. Assistance from family members, friends, paid care givers, and volunteers in the care of terminally ill patients. *N Engl J Med* 1999;**341**:956–63.

114 Christakis NA, Escarce JJ. Survival of Medicare patients after enrollment in hospice programs. *N Engl J Med* 1996; **335**:172–8.

115 Bergs D. 'The Hidden Client': women caring for husbands with COPD: their experience of quality of life. *J Clin Nurs* 2002;**11**:613–21.

116 Lynn J, Schuster JL, Kabcenell A. Offering end-of-life services to patients with advanced heart or lung failure. In: *Improving Care for the End of Life: a Sourcebook for Health Care Managers and Clinicians*. New York: Oxford University Press, 2000.

117 Meduri GU, Fox RC, Abou-Shala N, Leeper KV, Wunderink RG. Non-invasive mechanical ventilation via face mask in patients with acute respiratory failure who refused endotracheal intubation. *Crit Care Med* 1994;**22**:1584–90.

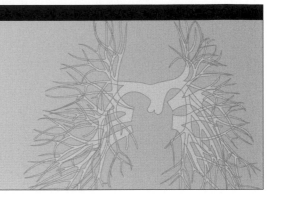

CHAPTER 64
Economic burden of COPD

David H. Au and Sean D. Sullivan

Chronic obstructive pulmonary disease (COPD) refers to a set of conditions made up primarily of chronic bronchitis and emphysema accompanied by permanent and not fully reversible airflow limitation. COPD is a prevalent and costly condition. As will be discussed in subsequent sections and based on current projections of disease prevalence, the full economic burden of COPD worldwide has yet to be appreciated. From the patients' perspectives, the economic burden of COPD will likely increase because of loss of productivity from themselves and/or family members. Independent of the health payer system, expenditure for patients is also likely to increase because of the costs of pharmaceutical therapies as well as inpatient and outpatient care. Because COPD is a chronic incurable illness, patients will also bear the burden of COPD on diminished health status and health-related quality of life. The prevalence of COPD is increasing worldwide and from a societal perspective, the economic burden from lost productivity, increased health-care expenditures and premature mortality will also increase. Within the constraints of budgetary limitations, the costs associated with technological and pharmaceutical therapies need to be balanced with their effectiveness. Many health payers base the decision to fund new therapies on their cost and cost effectiveness. If preventive measures were implemented today and were 100% effective, COPD would continue to contribute significant morbidity and mortality for decades to come. This article reviews our current understanding of the economic burden of COPD.

Epidemiology of COPD: prevalence and trends

Various survey designs that rely on patient self-report, presence of airflow limitation and physician diagnosis are likely to produce biased estimates of true disease prevalence [1]. A recent review of the literature found that among 32 studies representing 17 countries, COPD prevalence varied from 0.2% to 18.3% [2]. In the USA, the National Health Interview Survey estimated the prevalence of COPD in 2000 to be approximately 10.5 million persons based on patient self-reported affirmation that in the past 12 months a doctor or other health-care professional had told them that they had either emphysema or chronic bronchitis [3]. In contrast, as part of the National Health and Nutrition Examination Survey III (NHANES III) conducted between 1988 and 1994, a randomly selected subsample of patients performed spirometric evaluations without bronchodilatation [4]. For reporting purposes, airflow limitation was defined as a forced expiratory volume in 1 s to forced vital capacity (FEV_1/FVC) ratio of less than 70% and severity was determined by patients having mild obstruction if the FEV_1 was greater than 80% predicted, and moderate obstruction if the FEV_1 was less than 80% predicted. Using these definitions, Mannino *et al.* [5] reported that there were more than 24 million Americans who have some lung dysfunction, half having moderate obstruction. Recently, Confronting COPD, a study sponsored by GlaxoSmithKline, performed probability sampling in North America and the European Union which included more than 200 000 households [6]. Patients were considered to have COPD if they reported a physician diagnosis of emphysema or chronic bronchitis, were aged over 45 years and had smoked for more than 10 years. Results from this study suggest that the prevalence of COPD in Western industrialized countries in North America and Europe varied from 3.2% (France) to 5.4% (Netherlands). In Asia, reliable estimates of COPD prevalence are difficult to ascertain. In 1997, a survey suggested that the prevalence of COPD in Japan was only 0.2% [7]. A more recent estimate has suggested that the prevalence rate is closer to 8.5% among people over the age of 40 years [8]. Similarly, a study of the Korean population, which used a design similar to NHANES III and had a 50% response rate, estimated the prevalence of COPD to be 8.1% [9].

From an epidemiological standpoint, the definition used to identify patients with COPD directly affects the estimates of prevalence and burden of disease [1]. Even among well-respected societal recommendations, there is sufficient variation in definitions to lead to large disparities in estimates of COPD prevalence. For example, the American Thoracic Society (ATS) states that COPD is comprised of chronic bronchitis and emphysema that leads to irreversible loss of airflow [10]. The definition of chronic bronchitis and emphysema are defined on clinical and anatomical bases, respectively. The precise definition of irreversible airflow limitation was not defined, but was reviewed in another related ATS document on interpretation of pulmonary function testing [11]. The European Respiratory guidelines, although similar in requirement of irreversible airflow limitation, do not require that COPD be caused solely by chronic bronchitis and emphysema [12]. Recently, the GOLD guidelines published recommendations that a clinical history in conjunction with an FEV_1/FVC ratio of less than 70% was consistent with a diagnosis of COPD [13].

Risk factors for development of COPD

Tobacco smoke remains the leading risk factor for the development of COPD worldwide. International prevalence trends are consistent with those countries that have the greatest proportion of smokers also having the highest prevalence of COPD. Data from NHANES III demonstrated that among Caucasian men and women, current smokers had a prevalence of COPD of 14.2% and 13.6%, respectively; ex-smokers had a prevalence of 6.9% and 6.8%, respectively; and never smokers had a prevalence of 3.3% and 3.1%, respectively [14]. With changing behaviour patterns and an increase in consumption of tobacco by women, the prevalence of COPD among women and men are nearly equal in some industrialized countries [3,5,15]. Although not entirely clear, there is some evidence to suggest that women may be more susceptible to the effects of tobacco smoke than men [16,17]. Exposure to occupational dusts and chemicals or home biomass fuel used in cooking or home heating, in addition to or independent of tobacco smoke, has been associated with increased risk of COPD development [18–25].

Genetic factors, including gene–environment interactions, almost certainly play a significant part in the development of COPD [26–30] but which genetic factors lead to the development of COPD has not been elucidated. However, there is evidence to suggest that COPD risk may be higher in those with a previous family history of COPD. Some of these studies are difficult to interpret because of similar behaviour and exposures among family members. The most classic genetic factor is α_1-antitrypsin deficiency [30], which leads to panacinar emphysema.

Recently, the World Health Organization warned of the growing effects of non-communicable diseases. In 1990, COPD contributed to nearly 5% of deaths worldwide and was the fifth leading cause of death [31]. Likewise, there are a number of concerning statistics that have continued to emerge. Unlike every other major cause of morbidity and mortality in the USA, between 1965 and 1998, COPD mortality increased 163%. This is in contrast to coronary artery disease and cerebrovascular disease which demonstrated a 59% and 64% reduction in age-adjusted mortality, respectively [13,15]. Incidence of COPD in women has continued to rise and is comparable or higher than in men. Although reports have suggested that the prevalence of COPD in men may have plateaued, prevalence in women has steadily increased over the past two decades [5,32]. Moreover, in 2000, in the USA, women achieved the dubious distinction of surpassing men in the absolute number of COPD deaths (men vs women), although men still lead women in age-adjusted mortality [5]. Recent projections from the Netherlands suggest that by the year 2015, the prevalence of COPD will increase by 43% in men and 142% in women, after adjusting for projected decline in smoking status within the population [33]. Most of the projected prevalence of COPD will be from the direct effect of past smoking history. Even if there were no new smokers and all current smokers were to stop consuming tobacco products, 90% of the projected prevalence will be attributed to current and past use of tobacco [33,34].

Global burden of COPD

Costs associated with illnesses are often divided into those that result from direct management of disease, including medications, and clinical visits and indirect consequences, including work days lost, loss of productivity resulting from illness or premature death. The National Heart, Lung and Blood Institute (NHLBI) estimated that in 2002, the US total costs for patients with COPD was 32.1 billion dollars (Fig. 64.1) [35].

As demonstrated in Figure 64.1, direct costs represented approximately half of the total expenditures and, of these, 40.6% ($7.3 billion) of direct costs were related to hospital visits. Of the indirect costs, nearly 51.8% ($7.3 billion) were attributed to loss of income and productivity from early loss of life. In unadjusted dollars, this represents a relative increase of 34.3% in costs relative to 1993 when the total cost to treat COPD was $23.9 billion. The greatest increase cost was associated with premature mortality increasing from $4.5 billion to $7.3 billion. The results of this study are in agreement with other studies examining the cost of COPD. In the Netherlands, health-care costs for patients with COPD are projected to increase by 90% and possibly as much as 140% between 1994 and 2015 [33].

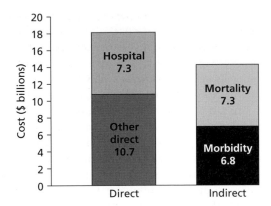

Figure 64.1 Costs in the USA associated with COPD in 2002.

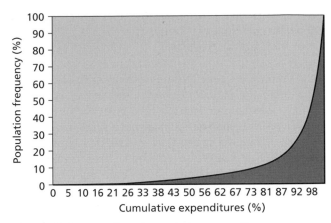

Figure 64.2 Proportion of cumulative expenditures as a percentage of the population. (From Strassels *et al.* [37] with permission.)

Women account for a larger proportion of the increase cost than men, mainly because of the relative increased prevalence of COPD in women. Hospital admission for patients with COPD is also a major contributor to costs in the USA, accounting for 45–68% of total expenditure [36–38]. Compared with patients of similar age and gender, patients with COPD consistently have more hospital admissions, longer lengths of hospital stay and 2–3 times the costs [39]. In other countries, the largest proportions of costs are associated with COPD treatment medications. For example, in the UK, 57% of costs are associated with medication use and only 17% are related to hospital admissions [40]. These are similar to a recent study which demonstrated that medications costs were similar to hospital admission costs in Germany [41]. Current predictions suggest that the importance of COPD to patient burden and economic significance is likely to continue to increase.

Costs of treatment and COPD severity

The greatest costs of COPD are associated with a relative minority of patients. At least three separate studies demonstrated that costs for COPD are not proportionally distributed among all patients with COPD, rather 10–20% of patients with COPD account for the majority (45–74%) of total direct expenditure (Fig. 64.2) [36–38].

One reason is that the relative distribution of costs changes with severity of illness. Several studies have demonstrated that there is a direct relationship between the severity of COPD, as measured by health status and/or airflow limitation, and the risk of COPD-related hospitalizations and mortality [39,42,43]. There is evidence that there is both a proportional increase in utilization of all medical care services, including proportional increases in pharmacy cost, outpatient and hospital care across COPD severity [42], as well as a non-proportional increase in severity-

related services including need for long-term oxygen therapy (LTOT) and hospitalizations [37,38,44,45].

There have been very few studies that have examined the indirect costs associated with COPD severity. In a Swedish study, the proportion of indirect costs relative to total costs increased generally with severity of disease [45]. For patients with the most severe to least severe disease (FEV_1 less than 40%, 40–59%, 60–79% and greater than 80%), indirect costs represented 58%, 68%, 52% and 28% of total costs in each stratum, respectively. Furthermore, total indirect costs for the most severe category were 89 times greater than those in the least severe stratum (at COPD risk), and 15 times greater than those with mild disease. The direct costs associated with COPD treatment also increase with severity and are reviewed in Figure 64.3 [44]. Several studies have demonstrated that direct costs increase mainly because of hospitalization (45–70% of total direct costs), medication acquisition (7–40%) and oxygen therapy (5–20%) [39,44].

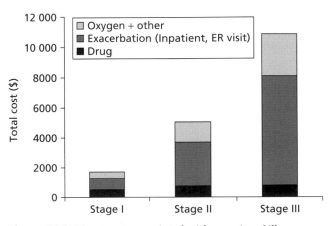

Figure 64.3 Direct costs associated with severity of illness.

Burden of disease from the patient's perspective

COPD represents a significant burden to the patient and their caregivers. From an economic standpoint, most studies have focused primarily on the perspective of the payer or society. Most cost-of-illnesses have not addressed the burden imposed by COPD from the patient's perspective. The direct costs of COPD to patients are likely to vary based on socioeconomic status and place of residence. In nations with national health coverage, direct medical costs will be generally limited. In countries such as the USA where there are multiple types of health-care payers, direct costs to the patient will vary based on coverage. For many patients with COPD over the age of 65, the Medicare programme provides coverage for outpatient and inpatient medical services; however, Medicare will not cover the majority of prescription-associated costs. Medicaid is available to those patients who are among the most socioeconomically challenged. Patients of higher economic status are more likely to be able to afford supplemental medication coverage or be covered by health plans that include medication coverage. A number of studies suggest that medication costs increase with severity of disease and the GOLD recommendations suggest that medications should be added with progressive symptoms [13]. A list of commonly used inhaled medications and charges are described in Table 64.1. Because

Table 64.1 Direct costs of commonly used inhaled therapy for COPD. (From www.drugstore.com [accessed 13 January 2004].)

Generic name	Brand name	MDI	Total cost ($)
β-Agonists			
Albuterol	Generic	×	13.99
	Airet		49.69
	Albuterol Sulfate		17.99
	Proventil HFA	×	38.47
	Ventolin HFA	×	38.99
Salmeterol	Serevent Diskus	×	80.99
Formoterol	Foradil		79.99
Metaproterenol	Metaproterenol Sulfate		33.99
	Alupent 0.65 mg/act	×	29.99
	Alupent 0.4% 2.5 mL		55.99
Anticholinergics			
Ipratropium bromide	Generic		11.99
	Atrovent 18 μg/act	×	50.99
	Atrovent 0.02% 2.5 mL		73.99
Combination therapy			
Albuterol and ipratropium bromide	Combivent	×	52.99
Fluticasone and salmeterol	Advair Diskus 100–50 μg/dose		106.99
	Advair Diskus 250–50 μg/dose		134.99
	Advair Diskus 500–50 μg/dose		184.99
Budesonide and formoterol*	Symbicort Turbuhaler 100 μg		80.00
	Symbicort Turbuhaler 200 μg		99.00
Inhaled corticosteroids			
Beclometasone	Beconase AQ	×	60.70
Triamcinolone	Azmacort	×	64.99
Flunisolide	Generic	×	37.99
	Aerobid-M	×	66.99
Fluticasone	Flovent 44 μg/act	×	52.99
	Flovent 110 μg/act	×	71.99
	Flovent 220 μg/act	×	106.99
Budesonide	Pulmicort Turbuhaler	×	122.99

* www.canadapharmacy.com (accessed 13 January 2004).
Act, actuation; MDI, metered dose inhaler.

15–40% of direct costs are derived from medications, patients who are economically disadvantaged and not covered by private health insurance or Medicaid, will be most directly affected by the costs associated with medication acquisition [39,44].

The effects of COPD on patients' health status and health-related quality of life (HRQoL) have been extensively reviewed [46]. In short, however, COPD has large detrimental effects on HRQoL using a variety of condition-specific and generic instruments. COPD has larger effects on HRQoL than other common chronic illness such as arthritis, prostate cancer, diabetes and hypertension. Confronting COPD demonstrated that 61% of patients with COPD reported that their health was fair to very poor [6]. Thirty per cent of patients reported that COPD affected their sex lives to a varying degree and 59% reported that COPD affected their normal physical exertion. Of patients under the age of 65, 45% reported that they had missed work because of COPD. Although COPD is a disease that affects many retired patients, 25% of patients over the age of 65 reported work loss secondary to COPD.

The disability adjusted life years was developed as part of the Global Burden of Disease Study as a composite measure of health status and health outcome that incorporates dimensions of premature life years lost and loss of productivity resulting from illness and injury [31]. In 1990, of the 30 most common disorders, COPD was the 12th leading cause of disability adjusted life years and sixth among non-infectious aetiologies. The effects of tobacco smoke will have the highest relative effects on non-third world countries, where the risk of mortality associated with infectious diseases are less apparent. Current projections suggest that COPD will rise from the 12th to the sixth leading cause of disability adjusted life years by the year 2020.

COPD exacerbations

Strategies to reduce costs associated with treatment of exacerbations

Because of the large proportion of costs associated with exacerbations, even strategies that have relatively small effects on COPD exacerbation rates may have large effects on reducing total costs [40]. Also, evidence would suggest that a large proportion of costs are associated with treatment failure. There have been a number of interventions that appear reasonable and effective and may lead to improvement in clinical outcomes and reduced costs. These interventions include non-invasive positive pressure ventilation (NIPPV), decreasing severity or managing patients outside of the hospital setting, and decisions about antibiotic use.

Controversy about antibiotics for treatment of acute exacerbations of COPD

Bacteria have clearly been implicated in the risk of COPD exacerbation; however, the use of antibiotics for all COPD exacerbations is probably not indicated [47,48]. An infectious aetiology in an acute exacerbation of COPD can be detected in 30–50% of cases and, of those with infectious aetiologies, viruses account for a significant proportion of these cases [49]. The best available evidence would suggest that antibiotics will most likely benefit those with severe exacerbations defined as a triad of worsening dyspnoea, increased sputum production and sputum volume [50]. A meta-analysis of antibiotics for COPD suggests a small but statistically significant benefit of using antibiotics for COPD exacerbations [10]. From a cost perspective, there are a number of important issues including prevention of relapse, need for hospitalization and the costs of antibiotic-resistant organisms in the community [51–53]. These issues have been reviewed in detail [51]. A recent economic analysis of resistance to medications, including antibiotics, suggested that the best policy may be to have a mixed treatment approach that may lessen the possibility of resistance to a single class of agents [52].

The issue of resistance and compliance with antibiotics also raises the question of the best choice of antibiotics for patients with COPD exacerbations. Currently, there is little evidence to support the choice of any specific antibiotic when considering clinical efficacy [54–60]. In a retrospective study of 60 patients with 224 exacerbations, Destache *et al.* [61] demonstrated that the initial costs of first-line antibiotic agents were significantly less than broader spectrum second- and third-line antibiotics, but may have less resource utilization. This study has significant methodological issues including no adjustments for prior COPD exacerbations and violations of independence in statistical analysis. Other studies have suggested that ciprofloxacin when compared to usual care may be cost-effective from the societal perspective ($18 588 per quality-adjusted life year [QALY]), however, there was no difference in time to resolution of symptoms [62]. Another study suggested that when comparing the macrolides azithromycin with clarithromycin among patients with lower respiratory track infections, patients taking azithromycin were able to return to work sooner, although there were no additional benefits in respect to clinical outcomes [63].

Mechanical ventilation and non-invasive positive pressure ventilation

Mechanical ventilation is costly for patients with severe COPD. In a secondary data analysis of the Study to Understand Prognoses and Preferences for Outcome and Risks of Treatment (SUPPORT), Ely *et al.* [64] compared patients requiring mechanical ventilation. In comparison to patients with other causes of respiratory failure, patients with COPD had similar length of stay (COPD 9 days), days of mechanical ventilation (COPD 5.5 vs other 5.0) and total hospital costs (COPD $24 217 vs other $27 672); however, they had appreciably more respiratory care costs (COPD $4064 vs other $2342). Of the median cost difference, 74% could be attributed to costs associated with bronchodilators and pulse oximetry. Despite the high costs associated with mechanical ventilation, Anon *et al.* [65] examined the cost–utility of mechanical ventilation for acute respiratory failure among 20 oxygen-dependant COPD patients. Despite having a high 1-year mortality of 75%, Anon *et al.* estimated that in the best and worse case scenarios the cost was $26 283/ QALY (US) and $44 602/QALY (US), respectively.

Interventions that reduce the need for invasive mechanical ventilation have been demonstrated to reduce hospital costs and mortality. Shortly after the introduction of NIPPV, there were concerns about its costs because of a lack of reimbursement from insurers [66] and clinical availability [67,68]. There is currently little doubt of the effectiveness of NIPPV, used in a select group of COPD patients with acute respiratory failure, as a therapeutic cost-saving strategy. There have now been several meta-analyses that consistently demonstrate that NIPPV reduces the odds of in-hospital mortality and mechanical ventilation when compared with standard therapy [69–71]. In addition, in one study the cost savings from a payer's perspective was $3244 (Canadian dollars, 1996) per patient hospitalization. Another study suggested that resource use, as measured by physician, respiratory therapist and nursing time, was similar to standard therapy for the first 48 h, but fell dramatically in favour of the NIPPV group after 48 h [69]. The use of NIPPV has risen dramatically, especially among patients with COPD [72]. Bilevel pressure-cycled ventilation has become the most common mode of ventilation.

Early discharge or avoiding hospitalizations by home management as a strategy to reduce costs

Hernadez *et al.* [73] recently described a randomized controlled trial of patients referred to an emergency room for COPD exacerbations. After excluding those who required imperative hospitalization, 222 patients were randomized to home hospitalization versus usual care. The programme consisted of a specialized team who encouraged immediate or early discharge, a comprehensive and tailored therapeutic approach to care, including education and a respiratory skilled nurse and/or a free-phone consultation. Treatment was considered to fail if a patient subsequently required hospitalization or had more than five home consultations with the nurse. The study was designed from the perspective of the payer. The costs associated with the intervention were nearly 60% of the usual care group (home hospitalization vs usual care: 1255.12 [95% CI 978.51–1568.04] vs 2033.51 [95% CI 1547.05–2556.81], in Euros, year 2000).

The number of days of hospitalization was significantly less in the intervention group. In addition, although there was no reduction in treatment failures that required hospitalization, there was a significant reduction in readmission to the emergency department for relapse and significant improvements in patient disease knowledge, home rehabilitation, inhalation technique and HRQoL. These results are supported by the results of Skwarska *et al.* [74], who demonstrated that supported discharge of selected patients resulted in fewer readmissions for treatment failure and a cost differential of 867 pounds/patient (home support 877 vs usual care 1753). In addition, observational data suggest that early outpatient follow-up visits after an emergency room visit was associated with a lower risk for repeat visits in the subsequent 90 days (hazard ratio 0.79; 95% CI 0.73–0.86) [75]. Also, interventions such as a home respiratory care visit after hospitalization may save as much as $2625/patient-hospitalization through reduced need for rehospitalization [76].

The home setting has also been employed to reduce COPD exacerbation relapse. In a recent study by Bourbeau *et al.* [77], patients who had COPD hospitalizations were randomized to an 8-week programme of weekly home visits followed by monthly telephone calls for 10 additional months to promote patient self-management. In this study, hospital admissions for COPD were reduced by 40%, with number of days/person in hospital decreasing by 42%. Unscheduled visits to primary care physicians and emergency room visits were reduced by 59% and 41%, respectively, while the number of scheduled visits to the primary care physician increased by 15%.

Long-term oxygen therapy

The beneficial effect on mortality of LTOT for patients with hypoxaemic respiratory failure has been clearly demonstrated [78,79]. However, LTOT is a major source of expenditure associated with outpatient therapy for COPD and is naturally associated with severity of illness. Based on COPD stage, Hilleman *et al.* [44] demonstrated that as a percentage of COPD costs, LTOT costs were associated with stage (0.0% cost for stage 1 disease, 13.8% for stage 2 disease and 18.6% of stage 3 disease). This is consistent with the results of others who have found that LTOT represented as much as 73% of outpatient expenditure for COPD [80]. The cost of LTOT in the USA in 1998, after mandated reductions in reimbursement, was 1.3 billion dollars or 28% of the durable medical equipment expenditure [81]. The Fifth Oxygen Consensus Conference made a number of recommendations that either reduced direct expenditure or improved the cost effectiveness of oxygen therapy. The most important of these focused on improving adherence to oxygen therapy [82]. Because many of the costs of LTOT are fixed, improving patient adherence would likely lead to improvements in cost effectiveness. Inappropriate use of oxygen may also be a source of potential cost savings.

Several studies have demonstrated that adherence to guidelines for LTOT is low [80,83,84]. These studies suggest that many patients who receive oxygen are not hypoxic. In addition, re-evaluation during a period of stability is recommended after the initial prescription for LTOT. In one study, only 19 of 226 patients had re-evaluation, 11 of whom were found not to need further LTOT [84]. Finally, several studies have examined the delivery of LTOT by cylinder or concentrator [80,85–87]. These studies together suggest that for patients who will likely need LTOT for a prolonged period of time (more than 3 months), oxygen concentrators are more cost effective.

Smoking cessation

Smoking cessation remains the most important therapy in COPD. It is the only therapy that has been definitively demonstrated to slow the progression of airflow limitation [16]. In addition to the effects on lung function, smoking cessation has immediate effects on cardiovascular disease and future risk of cancer. Independent of COPD in 1998, smoking-attributable medical expenditure was estimated by the Centers for Disease Control (CDC) at $75.5 billion. For the 46 million adult smokers in 1999, these costs were derived from $1760 for loss productivity and $1623 in excess medical expenditure [88]. In addition, smokers had greater absenteeism and less productivity at work but after smoking cessation had improvements in absenteeism and productivity [89]. Multiple studies have demonstrated the effectiveness of smoking cessation and smoking cessation programmes. A recent review summarized the findings from 157 studies, including 112 individual studies of adverse events, four systematic reviews, 17 economic studies and 13 individual studies of effectiveness [90]. Based on the literature contained in this review, the authors found that 1–3 life-years were saved per quitter. A decision model was built to compare the cost effectiveness of four smoking cessation interventions: counselling or advice about smoking cessation, advice plus nicotine replacement (NRT), advice plus bupropion SR and advice plus NRT and bupropion SR in combination. The incremental costs per quality of life-year saved was approximtaely £1000–2400 for NRT, £640–1500 for bupropion SR and £900–2000 for combination of NRT and bupropion SR. In a separate report by the same authors, when compared with counselling alone, they found similar results with incremental costs per life year saved was $1411–3455 for NRT, $920–2150 for bupropion and $1282–2836 for combination of NRT and bupropion SR [91]. Cornuz et al. [92] performed cost-effectiveness ratios for pharmacotherapies for nicotine dependence and found that that all first-line therapies for smoking cessation were cost effective, but the cost effectiveness varied widely by age and gender.

Coverage by health payers for tobacco cessation programmes has been a concern in part because of increased costs to the system. Fishman et al. [93] examined health-care expenditures in a non-for-profit mixed model Health Maintenance Organization (HMO) in western Washington State. This retrospective cohort study found that costs in the first year after cessation were higher for former smokers but that costs fell by the second year and were statistically not different for the subsequent 6 years. Cumulative health-care expenditure was lower for former smokers by the seventh year. This study supports the widely held notion adopted by the UK National Health Service programme that smoking cessation is cost effective not only the from the perspective of the individual, but also for the payer.

Pulmonary rehabilitation

Pulmonary rehabilitation is a multifaceted intervention that has been demonstrated to improve HRQoL, patient self-efficacy and exercise endurance [94,95]. The costs of these programmes are somewhat dependent on the provision in the rehabilitation programme. Goldstein et al. [96] reported the costs associated with a 6-month rehabilitation programme that included 2 months of inpatient hospitalization followed by 4 months of outpatient therapy. The incremental cost of this programme relative to usual care was $11 597 (Canadian). The proportion of patients who had a 0.5 point or more increase on each of the domains of the Chronic Respiratory Disease Questionnaire (CRQ) ranged between 0.23 and 0.39. On average, pulmonary rehabilitation lead to an improvement in 6-minute walk test of 38 m. Troosters et al. [95] performed a 6-month outpatient programme of exercise three times weekly for 3 months followed by twice weekly for the remainder of the programme. The mean cost of the intervention was $2615 ± 625 and resulted on average in an improvement of 52 m on 6-minute walk tests. Home rehabilitation produces similar effects on exercise endurance, but the effect may be more sustained than those in shorter inpatient or outpatient programmes [97,98]. From a cost-saving perspective, pulmonary rehabilitation has been demonstrated to decrease hospitalizations for COPD exacerbations, although this effect has not been consistently demonstrated in the literature.

Bronchodilators

Despite the fact that bronchodilators are the mainstay of therapy for patients with obstructive lung disease, there is a surprisingly sparse literature about the cost effectiveness of these medications. As demonstrated in Figure 64.3, medication acquisition costs as a function of COPD severity do not increase as rapidly as other costs. Thus, medication costs as a proportion of total of costs are least among patients with the most severe disease and greatest at the least severe stages.

Ipratropium bromide either alone or in combination with albuterol has been demonstrated to result in fewer health-care costs than either albuterol (cost over 85-day study period per patient: ipratropium $156; ipratropium plus albuterol $197; albuterol alone $269) [99], or theophylline alone (theophylline $121.40 per patient per therapy-month, ipratropium $84.56 per patient per therapy-month) [100]. In both studies, the reductions in cost were principally brought about by reductions in health-care utilization, including hospitalization, emergency room visits and unscheduled visits for COPD exacerbations.

There have been two studies to compare long-acting β-agonists with either usual care or ipratropium bromide. Jones *et al.* [101] recently reported that the addition of salmeterol to usual care had higher overall costs, but found that the addition of salmeterol had the incremental cost of £5.67 per symptom-free night. Hogan *et al.* [102] compared two doses of formoterol (12 and 24 μg) with ipratropium bromide with respect to the cost effectiveness on producing bronchodilatation (FEV_1) and quality of life. Ipratropium bromide had incremental cost effectiveness ratios that were more favourable than either doses of formoterol (increment of 0.137 L: ipratropium bromide $273.03/$FEV_1$; formoterol, 12 μg 1611.32/FEV_1 or 24 μg dominated) when compared with placebo. In contrast, when examining the effects on HRQoL, the 12 μg dose of formoterol appeared to be more effective ($25.20/change QoL score) than either the 24 μg dose of formoterol or ipratropium bromide (both dominated) when compared with placebo. More recently, Oostenbrink *et al.* [103] performed a prospective cost-effectiveness analysis along two 1-year randomized control trials of tiotropium compared with ipratropium bromide. Mean annual medical costs were 1721 euros for tiotropium and 1541 euros for ipratropium bromide. Of the higher costs of medication acqustion costs of tiotropium (cost difference 453 euros), 60% was offset by reductions in medical expenditures associated with fewer hospitalizations and unscheduled visits for COPD. The incremental cost-effectiveness ratio was 667 euros per exacerbation and 1084 euros per patient for clinically meaningful improvements in HRQoL. The cost and cost effectiveness presented in this study were likely conservative estimates given that indirect costs such as days of work missed were not included in the cost estimates.

Corticosteroids

Inhaled corticosteroids and risk of COPD exacerbation and mortality

The utility of inhaled corticosteroids among patients with COPD remains controversial. There have been four large well-performed randomized controlled trials that demonstrate no improvement in the rate of FEV_1 decline for patients with various degrees of COPD severity [104–107]. The medications included in these trials utilize inhaled corticosteroids of varying potency and include triamcinalone, fluticasone and budesonide. A recent meta-analysis identified nine randomized controlled trials of inhaled corticosteroids among patients with COPD [108]. Six of the nine trials reported risk of COPD exacerbations associated with inhaled corticosteroids in comparison with placebo. Two of the six reported no benefit in COPD exacerbation risk and when combined with the remaining four trials, inhaled corticosteroids were associated with a 30% reduction (RR, 0.70; 95% CI, 0.58–0.84) in exacerbation. Ayres *et al.* [109] have recently demonstrated that fluticasone in comparison with placebo had no effects on total costs (direct and indirect); however, they suggested that the incremental cost effectiveness may favour inhaled fluticasone with the cost of remaining exacerbation free estimated at £0.25/day from the payer's perspective. There have now been three trials that combine inhaled corticosteroids with long-acting β-agonists in comparison with individual components [110–112]. All trials examined the effects of combination therapy on exacerbation risk. The results of these trials consistently demonstrate that all treatment arms were better than placebo; however, these studies could not demonstrate consistent improvement in exacerbation risk between individual components and combinations.

In observational trials, the association of inhaled corticosteroids on risk of mortality has been mixed. In two observational trials, inhaled corticosteroids that were assessed at baseline and required limited exposure, defined as either single or three prescriptions for inhaled corticosteroids, were associated with a decreased risk of all-cause mortality as long as 3 years after exposure assessment [113,114]. These two trials have been questioned, largely because of the miminal exposure requirements and concern over immortal person time bias [115,116]. Two follow-up trials that utilized time-dependent exposures of inhaled corticosteroids assessments could not confirm a survival benefit associated with inhaled corticosteroids [115,116]. One of these trials used three methods to assess inhaled corticosteroid use and required at least 80% compliance with filling prescriptions for inhaled corticosteroids [115].

The GOLD COPD treatment guidelines endorse the use of inhaled corticosteroids for the treatment of moderate to severe COPD but also states that 'Prolonged treatment with inhaled glucocorticoids does not modify the long-term decline in FEV_1 in patients with COPD' [13]. Whether inhaled corticosteroids will be cost effective has yet to be determined; however, a clinical trial is currently underway to determine the effects of COPD exacerbation as a primary outcome. In one study, Sin *et al.* [117] examined the cost effectiveness of inhaled corticosteroids in treating COPD. Among patients with stage 2 or 3 disease, the cost effectiveness of the inhaled corticosteroids was $17 000/QALY. In contrast to prospective studies of cost effectiveness performed along clinical trials [103,118], assumptions about condition severity, treatment and outcomes were derived from a literature review that included heterogeneous patient populations, varying entry criteria and exclusions. In addition, the results appeared to be highly dependent upon the assumptions that inhaled corticosteroids would lead to a 16% reduction in mortality and that the effectiveness of inhaled corticosteroids (in contrast to the efficaciousness of inhaled corticosteroids) was 30% in reducing COPD exacerbations. The reliability of the estimates was also difficult to assess because of the lack of acceptability curves.

Lung volume reduction surgery

Although lung volume reduction surgery was not a new concept in 1994, Cooper *et al.* [119] reported beneficial effects of this operation on patients with severe emphysema. This and subsequent reports fuelled a prolific increase in the use of this procedure for emphysema. Early reports suggested improvement in pulmonary function tests, LTOT and HRQoL [120–128]. However, these reports were clouded by differential follow-up and reports of 1-year postoperative mortality of up to 17% [129]. In response to these lingering questions, the Health Care Financing Administration (HCFA) announced that it would no long reimburse for lung volume reduction surgery. At the same time, HCFA, along with the NHLBI and the Agency for Healthcare Research and Quality (AHRQ) announced plans for the National Emphysema Treatment Trial (NETT) [130]. This randomized clinical trial was designed to compare the best current medical therapy and best current medical therapy plus lung volume reduction surgery with all-cause mortality as the primary outcome measure. The trial enrolled 1358 patients from 17 medical centres. Interim analysis demonstrated that patients who had an FEV_1 of less than 20% predicted and either a DLCO less than 20% or homogeneous emphysema on chest computed tomography had excessive risk of mortality and were subsequently excluded from the trial [131]. Of the remaining 1218 patients, no benefit in mortality was detected at 24 months [132]. In *post hoc* subgroup analysis, it appeared that there was a potential benefit in survival, exercise capacity and HRQoL among those patients who had upper lobe emphysema and low exercise capabilities after pulmonary rehabilitation. A prospective cost-effectiveness analysis was also performed as part of this trial [118]. This trial used the societal perspective to determine the quality-adjusted life year gained. The Quality of Well Being scale was used to derive health state preferences, and cost estimates were calculated to be in 2002 dollars. Not surprisingly, in the first 12 months, hospital days, days of ambulatory care and nursing home admissions were greater in the surgical treatment group, but by 12–24 months there were more hospital admissions in the medical treatment group and no difference in any resource use between 24 and 36 months. Direct and total costs also followed similar trends, with the surgical arm having higher costs at 12 months (direct $61 415 vs 15 738 and total $71 515 vs 23 371), but having less direct and total cost at 13–24 months (direct $9474 vs 13 222, total $13 222 vs 21 319) and similar costs between 25 and 36 months (direct $10 199 vs 12 303, total $14 215 vs 17 870). The estimated quality-adjusted life year gained at 3 years after initiation was $190 000. Comparing direct cost only, the estimate quality-adjusted life year gained at 3 years was $193 000. Stratifying by those with upper lobe disease and exercise capacity, the cost-effectiveness ratio for those who had upper lobe disease and low exercise capacity was $98 000 at 3 years. The next most effective group, those who had upper lobe disease and high exercise capacity had a cost-effectiveness ratio of $240 000 at 3 years. Estimates of 10-year cost-effectiveness ratios was $53 000/QALY; however, the cost-effectiveness acceptability curves suggested significant instability in this estimate. In comparison to other common surgical procedures, medical therapy plus lung volume reduction surgery appears costly: coronary artery bypass graft $8300–64 000/QALY, lung transplantation $130 000–220 000/QALY, heart transplantation $65 000/QALY.

Conclusions

COPD is a prevalent problem and the economic effects are not isolated to Western countries. Worldwide, the prevalence of COPD will likely increase and outside the USA and western Europe, the cost of COPD has not been estimated. It is clear, however, that even if preventive measures were implemented today and were 100% effective, COPD will continue to contribute significant morbidity and mortality for decades to come.

Despite the substantial costs associated with the condition, there are surprisingly few data to support decision making for health payers on cost-effective therapy. Relative to effects of other conditions, research on COPD is underfunded [133]. Greater emphasis and a stronger commitment from non-commercial-based research are necessary to encourage significant advancements.

References

1 Mannino DM. COPD: epidemiology, prevalence, morbidity and mortality, and disease heterogeneity. *Chest* 2002;**121**:121–6S.

2 Halbert RJ, Isonaka S, George D *et al.* Interpreting COPD prevalence estimates: what is the true burden of disease? *Chest* 2003;**123**:1684–92.

3 National Health Interview Survey. Research for the 1995–2004 redesign. *Vital Health Stat 2* 1999;**126**:1–119.

4 Plan and Operation of the Third National Health and Nutrition Examination Survey, 1998–94: series 1; programs and collection procedures. *Vital Health Stat 1* 1994;**32**:1–407.

5 Mannino DM, Homa DM, Akinbami LJ *et al.* Chronic Obstructive Pulmonary Disease Surveillance: United States, 1971–2000. *MMWR Surveill Summ* 2002;**51**:1–16.

6 Rennard S, Decramer M, Calverley PM *et al.* Impact of COPD in North America and Europe in 2000: subjects' perspective of Confronting COPD International Survey. *Eur Respir J.* 2002;**20**(4):799–805.

7 Tatsumi K. Epidemiological survey of chronic obstructive pulmonary disease in Japan. *Respirology* 2001;**6**(Suppl):S27–33.

8 Teramoto S, Yamamoto H, Yamaguchi Y *et al.* Global burden of COPD in Japan and Asia. *Lancet* 2003;**362**:1764–5.

9 Committee TNCS. Nationwide Survey on the Prevalence of COPD in Korea. *Am J Respir Crit Care Med* 2003;**168**:A237.

10 ATS. Standards for the dragnosis and care of patients with chronic obstructive pulmonary disease. *Am J Respir Crit Care Med* 1995;**152**(5):577–121.

11 Lung function testing: selection of reference values and interpretive strategies. *Am Rev Respir Dis* 1991;**144**(5):1202–18.

12 Siafakas NM, Vermeire P, Pride NB *et al.* Optimal assessment and management of chronic obstructive pulmonary disease (COPD). The European Respiratory Society Task Force. *Eur Respir J* 1995;**8**:1398–420.

13 Consensus. Available at http://www.GOLDCOPD.com

14 Centers of Disease Control and Prevention. *Vital and Health Statistics: Currrent Estimates from the National Health Interview Survey, 1995.* DHHS Publication No. 96-1527, 1998.

15 National Heart, Lung, and Blood Institute. *Morbidity and Mortality: Chartbook on Cardiovascular, Lung and Blood Disease.* Bethesda, MD: US Department of Health and Human Services, Public Health Service, National Institutes of Health, 1998.

16 Anthonisen NR, Connett JE, Kiley JP *et al.* Effects of smoking intervention and the use of an inhaled anticholinergic bronchodilator on the rate of decline of FEV_1. The Lung Health Study. *JAMA* 1994;**272**:1497–505.

17 Xu X, Weiss ST, Rijcken B *et al.* Smoking, changes in smoking habits, and rate of decline in FEV_1: new insight into gender differences. *Eur Respir J* 1994;**7**:1056–61.

18 Samet JM, Marbury MC, Spengler JD. Health effects and sources of indoor air pollution. Part I. *Am Rev Respir Dis* 1987;**136**:1486–508.

19 Amoli K. Bronchopulmonary disease in Iranian housewives chronically exposed to indoor smoke. *Eur Respir J* 1998;**11**:659–63.

20 Behera D, Jindal SK. Respiratory symptoms in Indian women using domestic cooking fuels. *Chest* 1991;**100**:385–8.

21 Dennis RJ, Maldonado D, Norman S *et al.* Woodsmoke exposure and risk for obstructive airways disease among women. *Chest* 1996;**109**:115–9.

22 Dossing M, Khan J, al-Rabiah F. Risk factors for chronic obstructive lung disease in Saudi Arabia. *Respir Med* 1994;**88**:519–22.

23 Pandey MR. Prevalence of chronic bronchitis in a rural community of the IIill Region of Ncpal. *Thorax* 1984;**39**:331–6.

24 Pandey MR. Domestic smoke pollution and chronic bronchitis in a rural community of the Hill Region of Nepal. *Thorax* 1984;**39**:337–9.

25 Perez-Padilla R, Regalado J, Vedal S *et al.* Exposure to biomass smoke and chronic airway disease in Mexican women: a case–control study. *Am J Respir Crit Care Med* 1996;**154**:701–6.

26 Joos L, Pare PD, Sandford AJ. Genetic risk factors of chronic obstructive pulmonary disease. *Swiss Med Wkly* 2002;**132**:27–37.

27 Sandford AJ, Joos L, Pare PD. Genetic risk factors for chronic obstructive pulmonary disease. *Curr Opin Pulm Med* 2002;**8**:87–94.

28 Sandford AJ, Pare PD. Genetic risk factors for chronic obstructive pulmonary disease. *Clin Chest Med* 2000;**21**:633–43.

29 Sandford AJ, Chagani T, Weir TD *et al.* Susceptibility genes for rapid decline of lung function in the lung health study. *Am J Respir Crit Care Med* 2001;**163**:469–73.

30 Chen Y. Genetics and pulmonary medicine. 10: Genetic epidemiology of pulmonary function. *Thorax* 1999;**54**:818–24.

31 Murray CJ, Lopez AD. Mortality by cause for eight regions of the world. Global Burden of Disease Study. *Lancet* 1997;**349**:1269–76.

32 Soriano JB, Maier WC, Egger P *et al.* Recent trends in physician diagnosed COPD in women and men in the UK. *Thorax* 2000;**55**:789–94.

33 Feenstra TL, van Genugten ML, Hoogenveen RT *et al.* The impact of aging and smoking on the future burden of chronic obstructive pulmonary disease: a model analysis in the Netherlands. *Am J Respir Crit Care Med* 2001;**164**:590–6.

34 Rutten van-Molken MP, Feenstra TL. The burden of asthma and chronic obstructive pulmonary disease: data from the Netherlands. *Pharmacoeconomics* 2001;**19**(Suppl 2):1–6.

35 National Heart, Lung, and Blood Institute. *Morbidity and Mortality: 2002 Chartbook on Cardiovascular, Lung, and Blood Diseases.* Bethesda, MD: US Department of Health and Human Services, NIH, NHLBI. May 2002.

36 Grasso ME, Weller WE, Shaffer TJ *et al.* Capitation, managed care, and chronic obstructive pulmonary disease. *Am J Respir Crit Care Med* 1998;**158**:133–8.

37 Strassels SA, Smith DH, Sullivan SD *et al.* The costs of treating COPD in the United States. *Chest* 2001;**119**:344–52.

38 Yelin E, Trupin L, Cisternas M *et al.* A national study of medical care expenditures for respiratory conditions. *Eur Respir J* 2002;**19**:414–21.

39 Mapel DW, Hurley JS, Frost FJ *et al.* Health care utilization in chronic obstructive pulmonary disease: a case–control

study in a health maintenance organization. *Arch Intern Med* 2000;**160**:2653–8.

40 McGuire A, Irwin DE, Fenn P *et al.* The excess cost of acute exacerbations of chronic bronchitis in patients aged 45 and older in England and Wales. *Value Health* 2001;**4**:370–5.

41 Nowalk D, Oberender P, Spannheimer A *et al.* Cost of illness for COPD patients in Germany. *Am J Respir Crit Care Med* 2003;**167**:239A.

42 Miravitlles M, Murio C, Guerrero T *et al.* Pharmacoeconomic evaluation of acute exacerbations of chronic bronchitis and COPD. *Chest* 2002;**121**:1449–55.

43 Mapel DW, Picchi MA, Hurley JS *et al.* Utilization in COPD: patient characteristics and diagnostic evaluation. *Chest* 2000;**117**:346–53S.

44 Hilleman DE, Dewan N, Malesker M *et al.* Pharmaco-economic evaluation of COPD. *Chest* 2000;**118**:1278–85.

45 Jansson SA, Andersson F, Borg S *et al.* Costs of COPD in Sweden according to disease severity. *Chest* 2002;**122**:1994–2002.

46 Au DH, Curtis JR, Hudson LD. The assessment of health-related quality of life among patients with Chronic Obstructive Pulmonary Disease. *Lung Biology in Health and Disease*, Vol. 165, Clinical Management of Stable COPD. New York: Marcel Dekker, 2002.

47 Sethi S, Evans N, Grant BJ *et al.* New strains of bacteria and exacerbations of chronic obstructive pulmonary disease. *N Engl J Med* 2002;**347**:465–71.

48 Sethi S. The role of antibiotics in acute exacerbations of chronic obstructive pulmonary disease. *Curr Infect Dis Rep* 2003;**5**:9–15.

49 Bach PB, Brown C, Gelfand SE *et al.* Management of acute exacerbations of chronic obstructive pulmonary disease: a summary and appraisal of published evidence. *Ann Intern Med* 2001;**134**:600–20.

50 Anthonisen NR, Manfreda J, Warren CP *et al.* Antibiotic therapy in exacerbations of chronic obstructive pulmonary disease. *Ann Intern Med* 1987;**106**:196–204.

51 Saint S, Flaherty KR, Abrahamse P *et al.* Acute exacerbation of chronic bronchitis: disease-specific issues that influence the cost-effectiveness of antimicrobial therapy. *Clin Ther* 2001;**23**:499–512.

52 Laxminarayan R, Weitzman ML. On the implications of endogenous resistance to medications. *J Health Econ* 2002;**21**:709–18.

53 Howard D, Cordell R, McGowan JE Jr *et al.* Measuring the economic costs of antimicrobial resistance in hospital settings: summary of the Centers for Disease Control and Prevention–Emory Workshop. *Clin Infect Dis* 2001;**33**:1573–8.

54 Castaldo RS, Celli BR, Gomez F *et al.* A comparison of 5-day courses of dirithromycin and azithromycin in the treatment of acute exacerbations of chronic obstructive pulmonary disease. *Clin Ther* 2003;**25**:542–57.

55 DeAbate CA, Mathew CP, Warner JH *et al.* The safety and efficacy of short course (5-day) moxifloxacin vs. azithromycin in the treatment of patients with acute exacerbation of chronic bronchitis. *Respir Med* 2000;**94**:1029–37.

56 Umut S, Tutluoglu B, Aydin Tosun G *et al.* Determination of the etiological organism during acute exacerbations of COPD and efficacy of azithromycin, ampicillin-sulbactam, ciprofloxacin and cefaclor. Turkish Thoracic Society COPD Working Group. *J Chemother* 1999;**11**:211–4.

57 Hoepelman IM, Mollers MJ, van Schie MH *et al.* A short (3-day) course of azithromycin tablets versus a 10-day course of amoxycillin-clavulanic acid (co-amoxiclav) in the treatment of adults with lower respiratory tract infections and effects on long-term outcome. *Int J Antimicrob Agents* 1997;**9**:141–6.

58 Mertens JC, van Barneveld PW, Asin HR *et al.* Double-blind randomized study comparing the efficacies and safeties of a short (3-day) course of azithromycin and a 5-day course of amoxicillin in patients with acute exacerbations of chronic bronchitis. *Antimicrob Agents Chemother* 1992;**36**:1456–9.

59 Lorenz J, Thate-Waschke IM, Mast O *et al.* Treatment outcomes in acute exacerbations of chronic bronchitis: comparison of macrolides and moxifloxacin from the patient perspective. *J Int Med Res* 2001;**29**:74–86.

60 Hoepelman AI, Sips AP, van Helmond JL *et al.* A single-blind comparison of three-day azithromycin and ten-day co-amoxiclav treatment of acute lower respiratory tract infections. *J Antimicrob Chemother* 1993;**31**(Suppl E):147–52.

61 Destache CJ, Dewan N, O'Donohue WJ *et al.* Clinical and economic considerations in the treatment of acute exacerbations of chronic bronchitis. *J Antimicrob Chemother* 1999;**43**(Suppl A):107–13.

62 Grossman R, Mukherjee J, Vaughan D *et al.* A 1-year community-based health economic study of ciprofloxacin vs usual antibiotic treatment in acute exacerbations of chronic bronchitis: the Canadian Ciprofloxacin Health Economic Study Group. *Chest* 1998;**113**:131–41.

63 Sternon J, Leclerq P, Knepper C *et al.* Azithromycin compared with clarithromycin in the treatment of adult patients with acute purulent tracheobronchitis: a cost of illness study. *J Int Med Res* 1995;**23**:413–22.

64 Ely EW, Baker AM, Evans GW *et al.* The distribution of costs of care in mechanically ventilated patients with chronic obstructive pulmonary disease. *Crit Care Med* 2000;**28**:408–13.

65 Anon JM, Garcia de Lorenzo A, Zarazaga A *et al.* Mechanical ventilation of patients on long-term oxygen therapy with acute exacerbations of chronic obstructive pulmonary disease: prognosis and cost–utility analysis. *Intensive Care Med* 1999;**25**:452–7.

66 Criner GJ, Kreimer DT, Tomaselli M *et al.* Financial implications of noninvasive positive pressure ventilation (NPPV). *Chest* 1995;**108**:475–81.

67 Doherty MJ, Greenstone MA. Survey of non-invasive ventilation (NIPPV) in patients with acute exacerbations of chronic obstructive pulmonary disease (COPD) in the UK. *Thorax* 1998;**53**:863–6.

68 Vanpee D, Delaunois L, Lheureux P *et al.* Survey of non-invasive ventilation for acute exacerbation of chronic obstructive pulmonary disease patients in emergency departments in Belgium. *Eur J Emerg Med* 2002;**9**:217–24.

69 Keenan SP, Gregor J, Sibbald WJ *et al.* Non-invasive positive pressure ventilation in the setting of severe, acute exacerbations of chronic obstructive pulmonary disease: more effective and less expensive. *Crit Care Med* 2000;**28**:2094–102.

70 Lightowler JV, Wedzicha JA, Elliott MW *et al.* Non-invasive positive pressure ventilation to treat respiratory failure resulting from exacerbations of chronic obstructive pulmonary disease: Cochrane systematic review and meta-analysis. *BMJ* 2003;**326**:185.

71 Peter JV, Moran JL, Phillips-Hughes J *et al.* Non-invasive ventilation in acute respiratory failure: a meta-analysis update. *Crit Care Med* 2002;**30**:555–62.

72 Janssens JP, Derivaz S, Breitenstein E *et al.* Changing patterns in long-term non-invasive ventilation: a 7-year prospective study in the Geneva Lake Area. *Chest* 2003;**123**:67–79.

73 Hernandez C, Casas A, Escarrabill J *et al.* Home hospitalisation of exacerbated chronic obstructive pulmonary disease patients. *Eur Respir J* 2003;**21**:58–67.

74 Skwarska E, Cohen G, Skwarski KM *et al.* Randomized controlled trial of supported discharge in patients with exacerbations of chronic obstructive pulmonary disease. *Thorax* 2000;**55**:907–12.

75 Sin DD, Bell NR, Svenson LW *et al.* The impact of follow-up physician visits on emergency readmissions for patients with asthma and chronic obstructive pulmonary disease: a population-based study. *Am J Med* 2002;**112**:120–5.

76 Roselle S, D'Amico FJ. The effect of home respiratory therapy on hospital readmission rates of patients with chronic obstructive pulmonary disease. *Respir Care* 1982;**27**:1194–9.

77 Bourbeau J, Julien M, Maltais F *et al.* Reduction of hospital utilization in patients with chronic obstructive pulmonary disease: a disease-specific self-management intervention. *Arch Intern Med* 2003;**163**:585–91.

78 Medical Research Council Working Party. Long-term domiciliary oxygen therapy in chronic hypoxic cor pulmonale complicating chronic bronchitis and emphysema. *Lancet* 1981;**1**:681–6.

79 Nocturnal Oxygen Therapy Trial Group. Continuous or nocturnal oxygen therapy in hypoxemic chronic obstructive lung disease: a clinical trial. *Ann Intern Med* 1980;**93**:391–8.

80 Pelletier-Fleury N, Lanoe JL, Fleury B *et al.* The cost of treating COPD patients with long-term oxygen therapy in a French population. *Chest* 1996;**110**:411–6.

81 Dunne PJ. The demographics and economics of long-term oxygen therapy. *Respir Care* 2000;**45**:223–8; discussion 228–30.

82 Petty TL, Casaburi R. Recommendations of the Fifth Oxygen Consensus Conference. Writing and Organizing Committees. *Respir Care* 2000;**45**:957–61.

83 Shankar P, Muthiah MM. Audit on prescription of long-term oxygen treatment. *Clin Perform Qual Health Care* 2000;**8**:134–5.

84 Oba Y, Salzman GA, Willsie SK. Re-evaluation of continuous oxygen therapy after initial prescription in patients with chronic obstructive pulmonary disease. *Respir Care* 2000;**45**:401–6.

85 Strom K, Boe J, Herala M *et al.* Assessment of two oxygen treatment alternatives in the home. *Int J Technol Assess Health Care* 1990;**6**:489–97.

86 Lowson KV, Drummond MF, Bishop JM. Costing new services: long-term domiciliary oxygen therapy. *Lancet* 1981;**1**:1146–9.

87 McKeon JL, Saunders NA, Murree-Allen K. Domiciliary oxygen: rationalization of supply in the Hunter region from 1982–1986. *Med J Aust* 1987;**146**:73–8.

88 From the Centers for Disease Control and Prevention. Annual smoking attributable mortality, years of potential life lost and economic costs: United States, 1995–1999. *JAMA* 2002;**287**:2355–6.

89 Pronk NP, Goodman MJ, O'Connor PJ *et al.* Relationship between modifiable health risks and short-term health care charges. *JAMA* 1999;**282**:2235–9.

90 Woolacott NF, Jones L, Forbes CA *et al.* The clinical effectiveness and cost-effectiveness of bupropion and nicotine replacement therapy for smoking cessation: a systematic review and economic evaluation. *Health Technol Assess* 2002;**6**:1–245.

91 Song F, Raftery J, Aveyard P *et al.* Cost-effectiveness of pharmacological interventions for smoking cessation: a literature review and a decision analytic analysis. *Med Decis Making* 2002;**22**:S26–37.

92 Cornuz J, Pinget C, Gilbert A *et al.* Cost-effectiveness analysis of the first-line therapies for nicotine dependence. *Eur J Clin Pharmacol* 2003;**59**:201–6.

93 Fishman PA, Khan ZM, Thompson EE *et al.* Health care costs among smokers, former smokers, and never smokers in an HMO. *Health Serv Res* 2003;**38**:733–49.

94 Ries AL, Kaplan RM, Limberg TM *et al.* Effects of pulmonary rehabilitation on physiologic and psychosocial outcomes in patients with chronic obstructive pulmonary disease. *Ann Intern Med* 1995;**122**:823–32.

95 Troosters T, Gosselink R, Decramer M. Short- and long-term effects of outpatient rehabilitation in patients with chronic obstructive pulmonary disease: a randomized trial. *Am J Med* 2000;**109**:207–12.

96 Goldstein RS, Gort EH, Guyatt GH *et al.* Economic analysis of respiratory rehabilitation. *Chest* 1997;**112**:370–9.

97 Wijkstra PJ, Strijbos JH, Koeter GH. Home-based rehabilitation for patients with COPD: organization, effects and financial implications. *Monaldi Arch Chest Dis* 2000;**55**:130–4.

98 Ries AL, Kaplan RM, Myers R *et al.* Maintenance after pulmonary rehabilitation in chronic lung disease: a randomized trial. *Am J Respir Crit Care Med* 2003;**167**:880–8.

99 Friedman M, Serby CW, Menjoge SS *et al.* Pharmacoeconomic evaluation of a combination of ipratropium plus albuterol compared with ipratropium alone and albuterol alone in COPD. *Chest* 1999;**115**:635–41.

100 Jubran A, Gross N, Ramsdell J *et al.* Comparative cost-effectiveness analysis of theophylline and ipratropium bromide in chronic obstructive pulmonary disease: a three-center study. *Chest* 1993;**103**:678–84.

101 Jones PW, Wilson K, Sondhi S. Cost-effectiveness of salmeterol in patients with chronic obstructive pulmonary disease: an economic evaluation. *Respir Med* 2003;**97**:20–6.

102 Hogan TJ, Geddes R, Gonzalez ER. An economic assessment of inhaled formoterol dry powder versus ipratropium bromide pressurized metered dose inhaler in the treatment of chronic obstructive pulmonary disease. *Clin Ther* 2003;**25**:285–97.

103 Lung Health Study Research Group. Effect of inhaled

triamcinolone on the decline in pulmonary function in chronic obstructive pulmonary disease. *N Engl J Med* 2000; **343**:1902–9.

104 Burge PS, Calverley PM, Jones PW *et al*. Randomised, double blind, placebo controlled study of fluticasone propionate in patients with moderate to severe chronic obstructive pulmonary disease: the ISOLDE trial. *BMJ* 2000;**320**:1297–303.

105 Pauwels RA, Lofdahl CG, Laitinen LA *et al*. Long-term treatment with inhaled budesonide in persons with mild chronic obstructive pulmonary disease who continue smoking. European Respiratory Society Study on Chronic Obstructive Pulmonary Disease [see comments]. *N Engl J Med* 1999; **340**:1948–53.

106 Paggiaro PL, Dahle R, Bakran I *et al*. Multicentre randomised placebo-controlled trial of inhaled fluticasone propionate in patients with chronic obstructive pulmonary disease. International COPD Study Group. *Lancet* 1998;**351**:773–80.

107 Sin DD, McAlister FA, Man SF *et al*. Contemporary management of chronic obstructive pulmonary disease: scientific review. *JAMA* 2003;**290**:2301–12.

108 Ayres JG, Price MJ, Efthimiou J. Cost-effectiveness of fluticasone propionate in the treatment of chronic obstructive pulmonary disease: a double-blind randomized, placebo-controlled trial. *Respir Med* 2003;**97**:212–20.

109 Mahler DA, Wire P, Horstman D *et al*. Effectiveness of fluticasone propionate and salmeterol combination delivered via the Diskus device in the treatment of chronic obstructive pulmonary disease. *Am J Respir Crit Care Med* 2002;**166**: 1084–91.

110 Calverley P, Pauwels R, Vestbo J *et al*. Combined salmeterol and fluticasone in the treatment of chronic obstructive pulmonary disease: a randomised controlled trial. *Lancet* 2003;**361**:449–56.

111 Szafranski W, Cukier A, Ramirez A *et al*. Efficacy and safety of budesonide/formoterol in the management of chronic obstructive pulmonary disease. *Eur Respir J* 2003;**21**:74–81.

112 Sin DD, Tu JV. Inhaled corticosteroids and the risk of mortality and readmission in elderly patients with chronic obstructive pulmonary disease. *Am J Respir Crit Care Med* 2001;**164**:580–4.

113 Soriano JB, Vestbo J, Pride NB *et al*. Survival in COPD patients after regular use of fluticasone propionate and salmeterol in general practice. *Eur Respir J* 2002;**20**:819–25.

114 Fan VS, Bryson CL, Curtis JR *et al*. Inhaled corticosteroids in chronic obstructive pulmonary disease and risk of death and hospitalization: time-dependent analysis. *Am J Respir Crit Care Med* 2003;**168**:1488–94.

115 Suissa S. Effectiveness of inhaled corticosteroids in chronic obstructive pulmonary disease: immortal time bias in observational studies. *Am J Respir Crit Care Med* 2003;**168**:49–53.

116 Sin DD, Golmohammadi K, Jacobs P. Cost-effectiveness of inhaled corticosteroids for chronic obstructive pulmonary disease according to disease severity. *Am J Med* 2004;**116**: 325–31.

117 Ramsey SD, Berry K, Etzioni R *et al*. Cost effectiveness of

lung-volume-reduction surgery for patients with severe emphysema. *N Engl J Med* 2003;**348**:2092–102.

118 Oostenbrink JB, Rutten-van Molken MP, Al MJ *et al*. One-year cost-effectiveness of tiotropium versus ipratropium to treat chronic obstructive pulmonary disease. *Eur Respir J* 2004;**23**:241–9.

119 Cooper JD, Trulock EP, Triantafillou AN *et al*. Bilateral pneumonectomy (volume reduction) for chronic obstructive pulmonary disease. New York: 74th Annual Meeting of the American Association for Thoracic Surgery, 1994.

120 Miller JI Jr, Lee RB, Mansour KA. Lung volume reduction surgery: lessons learned. *Ann Thorac Surg* 1996;**61**:1464–8; discussion 1468–9.

121 Bagley PH, Davis SM, O'Shea M *et al*. Lung volume reduction surgery at a community hospital: program development and outcomes. *Chest* 1997;**111**:1552–9.

122 Bingisser R, Zollinger A, Hauser M *et al*. Bilateral volume reduction surgery for diffuse pulmonary emphysema by video-assisted thoracoscopy. *J Thorac Cardiovasc Surg* 1996; **112**:875–82.

123 Brenner M, Yusen R, McKenna R Jr *et al*. Lung volume reduction surgery for emphysema. *Chest* 1996;**110**:205–18.

124 Cooper JD, Patterson GA. Lung-volume reduction surgery for severe emphysema. *Chest Surg Clin North Am* 1995;**5**:815–31.

125 Cooper JD, Patterson GA, Sundaresan RS *et al*. Results of 150 consecutive bilateral lung volume reduction procedures in patients with severe emphysema. *J Thorac Cardiovasc Surg* 1996;**112**:1319–29; discussion 1329–30.

126 Cooper JD, Patterson GA. Lung volume reduction surgery for severe emphysema. *Semin Thorac Cardiovasc Surg* 1996; **8**:52–60.

127 Daniel TM, Chan BB, Bhaskar V *et al*. Lung volume reduction surgery: case selection, operative technique, and clinical results. *Ann Surg* 1996;**223**:526–31; discussion 532–533.

128 Kotloff RM, Tino G, Bavaria JE *et al*. Bilateral lung volume reduction surgery for advanced emphysema: a comparison of median sternotomy and thoracoscopic approaches. *Chest* 1996;**110**:1399–406.

129 Argenziano M, Moazami N, Thomashow B *et al*. Extended indications for lung volume reduction surgery in advanced emphysema. *Ann Thorac Surg* 1996;**62**:1588–97.

130 National Emphysema Treatment Trial Research Group. Rationale and design of the National Emphysema Treatment Trial: a prospective randomized trial of lung volume reduction surgery. *Chest* 1999;**116**:1750–61.

131 National Emphysema Treatment Trial Research Group. Patients at high risk of death after lung-volume-reduction surgery. *N Engl J Med* 2001;**345**:1075–83.

132 Fishman A, Martinez F, Naunheim K *et al*. A randomized trial comparing lung-volume-reduction surgery with medical therapy for severe emphysema. *N Engl J Med* 2003; **348**:2059–73.

133 Gross CP, Anderson GF, Powe NR. The relation between funding by the National Institutes of Health and the burden of disease. *N Engl J Med* 1999;**340**:1881–7.

CHAPTER 65
Pharmacoepidemiology of COPD

Joan B. Soriano

Pharmacoepidemiology is the study of the effects of drugs on disease and its determinants in large numbers of population by means of observational data. The pharmacoepidemiology of chronic obstructive pulmonary disease (COPD) has flourished recently, as a hypothesis-generating method. Ahead of ongoing randomized controlled trials, associations such as the increased mortality in COPD users of short-acting anticholinergics or the increased survival in COPD users of inhaled corticosteroids were formulated from pharmacoepidemiological studies. Standardization of methods and replication of single studies by independent investigators in other populations are needed. However, because of the absence of randomization intrinsic in any observational research, the advantages and limitations of these studies, and the interpretation of the direction and magnitude of their results are of great importance. Whenever possible, confirmation of results in carefully conducted randomized controlled trials in COPD patients is needed.

Introduction

Radical is the vision of Sackett *et al.* 'to keep up with the clinical literature, doctors should discard at once all articles on treatment that are not randomized trials' [1]. However, clinicians have long recognized the value of non-experimental research. Quoting Sir Austin Bradford Hill, one of the developers of the randomized trial methodology: 'Any belief that the randomized controlled trial (RCT) is the only way in medical research would mean not only that the pendulum had swung too far but that it had swung off its hook' [2]. The concordance of results of large clinical trials with well-conducted observational studies and meta-analyses of smaller RCTs, and its predictive power, has been the subject of recent reviews [3,4]. Some of the strengths of observational evidence versus RCTs include large numbers of real-life patients and not pure non-representative case

patients, and particularly the inclusion of elderly patients with additional comorbidities, often excluded in clinical research. Duration of follow-up can be also longer, and power to detect rare adverse events is greater.

Clinicians have often considered COPD as a 'Cinderella' disease, unattractive and self-inflicted, with little to offer and even less to expect. However, the contrary is true for respiratory epidemiologists, for whom COPD is indeed a 'dream' disease. COPD is a disease with a huge and increasing burden in society, affecting women as well as men, in developed and developing countries, and the age at COPD diagnosis is becoming younger. To date, respiratory epidemiology has not been as comprehensively developed as cancer or cardiovascular epidemiology. In clinical research, COPD has also been hindered by a shortage of large decisive trials involving tens of thousands of individuals. The clinical epidemiology of COPD is comprehensively presented elsewhere in this book (see Chapter 10); however, the study of beneficial effects (efficacy and effectiveness) and adverse effects (safety) of respiratory drugs in general, and of COPD drugs in particular, has not been well covered in respiratory clinical trials to date. Ultimate reasons for this are beyond the scope of this chapter, but most likely include: nihilism of the condition by patients and their doctors, an adaptation phenomenon in COPD patients similar to other long-lasting chronic conditions, the natural history of COPD *per se*, confusion regarding tobacco as the overwhelming cause but with other causative risk factors involved, and a difficulty to set thresholds for diagnosis and severity grading. Adding insult to injury, the historical lack of interest in COPD research is notorious compared with less severe, less common diseases of worldwide distribution. Gross *et al.* [5] identified COPD as an important example of the disproportionate lack of research funding provided by the US National Institutes of Health with relation to the burden of disease for society. Compared with AIDS, breast cancer, diabetes mellitus and dementia, all of which received relatively generous funding, research on perinatal conditions, peptic ulcer and COPD (the worst of them all) was underfunded.

Pharmacoepidemiology, the discipline that deals with the study of the effects of drugs in large numbers of individuals by means of observational data [6,7], seems to lead the way in COPD research ahead of largely absent or ongoing clinical trial data. In a recent comprehensive review of respiratory epidemiology in Europe [8], the term pharmacoepidemiology was not mentioned, and a search in Medline (October 2005) for the terms 'COPD' and 'pharmacoepidemiology' produced only four hits.

It has been difficult to study COPD medications until recently, as most drugs licensed for COPD are extensions of drugs developed to treat asthma or other conditions. Often, general practitioners apply sensible practical criteria when managing COPD patients. During the early 1990s, as no therapeutic options were available to manage their COPD patients other than advice to quit smoking, oxygen therapy and short-acting bronchodilators, general practitioners and primary care doctors started to try interventions that were successful in asthma. The pharmacoepidemiological study of this sensible approach by several research groups in different countries has created a recent effervescence of observational data in COPD and drugs. As highlighted in two recent editorials, observational studies are hypothesis-generating, and these hypotheses can be later confirmed (or rejected) in other observational independent studies or newly conducted trials [9,10]. Finally, RCTs are not unbiased, contrary to common assumptions. The recent large 1-year RCTs of combination therapy in COPD [11,12] have clearly shown differential drop-out rates, with large withdrawal numbers in placebo groups complicating interpretation and likely producing an underestimation of treatment effects. Therefore, pharmacoepidemiological studies, which allow for larger and more inclusive cohorts with longer durations of follow-up, could complement and help to interpret findings from RCTs. Consistency in the direction and magnitude of outcomes by independent researchers in different populations of patients is the real power of pharmacoepidemiology.

Asthma pharmacoepidemiology

To expand on COPD pharmacoepidemiology later, it is necessary to briefly mention that there is already extensive literature on the pharmacoepidemiology of asthma [13]. In spite of more than 30 years of asthma RCTs, some outcomes are difficult to assess with the RCT methodology [14]. In particular, asthma mortality and exacerbations have escaped trialists for years. It was not until recently that the beneficial effects of low-dose inhaled corticosteroids

(ICS) in preventing asthma deaths was demonstrated [15]. In addition to these Canadian findings, results have been replicated in the UK [16]. Similar beneficial results were also reported for use of low-dose ICS in preventing asthma hospitalizations [17–19]. The pharmacoepidemiology of asthma has recently been reviewed elsewhere [20].

Methodological issues when conducting/assessing COPD pharmacoepidemiology

To date, a number of databases have been explored to conduct COPD pharmacoepidemiology, including the Saskatchewan, Alberta and Ontario databases in Canada, the General Practice Research Database (GPRD) and UK Mediplus in the UK, Lovelace BCBS and Veteran Affairs in the USA, and Pharmo in the Netherlands. Collaborations pooling and comparing several of these databases are being established [21]. There are a number of challenges when conducting pharmacoepidemiological studies. Ideally, protocols with observational data should reflect the situation of a randomized clinical trial. A list of items (Table 65.1), not to be considered in comprehensive detail, should help the reader to develop greater awareness when conducting or assessing COPD pharmacoepidemiology.

Strategies of differential diagnosis of COPD/exclusion of asthma

The ability to differentiate COPD from asthma or other conditions is obviously critical. The effectiveness of ICS has been very well established in asthma, but it is the subject of debate in COPD. Thus, because the inclusion of asthma patients may exaggerate the effectiveness of respiratory medications in COPD studies, the study population must have clear criteria to identify COPD and exclude asthma

Table 65.1 Challenges when conducting/assessing COPD pharmacoepidemiology.

Strategies of differential diagnosis of COPD/exclusion of asthma
Confounding by indication
Reference groups: matching or restriction?
Time: date of clinical incidence of COPD, right- and left-truncation, censoring, rates, immortal time period
Drug exposure: onset, chronic, regular treatment
Dose–response relationships
Biases
Comorbidities
Main outcome and endpoints
Statistical analysis

patients. In particular, definitions and criteria based on physician's reported diagnosis, drug treatment and age must be carefully combined to optimize the diagnosis of COPD. GOLD and other COPD international guidelines use descriptions rather than definitions of COPD, and the challenge that a clinician faces with an individual patient is magnified when using observational data. However, some clinicians consider that the relevance of this misdiagnosis is exaggerated, as it seems much more likely that COPD patients may be classified as 'asthmatic' than asthmatics falsely being labelled as having COPD, although evidence to support this statement is scarce. Several strategies used to differentiate COPD from asthma in observational data research include: age restriction above 50 years or older thresholds; and primary care physician-diagnosed patients or patients discharged from hospital with a primary diagnosis compatible with COPD. However, it is important not to select a population with little resemblance to the target population, as the introduction of inappropriate exclusion criteria will create bias. Moreover, it is advisable to conduct validation studies of individual COPD definitions [22–25].

Confounding by indication

Confounding by indication is a major source of bias, perhaps the most important in pharmacoepidemiology. It is also referred to as confounding by severity, confounding by indication for a prescription, indication bias or channelling [26].

Confounding by indication is caused by the absence of randomization in the allocation of treatment, inherent in observational research. It exists when patients who receive different treatments also differ in their risk of adverse outcomes, independent of the treatment received [27]. In general, confounding by indication occurs when an observed association between a drug and an outcome is caused by the underlying illness or its severity, and not to any effect of the drug. In simple terms, patients with a disease who are treated with drug A would be expected to be sicker than those not so treated. In this case the risk factor under study is the drug and the outcome variable under study is the clinical variable that the drug is supposed to change.

In COPD, confounding by indication can be controlled by proper adjustment for underlying severity when available, such as previous use of health resources (i.e. history of COPD hospitalizations or emergency room visits), and the profile of use of other drugs for COPD.

Another type of bias, protopathic bias [28], can be found in COPD studies. Although related to confounding by indication, it is slightly different. It may occur when a particular manoeuvre is started, stopped or changed because of the baseline manifestation caused by a disease or other particular event. Then the event happens to be in the causal pathway between an exposure and the event. In COPD, protopathic bias occurs when a drug is used both as chronic and acute therapy. To avoid exposure misclassification in pharmacoepidemiological studies, some advocate using time-dependent analysis. However, respiratory drugs such as bronchodilators and steroids are also used during acute exacerbations. Thus, by using a time-dependent analysis, these drugs could be incorrectly shown to increase morbidity and mortality, which in reality is related to exacerbation itself.

Reference groups: matching or restriction?

It has been standard in respiratory epidemiology to compare users of one drug versus non-users of that drug, for instance COPD patients with or without prescriptions for ICS. However, it is possible that patients with a disease treated with drug A may be sicker than those not so treated with drug A. A partial solution is to compare patients with a disease who are treated with drug A versus those treated with drug B (i.e. the recommended treatment by COPD national or international clinical guidelines). Other solutions for the choice of reference groups are matching by demographic variables at baseline or restricting the analyses to only male, only older COPD patients or only those without a clinical suspicion of asthma, etc.

Time: date of clinical incidence of COPD, right- and left-truncation, censoring, rates, immortal time period

A recent report has underlined the major problems that can potentially occur when time to different events and outcomes, and different designs, are applied in COPD pharmacoepidemiology [29]. The issue on time control relates to the choice of design: cohort or case–control (Fig. 65.1). In addition, whether the events of interest are acute, or whether regular treatment is required to attain the effectiveness under study, needs to be considered with respect to drug exposure. Drug exposure also affects the choice of the reference group and whether this group can include patients who do not currently use a given drug but who used them previously, or patients who are restricted to other drugs or classes of drugs. With these classifications and the question of timing of use, one must then be concerned about issues of exposure misclassification. For instance, patients who are not using a drug might be wrongly classified as users and vice versa. The exposure and its timing will also relate to the analysis of the data and, particularly, whether exposure is fixed, such as for the intention-to-treat approach, or time-dependent, such as that used in nested case–control analysis.

The COPD patients under study may be incident (newly diagnosed patients) or prevalent (patients well into their

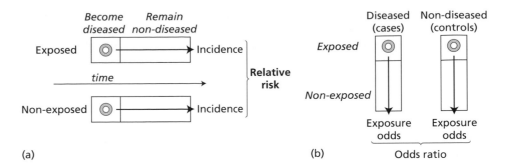

Figure 65.1 Basic analytical approach in: (a) cohort study; and (b) case–control study.

disease). It has to be determined whether patients at time zero already have had COPD for some time or have already been exposed to the drug under study. It may be preferable to use incident cohorts where new treatment or new disease defines time zero for the cohorts. If this is not possible, the duration of prior COPD or prior drug use should be examined and accounted for in the analysis. The choice of time zero is important and may be taken as the date of first COPD diagnosis, the date of the first hospitalization for COPD, the date of any hospitalization for COPD or the first time a drug was used. Finally, in all cohort studies that involve time-dependent exposure, immortal time should be explored. Immortal time periods, defined by follow-up times during which patients cannot, by definition, incur the outcome, have to be identified and accounted for with a proper analysis. In addition, studies that improperly exclude immortal time or do not account for it in the proper exposure group should be identified and assessed with respect to bias. As a rule of thumb, the duration of the immortal time period should equal the duration of the window of drug exposure.

Drug exposure: onset or chronic regular treatment

It is particularly relevant whether exposure is selected at cohort entry or at the time of the outcome under study. When studying harmful drug effects and acute events, the closer the assessment of drug exposure to the outcome under study seems fundamental, and a nested case–control is the design of choice. However, when searching for unanticipated beneficial effects of chronic regular drug treatment, the cohort design mirroring a RCT is to be considered first.

Dose–response relationship

Dose–response is one of the 10 Hill criteria for causality [30]. Ideally, once an association between a drug and a COPD outcome is considered causal, searching for a dose–response or a threshold indicates consistency and adds further evidence of causality.

Bias

There are three major types of bias in epidemiological research: selection bias, information bias and confounding. Selection bias includes referral bias, self-selection bias, prevalence study bias and protopathic bias. Information bias can be of differential misclassification (recall bias, detection bias) or non-differential misclassification; and there are many types of confounding. Confounding by indication will need to be tackled appropriately in any COPD pharmacoepidemiological study.

Comorbidity

Because COPD is not only a respiratory disorder but also a systemic disease, and because smoking has non-COPD effects, it is common that COPD patients have comorbid conditions associated. A modified Charlson comorbidity index helps quantitatively and qualitatively to assess imbalances in the distribution of comorbidities between drug exposure groups [31].

Main outcome and endpoints

To date, most RCTs in COPD have been powered to pulmonary function [32]. Observational studies permit observation of more relevant endpoints for the clinician and in particular to the patient, such as survival or time to next exacerbation.

Statistical analysis

The choice of statistical analysis, depending on the study design, cohort or case–control, is an important methodological aspect that requires extensive discussion [33].

Beneficial or adverse effects of COPD medications in epidemiological studies

A number of interventions in COPD have been assessed using pharmacoepidemiological methods. Outcomes of observational studies on antibiotics, oral theophyllines, anticholinergics, N-acetylcysteine, long-acting β_2-agonists (LABA), ICS and combination treatment are summarized below. It is important to note the scarcity of available data on COPD pharmacoepidemiology, most of which has only been available from the late 1990s.

Antibiotics

It is relatively surprising that after the original RCTs on the efficacy of antibiotics to treat or prevent exacerbations of COPD [34], little has been published regarding their effectiveness in the real world [35]. A recent report [36], from a population-based retrospective cohort study in Ontario, Canada, determined the association between outpatient use of oral antibiotics and 30-day all-cause mortality following hospitalization in a group of elderly COPD patients. Outpatient use of antibiotics was associated with a significant reduction in the 30-day mortality following hospitalization (odds ratio [OR] 0.83; 95% confidence interval [CI], 0.75–0.92). Use of macrolides had the lowest relative odds for mortality (OR 0.58; 95% CI, 0.47–0.73), while use of fluoroquinolones had the worst relative odds (OR 0.98; 95% CI, 0.84–1.15). However, another report from the same group identified an increased risk of COPD hospital readmission with antibiotic use (relative risk [RR] 1.17; 95% CI, 1.10–1.23) [37].

Oral theophyllines

Available evidence investigating the effect of oral theophyllines on COPD mortality, from well-conducted RCTs or from observational studies, is too scarce to draw any meaningful conclusions [38].

Anticholinergics

A paper by Benayoun *et al.* [39] on the concomitant use of ipratropium bromide and inhaled β_2-agonists in a single inhaler reported that it did not significantly alter the treatment of COPD and resulted in appreciable cost savings relative to using both drugs separately. Although an initial epidemiological study indicated an absence of increased mortality in COPD patients [40], there is open controversy regarding the safety of short-acting anticholinergics. Studies comparing short-acting combinations (ipratropium plus albuterol or metaproterenol) with short-acting β_2-agonists or anticholinergic monotherapies may have been too small or too short to conclude anything about COPD mortality and survival [41–43].

In UK patients with asthma and COPD [44], treatment with ipratropium bromide at discharge from hospital was associated with an increased risk of death from asthma (OR 4.04; 95% CI, 1.47–11.13) and from COPD (OR 7.75; 95% CI, 2.21–27.14), even after adjusting for peak flow, cardiovascular comorbidity, smoking history and age at onset of asthma. In Denmark [45], ipratropium bromide was associated with a relative risk of increased mortality of 2.0 (95% CI, 1.5–2.6) for COPD and 3.6 (95% CI, 1.8–7.1) for asthma patients. After adjustment for confounding factors, including forced expiratory volume in 1 s (FEV_1), smoking habits, asthma medication and presence of cor pulmonale, the relative risk for COPD remained increased at 1.6 for COPD (95% CI, 1.2–2.1) and 2.4 for asthma (95% CI, 1.2–5.0). A recent report from the 5-year Lung Health Study RCT [46], has shown that deaths and hospitalizations for cardiovascular disease and coronary artery disease were more common in the smoking intervention plus ipratropium bromide, than in the smoking intervention plus placebo inhaler group, and the differences approached statistical significance. Later correspondence has not yet clarified this finding [47,48]. Garcia-Aymerich *et al.* [49], in a prospective cohort of 340 COPD patients recruited during an admission for an exacerbation in four tertiary hospitals in Barcelona (Spain) followed for 1 year, reported that taking anticholinergic drugs was associated with an increased risk of COPD readmission of 1.81 (95% CI, 1.11–2.94). The authors concluded that the excess risk associated with anticholinergic drugs might be partially caused by confounding by indication. A recent reanalysis of this study with additional control for confounding by indication [50], reduced but did not negate this association. Residual confounding may still account for part of the remaining excess risk, but true adverse effects of this treatment cannot be excluded.

Regarding long-acting anticholinergics, five RCTs of the once-daily, inhaled long-acting anticholinergic bronchodilator tiotropium compared with either placebo or ipratropium bromide are available, including 3574 patients with moderate to severe COPD [51–55]. However, these trials are too short and underpowered to allow evaluation of the effect of tiotropium on all-cause mortality, and no observational studies are yet available.

N-acetylcysteine

Several epidemiological studies have assessed the effect of oral antioxidant N-acetylcysteine (NAC) in the prevention of rehospitalization for COPD exacerbations. In the Dutch Pharmo database [56], it was observed that NAC reduced the risk of COPD rehospitalization up to 1 year by approximately 30% and that this risk reduction was dose dependent. This positive result was consistent with three previous

6-month RCTs [57–59], and two recent meta-analyses of RCTs [60,61]. Methodological concerns about the account of immortal time and bias in the Pharmo study were recently raised [62]. The Bronchitis Randomized On NAC Cost-Utility Study (BRONCUS) [63] is an ongoing 3-year, randomized, double-blind, placebo-controlled, parallel group study in 10 European countries designed to assess the effectiveness of NAC in altering the decline in FEV_1, exacerbation rate and quality of life in patients with moderate to severe COPD.

Long-acting β₂-agonists

The use of LABAs has caused some concern about serious adverse events and mortality in COPD and in adult asthmatics [64]. Many COPD patients have a number of cardiovascular comorbidities, and the specificity of LABA effects in the β₂-adrenonoceptor is not so specific or selective in practice, and therefore could cause cardiac events.

Only one observational study, the Serevent Nationwide Surveillance Study [65], indicated a small non-significant trend towards increased mortality with salmeterol and this was in patients with asthma. However, in a posterior, large prescription-event monitoring study of 15 407 patients given salmeterol and observed for a minimum of 1 year [66], no evidence was found that salmeterol contributed to death in any of the patients. On careful examination of the clinical records, all deaths appeared to have been due to natural causes, suggesting that advanced age and severity of disease were the most likely factors contributing to mortality in the population studied.

In an UK GPRD study [67], salmeterol use was not associated with an increase in short-term mortality compared with ipratropium bromide and theophylline.

In a case–control study of admissions to the intensive care unit for asthma in 14 major hospitals within the Wessex region in 1992, the use of salmeterol by patients with chronic severe asthma or COPD was not associated with an increased risk of a near-fatal attack of asthma or COPD [68].

In a meta-analysis of all RCTs of salmeterol versus placebo in COPD [69], treatment with salmeterol ranging from 12 to 52 weeks showed no increased risk of cardiovascular adverse events compared with placebo (RR 1.03; 95% CI, 0.8–1.3), and both groups had a similar incidence of cardiovascular events (8%), including cardiovascular deaths. The conclusions that salmeterol does not increase mortality in patients with COPD was also shared in a recent review [70]. Finally, in another meta-analysis, the impact of LABAs as a drug class on COPD mortality was also assessed [71]. Nine randomized placebo-controlled trials of LABAs with 3-month or longer follow-up were identified,

including 4198 patients with moderate to severe COPD. No significant difference in all-cause mortality was observed (RR 0.76; 95% CI, 0.39–1.48).

Inhaled corticosteroids

Perhaps the most active area in pharmacoepidemiological research today is the study of the observational effects of ICS in COPD, involving several groups worldwide. Although all RCTs to date and most respiratory physicians are interested in lung function, COPD patients are not. As reviewed by van der Molen *et al.* [72], COPD patients are mainly interested in breathlessness in daily life, not being able to control breathlessness during an exacerbation, their symptoms getting worse, catching a cold and, above all, staying alive. It is appropriate to review randomized experimental evidence on exacerbations and survival at this point. A meta-analysis of published results of RCTs reported that there was a risk reduction in COPD exacerbation rate of 30% (RR 0.70; 95% CI, 0.58–0.74) and a 16% non-significant reduction in mortality in the five trials that measured this outcome (RR 0.84; 95% CI, 0.60–1.18) [73]. Although these trials were not designed or powered to detect differences in survival or COPD rehospitalization, this meta-analysis indicates a strong signal for unexpected beneficial effects of ICS on these outcomes.

Sin and Tu [37] used the Ontario health databases in Canada and found that elderly patients (65 years or older) who received at least one dispensation of ICS within 90 days of hospital discharge had a 26% lower adjusted risk for respiratory hospitalization and all-cause mortality than did those who did not receive these medications (RR 0.74; 95% CI, 0.71–0.78).

The results of Sin and Tu on reduced rehospitalization or death after a first COPD hospitalization associated with ICS were replicated in the UK GPRD population [74]. Additionally, an association with survival in COPD patients prescribed with combination treatment of fluticasone proprionate (an ICS) and salmeterol xinafoate (a LABA), was observed in UK COPD patients diagnosed at primary care [75]. Survival at year 3 was significantly greater in fluticasone proprionate and/or salmeterol users (78.6%) than in the reference group (63.6%). After adjusting for confounders, the survival advantage observed was highest in combined users of fluticasone proprionate and salmeterol (RR 0.48; 95% CI, 0.31–0.73), followed by users of fluticasone proprionate alone (RR 0.62; 95% CI, 0.45–0.85) and non-significantly by regular users of salmeterol alone (RR 0.79; 95% CI, 0.58–1.07) versus the reference group made up of users of short-acting bronchodilators.

In a second study from Sin and Man [76], administrative databases in Alberta, Canada were used to evaluate the

Table 65.2 Summary of methods in inhaled corticosteroids observational studies focused on survival.

	Sin & Tu [19]	Soriano et al. [75]	Sin & Man [76]	Soriano et al. [74]	Suissa [29], Bourbeau et al. [77] and Suissa [78]	Fan et al. [79]
n	22 620	4665	6740	4263	997, 1742 and 3524	8033
Period	1992–97	1990–98	1994–98	1990–98	1980–87, 1990–97 and 1990–97	1997–99
Source	Ontario, Canada	GPRD, UK	Alberta, Canada	GPRD, UK	Saskatchewan, Canada	ACQUIP trial, USA
Age	65+ years	50+ years	65+ years	50+ years	55+ years	45+ years
Design	Cohort	Cohort and nested case–control	Cohort	Cohort	Case–control and cohort	Cohort
Follow-up	1 year	3 years	3 years	1 year	1 year and 3 years	Mean of 544 days
COPD definition	ICD-9 codes with OLD	COPD compatible codes	ICD-9 codes with OLD	COPD compatible codes	Subjects newly treated for a likely COPD Dx	ICD-9 codes with OLD
Validation study	None	Yes	None	Yes	Yes	None
Asthma exclusion criteria	Did not include ICD-9 code 493	Confounding variable	Did not include ICD-9 code 493	Confounding variable	Asthma drugs prior 5-year	Only in sensitivity analysis, excluding all with an ICD-9 code for asthma (493.x) in the previous year
Drug exposure	One or more prescriptions of ICS within 90 days after discharge	3+ prescriptions of ICS within 6 months	None, low, medium and high ICS after discharge	One or more prescriptions of ICS within 90 days after discharge	Various	Various, including average, low and high dose, and recent use
Reference group	No ICS	Regular SABD/no ICS and no LABA	No ICS	Regular SABD/no ICS and no LABA	None (nested case–control), and regular SABD/no ICS	No ICS
Adjustment by COPD severity	Charlson comorbidity Use of other medications ER visits for COPD or asthma within last year	Charlson comorbidity Use of OCS	Charlson comorbidity Admission to ICU Use of other medications	Charlson comorbidity Use of OCS	Medications prior 1 year Number of CV risk factors Occurrence of COPD hospitalizations	Pulmonary medications prior 90 days Charlson comorbidity Prior outpatient visit for COPD Prior COPD hospitalizations
Immortal time period	Yes, all persons who died within 30 days after discharge	Yes, all deaths and COPD-rehospitalizations within 6 months after Dx	None	Yes, all deaths and COPD rehospitalizations within 90 days after discharge	None (nested case–control), and variable in other designs	Yes, all persons who died within 90 days after discharge
Smoking information	None	Current, ex- and non-smokers	None	Current, ex- and non-smokers	None	None

ACQUIP, Ambulatory Care Quality Improvement Project; CV, cardiovascular; Dx, diagnosis; ER, emergency room; GPRD, General Practice Research Database; ICS, inhaled corticosteroids; LABA, long-acting β_2-agonist; OCS, oral corticosteroids; OLD, obstructive lung disease; SABD, short-acting bronchodilators.

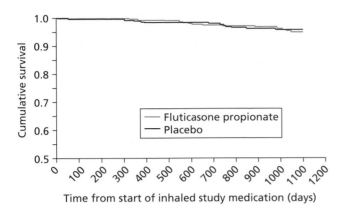

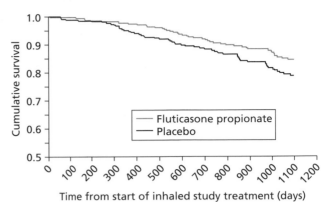

Figure 65.2 Survival in the Inhaled Steroids in Obstructive Lung Disease in Europe (ISOLDE) randomized controlled trial (RCT). Time to death during 3 years of follow-up of patients while receiving study treatment. (From Waterhouse *et al.* [82] [abstract], kindly forwarded from Professor S. Burge.)

Figure 65.3 Survival in the Inhaled Steroids in Obstructive Lung Disease in Europe (ISOLDE) randomized controlled trial (RCT). Time to death during 3 years of follow-up including all deaths obtained from UK central registers. (From Waterhouse *et al.* [82] [abstract], kindly forwarded from Professor S. Burge.)

long-term effects of ICS among elderly COPD patients and to determine whether the survival benefits were dose dependent. Patients who received at least one dispensation of ICS during follow-up (average follow-up 32 months) had a 25% relative reduction in the risk for all-cause mortality (RR 0.75; 95% CI, 0.68–0.82) compared with those who did not receive any ICS during follow-up. Patients on medium (501–1000 µg/day beclometasone equivalent) or high-dose therapy (more than 1 mg/day beclometasone) had lower risks for mortality than those on low doses (RR 0.77; 95% CI, 0.69–0.86 for low dose; RR 0.48; 95% CI, 0.37–0.63 for medium dose; and RR 0.55; 95% CI, 0.44–0.69 for high dose). The McGill group in Montreal has challenged these results [29,77,78] and found no association with survival, or mortality, of ICS in the Saskatchewan COPD population. Additionally, Fan *et al.* [79] reported in a time-dependent study of outpatients with COPD, adherence to ICS use was not associated with a decreased risk of mortality.

To date, groups determining outcomes of rehospitalization and mortality in COPD populations are using somewhat heterogeneous methods (Table 65.2). This heterogeneity might explain some or most of the differences in direction and magnitude of results. Nevertheless, any possible beneficial effects of ICS should be balanced against any adverse effects in the acute or long-term management in COPD [80].

Interestingly, no past RCTs mentioned in the meta-analysis of RCTs [73] had been powered to detect survival. However, reanalysis of old RCTs might provide further insights into the possible beneficial effects of ICS in COPD. In the Inhaled Steroids in Obstructive Lung Disease in Europe (ISOLDE) trial, the results of the 3-year study of 751 patients with moderate to severe COPD randomized

to the ICS fluticasone proprionate or placebo reported no differences in survival as per the protocol (Fig. 65.2) [81]. However, when an extensive search of life status for missing and withdrawn individuals from the protocol was undertaken, including searching national UK death registries, a survival advantage in the fluticasone proprionate arm was suggested, although not statistically significant ($P = 0.069$) (Fig. 65.3) [82].

To help settle the controversy on the effect of ICS and combination treatment in COPD survival, and in the absence of a higher level of evidence coming from new RCTs, yet more sophisticated analyses of old RCTs are worth exploring. Of interest, a new tool called patient-level pooled analysis is currently available. A pooled analysis follows the principle of traditional meta-analysis, but instead of grouping published results, it collects the raw data at the individual level, creates a new database, and analyses data as if they were a new RCT. Although patient-level pooled analyses are more difficult to conduct than those based on published data, they are more desirable, because patient-level pooled analyses are more powerful and less susceptible to methodological biases than those that rely exclusively on published reports [83]. Results of the pooled analysis known as Inhaled Steroid Effect Evaluation in COPD (ISEEC) have recently become available [84]. ISEEC aimed to re-analyse original data at the individual level from the seven available large long-term COPD RCTs with ICS or placebo that had life status recorded, including the Lung Health Study 2 (LHS-2), Copenhagen City Lung Study (CCLS), Inhaled Steroids in Obstructive Lung Disease in Europe (ISOLDE), European Respiratory Society Study on Chronic Obstructive Pulmonary Disease (EUROSCOP), TRial of Inhaled STeroids ANd long-acting β_2-agonists (TRISTAN), Szafranski's trial, and Calverley's trial. The most important and novel finding of ISEEC was that therapy with ICS was associated with a 27% reduction in all-cause mortality among individuals with stable COPD (adjusted hazard ratio [HR] 0.73; 95% CI, 0.55–0.96). The beneficial effects of these medications appeared to be especially pronounced in female COPD patients (adjusted HR 0.46), former smokers (adjusted HR 0.60) and in those with a baseline postbronchodilator FEV_1 of less than 60% predicted (adjusted HR 0.67). The findings of ISEEC might be considered surprising in terms of direction and magnitude, as each of the seven RCTs included did not identify this survival signal per se. ISEEC adds weight and consistency to the direction and magnitude of the hypothesis of beneficial associations of ICS in COPD formulated earlier via observational pharmacoepidemiological studies.

One important lesson for ongoing and future RCTs is that withdrawn individuals tend to be very informative. Past COPD RCTs did not study individuals withdrawn from study protocols as they were not contributing to respiratory function measurements. The Towards a Revolution in COPD Health (TORCH) study is an RCT designed to investigate the long-term effects of the salmeterol/fluticasone proprionate combination (Advair/Seretide) at a strength of 50/500 μg twice daily compared with salmeterol alone, fluticasone proprionate alone, or placebo, on survival of COPD subjects over 3 years of treatment [85]. The primary analysis is a difference in all-cause mortality rates in patients randomized to salmeterol/fluticasone proprionate combination versus placebo. The secondary efficacy endpoints include rate of COPD exacerbations and health status. Other secondary endpoints include other mortality and exacerbation endpoints, requirement for long-term oxygen therapy, and clinic lung function. Safety endpoints include adverse events, with additional information on bone fractures. TORCH is a multicentre randomized double-blind parallel-group placebo-controlled study conducted in 45 countries worldwide of approximately 6200 male and female outpatients aged 40–80 years with a baseline FEV_1 of less than 60% of predicted normal, an established clinical history of COPD (as per the European Respiratory Society [ERS] consensus statement), current or ex-smokers with a smoking history of at least 10 pack-years, poor reversibility of airflow obstruction (defined as less than 10% increase in FEV_1 as a percentage of normal predicted 30 min after inhalation of 400 μg salbutamol via metered dose inhaler [MDI] and spacer), and baseline FEV_1/forced vital capacity (FVC) ratio less than or equal to 70%. The first TORCH patient was recruited in September 2000, and results should be available early in 2006.

In 2002, it was announced a new large-scale 4-year study to look at the impact of long-term treatment with the long-acting anticholinergic bronchodilator tiotropium bromide (Spiriva) on lung function in COPD. The Understanding Potential Long-term Impacts on Function with Tiotropium (UPLIFT) trial will enrol up to 6000 patients in 37 countries and examine whether tiotropium bromide reduces the rate of lung function decline over time. It will also assess quality of life, exacerbations, hospitalizations and mortality [86]. The inclusion criteria of UPLIFT include a clinical diagnosis of COPD, age 40 years or older, smoking history of 10 pack-years or more, a maximal postbronchodilator FEV_1 of less than 70% of predicted and an FEV_1/FVC of less than 70%, and the ability to perform satisfactory spirometry. Patients are excluded if they had a respiratory infection or an exacerbation of COPD in the 4 weeks prior to screening, a history of asthma or pulmonary resection, used supplemental oxygen more than 12 h/day, or had a significant disease other than COPD that, in the opinion of the investigator, may influence the results of the study or the patient's ability to participate in the study. The presence or absence of reversibility to the bronchodilator was not an entry criterion in UPLIFT. Patients are permitted to continue using all previously prescribed respiratory medications other than inhaled anticholinergics, provided the prescriptions had not changed in the 6 weeks prior to randomization. Of interest, there are no restrictions for medications prescribed for treatment of exacerbations.

The ongoing TORCH and UPLIFT RCTs have a focus on mortality, the former being powered on it. Complete assessment of life status of all randomized patients during the entire period of follow-up is a necessity. Issues to interpret this intention-to-treat approach have been elegantly presented elsewhere and results are expected between 2006 and 2007 [87].

Future directions

Pharmacoepidemiology leads the way in COPD research, ahead of forthcoming COPD clinical trials data [33]. Data from clinical trials are classified as evidence A or B in the GOLD guidelines [88]. In the meantime, interpretation of pharmacoepidemiological studies, particularly on the direction and magnitude of survival results in COPD, has to be balanced with other sources of available data. The traditional skepticism towards observational evidence has to be put into perspective and its quality must be objectively assessed. Guidelines are now being presented on how to evaluate the quality of evidence from observational research [89]. To confirm or reject the effects of observational studies, standardization of methods, and of course independent replication by other researchers can help to clarify evidence C for GOLD and for the community. More good pharmacoepidemiology is needed, as well as more good RCTs. Eventually, randomized trials are the most robust tool to support and implement any medical intervention with solid experimental evidence. However, in COPD and other conditions, even with more and larger RCTs, outcomes in some disease endpoints and some rare adverse events will only be detected post-marketing by means of epidemiological and surveillance methods. The main problem interpreting pharmacoepidemiology – confounding by indication – will remain. It is a high price to pay but unavoidable because of the absence of randomization in observational research. Apart from the classic ways to deal with the problems described earlier, several alternative designs and analytical strategies have been proposed to deal with time-dependent variables, and specifically to avoid confounding by indication. Thus, case cross-over [90], G-estimation [91] and marginal structural [92] models might be considered for future studies in COPD patients. Other methods to be explored include multilevel analysis [93] and propensity score techniques [94]. On the latter, very recently a propensity score design within a UK pharmacoepidemniology cohort was reported [95] and its results add further evidence to the discussion on the effectiveness of ICS in COPD [96].

Future applications of meta-analysis [97] and pharmacogenetics [98] will still have a role in COPD. Short-term drug-associated serious events are more likely to be detected in selected COPD populations. Long-term genomics techniques can be incorporated into population data to map genetic risk factors for COPD and drug responses. Tissue specimens might be linked to clinical data in certain data resources like clinical trials, *ad hoc* cohorts, case registries, and cross-sectional and longitudinal population samples, giving a 'real world' perspective to COPD pharmacogenetics.

Finally, we must be aware that COPD pharmacoepidemiology is merely in its infancy, compared with a successful history in cardiovascular and cancer research for longer than 30 years, and even for at least 15 years in asthma pharmacoepidemiology. Most likely, old methods have to be adapted and perhaps new methods developed to study drugs in COPD by means of observational data. COPD has been a Cinderella disease for clinicians but should be considered a dream disease for respiratory epidemiologists. Perhaps, with time, COPD will be like Snow White. It has been kept in a long sleep by all sides, and now it is time to kiss it awake.

References

1 Sackett DL, Haynes RB, Guyatt GH, Tugwell PT. *Clinical Epidemiology: A Basic Science for Clinical Medicine*. Boston: Little Brown, 1985.

2 Hill AB. Reflections on the controlled trial. *Ann Rheum Dis* 1966;**25**:107–13.

3 Concato J, Shah N, Horwitz RI. Randomized, controlled trials, observational studies, and the hierarchy of research designs. *N Engl J Med* 2000;**342**:1887–92.

4 Benson K, Hartz AJ. A comparison of observational studies and randomized, controlled trials. *N Engl J Med* 2000;**342**:1878–86.

5 Gross CP, Anderson GF, Powe NR. The relation between funding by the National Institutes of Health and the burden of disease. *N Engl J Med* 1999;**340**:1881–7.

6 Strom BL. What is pharmacoepidemiology? In: Strom BL. *Pharmacoepidemiology*, 3rd edn. Chichester: John Wiley & Sons, 2000: 3–16.

7 Rothman KJ, Greenland S. *Modern Epidemiology*. Philadelphia: Lippincott-Raven, 1998.

8 Annesi-Maesano I, Gulsvik A, Viegi G, eds. Respiratory epidemiology in Europe. *Eur Respir Mon* 2000;**5**:15.

9 Vestbo J. Another piece of the inhaled corticosteroids-in-COPD puzzle. *Am J Respir Crit Care Med* 2001;**164**:514–5.

10 Calverley PM. Medical therapy for COPD: lessons from the real world. *Eur Respir J* 2002;**20**:797–8.

11 Calverley P, Pauwels R, Vestbo J *et al.* TRial of Inhaled STeroids ANd long-acting β$_2$-agonists study group. Combined salmeterol and fluticasone in the treatment of chronic obstructive pulmonary disease: a randomised controlled trial. *Lancet* 2003;**361**:449–56.

12 Szafranski W, Cukier A, Ramirez A *et al.* Efficacy and safety of budesonide/formoterol in the management of chronic obstructive pulmonary disease. *Eur Respir J* 2003;**21**:74–81.

13 Pearce N, Beasley R, Burgess C, Crane J, eds. *Asthma Epidemiology: Principles and Methods*. New York: Oxford University Press, 1998.

14 Van Ganse E. Use of computerized data in pharmacoepidemiology. *Therapie* 2000;**55**:123–6.

15 Suissa S, Ernst P, Benayoun S, Baltzan M, Cai B. Low-dose inhaled corticosteroids and the prevention of death from asthma. *N Engl J Med* 2000;**343**:332–6.

16 Lanes SF, Garcia Rodriguez LA, Huerta C. Respiratory medications and risk of asthma death. *Thorax* 2002;**57**:683–6.

17 Suissa S, Ernst P, Kezouh A. Regular use of inhaled corticosteroids and the long term prevention of hospitalisation for asthma. *Thorax* 2002;**57**:880–4.

18 Sin DD, Man SF. Low-dose inhaled corticosteroid therapy and risk of emergency department visits for asthma. *Arch Intern Med* 2002;**162**:1591–5.

19 Sin DD, Tu JV. Inhaled corticosteroid therapy reduces the risk of rehospitalization and all-cause mortality in elderly asthmatics. *Eur Respir J* 2001;**17**:380–5.

20 Suissa S, Ernst P. Inhaled corticosteroids: impact on asthma morbidity and mortality. *J Allergy Clin Immunol* 2001;**107**: 937–44.

21 van Staa TP, Cooper C, Leufkens HG, Lammers JW, Suissa S. The use of inhaled corticosteroids in the United Kingdom and the Netherlands. *Respir Med* 2003;**97**:578–85.

22 Rawson NS, Malcolm E. Validity of the recording of ischaemic heart disease and chronic obstructive pulmonary disease in the Saskatchewan health care datafiles. *Stat Med* 1995;**14**: 2627–43.

23 Barr RG, Herbstman J, Speizer FE, Camargo CA Jr. Validation of self-reported chronic obstructive pulmonary disease in a cohort study of nurses. *Am J Epidemiol* 2002;**155**:965–71.

24 Soriano JB, Maier WC, Visick G, Pride NB. Validation of general practitioner-diagnosed COPD in the UK General Practice Research Database. *Eur J Epidemiol* 2001;**17**:1075–80.

25 McKnight J, Scott A, Menzies D *et al*. A cohort study showed that health insurance databases were accurate to distinguish chronic obstructive pulmonary disease from asthma and classify disease severity. *J Clin Epidemiol* 2005;**58**:206–8.

26 Salas M, Hofman A, Stricker BH. Confounding by indication: an example of variation in the use of epidemiologic terminology. *Am J Epidemiol* 1999;**149**:981–3.

27 Collet JP, Boivin JF. Bias and confounding in pharmacoepidemiology. In: Strom BL, ed. *Pharmacoepidemiology*, 3rd edn. Chichester: John Wiley & Sons, 2000: 765–84.

28 Feinstein AR. *Clinical Epidemiology: The Architecture of Clinical Research*. Philadelphia, PA: Saunders, 1985.

29 Suissa S. Effectiveness of inhaled corticosteroids in COPD: immortal time bias in observational studies. *Am J Respir Crit Care Med* 2003;**168**:49–53.

30 Shakir SA, Layton D. Causal association in pharmacovigilance and pharmacoepidemiology: thoughts on the application of the Austin Bradford Hill criteria. *Drug Saf* 2002;**25**:467–71.

31 Deyo RA, Cherkin DC, Ciol MA. Adapting a clinical comorbidity index for use with ICD-9-CM administrative databases. *J Clin Epidemiol* 1992;**45**:613–29.

32 Fabbri L, Caramori G, Beghe B, Papi A, Ciaccia A. Chronic obstructive pulmonary disease international guidelines. *Curr Opin Pulm Med* 1998;**4**:76–84.

33 Burney P, Suissa S, Soriano JB *et al*. The pharmacoepidemiology of COPD: recent advances and methodological discussion. *Eur Respir J* 2003;**22**(Suppl 43):1–44.

34 Anthonisen NR, Manfreda J, Warren CP *et al*. Antibiotic therapy in exacerbations of chronic obstructive pulmonary disease. *Ann Intern Med* 1987;**106**:196–204.

35 Miravitlles M, Torres A. Antibiotics in exacerbations of COPD: lessons from the past. *Eur Respir J* 2004;**24**:896–7.

36 Sin DD, Tu JV. Outpatient antibiotic therapy and short-term mortality in elderly patients with chronic obstructive pulmonary disease. *Can Respir J* 2000;**7**:466–71.

37 Sin DD, Tu JV. Inhaled corticosteroids and the risk of mortality and readmission in elderly patients with chronic obstructive pulmonary disease. *Am J Respir Crit Care Med* 2001;**164**:580–4.

38 Ram FS, Jones PW, Castro AA *et al*. Oral theophylline for chronic obstructive pulmonary disease. *Cochrane Database Syst Rev* 2002:CD003902.

39 Benayoun S, Ernst P, Suissa S. The impact of combined inhaled bronchodilator therapy in the treatment of COPD. *Chest* 2001;**119**:85–92.

40 Sin DD, Tu JV. Lack of association between ipratropium bromide and mortality in elderly patients with chronic obstructive airway disease. *Thorax* 2000;**55**:194–7.

41 COMBIVENT Inhalation Aerosol Study Group. In chronic obstructive pulmonary disease, a combination of ipratropium and albuterol is more effective than either agent alone: an 85-day multicenter trial. *Chest* 1994;**105**:1411–9.

42 COMBIVENT Inhalation Solution Study Group. Routine nebulized ipratropium and albuterol together are better than either alone in COPD. *Chest* 1997;**112**:1514–21.

43 Tashkin DP, Ashutosh K, Bleecker ER *et al*. Comparison of the anticholinergic bronchodilator ipratropium bromide with metaproterenol in chronic obstructive pulmonary disease: a 90-day multi-center study. *Am J Med* 1986;**81**:81–90.

44 Guite HF, Dundas R, Burney PG. Risk factors for death from asthma, chronic obstructive pulmonary disease, and cardiovascular disease after a hospital admission for asthma. *Thorax* 1999;**54**:301–7.

45 Ringbaek T, Viskum K. Is there any association between inhaled ipratropium and mortality in patients with COPD and asthma? *Respir Med* 2003;**97**:264–72.

46 Anthonisen NR, Connett JE, Enright PL, Manfreda J. Hospitalizations and mortality in the Lung Health Study. *Am J Respir Crit Care Med* 2002;**166**:333–9.

47 Lanes S, Golisch W, Mikl J. Ipratropium and lung health study. *Am J Respir Crit Care Med* 2003;**167**:801.

48 Anthonisen NR, Manfreda J, Connett JE, Enright PL. Ipratropium and lung health study. *Am J Respir Crit Care Med* 2003;**167**:802.

49 Garcia-Aymerich J, Farrero E, Felez MA *et al*. Risk factors of readmission to hospital for a COPD exacerbation: a prospective study. *Thorax* 2003;**58**:100–5.

50 Garcia-Aymerich J, Marrades RM, Monso E *et al*. EFRAM Investigators. Paradoxical results in the study of risk factors of chronic obstructive pulmonary disease (COPD) re-admission. *Respir Med* 2004;**98**:851–7.

51 Casaburi R, Mahler DA, Jones PW *et al*. A long-term evaluation of once-daily inhaled tiotropium in chronic obstructive pulmonary disease. *Eur Respir J* 2002;**19**:217–24.

52 Donohue JF, van Noord JA, Bateman ED *et al*. A 6-month, placebo-controlled study comparing lung function and health status changes in COPD patients treated with tiotropium or salmeterol. *Chest* 2002;**122**:47–55.

53 Brusasco V, Hodder R, Miravitlles M *et al*. Health outcomes following treatment for six months with once daily tiotropium compared with twice daily salmeterol in patients with COPD. *Thorax* 2003;**58**:399–404.

54 van Noord JA, Bantje TA, Eland ME, Korducki L, Cornelissen PJ. A randomised controlled comparison of tiotropium and ipratropium in the treatment of chronic obstructive pulmonary disease: the Dutch Tiotropium Study Group. *Thorax* 2000;**55**:289–94.

55 Vincken W, van Noord JA, Greefhorst AP *et al*. Improved health outcomes in patients with COPD during 1 year's treatment with tiotropium. *Eur Respir J* 2002;**19**:209–16.

56 Gerrits CM, Herings RM, Leufkens HG, Lammers JW. *N*-acetylcysteine reduces the risk of re-hospitalisation among patients with chronic obstructive pulmonary disease. *Eur Respir J* 2003;**21**:795–8.

57 Boman G, Backer U, Larsson S, Melander B, Wahlander L. Oral acetylcysteine reduces exacerbation rate in chronic bronchitis: report of a trial organized by the Swedish Society for Pulmonary Diseases. *Eur J Respir Dis* 1983;**64**:405–15.

58 Rasmussen JB, Glennow C. Reduction in days of illness after long-term treatment with *N*-acetylcysteine controlled-release tablets in patients with chronic bronchitis. *Eur Respir J* 1988;**1**:351–5.

59 Pela R, Calcagni AM, Subiaco S *et al*. *N*-acetylcysteine reduces

the exacerbation rate in patients with moderate to severe COPD. *Respiration* 1999;**66**:495–500.

60 Grandjean EM, Berthet P, Ruffmann R, Leuenberger P. Efficacy of oral long-term *N*-acetylcysteine in chronic bronchopulmonary disease: a meta-analysis of published double-blind, placebo-controlled clinical trials. *Clin Ther* 2000;**22**: 209–21.

61 Stey C, Steurer J, Bachmann S, Medici TC, Tramer MR. The effect of oral *N*-acetylcysteine in chronic bronchitis: a quantitative systematic review. *Eur Respir J* 2000;**16**:253–62.

62 Ernst P, Suissa S. *N*-acetylcysteine is unlikely to reduce hospitalisation for chronic obstructive pulmonary disease. *Eur Respir J* 2003;**22**:865.

63 Decramer M, Dekhuijzen PN, Troosters T *et al*. The Bronchitis Randomized On NAC Cost-Utility Study (BRONCUS): hypothesis and design. BRONCUS Trial Committee. *Eur Respir J* 2001;**17**:329–36.

64 Martin RM, Shakir S. Age- and gender-specific asthma death rates in patients taking long-acting β_2-agonists: prescription event monitoring pharmacosurveillance studies. *Drug Saf* 2001; **24**:475–81.

65 Castle W, Fuller R, Hall J, Palmer J. Serevent Nationwide Surveillance Study: comparison of salmeterol with salbutamol in asthmatic patients who require regular bronchodilator treatment. *BMJ* 1993;**306**:1034–7.

66 Mann RD, Kubota K, Pearce G, Wilton L. Salmeterol: a study by prescription-event monitoring in a UK cohort of 15,407 patients. *J Clin Epidemiol* 1996;**49**:247–50.

67 Meier CR, Jick H. Drug use and pulmonary death rates in increasingly symptomatic asthma patients in the UK. *Thorax* 1997;**52**:612–7.

68 Williams C, Crossland L, Finnerty J *et al*. Case–control study of salmeterol and near-fatal attacks of asthma. *Thorax* 1998;**53**:7–13.

69 Ferguson GT, Funck-Brentano C, Fischer T, Darken P, Reisner C. Cardiovascular safety of salmeterol in COPD. *Chest* 2003;**123**:1817–24.

70 Gerber RB, Kavuru M. Does salmeterol increase mortality in patients with COPD? *Cleve Clin J Med* 2001;**68**:600–1.

71 Sin DD, McAlister FA, Man SF, Anthonisen NR. Contemporary management of chronic obstructive pulmonary disease: scientific review. *JAMA* 2003;**290**:2301–12.

72 Van der Molen T, Pieters W, Bellamy D, Taylor R. Measuring the success of treatment for chronic obstructive pulmonary disease: patient, physician and healthcare payer perspectives. *Respir Med* 2002;**96**(Suppl C):S17–21.

73 Alsaeedi A, Sin DD, McAlister FA. The effects of inhaled corticosteroids in chronic obstructive pulmonary disease: a systematic review of randomized placebo-controlled trials. *Am J Med* 2002;**113**:59–65.

74 Soriano JB, Kiri V, Pride NB, Vestbo J. Inhaled corticosteroids with/without long-acting beta agonists reduce the risk of rehospitalisation and death in COPD patients. *Am J Respir Med* 2003;**2**:67–74.

75 Soriano JB, Vestbo J, Pride NB *et al*. Survival in COPD patients after regular use of fluticasone propionate and salmeterol in general practice. *Eur Respir J* 2002;**20**:819–25.

76 Sin DD, Man SFP. Inhaled corticosteroids and survival in

COPD: does the dose of therapy matter? *Eur Respir J* 2003; **21**:260–7.

77 Bourbeau J, Ernst P, Cockcoft D, Suissa S. Inhaled corticosteroids and hospitalisation due to exacerbation of COPD. *Eur Respir J* 2003;**22**:286–9.

78 Suissa S. Inhaled steroids and mortality in COPD: bias from unaccounted immortal time. *Eur Respir J* 2004;**23**:391–5.

79 Fan VS, Bryson CL, Curtis JR *et al*. Inhaled corticosteroids in chronic obstructive pulmonary disease and risk of death and hospitalization: time-dependent analysis. *Am J Respir Crit Care Med* 2003;**168**:1488–94.

80 Bonay M, Bancal C, Crestani B. Benefits and risks of inhaled corticosteroids in chronic obstructive pulmonary disease. *Drug Saf* 2002;**25**:57–71.

81 Burge PS, Calverley PM, Jones PW *et al*. Randomised, double blind, placebo controlled study of fluticasone propionate in patients with moderate to severe chronic obstructive pulmonary disease: the ISOLDE trial. *BMJ* 2000;**320**:1297–303.

82 Waterhouse JC, Fishwick D, Burge PS, Calverley PMA, Anderson JA, on behalf of the ISOLDE Trial group: what caused death in the ISOLDE study? *Eur Respir J* 1999;**14** (Suppl 30):387S.

83 Blettner M, Sauerbrei W, Schlehofer B, Scheuchenpflug T, Friedenreich C. Traditional reviews, meta-analyses and pooled analyses in epidemiology. *Int J Epidemiol* 1999;**28**:1–9.

84 Sin DD, Wu L, Anderson JA *et al*. Inhaled corticosteroids and mortality in chronic obstructive pulmonary disease. *Thorax* 2005;**60**:992–7.

85 Vestbo J, TORCH Study Group. The TORCH (towards a revolution in COPD health) survival study protocol. *Eur Respir J* 2004;**24**:206–10.

86 Decramer M, Celli B, Tashkin DP *et al*. Clinical trial design considerations in assessing long-term functional impacts of tiotropium in COPD: the Uplift Trial. *J COPD* 2004;**1**:303–12.

87 Ware JH. Interpreting incomplete data in studies of diet and weight loss. *N Engl J Med* 2003;**348**:2136–7.

88 Pauwels RA, Buist AS, Calverley PM, Jenkins CR, Hurd SS, and the GOLD Scientific Committee. Global strategy for the diagnosis, management, and prevention of chronic obstructive pulmonary disease. NHLBI/WHO Global Initiative for Chronic Obstructive Lung Disease (GOLD) workshop summary. *Am J Respir Crit Care Med* 2001;**163**:1256–76.

89 Motheral B, Brooks J, Clark MA *et al*. A checklist for retrospective database studies: report of the ISPOR Task Force on Retrospective Databases. *Value Health* 2003;**6**:90–7.

90 Greenland S. Confounding and exposure trends in case-crossover and case-time-control designs. *Epidemiology* 1996; **7**:231–9.

91 Robins JM, Blevins D, Ritter G, Wulfsohn M. G-estimation of the effect of prophylaxis therapy for *Pneumocystis carinii* pneumonia on the survival of AIDS patients. *Epidemiology* 1992;**3**:319–36.

92 Hernán MA, Brumback B, Robins JM. Marginal structural models to estimate the causal effect of zidovudine on the survival of HIV-positive men. *Epidemiology* 2000;**11**:561–70.

93 Johnston SC. Combining ecological and individual variables to reduce confounding by indication: case study – subarachnoid hemorrhage treatment. *J Clin Epidemiol* 2000;**53**:1236–41.

94 Wang J, Donnan PT, Steinke D, MacDonald TM. The multiple propensity score for analysis of dose–response relationships in drug safety studies. *Pharmacoepidemiol Drug Saf* 2001; **10**:105–11.

95 Kiri VA, Pride NB, Soriano JB, Vestbo J. Inhaled corticosteroids in chronic obstructive pulmonary disease: results from two observational designs free of immortal time bias. *Am J Respir Crit Care Med* 2005;**172**:460–4.

96 Samet JM. Inhaled corticosteroids and chronic obstructive pulmonary disease: new and improved evidence? *Am J Respir Crit Care Med* 2005;**172**:407–8.

97 Ioannidis JP, Lau J. Heterogeneity of the baseline risk within patient populations of clinical trials: a proposed evaluation algorithm. *Am J Epidemiol* 1998;**148**:1117–26.

98 Jones JK. Pharmacogenetics and pharmacoepidemiology. *Pharmacoepidemiol Drug Saf* 2001;**10**:457–61.

CHAPTER 66
Social and behavioural impact of COPD – research opportunities

Suzanne S. Hurd and Claude Lenfant

Health-care professionals, patients, families, community leaders and policy makers struggle to understand interactions between health and behaviour and to use that knowledge to improve the health status of individuals and populations.

For patients with COPD, as with other chronic illnesses, health and behaviour are related in numerous ways, yet those interactions are neither simple nor straightforward. Psychosocial variables (e.g. depression, anxiety, self-esteem, optimism and social support), demographics (including age and socioeconomic status) and disease variables (such as dysponea, disease severity and functional status) all impact on quality of life for COPD patients.

Except for smoking cessation, factors in the development and manifestation of COPD have not received the attention of behavioural scientists or experts in health education that is warranted by the public health importance of this chronic lung disease. COPD management programmes are being implemented in several countries based on the Global Initiative for Chronic Obstructive Lung Disease (GOLD) [1] initiative, and much will be learned about how COPD patients can learn to cope with their disease in a variety of health-care settings.

This chapter describes some of the social and behavioural aspects of care that impact on COPD patients and areas where behavioural research is beginning to make a contribution, or where further research is warranted. For many years, health-care workers have had a rather nihilistic approach to care of COPD patients and to make a positive impact will require a modification of this negative approach. Effective management of COPD is no longer the responsibility of the pulmonary disease specialist alone, but requires a team approach that includes a variety of disciplines [2].

Behavioural impact of COPD

It is well documented that COPD patients experience gross difficulties in their emotional functioning, sleep and rest, physical mobility, social interaction, activities of daily living, recreation, work and finance. They frequently experience depression and anxiety and have a reduced quality of life [3]. In the early 1960s, it was reported that impairment of the psychosocial functioning and quality of life of the patient with COPD could exacerbate existing symptoms and decrease compliance with treatment [4]. In the 1980s, the Nocturnal Oxygen Therapy Trial (NOTT) [5] compared COPD patients with a group of healthy controls on four dimensions of life quality: emotional function, social role function, daily living activities and ability to engage in enjoyable hobbies and recreational pastimes. COPD patients were impaired in almost all respects: they were dissatisfied with life, tense, depressed, confused and socially withdrawn; quality of life was significantly related to severity of the disease. Study patients performed significantly worse on virtually all neuropsychological tests [5].

In 1983, another multicentre clinical trial, the Intermittent Positive Pressure Breathing Study (IPPB) [6], included patients with less severe COPD. Patients were between ages 30 and 74 years with prebronchodilator forced expiratory volume in 1 second (FEV_1) less than 60% predicted, and the patient group had a Pao_2 of 66 mmHg. Even though this group of patients was less physically limited than the patients in the NOTT study, they showed approximately equal impairment in psychosocial functioning, indicating that the degree of psychosocial limitation is not determined directly by the degree of pulmonary disease once COPD is present [6].

Since the publication of the NOTT and IPPB clinical trials, considerable research has been undertaken in the area of health and behaviour and the interplay between biological, behavioural and societal influences, although very little of this research is conducted specifically on COPD patients. Much of the current literature on chronic disease relates to cardiovascular diseases, cancer and musculoskeletal diseases (osteoarthritis), and it is expected that future research on COPD will benefit from the methodology developed from these investigations [7].

Studies on COPD patients have demonstrated that a comprehensive assessment of the effects of COPD requires a battery of instruments that not only tap the disease-specific effects, but also the overall burden of the disease on everyday functioning and emotional well-being [8]. However, many of these instruments have been developed to assess the severely impaired COPD patient.

In the GOLD guidelines [1], a classification of severity includes individuals "at risk" (Stage 0) for COPD as well as categories of mild (Stage 1), moderate (Stage 2), severe (Stage 3) and very severe disease (Stage 4). Including an "at risk" stage in this classification scheme was proposed to provide guidance for detection of early disease. However, to evaluate the impact of interventions, particularly at the early stages, it may be necessary to develop new outcome measures for use by health-care professionals, patients and health-care payers [9].

For example, it has been shown that quality of life is not significantly affected in patients with mild to moderate loss of pulmonary function, possibly because of coping and/or pulmonary reserve capacity [10]. This suggests that generic self-assessment questionnaires are of limited value, and that new measures need to be developed and evaluated to detect the early consequences of COPD. In later stages of the disease, however, current measures appear to be sensitive enough to discriminate between patients with different levels of pulmonary dysfunction [11], and it has been suggested that quality of life should be measured in these patients to evaluate the impact of therapeutic procedures on well-being from the patient's perspective [12].

Patients with endstage COPD have significantly impaired quality of life and emotional well-being [13]. COPD patients with recurrent exacerbations requiring emergency treatment show a significant association between treatment failure and anxiety and/or depression [14]. Poor emotional functioning of female patients with severe COPD at the time of prescription of long-term oxygen therapy (LTOT) was shown to be associated with increased mortality [15]. In one study, it was noted that emotional well-being of COPD patients may not be as well met in terms of medical and social care compared with those of patients with lung cancer [13]. In this study, both COPD and lung cancer patients reported a lack of information from professionals regarding diagnosis, prognosis and social support, although patients' information needs were disparate and often conflicting.

performing a particular behaviour, or set of behaviours) and social support (involving both benefits and costs) in predicting adjustment for COPD patients warrants further investigation [3]. This concept may be particularly important to study in COPD given the nihilistic approach to management of this illness that has permeated the health-care system.

Results from prospective longitudinal studies of breast cancer patients from diagnosis through treatment and recovery [16,17] have shown that successful coping is facilitated by optimism – the tendency to anticipate positive outcomes [7]. Through the use of strategies including acceptance, positive thinking and problem solving, optimism is associated with lower psychological distress (reduced symptoms of anxiety and depression). Conversely, pessimistic thinking is associated with avoidance and social withdrawal which are related to higher symptoms of anxiety and depression [16,17]. Patients who are more prone to poor coping have histories of social isolation, recent losses or multiple obligations [18].

Breast cancer patients who learn to use more direct and confrontational coping strategies are less distressed than those who use avoidance and denial [19]. Furthermore, a "fighting spirit" about the illness leads to a probability of longer survival [20,21]. Research suggests that belief one has control over the *cause* of the disease leads to poor outcome, whereas belief in control over the *course* of the disease leads to better outcome [21].

An interesting study comparing illness perceptions and coping strategies in patients with three different chronic diseases (rheumatoid arthritis, COPD and psoriasis) indicated a strong illness identity, passive coping, belief in a long illness duration, belief in more severe consequences and an unfavourable score on medical variables were associated with worse outcome on disease-specific measures of functioning and on general role and social functioning. Coping by seeking social support and a belief in being able to control or cure the disease were significantly related to better functioning [22]. The authors concluded that coping with illness by being active, expressive and thinking positively results in significantly higher levels of functioning, as well as more positive scores on clinical measures of disease.

Evaluation of COPD programmes in several countries will provide a spectrum of how various populations cope with COPD [12,23]. However, based on a growing literature from a number of chronic illnesses, it appears certain that a more optimistic approach to COPD outcomes by health professionals will lead to a better psychosocial adjustment.

Coping and COPD

Coping efforts are important in the process of adaptation to illness. Studies on the role of coping strategies, levels of self-efficacy (extent of the belief that one is, or is not capable of

Dysponea

Dysponea, a major symptom of COPD, is an important cause of suffering and disability in patients with advanced disease, and there are several methods to measure the impact of dysponea on daily living [24]. Although emotional factors are believed to influence the experience of dysponea, their role is unclear, as is the relationship between respiratory sensation and behavioural control of breathing. Very little is known about the effects of psychosocial stress on the immune system in COPD patients, exacerbations of the disease and the patient's perception of dysponea. Psychophysiologic studies of the relationship between respiratory sensation and the behavioural control of breathing may be useful in developing approaches to the management of dysponea.

An objective of current COPD management strategy is to identify individuals early in the course of disease. Individuals who experience dysponea may find themselves with a symptom of disease, but without a significant reduction in pulmonary function. Unfortunately, physicians may be inclined to inform the individual that there is simply no reason for the dysponea, and thus appropriate educational efforts for general practitioners are required. All patients with dysponea should remain physically active in the absence of a medical problem that prohibits it [25].

Prevention and risk factor reduction

The causal link between the chronic inhalation of tobacco smoke and COPD is beyond doubt, and smoking cessation remains the most important goal for patients. It has been well documented that the rate of decline in pulmonary function with increasing age is greater for smokers than for non-smokers. After cessation of smoking, the rate of decline gradually reverts to a more normal rate, although the function that has already been lost is not generally regained [26].

In 1994, the US Agency for Health Care Policy and Research provided clinical guidelines for effective smoking-cessation strategies that summarized the findings of 300 studies [27]. Some of the recommendations included the following:

• Effective smoking cessation treatments are available, and every patient who smokes should be offered one or more of these treatments. A combination of psychosocial counselling and nicotine replacement therapy appears to be the most effective strategy.
• Longer counselling sessions (more than 10 minutes) are more effective than shorter ones (less than 3 minutes). More sessions (more than eight) produce better results than do fewer (under four), but even fewer or shorter sessions still have a more substantial influence on smoking behaviour than do no sessions at all.
• Effective reduction of tobacco use requires that health-care systems make institutional changes that result in systematic identification of, and intervention with, all tobacco users at every visit.

It has been clearly demonstrated that smoking-cessation programmes are a cost-effective way to improve health [28], leading to the recommendation that physicians intervene by discussing smoking and potential treatment with every patient who smokes [29]. However, the trend in smoking-related research has been away from brief interventions studied sequentially to programmes that target smoking at the social, physiological and psychological levels [30]. Smoking cessation interventions targeted to specific needs, barriers and smoking patterns appear to be more effective in promoting higher cessation rates than standard (e.g. NCI Cancer Information Service quit smoking guide) interventions [31].

There are many barriers to effective prevention of COPD:
• Cost of implementation of smoking cessation programmes
• Difficulty in achieving smoking cessation
• Limited awareness of awareness of early signs and symptoms
• Lack of awareness of benefits of early treatment and risk factor modification
• Limited use of immunization for influenza
• Lack of patient knowledge, skills or motivation to follow management regimen
• Lack of knowledge by health-care providers

Although prevention of chronic diseases may be preferable from a public health point of view, current prospects for total elimination of chronic diseases are mostly unrealistic. For this reason, it is important to look at opportunities for preventing loss of physical functioning that often accompanies chronic diseases by identifying determinants of physical disabilities among chronically ill persons and by acting on those determinants [32,33]. For patients with COPD, this will depend not only on medical interventions, but will also require social and psychological interventions.

Rehabilitation programmes and health education

Rehabilitation forms an important component of the management of COPD. A Cochrane review concluded that rehabilitation relieves dysponea and fatigue and enhances patients' sense of control over their condition. Improvements in most studies were shown to be moderately large and clinically significant, although average improvements in exercise capacity are modest [34].

The optimal duration of pulmonary rehabilitation programmes remains the topic of many investigations. A 7-week course of pulmonary rehabilitation was shown to provide greater benefits to patients than a 4-week course in terms of improvements in health status [35]. A 6-week outpatient-based pulmonary rehabilitation programme appears to benefit quality of life in patients with moderate to severe COPD and benefit was still evident after 24 weeks [36]. Among patients who completed a 6-month programme, outpatient training resulted in significant and clinically relevant changes in 6-minute walking distance, maximal exercise performance, peripheral and respiratory muscle strength, and quality of life. Most of these effects persisted 18 months after initiation of the programme [37]. In another study, a simple home-based programme of exercise training achieved improvement in exercise tolerance, post-effort dysponea, basal dysponea and quality of life in COPD patients [38]. It will probably be necessary to examine the most effective – and cost effective – length and duration of outpatient rehabilitation programmes in relation to the appropriate health-care system.

An inpatient pulmonary rehabilitation programme led to improved endurance and functional ambulation, decreased supplemental oxygen use and fewer hospitalizations 1 year after discharge for patients with COPD [39]. However, long-term cost effectiveness and effects on mortality have yet to be elucidated [40].

Self-management education programmes for asthma have been proven to improve a wide range of measures of outcome [41] and are recommended for incorporation into routine asthma care [42]. However, a Cochrane analysis [43] concluded that data available are insufficient for forming recommendations regarding utilization of self-management for COPD and suggested that further research on the effectiveness of self-management programmes should be focused on behavioural change evaluated in well-designed randomized controlled trials with standardized outcomes designed for use in COPD patients, and with long follow-up time so that definite conclusions can be made [43].

Chronic diseases of adulthood have received the least systematic attention with respect to family-focused interventions. There have been many clinical reports and descriptive studies of interventions to assist families struggling with chronic disease. Most studies have been unsystematic and uncontrolled, but they indicate a growing recognition by the clinical community of the need to address family issues and of the utility of basing intervention in a family context [7].

Research opportunities

Because current treatments for COPD provide only modest benefit to the patient, substantial progress in COPD treatment may require the development of entirely new therapeutic approaches. Given the many important deficits of knowledge regarding the understanding of the disease process, and innovative approaches to modification of this process, an increase in basic and clinical research activities on COPD is sorely needed [44].

Research on molecular biology has received considerable attention in the scientific and lay communities as discoveries are made on genetic contributions to disease. Some are concerned that attention to molecular biology and genetics will lead to a growing chasm between social, behavioural and biomedical research [45]. However, health problems related to COPD – as in all complex chronic diseases – are brought about by an interaction of sociobehavioural and biological processes. Thus, research is required to understand the interactions in COPD patients between genetics and physiological processes with individual personalities, psychological characteristics, social status and relationships that affect health status.

Clinical trials are required to evaluate the value of behavioural and psychosocial interventions for COPD and the impact of these interventions on health, quality of life and longevity. Research has shown that behaviour can be changed, and that behavioural interventions can successfully teach new behaviours, and attenuate risky behaviours. However, maintaining behaviour change over time – essential for a disease like COPD – is a greater challenge.

Awareness of the signs and symptoms of COPD among the public and the health care community is a major goal of the GOLD programme. While spirometry is recommended to assess and monitor COPD, other measures need to be developed and evaluated in clinical practice.

Individual behaviour, family interactions, community and workplace relationships and resources, and public policy all contribute to health and influence behaviour change. Forming coalition groups at the local level to work with asthma patients has demonstrated that intervention at multiple levels (individual, family, community, society) are most likely to sustain behavioural change. Similar studies are required for patients with COPD. Such efforts should address the psychosocial factors associated with health status (including access to safe places to exercise, access to healthy foods) as well as individual behaviour (maintaining smoking cessation). Interventions aimed at increasing beliefs in personal control and changing beliefs about the course of illness could be associated with improvements in physical well-being and social functioning of patients with COPD [46].

References

1 Pauwels RA, Buist AS, Calverley PM *et al.* Global strategy for the diagnosis, management, and prevention of chronic obstructive pulmonary disease. NHLBI/WHO Global Initiative for Chronic Obstructive Lung Disease (GOLD) Workshop summary. *Am J Respir Crit Care Med* 2001;**163**:1256–76.
2 McSweeny AJ, Grant I, eds. *Chronic Obstructive Pulmonary Disease: A Behavioral Perspective.* New York: Marcel Dekker, 1988.
3 McCathie HC, Spence SH, Tate RL. Adjustment to chronic obstructive pulmonary disease: the importance of psychological factors. *Eur Respir J* 2002;**19**:47–53.

4 Dudley DL, Martin CJ, Holmes TH. Dyspnea: psychologic and physiologic observations. *J Psychosom Res* 1968;**11**:325–39.

5 Nocturnal Oxygen Therapy Trial Group. Continuous or nocturnal oxygen therapy in hypoxemic chronic obstructive lung disease: a clinical trial. *Ann Intern Med* 1980;**93**:391–8.

6 Intermittent positive pressure breathing therapy of chronic obstructive pulmonary disease: a clinical trial. *Ann Intern Med* 1983;**99**:612–20.

7 Health and behavior: The interplay of biological, behavioral, and societal influences. Washington, DC: Institute of Medicine, 2001: www.nap.edu

8 Engstrom CP, Persson LO, Larsson S *et al*. Health-related quality of life in COPD: why both disease-specific and generic measures should be used. *Eur Respir J* 2001;**18**:69–76.

9 Buist AS. Guidelines for the management of chronic obstructive pulmonary disease. *Respir Med* 2002;**96**(Suppl C):S11–6.

10 Engstrom CP, Persson LO, Larsson S *et al*. Functional status and well being in chronic obstructive pulmonary disease with regard to clinical parameters and smoking: a descriptive and comparative study. *Thorax* 1996;**51**:825–30.

11 Garrod R, Bestall JC, Paul EA *et al*. Development and validation of a standardized measure of activity of daily living in patients with severe COPD: the London Chest Activity of Daily Living scale (LCADL). *Respir Med* 2000;**94**:589–96.

12 Lisboa C, Villafranca C, Caiozzi G *et al*. [Quality of life in patients with chronic obstructive pulmonary disease and the impact of physical training.] *Rev Med Chil* 2001;**129**:359–66.

13 Gore JM, Brophy CJ, Greenstone MA. How well do we care for patients with end stage chronic obstructive pulmonary disease (COPD)? A comparison of palliative care and quality of life in COPD and lung cancer. *Thorax* 2000;**55**:1000–6.

14 Dahlen I, Janson C. Anxiety and depression are related to the outcome of emergency treatment in patients with obstructive pulmonary disease. *Chest* 2002;**122**:1633–7.

15 Crockett AJ, Cranston JM, Moss JR *et al*. The impact of anxiety, depression and living alone in chronic obstructive pulmonary disease. *Qual Life Res* 2002;**11**:309–16.

16 Carver CS, Pozo C, Harris SD *et al*. How coping mediates the effect of optimism on distress: a study of women with early stage breast cancer. *J Pers Soc Psychol* 1993;**65**:375–90.

17 Epping-Jordan JE, Compas BE, Osowiecki DM *et al*. Psychological adjustment in breast cancer: processes of emotional distress. *Health Psychol* 1999;**18**:315–26.

18 Rowland J. *Interpersonal resources: Coping*. New York: Oxford University Press, 1990.

19 Holland JC, Rowland JH, eds. *Handbook of Psychooncology: Psychological Care of the Patient with Cancer*. New York: Oxford University Press, 1990.

20 Green MA, Berlin MA. Five psychosocial variables related to the existence of post-traumatic stress disorder symptoms. *J Clin Psychol* 1987;**43**:643–9.

21 Watson M, Pruyn J, Greer S *et al*. Locus of control and adjustment to cancer. *Psychol Rep* 1990;**66**:39–48.

22 Scharloo M, Kaptein AA, Weinman J *et al*. Illness perceptions, coping and functioning in patients with rheumatoid arthritis, chronic obstructive pulmonary disease and psoriasis. *J Psychosom Res* 1998;**44**:573–85.

23 Yuet LM, Alexander M, Chun CJ. Coping and adjustment in Chinese patients with chronic obstructive pulmonary disease. *Int J Nurs Stud* 2002;**39**:383–95.

24 Hajiro T, Nishimura K, Tsukino M *et al*. Analysis of clinical methods used to evaluate dyspnea in patients with chronic obstructive pulmonary disease. *Am J Respir Crit Care Med* 1998;**158**:1185–9.

25 Dudley DL, Sitzman J. Psychobiological evaluation and treatment of COPD. In: McSweeny AJ, Grant I, eds. *Chronic Obstructive Pulmonary Disease: A Behavioral Perspective*. New York: Marcel Dekker, 1988: 183–235.

26 Anthonisen NR, Connett JE, Kiley JP *et al*. Effects of smoking intervention and the use of an inhaled anticholinergic bronchodilator on the rate of decline of FEV_1. The Lung Health Study. *JAMA* 1994;**272**:1497–505.

27 Agency for Health Care Policy and Research (AHCPR). The tobacco use and dependence clinical practice guideline panel, staff, and consortium representatives: a clinical practice guideline for treating tobacco use and dependence. *JAMA* 2000;**28**:3244–54.

28 Cromwell J, Bartosch WJ, Fiore MC *et al*. Cost-effectiveness of the clinical practice recommendations in the AHCPR guideline for smoking cessation. Agency for Health Care Policy and Research. *JAMA* 1997;**278**:1759–66.

29 Hughes JR, Goldstein MG, Hurt RD *et al*. Recent advances in the pharmacotherapy of smoking. *JAMA* 1999;**281**:72–6.

30 Schwartz JL. Methods of smoking cessation. *Med Clin North Am* 1992;**76**:451–76.

31 Orleans CT, Boyd NR, Bingler R *et al*. A self-help intervention for African American smokers: tailoring cancer information service counseling for a special population. *Prev Med* 1998;**27**(5 Pt 2):S61–70.

32 Mackenbach JP, Borsboom GJ, Nusselder WJ *et al*. Determinants of levels and changes of physical functioning in chronically ill persons: results from the GLOBE Study. *J Epidemiol Community Health* 2001;**55**:631–8.

33 Fries JF. Aging, natural death, and the compression of morbidity. *N Engl J Med* 1980;**303**:130–5.

34 Lacasse Y, Brosseau L, Milne S *et al*. Pulmonary rehabilitation for chronic obstructive pulmonary disease. *Cochrane Database Syst Rev* 2002: 3.

35 Green RH, Singh SJ, Williams J *et al*. A randomised controlled trial of four weeks versus seven weeks of pulmonary rehabilitation in chronic obstructive pulmonary disease. *Thorax* 2001;**56**:143–5.

36 Finnerty JP, Keeping I, Bullough I *et al*. The effectiveness of outpatient pulmonary rehabilitation in chronic lung disease: a randomized controlled trial. *Chest* 2001;**119**:1705–10.

37 Troosters T, Gosselink R, Decramer M. Short- and long-term effects of outpatient rehabilitation in patients with chronic obstructive pulmonary disease: a randomized trial. *Am J Med* 2000;**109**:207–12.

38 Hernandez MT, Rubio TM, Ruiz FO *et al*. Results of a home-based training program for patients with COPD. *Chest* 2000;**118**:106–14.

39 Stewart DG, Drake DF, Robertson C *et al*. Benefits of an inpatient pulmonary rehabilitation program: a prospective analysis. *Arch Phys Med Rehabil* 2001;**82**:347–52.

40 Faulkner MA, Hilleman DE. The economic impact of chronic obstructive pulmonary disease. *Expert Opin Pharmacother* 2002;**3**:219–28.

41 Wolf FM, Guevara JP, Grum CM *et al.* Educational interventions for asthma in children. *Cochrane Database Syst Rev* 2003: 1.

42 NHLBI/WHO Workshop Report. *Global strategy for asthma management and prevention*. Washington, DC: Department of Health and Human Services, 2002.

43 Monninkhof EM, van der Valk PD, van der Palen J *et al.* Self-management education for chronic obstructive pulmonary disease. *Cochrane Database Syst Rev* 2003: 1.

44 Croxton TL, Weinmann GG, Senior RM *et al.* Clinical research in chronic obstructive pulmonary disease: needs and opportunities. *Am J Respir Crit Care Med* 2003;**167**: 1142–9.

45 Anderson NB, Scott PA. Making the case for psychophysiology during the era of molecular biology. *Psychophysiology* 1999;**36**:1–13.

46 Petrie KJ, Weinman J, Sharpe N *et al.* Role of patients' view of their illness in predicting return to work and functioning after myocardial infarction: longitudinal study. *BMJ* 1996; **312**:1191–4.

CHAPTER 67
Guidelines

Peter M.A. Calverley

Chronic obstructive pulmonary disease is a complex disorder with many different aspects, as illustrated by the other chapters in this volume. As the management options for COPD have increased so has the perceived need for standardized care and this has led to the development of a series of COPD Guidelines. These documents have the difficult task of addressing the very different needs of those who wish to use them. For the research scientist, they should give a clear conceptual structure to the field of COPD. For the practising clinician, they should offer advice about diagnosis and the best way to manage patients, while for the health-care administrator they should give some indication of the likely costs of COPD care, either explicitly or, more commonly, implicitly by detailing what types of therapy are going to be available for what kinds of patients. COPD Guidelines should be regularly updated, otherwise they fossilize therapy instead of advancing it. As a result, this chapter is likely to be outdated in some specific areas by the time this book is published, let alone by the point at which you purchase your copy. None the less, there is some virtue in considering some of the general features that have affected the structure of these documents and which are likely to impact on future versions. Understanding some of these constraints may help the clinician reading this book to interpret the information with which they are provided.

COPD Guidelines – a brief history

Traditionally, most clinicians developed views about how to manage patients with COPD from discussion with senior colleagues and by reading textbooks and the medical literature. This undoubtedly led to a very fragmented approach to management of this disease, made worse by the historical distinctions of chronic bronchitis and emphysema which were thought of as separate illnesses requiring different treatment approaches. The recognition that these

differing pathologies could produce very similar clinical states occurred during the 1980s when interest moved from the management of very advanced disease with treatment such as domiciliary oxygen [1] to establishing a more rational basis for commonly used therapies such as bronchodilator drugs [2]. The perceived success of the introduction of systematized guidance for the management of asthma [3] led many people to consider undertaking this for patients with COPD. This was initially carried out on a national level, with Canada and Australia leading the way [4,5]. These documents were developed by expert consensus and focused on stating agreed care patterns for patients with COPD. As a result, they looked little different from information obtained in standard medical textbooks or review articles but they had the advantage of being approved by the national pulmonary societies and became a benchmark against which individual institutions could audit their care. This early function of guidelines remains one of the most important reasons for developing these documents.

Subsequently, larger international societies, particularly the American Thoracic Society (ATS), which had already considered in general standards of care for COPD [6,7], and then the European Respiratory Society (ERS) developed specific documents [8]. These differed in scope, content and constituency. The ERS Guidelines tried to encompass all physicians from those working in non-pulmonary specialist practice through to physicians working in large tertiary care institutions. A working definition of COPD was developed and more background to the impact and physiology of the degree of the disease was included. A novel feature of this document was the attempt to produce a series of flow charts, which might help in making specific management decisions. This, unfortunately, did not prove to be the case, largely because of the complexity of the algorithm but also because the charts themselves were never tested in practice before being included in the Guidelines. Thus, decision making at specific arbitrary cut points might appear to have been sensible in theory, but most clinicians found it hard to apply in those specific areas of practice.

The ATS Standards of Care document took a different approach, focusing much more on hospital-based practice and offering a detailed narrative review which provided ample information about certain areas of specialist care and was more comprehensive than its European counterpart. However, the resulting document was relatively long and difficult to access to discover the answers to specific questions without reading it in its entirety. Moreover, its limited scope restricted its usefulness to the non-pulmonary specialist. Throughout the late 1990s other national society documents were produced which drew similar conclusions to each of these preceding consensus statements but had the advantage of raising awareness of COPD in the individual country. One of the most important of these was the British Thoracic Society (BTS) Guidelines published in 1997 [9]. These were the first guidelines to draw in a wider constituency of interested people, including physicians in internal medicine, emergency medicine, family practice and those with nursing experience. The document was more didactic than others but had the advantage of being easier to read and clearer in its management recommendations. This was the first document to be developed with a specific programme for implementation, an area that remains difficult (see below).

The global scope of COPD and the progressively rising mortality and morbidity with which it is associated [10] led the National Institutes of Health (NIH) and World Health Organization (WHO) to convene a specific workshop group to develop global guidelines for COPD management. This resulted in the Global initiative for chronic Obstructive Lung Disease (GOLD), which produced its background documents and an executive summary in 2001 [11]. The principal aims of GOLD are summarized in Table 67.1 and progress to date suggests that at least some of these are now being met. Like its predecessors, GOLD was based around an expert group of pulmonary physicians and given the diversity of health-care systems it was attempting to address it was probably reasonable not to include individuals representing specific paramedical or patient groups. The intention was initially to establish a knowledge base, which could then be adapted locally for implementation, at which stage aspects specific to these other interested groups would be included. GOLD was the first guidelines to try and offer

Table 67.1 Global initiative for chronic Obstructive Lung Disease (GOLD): objectives.

Increase awareness of COPD among health professionals, health authorities and the general public
Improve diagnosis, management and prevention
Stimulate research

some grading of the strength of the evidence behind its recommendations and the grading system used is included in Tables 67.2 and 67.3. Although statements on evidence were based on only partial literature searching initially, subsequent review by other bodies suggest that no main clinical studies available at that time were omitted from the first GOLD review. None the less, the evidence gathering process was not as rigorous as has been undertaken subsequently by other organizations and by GOLD itself.

Two further features of the GOLD process are worth specific comment as neither has been fully addressed previously. From the outset, GOLD considered its role to be not just the formulation of an up-to-date evidence-based management plan, but also the dissemination of this information to as many countries as possible. By working with national opinion leaders and seeking approval for the programme from other interested parties, GOLD has developed rather specific coalitions that suit the general aim of standardizing COPD care but in very different health-care environments. The process of dissemination and implementation of the GOLD guidelines continues and is now moving towards building links with family medicine organizations and patient interest groups. If this can be achieved then an important and broadly based coalition for improving COPD care will have been developed. What is also clear is that specific countries, some of which have already developed perfectly serviceable and locally applicable guidelines, need to have a different approach in their relationships of GOLD from those where there has been no previous history of systematic COPD care. An equally important point is that there should be general agreement between the different guidelines about what COPD comprises. Needless revision of the content of guidelines, or rather futile arguments about the precise definition, are as likely to be counterproductive, especially for those doctors whose primary interest is not COPD. The second important contribution of GOLD has been to develop a mechanism for keeping itself up-to-date and this is discussed in detail below.

The beginning of the new century shows no sign of any reduction in the number of guidelines being produced and the ATS and ERS have now produced a joint guideline which is consensus-based but addresses some of the issues that require more detailed coverage than is possible in a document like that produced by the GOLD group [12]. The other novel aspect of this initative is its availability as a downloadable Web-based document, which can be used on a personal organizer or similar personal computer. This should help increase accessibility of the information provided and overcome the problem of excessive detail which dogged the original ATS Statement. In the UK the previous BTS guidance has been replaced by national guidelines developed in conjunction with the Government organisation the National Institute of Clinical Excellence (NICE) [13].

Table 67.2 National Instiitutes of Health (NIH)/Global initiative for chronic Obstructive Lung Disease (GOLD) evidence-based assessments.

Description of levels of evidence

Evidence category	Sources of evidence	Definition
A	RCTs Rich body of data	Evidence is from endpoints of well-designed RCTs that provide a consistent patternof findings in the population for which the recommendation is made. Category A requires substantial numbers of studies involving substantial numbers of participants
B	RCTs Limited body of data	Evidence is from endpoints of intervention studies that include only a limited number of patients, *post hoc* or subgroup analysis of RCTs, or meta-analysis of RCTs. In general, Category B pertains when few randomized trials exist, they are small in size, they were undertaken in a population that differs from the target population of the recommendation, or the results are somewhat inconsistent
C	Non-randomized trials Observational studies	Evidence is from outcomes of uncontrolled or non-randomized trials or from observational studies
D	Panel Consensus Judgement	This category is used only in cases where the provision of some guidance was deemed valuable but the clinical literature addressing the subject was deemed insufficient to justify placement in one of the other categories. The Panel Consensus is based on clinical experience or knowledge that does not meet the above-listed criteria

RCT, randomized controlled trial.

Table 67.3 UK evidence-based assessment.

Hierarchy of evidence		Grading of recommendations	
Ia	Evidence from meta analysis of randomized controlled trials	A	Based on category I evidence
Ib	Evidence from at least one randomized controlled trial		
IIa	Evidence from at least one controlled study without randomization	B	Based on category II evidence or extrapolated from category I
IIb	Evidence from at least one other type of quasi experimental study		
III	Evidence from non-experimental descriptive studies, such as comparative studies, correlation studies and case–control studies	C	Based on category III evidence or extrapolated from category I or II
IV	Evidence from expert committee reports or opinions and/or clinical experience of respected authorities	D	Directly based on category IV evidence or extrapolated from category I, II or III

RCT, randomized controlled trial.

These were the first guidelines based on systematic reviews of the evidence base with an external classification of the strength of the evidence, at least as judged by the quality of the studies (see Tables 67.2 and 67.3). They are a valuable resource for those surveying the COPD literature, saving much unnecessary labour as well as allowing easier updates in the future. Unfortunately what they have gained in com-prehensive coverage and evidence review has been lost in readability. In the end these guidelines have proven more important as a stimulus to political change in COPD care than as a practical management tool. Finally the GOLD guidance has come full circle and 2006 sees the launch of the second edition of the key resource document from which other guidance was abstracted in the original executive summary. This provides a chance to review all aspects of our current knowledge about COPD and not just the impact of new therapies.

Defining COPD

Several definitions of COPD have been proposed by the various guidelines and several of these are shown in Table 67.4. No specific ATS definition is given here as until recently this was based on the non-proportional Venn diagram developed by Snider to cope with the differential contributions of the underlying pathology to the individual COPD patient. The most important addition suggested in the recent ATS/ERS guidance is the inclusion of the statement that COPD is a preventable and treatable disorder before the definitions listed in Table 67.4. This is strictly speaking not a defining characteristic but is intended to re-dress the negative perception of COPD among clinicians and has now been adopted by the GOLD initiative as part of its revised definition. The problems of defining COPD are well known but one further aspect should be stressed here. The definition selected by all guidelines leans towards terms that can be applied practically. Hence, the emphasis is placed on airflow obstruction (reduced forced expiratory

---

Table 67.4 Definitions of chronic obstructive pulmonary disease (COPD).

European Respiratory Society 1995
COPD is a disorder characterized by reduced maximum expiratory flow and slow forced emptying of the lungs; features that do not change markedly over several months. Most of the airflow limitation is caused by varying combinations of airway disease and emphysema; the relative contribution of the two processes is difficult to define *in vivo*

British Thoracic Society 1997
COPD is a chronic, slowly progressive disorder characterized by airflow obstruction (reduced FEV_1 and FEV_1/FVC ratio) that does not change markedly over several months. Most of the lung function impairment is fixed, although some reversibility can be produced by bronchodilator (or other) therapy

GOLD 2001
COPD is a disease state characterized by airflow limitation that is not fully reversible. The airflow limitation is usually both progressive and associated with an abnormal inflammatory response of the lungs to noxious particles or gases

FEV_1, forced expiratory volume in 1 s; FVC, forced vital capacity.

---

volume in 1 s to forced vital capacity ratio [FEV_1/FVC] or, in the ERS version, slow forced emptying of the lungs) and lack of spontaneous variability (largely fixed in the BTS definition, not fully reversible in GOLD). Most definitions stress the progressive nature of the symptoms and physiological change, and GOLD emphasizes the key role of inhaled insults as a pathogenic mechanism. Based on these approaches, clinicians should be able to identify a patient with COPD and apply an appropriate management strategy. However, these definitions focus on the clinicophysiological outcomes of the processes that are occurring within the lower respiratory tract of the COPD patient. They are not the ideal way of identifying patients when a specific mechanism is to be studied (e.g. regulation of VGEF in the pulmonary endothelium as a mechanism promoting apoptosis in emphysema) [14]. They also do not account for the heterogeneity of the disease. Clearly, not all patients who meet the clinical definitions have a significant degree of emphysema. Thus, studies of this mechanism or indeed of agents to promote alveolar regeneration would not necessarily be appropriate in a clinically defined COPD population. We are still ignorant of the role of individual pathological phenotypes in the natural history of COPD, but the development of these mechanistic studies, together with the availability of quantitative computed tomography (CT) scanning may provide the necessary stimulus to initiate these longer-term investigations. Until such data are available, the definition of COPD will remain a compromise equivalent to that of 'cardiac failure' but without the specificity that allows us to subclassify cardiac dysfunction into systolic and diastolic or determine even more basic causes of the problem such as valvular abnormalities. Clearly, there is much work to be done in this area of COPD research.

Classifying disease severity

Clinicians look to guidelines to offer a practical approach to grade the severity of disease and relate this to management decisions. In asthma, this has been indirectly related to the patient's symptoms and is usually based on the amount of rescue medication they use and the type of treatment employed to control symptoms. Although, there is an approximate relationship of this empirical scheme to the diurnal variation to peak flow and/or histamine responsiveness, these measures have never been incorporated as primary outcomes in the staging of asthma severity [3].

A completely different approach has been used in COPD, which may not have always served patients well. Until recently, most guidelines based their staging on the FEV_1, making the generally reasonable assumption that the lower the FEV_1 as a percentage of predicted, then the greater the

Table 67.5 Spirometric classification of COPD severity.

	FEV$_1$ (% predicted)		
	Mild/stage I	Moderate/stage II	Severe/stage III
European Thoracic Society	>70	50–69	<50
American Thoracic Society	>50	35–49	<35
British Thoracic Society	60–79	40–59	<40
GOLD	>80	50–79 (A) 30–49 (B)	<30

FEV$_1$, forced expiratory volume in 1 s; GOLD, Global initiative for chronic Obstructive Lung Disease.

Old	0: At risk	I: Mild	II: Moderate		III: Severe
			IIA	IIB	
New	0: At risk	I: Mild	II: Moderate	III: Severe	IV: Very severe
Characteristics	• Chronic symptoms • Exposure to risk factors • Normal spirometry	• FEV$_1$/FVC < 70% • FEV$_1$ ≥ 80% • With or without symptoms	• FEV$_1$/FVC < 70% • 50% > FEV$_1$ < 80% • With or without symptoms	• FEV$_1$/FVC < 70% • 30% > FEV$_1$ < 50% • With or without symptoms	• FEV$_1$/FVC < 70% • FEV$_1$ < 30% or presence of chronic respiratory failure or right heart failure

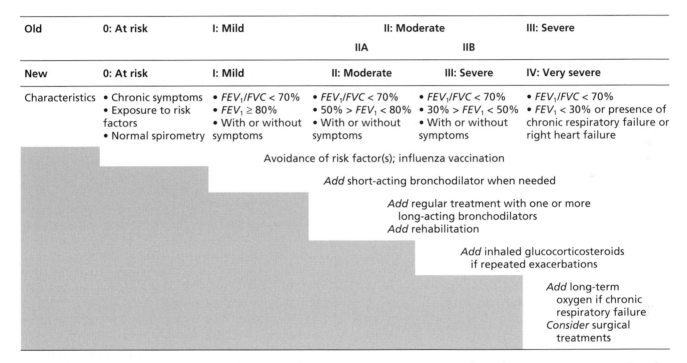

Avoidance of risk factor(s); influenza vaccination

Add short-acting bronchodilator when needed

Add regular treatment with one or more long-acting bronchodilators
Add rehabilitation

Add inhaled glucocorticosteroids if repeated exacerbations

Add long-term oxygen if chronic respiratory failure
Consider surgical treatments

Figure 67.1 The updated Global initiative for chronic Obstructive Lung Disease (GOLD) schema for COPD management. Note the inclusion of the former categorization and its revision. Therapy is cumulative although not all will be needed in any given patient even if they have a specified level of lung function impairment.

pathological and symptomatic severity. Some of the previous proposals about staging are shown in Table 67.5 and the most up-to-date version proposed by GOLD is included in Figure 67.1.

At least three problems limit this approach. The first is practical, as until recently spirometry has not been widely available, and this remains a problem especially in less developed countries and in primary care medicine. Improvements in spirometer design and software are making this measurement much easier to perform. More important is the arbitrary nature of the boundaries selected for the severity classification (see Table 67.5). Disease severity described spirometrically is a continuously distributed vari-

able in any COPD population and FEV$_1$ itself will show modest day-to-day variability. Patients who lie close to the selected boundary may therefore be reclassified as more or less severe if seen on a different day.

Most important of all is the relatively poor relationship between health status and spirometry, which means that an individual patient with an FEV$_1$ of 60% of predicted can be more symptomatic than one whose FEV$_1$ is 45% of predicted, despite the fact that both are given the same treatment. Because the benefits of bronchodilator therapy and rehabilitation are based on symptomatic improvement rather than altered lung mechanics, it is irrational to base management too precisely on a specified level of the FEV$_1$.

The authors of the GOLD Guidelines were aware of this dilemma when they produced their severity scheme. They allowed a wide range of spirometric abnormality to encompass symptomatic disease, now graded as moderate severity in the FEV_1 80–50% of predicted range. In addition they tried, less successfully than they originally anticipated, to stress that symptoms are the management driver in assessing which treatment should be selected. The practical value of identifying patients because they have symptoms is clear but the extension of this to include this 'stage' as an inevitable precursor of disease progression has not proven well founded [15]. As a result GOLD stage 0 is set to be downgraded to an at risk with symptoms category in the next version of the GOLD document. It will be interesting to see if the same happens to stage 1 where airflow obstruction is present down to 80% predicted. The NICE guidance opted not to use this stage as there is uncertainty about how closely symptoms relate to obstruction in this group and in how many cases disease progresses. More importantly there is a real problem in the elderly about applying a fixed FEV_1/FVC ratio to define obstruction [16]. Whether this matters clinically is less clear but the risk of over-diagnosis in the elderly can be minimised if only patients in stages II and above are accepted as having clinically important disease [17]. The most severe subgroup of COPD (less than 30% of predicted in GOLD and the forthcoming ATS/ERS scheme) are chosen to highlight a population where persistent daytime hypoxaemia is more likely to be found and hence where continuous domiciliary oxygen treatment is indicated. This clinical problem indicates the weakness of a purely symptom-based method of classifying COPD, as hypoxaemic patients are not necessarily more or less symptomatic than those without this important clinical complication.

Thus, classifying COPD for clinical rather than epidemiological purposes requires a hybrid approach. Several investigators are trying to develop scoring systems based on spirometry, assessment of dyspnoea (such as the Medical Research Council [MRC] dyspnoea scale), arterial oxygen tension, body mass index (an important prognostic sign in more severe disease), with or without some measurement of exercise capacity [18,19]. This approach provides better separation into groups with different prognoses but it is not clear yet whether changes in these indices give us a reliable surrogate endpoint for change in mortality, as blood pressure does in deaths from cerebrovascular disease.

Guidelines and management

Most guidelines clearly distinguish different phases of COPD care and the pattern used by GOLD now seems to be being adopted by other organizations. Thus, there is clear emphasis on issues related to diagnosis, prevention (which normally means reduction of risk factor exposure), management of stable disease and care of patients with exacerbations. Detailed consideration is given to each of these areas elsewhere in this book, but some general features about the rationale of guidelines is worth considering.

Despite the development of clear definitions (see above), there is still a legacy of confusion about what COPD really is and how it is best diagnosed. The simply message emphasized in GOLD that a diagnosis will normally involve a patient who presents with symptoms (cough, sputum production and/or breathlessness) who also has an appropriate risk factor (e.g. tobacco exposure). Such a patient should undergo spirometry to confirm the diagnosis. Difficulties about access to spirometry make this last step harder than it should be but it is really not acceptable to omit this step in developed countries where this relatively simple test can be easily undertaken. Difficulties, as usual, are made by specialists whose own clinical practice includes the most complex cases and where unrealistic concerns about 'missing asthma' have led to a very distorted picture of how patients should be diagnosed. Initial enthusiasm, exemplified in the original BTS Guidelines, for the diagnostic specificity and sensitivity of bronchodilator and corticosteroid treatment trials has now been tempered by experience [20,21] and modified in the subsequent NICE and GOLD recommendations. What these studies have shown is that a clinical diagnosis of COPD is a very good way of defining a population of people whose lung function declines more rapidly than expected over time and whose natural history is punctuated by exacerbations of disease and impaired health status. Reassuring doctors that they can make diagnosis of COPD easily is a major task for future generations of guideline writers.

The importance of smoking cessation is axiomatic in the management of COPD as is the prevention of smoking in the first place. In the Western world in particular, this is the dominant factor driving the incidence of new cases. However, even in these communities, it is not the only contributory factor and other well-established risk factors, including exposure to organic and inorganic dust and specific genetic predispositions, should also be considered. Sadly, removal of these factors will not cure COPD but serves to reduce the deterioration in lung function over time. Recognition that patients whose lungs have been damaged by these environmental and personal exposures will still need care is also an important feature for anyone writing guidelines, particularly thinking of their impact on the health-care provider audience. To date, this aspect has not been stressed sufficiently.

The management of stable disease can be usefully summarized in Figure 67.1, which is taken from the first update of the GOLD recommendations in July 2003. This scheme stresses that treatment is cumulative and can be broadly related to both the severity of spirometric impairment and the nature and impact of the disease's symptoms. Unsurprisingly, risk avoidance is a feature at all stages of disease severity as is the need to reduce the risk of having attacks of influenza. Although many organizations now advocate that pneumococcal vaccines should be routinely prescribed for COPD patients, this remains a contentious area because most of the data have been derived in younger adults and the efficacy of all the existing vaccines, both 7 and 23 valent forms, is much less documented in this specific group. There is reasonable evidence that the incidence of bacteraemia is reduced, although whether pneumococcal pneumonia, let alone COPD exacerbations, is less common is disputed [22], recent evidence suggesting benefit in those with most severe disease [23]. Given the ambivalent evidence, organizations such as GOLD have not chosen to recommend pneumococcal vaccination routinely but clearly local practice may vary depending upon the immunogeneity of the local strains of organism and there is evidence that community acquired pneumonia is prevented in those with more severe disease.

Within the GOLD classification there is now good evidence that a move to a long-acting inhaled bronchodilator is desirable for any patient with persistent symptoms. Those who have minor symptoms that are readily controlled by short-acting treatment do not need to take this step but this is not the case for most people with clinically important COPD. The more favourable risk–benefit profiles seen with these drugs compared with older therapy such as theophyllines have conditioned these recommendations. Likewise, the understanding that sustained bronchodilatation can itself reduce the number of exacerbations and improve health status over time has given much more confidence to this approach rather than short-acting therapy [24,25]. One further incidental conclusion is that studies in COPD of any medical treatment really need to extend to 1 year, if not longer, before the true impact of therapy can be evaluated. The role of inhaled corticosteroids is now much clearer and the current judgement is that it is only when patients are having frequent exacerbations that the addition of an inhaled corticosteroid to a long-acting bronchodilator can be justified [25,26]. This is quite a different view from the role of inhaled corticosteroids in bronchial asthma and emphasizes the need to actually make a diagnosis and not duck the issue. Although this particular recommendation is clearly linked to a specific level of lung functioning impairment, in practice patients with frequent exacerbations that require medical therapy will be those in whom this treatment is likely to be most effective [27].

Physical therapy is emphasized throughout COPD care and it is to be hoped that facilities for pulmonary rehabilitation will become more widespread and accessible as this undoubtedly produces a significant improvement that lasts between 12 and 18 months in most people. Maintaining this improvement for longer periods is still an unresolved problem. Likewise, other physical treatments such as oxygen are really confined to the most severely affected patients where they can be very valuable and prolong life. The grounds for surgical therapy with lung volume reduction surgery are now much clearer following the National Emphysema Treatment Trial (NETT) study [28] and this too has been incorporated within the most recent guidelines.

Managing exacerbations has undergone less change than other areas of treatment. An extensive systematic review has been conducted which identified a number of points in exacerbation care [29], all of which were highlighted in previous consensus-based guidelines. The place where care is delivered is clearly system specific and should be addressed in local modifications of these international documents. The initial care normally involves intensification of existing treatment and the addition of oral corticosteroids for which there is good evidence [30,31]. In hospitalized patients, the inability of the patient to cope in the community and their requirement for oxygen treatment often determines whether they are admitted to hospital, although newer approaches to care in the community for those who have been assessed in an emergency room are now available and appear to be acceptable to patients and doctor alike [32,33]. The availability of non-invasive ventilation, which can be conducted even on a general ward with appropriately trained staff [34], has helped to widen treatment opportunities in many communities for COPD patients. Issues about the patient's own wishes for continued intensive care, especially if that were to involve intubation, should be taken into account. This remains a cultural issue that can be best addressed in local variants of international guidelines. However, it is important that this is not omitted as it has major implications for the care of the individual who develops a COPD exacerbation. In all of these guidelines, details of ventilator care with a non-invasive or invasive are usually omitted as it is assumed that this will be undertaken in conjunction with individuals familiar with ICU management, an assumption that seems to be very reasonable.

One challenging area that has recently come to the fore is that of COPD comorbidity. Clinicians have become more aware of the impact of therapy on other systems (e.g. bruising with corticosteroids; tachycardia with β-agonists) but most now accept that loss of muscle bulk, especially in the legs, is a common disease-related feature in COPD. Impaired nutrition and reduced fat-free mass are also frequent once you start to look for them. It is now clear that the risk of cardiac disease including myocardial infarction, osteoporosis and lung cancer are increased in patients with COPD to levels above those seen in patients with comparable smoking histories. Finally the patient who has an unrelated illness which amplifies the effect of COPD on daily life (e.g. osteoarthritis, impaired vision or diabetes) has much more problems in coping with the difficulties COPD imposes. Thus far our evidence-based guidelines have addressed each condition in the same way so that a patient with four problems is manged by four different and occasionally conflicting sets of rules. The move to some form of more holistic guidance remains a challenge for all who believe in evidence-based care in the future.

Guidelines – practical issues

Several practical points are worth considering which apply to all management guidelines written to date. Each of these recommends management for the average patient who presents with the average symptoms and an average lung function abnormality. In practice, patients are individuals and doctors should still feel free to adapt the guidelines recommendations to individual care. A real danger in all of these documents is that they are seen as invariable patterns of practice, even if they are not always relevant to the specific patient. Clearly, most patients will benefit from following the steps laid out in roughly the order provided. One problem of the stepwise approach illustrated in Figure 67.1 is that it does rather imply that every patient requires every step. Fortunately, newer algorithms identifying specific aspects of patient care and promoting a specific evidence-based response have been developed and their use in the UK NICE Guidelines has been a promising start in this area.

The rise of evidence-based medicine has led to a number of misconceptions about guidelines in general. There seems to be a belief, largely amongst those unfamiliar with the data, that the answer to all questions can be obtained by objectively surveying the literature. This was never the intention of the pioneers of this field nor was the assumption that grade A evidence is necessarily more important than that based on a consensus [35]. It may be that it is not possible to do a randomized controlled trial and certainly none exists for the role of oxygen therapy in the management of severely hypoxaemic patients who exacerbate. None the less, few clinicians would decide not to give oxygen in these circumstances! Moreover, the interpretation of evidence, particularly in COPD, is as important as its collection and analysis. It is easy to look at the outcomes of treatment and say that one treatment is equivalent to another because it changes a commonly measured outcome (e.g. FEV_1). However, it may be that information from longer and larger studies, looking at other outcomes, clearly demonstrates superiority (e.g. the use of long-acting inhaled bronchodilators compared with short-acting ones). Merely aggregating the data without thinking carefully about what it means is unhelpful. This can have more subtle and potentially more important manifestations.

Patients who enter into randomized controlled trials, certainly those with COPD, are often a rather select group of people. Many COPD patients have significant comorbidities, which would lead to their exclusion from studies. Those entering a study that is planned to last for a year are often inadvertently selected by the investigators because the patient's prognosis is believed to be at least 12 months. As a result, the outcomes for patients who are recruited to studies of this kind are much better than those identified using pharmacoepidemiological techniques [36]. This issue is not often identified by those who conduct systematic reviews of literature, which should be sufficiently structured to pick up concerns of this sort. The controversy about simply pooling data in a meta-analysis continues, with the NIH and GOLD sceptical about the role of this form of analysis while Europeans and Canadians are much more enthusiastic. This too has implications in COPD as most of the data favouring the use of drugs, which are described as mucolytics, are based on meta-analysis of data in patients with chronic bronchitis. Those studies looking at COPD patients suggest some benefit but again their methodology is insufficiently strong to lead to a firm recommendation about use. The value of a large prospective trial where all patients belong to the same population at randomisation is clearly shown by the results of the BRONCUS study, which found an effect of the antioxidant/mucolytic drug N-acetyl cysteine on exacerbation frequency only in patients not receiving inhaled corticosteroids [37]. It will be interesting to see if other prospective trials, such as the soon to be published TORCH study, can do the same for the confusing data about the impact of inhaled corticosteroids on mortality in COPD.

A major concern in all COPD guidelines is how to keep the content up-to-date. Enormous efforts are required to survey the literature and particularly to meet the exacting standards of evidence-based review. This may explain why there are so few COPD-related studies available even on major government web sites (see www.ahrq.gov). The work of drafting these documents falls on a relatively few individuals and the composition of all of these committees is important as it can influence the shape of the resulting guideline. Having finally got the document to publication stage, it is understandable that most people are not enthusiastic about beginning to revise it again and yet the pace of medical advance is sufficiently fast to make this necessary. The best approach to doing this to date has been that adopted by the GOLD Science Committee which has been clearly detailed in an editorial [38]. Searching for specific terms that are COPD-related may mean that some studies are missed but it is hoped that the knowledge of an expert committee will be wide enough for important observations to be identified, even if conventional indexing misses them. Review by two independent individuals and discussion by a group of experts about the likely significance of any new data for the previous recommendations provides an important check on the relevance of the guidelines document. Use of the Internet to post the results of this in a planned fashion should allow wide access for all interested parties. The GOLD group are reviewing the whole document on a 5-yearly cycle but annual updates should permit the most up-to-date knowledge to be transmitted to interested parties.

Conclusions

COPD Guidelines continue to be developed, although it is hoped that some maturity in this field has now been reached. The level of evidence available to judge the claims of competing therapies is improving and there is now more openness about how that evidence has been collected and reviewed. The availability of new electronic means of communication has greatly improved accessibility of all guidelines and the concept that these could be downloaded to a pocket computer looks to be practical. Despite their limitations, guidelines provide a standard of care that can be assessed and reviewed. They present a view about COPD that can be tested and modified. As such, they are likely to continue to be an important part of our clinical management of these patients for the foreseeable future. More than this they provide the necessary tools to drive the implementation of COPD care. How best to do this is still debated and no single approach will work in all health care systems. However the group developing COPD guidance, specifically the ATS, ERS and GOLD, are now partners in the new Global Alliance against Respiratory Disease supported by the WHO and tasked with improving global respiratory care. Equally the existence of the NICE guidelines was a crucial step in persuading the UK government to develop a quality standards framework for COPD care, the first time a major developed country has identified the need to address the problems of COPD. Given these specific and political impacts we must be committed to make our guidance up to date, accurate and available to all; no small task for the years ahead.

References

1 Anonymous. Continuous or nocturnal oxygen therapy in hypoxemic chronic obstructive lung disease: a clinical trial. Nocturnal Oxygen Therapy Trial Group. *Ann Intern Med* 1980; **93**:391–8.

2 Hay JG, Stone P, Carter J *et al*. Bronchodilator reversibility, exercise performance and breathlessness in stable chronic obstructive pulmonary disease. *Eur Respir J* 1992;**5**:659–64.

3 Anonymous. The British guidelines on asthma management. 1995 review and position statement. *Thorax* 1997;**52**:i–S21.

4 Canadian Thoracic Society Workshop Group. Guidelines for the assessment and management of chronic obstructive pulmonary disease. *CMAJ* 1992;**147**:420–8.

5 Thoracic Society of Australia and New Zealand. Guidelines for the management of chronic obstructive pulmonary disease. *Mod Med Aust* 1995;**7**:132–46.

6 American Thoracic Society. Standards for the care of patients with chronic obstructive pulmonary disease (COPD) and asthma. *Am Rev Respir Dis* 1987;**136**:225–44.

7 American Thoracic Society. Standards for the diagnosis and care of patients with chronic obstructive pulmonary disease. *Am J Respir Crit Care Med* 1995;**152**:S77–120.

8 Siafakas NM, Vermeire P, Pride NB *et al*. Optimal assessment and management of chronic obstructive pulmonary disease (COPD). The European Respiratory Society Task Force. *Eur Respir J* 1995;**8**:1398–420.

9 Anonymous. BTS guidelines for the management of chronic obstructive pulmonary disease. The COPD Guidelines Group of the Standards of Care Committee of the BTS. *Thorax* 1997; **52**(Suppl 5):S1–28.

10 Murray CJ, Lopez AD. Global mortality, disability, and the contribution of risk factors: Global Burden of Disease Study. *Lancet* 1997;**349**:1436–42.

11 Pauwels RA, Buist AS, Calverley PMA, Jenkins CR, Hurd SS. Global strategy for the diagnosis, management and prevention of chronic obstructive pulmonary disease. *Am J Respir Crit Care Med* 2001;**163**:1256–76.

12 Celli BR, MacNee W. Standards for the diagnosis and treatment of patients with COPD: a summary of the ATS/ERS position paper. *Eur Respir J* 2004;**23**:932–46.

13 Chronic obstructive pulmonary disease. National clinical guideline on management of chronic obstructive pulmonary disease in adults in primary and secondary care. *Thorax* 2004;**59**(Suppl 1):1–232.

14 Kasahara Y, Tuder RM, Cool CD *et al*. Endothelial cell death and decreased expression of vascular endothelial growth factor and vascular endothelial growth factor receptor 2 in emphysema. *Am J Respir Crit Care Med* 2001;**163**:737–44.

15 Vestbo J, Lange P. Can GOLD Stage 0 provide information of prognostic value in chronic obstructive pulmonary disease? *Am J Respir Crit Care Med* 2002;**166**:329–32.

16 Hardie JA, Vollmer WM, Buist AS, Bakke P, Morkve O. Respiratory symptoms and obstructive pulmonary disease in a population aged over 70 years. *Respir Med* 2005;**99**: 186–95.

17 Celli BR, Halbert RJ, Isonaka S, Schau B. Population impact of different definitions of airway obstruction. *Eur Respir J* 2003;**22**:268–73.

18 Celli BR, Cote CG, Marin JM *et al*. The body-mass index, airflow obstruction, dyspnea, and exercise capacity index in chronic obstructive pulmonary disease. *N Engl J Med* 2004; **350**:1005–12.

19 Celli BR, Calverley PM, Rennard SI *et al*. Proposal for a multidimensional staging system for chronic obstructive pulmonary disease. *Respir Med* 2005;**99**:1546–54.

20 Calverley PMA, Burge PS, Spencer S, Anderson JA, Jones PW. Bronchodilator reversibility testing in chronic obstructive pulmonary disease. *Thorax* 2003;**58**:659–64.

21 Burge PS, Calverley PMA, Jones PW, Spencer S, Anderson JA. Prednisolone response in patients with chronic obstructive pulmonary disease: results from the ISOLDE study. *Thorax* 2003;**58**:654–8.

22 French N. Use of pneumococcal polysaccharide vacines:no simple answers. *J Infection* 2003;**46**:78–86.

23 Alfageme I, Vazquez R, Reyes N *et al.* Clinical efficacy of antipneumococcal vaccination in patients with COPD. *Thorax* 2006;**61**:189–95.

24 Vincken W, Van Noord JA, Greefhorst AP *et al.* Improved health outcomes in patients with COPD during 1 year's treatment with tiotropium. *Eur Respir J* 2002;**19**:209–16.

25 Calverley P, Pauwels R, Vestbo J *et al.* Combined salmeterol and fluticasone in the treatment of chronic obstructive pulmonary disease: a randomised controlled trial. *Lancet* 2003;**361**:449–56.

26 Szafranski W, Cukier A, Ramirez A *et al.* Efficacy and safety of budesonide/formoterol in the management of chronic obstructive pulmonary disease. *Eur Respir J* 2003;**21**:74–81.

27 Jones PW, Willits LR, Burge PS, Calverley PM. Disease severity and the effect of fluticasone propionate on chronic obstructive pulmonary disease. *Eur Respir J* 2003;**21**:68–73.

28 National Emphysema Treatment Trial Research Group. A randomized trial comparing lung-volume reduction surgery with medical therapy for severe emphysema. *N Engl J Med* 2003;**348**:2059–73.

29 Bach PB, Brown C, Gelfand SE, McCrory DC, American College of Physicians-American Society of Internal Medicine, American College of Chest Physicians. Management of acute exacerbations of chronic obstructive pulmonary disease: a summary and appraisal of published evidence. *Ann Intern Med* 2001;**134**:600–20.

30 Davies L, Angus RM, Calverley PMA. Oral corticosteroids in patients admitted to hospital with exacerbations of chronic obstructive pulmonary disease: a prospective randomised controlled trial. *Lancet* 1999;**354**:456–60.

31 Niewoehner DE, Erbland ML, Deupree RH *et al.* Effect of systemic glucocorticoids on exacerbations of chronic obstructive pulmonary disease. *N Engl J Med* 1999;**340**:1941–7.

32 Davies L, Wilkinson M, Bonner S, Calverley PMA, Angus RM. 'Hospital at home' versus hospital care in patients with exacerbations of chronic obstructive pulmonary disease: prospective randomised controlled trial. *BMJ* 2000;**321**:1265–8.

33 Skwarska E, Cohen G, Skwarski KM *et al.* Randomised controlled trial of supported discharge in patients with exacerbations of chronic obstructive pulmonary disease. *Thorax* 2000;**55**:907–12.

34 Lightowler JV, Wedzicha JA, Elliott MW, Ram FS. Noninvasive positive pressure ventilation to treat respiratory failure resulting from exacerbations of chronic obstructive pulmonary disease: Cochrane systematic review and meta-analysis. *BMJ* 2003;**326**:185.

35 Davidoff F, Haynes B, Sackett D, Smith R. Evidence based medicine. *BMJ* 1995;**310**:1085–6.

36 Soriano JB, Vestbo J, Pride NB *et al.* Survival in COPD patients after regular use of fluticasone propionate and salmeterol in general practice. *Eur Respir J* 2002;**20**:819–25.

37 Decramer M, Rutten-van Molken M, Dekhuijzen PN *et al.* Effects of *N*-acetylcysteine on outcomes in chronic obstructive pulmonary disease (Bronchitis Randomized on NAC Cost-Utility Study, BRONCUS): a randomised placebo-controlled trial. *Lancet* 2005;**365**:1552–60.

38 Fabbri LM, Hurd SS. Global Strategy for the Diagnosis, Management and Prevention of COPD: 2003 update. *Eur Respir J* 2003;**22**:1–2.

SECTION 7
Pharmacotherapy: developing therapies

CHAPTER 68
Protease inhibitors

Philip Davies, Malcolm MacCoss and Richard Mumford

Chronic obstructive pulmonary disease (COPD) results from the detrimental effects of inhaled toxic environmental stimuli on processes that maintain the normal function of the lung. The capacity of the host defence system, most obviously its innate component, to protect against toxic insults is remarkable. The development of COPD is insidiously slow and is manifested in only a minority of the population that exposes itself to stimuli such as cigarette smoke [1,2]. Effective host defence in the lung entails the recognition and removal of toxic stimuli by mechanisms that do not impact negatively on the physiological functions of the organ. Another essential aspect of host defence is the removal of damaged cells and extracellular matrices with initiation of repair mechanisms. Failure to fulfil these functions leads to persistent acute and chronic inflammation that can eventually lead to overt disease.

Appropriate expression and regulation of extracellular protease activity is essential for processes that maintain lung health. These functions include the extracellular breakdown and remodelling of damaged matrices as well as formation and inactivation of biologically active peptide and protein mediators. The activity of proteases is regulated by their maintenance as latent precursors, sequestration in intracellular compartments and inhibition by a wide variety of intra- and extracellular inhibitors. Genetically based defects in these regulatory mechanisms or inappropriate expression of protease activity can lead to pathological changes and overt disease. The observations by Laurell and Eriksson that a defect in α_1-antitrypsin, later shown to be a potent inhibitor of neutrophil elastase, is associated with the increased incidence of COPD led to the formulation of the protease–antiprotease hypothesis [3,4]. In a historical perspective published in 1991, Eriksson [3] concluded that 'Elastase may well be the causal agent in all cases of emphysema'. This conclusion was made with specific reference to neutrophil elastase. This hypothesis has been modified to include a number of other proteases with elastolytic activity. Moreover, it is likely that the inflammatory processes that lead to elastolysis associated with loss of lung function depend on cleavage of many substrates by both elastolytic and non-elastolytic enzymes. The activities of proteases in inflammation leading to COPD occur in the context of the interactions of recruited cells of the immune system with the local cells and the interstitial tissues of the lung. A total of 553 genes encoding proteases and their catalytically inactive homologues have been annotated in the human genome and many of these are expressed in the lung [5]. This number is significantly increased in COPD as cells of the immune system are recruited and local cells are activated in coordinated responses to inflammatory stimuli. These proteases fall into four distinct classes: the serine/threonine, metallo-, cysteine and aspartyl proteases. The classes that are of most obvious relevance to the pathology of COPD are also the most heavily populated; there are 186 metalloproteases, 176 serine proteases and 143 cysteine proteases.

Detailed knowledge of the three-dimensional structure and catalytic mechanism of these classes of proteases has allowed the development of prototypic inhibitors of great potency and often specificity to match. The challenge for medicinal chemists has been to identify compound classes with mechanistic, pharmacokinetic, pharmacodynamic and toxicological properties that are commensurate with safe long-term use in humans. These efforts have been extensively documented and reviewed [6–15]. Some of these inhibitors have advanced into clinical evaluation [13,16,17] yet there is no clear indication of disease-modifying efficacy for any of them. This is not surprising given the difficulty of establishing such parameters; the experience with evaluating the efficacy of replacement therapy with α_1-antitrypsin is salutary in this respect as disease progression is measured over a period of years and modification is correspondingly difficult to establish.

Strategies for the development of effective and safe protease inhibitors should benefit from an understanding of the physiological functions and role in host defence of their target enzyme(s) together with a definition of the shortfall of endogenous regulatory mechanisms that underlie their inappropriate activity in COPD. This knowledge will help define their pharmacological profile and their therapeutic index in the context of any mechanism-based toxicity that could occur during their extended use. Present concepts of inflammatory processes in COPD are discussed as they relate to proteases with a view to identifying how the spatial and temporal regulation of enzyme activity may be disrupted in the microenvironment of the lung during inflammatory responses to inhaled toxins (i.e. which activities of proteases are essential to lung health and which are in inappropriate locations at the wrong time thus leading to disease).

Because pharmacological inhibition of proteases will occur in the presence of endogenous inhibitors, measurements and correlation of the pharmacokinetic and pharmacodynamic properties of protease inhibitors are critical to ensure appropriate inhibition of the target enzyme(s). With this information in hand it will be more realistic to commit the resources required to determine whether pharmacological efficacy has clinical benefit based on the modification of chronic pathological changes. The elucidation of the precise role of individual proteases in COPD is exceedingly difficult, arguably best achieved by specific pharmacological approaches. The surprising robustness and relatively normal phenotype of mice in which a number of individual proteases have been genetically deleted [18,19] suggests that complete pharmacological inhibition of a protease-mediating pathology will not be accompanied by unacceptable mechanism-based toxicity.

Proteases with potential for involvement in inflammation and tissue damage leading to functional pathology in COPD

The irreversible consequences of the degradation of elastic tissue have provided a focus for research on proteases with elastinolytic activity. A number of these exist beyond the serine proteases, elastase, cathepsin G and protease 3 (PR3), which are present in large quantities in neutrophils. These include the cysteine cathepsins K, L and S [20,21], the matrix metalloproteases (MMP) MMP-2, MMP-7 [22–25], MMP-9 and MMP-12 [26–30]. These proteases are present in a variety of cells, most notably neutrophils and macrophages. Studies in gene-deleted and transgenic mice have provided a clear indication for the involvement of enzymes such as neutrophil elastase [31], MMP-12 [32,33] and MMP-9 [34] as well as cathepsins L and S [20] in certain aspects of the pathology of COPD.

Based on the complexity of the pathology of COPD, many elastolytic proteases are potential contributors to the disease. These activities are therefore key targets, especially for preservation of elastic recoil function. This is critical because elastic tissue constitutes only a small percentage of tissue mass and has very limited capacity for replacement based on calculations of the half-life of lung elastin [35]. Other non-elastolytic proteases acting on a variety of substrates have diverse and essential roles in mediating events leading to terminal elastolysis [28,29]. Many examples are emerging of how they can indirectly facilitate elastolytic activity, some of which are listed in Table 68.1.

Table 68.1 Elastolytic proteases and non-elastolysins that possess other activities which promote inflammation and tissue damage.

Enzyme	Elastolysin	Indirect effect	Ref.
Neutrophil elastase	Yes	Degradation of MMP inhibitors	[36]
		Stimulation of mucus secretion	[37]
		Cleavage of C3bi and CR1	[38]
		Transcriptional activation	[39]
MMP-2	Yes	Facilitation of aneurysm formation	[40,41]
MMP-7	Yes	Inactivation of α_1PI	[42]
		Release of active TNF from macrophages	[43]
MMP-9	No	Inactivation of α_1PI	[44]
MMP-12	Yes	Inactivation of α_1PI	[29]
		Chemotactic fragments from elastin	[32]
DPP1	No	Activation of neutrophil elastase, cathepsin G and PR3	[45]
Plasmin	No	Activation of pro-MMP-7	[24,46]
Cathepsin S	Yes	Antigen processing	[47]
Cathepsin L	Yes		

DPP1, dipeptidyl peptidase 1; MMP, matrix metalloprotease; PR3, protease 3; TNF, tumour necrosis factor.

This is not necessarily unidirectional because proteases sometimes have a negative modulatory effect on processes permissive to elastolysis. This can occur by degradation of peptide-based pro-inflammatory mediators or generation of anti-inflammatory peptides from endogenous substrates. The activity of these proteases is governed by a complex series of spatial and temporal considerations involving the release, activation of proenzymes, catalytic association with substrates and subsequent inactivation by natural inhibitors in the lung microenvironment. Some of the same principles apply to proteases derived from precursors involved in the activation of humoral pathways including the alternative–classical complement cascade, blood coagulation and processing of precursors of vasoactive peptides such as kinins, angiotensins and neurokinins. These will not be discussed further here although they are significant contributors to inflammation in the lung.

Innate immune responses, inflammation and tissue damage in COPD

COPD results from sustained self-perpetuating inflammation leading to tissue damage and structural changes in the lung. The disease is caused by a number of environmental stimuli of which cigarette smoke is the most common [1]. Many components of the humoral, innate and adaptive immune systems are activated in COPD and have been implicated in various aspects of its pathogenesis. This is to be expected given the complexity of cigarette smoke with its content of toxic substances and particles [48]. Tobacco contains more than 4500 compounds in its particulate and vapour phases. Many of these are biologically active, epitomized by nicotine [48]. Other components of cigarette smoke are pro-inflammatory and carcinogenic [48], which result in inflammation that persists for a long time after cessation of smoking [49,50].

Innate immunity is responsible for host responses against infectious and other exogenous agents together with the clearance of endogenous apoptotic cells and damaged tissue [51–54]. Its activation is dependent on genes coded by germline DNA in contrast to the gene rearrangements essential for adaptive immune responses. The convergence and synergies between innate and adaptive immunity has been recognized for over a century by the discoveries of the cellular basis of innate immunity and the role of antibodies as humoral effectors of adaptive immunity [53]. The function of the innate immune response is divided into afferent and efferent or sensing and effector arms, which in turn comprise cellular and humoral components. The cellular sensing functions are mediated through a series of specific receptors, notably the Toll-like receptors (TLR), of which at least 10 have now been identified [53]. They are derived from ancient precursors associated with host defence responses common to plants and animals and function either individually or in combination to recognize and respond to diverse stimuli. For example, TLR4 acts independently to recognize lipopolysaccharide (LPS), which is probably its only ligand. Other TLRs such as TLR1 and TLR6 can form complexes with TLR2 to broaden the function of TLR2 significantly [53–55]. Beyond the TLRs there exist structurally diverse receptors, loosely described as 'scavenger receptors', which recognize a wide variety of exogenous and endogenous ligands [56,57]. Examples with well-characterized endogenous ligands include Class A SR (modified low density lipoprotein), CD36 (modified lipids present on damaged cells), CD14 (LPS binding protein) and mannose receptor (lysosomal hydrolases, myeloperoxidase and other mannosyl/fucosyl glyconconjugates). The humoral arm of the innate immune system includes the well-characterized complement, vasoactive precursor and coagulation systems as well as the soluble products of acute phase responses.

Detailed information is not available on how these cellular receptors and humoral precursors recognize and respond to the components of cigarette smoke. However, the lack of major involvement of adaptive immunity in COPD is consistent with its pathogenesis being driven by aberrant function of the innate immune system. The activation of the humoral systems often requires regulated protease activity while activation of cellular receptors leads to signal transduction through a number of pathways including the MAP kinases, nuclear factor κB (NF-κB) and others that have been delineated in recent years [58] and shown to be important in host defence as well as homoeostasis. These signal transduction responses can facilitate the direct mobilization of intracellular stores of proteases by exocytosis, initiate the activation of latent precursors or the activation of gene programmes for the synthesis and release of new enzymes. It is not surprising that the pathology of COPD is complex because the multiple components of cigarette smoke probably activate several of these cellular receptors, triggering complex downstream responses and the generation of many mediators of inflammation and tissue injury.

While cells of the adaptive immune response have been implicated in various aspects of COPD [59–61], this discussion will pay particular attention to proteases of cells of the innate immune system, notably macrophages [28] and neutrophils [62]. The complex interactions between these two cell types that have evolved to protect the host against infectious agents are evident in COPD. It is ironic that our species has unknowingly or knowingly been unfortunate enough to expose itself to a wide range of non-infectious environmental stimuli that induce the spectrum of diseases that are recognized as the pneumoconioses and occupational lung diseases [63]. The lumen and interstitial tissues of the lung contain resident populations of macrophages. A primary function of these alveolar macrophages is to sequester and remove these stimuli without triggering tissue injurious inflammation. Lung washouts of smokers contain increased numbers of alveolar macrophages suggesting altered kinetics and transit into the lung of blood monocytes in response to cigarette smoke [19]. This new population of macrophages could include a subset of monocytes that home only to inflamed tissues. This possibility is illustrated by the preferential recruitment of a short-lived $CX_3CR1^{lo}CCR2^+Gr1^+$ subset of adoptively transferred monocytes into the inflamed peritoneal cavity of congenic mice [64]. It is unknown whether these recruited cells include those described as being enriched in serine proteases normally associated with neutrophils [25,65–67]. Alveolar macrophages from smokers appear morphologically activated and are laden with residues from cigarette smoke which they have endocytosed during their residence in the lung.

The understanding of the roles of macrophages in innate immune responses has led to a far better understanding of how neutrophils are recruited to the lungs of cigarette smokers. Neutrophils are rarely present in healthy extravascular tissues; the host probably has multiple mechanisms for ensuring that they are recruited from the circulation only when required. Innate immune responses have evolved in large part to protect against infectious agents and it is not surprising that macrophages normally resident in extravascular tissues have a considerable capacity to recruit and activate neutrophils when their receptors of innate immunity are triggered [68]. While the original protease–antiprotease hypothesis emphasized the role of neutrophil serine proteases in lung destruction, current thinking is much more focused on the role of the macrophage in recruiting neutrophils to the inflamed lung. This is most obviously facilitated by chemokines such as interleukin 8 (IL-8), leukotriene B_4 (LTB_4) and cytokines produced by macrophages in response to inflammatory stimuli. Tumour necrosis factor α (TNF-α) triggers the neutrophil to generate and release its mediators [69]. The severity of elastase-induced emphysema is reduced in double TNF-α receptor knockout mice [70], suggesting that this cytokine may have a key role. Furthermore, γ-interferon (IFN-γ) expressed as a transgene induces severe lung inflammation and destruction associated with the induction of a number of proteases [71], while overexpression of TNF-α leads to increases in lung volumes and pulmonary hypertension [72], confirming the role of inflammation.

The integrated cellular function of neutrophils is essential for protection against a wide range of infectious agents. Their bacteriostatic and bactericidal function is mediated by a powerful armamentarium of cidal molecules including hydroxyl radicals, singlet oxygen, oxygen halides, hydrogen peroxide [73] and nitrating agents together with antimicrobial peptides and, to some extent, proteases [74]. While these molecules are critical for protecting against infectious agents [75], they also have considerable potential for damaging the host. The capacity of neutrophil proteases, stored within azurophil granules in large amounts at millimolar concentrations [76], to cause acute lung damage is exemplified by diseases where they are released extracellularly in amounts in excess of available natural inhibitors. The presence of high concentrations of active neutrophil elastase in the sputum of cystic fibrosis patients can account in a number of ways for the extensive lung damage in this disease [38,77]. In acute exacerbations of Goodpasture syndrome [78], haemorrhagic immune complex-induced vasculitis results from gross destruction of alveolar basement membranes. This damage is probably mediated by the directed local activity of neutrophil serine proteases such as elastase, cathepsin G and PR3 following stimulation by engagement of Fc receptors by immune complexes formed in basement membranes [79,80]. This is consistent with inhibition of haemorrhage associated with immune complex formation in the lung by selective neutrophil elastase inhibitors [81]. This indicates how the persistence or release of proteases in inappropriate microenvironments in interstitial tissue, which excludes inhibitors, can rapidly lead to major tissue damage. It is noteworthy that patients with glomerulonephritis associated with Goodpasture syndrome are more likely to experience pulmonary haemorrhage if they smoke [82].

The potential of neutrophil serine proteases to cause catastrophic tissue damage is great. It is therefore all the more remarkable that the critical structures of the lung and other tissues are protected so well against these enzymes. Approximately 10^{10} neutrophils are released into the circulation every day and these cells spend half of their time in the pulmonary circulation with an even slower transit time during cigarette smoking [83]. These cells are efficiently cleared from the body with few emerging into extravascular tissues. In blood, α_2-macroglobulin and α_1-antitrypsin provide an excess of inhibitory capacity for any enzyme that may be released. This is indicated by the presence of α_1-antitrysin elastase complexes as well as specific cleavage products of plasma proteins as exemplified by the $A\alpha(Val^{360})$ neoepitope exposed on a 42-kd fragment of fibrinogen [84], even in plasma of healthy individuals. These markers are elevated in a variety of inflammatory diseases [84,85]. Interstitial tissues have their own complement of inhibitors for any released neutrophil proteases [62]. Also, there are very effective mechanisms in place for removal of neutrophils by macrophages that are specifically programmed to recognize and remove apoptotic cells

[86] to prevent further enzyme release if the cells were to disintegrate.

The alveolar macrophage removes ageing and damaged cells by various scavenger receptors such as CD36 and the phosphatidylserine receptor [86,87], which remove neutrophils before their proteases are released. This is important because neutrophil elastase cleaves the phosphatidylserine receptor [87] and inhibits the phagocytosis of apoptotic cells by alveolar macrophages. If, as suggested here, the role of the neutrophil to remove toxic constituents of cigarette smoke is not essential then containment and timely removal of its protease content is critical. The more efficiently that this end is achieved the less likely it is that the products of activated macrophages and neutrophils become misdirected against the host. It is significant that some of the same cytokines, such as TNF-α, IL-1β, IFN-γ and granulocyte–macrophage colony-stimulating factor (GM-CSF), that macrophages use to enhance the bactericidal activity of neutrophils are also strong inhibitors of apoptosis. These effects are mediated through a factor originally described as a growth factor for early stage B lymphocytes [88]. Decreased neutrophil apoptosis is seen in septic patients and a similar trend has been claimed in patients hospitalized with acute exacerbations of COPD [89] as well as in patients expressing the antiapoptotic molecule survivin in their neutrophils [90]. In view of this, mechanisms by which macrophages limit the recruitment of neutrophils to sites of inflammation and facilitate their removal may be important in limiting tissue damage. For example, the induction of CD36 function in alveolar macrophages by peroxisome proliferator activated receptor γ (PPARγ) agonism [91,92] could be a significant pharmacological target for enhancing clearance of apoptotic neutrophils.

Elucidation of the role of proteases in COPD

Robust surrogate markers of relevant activities of individual proteases in COPD are not available. While there have been many documented examples of elevated protease activity in the lung of COPD patients [93–97], these have not been definitively linked to degradation of critical substrates that lead to disease. The definition of the role of individual proteases in COPD would be greatly aided by the availability of proximal markers of their activity. Ideally, these would be unique soluble fragments (generated by the endogenous activity of a specific protease) that are readily measured in blood or urine. An alternative would be non-specific markers of the degradation of relevant substrates as exemplified by desmosine as a marker of elastic tissue damage. Failure to consistently detect specific breakdown products of elastin is not surprising given the relative paucity of this

substrate together with its longevity in the lung [35]. This is reminiscent of the difficulty in developing markers of cartilage breakdown in osteoarthritis [98]. This disease is characterized by the breakdown of type II collagen which, like elastin in the lung, is laid down only once and cannot be replaced in a fully functional form if damaged. Systemic measures of enzyme activation are seen with neutrophil elastase in a variety of diseases including cystic fibrosis and Acute Respiratory Distress Syndrome (ARDS) [85] but not reproducibly seen in COPD although this does not negate the role of the enzyme in the lung. Systemic measures of the consequence of ongoing local inflammation such as acute phase proteins have been used extensively in other diseases including atherosclerosis [99]. In COPD, robust increases of C-reactive protein levels are associated with exacerbations of diseases associated with infection [100] but are lower and highly variable in stable disease [101]. A possibility that remains to be fully explored is the generation of long-lived soluble neoepitopes measurable in plasma as exemplified by cleavage products of fibrinogen by neutrophil elastase [84] (see below).

Utility of animal models to study the role of proteases in COPD

The original protease–antiprotease concept led to widespread use and investigation of animal models of COPD based upon intratracheal administration of tissue-degrading enzymes [102], particularly elastases. In these models, immediate damage occurs, including the destruction of vascular basement membranes with consequent haemorrhage. A non-specific inflammatory response ensues, leading to damage resembling some aspects of emphysema. The initial effects of proteases lead to secondary changes which contribute to indices of subsequent alveolar destruction [70]. These models have utility for defining the pharmacodynamic properties of protease inhibitors [103]. However, they do not reflect the intricacies of damage caused by ongoing activity of multiple proteases in the microenvironments of the lung inflamed by cigarette smoke and have not been useful in delineating the role of individual proteases in COPD.

The development of technology to allow sustained exposure to and inhalation of cigarette smoke by mice [32] and other species [104,105] has allowed a more detailed evaluation of events leading to chronic pathological changes. Exposure of several animal species to cigarette smoke induces changes resembling emphysema-like loss of alveolar structural integrity and functional elasticity [104]. These studies have provided a much clearer understanding of how the innate immune response and its constituent proteases can mediate the irreversible changes brought about by loss of elastic tissue. A picture has emerged indicating a number of interdependent functions of macrophages and neutrophils involving their respective proteases in the inflammation and tissue destruction seen in this model.

The observation that deletion of the gene for MMP-12 in mice greatly reduces their susceptibility to cigarette smoke [32] led to a fundamental change in thinking about the protease–antiprotease hypothesis. This change continues as new observations are made in mice with specific genetic modifications related to protease function [19,28,29, 106–108]. Not only is the development of emphysema abolished in the smoke-exposed MMP-12 null mouse, but the recruitment of macrophages and neutrophils to the lung is also inhibited [32].

The decrease in experimental emphysema also observed in mice lacking neutrophil elastase has been attributed to multiple consequences of the absence of the enzyme [31,109]. These include inhibition of neutrophil recruitment, together with reductions in the inactivation of tissue inhibitor of metalloprotease 1 (TIMP1) and activation of the 55-kd latent precursor of MMP-12. In addition, higher levels of α_1-antitrypsin are present in lung tissue extracts from MMP-12 null mice exposed to cigarette smoke. This is attributed to lack of MMP-12 mediated degradation of the serine protease inhibitor. Alternatively, this could result from diminished consumption as a result of decreased release of elastase from activated neutrophils despite their recruitment in similar numbers as seen in MMP-12 sufficient mice. The failure of MMP-12 null macrophages to generate TNF-α, which in turn activates neutrophils to release elastase, would be consistent with this [110]. As commented on elsewhere [111,112], a series of studies by Churg *et al.* on the sequential events in the lungs of mice exposed to cigarette smoke have provided considerable insights into the phenotypes of the MMP-12 and neutrophil elastase null mice. Acute inhalation of cigarette smoke results in the recruitment of neutrophils [113], which is dependent both on MMP-12 [113,114] and TNF-α [110,114]. It is to be noted that the C57BL/6 mice used in these studies produce more TNF-α than the 129 strain used by Hautamaki *et al.* [32]. The acute damage is inhibited by α_1-antitrypsin [115,116], and in a similar model in guinea pigs, synthetic inhibitors of neutrophil elastase protect partially against emphysema development [105].

The relevance of these findings in humans remains to be clarified. The different activities of macrophage metalloelastases in the two species [24] raises significant questions regarding the role of MMP-12 compared with MMP-7 and MMP-9 in humans. Neutrophil elastase remains a target, with the potential role of PR3 [117] less clearly defined. Concerns remain, however, regarding the role of neutrophil serine proteases in host defence based on findings in

gene-deleted mice for elastase [118], dipeptidyl peptidase 1 (DPP1) [119] and the phenotype of Papillon–Lefèvre patients defective in DPP1 function [120]. All these studies suggest that strategies to regulate neutrophil elastase activity completely could be counterproductive.

Further insights into the potential function of individual proteases have been obtained when the genes for these molecules are conditionally up-regulated by cytokines and other endogenous molecules. In these instances, changes resembling COPD occur in the absence of an inducing stimulus in transgenic mice where molecules regulating protease activity are deleted or overexpressed. For example, the transgenic overexpression of IL-13 [121,122] results in aberrant expression of metalloproteases such as MMP-9 and MMP-12 and the cysteine proteases cathepsins K, L and S. Removal of the critical regulatory function of the integrin αv-$\beta 6$ [33] results in specific aberrant expression of MMP-12. Endogenously generated lung destruction can be induced by host defence mediators including cytokines such as IL-13, TNF-α and IFN-γ. Chemokines are also active in this respect as is illustrated by the significant protection of the IL-13 transgene-induced lung damage when present in mice lacking the chemokine receptor CCR2 [123] and CCR1 [124]. The phenotypes of these mice provide independent indications of the potential importance of alveolar macrophages to mediate lung destruction. Thus, intervention in pathology with protease inhibitors should not be targeted at endstage destructive processes alone. Consideration should also be given to the ability of proteases to generate biologically active molecules, or to degrade regulatory molecules, that contribute to inflammation and hence pathology. A summary of this work is provided in Table 68.2.

However, these findings cannot be directly extrapolated to humans. Overexpression of inducers of inflammatory cascades as exemplified by IL-13 will distort the natural inflammatory process by exaggerating the pattern of expression of pro-inflammatory proteases and anti-inflammatory protease inhibitors. This, together with differences in gene expression in humans compared with animal species, means that the molecular details of the pathogenic mechanisms of COPD in humans will be quite different from those being elucidated in mice and other species. This is the case for cystic fibrosis where deletion of the cystic fibrosis transmembrane conductance regulator (CFTR) channel is not sufficient for the development of lung disease in mice [143]. Comparative gene profiling should provide useful information and the basis for this is underway with the comparison of the human and murine degradomes [5]. Profiling of various sites of the inflamed lung at successive stages of disease progression in smokers, be they mice or men, will provide much information regarding the potential use of protease inhibitors.

Table 68.2 Genetic manipulation of protease genes and functions. Potential implications for pathogenesis of COPD.

Gene target	Phenotype	Challenge phenotype	Ref.
Serine proteases			
PMN elastase – deletion	Normal	Impaired cigarette smoke induced lung inflammation and emphysema	[31]
		Decrease in neutrophil recruitment, inactivation of TIMP, activation of MMP-12 precursor	[109]
		Decreased susceptibility to LPS	[125]
		Impaired host defence	[118]
Cathepsin G – deletion	Normal		[126]
		Decreased susceptibility to LPS	[125]
PMN elastase/cathepsin G – deletion	Normal	Decreased susceptibility to LPS	[125]
		Diminished bacterial clearance	[119]
SLPI – deletion	Normal	Increased susceptibility to LPS and sepsis – enhanced innate immune responses	[127]
Metalloproteases			
MMP-1 Overexpression under haptoglobin promoter	Enlarged airspace – not clear whether developmental		[128] [129]
MMP-2	Normal	Impaired allergic inflammation but increased susceptibility to asphyxiation	[130]
		Impaired tumour angiogenesis and growth	[131]
MMP-7		Impaired wound healing and host defence	[132]
		Impaired chemokine mobilization and neutrophil migration	[133]
MMP-9		No change in disease induction after cigarette smoke inhalation	[34]
		Decreased airspace enlargement in IL-13 transgenic mice	[121]
		Impaired cellular infiltration and hyperresponsiveness after allergen	[134]
		Diminished aortic aneurysm	[41]
		Decreased dendritic cell recruitment	[135]
MMP-12	Normal	Abolition of cigarette smoke induced emphysema	[32]
		Macrophages fail to penetrate basement membranes	[136]
MT1-MMP	Defect in skeletal development, dwarfism, osteopenia		[137,138]
TIMP 3	Spontaneous airway enlargement		[139]
αvβ6		Increased airspace enlargement. Specific increase in MMP-12 expression	[33]
Surfactant D	Increased MMP activation and emphysema		[140]
Cysteine proteases			
Cathepsin S		Decreased airspace enlargement in IL-13 transgenic mice	[121]
		Diminished vascular wall inflammation when crossed with LDL receptor null mice	[141]
DPP1	Normal		[45]
		Decrease in experimental arthritis	[142]
		Decreased susceptibility to caecal ligation induced sepsis	[119]
		Increased bacterial load	[119]

DPP1, dipeptidyl peptidase 1; IL, interleukin; LDL, low-density lipoprotein; LPS, lipopolysaccharide; MMP, matrix metalloprotease; PMN, polymorphonuclear neutrophil; SLPI, secretory leucoprotease inhibitor; TIMP, tissue inhibitor of metalloprotease.

Endogenous regulation of protease activity

While the profusion of information emerging from the studies described above gives an indication of the potential of these individual enzymes to cause tissue damage, it does not provide a clear picture of their role in human disease. This potential is governed by complex regulatory processes that limit protease activity. Prominent among these are the diverse families of natural protease inhibitors which regulate the function of proteases in various body compartments such as blood and in the microenvironments of cells and their pericellular environment in interstitial tissue and other extravascular sites. These inhibitors are diverse in their structure, specificity and mechanism. Each of the major families of the degradome have well-characterized inhibitors of varying specificity as exemplified by the serpins [144], cystatins [145] and TIMPs [6]. In addition, α_2-macroglobulin has a more global function as a paninhibitor of most proteases from every class [6]. Often, these inhibitors do not completely inactivate their target enzymes as is the case with α_2-macroglobulin and enzyme–inhibitor complexes may have distinct biological activities not seen with either free enzyme or inhibitor. This is exemplified by the chemotactic activity of α_1-protease inhibitor (α_1PI) which has been inactivated by mouse macrophage elastase [146]. The deficiency of α_1PI provides the most widely studied example of how the lack of a single inhibitor with considerable specificity has a clear association with increased susceptibility to COPD. The extensive experience with replacement therapy with this inhibitor is discussed in Vogelmeier et al. [147]. More limited experiences with replacement therapy with other serine protease inhibitors [147] will not be discussed further here. The clinical efficacy and usefulness of replacement therapy remains to be fully established [148].

Defects in metalloprotease inhibitors have not been widely described in humans. Genetic ablation of TIMP3 in mice leads to spontaneous airspace enlargement early in life with shortened life span [139]. Inflammation is not prominent in the lungs of these animals but they contain increased MMP activity as detected by zymography. It is therefore reasonable to consider the development and evaluation of protease inhibitors that not only replace deficient function of natural inhibitors but which will give qualitatively different profiles of activity. Such properties have the potential to be double-edged swords; on the one hand they can have beneficial effects on protease activity which drives pathology but on the other may interfere with essential biological functions of the protease themselves or their complexes with their natural inhibitors.

The complexities of the function of natural inhibitors and the consequences of their modification in the lung are illustrated by studies of natural inhibitor function in murine strains with defined differences in α_1PI function [149,150]. In the pa+/pa+ pallid mouse a nonsense mutation in the gene for a pallidin results in a 50% decrease in syntaxin13, a molecule with which it interacts to mediate vesicle docking and fusion to early recycling endosomes. This is associated with an inability to export α_1PI into the circulation and a decreased elastase inhibitory capacity. Significant differences in both the rate of onset and nature of smoking-induced emphysema are seen in these mice when compared with congenic C57 mice. In the pallid mouse, emphysema is panlobular but in congenic mice it is centrilobular in location, emphasizing the different function of the natural inhibitor in different regions of the lung. The onset of changes in pallid mice is more rapid and while increases in mean linear intercept are eventually seen in congenic mice, they are not accompanied by the changes in lung compliance seen in the pallid mice. This suggests that pathogenic mechanisms may differ in various parts of the lung, as may be the case with COPD patients with deficient and normal α_1PI phenotypes, a consideration to be borne in mind when studying novel therapeutics with specific mechanisms of action.

These multiple regulatory controls ensure that the activities of these proteases have stringent temporal and spatial restrictions for their activity. It is when these finely tuned regulatory mechanisms are disrupted that it becomes more likely that protease activity with potential for inducing pathology occurs. Examples where this is acute and potentially catastrophic in nature is exemplified by exacerbations of Goodpasture syndrome [78] where formation or deposition of immune complexes in basement membranes lead to the activation of complement, the recruitment of neutrophils and the release of their potent tissue destructive serine proteases.

Cell biological approaches to the definition of the role of proteases in COPD

The extracellular environment into which cellular proteases are released and activated differs greatly from the intravascular compartment to extravascular domains and, relevant to COPD, the lumen of the lung. It is only from the latter space that free active enzyme can be recovered in purulent sputum and fluids of cystic fibrosis [77] and acutely infected patients with bronchitis and pneumonia. However, in most instances, aberrant protease activity will be transient and spatially constrained as extracellular inhibitors gain access to the enzyme, making it difficult to quantify the extent and duration of enzyme activity.

The capacity of neutrophils to cause tissue damage is well established [79,151,152] based on the exocytosis of the proteases stored in active form at high concentrations in their granules. Cell biological systems have been developed that allow the demonstration and measurement of these activities. Campbell *et al.* [153] have used morphological approaches at the single-cell level to demonstrate the proteolysis associated with degranulation of neutrophils onto appropriately labelled substrates. They generated micrographical images of this phenomenon at the level of single cells. The quantal nature of the release of enzyme concentrated in the azurophil granules of the neutrophil [76,154–156] results in a concentration and time-defined transient proteolysis as the released enzyme is diluted and fluid phase inhibitors gain access to the cloistered pericellular environment. Subsequently, quantitative analyses of these striking images were made at the level of individual azurophil granules [76]. These established the dynamics of this rapidly changing environment to the point of equilibrium with extracellular inhibitors as exemplified by α_1-antitrypsin, α_2-macroglobulin, secretory leucocyte protease inhibitor and the small molecule elastase inhibitor ICI 200,335. In the presence of a physiological concentration of protease inhibitor, degradation of fluorescent labelled fibronectin occurred over an area approximately eight-fold that of the individual neutrophils under observation. Appropriate specificity controls with inhibitors and antioxidants as well as cells from chronic patients with granulomatous disease indicated that this process was specific for elastase and not dependent upon oxidative inactivation of inhibitors. This approach has allowed calculation of the extent and duration of enzyme activity [76,157] with the demonstration of increased activity when extracellular inhibitor activity is compromised as exemplified by PiZZ plasma [153].

The serine proteases of neutrophils constitute by far the highest level of circulating cellular proteases. For example, elastase is estimated to achieve millimolar concentrations in the azurophil granule [157] which is a hundred-fold that of its plasma inhibitors. When neutrophils are degranulated in human blood their serine proteases are complexed by α_1-antitrypsin and α_2-macroglobulin, which are present in approximately a thousand-fold excess (the volume of azurophil granules, the repository of the serine proteases, is tiny compared with that of plasma in blood). However, transient activity of these proteases, before they are sequestered by inhibitors, is demonstrable based on the cleavage of plasma substrates and generation of specific neoepitopes. The use of neoepitope specific antibodies has provided a novel way of measuring the transient catalytic activity of a protease before its inhibition by natural inhibitors. Nossel *et al.* [158] pioneered this approach with the development of an antibody specific for the C-terminus of fibrinopeptide A, a 16-residue fragment of the Aα chain of fibrinogen generated by thrombin. Weitz *et al.* [159] used this antibody for an indirect assay of the Aα(1-21) fragment of fibrinogen generated by neutrophil elastase.

This provided an opportunity to seek robust and specific direct assays for various degradation products of elastase. Mumford *et al.* [84,160] developed an antibody specific for the C-terminus of the Aα(1-21) peptide and used it to demonstrate the activity of elastase released from neutrophils degranulated in blood [161]. Stimulation with granule-releasing agents resulted in peptide formation in the face of the high amounts of natural inhibitors. As would be expected, this signal is considerably amplified in blood from PiZZ patients and is normalized by reconstitution of the patients with α_1-antitrypsin [162].

The claim that Aα(1-21) is elevated in plasma from PiZZ patients [163] has not been confirmed by others. Based on the rapid clearance of Aα(1-21) *in vivo* it is unlikely that these elevations are represented by this neoepitope. However, this approach has great potential to seek markers of *in vivo* activity when applied to neoepitopes with long *in vivo* half-lives. A systematic evaluation of fibrinogen in this respect yielded a number of cleavage sites to include one at the Val^{360}-Ser^{361} of the Aα chain of fibrinogen [84]. This releases a 250 residue C-terminal peptide leaving a 42-kd molecule with the Aα(Val^{360}) associated with the β and γ chain of fibrinogen. A specific antibody to this new C-terminus long-lived molecule of high molecular weight showed it to be present in the plasma of healthy individuals at approximately 4 nmol/L concentration and elevated in the plasma of cystic fibrosis patients up to 1000 nmol/L as well as in rheumatoid synovial fluid [84]. Thus, healthy individuals express neutrophil elastase activity sufficient to maintain circulating levels of this cleavage product. The significance of these products in health is unknown but their elevation in disease provides a sensitive and specific method for exploring the systemic activity of proteases such as neutrophil elastase. Evaluation of the levels of these long-lived neoepitopes in PiZZ and COPD patients will be informative. This approach also provides a sensitive and specific pharmacodynamic method for monitoring the activity of elastase inhibitors in various environments, both *in vitro* and *in vivo*.

These cell biological findings highlight the consideration of whether the design of a pharmacological inhibitor should allow the introduction of properties that inhibit enzymes under circumstances where endogenous inhibitors fail to do so. Pharmacological inhibitors have the potential to be effective in the presence of endogenous inhibitors which are often present in gross molar excess over their target enzymes. Assays that measure enzyme activity over brief periods of time in restricted spatial environments provide optimal demonstration of these activities. Such agents would supplement natural inhibitors that are either in deficit or inactivated (e.g. by oxidants or overwhelmed by abnormal release and activation of proteases).

Individual proteases implicated in COPD are in some

instances derived from more than one cell type, as exemplified by the presence of serine proteinases associated primarily with neutrophils in monocytes with a pro-inflammatory phenotype [66,67]. The complexities of establishing the role of individual proteases in COPD is exemplified by studies on the role of MMP-9, also known as gelatinase B, in lung remodelling [34]. This enzyme is present not only in macrophages (secreted as an inactive precursor), but also in a number of lung cells including epithelium, Clara cells, alveolar type II cells, fibroblasts and smooth muscle as well as neutrophil from which it is released as an active complex with lipocalin [34]. It has a wide range of natural substrates, including elastin, relevant to the inflammation and tissue damage of COPD. However, its genetic ablation does not change the susceptibility of mice to cigarette smoke [34], although the airspace enlargement seen in IL-13 transgenic mice is decreased in its absence. Its activation by MMP-3 and its ability to inactivate serine protease inhibitors [44] suggests that its contribution to tissue damage will be greatly influenced by multiple factors in its environment and that these are probably as important as its intrinsic activity in determining its contributions to pathology. This is illustrated by its interaction with MMP-2 in the development of aortic aneurysms [164].

As the role of individual enzymes in cell-based elastolysis is elucidated by various approaches in animal species, it is clear that these mechanisms are not necessarily of the same qualitative or quantitative relevance in humans. A premium is placed on the study of human cells by these species differences in the degradome [5,165] and phenotypic differences in integrated expression of multiple protease activity. For example, a defect in MMP-2 in humans causes severe osteolysis and arthritis [166] not seen in null mice [36,130].

The macrophage expresses an extensive repertoire of extracellular protease during tissue remodelling, cellular clearance after apoptosis and the débridement of injured tissue. Major species differences exist in the effector molecules for these functions. The up-regulation of proteases exemplified by MMP-12 in the mouse results in direct elastolysis as well as the generation of chemotactic stimuli and cytokines leading to pathology. As is discussed here and elsewhere, MMP-12 has been shown to have prominent activity, not only as an elastase, but in other aspects of the inflammatory process in the smoking mouse. These include the induction of TNF-α synthesis in the macrophage and subsequent activation and involvement of the neutrophil in the smoking mouse model of emphysema [110,114]. However, the demonstration of the elastolytic activity of this enzyme by human monocytes has been problematical despite clear evidence of its presence and activity [167–169]. Early studies showed that human

alveolar macrophages have considerable elastolytic activity when cultured in the presence of human serum [170,171], which was ascribed predominantly to cysteine proteases. Human blood monocytes can be cultured under conditions where they display elastolytic activity orders of magnitude greater than initially described [24]. Key to this finding is the mediation of elastolysis by plasmin-dependent activation of matrilysin (MMP-7), which does not occur in mouse macrophages. Human monocytes cultured in autologous serum show a 10-fold enhancement of elastin degradation in the presence of urinary plasminogen activator. This activity is mediated by a metalloprotease based on its sensitivity to inhibition by the non-specific MMP inhibitor BB94. Plasmin-dependent enhancement of elastolysis is not apparent when the cells are cultured on an extracellular matrix derived from MDCK cells, emphasizing how the matrix in which cells find themselves influence their secretion of proteases. Enzyme activity can also be up-regulated as illustrated by the induction of gelatinase B by substrate [172]. Under these conditions, the synthesis of matrilysin (MMP-7) is also suppressed but the elastolytic activity of the culture medium of these cells is reconstituted by addition of exogenous active enzyme without further enhancement by either MMP-9 or MMP-12. The activity of MMP-7 under these conditions is further enhanced by cysteine proteases such as cathepsins L and S [173], but probably not K [174], as indicated by studies with cells in which this gene has been inactivated. The activity of the cysteine proteases is probably restricted to the cell–substrate interface within an acidified vacuole dependent on H$^+$-ATPase activity. These findings suggest that human monocytes are dependent on members of several classes of proteases for their optimal elastinolytic activity – the serine protease plasmin, the MMP matrilysin and a subset of lysosomal cysteine proteases – leading to the conclusion that 'therapeutics aimed at select members of both (cysteine/MMP) gene families might be necessary to ameliorate elastolytic effects *in vivo*' [24]. The same conclusion is probably applicable to the role of proteases and other processes that sustain the inflammation in COPD. Matrilysin has a number of other significant properties which imply that it could contribute to the chronic inflammation in COPD. It is a product of healthy epithelium and in mice its deficiency results in significant defects in wound healing [40]. Moreover, it has a significant role in facilitating neutrophil egress during acute lung injury through cleavage of the heparin sulphate proteoglycan syndecan1, which forms chemotactic gradients by binding the chemokine KC [133].

Cell biological studies will therefore continue to provide insights on the complexities of protease function in health and disease and should provide a critical bridge in establishing the efficacy of protease inhibitors [175].

The development of protease inhibitors as drugs for chronic inflammatory diseases

An expert panel convened by the National Institutes of Health (NIH) in 2002 to consider the needs and opportunities for clinical research in COPD [176] suggested six potential new therapeutic approaches. The first advocates direct inhibition of protease activity. Several of the other approaches could have an impact on disease progression involving aberrant protease activity. These include the following:

• The inhibition of recruitment of inflammatory cells.
• Enhancement of the antioxidant capacity of the lung to prevent loss of activity of molecules that down-regulate protease activity in various ways [177] including the reduction of the inhibitory capacity of α_1-antitrypsin [178].
• Inhibition of apoptosis of pulmonary cells associated with the development of emphysema [97]. This process is critically dependent on the activity of the caspase family of cysteine protease [179].
• Inhibition of mucus secretion by goblet and glandular mucosal cells because neutrophil serine proteases are potent mucus secretagogues [37].

There are important examples of the successful use of protease inhibitors in the treatment of human disease. Angiotensin-converting enzyme (ACE) inhibitors have been used extensively to treat cardiovascular disease, while the introduction of inhibitors of the aspartyl protease of HIV has made major contributions to the treatment of AIDS [180]. Attempts to discover and develop protease inhibitors for the therapy of COPD have been guided by insights into the role of proteases in the pathogenesis of the disease. The original protease–antiprotease hypothesis led to extensive efforts on neutrophil elastase as a target [13]. Matrix metalloprotease inhibitors active against the endoproteolytic activity of a number of enzymes have been extensively evaluated for the treatment of a range of chronic diseases including cancer [181] and arthritis [6]. As it has become clear that some of the same enzymes may be significant mediators of the pathology of COPD, efforts have been initiated in this direction [7,10,29]. There have been no compelling therapeutic breakthroughs in the therapy of cancer and arthritis, suggesting that the understanding of the role of metalloproteases in these diseases remains to be elucidated.

Criteria for the design of low molecular weight protease inhibitors

While the search for protease inhibitors has yielded agents of great intrinsic potency and specificity, much less attention has been given to the requirements for these agents to be effective in the complex environment in which proteases function in health and disease. The intrinsic activities of proteases are extensively regulated in a variety of ways. These include sequestration in intracellular compartments, often as inactive precursors. Once synthesized and processed to an active form, functional latency can be maintained through storage in granules as exemplified by the high concentrations of serine proteases present in the specialized azurophilic lysosomes of myeloid leukocytes. When released from cells, these proteases face an environment containing specific and extremely potent natural inhibitors. This is exemplified in blood, which contains molar excesses of both α_2-macroglobulin and other more specific inhibitors for their target enzymes. The extracellular catalytic activity of the major classes of proteases have different functional requirements. Metalloproteases exist as pro-enzymes with specific activators. These activators are still not well defined and may be induced in pathological situations. Cysteine proteases act most effectively in an acidic environment created by exocytosis of lysosomes and lose activity with adjustment of pH towards physiological levels. Neutrophil serine proteinases are active within azurophilic granules. In blood, their extracellular environment contains very large molar excesses of inhibitors such as α_1-antitrypsin and α_2-macroglobulin, albeit at lower concentrations than that of the enzyme in granules, hence the brief activity seen in blood when cells are degranulated. It is possible that this activity can be further modulated by cytokines to increase the activity of neutrophil membrane associated enzyme [182, 183]. The synthesis and activity of natural inhibitors may be down-regulated during pathology. Indications of this are exemplified by the decrease in α_1-antitrypsin gene expression in IL-13 transgenic mice [123] and its inactivation by oxidative stress [177]. It is therefore critical that these requirements for activity be considered for inhibitor design.

Development of mechanism-based neutrophil elastase inhibitors exemplifies the demonstration of the biological activity of synthetic inhibitors in the presence of excess of natural inhibitors

The search for and development of protease inhibitors has been very much influenced by progress in the understanding of the biology of their target enzymes. This is illustrated by the series of lactam-based inhibitors of neutrophil elastase (Fig. 68.1) [85,103,184,185] culminating in the introduction into humans of a cell penetrant inhibitor L694458 (DMP 777) which provides long-lasting inhibition of the body load of the enzyme [16]. At the outset, such a compound was viewed as unlikely to be safe for introduction into humans because the physiological functions of neutrophil elastase were largely unknown. Subsequent biology has provided some insights in this respect, based both on gene knockouts in mice [45,118,125,126] and the

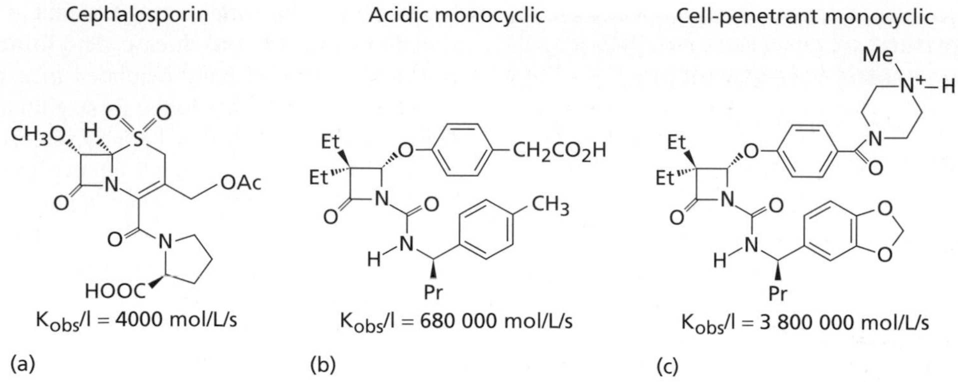

Cephalosporin   Acidic monocyclic   Cell-penetrant monocyclic

$K_{obs}/I = 4000$ mol/L/s $K_{obs}/I = 680\,000$ mol/L/s $K_{obs}/I = 3\,800\,000$ mol/L/s

(a)   (b)   (c)

Figure 68.1 Some properties of three representative lactam-based inhibitors of polymorphonuclear neutrophil (PMN) elastase. (a) Cephalosporin. Active by aerosol administration to inhibit PMN elastase-mediated lung damage in rats and hamsters. Not active systemically after oral administration. (b) Acidic monocyclic. Orally bioavailable in a number of species and systemically active to inhibit PMN elastase-mediated lung damage. (c) Cell-penetrant inhibitor which is orally bioavailable in a number of species. Causes rapid and long-lasting inhibition of PMN elastase in peripheral PMN in primates.

discovery of a genetic defect in humans of DPP1 [120], an enzyme that activates precursors of myeloid cell serine proteases [186] as they are packaged into storage granules in neutrophils, mast cells monocytes and natural killer (NK) cells. The development of the lactam-based inhibitors of neutrophil elastase shown in Figure 68.1 was initiated by a serendipitous observation with an inhibitor of a bacterial enzyme. Clavulanic acid is an acylating inhibitor of bacterial serine proteases but does not affect mammalian serine proteases. Doherty *et al.* [184] showed that the benzyl ester of clavulanic acid, while inactive against the bacterial enzyme, inhibits neutrophil elastase and other mammalian serine proteases. This provided a starting point for the development of a series of increasingly specific and potent lactam-based inhibitors [85,103].

The cephalosporin L658758, which by present-day standards is a modestly potent inhibitor of human neutrophil elastase, inhibits human neutrophil elastase-induced lung haemorrhage after intratracheal instillation to hamsters. The compound is not orally active because of metabolic instability. At the time of its development, it was already established that immune complexes cause degranulation of neutrophils [79] and it was thought that proteases such as elastase contributed to the damage seen in immune complex diseases. L658758 inhibited the haemorrhage associated with a reverse passive Arthus reaction in the rat lung. It prevented destruction of blood vessels associated with the basement membranes where immune complexes are deposited without significant effects on neutrophil recruitment [81]. Thus, the low molecular weight inhibitor was supplementing the activity of natural inhibitors of the target neutrophil serine proteases.

The studies of Owen *et al.* [156,182] lent a clear rationale for developing compounds that would be effective against

the local and transient activity of enzyme present at high concentration in exocytosed azurophil granules. Subsequent efforts sought orally active compounds and led to the development of more potent monolactam-based inhibitors of elastase as exemplified by L680833 (see Fig. 68.1) [103], which inhibited tissue damage by both exogenous and endogenous elastase. The availability of sensitive and specific neoepitope assays allowed the potency and activity of this family of compounds to be assayed in biological systems and it became clear that these agents inhibited the activity of elastase that escaped natural inhibitors [103,161]. The great intrinsic potency of L680833 against elastase [103] is considerably attenuated in the presence of physiological concentrations of natural inhibitors in blood. Approximately 10 μmol/L L680833 is required to inhibit by 50% the fibrinopeptide formation occurring when neutrophils are degranulated in the presence of 100 μmol/L or more of α_1PI and α_2-macroglobulin in blood [103].

Further enhancement of this potency was achieved by changing the physical properties of the inhibitors to allow them to penetrate into azurophil granules and inactivate the enzyme intracellularly. This is illustrated by the properties of L694458, which under the code name DMP 777 has been advanced to Phase II clinical studies in cystic fibrosis [16]. This compound inhibits the cellular pool of neutrophil elastase with an inhibitory concentration 50% (IC_{50}) close to the overall blood concentration of 100–200 nmol/L of the enzyme, indicating a very high efficiency of inhibition approaching unit stoichiometry. The detailed mechanism of action of this class of agents has been delineated with the identification of the precise nature of the complex and products of inactivated enzyme with parent inhibitor [187–190]. Using a combination of electrospray ionization mass spectrometry and two-dimensional nuclear magnetic

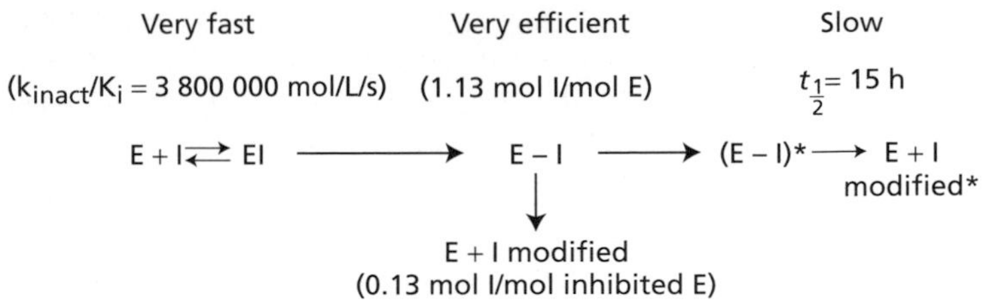

Figure 68.2 The potent and efficient inhibition of polymorphonuclear neutrophil (PMN) elastase by L694458.

Very fast   Very efficient   Slow

$(k_{inact}/K_i = 3\ 800\ 000\ mol/L/s)$ $(1.13\ mol\ I/mol\ E)$ $t_{\frac{1}{2}} = 15\ h$

$$E + I \rightleftharpoons EI \longrightarrow E - I \longrightarrow (E - I)^* \longrightarrow E + I\ \text{modified}^*$$

$$E + I\ \text{modified}$$
$$(0.13\ mol\ I/mol\ \text{inhibited}\ E)$$

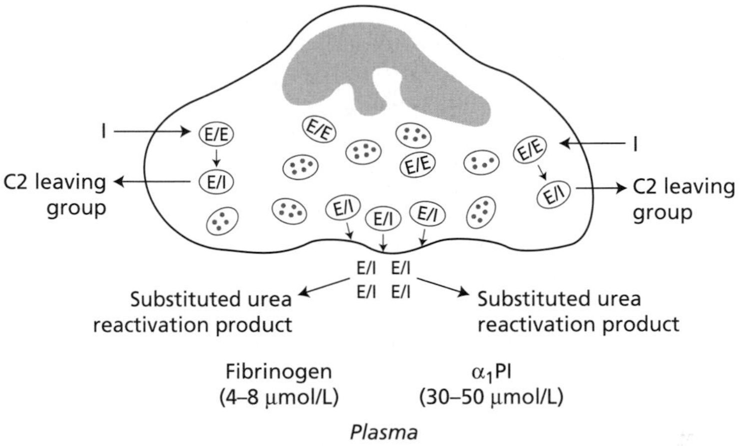

Figure 68.3 Schematic representation of inhibition of intracellular polymorphonuclear neutrophil (PMN) elastase by L694458 (DMP 777) in blood.

resonance (NMR) techniques, the precise molecular weights of enzyme–inhibitor complexes were determined with subsequent specific identification of reaction intermediates. With this information in hand, it was possible to develop a specific antibody to a substituted urea reactivation product (bottom right-hand side of monocyclic molecules in Fig. 68.1) that is uniquely derived from the stable enzyme–inhibitor complex [191]. Because the antibody has minimal cross-reactivity with parent inhibitor or enzyme, it is possible to measure formation of enzyme–inhibitor complexes in biological fluids containing excesses of either active enzyme or inhibitor. Figure 68.2 illustrates some of the general principles underlying this technology [191–197] using L694458 as an example. The compound is a very fast and efficient inhibitor of elastase, requiring only 1.13 mol to inhibit each mole of enzyme forming a complex of 25 560 Da with release of a 361-Da C2 leaving group (phenoxy group at top right part of the molecule, Fig. 68.1). This occurs extremely rapidly with a second-order rate constant, k_{inact}/K_i of 3 800 000 mol/s. The complex is stable with a $t_{1/2}$ of 15 h, which is well in excess of the half-life of circulating neutrophils. Slow reactivation of this complex, which can be accelerated to more rapid completion at elevated temperature, yields the substituted urea, which is not generated from the parent inhibitor [191].

Several complementary assays can be used to assay the potency of this type of inhibitor in neutrophils in blood or isolated from blood. These assays are useful for *in vitro* studies or for *in vivo* evaluation of compounds. They include:

• Hydrolysis of conventional synthetic substrates by neutrophils lysed after isolation from blood and washed to remove plasma inhibitors.

• LC-MS/MS quantitation of parent compound and C2 leaving group in blood and plasma to concentrations below 1 nmol/L.

• Immunoassay of specific fibrinogen cleavage products such as $A\alpha(1-21)$ and $A\alpha(Val^{360})$ formed in the presence of endogenous inhibitors after degranulation of neutrophils in blood.

• Immunoassay of α_1-antitrypsin–elastase complexes formed during the activation of neutrophils in blood. In the presence of inhibitor, lesser amounts of this natural complex are made.

• Immunoassay of the substituted urea leaving group derived from enzyme–inhibitor complex.

The diagram in Figure 68.3 illustrates how these assays can be used in one sample of human blood to characterize enzyme inhibition. In intact blood with no perturbation of neutrophils, the addition of inhibitor results in concentration-dependent release of equimolar amounts of the C2 leaving group and formation of complexes yielding the substituted urea. Close to maximum yield (in the range of several hundred nanomolar) of these require only approximately fivefold excess of parent compound, which is not detectable by LC-MS (less than 1 nmol/L) until this maximum is achieved, suggesting complete sequestration by intracellular enzyme. Neutrophils separated and lysed show the expected loss of activity against synthetic elastase substrate.

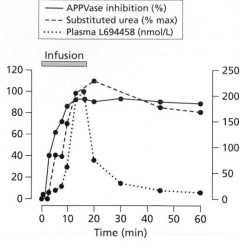

Figure 68.4 L694458 inhibits polymorphonuclear neutrophil (PMN) elastase *in vivo* rapidly and with great potency in chimpanzees. This figure shows an intravenous infusion (0.5 mg/kg) of L-694 458 (DMP 777) to a chimpanzee.

Inhibitor is totally consumed up to concentrations required to inhibit enzyme fully; the IC_{50} being approximately 100 nmol/L. Degranulation of neutrophils in blood allows access of elastase to substrates such as fibrinogen and high levels of 30–50 μmol of α_1PI. Catalytic activity against fibrinogen is evident by the formation of Aα(Val^{360}) [84] as is the formation of α_1PI–elastase complexes as the inhibitor gains access to the released enzyme. In the presence of L694458, formation of both fibrinopeptide and α_1PI–elastase complexes is inhibited with equal potency with IC_{50} of several hundred nanomolar [84]. This activity reflects the intracellular inhibition of enzyme.

Preclinical *in vivo* studies with L694458 are complicated by the fall in potency against elastase across species with second-order rate constants dropping from 2.4 to 1.6, and 0.059×10^6 mol/s from the chimpanzee, to the rhesus to the rat respectively. This necessitated the use of chimpanzees to model the *in vivo* pharmacodynamic properties of this compound. The potency of the compound predicted from *in vitro* studies is apparent *in vivo* (Fig. 68.4). A slow infusion of 0.5 mg/kg of L694458 over a period of approximately 20 min resulted in rapid inhibition of elastase in blood taken at various times after initiation of drug delivery. Within 10 min, with a total of 0.25 mg/kg of drug administered, complete inhibition was seen. Total inhibition of intracellular enzyme is achieved with plasma concentration of drug of 10 nmol/L as the drug rapidly penetrates cells and associates with intracellular enzyme. Based on the calculation of the amount of enzyme present in the body, only a 10- to 20-fold molar excess of drug is required to achieve this level of inhibition. Because the enzyme is sequestered in azurophil granules, which form only a tiny fraction of blood/whole body volume, the extreme tropism of L694458 for its target is again apparent.

These potent pharmacodynamic properties, combined with its good pharmacokinetic properties and safety profile, have provided the opportunity to evaluate the properties of L694458 (DMP 777) in humans [16]. Initial studies showed that these pharmacodynamic properties are observed in short-term studies in cystic fibrosis patients and controls. Close to full inhibition of elastase in lysates of neutrophils from patients receiving drug at single and multiple doses with inhibition of enzyme correlating with pharmacokinetic parameters including C_{max} and area under the curve (AUC). It is therefore clear that the combination of the extraordinary potency, amounting to almost stoichiometric inhibition of the enzyme, the ability to access intracellular enzyme and excellent pharmacokinetic properties allows this agent to inactivate the body load of elastase in humans.

The ability of the compound to prevent pathology in animal models has been demonstrated in the reverse passive Arthus in the rat, despite its far poorer potency ($k_{inact}/K_i = 59\,000$ mol/s) against elastase in this species. The compound has not been evaluated in the smoking mouse model. This should be possible based on the safety and efficacy in shorter term models in the mouse, despite relatively poor activity against the elastase of this species. The profile of the compound as compared with the elastase null mouse is not predictable. Confounding variables include possible effects on PR3 [185,192] which causes lung damage characteristic of other elastolysins [193] and functions that may not require catalytically active enzyme [74].

Another neutrophil elastase inhibitor, ZD 0892, an orally active trifluoromethyl ketone inhibitor, reduces cigarette smoke-induced emphysema in guinea pigs [105]. This agent inhibits both acute inflammation and chronic lung destruction. It effectively abolished increases in the chemokines MCP1 and MIP2 as well as reducing elevated plasma levels of TNF-α seen after 2 h exposure to cigarette smoke. On a longer term basis, decreases in desmosine, hydroxyproline and neutrophils in lung lavage fluid are observed while also reducing airspace enlargement by 45%. These findings were not complemented by measurement of surrogate markers of neutrophil elastase activity nor was there any information on the pharmacokinetics of the compound. However, if the effects were mechanism based then they give a clear indication that the neutrophil as well as TNF-α have significant roles in the inflammation and tissue damage seen in this model. Similar findings have been made with human α_1-antitrypsin administered to mice tolerized to this molecule by low level expression of a transgene for the human molecule [116].

What are the concerns regarding inhibition of elastase and other neutrophil serine proteases? The sophisticated biological mechanisms that regulate the extracellular activity of proteases *in vivo* place strict temporal and spatial restrictions on their activity. Yet it is clear that they allow these enzymes to be active against a wide range of endogenous substrates, including those that are targeted in destructive inflammatory diseases such as COPD. These activities are likely to mediate physiological tissue turnover and repair in many instances, particularly in the case of macrophages and connective tissue cells, probably less so in the case of the neutrophil. The boundary between these beneficial activities and aberrant activities that lead to pathology remain to be clearly defined and make it difficult to predict possible side-effects of inhibitors. This is particularly true if these agents also affect intracellular protease activity. The phenotype of mice in which individual serine proteases such as elastase and cathepsin G have been ablated give indications of specific defects in defences against some, but not all microorganisms [118,125,126]. Neutrophil elastase knockout mice have mild defects in host defence against specific infectious agents but animals appear phenotypically normal in the sheltered environment of protected animal housing. The realization that DPP1 (or cathepsin C) processes the precursors of serine proteases found in a number of myeloid cells including NK cells, mast cells and neutrophils and its deletion in mice [45] provided a broader perspective on the consequences of genetic ablation of not only neutrophil elastase but a number of other serine proteases. These findings have now been complemented by the discovery that the genetic defect underlying the juvenile periodontitis and plantar hyperkeratinization in Papillon–Lefèvre and Haim–Munk syndromes is caused by a loss of function of DPP1 [120]. The details of this genetic defect remain to be fully elucidated but the rare cases that have been described are characterized by early-onset periodontal disease, a phenomenon associated with other types of neutrophil dysfunction, but individuals with this defect survive into adulthood. Mice in which this gene is ablated appear to be normal in their protected environment and recent studies in a model of cecal ligation show that there is some protection to be derived from ablation of this gene [119]. This was associated with the loss of tryptase as a regulator of IL-6 and, while lethality was reduced, the clearance of the systemic bacterial load in these mice may have been hindered based on the increased bacterial count [119], which is consistent with the defects in certain aspects of host defence against specific organisms in neutrophil elastase knockout mice. These observations give an indication of the concerns about host defence that need to be registered about pharmacological inhibitors of this family of enzymes, particularly agents that give extensive coverage and are active against intracellular pools of these enzymes.

Other concerns regarding inhibition of extracellular

neutrophil elastase have been expressed [194,195] based on the exacerbation of lung damage seen in some pharmacodynamic models of elastase-induced lung haemorrhage used to evaluate competitive inhibitors that form reversible complexes with neutrophil elastase [196]. It was suggested that these reversible complexes are transported to sites where reactivated enzyme is not readily accessible to natural inhibitors [194,195].

A lack of neutrophil function has long been associated with marked defects in host defence function. Genetic defects in adhesion molecules such as CD18 and in the NADPH oxidase system have life-shortening consequences [73]. On the other hand, defects in the serine proteases have not been apparent until recently. Disordered intracellular trafficking of elastase has been associated with severe congenital neutropenia [197] while the cleavage by elastase of the fusion protein PML-RARα formed as a result of a chromosomal translocation in acute promyelocytic leukaemia has been associated with increased incidence of leukaemia [39]. In this instance, an elastase inhibitor has a beneficial effect on a transgenic mouse with a functional PML-RARα fusion protein [39]. Possible consequences of the pharmacological loss of function for neutrophil elastase on myelopoiesis in humans have not been determined.

Ohbayashi [13] has extensively reviewed neutrophil elastase inhibitors that are in development and the current status of a number of compounds brought forward into the clinic. At this time there is no documentation of the activity and clinical utility of these inhibitors. In many instances there is no demonstration that these inhibitors inactivate elastase that escapes inhibition by endogenous inhibitors. It is clear that while elastase on its own is not going to be solely responsible for the complex protease-mediated pathology in COPD, its interactions with other proteases, most notably cysteine and metalloproteases, will make the evaluation of its inhibition useful to determine whether it has a non-redundant role in the ongoing pathogenesis of COPD.

Matrix metalloproteases

The challenges for the development of MMP inhibitors for the therapy of chronic disease are reflected by the experiences in the cancer and arthritis fields [7,9,198]. Based on their up-regulation at affected sites, there is circumstantial evidence for a role of MMPs in tumour metastasis and in cartilage destruction in the arthritides. Clinical investigation of MMP inhibitors over the last 15 years has not yielded any conclusive evidence of clinical benefit. A number of issues stand in the way of gaining clear-cut knowledge and understanding of the potential of these agents. The complexity of the MMP family adds to the difficulty of designing specific, pharmaceutically and clinically acceptable compounds. Musculoskeletal side-effects, which are speculated to be mechanism based [198], have been observed with a number of non-specific inhibitors, such as the Roche MMP inhibitors [198] which have been taken forward to Phase II–III evaluation in arthritis. It is not clear whether any of these effects reflect the severe osteolysis and arthritis associated with MMP-2 deficiency in humans [166]. Development of more specific inhibitors such as prinomastat and tanomastat has not resolved these problems. Moreover, the complexity of the metalloprotease families with the emergence of the ADAM and ADAM-TS families makes it very difficult to evaluate broad-based specificity of inhibitors. Preclinical studies of MMP inhibitors have shown that the non-specific compound CP-471,474 attenuates the acute inflammation and emphysematous changes seen in guinea pigs exposed to cigarette smoke [199]. It is not clear which enzyme(s) is the target of the inhibitor.

The difficulty in developing MMP inhibitors is compounded by the lack of reliable biomarkers for MMP activity in disease. This has been a long-standing problem for COPD where reliable assays even for specific degradation products of elastic tissue are not available to allow development of markers of either individual proteases or as a collective indicator of accelerated elastic tissue turnover and degradation.

MMPs are maintained in a latent form until activated by physiological triggers or inappropriate signals at sites of pathology. Their activity is restricted to the pericellular environment by the activity of natural inhibitors. While increased levels of individual enzymes have been detected in lung fluids, good markers for their catalytic activity are not available. Unlike the serine proteases from neutrophils, which have well-validated markers such as specific cleavage products and their complexes with α_1PI, the metalloproteases are only available in small amounts which often serve physiological functions in the target tissue. Accordingly, direct catalytic activity is extremely difficult to measure. Local sampling for specific degradation products is also difficult and their release into the circulation results in their catabolism and/or dilution to undetectable levels so that they cannot be assayed in blood and urine.

Cysteine proteases

Cysteine proteases such as cathepsins L, S and K have been implicated in tissue injury and remodelling [20]. While cathepsin K is not obviously implicated in COPD, its genetic defect in humans [200] has provided a stimulus for seeking inhibitors that have beneficial effects on bone diseases. Cathepsin L and S both have significant elastolytic potency and there are indications that they may contribute to COPD

[20]. Design of inhibitors for cysteine proteases has proceeded the furthest with ICE, the IL-1 precursor processing enzyme [201]. Inhibitors for this enzyme have been taken forward to Phase II–III clinical studies in arthritis [202]. Other members of the ICE family, the caspases, have essential roles in apoptosis [179] and the progress in biology of this area may reveal rational targets in the context of cell death and removal that is such a critical part of lung host defence. Considerable interest in cathepsin S as a target has emerged, based on both its involvement in the immune response [47] as well as in vascular wall inflammation in genetically modified mice [141].

Conclusions

The clinical evaluation and development of protease inhibitors in COPD has only begun. The details of the proteome are now in hand [5] and intrinsically potent inhibitors of some of the individual enzymes are available. A handful of these have properties that have allowed their introduction into humans [13,16,17]. The rapidly evolving understanding of the biology of proteases in the healthy lung and in COPD will provide the basis for much further work in this area. This knowledge, together with the application of sensitive and specific tools for measuring the efficacy of candidate drugs against the irreversible damage to the lung, will provide the basis for determining whether they will be clinically useful.

Acknowledgements

We are grateful to Lorena Bennett for her assistance in the preparation of this chapter. We are appreciative of the many stimulating discussions with colleagues at Merck Research Laboratories regarding the subject matter of this chapter as well as their contributions to cited original work.

References

1 Calverley PMA, Walker P. Chronic obstructive pulmonary disease. *Lancet* 2003;**362**:1053–61.

2 Siafakas NM, Tzortzaki EG. Few smokers develop COPD: why? *Respir Med* 2002;**96**:615–24.

3 Eriksson S. Emphysema before and after 1963: historic perspectives. *Ann N Y Acad Sci* 1991;**624**:1–6.

4 Eriksson S. Pulmonary emphysema and α_1-antitrypsin deficiency. *Acta Med Scand* 1964;**175**:197–205.

5 Puente XS, Sanchez LM, Overall CM, Lopez-Otin C. Human and mouse proteases: a comparative genomic approach. *Nat Rev Genet* 2003;**4**:544–58.

6 Baker AH, Edwards DR, Murphy G. Metalloproteinase

inhibitors: biological actions and therapeutic opportunities. *J Cell Sci* 2002;**115**:3719–27.

7 Belvisi MG, Bottomley KM. The role of matrix metalloproteinases (MMPs) in the pathophysiology of chronic obstructive pulmonary disease (COPD): a therapeutic role for inhibitors of MMPs? *Inflamm Res* 2003;**52**:95–100.

8 Bernstein PR, Edwards PD, Williams JC. Inhibitors of human leukocyte elastase. *Prog Med Chem* 1994;**31**:60–120.

9 Coussens LM, Fingleton B, Matrisian LM. Matrix metalloproteinase inhibitors and cancer: trials and tribulations. *Science* 2002;**295**:2387–92.

10 Donnelly LE, Rogers DF. Antiproteases and retinoids for treatment of chronic obstructive pulmonary disease. *Expert Opin Ther Patents* 2003;**13**:1345–72.

11 Edwards PD, Bernstein PR. Synthetic inhibitors of elastase. *Med Res Rev* 1994;**14**:127–94.

12 Leung D, Abbenante G, Fairlie DP. Protease inhibitors: current status and future prospects. *J Med Chem* 2000;**43**:305–41.

13 Ohbayashi H. Neutrophil elastase inhibitors as treatment for COPD. *Expert Opin Investig Drugs* 2003;**11**:965–80.

14 Vender RL. Therapeutic potential of neutrophil–elastase inhibition in pulmonary disease. *J Invest Med* 1996;**44**: 531–9.

15 Ziedalski TM, Sankaranarayanan V, Chitkara RK. Advances in the management of chronic obstructive pulmonary disease. *Expert Opin Pharmacother* 2003;**4**:1063–82.

16 Vender RL, Burcham DL, Quon CY. DMP 777: a synthetic human neutrophil-elastase inhibitor as therapy for cystic fibrosis. *Pediatr Pulmonol* 1998;**17**:136–7.

17 Shah PL. Update on clinical trials in the treatment of pulmonary disease in patients with cystic fibrosis. *Expert Opin Investig Drugs* 1999;**8**:1917–27.

18 Shapiro SD. Animal models for chronic obstructive pulmonary disease: age of Klotho and Marlboro mice. *Am J Respir Cell Mol Biol* 2000;**22**:4–7.

19 Shapiro SD. Chronic obstructive pulmonary disease: evolving concepts in the pathogenesis of chronic obstructive pulmonary disease. *Clin Chest Med* 2000;**21**:621–32.

20 Chapman HA Jr, Shi G-P. Protease injury in the development of COPD. *Chest* 2000;**117**:295S–8S.

21 Russell REK, Thorley A, Culpitt SV *et al.* Alveolar macrophage-mediated elastolysis: roles of matrix metalloproteinases, cysteine, and serine proteinases. *Am J Physiol Lung Cell Mol Physiol* 2002;**283**:L867–3.

22 Busiek DF, Baragi V, Nehring LC, Parks WC, Welgus HG. Matrilysin expression by human mononuclear phagocytes and its regulation by cytokines and hormones. *J Immunol* 1995;**154**:6484–91.

23 Busiek DF, Ross FP, McDonnell S *et al.* The matrix metalloprotease matrilysin (PUMP) is expressed in developing human mononuclear phagocytes. *J Biol Chem* 1992;**267**:9087–92.

24 Filippov S, Caras I, Murray R *et al.* Matrilysin-dependent elastolysis by human macrophages. *J Exp Med* 2003;**198**: 925–35.

25 Campbell EJ, Cury JD, Shapiro SD, Goldberg GI, Welgus HG. Neutral proteinases of human mononuclear phagocytes: cellular differentiation markedly alters cell phenotype for serine proteinases, metalloproteinases, and tissue inhibitor of metalloproteinases. *J Immunol* 1991;**146**:1286–93.

26 Parks WC, Shapiro SD. Matrix metalloproteinases in lung biology. *Respir Res* 2001;**2**:10–9.

27 Senior RM, Connolly NL, Cury JD, Welgus HG, Campbell EJ. Elastin degradation by human alveolar macrophages. *Am Rev Respir Dis* 1989;**139**:1251–6.

28 Shapiro SD. The macrophage in chronic obstructive pulmonary disease. *Am J Respir Crit Care Med* 1999;**160**:S29–32.

29 Shapiro SD. Matrix metalloproteinase degradation of extracellular matrix: biological consequences. *Curr Opin Cell Biol* 1998;**10**:602–8.

30 Welgus HG, Campbell EJ, Cury JD *et al.* Neutral metalloproteinases produced by human mononuclear phagocytes: enzyme profile, regulation, and expression during cellular development. *J Clin Invest* 1990;**86**:1496–502.

31 Shapiro SD, Goldstein NM, Houghton AM *et al.* Neutrophil elastase contributes to cigarette smoke-induced emphysema in mice. *Am J Pathol* 2003;**163**:2329–35.

32 Hautamaki RD, Kobayashi DK, Senior RM, Shapiro SD. Requirement for macrophage elastase for cigarette smoke-induced emphysema in mice. *Science* 1997;**277**:2002–4.

33 Morris DG, Huang X, Kaminski N *et al.* Loss of integrin $\alpha v\beta 6$-mediated TGF-β activation causes MMP-12-dependent emphysema. *Nature* 2003;**422**:169–73.

34 Atkinson JJ, Senior RM. Matrix metalloproteinase-9 in lung remodeling. *Am J Respir Crit Care Med* 2003;**28**:12–24.

35 Shapiro SD, Endicott SK, Province MA, Pierce JA, Campbell EJ. Marked longevity of human lung parenchymal elastic fibers deduced from prevalence of D-aspartate and nuclear weapons-related radiocarbon. *J Clin Invest* 1991;**87**:1828–34.

36 Itoh Y, Nagase H. Preferential inactivation of tissue inhibitor of metalloproteinases-1 that is bound to the precursor of matrix metalloproteinase 9 (progelatinase B) by human neutrophil elastase. *J Biol Chem* 1995;**270**:16518–21.

37 Fischer BM, Voynow JA. Neutrophil elastase induces MUC5AC gene expression in airway epithelium via a pathway involving reactive oxygen species. *Am J Respir Crit Care Med* 2002;**26**:447–52.

38 Tosi MF, Zakem H, Berger M. Neutrophil elastase cleaves C3bi on opsonized *Pseudomonas* as well as CR1 on neutrophils to create a functionally important opsonin receptor mismatch. *J Clin Invest* 1990;**86**:300–8.

39 Lane AA, Ley TJ. Neutrophil elastase cleaves PML-RARα and is important for the development of acute promyelocytic leukemia in mice. *Cell* 2003;**115**:305–18.

40 Parks WC. A confederacy of proteinases. *J Clin Invest* 2002; **110**:613–4.

41 Pyo R, Lee JK, Shipley JM *et al.* Targeted gene disruption of matrix metalloproteinase-9 (gelatinase B) suppresses development of experimental abdominal aortic aneurysms. *J Clin Invest* 2000;**105**:1641–9.

42 Sires UI, Murphy G, Baragi VM *et al.* Matrilysin is much more efficient than other matrix metalloproteinases in the proteolytic inactivation of α_1-antitrypsin. *Biochem Biophys Res Commun* 1994;**204**:613–20.

43 Haro H, Crawford HC, Fingleton B *et al.* Matrix metalloproteinase-7-dependent release of tumor necrosis factor-α in a model of herniated disc resorption. *J Clin Invest* 2000;**105**:143–50.

44 Liu Z, Zhou X, Shapiro SD *et al*. The serpin α_1-proteinase inhibitor is a critical substrate for gelatinase B/MMP-9 *in vivo*. *Cell* 2000;**102**:647–55.

45 Pham CT, Ley TJ. Dipeptidyl peptidase I is required for the processing and activation of granzymes A and B *in vivo*. *Proc Natl Acad Sci USA* 1999;**96**:8627–32.

46 Carmeliet P, Moons L, Lijnen R *et al*. Urokinase-generated plasmin activates matrix metalloproteinases during aneurysm formation. *Nat Genet* 1997;**17**:429–44.

47 Honey K, Rudensky AY. Lysosomal cysteine proteases regulate antigen presentation. *Nat Rev Immunol* 2003;**3**:472–82.

48 Sopori M. Effects of cigarette smoke on the immune system. *Nat Rev Immunol* 2002;**2**:372–7.

49 Shapiro SD. End-stage chronic obstructive pulmonary disease: the cigarette is burned out but inflammation rages on. *Am J Respir Crit Care Med* 2001;**164**:339–40.

50 Retamales I, Elliott WM, Meshi B *et al*. Amplification of inflammation in emphysema and its association with latent adenoviral infection. *Am J Respir Crit Care Med* 2001; **164**:469–73.

51 Janeway C Jr, Medzhitov R. Innate immune recognition. *Annu Rev Immunol* 2002;**20**:197–216.

52 Medzhitov R, Janeway C Jr. Innate immunity. *N Engl J Med* 2000;**343**:338–44.

53 Beutler B. Innate immunity: an overview. *Mol Immunol* 2004;**40**:845–59.

54 Beutler B, Hoffman J. Innate immunity. *Curr Opin Immunol* 2004;**16**:1–3.

55 Ozinsky A, Underhill DM, Fontenot JD *et al*. The repertoire for pattern recognition of pathogens by the innate immune system is defined by cooperation between Toll-like receptors. *Proc Natl Acad Sci U S A* 2000;**97**:13766–71.

56 Gordon S. Pattern recognition receptors: doubling up for the innate immune response. *Cell* 2002;**111**:927–30.

57 Underhill DM, Ozinsky A. Phagocytosis of microbes: complexity in action. *Annu Rev Immunol* 2002;**20**:825–52.

58 Dong C, Davis RJ, Flavell RA. MAP kinases in the immune response. *Annu Rev Immunol* 2002;**20**:55–72.

59 Saetta M, Mariani M, Panina-Bordignon P *et al*. Increased expression of the chemokine receptor CXCR3 and its ligand CXCL10 in peripheral airways of smokers with chronic obstructive pulmonary disease. *Am J Respir Crit Care Med* 2002;**165**:1404–9.

60 Leckie MJ, Jenkins GR, Kahn J *et al*. Sputum T lymphocytes in asthma, COPD and healthy subjects have the phenotype of activated intraepithelial T cells (CD69+ CD103+). *Thorax* 2003;**58**:23–9.

61 Hogg JC, Chu F, Utokaparch S *et al*. The nature of small-airway obstruction in chronic obstructive pulmonary disease. *N Engl J Med* 2004;**350**:2645–53.

62 Stockley RA. Cellular mechanisms in the pathogenesis of COPD. *Eur Respir Rev* 1996;**6**:264–96.

63 Spencer H. The pneumoconioses and other occupational lung diseases. In: *Pathology of the Lung*. New York: Pergamon, 1985: 413–50.

64 Geissmann F, Jung S, Littmann DR. Blood monocytes consist of two principal subsets with distinct migratory properties. *Immunity* 2003;**19**:71–82.

65 Campbell EJ, Silverman EK, Campbell MA. Elastase and cathepsin G of human monocytes: quantification of cellular content, release in response to stimuli, and heterogeneity in elastase-mediated proteolytic activity. *J Immunol* 1989;**143**:2961–8.

66 Owen CA, Campbell MA, Boukedes SS, Campbell EJ. Monocytes recruited to sites of inflammation express a distinctive proinflammatory (P) phenotype. *Am J Physiol* 1994;**267**:L786–96.

67 Owen CA, Campbell MA, Boukedes SS, Stockley RA, Campbell EJ. A discrete subpopulation of human monocytes expresses a neutrophil-like proinflammatory (P) phenotype. *Am J Physiol* 1994;**267**:L775–85.

68 Rot A, Von Andrian UH. Chemokines in innate and adaptive host defense: basic chemokinese grammar for immune cells. *Annu Rev Immunol* 2004;**22**:891–928.

69 Nathan CF. Neutrophil activation on biological surfaces: massive secretion of hydrogen peroxide in response to products of macrophages and lymphocytes. *J Clin Invest* 1987;**80**:1550–60.

70 Lucey EC, Keane J, Kuang PP, Snider GL, Goldstein RH. Severity of elastase-induced emphysema is decreased in tumor necrosis factor α and interleukin-1β receptor-deficient mice. *Lab Invest* 2002;**82**:79–85.

71 Wang Z, Zheng T, Zhu Z *et al*. Interferon gamma induction of pulmonary emphysema in the adult murine lung. *J Exp Med* 2000;**192**:1587–99.

72 Fujita M, Shannon JM, Irvin CG *et al*. Overexpression of tumor necrosis factor-α produces an increase in lung volumes and pulmonary hypertension. *Am J Physiol Lung Cell Mol Physiol* 2001;**280**:L39–49.

73 Babior BM. NADPH oxidase. *Curr Opin Immunol* 2004;**16**:42–7.

74 Elsbach P, Weiss J. Oxygen-independent antimicrobial systems in phagocytes in inflammation. In: Gallin JI, Goldstein IM, Snyderman R, eds. *Inflammation, Basic Principles and Clinical Correlates*, 2nd edn. New York: Raven Press, 1992: 603–36.

75 Segal BH, Leto TL, Gallin JI, Malech HL, Holland SM. Genetic, biochemical, and clinical features of chronic granulomatous disease. *Medicine (Baltimore)* 2000;**79**:170–200.

76 Liou TG, Campbell EJ. Quantum proteolysis resulting from release of single granules by human neutrophils. *J Immunol* 1996;**157**:2624–31.

77 O'Connor CM, Gaffney K, Keane J *et al*. α_1-Proteinase inhibitor, elastase activity, and lung disease severity in cystic fibrosis. *Am Rev Respir Dis* 1993;**148**:1665–70.

78 Lan HY, Paterson DJ, Hutchinson P, Atkins RC. Leukocyte involvement in the pathogeneis of pulmonary injury in experimental Goodpasture's syndrome. *Lab Invest* 1991;**64**:330–8.

79 Henson PM, Henson JE, Fittschen C, Bratton D, Riches DWH. Degranulation and secretion by phagocytic cells. In: Gallin JI, Goldstein IM, Snyderman R, eds. *Inflammation, Basic Principles and Clinical Correlates*, 2nd edn. New York: Raven Press, 1992: 511–39.

80 Ravetch JV. A full complement of receptors in immune complex diseases. *J Clin Invest* 2002;**110**:1759–61.

81 Fletcher D, Osinga DG, Keenan K *et al*. An inhibitor of

leukocyte elastase prevents immune complex-mediated hemorrhage in the rat lung. *J Pharmacol Exp Ther* 1995; **274**:548–54.

82 Donaghy M, Rees AJ. Cigarette smoking and lung haemorrhage in glomerulonephritis caused by autoantibodies to glomerular basement membrane. *Lancet* 1983;**2**:1390–3.

83 MacNee W, Wiggs B, Belzberg AS, Hogg JC. The effect of cigarette smoking on neutrophil kinetics in human lungs. *N Engl J Med* 1989;**321**:924–8.

84 Humes JL, Mumford RA, Davies DTP, Dahlgren ME, Boger JS. Inventors: assay for marker of human polymorphonuclear leukocyte elastase activity. *USA patent 6, 124, 107*, 2000.

85 Davies P, Ashe BM, Bonney RJ *et al.* The discovery and biologic properties of cephalosporin-based inhibitors of PMN elastase. *Ann N Y Acad Sci* 1991;**624**:219–29.

86 Savill J, Hogg N, Ren Y, Haslett C. Thrombospondin cooperates with CD36 and the vitronectin receptor in macrophage recognition of neutrophils undergoing apoptosis. *J Clin Invest* 1992;**90**:1513–22.

87 Vandivier RW, Fadok VA, Hoffmann PR *et al.* Elastase-mediated phosphatidylserine receptor cleavage impairs apoptotic cell clearance in cystic fibrosis and bronchiectasis. *J Clin Invest* 2002;**109**:661–70.

88 Jia SH, Li Y, Parodo J *et al.* Pre-B cell colony-enhancing factor inhibits neutrophil apoptosis in experimental inflammation and clinical sepsis. *J Clin Invest* 2004;**113**:1318–27.

89 Pletz MW, Ioanas M, de Roux A, Burkhardt O, Lode H. Reduced spontaneous apoptosis in peripheral blood neutrophils during exacerbation of COPD. *Eur Respir J* 2004; **23**:532–7.

90 Altznauer F, Martinelli S, Yousefi S *et al.* Inflammation-associated cell cycle-independent block of apoptosis by surviving in terminally differentiated neutrophils. *J Exp Med* 2004;**199**:1343–54.

91 Asada K, Sasaki S, Suda T, Chida K, Nakamura H. Anti-inflammatory roles of peroxisome proliferator-activated receptor gamma in human alveolar macrophages. *Am J Respir Crit Care Med* 2004;**169**:195–200.

92 Riches DW. Peroxisome proliferator-active receptor gamma: a legitimate target to control pulmonary inflammation? *Am J Respir Crit Care Med* 2004;**169**:145–6.

93 Dimakou K, Bakakos P, Rassidakis A *et al.* Neutrophil elastase concentration and α_1-proteinase inhibitor in serum of patients with COPD during and after exacerbation. *Am J Respir Crit Care Med* 1999;**159**:A809.

94 Finlay GA, O'Driscoll LR, Russell KJ *et al.* Matrix metalloproteinase expression and production by alveolar macrophages in emphysema. *Am J Respir Crit Care Med* 1997;**156**:240–7.

95 Finlay GA, Russell KJ, McMahon KJ *et al.* Elevated levels of matrix metalloproteinases in bronchoalveolar lavage fluid of emphysematous patients. *Thorax* 1997;**52**:502–6.

96 Imai K, Dalal SS, Chen ES *et al.* Human collagenase (matrix metalloproteinase-1) expression in the lungs of patients with emphysema. *Am J Respir Crit Care Med* 2001;**163**:786–91.

97 Segura-Valdez L, Pardo A, Gaxiola M *et al.* Upregulation of gelantinases A and B, collagenases 1 and 2, and increased parenchymal cell death in COPD. *Chest* 2000;**117**:684–94.

98 Poole RA. Can serum biomarker assays measure the progression of cartilage degeneration in osteoarthritis? *Arthritis Rheum* 2002;**46**:2549–52.

99 Danesh J, Wheeler JG, Hirschfield GM *et al.* C-reactive protein and other circulating markers of inflammation in the prediction of coronary heart disease. *N Engl J Med* 2004;**350**:1387–97.

100 Dev D, Wallace E, Sankaran R *et al.* Value of C-reactive protein measurements in exacerbations of chronic obstructive pulmonary disease. *Respir Med* 1998;**92**:664–7.

101 Dentener MA, Creutzberg EC, Schols AM *et al.* Systemic anti-inflammatory mediators in COPD: increase in soluble interleukin 1 receptor II during treatment of exacerbations. *Thorax* 2001;**56**:721–6.

102 Gross PE, Pfitzer E, Tolker M, Babyak M, Kaschak M. Experimental emphysema: its production with papain in normal and silicotic rats. *Arch Environ Health* 1965;**11**:50–8.

103 Doherty JB, Shah SK, Finke PE *et al.* Chemical, biochemical, pharmacokinetic, and biological properties of L-680,833: a potent, orally active monocyclic β-lactam inhibitor of human polymorphonuclear leukocyte elastase. *Proc Natl Acad Sci USA* 1993;**90**:8727–31.

104 Wright JL, Churg A. A model of tobacco smoke induced airflow obstruction in the guinea pig. *Chest* 2002;**121**:188S–90S.

105 Wright JL, Farmer SG, Churg A. Synthetic serine elastase inhibitor reduces cigarette smoke-induced emphysema in guinea pigs. *Am J Respir Crit Care Med* 2002;**166**:954–60.

106 Shapiro SD. Proteinases in chronic obstructive pulmonary disease. *Biochem Soc Trans* 2002;**30**:98–102.

107 Tetley TD. Macrophages and the pathogenesis of COPD. *Chest* 2002;**121**:156S–9S.

108 Tetley TD. Neutrophil- and macrophage-derived proteases in chronic obstructive pulmonary disease and acute respiratory distress syndrome. In: Bellingan GJ, Lauren GJ, eds. *Acute Lung Injury: From Inflammation to Repair*. Amsterdam: IOS Press, 2000: 129–42.

109 Young RE, Thompson RD, Larbi KY *et al.* Neutrophil elastase (NE)-deficient mice demonstrate a non-redundant role for NE in neutrophil migration, generation of proinflammatory mediators, and phagocytosis in response to zymosan particles *in vivo*. *J Immunol* 2004;**172**:4493–502.

110 Churg A, Dai J, Tai H, Xie C, Wright JL. Tumor necrosis factor-α is central to acute cigarette smoke-induced inflammation and connective tissue breakdown. *Am J Respir Crit Care Med* 2002;**166**:849–54.

111 Stockley RA. Knock-out mouse: down but not out. *Am J Respir Crit Care Med* 2003;**168**:145–6.

112 Snider GL. Understanding inflammation in chronic obstructive pulmonary disease. *Am J Respir Crit Care Med* 2003;**167**:1045–9.

113 Churg A, Zay K, Shay S *et al.* Acute cigarette smoke-induced connective tissue breakdown requires both neutrophils and macrophage metalloelastase in mice. *Am J Respir Cell Mol Biol* 2002;**27**:368–74.

114 Churg A, Wang R, Tai H *et al.* Macrophage metalloelastase mediates acute cigarette smoke-induced inflammation via tumor necrosis factor-α release. *Am J Respir Crit Care Med* 2003;**167**:1083–9.

115 Dhami R, Gilks B, Xie C *et al.* Acute cigarette smoke-induced connective tissue breakdown is mediated by neutrophils and prevented by α₁-antitrypsin. *Am J Respir Cell Mol Biol* 2000;**22**:244–52.

116 Churg A, Wang RD, Xie C, Wright JL. α₁-Antitrypsin ameliorates cigarette smoke-induced emphysema in the mouse. *Am J Respir Crit Care Med* 2003;**168**:199–207.

117 Danel C, Motocescu C, Riguet M, Dusser DJ. Proteinase 3, neutrophil elastase and secretory leukocyte proteinase inhibitor in airway mucosa of patients with COPD. *Am J Respir Crit Care Med* 1999;**159**:A801.

118 Belaaouaj A, McCarthy R, Baumann M *et al.* Mice lacking neutrophil elastase reveal impaired host defense against gram negative bacterial sepsis. *Nat Med* 1998;**4**:615–8.

119 Mallen-St. Clair J, Pham CTN, Villalta SA, Caughey GH. Mast cell dipeptidyl peptidase I mediates survival from sepsis. *J Clin Invest* 2004;**113**:628–34.

120 Toomes C, James J, Wood AJ *et al.* Loss-of-function mutations in the cathepsin C gene result in periodontal disease and palmoplantar keratosis. *Nat Genet* 1999;**23**:421–4.

121 Zheng T, Zhu Z, Wang Z *et al.* Inducible targeting of IL-13 to the adult lung causes matrix metalloproteinase- and cathepsin-dependent emphysema. *J Clin Invest* 2000;**106**:1081–93.

122 Zhu Z, Homer RJ, Wang Z *et al.* Pulmonary expression of interleukin-13 causes inflammation, mucus hypersecretion, subepithelial fibrosis, physiologic abnormalities, and eotaxin production. *J Clin Invest* 1999;**103**:779–88.

123 Zhu Z, Ma B, Zheng T *et al.* IL-13-induced chemokine responses in the lung: role of CCR2 in the pathogenesis of IL-13-induced inflammation and remodeling. *J Immunol* 2002;**168**:2953–62.

124 Ma B, Zhu Z, Homer RJ *et al.* The C10/CCL6 chemokine and CCR1 play critical roles in the pathogenesis of IL-13-induced inflammation and remodeling. *J Immunol* 2004;**172**:1872–81.

125 Tkalcevic J, Novelli M, Phylactides M *et al.* Impaired immunity and enhanced resistance to endotoxin in the absence of neutrophil elastase and cathepsin G. *Immunity* 2000;**12**:201–10.

126 MacIvor DM, Shapiro SD, Pham CT *et al.* Normal neutrophil function in cathepsin G-deficient mice. *Blood* 1999;**94**:4282–93.

127 Nakamura A, Mori Y, Hagiwara K *et al.* Increased susceptibility to LPS-induced endotoxin shock in secretory leukoprotease inhibitor (SLPI)-deficient mice. *J Exp Med* 2003;**197**:669–74.

128 D'Armiento J, Dalal SS, Okada Y, Berg RA, Chada K. Collagenase expression in the lungs of transgenic mice causes pulmonary emphysema. *Cell* 1992;**71**:955–61.

129 Foronjy RF, Okada Y, Cole R, D'Armiento J. Progressive adult-onset emphysema in transgenic mice expressing human MMP-1 in the lung. *Am J Physiol Lung Cell Mol Physiol* 2003;**284**:L727–37.

130 Corry DB, Rishi K, Kanellis J *et al.* Decreased allergic lung inflammatory cell egression and increased susceptibility to asphyxiation in MMP2-deficiency. *Nat Immunol* 2002;**3**:347–53.

131 Itoh T, Tanioka M, Yoshida H *et al.* Reduced angiogenesis and tumor progression in gelatinase A-deficient mice. *Cancer Res* 1998;**58**:1048–51.

132 Wilson CL, Ouellette AJ, Satchell DP *et al.* Regulation of intestinal alpha-defensin activation by the metalloproteinase matrilysin in innate host defense. *Science* 1999;**286**:113–7.

133 Li Q, Park PW, Wilson CL, Parks WC. Matrilysin shedding of syndecan-1 regulates chemokine mobilization and transepithelial efflux of neutrophils in acute lung injury. *Cell* 2002;**11**:635–46.

134 Cataldo DD, Tournoy KG, Vermaelen KY *et al.* Matrix metalloproteinase-9 deficiency impairs cellular infiltration and bronchial hyperresponsiveness during allergen-induced airway inflammation. *Am J Pathol* 2002;**161**:491.

135 Vermaelen KY, Cataldo D, Tournoy K *et al.* Matrix metalloproteinase-9-mediated dendritic cell recruitment into the airways is a critical step in a mouse model of asthma. *J Immunol* 2003;**171**:1016–22.

136 Shipley JM, Wesselschmidt RL, Kobayashi DK, Ley TJ, Shapiro SD. Metalloelastase is required for macrophage-mediated proteolysis and matrix invasion in mice. *Proc Natl Acad Sci USA* 1996;**93**:3942–6.

137 Bartlett JD, Zhou Z, Skobe Z, Dobeck JM. Delayed tooth eruption in membrane type-1 matrix metalloproteinase deficient mice. *Connect Tissue Res* 2003;**44**:300–4.

138 Shankavaram UT, Lai W-C, Netzel-Arnett S *et al.* Monocyte membrane type 1-matrix metalloproteinase. *J Biol Chem* 2001;**276**:19027–32.

139 Leco KJ, Waterhouse P, Sanchez OH *et al.* Spontaneous air space enlargement in the lungs of mice lacking tissue inhibitor of metalloproteinases-3 (TIMP-3). *J Clin Invest* 2001;**108**:817–29.

140 Wert SE, Yoshida M, LeVine AM *et al.* Increased metalloproteinase activity, oxidant production, and emphysema in surfactant protein D gene-inactivated mice. *Proc Natl Acad Sci USA* 2000;**97**:5972–7.

141 Sukhova GK, Zhang Y, Pan J-H *et al.* Deficiency of cathepsin S reduces atherosclerosis in LDL receptor-deficient mice. *J Clin Invest* 2003;**111**:897–906.

142 Adkison AM, Raptis SZ, Kelley DG, Pham CT. Dipeptidyl peptidase I activates neutrophil-derived serine proteases and regulates the development of acute experimental arthritis. *J Clin Invest* 2004;**109**:363–71.

143 Kent G, Iles R, Bear CE *et al.* Lung disease in mice with cystic fibrosis. *J Clin Invest* 1997;**100**:3060–9.

144 Carrell RW, Lomas DA. α₁-Antitrypsin deficiency: a model for conformational diseases. *N Engl J Med* 2002;**346**:45–53.

145 Abrahamson M, Alvarez-Fernandez M, Nathanson CM. Cystatins. *Biochem Soc Symp* 2003;**70**:179–99.

146 Banda MJ, Rice AG, Griffin G, Senior RM. α₁-Proteinase inhibitor is a neutrophil chemoattractant after proteolytic inactivation by macrophage elastase. *J Biol Chem* 1988;**263**:4481–4.

147 Vogelmeier C, Buhl R, Hoyt RF *et al.* Aerosolization of recombinant SLPI to augment antineutrophil elastase protection of pulmonary epithelium. *J Appl Physiol* 1990;**69**:1843–8.

148 Abboud RT, Ford GT, Chapman KR. α₁-Antitrypsin deficiency: a position statement of the Canadian Thoracic Society. *Can Respir J* 2001;**8**:81–8.

149 Cavarra E, Bartalesi B, Lucattelli M *et al.* Effects of cigarette smoke in mice with different levels of α_1-proteinase inhibitor and sensitivity to oxidants. *Am J Respir Crit Care Med* 2001;**164**:886–90.

150 Takubo Y, Guerassimov A, Ghezzo H, Triantafillopoulos A, Bates JHT. α_1-Antitrypsin determines the pattern of emphysema and function in tobacco smoke-exposed mice: parellels with human disease. *Am J Respir Crit Care Med* 2002;**166**:1596–603.

151 Janoff A. Elastase in tissue injury. *Annu Rev Med* 1985;**36**:207–16.

152 Weiss SJ. Tissue destruction by neutrophils. *N Engl J Med* 1989;**320**:365–76.

153 Campbell EJ, Campbell MA, Boukedes SS, Owen CA. Quantum proteolysis by neutrophils: implications for pulmonary emphysema in α_1-antitrypsin deficiency. *J Clin Invest* 1999;**104**:337–44.

154 Campbell EJ, Campbell MA. Pericellular proteolysis by neutrophils in the presence of proteinase inhibitors: effects of substrate opsonization. *J Cell Biol* 1988;**106**:667–76.

155 Owen CA, Campbell EJ. The cell biology of leukocyte-mediated proteolysis. *J Leukoc Biol* 1999;**65**:137–50.

156 Owen CA, Campbell EJ. Neutrophil proteinases and matrix degradation: the cell biology of pericellular proteolysis. *Semin Cell Biol* 1995;**6**:367–76.

157 Liou TG, Campbell EJ. Non-isotropic enzyme-inhibitor interactions: a novel non-oxidative mechanism for quantum proteolysis by human neutrophils. *Biochemistry* 1995;**34**:16171–7.

158 Nossel HL, Yudelman I, Canfield RE *et al.* Measurement of fibrinopeptide A in human blood. *J Clin Invest* 1974;**54**:43–53.

159 Weitz JI, Landman SL, Crowley KA, Birken S, Morgan FJ. Development of an assay for *in vivo* human neutrophil elastase activity: increased elastase activity in patients with α_1-proteinase inhibitor deficiency. *J Clin Invest* 1986;**78**:155–62.

160 Mumford RA, Williams H, Mao J *et al.* Direct assay of Aα(1–21), a PMN elastase-specific cleavage product of fibrinogen, in the chimpanzee. *Ann N Y Acad Sci* 1991;**624**:167–78.

161 Pacholok SG, Davies P, Dorn CP Jr *et al.* Formation of polymorphonuclear leukocyte elastase: α_1-proteinase inhibitor complex and Aα(1–21) fibrinopeptide in human blood stimulated with the calcium ionophore A23187. A model to characterize inhibitors of polymorphonuclear leukocyte elastase. *Biochem Pharmacol* 1995;**49**:1513–20.

162 Mumford RA, Williams H, Mao J *et al.* Production of Aα (1–21), the human PMN elastase cleavage product of fibrinogen, in PiZZ individual blood stimulated by calcium inophore (A23187) before and after reconstitution therapy with α_1-antitrypsin (α1AT). *Am Rev Respir Dis* 1990;**141**:A111.

163 Weitz JI, Silverman EK, Thong B, Campbell EJ. Plasma levels of elastase-specific fibrinopeptides correlate with proteinase inhibitor phenotype: evidence for increased elastase activity in subjects with homozygous and heterozygous deficiency of α_1-proteinase inhibitor. *J Clin Invest* 1992;**89**:766–73.

164 Longo GM, Xiong W, Greiner TC *et al.* Matrix metallo-proteinases 2 and 9 work in concert to produce aortic aneurysms. *J Clin Invest* 2002;**110**:625–32.

165 Lopez-Otin C, Overall CM. Protease degradomics: a new challenge for proteomics. *Nat Rev Cell Biol* 2002;**3**:509–19.

166 Martignetti JA, Aqeel AA, Sewairi WA *et al.* Mutation of the matrix metalloproteinase 2 gene (MMP-2) causes a multicentric osteolysis and arthritis syndrome. *Nat Genet* 2001;**28**:261–5.

167 Mecham RP, Broekelmann TJ, Fliszar CJ *et al.* Elastin degradation by matrix metalloproteinases: cleavage site specificity and mechanisms of elastolysis. *J Biol Chem* 1997;**272**:18071–6.

168 Gronski TJ Jr, Martin RL, Kobayashi DK *et al.* Hydrolysis of a broad spectrum of extracellular matrix proteins by human macrophage elastase. *J Biol Chem* 1997;**272**:12189–94.

169 Belaaouaj A, Shipley JM, Kobayashi DK *et al.* Human macrophage metalloelastase: genomic organization, chromosomal location, gene linkage and tissue-specific expression. *J Biol Chem* 1995;**270**:14568–75.

170 Chapman HA Jr, Stone OL. Comparison of live human neutrophil and alveolar macrophage elastolytic activity *in vitro*: relative resistance of macrophage elastolytic activity to serum and alveolar proteinase inhibitors. *J Clin Invest* 1984;**74**:1693–700.

171 Chapman HA Jr, Stone OL, Vavrin Z. Degradation of fibrin and elastin by intact human alveolar macrophages *in vitro*: characterization of a plasminogen activator and its role in matrix degradation. *J Clin Invest* 1984;**73**:806–15.

172 Bannikov GA, Karelina TV, Collier LE, Marmer BL, Goldberg GI. Substrate binding of gelatinase B induces its enzymatic activity in the presence of intact propeptide. *J Biol Chem* 2002;**277**:16022–7.

173 Reddy VY, Zhang QY, Weiss SJ. Pericellular mobilization of the tissue-destructive cysteine proteinases, cathepsins B, L, and S, by human monocyte-derived macrophages. *Proc Natl Acad Sci USA* 1995;**92**:3849–53.

174 Punturieri A, Filippov S, Allen E *et al.* Regulation of elastinolytic cysteine proteinase activity in normal and cathepsin K-deficient human macrophages. *J Exp Med* 2000;**192**:789–99.

175 Sternlicht MD, Werb Z. How matrix metalloproteinase regulate cell behaviour. *Annu Rev Cell Dev Biol* 2001;**17**:463–516.

176 Croxton TL, Weinmann GG, Senior RM *et al.* Clinical research in chronic obstructive pulmonary disease: needs and opportunities. *Am J Respir Crit Care Med* 2003;**167**:1142–9.

177 Repine JE, Bast A, Lankhorst I. Oxidative stress in chronic obstructive pulmonary disease. *Am J Respir Crit Care Med* 1997;**156**:341–57.

178 Ogushi F, Hubbard RC, Vogelmeier C, Fells GA, Crystal RG. Risk factors for emphysema: cigarette smoking is associated with a reduction in the association rate constant of lung α_1-antitrypsin for neutrophil elastase. *J Clin Invest* 1991;**87**:1060–5.

179 Nicholson DW, Thornberry NA. Apoptosis: life and death decisions. *Science* 2003;**299**:214–5.

180 Palella FJ Jr, Delaney KM, Moorman AC *et al.* Declining morbidity and mortality among patients with advanced

human immunodeficiency virus infection. *N Engl J Med* 1998;**338**:853–60.

181 Egeblad M, Werb Z. New function for the matrix metalloproteinases in cancer progression. *Nature Rev Cancer* 2002; **2**:161–74.

182 Owen CA, Campbell MA, Boukedes SS, Campbell EJ. Cytokines regulate membrane-bound leukocyte elastase on neutrophils: a novel mechanism for effector activity. *Am J Physiol Lung Cell Mol Physiol* 1997;**272**:L385–93.

183 Owen CA, Campbell MA, Sannes PL, Boukedes SS, Campbell EJ. Cell surface-bound elastase and cathepsin G on human neutrophils: a novel, non-oxidative mechanism by which neutrophils focus and preserve catalytic activity of serine proteinases. *J Cell Biol* 1995;**131**:1–15.

184 Doherty JB, Ashe BM, Argenbright LW *et al*. Cephalosporin antibiotics can be modified to inhibit human leukocyte elastase. *Nature* 1986;**322**:192–4.

185 Mumford RA, Chabin R, Chiu S *et al*. A cell-penetrant monocyclic β-lactam inhibitor (MBI) which inactivates elastase (E) within PMN *in vitro* and *in vivo*. *Am J Respir Crit Care Med* 1995;**151**:A532.

186 McGuire MJ, Lipsky PE, Thiele DL. Generation of active myeloid and lymphoid granule serine proteases requires processing by the granule thiol protease dipeptidyl peptidase I. *J Biol Chem* 1993;**268**:2458–67.

187 Knight WB, Green BG, Chabin RM *et al*. Specificity, stability, and potency of monocyclic β-lactam inhibitors of human leucocyte elastase. *Biochemistry* 1992;**31**:8160–70.

188 Knight WB, Swiderek KM, Sakuma T *et al*. Electrospray ionization mass spectrometry as a mechanistic tool: mass of human leucocyte elastase and a β-lactam-derived E-I complex. *Biochemistry* 1993;**32**:2031–5.

189 Green BG, Chabin R, Mills S *et al*. Mechanism of inhibition of human leucocyte elastase by β-lactams. 2. Stability, reactivation kinetics, and products of β-lactam-derived E-I complexes. *Biochemistry* 1995;**34**:14331–43.

190 Underwood DJ, Green BG, Chabin R *et al*. Mechanism of inhibition of human leucocyte elastase by β-lactams. 3. Use of electrospray ionization mass spectrometry and two-dimensional NMR techniques to identify β-lactam-derived E-I complexes. *Biochemisty* 1995;**34**:14344–55.

191 Finke PE, Hagmann WK, Hanlon WA *et al*. Inventors: urea derived haptens, an assay for evaluating inhibition of polymorphonuclear leukocyte elastase by N-substituted azetidinones. *Br UK* 1993.

192 Campanelli D, Melchior M, Fu Y *et al*. Cloning of cDNA for proteinase 3: a serine protease, antibiotic, and autoantigen from human neutrophils. *J Exp Med* 1990;**172**:1709–15.

193 Kao RC, Wehner NG, Skubitz KM, Gray BH, Hoidal JR. Proteinase 3: a distinct human polymorphonuclear leukocyte proteinase that produces emphysema in hamsters. *J Clin Invest* 1988;**82**:1963–73.

194 Stone PJ, Lucey EC, Snider GL. Induction and exacerbation of emphysema in hamsters with human neutrophil elastase inactivated reversibly by a peptide boronic acid. *Am Rev Respir Dis* 1990;**141**:47–52.

195 Travis J, Fritz H. Potential problems in designing elastase inhibitors for therapy. *Am Rev Respir Dis* 1991;**143**:1412–5.

196 Williams JC, Falcone RC, Knee C *et al*. Biologic characterization of ICI 200,880 and ICI 200,355, novel inhibitors of human neutrophil elastase. *Am Rev Respir Dis* 1991;**144**:875–83.

197 Benson KF, Li F-Q, Person RE *et al*. Mutations associated with neutropenia in dogs and humans disrupt intracellular transport of neutrophil elastase. *Nat Genet* 2003;**35**:90–6.

198 Murphy G, Knauper V, Atkinson S *et al*. Matrix metalloproteinases in arthritic disease. *Arthritis Res* 2002;**4**:S39–49.

199 Selman M, Cisneros-Lira J, Gaxiola M *et al*. Matrix metalloproteinases inhibition attenuates tobacco smoke induced emphysema in guinea pigs. *Chest* 2003;**123**:1633–41.

200 Motyckova G, Fisher DE. Pycnodysostosis: role and regulation of cathepsin K in osteoclast function and human disease. *Curr Mol Med* 2002;**2**:407–21.

201 Randle JC, Harding MW, Ku G, Schonharting M, Kurrle R. ICE/Caspase-1 inhibitors as novel anti-inflammatory drugs. *Expert Opin Investig Drugs* 2001;**10**:1207–9.

202 Siegmund B, Zeitz M. Pralnacasan (vertex pharmaceuticals). *IDrugs* 2003;**6**:154–8.

CHAPTER 69
Retinoids

Stephen R. Tudhope

Emphysema is caused by the destruction of alveolar walls leading to a loss of elastic recoil and small airway closure in addition to loss of alveolar surface area for gas exchange [1]. Emphysema, which is a component of chronic obstructive pulmonary disease (COPD), is thought to result from the action of proteases [2], reactive oxygen species and cytotoxic T lymphocytes [3]. While the majority of pharmaceutical research effort is currently focused on inhibiting the inflammatory response in COPD or targeting proteases involved in lung destruction, the 'holy grail' of therapeutics for the treatment of emphysema is undoubtedly an agent that will regenerate damaged lung tissue. Retinoids hold that promise.

The term retinoids refers to the natural and synthetic derivatives of vitamin A (retinol). While retinol is required for reproduction and its metabolite retinaldehyhde for vision, it is another metabolite, all-*trans*-retinoic acid (ATRA) that is the focus of this chapter. The discovery that ATRA is a powerful and important morphogen involved in cell differentiation and branching pattern formation during embryonic development triggered the so-called 'retinoid revolution' of the 1980s [4]. ATRA was also found to be critical for the development of pulmonary alveoli and the discovery in 1997 that it could induce alveolar repair in an animal model of emphysema [5] appears to have triggered a new retinoid revolution.

This chapter reviews the role of retinoids in alveolar formation and models of emphysema as well as briefly considering some potentially related repair models. It also considers gene products that may be involved in retinoid-induced repair and assesses the clinical promise of retinoids for the treatment of emphysema.

Retinoid receptors

Retinoids exert their biological effects by directly regulating gene expression, their receptors belonging to the super-family of nuclear hormone receptors. These include steroid, thyroid and vitamin D_3 receptors [6]. There are two major classes of retinoid receptors, retinoic acid receptors (RARs) and retinoid X receptors (RXRs), each with three subtypes (α, β and γ) and various isoforms arising from differential gene splicing. RARs and RXRs bind to specific DNA sequences known as response elements (RAREs and RXREs, respectively) (Fig. 69.1). These receptors typically suppress gene transcription in the absence of retinoids and induce it in the presence of retinoid agonists [7]. Although RARs and RXRs can homodimerize, heterodimerization increases the efficiency of binding to the response elements and generates combinatorial diversity [8].

The response elements usually consist of direct repeats of the sequence AGGTCA separated by a defined number of nucleotides, although palindromes and complex elements with little consensus structure have also been shown to bind. RARs usually associate with direct repeats separated by a spacer of five nucleotides, whereas RXRs generally bind to

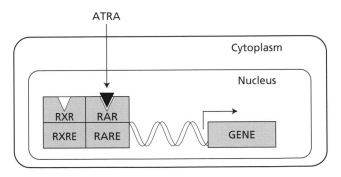

Figure 69.1 All-*trans*-retinoic acid (ATRA) signal transduction: The retinoic acid receptor (RAR) dimerizes with the retinoid X receptor (RXR) and associates with the retinoid response elements (RARE and RXRE) on DNA. ATRA activation of RAR induces gene transcription.

Compound	Structure	RAR selectivity
ATRA	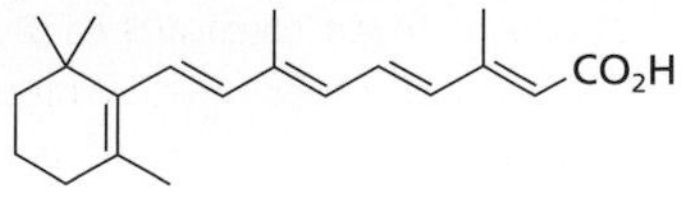	α, β, γ
TTNPB	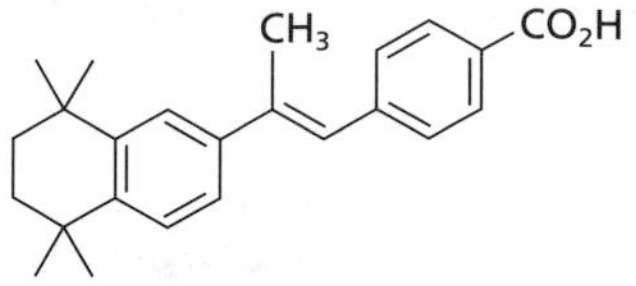	α, β, γ
Am580	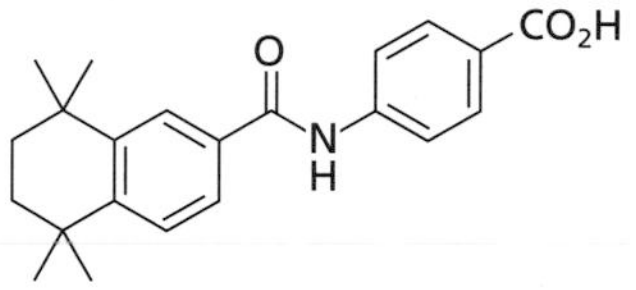	α
CD2019	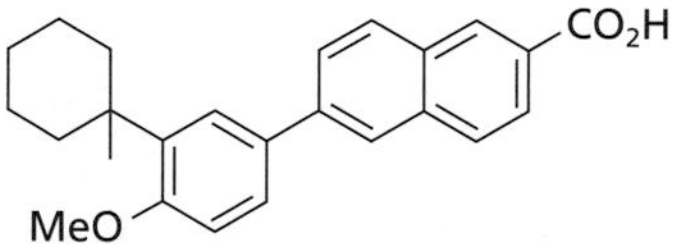	β
CD666	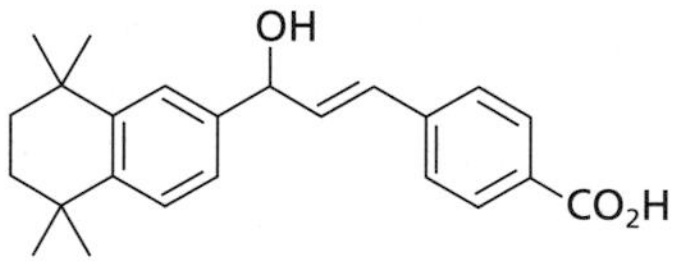	γ
Ro444753	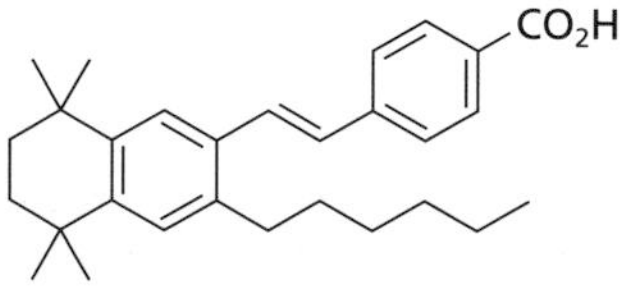	γ

Figure 69.2 Structures and selectivity profiles of retinoid agonists.

Compound	Structure	RAR selectivity
AGN193109	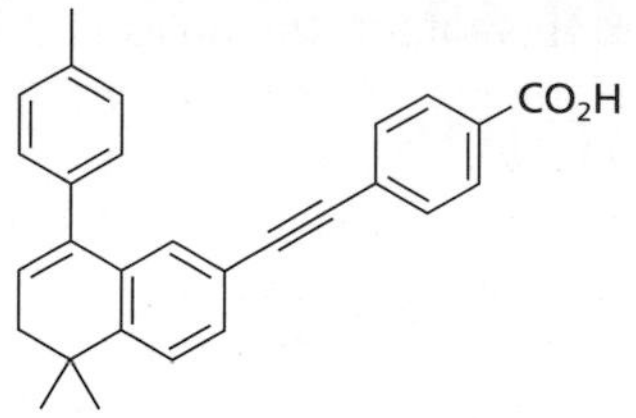	α, β, γ
AGN194301	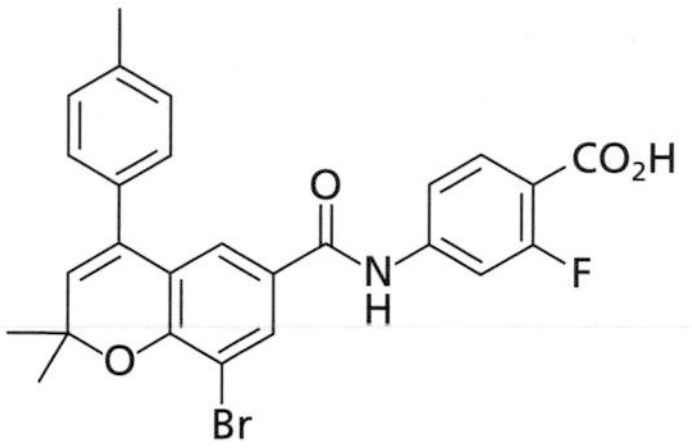	α

Figure 69.3 Structures and selectivity profiles of retinoid antagonists.

direct repeats with a spacer of one nucleotide [9]. There is, however, a degree of promiscuity between the response elements such that a particular response element may be activated by more than one member of the nuclear receptor superfamily. In addition, there is some tolerance for nucleotide substitution in the consensus sequence, leading to a range of binding affinities and therefore potentially different levels of retinoid responsiveness for different genes [9].

ATRA is the physiological hormone for RARs, binding with approximately equal affinity to the three subtypes, but has low affinity for RXRs. An isomer of ATRA, 9-*cis*-retinoic acid, which binds equally to RARs and RXRs, has been proposed as the physiological hormone for RXR activation, although this is still a matter of debate [10]. In the context of RAR/RXR heterodimers, activation is achieved by RAR agonists, although RXR agonists have been shown to enhance their effects in cellular assays [11,12]. RXRs also serve as heterodimeric partners to other nuclear receptors including the vitamin D, thyroid hormone and peroxisome proliferator-activated receptors (PPARs). Thus, RXRs are functionally different to RARs and appear to act as a master partner for nuclear receptor signalling, albeit usually a silent one.

There is a remarkably high degree of conservation between mouse and human RAR subtypes, suggesting that each subtype may have important and distinct physiological roles [13]. In addition, the spatiotemporal expression pattern of the RAR subtypes in mouse and human is also highly conserved. In adult mice and humans, RARα is ubiquitous, RARβ is highly expressed in the heart, lung and spleen, while RARγ is confined to lung and skin [14–16]. This suggests that selective RAR agonists may provide a way to target specific tissues and minimize the side-effects associated with non-selective retinoids.

Through decades of retinoid research, mainly pioneered by companies interested in their dermatological and oncological effects, there are now many synthetic retinoids reported with varying degrees of selectivity for retinoid receptor subtypes. TTNPB, for example, is a synthetic retinoid activating all three RAR subtypes but not RXRs [17]. AM580 is selective for the RARα receptor subtype [18], CD2019 preferentially binds to the RARβ receptor [19] and CD666 is RARγ selective (Fig. 69.2) [20]. Antagonists have also been reported, such as AGN 193109, a pan-RAR antagonist [21] and the RARα selective retinoid antagonist AGN 194301 (Fig. 69.3) [22]. Using such pharmacological tools, RAR subtype-specific effects are being identified.

Retinoids in alveolar formation

Studies utilizing vitamin A deficiency, RAR mutations and lung explants have demonstrated that ATRA is essential for lung development [23]. During the pseudoglandular stage of lung development, retinoid signalling promotes formation of conducting airways and later promotes formation of the primary lung buds [24]. Retinoids also have a critical role in the development of alveoli by a process known as septation, where lung saccules constituting the gas exchange region of the immature lung subdivide to increase the available surface area for gas exchange. Septation mostly occurs postnatally in mammalian species beginning around the fourth postnatal day in rats and mice and completed by the fourteenth. In humans, the process begins during the last month of gestation and continues at least through the first few postnatal years.

There is a critical window for septation in rats and mice, which if inhibited – for example, by the administration of the synthetic glucocorticosteroid dexamethasone – prevents normal alveolar formation and the lung takes on a permanent emphysematous-like appearance [25]. The septation period in rats is associated with low serum levels of natural glucocorticosteroid hormones [26,27], an abundance of pulmonary lipofibroblasts (LIFs) [28] and high lung levels of a retinoid binding protein CRBP1 [29].

The LIFs appear to act as retinoid storage cells, containing abundant stores of retinol and ATRA prior to septation that are depleted post-septation. LIFs also secrete tropoelastin, the precursor to cross-linked elastin that provides the support and elasticity essential for lung function. Studies with rat fetal lung explants showed that inhibiting the metabolism of retinyl esters reduced elastin gene expression in culture, whereas supplementation with ATRA increased elastin gene expression [30]. Expression of RARβ and RARγ was shown to increase in LIFs at birth, at the same time that these cells contain their maximal amount of ATRA. The RARγ expression level declines again after the second postnatal day, as ATRA levels also decrease. These associations strongly implicate retinoids with the processes of septation and elastin synthesis.

Investigating the role of ATRA in septation, Massaro and Massaro [31] demonstrated that treatment of normal neonatal rat pups with ATRA induced the formation of additional septa compared with untreated animals. An increased rate of septation was also observed in RARβ knockout mice [32], suggesting that signalling through RARβ inhibited septation. This was confirmed by the use of an RARβ selective agonist [32]. McGowan *et al.* [33] discovered a decrease in the numbers of alveoli and alveolar surface area in RARγ knockout mice, suggesting that RARγ signalling is the trigger for septation. This proposal is supported by the finding that only RARγ agonists stimulated elastin synthesis in pulmonary fibroblasts [34].

Although septation is the primary means to generate alveoli in the developing lung, there appears to be another, less understood process by which alveoli are formed during post-neonatal lung growth. This process does not occur by subdivision of saccules [35] and appears to be regulated by RARα signalling [36]. Taken together, these studies demonstrate a crucial role for retinoids in mediating alveolar formation, implicating RARγ as the trigger for septation with RARβ acting as a brake to prevent excessive subdivision and RARα mediating slower alveolar formation to synchronize with lung growth.

Retinoids in models of emphysema

Dexamethasone model

Treatment of neonatal rodents with dexamethasone during the critical period of septation results in an emphysematous-like lesion. However, as the alveoli have not yet formed and emphysema is defined as alveolar destruction, it is more correct to call this a model of impaired septation rather than emphysema. Nevertheless, the lungs do not spontaneously regenerate and adult animals have larger and fewer alveoli than untreated littermates (Fig. 69.4) [37,38]. Concomitant treatment with ATRA during the dexamethasone treatment period was found to reverse or block the inhibition of septation [31]. This effect could, however, be caused by inhibition of the steroid at a molecular level rather than overcoming its effect.

In adult rats with dexamethasone-impaired septation, ATRA induced the formation of smaller and more numerous alveoli [39], presumably by initiating septation, although the repair was only partial compared with control animals. This remarkable result has been confirmed in mice [40], demonstrating that ATRA can induce alveolar formation in adult animals at a time when alveoli do not normally form.

Elastase model

Many different proteases have been shown to induce an emphysematous condition when instilled into the lungs of animals. These include papain [41,42], neutrophil elastase [43] and trypsin [44], although the most frequently employed agent is porcine pancreatic elastase (subsequently referred to as elastase). A single administration of elastase has been shown to induce a condition that is functionally and morphologically similar to human panacinar emphysema [45].

Following their studies implicating ATRA in developmental alveolar formation, Massaro and Massaro [5] discovered that following elastase-induction of emphysema in rats, daily intraperitoneal injections of ATRA over 12 days resulted in a marked improvement in lung morphometry. This is consistent with formation of new alveoli by septation and the authors suggested that ATRA may have

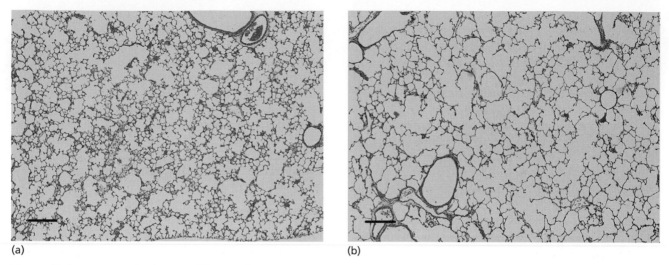

(a)   (b)

Figure 69.4 Representative images of dexamethasone-impaired septation in rats. (a) Daily treatments from age 4 to 13 days with saline. (b) Daily treatments from age 4 to 13 days with 0.25 µg dexamethasone in saline. Lungs were harvested at age 60 days, fixed at a transpulmonary pressure of 20 cm H_2O, sectioned and stained with haematoxylin and eosin. Scale bars 200 µm.

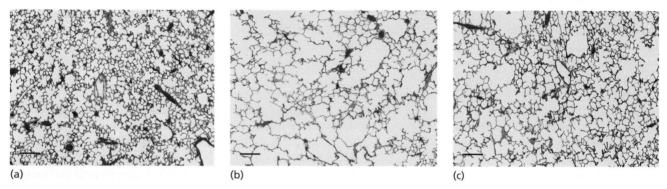

(a)   (b)   (c)

Figure 69.5 Representative images of the effect of all-*trans*-retinoic acid (ATRA) on elastase-induced emphysema in rats. (a) Animals instilled with saline on day 0 and cottonseed oil daily from day 24. (b) Animals instilled with elastase (2 units/g) on day 0 and cottonseed oil daily from day 24. (c) Animals instilled with elastase (2 units/g) on day 0 and ATRA (0.5 mg/kg) in cottonseed oil daily from day 24. Lungs were harvested on day 37, fixed at a transpulmonary pressure of 20 cm H_2O, sectioned and stained with haematoxylin and eosin. Scale bars 200 µm.

'turned back the clock' to induce gene expression patterns associated with early lung development and the formation of alveoli in the immature lung. We have corroborated these findings and representative lung images are presented in Figure 69.5 [38].

A major question regarding this ATRA-induced alveolar regeneration was whether the newly regenerated lung was 'normal' and contributed to gaseous exchange. Using physiological measurements of lung function, Tepper *et al.* [46] demonstrated that treatment with ATRA reversed the elastase-induced increase in Pause (a measurement reflecting airflow obstruction) and the lung volume parameters TLC (total lung capacity) and RV (residual volume). This suggested that the ATRA-induced regeneration of alveoli in

the elastase model of emphysema resulted in the formation of normal functional alveoli.

These findings have been substantiated by Belloni *et al.* [47] who reported that ATRA induced a 50% reversal of elastase-induced lung damage in rats. Furthermore, in the same model, the RARγ-selective agonist Ro444753 (see Fig. 69.2) induced lung repair by approximately 40% and improved some lung function parameters [48].

However, not all workers have been able to reproduce Massaro and Massaro's findings. March *et al.* [49] found no significant effect of ATRA on Lm (a measure of alveolar size) in a rat model of elastase-induced emphysema and Lucey *et al.* [50] found the same lack of statistical significance in a mouse model. In both studies, however, ATRA reduced the mean Lm by approximately 20%, which was similar to our own finding, although the data we obtained were statistically significant [38]. These contradicting results may stem from different techniques used to assess lung morphometry including their sensitivity to change [51] or from using different strains, species or dosing regimen [49,50].

Smoking model

It is well established that cigarette smoking can cause emphysema in humans [52]. In laboratory animals, cigarette smoke exposure has also been shown to induce emphysema in mice [53], rats [54] and guinea pigs [55].

In a rat model of smoke-induced emphysema, ATRA and Ro444753, administered daily for 1 month following the induction of emphysema, decreased elastin breakdown products and improved lung morphometry by 74% and 75%, respectively [56]. However, ATRA was found to be ineffective in guinea pig [57] and mouse [49] smoking models, although the guinea pig study was atypical as ATRA was administered during the smoke-induction of emphysema. The lack of effect of ATRA in mice, compared with the similarly conducted rat study, may result from differences in species, dosing regimen or the severity of emphysema [49].

Genetic models

Tight skinned (Tsk) mice [58], which contain a tandem duplication within the fibrillin-1 gene [59], fail to septate, resulting in an emphysematous-like condition [60,61]. Treatment of adult Tsk mice with daily injections of ATRA over 12 days was found to induce septation, resulting in 3.5 times more alveoli that on average were 2.7 times smaller compared with control animals [39].

The blotchy mouse is another example of disrupted lung matrix formation resulting in the development of an emphysematous-like condition [62]. In this case, altered copper transport effects lysyl oxidase activity [63] that is essential for the synthesis of mature cross-linked elastin [64]. The effect of retinoids in this model has yet to be reported.

Knockout models

The genetic models previously described suggest that defects in lung matrix deposition can lead to the inhibition of septation and altered lung morphology [65]. Elastin is possibly the most crucial of these proteins and its synthesis has been suggested to be the driving force behind alveogenesis [66–68]. Knockout mice lacking elastin die shortly after birth and display disruption of terminal airway branching

and fewer distal air sacs, indicating that elastin is essential for terminal airway development [69].

Mice lacking the growth factor PDGF-α survive birth and have normal lungs until the onset of septation [70]. Thereafter they develop an emphysematous morphology consistent with failed septation, undergo collapse of the lung parenchyma within a few weeks and die [71]. In these PDGF-α knockout mice, alveolar myofibroblasts fail to proliferate and spread, resulting in reduced elastin synthesis in the lung parenchyma. ATRA has been shown, *in vitro*, to stimulate postnatal rat lung fibroblast proliferation via a PDGF-mediated autocrine mechanism [72], suggesting that PDGF-α is a crucial downstream signalling molecule for ATRA-induced septation. These results also reinforce the central role of fibroblasts in lung septation.

A milder form of impaired septation is seen in a double knockout mouse model lacking the fibroblast growth factor receptors FGFR3 and FGFR4 [73]. However, in this knockout, elastin synthesis is apparently normal during the usual septation period although septation does not occur. The authors suggest that, besides elastin synthesis, a cellular differentiation step, blocked by the deletion of these receptors, is equally crucial for septation [73].

Angiogenesis models

Contrary to the widely held belief that the sole cause of emphysema is proteolytic injury to the lung extracellular matrix, Kasahara *et al.* [74] demonstrated that antagonism of the VEGF receptor VEGFR-2 induced emphysema in adult rats by an apoptosis-dependent mechanism with an absence of inflammatory cells. VEGF signalling through VEGFR-2 is necessary for maintenance of endothelial cells and angiogenesis. An antibody to PECAM-1, another effector of angiogenesis, was found to inhibit septation in rat pups, suggesting that angiogenesis also has an essential role in alveolar formation [75]. These novel findings revived the largely forgotten hypothesis of Liebow [76], which, based on histological examination of emphysematous lungs, proposed that vascular atrophy may initiate the loss of alveolar septa. Further support to this theory came from the observation that smokers with emphysema, but not healthy smokers, have decreased levels of VEGF, VEGFR-2 and increased lung endothelial and epithelial cell apoptosis [77]. This exciting new model of emphysema raises many questions, including whether or not the animals spontaneously repair following removal of the VEGFR-2 antagonist and whether ATRA can induce alveolar repair.

Hyperoxic lung injury

Exposure of neonatal animals to hyperoxic conditions during the period of septation inhibits the formation of alveoli

[78]. This inhibition of septation is similar to that seen with dexamethasone and is a feature of human bronchopulmonary dysplasia (BPD) seen in low birthweight infants supplemented with oxygen [79]. Although still a matter of controversy, treatment of vitamin A deficient, low birthweight infants with retinol has been reported to reduce the incidence of BPD [80], suggesting that retinol or a related metabolite may protect against the inhibition of septation caused by hyperoxia. Exposure of newborn rats to hyperoxic conditions and ATRA from age 3 to 14 days showed that unlike dexamethasone-impaired septation, ATRA had no effect on alveolar formation at this time [81]. However, following weaning to room air, examination of the lungs at age 42 days revealed that ATRA-treated animals had smaller alveoli and increased gas-exchange surface area relative to control hyperoxic lungs [82]. This suggests that ATRA protected against the hyperoxic-induced lung injury although the effect was only observed when a larger gas-exchange area was required for breathing normal air.

Calorific restriction

A possibly related model is that of calorific restriction, which supports a reversible link between lung architecture and an animal's oxygen demand [83]. In all mammals, there is a direct linear relationship between alveolar surface area and oxygen uptake [84]. During periods of starvation an animal's metabolic rate drops, lowering the oxygen demand [85] and in an apparent attempt to redress the balance between oxygen demand and alveolar surface area, calorific restriction results in an emphysematous morphology, which is returned to normal following refeeding [86]. This spontaneously regenerating model may throw new light on the natural mechanisms of alveolar destruction and regeneration, which could be involved in development of emphysema.

Associated models of regeneration

The mechanism of retinoid-induced alveolar regeneration may be related to the capacity of some species for compensatory organ growth and limb regeneration.

Compensatory lung growth

Spontaneous lung growth following partial lung resection has been documented in many species including dogs [87], ferrets [88], mice [89] and rats [90]. It also occurs in humans under the age of 4 years [91] and to a lesser extent up to the age of 20 years [92]. The rat model of compensatory lung growth post-pneumonectomy has been extensively studied, where, following pneumonectomy, the remaining lung undergoes expansion and remodelling to compensate for the loss of lung capacity. The 'new' lung has normal morphology, implying that alveolar formation occurs together with lung growth [93]. This post-pneumonectomy lung growth is modulated by the hormonal status of the animal, proceeding more rapidly in adrenalectomized animals and can be inhibited by administration of adrenal corticosteroid [94]. It is tempting to speculate that dexamethasone may also inhibit post-pneumonectomy alveolar formation akin to inhibition of septation during development. In addition, ATRA has been reported to enhance lung growth following pneumonectomy [95], which further supports a link between neonatal alveolar development and compensatory lung growth.

Limb regeneration

Amphibians of the order Urodela such as the Axolotl have the remarkable ability to regenerate limbs and other large sections of body following wounding or amputation. The effect of retinoids is to enhance the process in a proximal manner. That is, following amputation of an Axolotl forearm and treatment with ATRA, a complete limb from the shoulder level onwards can regenerate from the forearm [96]. Frog tadpoles, which can regenerate tails following amputation, may be induced to regenerate hindlimbs from amputated tail stumps by treatment with ATRA [97]. This 'proximalizing' effect of ATRA has also been observed in developing mammalian lungs *in vitro* [98,99], where ATRA was found to suppress the development of distal epithelial buds in favour of proximal airways.

MRL mouse model

The MRL/MpJ strain of mice, originally bred for their susceptibility to autoimmune disorders, have the remarkable ability to heal ear hole punctures [100]. This repair of a through-and-through hole is more like tissue regeneration than wound healing, as it is associated with complete recovery of normal architecture and a lack of scarring. Their regenerative capacity is not limited to the skin, however, and has also been demonstrated in the hearts of adult MRL mice [101]. Scarless wound healing is a trait usually associated with fetal rather than adult animals and has been linked to the lack of development of the immune system, particularly T lymphocytes. However, analysis of the genetic trait responsible for the regenerative capacity of MRL mice showed no overlap with the autoimmune phenotype. Instead, the researchers found a number of genetic loci that in combination led to the healing phenotype. Candidate genes associated with these loci include

*RAR*γ, *PDGF*, *FGFR4*, *TGF*β-*3* and *hox8* amongst others [102]. This discovery demonstrates that far from being restricted to amphibians, spontaneous tissue regeneration is also possible in adult mammals and may require a multitude of factors.

Although there are obvious differences between limb regeneration, scarless wound repair, compensatory lung growth, alveolar development and alveolar regeneration, there are also some striking similarities, especially in the context of pattern formation and signalling pathways [103].

Retinoid-responsive genes

Some retinoid-responsive genes are listed in Table 69.1. Many of these are known to be involved in early lung branching morphogenesis, such as *Shh*, *Hox*, growth factors and matrix proteins [153]. Some of these genes are also likely to be required for alveolar formation. These include: matrix proteins, particularly tropoelastin, essential for the formation of alveolar septa; growth factors and their receptors such as EGF, PDGF and TGF-β, required for cell differentiation and proliferation; and proteases and cell adhesion proteins required for cell migration. ATRA also regulates genes associated with retinoid activity, such as retinoid receptors, binding proteins and catabolic enzymes that may have a role in retinoid self-regulation.

Table 69.2 lists some further gene products associated with developmental or regenerative models. Although these genes are not known to be directly regulated by ATRA, by association with these models they may be regulated by downstream factors following retinoid activation. The list again includes matrix proteins and growth factors, as well as enzymes and hormones. It seems likely that a conserved mechanism exists for the formation and regeneration of pulmonary alveoli and therefore comparing gene expression in the different models may lead to a better understanding of this process [165].

Retinoids in clinical development for emphysema

Retinoids are currently used in the clinic for treatment of skin disorders and particular forms of cancer [166]; however, only limited studies have been undertaken in emphysema. In 2002, a group from the UCLA reported the results of a pilot study to assess the effects of ATRA in human emphysema [167]. This small study of 20 patients with severe emphysema showed no clinical benefits on pulmonary lung function or by computerized tomography imaging following a 3-month cross-over treatment with ATRA. A larger, five-centre study, sponsored by the National Heart, Lung and Blood Institute (NHLBI) using a 6-month treatment time followed by a 3-month crossover phase commenced in 1999 [168,169] and the results are expected in 2006.

Although ATRA was well tolerated in the UCLA study, mild side-effects including skin changes, transient headache, hyperlipidaemia and musculoskeletal pains were reported. Such side-effects may prove to be dose limiting. An alternative approach is to use selective retinoids targeting a single receptor subtype, which may have a more favourable therapeutic ratio. Roche [170,171] have released press reports on a selective RARγ agonist (R667), which is currently in phase II clinical development for the treatment of emphysema. The results of these clinical trials are expected in 2006.

Discussion

It has been demonstrated that retinoids not only promote alveolar formation during the neonatal period, but can also induce alveolar regeneration in adult emphysematous disease models. These include genetic dysfunction and protease or cigarette smoke induced lung destruction, although results in the latter models remain controversial and may be species or strain dependent.

Retinoids induce gene expression by activation of RARs and it is most likely that activation of specific RARs in particular cells underlie the effects discussed so far. Alternative mechanisms are inhibition of gene transcription by association with other transcription factors and indirect antioxidant effects; neither of which would appear to lend the required complexity to direct morphogenesis.

Although the exact mechanism of retinoid-induced alveolar formation remains a mystery, genetic models and knockouts have implicated a number of essential gene products in the process. These include the matrix proteins fibrillin-1 and tropoelastin; lysyl oxidase, to cross-link and produce mature elastin fibres; growth factor PDGF-α and fibroblast growth factors acting through FGFR3 and FGFR4. In addition, angiogenic factors such as VEGF and PECAM-1 may also have a pivotal role. That ATRA can induce alveolar formation and repair implicates it as a master morphogen, being able to initiate a cascade of controlled gene signalling resulting in coordinated lung growth.

Associated spontaneous repair models such as amphibian limb regeneration, mammalian compensatory lung growth, calorific restriction and scarless wound healing may also share repair pathways with the retinoids. Elucidating the mechanisms of these processes will enhance our understanding of natural tissue regeneration and may shed further light on retinoid mechanisms.

Table 69.1 All-*trans*-retinoic acid (ATRA)-responsive genes. Table represents gene products induced (↑) or inhibited (↓) by ATRA, grouped by function.

Gene family and product	Regulated	Mode*	System†	Refs
Matrix components				
Tropoelastin	↑	Indirect	D,C	[30,93,104]
Type 1 procollagen	↑	Indirect	D,C	[81,93,105]
Laminin B1	↑	Direct	–	[106]
MMP-1	↓	Direct	–	[107]
MMP-3	↓	–	–	[108]
MMP-7	↓	–	–	[109]
MMP-9	↓	Indirect	–	[110,111]
MMP-11	↑↓	Direct	–	[112,113]
TIMP1	↑	Indirect	–	[111,114]
Cell adhesion				
Galectin-1	↑	–	–	[115]
Galectin-3	↓	–	–	[115]
LAMP	↑	–	–	[115]
Transglutaminase C	↑	–	–	[116,117]
Growth factors and receptors				
IGF-2	↑	Direct	–	[118]
IGFBP-3	↑	Direct	–	[119]
IGFBP-6	↑	Direct	–	[120,121]
IGF-1R	↑	–	–	[122]
EGFR	↑	Indirect	D,C	[95,123,124]
FGF-8	↑	Direct	–	[125]
FGF-BP	↓	–	–	[126]
PDGF	↑	Indirect	D,C	[71,72,127]
PDGFRs	↑	–	–	[128]
TGF-β1	↓	–	–	[129]
TGF-β2	↑	–	–	[130]
TGF-β3	↑	–	–	[130]
TGF-βRs	↑	–	–	[131]
NGF	↑	–	–	[132]
NGFR	↑	Direct	–	[133,134]
Midkine	↑	Direct	D	[135,136]
Enzymes				
Cathepsin D	↑	–	–	[137]
Transcription factors				
Ets-1	↑	Direct	–	[138]
HNF-3α	↑	Direct	–	[139]
Receptors				
RARβ	↑	Direct	–	[140]
β1-AR	↑	Direct	–	[141]
Pattern genes				
Hoxa-1,2,7	↑	Direct	D	[142–144]
Hoxb-1,5,6,8	↑	Direct	D	[143,145,146]
Hoxd-4	↑	Direct	D	[147]
Shh	↑	–	D	[143]
Other				
SPB	↑	Direct	–	[148]
CRBPI	↑	Direct	D	[149,150]
CRBPII	↑	Direct	–	[151]
P450RAI	↑	Direct	–	[152]

* The mode of regulation is direct if the presence of a RARE or direct gene modulation has been demonstrated. Indirect means that protein synthesis is required before modulation of gene transcription is observed.
† D, developmentally regulated gene; C, regulated during compensatory lung growth; –, information not available.

Table 69.2 Other gene products associated with developmental or regenerative models. Table represents gene products positively ($\uparrow$) or negatively ($\downarrow$) regulated, grouped by function.

Gene family and product	Regulated	System*	Refs
Matrix components			
Fibrillin-1	$\uparrow$	D	[154]
Growth factors and receptors			
IGF-1	$\uparrow$	C	[155,156]
HGF	$\uparrow$	C	[157]
EGF	$\uparrow$	D	[158]
FGFs	$\uparrow$	D,C	[153,159]
FGFRs	$\uparrow$	D	[73]
VEGF	$\uparrow$	D	[160]
Hormones			
Thyroid (T_3)	$\uparrow$	D,L	[97,161]
Corticosteroids	$\downarrow$	D,C	[37,94]
Enzymes			
ENOS	$\uparrow$	C	[89]
Lysyl oxidase	$\uparrow$	D,C	[162]
Transcription factors			
Egr-1	$\uparrow$	C	[163]
Nurr77	$\uparrow$	C	[163]
Tristetrapolin	$\uparrow$	C	[163]
I kappa B-alpha	$\uparrow$	C	[163]
GKLF	$\uparrow$	C	[163]
LRG-21	$\uparrow$	C	[163]
Other			
PECAM-1	$\uparrow$	D	[164]

* The gene product may be associated with developmental alveolar formation (D), compensatory lung growth (C) or limb regeneration (L).

Conclusions

Until recently, there has been little optimism for finding therapeutic treatments to promote alveolar repair. However, the discoveries surrounding the effects of retinoids on lung morphogenesis are now changing the dogma that the adult mammalian lung is non-repairable. With clinical studies ongoing to test the efficacy of ATRA and selective retinoid agonists in human pulmonary emphysema, it will soon be known whether retinoids can deliver their promise. In addition, further work to understand the mechanism of retinoid-induced alveolar repair in animal models may provide insight into alternative therapeutic approaches for the treatment of human emphysema.

Acknowledgements

The author would like to thank Mary Fitzgerald, Craig Fox and Sarah Lewis from Argenta Discovery and Guenter Benz from Bayer AG for kind permission to include unpublished work. Many thanks also to Mark Giembycz and Louise Donnelly from the Department of Thoracic Medicine, National Heart and Lung Institute, Imperial College and Craig Fox from Argenta Discovery for their critical review of this manuscript.

References

1 Snider GL, Kleinerman J, Thurlbeck WM, Bengali Z. The definition of emphysema: Report of a National Heart, Lung and Blood Institute, Division of Lung Diseases Workshop. *Am Rev Respir Dis* 1985;**132**:182–5.

2 Gadek JE, Pacht ER. The protease–antiprotease balance within the human lung: implications for the pathogenesis of emphysema. *Lung* 1990;**168**(Suppl):552–64.

3 Barnes PJ. New concepts in chronic obstructive pulmonary disease. *Annu Rev Med* 2003;**54**:113–29.

4 Chytil F. Retinoids in lung development. *FASEB J* 1996;**10**: 986–92.

5 Massaro GD, Massaro D. Retinoic acid treatment abrogates elastase-induced pulmonary emphysema in rats. *Nat Med* 1997;**3**:675–7.

6 Chambon P. A decade of molecular biology of retinoic acid receptors. *FASEB J* 1996;**10**:940–54.

7 Lin BC, Hong SH, Krig S, Yoh SM, Privalsky ML. A conformational switch in nuclear hormone receptors is involved in coupling hormone binding to corepressor release. *Mol Cell Biol* 1997;**17**:6131–8.

8 Leid M, Kastner P, Chambon P. Multiplicity generates diversity in the retinoic acid signalling pathways. *Trends Biochem Sci* 1992;**17**:427–33.

9 Mangelsdorf DJ, Umesono K, Evans RM. The retinoid receptors. In: Sporn MB, Roberts AB, Goodman DS, eds. *The Retinoids: Biology, Chemistry and Medicine*. New York: Raven Press, 1994: 319–49.

10 Nagpal S, Chandraratna RA. Recent developments in receptor-selective retinoids. *Curr Pharm Des* 2000;**6**:919–31.

11 Botling J, Castro DS, Oberg F, Nilsson K, Perlmann T. Retinoic acid receptor/retinoid X receptor heterodimers can be activated through both subunits providing a basis for synergistic transactivation and cellular differentiation. *J Biol Chem* 1997;**272**:9443–9.

12 Minucci S, Leid M, Toyama R *et al.* Retinoid X receptor (RXR) within the RXR-retinoic acid receptor heterodimer binds its ligand and enhances retinoid-dependent gene expression. *Mol Cell Biol* 1997;**17**:644–55.

13 Chambon P. The retinoid signaling pathway: molecular and genetic analyses. *Semin Cell Biol* 1994;**5**:115–25.

14 Elder JT, Fisher GJ, Zhang QY *et al*. Retinoic acid receptor gene expression in human skin. *J Invest Dermatol* 1991;**96**:425–33.

15 Rees J. The molecular biology of retinoic acid receptors: orphan from good family seeks home. *Br J Dermatol* 1992;**126**:97–104.

16 Fisher GJ, Talwar HS, Xiao JH *et al*. Immunological identification and functional quantitation of retinoic acid and retinoid X receptor proteins in human skin. *J Biol Chem* 1994;**269**:20629–35.

17 Beard RL, Colon DF, Song TK *et al*. Synthesis and structure–activity relationships of retinoid X receptor selective diaryl sulfide analogs of retinoic acid. *J Med Chem* 1996;**39**: 3556–63.

18 Kagechika H, Kawachi E, Hashimoto Y, Himi T, Shudo K. Retinobenzoic acids. I. Structure–activity relationships of aromatic amides with retinoidal activity. *J Med Chem* 1988; **31**:2182–92.

19 Martin B, Bernardon JM, Cavey MT *et al*. Selective synthetic ligands for human nuclear retinoic acid receptors. *Skin Pharmacol* 1992;**5**:57–65.

20 Bernard BA, Bernardon JM, Delescluse C *et al*. Identification of synthetic retinoids with selectivity for human nuclear retinoic acid receptor gamma. *Biochem Biophys Res Commun* 1992;**186**:977–83.

21 Klein ES, Pino ME, Johnson AT *et al*. Identification and functional separation of retinoic acid receptor neutral antagonists and inverse agonists. *J Biol Chem* 1996;**271**: 22692–6.

22 Johnson AT, Klein ES, Gillett SJ *et al*. Synthesis and characterization of a highly potent and effective antagonist of retinoic acid receptors. *J Med Chem* 1995;**38**:4764–7.

23 Masuyama H, Hiramatsu Y, Kudo T. Effect of retinoids on fetal lung development in the rat. *Biol Neonate* 1995;**67**:264–73.

24 Mollard R, Ghyselinck NB, Wendling O, Chambon P, Mark M. Stage-dependent responses of the developing lung to retinoic acid signaling. *Int J Dev Biol* 2000;**44**:457–62.

25 Sahebjami H, Domino M. Effects of postnatal dexamethasone treatment on development of alveoli in adult rats. *Exp Lung Res* 1989;**15**:961–73.

26 Henning SJ. Plasma concentrations of total and free corticosterone during development in the rat. *Am J Physiol* 1978; **235**:E451–6.

27 Jones CT. Corticosteroid concentrations in the plasma of fetal and maternal guinea pigs during gestation. *Endocrinology* 1974;**95**:1129–33.

28 Vaccaro C, Brody JS. Ultrastructure of developing alveoli. I. The role of the interstitial fibroblast. *Anat Rec* 1978;**192**: 467–79.

29 Ong DE, Chytil F. Changes in levels of cellular retinol- and retinoic-acid-binding proteins of liver and lung during perinatal development of rat. *Proc Natl Acad Sci USA* 1976;**73**: 3976–8.

30 McGowan SE, Doro MM, Jackson SK. Endogenous retinoids increase perinatal elastin gene expression in rat lung fibroblasts and fetal explants. *Am J Physiol* 1997;**273**:L410–6.

31 Massaro GD, Massaro D. Postnatal treatment with retinoic acid increases the number of pulmonary alveoli in rats. *Am J Physiol* 1996;**270**:L305–10.

32 Massaro GD, Massaro D, Chan WY *et al*. Retinoic acid receptor-beta: an endogenous inhibitor of the perinatal formation of pulmonary alveoli. *Physiol Genomics* 2000;**4**:51–7.

33 McGowan S, Jackson SK, Jenkins-Moore M *et al*. Mice bearing deletions of retinoic acid receptors demonstrate reduced lung elastin and alveolar numbers. *Am J Respir Cell Mol Biol* 2000;**23**:162–7.

34 Belloni PN, Klaus M. Treatment of emphysema using RAR selective retinoid agonists. F Hoffmann-La Roche Ltd: Patent WO0130326 2001.

35 Blanco LN, Massaro D, Massaro GD. Alveolar size, number, and surface area: developmentally dependent response to 13% O_2. *Am J Physiol* 1991;**261**:L370–7.

36 Massaro GD, Massaro D, Chambon P. Retinoic acid receptor-alpha regulates pulmonary alveolus formation in mice after, but not during, perinatal period. *Am J Physiol Lung Cell Mol Physiol* 2003;**284**:L431–3.

37 Massaro D, Teich N, Maxwell S, Massaro GD, Whitney P. Postnatal development of alveoli: regulation and evidence for a critical period in rats. *J Clin Invest* 1985;**76**:1297–305.

38 Tudhope SR, Fox JC, Lewis S, Fitzgerald MF. Unpublished data.

39 Massaro GD, Massaro D. Retinoic acid treatment partially rescues failed septation in rats and in mice. *Am J Physiol Lung Cell Mol Physiol* 2000;**278**:L955–60.

40 Hind M, Maden M. Retinoic acid induced neoalveogenesis in the adult mouse lung. *Thorax* 2001;**56**:iii2.

41 Gross P, Pfitzer E, Tolker E, Babyak M, Kaschak M. Experimental emphysema: its production with papain in normal and silicotic rats. *Arch Environ Health* 1965;**11**:50–8.

42 Colombo C, Steinetz BG. Lung enzymes in emphysematous rats: effects of progestagens, antiphlogistics and metabolic inhibitors. *Arch Int Pharmacodyn Ther* 1975;**216**:86–96.

43 Senior RM, Tegner H, Kuhn C *et al*. The induction of pulmonary emphysema with human leukocyte elastase. *Am Rev Respir Dis* 1977;**116**:469–75.

44 Reichart E, Boerkmann P, Plenat F. Trypsin-triggered emphysema: an established model in rats. *Respir Med* 1994; **88**:701–2.

45 Snider GL, Lucey EC, Stone PJ. Animal models of emphysema. *Am Rev Respir Dis* 1986;**133**:149–69.

46 Tepper J, Pfeiffer J, Aldrich M *et al*. Can retinoic acid ameliorate the physiologic and morphologic effects of elastase instillation in the rat? *Chest* 2000;**117**(Suppl 1):242S–4S.

47 Belloni PN, Garvin L, Mao CP, Bailey-Healy I, Leaffer D. Effects of all-*trans*-retinoic acid in promoting alveolar repair. *Chest* 2000;**117**(Suppl 1):235S–41S.

48 Mao CP, Bailey-Healy I, Gater PR, Belloni PN. Effects of Ro444753, a synthetic retinoid agonist, on morphologic and lung function changes in a rat model of emphysema. *Am J Respir Crit Care Med* 2002;**165**:A825.

49 March TH, Cossey PY, Wayne BJ, Esparza DC, Bowen LE. All *trans*-retinoic acid (ATRA) administered by inhalation or injection does not ameliorate pulmonary emphysema in two animal models. *Am J Respir Crit Care Med* 2003;**167**:A317.

50 Lucey EC, Goldstein RH, Breuer R *et al*. Retinoic acid does not affect alveolar septation in adult FVB mice with elastase-induced emphysema. *Respiration* 2003;**70**:200–5.

51 Fox JC, Tudhope SR, Meshi B, Hogg JC, Stockley RA. Development of a computer-based image analysis technique for the detection of emphysematous lung morphology in animal models. *Am J Respir Crit Care Med* 2003;**167**:A744.

52 Petty TL. COPD in perspective. *Chest* 2002;**121**(Suppl): 116S–20S.

53 Hautamaki RD, Kobayashi DK, Senior RM, Shapiro SD. Requirement for macrophage elastase for cigarette smoke-induced emphysema in mice. *Science* 1997;**277**:2002–4.

54 Ofulue AF, Ko M, Abboud RT. Time course of neutrophil and macrophage elastinolytic activities in cigarette smoke-induced emphysema. *Am J Physiol* 1998;**275**:L1134–44.

55 Wright JL, Churg A. Cigarette smoke causes physiologic and morphologic changes of emphysema in the guinea pig. *Am Rev Respir Dis* 1990;**142**:1422–8.

56 Ofulue AF, Xiang Y, Yang N, Belloni PN. Retinoids reverse cigarette smoke-induced emphysema in rats. *Am J Respir Crit Care Med* 2002;**165**:B7.

57 Meshi B, Vitalis TZ, Ionescu D *et al*. Emphysematous lung destruction by cigarette smoke: the effects of latent adenoviral infection on the lung inflammatory response. *Am J Respir Cell Mol Biol* 2002;**26**:52–7.

58 Green MC, Sweet HO, Bunker LE. Tight-skin, a new mutation of the mouse causing excessive growth of connective tissue and skeleton. *Am J Pathol* 1976;**82**:493–512.

59 Siracusa LD, McGrath R, Ma Q *et al*. A tandem duplication within the fibrillin 1 gene is associated with the mouse tight skin mutation. *Genome Res* 1996;**6**:300–13.

60 Martorana PA, van Even P, Gardi C, Lungarella G. A 16-month study of the development of genetic emphysema in tight-skin mice. *Am Rev Respir Dis* 1989;**139**:226–32.

61 Starcher B, James H. Evidence that genetic emphysema in tight-skin mice is not caused by neutrophil elastase. *Am Rev Respir Dis* 1991;**143**:1365–8.

62 McCartney AC, Fox B, Partridge TA *et al*. Emphysema in the Blotchy mouse: a morphometric study. *J Pathol* 1988;**156**: 77–81.

63 Starcher B, Madaras JA, Fisk D, Perry EF, Hill CH. Abnormal cellular copper metabolism in the blotchy mouse. *J Nutr* 1978;**108**:1229–33.

64 Fisk DE, Kuhn C. Emphysema-like changes in the lungs of the blotchy mouse. *Am Rev Respir Dis* 1976;**113**:787–97.

65 Starcher BC. Lung elastin and matrix. *Chest* 2000;**117**(Suppl 1):229S–34S.

66 Burri PH, Weibel ER. Ultrastructure and morphometry of the developing lung. In: Hodson WA, ed. *Development of the Lung, Part 1: Structural Development*. New York: Marcel Dekker, 1977: 215–68.

67 Emery JL. The postnatal development of the human lung and its implications for lung pathology. *Respiration* 1970;**27**: Suppl 50.

68 Noguchi A, Reddy R, Kursar JD, Parks WC, Mecham RP. Smooth muscle isoactin and elastin in fetal bovine lung. *Exp Lung Res* 1989;**15**:537–52.

69 Wendel DP, Taylor DG, Albertine KH, Keating MT, Li DY. Impaired distal airway development in mice lacking elastin. *Am J Respir Cell Mol Biol* 2000;**23**:320–6.

70 Lindahl P, Karlsson L, Hellstrom M *et al*. Alveogenesis failure in PDGF-A-deficient mice is coupled to lack of distal spreading of alveolar smooth muscle cell progenitors during lung development. *Development* 1997;**124**:3943–53.

71 Bostrom H, Willetts K, Pekny M *et al*. PDGF-A signaling is a critical event in lung alveolar myofibroblast development and alveogenesis. *Cell* 1996;**85**:863–73.

72 Liebeskind A, Srinivasan S, Kaetzel D, Bruce M. Retinoic acid stimulates immature lung fibroblast growth via a PDGF-mediated autocrine mechanism. *Am J Physiol Lung Cell Mol Physiol* 2000;**279**:L81–90.

73 Weinstein M, Xu X, Ohyama K, Deng CX. FGFR-3 and FGFR-4 function cooperatively to direct alveogenesis in the murine lung. *Development* 1998;**125**:3615–23.

74 Kasahara Y, Tuder RM, Taraseviciene-Stewart L *et al*. Inhibition of VEGF receptors causes lung cell apoptosis and emphysema. *J Clin Invest* 2000;**106**:1311–9.

75 Savani RC, Zaman A, Pooler PM *et al*. Angiogenesis driving alveolization: the role of PECAM-1 in alveolar septation. *Am J Respir Crit Care Med* 2000;**161**:A521.

76 Liebow AA. Pulmonary emphysema with special emphasis to vascular changes. *Am Rev Respir Dis* 1959;**80**:67–93.

77 Kasahara Y, Tuder RM, Cool CD *et al*. Endothelial cell death and decreased expression of vascular endothelial growth factor and vascular endothelial growth factor receptor 2 in emphysema. *Am J Respir Crit Care Med* 2001;**163**:737–44.

78 Blanco LN, Frank L. The formation of alveoli in rat lung during the third and fourth postnatal weeks: effect of hyperoxia, dexamethasone, and deferoxamine. *Pediatr Res* 1993; **34**:334–40.

79 Northway WH Jr, Moss RB, Carlisle KB *et al*. Late pulmonary sequelae of bronchopulmonary dysplasia. *N Engl J Med* 1990;**323**:1793–9.

80 Shenai JP, Kennedy KA, Chytil F, Stahlman MT. Clinical trial of vitamin A supplementation in infants susceptible to bronchopulmonary dysplasia. *J Pediatr* 1987;**111**:269–77.

81 Veness-Meehan KA, Bottone FG Jr, Stiles AD. Effects of retinoic acid on airspace development and lung collagen in hyperoxia-exposed newborn rats. *Pediatr Res* 2000;**48**: 434–44.

82 Veness-Meehan KA, Pierce RA, Moats-Staats BM, Stiles AD. Retinoic acid attenuates O_2-induced inhibition of lung septation. *Am J Physiol Lung Cell Mol Physiol* 2002;**283**: L971–80.

83 Massaro D, Massaro GD. Invited review: pulmonary alveoli: formation, the 'call for oxygen', and other regulators. *Am J Physiol Lung Cell Mol Physiol* 2002;**282**:L345–58.

84 Tenney SM, Remmers JE. Comparative quantitative morphology of the mammalian lung diffusing area. *Nature* 1963;**197**:54–6.

85 Munch IC, Markussen NH, Oritsland NA. Resting oxygen consumption in rats during food restriction, starvation and refeeding. *Acta Physiol Scand* 1993;**148**:335–40.

86 Massaro GD, Radaeva S, Clerch LB, Massaro D. Lung alveoli: endogenous programmed destruction and regeneration. *Am J Physiol Lung Cell Mol Physiol* 2002;**283**:L305–9.

87 Hsia CC, Herazo LF, Fryder-Doffey F, Weibel ER. Compensatory lung growth occurs in adult dogs after right pneumonectomy. *J Clin Invest* 1994;**94**:405–12.

88 McBride JT. Lung volumes after an increase in lung distension in pneumonectomized ferrets. *J Appl Physiol* 1989;**67**: 1418–21.

89 Leuwerke SM, Kaza AK, Tribble CG, Kron IL, Laubach VE. Inhibition of compensatory lung growth in endothelial nitric oxide synthase-deficient mice. *Am J Physiol Lung Cell Mol Physiol* 2002;**282**:L1272–8.

90 Fisher JM, Simnett JD. Morphogenetic and proliferative changes in the regenerating lung of the rat. *Anat Rec* 1973; **176**:389–95.

91 Nakajima C, Kijimoto C, Yokoyama Y *et al*. Longitudinal follow-up of pulmonary function after lobectomy in childhood: factors affecting lung growth. *Pediatr Surg Int* 1998; **13**:341–5.

92 Laros CD, Westermann CJ. Dilatation, compensatory growth, or both after pneumonectomy during childhood and adolescence: a thirty-year follow-up study. *J Thorac Cardiovasc Surg* 1987;**93**:570–6.

93 Koh DW, Roby JD, Starcher B, Senior RM, Pierce RA. Postpneumonectomy lung growth: a model of reinitiation of tropoelastin and type I collagen production in a normal pattern in adult rat lung. *Am J Respir Cell Mol Biol* 1996; **15**:611–23.

94 Rannels DE, Stockstill B, Mercer RR, Crapo JD. Cellular changes in the lungs of adrenalectomized rats following left pneumonectomy. *Am J Respir Cell Mol Biol* 1991;**5**:351–62.

95 Kaza AK, Kron IL, Kern JA *et al*. Retinoic acid enhances lung growth after pneumonectomy. *Ann Thorac Surg* 2001;**71**: 1645–50.

96 Maden M. Vitamin A and pattern formation in the regenerating limb. *Nature* 1982;**295**:672–5.

97 Maden M, Corcoran J. Role of thyroid hormone and retinoid receptors in the homeotic transformation of tails into limbs in frogs. *Dev Genet* 1996;**19**:85–93.

98 Cardoso WV, Williams MC, Mitsialis SA *et al*. Retinoic acid induces changes in the pattern of airway branching and alters epithelial cell differentiation in the developing lung *in vitro*. *Am J Respir Cell Mol Biol* 1995;**12**:464–76.

99 Packer AI, Mailutha KG, Ambrozewicz LA, Wolgemuth DJ. Regulation of the *Hoxa4* and *Hoxa5* genes in the embryonic mouse lung by retinoic acid and TGFβ1: implications for lung development and patterning. *Dev Dyn* 2000;**217**: 62–74.

100 Clark LD, Clark RK, Heber-Katz E. A new murine model for mammalian wound repair and regeneration. *Clin Immunol Immunopathol* 1998;**88**:35–45.

101 Leferovich JM, Bedelbaeva K, Samulewicz S *et al*. Heart regeneration in adult MRL mice. *Proc Natl Acad Sci USA* 2001;**98**:9830–5.

102 McBrearty BA, Clark LD, Zhang XM, Blankenhorn EP, Heber-Katz E. Genetic analysis of a mammalian wound-healing trait. *Proc Natl Acad Sci USA* 1998;**95**:11792–7.

103 Gilbert KA, Rannels DE. From limbs to lungs: a new perspective on compensatory lung growth. *News Physiol Sci* 1999;**14**:260–7.

104 Bruce MC, Honaker CE. Transcriptional regulation of tropoelastin expression in rat lung fibroblasts: changes with age and hyperoxia. *Am J Physiol* 1998;**274**:L940–50.

105 Federspiel SJ, DiMari SJ, Guerry-Force ML, Haralson MA. Extracellular matrix biosynthesis by cultured fetal rat lung epithelial cells. II. Effects of acute exposure to epidermal growth factor and retinoic acid on collagen biosynthesis. *Lab Invest* 1990;**63**:455–66.

106 Vasios G, Mader S, Gold JD *et al*. The late retinoic acid induction of laminin B1 gene transcription involves RAR binding to the responsive element. *EMBO J* 1991;**10**:1149–58.

107 Pan L, Eckhoff C, Brinckerhoff CE. Suppression of collagenase gene expression by all-*trans* and 9-*cis* retinoic acid is ligand dependent and requires both RARs and RXRs. *J Cell Biochem* 1995;**57**:575–89.

108 Zhu YK, Liu X, Ertl RF *et al*. Retinoic acid attenuates cytokine-driven fibroblast degradation of extracellular matrix in three-dimensional culture. *Am J Respir Cell Mol Biol* 2001; **25**:620–7.

109 Yamamoto H, Itoh F, Hinoda Y, Imai K. Suppression of matrilysin inhibits colon cancer cell invasion *in vitro*. *Int J Cancer* 1995;**61**:218–22.

110 Tsang KJ, Crowe DL. Retinoic acid and extracellular matrix inhibition of matrix metalloproteinase 9 expression is mediated by the mitogen activated protein kinase pathway. *Int J Oncol* 2001;**18**:369–74.

111 Frankenberger M, Hauck RW, Frankenberger B *et al*. All *trans*-retinoic acid selectively down-regulates matrix metalloproteinase-9 (MMP-9) and up-regulates tissue inhibitor of metalloproteinase-1 (TIMP-1) in human bronchoalveolar lavage cells. *Mol Med* 2001;**7**:263–70.

112 Anglard P, Melot T, Guerin E, Thomas G, Basset P. Structure and promoter characterization of the human stromelysin-3 gene. *J Biol Chem* 1995;**270**:20337–44.

113 Anderson IC, Sugarbaker DJ, Ganju RK *et al*. Stromelysin-3 is overexpressed by stromal elements in primary non-small cell lung cancers and regulated by retinoic acid in pulmonary fibroblasts. *Cancer Res* 1995;**55**:4120–6.

114 Bigg HF, McLeod R, Waters JG, Cawston TE, Clark IM. Mechanisms of induction of human tissue inhibitor of metalloproteinases-1 (TIMP-1) gene expression by all-*trans* retinoic acid in combination with basic fibroblast growth factor. *Eur J Biochem* 2000;**267**:4150–6.

115 Lu Y, Amos B, Cruise E, Lotan D, Lotan R. A parallel association between differentiation and induction of galectin-1, and inhibition of galectin-3 by retinoic acid in mouse embryonal carcinoma F9 cells. *Biol Chem* 1998;**379**:1323–31.

116 Antonyak MA, McNeill CJ, Wakshlag JJ, Boehm JE, Cerione RA. Activation of the Ras-ERK pathway inhibits retinoic acid-induced stimulation of tissue transglutaminase expression in NIH3T3 cells. *J Biol Chem* 2003;**278**:15859–66.

117 Mahoney SA, Wilkinson M, Smith S, Haynes LW. Stabilization of neurites in cerebellar granule cells by transglutaminase activity: identification of midkine and galectin-3 as substrates. *Neuroscience* 2000;**101**:141–55.

118 Matsumoto K, Gaetano C, Daughaday WH, Thiele CJ. Retinoic acid regulates insulin-like growth factor II expression in a neuroblastoma cell line. *Endocrinology* 1992;**130**:3669–76.

119 Shang Y, Baumrucker CR, Green MH. Signal relay by retinoic acid receptors alpha and beta in the retinoic acid-induced expression of insulin-like growth factor-binding protein-3 in breast cancer cells. *J Biol Chem* 1999;**274**:18005–10.

120 Sueoka N, Lee HY, Walsh GL *et al.* Insulin-like growth factor binding protein-6 inhibits the growth of human bronchial epithelial cells and increases in abundance with all-*trans*-retinoic acid treatment. *Am J Respir Cell Mol Biol* 2000;**23**:297–303.

121 Dailly YP, Zhou Y, Linkhart TA, Baylink DJ, Strong DD. Structure and characterization of the human insulin-like growth factor binding protein (IGFBP)-6 promoter: identification of a functional retinoid response element. *Biochim Biophys Acta* 2001;**1518**:145–51.

122 Moreno B, Rodriguez-Manzaneque JC, Perez-Castillo A, Santos A. Thyroid hormone controls the expression of insulin-like growth factor I receptor gene at different levels in lung and heart of developing and adult rats. *Endocrinology* 1997;**138**:1194–203.

123 Schuger L, Varani J, Mitra R Jr, Gilbride K. Retinoic acid stimulates mouse lung development by a mechanism involving epithelial–mesenchymal interaction and regulation of epidermal growth factor receptors. *Dev Biol* 1993;**159**:462–73.

124 Oberg KC, Carpenter G. Dexamethasone and retinoic acid regulate the expression of epidermal growth factor receptor mRNA by distinct mechanisms. *J Cell Physiol* 1991;**149**:244–51.

125 Brondani V, Klimkait T, Egly JM, Hamy F. Promoter of FGF8 reveals a unique regulation by unliganded RARα. *J Mol Biol* 2002;**319**:715–28.

126 Aigner A, Malerczyk C, Houghtling R, Wellstein A. Tissue distribution and retinoid-mediated downregulation of an FGF-binding protein (FGF-BP) in the rat. *Growth Factors* 2000;**18**:51–62.

127 Yuan S, Hannam V, Belcastro R *et al.* A role for platelet-derived growth factor-BB in rat postpneumonectomy compensatory lung growth. *Pediatr Res* 2002;**52**:25–33.

128 Mercola M, Wang CY, Kelly J *et al.* Selective expression of PDGF A and its receptor during early mouse embryogenesis. *Dev Biol* 1990;**138**:114–22.

129 Danielpour D, Kim KY, Winokur TS, Sporn MB. Differential regulation of the expression of transforming growth factor-β s 1 and 2 by retinoic acid, epidermal growth factor, and dexamethasone in NRK-49F and A549 cells. *J Cell Physiol* 1991;**148**:235–44.

130 Glick AB, McCune BK, Abdulkarem N *et al.* Complex regulation of TGF β expression by retinoic acid in the vitamin A-deficient rat. *Development* 1991;**111**:1081–6.

131 Yoshizawa M, Miyazaki H, Kojima S. Retinoids potentiate transforming growth factor-β activity in bovine endothelial cells through up-regulating the expression of transforming growth factor-β receptors. *J Cell Physiol* 1998;**176**:565–73.

132 Wion D, Houlgatte R, Barbot N *et al.* Retinoic acid increases the expression of NGF gene in mouse L cells. *Biochem Biophys Res Commun* 1987;**149**:510–4.

133 Haskell BE, Stach RW, Werrbach-Perez K, Perez-Polo JR. Effect of retinoic acid on nerve growth factor receptors. *Cell Tissue Res* 1987;**247**:67–73.

134 Metsis M, Timmusk T, Allikmets R, Saarma M, Persson H. Regulatory elements and transcriptional regulation by testosterone and retinoic acid of the rat nerve growth factor receptor promoter. *Gene* 1992;**121**:247–54.

135 Pedraza C, Matsubara S, Muramatsu T. A retinoic acid-responsive element in human midkine gene. *J Biochem (Tokyo)* 1995;**117**:845–9.

136 Matsuura O, Kadomatsu K, Takei Y *et al.* Midkine expression is associated with postnatal development of the lungs. *Cell Struct Funct* 2002;**27**:109–15.

137 Ju BG, Kim WS. Upregulation of cathepsin D expression in the dedifferentiating salamander limb regenerates and enhancement of its expression by retinoic acid. *Wound Repair Regen* 1998;**6**:349–57.

138 So EN, Crowe DL. Characterization of a retinoic acid responsive element in the human ets-1 promoter. *IUBMB Life* 2000;**50**:365–70.

139 Jacob A, Budhiraja S, Reichel RR. The HNF-3α transcription factor is a primary target for retinoic acid action. *Exp Cell Res* 1999;**250**:1–9.

140 de The H, Vivanco-Ruiz MM, Tiollais P, Stunnenberg H, Dejean A. Identification of a retinoic acid responsive element in the retinoic acid receptor beta gene. *Nature* 1990;**343**:177–80.

141 Bahouth SW, Beauchamp MJ, Park EA. Identification of a retinoic acid response domain involved in the activation of the β1-adrenergic receptor gene by retinoic acid in F9 teratocarcinoma cells. *Biochem Pharmacol* 1998;**55**:215–25.

142 Frasch M, Chen X, Lufkin T. Evolutionary-conserved enhancers direct region-specific expression of the murine Hoxa-1 and Hoxa-2 loci in both mice and *Drosophila*. *Development* 1995;**121**:957–74.

143 Cardoso WV, Mitsialis SA, Brody JS, Williams MC. Retinoic acid alters the expression of pattern-related genes in the developing rat lung. *Dev Dyn* 1996;**207**:47–59.

144 Kim MH, Shin JS, Park S *et al.* Retinoic acid response element in HOXA-7 regulatory region affects the rate, not the formation of anterior boundary expression. *Int J Dev Biol* 2002;**46**:325–8.

145 Huang D, Chen SW, Gudas LJ. Analysis of two distinct retinoic acid response elements in the homeobox gene Hoxb1 in transgenic mice. *Dev Dyn* 2002;**223**:353–70.

146 Oosterveen T, Niederreither K, Dolle P *et al.* Retinoids regulate the anterior expression boundaries of 5' Hoxb genes in posterior hindbrain. *EMBO J* 2003;**22**:262–9.

147 Nolte C, Amores A, Nagy KE, Postlethwait J, Featherstone M. The role of a retinoic acid response element in establishing the anterior neural expression border of Hoxd4 transgenes. *Mech Dev* 2003;**120**:325–35.

148 Yan C, Ghaffari M, Whitsett JA *et al.* Retinoic acid-receptor activation of SP-B gene transcription in respiratory epithelial cells. *Am J Physiol* 1998;**275**:L239–46.

149 Smith WC, Nakshatri H, Leroy P, Rees J, Chambon P. A retinoic acid response element is present in the mouse cellular retinol binding protein I (mCRBPI) promoter. *EMBO J* 1991;**10**:2223–30.

150 Whitney D, Massaro GD, Massaro D, Clerch LB. Gene expression of cellular retinoid-binding proteins: modulation

by retinoic acid and dexamethasone in postnatal rat lung. *Pediatr Res* 1999;**45**:2–7.

151 Mangelsdorf DJ, Umesono K, Kliewer SA *et al*. A direct repeat in the cellular retinol-binding protein type II gene confers differential regulation by RXR and RAR. *Cell* 1991; **66**:555–61.

152 Loudig O, Babichuk C, White J *et al*. Cytochrome P450RAI (CYP26) promoter: a distinct composite retinoic acid response element underlies the complex regulation of retinoic acid metabolism. *Mol Endocrinol* 2000;**14**:1483–97.

153 Warburton D, Schwarz M, Tefft D *et al*. The molecular basis of lung morphogenesis. *Mech Dev* 2000;**92**:55–81.

154 Quondamatteo F, Reinhardt DP, Charbonneau NL *et al*. Fibrillin-1 and fibrillin-2 in human embryonic and early fetal development. *Matrix Biol* 2002;**21**:637–46.

155 McAnulty RJ, Guerreiro D, Cambrey AD, Laurent GJ. Growth factor activity in the lung during compensatory growth after pneumonectomy: evidence of a role for IGF-1. *Eur Respir J* 1992;**5**:739–47.

156 Nobuhara KK, DiFiore JW, Ibla JC *et al*. Insulin-like growth factor-I gene expression in three models of accelerated lung growth. *J Pediatr Surg* 1998;**33**:1057–60.

157 Sakamaki Y, Matsumoto K, Mizuno S *et al*. Hepatocyte growth factor stimulates proliferation of respiratory epithelial cells during postpneumonectomy compensatory lung growth in mice. *Am J Respir Cell Mol Biol* 2002;**26**:525–33.

158 Foster DJ, Yan X, Bellotto DJ *et al*. Expression of epidermal growth factor and surfactant proteins during postnatal and compensatory lung growth. *Am J Physiol Lung Cell Mol Physiol* 2002;**283**:L981–90.

159 Kaza AK, Kron IL, Leuwerke SM, Tribble CG, Laubach VE. Keratinocyte growth factor enhances post-pneumonectomy lung growth by alveolar proliferation. *Circulation* 2002;**106** (Suppl 1):I120–4.

160 Greenberg JM, Thompson FY, Brooks SK *et al*. Mesenchymal expression of vascular endothelial growth factors D and A defines vascular patterning in developing lung. *Dev Dyn* 2002;**224**:144–53.

161 Massaro D, Teich N, Massaro GD. Postnatal development of pulmonary alveoli: modulation in rats by thyroid hormones. *Am J Physiol* 1986;**250**:R51–5.

162 Brody JS, Kagan H, Manalo A. Lung lysyl oxidase activity: relation to lung growth. *Am Rev Respir Dis* 1979;**120**: 1289–95.

163 Landesberg LJ, Ramalingam R, Lee K, Rosengart TK, Crystal RG. Upregulation of transcription factors in lung in the early phase of postpneumonectomy lung growth. *Am J Physiol Lung Cell Mol Physiol* 2001;**281**:L1138–49.

164 Healy AM, Morgenthau L, Zhu X, Farber HW, Cardoso WV. VEGF is deposited in the subepithelial matrix at the leading edge of branching airways and stimulates neovascularization in the murine embryonic lung. *Dev Dyn* 2000;**219**:341–52.

165 Pierce RA, Tudhope S, Moore C *et al*. Transcriptome analysis of alveolar development. *Am J Respir Crit Care Med* 2003; **167**:A381.

166 Sun SY. Recent developments of retinoids as therapeutic agents. *Expert Opin Ther Patents* 2002;**12**:529–42.

167 Mao JT, Goldin JG, Dermand J *et al*. A pilot study of all-*trans*-retinoic acid for the treatment of human emphysema. *Am J Respir Crit Care Med* 2002;**165**:718–23.

168 Feasibiility of Retinoic Acid Treatment in Emphysema (FORTE). http://clinicaltrials.gov/show/NCT00000621

169 The FORTE Study. http://www.lung.med.ucla.edu/ clinicalresearch/FORTE/patientinfo.html

170 Roche R&D Day. 2002. http://www.rocheusa.com/ newsroom/current/2002/pr2002043002.html

171 Roche R&D Day 2004. http://www.rocheusa.com/ newsroom/current/2004/pr2004050502.html

CHAPTER 70
Chemokines in COPD

Peter J. Barnes

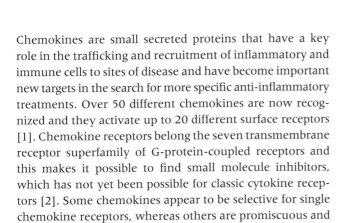

Chemokines are small secreted proteins that have a key role in the trafficking and recruitment of inflammatory and immune cells to sites of disease and have become important new targets in the search for more specific anti-inflammatory treatments. Over 50 different chemokines are now recognized and they activate up to 20 different surface receptors [1]. Chemokine receptors belong the seven transmembrane receptor superfamily of G-protein-coupled receptors and this makes it possible to find small molecule inhibitors, which has not yet been possible for classic cytokine receptors [2]. Some chemokines appear to be selective for single chemokine receptors, whereas others are promiscuous and mediate the effects of several related chemokines.

Four different families of chemokines are now differentiated, based on differences in the position of critical cysteine residues: CC, CXC, C and CX_3C chemokines are recognized. Each chemokine molecule binds to a single or several receptors expressed on target inflammatory cells, resulting in the activation of signal transduction pathways that then result in chemotaxis or other cellular activities that include proliferation, differentiation and survival. Chemokines appear to act in sequence in determining the final inflammatory response and so inhibitors may be more or less effective depending on the kinetics of the response [3].

Chemokines have a critical role in orchestrating inflammatory and immune responses by regulating the trafficking of inflammatory and immune cells to target organs [4]. Several chemokines are involved in the recruitment of inflammatory cells in COPD [5]. There is considerable interest in identifying the critical chemokines as small molecule chemokine receptor inhibitors are now in development for COPD [6,7].

The inflammation in COPD is characterized by a marked increase in numbers of macrophages, which are derived from blood monocytes, neutrophils and T lymphocytes with a predominance of cytotoxic (CD8+) cells over helper (CD4+) cells [8,9]. All of these cells are derived from the circulation and it is therefore likely that chemokines have an import-

ant role in the migration of these cells into small airways and the lung parenchyma where the inflammation in COPD predominates.

CXC chemokines

Interleukin 8

The CXC chemokine interleukin 8 (IL-8) (CXCL8) is a potent chemoattractant of neutrophils and it is not surprising that it has been implicated in COPD as there is a marked increase in neutrophils in airway secretions. IL-8 levels are markedly increased in induced sputum of patients with COPD and correlate with the increased proportion of neutrophils [10,11]. The concentrations of IL-8 are even more elevated in patients with emphysema resulting from α_1-antitrypsin deficiency [12] and during exacerbations [13]. Anti-IL-8 antibodies have an inhibitory effect on the chemotactic response to COPD sputum, indicating that IL-8 contributes to neutrophil chemotaxis into the airways [14,15]. The concentrations of IL-8 in induced sputum are further increased during acute exacerbations, which presumably contributes to the increased numbers of neutrophils and the increased purulence of the sputum [13,16,17]. There is a correlation between IL-8 concentrations and the bacterial colony count in sputum, indicating that bacterial infection may induce neutrophilic inflammation, at least in part, via induction of IL-8 release in the airways [18,19]. IL-8 is also increased in bronchoalveolar lavage (BAL) fluid of patients with COPD and correlates with numbers of neutrophils [20,21]. The concentrations of IL-8 are significantly higher in smokers with emphysema than in matched smokers without airflow limitation, whereas the concentrations of other CXC chemokines in BAL do not appear to discriminate between these groups [22].

The cellular source of IL-8 in COPD is not completely certain. Airway epithelial cells secrete IL-8 in response to

859

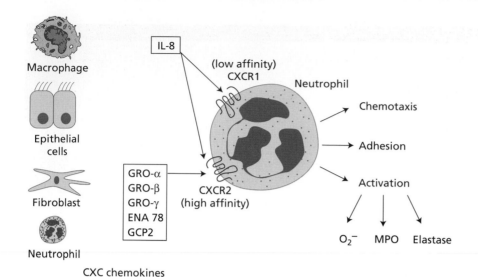

Figure 70.1 CXC chemokine receptors on neutrophils. Interleukin 8 (IL-8) binds with low affinity to CXCR1, resulting in adhesion and activation and to CXCR2 with high affinity resulting in chemotaxis. CXCR2 is also activated by other CXC chemokines, including growth-related oncogene α (GRO-α), β and γ, epithelial cell-derived neutrophil-activating peptide of 78 kD (ENA-78) and granulocyte chemotactic protein-2 (GCP-2). MPO, myeloperoxidase.

several stimuli, including tumour necrosis factor-α (TNF-α) and cigarette smoke extract [23–25]. IL-8 protein and mRNA are increased in bronchiolar epithelial cells of patients with COPD [26] and there is increased basal release of IL-8 from airway epithelial cells of patients with COPD [27,28]. Alveolar macrophages also secrete IL-8 in response to the same stimuli and cells derived from patients with COPD secrete more IL-8 than those from normal smokers, who in turn secrete more macrophages than normal non-smokers [29]. Neutrophils also release IL-8 and attract more neutrophils, so that a self-perpetuating inflammatory state may be established [30]. The secretion of IL-8 is regulated transcriptionally by several transcription factors, amongst which nuclear factor-κB (NF-κB) is predominant. NF-κB is activated in alveolar macrophages of patients with COPD and is further activated during exacerbations [31,32].

Neutralization of IL-8 with a blocking antibody significantly reduces the neutrophil chemotactic activity of sputum from patients with COPD [15,17]. However, the reduction in neutrophil chemotactic activity is only of the order of approximately 30%, indicating that other neutrophil chemotactic factors are also involved and that blocking IL-8 alone may be insufficient as a therapeutic strategy to reduce neutrophil inflammation in the respiratory tract.

IL-8 acts via two receptors: CXCR1, which is a low affinity receptor that is specific for IL-8; and CXCR2, which has high affinity and is shared by other CXC chemokines (Fig. 70.1). It is likely that CXCR2 mediates the chemotactic response of neutrophils and monocytes to IL-8, whereas CXCR1 may mediate the effects of IL-8 on release of mediators and proteases. There is a marked up-regulation of CXCR2 in airway epithelial cells during acute exacerbations of COPD and this is correlated with the increased numbers of neutrophils in the airway [33].

Other CXC chemokines

GRO-α

Growth-related oncogene-α (GRO-α, CXCL1) is another CXC chemokine that is likely to be involved in COPD. GRO-α activates neutrophils, monocytes, basophils and T lymphocytes via CXCR2 [34]. The concentrations of GRO-α is markedly elevated in induce sputum and BAL of patients with COPD compared with normal smokers and non-smokers (Fig. 70.2) [35]. GRO-α selectively activates

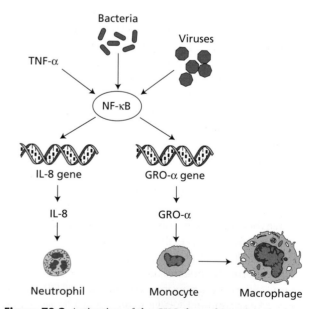

Figure 70.2 Activation of the CXC chemokines interleukin 8 (IL-8) and growth-related oncogene α (GRO-α) via nuclear factor-κB (NF-κB) after stimulating with tumour necrosis factor α (TNF-α), bacteria and viruses. This results in chemotaxis of neutrophils and monocytes that differentiate into alveolar macrophages.

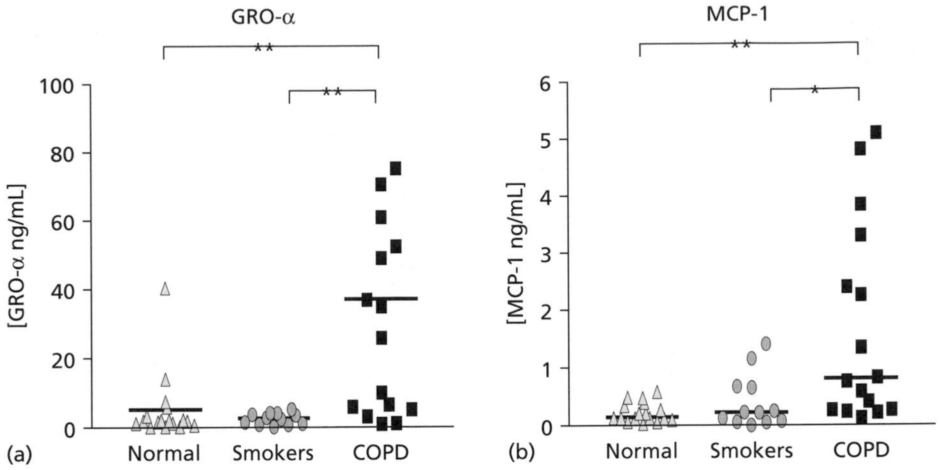

Figure 70.3 Elevated concentrations of: (a) growth-related oncogene α (GRO-α); and (b) monocyte chemotactic protein-1 (MCP-1) in induced sputum of patients with COPD. (From Traves *et al.* [35] with permission.)

CXCR2 and is chemotactic for neutrophils and monocytes. There is an increase in the monocytes' chemotactic response to GRO-α in COPD patients and this may be related to increased turnover of CXCR2 on monocytes of COPD patients [36]. It is possible that the increased chemotactic response of monocytes to GRO-α is one of the mechanisms leading to increased numbers of alveolar macrophages in the lungs of patients with COPD (Fig. 70.3) [37] and could be one of mechanisms of susceptibility to cigarette smoking.

ENA-78

Epithelial cell-derived neutrophil-activating peptide-78 (ENA-78, CXCL5) is derived predominantly from epithelial cells and also activates CXCR2, although monocytes do not appear to show an increased chemotactic response to this chemokine as they do to GRO-α [36]. ENA-78 is increased in BAL fluid of COPD patients compared with normal subjects, but there is no difference between patients with emphysema and normal smokers [22]. A marked increase in expression of ENA-78 has been reported in epithelial cells during exacerbations of COPD [33].

CXCR2 antagonists

The involvement of several CXC chemokines in COPD and the involvement of CXCR2 in chemotactic responses of neutrophils and monocytes indicates that CXCR2 antagonists may have therapeutic potential in inhibiting recruitment of monocytes and neutrophils. Potent small molecule inhibitors of CXCR2, such as SB 225002, have now been developed that block the chemotactic response of neutrophils to IL-8 and GRO-α [38,39]. This antagonist has a significant inhibitory effect on the chemotactic response to COPD sputum. Concentrations of GRO-α are also elevated in induced sputum of patients with COPD and this mediator has a chemotactic effect on neutrophils and monocytes [35]. CXCR2 antagonists may therefore also reduce monocyte chemotaxis and the accumulation of macrophages in COPD patients.

CXCR3

The mechanisms by which CD8[+], and to a lesser extent CD4[+] cells, accumulate in the airways and lungs of patients with COPD is not yet understood. However, homing of T cells to the lung must depend upon some initial activation then adhesion and selective chemotaxis. T cells in peripheral airways of COPD patients show increased expression of CXCR3, a receptor activated by γ-interferon inducible protein of 10 kDa (IP-10, CXCL10), monokine induced by γ-interferon (Mig, CXCL9) and interferon-inducible T cell-α chemoattractant (I-TAC, CXCL11). All three chemokines activate CXCR3, although I-TAC has the highest affinity [40]. CXCR3 is expressed on T lymphocytes, particularly of the CD8[+] subtype. There is increased expression of IP-10 by bronchiolar epithelial cells and this could therefore contribute to the accumulation of CD8[+] cells, which preferentially express CXCR3 [41]. It is of interest that γ-interferon (IFN-γ) stimulates dendritic cells to produce IP-10 and Mig which then enhances their ability to attract CD8[+] cells [42]. Alveolar macrophages also have the capacity to produce IP-10 and Mig and result in attraction of CD8[+] T cells [43]. Because CD8[+] Tc1 cells produce IFN-γ this provides a potential feed-forward amplification loop. The role of CD8[+] T cells in COPD is not yet certain, but as they have the capacity to produce perforins and granzyme B they might induce apoptosis in alveolar epithelial and endothelial cells, thereby contributing to emphysema [44,45]. This suggests that blocking CXCR3 might be beneficial in the treatment of COPD (Fig. 70.4).

CC chemokines

CCR2

Monocyte chemotactic protein-1 (MCP-1, CCL2) is a CC chemokine that activates CCR2 on monocytes and T

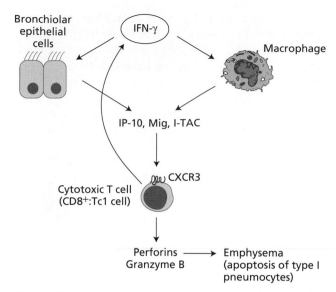

Figure 70.4 Chemotaxis of cytotoxic (CD8+) T lymphocytes via activation of CXCR3 by the CXC chemokines γ-interferon inducible protein of 10 kDa (IP-10), monokine induced by γ-interferon (Mig) and interferon-inducible T-cell-α chemoattractant (I-TAC). CD8+ cells may release perforins and granzyme B which may induce apoptosis in alveolar cells and release γ-interferon (IFN-γ), which in turn activates the release of these chemokines.

lymphocytes. CCR2 may have a role in COPD, as MCP-1 levels are increased in sputum, BAL fluid and lungs of patients with COPD (see Fig. 70.3) and MCP-1 is expressed in alveolar macrophages and epithelial cells [26,35,46]. MCP-1 is a potent chemoattractant of monocytes and may therefore be involved in the recruitment of macrophages in COPD. Indeed, the chemoattractant effect of induced sputum from patients with COPD is abrogated by an antibody to CCR2. Because macrophages appear to have a critical role in COPD as a source of elastases and neutrophil chemo-attractants, blocking CCR2 may be a therapeutic strategy in COPD and small molecule inhibitors are in development.

CCR3

CCR3 are predominantly expressed on eosinophils and therefore have an important role in asthma. In COPD there is a small increase in eosinophils and eosinophil basic pro-teins in induced sputum and BAL fluid and an increase in eosinophils has been described in exacerbations of chronic bronchitis [10,47,48]. This suggests that eosinophil chemo-attractants may play some part. RANTES (released by activated normal T cells expressed and secreted, CCL5) activates CCR3 and is strongly expressed in airway epithe-lial cells of patients with chronic bronchitis exacerbations [49]. Eotaxin (CCL*) and CCR3 show increased expression

in the bronchi of patients with exacerbations of chronic bronchitis and are correlated with increased numbers of eosinophils [50].

Other CC chemokine receptors

CCR4 and CCR8 are selectively expressed on Th2 cells and are activated by the chemokines macrophage-derived chemokine (MDC, CCL22) and thymus and activation dependent chemokine (TARC, CCL17) [51]. However, Th2 cells are not prominent in COPD so it is unlikely that these receptors are relevant.

CCR7 has a role in the migration of dendritic cells to regional lymph nodes and therefore blocking this receptor might suppress antigen presentation [52]. There is an in-crease in the number of dendritic cells in rat lungs exposed to cigarette smoke [53,54] and in the airways and alveolar walls of smokers [55,56], but the chemotactic factors involved have not yet been determined. MIP-3α (CCL20), which acts on CCR6 that is expressed by immature dendritic cells, is potent chemoattractant of dendritic cells and is expressed by airway epithelial cells in response to IFN-γ [57].

CX₃C chemokines

The unique CX_3C chemokine fractalkine, which is tethered to cell surfaces, shows increased expression in human air-way epithelial cells after stimulation with IFN-γ and may be involved in recruitment and adhesion of monocytes, T lym-phocytes and natural killer cells to epithelial surfaces [58]. Whether fractalkine or its receptor CX_3CR1 are increased in COPD is not yet known.

Therapeutic implications

Chemokine receptor antagonists

Many new approaches to the treatment of inflammation ion COPD are now under consideration [7]. Chemokine receptor antagonists are an attractive approach to the ther-apy of COPD because chemokines have a critical role in the recruitment of the key inflammatory cells, including macrophages (and monocytes), neutrophils and T lympho-cytes. However, there is considerable redundancy in the system, so that blocking a specific chemokine receptor may not inhibit the chemotactic response as other chemokine receptors and other classes of chemotactic mediator also aid in recruitment. However, in COPD, a critical feature of the disease is an amplification of the inflammatory response seen in normal smokers, so that the aim of therapy is not to abolish the inflammatory cells but to reduce them to the numbers seen in normal smokers. No chemokine receptor antagonists have so far been studied in COPD patients and it is only when clinical trials are conducted that the size of the clinical effect can be determined. Studies involving neutralization of IL-8 in sputum indicate that this chemokine accounts for only approximately 30% of the neutrophil chemotactic activity of sputum in COPD patients [15], and that leukotriene B_4 (LTB$_4$) accounts for a similar proportion, so that when these two chemotactic agents are blocked there is still approximately 50% of the chemotactic activity remaining. Whether this is sufficient to have an impact on clinical parameters such as exacerbation frequency or disease progression will only be determined by expensive clinical trials in relatively large numbers of patients.

Chemokine receptors are an attractive therapeutic target as small molecule inhibitors can be identified by screening and in the future by molecular design as each G-protein coupled receptor has a defined binding cleft for ligand interaction [2]. Several small molecule inhibitors have now been developed but so far none has reached the clinic. Another approach is the use of monoclonal antibodies directed at either the chemokine receptor (preferably) or the chemokine. An antibody to IL-8 has been developed [59] and has recently been in clinical trials in COPD, but the results have not yet been reported.

Chemokine synthesis inhibitors

Another approach to reduce chemotaxis is to inhibit the production of chemokines, although this approach is not specific. Corticosteroids inhibit the transcription of many chemokines through inhibiting the transcription factor NF-κB. However, there appears to be a resistance to the anti-inflammatory effects of corticosteroids in patients with COPD, so that even high doses of inhaled or oral corticosteroids do not reduce the elevated concentrations of IL-8 in sputum [60,61]. Alveolar macrophages from patients with COPD are also steroid resistant and even high concentrations of corticosteroids do not inhibit the baseline or cigarette smoke-stimulated release of IL-8 [29]. The mechanism for this molecular resistance to corticosteroids is not yet certain, but there is a decrease in the expression of histone deacetylase-2, an enzyme that is critical for switching off inflammatory genes by corticosteroids [62–65].

Theophylline is a bronchodilator through inhibition of phosphodiesterases (PDE) in airway smooth muscle, but at lower concentrations acts as an anti-inflammatory agent through a novel molecular mechanism that involves activation of histone deacetylases [66]. This results in reduced expression of IL-8 in macrophages and epithelial cells. This also leads to increased responsiveness to corticosteroids,

raising the possibility that theophylline may reduce the apparent steroid resistance seen in COPD [67]. Theophylline in low concentrations reduces both neutrophil numbers and IL-8 concentrations in patients with COPD [68], indicating that unlike corticosteroids it has a useful anti-inflammatory action.

Selective inhibitors of PDE4 are now in development as anti-inflammatory therapy for COPD and are effective in inhibiting the synthesis of chemokines such as IL-8 in airway cells. PDE4 inhibitors markedly suppress IL-8 release from human neutrophils [69]. Unexpectedly, IL-8 release from epithelial cells and sputum cells from patients with COPD was not inhibited by a PDE4 inhibitor cilomilast that was effective in reducing TNF-α release [28], indicating that this therapy may not be effective in reducing chemokine expression. Indeed, a recent clinical trial of cilomilast in COPD showed no reduction in IL-8 expression in bronchial epithelial cells [70].

The p38 MAP kinase pathway is involved in expression of many chemokines, including IL-8 [71,72]. Non-peptide inhibitors of p38 MAP kinase, such as SB 203580, SB 239063 and RWJ 67657, have now been developed and these drugs have a broad range of anti-inflammatory effects [73], but they have not been tested in clinical trials in COPD. P38 MAP kinase inhibitors reduce IL-8 expression by epithelial cells by a post-transcriptional mechanism as they do not reduce its gene expression [74].

NF-κB regulates the expression of IL-8 and other chemokines. NF-κB is activated in macrophages and epithelial cells of COPD patients, particularly during exacerbations [31,32]. There are several possible approaches to inhibition of NF-κB, including gene transfer of the inhibitor of NF-κB (IκB), a search for inhibitors of IκB kinases (IKK), NF-κB-inducing kinase (NIK) and IκB ubiquitin ligase, which regulate the activity of NF-κB, and the development of drugs that inhibit the degradation of IκB [75]. The most promising approach may be the inhibition of IKK-2 by small molecule inhibitors which are now in development [76]. A small molecule IKK-2 inhibitor suppresses the release of IL-8 from alveolar macrophages [77] and might be effective in COPD when alveolar macrophages appear to be resistant to the anti-inflammatory actions of corticosteroids [29].

Resveratrol is a phenolic component of red wine that has anti-inflammatory and antioxidant properties. It has a marked inhibitory effect on IL-8 release from alveolar macrophages from COPD patients who show little or no response to corticosteroids [78]. The molecular mechanism for this action is currently unknown, but identification of the cellular target for resveratrol may lead to the development of a novel class of anti-inflammatory compounds. Resveratrol itself has a very low oral bioavailability so related drugs will need to be developed.

References

1 Rossi D, Zlotnik A. The biology of chemokines and their receptors. *Annu Rev Immunol* 2000;**18**:217–42.

2 Proudfoot AE. Chemokine receptors: multifaceted therapeutic targets. *Nat Rev Immunol* 2002;**2**:106–15.

3 Gutierrez-Ramos JC, Lloyd C, Kapsenberg ML, Gonzalo JA, Coyle AJ. Non-redundant functional groups of chemokines operate in a coordinate manner during the inflammatory response in the lung. *Immunol Rev* 2000;**177**:31–42.

4 Olson TS, Ley K. Chemokines and chemokine receptors in leukocyte trafficking. *Am J Physiol Regul Integr Comp Physiol* 2002;**283**:R7–28.

5 Lukacs NW. Role of chemokines in the pathogenesis of asthma. *Nat Rev Immunol* 2001;**1**:108–16.

6 Panina-Bordignon P, D'Ambrosio D. Chemokines and their receptors in asthma and chronic obstructive pulmonary disease. *Curr Opin Pulm Med* 2003;**9**:104–10.

7 Barnes PJ. New treatments for COPD. *Nat Rev Drug Discov* 2002;**1**:437–45.

8 Barnes PJ. New concepts in COPD. *Ann Rev Med* 2003;**54**:113–29.

9 Barnes PJ, Shapiro SD, Pauwels RA. COPD: molecular and cellular mechanisms. *Eur Respir J* 2003;**22**:672–88.

10 Keatings VM, Collins PD, Scott DM, Barnes PJ. Differences in interleukin-8 and tumor necrosis factor-α in induced sputum from patients with chronic obstructive pulmonary disease or asthma. *Am J Respir Crit Care Med* 1996;**153**:530–4.

11 Yamamoto C, Yoneda T, Yoshikawa M *et al.* Airway inflammation in COPD assessed by sputum levels of interleukin-8. *Chest* 1997;**112**:505–10.

12 Woolhouse IS, Bayley DL, Stockley RA. Sputum chemotactic activity in chronic obstructive pulmonary disease: effect of α_1-antitrypsin deficiency and the role of leukotriene B_4 and interleukin 8. *Thorax* 2002;**57**:709–14.

13 Aaron SD, Angel JB, Lunau M *et al.* Granulocyte inflammatory markers and airway infection during acute exacerbation of chronic obstructive pulmonary disease. *Am J Respir Crit Care Med* 2001;**163**:349–55.

14 Hill AT, Bayley D, Stockley RA. The interrelationship of sputum inflammatory markers in patients with chronic bronchitis. *Am J Respir Crit Care Med* 1999;**160**:893–8.

15 Beeh KM, Kornmann O, Buhl R *et al.* Neutrophil chemotactic activity of sputum from patients with COPD: role of interleukin 8 and leukotriene B_4. *Chest* 2003;**123**:1240–7.

16 Gompertz S, O'Brien C, Bayley DL, Hill SL, Stockley RA. Changes in bronchial inflammation during acute exacerbations of chronic bronchitis. *Eur Respir J* 2001;**17**:1112–9.

17 Crooks SW, Bayley DL, Hill SL, Stockley RA. Bronchial inflammation in acute bacterial exacerbations of chronic bronchitis: the role of leukotriene B_4. *Eur Respir J* 2000;**15**:274–80.

18 Hill AT, Campbell EJ, Hill SL, Bayley DL, Stockley RA. Association between airway bacterial load and markers of airway inflammation in patients with stable chronic bronchitis. *Am J Med* 2000;**109**:288–95.

19 Patel IS, Seemungal TA, Wilks M *et al.* Relationship between bacterial colonisation and the frequency, character, and severity of COPD exacerbations. *Thorax* 2002;**57**:759–64.

20 Nocker RE, Schoonbrood DF, Van de Graaf EA *et al.* Interleukin-8 in airway inflammation in patients with asthma and chronic obstructive pulmonary disease. *Int Arch Allergy Immunol* 1996;**109**:183–91.

21 Soler N, Ewig S, Torres A *et al.* Airway inflammation and bronchial microbial patterns in patients with stable chronic obstructive pulmonary disease. *Eur Respir J* 1999;**14**:1015–22.

22 Tanino M, Betsuyaku T, Takeyabu K *et al.* Increased levels of interleukin-8 in BAL fluid from smokers susceptible to pulmonary emphysema. *Thorax* 2002;**57**:405–11.

23 Nakamura H, Yoshimura K, Jaffe HA, Crystal RG. Interleukin-8 gene expression in human bronchial epithelial cells. *J Biol Chem* 1991;**266**:19611–7.

24 Nakamura H, Yoshimura K, Jaffe HA, Crystal RG. Transcriptional regulation of interleukin-8 gene expression by tumor necrosis factor-α in bronchial epithelial cells. *Am Rev Respir Dis* 1991;**143**:A201.

25 Kwon OJ, Au BT, Collins PD *et al.* Tumor necrosis factor-induced interleukin 8 expression in cultured human epithelial cells. *Am J Physiol* 1994;**11**:L398–405.

26 de Boer WI, Sont JK, van Schadewijk A *et al.* Monocyte chemoattractant protein 1, interleukin 8, and chronic airways inflammation in COPD. *J Pathol* 2000;**190**:619–26.

27 Schulz C, Wolf K, Harth M *et al.* Expression and release of interleukin-8 by human bronchial epithelial cells from patients with chronic obstructive pulmonary disease, smokers, and never-smokers. *Respiration* 2003;**70**:254–61.

28 Profita M, Chiappara G, Mirabella F *et al.* Effect of cilomilast (Ariflo) on TNF-α, IL-8, and GM-CSF release by airway cells of patients with COPD. *Thorax* 2003;**58**:573–9.

29 Culpitt SV, Rogers DF, Shah P *et al.* Impaired inhibition by dexamethasone of cytokine release by alveolar macrophages from patients with chronic obstructive pulmonary disease. *Am J Respir Crit Care Med* 2003;**167**:24–31.

30 Bazzoni F, Cassatella MA, Rossi F *et al.* Phagocytosing neutrophils produce and release high amounts of the neutrophil-activating peptide 1/interleukin 8. *J Exp Med* 1991;**173**:771–4.

31 Di Stefano A, Caramori G, Capelli A *et al.* Increased expression of NF-κB in bronchial biopsies from smokers and patients with COPD. *Eur Respir J* 2002;**20**:556–63.

32 Caramori G, Romagnoli M, Casolari P *et al.* Nuclear localisation of p65 in sputum macrophages but not in sputum neutrophils during COPD exacerbations. *Thorax* 2003;**58**:348–51.

33 Qiu Y, Zhu J, Bandi V *et al.* Biopsy neutrophilia, chemokine and receptor gene expression in severe exacerbations of COPD. *Am J Respir Crit Care Med* 2003;**168**:968–75.

34 Geiser T, Dewald B, Ehrengruber MU, Clark-Lewis I, Baggiolini M. The interleukin-8-related chemotactic cytokines GROα, GROβ, and GROγ activate human neutrophil and basophil leukocytes. *J Biol Chem* 1993;**268**:15419–24.

35 Traves SL, Culpitt S, Russell REK, Barnes PJ, Donnelly LE. Elevated levels of the chemokines GRO-α and MCP-1 in sputum samples from COPD patients. *Thorax* 2002;**57**:590–5.

36 Traves SL, Smith SJ, Barnes PJ, Donnelly LE. Increased migration of monocytes from COPD patients towards GROα is not mediated by an increase in CXCR2 receptor expression. *Am J Respir Crit Care Med* 2003:A824.

37 Retamales I, Elliott WM, Meshi B *et al*. Amplification of inflammation in emphysema and its association with latent adenoviral infection. *Am J Respir Crit Care Med* 2001;**164**:469–73.

38 White JR, Lee JM, Young PR *et al*. Identification of a potent, selective non-peptide CXCR2 antagonist that inhibits interleukin-8-induced neutrophil migration. *J Biol Chem* 1998;**273**:10095–8.

39 Hay DWP, Sarau HM. Interleukin-8 receptor antagonists in pulmonary diseases. *Curr Opin Pharmacol* 2001;**1**:242–7.

40 Clark-Lewis I, Mattioli I, Gong JH, Loetscher P. Structure–function relationship between the human chemokine receptor CXCR3 and its ligands. *J Biol Chem* 2003;**278**:289–95.

41 Saetta M, Mariani M, Panina-Bordignon P *et al*. Increased expression of the chemokine receptor CXCR3 and its ligand CXCL10 in peripheral airways of smokers with chronic obstructive pulmonary disease. *Am J Respir Crit Care Med* 2002;**165**:1404–9.

42 Padovan E, Spagnoli GC, Ferrantini M, Heberer M. IFN-α2a induces IP-10/CXCL10 and MIG/CXCL9 production in monocyte-derived dendritic cells and enhances their capacity to attract and stimulate CD8$^+$ effector T cells. *J Leukoc Biol* 2002;**71**:669–76.

43 Agostini C, Facco M, Siviero M *et al*. CXC chemokines IP-10 and Mig expression and direct migration of pulmonary CD8$^+$/CXCR3$^+$ T cells in the lungs of patients with HIV infection and T-cell alveolitis. *Am J Respir Crit Care Med* 2000;**162**:1466–73.

44 Majo J, Ghezzo H, Cosio MG. Lymphocyte population and apoptosis in the lungs of smokers and their relation to emphysema. *Eur Respir J* 2001;**17**:946–53.

45 Cosio MG, Majo J, Cosio MG. Inflammation of the airways and lung parenchyma in COPD: role of T cells. *Chest* 2002;**121**:160S–5S.

46 Capelli A, Di Stefano A, Gnemmi I *et al*. Increased MCP-1 and MIP-1b in bronchoalveolar lavage fluid of chronic bronchitis. *Eur Respir J* 1999;**14**:160–5.

47 Pesci A, Balbi B, Majori M *et al*. Inflammatory cells and mediators in bronchial lavage of patients with chronic obstructive pulmonary disease. *Eur Respir J* 1998;**12**:380–6.

48 Saetta M, Distefano A, Maestrelli P *et al*. Airway eosinophilia in chronic bronchitis during exacerbations. *Am J Respir Crit Care Med* 1994;**150**:1646–52.

49 Zhu J, Qiu YS, Majumdar S *et al*. Exacerbations of bronchitis: bronchial eosinophilia and gene expression for interleukin-4, interleukin-5, and eosinophil chemoattractants. *Am J Respir Crit Care Med* 2001;**164**:109–16.

50 Bocchino V, Bertorelli G, Bertrand CP *et al*. Eotaxin and CCR3 are up-regulated in exacerbations of chronic bronchitis. *Allergy* 2002;**57**:17–22.

51 Lloyd CM, Delaney T, Nguyen T *et al*. CC chemokine receptor (CCR)3/eotaxin is followed by CCR4/monocyte-derived chemokine in mediating pulmonary T helper lymphocyte type 2 recruitment after serial antigen challenge *in vivo*. *J Exp Med* 2000;**191**:265–74.

52 Sallusto F, Lanzavecchia A. Understanding dendritic cell and T-lymphocyte traffic through the analysis of chemokine receptor expression. *Immunol Rev* 2000;**177**:134–40.

53 Zeid NA, Muller HK. Tobacco smoke induced lung granulomas and tumors: association with pulmonary Langerhans cells. *Pathology* 1995;**27**:247–54.

54 D'Hulst A, Vermeulen KY, Pauwels RA. Cigarette smoke exposure causes increase in pulmonary dendritic cells. *Am J Respir Crit Care Med* 2002;**164**:A604.

55 Casolaro MA, Bernaudin JF, Saltini C, Ferrans VJ, Crystal RG. Accumulation of Langerhans' cells on the epithelial surface of the lower respiratory tract in normal subjects in association with cigarette smoking. *Am Rev Respir Dis* 1988;**137**:406–11.

56 Soler P, Moreau A, Basset F, Hance AJ. Cigarette smoking-induced changes in the number and differentiated state of pulmonary dendritic cells/Langerhans cells. *Am Rev Respir Dis* 1989;**139**:1112–7.

57 Reibman J, Hsu Y, Chen LC, Bleck B, Gordon T. Airway epithelial cells release MIP-3a/CCL20 in response to cytokines and ambient particulate matter. *Am J Respir Cell Mol Biol* 2003;**28**:648–54.

58 Fujimoto K, Imaizumi T, Yoshida H *et al*. Interferon-γ stimulates fractalkine expression in human bronchial epithelial cells and regulates mononuclear cell adherence. *Am J Respir Cell Mol Biol* 2001;**25**:233–8.

59 Yang XD, Corvalan JR, Wang P, Roy CM, Davis CG. Fully human anti-interleukin-8 monoclonal antibodies: potential therapeutics for the treatment of inflammatory disease states. *J Leukoc Biol* 1999;**66**:401–10.

60 Keatings VM, Jatakanon A, Worsdell YM, Barnes PJ. Effects of inhaled and oral glucocorticoids on inflammatory indices in asthma and COPD. *Am J Respir Crit Care Med* 1997;**155**:542–8.

61 Culpitt SV, Nightingale JA, Barnes PJ. Effect of high dose inhaled steroid on cells, cytokines and proteases in induced sputum in chronic obstructive pulmonary disease. *Am J Respir Crit Care Med* 1999;**160**:1635–9.

62 Ito K, Barnes PJ, Adcock IM. Glucocorticoid receptor recruitment of histone deacetylase 2 inhibits IL-1b-induced histone H4 acetylation on lysines 8 and 12. *Mol Cell Biol* 2000;**20**:6891–903.

63 Barnes PJ, Adcock IM. How corticosteroids switch off inflammation in asthma. *Ann Intern Med* 2003;**139**:359–70.

64 Ito K, Lim S, Caramori G *et al*. Cigarette smoking reduces histone deacetylase 2 expression, enhances cytokine expression and inhibits glucocorticoid actions in alveolar macrophages. *FASEB J* 2001;**15**:1100–2.

65 Barnes PJ, Ito K, Adcock IM. Corticosteroid resistance in chronic obstructive pulmonary disease: inactivation of histone deacetylase. *Lancet* 2004;**363**:731–3.

66 Ito K, Lim S, Chung KF, Barnes PJ, Adcock IM. Theophylline enhances histone deacetylase activity and restores glucocorticoid function during oxidative stress. *Am J Respir Crit Care Med* 2002;**165**:A625.

67 Barnes PJ. Theophylline: new perspectives on an old drug. *Am J Respir Crit Care Med* 2003;**167**:813–8.

68 Culpitt SV, de Matos C, Russell RE *et al.* Effect of theophylline on induced sputum inflammatory indices and neutrophil chemotaxis in COPD. *Am J Respir Crit Care Med* 2002;**165**: 1371–6.

69 Au BT, Teixeira MM, Collins PD, Williams TJ. Effect of PDE4 inhibitors on zymosan-induced IL-8 release from human neutrophils: synergism with prostanoids and salbutamol. *Br J Pharmacol* 1998;**123**:1260–6.

70 Gamble E, Grootendorst DC, Brightling CE *et al.* Anti-inflammatory effects of the phosphodiesterase 4 inhibitor cilomilast (Ariflo) in COPD. *Am J Respir Crit Care Med* 2003; **168**:976–82.

71 Carter AB, Monick MM, Hunninghake GW. Both erk and p38 kinases are necessary for cytokine gene transcription. *Am J Respir Cell Mol Biol* 1999;**20**:751–8.

72 Meja KK, Seldon PM, Nasuhara Y *et al.* p38 MAP kinase and MKK-1 co-operate in the generation of GM-CSF from LPS-stimulated human monocytes by an NF-κB-independent mechanism. *Br J Pharmacol* 2000;**131**:1143–53.

73 Lee JC, Kumar S, Griswold DE *et al.* Inhibition of p38 MAP kinase as a therapeutic strategy. *Immunopharmacology* 2000; **47**:185–201.

74 Li J, Kartha S, Iasvovskaia S *et al.* Regulation of human airway epithelial cell IL-8 expression by MAP kinases. *Am J Physiol Lung Cell Mol Physiol* 2002;**283**:L690–9.

75 Delhase M, Li N, Karin M. Kinase regulation in inflammatory response. *Nature* 2000;**406**:367–8.

76 Kishore N, Sommers C, Mathialagan S *et al.* A selective IKK-2 inhibitor blocks NF-κB-dependent gene expression in IL-1b stimulated synovial fibroblasts. *J Biol Chem* 2003;**278**:32861–71.

77 Jazrawi E, Cosio BG, Barnes PJ, Adcock IM. Inhibition of IKK2 and JNK differentially regulates GM-CSF and IL-8 release in epithelial cells and alveolar macrophages. *Am J Respir Crit Care Med* 2003;**167**:A798.

78 Culpitt SV, Rogers DF, Barnes PJ, Donnelly LE. Resveratrol has a greater inhibitory effect than corticosteroids in inhibiting alveolar macrophages from COPD patients. *Am J Respir Crit Care Med* 2003;**167**:A91.

Index